Part A Nov 2018 – Nov 2014

Qs with Explanations

2 Vol. Set

9th Edition

PGI CHANDIGARH

Postgraduate Medical Entrance Examination

Self-Assessment & Review

Dr Manoj Chaudhary

MBBS MD

Dr Hemlata Patel Chaudhary

MS (Obstetrics & Gynecology) BHU

Special Thanks to

Dr Rajiv Dagar

CMO, M/H Defence Colony, SDMC, New Delhi

Contributors

Dr OP Singh *MBBS, MD*

ESI Hospital, Jamshedpur, Jharkhand

Dr Pankaj Nagar *MBBS, UCMS SR*

Shri Dada Dev Matri Avum Shishu Chikitsalaya, New Delhi

Dr Sulekha Saxena

Assistant Professor

ICU, KGMU, Lucknow

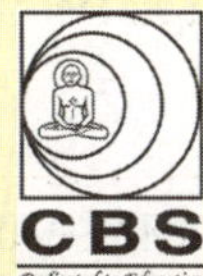

CBS Publishers & Distributors Pvt Ltd

• New Delhi • Bengaluru • Chennai • Kochi • Mumbai

• Hyderabad • Kolkata • Patna • Vijayawada

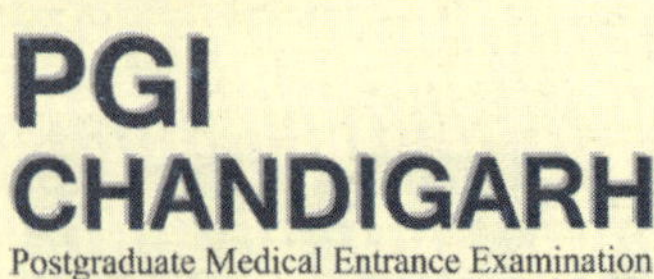

DISCLAIMER

This book contains questions based upon the topics which have been most frequently asked in Pre PG Medical entrance examinations throughout the world. We do not claim the material and question present in this book to be exactly the same, duplicated or reproduced from any examination conducted by any Board or Authority, statutory or nonstatutory in India or outside India. We declare that this book is neither sponsored nor related to any board or authority of Government (statutory or nonstatutory) and Neither it contains any Proprietary material of any board nor authority of Government (statutory or non- statutory). The questions in this book are purely the work of our author, however medical science is a generic knowledge and creating similar material by authors is not uncommon. Any resemblance to them is purely a coincidence and by chance.

Copying and reproducing any of the material of this book in any form completely or partially is prohibited under copyright act and is binding by law.

ISBN: 978-93-88108-79-9

Ninth Edition: 2018-19

Published by **Satish Kumar Jain** and produced by **Varun Jain** for **CBS Publishers and Distributors Pvt Ltd**

4819/XI Prahlad Street, 24 Ansari Road, Daryaganj, New Delhi 110 002, India.
Ph: +91-11-23289259, 23266861, 23266867 Website: www.cbspd.com
Fax: 011-23243014
e-mail: delhi@cbspd.com; cbspubs@airtelmail.in.

Corporate Office: 204 FIE, Industrial Area, Patparganj, Delhi 110 092
Ph: +91-11-4934 4934 Fax: 4934 4935
e-mail: feedback@cbspd.com; bhupesharora@cbspd.com

Branches

- **Bengaluru:** Seema House 2975, 17th Cross, K.R. Road, Banasankari 2nd Stage, Bengaluru 560 070, Karnataka
  Ph: +91-80-26771678/79 Fax: +91-80-26771680 e-mail: bangalore@cbspd.com
- **Chennai:** 7, Subbaraya Street, Shenoy Nagar, Chennai 600 030, Tamil Nadu
  Ph: +91-44-26680620, 26681266 Fax: +91-44-42032115 e-mail: chennai@cbspd.com
- **Kochi:** Ashana House, No. 39/1904, AM Thomas Road, Valanjambalam, Ernakulam 682 018, Kochi, Kerala
  Ph: +91-484-4059061-65 Fax: +91-484-4059065 e-mail: kochi@cbspd.com
- **Kolkata:** 6/B, Ground Floor, Rameswar Shaw Road, Kolkata-700 014, West Bengal
  Ph: +91-33-22891126, 22891127, 22891128 e-mail: kolkata@cbspd.com
- **Mumbai:** 83-C, Dr E Moses Road, Worli, Mumbai-400018, Maharashtra
  Ph: +91-22-24902340/41 Fax: +91-22-24902342 e-mail: mumbai@cbspd.com

Representatives

- **Hyderabad** +91-9885175004
- **Patna** +91-9334159340
- **Vijayawada** +91-9000660880
- **Mangalore** +91-9741432102

Printed At : Goyal Offset Printers

This Book is Dedicated to

Jawahar Navodaya Vidyalaya

A Unique Institution

Which shaped my future and continues shaping futures of hundreds of thousand students across India, especially from rural background

Congratulations to all the Contributors...

Congratulations to all the contributors for providing recent questions for PGI Nov 2018 paper.
I am happy to give your name here and will send you
free complementary copy along with the CBS free book voucher.

Dr OP Singh *MBBS, MD*
ESI Hospital, Jamshedpur, Jharkhand

Dr Pankaj Nagar *MBBS, UCMS SR*
Shri Dada Dev Matri Avum Shishu Chikitsalaya, New Delhi

Dr Avinash Dhakad *MBBS*
Netaji Subhash Chandra Bose Medical College
Jabalpur, Madhya Pradesh

Dr Md Irfan Ul Hasan *MBBS*
AIIMS Patna, Bihar

Dr Mehak Trehan *MBBS*
Government Medical College and Hospital, Chandigarh

Dr Rachit Singhania *MBBS*
North Bengal Medical College and Hospital
Darjeeling, West Bengal

Dr Rekha Jakhar *MBBS*
Pandit Bhagwat Dayal Sharma Post Graduate
Institute of Medical Sciences, Rohtak, Haryana

Dr Praveen. B *MBBS*
Government Thiruvarur Medical College
Thiruvarur, Tamil Nadu

Dr Swapnil *MBBS*
RMC Maharashtra

Dr Vignesh Kumar *MBBS*
Thoothukudi Government Medical College
Thoothukudi, Tamil Nadu

Dr Sunil *MBBS*

Golden Opportunity
to Win Cash Prizes/Gift Vouchers
(Worth ₹50,000/- in total sum among top 10 contributors)

Dear students, contribute recent questions of upcoming exams along with options in the book.

The top 10 contributors will get a chance to win cash prizes/gift vouchers of worth ₹50,000/- in total.

For details please contact author on his email ID pgichdreview@gmail.com

---

Join me on facebook page **facebook.com/PGI Chandigarh Book lovers**

All Readers are requested to share their valuable feedback & suggestions to make this book more authentic and valuable at my email id: pgichdreview@gmail.com

In the next edition Top 10 Questions contributors will find him/her name on this page along with free complementary copy and CBS book voucher.

Preface

It is great pride and pleasure to present the book **"PGI CHANDIGARH Self-Assessment & Review, 9th edition Part A Nov 2018–Nov 2014"** to all the postgraduate aspirants.

I tried my best to give you all relevant matter regarding the topic from authentic sources, so that you can get much help for forthcoming exams. The text has been prepared so as to provide with all the relevant information on old and repeated questions as well as guidelines to solve the newer ones. The explanations have been enriched with relevant flowcharts, tabulations, diagrams and mnemonics to make it easy to learn and yet, at same time, not compromising the quality of information.

In the last I would like to say to all that -

Don't Give Up

Don't give up and don't give in
It's all in the Lord's hand
No matter what you're facing
He is the one who can
In any situation
His grace can turn it around
So you can be victorious
As his love does abound
The beginning and the end he knows
And all that's in between
So put your total trust in him
To him it's all foreseen.
He knows about your struggles
He knows about your pain
Your hardship and your sorrows
And he will help you to reign
So don't give up and don't give in
Don't quit before it's time
God's grace will give you power
To make it to the finish line
In his way and time !!!

Dr Manoj Chaudhary
Dr Hemlata Patel Chaudhary
Email: pgichdreview@gmail.com

Join me on facebook page facebook.com/PGI Chandigarh Book Lovers

All Readers are requested to share their valuable feedback & suggestions to make this book more authentic and valuable. I also request students to contribute the recent questions of upcoming exams along with options at our email id's:
pgichdreview@gmail.com

Acknowledgments

Though the words are too feeble to express gratitude and thankfulness to all of those who helped us in the process of writing this book

I want to give special thanks to Asha Meena, Dr Ashok Singh (Globe Hospital, Lucknow), Ms Preeti (Noida), Dr Reeta, Dr Kanchan, Dr Nidhi, Dr Rinku, Dr Lalrinpuii (M/H Defence Colony SDMC, Delhi), Mrs Monu Sharma, Dr Pankaj Nagar (MBBS, UCMS), Mr Shrikant Srivastava, Dr Yogesh Goyal, SR, Opthalmology, New Delhi), Alok Singh (Lucknow), Dr Ankur Chakraborty, Mr Shashank Gupta, Mrs Neha Gangwar, Dr Mayank Singh, Ashish Kr Mishra (HC/NA BSF - Hazaribagh), BD Mahto (HC/NA BSF - Hazaribagh), Dr Debjyoti Dutta (MD, Anesthesia, Pain Specialist, Kolkatta), Dr Kajal Gupta (MD, Anesthesia, Kanpur), Manoj Maurya, Dr Debjyoti Dutta (MD, Asth, Calcutta), Dr Rahul Saha (SR, Psychiatry, RML New Delhi), Dr Rajesh Yadav (SR, Paediatrics, MLBMC Jhansi), Dr Sameer Saraf (MD, Medicine KGMU) & Dr Naveen Chaudhary (MBBS, KGMC), Dr Saurabh (MBBS, KGMC), Dr Sandeep Kumar (SR, Skin, Ambedkar Hospital, New Delhi), Dr Poonam Gangwar (MO, ESI Rohini), Sapna, Arpita, Pranav, Himanshu Pansaria, Jassi, Aarti and Hina for their support.

I offer cordial thanks to staff members and other employees of M/H Defence Colony, SDMC, New Delhi. Nand Kishore, Sushma Rani, Lily Mary Ekka, Rumana Javed, Sateshwari Noutiyal, Suman Gil, Chanu Kumari, Sunil Singh Rawat, Vijay Kumar, Monu Sharma, Shweta, Preeti Ahlawat, Etti Chhikara, Anjani Kumar Pandey, Ashok Kumar, Mamta Kumari, Pramod, Preeti Verma and Sateshwari.

I offer cordial thanks to my NGO members for their kind initiatives- Uday Kumar Singh, Manilal Patidar, Dr Arvind Namdeo, Laxmikant Mani Tripathi, Sipra Sarkar, Reema Bajaj, Ajithesh sagar, Amit Kumar, Gaurav Maurya, Niharika, Ravi Prabhat, Ashish Vashney, Ashok Sharma, Prashun Lal, Amit Raj, Gaurav Prakash, Sunil, Deepak Namdeo, Madhulika Chaudhary, Padam Dhuman, Aditya Rajput, Ramchandra Kumar, Pawan Pandey, Manvendra Singh, Zahid Khan, Sahid Khan, Wahid Khan, Dharmendra Kumar, Rahul Arora, Mukesh Kumar & Prakash Ji.

I am thankful to our ALS friends for their moral support— Vijay Murthi, Ashutosh, Lucy, Rahman, Hemendra Gurjar, Roshan Gul, Vivek, Alok, Ramiz, Jyoti Chaube, Bhola Tiwari, Shivang Yadav, Sweta, Dr Abhay Pratap Singh, Konark, Dr Suman, Rahul, Parul chaudhary, Priyaka, Prakash Gupta, Rajneesh, Vivek Tripathi, Rem Sevak & all others.

I am also thankful to Dr OP Singh (MBBS, DMCH, Darbhanga), Dr Amit Gupta (MD, Anesthesia, SNMC, Agra), Dr Kapil Rastogi (MBBS, GSVMC, Kanpur), Dr Nikhil Malhotra (MBBS, GMC, Nagpur), Dr Amit Ojha (MBBS, GMC, Nagpur) Dr Saurabh Mishra (MBBS, GSVM, Kanpur) Dr Durgesh Pandey (MBBS, GSVM, Kanpur) Dr Jitendra Rai (MBBS, MLNMC, Allahabad for contributing questions for this book.

I would also like to thank Dr Chakrapani Awasthi, Dr Pradeep Khariya, Dr Jitendra Jakhar, Dr Anand Gautam, Dr Chandraprakash, Dr Vinay Shukla, Dr Sunil Madhesia, Dr Avinash Gupta, Dr Yadunath, Dr Md. Azhar, Dr Obadul, Dr Adarsh Shrivastav, Dr Santosh Yadav, Dr Rahul Bajaj, Dr Laxmi Prasad Sonkar, Dr Dhananjay (MBBS, MLBMC, Jhansi).

My special thanks to **Mr Satish Kumar Jain (Chairman)** and **Mr Varun Jain (Managing Director)**, M/s CBS Publishers and Distributors Pvt Ltd for their wholehearted support in publication of this book. We have no words to describe the role, efforts, inputs and initiatives undertaken by **Mr Bhupesh Arora, Vice-President (Publishing and Marketing)**, PGMEE and Nursing Division for helping and motivating us.

I would like to thank Dr Mrinalini Bakshi (Editorial Head and Content Strategist) for her editorial support on this project. I personally thank Ms Nitasha Arora (Production Head and Content Strategist), Dr Anju Dhir (Senior Scientific Coordinator/Editor), Mr Nitish K Dubey (Senior Editor) and all the production team members Mr Ashutosh Pathak, Mr Bunty Kashyap, Mr Phool Kumar, Mr Prakash Gaur, Mr Chaman Lal, Ms Tahira Parveen, Ms Babita Verma, Mr Chander, Ms Manorama, Mr Raju Sharma, Mr Vikram Chaudhary, Mr Manoj Chaudhary, Mr Manoj Malakar, and Arun Kumar for devoting laborious hours in designing and type-setting of the book.

Contents

Questions with Answers & Explanations
Nov 2018–Nov 2014

May 2015

November 2014

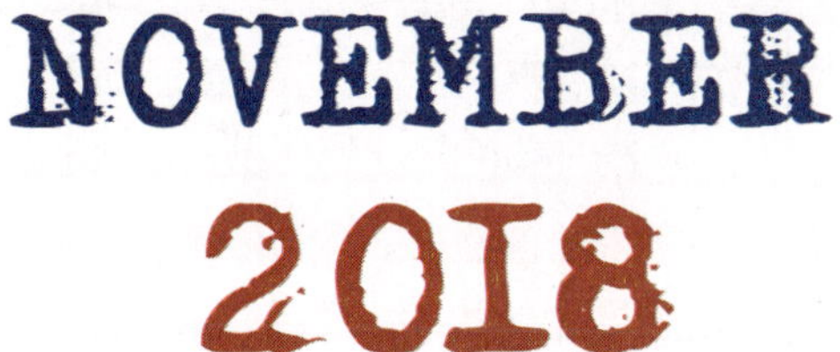

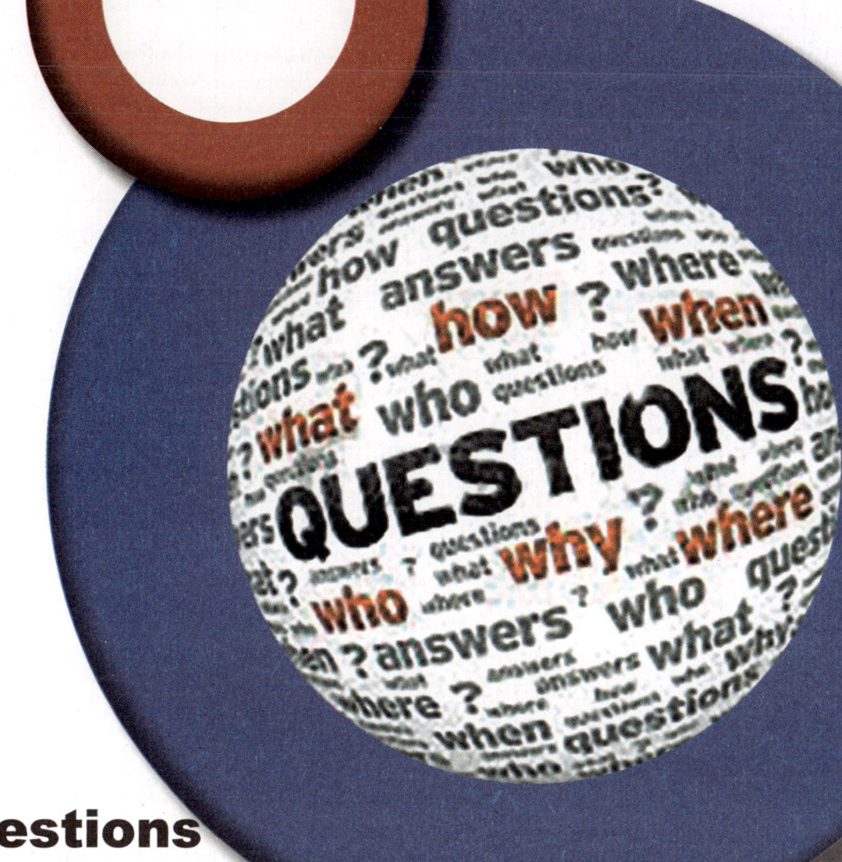

Multiple Choice Questions
Answers & Explanations

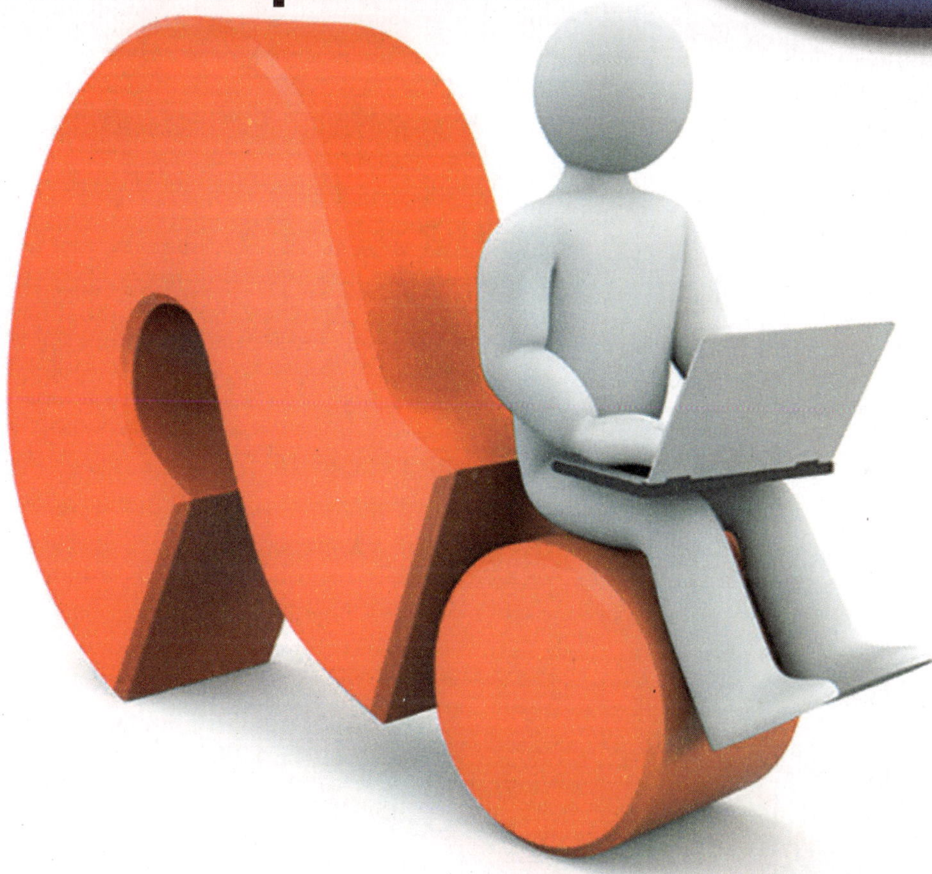

NOVEMBER 2018 MULTIPLE CHOICE QUESTIONS

ANATOMY

1. **Stability of pelvic ring is/are maintained by:**
   a. Sacroiliac ligaments
   b. Pubis symphysis
   c. Inguinal ligament
   d. External oblique aponeurosis
   e. Iliolumber ligament
2. **Nasal septum is/are formed by all except:**
   a. Vomer bone
   b. Lacrimal bone
   c. Perpendicular plate of Ethmoid
   d. Greater wing of sphenoid
   e. Septal (quadrilateral) cartilage
3. **Structure(s) not passing through aortic opening of diaphragm:**
   a. Aorta
   b. Inferior vena cava
   c. Vagus nerve
   d. Phrenic nerve
   e. Azygous vein
4. **True about blood supply of conducting system of heart:**
   a. SA Node is supplied by right coronary artery in majority of cases
   b. SA Node is also supplied by circumflex branch of left coronary artery
   c. Whole conducting system is supplied by left coronary artery
   d. AV node is supplied mainly by left coronary artery
   e. Left bundle branch is supplied by both right & left coronary artery
5. **Root value of long thoracic nerve (Nerve of bell):**
   a. C_5
   b. C_4
   c. C_6
   d. C_7
   e. T_1
6. **All are true regarding erb's palsy except:**
   a. Deformity is adduction and medial rotation of arm
   b. Nerve root involved is *C5 & C6*
   c. Difficulty in supination of forearm
   d. Associated with birth injury
   e. Ulnar nerve is affected
7. **Which of the muscle is/are elevater of nose:**
   a. Depressor septi
   b. Alar nasalis
   c. Orbicularis oris
   d. Zygomaticus minor
   e. Levator labii superioris alaeque nasi
8. **Prostate is/are supplied by:**
   a. Inferior vesicle artery
   b. Middle rectal artery
   c. Superior vesicle artery
   d. Internal pudendal artery
9. **True about epiglottis:**
   a. Contains serous gland
   b. Contains mucous secreting glands
   c. It is oval shaped
   d. Made up of elastic cartilage
   e. Has bilateral lymphatic supply
10. **Superficial vein thrombosis involves cerebral white matter while deep thrombosis involving gray matter in:**
    a. Thalamus
    b. Internal capsule
    c. Basal ganglia
    d. Cerebellum
    e. Optic chiasma
11. **Which of the following statement(s) is/are true regarding development of urogenital system:**
    a. Differentiation of genital ridge into lineage of female or male gonads occurs at 10 weeks
    b. Urinary bladder trigone is derived from vesicourethral canal
    c. Metanephric duct forms glomerulus
    d. Nephrons are formed from metanephros
    e. Collecting duct develop from mesonephric duct

PHYSIOLOGY

12. **Factor affecting viscosity of blood:**
    a. RBCs
    b. Temperature
    c. Plasma protein
    d. Flow rate
    e. Infection
13. **True about Methemoglobinemia:**
    a. Seen in Carbon monoxide poisoning
    b. Causes anemia
    c. Cyanosis is observed
    d. Caused by Nitrate and nitrite compounds
    e. Methylene blue is used for therapy
14. **True about Brown-Sequard Syndrome:**
    a. Ipsilateral loss of pain & temperature
    b. Contralateral loss of pain & temperature
    c. Ipsilateral motor loss
    d. Contralateral loss of proprioception & touch
    e. Ipsilateral loss of discriminative touch

Answer

1. a, b, e	2. b, d.	3. b, c, d.	4. a, b, e.	5. a, c, d.	6. e.	7. b, e.
8. a, b, d.	9. b, d, e.	10. a, c.	11. a, c, d, e.	12. a, b, c, d, e.	13. b, c, d, e.	14. b, c, e.

15. **Which of the following dyads of fiber types & function is/are true:**
   a. Aα – Proprioception b. Aβ → Touch & pressure
   c. Aγ → Pain and temperature d. Aδ → Pain & temperature
   e. C →Proprioception
16. **Secondary lymphoid organ is/are:**
   a. Spleen b. Bone marrow
   c. Lymph node d. Liver
   e. Mucosa associated lymphoid tissue (MALT)
17. **All are true about SIADH except:**
   a. Hyponatremia
   b. Decrease osmolality of plasma
   c. Natriuresis
   d. May be associated with internal malignancy
   e. Plasma osmolality higher than urine osmolality
18. **Substance used for GFR estimation:**
   a. Inulin b. Iohexol
   c. Creatinine d. Tc99m-DTPA
   e. MUGA
19. **Right combination of velocity (*m/s*) and pacemaker conduction (beats/minute) for different parts of cardiac conduction system is/are:**
   a. AV node -0.02.0.05 m/s & 40-55 b/m
   b. SA node-0.05 m/s & 60-100 b/m
   c. Atrial myocardium – 1-1.2 m/s & 25-40 b/m
   d. Bundle of His – 1.2-2 m/s & 25-40 b/m
   e. Ventricular myocardium – 0.3-1.0 m/s & nil
20. **Increased PR interval is seen in:**
   a. First degree AV block
   b. Second degree Mobitz type 1 AV block
   c. Second degree Mobitz type 2 AV block
   d. Third degree AV block
   e. Ventricular tachycardia
21. **Oxygen content of the arterial blood depends upon:**
   a. Hemoglobin concentration
   b. Oxygen saturation in mixed venous blood
   c. PaO_2 in arterial blood
   d. RBC volume
   e. Cardiac output
22. **Hypothalamic pituitary axis (HPA) controls all except:**
   a. Thyroid b. Parathyroid
   c. Pancreas d. Testis
   e. Adrenals
23. **Which of the following are true with respect to red pulp of spleen:**
   a. It has B cell rich lymphoid tissues
   b. Composed of splenic cords and sinusoids
   c. It has T cell rich periarticular lymphatic sheath
   d. Perisinusoidal macrophages are present
   e. Removes senescent erythrocytes from circulation

BIOCHEMISTRY

24. **Which of the following lipoprotein has highest content of triglycerides:**
   a. Chylomicron b. VLDL
   c. HDL d. LDL
   e. Intermediate DL
25. **Example(s) of Polyunsaturated fatty acid (PUFA):**
   a. Folic acid
   b. Linoleic acid
   c. Stearic acid
   d. Linolenic acid
   e. Palmitoleic acid
26. **Main enzyme responsible for Classical Galactosemia is:**
   a. Galactose-1-phosphateuridyltransferase (GALT) deficiency
   b. Galactokinase deficiency
   c. Uridine diphosphate galactose 4-epimerase deficiency
   d. Hexokinase
27. **Example of ketogenic amino acid is/are:**
   a. Leucine b. Lysine
   c. Phenylalanine d. Arginine
   e. Aspartate
28. **Folate deficiency causes decrease in all of the following processes except:**
   a. Homocysteine to methionine
   b. All pyrimidine synthesis during RNA formation
   c. Synthesis of N-formylmethionine
   d. Conversion of creatine phosphate to creatinine
   e. Serine to glycine conversion
29. **Which of the following is/true about Recommended daily allowance(RDA) by ICMR of Vitamin A(Retinol)in different age groups:**
   a. Infant-350 μg b. Adolescent- 600 μg
   c. Adult male-600 μg d. Pregancy-950 μg
   e. Lactating mother-800 μg
30. **Which of the following is/are enzyme(s) of urea cycle:**
   a. Ornithine transcarbamoylase
   b. Argi nosuccinic acid synthetase
   c. Arginase
   d. Aspartase
   e. Carbamoyl phosphate synthetase I
31. **Hyperuricemia is/are seen in:**
   a. HGPRT deficiency
   b. Glucose-6-phosphatase deficiency
   c. HGPRT over activity
   d. Glucose-6-phosphatase over activity
   e. Phosphoribosyl pyrophosphate (PRPP) synthetase deficiency

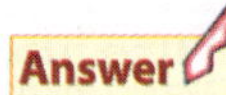

Answer

15. a, b, d.	16. a, c, e.	17. e.	18. a, b, c, d.	19. a, b, d, e.	20. a, b.	21. a, c.
22. b, c.	23. b, d, e.	24. a.	25. b, d.	26. a.	27. a, b, c	28. b, d.
29. a, b, c.	30. a, b, c, e.	31. a, b.				

32. Daily use of 100 mg of which of the following vitamin can cause toxicity:
a. Vitamin A b. Thiamine
c. Vitamin D d. Vitamin C
e. Vitamin E

33. True about ubiquitin-proteasome system of protein degradation:
a. ATP is required
b. Degradation occurs after ubiquitination of the target substrate
c. Regulation by Heat stroke protein (HSP)
d. ATP independent
e. Ubiquitins are recycled

34. Chronic use of alcohol intake causes:
a. Hyperglycemia b. Hypoglycemia
c. Thiamine deficiency d. Lactic acidosis

35. Enzyme(s) with same metallic cofactor are all except:
a. Isocitrate dehydrogenase
b. Pyruvate dehydrogenase
c. Glutamate dehydrogenase
d. Glucose-6-phophatase
e. G6-Phosphate dehydrogenase

36. Non-polar amino acids are:
a. Proline b. Lysine
c. Isoleucine d. Arginine
e. Asparagine

37. True regarding glutathione conjugation :
a. Cannot occur without N-acetylglutamate synthase (NAGS) enzyme
b. N-glutathione transferase enzyme is the most important enzyme
c. High expression of enzymes leads to decrease activity of anticancer drugs
d. Glutathione transferase enzyme constitutes about 10% of soluble proteins in liver cells
e. An increased GSSG-to-GSH ratio is indicative of oxidative stress

38. Endoplasmic reticular proteins which causes folding of protein:
a. ERp57 b. Cytochrome 450
c. Insulin receptors
d. Protein disulfide isomerase
e. Glucose related protein(GRP)

39. Which of the following enzyme(s) is/are involved in fatty acid synthesis:
a. Glycerol-3-phosphate hydrogenase
b. Acetyl Co-A carboxylase
c. ATP -citrate lyase
d. Acetyl transacylase
e. Glycerol kinase

40. Mitochondrial matrix contain enzyme(s) of:
a. Beta oxidation b. ATP synthase
c. TCA cycle d. Pyruvate dehydrogenase
e. Acyl CoA synthetase

IMMUNOGENETICS & MOLECULAR BIOLOGY

41. Total number of base pairs in human DNA genome:
a. 1 billion b. 1.2 billion
c. 2 billion d. 3 billion
e. 5.6 billion

42. What is the percentage of mitochondrial DNA in total DNA:
a. 1% b. 2%
c. 2.5% d. 3.5%
e. 4%

43. Not true about structure of DNA:
a. Adenine is paired to thymidine, and guanine is paired to cytosine
b. Deoxyribose phosphate forms the backbone of helix
c. Has uracil (U) as base pair
d. Absent phosphodiester bond
e. Amount of adenine equals the amount of cytosine & the amount of guanine equals the amount of thymine

44. True about DNA polymerase I:
a. Has 3' exonuclease
b. Has 5' exonuclease
c. Help in DNA proofreading
d. Help in synthesis of DNA only in 3'→5' direction
e. Help in DNA repair

45. Incorrect statement(s) about transcription in prokaryotes:
a. Synthesis of RNA done by RNA polymerase
b. Inhibited by rifabutin
c. Translation occur after transcription
d. Formation of complementary RNA copy of the DNA template strand
e. RNA is synthesized in 3→5 direction

46. Stop codon is/are:
a. AUG b. UAG
c. UAA d. AAG
e. UGA

47. Step(s) which is/are common between eukaryotic and bacterial transcription:
a. 5' capping
b. Binding to the promoter region
c. DNA dependent RNA polymerase enzyme involvement
d. Poly A-tail addition
e. One species of RNA polymerase synthesizes all of the RNA

Answer

32. a, d.	33. a, b, c, e.	34. b, c, d.	35. c.	36. a, c.	37. b, c, e.	38. a, d, e.
39. b, c, d.	40. a, c, d.	41. d.	42. a.	43. c, d, e.	44. a, b, c, e.	45. e.
46. b, c, e.	47. b, c.					

PATHOLOGY

48. Which of the following pair of chromosomal translocation is/are correctly matched:
- a. Chronic myeloid leukemia (CML) →t(15:17)
- b. Ewing sarcoma →t(8:21)
- c. Synovial sarcoma →t(X:18)
- d. Acute lymphocytic leukemia→ t(9;22)
- e. Burkitt's lymphoma → t(8;14)

49. Marker(s) of pancreatic cancer:
- a. CA-19-9
- b. HCG
- c. CA-125
- d. Carcinoembryonic antigen (CEA)
- e. CA-19-9

50. Which of the following immunostain is positive for sarcoma:
- a. Pankeratin
- b. Desmin
- c. Vimentin
- d. Glial fibrillary acidic protein (GFAP)
- e. Neurofilaments

51. Anti-apoptotic factor(s) is/are:
- a. BCL2
- b. BCL-XL
- c. MCL1
- d. BAK
- e. BAX

52. Which is/are correct pair of trisomy:
- a. Edward syndrome – Chromosome 13
- b. Edward syndrome – Chromosome 15
- c. Down syndrome-Chromosome 21
- d. Down syndrome occurs due to non-disjunction of chromosome
- e. Patau syndrome- Chromosome 18

53. True about Down syndrome:
- a. Paternal age more than 35 is a risk factor
- b. Maternal age more than 35 is a risk factor
- c. Paternal trisomy is most common cause
- d. Occur due to meiotic nondisjunction of chromosome 21
- e. Most commonly due to translocation of chromosome 21

54. Feature(s) of Down syndrome:
- a. Furrowed protruding tongue
- b. Small nose
- c. Intellectual impairment
- d. Broad ears
- e. Short & broad hand

55. True about acute graft rejection in organ transplantation :
- a. Higher mortality & morbidity than hyper-acute graft rejection
- b. Mainly mediated by anti-HLA antibodies
- c. Most common cause of graft failure
- d. Can be reversed by increasing dose of corticosteroid
- e. Predictor of chronicity

56. Function of suppressor T cells:
- a. Prevent reactions against self-antigens
- b. Primary function is to suppress immune system
- c. Carry CD8 molecule on their surface
- d. Stimulate B lymphocytes
- e. Kill infected cells

57. Schistocyteis/are seen in all except:
- a. Liver failure
- b. Hemolytic uremic syndrome (HUS)
- c. Severe burn
- d. Thrombotic thrombocytopenic purpura (TTP)
- e. Prosthetic heart valve

58. True about cystic fibrosis:
- a. Bath restrictive and obstructive symptoms are present
- b. Autosomal dominant inheritance
- c. Viscous mucus secretion
- d. Lung transplantation is a therapeutic option in case of pulmonary failure
- e. Recombinant human deoxyribonuclease (rhDNAase) is useful to decrease sputum viscosity

59. Feature(s) of DiGeorge syndrome includes all except:
- a. Hyperparathyroidism
- b. Hypocalcemia
- c. Hyperthyroidism
- d. Thymic hyperplasia
- e. Thymic hypoplasia

60. Luminal A & B classification is used for:
- a. Breast cancer
- b. Lung cancer
- c. Liver cancer
- d. Ovarian cancer
- e. Colon cancer

61. Immunodeficiency of B cells is/are seen in:
- a. DiGeorge syndrome
- b. Wiskott-Aldrich syndrome
- c. Severe combined immunodeficiency
- d. Ataxia telangiectasia
- e. Common variable immunodeficiency

62. True about metastatic bone tumor:
- a. Bone pain is most frequent symptom
- b. Prostate & lung carcinoma are common source of metastasis
- c. Increase chance of pathological fracture
- d. Higher serum levels of alkaline phosphatase
- e. Majority of bone secondaries are osteoblastic

63. Which of the blood component is/are stored at room temperature:
- a. Packed RBC
- b. Platelet
- c. Fresh Frozen Plasma(FFP)
- d. Leucocyte concentrate
- e. Whole blood

64. All are true about Pulmonary alveolar proteinosis except:
- a. Occur due to pulmonary macrophage dysfunction
- b. Deposition of PAS positive amorphous material in lung alveoli
- c. Whole-lung lavage is used for treatment
- d. More common in females
- e. Antibodies to GM-CSF

MCQs

Answer

48. c, d, e. 49. a, d. 50. b, c. 51. a, b, c. 52. c, d. 53. b, d. 54. a, b, c, e.
55. d, e. 56. c, e. 57. a. 58. a, c, d, e. 59. a, c, d. 60 a. 61. b, c, e.
62. a, b, c, d. 63. b, d. 64. d.

65. **True about Hemophilia:**
   a. Hemophilia A constitute 80-85%
   b. Cryoprecipitate is used for treatment of Hemophilia B
   c. Hemophilia B is classified as severe when factor IX residual activity <5%
   d. Prolonged PTT with normal PT
   e. Autosomal recessive inheritance in Hemophilia B

66. **Secondary amyloidosis is/are seen in:**
   a. Bronchiectasis
   b. Pulmonary TB
   c. Chronic osteomyelitis
   d. Idiopathic pulmonary fibrosis
   e. Primary pulmonary hypertension

67. **Microcytic hypochromic picture is/are seen in:**
   a. Sideroblastic anemia b. Lead poisoning
   c. Occult blood loss d. Atransferrinemia
   e. Thalassemia

68. **According to WHO classification of brain tumor, meningioma type I include(s):**
   a. Clear cell b. Secretary
   c. Microcystic d. Transitional
   e. Papillary

69. **Which of following is not classified as primitive neuroectodermal tumour (PNET):**
   a. Retinoblastoma b. Medulloblastoma
   c. Rhabdomyosarcoma d. Ewing sarcoma
   e. Carcinoid tumour

70. **Feature(s) of Noonan syndrome are all except:**
   a. Short stature
   b. Shield chest
   c. Hypertrophic cardiomyopathy
   d. Wide carrying angle
   e. PTPN11 gene association

71. **All are true about proto-oncogene except:**
   a. P53 is an important oncogene
   b. Point mutation activates RAS
   c. Need some stimuli to get activated
   d. Responsible for normal cell proliferation
   e. Single mutation is sufficient for cancer

72. **Correct match of stain with structure is/are:**
   a. Von Kossa-collagen b. Sudan III-fat
   c. Oil red O-calcium d. PAS-glycogen
   e. Gomori stain- fungus

73. **In hereditary spherocytosis, which of the following is/are increased:**
   a. Haptoglobin
   b. Urine urobilinogen
   c. MCHC
   d. MCV
   e. LDH

74. **Cytokines induced rise in body temperature is/are seen in:**
   a. Malignant neuroleptic syndrome
   b. Heat stroke
   c. Thyroid storm
   d. Viral fever
   e. Lymphoma

75. **Superior vena cava syndrome is/are commonly seen in:**
   a. Small cell carcinoma lung
   b. Squamous cell carcinoma lung
   c. Lymphoma
   d. Multiple myeloma
   e. Scleroderma

76. **True about Osteitis fibrosa cystica:**
   a. ↑ Parathyroid hormone
   b. Increase in the giant multinucleated osteoclasts
   c. Generalized bone resorption
   d. ↓ Serum calcium

PHARMACOLOGY

77. **A man ingested 15 gram of paracetamol tablet & he is also chronic alcoholic. Which of the following is/are true:**
   a. Gastric lavage is done to prevent absorption
   b. Activated charcoal is used in lavage
   c. N- acetyl cysteine is antidote
   d. No role of N-Acetylcysteine after 24 hours
   e. Death may occur

78. **Which of the following is/are true regarding paracetamol poisoning in children:**
   a. Deranged hepatic function
   b. N- acetyl cysteine is antidote
   c. Increased serum amylase
   d. Abnormal renal function

79. **All are true about mechanism of action of vinblastine:**
   a. Acts on M phase of cell cycle
   b. Cell cycle specific
   c. Act on tubulin
   d. Enhances polymerization of mitotic spindle
   e. Decreases polymerization of mitotic spindle

80. **Which of the following is/are alkylating agent(s) except:**
   a. Cyclophosphamide b. Vinorelbine
   c. Carmustine d. Azathioprine
   e. Cisplatin

81. **True about use of silver nitrate cream in Burns:**
   a. Doesn't cause black stain on skin
   b. Topically used every 2-4 hours
   c. Causes metabolic acidosis
   d. Effective against pseudomonas
   e. May cause methemoglobinemia

Answer

65. a, d.	66. a, b, c.	67. a, b, d, e.	68. b, c, d.	69. a, c, d, e.	70. b.	71. a.
72. b, d, e.	73. b, c, e.	74. d, e.	75. a, b, c.	76. a, b, c.	77 a, b, c, e.	78. a, b, d.
79. d.	80. b, d, e.	81. d, e.				

82. Proteus mirabilis is/are intrinsic resistant to which antibiotic(s):
a. Nitrofurantoin
b. Cephalosporins
c. Tetracycline
d. Ampicillin
e. Ampicillin-sabbatum

83. For extensive tinea infection in pregnancy, which of the following antifungal drug can be used:
a. Terbinafine
b. Fluconazole
c. Lamivudine
d. Griseofulvin
e. Itraconazole

84. According to NACO guideline, first line anti- HIV drug(s) is/are all except:
a. Tenofovir
b. Efavirenz
c. Lamuvidine
d. Zidovudine
e. Ritonavir

85. Both CCR5 & CCR2 receptor antagonist is/are:
a. Maraviroc
b. Vicriviroc
c. Aplaviroc
d. Cenicriviroc
e. None of the above

86. Regarding 1st order drug kinetics, which of the following is/are true:
a. Constant fraction of drug is eliminated per unit time
b. Rate of elimination inversely proportional to dose
c. As concentration of drugs increases, rate of elimination increases
d. Elimination half-life is dose dependent
e. Clearance (CL) is dependent on dose

87. All are short Acting Insulin Except:
a. Glargine
b. Aspart
c. Lispro
d. Degludec
e. Glulisine

88. Uricosuric drug(s) is/are:
a. Probenecid
b. Allopurinol
c. Febuxostat
d. Sulfinpyrazone

89. True about effect of Milrinone:
a. ↑ Systemic BP
b. ↑ Stroke volume
c. ↑ Cardiac output
d. ↑ Pulmonary hypertension

90. For opioid overdose, naloxone is given through which route:
a. IV
b. IM
c. Oral
d. Subcutaneous
e. Per rectal

91. Which of the following pair of drug-receptor/target is/are correctly matched:
a. Cetuximab – VEGF
b. Muromonab – RANK
c. Bevacizumab – CD3
d. Gemtuzumab- CD33
e. Trastuzumab- HER2/neu

92. Side effect of isoniazid include(s):
a. GIT upset
b. Memory impairment
c. Optic neuritis
d. Peripheral neuropathy
e. Hepatitis

93. 3rd generation beta blocker cause vasodilation by:
a. Carvedilol – β_2 agonistic activity
b. Celiprolol – Potassium channel blocker
c. Lebetalol –enhance NO production
d. Nebivolol– enhance NO production
e. Bopindolol- Calcium channel blockage

94. True regarding ketotifen:
a. Given orally
b. Bronchodilator
c. Used prophylactically
d. Prevents release from mast cells
e. Dry mouth is a side-effect

95. Which of the following is/are not Bacteriostatic drug:
a. INH
b. Pyrazinamide
c. Streptomycin
d. Rifampicin
e. Ethambutol

96. Management for diazepam overdose includes:
a. Blood glucose test
b. Blood urea test
c. Mechanical ventilation
d. Single large dose of activated charcoal
e. Flumazenil as antidote

Answer

82. a, c.	83. a.	84. e.	85. d.	86. a, c.	87. a, d.	88. a, d.
89. b, c.	90. a, b, d.	91. d, e.	92. a, b, c, d, e.	93. d.	94 a, c, d, e.	95. a, b, c, d.
96. a, b, c, d, e.						

MICROBIOLOGY

97. **True about Cytomegalovirus infection:**
   a. May be associated with GBS syndrome
   b. Ganciclovir and valacyclovir are given for prophylaxis only in immunocompromised patients and not for treatment of symptomatic immunocompetent patients
   c. Virus can be isolated from body secretions
   d. Severe birth defects may occur
   e. Hepatosplenomegaly is the common feature of congenital CMV infection

98. **All are true about kala-azar except:**
   a. Transmitted by female sand fly
   b. Endemic in African
   c. Rapid diagnostic kit is available
   d. Indian kala–azar is a zoonotic disease
   e. Two peak in a year

99. **Which of the following is/are example of superantigens:**
   a. Toxic shock syndrome toxin (TSST)
   b. Cholera toxin
   c. Group A streptococcal pyrogenic exotoxin
   d. Staphylococcal enterotoxins
   e. Diphtheria toxin

100. **True about Superantigens:**
   a. Polyclonal T-lymphocyte activation
   b. Releases large amount of cytokines
   c. Bind TCRβ and class II MHC molecule
   d. Need no processing
   e. Require antigen specificity

101. **True about microbial sterilization techniques:**
   a. Kills both vegetative and spore forms of bacteria
   b. Kill vegetative but not spore forms of bacteria
   c. Can be used only for living surface
   d. CO_2 can be used for sterilization
   e. Water can be disinfected by chlorination

102. **Non-sporing anaerobic bacteria is/are:**
   a. Peptostreptococcus b. Propionibacterium
   c. Clostridium d. Anthrax
   e. Bacteroides

103. **Anaerobic gram positive bacilli is/are:**
   a. Actinomyces b. Lactobacillus
   c. Bacteroides d. Veillonella
   e. Clostridium

104. **Leprosy is zoonosis in:**
   a. Nine banded armadillos b. Nude mice
   c. Mangabey monkey d. Chimpanzee
   e. European hedgehog

105. **Which of the following is/are not feature of Weil's disease:**
   a. Uveitis b. Renal failure
   c. Jaundice d. Icterohemorrhagic fever
   e. Ecchymosis and petechiae

106. **True about Category A bioweapon agents except:**
   a. May cause life threatening infection
   b. Easily transmitted from person to person
   c. Potential for major public health impact
   d. Brucellosis is an example
   e. Require special action for public health preparedness

107. **Match the correct dyads of rickettsial disease with their causative agents:**
   a. Endemic typhus- R. typhi
   b. Rickettsial pox- R. akari
   c. Q fever: Coxiella burnetii
   d. Epidemic typhus: R. prowazekii
   e. Rocky Mountain spotted fever- Orientia tsutsugamushi

108. **Feature(s) of scrub typhus:**
   a. Transmitted by rat flea
   b. Caused by *R. prowazekii*
   c. Black eschar
   d. Doxycycline is used for treatment
   e. Rats are the reservoir

109. **To screen congenital syphilis, which of the following test(s) is/are done:**
   a. VDRL b. Rapid plasma Reagin (RPR)
   c. THPP d. TPHA
   e. Dark field microscopy

110. **Non-treponemal test includes:**
   a. TPHA b. RPR
   c. TPI d. VDRL
   e. FTA-ABS

111. **Which of the following is/are not feature of chancroid:**
   a. Caused by H.ducreyi b. Painful ulcer
   c. Ulcer bleeds easily d. Bubo formation
   e. Typically indurated

112. **Maximum accepted contamination rate for a blood culture is:**
   a. 1%
   b. 2%
   c. 3%
   d. 6%
   e. 10%

113. **Sample for routine anaerobe culture can be taken from:**
   a. Tissue specimen b. Blood
   c. Vaginal swab d. Bone marrow
   e. Sputum

114. **New Delhi ambler class B metallo-beta lactamase *(NDM)* mediated carbapenem resistance is seen in:**
   a. Citrobacter freundii
   b. E. coli
   c. P. aeruginosa
   d. K. pneumoniae
   e. Acinetobactor baumannii

Answer

97. a, c, d, e.	98. d.	99. a, c, d.	100. a, b, c, d.	101. a, d, e.	102. a, b, e.	103. a, b, e.
104. a, c, d.	105. None	106. d.	107. a, b, c, d.	108. c, d, e.	109. a, b.	110. b, d.
111. e.	112. c.	113. a, b, d.	114. a, b, d, e.			

FORENSIC MEDICINE

115. True about dactylography:
a. Also *k/a* Fingerprint system
b. Also k/a Foot print system
c. Almost reliable method for identification
d. Lip printing
e. Palatal print

116. Abrasion collar may be associated with:
a. Entry wound of rifled arms
b. Exit wound of rifled arms
c. Railway accident
d. Strangulation's neck mark
e. Postmortem lividity

117. In which of the following condition(s) stiffening of muscles occur without primary relaxation:
a. Rigor mortis
b. Cadaveric spasm
c. Cadaveric rigidity
d. Cold stiffening
e. Heat stiffening

118. All are true about abrus precatorius except:
a. Contains active principle ricin
b. Contains active principle abrin
c. Used as abortifacient
d. Also k/a rati
e. Sui are fine needle

119. Saturated NaCl is/are not used in preservation of viscera in which of the following poisoning:
a. Carbolic acid
b. Aconite
c. Sodium hydroxide
d. Sulfuric acid

120. Age determination by elbow X-ray is done at:
a. 11-12 yr
b. 12-13 yr
c. 13-14 yr
d. 14-15 yr
e. 15-16 yr

121. True about Gustafson's method:
a. Useful in dead person
b. Useful in living person
c. Attrition of teeth is component
d. Used for identification of sex
e. Used for age estimation

PSM

122. Primary prevention for hypertension include(s):
a. Weight reduction
b. Low sodium diet
c. Low potassium diet
d. Regular exercise
e. Low fat diet

123. KIT 1 for cervical discharge/anorectal discharge/cervicitis contain(s):
a. Azithromycin
b. Erythromycin
c. Cefixime
d. Ceftriaxone
e. Doxycycline

124. Which of the following is/are true regarding RNTCP changes:
a. Active case finding
b. Thrice weekly regimen
c. Focus to improve outcome of TB care in the private sector
d. To achieve 90% success rate for all new cases and 85% for retreatment cases
e. Involvement of NGOs

125. True about incidence:
a. Number of new cases
b. New plus old cases
c. Depends on duration of disease
d. Used as tool for measurement of morbidity
e. Only used for chronic disease

126. True about case control study:
a. Prospective study
b. Suitable for study of rare disease
c. Time consuming
d. Incidence rate can be calculated
e. Expensive

127. Mass chemoprophylaxis is/are given for all except:
a. Deworming
b. Lymphatic filariasis
c. Trachoma
d. Vitamin A deficiency
e. Scabies

128. According to Article 246(7th Schedule) of the Constitution of India, which of the following is/are part of state list:
a. Port quarantine
b. Higher education
c. Public health and sanitation; hospitals and dispensaries
d. Adulteration of foodstuffs and other goods
e. Land revenue

129. Which of the following can be calculated from Screening test:
a. Sensitivity
b. Specificity
c. Positive predictive value (PPV)
d. Negative predictive value (NPV)
e. Prevalence

130. False about pasteurization of milk:
a. Methylene blue test is used to detect microorganism in milk
b. Phosphatase test is used to detect the efficiency of pasteurization
c. In Standard plate count, limit of bacteria is 30000 bacteria/ml
d. Kills 100% bacteria
e. Milk is heated to 125 degree in ultra-high temperature method

131. Criteria for drinking water quality recommended by WHO includes:
a. Chloride 200 mg/litre
b. pH 6.5-8.5/ litre
c. Fe- 3 mg/litre
d. Manganese - 1 mg/litre

Answer

115. a, c. 116. a. 117. b, d, e. 118. a. 119. b, c, d. 120. c, d, e. 121. a, c, e.
122. a, b, d, e. 123. a, c. 124. a, c, d, e. 125. a, d. 126. b. 127. e. 128. c, e.
129. a, b, c, d. 130. d. 131. a, b.

OPHTHALMOLOGY

132. Gradual painless loss of vision is/are seen in:
a. Senile cataract
b. Iridocyclitis
c. Pterygium
d. Diabetic retinopathy
e. Optic neuritis

133. All are true about pterygium except:
a. More common on temporal side
b. Wing shaped degeneration of conjunctiva
c. May cause diminution of vision
d. More common in elderly male
e. More common in tropical region

134. Blood supply of optic chiasm is/are by:
a. Middle cerebral artery
b. Internal carotid artery
c. Anterior cerebral artery
d. Posterior cerebral artery
e. Basilar artery

135. True about Iridocyclitis:
a. It is part of anterior uveitis
b. No risk of phthisis bulbi
c. Keratic precipitates may be found
d. Steroids are used for treatment
e. May be associated with ankylosing spondylitis

136. All are true about Macular corneal opacity except:
a. Diminished vision
b. Penetrating keratoplasty is used for treatment
c. Autosomal dominant inheritance
d. Mucopolysaccharide deposits on cornea
e. Often bilateral

137. Ophthalmic feature of Wilson's disease include(s):
a. Stocker's line
b. Kayser-Fleischer ring in cornea
c. Arcus Senilis
d. Sunflower cataract
e. Ferry's line

138. Causes of lens dislocation:
a. Down syndrome
b. Turner syndrome
c. Sulfite oxidase deficiency
d. Homocystinuria
e. Ehlers-Danlos syndrome

139. Dye used for corneal examination:
a. Fluorescein stain
b. Rose Bengal
c. Indian ink
d. Lissamine green
e. Masson's trichrome

140. Optic neuropathy is associated with:
a. Retinal microaneurysm
b. Neuroretinitis
c. Papilitis
d. Retrobulbar neuritis
e. Hypertension retinopathy

141. Nuclear drop is seen in:
a. Posterior polar cataract
b. Posterior subcapsular cataract
c. Cortical cataract
d. Traumatic cataract
e. Anterior polar cataract

142. True regarding right eye exotropia is/are:
a. Outward deviation of eye
b. Inward deviation of eye
c. Associated with left side hypertrophia
d. Diplopia may occur
e. Sometimes a/w amblyopia

143. Which of the following vitamin deficiency can cause centrocecal scotoma:
a. Vit A
b. Vit E
c. B6
d. B2
e. B12

ENT

144. True about Ludwig angina:
a. Pus formation
b. Spread of infection to parapharyngeal and retropharyngeal space
c. Tongue is pushed upward
d. Presents with painful neck swelling below the mandible
e. Inflammation of floor of mouth

145. Trotter's triads of nasopharyngeal cancer consists of:
a. Palatal palsy
b. Conductive deafness
c. Facial nerve palsy
d. Temporoparietal neuralgia
e. SNHL

146. True about malignant otitis externa:
a. More common in diabetics
b. Pseudomonas is causative organism
c. Granulation tissue formation
d. May involve facial nerve
e. Associated with squamous cell carcinoma

147. All are true about laryngeal carcinoma except:
a. Supraglottic cancer is most common variety
b. Early detected subglottic carcinoma can be treated by radiotherapy
c. Tobacco consumption is a risk factor
d. Hoarseness of voice is a clinical feature
e. Associated with Human papillomavirus (HPV) 16 and 18

148. True about apical petrositis:
a. 6th CN palsy
b. 7th CN palsy
c. Post auricular pain
d. Vertigo
e. Retro-orbital pain

149. Vertigo associated with hearing loss is/are seen in:
a. Meniere's disease
b. Labyrinthitis
c. Vestibular neuritis
d. Acoustic neuroma

Answer

132. a, c, d.	133. a.	134. b, c.	135. a, c, d, e.	136. c.	137. b, d.	138. c, d, e.
139. a, b, d.	140. b, c, d.	141. a.	142. a, d, e.	143. e.	144. b, c, d, e.	145. a, b, d.
146. a,b, c, d.	147. a.	148. a, b, d, e.	149. a, b, d.			

150. True statement(s) about Olfactory system :
- a. Olfactory mucosa cover upper 1/3 of nasal cavity
- b. Olfactory pathway passes via thalamus to orbitofrontal cortex
- c. Adaptation to odour develop only after 1–2 minutes
- d. Olfactory receptors act via cAMP
- e. Rate of olfactory nerve impulses change approximately in proportion to the logarithm of stimulus strength

151. Feature(s) of Scheibe's syndromeis/are:
- a. Semicircular canal fistula
- b. Abnormality in bony labyrinth
- c. Dysplasia of cochlea
- d. Middle ear anomaly

MEDICINE

152. Which of the following is/are not primary headache:
- a. Intracranial hemorrhage
- b. Cluster headache
- c. Migraine
- d. Tension-type headache
- e. High altitude headache

153. Pulsus Bisferiens is/are not seen in:
- a. Severe Aortic stenosis
- b. HOCM
- c. Severe Mitral stenosis
- d. Chronic Aortic regurgitation
- e. Aortic dissection

154. True statement(s) about multiple sclerosis:
- a. Relapsing and remitting symptoms
- b. Autoimmune disease
- c. Steroid is useful during attack
- d. Dawson fingers is characteristic MRI finding
- e. Peginterferon beta-1a reduces severity of attack

155. Metabolic syndrome is/are associated with:
- a. Hypertension
- b. ↑HDL
- c. Hypertriglyceridemia
- d. Increased glucose
- e. PCOS

156. Major criteria of Tuberous sclerosis complex include(s):
- a. Cardiac rhabdomyoma
- b. Confetti skin lesions
- c. Multiple renal cysts
- d. Shagreen patch
- e. Multiple retinal hamartomas

157. True about Gene Xpert:
- a. Rapidly detect Mycobacterium tuberculosis and rifampicin resistance
- b. Use nucleic acid amplification tests (NAAT) technique
- c. Useful to diagnose HIV, hepatitis and TB
- d. Uses real time PCR
- e. Software for gene development

158. Cause(s) of non-anion gap acidosis:
- a. Starvation
- b. Salicylate poisoning
- c. Diarrhea
- d. Ketoacidosis
- e. Type 4 RTA

159. Diagnostic Criteria of Behçet's syndrome include(s):
- a. Recurrent genital ulceration
- b. Recurrent oral ulcers
- c. Uveitis
- d. Negative pathergy test
- e. Conjunctivitis

160. Which of the following is/are true about revised jones criteria 2015 of AHA for diagnosis of acute rheumatic fever:
- a. Monoarthritis is a major criteria in a moderate and high risk population
- b. Single criteria is used all over with one pathway
- c. Fever > 38.5^{0}C is a major criteria
- d. Echocardiography is indicated in all suspected and confirmed cases
- e. In low risk areas incidence of ARF is < 1 per 100,000 school aged children per year

161. Criteria for defining systemic inflammatory response syndrome (SIRS) include(s):
- a. Temperature >40°C
- b. >10% Band form
- c. Tachycardia
- d. Leukopenia (<4,000/ μL)
- e. Tachypnea (>24 breaths/min)

162. True statement(s) about myotonic dystrophy:
- a. Facial sparing
- b. Diaphragm and intercostal muscle weakness result in ventilatory insufficiency
- c. Autosomal recessive inheritance
- d. Heart block may present
- e. Autosomal dominant inheritance

163. Friedrich ataxia is characterised by:
- a. Upper limbs involve more than lower limb
- b. GAA triplet repeats
- c. Absent deep tendon reflexes
- d. Flexor plantar responses
- e. Autosomal recessive inheritance

164. Cause(s) of exudative pleural effusion :
- a. Pancreatitis
- b. Esophageal perforation
- c. Urinothorax
- d. Peritoneal dialysis
- e. Pulmonary embolism

165. Treatment option for malignant pleural effusion include(s):
- a. Pleurodesis
- b. Thoracentesis
- c. Chemotherapy
- d. Radiotherapy
- e. Indwelling Pleural Catheters

Answer

150. a, b, d, e.	151. c.	152. a, e.	153. c.	154. a, b, c, d, e.	155. a, c, d, e.	156. a, d, e.
157. a, b, d.	158. c, e.	159. a, b, c.	160. a, d.	161. b, c, d, e.	162. b, d, e.	163. b, c, e.
164. a, b, e.	165. a, b, c, d, e.					

166. Cause(s) of neutropenia is/are:
a. EBV infection b. Kostmann's syndrome
c. Chediak Higashi syndrome
d. Vitamin B12 deficiency e. Cyclic neutropenia

167. Kussmaul sign is/are seen in:
a. COPD b. Constrictive pericarditis
c. Tension pneumothorax d. HOCM
e. Sometime in Cardiac tamponade

168. Clinical features of MEN 2B syndrome includes:
a. Pheochromocytoma b. Mucosal neuroma
c. Hyperparathyroidism d. Marfanoid features
e. Medullary carcinoma thyroid

SURGERY

169. Intravesicular therapy for non muscle-invasive bladder cancer include(s):
a. BCG b. Interferon
c. Mitomycine C d. Actinomycin D
e. Thiotepa

170. True statements regarding cellulitis:
a. Skin breach is route of entry of microorganisms
b. Staphylococcus & streptococcus are most common microbe
c. Involves skin and Subcutaneous tissue
d. Commonly affects lower limbs
e. Sharp demarcation seen

171. All are true about papillary carcinoma of thyroid except:
a. Homogeneous spread is common
b. Better prognoses than follicular carcinoma
c. May spread to Delphian node
d. More common than follicular carcinoma
e. Capsular invasion is characteristic

172. Treatment modalities for differentiated thyroid carcinoma include(s):
a. Radiotherapy b. Surgery
c. Chemotherapy d. TSH suppression therapy
e. Radioiodine ablation

173. Risk Factors for Squamous cell carcinoma of esophagus include(s)
a. Barret's esophagus b. Hot tea ingestion
c. Alcohol consumption d. Paterson Kelly Syndrome
e. H. Pylori

174. True about Pagett's disease of nipple:
a. Named after 1st patient
b. Confirmed from studying cells from nipple discharge
c. Resembles eczema
d. Melanoma of nipple
e. Superficial manifestation of an underlying breast carcinoma

175. True regarding nipple discharge is/are:
a. Most bilateral discharges are due to benign breast diseases
b. Most common cause of nipple discharge is breast carcinoma in a non-lactating female
c. Purulent discharge can be due to subareolar abscess
d. Duct ectasia presents with palpable indurated mass and green discharge
e. Most common cause of malignant discharge is breast cancer

176. True about splenic rupture:
a. Radiating left shoulder pain
b. Shifting dullness present
c. Secondary to blunt trauma
d. All hemodynamically unstable patients need urgent laparotomy
e. USG is best investigation

177. Management of stage I seminoma involve(s):
a. High inguinal orchidectomy
b. Scrotal orchidectomy
c. Radiotherapy
d. Chemotherapy
e. Retroperitoneal lymphadenectomy (RPLND)

178. True about Direct inguinal hernia:
a. Pass medial to inferior epigastric Artery
b. Occur due to defect in floor of inguinal canal
c. More common in Children
d. Direct hernias are less likely to become strangulated
e. Strangulates more commonly than femoral hernia

179. True statement(s) about umbilical hernia in adults:
a. More common in male
b. Occur due to increased intra-abdominal pressure
c. High risk of strangulation seen in umbilical hernia containing Bowel
d. Mayo repair is done
e. Defect <2 cm can be repaired by sutures alone without mess

180. Fluid calculation in burn patient is/are done by:
a. Parkland Formula
b. Clark Formula
c. Brooke Formula
d. Rule of 9
e. Henderson-Hasselbalch equation

181. Cause of unilateral leg edema include(s):
a. Myxedema
b. Deep vein thrombosis
c. Nephrotic syndrome
d. Compartment syndrome
e. CHF

Answer

166. a, b, c, d, e.	167. b, d, e.	168. a, b, d, e.	169. a, b, c, d, e.	170. a, b, c, d.	171. a, e.	172. a, b, c, d, e.
173. b, c, d.	174. b, c, e.	175. a, c, d, e.	176. a, b, c, d.	177. a, c, d.	178 a, b, d.	179 b, c, d, e.
180 a, c.	181 b, d.					

182. Differential diagnosis of Torsion testis include(s):
a. Appendicitis
b. Hydrocele
c. Viral orchitis
d. Strangulated inguinal hernia
e. Acute epididymo orchitis

183. True about acute Subdural hematoma:
a. Lucid interval seen
b. Due to rupture of middle meningeal artery
c. Immediate evacuation is needed
d. Concave appearance on CT scan
e. Burr hole procedure is treatment option

184. True about Varicocele:
a. Associated with oligospermia
b. Dilatation of pampiniform plexus of veins
c. More common on left side
d. In renal cell cancer, varicocele does not decompress in the supine position
e. Valsalva manoeuver decrease swelling

185. True statement about Cleft Lip and Palate:
a. Isolated Cleft palate is more common than cleft lip alone
b. Unilateral Cleft lip more common on right side
c. Cleft palate doesn't involves soft palate
d. Associated with Sensorineural hearing loss
e. MC syndrome associated with Pierre Robin syndrome

186. True about acute cholecystitis:
a. Pain in right upper quadrant and radiating to scapular area
b. <50% is associated with stone
c. Interval cholecystectomy is better than early cholecystectomy
d. Murphy's sign is positive
e. Tokyo guidelines is used for diagnosis & severity grading

187. False regarding prostate specific antigen (PSA):
a. PSA is organ specific but not cancer specific
b. Cannot be used for screening of prostate cancer
c. Level is high in all patient of prostate carcinoma
d. Normal cutoff value is <4 ng/mL
e. It is age specific

188. True about indications of sentinel lymph node Biopsy in breast cancer:
a. Clinically negative axillary nodes
b. Clinically positive axillary nodes
c. To prevent lymphedema by avoiding unwanted surgery
d. Multifocal breast carcinoma is contraindication
e. Contraindicated in Pregnancy

189. True about clinical feature of Caecal Carcinoma:
a. Generalized weakness
b. Iron deficiency anemia
c. Tenesmus
d. Hematochezia
e. Apple core lesion on radiography

190. True about rectal prolapse:
a. Full thickness is most common in adult
b. Mucosal prolapse is most common in children
c. Diarrhoea in children may be precipitating factor for mucosal prolapse
d. Mucosal prolapse is most common in adult
e. Rectal prolapse in adults is often associated with third-degree haemorrhoids

191. True regarding anal fissure is/are:
a. Up to 5 mm in width
b. Most commonly located anteriorly in midline
c. Usually diagnosed by anoscopy
d. Conservative management is done initially
e. In chronic and recurrent cases lateral internal sphincterotomy is helpful

192. True about spontaneous bacterial peritonitis:
a. Mostly asymptomatic
b. Fever and abdominal pain are common presentation
c. High risk of mortality
d. Antibiotics may be given prior to bacterial culture report
e. Leukocytosis

193. Achalasia cardia is characterized by all except:
a. Regurgitation
b. Difficulty in swallowing
c. Loss of appetite
d. Hematesis
e. Ulcerations

194. All of the following are good prognostic factors for seminoma testis except:
a. Nonpulmonary visceral metastases
b. Primarily retroperitoneal
c. Primarily gonadal
d. AFP more than 10,000 ng/ml
e. hCG more than 50,000 IU/ml

195. True about physiological hernia
a. Herniation of Foregut
b. Herniation of Foregut + midgut
c. Herniation of Midgut
d. Goes back around 4 week after herniation
e. Goes back around 10 week of fetus age

OBSTETRICS & GYNECOLOGY

196. Subtype included in type II endometrial carcinoma:
a. Clear cell
b. Mixed mullerian
c. Mucinous
d. Serous
e. Endometrioid

Answer

182. c, d, e. 183. c, d, e. 184. a, b, c, d. 185. a, d, e. 186. a, d, e. 187. b, c. 188. a, c, d, e.
189. a, b, e. 190. a, b, c, e. 191. a, d, e. 192. b, c, d, e. 193. d. 194 a. 195. c, d, e.
196. a, b, d.

197. Not a risk factor for endometrial carcinoma:
a. OCP b. Tamoxifen
c. Early menarche d. Infertility
e. Nulliparity

198. Which of the following cervical length is predictor of preterm labour:
a. ≤2.5 cm b. ≤3.0 cm
c. ≤3.5 cm d. ≤4.0 cm
e. ≤4.5 cm

199. Incorrect statement (s) about menstrual cycle:
a. Luteal phase is constant
b. Follicular phase is constant
c. Onset of LH surge occur 36 hr before ovulation and peak 12 hr before ovulation
d. Ovulation occur after 14 day of menstruation
e. Ovulation occur 14 day before next menstruation

200. Ultrasonographic finding of intrauterine pregnancy in first trimester include (s):
a. Pseudogestational sac b. True gestational sac
c. Corpus luteum in ovary d. Fetal pole
e. Yolk sac

201. Karyotype of complete hydatidiform mole is/are:
a. 46 XX b. 46 XY
c. 45XX d. 69XXX
e. 69XXY

202. Feature (s) of magnesium toxicity in pregnancy:
a. Loss of deep tendon reflex b. Decreased respiratory rate
c. Decreased urine output d. Hypertension
e. Increased heart rate

203. Stage 3 carcinoma cervix (FIGO staging) involves:
a. Lower 1/3rd of vagina
b. Lower 2/3rd of vagina
c. Medial 1/3rd of parametrium
d. Complete parametrium
e. Pelvis wall

204. All are true about Ashermann syndrome except:
a. Due to tubercular pathology
b. Causes primary amenorrhoea
c. Curettage can be a cause
d. Can be viewed by hsyterogram
e. All of the above

205. True about varicella zoster in pregnancy:
a. Congenital anomalies are more common when the infection occurs during 12-20 weeks of gestation
b. Congenital anomalies are more common when the infection occurs after 20 weeks of gestation
c. Immunoglobulins can be given to the neonates whose mother had varicella 5 days before to 2 days after the delivery
d. Acyclovir is unsafe in pregnancy
e. Varicella vaccine is given in pregnancy

206. False statement (s) about PCOS:
a. Prevalence is >5% in Chinese population
b. Rotterdam criteria decreases the prevalence in the population
c. More in Caucasian as compared to Asian
d. Prevalence of PCOS varies in different population due to use of different diagnostic criteria
e. More common in monozygotic twins

207. Management options of HSIL on pap smear include (s)
a. Liquid based cytology b. Colposcopy & biopsy
c. HPV DNA testing d. HPV vaccination
e. Hysterectomy

208. Post-coital contraceptive used to prevent pregnancy is/are:
a. LNG
b. CuT < 5 days of unprotected sex
c. Progesterone only pill d. Progesterone and estrogen pill
e. None of the above

209. Rh immunization is/are diagnosed by:
a. Increase in Middle cerebral artery Peak systolic velocity
b. By platting Lilly zone graph
c. Doppler flow velocity waveforms in umbilical artery
d. Disproportionate growth on USG
e. None of the above

210. Mechanisms of action of depot medroxyprogesterone (DMPA) include all except:
a. Thinning of inner uterine layer
b. Thickening of cervical mucosa
c. Immobilization of sperms
d. Inhibition of ovulation
e. Decreased entry of sperms in uterus

211. Following is true regarding immunoprophylaxis of Hepatitis B in pregnancy:
a. A combination of hepatitis B immune globulin (HBIG) and hepatitis B vaccination should be initiated within 24 hours of delivery
b. HBIG can be given up to 72 hours after birth
c. In mothers with an unknown HBsAg positivity status at delivery, the birth dose of hepatitis B vaccine can be delayed up to >24 hours of birth
d. In the case of preterm babies of HBsAg positive mothers, the birth dose is indicated only if the baby weighs more than 2 kilograms
e. 4 doses of vaccine should be given postnatally

PAEDIATRICS

212. True regarding typical absence seizure:
a. Most common age group is 5-10 yr
b. Generally last more 30 seconds
c. Post seizure confusion present
d. Leaves children unaware
e. Precipitated by hyperventilation

Answer

197. a.	198. a.	199. b, d.	200. b, c, d, e.	201. a, b.	202. a, b, c.	203. a, e.
204. b.	205. a, c.	206. b, c.	207. b, e.	208. a, b, c, d.	209. a, b, c, d.	210. c.
211. a, b, e.	212. a, d, e.					

213. Which of the following is/are found in neonatal lupus:
a. Anti-ds DNA antibody
b. Anti-histone antibody
c. Anti-La (SS-B)
d. Anti-Ro (SSA)
e. Anti-U1RNP

214. Which of the following surgeries are used for TOF:
a. Modified Blalock–Taussig shunt
b. Waterston-Cooley shunt
c. Potts shunt
d. Aortoplasty
e. Cutting & end to end anastomosis of aorta

215. Lanugo hair occur in:
a. Preterm baby
b. Post term baby
c. Shoulder
d. Fetus
e. Palm

216. Craniosynostosis is/are seen in:
a. Crouzon syndrome
b. Carpenter syndrome
c. Pfeiffer syndrome
d. Down syndrome
e. Pierre Robin syndrome

217. True about Wilms' Tunor:
a. Associated with aniridia
b. Mostly unilateral
c. Surrounded by pseudocapsule
d. Most commonly presents in neonate
e. Associated with palpable abdominal mass

218. Which of the following statement (s) is/are true about ventilatory support for ARDS in infants:
a. High FiO_2
b. Low respiratory rate
c. High positive end expiratory pressure (PEEP)
d. Long inspiration time
e. Low tidal volume

219. Difficult airway in child is associated with:
a. Fragile-X syndrome
b. Pierre-Robin syndrome
c. Turner syndrome
d. De-George syndrome
e. Choanal atresia

220. An infant presented with sparse, curly, hypopigmented hair with failure to thrive. There is history of seizures & frequent fractures. Genetic analysis shows- positive for ATP7A gene. Following is/are also associated with the condition:
a. Also k/a kinky hair disease
b. Hypotonia
c. Mental retardation
d. Increased circulating ceruloplasmin
e. Trichorhexis nodosa

ORTHOPAEDICS

221. Absolute indications of open reduction:
a. Long bone fractures
b. Failed closed reduction
c. Non-union of old fracture
d. Displaced intra-articular fractures
e. Fracture of lateral condyle of humerus in children

222. A 20 year old man's X-ray of lower end femur shows periosteal reaction & codman triangle. Which of the following investigation is/are required for further management of this person:
a. Bone scan
b. Bone biopsy
c. CT scan
d. MRI scan
e. PET

223. Ivory vertebrae is/are seen in:
a. Sickle cell anaemia
b. Osteoporosis
c. Osteoblastic metastasis
d. Paget's disease of bone
e. Lymphoma

224. True statement (s) about Triple deformity of knee:
a. Flexion at the knee, posterior subluxation & external rotation of tibia
b. Extension at the knee, posterior subluxation & external rotation of tibia
c. Flexion at the knee, posterior subluxation & internal rotation of tibia
d. Extension at the knee, posterior subluxation & internal rotation of tibia
e. Seen in TB

225. Joint involved in triple arthrodesis:
a. Subtalar joint
b. Cuboideonavicular joint
c. Calcaneocuboid joint
d. Talonavicular joint
e. Naviculocuneiform joint

226. Injuries with high risk of developing compartment syndrome:
a. Closed tibial fractures
b. Supracondylar fracture of humerus
c. Forearm bone fractures
d. Femur fracture
e. Pelvic fracture

227. True about Ewing sarcoma:
a. Common in old age
b. Classical cytogenetic abnormality is t (14:7)
c. Chemotherapy is of no use
d. Highly radiosensitive tumour
e. Very aggressive tumor

Answer

213. c, d, e. 214. a, b, c. 215. a, c, d. 216. a, b, c. 217. a, b, c, e. 218. c, d, e. 219. a, b, c, d, e.
220. a, b, c, e. 221. b, c, d. 222. a, b, c, d. 223. a, c, d, e. 224. a, e. 225. a, c, d. 226. a, b, c.
227. d, e.

228. **Common feature of Ewing sarcoma and chronic osteomyelitis:**
   a. Periosteal reaction b. New bone formation
   c. Sunburst appearance d. Location at metaphysic
   e. Fever

229. **A young patient presented with left knee and right ankle swelling and pain. On examination there were yellowish brown keratotic papules present on palm & soles and erythema with pain in the eye. There is h/o burning micturition and urethral discharge. Most likely diagnosis is:**
   a. Behçet' disease b. Reactive arthritis
   c. Psoriasis d. Secondary syphilis
   e. Rheumatoid arthritis

ANESTHESIA

230. **True regarding anesthesia in an obstetric female:**
   a. Epidural is contraindicated in HELLP syndrome
   b. Risk of aspiration is increased as lower oesophageal sphincter tone is reduced due to progesterone
   c. General anesthesia is preferred in every caesarean
   d. Dose of local anesthesia is decreased while giving epidural anesthesia for caesarean
   e. General anesthesia is preferred only for emergency caesarean

231. **True about paediatric anesthesia:**
   a. Spinal anaesthesia in < 6 month child is contraindicated
   b. ETT size is calculated according to weight
   c. For post-operative pain caudal block is used
   d. Low dose of drug is required as compared to adult in regional anaesthesia
   e. Abdominal surgeries preferred in general anaesthesia

232. **True about ketamine:**
   a. Deceases ICT
   b. Bronchodilator
   c. Choice in day care surgery
   d. Bradycardia
   e. Bronchoconstrictor

233. **Agent used for spinal anesthesia:**
   a. Bupivacaine 0.5% b. Bupivacaine 1%
   c. Lidocaine 1% d. Lidocaine 2.5
   e. Lidocaine 5%

234. **Which of the following drug (s) is/are mainly metabolized extra-hepatically in plasma:**
   a. Halothane
   b. Propofol
   c. Lignocaine
   d. Atracurium
   e. None of the above

SKIN

235. **False regarding Dermatitis herpetiformis:**
   a. Associated with gluten-sensitive enteropathy
   b. Caused by Herpes simplex virus 6 & 7
   c. Dapsone is used for treatment
   d. Deposition of IgG in dermis
   e. Lesion common on flexure surfaces

236. **Nail changes in psoriasis is/are:**
   a. Onycholysis b. Oil drop discolouration
   c. Subungual hyperkeratosis d. Nail pitting
   e. Pterygium formation

PSYCHIATRY

237. **True regarding lucid interval:**
   a. Common in extradural hemorrhage
   b. Period of sanity
   c. Occur in subarachnoid hemorrhage
   d. Occur in mania
   e. None of the above

238. **Which of the following is/are given in treatment of OCD except:**
   a. Cyclophosphamide b. Azathioprine
   c. SSRIs d. Anti-psychotic drugs
   e. Behaviour therapy

239. **Which of the following drug is/are serotonin and noradrenaline reuptake inhibitor (SNRI):**
   a. Paroxetine b. Fluoxetine
   c. Duloxetine d. Venlafaxine
   e. Desvenlafaxine

240. **Kurt Schneider 1st rank symptom include (s) all except:**
   a. Third person auditory hallucination
   b. Through insertion
   c. Somatic passivity phenomenon
   d. Perplexity
   e. Delusional perceptions

241. **True about acute and transient psychosis disorder (ATPD):**
   a. Acute onset
   b. Variation in symptom & severity
   c. Present for long duration
   d. Presence of predisposing factor
   e. Good prognosis

242. **Drug (s) which are used as anti-craving agent in alcohol:**
   a. Acamprosate b. Naloxone
   c. Naltrexone d. Disulfiram

243. **Cannabis abuse may be associated with:**
   a. OCD b. Schizophrenia
   c. Anxiety d. Flash-back
   e. Psychosis

Answer

228. a, b, e. 229. b. 230. a, b, d, e. 231. c, d, e. 232. b. 233. a, e. 234. d.
235. b, d, e. 236. a, b, c, d. 237. a, b, d. 238. a, b. 239. c, d, e. 240 d. 241. a, b, d, e.
242. a, c, d. 243. b, c, d, e.

244. According to latest update, which of the following is true about suicide:
a. Attempted suicide is now decriminalized
b. More common in depression
c. Related to substance abuse
d. Elderly people are more predisposed
e. No relation with personality traits

RADIOLOGY

245. Telltale triangle radiographic sign is/are seen in:
a. Pleural effusion
b. Pericardial effusion
c. Pneumothorax
d. Pneumoperitoneum
e. Pneumoediastinum

246. Minimum pleural effusion is/are detected by:
a. X-ray PA view
b. X-ray AP view
c. X-ray lateral view
d. USG
e. Lateral decubitus

247. True about 'Technetium 99m' (99mTc):
a. Half-life 6 hr
b. Most commonly used radionuclide
c. Can detect ectopic gastric tissue
d. Generator originated nuclide
e. Emit beta & alpha rays

248. True statement about MRI:
a. Less radiation exposure
b. Oxygen cylinder should not take inside of MRI room
c. MR scanner installation is enclosed in a lead shield
d. No influence from radiofrequency signals
e. MR scanner installation enclosed in Faraday cage

249. True about left atrial enlargement:
a. Double atrial shadow
b. Downward & outward extension of the apex
c. Associated with mitral stenosis
d. Splaying of the carina
e. Posterior displacement of left upper lobe bronchus

250. Radioactive isotopes of iodine are all except:
a. I 123
b. I 125
c. I 127
d. I 124
e. I 131

Answer

244. a, b, c, d. 245. d. 246. d>e. 247. a, b, c, d. 248. b, e. 249. a, c, d, e. 250. c.

NOVEMBER 2018 ANSWERS & EXPLANATIONS

ANATOMY

1. Ans. a. Sacroiliac ligaments, b. Pubis symphysis, e. Iliolumber ligament

[Ref: Maheshwari 6th/123; BDC 7th/Vol. II 460-62;Campbell 11th/3339-42; Snell's 9th/ 241-42; Apley 9th/829]

- ***Inguinal ligament & External oblique aponeurosis play no role in providing stability to pelvic ring***

Pelvic Ring

◈ *Maheshwari 6th/123; Apley 9th/829*

- Pelvic ring is formed, in continuity from the front, by pubic symphysis, pubic crest, pectineal line of pubis, arcuate line of the ileum & ala & promontory of the sacrum
- **Stability of pelvic ring** *depends, posteriorly on* ***sacro-iliac joints*** *& anteriorly on the* ***symphysis pubis.***
- *The* **sacroiliac-iliac joints** *are bound in front & behind by the strong, band like,* ***sacroiliac ligaments.***
- *The* **pubic symphysis** *is reinforced by ligaments of the pelvis, such as* ***ilio-lumbar ligaments*** *& sacrospinous ligaments, provide additional stability of the ring.*

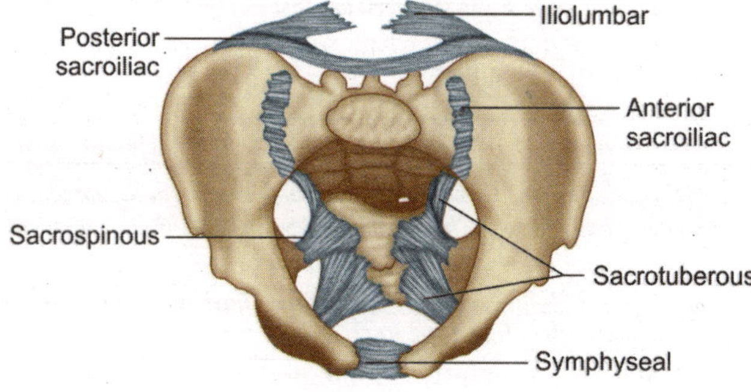

Fig: (*Apley 9th/829*): Ligaments supporting the pelvis

2. Ans. b. Lacrimal bone, d. Greater wing of spenoid

[Ref: Dhingra 7th/165; Grays 40th/471; ENT by Hazarika 3rd/231; L & T 11th/5; BDC 7th/28]

Lacrimal Bone: Forms Medial Wall of Orbit

◈ *BDC 7th/28*

Nasal Septum

◈ *Dhingra 7th/165; Grays 40th/471*

The nasal septum is the median osteocartilaginus partition b/w two halves of nasal cavity

Nasal Septum Consists of 3 Part

- Columellar Septum - It is formed by columella, containing the medial crura of alar cartilage.
- Membranous Septum - It consists of double longer of skin with no bony or cartilaginous support. It lies b/w columella & caudal border of septal cartilages.
- Septum proper - It consists of osteocartilaginous framework. It has 2 part: bony & cartilaginous

Bony part

- *Mainly by – Vomer; Perpendicular plate of ethmoid*
- *Also by- Nasal spine of frontal bone; Rostrum of sphenoid; Nasal crests of nasal; Palatine bone; Maxillary bone*

Cartilaginous part - ***Septal cartilage (Quadrilateral);*** *Septal processes of Inferior nasal*

The septum has 4 borders-Superior, Inferior, anterior & posterior, two surfaces-right & Left.

Nasal Septum Proper: Principle Constituents are

◈ *Hazarika 3rd/231*

- Perpendicular plate of ethmoid
- Vomer
- Large septal (quadrilateral) cartilage
- *Small contribution from: crests of nasal bones, nasal spine of frontal bone,* ***rostrum of sphenoid****, crest of palatine bones, crest of maxilla, anterior nasal spine of maxilla etc*

3. Ans. b. Inferior vena cava, c. Vagus nerve, d. Phrenic nerve

[Ref: BDC 7th/ Vol.I 201-02; Snell 9th/46; Gray's 40th/1007-08]

Table: Major opening in Diaphragm

Opening	Situation	Shape	Structures passing	Effect on contraction
Vena cava	T8, junction of right and median leaflet of central tendon	Quadrilateral	IVC Right phrenic nerve Lymphatic of liver	Dilation
Oesophageal	T10, splitting of right crus	Elliptical	Oesophagus, Both vagal trunks, Left gastric vessel	Constriction
Aortic	T12, behind median arcuate ligament	Rounded	Aorta , Thoracic duct, Azygos vein	No change

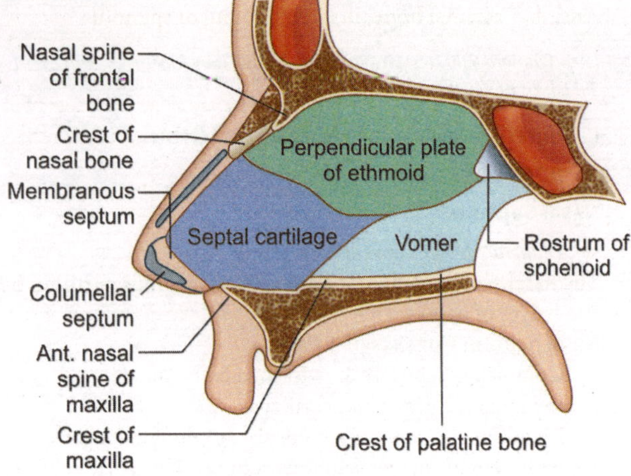

Fig: Anatomy of nasal septum

4. **Ans. a. SA Node is supplied by right coronary artery in majority of cases, b. SA Node is also supplied by …, e. Left bundle branch is supplied by both right & left coronary artery**

[Ref: BDC 7th/Vol.I 279;Gray's 40th/ 979-80; Snell's 9th/86-87]

- **Whole(almost) conducting system is supplied by right coronary artery**
- **AV node is supplied mainly by right coronary artery**

Right Coronary Artery

◈ *BDC 7th/Vol.I 279*
- Whole of the conducting system of the heart except a part of the left branch of the AV bundle(left coronary artery)
- The SA node is supplied by the left coronary artery in about 40% of cases

Right Coronary Artery

◈ *Snell's 9th/86-87*
- *A large septal branch(of posterior interventricular artery) supplies the* **atrioventricular node***(In 10% of individuals, the posterior interventricular artery is replaced by a branch of left coronary artery)- Snell's 9th/87*
- Artery of the sinuatrial node(SA) supplies SA node(In 35% of individuals it arises from the left coronary artery-Circumflex branch)

"**Left coronary artery**: *Supplies* ***Right bundle branch(RBB) & Left bundle branch(LBB)***"*- Snell's 9th/88*

"**Right coronary artery**: *Supplies* ***SA node, AV node & bundle. LBB also receives small branches***"*- Snell's 9th/88*

Cardiac dominance: *The artery which gives posterior interventricular branch is dominant artery(85-90% cases: RCA; 10-15% cases: Circumflex artery-LCA)*

5. **Ans. a. C_5, c. C_6, d. C_7**

[Ref: BDC 7th/Vol. I 58; Snell's 9th/ 352;Gray's 39th/846]

"Root value of **long thoracic nerve** (Nerve to serratus anterior/ Nerve of Bell): ***C 5, 6, 7***"*-BDC 7th/Vol. I 58; Snell's 9th/ 352*

Root Value

◈ *BDC 7th/Vol. I 58*
- Ulnar nerve: C7, 8 T1
- Radial nerve C5-8, T1
- Axillary nerve: C5, 6
- Brachial plexus: C5, 6, 7, 8, T1

6. **Ans. e. Ulnar nerve is affected**

[Ref: BDC 7th/Vol.I 59; Snell's 9th/429]

Erb's Paralysis

◈ *BDC 7th/Vol.I 59*
- *Cause of injury:* ***Birth injury****, fall on the shoulder & during anesthesia*
- *Nerve root involved:* ***Mainly C5 & partly C6***
- Ulnar nerve(C7-8,T1) is not involved
- **Muscle paralysed:** Mainly biceps brachii, deltoid, brachialis & brachioradialis. Partly supraspinatus, infraspinatus & supinator
- Deformity
  - *Arms: Hangs by side; it is* ***adducted & medially rotated***
  - *Forearm: Extended & pronated*
- Disability
  - Abduction & lateral rotation of the arm at shoulder joint
  - Flexion & supination of the forearm
  - Biceps & supinator jerk are lost
  - Sensation are lost over a small area over the lower part of the deltoid

7. **Ans. b. Alar nasalis, e. Levator labii superioris alaeque nasi**

[Ref: BDC 7th/Vol. III 66-67; Gray's 40th/548-49; The Cyclopedia of Anatomy and Physiology by Robert Bentley Todd Vol. II /222; theodora. com]

- ***Levator labii superioris alaeque nasi & Alar nasalis elevates the alae of the nose***

Levator labii superioris alaeque nasi: It is the muscle that ***elevates the upper lip and the alae of the nose***, allowing the nostrils to dilate in a sneering expression- *thefreedictionary.com*

Nose Muscles

◈ *en.wikipedia.org*
- The **elevator muscle group** includes the procerus muscle that helps to flare the nostrils; and ***the levator labii superioris alaeque nasi muscle***, which ***lifts the upper lip and the alae.***
- The **depressor muscle group** includes the alar nasalis muscle and the depressor septi nasi muscle.
- The **compressor muscle group** includes the transverse nasalis muscle.
- The **dilator muscle group** includes the dilator naris muscle that expands the nostrils; it is in two parts: (i) the dilator naris anterior muscle, and (ii) the dilator naris posterior muscle

Alar Nasalis

◈ *Robert Bentley Todd Vol. II /222*
- Thin, long & triangular muscle
- Action: ***To raise the ala of the nose*** & the adjacent part of the upper lip; in doing so it dilates also the nostril & become a muscle of inspiration. When strongly thrown into action, it corrugates the skin of the nose transversely

"**Orbicularis oris**: It is situated around lip. Action- Closes lips & protrudes lips, numerous extrinsic muscles make it most versatile for various types of grimaces"- *BDC 7th/Vol. III 66*

"**Zygomatic minor**: It is around around lip. Action- Elevates the upper lip"- *BDC 7th/Vol. III 66*

"**Levator labii superioris**: It is muscle around lip. Action- Elevates the upper lip, forms nasolabial groove"- *BDC 7th/Vol. III 66*

Muscles Around Nasal Opening

◈ *BDC 7th/Vol. III 66; Gray's 40th/548-49*

- Procerus: Cause transverse wrinkles
- Compressor naris: Nasal aperture compressed
- Dilator naris:Nasal aperture dilated
- Depressor septi: Nose pulled inferiorly

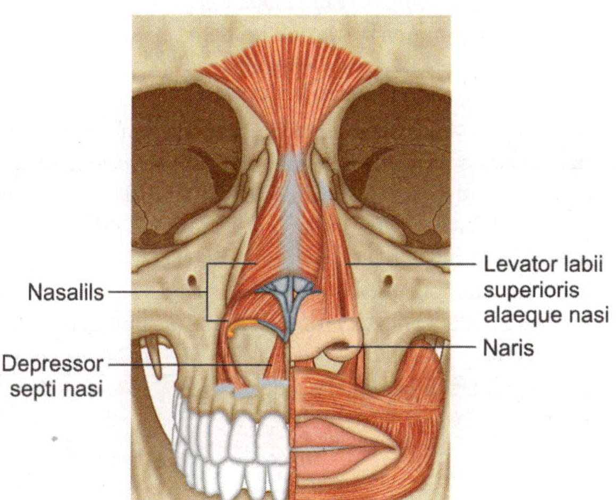

Fig: *(Gray's 40th/548):* The nasal musculature

8. Ans. a. Inferior vesicle artery, b. Middle rectal artery, d. Internal pudendal artery

[Ref: BDC 7th/Vol. II 437; Snell's 9th/277]

Blood Supply of Prostate

◈ *BDC 7th/Vol. II 437*

- Inferior vesicle
- Middle rectal
- ***Internal pudendal artery***
- Branches of these arteries form a large outer or subscapular plexus & a small inner or periurethral plexus. The greater part of the gland is supplied by the subcapsular plexus

9. Ans. b. Contains mucous secreting glands, d. Made up of elastic cartilage, e. Has bilateral lymphatic supply

[Ref: BDC 7th/ Vol. III 264; Snell's 8th/ 802; Moore 2nd/628; Gray's 40th/ 577-78, 588; Dhingra 6th/283-85; H and N Cancer by Louis B Harrison 3rd/368; H and N Surgery by Robert Satalof 1st /693]

Epiglottis/Epiglottic Cartilage

◈ *BDC 7th/ Vol. III 264*

- The epiglottis is a *leaf-shaped structure.*
- It is a flap that is made of ***elastic cartilage*** tissue covered with a mucous membrane, attached to the entrance of the larynx.
- The epiglottis is one of nine cartilaginous structures that make up the larynx (voice box). While one is breathing, it lies completely within the pharynx. When one is swallowing it serves as part of the anterior of the larynx.
- The epiglottis has two surfaces, a lingual and a laryngeal surface, related to the oral cavity and the larynx respectively
- The entire lingual surface and the apical portion of the laryngeal surface (since it is vulnerable to abrasion due to its relation to the digestive tract) are covered by *a stratified squamous non-keratinized epithelium.*
- The rest of the laryngeal surface on the other hand, which is in relation to the respiratory system, has respiratory epithelium: pseudostratified, ciliated columnar cells and ***mucus secreting Goblet cells.***

Lymphatic Drainage

◈ *Gray's 40th/ 588; Moore 2nd/628*

- The vocal cords, with their firmly bound mucosa and paucity of lymphatics, provide a clear demarcation between the upper and lower areas of the larynx.
- **Above the vocal cords**, the lymph vessels draining the supraglottic part of the larynx accompany the superior laryngeal artery, pierce the thyrohyoid membrane, and end in the upper deep cervical lymph nodes, ***often bilaterally.*** The supraglottic lymphatics also communicate with those at the base of the tongue. (Note: ***Epiglottis is supraglottic part of larynx***- *Dhingra 6th/283*)
- **Below the vocal cords**, some of the lymph vessels pass through the conus elasticus to reach the prelaryngeal

(Delphian) and/or pretracheal and paratracheal lymph nodes, while others accompany the inferior laryngeal artery and join the ***lower deep cervical nodes.***

"The supraglottis has **extensive bilateral network** of lymphatics that result in frequent regional metastases"-*H and N Cancer by Louis B Harrison 3rd/368*

*"Unlike the other two anatomic sites (glottis and subglottis) of the larynx, the supraglottis is formed without midline union and consequently has **bilateral lymphatic drainage**"-H and N Surgery by Robert Satalof 1st /693*

10. Ans. a. Thalamus & c. Basal..

[Ref: Harrison 18th/2170-76; CSDT 11th/875-76; radiographics.rsna.org/ content /31/1/5. full; www.ajronline.org]

"Deep venous thrombosis typically results in bilateral *symmetric involvement of the thalami and occasionally the basal ganglia. The causes include pregnancy, oral contraceptives, infection, trauma, and dehydration,* but the cause is undetermined in 20–25% of patients. An abnormally hyperdense vein may be seen

on CT scans, and corresponding T1 hyperintensity from clot in the sinuses may be seen on MR images" *(radiographics. rsna.org/ content/31/1/5. full)*

Deep Cerebral Venous Thrombosis

◈ *www.ajronline.org/content/192/2/W53.full*

- Cerebral venous thrombosis (CVT) is usually associated with risk factors such as a hypercoagulable state during pregnancy or puerperium, use of oral contraceptives, vasculitis, and intracranial or systemic infections.
- Thrombosis of the **superficial dural sinus system** (the superior and inferior sagittal sinuses, transverse sinuses, and cortical veins) typically results in cerebral edema and venous infarction of the ***cerebral cortex*** near the vertex.
- However, involvement of the deep venous system (the *internal cerebral vein, vein of Galen, and straight sinus*) can result in a different distribution of venous hypertension.
- Deep CVT often occurs as an extension of widespread superficial dural sinus CVT; in rare instances, however, it may occur in isolation, with bilateral involvement of the *thalamus and basal ganglia* without cerebral lobar venous infarction
- Patients present with acute headache, nausea, vomiting, seizures, and altered mental status.
- Focal neurologic deficits, coma, and death may ensue in severe cases

11. Ans. a. Differentiation of genital ridge into lineage of female or male gonads occurs at 10 weeks, c. Metanephric duct forms glomerulus, d. Nephrons are formed from metanephros, e. Collecting duct develop from mesonephric duct

[Ref: Gray's 40th/ 1307;I.B.Singh 11th/265-68;Langman 11th/235-37]

*The **urinary bladder** (except trigone) is derived from vesicourethral canal, cranial part of urogenital sinus(endodermal). **Trigone** is derived from absorbed part of **Wolfian duct/mesonephric duct(mesodermal)**"- I.B.Singh 11th/271*

*"Differentiation of genital ridge into lineage of female or male gonads(ovary or testes) occurs at **6-10 weeks.** By **12 weeks** this differentiation has occurred in all foetuses"- I.B.Singh 11th/286-87*

*"The **kidney** develops from two source. The **excretory tubules (nephrons)** are derived from the **metanephros** (=lowest part of nephrogenic cord which is derived from intermediate mesoderm). The **collecting part** is formed by ramification of the ureteric bud (which arise from the **mesonephric duct**)- I.B.Singh 11th/264*

Metanephric mesenchyme *• Metanephric blastema → Solid clump • Vesicle→ Pear shaped(Comma C stage) vesicle • S Stage vesicle → Distal end of vesicle invaginated by a tuft of capillaries •**Glomerulus**- I.B.Singh 11th/267-68*

Uretric bud→ Ampula • Pelvis of kidney → Major calyces • minor calyces & collecting tubules-I.B.Singh 11th/266-67

PHYSIOLOGY

12. Ans. a. RBCs, b. Temperature, c. Plasma protein, d. Flow rate, e. Infection

[Ref: Ganong 25th/573-74; Guyton 13th(2nd SAE)/234-35; A.K. Jain 6th/316]

Factor Affecting Viscosity of Blood

◈ *A.K. Jain 6th/316*

- Viscosity of blood inversely proportional to:
  - ***Temperature*** *within limit*
  - Flow rate
- **Viscosity of blood directly proportional to:**
  - ***Haematocrit*** *i.e, packed cell volume(PCV) or* ***volume of blood occupied by red blood cells.***
  - *Concentration of **plasma proteins,** especially increase in high molecular weight proteins e.g, Ig*
  - *Diameter of vessel wall*

Malaria: The analysis of blood viscosity for shear rates revealed that the blood viscosity of the infected patients was significantly greater than that of the non-infected individuals. The ***viscosity of the blood was greater in the infected individuals than in the non-infected subjects***"- www.sciencedirect.com

"Clinically significant increases in viscosity are seen in diseases in which ***plasma proteins*** such as the immunoglobulins are markedly elevated as well as when ***red blood cells*** are abnormally rigid (hereditary spherocytosis)"- *Ganong 25th/573-74*

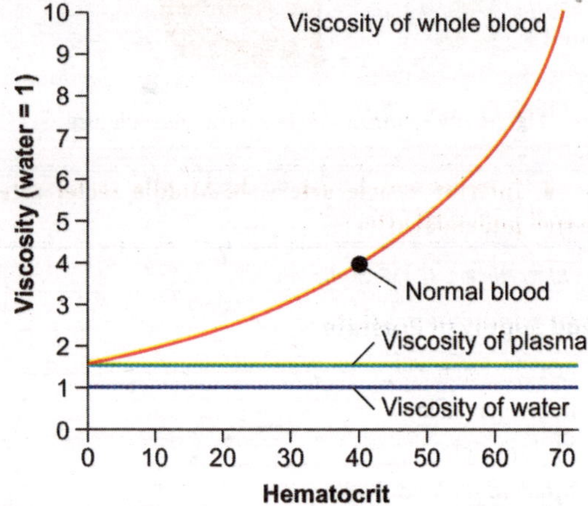

Fig: *(Guyton 13th(2nd SAE)/234):* Effect of Hematocrit on Blood Viscosity

13. Ans. b. Causes anemia, c. Cyanosis is observed, d. Caused by Nitrate and nitrite compounds, e. Methylene blue is used for therapy

[Ref: Ganong 25th/ 556-57; A.K. Jain 6th/59; Harrison 20th/695,236]

Carbon monoxide(CO) *react with Hb to form carboxy haemoglobin or* ***carbon monoxy haemoglobin***- *A.K. Jain 6th/59*
Carbon dioxide *reacts with Hb to form* ***carbamino-haemoglobin***- *A.K. Jain 6th/59*

"**Cyanosis** is also observed when non-functional hemoglobin, such as ***methemoglobin*** (consequential or acquired) or sulfhemoglobin, is present in blood"-*Harrison 20th/236*

"**Cyanosis** refers to a bluish color of the skin and mucous membranes resulting from an increased quantity of reduced hemoglobin (i.e., deoxygenated hemoglobin) or of hemoglobin derivatives (e.g., ***methemoglobin*** or sulfhemoglobin) in the small blood vessels of those tissues. ***A cherry-colored flush, rather than cyanosis, is caused by COHb***"-*Harrison 20th/236*

Methemoglobinemias

◈ *Harrison 20th/695*

- Methemoglobin is generated by oxidation of the ***heme iron moieties to the ferric state***, causing a characteristic ***bluish-brown muddy color*** resembling cyanosis.
- Methemoglobin has such high oxygen affinity that virtually no oxygen is delivered.
- Levels >50–60% are often fatal.
- Congenital methemoglobinemia arises from globin mutations that stabilize iron in the ferric state (e.g., HbM Iwata [α87His→Tyr], or from mutations that impair the enzymes that reduce methemoglobin to hemoglobin (e.g., methemoglobinreductase, NADP diaphorase).
- Acquired methemoglobinemia is caused by toxins that oxidize heme iron, notably ***nitrate and nitrite***-containing compounds, including drugs commonly used in cardiology and anesthesiology.
- Methemoglobinemia often causes symptoms of cerebral ischemia at levels >15%; levels >60% are usually lethal.
- Intravenous injection of 1 mg/kg of methylene blue is effective emergency therapy. Milder cases and follow-up of severe cases can be treated orally with methylene blue or ascorbic acid (300–600 mg/d).
- Congenital methemoglobinemia does not usually require treatment other than avoidance of oxidative drugs or agents.

14. Ans. b. Contralateral loss of pain & temperature, c. Ipsilateral motor loss, e. Ipsilateral loss of discriminative touch

[Ref: Ganong 25th/172;Harrison 20th/3173-74; A K Jain 6th/934-35]

Brown-Séquard Hemicord Syndrome

◈ *Harrison 20th/3173-74*

- This consists of **ipsilateral** ***weakness (corticospinal tract) and loss of joint position and vibratory sense*** (posterior column), with **contralateral** loss of ***pain and temperature sense*** (spinothalamic tract) one or two levels below the lesion.
- Segmental signs, such as radicular pain, muscle atrophy, or loss of a deep tendon reflex, are unilateral. Partial forms are more common than the fully developed syndrome
- "**Below the level of the lesion**, on the ***same side, there is extensive motor loss*** but little sensory loss; while on the ***opposite side there is extensive sensory loss but little motor loss***"- A K Jain 6th/935

Brown-Séquard Syndrome

◈ *Ganong 25th/172*

- A functional hemisection of the spinal cord causes a characteristic and easily recognized clinical picture that reflects damage to ascending sensory (dorsal column pathway, ventrolateral spinothalamic tract) and descending motor (corticospinal tract) pathways, which is called the Brown Séquard syndrome.
- The lesion to fasciculus gracilus or fasciculus cuneatus leads to ***ipsilateral loss of discriminative touch, vibration, and proprioception*** below the level of the lesion.
- The loss of the spinothalamic tract leads to ***contralateral loss of pain and temperature sensation*** beginning one or two segments below the lesion.
- Damage to the corticospinal tract produces ***weakness and spasticity in certain muscle groups on the same side of the body.***
- Although a precise spinal hemisection is rare, the syndrome is fairly common because it can be caused by a spinal cord tumor, spinal cord trauma, degenerative disk disease, and
- ischemia.
- ***Pyramidal tract includes*** **corticospinal tract and corticobulbar tract**

15. Ans. a. Aα → Proprioception, b. Aβ → Touch & pressure, d. Aδ → Pain & temperature

[Ref: Ganong 25th/94]

Nerve Fiber Types & Function

◈ *Ganong 25th/94*

- Mammalian nerve fibers are divided into ***A, B, and C groups***
- A group can be subdivided into ***α, β, γ, and δ fibers.***
- In general, the greater the diameter of a given nerve fiber, the greater its speed of conduction.
- The **large axons** are concerned primarily with proprioceptive sensation, somatic motor function, conscious touch, and pressure, while the **smaller axons** subserve pain and temperature sensations and autonomic function.

Table: *(Ganong 25th/94)*: **Types of mammalian nerve fibers**

Fiber Type	Function	Fiber Diameter (μm)	Conduction Velocity (m/s)	Spike Duration (ms)	Absolute Refract Period (ms)
Aα	Proprioception; somatic: motor	12–20	70–120		
Aβ	Touch, pressure	5–12	30–70	0.4–0.5	0.4–1

Contd...

Fiber Type	Function	Fiber Diameter (μm)	Conduction Velocity (m/s)	Spike Duration (ms)	Absolute Refract Period (ms)
AY	Motor to muscle spindles	3–6	15–30		
Aδ	Pain, temperature	2–5	12–30		
B	Preganglionic autonomic	< 3	3–15	1.2	1.2
C, Dorsal root	Pain, temperature	0.4–1.2	0.5–2	2	2
C, Sympathetic	Postganglionic sympathetic:	0.3–1.3	0.7–23	2	2

16. Ans. a. Spleen, c. Lymph node, e. Mucosa associated lymphoid tissue (MALT)

[Ref: Robbins 9th/193-94; Harrison 19th/2469; A.K. Jain 6th/115]

Tissues of the Immune System

◈ *Robbins 9th/193-94*

- The tissues of the immune system consist of the *generative* (also called *primary*, or *central*) lymphoid organs, in which T and B lymphocytes mature and become competent to respond to antigens, and the *peripheral* (or *secondary*) lymphoid organs, in which adaptive immune responses to microbes are initiated.
- **Generative lymphoid organs.** The principal generative lymphoid organs are the thymus, where T cells develop, and the bone marrow, the site of production of all blood cells and where B lymphocytes mature.
- **Peripheral lymphoid organs.** The peripheral lymphoid organs are:lymph nodes, spleen, and the mucosal and cutaneous lymphoid tissues.
- The cutaneous and mucosal lymphoid systems: Pharyngeal tonsils and Peyer's patches of the intestine are two anatomically defined mucosal lymphoid tissues.

"**Secondary lymphoid organs** (SLOs) include lymph nodes (LNs), spleen, Peyer's patches (PPs) and mucosal tissues- the nasal associated lymphoid tissue (NALT), adenoids, and tonsils"-*www.ncbi.nlm.nih.gov; Harrison 19th/2469*

Secondary lymphoid tissues includes: **lymph nodes, tonsils, spleen, Peyer's patches** and **mucosa associated lymphoid tissue (MALT)**"- *www.histology.leeds.ac.uk*

17. Ans. e. Plasma osmolality higher than urine osmolality

[Ref: Harrison 20th/2689-91; Ganong 25th/698; A K Jain 6th/ 673-74]

Syndrome of Inappropriate Antidiurectic Hormone (SIADH)

◈ *Ganong 25th/698*

- The syndrome of "inappropriate" hypersecretion of antidiuretic hormone (SIADH) occurs when ***vasopressin is inappropriately high relative to serum osmolality.***
- Vasopressin is responsible not only for ***dilutional hyponatremia***(serum sodium < 135 mmol/L) but also for ***loss of salt in the urine*** when water retention is sufficient to expand the ECF volume, reducing aldosterone secretion

SIADH

◈ *A K Jain 6th/ 673-74*

- *Hyposmolality of plasma*
- *↑ed urine osmolality*
- *Urine osmolality becomes higher than plasma osmolality*
- *Urinary Na+ exceeds 20 mEq/L*

"In SIADH, the inappropriate secretion of AVP can have many different causes. They include ectopic production of AVP by ***lung cancer or other neoplasms;*** eutopic release induced by various diseases or drugs; and exogenous administration of AVP, DDAVP, or large doses of oxytocin. The ectopic forms result from abnormal expression of the *AVP-NPII* gene by primary or metastatic malignancies"- *Harrison 20th/2689*

Table: *(Harrison 20th/2691):* **Differential Diagnosis of Hyponatremia Based on Clinical Assessment of Extracellular Fluid Volume (ECFV)**

Clinical findings	Siadh and siad euvolemic
History	No
CHF, cirrhosis, or nephrosis	No
Salt and water loss	No
ACTH–cortisol deficiency and/ or nausea and vomiting	
Physical examination	
Generalized edema, ascites	No
Postural hypotension	No
Laboratory	
BUN, creatinine	Low-normal
Uric acid	Low-normal
Serum potassium	Normal
Serum urate	Low
Serum albumin	Normal
Serum cortisol	Normal
Plasma renin activity	Low
Urinary sodium (meq per unit of time)	High

18. Ans. a. Inulin, b. Iohexol, c. Creatinine, d. Tc99m-DTPA

[Ref: Ganong 25th/ 677; A.K. Jain 6th/535,570; Vasudevan 5th/503; radiopaedia.org]

"Radionuclide ventriculography (RVG, RNV) or radionuclide angiography (RNA) is often referred to as a **MUGA (multiple-gated acquisition)** scan. It is a type of nuclear imaging test. This scan shows how well your heart is pumping"- *www.heart.org*

Ideal Substance used to Measure GFR

◈ *A.K. Jain 6th/535,570*

- *Inulin*
- *Creatinine*

- *Sodium ferrocyanides*
- *Mannitol*
- *Sorbitol*
- *Sucrose*
- *Radioactive cobalt labelled Vit. B12*
- *51Cr-labelled EDTA*
- *Radio iodine labelled hypaque*
- **Tc-99m DTPA (diethylene-triamine-pentaacetate)** is one of the technetium radiopharmaceuticals used in renal imaging and primarily used to measure ***the glomerular filtration rate (GFR)***- *radiopaedia.org*
- *Inulin & creatinine clearance test is commonly used to measure GFR*

"Isotopic (^{125}I-iothalamate, ^{51}Cr-EDTA or ^{99}Tc-DTPA) or non-isotopic (***iohexol*** or iothalamate) ia used to measure GFR"- *academic.oup.com*

19. Ans. a. AV node -0.02.0.05 m/s & 40-55 b/m, b. SA node-0.05 m/s & 60-100 b/m, d. Bundle of His – 1.2-2 m/s & 25-40 b/m, e. Ventricular myocardium – 0.3-1.0 m/s & nil

[Ref: Ganong 25th/ 522-24; Guyton 13th (2nd SAE)/191-92; ECG Made Easy 8th/105-24; A.K. Jain 6th/292; www.vhlab.umn.edu]

Table: *(Ganong 25th/ 522; www.vhlab.umn.edu):* **Conduction speeds in cardiac tissue**

Cardiac tissue	Conduction velocity (meter/second)	Rate of impulse generation
SA node	0.05 (<0.1)	60-100/minute
Atrial muscle	1-1.2	None
AV node	0.02-0.05	40-55/minute
Bundle of His	1.2-2.0	25-40/min
Bundle branches	2-4	25-40/min
Purkinje system	2.0-4.0	25-40/min
Ventricular muscles	0.3-1.0	None

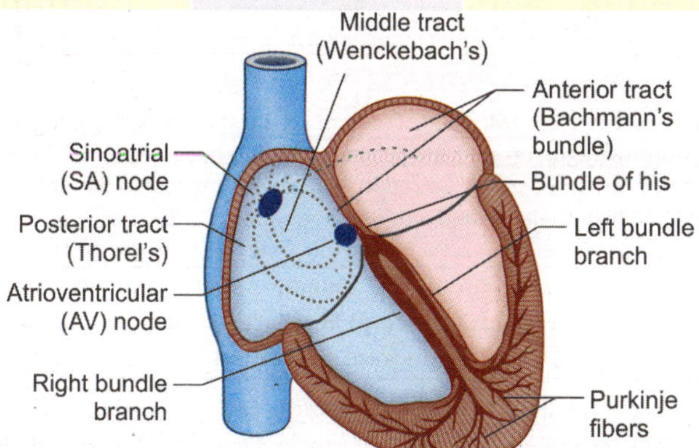

Fig: The conduction system of the heart: Normal excitation originates in the sinoatrial (SA) node, then propagates through both atria (internodal tracts shown as dashed lines). The atrial depolarization spreads to the atrioventricular (AV) node, passes through the bundle of His (not labeled), and then to the Purkinje fibers which make up the left and right bundle branches; subsequently all ventricular muscle becomes activated.

20. Ans. a. First degree AV block, b. Second degree Mobitz type 1 AV block

[Ref: ECG Made Easy by Hampton 8th/37-38,112Harrison l8th/1891]

- In Second degree Mobitz type 2 AV block , ***PR interval in conducted beats are constant***
- ***P waves are absent in ventricular tachycardia therefore PR interval cannot be measured.***

Differential of a prolonged PR interval is based on the ECG and can be divided into: *ECG Made Easy by Hampton 8th/37-38*

- ***First Degree Heart Block: Prolonged PR interval***
- ***Second Degree Heart Block (Higher grade AV block): Mobitz Type I (Progressive lengthening of PR interval), Mobitz Type II (PR interval in conducted beats are constant)***

Third-degree AV block **(as third-degree heart block or complete heart block is electrocardiographically characterized by:**

- Regular P-P interval
- Regular R-R interval
- Lack of an apparent relationship between the P waves and QRS complexes
- The ***PR interval will be variable***, as the hallmark of complete heart block is lack of any apparent relationship between P waves and QRS complexes.
- More P waves are present than QRS complexes.

PR interval

◈ *ECG Made Easy by Hampton 8th/6-7*

- The **PR interval** is the period, measured in milliseconds, that extends from the beginning of the P wave (the onset of atrial depolarization) until the beginning of the ORS complex (the onset of ventricular depolarization); it is ***normally between 120 and 200 ms in duration (3-5 small squares).***

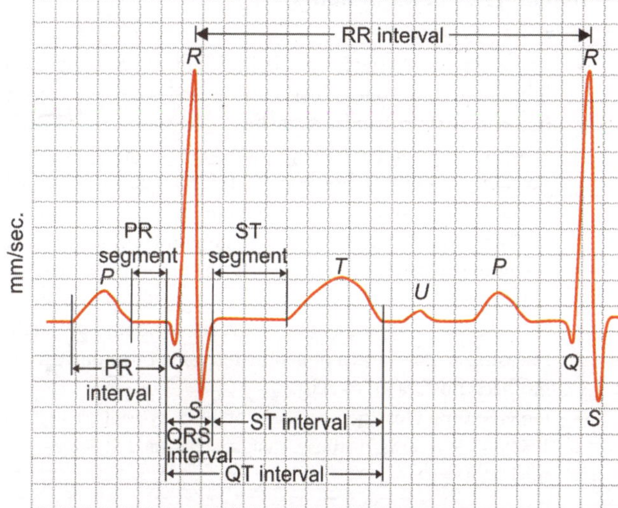

- A short PR interval (of less than 120ms) may be associated with an atrioventricular reentrant tachycardia (such as Wolff Parkinson-White syndrome or Lown-Ganong-Levine syndrome) or junctional rhythm.

21. Ans. a. Hemoglobin concentration, c. PaO_2 in arterial blood

[Ref: A.K. Jain 6th/429-30; Guyton 13th/371-73; Ganong 25th/639-40; breathe.ersjournals.com]

- Delivery of oxygen(not oxygen content) is depends upon ***cardiac output***
- ***It is not RBC volume(rather Hb concentration) which determines oxygen content***

"**Amount of dissolve oxygen** increases in ***linearity with arterial pO2***"- A.K. Jain 6th/429

"The **oxygen concentration** (usually termed "**oxygen content**") of systemic arterial blood depends on several factors, including the ***partial pressure of inspired oxygen, the adequacy of ventilation and gas exchange, the concentration of haemoglobin and the affinity of the haemoglobin molecule for oxygen***. Of the oxygen transported by the blood, a very small proportion is dissolved in simple solution, with the great majority chemically bound to the haemoglobin molecule in red blood cells, a process which is reversible"- *breathe.ersjournals.com*

"Although oxygen dissolves in blood, only a small amount of oxygen is transported this way. Only 1.5 percent of oxygen in the blood is dissolved directly into the blood itself. Most oxygen—98.5 percent—is bound to a protein called **hemoglobin** and carried to the tissues"- *courses.lumenlearning.com*

"**Global oxygen delivery** describes the amount of oxygen delivered to the tissues in each minute and is a product of the ***cardiac output*** and arterial oxygen content"- academic.oup.com

22. Ans. b. Parathyroid, c. Pancreas

[Ref: Ganong 25th/308-14; Harrison 19th/401e-2]

Hypophysiotropic Hormones

◈ *Ganong 25th/314*

- There are six established hypothalamic releasing and inhibiting hormones: corticotropin-releasing hormone (CRH); **thyrotropin-releasing hormone (TRH);** growth hormone–releasing hormone (GRH); growth hormone–inhibiting hormone (GIH, now generally called somatostatin); luteinizing hormone–releasing hormone (LHRH, now generally known as **gonadotropin-releasing hormone** [**GnRH**]); and prolactin-inhibiting hormone (PIH).
- In addition, hypothalamic extracts contain prolactin releasing activity, and a prolactin-releasing hormone (PRH) has been postulated to exist.
- GnRH stimulates the secretion of FSH as well as that of LH, and it seems unlikely that a separate FSH-releasing hormone exists.

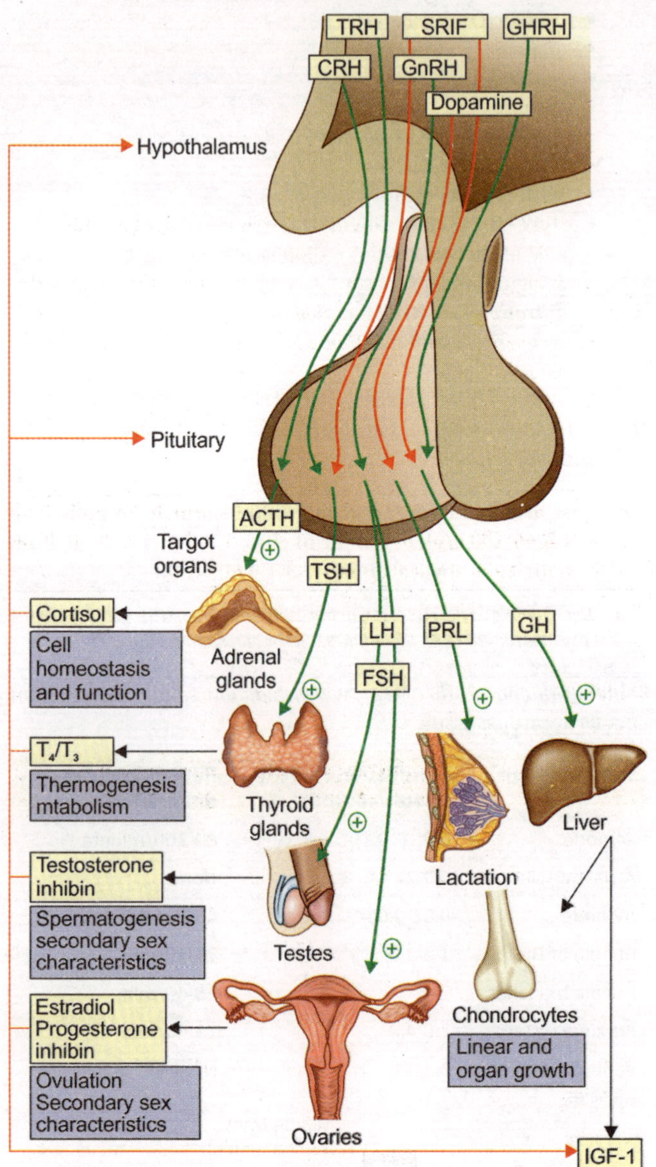

Fig: *(Harrison 19th/401e-2):* Diagram of pituitary axis. Hypothalamic hormones regulate anterior pituitary trophic hormones that in turn determine target gland secretion. Peripheral hormones feedback to regulate hypothalamic and pituitary hormones

23. Ans. b. Composed of splenic cords and sinusoids; d. Perisinusoidal macrophages are present; e. Removes senescent erythrocytes from circulation

[Ref: BDC 7th/ Vol. II 325; Guyton 13th (SAE) /252; A.K. Jain 6th/116;Gray's 40th/1193; Harshmohan 7th/366-67; Schwartz 10th/1425–26]

- B and T cells (option a and c) are component of white pulp

"**White pulp**: *It consists of **lymphatic nodules arranged around an arteriole called malpighian corpuscle***"- *BDC 7th/ Vol. II 325*

Red pulp: *Formed by collection of cells in the interstices of reticulum, in b/w the* ***sinusoids****. It consists of* ***fixed and free macrophages****"-BDC 7th/ Vol. II 325*

Spleen

◈ *Schwartz 10th/1425-26*

Red Pulp

- The **red pulp** is comprised of large numbers of **venous sinuses (Sinusoids),** which ultimately drain into tributaries of the splenic vein.
- The sinuses are surrounded and separated by a fibrocellular network, called the reticulum, consisting of collagen fibers and fibroblasts. Within this network or mesh lie ***splenic macrophages***. These intersinusoidal regions appear as ***splenic cords.***
- The red pulp serves as a dynamic filtration system, enabling ***macrophages to remove microorganisms, cellular debris, antigen/antibody complexes and senescent erythrocytes from circulation.***

White Pulp

- Around the terminal millimeters of splenic arterioles, a ***periarticular lymphatic sheath*** replaces the native adventitia of the vessel.
- The sheath is ***comprised of T lymphocytes and intermittent aggregations of B lymphocytes or lymphoid follicles.***
- When antigenically stimulated, the follicles, which are centers of lymphocyte proliferation, develop germinal centers

BIOCHEMISTRY

24. Ans. a. Chylomicron

[Ref: Harper 31st/ 237; Lippincott 7th/227;Biochemistry by Dinesh Puri 4th/192]

Lipoproteins

◈ *Dinesh Puri 4th/192*

Chylomicron- *Highest triglyceride*
HDL-*Highest phospholipid, protein*
LDL- *Highest cholesterol*

Table: *(Dinesh Puri 4th/192):* **Lipoproteins**

Composition (%)	Chylomicrons	VLDL	LDL	HDL
TAG(Triglyceride)	84-89	50-65	7-10	3-5
Protein	1.5-2.5	5-10	20-25	40-55
Cholesterol	4-8	15-23	40-50	15-18
Phospholipids	7-9	15-20	15-20	20-35

"**Chylomicrons** are the lipoprotein particles lowest in density and largest in size, and contain the highest percentage of lipid and the lowest percentage of protein. **VLDLs and LDLs** are successively denser, having higher ratios of protein to lipid. **HDL** particles are the densest"- *Lippincott 7th/227*

Four Major Groups of Plasma Lipoproteins Have Been Identified

◈ *Harper 31st/ 237*

- Since fat is less dense than water, the density of a lipoprotein decreases as the proportion of lipid to protein increases
- Four major groups of lipoproteins have been identified that are important physiologically and in clinical diagnosis.
- These are (1) **chylomicrons,** derived from intestinal absorption of triacylglycerol and other lipids; (2) **very low density lipoproteins**(VLDL), derived from the liver for the export of triacylglycerol; (3) **low-density lipoproteins** (LDL), representing a final stage in the catabolism of VLDL; and (4) **high density lipoproteins**(HDL), involved in cholesterol transport and also in VLDL and chylomicron metabolism.
- ***Triacylglycerol is the predominant lipid in chylomicrons and VLDL***, whereas cholesterol and phospholipid are the predominant lipids in LDL and HDL, respectively

Table: *(Harper 31st/ 237):* **Composition of the Lipoproteins in Plasma of Humans**

Lipoprotein	Source	Diameter (nm)	Density (g/mL)	Composition		Main lipid components	Apolipoproteins
				Protein (%)	Lipid (%)		
Chylomicrons	Intestine	90-1000	<0.95	1-2	98-99	Triacylglycerol	A-I, A-II, A-IV,2 B-48, C-I, C-II, C-III, E
Chylomicron remnants	Chylomicrons	45-150	<1.006	6-8	92-94	Triacylglycerol, phospholipids, cholesterol	B-48, E
VLDL	Liver (Intestine)	30-90	0.95-1.006	7-10	90-93	Triacylglycerol	B-100, C-I, C-II, C-III,
IDL	VLDL	25-35	1.006-1.019	11	89	Triacylglycerol, cholesterol	B-100, E
IDL	VLDL	25-35	1,006-1.019	11	89	Triacylglycerol, cholesterol	B-100, E
LDL	VLDL	20-25	1.019-1.063	21	79	Cholesterol	B-100
HDL	Liver, intestine, VLDL, chylomicrons					Phospholipids, cholesterol	A-I, A-II, A-IV, C-I, C-II, C-III, D,[b] E
HDL_1		20-25	1.019-1.063	32	68		
HDL_2		10-20	1.063-1.125	33	67		
HDL_3		5-10	1.125-1.210	57	43		

25. **Ans.** **b. Linoleic acid, d. Linolenic acid**

[Ref: Harper 31st/ 197;Satyanarayan 4th/ 30]

- **Folic acid is a vitamin**

Unsaturated Fatty Acids Contain one or MoreDouble Bonds

◈ *Harper 31st/ 197*

Unsaturated fatty acids may be further subdivided as follows:

- **Monounsaturated** (monoethenoid, monoenoic) acids, containing one double bond.
- **Polyunsaturated** (polyethenoid, polyenoic) acids, containing two or more double bonds.
- **Eicosanoids:** These compounds, derived from eicosa (20-carbon) polyenoic fatty acids, comprise the **prostanoids, leukotrienes (LTs)**, and **lipoxins (LXs)**. Prostanoids include **prostaglandins (PGs), prostacyclins (PGIs)**, and **thromboxanes (TXs)**.

Table: *(Harper 31st/197):* **Unsaturated Fatty Acids of Physiologic and Nutritional Significance**

Number of C Atoms and Number and Position of Common Double Bonds	Family	Common Name
Monoenoic acids (one double bond)		
16:1; 9	ω7	Palmitoleic
18:1; 9	ω9	Oleic
18:1; 9	ω9	Elaidic
Dienoic acid (two double bonds)		
18:2; 9, 12	ω6	Linoleic
Trienoic acids (three double bonds)		
18:3; 6, 9, 12	ω6	γ-Linolenic
18:3; 9, 12, 15	ω3	α-Linolenic
Tetraenoic acids (four double bonds)		
20:4, 5, 8, 11, 14	ω6	Arachidonic
Pentaenoic acids (five double bonds)		
20:5; 5, 8, 11, 14, 17	ω3	Timnodonic
Hexaenoic acids (six double bonds)		
22:6; 4, 7, 10, 13, 16, 19	ω3	Cervonic

Table: *(Harper 31st/ 197):* **Saturated Fatty acids**

Common Name	Number of C atoms
Acetic	2
Butyric	4
Valeric	5
Caproic	6
Lauric	12
Myristic	14
Palmitic	16
Stearic	18

Contd...

26. **Ans. a. Galactose-1-phosphateuridyltransferase (GALT) deficiency**

[Ref: Harper 31st/ 191; Harrison 20th/3012; Vasudevan5th/125; O.P. Ghai 8th/655-56]

Enzyme Deficiencies in the Galactose Pathway Cause Galactosemia

◈ *Harper 31st/ 191*

- Inability to metabolize galactose occurs in the **galactosemias,** which may be caused by inherited defects of galactokinase, uridyltransferase, or 4-epimerase, though deficiency of **uridyl transferase** is best known.
- Galactose is a substrate for aldose reductase, forming galactitol, which accumulates in the lens of the eye, causing cataract.
- The condition is more severe if it is the result of a defect in the uridyl transferase since galactose-1-phosphate accumulates and depletes the liver of inorganic phosphate.
- Ultimately, liver failure and mental deterioration result. In uridyl transferase deficiency, the epimerase is present inadequate amounts, so that the galactosemic individual can still form UDP Gal from glucose. This explains how it is possible for normal growth and development of affected children to occur despite the galactose-free diets used to controlthe symptoms of the disease.

Galactosemia

◈ *O.P .Ghai 8th/655-56*

- There are three disorders of galactose metabolism, but it is the deficiency of the enzyme **galactose-1-phosphateuridyltransferase (GALT),** that is referred to as galactosemia
- Deficiency of GALT results in accumulation of galactose-1-phosphate & metabolites (e.g. galactitol)
- Patients appear normal at birth, but by 3-4 days of breastmilk or formula feeding life-threatening disease

TABLE: *(Harrison 20th/3012):* **Features of Galactose Disorders**

Type/common name	Basic defect	Clinical features	Comments
• Galactosemia with uridy ltransferase deficiency	Galactose 1-phosphate uridyl transferase	Vomiting, hepatomegaly, jaundice, cataracts, amino aciduria, failure to thrive	Long-term complications exist despite early diagnosis and treatment.
• Galactokinase deficiency	Galactokinase	Cataracts	Benign
• Uridine diphosphategalactose 4-epimerase deficiency	Uridine diphosphategalactose 4-epimerase	Similar to transferase deficiency with additional findings of hypotonia and nerve deafness	Benign variant exists.

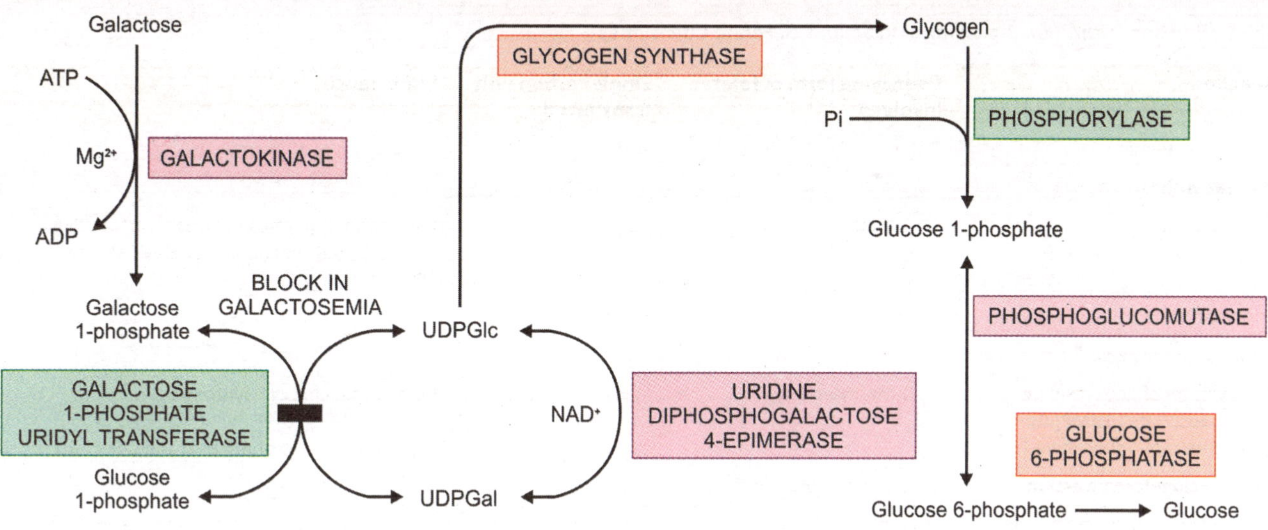

Fig: Pathway of conversion of galactose to glucose in the liver

27. Ans. a. Leucine, b. Lysine, c. Phenylalanine

[Ref: Lippincott 7th/262; Satyanarayan 4th/48]

Ketogenic Amino Acids

◈ *Lippincott 7th/262*

- Amino acids whose catabolism yields either acetoacetate or one of its precursors (acetyl CoA or acetoacetyl CoA) are termed **ketogenic**
- Acetoacetate is one of the ketone bodies, which also include 3-hydroxybutyrate and acetone
- ***Leucine and lysine are the only exclusively ketogenic amino acids found*** in proteins. Their carbon skeletons are not substrates for gluconeogenesis and, therefore, cannot give rise to the net formation of glucose.

	Glucogenic	Glucogenic and ketogenic	Ketogenic
Nonessential	Alanine Arginine Asparagine Aspartate Cysteine Glutamate Glutamine Glycine Proline Serine	Tyrosine	
Essential	Histidine Methionine Threonine Valine	Isoleucine Phenylalanine Tryptophan	Leucine Lysine

Fig: *(Lippincott 7th/262):* Classification of amino acids

28. Ans. b. All pyrimidine ..., d. Conversion of creatine ...

[Ref: Harper 31st/537-38; Lippincott 7th/378; Dinesh Puri 4th/341-43]

- Conversion of creatine phosphate to creatinine: no role of folic acid
- Homocysteine to methionine: 5-Methyl(M)THF is required
- Pyrimidine in RNA: cytosine & uracil
- Pyrimidine in DNA: thymine & cytosine

Role of Folic Acid (asTHF)

◈ *Dinesh Puri 4th/3412*

- *DNA & RNA synthesis:* ***Purine ring synthesis & thymidylate synthesis***
- Amino acid metabolism: Synthesis of serine, glycine etc
- *Protein synthesis: Formation of initiator amino acid,* ***N-formylmethionine***

Folic Acid

◈ *Lippincott 7th/378; Harper 31st/537-38*

- Folic acid (or folate), which plays a key role in one-carbon metabolism, is essential for the biosynthesis of several compounds
- The ***active form of folic acid (pteroyl glutamate) is tetrahydrofolate***
- Tetrahydrofolate (reduced folate) receives one-carbon fragments from donors such as serine, glycine, and histidine and transfers them to intermediates in the ***synthesis of amino acids, purines, and thymidine monophosphate (TMP)-a pyrimidine found in DNA***
- A primary result of folic acid deficiency is ***megaloblastic anemia***, caused by diminished synthesis of purines and TMP, which leads to an inability of cells (including red cell precursors) to make DNA and, therefore, they cannot divide.
- **Note:** It is important to evaluate the cause of the megaloblastic anemia prior to instituting therapy, because vitamin B12 deficiency indirectly causes symptoms of this disorder
- Folic acid supplementation before conception and during the first trimester has been shown to significantly reduce the **neural tube defects in the fetus**
- Inhibitors of Folate Metabolism provide Cancer Chemotherapy, Antibacterial, & Antimalarial Drugs
- Vitamin B12 Deficiency Causes Functional Folate Deficiency-the "Folate Trap"

Table: *(Harrison 20th/700):* **Biochemical Reactions of Folate Coenzymes**

Reaction	Coenzyme form of folate involved	Single carbon unit transferred	Importance
Formate activation	THF	–CHO	Generation of 10-formyl-THF
Purine synthesis			
Formation of glycinamideribonucleotide	5,10-Methylene-THF	–CHO	Formation of purines needed for DNA, RNA synthesis, but reactions probably not rate-limiting
Formylation of aminoimidazolecarboxamideribonucleotide (AICAR)	10-Formyl (CHO)THF		
Pyrimidine synthesis			
Methylation of deoxyuridine monophosphate (dUMP) to thymidine monophosphate (dTMP)	5,10-Methylene-THF	$-CH_3$	Rate limiting in DNA synthesis Oxidizes THF to DHF Some breakdown of folate at the C-9–N-10 bond
Amino acid interconversion			
Serine–glycine interconversion	THF	$=CH_2$	Entry of single carbon units into active pool
Homocysteine to methionine	5-Methyl(M)THF	$-CH_3$	Demethylation of 5-MTHF to THF; also requires cobalamin, flavine adenine dinucleotide, ATP, and adenosylmethionine

29. Ans. a. Infant-350 µg, b. Adolescent- 600 µg, c. Adult male-600 µg

[Ref: Park 25th/673; Dinesh Puri 4th/333]

Table: **(***Park 25th/673***): Daily intake of vitamin A recommended by ICMR (2010)**

Group		Retinol (µg)	β-carotene (µg)*
Adults	Man	600	4,800
	Woman	600	4,800
	Pregnancy	800	6,400
	Lactation	950	7,600
Infants	0 to 6 months	350	–
	6 to 12 months	350	2800
Children	1 to 6 years	400	3,200
	7 to 9 years	600	4,800
Adolescents	10 to 17 years	600	4,800

* A Conversion ratio of 1: 8 is used

30. Ans. a. Ornithine transcarbamoylase, b. Argininosuccinic acid synthetase, c. Arginase, e. Carbamoyl phosphate synthetase I

[Ref: Harper 30th/290-96, 29th/274-88; Lippincott 6th/ 253-55; Shinde 7th/450-51; Vasudevan 5th/180-81]

Urea cycle: 5 steps *(Shown in Figure)*

1. Synthesis of carbamoyl-phosphate
2. Synthesis of citrulline
3. Synthesis of arginine succinate
4. Cleavage of arginine succinate
5. Cleavage of arginine to form ornithine & urea

Note: "Rate-limiting enzyme (pacemaker enzyme) of Urea cycle*: Carbamoyl phosphate synthetase I (CPS II is involved in pyrimidine synthesis)" (Harper 29th/274)*

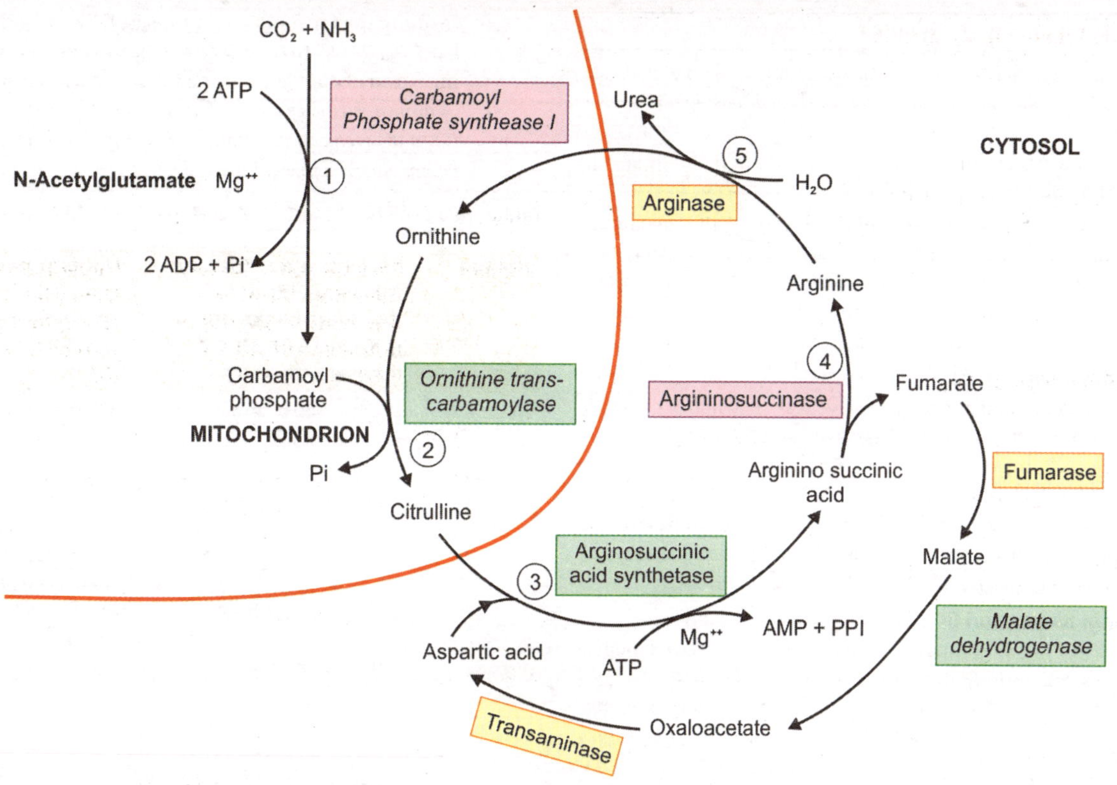

Fig: Biosynthesis of urea of ornithine-urea cycle

31. Ans. a. HGPRT deficiency, b. Glucose-6-phosphatase deficiency

[Ref: Harrison 20th/2998; Harper 31st/334-35; Lippincott 7th/299; Satyanarayan 4th/394-95]

Table: *(Harrison 20th/2998):* **Hyperuricemia (Partial list)**

Urate Overproduction
HPRT (Hypoxanthine phosphoribosyltransferase) deficiency PRPP (phosphoribosylpyrophosphate) synthetase overactivity
Urate Overproduction & Decreased Uric Acid Excretion
Glucose-6-phosphatase deficiency Fructose-1-phosphate Aldolase deficiency

Primary Gout (Overproduction of Uric Acid): Important Metabolic Defects (Enzymes)

Satyanarayan 4th/394-95

- **PRPP synthetase**: *Increased production of purines*
- *PRPP glutamyl amido transferase: Increased production of purines*
- ***HGPRT deficiency*** *(as seen in Lesch-Nyhan syndrome): Increased production of purines*
- ***Glucose 6-phosphatase deficiency****: Purine overproduction*
- *Elevation of glutathione reductase*

TABLE: ***(Harrison 20th/2998):*** **Inborn Errors of Purine Metabolism**

Enzyme	Activity	Inheritance	Clinical features	Laboratory features
Hypoxanthine phosphoribosyl transferase (HPRT)	Complete deficiency	X-linked	Self-mutilation, choreoathetosis, gout, and uric acid lithiasis	Hyperuricemia, hyperuricosuria
Phosphoribosyl pyrophosphate synthetase (PRPPS)	Overactivity	X-linked	Gout, uric acid lithiasis, and deafness	Hyperuricemia, hyperuricosuria
Adenine phosphoribosyl transferase	Deficiency	Autosomal recessive	2,8-Dihydroxyadenine lithiasis	—
Xanthine oxidase	Deficiency	Autosomal recessive	Xanthinuria and xanthine lithiasis	Hypouricemia, hypouricosuria

32. Ans. a. Vitamin A, d. Vitamin C

[Ref: Harrison 20th/ 2313-17; Harper 31st/540; Harper 30th/548; Lippincott 7th/392; Satyanarayan 4th/129; Dinesh Puri 4th/335; www.webmd.com]

- Vitamin A & Vitamin D are toxic on daily intake of >100mg/d (see explanation)

"The **UL (Tolerable upper intake level)** is the maximum amount of daily vitamins and minerals that you can safely take without risk of an overdose or serious side effects. For certain nutrients, the higher you go above the UL, the greater the chance you›ll have problems"- *www.webmd.com*

Vitamin A (Option A)

- "The acute toxicity of vitamin A was first noted in Arctic explorers who ate polar bear liver and has also been seen after administration of ***150 mg to adults or 100 mg to children***"-*Harrison 20th/ 2313*
- **"A large single dose of 300 mg or more commonly chronic ingestion of amounts grossly in excess of requirements, leads to toxic effect"**-*Dinesh Puri 4th/349-50*

Vitamin B1 (Option B)

- *"Excess intake of* **thiamine**, *like that of other water soluble vitamins,* ***usually not toxic*** *because it is promptly excreted in urine. However, it has been recorded that chronic intake of thiamine in excess of* ***3g/d*** *is toxic to adults"- Dinesh Puri 4th/335*

Vitamin D (Option C)

- "**Vit D Toxicity:** The upper limit of intake has been set at 4000 IU/d(**100μg/d).** Contrary to earlier beliefs, acute vitamin D intoxication is rare and usually is caused by the uncontrolled and excessive ingestion of supplements or by faulty food fortification practices"- *Harrison 20th/ 2316*
- "Upper limit of toxicity is ***100μg/d(4000IU/d)*** for individual ages 9 yr or older"-*Lippincott 7th/392*

Vitamin C (Option D)

- "***Taking >2 g of vitamin C*** in a single dose may result in abdominal pain, diarrhea, and nausea. Since vitamin C may be metabolized to oxalate, it is feared that chronic high-dose vitamin C supplementation could result in an increased prevalence of kidney stones. However, except in patients with preexisting renal disease, this association has not been borne out in several trials"-*Harrison 20th/ 2313*
- "***Megadose(1-4gm/d***) of vitamin are still used in common cold, wound healing, trauma etc"-*Satyanarayan 4th/134*

Vitamin E (Option E)

- All forms of vitamin E are absorbed and could contribute to toxicity; however, the toxicity risk seems to be rather low as long as liver function is normal. ***High doses of vitamin E (>800 mg/d)*** may reduce platelet aggregation and interfere with vitamin K metabolism and are therefore contraindicated in patients taking warfarin and antiplatelet agents (such as aspirin or clopidogrel). Nausea, flatulence, and diarrhea have been reported at doses >1 g/d"- *Harrison 20th/ 2317*
- **"Among the fat soluble vitamins (ADEK)** ***vitamin E is the least toxic.*** **No toxic effect has been reported even after ingestion of *300mg/day* for 23 years"**-*Satyanarayan 4th/129*
- *"Vitamin E is least toxic of all fat- soluble vitamins-even 50 times the recommended intake(**8-12mg**) has been reported to be non-toxic"-Dinesh Puri 4th/354*

Table: *(www.webmd.com)*: **RDA & Upper Tolerable Limit**

Vitamin	Recommended Dietary Allowance (RDA) or Adequate Intake (AI) *Nutrients with AIs are marked with an (*)*	Upper Tolerable Limit (UL) *The highest amount you can take without risk*
Vitamin A	• *Men*: 900 mcg/day • *Women*: 700 mcg/day	3,000 mcg/day
Vitamin B3 (Niacin)	• *Men*: 16 mg/day • *Women*: 14 mg/day	35 mg/day *This applies only to niacin in supplements or fortified foods. There is no upper limit for niacin in natural sources.*
Vitamin B6	• *Men age 19-50*: 1.3 mg/day • *Men age 51 up*:1.7 mg/day • *Women age 19-50*: 1.3 mg/day • *Women age 51 up*: 1.5 mg/day	100 mg/day
Vitamin C	• *Men*: 90 mg/day • *Women*: 75 mg/day	2,000 mg/day
Vitamin D (Calciferol)	• *Age 1-70*: 15 mcg/day • (600 IU, or international units) * • *Age 70 and older*: 20 mcg/day (800 IU) *	100 mcg/day (4,000 IU)
Vitamin E (alpha-tocopherol)	• 22.4 IU/day • (15 mg/day)	1,500 IU/day (1,000 mg/day) *This applies only to vitamin E in supplements or fortified foods. There is no upper limit for vitamin E from natural sources.*

33. Ans. a. ATP is required, b. Degradation occurs after ubiquitination of the target substrate, c. Regulation by Heat stroke protein (HSP), e. Ubiquitins are recycled

[Ref: Harper 31st/585; Lippincott 7th/246-47,20]

"**Protein degradation:** There are two major enzyme systems responsible for degrading damaged or unneeded proteins: the ***ATP-dependent ubiquitin-proteasome system*** of the cytosol, and the ATP-independent degradative enzyme system of the lysosome"- *Lippincott 7th/246*

Ubiquitin-Proteasome Proteolytic Pathway

◈ *Lippincott 7th/247*

- Proteins selected for degradation by the ubiquitin-proteasome system are ***first covalently attached to ubiquitin***, a small, globular, non-enzymic protein.
- **Ubiquitination of the target** substrate occurs through linkage of the α-carboxyl group of the C-terminal glycine of ubiquitin to the ε-amino group of a lysine on the protein substrate by a three-step, enzyme-catalyzed, ATP-dependent process.
- The consecutive addition of ubiquitin moieties generates a polyubiquitin chain. Proteins tagged with ubiquitin are then recognized by a large, barrel-shaped, macromolecular, proteolytic complex called a **proteasome**, which functions like a garbage disposal
- The proteasome unfolds, deubiquitinates, and cuts the target protein into fragments that are then further degraded to amino acids, which enter the amino acid pool. [Note: The ubiquitins are recycled.]
- It is noteworthy that the selective degradation of proteins by the ubiquitin-proteosome complex (unlike simple hydrolysis by proteolytic enzymes) ***requires energy in the form of ATP***

"Proteasomal degradation of oxidized proteins is a crucial mechanism to prevent the accumulation of cellular damage. **Heat shock proteins (Hsp)** as molecular chaperones are involved in the folding, activation and assembly of a variety of proteins. Among these Hsp40, Hsp70 and Hsp90 are believed to act as a chaperone system to regulate the ***proteasomal degradation***"- *www.ncbi.nlm.nih.gov*

Ubiquitinated Proteins Are Degraded in Proteasomes

◈ *Harper 31st/585*

- Polyubiquitinated target proteins enter **proteasomes** located in the cytosol. Proteasomes are protein complexes with a relatively **large cylindrical structure** and are composed of four rings with a hollow **core** containing the protease active sites, and one or two **caps** or **regulatory particles** that recognize the polyubiquinated substrates and initiate degradation.
- Target proteins are unfolded by ATPases present in the proteasome caps. Proteasomes can hydrolyze a very wide variety of peptide bonds. Target proteins pass into the core to be degraded to small peptides, which then exit the proteasome to be further degraded by cytosolic peptidases.
- Both ***normally and abnormally folded proteins are substrates for the proteasome.*** Liberated ubiquitin molecules are recycled.
- The proteasome plays an important role in **presenting small peptides** produced by **degradation of various viruses** and other molecules to **MHC class I molecules,** a key step in antigen presentation to T lymphocytes.

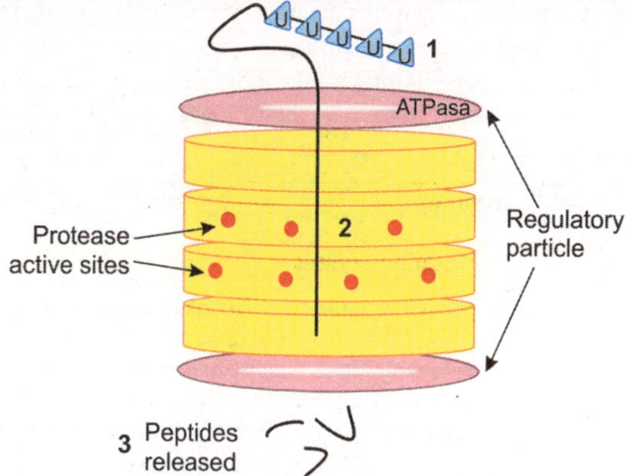

Fig: *(Harper):* **Protein degradation in the proteasome.** 1. The regulatory particle recognizes the ubiquitinated protein which are unfolded by ATPases present in the regulatory particles or caps. 2. Protease active sites in the core of the proteosome attack peptide bonds and degrade the protein. 3. Peptides are released into the cytosol for further degradation by cytosolic peptidases.

34. Ans. b. Hypoglycemia, c. Thiamine deficiency, d. Lactic acidosis

[Ref: Lippincott 7th/110,317-18; Robbins 9th/418-19;Kaplon & Saddock 11th/628]

Alcohol consumption can produce ***hypoglycaemia*** (especially who depleted their stores of liver glycogen)"- *Lippincott 7th/318*

"Alcohol oxidation by alcohol dehydrogenase causes the reduction of nicotinamide adenine dinucleotide (NAD) to NADH, with a consequent decrease in NAD and increase in NADH. NAD is required for fatty acid oxidation in the liver and for the conversion of lactate into pyruvate. Its deficiency is a main cause of the accumulation of fat in the liver of alcoholics. The increase in the NADH/NAD ratio in alcoholics also causes lactic acidosis"-Robbins 9th/418

"*Thiamine (vitamin B1) deficiency* is common in chronic alcoholics. The principal lesions resulting from this deficiency are *peripheral neuropathies* and the *Wernicke-Korsakoff syndrome;* cerebral atrophy, cerebellar degeneration, and optic neuropathy may also occur"-Robbins 9th/419

"In alcohol abuse, ***thiamine deficiency*** may be seen"- *Lippincott 7th/110*

"Chronic alcoholism is also associated with an increased incidence of hypertension, and heavy alcohol consumption, with attendant liver injury, results in decreased levels of HDL, increasing the likelihood of coronary heart disease"-Robbins 9th/419

35. Ans. c. Glutamate dehydrogenase

[Ref: Lippincott 7th/405,401;Satyanarayan 4th/404,135-39 :Shinde 7th/587;Dinesh Puri 4th/334-37;Shinde 7th/166-67; Essential of biochemistry/ 128]

- Glutamate dehydrogenase uses zinc as a cofactor whereas all other mentioned options use magnesium as co factor.

Metalloenzymes (Cofactors): The enzymes that require ***inorganic metal ions*** as their cofactor are termed as metalloenzymes

Table: Metalloenzymes

Metal	Metalloenzymes
Magnesium	Hexokinase, phosphofructokinase, ***glucose-6-phosphatase***, enolase, creatinine kinase, ***Pyruvte dehydrogenase, Isocitrate dehydrogenase***, **Phosphatases, Kinases**, Creatine kinase, adenylate cclase, glutamine synthase, thiokinase, squalene synthase, ***glutathione synthase, Glucose-6-phosphate dehydrogenase***
Copper	**Cytochrome oxidase,** Tyrosinase, **Lysyl oxidase,** superoxide dismutase, **Ascorbic acid oxidase,** Ferroxidase **(ceruloplasmin)**
Iron	Cytochrome oxidase, **Xanthine oxidase**, Catalase, Peroxidase
Zinc	**Carbonic anhydrase, alkaline phosphatase,** RNA polymerase, **alcohol dehydrogenase, Carboxypeptidase**, Prophobilinogen synthase, ***glulamate dehydrogenase*, lactate dehydrogenase, superoxide dismutase**
Calcium	Lipase, Lecithinase
Maganese	Arginase, Pyruvate carboxylase, Phosphoglucomutase, Glycosyl transferase, Hexokinase, Enolase
Potassium	Pyruvate kinase
Selenium	Glutathione peroxidase
Nickle	Urease
Molybdenum	Xanthine oxidase, sulfite oxidase

Also Know

TPP is Coenzyme for

◈ *Satyanarayan 4th/135; Shinde 7th/166-67*

- Pyruvate dehydrogenase
- α-ketoglutarate dehydrogenase
- **Pyruvate carboxylase**
- Branched chain α-ketoacid decarboxylase (dehydrogenase)
- Transketolase

FAD Linked Enzymes

◈ *Dinesh Puri 4th/336; Satyanarayan 4th/139*

- Pyruvate dehydrogenase
- α-ketoglutarate dehydrogenase
- Succinate dehydrogenase
- Acyl-CoA dehydrogenase
- Xanthine oxidase

NAD+ Linked Enzymes

◈ *Dinesh Puri 4th/337; Satyanarayan 4th/142*

- Pyruvate dehydrogenase
- α-ketoglutarate dehydrogenase
- Isocitrate dehydrogenase
- Succinate dehydrogenase
- Glutamate dehydrogenase
- Lactate dehydrogenase
- Branched chain α-ketoacid dehydrogenase
- Glyceraldehyde 3-phosphate dehydrogenase

NADP+ Linked Enzymes

◈ *Dinesh Puri 4th/337*

- Isocitrate dehydrogenase
- G6-Phosphate dehydrogenase
- Malic enzymes

"Isocitrate dehydrogenase coenzyme: NAD+ & NADP+"- *Dinesh Puri 4th/337*

36. Ans. a. Proline, c. Isoleucine

[Ref: Harper 30th/16-22; Lippincott 6th/1-9; Satyanarayan 4th/ 48]

Polar Amino Acids with Polar Side Chains

Acidic and Polar Side Chains

Aspartic Acid

- Glutamic Acid

Basic and Polar Side Chains

- ***Arginine***
- ***Lysine***
- *Histidine*

Uncharged & Polar Side Chains

- ***Asparginine***
- Glutamine
- Serine
- Threonine
- Tyrosine

Note: *Carboxyl side chains are associated with Acidic amino acids while Amino side chains are associated with Basic Amino acids, both of which are 'Polar' molecules.*

Non Polar Amino Acids with Non Polar side chains

- Glycine
- *Alanine*
- *Valine*
- *Leucine*
- ***Isoleucine***
- ***Proline***

37. Ans. b. N-glutathione transferase enzyme is the most important enzyme, c. High expression of enzymes leads to decrease activity of anticancer drugs, e. An increased GSSG-to-GSH ratio is indicative of oxidative stress

[Ref: www.herbaltransition.com; KDT 8th/31;Shinde 7th/478-80]

Glutathione Conjugation

◈ *www.herbaltransition.com*

- Glutathione transferases (GSTs) are often upregulated in tumors and have been suggested to play an important role in multiple drug resistance in cancer chemotherapy
- Glutathione-S-transferase (GST) Enzyme family is necessary for glutathione conjugation

- ***N-acetylglutamat synthase (NAGS)*** *is an enzyme that catalyses the production of N-Acetylglutamate (NAG) from glutamate and acetyl-CoA.* ***It is an urea cycle enzyme and not associate with glutathione conjugation***
- In humans and rodents, the soluble GSTs are collectively expressed in relatively large amounts, and ***may comprise as much as 4% of total soluble protein in the liver***
- In healthy cells and tissue, more than 90% of the total glutathione pool is in the reduced form (GSH) and less than 10% exists in the disulfide form (GSSG). ***An increased GSSG-to-GSH ration is considered indicative of oxidative stress.***

Glutathione is also an Important Antioxidant

◈ *www.sciencedirect.com*

- Glutathione is one of the most important ***anti-carcinogens and antioxidants*** in our cells, which means that a deficiency is cause of serious liver dysfunction and damage.
- Exposure to high levels of toxins depletes glutathione faster than it can be produced or absorbed from the diet. This results in increased susceptibility to toxin-induced diseases, such as cancer.
- Health conditions like mold susceptibility (CIRS due to water-damaged buildings), Parkinson's and Alzheimer's have been linked to glutathione deficiency.
- **Glutathione** is needed to protect us from damage due to cigarette smoke, radiation exposure, and alcohol to name a few issues.
- Glutathione provides the major intracellular defense against mercury-induced neurotoxicity.

38. Ans. a. ERp57. d. Protein disulfide isomerase, e. Glucose related protein (GRP)

[Ref: Lippincott 7th/20; Harper 31st/41-42, 551-52; Shinde 5th/e p. 235; Vasudevan 5th/ 17]

Option a, d & e

◈ *(Harper 31st/41-42,551-52)*

- Protein disulfide isomerase, or PDI, is an enzyme in the endoplasmic reticulum (ER) in eukaryotes and the periplasm of bacteria that allows proteins to quickly find the correct arrangement of disulfide bonds in their fully folded state, and therefore the enzyme acts to caalyze protein folding.
- ***GRP78 and GRP94*** *Junction as molecular chaperones and can bind to mafolded proteins and unassembled complexes.*
- *The* ***ER foldase ERp57*** *(also known as Grp58) is a disulfide isomerase involved in the folding of a subset of glycoproteins in the ER aspart of the calnexin/ calreticulin cycle*

Option b&c

- *The* ***insulin receptor (IR)*** *is a transmembrane receptor that is activated by insulin, IGF-1, IGF-II and belongs to the large class of tyrosine kinase receptors. Metabolically, the insulin receptor plays a key role in the regulation of glucose homeostasis.*
- ***Cytochrome P450*** *enzymes are present in most tissues of the body, and play important roles in hormone synthesis and breakdown (including estrogen and testosterone synthesis and metabolism), cholesterol synthesis, and vitamin D metabolism. Cytochrome P450 enzymes also junction to metabolize potentially toxic compounds, including drugs and products of endogenous metabolism such as bilirubin, principally in the liver.*

Some Chaperones and Enzymes Involved in Folding that are Located in the Rough Endoplasmic Reticulum

◈ *Harper 31st/584*

- BiP (immunoglobulin heavy chain binding protein)
- General chaperones: GRP78/BiP, GRP94, GRP170 (glucose-regula ted protein)
- Lectin chaperones: - Calnexin, Calreticulin
- Non-classical molecular chaperones: HSP47 and ERp29
- Alpha-lytic protease, subtilisin (intramolecular chaperones)
- Hsp60, Hsp70, Hsp90, HsplOO
- Folding chaperones:-
- PDI (protein disulfide isomerase)
- PPI (peptidyl prolyl-cis-trans isomerase)
- ERp57

39. Ans. b. Acetyl Co-A carboxylase, c. ATP-citrate lyase, d. Acetyl transacylase

[Ref Harper 31st/216-20,153-55,216; 30th/233&; Satyanarayan 4 th/302]

Option b, c & d

- ***Production of malonyl-CoA from acetyl-CoA is the initial and rate limiting step in fatty acid synthesis. The reaction is catalyzed by acetyl-CoA carboxylase***
- Acetyl-CoA is the immediate substrate for fatty acid synthesis. ***In cytosol, citrate is cleaved by ATP-citrate lyase to oxaloacetate and acetyl-CoA .*** Acetyl-CoA enters into fatty acid synthesis.
- **Malonyl acetyl transferase (MAT)** is a part of multienzyme complex -**Fatty acid synthase.**
  It has two activities:-
  - Acetyl transferase or acetyl transacylase (E1).
  - ***Malonyl transferase or malonyl transacylase*** *(E2).*

Options a & e

These two enzymes are involved in triglyceride synthesis from glycerol and fatty acids.

Fatty Acids Synthesis

- Fatty acid synthesis **takes place** in **cytosol. Acetyl-CoA is the immediate substrate for lipogenesis and synthesis always ends in formation of palmitic acid.**
- In humans; ***liver and lactating mammary glands are the main organs for lipogenesis.*** Although ***kidney, brain, lungs and adipose tissue*** are also involved, to a lesser extent.
- **Cofactor** requirements for fatty acid synthesis are ***NADPH, ATP, Mn+2, biotin and HCO3- (as a source of CO_2).***
- The biosynthetic pattway occurs in 3 stages :
  - Transport of acetyl-CoA to cytosol
  - Conversion of acetyl-CoA to malonyl-CoA *by carboxylation*
  - Reaction of fatty acid synthase complex.

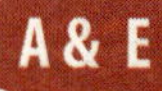

- **Transport of acetyl-CoA to cytosol**
  - ***Glucose is the primary substrate for lipogenesis and acetyl-CoA (immediate substrate for fatty acid synthesis)*** is formed from glucose via oxidation of pyruvate within the mitochondria.
  - However, acetyl-CoA cannot penetrate inner mitochondrial membrane. Therefore it is transferred in the form of **citrate.**
  - In **cytosol. citrate is cleaved by *ATP-citrate lyase to oxaloacetate and acetyl-CoA.***
- **Conversion of Acetyl CoA to Malonyl CoA**
  - ***Production of malonyl-CoA is the initial and rate limiting step*** in fatty acid synthesis.
- **Reactions catalyzed by fatty acid synthase**
  - All other enzymes (beside acetyl-CoA carboxylase) required for fatty acid synthesis are present in the form of **multienzyme complex, called as fatty acid synthase.**
  - Fatty acid synthase is made up of two identical subunits, each subunit contains ***seven enzymes*** and an ***acyl carrier protein (ACP).*** ACP contains the vitamin **pantothenic acid** in the form of 41- phosphopantetheine. The enzymes present in each unit are (1) El: *Acy/ transacylase (AT);* (2) E2: malonyl transacylase (MT); (3) E3: ketoacyl synthase; (4) E4: ketoacyl reductase; (5) E5: Hydratase; (6) E6: Enoyl reductase; and (7) E7: Thioesterase.

40. Ans. a. Beta oxidation, c. TCA cycle, d. Pyruvate dehydrogenase

[Ref: Harper 31st/576-77,30th/ 127; Lippincott 7th/74]

Option b & e

◈ *Lippincott 7th/74*

- *ATP synthase - inner membrane*
- *Acyl CoA synthatase - outer membrane*

Mitochondrial Matrix

◈ *Lippincott 7th/74; Harper 31st/576-77*

- The mitochondrion consists of an outer membrane, an inner membrane, and a gel-like material called the matrix. This **matrix** is more viscous than the cell's cytoplasm as it contains less water. The mitochondrial matrix has several functions.
- It is where the ***citric acid cycle*** takes place.
- Mitochondrial matrix also contains soluble enzymes, small organic molecules and nucleotide cofactors. **The *enzymes in the matrix facilitate reactions responsible for the production of ATP, such as the citric acid cycle, oxidative phosphorylation, oxidation of pyruvate and the beta oxidation of fatty acids.***

Enzymes in Matrix

- Enzymes from processes that take place in the matrix are:
  - ***The Citric Acid Cycle*** is facilitated by ***Pyruvate dehydrogenase,*** Citrate synthase, Aconitase, Isocitrate dehydrogenase, α-ketoglutarate dehydrogenase, Succinyl-CoA Synthetase, Fumarase, and Malate dehydrogenase.
  - The Urea Cycle is facilitated by Carbamoyl phosphate synthetase I and Ornithine transcarbamylase.
  - ***β-Oxidation*** uses pyruvate carboxylase, Acyl-CoA dehydrogenase, and β-Ketothiolase.
  - Amino acid production is facilitated by transaminases

IMMUNOGENETICS & MOLECULAR BIOLOGY

41. Ans. d. 3 billion

[Ref: Harrison 20th/3347;Harper 31st/349;Robbins 9th/1]

"Human DNA consists of ~***3 billion base pairs*** (bp) of DNA per haploid genome, which is nearly 1000-fold greater than that of the *Escherichia coli* genome"- *Harrison 20th/3347*

The ***3 billion base pairs of DNA*** that compose the haploid genome of humans are divided uniquely between 23 linear DNA units, the chromosomes. humans, being diploid, have 23 pairs of chromosomes: 22 autosomes and two sex chromosomes- *Harper 31st/349*

"Current estimates predict roughly ***20,000 protein-coding genes*** in the human genome with an average of about four different coding transcripts per gene. Remarkably, the exome only constitutes 1.14% of the genome. Of note, the number of transcripts is close to 200,000 and includes thousands of noncoding transcripts (RNAs of various length such as microRNAs [miRNA] and long noncoding RNAs [lncRNA])"- *Harrison 20th/3349*

42. Ans. a. 1%

[Ref: Harper 31st/358;Harrison 20th/3476-77]

One Percent of Cellulardna is in Mitochondria

◈ *Harper 31st/358*

- The majority of the polypeptides in mitochondria (about 54 outof 67) are encoded by nuclear genes, while the rest are coded bygenes found in mitochondrial (mt) DNA.
- Human mitochondria contains 2 to 10 copies of a small circular ~16 kbpds DNA molecule that makes up approximately ***1% of total cellular DNA***
- This mtDNA codes for mt-specific ribosomal and transfer

Mitochondrial DNA

◈ *Harrison 20th/3476*

- The integrated activity of estimated ***1500 gene*** products is required for normal mitochondrial biogenesis, function, and integrity.
- Aside from the 37 genes that comprise the mitochondrial DNA (mtDNA)molecule, the remaining 1400+ gene products are encoded by nuclear genes (referred to as nDNA) and thus follow the rules and patterns of nuclear genomic inheritance
- In addition, the mitochondria contain their own small genome consisting of numerous copies (polyploidy) per

mitochondrion of a circular, double-strand mitochondrial DNA (mtDNA) molecule comprising ***16,569 nucleotides.***

- This mtDNA sequence (also known as the "mitogenome") might represent the remnants of endosymbiotic prokaryotes from which mitochondria are thought to have originated.
- The mtDNA sequence contains a **total of 37 genes,** of which 13 encode mitochondrial protein components of the ETC.
- The remaining 22 tRNA- and 2 rRNA-encoding genes are mitochondria-specific and dedicated to the process of translating the 13 mtDNA-encoded proteins.

43. Ans. c. Has uracil (U) as base pair, d. Absent phosphodiester bond, e. Amount of adenine equals the amount of cytosine & the amount of guanine equals the amount of thymine

[Ref: Lippincott 6th/396-98;Harrison 20th/3348]

Structure of DNA

◈ *Harrison 20th/3348*

- DNA is a double-stranded helix composed off four different bases: adenine (A), thymidine (T), guanine (G), and cytosine (C).
- ***Adenine is paired to thymidine, and guanine is paired to cytosine***, by hydrogen bond interactions that span the double helix
- DNA is a polymer of deoxyribonucleoside monophosphates covalently linked by ***3'→5'–phosphodiester bonds.***
- Phosphodiester bonds join the 3'-hydroxyl group of the deoxypentose of one nucleotide to the 5'-hydroxyl group of the deoxypentose of an adjacent nucleotide through a phosphate group
- In the double helix, the two chains are coiled around a common axis called the axis of symmetry. The chains are paired in an antiparallel manner, that is, the 5'-end of one strand is paired with the 3'-end of the other strand.
- In the **DNA helix,** the ***hydrophilic deoxyribose–phosphate backbone of each chain*** is on the outside of the molecule, whereas the hydrophobic bases are stacked inside. The overall structure resembles a twisted ladder.
- **Chargaff Rule**: In any sample of dsDNA, the ***amount of adenine equals the amount of thymine, the amount of guanine equals the amount of cytosine***, and the ***total amount of purines equals the total amount of pyrimidines.***
- The base pairs are held together by **hydrogen bonds**: two between A and T and three between G and C. These hydrogen bonds, plus the hydrophobic interactions between the stacked
- Bases, stabilize the structure of the double helix.
- **Structural forms of the double helix:** There are three major structural forms of DNA: the B form, described by Watson and Crick in 1953, the A form, and the Z form

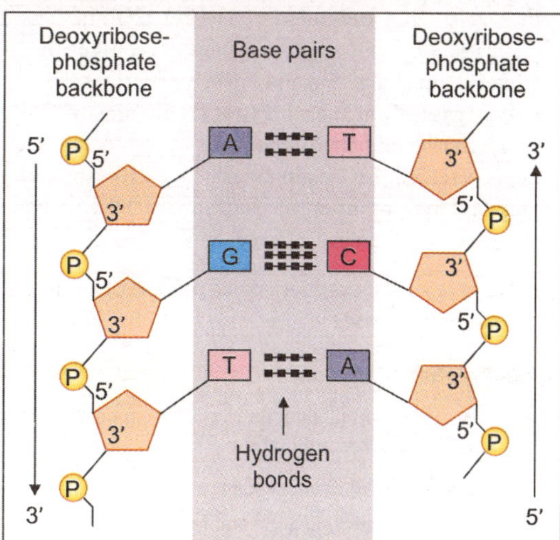

Fig: *(Lippincot 6th/397):* Two complementary DNA

44. Ans. a. Has 3' exonuclease, b. Has 5' exonuclease, c. Help in DNA proofreading, e. Help in DNA repair

[Ref: Harper 31st/363-64; Lippincott 7th/418;Biochemistry by Dinesh Puri 4th/400-401]

Table: *(Dinesh Puri 4th/400):* **Comparison of DNA polymerases (DNAP)**

	DNAP I	DNAP II	DNAP III
Subunits	1	4	8
3'-Exonuclease	Yes	Yes	Yes
5'-Exonuclease	Yes	No	Yes
Speed (bases per second)	16-20	<7	600-1000
Processivity	3-200	~10,000	~500,000
Molecules per cell	400	100	15

The DNA polymerase Complex

◈ *Harper 31st/363*

- A number of different DNA polymerase molecules engage in DNA replication. These share three important properties: (1) **chain elongation,** (2) **processivity,** and (3) **proofreading.**
- Chain elongation accounts for the rate (in **nucleotides per second; nt/s**) at which polymerization occurs.
- Processivity is an expression of the number of nucleotides added to the nascent chain before the polymerase disengages from the template.
- The proofreading function identifies copying errors and corrects them.

- In *E coli,* **DNA polymerase III (pol III)**functions at the replication fork. Of all polymerases, it catalyzes the highest rate of chain elongation and is the most processive.
- **Polymerase I (pol I) and II (pol II)** are mostly involved in ***proofreading and DNA repair***.
- Eukaryotic cells have counterparts for each of these enzymes plus a large number of additional DNA polymerases primarily involved in DNA repair.

Table: *(Harper 31st/364):* **Comparison of prokaryotic and Eukaryotic DNA polymerases**

E coli	Eukaryotic	Function
I		Gap filling following DNA replication, repair & recombination
II		DNA proof reading and repair
	β	DNA repair
	γ	Mitochondrial DNA synthesis
III	α	Primase
	d	Processive lagging strand synthesis

Direction of DNA Replication

◈ *Lippincott 7th/418*

- The **DNA polymerases** responsible for copying the DNA templates are only able to "read" the parental nucleotide sequences in the 3'→5' direction, and they ***synthesize the new DNA strands only in the 5'→3' (antiparallel) direction***. Therefore, beginning with one parental double helix, the two newly synthesized stretches of nucleotide chains must grow in opposite directions—one in the 5'→3' direction toward the replication fork and one in the 5'→3' direction away from the replication fork.
- **Leading strand:** The strand that is being copied in the direction of the advancing replication fork is called the leading strand and is synthesized ***continuously.***
- **Lagging strand:** The strand that is being copied in the direction away from the replication fork is synthesized ***discontinuously,*** with small fragments of DNA being copied near the replication fork.
- These short stretches of discontinuous DNA, termed ***Okazaki fragments***, are eventually joined (ligated) to become a single, continuous strand. The new strand of DNA produced by this mechanism is termed the lagging strand

45. Ans. e. RNA is synthesized in 3→5 direction

[Ref: Lippincott 7th/435-36;Harrison 20th/3348; KDT 8th/822]

Transcription in Prokaryotes

◈ *Lippincott 7th/435-36*

- In ***bacteria, one species of RNA polymerase synthesizes all of the RNA*** except for the short RNA primers needed for DNA replication(RNA primers are synthesized by a specialized enzyme, primase)
- RNA polymerase is a multisubunit enzyme that recognizes a nucleotide sequence (the promoter region) at the beginning of a length of DNA that is to be transcribed.
- It next makes a ***complementary RNA copy of the DNA template strand***, and then recognizes the end of the DNA sequence to be transcribed (the termination region).
- ***RNA is synthesized from its 5'-end to its 3'-end***,antiparallel to its DNA template strand
- The template is copied as it is in DNA synthesis, in which a G on the DNA specifies a C in the RNA, a C specifies a G, a T specifies an A, but an A specifies a U instead of a T
- The ***RNA, then, is complementary to the DNA template*** (antisense) strand and identical to the coding (sense) strand, with U replacing T.
- Within the DNA molecule, regions of both strands can serve as templates for transcription. For a given gene, however, only one of the two DNA strands can be the template. Which strand is used is determined by the location of the promoter for that gene.
- Transcription by RNA polymerase involves a core enzyme and several auxiliary proteins
- The process of transcription of a typical gene of E. coli can be divided into three phases: initiation, elongation, and termination.
- A transcription unit extends from the promoter to the termination region, and the initial product of transcription by RNA polymerase is termed the primary transcript
- As with replication, ***transcription is always in the 5'→3' direction.***
- In contrast to DNA polymerase, RNA polymerase does not require a primer and does ***not appear to have proofreading activity.***
- **Rifampin** inhibits the initiation of transcription by binding to the β subunit of ***prokaryotic RNA* polymerase**
- Mechanism of action of ***rifabutin*** is like rifampin-KDT 8th/822

46. Ans. b. UAG, c.UAA, e. UGA

[Ref: Harper 31st/394; Shinde 7th/250; Lippincott 7th/448-49]

Stop codon are: ***UAA, UAG & UGA***- *Shinde 7th/250*

Codons

◈ *Lippincott 7th/448-49*

- Codons are presented in the mRNA language of adenine (A), guanine (G), cytosine (C), and uracil (U). Their nucleotide sequences are always written from the 5'-end to the 3'-end. The four nucleotide bases are used to produce the three-base codons. There are, therefore, 64 different combinations of bases, taken three at a time (a triplet code)
- AUG is the initiation (start) codon for translation.
- **Termination ("stop" or "nonsense") codons:** Three of the codons, ***UAG, UGA, and UAA,*** do not code for amino acids, but rather are termination codons. When one of these codons appears in an mRNA sequence, synthesis of the polypeptide coded for by that mRNA stops

47. Ans. b. Binding to the promoter region, c. DNA dependent RNA polymerase enzyme involvement

[Ref: Vasudevan 5th/426; Lippincott 7th/441-42; Molecular Biology by Lodish 6th/348]

- *Poly-A tail addition & 5' capping are* **Post-transcriptional Modification found only in eukaryotes, as in prokaryotes primary transcript of mRNA is functional**
- Binding to the promoter region & DNA dependent RNA polymerase enzyme involvement occur in both
- One species of RNA polymerase synthesizes all of the RNA only in prokaryotes

Post-transcriptional Modification in Eukaryotes

◈ *Vasudevan 5th/426; Lippincott 7th/441-42*

- ***Poly-A tailing***
- ***5' capping***
- *Methylation*
- *Removal of introns*
- *Spicing of exons (connect together)*
- *Endonuclease cleavage*

"In bacteria(Prokaryotes), **one species of RNA polymerase** synthesizes all of the RNA except for the short RNA primers needed for DNA replication (RNA primers are synthesized by a specialized enzyme, primase)"- *Lippincott 7th/435*

"The transcription of eukaryotic genes is a far more complicated process than transcription in prokaryotes. ***Eukaryotic transcription involves separate polymerases for the synthesis of rRNA, tRNA, and mRNA.*** In addition, a large number of proteins called transcription factors (TFs) are involved. TFs bind to distinct sites on the DNA—either within the core promoter region, close (proximal) to it, or some distance away (distal). [**Note:** Each eukaryotic RNA polymerase has its own promoters and TFs.]"-*Lippincott 7th/438*

PATHOLOGY

48. Ans. c. Synovial sarcoma →t(X:18), d. Acute lymphocytic leukemia→ t(9;22), e. Burkitt's lymphoma → t(8;14)

[Ref: Harrison 20th/591;Robbins 9th/1219; Harshmohan 8th/397]

Burkit's lymphoma *typical cytological abnormalities: t(8;14) & t(8;22)"-Harshmohan 8th/397*

"**Synovial sarcoma:** *Translocation t(X;18)(p11;q11) & SS18-SSX1 fusion gene"- Harshmohan 8th/914*

Acute Lymphocytic Leukemia (ALL)

◈ *Harrison 20th/759,775; Harshmohan 8th/393*

- Ph+ ALL, with the chromosomal translocation ***t(9;22)*** (q34;q11) with corresponding
- *BCR-ABL1* gene rearrangement.
- t(4;11)(q21;q23)/*MLL-AFA4*, abn11q23/*MLL*, and t(1;19) (q23;p13)/*PBX-E2A*.

Table: *(Harrison 20th/454):* **Representative Oncogenes at Chromosomal Translocations**

Gene (chromosome)	Translocation	Malignancy
BCR-ABL	(9;22)(q34;q11)	Chronic myeloid leukemia
BCL1 (11q13.3)–*IgH* (14q32)	(11;14)(q13;q32)	Mantle cell lymphoma
BCL2 (18q21.3)–*IgH* (14q32)	(14;18)(q32;q21)	Follicular lymphoma
FLI-EWSR1	(***11;22***)(q24;q12)	Ewing's sarcoma
LCK –TCRB	(1;7)(p34;q35)	T-cell acute lymphocytic leukemia
PAX3–FOXO1	(2;13)(q35;q14)	Rhabdomyosarcoma
PAX8-PPARG	(2;3)(q13;p25)	Thyroid
IL21R-BCL6	(3;16)(q27;p11)	Non-Hodgkin's lymphoma
TAL1–TCTA	(1;3)(p34;p21)	Acute T cell leukemia
TMPRSS2-ERG	Rearrangement on Chr21q22	Prostate

Table: *(Robbins 9th/1219):* **Chromosomal Abnormalities in Soft tissue Tumors**

Tumor	Cytogenetic Abnormality	Gene fusion	Proposed function
Ewing sarcoma family tumors Extraskeletalmyxoid chondrosarcoma Desmoplastic small round-cell tumor Clear-cell sarcoma	t (11;22)(q24;q12) t(21;22)(q22;q12) t(9;22) (q22;q12) t(11;22)(p13;q12) t(2;22)(q13;q12)	EWS-FLI1 EWS-ERG EWS-CHN EWS-WT1 EWS-ATF1	Disordered protein with multiple functions, including aberrant transcription, cell cycle regulation. RNA spicing and telomerase
Liposarcoma-myxoid and round-cell type	t(12;16)(q13:p11)	FUS-DDIT3	Arrests adipocytic differentiation.
Synovial sarcoma	t(x;18)(p11;q11) SS18-SSx2 SS18-SSx4	SS18-SSX1	Chimeric transcription factors, interrupts cell cycle control
Rhabdomyosarcoma -alveolar type	t(2;13)(q35;q14) t(1;13)(o36;q14)	PAX3-FOX01 PAX7-FOX01	Chimeric transcription factors, disrupt skeletal muscle differentiation
Dermatofibrosarcoma protuberans	t(17;22)(q11.2;q25)	COLA1-PDGFB	Promoter driven overexpression of PDGF-β autocrine stimulation
Alveolar soft-part sarcoma	t(x;17)(p11.2; q25)	TFE3-ASPL	Unknown

Contd...

Tumor	Cytogenetic Abnormality	Gene fusion	Proposed function
Infantiefibrosarcoma	t(12;15)(p13;q23)	ETV6-NTRK3)	Chimeric tyrosine kinase leads to constitutively active Ras/ MAPK pathway
Nodular fasciitis	T(22;17)	MYH9-USP6	Unknown

49. Ans. a. CA-19-9, d. Carcinoembryonic antigen (CEA)

[Ref: Harrison 20th/591; Harshmohan 8th/674;Robbins 9th/337]

Tumor Marker

◈ *Robbins 9th/337(Table)*

- ***CA-19-9**: **Pancreatic cancer**; colon cancer*
- CA-125: Ovarian cancer
- CA-15-3: Breast cancer
- ***Carcinoembryonic antigen (CEA)**: Cacinoma of colon, **pancrease**, lung, stomach & heart*
- Human chorionic gonadotropin (HCG): Trophoblastictumors, nonseminomatous testicular tumors

Table: *(Harrison 20th/591):* **Germ-line Mutations, Their Familial Cancer Syndrome, and Fold Risk of Pancreatic Cancer**

Germ-line mutation	Familial cancer syndrome	Estimated increased risk (fold) of pancreatic cancer
Brca2a	Familial breast/ovarian cancer	3.5–10
Palb2 (partner and localizer of brca2)	Familial breast cancer and others	~Six fold
P16/cdkn2a	Familial atypical multiple mole melanoma (fammm)	13–38
Stkii (lkb1)	Peutz-jeghers syndrome	132
Prss1 or spin11b	Hereditary (familial) pancreatitis	53
Atm	Ataxia-telangiectasia	Not yet established
Mlh1, msh2, msh6, Pms2	Heredity nonpolyposis colorectal syndrome or lynch syndrome	9–30

50. Ans. b. Desmin, c. Vimentin

[Ref: Harshmohan 8th/244]

Table: *(Harshmohan 8th/244):* **Common panel of immunohistochemical stains for tumors of uncertain origin**

Tumour	Immunostain
• Epithelial tumours (carcinomas)	• ***Pankeratin*** (fractions: high and low molecular weight keratins (HMW-K, LMW-K)] • Epithelial membrane antigen (EMA) • Carcinoembryonic antigen (CEA) • Neuron-specific enolase (NSE)

Contd...

Tumour	Immunostain
• Mesenchymal tumours (sarcomas)	• ***Vimentin*** (general mesenchymal) • ***Desmin*** (for general myogenic) • Muscle specific actin (for general myogenic) • Myoglobin (for skeletal myogenic) • α-1 anti-chymotrypsin (for malignant fibrous histiocytoma) • Factor VIII (for vascular tumours) • CD34 (endothelial marker)
• Special groups ▪ Melanoma	• HMB-45 (most specific) • Vimentin • S-100
▪ Lymphoma	• Leucocyte common antigen (LACA/CD45) • Pan-B (Immunoglobulins CD20) • Pan-T (CD3) • CD 15, CD 30, (RS cell marker for Hodgkin's)
▪ Neural and neuroendocrine tumours	• ***Neurofilaments*** (NF) • Neuron-specific enolase (NSE) • ***Glial fibrillary acidic protein*** (GFAP) (for glial tumours) • Chromogranin (for neuroendocrine)

51. Ans. a. BCL2 b. BCL-XL, c. MCL1

[Ref: Robbins 9th/55;Harshmohan 8th/58]

Proapoptotic or Antiapoptotic

◈ *Robbins 9th/55*

- There are more than 20 members of the *BCL* family, which can be divided into three groups based on their pro-apoptotic or antiapoptotic function and the BCL2 homology (BH) domains they possess
- **Antiapoptotic**: ***BCL2, BCL-XL, and MCL1*** are the principal members of this group; they possess four BH domains (called BH1-4). These proteins reside in theouter mitochondrial membranes as well as the cytosol and ER membranes. By keeping the mitochondrial outer membrane impermeable they prevent leakage of cytochrome c and other death-inducing proteins into the cytosol
- **Proapoptotic**: ***BAX and BAK*** are the two prototypic members of this group. Like their anti-apoptotic cousins they also have four BH domains. Upon activation, BAX and BAK oligomerize within the outer mitochondrial protein and promote mitochondrial outer membrane permeability. The precise mechanism by which Bax-Bakpermeabilize membranes is not settled.
- **Sensors:** Members of this group, including ***BAD, BIM, BID, Puma, and Noxa,*** contain only one BH domain, the third of the four BH domains, and hence are sometimes called BH3-only proteins. BH3-only proteins act as sensors of cellular stress and damage, and regulate the balance between the other two groups, thus acting as arbiters of apoptosis

52. Ans. c. Down syndrome-Chromosome 21, d. Down syndrome occurs due to non-disjunction of chromosome

[Ref: Robbins 9th/ 161;Harshmohan 8th/289;Davidson 23rd/44]

"**Trisomy 21 (Down Syndrome)**: Down syndrome is the most common of the chromosomal disorders and is a major cause of mental retardation"- *Robbins 9th/ 161*

Down syndrome: Due to Nondisjunction of Chromosome

◈ *Harshmohan 8th/289*

"A variety of other trisomies involving chromosomes 8, 9, 13, 18, and 22 have been described. Only ***trisomy 18 (Edwards syndrome) and trisomy 13 (Patau syndrome)*** are common enough to merit brief mention here"- *Robbins 9th/ 163*

Table: *(Davidson 23rd/44)*: **Chromosome disorder**

Disease	Locus	Incidence	Clinical features
Numerical chromosomal	Abnormalities		
Down's syndrome (Trisomy 21)	47, XY, +21 OR 47, XX+21	1:800	Characteristic, facies, IQ usually < 50, congenital heart disease, reduced life expectancy.
Edwards syndrome (trisomy 18)	47, XY,+18 OR 47, XX, +18	1:6000	Early lethality, characteristic skull and facies, frequent malformations of heart, kidney and other organs
Patau's syndrome (trisomy 13)	47,XY, +13 or 47, XX, +13	1:15000	Early lethality, cleft lip and palate, polydactyly, small head, frequent congenital heart disease
Klinefelter's syndrome	47, XXY	1:1000	Phenotypic male, infertility, gynaecomastia, small testes
XYY	47, XYY	1:1000	Usually asymptomatic, some impulse control problems
Triple X syndrome	47, XXX	1:1000	Usually asymptomatic, may have reduced IQ
Tuner's syndrome	45, X	1:5000	Phenotypic female, short stature, webbed neck, coarctation of the aorta, primary amenorrhoea

53. Ans. b. Maternal age more than 35 is a risk factor, d. Occur due to meiotic nondisjunction of chromosome 21

[Ref: Davidson 23rd/44; Robbins 9th/161; O.P. Ghai 8th/637-38]

Trisomy 21 (Down Syndrome)

◈ *Robbins (SEA) 9th/ 161*

- Down syndrome is the most common of the chromosomal disorders and is a major cause of mental retardation.
- **Approximately 95%** of affected ***individuals have trisomy 21***
- **Maternal age** has a strong influence on the incidence of trisomy 21. It occurs once in 1550 live births in women under age 20, in contrast to 1 in 25 live births for mothers older than age 45. The correlation with **maternal age** suggested that ***most cases the meiotic nondisjunction of chromosome 21 occurs in the ovum.***
- Indeed, studies in which DNA polymorphisms were used to trace the parental origin of chromosome 21 have revealed that in ***95% of the cases with trisomy 21 the extra chromosome is of maternal origin.***

Trisomy 21 (Down Syndrome)

◈ *O.P. Ghai 8th/637-38*

- *Chromosome no. 21 is present in triplicate, the origin of extra chromosome 21 being* ***either maternal or paternal***
- ***In most cases the extra chromosome from the mother***
- Trisomy is found in 94% cases.
- *Approx. 1% of cases are mosaic and* ***rest (5%) are due to translocations, most commonly involving chromosome 21 and 14***

54. Ans. a. Furrowed protruding tongue b. Small nose, c. Intellectual impairment, e. Short & broad hand

[Ref: Robbins (SEA) 9th/ 161-63; O.P.Ghai 9th/635-37; Harrison 19th/83e1-4; Nelson 18th/508; Davidson 23rd/44]

Down Syndrome

◈ *O.P.Ghai 9th/635*

- Furrowed protruding tongue
- ***Small nose*** *with flat nasal bridge*
- Small & dysplastic ear
- Upward slant of eye
- Narrow short palate with small teeth
- Short & broad hand
- Epicanthic fold
- Down syndrome is a major cause of ***mental retardation***- *Robbins (SEA) 9th/ 161*

Systemic Abnormalities in Down Syndrome

◈ *Nelson 18th/508*

- **GIT:** ***Duodenal, ileal and jejunal atresia***, tracheoesophogeal fistula, Hirschsprung's disease, Meckel's diverticulum, imperforate anus, omphalocele.
- **Eye:** Brushfield spot, ↑ed risk of cataract, nystagmus and squint.
- **CVS:** Endocardial cushion defect (MC), VSD, Ostium primum ASD and AV valve malformation
- **Hearing defects:** Serous otitis media; conductive and/or ***sensorineural hearing loss*** (Nelson 18th/508)
- **Thyroid-dysfunction:** Hypothyroidism

- Atlanto-occipital dislocation/subluxation
- **Malignancy:** ↑ed risk of AML and ALL
- Early onset of Alzheimer disease
- Abnormal immune response

55. Ans. d. Can be reversed by increasing dose of corticosteroid, e. Predictor of chronicity

[Ref: Robbins 9th/ 233-34,237; L & B 27th/1535-36; Harshmohan 8th/130]

- Hyperacute rejection carries high morbidity and mortality
- Hyperacute rejection is HLA mediated
- MC cause of graft failure is chronic rejection

"The single most important risk factor for **chronic rejection** after kidney transplantation is ***acute rejection*** (with vascular inflammation) and recurrent episodes of acute rejection"- *L & B 27th/1536; Harshmohan 8th/130*

"In recent years, acute rejection has been significantly controlled by immunosuppressive therapy(including ***steroids***), and chronic rejection has emerged as an important cause of graft failure"- *Robbins 9th/ 234*

Types of Graft Rejection

◈ *L & B 27th/1535*

- **Hyperacute rejection**
  - Immediate graft destruction due to ABO or ***preformed anti-HLA antibodies***
  - Characterised by intravascular thrombosis and interstitial haemorrhage
- **Acute rejection**
  - Usually occurs during first six months
  - T cell dependent
  - May be cell-mediated, antibody-mediated or both
  - Usually reversible
- **Chronic rejection**
  - Occurs after first six months
  - Most common cause of graft failure
  - Antibodies play an important role
  - Non-immune factors contribute to pathogenesis
  - Characterized by myointimal proliferation in graft arteries leading to ischaemia and fibrosis

Acute Rejection L & B

◈ *27th/1536*

- This usually occurs during the first six months of transplantation but may occur later.
- *It is* **mediated predominantly** *by* ***T lymphocytes****, but alloantibodies may also play an important role.*
- Acute rejection is characterised by mononuclear cell infiltration of the graft
- The mononuclear cell infiltrate is heterogeneous and includes cytotoxic T cells, B cells, NK cells and activated macrophages.
- Antibody-mediated damage may also be present as evidenced by the deposition of the complement component C4d within the graft microvasculature
- *All types of organ allograft are susceptible to acute rejection, and although relatively common (typically occurring in around 20–30 per cent of grafts),* ***most episodes of acute rejection can be reversed by additional immunosuppressive therapy****.*

56. Ans. c. Carry CD8 molecule on their surface, e. Kill infected cells

[Ref: Harrison 20th/2451,2467-68; Harshmohan 8th/125; Robbins 9th/190]

T Lymphocytes

◈ *Robbins 9th/190*

- There are three major populations of T cells, which serve distinct functions.
- **Helper T lymphocytes** stimulate B lymphocytes to make antibodies and activate other leukocytes (e.g., phagocytes) to destroy microbes
- **Cytotoxic T lymphocytes** (CTLs; a/k **suppressor T cell**) kill ***infected cells***
- **Regulatory T lymphocytes** limit immune responses and prevent reactions against self-antigens

T lymphocyte

◈ *Harrison 20th/2451*

- **CD4 T cell:** T lymphocyte subset that participates in adaptive immunity and helps B cells make antibody.
- **CD8 T cell:** Cytotoxic T lymphocyte subset that destroys tumor cells and ***cells infected with intracellular pathogens.***

Suppresor T Cell

◈ *Harshmohan 8th/125*

- Carry CD8 molecule on their surface & hence also called CD8+ cells
- CD+ cells in circulation are about half the number of CD+ cells(Helper T cell)
- Compared to CD+ cells which act by elaboration of cytokines, CD+ are directly cytotoxic to antigen
- Particularly involved in destroying cells infected with virus, foreign cells & tumor cells

57. Ans. a. Liver failure

[Ref: Harrison 20th/2105,379,827;Harshmohan 8th/308]

"Schistocytes are helmet-shaped cells that reflect ***microangiopathic haemolytic anemia or fragmentation on an artificial heart valve****"-Harrison 20th/380*

"Schistocytosis is identified by fragmentation of erythrocytes. **Schistocytes** *are found in thalassemia, hereditary elliptocytosis, megaloblastic anaemia, iron deficiency anaemia, microangiopathic haemolytic anaemia & in* ***severe burn****"-Harshmohan 8th/308*

TTP/HUS: ***Schistocytes on peripheral blood smear***, elevated LDH, anemia, thrombocytopenia- *Harrison 20th/2105*

RBC: Inclusion Bodies & Different Shape

◈ *Harrison 20th/379-80*

- *Basophilic stippling*: lead poisoning
- *Howell-Jolly bodies*: defective splenic function
- *Spherocytes*: hereditary spherocytosis,

- *Dacrocytes*: hemolyticanemias, severe iron deficiency, thalassemias, myelofibrosis, and myelodysplastic syndromes.
- *Echinocytes*: renal failure and malnutrition and are often reversible.
- *Acanthocytes*: renal disease, abetalipoproteinemia, or splenectomy.
- *Elliptocytes*: iron deficiency, myelodysplastic syndromes, megaloblastic anemia, and thalassemias.
- *Stomatocytes*: inherited red cell membrane defect, alcoholism.
- *Target cells*: thalassemia, iron deficiency, ***cholestatic liver disease***, and some hemoglobinopathies.

58. Ans. a. Bath restrictive and obstructive symptoms are present, c. Viscous mucus secretion, d. Lung transplantation is a therapeutic option in case of pulmonary failure, e. Recombinant human deoxyribonuclease (rhDNAase) is useful to decrease sputum viscosity

[Ref: Harrison 20th/1986-90; CMDT 2019/276-77; Robbins 9th/470]

"Pulmonary function studies show a ***mixed obstructive and restrictive pattern.*** There is a reduction in FVC, airflow rates, and TLC. Air trapping (high ratio of RV to TLC) and reduction in pulmonary diffusing capacity are common"-*CMDT 2019/276*

"**Cystic fibrosis (CF)** is an ***autosomal recessive*** exocrinopathy affecting multiple epithelial tissues. The gene product responsible for CF (the cystic fibrosis transmembrane conductance regulator [CFTR]) serves as an anion channel in the apical (luminal) plasma membranes of epithelial cells and regulates volume and composition of exocrine secretion"-*Harrison 20th/1986*

Respiratory manifestations: The major morbidity and mortality associated with CF is attributable to respiratory compromise, characterized by ***copious hyperviscous and adherent pulmonary***secretions that ***obstruct small and medium-sized airways.*** CF airway secretions are exceedingly difficult to clear, and a complex bacterial flora that includes *Staphylococcus aureus, Haemophilus influenzae*, and *Pseudomonas aeruginosa* (among other pathogens) is routinely cultured from CF sputum"- *Harrison 20th/1986*

"**Considerations regarding lung transplantation:** In the setting of end-stage CF pulmonary failure, lung transplantation is a viable therapeutic option with 5-year survival rates on the order of 60% and median survival >8 years"- *Harrison 20th/1988*

"**Lung transplantation** is currently the only definitive treatment for advanced cystic fibrosis. Double-lung or heart-lung transplantation is required"-*CMDT 2019/276*

"**Inhaled recombinant human deoxyribonuclease (rhDNase,** dornase alpha) cleaves extracellular DNA in sputum(degraded DNA strand contribute to mucus viscosity); when administered long-term at a daily nebulized dose of 2.5 mg, this therapy leads to improved FEV1 and reduces the risk of cystic fibrosis–related respiratory exacerbations and the need for intravenous antibiotics"-*CMDT 2019/276; Harrison 20th/1988*

Table: *(Robbins 9th/470, 8th/470)*: **Clinical Features of Cystic Fibrosis**

***Chronic sinopulmonary disease* manifested by**
• Persistent colonization/infection with typical cystic fibrosis *pathogens, including Staphylococcus aureus, nontypeable Hemophilusinfluenzae*, mucoid and nonmucoid*Pseudomonas aeruginosa, Burkholderiacepacia*
• Chronic cough and sputum production
• Persistent chest radiograph abnormalities (*e.g.,* bronchiectasis, atelectasis, infiltrates, hyperinflation)
• Airway obstruction manifested by wheezing and air trapping
• Nasal polyps; radiographic or computed tomographic abnormalities of paranasal sinuses
• Digital clubbing
***Gastrointestinal and nutritional abnormalities*, including**
• **Intestinal:** Meconium ileus, distal intestinal obstruction syndrome, rectal prolapsed
• **Pancreatic:** Pancreatic insufficiency, recurrent pancreatitis
• **Hepatic:** chronic hepatic disease manifested by clinical or histologic evidence of focal biliary cirrhosis, or multilobular cirrhosis
• **Nutritional:** Failure to thrive (protein-calorie malnutrition), hypoproteinemia, edema, complications secondary to fat-soluble vitamin deficiency

59. Ans. a. Hyperparathyroidism, c. Hyperthyroidism, d. Thymic hyperplasia

[Ref: Robbins 9th/241;Harshmohan 8th/130-31; CMDT 2019/1163;Ananthanarayan 10th/175]

"**Hypoparathyroidism** may also be seen in DiGeorge syndrome, along with congenital cardiac and facial anomalies; ***hypocalcemia usually presents*** with tetany in infancy, but some cases are not detected until adulthood"- *CMDT 2019/1163;Harrison 20th/2937*

DiGeorge Syndrome (Thymic Hypoplasia)

◈ *Robbins 9th/241*

- **DiGeorge syndrome is a T-cell deficiency that results from failure of development of the third and fourth pharyngeal pouches**. The latter give rise to the thymus, the parathyroids, some of the C cells of the thyroid, and the ultimobranchial body.
- Thus, individuals with this syndrome have a variable loss of T cell–mediated immunity(resulting from hypoplasia or lack of the thymus), tetany(resulting from ***lack of the parathyroids***), and congenital defects of the heart and great vessels.
- In addition, the appearance of the mouth, ears, and facies may be abnormal.
- Absence of cell-mediated immunity is caused by low numbers of T lymphocytes in the blood and lymphoid

tissues and poor defense against certain fungal and viral infections.

- The T-cell zones of lymphoid organs—paracortical areas of the lymph nodes and the periarteriolar sheaths of the spleen—are depleted. Ig levels may be normal or reduced, depending on the severity of the T-cell deficiency.
- In many cases, DiGeorge syndrome is not a familial disorder. It results from a deletion that maps to chromosome 22q11. This deletion is seen in more than 50% of patients, and DiGeorge syndrome is now considered a component of the *22q11 deletion syndrome*

60. Ans. a. Breast cancer

[Ref: Schwartz 10th/536; Sabiston 19th/846; ww5.komen.org; www.breastcancer.org; www.mayoclinic.org]

Five Main Intrinsic or Molecular Subtypes of Breast Cancer

◈ *www.breastcancer.org*

- **Luminal A** breast cancer is hormone-receptor positive (estrogen-receptor and/or progesterone-receptor positive), HER2 negative, and has low levels of the protein Ki-67, which helps control how fast cancer cells grow. Luminal A cancers are low-grade, tend to grow slowly and have the best prognosis.
- **Luminal B** breast cancer is hormone-receptor positive (estrogen-receptor and/or progesterone-receptor positive), and either HER2 positive or HER2 negative with high levels of Ki-67. Luminal B cancers generally grow slightly faster than luminal A cancers and their prognosis is slightly worse.
- **Triple-negative/basal-like** breast cancer is hormone-receptor negative (estrogen-receptor and progesterone-receptor negative) and HER2 negative. This type of cancer is more common in women with *BRCA1* gene mutations.
- **HER2-enriched** breast cancer is hormone-receptor negative (estrogen-receptor and progesterone-receptor negative) and HER2 positive.
- **Normal-like** breast cancer is similar to luminal A disease: hormone-receptor positive (estrogen-receptor and/or progesterone-receptor positive), HER2 negative, and has low levels of the protein Ki-67, which helps control how fast cancer cells grow.

Table: Molecular subtypes of breast cancer

	Luminal A	Luminal B	Her-2/neu	Basal-like
		Luminal B tends to be higher histological grade than luminal A	TPS3 mutation common More likely to be high grade and node positive	TP53 mutation common BRCA-1 dysfunction (germine sporadic)
Histological correlation	Tubular carcinoma cribriform carcinoma Low grade (DC(NOS) lobular carcinoma	IDC (NOS) Micropapillary carcinoma	High grade IDC (NOS)	High grade IDC(NOS) Metaplastic carcinoma Medullary carcinoma
Treatment	Respond to endocrine therapy	Respond to endocrine therapy (tamoxifen & aromatase inhibitors)	Respond to trastuzumab	No response to Endorcine therapy and trastuzumab
Response to chemotherapy	Variable	Variable (>in luminal A)	Good (anthracycline based chemotherapy)	Good (platinum-based chemotherapy)
Prognosis	Good prognosis	Prognosis not as good as for luminal A	Generally poor prognosis	Generally poor prognosis

61. Ans. b. Wiskott-Aldrich syndrome, c. Severe combined immunodeficiency, e. Common variable immunodeficiency

[Ref: Ananthanarayan 10th/174; Robbins 9th/239-43; Harshmohan 7th/51]

Table: *(Ananthanarayan 10th/174)*: **Classification of primary immunodeficiency syndrome**

Disorders of specific Immunity

- **Humoral immunodeficiencies (B cell defects)**
  - X-Linked agammaglobulinemia
  - Transient hypogammaglobullnernia of Infancy
  - ***Common variable immunodeficiency*** (late onset hypogammaglobulinemia)
  - Selective immunoglobulin deficiencies (IpA IgM or IgG subclasses)
  - Immunodeficiency with hyper-IgM
  - Transcobalamin II deficiency

Contd...

- **Cellular immunodeficiencies (T cell defects)**
  - Thymic hypoplasia (DiGeorge syndrome)
  - Chronic mucocutaneouscandidosis
  - Purine nucleoside phosphorylase (PNP) deficiency
- **Combined immunodeficiencies (B and T cell defects)**
  - Cellular Immunodeficiency with abnormal immunoglobulin synthesis (Nezelof syndrome)
  - ***Ataxia telangiectasia***
  - ***Wiskott-Aldrich syndrome***
  - Immunodeficiency with thymoma
  - Immunodeficiency with short-limbed dwarfism
  - Episodic lymphopenla with lymphocytotoxin
  - **Severe combined immunodeficiency**

'Swiss type' agammaglobulinemia 1.
Reticular dysgenesis of de Vaal 2.
3. ***Adenosine deaminase (ADA) deficiency***

Contd...

- **Disorders of complement**
  - Complement component deficiencies
  - Complement inhibitor deficiencies
- **Disorders of phagocytosis**
  - Chronic granulomatous disease
  - Myeloperoxidase deficiency
  - Chediak-Higashi syndrome
  - Leukocyte GOPD deficiency
  - Job's syndrome
  - Tuftsin deficiency
  - Lazy leukocyte syndrome
  - Hyper-IgE syndrome
  - Actin binding protein deficiency
  - Shwachman's disease

62. Ans. a. Bone pain is most frequent symptom, b. Prostate & lung carcinoma are common source of metastasis, c. Increase chance of pathological fracture, d. Higher serum levels of alkaline phosphatase

[Ref: Harrison 20th/657;Robbins 9th/1207;Harshmohan 8th/892;Maheshwari 6th/246-47]

Clinical Feature of Metastasis in Bone: Patient with known Primary/Not a known Case of Primary Malignancy

◈ *Maheshwari 6th/246-47*

- Bone pain
- Pathological fracture

Tumors Metastatic to Bone

◈ *Harrison 20th/657*

- Bone metastases may be asymptomatic or may produce pain, swelling, nerve root or spinal cord compression, pathologic fracture, or myelophthisis (replacement of the marrow).
- Symptoms of hypercalcemia may be noted in cases of bony destruction.
- ***Pain is the most frequent symptom***. It usually develops gradually over weeks, is usually localized, and often is more severe at night.
- When patients with back pain develop neurologic signs or symptoms, emergency evaluation for spinal cord compression is indicated
- Cancer in the bone may produce osteolysis, osteogenesis, or both.
- Osteoblastic lesions are associated with ***higher serum levels of alkaline phosphatase and***, if extensive, may produce hypocalcemia.
- Although some tumors may produce mainly osteolyticlesions (e.g., kidney cancer) and others mainly osteoblastic lesions (e.g., prostate cancer), most metastatic lesions produce both types of lesion and may go through stages where one or the other predominates.

Metastatic in Bone

◈ *Maheshwari 6th/246-47*

- Metastatic tumors in the bone are commoner than the primary bone tumors
- ***Carcinoma of the prostate*** in males & carcinoma of breast in females are the commonest tumors to give rise to scelerotic bone secondaries in the bone
- In adults more than 75% of skeletal metastasis originates from cancers of ***prostate, breast, kidney & lung***.
- In children, metastases to bone originate from neuroblastoma, Wilms tumor, osteosarcoma, Ewingsarcoma, and rhabdomyosarcoma.
- ***Majority of bone secondaries are osteolytic***, but a few are osteoblastic
- Metastatic bone tumors are exceeded in frequency by only 2 other organs-lung & liver-*Harshmohan 8th/892*
- Vertebral bodies are affected most frequently
- Other common sites are: ribs, pelvis,humerus& femur
- Metastases to the small bones of the hands and feet are uncommon and usually originate from cancers ofthe lung, kidney, or colon.

63. Ans. b. Platelet, d. Leucocyte concentrate

[Ref: Harrison 20th/811; Davidson 23rd/ 930; Wintrobe's Clinical Hematology 12th/Chap 23]

"**Whole blood** is stored at ***4°C*** to maintain erythrocyte viability, but platelet dysfunction and degradation of some coagulation factors occur"- *Harrison 20th/811*

"**PRBC:** This product increases oxygen-carrying capacity in the anemic patient. PRBC are stored in additive solution up to ***35–42 days at 4°C***"-*Harrison 20th/811*

"**Platelets** are *stored in plasma or in additive solution up to* ***5–7 days at 20–24°C*** *and under permanent motion"-Harrison 20th/812*

Blood component	Temperature for storage	Shelf life
Albumin	Room temperature	3 years
Cryoprecipitate *Frozen *Thawed	 –30C 1 to 6C	 1 year 4 hours
FFP *Frozen *Thawed	 –30C 1 to 6C	 1 year 1 day
Platelets	20 to 24 C	5 day
Leukocyte concentrate	20 to 24 C	1 day
Packed RBC		42 days
Whole blood	1 to 6 C	35 days
Leucocyte reduced RBCs	1 to 6 C	1 day

Blood Storage

◈ *Wintrobe's Clinical Hematology 12th/Chap 23*

- **Red cells** collected in any of the anticoagulants and preservatives must be stored at 1 to 6°C to maintain optimum function
- **Platelet products** must be kept under specific conditions to ensure optimal recovery and function after transfusion. Unlike red cells, platelets stored at 4°C undergo shape changes and lose their viability; platelet survival and

function are optimized ***by storage at room temperature (20 to 24°C)***

- **FFP** is prepared by separating citrated plasma from whole blood and freezing it within 8 hours of collection or by freezing citrated apheresis plasma within 6 hours of collection. FFP may be stored at -18°C or below for up to 1 year.
- **Plasma, Cryoprecipitate-Reduced**: This is the supernatant remaining after removal of cryoprecipitate from FFP . Storage conditions are the same as for FFP.
- Although **granulocyte storage** is ***permitted for up to 24 hours at room temperature***, transfusion within 8 hours of collection is recommended. Effective storage may be possible for up to 48 hours at 10°C

Table: (Harrison 20th/811): Blood components

Component	Volume, Ml	Content	Clinical response
PRBC	250-300 (including additive solution)	RBCs with variable leukocyte content and small amount of plasma	Increase hemoglobin 10 g/L and hematocrit 3%
Platelets (from whole blood)	50-70/RD unit pool of 4 to 6 RD unit	5.5 X 10^{10} /RD Unit	Increase platelet count 5000-10000/µL/ RD unit
Platelets (from apheresis)	200-400	$\geq 2 \times 10^{11}$/SDAP product	For pooled RD and SDAP CCI $\geq 10 \times 10^9$/L within 1 h and,$\geq 7.5 \times 10^9$/L within 24 h Postinfusion
FFP	200-250	Plasma protein-coagulation factors, proteins C and S antithrombin	Increases coagulation factors about 2%
Cryoprecipitate (may be used as topical fibrin glue as well)	10-15 /unit, pool of 4 to 5 unit	Cold-insoluble plasma, proteins fibrinogen, factor, VIII factor XIII vWF fibronectin	Increased plasma fibrinogen 0.3-1 g/L increased factor VIII

64. Ans. d. More common in females

[Ref: Harrison 19th/1714; Robbins 9th/696; CMDT 2019/304-05; Harshmohan 8th/518-19]

"Characteristic biopsy findings show filling of the alveoli (and sometimes terminal bronchioles) with an ***amorphous eosinophilic material***, which stains strongly positive on PAS stain and the PAS diastase stain"- emedicine.medscape.com

Pulmonary Alveolar Proteinosis

◈ *Robbins 9th/696*

- Pulmonary alveolar proteinosis (PAP) is a rare disease caused by defects related to granulocyte-macrophage colony-stimulating factor (GM-CSF) or ***pulmonary macrophage dysfunction*** that results in the accumulation of surfactant in the intra-alveolar and bronchiolar spaces.
- PAP is characterized radiologically by bilateral patchy asymmetric pulmonary opacifications.
- There are three distinct classes of disease—autoimmune (formerly called acquired), secondary, and congenital—each with a similar spectrum of histologic changes.
- *Autoimmune PAP* is caused by circulating neutralizing ***antibodies specific for GM-CSF***. It occurs primarily in adults, represents 90% of all cases of PAP
- *Secondary PAP* is uncommon and is associated with diverse diseases
- *Hereditary PAP* is extremely rare, occurs in neonates and is caused by mutations that disrupt genes involved in GM-CSF signalling (GM-CSF and GM-CSF receptor gene mutations).
- Adult patients, for the most part, present with cough and abundant sputum that often contains chunks of gelatinous material.
- Progressive dyspnoea, cyanosis, and respiratory insufficiency may occur, but other patients follow a benign course, with eventual resolution of the lesions.
- ***Whole-lung lavage*** is the standard of care and provides benefit regardless of the underlying defect.
- GM-CSF therapy is safe and effective

Pulmonary Alveolar Proteinosis

◈ *Harrison 19th/1714*

- Cause interstitial lung disease- *Harrison 19th/1708*
- There are three distinct classes of PAP: acquired (>90% of all cases), congenital, and secondary.
- The typical age of ***presentation is 30–50 years***, and ***males predominate.***
- Polycythemia, hypergammaglobulinemia, and increased LDH levels are common.
- Markedly elevated serum levels of lung surfactant proteins A and D have been found in PAP.
- Radiographically, bilateral symmetric alveolar opacities located centrally in middle and lower lung zones result in a "bat-wing"distribution.
- HRCT shows a ground-glass opacification and thickened intralobular structures and interlobular septa.

65. Ans. a. Hemophilia A constitute 80-85%, d. Prolonged PTT with normal PT

[Ref: Harrison 20th/830-33;Robbins 9th/663; Davidson 22nd/1051-52]

◈ *Cryoprecipitate is used for treatment of Hemophilia A(Factor 8)*

Hemophilia B (Christmas Disease, Factor IX Deficiency)

◈ *Robbins 9th/663*

- Severe factor IX deficiency produces a disorder clinically indistinguishable from factor VIII deficiency (haemophilia A). Like hemophilia A, it is inherited as an ***X-linked recessive*** trait and shows variable clinical severity.
- In about 15% of these patients, factor IX protein is present but is nonfunctional. As with hemophilia A, the ***PTT is prolonged and the PT is normal.***
- Diagnosis of Christmas disease (named after the first patient identified with this condition, and not the holiday) is possible only by assay of the factor levels.
- The disease is treated with infusions of ***recombinant factor IX***
- ***FFP or plasma enriched with factor IX is used for treatment-*** *Harshmohan 8th/352*

Hemophilia

◈ *Harrison 20th/830-33*

- Hemophilia is an X-linked recessive hemorrhagic disease due to mutations in the *F8* gene (hemophilia A or classic hemophilia) or *F9* gene (hemophilia B).
- The disease affects 1 in 10,000 males worldwide, in all ethnic groups; ***hemophilia A represents 80% of all cases.***
- ***Male subjects are clinically affected***; women, who carry a single mutated gene, are generally asymptomatic.
- Family history of the disease is absent in ~30% of cases, and in these cases, 80% of the mothers are carriers of the de novo mutated allele..
- Clinically, hemophilia A and hemophilia B are indistinguishable.
- The disease phenotype correlates with the residual activity of FVIII or FIX and can be classified as ***severe (<1%), moderate (1–5%), or mild (6–30%).***
- In the severe and moderate forms, the disease is characterizedby bleeding into the joints (hemarthrosis), soft tissues, and muscles after minor trauma or even spontaneously. Patients with mild disease experience infrequent bleeding that is usually secondary to trauma.
- ***Patients with hemophilia have normal bleeding times and platelet counts.*** The diagnosis is made after specific determination of FVIII or FIX clotting activity
- **Cryoprecipitate is enriched with FVIII protein** (each bag contains ~80 IU of FVIII) is commonly used for the treatment of haemophilia A
- *DDAVP (1-Amino-8-d-Arginine Vasopressin)* DDAVP is a synthetic vasopressin analog that causes a transient rise in FVIII and von Willebrand factor (VWF), but not FIX
- Gene therapy trials for hemophilia A and B using adenoassociated viral vectors are ongoing

66. Ans. a. Bronchiectasis, b. Pulmonary TB. c. Chronic osteomyelitis

[Ref: Harrison 20th/804-07;Robbins 9th/258-60;Harshmohan 8th/154]

Amyloidosis

◈ *Robbins 9th/258*

- On clinical grounds, the systemic, or generalized, pattern is sub-classified into ***primary amyloidosis,*** when it is associated with some plasma cell disorder, or ***secondary amyloidosis,*** when it occurs as a complication of an underlying chronic inflammatory or tissue-destructive process.
- ***Hereditary* or *familial amyloidosis*** constitutes a separate, albeit heterogeneous group, with several distinctive patterns of organ involvement.

Reactive Systemic Amyloidosis

◈ *Robbins 9th/258-59*

- The amyloid deposits in this pattern are systemic in distribution and are composed of AA protein. This category was previously referred to as *secondary amyloidosis* because it is secondary to an associated inflammatory condition.
- At one time, ***tuberculosis, bronchiectasis, and chronic osteomyelitis*** were the most important underlying conditions, but with the advent of effective antimicrobial chemotherapy the importance of these conditions has diminished.
- More commonly now, ***reactive systemic amyloidosis complicates rheumatoid arthritis, other connective tissue disorders such as ankylosing spondylitis, and inflammatory bowel disease, particularly Crohn disease and ulcerative colitis.*** Among these the most frequent associated condition is rheumatoid arthritis.
- The chronic skin infections associated with "skin-popping" of narcotics seem to be responsible for the amyloidosis.
- Reactive systemic amyloidosis may also occur in association with solid tumors, the most common being ***renal cell carcinoma and Hodgkin lymphoma.***

AA AMYLOIDOSIS

◈ *Harrison 20th/807*

- AA amyloidosis can occur in association with almost any chronic inflammatory state (e.g., ***rheumatoid arthritis, inflammatory bowel disease, familial Mediterranean fever***or other periodic fever syndromes) or chronic infections such as ***tuberculosis or subacute bacterial endocarditis.***
- It has also been described in association with Castleman's disease, lymphomas, renal cell carcinoma, emphasizing the diagnostic importance of CT scanning to look for such tumors as well as serologic and microbiologic studies.

Table: (Harrison 20th/804): Amyloid Precursor Proteins and Their Clinical Syndromes

Designation	Precursor	Clinical syndrome	Clinical involvement
Systemic Amyloidosis			
AL	Immunoglobulin light chain	Primary or myeloma-associated	Any
AH	Immunoglobulin heavy chain	Rare variant of primary or myeloma-associated	Any

Contd...

Designation	Precursor	Clinical syndrome	Clinical involvement
AA	Serum amyloid A protein	Secondary reactive	Renal, heart, other
Aβ	β Microglobulin	Hemodialysis-associated	Synovial tissue, bone
ATTR		Familial (mutant)	Cardiac, peripheral and autonomic nerves
		Age-related (wild type)	
AApoAI	Apolipoprotein AI	Familial	Hepatic
AApoAII	Apolipoprotein AII	Familial	Renal
AGel	Gelsolin	Familial	Cornea, cranial nerves, skin, renal
AFib	Fibrinogen Aα	Familial	Renal
Alys	Lysozyme	Familial	Renal, hepatic
ALECT2	Leukocyte chemotactic factor 2	Undefined	Renal
Localized Amytoidoses			
Aβ	Amyloid β protein	Alzhemier's disease: Down's syndrome	Central nervous system
ACys	Cystatin C	Cerebral amyloid Angiopathy	Central nervous system vascular
APrP	Prion protein	Spongiform Encephalopathies	Central nervous system
AIAPP	Islet amyloid polypeptide (amylin)	Diabetes-associated	Pancreas
ACal	Calcitonin	Medullary carcinoma of the thyroid	Thyroid
AANF	Atrial natriuretic factor	Atrial fibrillation	Cardiac atria
Apro	Prolactin	Endocrinopathy	Pituitary
ASgi	Semenogelin I	Age-related; incidental autopsy or biopsy finding	Seminal vesicles

67. Ans. a. Sideroblastic anemia, b. Lead poisoning, d. Atransferrinemia, e. Thalassemia

[Ref: Harrison 20th/687;Robbins 9th/652; Harshmohan 8th/313-15]

Microcytic hypochromic: *MCV,MCH,MCHC are all reduced e.g in iron deficiency anaemia & in certain non-iron deficient anaemias(sideroblastic anaemia, thalassaemia, anaemia of chronic disorders)- Harshmohan 8th/309*

"**Atransferrinemia** *causes* ***hypochromic, microcytic anaemia***"*-rarediseases.org*

"**Normocytic,normochrmic**: *after* ***acute blood loss****, haemolytic anaemia, bone marrow failure"- Harshmohan 8th/309*

Sideroblastic anaemia: ***Hypochromic anaemia which may be microcytic*** *or there may be some normocytic red cell as well(dimorphic)- Harshmohan 8th/315; Harshmohan 8th/313*

Lead poisoning: *Hemolytic anaemia from direct toxic effect;* ***basophilic stippling*** *of red blood cells- Harshmohan 8th/328*

"**Microcytic, hypochromic anemia** can be caused by ***lead toxicity***, chronic disease, thalassemia and hemoglobin E disorder"-*medicalnewstoday.com*

Table: *(Harrison 20th/687):* **Diagnosis of Microcytic Anemia**

Tests	Iron deficiency	Inflammation	Thalassemia	Sideroblastic anemia
Smear	Micro/hypo	Normal micro/hypo	Micro/hypo with targeting	Variable
Serum iron (μg/dL)	<30	<50	Normal to high	Normal to high
TIBC (μg/dL)	>360	<300	Normal	Normal
Percent saturation	<10	10-20	30-80	30-80
Ferritin (μg/dL)	<15	30-200	50-300	50-300
Hemoglobin pattern on electrophoresis	Normal	Normal	Abnormal with β thalassemia; can be normal with α thalassemia	Normal

68. Ans. b. Secretary, c. Microcystic d. Transitional

[Ref: www.aans.org; Harrison 20th/648; Robbins 9th/1315]

Types and Classification of Meningioma

◈ *www.aans.org*

- WHO classification of brain tumors is the most widely utilized tool in grading tumor types.
- The WHO classification scheme recognizes 15 variations of meningiomas according to their cell type as seen under a microscope.
- These variations are called **meningioma subtypes**; the technical term for these cell variations is histological subtypes.

Table: *(www.aans.org)*: **Classification of Meningioma**

WHO Grade I-Benign	WHO Grade II – Atypical	WHO Grade III-Malignant
• Meningothelial	• Chordoid	• Papillary
• Fibrous (fibroblastic)	• Clear Cell	• Rhabdoid
• Transitional (mixed)	• Atypical	• Anaplastic
• Psammomatous		
• Anglomatous		
• Microcystic		
• Secretory		
• Lymphoplasmacyte-rich		
• Metaplastic		

Meningiomas

◈ *Robbins 9th/1315*

- Most meningiomas have a relatively low risk of recurrence or aggressive growth, and so are considered **WHO grade I/IV**
- These include
  - **Syncytial** ("meningothelial"), appropriately named for the whorled clusters of cells that sit in tight
  - Groups without visible cell membranes;
  - **Fbroblastic**, with elongated cells and abundant collagen deposition between them;
  - **Transitional**, which share features of the syncytial and fbroblastic types;
  - **Psammomatous**, with psammoma bodies, apparently formed from calcifcation of the syncytial nests of meningothelial cells
  - **Secretory**, with PAS-positive intracytoplasmic droplets and intracellular lumens by electron microscopy;
  - **Microcystic**, with a loose, spongy appearance.
- **Atypical meningiomas (WHO grade II/IV)** are lesions with a higher rate of recurrence and more aggressive local growth, and may require radiation therapy in addition to surgery. It includes: **clear cell** and **chordoid**
- **Anaplastic (malignant) meningioma** (**WHO grade III/IV**) is a highly aggressive tumor. It includes: **Papillary** meningioma (with pleomorphic cells arranged around fbrovascular cores) and **rhabdoid** meningioma

69. Ans. a. Retinoblastoma, c. Rhabdomyosarcoma, d. Ewing sarcoma, e. Carcinoid tumour

[Ref: radiopaedia.org; Nelson (SAE) 20th/ 2458; Danhert Radiology 7th/327;Harshmohan 7th/483-84,839-40;emedicine.medscape.com]

Ewing's sarcoma is closely related to PNET, but not PNET *(Robbins and Schwartz)*

"Embryonal tumors or **primitive neuroectodermaltumors (PNET)** are the most common group of malignant CNS tumors of childhood, accounting for 20–25% of pediatric CNS tumors. These tumors have the potential to metastasize to the neuraxis. This group includes ***medulloblastoma, supratentorial PNET, ependymoblastoma, medulloepithelioblastoma, and atypical teratoid/rhabdoid tumor (ATRT),*** all of which are histologically classified as WHO grade IV tumors"- *Nelson (SAE) 20th/ 2458*

Ewing Sarcoma Family Tumors: **Ewing sarcoma** is a malignant bone tumor characterized by primitive round cells without obvious differentiation. Recently, Ewing sarcoma and **primitive neuroectodermaltumor**(PNET) have been unified into a single category: **Ewing sarcoma family tumors**(ESFT) based on shared clinical, morphologic, biochemical and molecular features. Although PNET demonstrates more neuroectodermal differentiation than Ewing sarcoma, the distinction is not clinically significant"- *Robbins 9th/1203*

"PNETs (***neuroblastomas, ganglioneuroblastomas, and ganglioneuromas***) derive from primordial neural crest cells that migrate from the mantle layer of the developing spinal cord. ***Ewing's sarcoma and Askin's tumour are closely related to PNET***. Histologically, PNETs and Ewing's sarcomas are small, round cell tumors."-Schwartz 9th/565

"**Medulloblastoma** (an infratentorial PNET)"- *L and B 26th/616*

70. Ans. b. Shield chest

[Ref: Harrison 20th/ 1832; CPDT 17TH/1075;Davidson 23rd/;Robbins 9th/ 532]

- Shield chest occur in Turner's syndrome

"**Turner's syndrome:** A broad chest with widely spaced nipples may occur, which is sometimes referred to as "***shield chest***"- rarediseases.org

"**Noonan syndrome**- pulmonary valve stenosis, VSD, ***hypertrophic cardiomyopathy***. Associated genes are:***PTPN1***1, KRAS & SOS1"-*Robbins 9th/ 532*

"Patients with **Noonan syndrome** commonly have a dysplastic pulmonary valve and have facial and lymphatic abnormalities. Several defects in specific genes have been associated with Noonan syndrome, most notably ***PTPN11"***- *Harrison 20th/ 1832*

Noonan Syndrome

◈ *CPDT 17TH/1075*

- Noonan syndrome is an autosomal dominant disorder characterized by ***short stature, congenital heart disease, abnormalities of cardiac conduction and rhythm, webbed neck, down-slanting palpebral fissures, and low-set ears.***
- Affected children may be large at birth and have mild subcutaneous edema. The phenotype evolves with age and may be difficult to recognize in older relatives.
- Mild developmental delays are often present.

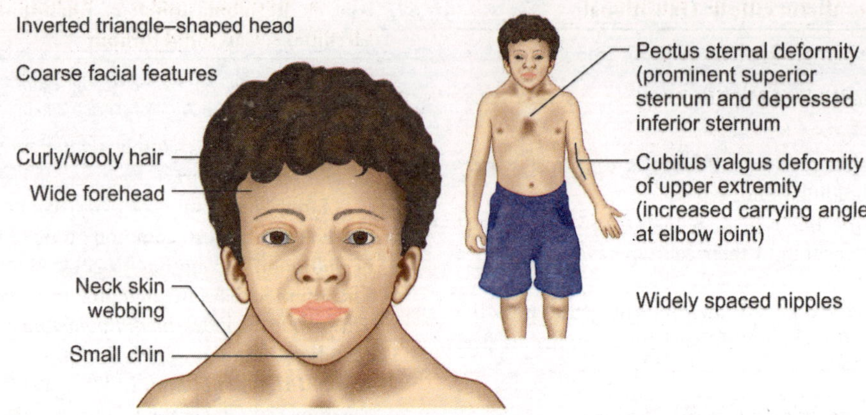

Fig. *(www.aafp.org):* Child/adolescent with Noonan syndrome

71. Ans. a. P53 is an important oncogene

[Ref: Robbins 9th/283-90, 8th/ 279-80;Sabiston 18th/36; Harriosn 19th/101-e2; Devita 7th/90; Manual of Onacology by Casciato 5th/22, 25]

- *P53 is a tumor suppressor gene*
- *Oncoproteins are specific proteins encoded by oncogenes*
- *Proto-oncogenes are required for normal growth & proliferation*
- *RAS is best example of proto-oncogenes activated by point mutation*

"**Point mutations of *RAS* family genes constitute the most common type of abnormality involving proto-oncogenes in human tumors.** Approximately 15% to 20% of all human tumors express mutated RAS proteins, but in some types of cancers the frequency of **RAS mutations** is much higher."- *Robbins 9th (SAE)/286*

"The genes encoding cell cycle regulatory proteins are often targets of mutation during neoplastic transformation. If the mutated gene is cancer causing, it is referred to as an ***oncogene and its normal counterpart is called a proto-oncogene.*** Many *proto-oncogenes* have been identified and they are typically involved in relay of stimulatory signals from growth factor receptors to the nucleus. They include the intracellular signalling protein RAS, as well as the cell cycle regulatory protein cyclin D1. ***Mutation of a single copy of a proto-oncogene is sufficient to bring about increased cellular proliferation, one of the hallmarks of cancer***"- *Sabiston 18th/36*

Protooncogenes, Oncogenes, and Oncoproteins

◈ *Robbins 9th/283-90, 8th/ 279-80.*

- Because they were discovered initially as viral genes, these protooncogenes were named after their viral homologues.
- One consequence of proviral insertion near a protooncogene is to induce a structural change in the cellular gene, thus converting it into a cellular oncogene (*c-onc, or onc*). This mode of protooncogene activation is called *insertional mutagenesis.* Alternatively, strong retroviral promoters inserted in the vicinity of the protooncogenes lead to dysregulated expression of the cellular gene.
- A large number of protooncogenes have been identified during the past 20 years, most of which do not have a viral counterpart.
- Protooncogenes have multiple roles, ***participating in cellular functions related to growth and proliferation.***
- ***Proteins encoded by protooncogenes may function as growth factor*** ligands and receptors, signal transducers, transcription factors, and cell-cycle components.
- Oncoproteins encoded by oncogenes generally serve similar functions as their normal counterparts. However, because they are constitutively expressed, oncoproteins endow the cell with self-sufficiency in growth.
- *This is the **most common form of oncogene in human tumors**, the abnormality being induced by point mutation in RAS gene- Harshmohan 7th/203-04*

72. Ans. b. Sudan III-fat, d. PAS-glycogen, e. Gomori stain-fungus

[Ref: bitesizebio.com bitesizebio.com; www.ivyroses.com]

Option a-e

- ***Gomori Methenamine Silver (GMS) is used to stain fungi***
- **Oil red O, *Sudan black and Sudan* III *& IV are used to stain lipids.***
  - PAS stain is used for glycogen and fungi
  - ***Collagen** is **stained with Picrosirius Red (polarised)***
  - Calcium is stained with Von kossa

Important Stains and Structures they Stain

- Acid Fast Stain - Mycobacterial organisms and other Acid Fast Orgaisms
- **Acridine orange - Acid mucin, nucleic acid**
- Alician Blue - Mucins and Muco-substances
- Cajal Stain - Nervous Tissue
- Congo Red -Amyloid
- **Fontana Masson's - Melanin and Argentaffin Cells**
- **Gomori Methenamine Silver (GMS) - Fungi**
- Masson's Trichrome - Connective tissue, Collagen

- Mucicarmine - Epithelial Mucin
- Oil-Red-O (On Frozen Section) -Lipid
- Orcien Stain - Elastin fibers
- Osmium Tetroxide - Lipids
- **Periodic Acid-Schiff (PAS) - Glycogen. Fungi**
- **Pho**photungstic Acid-Haematoxylin Fibrin, Cross Striations of skeletal Muscle Fibres
- Picro irius Red (polarised) - Collagen

Table: *(www.ivyroses.com):* **Histology stain**

Masson trichrome	• Trichrome histology stains are formed from a mixture of three dyes • Can be used to distinguish between cellular items and extracellular items • Can be used on connective tissue
Von kossa stain	• Used to indicate calcium and calcium deposits
Periodic Acid Schiff (PAS)	• A Mucin stain (listed above) • Used for staining glycogen and other carbohydrates • Used to show glomeruli, basement membranes, and glycogen in the liver
Perl's Iron stain	• Can be used to reveal the presence of iron in biological tissues.
Gomori trichrome	• Trichrome histology stains are formed from a mixture of three dyes • Gomoril's trichrome stains connective tissue and collagen (green or blue), muscle, keratin and cytoplasm (red) and nuclei (grey/blue/black)
Orcien stain	• Can be used to stain for elastin fibres

73. Ans. b. Urine urobilinogen, c. MCHC, e. LDH

[Ref: Robbins (SAE) 9th/633-34; Harrison 19th/649; Davidson 23rd/947-48]

In HS: ***MCV is usually normal or slightly decreased***-*Harshmohan 7th/292*

Hereditary Spherocytosis (HS)

◈ *Harrison 19th/651-52*

- The presence of *osmotic fragility* is the main diagnostic test for HS.
- The main clinical findings are jaundice, ***an enlarged spleen*** and often gallstones; indeed, it may be the finding of gallstones in a young person that triggers diagnostic investigations.
- An **increased mean corpuscular haemoglobin concentration (MCHC)** on an ordinary blood count report should raise the suspicion of HS, because HS is almost the only condition in which this abnormality occurs.

Hereditary Spherocytosis

◈ *Robbins (SAE) 9th/633-34*

- **It is caused by intrinsic defects in the red cell membrane skeleton**
- The characteristic clinical features are *anemia, splenomegaly and jaundice.* The generally stable clinical course is sometimes punctuated by *aplastic crises,* usually triggered by an acute parvovirus infection.
- Gallstones, found in many patients, can also produce symptoms.
- Splenectomy treats the anemia and its complications, but brings with it an increased risk of sepsis, since the spleen acts as an important filter for blood borne bacteria

Features Common to Most Patients with a Hemolytic Disorder (Including HS)

◈ *Harrison 19th/649*

General examination	Jaundice, pallor
Other physical findings	Spleen may be enlarged; bossing of skull in severe congenital cases
Hemoglobin level	From normal to severely reduced
MCV, MCH	Usually increased
Reticulocytes	Increased
Bilirubin	Increased (mostly unconjugated) ***Urine urobilinogen increased***
LDH	Increased (up to 10 time normal with intravascular hemolysis)
Haptoglobin	Reduced to absent

74. Ans. d. Viral fever, e. Lymphoma

[Ref: academic.oup.com;www.ncbi.nlm.nih.gov]

- Viral fever & neoplastic fever are due to cytokine induced rise in temperature.

Fever/hyperpyrexia (cytokine induced)	Hyperthermia (externally induced)
• Infections (bacterial, ***viral***, and parasitic) • Intracranial hemorrhage (me cause of hyperpyrexia) • Sepsis • Kawasaki syndrome • Druginduced (Malignant hyperpyrexia) • ***Tumors***	• ***Heat stroke*** • Malignant hyperthermia • ***Neuroleptic syndrome*** • ***Thyroid storm*** • Propofol infusion syndrome • Stimulants such as substituted amphetamines and cocaine, • Idiosyncratic drug reactions

"**Hyperthyroidism** *is associated with hyperthermia; patients with* **thyroid storm** *have an average body temperature of 38.0 °C; temperatures above 41 °C have been reported. The mechanism of thermogenesis is not clear; the classical view is that metabolism of peripheral tissues increases through a peripherally mediated pathway. Recent work suggests that thyroid hormones may instead act centrally to increase the hypothalamic 'set-point', and that centrally driven neurogenic activation of uncoupling protein-1 acting on brown adipose tissue may instead be responsible for the thermogenesis"www.ncbi.nlm.nih.gov*

"Fever in patients with malignancy *is reported to be sepsis related in around two thirds of cases. The tumour is the direct cause of fever in less than 10 % of febrile episodes;* ***tumour necrosis and production of pyrogenic cytokines is the likely pathogenesis."***-ncbi.nlm.nih.gov

75. Ans. a. Small cell carcinoma lung, b. Squamous cell carcinoma lung, c. Lymphoma

[Ref: Harrison 20th/511; Schwartz 8th/562; Robbins 9th/515;CMDT 2019/502]

Superior Vena Cava Syndrome

◈ *Harrison 20th/511; CMDT 2019/502*

- Superior vena cava syndrome (SVCS) is the clinical manifestation of superior vena cava (SVC) obstruction, with severe reduction in venous return from the head, neck, and upper extremities.
- Malignant tumors, such as ***lung cancer, lymphoma**, and metastatic tumors,* are responsible for the majority of SVCS cases.
- ***Lung cancer, particularly of small cell and squamous cell** histologies,* accounts for approximately 85% of all cases of malignant origin.
- In young adults, ***malignant lymphoma*** is a leading cause of SVCS. *Hodgkin's lymphoma involves the mediastinum more commonly than other lymphomas but rarely causes SVCS.*
- When SVCS is noted in a young man with a mediastinal mass, the differential diagnosis is lymphoma vs primary mediastinal germ cell tumor.
- Metastatic cancers to the mediastinum, such as *testicular and breast carcinomas,* account for a small proportion of cases. Other causes include benign tumors, aortic aneurysm, thyromegaly, thrombosis, and fibrosing mediastinitis from prior irradiation or histoplasmosis.
- Characteristic physical findings are dilated neck veins, increased number of collateral veins covering the anterior chest wall, cyanosis, edema of forearms & chest
- *Most significant chest radiographic finding is widening of superior mediastinal (MC on right side)*
- Most reliable diagnostic test is CT scan
- Life threatening complication of superior mediastinal mass is tracheal obstruction

Underlying cause of SVC syndrome	Treatment
Non-small cell lung cancer & other metastatic tumors	Radiation
Small cell lung cancer or lymphoma	Chemotherapy
All other cases	Surgery

76. Ans. a. ↑ Parathyroid hormone, b. Increase in the giant multinucleated osteoclasts, c. Generalized bone resorption

[Ref: Harrison 20th/2927; Davidson 23rd/418-19; Robbins 9th/1102, 1192]

Osteitis Fibrosa Cystica

◈ *Harrison 20th/2927; www.hindawi.com*

- The distinctive bone manifestation of ***hyperparathyroidism*** is *osteitis fibrosa cystica*, which occurred in 10–25% of patients in series reported 50 years ago.
- Histologically, the pathognomonic features are ***an increase in the giant multinucleated osteoclasts*** in scalloped areas on the surface of the bone (Howship's lacunae) and a replacement of the normal cellular and marrow elements by fibrous tissue.
- X-ray changes include resorption of the phalangeal tufts and replacement of the usually sharp cortical outline of the bone in the digits by an irregular outline (subperiosteal resorption).
- In recent years, osteitis fibrosa cystica is very rare in primary HPT, probably due to the earlier detection of the disease
- Caused by a ***surplus of parathyroid hormone (PTH)*** from overactive parathyroid gland
- The symptoms of the disease are the consequences of both the general softening of the bones and the ***excess calcium in the blood*** and include bone fractures, kidney stones, nausea, peptic ulcers, appetite loss, and weight loss-"bones, stones, abdominal groans and psychic overtones
- Women are more often affected than men, and it occurs more frequently in the 5th and 6th decades.
- The ***serum calcium*** (8.4–10.2 mg/dL), ***PTH*** (15–65 pg/mL), and ***alkaline phosphatase*** (20–140 IU/L) are ***usually elevated.***
- Plain radiographs distinctly ***show resorption***, and the skull depicts the "***ground glass"/"salt and pepper" appearance.***

PHARMACOLOGY

77. Ans. a. Gastric lavage is done to prevent absorption, b. Activated charcoal is used in lavage, c. N- acetyl cysteine is antidote, e. Death may occur

[Ref: K. D. T 8th/223-24; Nelson (SAE) 20th/456-57, 453; Katzung 13th/1006-07]

- ***Even after 24 hours, N-Acetylcysteine has some role*** in paracetamol poisoning

*"In **chronic alcoholic even 5 g taken** in one day can result in hepatotoxicity"- K. D. T 8th/224*

"If patient is brought early, vomiting should be induced or gastric lavage done. ***Activated charcoal** is given orally or through the tube to prevent further absorption"- K. D. T 8th/224*

Acetaminophen

◈ *Nelson(SAE) 20th/456-57*

- Acetaminophen intoxication is a common cause of acute liver failure in adolescents and adults.
- Acetaminophen toxicity results from the formation of a highly reactive intermediate metabolite, ***N-acetyl-p-benzoquinoneimine (NAPQI).***
- When hepatic stores of glutathione are depleted to <70% of normal, the NAPQI metabolite can combine with hepatic macromolecules to produce hepatocellular damage.
- The acute toxic dose of acetaminophen is generally considered to be ***>200 mg/kg in children younger than 12 yr of age***; a single ingestion of >7.5 g is considered a minimum toxic dose in adolescents and adults.
- ***Adolescents have a higher incidence of toxic plasma concentrations after ingestion than do children***, and their

exposures are often associated with intentional overdose. If untreated, patients with an acute overdose may pass through the 4 stages of acetaminophen toxicity

- The antidote for acetaminophen poisoning is NAC
- ***NAC therapy is most effective when initiated early in the course of intoxication (within 8 hr), but may have value even if started 24–36 hr after the ingestion in severe cases.***

Paracetamol: Adverse Effects

◈ *Katzung 13th/1006-07*

- In therapeutic doses, a mild ***increase in hepatic enzymes*** may occasionally occur in the absence of jaundice; this is reversible when the drug is withdrawn. With larger doses, dizziness, excitement, and disorientation can be seen.
- ***Ingestion of 15 g of acetaminophen may be fatal***, death being caused by ***severe hepatotoxicity with centrilobular necrosis, sometimes associated with acute renal tubular necrosis***.
- Doses greater than 4–6 g/d are not recommended and a ***history of alcoholism contraindicates*** even this dose.
- Early symptoms of hepatic damage include nausea, vomiting, diarrhea, and abdominal pain.
- ***Cases of renal damage without hepatic damage have occurred***, even after usual doses of acetaminophen.
- Hemolyticanemia and methemoglobinemia are very rare adverse events. ***Interstitial nephritis and papillary necrosis***-serious complications of phenacetin—have not occurred nor has gastrointestinal bleeding.

78. Ans. a. Deranged hepatic function, b. N-acetyl cysteine is antidote, d. Abnormal renal function

[Ref: K. D. T 8th/223-24; Nelson (SAE) 20th/456-57, 453; Katzung 13th/1006-07]

Refer to explanation of above Q

Table: *(Nelson (SAE) 20th /456)*: **Classic stage in the clinical course of acetaminophen toxicity**

Stage	Time after ingestion	Characteristics
I	0.5-24 hr	Anorexia, vomiting, malaise, Labs typically normal except for acetaminophen level
Ii	24-48 hr	Resolution of earlier symptoms, right upper quadrant abdominal pain and tenderness, elevated ***hepatic transaminases*** (aspartate aminotransferase> alanine aminotransferase) Elevated INR
Iii	3-5 days	Peak transaminase elevations; *development of **liver failure***, multi organ-system failure, death or recovery begins.
Iv	4 days – 2 wk	Resolution of liver function abnormalities, Clinical recovery precedes histologic recovery

79. Ans. d. Enhances polymerization of mitotic spindle

[Ref: K. D. T 8th/924; Katzung 13th/931-32;Satoskar Pharma 25th/834]

Paclitaxel *(a taxane) enhances tubulin polymerization, a mechanism opposite to that of vinca alkaloid- K. D. T 8th/925*

Vincaalkaloids (Vinblastine, vincristine, vindesine, vinorelbine) are cell-specific agents (act on M phase)-*Katzung 13th/921*

Vinblastine

◈ *Katzung 13th/931-32*

- Vinblastine is an alkaloid derived from the periwinkle plant Vincarosea.
- Its mechanism of action involves ***inhibition of tubulin polymerization***, which ***disrupts assembly of microtubules***, an important part of the cytoskeleton and the mitoticspindle.
- This inhibitory effect results in ***mitotic arrest in metaphase***, bringing cell division to a halt, which then leads to cell death.
- Vinblastine and other vinca alkaloids are metabolized by the liver P450 system, and the majority of the drug is excreted in feces via the biliary system. As such, dose modification is required in the setting of liver dysfunction.
- The main adverse effects include nausea and vomiting, bone marrow suppression, and alopecia. This agent is also a potent vesicant, and care must be taken in its administration.
- It has clinical activity in the treatment of Hodgkin's and non-Hodgkin's lymphomas, breast cancer, and germ cell cancer.

Vincristine

◈ *Katzung 13th/932*

- Vincristine is an alkaloid derivative of Vincarosea and is closely related in structure to vinblastine. Its mechanism of action, mechanism of resistance, and clinical pharmacology are identical to those of vinblastine.
- Despite these similarities to vinblastine, vincristine has a strikingly different spectrum of clinical activity and safety profile

80. Ans. b. Vinorelbine, d. Azathioprine, e. Cisplatin

[Ref: K. D. T 8th/916; Katzung 13th/928]

Table: *(Katzung 13th/921)*: **Cell cycle effects of major classes of anticancer drugs**

Cell cycle- specific agents	Cell cycle–nonspecific agents
Antimetabolites (S phase)	**Alkylating agents**
Capecitabine	Altretamine
Cladribine	Bendamustine
Clofarabine	Busulfan
Cytarabine (ara-C)	*Carmustine*
Fludarabine	Chlorambucil
5-Fluorouracil (5-FU)	*Cyclophosphamide*
Gemcitabine	Dacarbazine
6-Mercaptopurine (6-MP)	Procarbazine
Methotrexate (MTX)	Lomustine
6-Thioguanine (6-TG)	Mechlorethamine
Azathioprine	Melphalan
	Temozolomide
	Thiotepa

Contd...

Cell cycle- specific agents	Cell cycle–nonspecific agents
Epipodophylloxtoxin (toposiomerase II inlibitor) (G1 – S phase) Etoposide	**Platinum analogs** Carboplatin Cisplatin Oxaliplatin
Taxanes (M phase) Albumin-bound paclitaxel Docetaxel Paclitaxel	**Anthracyclines** Daunorubicin Doxorubicin Epirubicin Idarubicin Mitoxantrone
Vinca alkaloids (M phase) Vinblastine vincristine Vinorelbine	**Antitumor antibiotics** Dactinomycin Mitomycin
Antimicrotubule inhibitor (M phase) Ixabepilone	**Camptothecins (topoisomerase I inhibitors)** Irinotecan Topotecan
Antitumor antibiotics (G2 – M phase) Bleomycin	

81. Ans. d. Effective against pseudomonas, e. May cause methemoglobinemia

[Ref: K. D. T 8th/961; Katzung 13th/871; Satoskar Pharma 25th/851; Sabiston 19th/530-34]

- Metabolic acidosis is caused by mafenide acetate cream(***not silver nitrate***)
- Applies 2-3 times/week

"**Silver nitrate Topical solution:** Apply a cotton applicator dipped in solution/ointment on the affected area ***2-3 times per week for 2-3 weeks***"- reference.medscape.com

"**Silver nitrate:** It has now been reinstated as a 0.5% solution, which is non-toxic, does not injure regenerating epithelium in the wound and is ***bacteriostatic against S. aureus, E. coli, and P. aeruginosa***. *Klebsiellaspp., Providencia spp., and other Enterobacteriaceae are not as susceptible* to $AgNO_3$ 0.5% solution as other bacteria. Because it is hypotonic in nature it can cause osmolar dilution, resulting in hyponatremia and hypochloremia"- www.sciencedirect.com

Silver Nitrate

◈ *Sabiston 19th/534*

- Silver nitrate has the advantage of being painless on application and having complete antimicrobial effectiveness.
- Its disadvantages include ***staining of surfaces to a dull gray or black*** when the solution dries. This can become problematic in deciphering wound depth during excision of burns and in keeping the patient and surroundings clean of the black staining.
- The solution is hypotonic as well, and continuous use can cause electrolyte leaching, with rare ***methemoglobinemia*** as another complication.

"**0.5% Silver nitrate**: Effective against all microorganisms; ***stains contacted areas***; leaches sodium from wounds; may cause ***methemoglobinemia***"-Sabiston 19th/533

Mafenide acetate is another topical agent with a broad spectrum of activity because of its sulfa moiety. It is particularly useful against resistant *Pseudomonas* and *Enterococcus* species. It can also penetrate eschar, which silver sulfadiazine cannot. Disadvantages include painful application on skin, such as in second-degree wounds. It can also cause an allergic rash, and it has carbonic anhydrase inhibitory characteristics that can result in ***metabolic acidosis*** when applied over large surfaces."-Sabiston 19th/533

82. Ans. a. Nitrofurantoin, c. Tetracycline

[Ref: Harrison 20th/1156;K. D. T 8th/773,761; Jawetz 27th/379; Ananthanarayan 10th/289]

P.mirabilis *is sensitive to* ***ampicillin & cephalosporins****-Ananthanarayan 10th/289*

Resistance of *P. mirabilis*

◈ *Harrison 20th/1156*

- The **intrinsic resistance** of *P. mirabilis* to ***tetracyclines,*** cefazolin, ***nitrofurantoin,*** polymyxins, and tigecycline renders treatment of XDR isolates problematic.
- Acquired resistance to ampicillin (prevalence range, 15–60%), ***fluoroquinolones*** (11–55%), and TMP-SMX (20–50%) is common.
- **Ampicillin-sulbactam** tends to be more active, with resistance prevalences of 6–18%.
- In the United States and Canada, the prevalence of ESBL production by *P. mirabilis* remains low (generally <5%). However, rates as high as 60% have been reported from Asia. Isolates of *P. mirabilis* that produce CTX-M
- ESBLs have been recovered from ambulatory patients with no recent health-care contact (see the section on the treatment of extraintestinal *E. coli* infections for treatment considerations). *P. vulgaris* and *P. penneri* exhibit more extensive drug resistance than does *P. mirabilis*, and induction or selection of *P. vulgaris* variants with stable derepression of chromosomal AmpC®-lactamase may occur.
- For critically ill patients, carbapenems, fourth-generation cephalosporins (e.g., cefepime), ceftazidime-avibactam, ceftolozane-tazobactam, and amikacin generally display **excellent activity** against *Proteus* species (90–100% of isolates susceptible).

P. mirabilis

◈ *Jawetz 27th/379*

- **Drug of first choice-*Ampicillin***
- **Alternative drugs:**An aminoglycoside, TMP-SMZ, a fluoroquinolone(Ciprofloxacin has the best activity against *P aeruginosa)* a cephalosporin,imipenem, meropenem, ertapenem, ticarcillin-clavulanate, piperacillin-tazobactam, chloramphenicol

83. Ans. a. Terbinafine

[Ref: K. D. T 8th/847; Harrison 20th/1546; Satoskar Pharma 25th/713; Ananthanarayan 10th/600]

- According to FDA, drug risk category , Terbinafine is safest drug(Category B). All other options in Q are category C drugs (less safer)

Table: *(academic.oup.com):* **Antifungal drugs and risk category in pregnancy**

Drug	Designation
Ketoconazole	C
Fluconazole	C (low dose); D (high dose)
Itraconazole	C
Terbinafine	B
Griseofulvin	C

Table: Classification of prescription drugs by the US FDA according to the risk in pregnancy (academic.oup.com)

Pregnancy risk category	Description
A	Controlled studies of women failed to demonstrate a risk to the fetus in the first trimester, and the possibility of fetal harm appears remote
B	Either animal studies do not indicate a risk to the fetus and there have been no controlled studies in pregnant women, or animal studies have indicated fetal risk but controlled studies of pregnant women failed to demonstrate a risk
C	Either animal studies indicate a fetal risk and there have been no controlled studies of women, or there are no available reports of studies of women or animals
D	There is positive evidence of fetal risk, but there may be certain situations where the benefit may outweigh the risk (e.G. Life-threatening or serious diseases for which other drugs are ineffective or carry a greater risk)
X	There is definite fetal risk, according to studies of animals or humans or on the basis of human experience, and the risk clearly outweighs any benefit in pregnant women.

Terbinafine: Used for tinea capitis- *K. D. T 8th/847;Satoskar Pharma 25th/717*

All azoles(e.g ketoconazole, itraconazole) are potentially embryotoxic& teratogenic & should be avoided during pregnancy & lactation- *Satoskar Pharma 25th/715*

Fluconazole is not recommended in pregnant & lactating women- *K. D. T 8th/845*

Dermatophytosis*(commonly called* ***tinea*** *or ringworm) refer to infection caused by a group of keratinophilic fungi called the dermatophytes-Ananthanarayan 10th/600*

Griseofulvin is used orally only for dermatophytosis- *K. D. T 8th/842*

Griseofulvin has made clinical control of some chronic resistant ringworm infection possible-*Satoskar Pharma 25th/713*

Orally administered ketoconazole is effective in dermatophytosis- *K. D. T 8th/844*

Table: *(Harrison 20th/1546):* **Antifungal drugs used for Extensive Tinea Infection**

Terbinafine	Adverse reactions minimal with short treatment period
Itraconazole	Adverse reactions minimal with short treatment period except for drug interactions

Tinea cruris: When patients have extensive skin lesions, oral itraconazole or terbinafine can hasten resolution. ***Terbinafine*** interacts with fewer drugs than itraconazoleand is generally the first-line agent"- Harrison 20th/1546

Dermatophyte infection of the skin is often called ***ringworm***. This term is confusing because worms are not involved. ***Tinea,*** the Latin word for *worm*, describes the serpentine nature of the skin lesions and is a less confusing designation that is used in conjunction with the name of the body part affected—e.g., tinea capitis (head), tinea pedis (feet), tinea corporis (body), tinea cruris (crotch), and tinea unguium (nails, although infection at this site is more often termed *onychomycosis*)- Harrison 20th/1546

84. Ans. e. Ritonavir

[Ref: K. D. T 8th/868-70; Park 25th/381]

- NACO follows WHO recommendation- K. D. T 8th/868

Table: *(K. D. T 8th/869):* **WHO (2016) ART recommendation**

First-line antiretroviral regimens for adults and adolescents
Preferred regimen
• ***Tenofovir + Lamivudine + Efavirenz***
• Tenofovir + Emtricitabine + Efavirenz
Alternative regimens
• Zidovudine + Lamivudine + Efavirenz
• Zidovudine + Lamivudine + Nevirapine
• Tenofovir + Lamivudine + Dolutegravir
• Tenofovir + Emtricitabine + Dolutegravir
• Tenofovir + Lamivudine + Nevirapine
• Tenofovir + Emtricitabine + Nevirapine.

Table: Choice of 2nd line ART regimens (NACO 2013) *K. D. T 8th/870*

Failed 1st line regimens	Second-line regimens	
	NRTI component	PI component
• ***Zidovudine + Lamivudine*** + Nevirapine/Efavirenz • Tenofovir + Lamivudine + Nevirapine	Choices *1st:* Tenofovir + Abacavir *2nd:* Didanosine + Abacavir *3rd:* Tenofovir + Zidovudine ± Lamivudine (continued)	Choices *1st:* Atazanavir/r *2nd:* Lopinavir/r *3rd:* Saquinavir/r *4th:* Indinavir/r *5th:* Nelfinavir

Note: r=low dose ritonavir boosted;PI-Protease inhibitors

85. Ans. d. Cenicriviroc

[Ref: K. D. T 8th/861; Katzung 13th/842-55; Satoskar Pharma 25th/747; Park 24th/369]

"Dual CCR5/CCR2 antagonist: Cenicriviroc" *-www.ncbi.nlm.nih.gov*

*"**Aplaviroc, Vicriviroc & Maraviroc** are **only CCR5 antagonist**"-www.ncbi.nlm.nih.gov*

Anti-Retrovirus Drug

◈ *K. D. T 8th/861; Katzung 13th/842-55*

- Nucleoside reverse transcriptase inhibitors (NRTIs): Zidovudine, Didanosine, Stavudine Lamivudine, Abacavir, Emtriitabine, Tenofovir (Nt RTI)
- Nonnucleoside reverse transcriptase inhibitors (NNRTIs): ***Nevirapine***, Efavirenz, Delavirdine, Etravirine, Rilpivirine
- Protease inhibitor: Ritonavir**,** Atazanair, ***Indinavir***, Nelfinavir, Saquinavir, Amprenavir, Lopinavir ***Darunavir***, Fosamprenavir,Tipranavir
- **Entry (fusion) inhibitor**: Enfuvirtide
- **CCR5 receptor inhibitor**: ***Maraviroc***
- **Integrase inhibitor**: ***Raltegravir***, Elvitegravir, Dolutegravir

Cenicriviroc (TAK-652, TBR-652)

- It is an experimental drug candidate for the treatment of HIV infection.
- ***Cenicriviroc is an inhibitor of* CCR2 *and CCRS receptors,*** allowing it to function as an entry inhibitor which prevents the virus from entering into a human cell. Inhibition of CCR2 may have an anti-inflammatory effect.

Maraviroc

- It is an antiretroviral drug in the CCR5 receptor antagonist class used in the treatment of HIV infection.
- It is also classed as an entry inhibitor.
- Specifically, maraviroc is a negative allosteric modulator of the CCRS.receptor.

Vicriviroc

- It has an excellent selectivity for CCR5 receptors. Phase I clinical trial of vicriviroc gave promising results, so a phase II study in the treatment o£ nalve patients was initia,ted. The phase II study was discontinued since there was a viral breakthrough in the vicriviroc group compared to the control group

Aplaviroc

- The lead compound showed *good potency in blocking CCR5* in a number of RS HIV strains and against multi-drug resistant strains.
- Unfortunately , despite the promising preclinical and early clinical results, some severe liver toxicity was observed in the treatment of naive and treatment-experienced patients that led to the discontinuation in further development of aplaviroc.

86. Ans. a. Constant fraction of drug is eliminated per unit time, c. As concentration of drugs increases, rate of elimination increases

[Ref: K. D. T 8th/38-39, 7th/30-31; SatoskarPharma 24th/22-23]

First Order Kinetic

◈ *K. D. T 8th/38-40, 7th/30-31*

- The **rate of elimination** is ***directly proportional to the drug concentration, CL (clearance) remain constant;*** or a ***constant fraction of the drug present in the body is-eliminated in unit time***
- This ***applied to majority of drugs*** which do not saturate the elimination processes (transporters, enzymes, blood flow etc.) over the therapeutic concentration range
- However, if the dose is high enough, elimination pathways of all drugs will get saturated
- ***T1/2 remain constant*** because V (volume of distribution) and ***CL (clearance) do not change with dose***

Zero Order Kinetic

◈ *K. D. T 8th/38-39, 7th/31*

- ***Few drugs*** normally saturate eliminating mechanisms and handled by zero order kinetics
- The ***rate of elimination remain constant irrespective of the drug concentration***, CL decreases with increase in concentration; or a *constant amount is eliminated in unit time*

87. Ans. a. Glargine, d. Degludec

[Ref: Harrison 20th/2863;K. D. T 8th/285; Katzung 13th/728;Satoskar Pharma 25th/893]

Table: *(Harrison 20th/2863):* **Insulin preparation**

Short-acting
Aspart
Glulisine
Lispro
Regular
Inhaled human insulin
Long-acting
Degludec
Detemir
Glargine
NPH

Table: *(Satoskar Pharma 24th/893):* **Currently available human insulins**

- **Standard Recombinant (SR) insulins:**
  - Rapid acting regular (Actrapid)
  - Intermediate acting (NPH, Insulatard)
  - Premade mixture of (a) and (b) (Mixtard)
- **Human Insulin analogues, recombinant:**
  - Very Rapid Acting (VRA): Lispro; (Humalog); Aspart
  - Glulisine
  - Intermediate acting premade mixtures; Lispro-protamine +
  - Lispro (Humalog Mix); Aspart-protamine + Aspart (Novolog Mix)
  - Long acting insulins: ***Glargine; Detemir***
  - Ultra-long acting insulin: Insulin ***Degludec***

88. Ans. a. Probenecid, d. Sulfinpyrazone

[Ref: K. D. T 8th/231]

Drug for Gout

◈ *K. D. T 8th/231*

- Acutegoutyarthritis:NSAIDS,colchicines&glucocorticoides
- Chronic gout/Hyperuricaemia
  - Uricosurics: *Probenecid, sulfinpyrazone*
  - Synthesis inhibitors: Allopurinol, febuxosat

89. Ans. b. ↑ Stroke volume, c. ↑ Cardiac output

[Ref: K. D. T 8th/568; Katzung 13th/216; Satoskar Pharma 25th/467]

Milrinone & Amrinone

◈ *K. D. T 8th/568*

- Two most important action: positive inotropy & direct vasodilation
- It increases cardiac output & decreases peripheral vascular resistance, CVP & left ventricular end diastolic volume, accompanied by mild tachycardia & slight fall in BP
- ***"Milrinone caused heart rate & stroke volume*** to increase, and systemic vascular resistance to decrease in a concentration-related manner."- ncbi.nlm.nih.gov
- Inamrinone (previously called amrinone) and milrinone are bipyridine compounds that inhibit phosphodiesterase isozyme 3 (PDE-3). They are active orally as well as parenterally but are available only in parenteral forms. They have elimination half lives of 3–6 hours, with 10–40% being excreted in the urine-*Katzung 13th/216*

Milrinone & Amrinone

◈ *G & G 2008/575*

- These drugs cause direct stimulation of myocardial contractilityand acceleration of myocardial relaxation.
- In addition, they cause balanced arterial andvenous dilation with a consequent ***fall in systemic and pulmonary vascular resistances***, and left andright heart filling pressures.
- ***Cardiac output increases*** due to the stimulation of myocardial contractilityand the decrease in left ventricular afterload. As a result of this dual mechanism of action, theincrease in cardiac output with milrinone is greater than that seen with nitroprusside at doses thatcomparably reduce systemic resistance.
- Conversely, the arterial and venous dilator effects of milrinoneare greater than those of dobutamine at doses that produce comparable increases in cardiacoutput

90. Ans. a. IV, b. IM, d. Subcutaneous

[Ref: K. D. T 8th/; Katzung 13th/550; Satoskar Pharma 25th/164-65]

Naloxone

◈ *Satoskar Pharma 25th/164*

- It is administered as IV bolus
- It can be administered intramuscularly or subcutaneously

Naltrexone

◈ *Katzung 13th/550; Katzung 13th/398*

- Oral: 50 mg tablets
- Parenteral: 380 mg suspension for injection
- Parenteral : 380 mg for IM injection once per month

91. Ans. d. Gemtuzumab- CD33, e. Trastuzumab- HER2/neu

[Ref: K. D. T 8th/; Katzung 13th/960-61;Satoskar Pharma 25th/1060]

Table: *(Satoskar Pharma 25th/1060)*: **Monoclonal antibodies for clinical use**

Generic Name	Target/Receptor	Indications
Muromonab	CD3 (T cell)	Graft rejection
Basiliximab, daclizumab	CD25 (IL-2 receptor)	-Do-
Alemtuzumab	CD52	Graft rejection; CLL
Infliximab, adalimumab	TNF-alpha	RA;Crohn's disease
Trastuzumab	HER2/neu	Breast cancer
Rituximab	CD20 (B cell)	Lymphoma; CLL
Abciximab	GpIIb/IIIa	Antiplatelet
Palivizumab	Fusion protein	Anti Resp. syncytial virus
Gentuzumab	CD33	AML
Cetuximab, panitumumab	EGFR	Colorectal cancer; NSCLC
Efalizumab	$CD11_a$ (LFA-1)	Psoriasis
Bevacizumab	VEGF neovascular AMD	Colorectal, lung cancer;
Ranibizumab	VEGF	Neovascular AMD
Eculizumab	Complement protein C5	Paroxymal nocturnal haemoglobinuria
Omalizumab	IgE receptor	Bronchial asthma
Natalizumab	Integrin	Crohn disease; MS
Certolizumab	TNF-alpha	Crohn disease

"**Bevacizumab** is a humanized IgG1 monoclonal antibody that binds to vascular endothelial growth factor (VEGF) and inhibits VEGF from binding to its receptor, especially on endothelial cells. It is an antiangiogenic drug that has been shown to inhibit growth of blood vessels (angiogenesis) in tumors"-*Katzung 13th/960*

"**Cetuximab**is a human-mouse chimeric monoclonal antibody that targets epidermal growth factor receptor (EGFR). Binding of cetuximab to EGFR inhibits tumor cell growth by a variety of mechanisms, including decreases in kinase activity, matrix metalloproteinase activity, and growth factor production, and increased apoptosis. It is indicated for use in patients with metastatic colorectal cancer whose tumors overexpress EGFR"-*Katzung 13th/961*

"**Gemtuzumab** is a humanized IgG4 monoclonal antibody with a kappa light chain specific for CD33, a sialo adhesion protein found on leukemic blast cells in 80–90% of patients with acute myelogenous leukemia (AML)"-*Katzung 13th/961*

"**Trastuzumab** is a recombinant DNA-derived, humanized monoclonal antibody that binds to the extracellular domain of the human epidermal growth factor receptor HER-2/neu"-. *Katzung 13th/961*

92. Ans. a. GIT upset, b. Memory impairment, c. Optic neuritis, d. Peripheral neuropathy, e. Hepatitis

[Ref: K. D. T 8th/817-18; Katzung 13th/817; Satoskar Pharma 25th/752]

Isoniazid: Adverse Reactions

◈ *Katzung 13th/817*

- ***Isoniazid-induced hepatitis*** is the most common major toxic effect of isoniazid.
- Clinical hepatitis with ***loss of appetite, nausea, vomiting***, jaundice, and right upper quadrant pain occurs in 1% of isoniazid recipients and can be fatal, particularly if the drug is not discontinued promptly.
- ***Peripheral neuropathy*** is observed in 10–20% of patients given dosages greater than 5 mg/kg/d.
- Neuropathy is due to a relative pyridoxine deficiency. Isoniazid promotes excretion of pyridoxine, and this toxicity is readily reversed by administration of pyridoxine in a dosage as low as 10 mg/d.
- Central nervous system toxicity, which is less common, includes ***memory loss***, psychosis, and seizures. These may also respond to pyridoxine.
- Miscellaneous other reactions include hematologic abnormalities, provocation of pyridoxine deficiency anemia, tinnitus, and ***gastrointestinal discomfort***. Isoniazid can reduce the metabolism of phenytoin, increasing its blood level and toxicity
- Fever and skin rashes are occasionally seen. Drug-induced systemic lupus erythematosus has been reported.
- Lethargy, rashes, mild anaemia & arthralgia are also side-effect-*K. D. T 8th/818*
- *Rarely* **optic neuritis** *leading to atrophy may develop; hence it* ***should be discontinued if visual disturbances develop***-*Satoskar Pharma 25th/752*

93. Ans. d. Nebivolol– enhance NO production

[Ref: K. D. T 8th/165; Katzung 13th/160;Satoskar Pharma 25th/284; spo.escardio.org]

"3rd generation beta blockers have additional vasodilator property"- *spo.escardio.org*

"Celiprolol*-Third generation selective β_1 blocker having* ***additional β_2 agonistic activity*** *which reduces vascular resistance & holds promise of safety in asthmatics"- K. D. T 8th/163*

"**Nevivolol**-It activates endothelial nitric oxide (NO) synthase & enhance ***NO production***"-*K. D. T 8th/163*

"Carvedilol: Produce vasodilation by α1 blockade as well as calcium channel blockade"- *K. D. T 8th/****165***

Lebetalol: ***Fall in BP is due to α1 & β1 blockade as well as β2 agonism***-*K. D. T 8th/165*

"**Bopindolol**- Cause vasodilation by partial ***β2 agonistic activity***"- *Katzung 13th/162*

Betablockers with Vasodilator Property

Alpha blockade	Beta 2 agonism	CCB action	K+ Channel opening	No production	Anti oxidant
Labetalol	Celiprolol	Betaxolol	Tilisolol	Celiprolol	Carvedilol
Carvedilol	Carteolol	Bevantolol		Carteolol	
Bucindolol	Bopindolol	Carvedilol		Bopindolol	
Bevantolol				Nipradilol	
Nipradilol				Nebivolol	

94. Ans. a. Given orally, c. Used prophylactically, d. Prevents release from mast cells, e. Dry mouth is a side-effect

[Ref: KDT 8th/249]

Ketotifen

◈ *KDT 8th/249*

- *It prevent release of mediators from mast cell(mast cell stabilizer)*
- *It is* ***not a bronchodilator***
- *After prolonged use, modest symptomatic relief may occur in some patients of bronchial asthma, atopic dermatitis, perennial rhinitis, conjunctivitis, urticaria & food allergy*
- *Used as* ***tablet, syrup*** *or eye drop*
- It is generally well tolerated. Sedation & dry mouth are common
- Other side-effects are dizziness, nausea & weight gain

95. Ans. a. INH, b. Pyrazinamide, c. Streptomycin, d. Rifampicin

[Ref: KDT 8th/816-19; Park 25th/199-200]

"**Bactericidal drugs** *are: Rifampicin (R), Isoniazid (INH), Streptomycin (S) & Pyrazinamide (Z)"-Park 25th/199*

"**Bacteriostatic drugs** are: *Ethambutol (E) & Thioacetazone (Tzn)"- Park 25th/199-200*

96. Ans. a. Blood glucose test, b. Blood urea test, c. Mechanical ventilation, d. Single large dose…, e. Flumazenil as antidote

[Ref: CMDT 2019/1598;Emergency Medicine by S N Chugh 4th/479; Reddy 34th/554;K. D. T 8th/431,383-84; Katzung 13th/382;Satoskar Pharma 25th/119,317]

Flumazenil: *Antagonist of benzodiazepines (including diazepam)- K. D. T 8th/435*

Diazepam overdose: *Drowsiness, mental confusion, dizziness, coma etc may occur- S N Chugh 4th/479*

"**Diazepam side effect** on Urogenital System: incontinence, changes in libido, urinary retention"- www.rxlist.com (so ***blood urea estimation may be needed***)

Management of Benzodiazepines (Including Diazepam)

- *S N Chugh 4th/479*
- Removal of unabsorbed drug by ***repeated gastric lavage*** & ***administration of activated charcoal***
- ***"Administer activated charcoal if the patient has ingested a massive dose & the airway is protected***-*CMDT 2019/1598*
- **Respiratory support:** Supplement oxygen, maintain the airway & intubate(***mechanical ventilation***) if there is altered sensorium & /or respiratory depression
- Use of an antidote: **flumazenil**

Management of Benzodiazepine Overdose

- *ncbi.nlm.nih.gov*
- Before any diagnostic tests are ordered in the patient presenting with altered mental status with suspected overdose or toxicity; any respiratory or abnormal vital signs should be addressed first.
- ***Mechanical ventilation may be required to address respiratory compromise*** and IV fluids administered to address hemodynamic instability.
- In terms of general diagnostic testing, routine testing for the acutely poisoned patient should include a ***finger stick glucose to immediately rule out and address hypoglycemia as the cause of altered mental status.***
- The mainstay treatment for acute benzodiazepine toxicity is supportive care which may include endotracheal intubation to provide definitive airway management.
- While the mainstay treatment of acute benzodiazepine toxicity or overdose is **supportive care**, there is, however, an "antidote" that may be used in limited situations.
- **Flumazenil is** a nonspecific competitive antagonist at the benzodiazepine receptor that can reverse BZD induced sedation.
- **Supportive care** in a patient with benzodiazepine overdose includes close monitoring, preferably in the drainage position. If hypotension or prolonged eNS depression occurs, intravenous fluids should be administered.
- Occasionally, ***gastric lavage and administration of activated charcoal is indicated, but only if the patient is awake and potentially sensitive to benzodiazepines and if a large dose has been ingested within the last 1 to 2 hours*** link.springer.com

MICROBIOLOGY

97. Ans. a. May be associated with GBS syndrome, c. Virus can be isolated from body secretions, d. Severe birth defects may occur, e. Hepatosplenomegaly is the common feature of congenital CMV infection

[Ref: Harrison 20th/3225,1364;Ananthanarayan 10th/479-80;Baveja Micro 5th446-47;Jawetz 27th/470-74]

- *GBS may be preceded by CMV infection*
- Ganciclovir and valacyclovir are given for both-prophylaxis in immunocompromised patients and for treatment of symptomatic immunocompetent patients

Antecedent Events in GBS: Approximately 70% of cases of GBS occur 1–3 weeks after an acute infectious process, usually respiratory or gastrointestinal. *Campylobacter jejuni*, human herpes virus infection, often **CMV,** Epstein-Barr virus, HIV, hepatitis E, Zika, *Mycoplasma pneumoniae* have been identified as agents involved in antecedent infections"- *Harrison 20th/3225*

"**CMV can be isolated** *from urine, saliva, breast milk, semen,* ***cervical secretions*** *and blood leukocytes"- Baveja Micro 5th447*

"**Congenital CMV Infection:** Petechiae, ***hepatosplenomegaly***, and jaundice are the most common presenting features (60–80% of cases). Microcephaly with or without cerebral calcifications, intrauterine growth retardation, and prematurity are reported in 30–50% of cases. Inguinal hernias and chorioretinitis are less common"-Harrison 20th/1362-63

Acyclovir is useful in prophylaxis but not in treatment. ***Ganciclovir*** *and foscarnet have been found to be effective and are used for the treatment of CMV disease in patients with AIDS- Ananthanarayan 10th/480*

"**Prophylaxis**: *Indicated only in high risk case such as organ transplant, premature infants and* ***immunodeficient persons.*** *CMV immunoglobulins and acyclovir is useful in prophylaxis"- Baveja Micro 5th447*

"For treatment of severe CMV infections, ***ganciclovir*** *is the drug of choice"- Baveja Micro 5th447*

- **CMV** *Harrison 20th/1364*
- ***Ganciclovir*** is a guanosine derivative that has considerably more activity against CMV than its congener acyclovir. It is used for ***CMV retinitis or colitis.*** In severe infections (e.g., CMV pneumonia in hematopoietic stem cell transplant recipients), ganciclovir is sometimes combined with CMV immune globulin.
- **Prophylactic or suppressive ganciclovir** may be useful in high-risk hematopoietic stem cell or organ transplant recipients (e.g., those who are CMV-seropositive before transplantation).

- **Prevention** ***Harrison 20th/1364***
- Prevention of CMV infection and disease in organ and hematopoietic stem cell transplant recipients is usually based on one of two methods: universal prophylaxis or preemptive therapy.
- With universal prophylaxis, antiviral drugs are used for a defined period, often 3 or 6 months.
- Letermovir, which has recently been approved, allows prophylaxis in higher-risk patients.
- ***Primary prophylaxis with ganciclovir or valganciclovir is not recommended.***
- **Prophylactic acyclovir or valacyclovir** at high doses may reduce rates of CMV infection and disease in renal transplant recipients; neither drug is effective in the treatment of active CMV disease.

Cytomegalovirus (Human Herpes Virus Type 5)

- *Harrison 20th/1362-63; Ananthanarayan 10th/479-80*

- It is cytomegalic (***not lymphoproliferative***, which occur in HHV4, 6 and 7)
- Characterized by ***enlargement of infected cells***
- **Cytomegalic cells: *"owl's eye" appearance.***
- Congenital infection- Intrauterine infection leads to ***fetal death or cytomegalic inclusion disease of newborn which is often fatal***
- In addition to inducing ***severe birth defects***, CMV causes a wide spectrum of disorders in older children and adults, ranging from an asymptomatic subclinical infection to a *mononucleosis syndrome*
- The hallmark of such infection is the appearance of ***atypical lymphocytes in the peripheral blood; these cells are predominantly activated CD8+ T lymphocytes.***

98. Ans. d. Indian kala-azar is a zoonotic disease

[Ref: Park 25th/331-35; Harrison 20th/1594-98;Panikar 7th/50-54]

VL: Endemic in many places in ***India, China, Africa, Southern Europe, South America and Russia***-Chatterjee Parasitology 13th/67

"The majority of the leishmaniasis are zoontotic involving wild or domestic mammals(rodents, cannines). Some forms(e.g, ***Indian kala-azar are considered to be nonzoonotic infection****"- Park 25th/331*

*"**Season:** In past epidemics, **two peaks,** one in November and another in March-April were reported. Generally there is high prevalence during and after rains"- Park 25th/333*

Vl (Kala-Azar/"Black Fever")

◈ *Harrison 20th/1594*

- It is caused by the *Leishmania donovani* complex, which includes *L. donovani* and *Leishmania infantum* (the latter designated *Leishmania chagasi* in the New World);these species are responsible for anthroponotic and zoonotic transmission, respectively.
- India and neighboring Bangladesh, Sudan and neighboring ***South Sudan, Ethiopia***, and Brazil are the four largest foci of VL and account for 90% of the world's VL burden.
- In Sudan and South Sudan, large outbreaks are thought to be anthroponotic, although zoonotic transmission also occurs. VL is rare in West and sub-Saharan Africa
- "Major epidemic of disease are currently found in- ***India, Brazil and Sudan***"- *Panikar 7th/50*

Leishmaniasis

◈ *Park 25th/331-33; Panikar 7th/50-55*

- Occur in 3 forms- Kala-azar(VL), cutaneous leishmaniasis and muco-cutaneous leishmaniasis
- *"In India, kala-azar is transmitted from person to person by the bite of the* ***female phlebotomine*** *sandfly, P.argentipes"- Park 25th/333*
- "The **rapid diagnostic kit(rk39)** has become the mainstay in the serological diagnosis of Kala-azar and is the method of choice for diagnosis of disease"-Park 25th/333
- Splenomegaly- early, progressive and massive
- Hepatomegaly and lymphadenopathy- also occur but not so prominent
- Skin: Dry, rough and darkly pigmented
- Demonstration of amastigotes in smears of tissue aspirates: gold standard for diagnosis of VL

99. Ans. a. Toxic shock syndrome toxin (TSST), c. Group A streptococcal pyrogenic exotoxin, d. Staphylococcal enterotoxins

[Ref: Ananthanarayan 10th/93,204; Jawetz 27th/135,206;Baveja 5th/95]

*"**Staphylococcal enterotoxins, Streptococcal pyrogenic exotoxin (SPE), Toxic shock syndrome toxin(TSST)** are superantigens"- Ananthanarayan 10th/204,214*

Examples of superantigens include certain bacterial toxins, including the ***staphylococcal enterotoxins, toxic shock syndrome toxin, and group A streptococcal pyrogenic exotoxin A***"- *Jawetz 27th/135*

"A superantigenic toxin, *Y. pseudotuberculosis* mitogen (YPM) is produced by strains seen in eastern Russia in association with Far Eastern scarlet-like fever, a childhood illness with desquamating rash, arthralgia, and toxic shock"-*Harrison 20th/1207*

Table *(Ananthanarayan 10th/93)*: **Human disease associated with superantigens**

Organism	Superantigen	Disease
Staphylococcus aureus	Enterotoxins	Food poisoning Toxic shock syndrome Multiple sclerosis
Group A streptococci	Pyrogenic exotoxins	Shock Psoriasis Rheumatic heart disease
Mycobacterium tuberculosis	Not identified	Tuberculosis
HIV	Nef (negative regulatory factor)	AIDS
Rabies virus	Nucleocapsid protein	Rabies
Epstein-Barr virus	Not identified	B cell lymphoma

Table *(Kuby Immunology 6th/260)*: **Exogens Superantigen**

Exogens Superantigen	Disease
Staphylococcal enterotoxins - SEA, SEB, SEC1, SEC2, SEC3, SED, SCE	Food poisoning
Toxic Shock Syndrome Toxin 1	Toxic shock syndrome
Exfoliative dermatitis toxin (EXFT)	Scalded skin Syndrome
Mycoplasma arthritidis Supernatant (MAS)	Arthritis, shock
Streptococcal pyrogenic exotoxins (SPE-A, B, C, D)	Rheumatic fever, shock

100. Ans. a. Polyclonal T-lymphocyte activation, b. Releases large amount of cytokines, c. Bind TCRβ and class II MHC molecule, d. Need no processing

[Ref: Ananthanarayan 10th/93, 204; Jawetz 27th/135,206; Greenwood 16th/92;Baveja 5th/95; Immunology by David Male 7th/272-273; Kuby Immunology 6th/260-261]

*"Superantigens are **polyclonal T-lymphocyte activators** and **releases cytokines**"-Robbins 9th/133*

"Superantigens activate large populations of T cells that express particular subsets of the T cell receptor ® protein, causing massive cytokine release and subsequent host reactions'-Harrison 20th/873

"Superantigens, stimulating certain T cells to proliferate without processing of the protein toxin by antigen-presenting cells. Part of this process involves stimulation of the antigen-presenting cells to produce IL-1 and TNFα, which have been implicated in many clinical features of diseases like toxic shock syndrome and scarlet fever"- Harrison 20th/876

Superantigen

◈ *Jawetz 27th/135*

- **"Microbial superantigens,** such as staphylococcal protein A and staphylococcal enterotoxins, are substances that can stimulate a ***broad range of T and B cells*** through specific interactions with selected families of immune receptors, irrespective of their antigen specificity"- Harrison 20th/2510
- "Some **superantigens** are able to bind to MHC molecules outside the peptide-binding cleft. One consequence is that whereas an individual peptide complexed to an MHC molecule will normally stimulate only a small percentage of the T cells in an individual, ***superantigens cause up to 10% of T cells to be nonspecifically activated.***
- Superantigens binds directly to the *lateral portion of TCRβ chain and MHC class II βchain* (c.f. conventional antigens bind to MHC class I or II molecules in the groove of the α β heterodimer and bind to T cell via the V region of TCR α and β chains)- *Immunology by David Male/7th*
- It is the release of ***large amounts of cytokines*** from stimulation of a high percentage of the pool of T lymphocytes that explains to a large extent the pathogenesis of diseases caused by organisms expressing superantigens
- Superantigen induce apoptotic death of mature CD4+ and CD8+ T cells.

101. Ans. a. Kills both vegetative and spore forms of bacteria, d. CO_2 can be used for sterilisation, e. Water can be disinfected by chlorination

[Ref: Ananthanarayan 10th/28-37;Park 25th/774;Jawetz 27th/63]

Supercritical carbon dioxide: Supercritical carbon dioxide (sCO_2) is a fluid state of carbon dioxide **where it is held at or above its** critical temperature **and** critical pressure. It is ***used for sterilization*** of heat-sensitive or porous materials or devices, such as endoscopes, porous implants, liquid foodstuff, and liquid medicine"- *www.sciencedirect.com*

Sterilization Techniques

◈ *Ananthanarayan 10th/28-37*

- ***Sterilisation** is defined as the process by which an **article, surface or medium is freed of all living microorganism either in the vegetative or spore state**- Ananthanarayan 10th/28*
- ***Disinfection** is destruction of all pathogenic organisms*
- ***Antisepsis** are agents that can be safely applied on the skin or mucous membrane to prevent infection by inhibiting the growth of bacteria*
- *Chlorine and its compound hypochlorite have been used as disinfectants over time. They are markedly **bactericidal and virucidal**- Ananthanarayan 10th/34*
- Chlorination: Kills pathogenic bacteria, but it has no effect on spores and certain viruses(e.g polio, viral hepatitis"-Park 25th/774

Table *(Ananthanarayan 10th/28)*: **Sterilising agents**

Methods used for sterilising an object are:
• **Physical agents** ▪ Dry heat: By flaming, incineration or using hot air ▪ Moist heat: By boiling, steam at atmospheric pressure, steam above atmospheric pressure ▪ Filtration: Using candles, asbestos pads, membranes ▪ Radiation • **Chemical agents** ▪ Alcohols: ethyl, isopropyl, trichlorobutanol ▪ Aldehydes: formaldehyde, glutaraldehyde ▪ Orthophthalaldehyde ▪ Peracetic acid ▪ Hydrogen peroxide ▪ Hypochlorous acid ▪ Dyes ▪ Halogens ▪ Phenols ▪ Surface-active agents ▪ Metallic salts

102. Ans. a. Peptostreptococcus, b. Propionibacterium, e. Bacteroides

[Ref: Ananthanarayan 10th/273;Baveja 5th/238]

- ***Peptostreptococcus is non-sporing anaerobe***

Bacillus anthracis*: It is* ***aerobic. Spores*** *are central or subterminal, elliptical or oval in shape"- Ananthanarayan 10th/249*

Anaerobic Bacilli

◈ *Ananthanarayan 10th/273*

- **Endoscope forming: *Clostridia***
- **Non-sporing**
- Gram-positive
  - Eubacterium
  - Propionibacterium
  - Lactobacillus
  - Mobiluncus
  - Bifidobacterium
  - Actinomyces

- Gram-negative
  - Bacteroides
  - Prevotella
  - Porphyromonas
  - Fusobacterium
  - Leptotrichia

Anaerobic Cocci (Nonsporing)

◈ *Ananthanarayan 10th/273*

- Gram positive
  - Peptostreptococcus
  - Peptococcus
  - Blantia
- Gram negative
  - Veillonella
  - Megasphaera

103. Ans. a. Actinomyces, b. Lactobacillus, e. Clostridium

[Ref: Above Q explanation; Ananthanarayan 10th/273-74,257]

- ***Clostridium is a sporeforming gram positive anaerobic bacilli whereas Lactobacillus and Actinomyces are non sporeforming gram positive anaerobic bacilli.***
- ***Valionella is a gram negative anaerobic cocci.***
- ***Bacteroides is a gram negative anaerobic bacilli.***

104. Ans. a. Nine banded armadillos, c. Mangabey monkey, d. Chimpanzee

[Ref: Park 25th/344; Ananthanarayan 10th/372; Baveja Micro 5th/353;Jawetz 27th/319;Greenwood 16th/210]

- *Although* **European hedgehog and Nude mice** are used for ***experimental infection with M.Leprae, natural infection do not occur (hence not zoonosis)***

  "Until recently man was considered to be the only host and source of infection. There is now evidence that natural infections with M.leprae are present in wild animals, e.g, ***armadillos, mangabey monkeys and chimpanzees****"-Park 25th/344*

  "*M. leprae* causes disease primarily in humans. However, in Texas and Louisiana, 15% of ***nine-banded armadillos*** are infected, and armadillo contact occasionally results in human disease"- *Harrison 20th/1261*

  When bacilli from human leprosy (ground tissue nasal scrapings) are inoculated into footpads of ***mice***, local granulomatous lesions develop with limited multiplication of bacilli. ***Inoculated armadillos*** develop extensive lepromatous leprosy, and ***armadillos naturally infected*** with leprosy have been found in Texas and Mexico. - *Jawetz 27th/319*

Following Animals have been used for Experimental Infection with M.Leprae

◈ *Baveja Micro 5th/353*

- Mouse (foot-pad)
- ***Nine-banded armadillos***
- ***Chimpanzees,***
- ***Monkeys***
- Slender loris
- Indian pangolin
- Chipmunks
- Golden hamsters
- ***European hedgehog.***

- Among these animals, the most important are ***mouse and nine-banded armadillos***

105. Ans. None

[Ref: Harrison 20th/1292-93;Ananthanarayan 10th/387-91]

All mentioned features are found in Weil's disease

Icterohemorrhagiae *serogroup of L.interrogans cause* ***Weil's disease(Fever, jaundiceand haemorrhages)****- Ananthanarayan 10th/388-89*

*Severe leptospirosis(****Weil's disease****) is associated with* ***fever, conjunctivitis, albuminuria, jaundice and haemorrhage****- Baveja Micro 5th/370*

"**Leptospiral uveitis** commonly affects the young and middle-aged patients, men more often than women, mainly because of the increased chance of exposure to leptospiral-contaminated water or soil. Leptospiral uveitis was first reported by Weil in 1866 in his original article and subsequently, several authors found its varying presentations. The precise incidence of uveitis in systemic leptospirosis is not known and it ranges from 3% to 92%"- *www.jpgmonline.com*

Severe Leptospirosis

◈ *Harrison 20th/1293*

- Although the onset of severe leptospirosis may be no different from that of mild leptospirosis, severe disease is often rapidly progressive and is associated with a case–fatality rate ranging from 1 to 50%.
- Higher mortality rates are associated with an age >40, altered mental status, ***acute renal failure***, respiratory insufficiency, hypotension, and arrhythmias.
- The classic presentation, often referred to as Weil's syndrome, encompasses the triad of hemorrhage ,jaundice, and acute kidney injury
- Patients die of septic shock with multi organ failure and/ or severe bleeding complications that most commonly involve the lungs (pulmonary hemorrhage), gastrointestinal tract (melena, hemoptysis), urogenital tract (hematuria), and skin (***petechiae, ecchymosis,*** and bleeding from venipuncture sites).
- **Pulmonary hemorrhage (with or without jaundice)** is now recognized as a widespread public health problem, presenting with cough, chest pain, respiratory distress, and hemoptysis that may not be apparent until patients are intubated
- ***Jaundice occurs in 5–10% of all patients*** with leptospirosis; it can be profound and give an orange cast to the skin but usually is not associated with fulminant hepatic necrosis.

Mild Leptospirosis

◈ *Harrison 20th/1293*

- ***Mild symptomatic leptospirosis usually presents as a flu-like illness of sudden onset, with fever, chills, headache,***

nausea, vomiting, abdominal pain, conjunctival suffusion(redness without exudate), and myalgia.

- Muscle pain is intense and especially affects the calves, back, and abdomen. The headache is intense, localized to the frontal or retroorbital region (resembling that occurring in dengue), and sometimes accompanied by photophobia.
- Physical examination may include any of the following findings, none of which is pathognomonic for leptospirosis: *fever, conjunctival suffusion, pharyngeal injection, muscle tenderness, lymphadenopathy ,rash, meningismus, hepatomegaly, and splenomegaly.*

106. Ans. d. Brucellosis is an example

[Ref: Harrison 19th/261e-1; Ananthanarayan 10th/662; Jawetz 27th/417-18]

CDC Category A, B, and C Agents

- *Harrison 19th/261e-1and2*
- The U.S. Centers for Disease Control and Prevention (CDC) classifies potential biologic threats into three categories: A, B, and C.
- Category A agents are the highest-priority pathogens. They pose the greatest risk to national security because they (1) can be easily disseminated or transmitted from ***person to person***, (2) result in ***high mortality rates*** and have the ***potential for major public health impact***, (3) might cause public panic and social disruption, and (4) ***require special action for public health preparedness.***
- **Category B agents** are the second highest priority pathogens and include those that are moderately easy to disseminate, result in moderate morbidity rates and low mortality rates, and require specifically enhanced diagnostic capacity.
- **Category C agents** are the third highest priority.
- It should be pointed out, however, that these A,B, and C designations are empirical and, depending on evolving circumstances such as intelligence-based threat assessments, the priority rating of any given microbe or toxin could change.

Key Features of Biologic agents used as Bioweapons

- *Harrison 19th/261e-1*
- High morbidity and mortality rates
- Potential for person-to-person spread
- Low infective dose and highly infectious by aerosol
- Lack of rapid diagnostic capability
- Lack of universally available effective vaccine
- Potential to cause anxiety
- Availability of pathogen and feasibility of production
- Environmental stability
- Database of prior research and development
- Potential to be "weaponized"

Table: CDC Category A, B, and C Agents *(Harrison 19th/261e-1)*

Category A
Anthrax (***Bacillus anthracis***) Botulism (***Clostridium botulinum***toxin) Plague (***Yersinia pestis***) Smallpox (*Variola major*) Tularemia (*Francisellatularensis*) Viral hemorrhagic fevers **Arenaviruses:** Lassa, New World (Machupo, Junin,Guanarito, and Sabia) **Bunyaviridae:** Crimean-Congo, Rift Valley **Filoviridae:** Ebola, Marburg
Category B
Brucellosis (*Brucella*spp.) Epsilon toxin of *Clostridium perfringens* Food safety threats (e.g., *Salmonella* spp., *Escherichia coli* 0157:H7, *Shigella*) Glanders (*Burkholderia mallei*) Melioidosis (*B. pseudomallei*) Psittacosis (*Chlamydophilapsittaci*) Q fever (*Coxiellaburnetii*) Ricin toxin from *Ricinuscommunis*(castor beans) Staphylococcal enterotoxin B Typhus fever (*Rickettsia prowazekii*) Viral encephalitis [alphaviruses (e.g., Venezuelan, eastern, and western equine encephalitis)] Water safety threats (e.g., *Vibrio cholerae, Cryptosporidium parvum*)
Category C
Emerging infectious diseases threats such as Nipah, hantavirus, SARS or MERS coronavirus, and pandemic influenza.

107. Ans. a. Endemic typhus- R.typhi, b. Rickettsial pox- R.Akari, c. Q fever: Coxiella burnetii, d. Epidemic typhus: R. prowazekii

[Ref: Ananthanarayan 10th/413; Harrison 20th/1304]

Table *(Ananthanarayan 10th/413, Harrison 20th/1304)*: **Disease caused by Rickettsia and Orientia species**

Disease	Species	Vector
Rocky Mountain spotted fever	*Rickettsia rickettsii*	Tick
Rickettsial pox	R.Akari	Mite
Scrub typhus	*Orientia tsutsugamushi*	Mite
Q fever	*Coxiella burnetii*	*Inhalation of aerosolsof infected parturitionmaterial, ingestion of infected milkor milk products*

Contd...

Disease	Species	Vector
Epidemic typhus	*R. prowazekii*	Louse
Endemic typhus	R.typhi	Rat flea

108. Ans. c. Black eschar, d. Doxycycline is used for treatment, e. Rats are the reservoir

[Ref: Ananthanarayan 10th/415-16; Park 25th/327;Harrison 20th/1309-10; Jawetz 27th/342]

*"**Scrub typhus:** One typical feature is the punched-out ulcer covered with a **blackened scab(eschar)** which indicates the location of **mite bite**"- Park 25th/327*

*"**Scrub typhus**: Most travel-acquired cases occur during visits to **rural areas** in endemic countries for activities such as **camping, hiking or rafting**, but urban cases have also been described. **Tetracycline is drug of choice**"- Park 25th/327*

*"**Scrub typhus,** originally found in scrub jungles, has also been identified in a variety of other habitats, such as sandy beaches, **mountain deserts** and equatorial rain-forests"- Ananthanarayan 10th/415*

Scrub Typhus

◈ *Ananthanarayan 10th/415-16*

- *The vectors are **trombiculid mites** of genus Leptotrombidium*
- ***Incubation period is 1-3 week***
- *Originally found in scrub jungles, has also been identified in a variety of other habitats, such as **sandy beaches, mountain deserts and equatorial rain-forests***
- "Human beings are infected *when they are beaten by the mite larva(chigger). Adult mites feed only on plant"*
- "Zoonotic tetrad of Scrub typhus: *It consists of Orientatsutsugamushi, chiggers, rats, secondary or transitional forms of vegetation"*
- "Three major antigenic types have been recognized-Gilliam, Karp and Kato"

Scrub Typhus (Chigger-borne Typhus)

◈ *Harrison 20th/1309-10*

- *Illness varies from mild and self-limiting to fatal. After an incubation period of 6–21 days, onset is characterized by fever, headache, myalgia, cough, and gastrointestinal symptoms.*
- Patients are treated with ***doxycycline, azithromycin, or chloramphenicol***

Table *(Jawetz 27th/342)*: **Scrub typhus**

Organism	Disease	Geographic Distribution	Vector	Mammalian Resevoir	Clinical Features
Orientia tsutsugamushi	Scrub typhus	Asia, South Pacific, Northern Australia	Mite	Rodents, birds	Fever, headache, rash (50% have eschar), lymphadenopathy, atypical lymphocytes

109. Ans. a. VDRL, b. Rapid plasma Reagin (RPR)

[Ref: Ananthanarayan 10th/383; Harrison 20th/2283; Dutta Obs 9th/276;O.P.Ghai 9th/265;Nelson 20th/1473;Baveja Micro 5th/366]

Congenital Syphilis

◈ *medind.nic.in*

- A national strategy for India "toward elimination of parent-to child transmission (E-PTCT) of syphilis" was launched in February 2015 by NACO under Ministry of Health and Family Welfare and World Health Organization (WHO).
- This strategy emphasizes the management of syphilis among pregnant women through a functional convergence approach
- At health care points without laboratories, ANC attendees have to be screened using point-of-care (POC) test.
- At healthcare service points with laboratory support, ANC attendees can be **screened** using the ***RPR or VDRL test.***
- When the screening test is an RPR/VDRL test, a treponema pallidum hemagglutination assay may be conducted, if available, to confirm active syphilis.

Syphilis in Pregnancy

◈ *Dutta Obs 9th/276*

- ***VDRL is commonly done for screening***
- *A positive VDRL test has to be confirmed by FTA-ABS and MHA-TP*

Table *(Baveja Micro 5th/366)*: **Diagnostic methods in Syphilis**

Demonstration of Treponemes	• Dark ground microscopy • Direct fluorescent antibody staining for *T. pallidum* (DFA-TP) • Treponemes in tissue ▪ Silver impregnation method (Levaditi stain) ▪ Immunofluorescence staining
Serological tests Non-treponemal tests	• VDRL • RPR
Treponemal tests	• FTA, FTA-ABS (using killed *T. pallidum*) • TPHA, MHA-TP, TP-PA (using *T. pallidum extract*) • TPI test (using live *T. pallidum*)

110. Ans. b. RPR, d. VDRL

[Ref: Ananthanarayan 10th/383; Harrison 20th/2283; Dutta Obs 9th/276;O.P.Ghai 9th/265;Nelson 20th/1473;Baveja Micro 5th/366; CMDT 2016/1464]

Serologic Tests for Syphilis

◈ *CMDT 2016/1464 There are two general categories of serologic tests for syphilis:*

- **Nontreponemal tests** detect antibodies to lipoidal antigens present in the host after modification by *T pallidum.*

- **Treponemal tests** use live or killed *T pallidum* as antigen to detect antibodies specific for pathogenic treponemes.

Serologic Tests for Syphilis

◈ *Harrison 20th/2283, 19th/1137-38*

- The most widely used **nontreponemal antibody tests** for syphilis are the ***rapid plasma reagin (RPR) and Venereal Disease Research Laboratory (VDRL) tests***, which measure IgG and IgM directed against a cardiolipin-lecithincholesterol antigen complex
- **Treponemal tests** measure antibodies to native or recombinant *T. pallidum* antigens and include the ***fluorescent treponemal antibody-absorbed (FTA-ABS) test and the T. pallidum particle agglutination (TPPA) test***, both of which are more sensitive for primary syphilis than the previously used hemagglutination tests.
- *When used to confirm positive nontreponemal test results, treponemal tests have a very high positive predictive value* for diagnosis of syphilis. In a screening setting, however, these tests give false-positive results at rates as high as 1–2%.
- Treponemal tests are likely to remain reactive even after adequate treatment and cannot differentiate past from current *T. pallidum* infection.

111. Ans. e. Typically indurated

[Ref: Ananthanarayan10th/337; Harrison 19th/880, 1012-13]

"**Inguinal and femoral buboes** are localized enlargements of the lymph nodes in the groin area, which are painful and may be fluctuant. They are frequently associated with LGV and ***chancroid***"- www.sciencedirect.com

Chancroid or Soft Sore

◈ *Harrison 19th/1012-13; Ananthanarayan10th/337*

- *Characterized by **tender non-indurated irregular ulcers on the genitalia***
- *The infection remains localized, spreading only to the regional **lymph nodes which are enlarged and painful***
- ***Incubation period is 4–7 days***
- The ***ulcers are painful and bleed easily***
- Approximately half of patients develop ***enlarged, tender inguinal lymph nodes***, which frequently become fluctuant and spontaneously rupture.
- An **accurate diagnosis** of chancroid relies on ***culture of H. ducreyi*** from the lesion or from an aspirate of suppurative lymph nodes.
- A **probable diagnosis** of chancroid can be made when the following criteria are met: *(1) one or more painful genital ulcers; (2) no evidence of Treponema pallidum infection by dark-field examination of ulcer exudate or by a negative serologic test for syphilis performed at least 7 days after ulcer onset; (3) a typical clinical presentation for chancroid; and (4) a negative test for herpes simplex virus in the ulcer exudate*

Table *(Harrison 19th/880)*: **Clinical Features of Genital Ulcer**

Feature	Syphilis	Herpes	Chancroid	Lymphogranuloma Venereum	Donovanosis
Incubation period	9–90 day	2–7 days	***1–14 days***	3 day–6 weeks	1–4 weeks (up to 6 months)
Early primary lesion	Papule	Vesicle	Pustule	Papule, pustule, or vesicle	Papule
No. of lesion	Usually one	Multiple	Usually multiple, may coalesce	Usually one; often not detected, despite lymphadenopathy	Variable
Diameter	5–15 mm	1–2 mm	Variable	2–10 mm	Variable
Edges	Sharply demarcated, elevated, round, or oval	Erythematous	***Undermined, ragged, irregular***	Elevated, round or oval	Elevated irregular
Depth	Superficial or deep	Superficial	Excavated	Superficial or deep	Elevated
Base	Smooth, non-purulent, relatively nonvascular	Serous, erythematous nonvascular	Purulent, bleeds easily	Variable, nonvascular	Red and velvety bleeds readily
Induration	Firm	None	Soft	Occasionally firm	Firm
Pain	Uncommon	Frequent tender	***Usually very tender***	Variable	Uncommon
Lymphadenopathy	Firm, nontender, bilateral	Firm,tender,often bilateral with initial episode	***Tender, may suppurate, loculated, usually unilateral***	Tender, may suppurate, loculated, usually unilateral	None; pseudobuboes

112. Ans. c. 3%

[Ref: jamanetwork.com; www.jpsiconline.com; www.ncbi.nlm.nih.gov]

"According to the clinical and Laboratory Standards Institute guidelines, the ***maximum acceptable percentage*** *of contaminated blood culture in any healthcare facility is* ***3%.****"-www.jpsiconline.* com; jamanetwork.com

"The **acceptable blood contamination** *rate benchmark is* **2-3%,** *with rates ranging from* ***1% to 9%.****"- www.ncbi.nlm.nih.gov*

"While target rates for contamination have been set at 2 to 3%, actual rates seem to vary widely between institutions, from as little as 0.6% to over 6%"-cbi.nlm.nih.gov

113. Ans. a. Tissue specimen, b. Blood, d. Bone marrow

[Ref: Anathanarayan 10th/695; Clinical microbiology 2nd/812; Essentials of microbiology/224]

"Some types of specimens should always be cultured for anaerobes if an infection is suspected. *These include* ***abscesses, bites, blood, cerebrospinal fluid and exudative body fluids, deep wounds, and dead tissues****"- www.surgeryencyclopedia.com*

"Because of resident anaerobic flora, the ***following sites are inappropriate for anaerobic cultures*** *and will be rejected: throat and nasopharynx,* ***sputum****, bronchoscopy specimens, gastrointestinal contents, voided or catheterized urine,* ***urogenital swabs (eg, vaginal and/or cervical)****, and specimens from superficial wounds"- www.labcorp.com*

Some Specimens from which Anaerobes are Likely to be Isolated

◈ *www.urmc.rochester.edu*

- Bile
- Blood
- ***Bone marrow***
- Cerebrospinal fluid
- Direct lung aspirate
- ***Tissue biopsy*** from a normally sterile site
- Fluid from a normally sterile site (like a joint)
- Dental abscess
- Abdominal or pelvic abscess
- Knife, gunshot, or surgical wound
- Severe burn

114. Ans. a. Citrobacter freundii, b. E. coli, d. K. pneumoniae, e. Acinetobactor baumannii.

[Ref: www.ncbi.nlm.nih.gov; academic.oup.com]

Carbapenem Resistance

◈ *academic.oup.com*

- β-Lactamases are the primary cause of bacterial resistance to β-lactam antibiotics.
- The most widely used classification of β-lactamases is the Ambler classification that divides β-lactamases into **four classes (A, B, C and D)** based upon their amino acid sequences.
- Ambler originally specified two classes: class A, the active-site serine β-lactamases; and ***class B, the metallo-β-lactamases*** that require a bivalent metal ion, usually Zn^{2+}, for activity.
- ***NDM belongs to Ambler B class of carbapenemases***

"NDM-1 has now spread worldwide, and it is one of the most common carbapenemases in all *Enterobacteriaceae* and in ***A. baumannii****"- www.sciencedirect.com*

"Carbapenem-resistant **Citrobacter freundii** isolated in Spain from 2013 to 2015 produced a variety of carbapenemases including VIM-1, OXA-48, KPC-2, ***NDM-1*** and VIM-2"- www.ncbi.nlm.nih.gov

"The NDM-1 was found in many species of bacteria, predominantly ***K. pneumoniae*** **and** ***Escherichia coli,*** collected in an extended survey in the UK, India"- www.ncbi.nlm.nih.gov

"The NDM-1 enzyme was named after New Delhi, the capital city of India, as it was first described by Yong et al. in December 2009 in a Swedish national who fell ill with an antibiotic-resistant bacterial infection that he acquired in India.The infection was identified as a carbapenem-resistant ***Klebsiella pneumoniae*** strain bearing the novel gene bla_{NDM-1} "-*wiki*

"In July 2010, a team in New Delhi reported a cluster of three cases of ***Acinetobacter baumannii*** bearing bla_{NDM-1} that were found in the intensive care unit of a hospital in Chennai"-wiki

Table *(www.ncbi.nlm.nih.gov)*: **Initial reports of the NDM-1 and its variant**

Genotyping	Organism	Country	Travel and healthcare history
NDM-1	*K. pneumonia,* *E. coli*	India	Travelled to India and hospitalized in Ludhiana, Punjab and New Delhi
NDM-2	*A. baumannii*	Egypt	Transferred from a hospital in Egypt to Germany
NDM-3	*E. coli*	Australia	The patient returned from travel to India a few days earlier
NDM-4	*E. coli*	India	Previously hospitalized in India
NDM-5	*E. coli*	UK	A recent history of hospitalization in India
NDM-6	*E. coli*	New Zealand	NZ resident hospitalized in New Delhi With pneumonia

FORENSIC MEDICINE

115. Ans. a. Also k/a Fingerprint system, c. Almost reliable method for identification

[Ref: Parikh 7th/67-68; Reddy 34th/82-84; Pillay Forensic 18th/102]

"Rugoscopy: ***Palatal rugae*** *are as unique to each individual as are lips prints"- Pillay Forensic 18th/107*

Lip print (Cheiloscopy): *The fissures and grooves on the lips are claimed to be characteristic of the individual"- Reddy 34th/85*

Footprints (Podogram)

- *Reddy 34th/85*
- *The skin patterns of toes and heels are distinct and permanent as those of fingers*
- *Footprints of newborn infants are used to prevent exchange or substitution of infants*
- *Evidential value of footprint in criminology is less than that of fingerprints- Parikh 7th/70*

Dactylography

- *Reddy 34th/82-84; Parikh 7th/67-68*
- *Also k/a* ***Fingerprint system or Dermatoglyphics or Galton-Henry system***
- *The fingerprint patterns are distinctive and permanent in individuals*
- *The fingerprint system is the* ***only guide to identity, which is unfailing in practice***
- *They form patterns that are absolutely individual. They are not entirely alike, even identical twins- Parikh 7th/67*
- *Fingerprint pattern are classified on basis of arrangement of ridges into four main types- loops, whorls, arches and composite or compound*
- *Fingerprints can also be obtained even from putrefied bodies*

Dactylography: Classification

- *Reddy 33th/85-86*
- ***Loops:*** *Radial, ulnar*
- ***Whorls:*** *Concentric, spiral, double spiral, almond shaped*
- ***Arches:*** *Plain, tented, exceptional*
- ***Composite:*** *Central pocket loops, lateral pocket loops, twined loop, accidental*

116. Ans. a. Entry wound of rifled arms

[Ref: Parikh 7th/249-53; Reddy 34th/ 213-34;Forensic Anthropology by Steven Byers 4th/256]

Abrasion Collar (Marginal Abrasion)

- *Reddy 34th/ 214*
- *Abrasion collar surrounds the dirt collar.*
- The skin is abraded (***abrasion collar***) around bullet(***like of rifled arm***) hole due to rubbing of the gyrating body of bullet against the inverted epidermis and heat of the bullet
- *The abraded collar is reddish at first, but becomes reddish brown as it dries. Some contusion is present in abraded collar and as such, it is also called "contusion collar*
- *These two features are proof of an* ***entrance firearm wound***
- *Abrasion collar may be absent when the tissues are soft and yielding, e.g, in the abdomen or buttocks*

Smudge Ring/Lead Ring/Grease Collar/Dirt Collar

- *Parikh 7th/ 249-50; Reddy 34th/ 213*
- *This is* ***due to the wipe of the soft metal of the bullet****, or dirt present on it, or grease carried from the barrel and is deposited round the entrance wound internal to the abraded collar*
- *The smudge ring may therefore be absent when the jacketed bullet has passed through clothing*
- The smudging in case of lead shot or unjacketed bullets can be detected micro-chemically on the target (skin/cloth)
- The forensic value of bullet wipe is to establish a hole as a bullet hole, to determine the entry site, and on occasion the sequence of shots or bullet's passage through multiple objects

117. Ans. b. Cadaveric spasm, d. Cold stiffening, e. Heat stiffening

[Ref: Parikh 7th/147-49; Reddy 34th/ 152-54; Pillay Forensic 18th/155-57]

- *Primary relaxation of muscles occur only in rigor mortis(cadaveric rigidity). In all other options, muscles directly go into stiffening*

Rigor Mortis Pillay

- *Forensic 18th/155-57*
- *Death → Primary relaxation of muscles → Stiffening of muscle (Rigor mortis) → Secondary relaxation → Decomposition*
- Cadaveric spasm: *No primary flaccidity of muscle; muscles go into sudden state of stiffening. Usually seen in violent death associated with emotional disturbances at time of death, as in drowning, suicide by shooting*
- *Other conditions that result in the body becoming stiff after death include:*
  - *Heat stiffening:* Pugilistic attitude
  - *Cold stiffening*
  - *Putrefaction: Gas stiffening*

Rigor mortis (death stiffening; cadaveric rigidity) *is a state of stiffening of muscles, sometimes with slight shortening of the fibres- Reddy 34th/ 152*

Conditions Simulating Rigor

- *Reddy 34th/ 154; Parikh 7th/149*
- *Heat stiffening*
- *Cold stiffening*
- *Cadaveric spasm or Instantaneous rigor*
- *Putrefaction*

Livor mortis: This is bluish-purple or purplish-red discolouration- Reddy 34th/ 147

Algor mortis*- It is postmortem cooling of body- Reddy 34th/ 145*

118. Ans. a. Contains active principle ricin

[Ref: Parikh 7th/566-67; Reddy 34th/516]

Ricin *is active principle of Ricinus communis (castor plant, Arandi)- Reddy 34th/515*

Abrus Precatorius (Rati or Gunja or Indian liquorice)

◈ *Reddy 34th/516*

- *Seeds contain active principle* ***abrin. Also contains abrine*** *and abralin*
- ***Suis or needles*** *or sharp-pointed spikes; Used for killing cattle*
- ***Suis are fine needles prepared by decorticating the seeds, powdering and mixing with opium, onion, dhatura and spirit or water****- Parikh 7th/567*
- *Seeds are used for killing cattles*
- *Animal poisoning: The symptoms resemble those of viperine snake bite*
- *Seeds are used as an abortifacient*

119. Ans. b. Aconite, c. Sodium hydroxide, d. Sulfuric acid

[Ref: Reddy 33rd/124; Parikh 7th/108-09]

"In all cases of poisoning, ***inclusive of carbolic acid*** *but exclusive of other acids, saturated solution of common salt should be used"- Parikh 7th/108*

Sulphuric acid is a corrosive acid*- Reddy 33rd/530*

*"****Sodium hydroxide is an alkali****"- Reddy 33rd/536*

Preservatives

◈ *Reddy 33rd/124*

- Saturated **sodium chloride** solution, ***except in poisoning from corrosive acids, alkalis, corrosive sublimate*** **(mercuric chloride),** ***and aconite.***
- **Rectified spirit**, except in cases of suspected poisoning by (a) alcohol, kerosene, (b) chloroform, ether, (c) chloral hydrate, (d) formic acid, (e) formaldehyde, acetic acid, (f) phenol, (g) phosphorus, and h) paraldehyde, because the organic acids and paraldehyde are soluble in alcohol and the phosphorescence of phosphorus is diminished by alcohol.
- Ten. mg./ml of sodium or **potassium fluoride**. (prevents glycolysis, inhibits enzyme enolase and inhibits bacterial growth) and 3 mg. potassium oxalate (anti-coagulant) should be used for preserving blood.
- Fluoride should also be added to urine, CSF, and vitreous humour if alcohol estimation is required, and also to samples for analysis for cocaine, cyanide and CO.
- In poisoning by oxalic acid, ethylene glycol, fluoride and CO, 30 mg. sodium citrate should be added for 10 ml. of blood as preservative.
- One ml of concentrated hydrochloric acid or 100 mg. of thymol or 100 mg. of sodium fluoride can be used for 10 ml urine as a preservative. Toluene is better.
- Preservative is not necessary if (1) viscera can be analysed within 24 hours, (2) if sample can be kept in a refrigerator or ice box, (3) bone, hair, nails, (4) lung for detecting inhaled poisons.
- N.B. The viscera **should not be preserved in formaldehyde** because extraction of poison, especially non-volatile organic compounds becomes difficult

120. Ans. c. 13-14 yr, d. 14-15 yr, e. 15-16 yr

Radiology for Estimation of Age b/w 13 to 16 years: ***X-ray of elbow joint****- Reddy 34th/79*

Fusion of Bones/Joints in Male at 16 years: ***Elbow joint****- Reddy 34th/79*

Region *(Parikh 7th/62)*	Girls	Boys
Elbow	13-14	15-17
Wrist	16-17	18-19
Shoulder	17-18	19-20
Crest of ilium	18-19	20-21
Ischial tuberosity	21-22	23-24
Inner end of clavicle	21-22	23-24

121. Ans. a. Useful in dead person, c. Attrition of teeth is component, e. Used for age estimation

[Ref: Reddy 34th/67; Parikh 7th/60; V V Pillay 18th/87; Principles of Forensic Medicine and Toxicology By Rajesh Bardale 1st/64-65]

Disadvantage of gustafson's method: cannot be used in living person"- *www.ijahs.net*

Advantage of Gustafson's Method

◈ *Rajesh Bardale 1st/64*

- Useful in adult population
- Fairly reliable method

Disadvantage of Gustafson's Method

◈ *Rajesh Bardale 1st/64-65*

- ***It cannot be used in living person; only in dead when extraction of a tooth is allowed***
- Too many age related changes needed to be considered making the method time-consuming
- The assessment of the scores is the result of a subjective evaluation of the changes

Gustafson's Method

◈ *Parikh 7th/60, Reddy 34th/67*

- ***Age estimation of adult over 21 years*** depends on the physiological age changes in each of the dental tissues
- **Components includes**
  - Attrition (A)
  - Periodontosis (P)
  - Secondary dentine (S)
  - Cementum apposition (C)
  - Root resorption (R)
  - Transparency of the root (T)

Total score = A+P+S+C+R+T (a ranking scale 0–3 is given to each criteria)

Estimated age (years) = 11.43 + 4.56 × (Total score)

The transparency of root and secondary dentine have the highest correlation with age- *V V Pillay 18th/87*

The ***transparency of root is most reliable of all criteria****- Reddy 34th/69*

If the eruption order of teeth could help determine the age up to 25 years, Gustafson's method is helpful in determining the ages beyond 25 years- www.doctoralerts.com, *V V Pillay 18th/87*

122. Ans. a. Weight reduction, b. Low sodium diet, d. Regular exercise, e. Low fat diet

[Ref: Park 25th/406; Community Medicine by Piyush Gupta 1st/490]

Primary prevention: *Modify diet to* ***reduce salt intake*** *(less than 2000 mg of sodium or 5 grams of salt) as much as possible and* ***increase food intake of items rich in potassium****(at least 3510 mg of potassium/day)-Piyush Gupta 1st/490;*

Primary Prevention

- *Park 24th/394*
- Defined as: ***all measures to reduce the incidence of disease*** in a population by reducing the risk of onset
- In connection with primary prevention terms such as **population strategy and High-risk strategy** have become established. WHO has recommended these approaches in the prevention of hypertension. Both the approaches are complementary

Table *(Park 25th/406)*: **Lifestyle modifications to manage hypertension (HTN)**

Modification	Recommendation (Reduction Range)	Approximate systolic BP
Weight reduction	***Maintain normal body weight*** (BMI 18.5 – 24.9)	5-20 mm Hg/10 kg weight loss
Adopt DASH (Dietary approaches to stop HTN) eating plan	Consume a diet rich in fruits, vegetables and ***low-fat dairy products*** with a reduced content of saturated fat and total fat	8-14 mm Hg
Dietary sodium reduction	***Reduce dietary sodium intake*** to no more than 100 mEq/d (2.4 g sodium or 6 g sodium chloride)	2-8 mm Hg
Physical activity	Engage in regular aerobic physical activity such as brisk walking (at least 30 minutes per day, most days of the week)	4-9 mm Hg
Moderation of alcohol consumption	Limit consumption to no more than two drinks per day in most men and no more than one drink per day in women and lighter width persons	2-4 mm Hg

123. Ans. a. Azithromycin, c. Cefixime

[Ref: Park 25th/472; Community Medicine with recent Advances by Suryakantha 4th/494]

Pre-Packed STI/RTI Color Coded Kits

- *These kits are provided for free supply to all designated STI/RTI clinics*
- *They procured centrally and supplied to all states AIDS control societies*

Table *(Suryakantha 4th/494)*: **Seven Pre-packed kit**

Kit No.	Syndrome	Color	Contents
Kit 1	UD (Urethral discharge)ARD (Anorectal discharge), Cervicitis	Gray	Tab. ***Azithromycin 1 G (1) and Tab. Cefixime 400 mg (1)***
Kit 2	Vaginitis	Green	Tab. Secnidazole 2 g (1) and Tab. Fluconazole 150 mg (1)
Kit 3	GUD (Genital ulcer disease Non herpetic	White	Inj. Benzathine penicillin 2.4 MU (1) and Tab. Azithromycin 1 g(1) and Disposable syringe 10 mL with 21 gauge needle (1) and sterile water 10 mL (1)
Kit 4	GUD (Genital ulcer disease Non herpetic	Blue	Tab. ***Doxycycline*** 100 mg (30) and Tab. Azithromycin 1 g (1)
Kit 5	GUD (Genital ulcer disease Non herpetic	Red	Tab. Acyclovir 400 mg (21)
Kit 6	LAP (Lower abdominal pain)	Yellow	Tab. Cefixime 400 mg (1) and Tab. Metronidazole 400 mg (28) and Cap. Doxycycline 100 mg (42) and Tab Azithromycin 1 g (1)
Kit 7	IB (Inguinal bubo)	Black	Tab. Doxycycline 100 mg (42) and tab Azithromycin 1 g (1)

124. Ans. a. Active case finding, c. Focus to improve outcome of TB care in the private sector, d. To achieve 90% success rate for all new cases and 85% for retreatment cases, e. Involvement of NGOs

[Ref: Park 25th/457-64; Community Medicine by Piyush Gupta 1st/826-30; Community Medicine with recent Advances by Suryakantha 4th/921-23]

Newer Initiatives

◈ *Park 25th/461*

- ***Daily regimen for all forms of TB in country***
- Daily regimen for paediatric TB
- Campaign mode: ***Active case finding***
- Bedaquiline conditional access programme
- Pilots for universal access to TB cases

New Initiatives

◈ *Park 25th/460*

- *NIKSHAY*
- *TB notification*
- *Ban on TB serology*
- *Direct benefit transfer schemes*

National Strategic Plan (2017-25) for TB Elimination: Key Strategies

◈ *Park 25th/464*

- ***Private sector engagement***
- ***Active case finding***
- *Community engagement and multisectoral approach*

RNTCP Under 12th 5-year Plan (2012-17)

◈ *Piyush Gupta 1st/829*

- ***To achieve 90% success rate for all new cases and 85% for retreatment cases***
- ***To improve outcome of TB care in the private sector***

Revised National Tuberculosis Control Programme (RNTCP)

◈ *Park 24th/427*

The government of India, WHO and World Bank together reviewed the NTP (Operated since 1962) in the year 1992

The salient features are:

- Achievement of ***at least 85% cure rate*** of infectious cases through the supervised short course chemotherapy involving peripheral health functionaries.
- Augmentation of ***case finding activities*** through high quality sputum microcopy to detect at ***least 70%*** estimated cases.
- Involvement of ***NGOs***, information, education and communication and improved operational research. • Direct observed therapy short-term (DOTS)- a community based TB treatment and care strategy

Note:

- ***The RNTCP covers the whole country since March 2006***
- ***DOTS-Plus is a strategy under development for the management of multi-drug resistant TB (MDR-TB)***
- *The first phase of the World Bank assisted RNTCP ended on 30th Sept. 2006. The second phase of the project has started on 1st Oct. 2006 for a further period of 5 years*

125. Ans. a. Number of new cases, d. Used as tool for measurement of morbidity

[Ref: Park 25th/68; Community Medicine by Piyush Gupta 1st/27; Community Medicine with recent Advances by Suryakantha 4th/]

Measurement of morbidity: Three aspects of morbidity are commonly measured by morbidity rates or morbidity ratios, namely frequency, duration and severity. ***Disease frequency is measured by incidence*** and prevalence rates"-Park 25th/68

Incidence

◈ *Park 25th/68*

- *Incidence measures the rate at which **new cases** are occurring in a population. It is **not influenced by the duration of disease***
- *The use of incidence is **generally restricted to acute conditions***
- *Incidence rate refers to*
  - ***Only to new cases***
  - ***During a given period** (usually one year)*
- *Use: Useful for taking action*
  - *To control disease*
  - *For research into aetiology and pathogenesis, distribution of disease and efficacy of preventive and therapeutic measures*

Table *(Piyush Gupta 1st/27)*: **Comparison of incidence and prevalence rate**

Incidence	Prevalence
• Includes new cases only	• Includes both new and old cases
• It is a direct measure of risk	• Does not necessarily signify high risk
• Estimation requires exact knowledge of time of onset of disease	• Such knowledge is not required
• Mainly used for etiological studies of both acute and Chronis diseases	• Mainly used for studying the magnitude of the disease in community
• Estimation by longitudinal studies	• Estimation by cross sectional studies

126. Ans. b. Suitable for study of rare disease

[Ref: Park 25th/79-82; Community Medicine by Piyush Gupta 1st/585]

Case Control Study

◈ *Park 25th/79,82*

- ***Case control studies, often called retrospective studies:** No attrition problems, because case control studies **do not require follow-up** of individual into the future*
- *Generally yields only **estimate of relative risk (odd ratio)***
- ***Suitable for study of rare disease***
- ***Rapid and inexpensive (compared with cohort studies)***
- ***Yiels relatively quick results**- Park 25th/87*

Characteristics	Cohort studies	Case Control Studies	Cross Sectional Studies
Design	Prospective	***Retrospective***	One point in time
Incidence Rate	Estimated	***Not Estimated***	Not Estimated

Contd...

Characteristics	Cohort studies	Case Control Studies	Cross Sectional Studies
Prevalence Rate	Not Estimated	Not Estimated	Estimated
Causality	May be estimated	May be estimated	Not estimated
Calculations	Incidence Rates Relative Risk Attributable risk	Odds Ratio (This gives on estimate of relative risk)	

127. Ans. e. Scabies

[Ref: Park 25th/299,268]

For **scabies,** ***mass prophylaxis is not required*** *(only treatment of family members/close contact is required)*

Lymphatic Filariasis

- Large scale treatment involves a single dose of 2 medicines (albendazole andivermectin/ diethylcarbamazine) given annually to an entire at-risk population- *Park 25th/299*
- DEC medicated salt: special form of mass treatment- *Park 25th/300*

Deworming (To control helminthic infection*)***:** WHO recommends ***periodic deworming*** without previous individual diagnosis to all at-risk people living in endemic areas- *Park 25th/268*

Trachoma: A prevalence of more than 5% severe and moderate trachoma in children under 10 years is an indication for ***mass or blanket treatment*** *-Park 25th/337*

"**National programme for prevention of nutritional blindness**: Administration of massive dose of Vitamin A ***up to five years.*** First dose of 100000 IU with measles vaccination at nine monthsand subsequent doses of 200000 IU each, every six months up to age of 5 years"- *Park 25th/337*

128. Ans. c. Public health and sanitation; hospitals and dispensaries, e. Land revenue

[Ref: www.constitution.org; indiankanoon.org]

Option (a): ***Port quarantine, including hospitals connected therewith; seamen's and marine hospitals (Union list)***

Option (b): ***Education, including technical education, medical education and universities, subject to the provisions of entries 63, 64, 65 and 66 of List I; vocational and technical training of labour (Concurrent list)***

Option (c): ***Public health and sanitation; hospitals and dispensaries (State list)***

Option (d): ***Adulteration of foodstuffs and other goods (Concurrent list)***

Option (e): ***Land revenue***, including the assessment and collection of revenue, the maintenance of land records, survey for revenue purposes and records of rights, and alienation of revenues.**(State list)**

Article 246 in The Constitution Of India indiankanoon.org

246. Subject matter of laws made by Parliament and by the Legislatures of States

- **(1)** Notwithstanding anything in clauses (2) and (3), Parliament has exclusive power to make laws with respect to any of the matters enumerated in List I in the Seventh Schedule (in this Constitution referred to as the **Union List**)
- **(2)** Notwithstanding anything in clause (3), Parliament, and, subject to clause (1), the Legislature of any State also, have power to make laws with respect to any of the matters enumerated in List III in the Seventh Schedule (in this Constitution referred to as the **Concurrent List**)
- **(3)** Subject to clauses (1) and (2), the Legislature of any State has exclusive power to make laws for such State or any part thereof with respect to any of the matters enumerated in List II in the Seventh Schedule (in this Constitution referred to as the "**State List**")
- **(4)** Parliament has power to make laws with respect to any matter for any part of the territory of India not included (in a State) notwithstanding that such matter is a matter enumerated in the State List
- The legislative powers revolve around the scheme of distribution of powers between the union and state legislature which is provided in the three lists under the 7th schedule of the constitution which entails.

129. Ans. a. Sensitivity, b. Specificity, c. Positive predictive value (PPV), d. Negative predictive value (NPV)

[Ref: Park 25th/148-52; Community Medicine by Piyush Gupta 1st/593]

- *Although positive predictive is mainly dependent on prevalence of a disease but prevalence cannot be calculated from a screening test*
- *All others given in option can be calculated from screening test*

Table *(Park 24th/149)*: **Screening test result by diagnosis**

Screening test result	Diagnosis		Total
	Disease	Not disease	
Positive	A (true positive)	B (False positive)	A + B
Negative	C (False Negative)	D (True negative)	C + D)
Total	A + C B + D	D (True negative)	A + B + C+ D

Sensitivity = A/(A+C) X 100
Specificity = D/(B+D) X 100
Predictive value of positive test = A/(A+B) X 100
Predictive value of negative test = D/(C+D) X 100
Percentage of false negative = C/(A+C) X 100
Percentage of false positive = B/(B+D) X 100

Sensitivity

◈ *Park 24th/149*

- The term **sensitivity** was introduced by Yerushalmy in 1940s as a statistical index of diagnostic accuracy. It has been defined as the ability of a test to identify correctly all those who have the disease, that is "true-positive".

- A 90 per cent of the diseased people screened by the test will give a "true-positive" result and the remaining 10 per cent a "false-negative" result.
- *"An ideal screening test should be both 100 percent sensitive and 100 percent specific. Practically, this is never the case"- Piyush Gupta 1st/593*

Specificity

◈ *Park 24th/149*

- It is defined as the ability of a test to identify correctly those who do not have the disease, that is, "true-negatives".
- A 90 per cent specificity means that 90 per cent of the non-diseased persons will give "true-negative" result, 10 per cent of non-diseased people screened by the test will be wrongly classified as "diseased" when they are not.

130. Ans. d. Kills 100% bacteria

[Ref: Park 25th/711-12; Community Medicine with Recent Advances by Suryakantha 4th/186]

Test of Pasteurized Milk

◈ *Park 25th/712; Suryakantha 4th/186*

Phosphatase test: This test is widely used to check the efficiency of pasteurization. This test is based on the fact that raw milk contains an enzyme called phosphatase which is destroyed on heating at a temperature which corresponds closely with the standard time and temperature required for pasteurization

Standard plate count: The bacteriolocial quality of pasteurized milk is determined by the standard plate count. Most countries in the west enforce a ***limit of 30,000 bacterial count per ml*** of pasteurized milk

Coliform count: Coliform organism is usually completely destroyed by pasteurization

Methylene blue test: Indirect method to detect microorganism in milk

Pasteurization of Milk

◈ *Park 25th/711*

- It kills nearly 90% of the bacteria in milk including the more heat-resistant tubercle bacillus and the Q fever organisms. But it will not kill thermoduric bacteria nor the bacterial spores
- **Three methods are commonly used for pasteurization**
  - Holder (Vat method)
  - High temperature and short time method (HTST)
  - Ultra high temperature: Milk is heated in usually 2 stages (the second stage usually being under pressure) to 125 °C for a few seconds. It is then rapidly cooled and bottled as quickly as possible

131. Ans. a. Chloride 200 mg/litre, b. pH 6.5-8.5/ litre

[Ref: Park 25th/779-81;Piyush Gupta 1st/88]

"**Chloride**: *The standard prescribed for chloride is 200 mg/litre. The maximum permissible limit is 600mg/litre"- Park 25th/779*

*"**pH:** An acceptable pH of drinking water is b/w 6.5 and 8.5"- Park 25th/780*

*"**Iron:** At level above 0.3 mg/litre, iron stains laundry and plumbing fixtures"- Park 25th/780*

*"**Manganese:** Mn concentration below 0.1 mg/litre are usually acceptable to consumers"- Park 25th/780*

Guidelines for Drinking Water

◈ *Park 25th/779-81; Piyush Gupta 1st/88*

- **Colour< 15 true colour units (TCU)**
- **Turbidity < 1 nephlometric turbidity units (NTU)**
- Hardness < 100 – 300 mg/litre calcium ion
- ***pH: 6.5 – 8.5***
- Total dissolved solids (TDS) < 600 mg/liter
- **Chloride 200 – 600 mg/L**
- H_2S < 0.05 mg/L
- ***Iron < 0.3 mg/L***
- Sodium < 200 mg/L
- Sulphate< 250 mg/L
- **Zinc < 4 mg/L**
- **Manganess – 0.1 mg/liter**
- **NH3 < 1.50 mg/L**
- **Fluorine < 1.5 ppm (0.5 – 0.8 ppm: Optimum level)**
- **Nitrates < 50 mg/liter**
- **Nitrites < 3 mg/liter**
- Gross alpha radiological activity < 0.5 Bq/liter
- Gross beta radiological activity < 1.0 Bq/liter
- Zero pathogenic microorganisms
- Zero infectious viruses
- Absence of pathogenic protozoa and infective stages of helminthes
- **Dissolved O_2 has indirect effect, level is not specified**
- Nitrite in water indicates recent contamination, whereas nitrate indicates past (remote) contamination

OPHTHALMOLOGY

132. Ans. a. Senile cataract, c. Pterygium, d. Diabetic retinopathy

[Ref: A.K.Khurana 7th/514]

Gradual Painless Defective Vision

◈ *A.K.Khurana 7th/514*

- Progressive ***pterygium*** involving pupillary area
- Corneal degenerations
- Corneal dystrophies
- Developmental cataract
- ***Senile cataract***
- Optic atrophy
- Chorioretinal degenerations
- Age-related macular degeneration
- ***Diabetic retinopathy***
- Refractive errors

Sudden Painless Loss of Vision

◈ *A.K. Khurana 7th/514*

- Central retinal artery occlusion
- Massive vitreous haemorrhage
- Retinal detachment involving macular area
- Ischacmic central retinal vein occlusion

Sudden Painless Onset of Defective Vision

- *A.K.Khurana 7th/514*
- Central serous retinopathy
- ***Optic neuritis***
- Methyl alcohol amblyopia
- Non-ischacmic central retinal vein occlusion

Sudden Painful Loss of Vision

- *A.K.Khurana 7th/514*
- Acute congestive glaucoma
- ***Acute iridocyclitis***
- Chemical injuries to the eyeball
- Mechanical injuries to the eyeball

Gradual Painful Defective Vision

- *A.K.Khurana 7th/514*
- ***Chronic iridocyclitis***
- Corneal ulceration
- Chronic simple glaucoma

133. Ans. a. More common on temporal side

[Ref: A.K.Khurana 7th/89-90; Parson 22nd/184-85; Oxford Handbook of Ophthalmology 3rd/207]

Pterygium

- *A.K.Khurana 7th/89-90*
- Pterygium (L. Pterygion = a wing) is a ***wing-shaped fold of conjunctiva*** encroaching upon the cornea from either side within the interpalpebral fissure.
- Etiology of pterygium is not definitely known. But the disease is ***more common in people living in hot climates.*** Therefore, the most accepted view is that it is a response to prolonged effect of environmental factors such as exposure to sun (ultraviolet rays), dry heat, high wind and abundance of dust.
- It is ***common in tropical region***-www.up todate.com
- Pathologically pterygium is a degenerative and hyperplastic condition of conjunctiva. The subconjunctival tissue undergoes elastotic degeneration and proliferates as vascularized granulation tissue under the epithelium, which ***ultimately encroaches the cornea.*** The corneal epithelium, Bowman's layer and superficial stroma are destroyed.
- Pterygium is ***more common in elderly males*** doing outdoor work. It may be unilateral or bilateral.
- It presents as a triangular fold of conjunctiva encroaching the cornea in the area of palpebral aperture, ***usually on the nasal side***, but ***may also occur on the temporal side.***
- Deposition of iron seen sometimes in corneal epithelium anterior to advancing head of pterygium is called ***stocker's line.***
- ***Parts:*** Three parts
    - *Head* (apical part present on the cornea),
    - *Neck* (limbal part), and
    - *Body* (scleral part) extending between limbus and the canthus.
- ***Types:*** Depending upon the progression it may be progressive or regressive pterygium.
- *Progressive pterygium* is thick, fleshy and vascular with a few infiltrates in the cornea, in front of the head of the pterygium (called cap of pterygium).
- *Regressive pterygium* is thin, atrophic, attenuated with very little vascularity. There is no cap. Ultimately it becomes membranous but never disappears.
- Pterygium is an asymptomatic condition in the early stages, except for *cosmetic intolerance.*
- ***Visual disturbances*** occur when it ***encroaches the pupillary area or due to corneal astigmatism*** induced due to fibrosis in the regressive stage.
- Occasionally *diplopia* may occur due to limitation of ocular movements.
- ***Complications*** like cystic degeneration and infection are infrequent. Rarely, neoplastic change to epithelioma, fibrosarcoma or malignant melanoma, may occur.

134. Ans. b. Internal carotid artery, c. Anterior cerebral artery

[Ref: Gray's 40th/253; Oxford Handbook of Ophthalmology 3rd/652; Review of Ophthalmology by William B. Trattler 2nd/49,51]

"The blood supplies of the optic chiasma, tract and radiation are of considerable clinical importance. The **chiasma** is supplied in part by the ***anterior cerebral arteries*** but its median zone depends upon rami from the ***internal carotid arteries*** reaching it via the stalk of the hypophysis. The anterior choroidal and posterior communicating arteries supply the **optic tract, and the optic radiation** receives blood through deep branches of the *middle and posterior cerebral arteries*"-*Gray's 40th/253*

Optic Chiasm

- *Trattler 2nd/49*
- 10 mm above pituitary gland
- ***55% of optic nerve fibers cross in chiasm:*** nasal retinal fibers cross in chiasm to contralateral optic tract (decussating nasal fibers); temporal fibers remain uncrossed; macular fibers run posteriorly (posterior compression leads to bitemporal defect)
- ***Blood supply: ICA; occasionally by anterior cerebral and anterior communicating arteries***

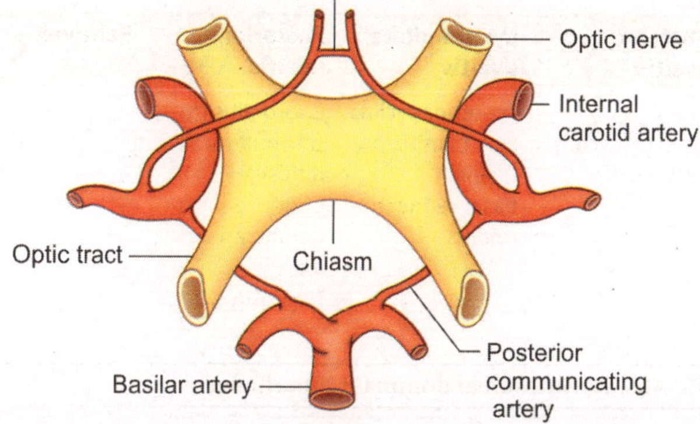

Fig: *(Trattler 2nd/51):* Relationship of the optic chiasm, optic nerves, and optic tracts to the arterial circle of Willis. The chiasm passes through the circle of Willis and receives its arterial supply from the anterior cerebral and communicating arteries from above, and the posterior communicating, posterior cerebral, and basilar arteries from below

135. Ans. a. It is part of anterior uveitis, c. Keratic precipitates may be found, d. Steroids are used for treatment, e. May be associated with ankylosing spondylitis

[Ref: A.K.Khurana 7th/158-65; Parson 22nd/237-38; Oxford Handbook of Ophthalmology 3rd/422-26]

Anterior Uveitis: Depending upon clinical presentation, it can be categorized into iritis, cyclitis or iridocyclitis- *Parson 22nd/235; Oxford Handbook of Ophthalmology 3rd/410*

Ankylosing spondylitis: Acute, recurrent iridocyclitis is part of the syndrome (25% of patients)- *Parson 22nd/250*

Corticosteroids, administered locally, are very effective in cases of iridocyclitis. When administered systemically they have a definite role in non-granulomatous iridocyclitis- *A.K.Khurana 7th/165*

Chronic Iridocyclitis

◈ *Parson 22nd/238*

- The ***keratic precipitates***, which may be the only obviousevidence of the disease, are sometimes scattered over a triangulararea in the lower pan of the cornea (***Arlt triangle***),due to convection currents in the aqueous and gravitationof the particles towards the bottom of the anterior chamber
- After many years, the eye may finally become soft and tender and enter into the condition of ***phthisis bulbi.***
- An important and not uncommon complication is a rise of intraocular pressure in the course of the disease to constitute the clinical syndrome of ***hypertensive iridocyclitic crisis***
- *"Granulomatous iridocyclitis: It* is characterized by the presenceof large, greasy ***'mutton fat' keratic precipitates***, which are deposits of white bloodcells (mainly lymphocytes) derived from the aqueous,on the corneal endothelium and dense posterior synechiaewith clusters of inflammatory cells on the pupillary border Koeppe nodules or on theperipheral part of the anterior surface of the iris (***Busacca nodules***)"- *Parson 22nd/233*

Table *(Parson 22nd/233)*: **Classification of uveitis Based on predominant anatomical site affected**

Anterior uveitis	Intermediate uveitis	Posterior uveitis	Panuveitis
Iritis Anterior cyclitis Iridocyclitis	Posterior cyclitis Pars planitis Hyalitis Basal retinochoroiditis	Choroiditis (focal/multifocal/diffuse) Chorioretinitis Retinochoroiditis Neuro-uveitis	-

136. Ans. c. Autosomal dominant inheritance

[Ref: A.K.Khurana 7th/138-39; Parson 22nd/194-95; Review of Ophthalmology by William B. Trattler 2nd/215]

Macular Corneal Opacity

◈ *Trattler 2nd/215*

- ***AR inheritance***; Mapped to chromosome 16q22
- ***Bilateral(often asymmetric)***-Oxford Opthalmology 3rd/272
- Error in synthesis of keratan sulfate
- ***Most severe*** but least common of the 3 classic stromal dystrophies
- Deposits present in 1st decade of life
- **Symptoms: *Decreased vision*** in 1st–2nd decade of life
- **Findings:** gray-white stromal opacities at all levels extending to periphery with diffuse clouding (no intervening clear spaces), central thinning; may have guttata
- **Pathology:** Mucopolysaccharide deposits, stain with Alcian blue and colloidal iron
- **Treatment: *Penetrating keratoplasty;*** PTK (less useful, lesions extend though entire stroma and erosions rare

Corneal Opacities

◈ *A.K.Khurana 7th/138-39*

Causes

- Congenital opacities may occur as developmental anomalies or following birth trauma.
- Healed corneal wounds.
- Healed corneal ulcers.

Clinical features: A corneal opacity may produce loss of vision (when dense opacity covers the pupillary area) or blurred vision (due to astigmatic effect)

Types of corneal opacity: Depending on the density, corneal opacity is graded as nebula, macula and leucoma.

- *Nebular corneal opacity*
- *Macular corneal opacity.* It is a semi-dense opacity produced when scarring involves about half the corneal stroma
- *Leucomatous corneal opacity* (leucoma simplex)
- *Adherent leucoma*
- *Corneal facet*
- *Kerectasia*
- *Anterior staphyloma*

Secondary changes in corneal opacitywhich may be seen in long-standing cases include: hyaline degeneration, calcareous degeneration, pigmentation and atheromatous ulceration.

Treatment

- *Optical iridectomy*
- *Keratoplasty provides good visual results* in uncomplicated cases with corneal opacities, where optical iridectomy is not of much use.
- *Phototherapeutic keratectomy* (PTK)
- *Cosmetic coloured contact lens*
- *Tattooing of scar*

137. Ans. b. Kayser-Fleischer ring in cornea, d. Sunflower cataract

[Ref: A.K.Khurana 7th/200; Parson 22nd/214;Review of Ophthalmology by William B. Trattler 2nd/207]

"**Arcus senilis** refers to an annular lipid infiltration of corneal periphery. This is an age-related change occurring bilaterally in 60 percent of patients between 40 and 60 years of age and in nearly all patients over the age of 80. The ring of opacity is about 1-mm wide and is separated from the limbus by a clear zone (lucid interval of Vogt)"-*A.K.Khurana 7th/126; Parson 22nd/214*

Cataract Due to Error of Copper Metabolism

◈ *A.K.Khurana 7th/200*

- Inborn error of copper metabolism results in Wilson's disease (***hepatolenticular degeneration***).
- The green *'sunflower cataract'* may be observed rarely in such patients.
- The more commonly observed ocular feature of Wilson's disease is '***Kayser-Fleischer ring' (KF ring) in the cornea***

Wilson's Disease (Hepatolenticular Degeneration)

◈ *Trattler 2nd/207*

- Increased copper levels due to deficiency in ceruloplasmin
- Copper deposition in ***Eye: Kayser-Fleischer ring*** (copper deposition in peripheral Descemet's; starts superiorly, then inferiorly, medially, and temporally); ***sunflower cataract***
- **Treatment:** Oral tetrathiomolybdate (penicillamine), followed by oral zinc maintenance; Kayser Fleischer rings resolve with adequate treatment

Lines & Rings in Ophthalmology

◈ *www.slideshare.net*

- Arlt's Line = conjunctival scar in sulcus subtarsalis in Trachoma.
- Ehrlich-Turck Line = linear deposition of KPs in uveitis
- **Ferry's Line** = corneal epithelial iron line at the edge of filtering blebs.
- Hudson-Stahil Line= Horizonatl corneal epithelial iron line at the inferior one third of cornea due to aging.
- Khodadoust Line = corneal graft endothelial rejection line composed of inflammatory cells.
- Paton's Line = Circumferential retinal folds due to optic nerve edema.
- Sampaoelesi line = Increased pigmentation anterior to Schwalbe's line in pseudoexfoliation syndrome.
- Zentmeyer line (Scheie's Line): on the equatorial surface of the lens pigment dispersion syndrome
- Schwalbe's Line = Angle structure representing peripheral edge of Descemets membrane.
- **Stockers Line** = Corneal epithelial iron line at the edge of pterygium
- White lines of Vogt = Sheathed or sclerosed vessels seen in Lattice degeneration
- Fingerprint lines: The map-dot fingerprint dystrophy

138. Ans. c. Sulfite oxidase deficiency, d. Homocystinuria, e. Ehlers-Danlos syndrome

[Ref: A.K.Khurana 7th/222-23; Parson 22nd/275]

Displacement of the Lens

◈ *A.K.Khurana 7th/222-23*

Displacement of the lens from its normal position (in patellar fossa) results from partial or complete rupture of the lens zonules.

Clinico-Etiological Types

- **Congenital displacements**
  - ***Simple ectopialentis***
  - ***Ectopialentis et pupillae***
  - ***Ectopialentis with systemic anomalies***
- ***Marfan's syndrome.*** It is an autosomal dominant mesodermal dysplasia. In this condition lens is displaced upwards and temporally (bilaterally symmetrical)
- ***Homocystinuria.*** It is an autosomal recessive, inborn error of metabolism. In it the lens is usually subluxated downwards and nasally.
- ***Weil-Marchesani syndrome***
- ***Ehlers-Danlos syndrome.*** In it the *ocular features* are subluxation of lens and blue sclera.
- ***Hyperlysinaemia***
- ***Stickler syndrome***
- ***Sulphite oxidase deficiency.*** It is a very rare autosomal recessive disorder of sulphur metabolism.

139. Ans. a. Fluorescein stain, b. Rose Bengal, d. Lissamine green

[Ref: Khurana 6th/517-18; Parson 22nd/142-43;catalog.hardydiagnostics.com;medlineplus.gov]

Corneal staining (Dye used): ***Fluorescein, rose Bengal and lissamine green***"-www.sciencedirect.com

"**India Ink** is recommended for use in the identification of ***Cryptococcus neoformans***" *-catalog.hardydiagnostics.com*

"**Masson's trichrome is a three-colour** staining **protocol used in** histology. It is used for distinguishing cells **from surrounding** connective tissue. Most recipes produce red keratin **and** muscle fibers, blue or green ***collagen*** and bone, light red or pink cytoplasm, and dark brown to black cell nuclei."-wikipedia

Fluorescein eye stain: This is a test that uses orange dye (fluorescein) and a blue light to detect foreign bodies in the eye. This test can also ***detect damage to the cornea***. The cornea is the outer surface of the eye"- *medlineplus.gov; www.jcor.in/article.as*

"**Rose Bengal:** Rose bengal is actually a derivative of fluorescein. It's been used for the evaluation of numerous other ocular pathologies including herpetic ***corneal epithelial dendrites, superficial punctate keratitis***, and dysplastic or squamous metaplastic cells of conjunctival squamous neoplasms"- www.jcor.in

140. Ans. b. Neuroretinitis, c. Papilitis, d. Retrobulbar neuritis

[Ref: A.K.Khurana 7th/281-85; Parson 22nd/311-12; Oxford Handbook of Ophthalmology 3rd/564-65]

Retinal microaneurysm may occur in diabetes & in *chronic hypertension*"- *Oxford Handbook of Ophthalmology 3rd/564*

Hypertension retinopathy is associated with focal attenuation of a major retinal arteriole is one the earliest sign. Diffuse arteriolar attenuation, broadening of the arteriolar light reflex & arteriovenous crossing changes may also occur- *A.K.Khurana 7th/281*

"Optic neuropathy **is damage to the optic nerve from any cause. Damage and death of these nerve cells, or neurons, leads to characteristic features of optic neuropathy"**- *A.K.Khurana 7th/432*

Optic Neuritis

◈ *A.K.Khurana 7th/330*

Can be classified into three anatomical types:

- ***Papillitis.*** It refers to involvement of the optic disc in inflammatory and demyelinating disorders. This condition is usually unilateral but sometimes may be bilateral.

- ***Neuroretinitis*** refers to combined involvement of optic disc and surrounding retina in the macular area.
- ***Retrobulbar neuritis*** is characterized by involvement of optic nerve behind the eyeball.

141. Ans. a. Posterior polar cataract

[Ref: www.ncbi.nlm.nih.gov; bjo.bmj.com]

Nuclear Drop

◈ *Www.ncbi.nlm.nih.gov*

- Nuclear drop or dropped lens is a complication of cataract surgery.
- During cataract surgery there may be tear in posterior capsule causing dropping of lens in vitreous
- ***"The importance of posterior polar cataract lies in its higher risk of complications - posterior capsular tear and possible nucleus drop during surgery".***

Nuclear Drop

◈ *Bjo.bmj.com*

- Dislocation of the lens nucleus into the vitreous cavity is one of the most severe complications in cataract surgery.
- Incidence of nucleus drop into the vitreous cavity for phacoemulsification surgery varies between 0.3% and 1.1% depending on the surgeon's experience.1–3 Retained nuclear material in the vitreous cavity can lead to severe complications like severe inflammation, intraocular pressure increase, cystoid macular oedema and retinal detachment.
- **Risk factors for dropped nuclear** fragments include: inexperienced surgeon, advanced age, undilated pupil, increased axial length, ***posterior polar cataract***, hollow orbit, pseudoexfoliation, previous trauma and previous vitrectomy surgery

142. Ans. a. Outward deviation of eye, d. Diplopia may occur, e. Sometimes a/w amblyopia

[Ref: A.K.Khurana 7th/363-64; Oxford Handbook of Ophthalmology 3rd/750-51; Yanoff 2014/156]

- **Hypertropia:** There is no association with exotropia
- **Strabismus:** Inward deviation (esotropia) or outward deviation (exotropia) or vertical deviation (hypertropia)

Exotropia (**Divergent strabismus, external strabismus, "walleye"**) *Yanoff 2014/156*

Definition

Strabismus in which manifest deviation of the visual axis of one eye occurs away from that of the other eye, resulting in ***diplopia.***

Symptoms

- Asthenopia (headaches, irritability, visual discomfort): with onset of strabismus
- *Probable loss of stereoscopic ability*: when strabismic
- Possible cosmetic deformity
- Children less than 7–9 years of age who are binocular will develop sensory adaptations of suppression and anomalous retinal correspondence. They will also be asymptomatic.
- Children less than 7–9 years of age who are binocular will develop diplopia and visual confusion.

Signs

- *Intermittent or constant outward deviation of the visual axes*: especially when tired or ill
- *Squinting or rubbing of one or both eyes*: especially in bright sunlight.

Complications

- ***Amblyopia:*** If exotropia is not alternating and age of onset is less than 5 years
- Probable loss of stereoptic ability while eyes are strabismic
- **Cosmetic deformity**

143. Ans. e. B12

[Ref: Harrison 19th/197 www.medmerits.com/index.php; doctorsjunction.blogspot.in]

"**Centrocecal or cecocentral scotoma**: Field defect involving both the macula and the blind spot; seen in optic nerve disease, such as Leber's hereditary optic neuropathy, toxic or ***nutritional optic neuropathies*** (said to be typical of ***vitamin B12 deficiency optic neuropathy***), sometimes in optic neuritis" *(doctorsjunction. blogspot.in)*

Ophthalmologic Manifestations

◈ *www.medmerits.com/index*

- An unusual but well-documented manifestation of ***cobalamin deficiency is optic neuropathy***. This may present as a sub acutely progressive decrease in visual acuity with a ***cecocentral scotoma*** (i.e., a scotoma obscuring central vision and enlarging the blind spot).
- The condition known as tobacco-ethanol amblyopia is similar, and may, at least in part, depend on cobalamin deficiency.

ENT

144. Ans. b. Spread of infection to parapharyngeal and retropharyngeal space, c. Tongue is pushed upward, d. Presents with painful neck swelling below the mandible, e. Inflammation of floor of mouth

[Ref: Dhingra 7th/297-98; Logan and Turner 10th / 264-65; ENT by Hazarika3rd/497-98; Ballenger H and NSurgery 16th/1039]

Ludwig Angina

◈ *Dhingra 7th/297-98; ENT by Hazarika3rd/497-98*

- It is infection of submandibular space.
- Submandibular space consists of two compartment: Sub-lingual compartment (above mylohyoid) and submaxillary and submental compartment (above mylohyoid)
- ***Unlike other neck infection where the abscess formation is the rule,*** here in Ludwig's angina, it has characteristic cellulitis without lymphatic involvement causing massive swelling of the tongue and floor of the mouth- *ENT by Hazarika3rd/497*
- ***Usually there is cellulitis of the tissue rather than frank abscess****-Dhingra 7th/298*
- ***Tongue is progressively pushed upwards and backwards*** threatening the airway

- ***Presents with painful neck swelling in the region below the mandible***
- Complication: ***Spread of infection to parapharyngealand retropharyngeal space***
- Treatment- Surgical drainage: ***Pus is often not seen*** as seen in other abscess rather edematous fluid collection may be drained

145. Ans. a. Palatal palsy, b. Conductive deafness, d. Temporoparietal neuralgia

[Ref: Dhingra 7th/ 285,511; ENT by Hazarika3rd/527]

Trotter's Triad

◈ *Dhingra 7th/ 285*

- Occurs in nasopharyngeal cancer
- It includes *conductive deafness (eustachanian tube blockage), ipsilateral temporoparietal neuralgia (involvement of CN V) and palatal paralysis(CN X)*

Trotter's Triad: It consists of *simple-med.blogspot.com*

- *Unilateral conductive hearing loss (secretory otitis media).*
- *Ipsilateral earache and facial pain (trigeminal nerve).*
- *Ipsilateral paralysis of the soft palate.*

146. Ans. a. More common in diabetics, b. Pseudomonas is causative organism, c. Granulation tissue formation, d. May involve facial nerve

[Ref: Dhingra 7th/55; Current Diagnosis and Treatment in Otolaryngology 3rd/652]

Malignant Otitis Externa

◈ *Dhingra 7th/55*

- *Caused by pseudomonas infection usually in elderly diabetics*
- *Granulations in the ear canal*
- *Facial paralysis is common*

Malignant Otitis Externa (Necrotizingexternal Otitis)

◈ *Current Diagnosis and Treatment in Otolaryngology 3rd/652*

- Skull base osteomyelitis, also known as malignant otitis externa or necrotizing otitis externa (NOE), is a bacterial infection of the EAC and skull base.
- This disease process is most frequently seen in ***elderly diabetics*** and immunocompromised patients.
- It most commonly begins as an external otitis that progresses to involve the temporal bone, and may progress to fatal meningitis, sepsis, and death if unrecognized or untreated
- As this progresses along the base of the skull, the ***facial nerve*** (stylomastoid foramen), hypoglossal nerve (hypoglossal canal), the abducens and trigeminal nerves (petrous apex), the glossopharyngeal, vagus, and spinal accessory nerves (jugular foramen) may be involved.
- The ***most frequently isolated causative organism is P aeruginosa,*** which may exhibit high levels of antibiotic resistance. *Aspergillus* may also be an etiologic organism and is thought to originate from the middle ear or mastoid.
- **Elderly diabetics** are thought to be particularly susceptible because of the microangiopathic changes that blunt an already attenuated immune response.
- The cerumen of ***diabetic patients***has also been described to be more acidic in nature, further contributing to their susceptibility.
- Patients may present with ***intense otalgia, otorrhea, aural fullness, pruritus, and hearing loss.***
- As the disease advances to involve the temporal bone, granulation tissue is seen on the floor of the EAC at the osteocartilaginous junction. Bony sequestra can also be found in the EAC.
- Edema, periaural lymphadenopathy, and trismus may be present.
- Cranial neuropathies occur in more advanced presentations of disease, and the ***facial nerve is the most frequently affected cranial nerve***.
- Further progression may lead to sigmoid sinus thrombosis, meningitis, sepsis, and death.
- Long-term parenteral antibiotics are the treatment of choice

147. Ans. a. Supraglottic cancer is most common variety

[Ref: Dhingra 7th/352,347; Ballenger H and N Surgery 16th/1258; Current Diagnosis and Treatment in Otolaryngology 3rd/456-65]

- Glottic cancer is most common variety

Laryngeal Carcinoma

◈ *Dhingra 7th/347-55*

- *Curative radiotherapy is reserved for early lesions which neither impair cord mobility nor invade cartilage or cervical nodes*
- ***Early lesion of T1 and T2 are treated by radiotherapy.*** T3 and T4 lesions require total laryngectomy and postoperative radiation"-*Dhingra 7th/352*
- *"Both **tobacco and alcohol** are well established risk factor in laryngeal cancer"- Dhingra 7th/347*

Etiologic Factors

◈ *Ballenger H and NSurgery 16th/1258*

- By far, **smoking tobacco** has been implicated as the prime factor in causing laryngeal cancer. Cigarette, pipe, and cigar smoking are all considered risk factors, with cigarette smoking posing the greatest risk.
- Only about 1% of larynx cancer occurs in nonsmokers
- **Alcoholics** who smoke are thought to carry a 25- to 50-fold increase in risk of laryngeal cancer over nonsmokers.
- Other etiologic factors include gastroesophageal reflux16 and exposure to wood dust, asbestos, volatile chemicals, nitrogen mustard, and ionizing radiation.
- **Human papillomavirus (HPV)** is also considered to be an important cofactor in the development of laryngeal cancers. The ***strains of HPV 16 and 18*** have been most frequently demonstrated in laryngeal squamous carcinomas by using probes for HPV deoxyribonucleic acid (DNA)

Laryngeal Carcinoma

◈ *Current Diagnosis and Treatment in Otolaryngology 3rd/456*

- The larynx can be divided into three parts: the supraglottis, the glottis, and the subglottis.
- The **supraglottic larynx** extends from the tip of the epiglottis and vallecula superiorly to the ventricle and

undersurface of the "false" cords inferiorly; it includes the arytenoid cartilages, the aryepiglottic folds, the false vocal cords, and the epiglottis.

- The **glottic larynx** encompasses the "true" vocal cords, extending from the ventricle between the true and false cords to 0.5 cm below the free edge of the true cords, including the anterior commissure and interarytenoid area.
- The **subglottic larynx** extends from the inferior extent of the glottis to the inferior edge of the cricoid cartilage
- Signs and symptoms of malignant laryngeal lesions include ***hoarseness,*** dysphagia, hemoptysis, a mass in the neck, throat pain, ear pain, airway compromise, and aspiration

Incidence of Larynx Cancer by Site Current Diagnosis and Treatment in Otolaryngology 3rd/459

Supraglottic*—40%*

Glottic*—59%*

Subglottic*—1%*

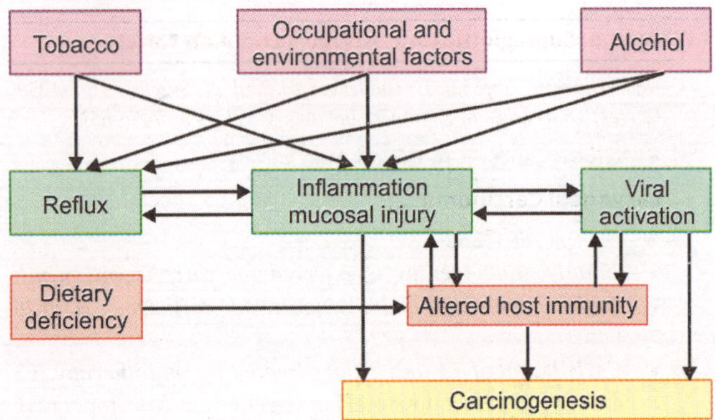

Fig: *(Ballenger H and NSurgery 16th/1258):* A multifactorial model for the development of laryngeal cancer

148. Ans. a. 6th CN palsy, b. 7th CN palsy, d. Vertigo, e. Retro-orbital pain

[Ref: Dhingra 7th/87-88; Logan and Turner 10th /426;Current Diagnosis and Treatment in Otolaryngology 3rd/679]

- ***Post auricular pain is feature of mastoiditis****- Dhingra 7th/87*

Petrositis

- *Dhingra 7th/87-88*
- Gradenigo's syndrome: Triad of ***external rectus palsy****(VI* ***nerve palsy****)*, deep-seated ear or ***retro-orbital pain*** and persistent ear discharge. It is uncommon to see the full triad these days
- Fever, headache, vomiting and sometimes neck rigidity may also be associated
- Some patients may get facial paralysis and recurrent ***vertigo*** due to involvement of facial and statoacoustic nerves
- Diagnosis of petrous apicitis requires both CT scan and MRI

Petrositis

- *Current Diagnosis and Treatment in Otolaryngology 3rd/679*
- Although exceptionally rare, petrositis is a known complication of AOM.
- Petrositis occurs when infection spreads within the temporal bone into the petrous apex.
- The classic triad, or Gradenigo's syndrome, is rare and characterized by retroorbital pain, AOM, and ipsilateral abducens nerve paresis.
- In conjunction with the clinical triad, diagnosis is confirmed with radiographic findings of bony destruction of the petrous apex

149. Ans. a. Meniere's disease, b. Labyrinthitis, d. Acoustic neuroma

[Ref: Dhingra 7th/47,88; Logan and Turner 10th /466]

- ***Hearing loss is not seen in Vestibular neuritis (= Labyrinthitis-hearing loss)***

"Disorder of vestibular system *cause vertigo and divided into: Peripheral(which involves vestibular end organs and their first order neurons i,e. vestibular nerve) andCentral(which involves central nervous system)"-Dhingra 7th/47*

Meniere's disease: *It is characterized by vertigo, fluctuating hearing loss, tinnitus and sense of pressure in the involved ear"- Dhingra 7th/47*

"Acoustic neuroma: *Progressive unilateral sensorineural hearing loss, often accompanied by tinnitus, is the presenting symptom in majority of cases"- Dhingra 7th/125*

"The term labyrinthit *is should be reserved for cases where there is simultaneous vestibular and sensorineural hearing loss"- Logan and Turner 10th /466*

"**Vestibular neuritis and labyrinthitis** are closely related disorders. **Vestibular neuritis** involves swelling of a branch of the vestibulocochlear nerve (the vestibular portion) that affects balance. **Labyrinthitis** involves the swelling of both branches of the vestibulocochlear nerve (the vestibular portion and the cochlear portion) that affects balance and ***hearing.*** The symptoms of labyrinthitis are the same as vestibular neuritis plus the additional symptoms of tinnitus (ringing in the ears) and/or ***hearing loss***"- my.clevelandclinic.org

Table *(Dhingra 7th/47)*: **Vestibular disorders**

Peripheral (Lesions of end organs vestibular nerve)	Central (Lesions of brainstem and central connections)
• Meniere's disease • Benign paroxysmal positional vertigo • Vestibular neuronitis • Labyrinthitis • Vestibulotoxic drugs • Head trauma • Perilymph fistula • Syphilis • Acoustic neuroma	• Vertebrobasilar insufficiency • Posterior inferior cerebellar artery syndrome • Basilar migraine • Cerebellar disease • Multiple sclerosis • Tumours of brainstem and forth ventricle • Epilepsy • Cervical vertigo

150. Ans. a. Olfactory mucosa cover upper 1/3 of nasal cavity, b. Olfactory pathway passes d. Olfactory receptors act via cAMP, e. Rate of olfactory nerve impulses...

[Ref: BDC 7th/Vol. IV 248; A.K. Jain 6th/1055-59; Guyton 12th/716-20; Ganong 25th/217-21;Dhingra 6th/142; L and T 10 th/10-11]

*"The olfactory receptors **adapt about 50% in the first second or so after stimulation**. Thereafter, they adapt very little and very slowly"- Guyton 12th/718*

*"**Adaptation**: It develops within **seconds or minutes**, depending on the nature of the substance"- A.K. Jain 6th/1058*

"Over a wide range, the ***rate of olfactory nerve impulses change approximately in proportion to the logarithm of stimulus strength***, which states that the olfactory receptors obey principles of transduction similar to those of other sensory receptors"- *Guyton 12th/718*

"**Webner-Fechner Law** states that the subjective sensation(of odor, sound or light intensity) is ***proportional to the logarithm of the stimulus intensity***"- books.google.co.in/books

"There are **3 olfactory pathway**: the Very Old, the Less Old, and the Newer Olfactory Pathways into the Central Nervous System. The *very old* olfactory system subserves the basic olfactory reflexes, a *less old* system provides automatic but partially learned control of food intake and aversion to toxic and unhealthy foods, and a *newer* system is comparable to most of the other cortical sensory systems and is used for conscious perception and analysis of olfaction.The ***newer olfactory pathway passes through the thalamus***, passing to the ***dorsomedial thalamic nucleus*** and then to the lateroposterior quadrant of the orbitofrontale cortex. Based on studies in monkeys, this newer system probably helps in the conscious analysis of odor"- *Guyton 12th/718*

*"The receptor for smell are placed in **upper one-third of the nasal cavity** including the roof formed by cribriform plate and the medial and lateral walls up to the level of the superior concha. This part is lined by olfactory mucosa. The rest of the nasal cavity is lined by respiratory mucosa"- BDC 7th/Vol. IV 248*

*"The **receptor in the olfactory mucous membrane are coupled to G-proteins**. Some act via adenyl cyclase and cAMP and others act via phospholipase C. All of them are cation channels causing Na+ and Ca2+ influx"-A.K. Jain 6th/1058*

"Adaptation: The first step may be mediated by a calcium-binding protein (calcium/calmodulin) that binds to the receptor channel protein to lower its affinity for cyclic nucleotides. The next step is called **short-term adaptation, *which occurs in response to cAMP*** and implicates a feedback pathway involving calcium/calmodulin-dependent protein kinase II acting on adenylyl cyclase. The next step is called **long-term adaptation,** which includes activation of ***guanylyl cyclase and cGMP production***. A Na+/Ca2+ exchanger to restore ion balance also contributes to long-term adaptation"- *Ganong 25th/221*

Olfactory region: *Upper 1/3 of lateral wall* *(up to superior concha), corresponding part of the nasal septum and the roof of nasal cavity from the olfactory region. Here, mucous membrane is paler in color"-Dhingra 6th/138*

151. Ans. c. Dysplasia of cochlea

[Ref: Dhingra 6th/115;ENT by P.Hazarika 3rd/81]

Scheibe's Syndrome or Dysplasia

◈ *Dhingra 6th/115*

- *It is most common **inner ear anomaly***
- ***Bony labyrinth is normal***
- *Superior part of membranous labyrinth (utricle and **semicircular canal ducts) is also normal***
- ***Dysplasia is seen in the cochlea and saccule**; hence also called cochleosaccular dysplasia*
- *It is inherited as an autosomal recessive nonsyndromic trait*

Scheibe's syndrome: Cochleosaccular aplasia with normal bony labyrinth" *(ENT by P.Hazarika 3rd/81)*

MEDICINE

152. Ans. a. Intracranial hemorrhage, e. High altitude headache

[Ref:Harrison 20th/85; Davidson 23rd/185:CMDT 2019/990]

High altitude headache is a type of ***secondary headache*** (d/t hypoxia)- *err.ersjournals.com*

Headache

◈ *Harrison 20th/85*

- *Primary headaches* are those in which headache and its associated features are the disorder itself, whereas *secondary headaches* are those caused by exogenous disorders (Headache Classification Committee of the International Headache Society,2018).
- Primary headache often results in considerable disability and a decrease in the patient's quality of life.
- Mild secondary headache, such as that seen in association with upper respiratory tract infections, is common but rarely worrisome.
- Life-threatening headache is relatively uncommon, but vigilance is required in order to recognize and appropriately treat such patients

Table *(Davidson 23rd/185)*: **Primary and secondary headache syndromes**

Primary headache syndromes	Secondary causes of headache
• ***Migraine (with or without aura)***	• Medication overuse headache (chronic daily headache)
• ***Tension-type headache***	• ***Intracerebral bleeding*** (subdural haematoma, subarachnoid or intracerebral haemorrhage)
• Trigeminal autonomic cephalalgia (including ***cluster headache***)	• Raised intracranial pressure (brain tumour, idiopathic intracranial hypertension)
• Primary stabbing/coughing/ exertional/sex-related headache	• Infection (meningitis, encephalitis, brain abscess)
• Thunderclap headache	• Inflammatory disease (temporal arteritis, other vasculitis, arthritis)
• New daily persistent headache syndrome	• Referred pain from other structures (orbit, temporo-mandibular joint, neck)

Table *(Harrison 20th/85)*: **Common Causes of Headache**

Primary Headache		Secondary Headache	
Type	%	Type	%
Tension-type	69	Systemic infection	63
Migraine	16	Head injury	4
Idiopathic stabbing	2	Vascular disorders	1
Exertional	1	Subarachnoid hemorrhage	<1
Cluster	0.1	Brain tumor	0.1

153. Ans. c. Severe Mitral stenosis

[Ref:Harrison 20th/1670; Davidson 23rd/; P.J.M 20th/40-42; Kundu 4th/295-97;CMDT2016/414]

Pulsus bisferiens or double pulse refers to a wave pattern where there is the presence of two systolic peaks that can be seen in pressure tracings of the ascending aorta, the aortic arch, and the carotid artery.

Pulsus bisferiens: Occur in

- *radiopaedia.org*
- Aortic valve pathology: ***aortic regurgitation with or without concurrent aortic stenosis***
- ***Severe obstructive hypertrophic cardiomyopathy.***
- ***Aortic dissection***

"Some patients with **advanced AR** may have a bifid or bisferiens pulse, in which two systolic peaks can be appreciated. A bifid pulse is also described in patients with hypertrophic obstructive cardiomyopathy **(HOCM),** with inscription of percussion and tidal waves. A bifid pulse is easily appreciated in patients on ***intraaortic balloon counterpulsation*** (IABP), in whom the second pulse is diastolic in timing"- *Harrison 20th/1670*

"In some patients with ***AR or with combined AS and AR***, the carotid arterial pulse may be bisferiens "-*Harrison 20th/1811; Braunwald 8th/Chap 65*

Table *(P.J.M 20th/40-42; Kundu 4th/295-97)*: **Different Types of Pulses**

Pulse type	Condition
Anacrotic pulse	*Aortic stenosis*
Pulsus bisferiens	*Idiopathic hypertrophic subaortic stenosis;* ***Severe AR with mild AS***
Dicrotic pulse	*Fever like typhoid fever, congestive cardiac failure, cardiac temponade, following open heart surgery*
Pulsus parvus Et Tardus	*Severe AS*
Pulsus alternans	*LVF, Toxic myocarditis, Paroxymal tachycardias*
Pulsus paradoxus	*SVC obstruction; Lung conditions asthma,emphysema, airway obstruction; Cardiac- pericardial effusion, constrictive pericarditis, severe CCF*
Pulsus bigeminus	*A.V block, sinoatrial block with ventricular escape*
Thready pulse	*Shock especially cardiogenic*
Waterhammer pulse (High volume collapsing pulse)	*High output states like anaemia, beri beri, thyrotoxicosis; Cardiac lesions- AR, PDA, Rupture of sinus of valsalva into the heart chambers,aortopulmonary window*

154. Ans. a. Relapsing and remitting symptoms, b. Autoimmune disease, c. Steroid is useful during attack, d. Dawson fingers is characteristic MRI finding, e. Peginterferon beta-1a reduces severity of attack

[Ref:Harrison 20th/3188-98; Davidson 23rd/1107-09;Robbins 9th/1283-85; CMDT 2016/1007]

Option a-e

- *It is an* ***autoimmune disorder***
- *MS is* ***relapsing-remitting*** *MS (RRMS) type in approximately 85% of cases*
- *Typical lesions on MR are periventricular nodular hyperintense ovoid lesion on T2 images with long axis oriented perpendicular to ventricular wall creating finger like appearance, i.e.,* ***Dawson fingers***
- ***Peginterferon beta-1a*** *is a disease-modifying drug that have shown beneficial effects in patients with relapsing MS, including reduced frequency and severity of clinical attacks*
- ***Glucocorticoids are used to manage either first attacks or acute exacerbations***

Multiple Sclerosis (MS)

- *Harrison 20th/3188-98; Robbins 9th/1284*
- **MS is an autoimmune disease** of the central nervous system (CNS) characterized by chronic inflammation, demyelination, gliosis (plaques or scarring), and neuronal loss; the course can be ***relapsing or progressive.***
- *Multiple sclerosis is a neurodegenerative disease.*
- The disease may become clinically apparent at any age, although onset in childhood or after age 50 years is relatively rare.
- Women are affected twice as often as are men.
- In most individuals with MS, the clinical course takes the form of ***relapsing and remitting episodes*** of variable duration (weeks to months to years) marked by neurologic defects, followed by gradual, partial recovery of neurologic function.
- In the fresh state, the lesions are firmer than the surrounding white matter **(sclerosis)** and appear as well circumscribed, somewhat depressed, glassy, gray-tan, irregularly shaped **plaques**
- MRI has revolutionized the diagnosis and management of MS; characteristic abnormalities are found in >95% of patients, although >90% of the lesions visualized by MRI are asymptomatic
- **MRI findings of MS:** Typical lesions are ***periventricular nodular hyperintense ovoid lesions*** on T2 images with long axis oriented perpendicular to ventricular wall creating finger like appearance, i.e., ***Dawson fingers***

- Therapy for MS can be divided into several categories: (1) treatment of acute attacks, (2) treatment with disease-modifying agents that reduce the biologic activity of MS, and (3) symptomatic therapy.
- ***Glucocorticoids are used to manage either first attacks or acute exacerbations.***
- ***Plasma exchange (plasmapheresis)*** can be used short term for severe attacks if steroids are contraindicated or ineffective.
- ***Immunomodulatory Therapy forRelapsing-Remitting MS***
- Disease –modifying therapies have shown beneficial effects in patients with relapsing MS, including ***reduced frequency and severity of clinical attacks***. These agents appear to slow the progression of disability and the reduce accumulation of lesions within the brain and spinal cord. The disease-modifying agents for MS (DMAMS) currently approved for use by the US food and drug administration (FDA) include the following:
  - ***Interferon beta-1a***
  - ***Interferon beta-1b***
  - Peginterferon beta-1a
  - Glatiramer acetate
  - Natalizamab
  - Mitoxantrone
  - Fingolimod
  - Teriflunomide
  - Dimethyl fumarate
  - Alemtuzumab
  - Daclizumab
  - Ocrelizumab

Clinical features of multiple sclerosis *Davidson 23rd/1108*

Common presentations of multiple sclerosis
- Optic neuritis
- Relapsing/remitting sensory symptoms
- Subacute painless spinal cord lesion
- Acute brainstem syndrome
- Subacute loss of function of upper limb (dorsal column deficit)
- 6th cranial nerve palsy

Other symptoms and syndromes suggestive of CNS demyelination
- Afferent pupillary defect and optic atrophy (previous optic neuritis)
- Lhermitte's symptom (tingling in spine or limbs on neck flexion)
- Progressive non-compressive paraparesis
- Partial Brown–Séquard syndrome
- Internuclear ophthalmoplegia with ataxia
- Postural ('rubral', 'Holmes') tremor
- Trigeminal neuralgia under the age of 50
- Recurrent facial palsy

155. Ans. a. Hypertension, c. Hypertriglyceridemia, d. Increased glucose, e. PCOS

[Ref: Harrison 20th/ 2903; Davidson 23rd/730-31; CMDT 2019/795]

"**PCOS**: Women with PCOS are at increased risk of DM 2 and **metabolic syndrome**"-*CMDT 2019/795*

"The **metabolic syndrome** (syndrome X, insulin resistance syndrome) consists of a constellation of metabolic abnormalities that confer increased risk of cardiovascular disease (CVD) and diabetes mellitus. The major features of the metabolic syndrome include ***central obesity, hypertriglyceridemia, low levels of high-density lipoprotein (HDL) cholesterol, hyperglycemia, and hypertension***"- Harrison 20th/ 2903; Davidson 23rd/730-31

Table *(Harrison 20th/ 2903)*: **NCEP: ATPIII 2001 Criteria for the Metabolic Syndrome**

NCEP: ATPIII 2001

Three or more of the following:
- Central obesity. Waist circumference >102 cm (M), >88 cm (F)
- ***Hypertriglyceridemia:*** Triglyceride level ≥150 mg/dL or specific medication
- ***Low HDL cholesterol***: <40 mg/dL and <50 mg/dL for men and women, respectively, or specific medication
- ***Hypertension:*** Blood pressure ≥130 mmHg systolic or ≥85 mmHg diastolic or specific medication
- ***Fasting plasma glucose level ≥100 mg/dL*** or specific medication or previously diagnosed type 2 diabetes

156. Ans. a. Cardiac rhabdomyoma, d. Shagreen patch, e. Multiple retinal hamartomas

[Ref: Harrison 20th/2154-55; Davidson 23rd/1264; CMDT 2019/1023; www.ncbi.nlm.nih.gov]

Updated Diagnostic Criteria for Tuberous Sclerosis Complex 2012

www.ncbi.nlm.nih.gov

- **Genetic diagnostic criteria**
  The identification of either a TSC1 or TSC2 pathogenic mutation in DNA from normal tissue is sufficient to make a definite diagnosis of tuberous sclerosis complex (TSC).
- **Clinical diagnostic criteria**
  - Major features
    - Hypomelanotic macules (≥3, at least 5-mm diameter)
    - Angiofibromas (≥3) or fibrous cephalic plaque
    - Ungual fibromas (≥2)
    - ***Shagreen patch***
    - ***Multiple retinal hamartomas***
    - Cortical dysplasias
    - Subependymal nodules
    - Subependymal giant cell astrocytoma
    - ***Cardiac rhabdomyoma***
    - Lymphangioleiomyomatosis (LAM)
    - Angiomyolipomas (≥2)
  - **Minor features**
    - ***"Confetti" skin lesions***
    - Dental enamel pits (>3)
    - Intraoral fibromas (≥2)
    - Retinal achromic patch
    - ***Multiple renal cysts***
    - Nonrenal hamartomas

Tuberous Sclerosis

◈ *Davidson 23rd/1264; Harrison 20th/2154-55*

- This is an autosomal dominant condition, with two genetic loci identified: *TSC-1* (chromosome 9), encoding hamartin, and *TSC-2* (chromosome 16), encoding tuberin.
- The hallmark is of hamartomas in many systems.
- The classic triad of clinical features comprises ***learning disability, epilepsy and skin lesions*** but there is marked heterogeneity in clinical features.
- Skin changes include pale oval (ash leaf) macules that occur in early childhood; yellowish/pink papules in the mid-face (angiofibromas, 'adenoma sebaceum'), occurring in adolescence; periungual and subungual fibromas; and connective tissue naevi (***shagreen patches***, often on lower back).
- Gum hyperplasia, retinal phakomas (fibrous overgrowths), renal, lung and heart tumours, cerebral gliomas and calcified basal ganglia may also occur.

157. Ans. a. Rapidly detect Mycobacterium tuberculosis and rifampicin resistance, b. Use nucleic acid amplification tests (NAAT) technique, d. Uses real time PCR

[Ref: Harrison 20th/ 1247; Park 25th/197; who.int/tb/laboratory]

Gene Xpert MTB/RIF

◈ *Park 25th/197; Harrison 20th/ 1247*

- The *Xpert MTB/RIF* is a cartridge-based, automated diagnostic test that can *identify* ***Mycobacterium tuberculosis (MTB) and resistance to rifampicin (RIF)***
- In December 2010, the World Health Organization (WHO) endorsed the Xpert MTB/RIF for use in TB endemic countries and declared it a major milestone for global TB diagnosis.
- It detects *DNA sequences specific for* ***Mycobacterium tuberculosis and rifampicin resistance*** *by* ***polymerase chain reaction.***
- It is based on the Cepheid GeneXpert system, a platform for rapid and simple-to-use ***nucleic acid amplification tests (NAAT).***
- It purifies and *concentrates* ***Mycobacterium tuberculosis*** *bacilli from sputum samples, isolates genomic material from the captured bacteria by sonication and subsequently amplifies the genomic* ***DNA by PCR*** *and identifies all the clinically relevant* ***Rifampicin resistance*** *inducing mutations in the RNA polymerase beta (rpoB) gene in the Mycobacterium tuberculosis genome in a* ***real time format*** *using fluorescent probes called molecular beacons.*
- Results are obtained from unprocessed sputum samples in 90 minutes, with minimal biohazard and very little technical training required to operate.
- This test was developed as an on-demand near patient technology which could be performed even in a doctor's office if necessary.
- Some concerns have been raised about the Xpert MTB/RIF, including minor operational issues and cost

"The **Xpert MTB/Rif test** is a cartridge-based ***fully automated NAAT*** (nucleic acid amplification test) for TB case detection and rifampicin resistance testing, suitable for use in disease-endemic countries. It purifies, concentrates, amplifies (***by rapid, real-time PCR***) and identifies targeted nucleic acid sequences in the TB genome, and provides results from unprocessed sputum samples in ***less than 2 hours***, with minimal hands-on technical time"- www.who.int

158. Ans. c. Diarrhea, e. Type 4 RTA

[Ref: Harrison 20th/317; Davidson 23rd/365]

Starvation, Salicylate poisoning and Ketoacidosis cause high anion gap acidosis

Table *(Harrison 20th/317)*: **Causes of HIGH-ANION GAP ACIDOSES**

Lactic acidosis	**Toxins**
Ketoacidosis	Ethylene glycol
Diabetic	Methanol
Alcoholic	Salicylates
Starvation	Propylene glycol
	Pyroglutamic acid
	Renal failure (acute and chronic)

Causes of Non–Anion Gap Acidosis(Harrison 19th/320)

- Gastrointestinal bicarbonate loss
  - ***Diarrhea***
  - External pancreatic or small-bowel drainage
  - Ureterosigmoidostomy, jejunal loop, ileal loop
  - Drugs
    - Calcium chloride (acidifying agent)
    - Magnesium sulfate (diarrhea)
    - Cholestyramine (bile acid diarrhea)
- Renal acidosis
  - Hypokalemia
    - Proximal RTA (type 2)
      Drug-induced: acetazolamide, topiramate
    - Distal (classic) RTA (type 1)
      Drug induced: amphotericin B, ifosfamide
  - Hyperkalemia
    - Generalized distal nephron dysfunction (***type 4 RTA***)
      - Mineralocorticoid deficiency
      - Mineralocorticoid resistance (PHA I, autosomal dominant)
      - Voltage defect (PHA I, autosomal recessive, and PHA II)
      - Tubulointerstitial disease
  - Normokalemia
    - Chronic progressive kidney disease
- Drug-induced hyperkalemia (with renal insufficiency)
  - Potassium-sparing diuretics (amiloride, triamterene, spironolactone, eplerenone)
  - Trimethoprim
  - Pentamidine
  - ACE-Is and ARBs
  - Nonsteroidal anti-inflammatory drugs
  - Calcineurin inhibitors
- Other
  - Acid loads (ammonium chloride, hyperalimentation)
  - Loss of potential bicarbonate: ketosis with ketone excretion

- Expansion acidosis (rapid saline administration)
- Hippurate
- Cation exchange resins

159. Ans. a. Recurrent genital ulceration, b. Recurrent oral ulcers, c. Uveitis

[Ref: Harrison 20th/2589-90; Davidson 23rd/ 1043-44; CMDT 2019/876]

◈ *Conjunctivitis is not a feature of Behçet's syndrome*

Table *(Harrison 20th/2589)*: **Diagnostic Criteria of Behçet's Disease**

Recurrent oral ulceration plus two of the following:
• ***Recurrent genital ulceration***
• ***Eye lesions(Uveitis)***
• ***Skin lesions***
• ***Positive Pathergy test***

Behçet Syndrome

◈ *CMDT 2019/876*

- **Essentials of Diagnosis:** Recurrent, ***painful aphthous ulcers of the mouth and genitals***; additional cutaneous findings include *erythema nodosum*–like lesions, a follicular rash, and the ***"pathergy" phenomenon*** (formation of a sterile pustule at the site of a needle stick).
- **Either anterior or posterior uveitis** may be asymptomatic until significant damage to the retina has occurred

Behçet Syndrome

◈ *Harrison 20th/2589-90*

- The hallmark of Behçet disease is ***painful aphthous ulceration in the mouth.*** These lesions, which usually occur multiply, may be found on the tongue, gums, and inner surfaces of the oral cavity
- Genital lesions, similar in appearance, are also common but do not occur in all patients.
- The **pathergy phenomenon** is frequently underappreciated (unless the patient is asked); in this phenomenon, sterile pustules develop at sites where needles have been inserted into the skin (*e.g.,* for phlebotomy) in some patients
- Eye involvement with scarring and bilateral ***panuveitis*** is the most dreaded complication, since it occasionally progresses rapidly to blindness. Uveitis occurs in 10–15% of patients, primarily in males
- Non-deforming **arthritis or arthralgias** are seen in 50% of patients and affect mostly the knees and ankles
- Superficial or deep peripheral vein thrombosis is seen in 30% of patients
- **Skin involvement** is observed in 80% of patients and includes folliculitis, erythema nodosum, acne-like rashes, and, infrequently, vasculitis, Sweet syndrome, and pyoderma gangrenosum.

160. Ans. a. Monoarthritis is a major criteria in a moderate and high risk population, d. Echocardiography is indicated in all suspected and confirmed cases

[Ref: Harrison 20th/2542-44; CMDT 2019/436]

Rheumatic Fever – New Diagnostic Criteria (2015)

◈ *www.ncbi.nlm.nih.go*

- The last revision of the Jones criteria consists mainly in the supplementation of the major criteria with **echocardiographic examination,** the introduction of a concept of subclinical carditis and ***the isolation of low, medium and high risk populations among the patients (i.e two pathway- low and medium/high risk)***
- AHA recommends that ***all the patients with suspected RF undergo Doppler echocardiographic*** examination after the Jones criteria have been verified, even if no clinical signs of carditis are present.
- Low-risk populations are those with ***ARF incidence ≤2 per 100,000 school-age children*** or all-age rheumatic heart disease prevalence of ≤1 per 1000 population per year.

Table *(Harrison 20th/2544; CMDT 2019/436)*: **2015 Revised Jones Criteria**

A. For All Patient Populations with Evidence of Preceding Group A Streptococcal Infection	
Diagnosis: initial ARF	2 major manifestations or 1major plus 2 minor manifestations
Diagnosis: recurrent ARF	2 major or 1major and 2 minor or 3 minor
B. Major Criteria	
Low-risk populations[a]	**Moderate and high-risk populations**
Carditis[b]	Carditis
• Clinical and/or subclinical	• Clinical and/or subclinical
Arthritis	Arthritis
• Polyarthrits only	• ***Monoarthritis or polyarthritis***
• Polyarthralgia[c]	
Chorea	Chorea
Erythema marginatum	Erythema marginatum
SC nodules	SC nodules
C. Minor Criteria	
Low-risk populations[a]	**Moderate- and high-risk populations**
Polyarthralgia	Monoarthralgia
Fever (≥38.5°C)	Fever (≥38°C)
ESR ≥60 mm in the first hour and/ or CRP ≥3.0 mg/dL[d]	ESR ≥30 mm/h and/or CRP ≥3.0 mg/dL[d]
Prolonged PR interval, after accounting for age variability (unless carditis is a major criterion)	Prolonged PR interval, after accounting for age variability (unless carditis is a major criterion)

[a] Low-risk populations are those with ARF incidence ≤2 per 100,000 school-age children or all-age rheumatic heart disease prevalence of ≤1 per 1000 population per year.

[b] Subclinical carditis indicates echocardiographic valvulitis.

[c] Polyarthralgia should only be considered as a major manifestation in moderate- to high-risk populations after exclusion of other causes. As in past versions of the criteria, erythema marginatum and SC nodules are rarely "stand alone" major criteria. Additionally, joint manifestations can only be considered in either the major or minor categories but not both in the same patient. (See source document for more information.)
[d]CRP value must be greater than upper limit of normal for laboratory. Also, because ESR may evolve during the course of ARF, peak ESR values should be used.

161. Ans. b. >10% Band form, c. Tachycardia, d. Leukopenia (<4,000/ µL), e. Tachypnea (>24 breaths/min)

[Ref: CMDT2019/506;Harrison 19th/1751; L and B 27th/51]

Table *(Harrison 19th/1751)*: **Definitions Used to Describe SIRS**

Systemic inflammatory response syndrome (SIRS)	Two or more of the following conditions: (1) fever (oral temperature >38°C) or hypothermia (<36°C); (2) tachypnea (>24 breaths/min); (3) tachycardia (heart rate >90 beats/min); (4) leukocytosis (>12,000/µL), leukopenia (<4,000/µL), or >10% bands; may have a noninfectious etiology

Table *(L and B 27th/51)*: **Definitions of systemic inflammatory response syndrome (SIRS)**

SIRS is ***Two of:***
- Hyperthermia (>38°C) or hypothermia (<36°C)
- Tachycardia (>90/min, no _-blockers) or tachypnoea (>20/min)
- White cell count >12 × 109/l or <4 × 109/l

162. Ans. b. Diaphragm and intercostal muscle weakness result in ventilatory insufficiency, d. Heart block may present, e. Autosomal dominant inheritance

[Ref: Harrison 20th/3248;CMDT 2019/1060-61;Davidson 23rd/1143; Robbins 9th/ 1243-44]

"**Myotonic dystrophy**: ***Autosomal dominant*** inheritance- *CMDT 2019/1061; Robbins 9th/ 1243*

Myotonic Dystrophy

◈ *Harrison 20th/3248*
- There are two distinct forms of myotonic dystrophy (*dystrophia myotonica* or DM), namely myotonic dystrophy type 1 (DM1), and myotonic dystrophy type 2 (DM2) also called *proximal myotonic myopathy* (PROMM).

Clinical Expression of Myotonic Dystrophy Type 1 (DM1)

- The clinical expression of DM1 varies widely and involves many systems other than muscle. Affected patients may have a "**hatchet-faced**" appearance due to ***temporalis, masseter, and facial muscle atrophy and weakness.***
- Frontal baldness is frequent.
- Weakness of wrist and fingers occurs early as does foot drop.
- ***Proximal muscles are less affected.***
- Palatal, pharyngeal, and tongue involvement can lead to dysarthria and dysphagia.
- Some patients have ***diaphragm and intercostal muscle weakness, resulting in ventilatory insufficiency.***
- Myotonia is usually apparent by the age of 5 years and is best demonstrable by percussion of the thenar eminence or asking patients to close their fingers very tightly and then relax.
- ECG abnormalities include ***first-degree heart block*** and more extensive conduction system involvement. Complete heart block and sudden death can occur.
- **Congestive heart failure** occurs infrequently but may result from cor pulmonale secondary to respiratory failure.
- Other associated features include intellectual impairment, hypersomnia, posterior subcapsular cataracts, gonadal atrophy, insulin resistance, and decreased esophageal and colonic motility.
- ***Congenital myotonic dystrophy*** is a more severe form of DM1 and occurs in ~25% of infants of affected mothers. It is characterized by severe facial and bulbar weakness, transient neonatal respiratory insufficiency, and mental retardation.

Clinical Expression of Myotonic Dystrophy Type 2 (DM2)

- DM2 or PROMM ***involves mainly proximal muscles***.
- Other features of the disease overlap with DM1, including cataracts, testicular atrophy, insulin resistance, constipation, hypersomnia, and cognitive defects.
- Cardiac conduction defects occur but are less common. The hatchet face and frontal baldness are also less consistent features.
- A very striking difference is the failure to clearly identify a congenital form of DM2.

163. Ans. b. GAA triplet repeats, c. Absent deep tendon reflexes, e. Autosomal recessive inheritance

[Ref: Harrison 20th/3157; CMDT 2019/1049]

"**Friedrich ataxia: *This disorder, the only known autosomal recessive trinucleotide repeat disease, is caused by expansion of a poly-GAA locus in the gene for frataxin on chromosome 9***"- CMDT 2019/1049

"The classic form of Friedreich's ataxia has been mapped to 9q13- q21.1, and the mutant gene, *frataxin*, contains expanded ***GAA triplet repeats*** in the first intron. There is homozygosity for expanded GAA repeats in >95% of patients. Normal persons have 7–22 GAA repeats, and patients have 200–900 GAA repeats."- Harrison 20th/3157

Friedreich's Ataxia

◈ *Harrison 20th/3157*
- This is the most common form of inherited ataxia, comprising one-half of all hereditary ataxias.
- It can occur in a classic form or in association with a genetically determined vitamin E deficiency syndrome; the two forms are clinically indistinguishable.
- Friedreich's ataxia presents before 25 years of age with progressive staggering gait, frequent falling, and titubation.
- The ***lower extremities are more severely involved than the upper ones.***
- Dysarthria occasionally is the presenting symptom; rarely, progressive scoliosis, foot deformity, nystagmus, or cardiopathy is the initial sign.

- The neurologic examination reveals nystagmus, loss of fast saccadic eye movements, truncal titubation, dysarthria, dysmetria, and ataxia of trunk and limb movements.
- ***Extensor plantar responses*** (with normal tone in trunk and extremities***), absence of deep tendon reflexes***, and weakness (greater distally than proximally) are usually found.
- Loss of vibratory and proprioceptive sensation occurs.
- The median age of death is 35 years.
- Women have a significantly better prognosis than men.
- Cardiac involvement occurs in 90% of patients. Cardiomegaly, symmetric hypertrophy, murmurs, and conduction defects are reported.
- Moderate mental retardation or psychiatric syndromes are present in a small percentage of patients.
- A high incidence of diabetes mellitus (20%) is found
- Musculoskeletal deformities are common and include pes cavus, pes equinovarus, and scoliosis.

164. Ans. a. Pancreatitis, b. Esophageal perforation, e. Pulmonary embolism

[Ref:Harrison 20th2007-08; CMDT 2019/323;Robbins 9th/722]

Pleural Effusions

◈ *Harrison 20th2007*

- Transudative and exudative pleural effusions are distinguished by measuring the lactate dehydrogenase (LDH) and protein levels in the pleural fluid.
- Exudative pleural effusions meet at least one of the following criteria, whereas transudative pleural effusions meet none:
  - *Pleural fluid protein/serum protein >0.5*
  - *Pleural fluid LDH/serum LDH >0.6*
  - *Pleural fluid LDH more than two-thirds the normal upper limit for serum*
- These criteria misidentify ~25% of transudates as exudates.

Table *(Harrison 20th/2008)*: **Differential Diagnoses of Pleural Effusions**

Transudative Pleural Effusions

- Congestive heart failure
- Cirrhosis
- Nephrotic syndrome
- ***Peritoneal dialysis***
- Superior vena cava obstruction
- Myxedema
- ***Urinothorax***

Exudative Pleural Effusions

- Neoplastic diseases
  - Metastatic disease
  - Mesothelioma
- Infectious diseases
  - Bacterial infections
  - Tuberculosis
  - Fungal infections
  - Viral infections
  - Parasitic infections
- ***Pulmonary embolization***
- Gastrointestinal disease
  - ***Esophageal perforation***
  - ***Pancreatic disease***
  - Intraabdominal abscesses
  - Diaphragmatic hernia
  - After abdominal surgery
  - Endoscopic variceal sclerotherapy
  - After liver transplant
- Collagen vascular diseases
  - Rheumatoid pleuritis
  - Systemic lupus erythematosus
  - Drug-induced lupus
  - Sjögren syndrome
  - Granulomatosis with polyangiitis (Wegener)
  - Churg-Strauss syndrome
- Post-coronary artery bypass surgery
- Asbestos exposure
- Sarcoidosis
- Uremia
- Meig's syndrome
- Yellow nail syndrome
- Drug-induced pleural disease
  - Nitrofurantoin
  - Dantrolene
  - Methysergide
  - Bromocriptine
  - Procarbazine
  - Amiodarone
  - Dasatinib
- Trapped lung
- Radiation therapy
- Post-cardiac injury syndrome
- Hemothorax
- Iatrogenic injury
- Ovarian hyperstimulation syndrome
- Pericardial disease
- Chylothorax

165. Ans. a. Pleurodesis, b. Thoracocentesis, c. Chemotherapy, d. Radiotherapy, e. Indwelling Pleural Catheters

[Ref: L and B 27th/921-23; CMDT 2019/323-24; www.cancertm.com]

Malignant Pleural Effusion

◈ *L and B 27th/921-23*

Pleural effusion is a common complication of cancer. This may be due to:

- Lung cancer
- Pleural involvement with primary or secondary malignancy; mediastinal lymphatic involvement.

Malignant Pleural Effusion

◈ *CMDT 2019/323-24*

- ***Chemotherapy or radiation therapy*** or both offer temporary control in some malignant effusions but are generally ineffective in lung cancer in the pleural space except for small cell lung cancer.
- Asymptomatic malignant effusions usually do not require specific treatment.

- Symptomatic patients should have a ***therapeutic thoracentesis***. If symptoms are relieved but the effusion returns, the options are serial thoracenteses, ***attempted pleurodesis, or placement of an indwelling drainage catheter*** that the patient can access at home.

Treatment of Malignant Pleural Effusion (MPE)

- *www.cancertm.com*
- **Thoracentesis,** guided by ultrasound (US) with experienced physicians, is a diagnostic and therapeutic option for MPE.
- **IPCs (Indwelling Pleural Catheters)** have become widely used for the palliative treatment of recurrent MPE.
- **Pleurodesis** is a better option for recurrent MPE than thoracocentesis unless the patient has a very poor performance status, or a short life expectancy, or a trapped lung.
- **Intrapleural chemotherapeutic agents** (e.g., 5-fluorouracil [5-FU], cisplatin, etoposide, paclitaxel, carboplatin, cytarabine, and docetaxel) have been demonstrated safe by several Phase I and II studies.
- **Gene therapy** is a promising option for local intrapleural therapy, which includes inserting a therapeutic gene into tumor cells via viral and nonviral gene transfer vectors, thus modifying a noncytotoxic drug into a cytotoxic and arresting uncontrolled cell proliferation
- **Intrapleural fibrinolytics** can break the locules and improve pleural fluid drainage. Thus it is recommended for patients with multiloculated malignant effusion
- **Prophylactic radiotherapy:** Up to 40% of patients with mesothelioma can develop needle tract metastasis (NTM) after pleural interventions, especially tube thoracostomy and thoracoscopy. However, it can be prevented by local radiation at the access sites within 2 weeks.
- **Pleuroperitoneal Shunting (PPS)** is an alternative approach to control MPEs for patients with a trapped lung that cannot undergo pleurodesis, or failed pleurodesis, or patients with large loculated effusions

166. Ans. a. EBV infection, b. Kostmann's syndrome, c. Chediak Higashi syndrome, d. Vitamin B12 deficiency, e. Cyclic neutropenia

[Ref: Harrison 20th/398-99; CMDT 2018/528-29]

Causes of Neutropenia

- *www.luriechildrens.org*
- ***Cyclic neutropenia***–Characterized by cycling of the neutrophil count
- ***EBV infection***
- ***Kostmann's syndrome*** (a disorder involving low production of neutrophils)

Table *(Harrison 20th/398)*: **Causes of Neutropenia**

Decreased production
Drug-induced—alkylating agents (nitrogen mustard, busulfan, chlorambucil, cyclophosphamide); antimetabolites (methotrexate, 6-mercaptopurine, 5-flucytosine); noncytotoxic agents (antibiotics [chloramphenicol, penicillins, sulfonamides], phenothiazines, tranquilizers [meprobamate], anticonvulsants [carbamazepine], antipsychotics [clozapine], certain diuretics, anti inflammatory agents, antithyroid drugs, many others)
Hematologic diseases—idiopathic, cyclic neutropenia, Chédiak-Higashi syndrome, aplastic anemia, infantile genetic disorders
Tumor invasion, myelofibrosis
Nutritional deficiency—***vitamin B12,*** folate (especially alcoholics)
Infection—tuberculosis, typhoid fever, brucellosis, tularemia, measles, infectious mononucleosis, malaria, viral hepatitis, leishmaniasis, AIDS
Peripheral Destruction
Antineutrophil antibodies and/or splenic or lung trapping
Autoimmune disorders—Felty's syndrome, rheumatoid arthritis, lupus erythematosus
Drugs as haptens—aminopyrine, phenylbutazone, mercurial diuretics, some phenothiazines
Granulomatosis with polyangiitis (Wegener's)
Peripheral Pooling (Transient Neutropenia)
Overwhelming bacterial infection (acute endotoxemia)
Hemodialysis
Cardiopulmonary bypass

167. Ans. b. Constrictive pericarditis, d. HOCM, e. Sometime in Cardiac tomponade

[Ref: Harrison 20th/1669;CMDT 2019/383,441; usmlechannel.blogspot.com]

Kussmaul Sign

- *usmlechannel.blogspot.com*
- *Severe Rt. Sided Heart failure*
- *Tricuspid Atresia*
- *Chronic Constrictive Pericarditis*
- *Restrictive Pericarditis*
- *Cardiac Temponade (Sometimes)*

Kussmaul Sign

- *H20/1669*
- Normally, during inspiration, there is an increase in the *a* wave of the JVP but a decrease in the mean JVP as a result of the increased filling of the right-sided chambers associated with the decrease in intrathoracic pressure.

- *Kussmaul sign* denotes an inspiratory increase in the venous pressure, which can occur in patients with ***severe constrictive pericarditis*** when the heart is unable to accept the increase in RV volume without a marked increase in the filling pressure.
- Although Kussmaul sign was first described in patients with constrictive pericarditis, its most common cause is ***severe right-sided heart failure,*** regardless of etiology.
- The presence of Kussmaul sign is also useful in the diagnosis of ***RV infarction***

168. Ans. a. Pheochromocytoma, b. Mucosal neuroma, d. Marfanoid features e. Medullary carcinoma thyroid

[Ref: Harrison 20th/2747,2752; CMDT 2019/1198;Robbins 9th/1134]

"Unlike in MEN-2A, ***primary hyperparathyroidism is not present***"- Robbins 9th/1137

Clinical Manifestations

◈ *Harrison 20th/2752*

- MEN type 2 (MEN 2), which is also called Sipple's syndrome, is characterized by the association of medullary thyroid carcinoma (MTC), pheochromocytomas, and parathyroid tumors
- Three clinical variants of MEN 2 are recognized: MEN 2A, MEN 2B, and MTC only.
- **MEN 2A**, which is often referred to as MEN 2, is the most common variant. In MEN 2A, MTC is associated with pheochromocytomas in 50% of patients (may be bilateral) and with parathyroid tumors in 20% of patients.
- **MEN 2A** may rarely occur in association with Hirschsprung's disease, caused by the absence of autonomic ganglion cells in the terminal hindgut, resulting in colonic dilatation, severe constipation, and obstruction. MEN 2A may also be associated with cutaneous lichen amyloidosis, which is a pruritic lichenoid lesion that is usually located on the upper back.
- **MEN 2B**, which is also referred to as MEN 3, represents 5% of all cases of MEN 2 and is characterized by the occurrence of ***MTC and pheochromocytoma*** in association with a ***Marfanoid habitus; mucosal neuromas*** of the lips, tongue, and eyelids; medullated corneal fibers; and intestinal autonomic ganglion dysfunction leading to multiple diverticulae and megacolon.
- ***Parathyroid tumors do not usually occur in MEN 2B.***
- MTC only (FMTC) is a variant in which MTC is the sole manifestation of the syndrome.

Table *(Harrison 20th/2747)*: **Multiple Endocrine Neoplasia (MEN) Syndromes**

Type	Tumors (Estimated Penetrance)
MEN 1	Parathyroid adenoma (90%) Enteropancreatic tumor (30–70%) • Gastrinoma (>50%) • Insulinoma (10–30%) • Nonfunctioning and PPoma (20–55%) • Glucagonoma (<3%) • VIPoma (<1%) Pituitary adenoma (15–50%) • Prolactinoma (60%) • Somatotrophinoma (25%) • Corticotropinoma (<5%) • Nonfunctioning (<5%) Associated tumors • Adrenal cortical tumor (20–70%) • Pheochromocytoma (<1%) • Bronchopulmonary NET (2%) • Thymic NET (2%) • Gastric NET (10%) • Lipomas (>33%) • Angiofibromas (85%) • Collagenomas (70%)
MEN 2A	MTC (90%) Pheochromocytoma (>50%) Parathyroid adenoma (10–25%)
MEN 2B (also known as MEN 3)	MTC (>90%) Pheochromocytoma (>50%) Associated abnormalities (40–50%) • Mucosal neuromas • Marfanoid habitus • Medullated corneal nerve fibers • Megacolon
MEN 4	Parathyroid adenoma Pituitary adenoma Reproductive organ tumors (e.g., testicular cancer, neuroendocrine cervical carcinoma) ?Adrenal + renal tumors

SURGERY

169. Ans. a. BCG, b. Interferon, c. Mitomycine C, d. Actinomycin D, e. Thiotepa

[Ref: L and B 27th/1447-48; CSDT 14th/1000-03; Campbell-Walsh Urology, 9th/Chap 75]

Intravesical Therapy

◈ *CSDT 14th/1002-03*

- A variety of chemotherapeutic agents have been used in patients with recurrent low-grade, low-stage tumors.
- Immunotherapeutic drugs, which include ***BCG***, are effective in prophylaxis (60%) of ***recurrent papillary tumors*** and curative (70%) in carcinoma *in situ*, a highly malignant lesion less responsive to the cytotoxic agents described earlier.
- ***Intravesical BCG is the gold-standard first line therapy for carcinoma in situ of the bladder.***
- The combination of ***BCG and interferon alpha*** has shown nearly 50% response rates and is occasionally used in patients who have failed BCG.
- "Those patients with high-grade disease or recurrent tumors can be treated with intravesical agents such as ***bacilli Calmette-Guerin or mitomycin C***"- Schwartz 10th/1654

Table: *(Campbell-Walsh Urology, 9th/Chap 75):* **Comparisons between Intravesical Agents**

Agent	Peri-op Use	Risk Group	Cystitis (%)	Other Toxicity
Doxorubicin (Adriamycin)	Yes	Low-Intermediate	20-40	Fever, allergy, contracted bladder, 5%
Epirubicin	Yes	Low-Intermediate	10-30	Contracted bladder rare
Thiotepa	Yes	Low-Intermediate	10-30	Myelosuppression 8%-19%
Mitomycin	Yes	Low-Intermediate	30-40	Rash 8%-19%, contracted bladder 5%
BCG	No	Intermediate-High	60-80%	Serious infection, 5%
Interferon	No	Salvage	<5%	Flu-like symptoms 20%
Gemcitabine	Yes	Salvage	Mild	Occasional nausea

170. Ans. a. Skin breach is route of entry of microorganisms, b. Staphylococcus & streptococcus are most common microbe, c. Involves skin and Subcutaneous tissue, d. Commonly affects lower limbs

[Ref: L and B 27th/48-49; Harrison 20th/936;Manipal Surgery 4th/15-16]

"**Cellulitis *usually affects the skin on the lower legs***, but it can occur in the face, arms and other areas. Cellulitis occurs when bacteria, most commonly ***streptococcus and staphylococcus***, enter ***through a crack or break in your skin.*** The incidence of a more serious staphylococcus infection called methicillin-resistant Staphylococcus aureus (MRSA) is increasing"-.www.mayoclinic.org

Table: *(Manipal Surgery 4th/16):* **Cellulitis & abscess**

Cellulitis	Abscess
No edge(diffuse swelling)	Well-circumscribed, has an edge
No limit	Limit is present
No pus	Pus is present
No fluctuation	Fluctuation is positive

Cellulitis

◈ *L and B 27th/48-49*

- Cellulitis is the ***non-suppurative*** invasive infection of tissues.
- There is ***poor localisation*** in addition to the cardinal signs of inflammation.
- Spreading infection presenting in surgical practice is typically caused by organisms such as ***β-haemolytic streptococci , staphylococci and C. perfringens***.
- Tissue destruction, gangrene and ulceration may follow, which are caused by release of proteases.
- Systemic signs (the old-fashioned term toxaemia) are common, with chills, fever and rigors. These follow the release of toxins into the circulation

Cellulitis

◈ *L and B 27th/49; Manipal Surgery 4th/16*

- Non-suppurative, poorly localised
- Commonly caused by streptococci, staphylococci or clostridia
- Blood cultures are often negative
- Common site- lower limb, face & scrotum- *Manipal Surgery 4th/16*
- *It affects **skin & subcutaneous tissue***

Cellulitis

◈ *Harrison 20th/936*

- Cellulitis is an acute inflammatory condition of the skin that is characterized by localized pain, erythema, swelling, and heat.
- It may be caused by indigenous flora colonizing the skin and appendages (e.g., ***S. aureus and S. pyogenes)*** or by a wide variety of exogenous bacteria.
- Bacteria may gain access to the ***epidermis through cracks in the skin,*** abrasions, cuts, burns, insect bites, surgical incisions, and IV catheters.

171. Ans. a. Homogeneous spread is common, e. Capsular invasion is characteristic

[Ref: L and B 27th/818-22; Harrison 20th/2715;Manipal Surgery 4th/339-45; Sabiston 19th/904-11;Schwartz 9th/1363]

"The **Delphian (prelaryngeal/precricoid) node** is one of the cervical lymph node groups that comprise level VI cervical lymph nodes and is not routinely excised in radical neck dissections.

Thyroid carcinomas may also involve this node, in which case it usually signifies disease spread to the central and lateral cervical lymph nodes"- radiopaedia.org

Follicular carcinoma: *Capsular invasion* & vascular invasion- *Manipal Surgery 4th/350*

Prognosis: *Papillary-excellent;* *Follicular-good; medullary-bad & anaplastic-worst"- Manipal Surgery 4th/350*

Papillary Carcinoma

◈ *L and B 27th/818*

- Histologically the tumour shows papillary projections and characteristic pale, empty nuclei (Orphan Annie-eyed nuclei).
- Papillary carcinomas are ***very seldom encapsulated.***
- Multiple foci may occur in the same lobe as the primary tumour or, less commonly, in both lobes.
- They may be due to lymphatic spread in the rich intrathyroidal lymph plexus, or to multicentric growth.
- Spread to the lymph nodes is common, but blood-borne metastases are unusual unless the tumour is extrathyroidal.

- *"Irradiation to the neck during childhood increases the risk of papillary carcinoma"- Manipal Surgery 4th/339*
- "**Follicular carcinomas** account for 10% of thyroid cancers and occur more commonly in ***iodine-deficient areas***"- *Schwartz 9th/1363*

Papillary Carcinoma

◈ *Harrison 20th/2715*

- ***PTC is the most common type of thyroid cancer,*** accounting for 80–85% of well-differentiated thyroid malignancies.
- *PTC may be multifocal and invade locally within the thyroid gland as well as through the thyroid capsule and into adjacent structures in the neck.*
- ***It has a propensity to spread via the lymphatic system but can metastasize hematogenously as well***, particularly to bone and lung.

Table: *(L and B):* **Major differences between papillary and follicular carcinoma**

	Papillary (%)	Follicular (%)
Male incidence	22	35
Lymph node metastases	35	13
Blood vessel invasion	40	60
Recurrence rate	19	29
Overall mortality rate	11	25
Lactation of recurrent carcinoma		
Distant metastases	45	75
Nodal metastases	34	12
Local recurrence	20	12

172. Ans. a. Radiotherapy, b. Surgery, c. Chemotherapy, d. TSH suppression therapy, e. Radioiodine ablation

[Ref: L and B 27th/819-20; Manipal Surgery 4th/338; Schwartz 10th/1546-48; Harrison 20th/2716]

According to the classification of the WHO, **differentiated thyroid carcinoma** can be subdivided into ***papillary and follicular thyroid carcinoma.***

Surgical Treatment for Differentiated Thyroid Carcinoma

◈ *L and B 27th/819-20*

- Patients with large, locally aggressive or metastatic differentiated thyroid cancer (DTC) require ***total thyroidectomy***, with excision of adjacent involved structures if necessary, and appropriate ***nodal surgery*** followed by ***radioiodine ablation*** with ***long-term TSH suppression***.
- Such 'high risk' patients however are in the minority and there is continuing disagreement on the most appropriate operation for '**low risk' differentiated thyroid carcinoma,** particularly with the increase in diagnosis of incidental microcarcinomas of less than 1 cm.
- Current guidelines advocate routine ***total thyroidectomy***, often necessitating early reoperation and second lobectomy following a diagnostic first lobectomy with routine ***central compartment node dissection*** for all tumours greater than 1 cm.

Postoperative Management of Differentiated Thyroid Cancer

◈ *Schwartz 10th/1546-48*

- ***Radioiodine Therapy:*** RAI therapy reduces recurrence and provides a small improvement in survival, even in low-risk patients.
- ***External-Beam Radiotherapy and Chemotherapy:*** External beam radiotherapy is occasionally required to control unresectable, locally invasive or recurrent disease and to treat metastases in support bones to decrease the risk of fractures. Doxorubicin (Adriamycin) and paclitaxel (Taxol) are the most frequently used agents for chemotherapy . The former acts as a radiation sensitizer and should be considered in patients undergoing external-beam radiation.
- ***Thyroid Hormone:*** T4 is necessary as replacement therapy in patients after total or near-total thyroidectomy, and also has the additional effect of **suppressing TSH** and reducing the growth stimulus for any possible residual thyroid cancer cells.

173. Ans. b. Hot tea ingestion, c. Alcohol consumption, d. Paterson Kelly Syndrome

[Ref: L and B 27th/1085-86; Sabiston 19th/1050-51; CSDT 14th/474; Harrison 20th/566-67]

- Barret's is a risk factor for adenocarcinoma

Some Etiologic Factors Associated with Squamous Cell Cancer of the Esophagus

◈ *Harrison 20th/566*

- Excess alcohol consumption
- Cigarette smoking
- **Other ingested carcinogens:** Nitrates (converted to nitrites), Smoked opiates, Fungal toxins in pickled vegetables
- Mucosal damage from physical agents: Hot tea, ***Lye ingestion***, Radiation-induced strictures,
- Chronic achalasia
- Host susceptibility
- **Esophageal web** with glossitis and iron deficiency (i.e., ***Plummer-Vinson or Paterson-Kelly syndrome***)
- Congenital hyperkeratosis and pitting of the palms and soles (i.e., tylosispalmarisetplantaris)
- ? Dietary deficiencies of selenium, molybdenum, zinc, and vitamin A

Table: *(Maingot's Abdominal Operations – Chapter 9):* **Factors Associated with Pathogenesis of Esophageal Cancer**

Factor	Squamous Cell	Adenocarcinoma
Smoking	+++	+
Alcohol consumption	+++	-
Hot beverages	+	-
N-nitroso compounds (e.g., pickled vegetables)	+	-
Betel nut chewing	+	-
Mate drinking	+	-

Contd...

Factor	Squamous Cell	Adenocarcinoma
Deficiencies of green vegetables and vitamins	+	-
Low socioeconomic class	+	-
Fungal toxin or virus	+	-
History of radiation to the mediastinum	+	+
Lye corrosive stricture	+	-
History of aerodigestive malignancy	+++	-
Plummer-Vinson syndrome	+	-
Obesity	-	++
Achalasia	+	-
Gastroesophageal reflux	-	+++
Barrett's esophagus	-	++++

"These results suggest that ***Helicobacter pylori is not an etiological factor*** in patients with esophageal squamous cell carcinoma. We found a statistically significant ***negative correlation*** between esophageal squamous cell cancer and Helicobacter pylori infection"- www.ncbi.nlm.nih.gov

174. Ans. b. Confirmed from studying cells from nipple discharge, c. Resembles eczema, e. Superficial manifestation of an underlying breast carcinoma

[Ref: L and B 27th/873; Sabiston 19th/885; S.Das 5th/716]

"Paget's disease of the nipple: It was first described by Sir James Paget, a English surgeon, in 1874"-wikipedia

Paget's Disease of the Nipple

◈ *L and B 27th/873*

- Paget's disease of the nipple is a ***superficial manifestation of an underlying breast carcinoma***. It presents as an ***eczema-like condition of the nipple and areola,*** which persists despite local treatment.
- The nipple is eroded slowly and eventually disappears. If left, the underlying carcinoma will sooner or later become clinically evident. Nipple eczema should be biopsied if there is any doubt about its cause.
- **Microscopically,** Paget's disease is characterised by the *presence of large, **ovoid cells with abundant, clear, pale-staining cytoplasm** in the Malpighian layer of the epidermis.*

"The most common test used **to diagnose Paget's disease** is the biopsy, removal of a tissue sample from the affected area which is then examined under the microscope by a pathologist, who distinguishes Paget cells from other cell types by staining tissues to identify specific cells (immunohistochemistry). ***Samples of nipple discharge*** may also be examined ***under the microscope*** to determine whether Paget cells are present"- www.cancer.gov

175. Ans. a. Most bilateral discharges are ..., c. Purulent discharge can be due..., d. Duct ectasia presents with..., e. Most common cause of malignant ...

[Ref: L and B 27th/864,867-68; Sabiston 19th/828; Manipal Surgery 4th/391]

- **Most common cause** of nipple discharge in a non lactating female is **benign conditions(rarely cancer)**
- **Purulent discharge** can be due to underlying infection (***subareolar abscess***)

"Duct ectasia/periductal mastitis: The classical description of the pathogenesis of duct ectasia asserts that the first stage in the disorder is a dilatation in one or more of the larger lactiferous ducts, which fill with a stagnant ***brown or green secretion***. In some cases, a ***chronic indurated mass forms*** beneath the areola, which mimics a carcinoma"- *L and B 27th/867*

"The most common malignancy associated with nipple discharge in absence of other findings is DCIS"- ncbi.nlm.nih.gov

"The most common cause of pathological nipple discharge is papilloma(benign condition)"- www.mayoclinic.org

Nipple Discharge

◈ *Sabiston 19th/828*

- The appearance of a discharge from the nipple of a nonlactating woman is frightening out of proportion to its medical significance. *Nipple discharge is common and is **rarely associated with an underlying carcinoma***
- *The most common cause of* **spontaneous nipple discharge** *from a single duct is a* ***solitary intraductal papilloma*** *in one of the large subareolar ducts under the nipple.*
- Subareolar duct ectasia producing inflammation and dilation of large collecting ducts under the nipple is common and usually involves discharge from multiple ducts. Cancer is a very unusual cause of discharge in the absence of other signs.
- In summary, nipple discharge that is bilateral and comes from multiple ducts is not usually a surgical problem. Bloody discharge from a single duct, does require surgical biopsy to establish a diagnosis. Intraductal papilloma is found in most of these cases.
- **Unilateral, nonmilky discharge** coming from one duct orifice is surgically significant and warrants special attention. However, the underlying cause is rarely a breast malignancy.

Discharges from the Nipple

◈ *L and B 27th/864*

Discharge from a Single Duct

Blood-stained: Intraduct papilloma, Intraduct carcinoma, Duct ectasia

Serous (any colour): Fibrocystic disease,Ductectasia, Carcinoma

Discharge from More than One Duct

Blood-stained: Carcinoma, Ectasia, Fibrocystic disease

Black or green: Duct ectasia

Purulent: Infection

Serous: Fibrocystic disease, Duct ectasia, Carcinoma

Milk: Lactation, Rare causes (hypothyroidism, pituitary tumour)

Finding	Significance
Serous	Most likely benign FCC(fibrocystic condition), ie, duct ectasia
Bloody	More likely neoplastic-papilloma, carcinoma

Contd...

Finding	Significance
Associated mass	More likely neoplastic
Unilateral	Either neoplastic or non-neoplastic
Bilateral	Most likely non-neoplastic
Single duct	More likely FCC
Milky	Endocrine disorders, medications
Spontaneous	Either neoplastic or non-neoplastic
Produced by pressure at single site	Either neoplastic or non-neoplastic

176. Ans. a. Radiating left shoulder pain, b. Shifting dullness present, c. Secondary to blunt trauma, d. All hemodynamically unstable patients need urgent laparotomy

[Ref: L and B 27th/374; Schwartz 10th/1644; CSDT 14th/213; Sabis.ton 19th/1147; emedicine.medscape. com]

- Unilateral Shifting dullness known as **Balance Sign** seen in Splenic Trauma

"The ***spleen is the most commonly injured organ in cases of blunt abdominal trauma***"-CSDT 14th/213

"Although protected under the bony rib cage, ***the spleen remains the most commonly affected organ in blunt injury to the abdomen in all age groups***"- emedicine.medscape.com

Option a, b, d & e

- *There is a* ***sharp radiating left shoulder pain*** *(known as Kehr's sign).*
- *Often there is dullness to percussion in the left flank LUQ and shifting dullness to percussion in the right flank (Ballance's sign).*
- *FAST ultrasound of the abdomen is usually the first method of evaluation in splenic rupture but* ***Computed tomography*** *with IV contrast is the preferred imaging study as it can provide high quality images of the full peritoneal cavity.*
- Patients who are haemodynamically unstable or with a grade 5 injury (a shattered spleen or major hilar vascular injury) need urgent laparotomy

Splenic Rupture

- Splenic rupture is a potentially life-threatening condition, often associated with chest or abdominal trauma.
- Etiology
  - Trauma
    - Blunt trauma (MC cause).
    - Penetrating trauma (eg, gun shot wounds, knife wounds) may involve the spleen, the incidence of injury is well below that of the small and large intestine.
    - Explosive type injuries, as seen in warfare and civilian bombing.
  - Non-traumatic causes (less common) include infectious diseases, medical procedures such as colonoscopy, haematological diseases, medications, and pregnancy.

Presentation

- The clinical presentation of splenic injury is highly variable. Most patients with minor focal injury to the spleen complain of left upper quadrant abdominal tenderness.
- ***Left shoulder tenderness*** may also be present as a result of sub-diaphragmatic nerve root irritation by free blood with referred pain . Often there is a sharp radiating left shoulder pain, (known as ***Kehr's sign***).
- With free intraperitoneal blood, diffuse abdominal pain, peritoneal irritation, and rebound tenderness are more likely.
- Often there is dullness to percussion in the left flank LUQ and shifting dullness to percussion in the right flank (***Ballance's sign***).
- **Hypotension** in a patient with a suspected splenic injury, especially if young and previously healthy, is a grave sign and a surgical emergency.

Investigation

- Splenic rupture is usually evaluated by ***FAST ultrasound*** of the abdomen.
- Computed tomography with IV contrast is the preferred imaging study as it can provide high quality images of the full peritoneal cavity
- Patients who are haemodynamically unstable with peritonism following trauma have abdominal bleeding until proven otherwise and require immediate laparotomy.
- The American Association for the Surgery of Trauma (AAST) splenic injury scale is the most commonly used system for grading splenic trauma and as help guide for management.

Treatment

- Ali patients with suspect splenic injury should be assessed, resuscitated, and treated according to ATLS principles .
- **Patients who are haemodvnamically unstable** *or with a grade 5 injury (a shattered spleen or ma jor hilar vascular injury)* ***need urgent laparotomy.***
- **Haemodynamically stable patients** with grade 1-3 injuries without active extravasation can be treated conservatively.

Grading of Splenic Injuries

◈ *Schwartz 10th/1644*

Grade I: Subcapsular hematoma, <10% surface area capsular tear, <1 cm in depth

Grade II: Subcapsular hematoma, nonexpanding, 10%–50% surface area; intraparenchymal hematoma, nonexpanding, <2 cm in diameter; capsular tear, active bleeding, 1–3 cm, does not involve trabecular vessel

Grade III: Subcapsular hematoma, >50% surface area or expanding; intraparenchymal hematoma, >2 cm or expanding; laceration >3 cm in depth or involving trabecular vessels

Grade IV: Ruptured intraparenchymal hematoma with active bleeding; laceration involving segmental or hilar vessels producing major devascularization (>25% of spleen)

Grade V: Shattered spleen; hilar vascular injury which devascularizes spleen

177. Ans. a. High inguinal orchidectomy, c. Radiotherapy, d. Chemotherapy

[Ref: L and B 27th/1506-09; Manipal Surgery 4th/994-99; Robbins 9th/975-79;Schwartz 9th/1462; Sabiston 19th/2077]

Retroperitoneal lymlymphadenectomy(RPLND) is done in ***non-seminomatous tumor***- *Sabiston 19th/2077*

Treatment of Stage I Seminoma

◈ *Manipal Surgery 4th/994*

- Radical inguinal orchidectomy is the treatment of choice in all testicular tumors irrespective of the histological type & stage
- *Stage I-IIA:* ***Radiotherapy to retroperitoneum*** *is treatment of choice. Relapse after radiotherapy is managed by* ***chemotherapy***

"The standard initial treatment for all testicular tumor is ***Radical inguinal orchidectomy****. Further treatment of seminoma I includes:* ***radiation to regional L.N or limited prophylactic chemotherapy****"- Sabiston 19th/2077*

Stage I Tumours

◈ *L and B 27th/1508-09*

- Seminomas are ***radiosensitive*** and for many years ***adjuvant radiotherapy to the para-aortic nodes*** was the mainstay of treatment for stage I disease.
- Some years ago, the excellent response to ***platinum-based chemotherapy*** led to chemotherapy being introduced for most men with stage 1 seminoma.
- However, current practice uses ***CT and tumour marker-based surveillance protocols*** with chemotherapy being reserved for men who demonstrate relapse

Stage II–IV Tumours

◈ *L and B 27th/1509*

- Combination BEP **chemotherapy** is the mainstay of treatment for stages II–IV seminoma and NSGCT.
- **Retroperitoneal lymph node dissection** is sometimes needed in some cases of NSGCT when retroperitoneal masses remain after chemotherapy.

Table: *(CSDT 14th/1009):* **Treatment and prognosis of testicular cancer related to tumor stage**

Conventional stage	TNM stage	Clinical findings	Treatment	Five-Year Survival (%)
I	T1	Confined to testicle	Nonseminoma: RPLND vs. Surveillance; ***Seminoma: irradiation***	>95
IIA	N1	Regional nodes <2cm	Adjuvant chemotherapy Nonseminoma: RPLND or chemotherapy; Seminoma: XRT or chemotherapy	>90
IIB	N2	Nodes 2-5 cm	Adjuvant chemotherapy Nonseminoma; RPLND or adjuvant chemotherapy; Seminoma: XRT or chemotherapy	>85
IIC III	N3 M+	Nodes > 5 cm Distant metastases	Chemotherapy followed by resection of residual disease	~70

178. Ans. a. Pass medial to inferior epigastric Artery, b. Occur due to defect in floor of inguinal canal, d. Direct hernias are less likely to become strangulated

[Ref: L and B 27th/1029-31; CSDT 14th/768-70Manipal Surgery 4th/845-46; Sabiston 19th/1856, 1114; Schwartz 9th/ 144-45, 1340-41]

"Femoral hernia: Because its borders are distinct and unyielding, a ***femoral hernia has the highest risk of incarceration and strangulation of groin hernias***"*-CSDT 14th/769*

"Direct or medial inguinal hernia: It is acquired. It is a result of stretching and weakening of the abdominal wall just ***medial to the inferior epigastric (IE) vessels***. Looked at from within the abdominal cavity, there is a triangle referred to as **Hasselbach's triangle,** whose three sides are the **IE vessels laterally**, the lateral edge of the rectus abdominus muscle medially and the pubic bone below (the iliopubic tract). A direct, medial hernia is more likely in elderly patients. ***It is broadly based and therefore unlikely to strangulate"****- L and B 27th/1029-31*

Inguinal Hernia

◈ *Sabiston 19th/1856; CSDT 14th/769*

- ***Virtually all IHs in children are indirect and congenital in origin.***
- ***Males are affected about six times more often than females.***
- The ***right side is involved in 60% and the left in 30% of patients***; bilateral hernias are seen in 10%.
- "In general, ***direct hernias produce fewer symptoms than indirect inguinal*** hernias and are less likely to become ***incarcerated or strangulated***"*-CSDT 14th/770*
- "In the groin, an **indirect inguinal hernia** results ***when obliteration of the processus vaginalis***, the peritoneal extension accompanying the testis in its descent into the scrotum, fails to occur. The resultant hernia sac passes through the internal inguinal ring, a ***defect in the transversalis fascia*** halfway between the anterior iliac spine and the pubic tubercle"*-CSDT 14th/768*
- The **Hesselbach triangle** is bounded by the inguinal ligament, the inferior epigastric vessels, and the lateral border of the rectus muscle. ***A weakness or defect in the transversalis fascia, which forms the floor of this triangle, results in a direct inguinal hernia.***

"***Nearly all inguinal hernias in infants, children, and young adults are indirect inguinal hernias***. Although these"congenital" hernias most often present during the first year of life, the first clinical evidence of hernia may not appear until middle or old age, when increased intra-abdominal pressure and dilation of the internal inguinal ring allow abdominal contents to enter the previously empty peritoneal diverticulum"*-CSDT 14th/769*

179. Ans. b. Occur due to increased intra-abdominal pressure, c. High risk of strangulation seen in umbilical hernia containing Bowel, d. Mayo repair is done, e. Defect <2 cm can be repaired by sutures alone without mess

[Ref: L and B 27th/1036-38; Manipal Surgery 4th/863-65; Schwartz 10th/1631]

Umbilical Hernia in Adults

◈ L and B 27th/1036-38

- Conditions which cause stretching and thinning of the midline raphe (linea alba), such as pregnancy, obesity and liver disease with cirrhosis, predispose to reopening of the umbilical defect.
- Small umbilical hernias often contain extraperitoneal fat or omentum.
- Larger hernias can contain small or large bowel but, even when very large, the neck of the sac is narrow compared with the volume of its contents. ***As a result, in adults, umbilical hernias which include bowel are prone to become irreducible, obstructed and strangulated.***
- Patients are commonly overweight with a thinned and attenuated midline raphe. ***The bulge is typically slightly to one side of the umbilical depression,*** creating a crescent-shaped appearance to the umbilicus
- Women are affected more than men.
- Most patients complain of pain due to tissue tension or symptoms of intermittent bowel obstruction.
- In large hernias, the overlying skin may become thinned, stretched and develop dermatitis.
- **Very small defects less than 1 cm** in size may be closed with a simple figure-of-eight suture, or repaired by a darn technique where a non-absorbable, monofilament suture is criss-crossed across the defect and anchored firmly to the fascia all around.
- **Defects up to 2 cm** in diameter may be sutured primarily with minimal tension, although the larger the defect, the more tension and the more likely it is that mesh reinforcement will be beneficial. The ***classical repair was described by Mayo.***
- ***For defects larger than 2 cm in diameter, mesh repair is recommended.*** The mesh may be placed in one of several anatomical planes:

180. Ans. a. Parkland Formula, c. Brooke Formula

[Ref: L and B 27th/624; Sabiston 19th/530; Schwartz 10th/230]

Table: *(Sabiston 19th/530):* **Resuscitation Formulas**

Formula	Crystalloid volume	Colloid volume	Free water
Parkland	4 mL/kg per % TBSA burn	None	None
Brooke	1.5 mL/kg per % TBSA burn	0.5 mL/kg per % TBSA burn	2.0 L
Galveston (pediatric)	5000 mL/m^2 burned area + 1500 mL/m^2 total area	None	None

"There are three types of fluid used. The most common is Ringer's lactate or Hartmann's solution; some centres use human albumin solution or fresh-frozen plasma, and some centres use hypertonic saline.

Perhaps the simplest and most widely used formula is the Parkland formula. This calculates the fluid to be replaced in the first 24 hours by the following formula: total percentage body surface area × weight (kg) × 4 = volume (mL). Half this volume is given in the first 8 hours and the second half is given in the subsequent 16 hours"- *L and B 27th/624*

"The **rule of nines,** which states that each upper limb is 9 per cent TBSA, each lower limb 18 per cent, the torso 18 per cent each side and the head and neck 9 per cent, can be used as a rough guide to TBSA outside the hospital environment"- *L and B 27th/624*

181. Ans. b. Deep vein thrombosis, d. Compartment syndrome

[Ref: wikem.org; L and B 27th/987,998; CSDT 14th/849,837-38]

"**Unilateral leg swelling** can result from DVT, *lymphedema, obstruction of the popliteal vein by Baker cyst, or obstruction of the iliac vein by retroperitoneal mass or idiopathic fibrosis.* ***Bilateral leg edema*** *suggests heart, liver, or kidney failure or IVC obstruction by tumor or pregnancy*"- CSDT 14th/837-38

"A variety of diseases can result in **bilateral lower extremity edema**. These include congestive heart failure, pulmonary hypertension, chronic renal or hepatic insufficiency, and hypoproteinemia. In patients with **unilateral leg edema**, differential diagnosis includes congenital ***vascular malformations, chronic venous insufficiency,*** *and reflex sympathetic dystrophy*"- CSDT 14th/849

Unilateral Leg Swelling

◈ *wikem.org*

- Gravitational
- Venous insufficiency
- Thrombophlebitis
- Lymphedema
- Medications
  - NSAIDS
  - Birth control
  - Steroids
- ***Deep venous thrombosis*** (uncomplicated)
  - Phlegmasia alba dolens
  - Phlegmasia cerulea dolens
- Leg or foot infection
  - Cellulitis
  - Necrotizing fasciitis
  - Septic Joint
- Fracture
- Compartment syndrome
- Limb hypertrophy
  - Hypertrophy of soft tissue or bone (Klippel-Trenaunay syndrome)
  - Overgrowth of body part (Proteus Syndrome)
- Lipedema
- Tumor
- Post-thrombotic Syndrome

Bilateral Leg Swelling

◈ *wikem.org*

- ***CHF***
- ***Pretibial myxedema***
- ***Renal failure***
- ***Nephrotic syndrome***
- ***Liver failure***
- ***Hypoalbuminemia***

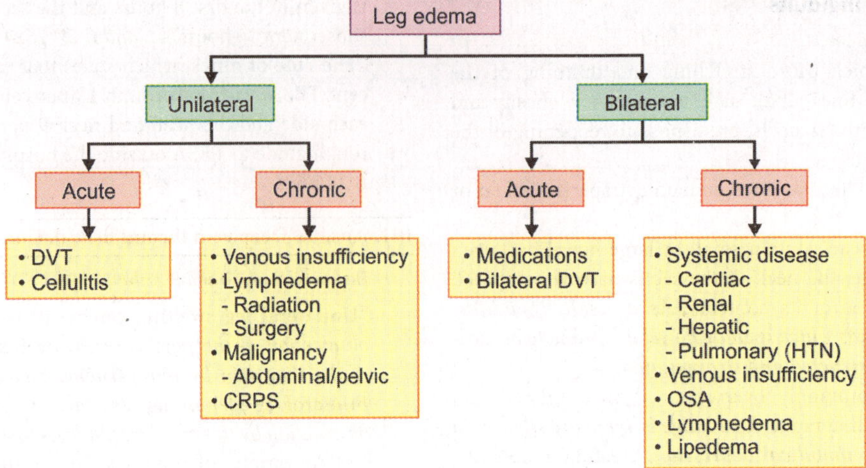

182. Ans. c. Viral orchitis, d. Strangulated inguinal hernia, e. Acute epididymo orchitis

[Ref: L and B 27th/1500-01; CSDT 14th/982]

Differential Diagnosis of Torsion Testis

- *L and B 27th/1500-01*
- Acute Epididymo-orchitis
- Torsion of Appendage of testis (MC hydatid of Morgagni) Conservative treatment
- Mumps orchitis
- Idiopathic Scrotal edema (Allergic, Bilateral)
- Small tense strangulated inguinal hernia

Differential Diagnosis of Torsion Testis

- *online.epocrates.com & emedicine.medscape.com*
- These above internet links also included ***appendicitis & hydrocele*** in D/D of torsion of testis
- But these are not mentioned in standard textbooks(so not included in answer)

183. Ans. c. Immediate evacuation is needed, d. Concave appearance on CT scan, e. Burr hole procedure is treatment option

[Ref: L and B 27th/334-35; Danhert Radiology 7th/290; Harrison 20th/3184]

- Lucid interval seen in EDH

Acute Subdural Haematoma

- *L and B 27th/334*
- Acute subdural bleeding arises from ***rupture of cortical vessels.***
- In contrast to extradural haematoma (and chronic subdural haematoma), acute subdural haematoma is ***usually associated with a high energy injury mechanism*** and significant primary brain injury. Conscious level is usually therefore impaired at presentation, but may deteriorate further as the haematoma expands.
- Since the dura is not adherent to the brain as it is to the skull, subdural blood is free to expand across the brain surface giving a ***diffuse concave appearance.***
- Acute subdural bleeds of significant size or with significant associated midline shift ***require evacuation***, and the cumulative mortality in this group is about 50 per cent. Smaller bleeds in neurologically stable patients may be managed conservatively, with ICP monitoring, in a neurosurgical unit

Subdural Haemorrhage

- *L and B 27th/335*
- Relatively severe trauma
- No lucid interval
- Diffuse concave lesion on computed tomography
- Require immediate transfer to a neurosurgical unit for decision on evacuation
- 50 per cent mortality

Extradural Hematoma	Subdural Hematoma
• Biconvex or lenticular	• Diffuse and concave
• Temporal or temporoparietal	• Entire surface of brain
• ***Middle meningeal artery***	• ***Tearing of bridging veins***
• 0.5% of all head injured patients	• 30% of severe head injuries
• ***"Lucid" Interval classically***	• Underlying brain damage more severe
• Outcome related to status prior to surgery	• Prognosis is worse than extradural

Neurosurgeons may perform a burr hole procedure to relieve pressure around the brain due to: *hopkinsmedicine.org*

- A ***sudden (acute) subdural hematoma***
- An ongoing (chronic) subdural hematoma
- An epidural hematoma
- Certain kinds of brain cancer
- Buildup of pus around the meninges
- Hydrocephalus
- Certain kinds of bleeds from the brain itself (rare)

184. Ans. a. Associated with oligospermia, b. Dilatation of pampiniform..., c. More common on left side, d. In renal cell cancer, varicocele does not decompress in the supine position

[Ref: L and B 27th/1501-02; Sabiston 19th/2056; Manipal Surgery 4th/993]

"**Valsalva manoeuver:** On blowing(blow test) fluid thrill may be felt. It ***may increase in size***"- *Manipal Surgery 4th/993*
"Asymptomatic varicocele is best untreated unless it is a suspected factor in ***male infertility***"-CSDT 14th/1015
"**Complication of varicocele:** ***Oligospermia,*** hydrocele & recurrence"- *Manipal Surgery 4th/994*

Varicocele

◈ *L and B 27th/1501-02*

- A varicocele is a varicose ***dilatation of*** pampiniform plexus
- Varicocele is a common condition and ***90% are left sided***
- Development of a left-sided varicocele in later life may indicate the ***presence of a renal tumour***
- They are usually asymptomatic and as such rarely need treatment
- First-line treatment is embolisation in symptomatic cases
- Varicoceles often recur, even after surgical treatment
- The association of varicoceles with subfertility is controversial

185. Ans. a. Isolated Cleft palate is more common than cleft lip alone, d. Associated with Sensorineural hearing loss, e. MC syndrome associated with Pierre Robin syndrome

[Ref: L and B 27th/686-90; CSDT 11th/1257-58; Sabiston 18th/2138; Manipal Surgery 4th/297]

- Unilateral cleft lip is common on left side (60%)
- Plerre Robin sequence-most common syndrome associated
- ***Sensorneural and conductive loss*** is associated with cleft lip and palate

Cleft Lip and Palate

◈ *L and B 27th/686-90*

- The incidence of cleft lip and palate is 1:600 live births and of isolated cleft palate is 1:1000 live births.
- Although cleft lip and palate is an extremely diverse and variable congenital abnormality, several distinct subgroups exist, namely cleft lip with/without cleft palate (CL/P), cleft palate
- (CP) alone and submucous cleft palate (SMCP).
- **The typical distribution of cleft types is:**
- **Cleft lip alone: 15 per cent;**
- **Cleft lip and palate: 45 per cent;**
- **Isolated cleft palate: 40 per cent.**
- Cleft lip/palate predominates in males, whereas cleft palate alone appears to be more common in females.
- ***In unilateral cleft lip, the deformity affects the left side in 60 per cent of cases.***
- Although most clefts of the lip and palate occur as an isolated deformity, ***Pierre Robin sequence*** remains the most common syndrome. This syndrome comprises isolated cleft palate, retrognathia and a posteriorly displaced tongue (glossoptosis), which is associated with early respiratory and feeding difficulties.
- **Isolated cleft palate** is more commonly associated with a syndrome than cleft lip/palate and cleft lip alone. Over 150 syndromes are associated with cleft lip and palate, although Stickler's (ophthalmic and musculoskeletal abnormalities), Shprintzen's (cardiac anomalies), Down's, Apert's and Treacher Collins' syndromes are most frequently encountered
- Cleft palate results in failure of fusion of the two palatine shelves. This failure may be confined to the ***soft palate alone or involve both hard and soft palate.*** When the cleft of the hard palate remains attached to the nasal septum and vomer, the cleft is termed **incomplete**. When the nasal septum and vomer are completely separated from the palatine processes, the cleft palate is termed **complete**
- C. lip results from abnormal development of the median nasal & maxillary process

186. Ans. a. Pain in right upper quadrant and radiating to scapular area, d. Murphy's sign is positive, e. Tokyo guidelines is used for diagnosis & severity grading

[Ref: Manipal Surgery 4th/556-60; Harrison 20th/2427-28]

- Early cholecystectomy is advised nowadays in 5-7 days and better than delayed interval cholecystectomy

"The **Tokyo Guidelines 2013** (TG13) diagnostic criteria and severity grading- is used for ***acute cholecystitis***"- onlinelibrary.wiley.co

Acute Cholecystitis

◈ *Harrison 20th/2427-28*

- Acute cholecystitis often begins as an attack of biliary pain that progressively worsens. Approximately 60–70% of patients report having experienced prior attacks that resolved spontaneously.
- As the episode progresses, however, the pain of acute cholecystitis becomes more generalized in the ***right upper abdomen.*** As with biliary colic, the pain of cholecystitis ***may radiate to the interscapular area, right scapula, or shoulder.***
- Vomiting is relatively common
- Jaundice is unusual early in the course of acute cholecystitis but may occur when edematous inflammatory changes involve the bile ducts and surrounding lymph nodes.
- ***A low-grade fever is characteristically present,*** but shaking chills or rigors are not uncommon.
- The RUQ of the abdomen is almost invariably tender to palpation. An enlarged, tense gallbladder is palpable in 25–50% of patients. Deep inspiration or cough during subcostal palpation of the RUQ usually produces increased pain and inspiratory arrest (***Murphy's sign***).
- ***The triad of sudden onset of RUQ tenderness, fever, and leukocytosis is highly suggestive.***
- ***Ultrasound will demonstrate calculi in 90–95% of cases and is useful for detection of signs of gallbladder inflammation*** *including thickening of the wall,* pericholecystic fluid, and dilatation of the bile duct.
- The radionuclide (e.g., HIDA) biliary scan may be confirmatory if bile duct imaging is seen without visualization of the gallbladder.
- ***In view of the natural history of the disease, acute cholecystitis is best treated by early surgery whenever possible.***

- Mirizzi's syndrome is a rare complication in which a gallstone becomes impacted in the cystic duct or neck of the gallbladder causing compression of the CBD, resulting in CBD obstruction and jaundice.
- ***The complication rate is not increased in patients undergoing early as opposed to delayed (>6 weeks after diagnosis) cholecystectomy***
- ***Early cholecystectomy (within 72 h) is the treatment of choice for most patients with acute cholecystitis.***
- **Laparoscopic cholecystectomy** is a minimal-access approach for the removal of the gallbladder together with its stones. ***Conversion to laparotomy occurs in 5%***
- ***Laparoscopic cholecystectomy has become the "gold standard" for treating symptomatic cholelithiasis.***

187. Ans. b Cannot be used for screening of prostate cancer, c. Level is high in all patient of prostate carcinoma

[Ref: L and B 27th/1469; Robbins 9th/988-89; Manipal Surgery 4th/977:Schwartz 9th/256]

"20% to 40% of patients with organ-confined prostate cancer have a PSA value of 4.0 ng/mL or less- *Robbins 9th/988*

Screening for Prostate Cancer

◈ *L and B 27th/1469*

- The ***cancer detection rate using measurement of PSA is between 2 and 4 per cent,*** and approximately 30 per cent of men with an elevated PSA will have prostate cancer confirmed by biopsy.
- Unfortunately, ***20 per cent of men with clinically significant prostate cancer will have PSA values within the normal range.*** There is therefore controversy over the usefulness of PSA alone as a screening procedure.

PSA

Robbins 9th/988-89

- ***PSA is organ specific but not cancer specific.***
- A significant rise in serum PSA levels, despite the latest serum PSA test being below the normal ***cutoff (<4 ng/mL),*** is abnormal and should prompt a work-up.
- Furthermore, it appears that per cent free PSA is most valuable in discriminating between benign and malignant disease when the total PSA level is in the "gray zone" of 4 to 10 ng/mL. *When per cent free PSA is higher than 25%, it indicates a lower risk of cancer, whereas per cent free PSA values of less than 10% are worrisome for cancer*

PSA

◈ *Manipal Surgery 4th/977*

>4 nmol/ml: carcinoma to be suspected
10 nmol/ml: suggestive of prostatic cancer
35 nmol/ml: disseminated carcinoma

Prostate-Specific Antigen

◈ *CSDT 14th/1004-05*

- PSA is elevated in the serum of most men with prostate cancer, but high-grade (Gleason 8-10) cancers and ductal variant adenocarcinomas can present with normal PSA levels.
- ***Values above 4 ng/mL are considered abnormal*** but rise normally with age and significant benign prostatic hypertrophy.
- **Methods for enhancing PSA specificity** include the following: (1) **age-specific PSA** (younger men [< age 50 years], normal < 2.5 ng/mL; older men [> age 70 years], normal > 6.5 ng/mL); (2) **PSA density** (PSA divided by prostate volume), where less than 0.15 ng/mL suggests cancer; (3) **percent-free PSA** (total PSA minus complexed PSA), where lower values signify an increased risk of cancer (useful for total PSA levels between 4 and 10).
- ***While total PSA is useful for staging, it is not absolute.*** PSA appears to be ***most helpful in following up on patients after treatment, as levels fall to undetectable after surgery and decrease dramatically after radiation*** therapy when there is a complete response.

Prostate-Specific Antigen

◈ *Schwartz 9th/256*

Prostate-specific antigen (PSA) is an androgen-regulated serine protease ***produced by the prostate epithelium.***

PSA levels have been shown to be ***useful in evaluating the effectiveness of prostate cancer treatment*** and ***monitoring for recurrence after therapy.*** In ***monitoring for recurrence, a trend of increasing levels is considered more significant than a single absolute elevated value.***

Table: Schwartz 9th/255

Marker	Cancer	Sensitivity (%)	Specificity
PSA (4 g/L)	Prostate	57–93	55–68

188. Ans. a. Clinically negative axillary nodes, c. To prevent lymphedema by avoiding unwanted surgery, d. Multifocal breast carcinoma is contraindication, e. Contraindicated in Pregnancy

[Ref: L and B 27th/877; Sabiston 19th/854; Manipal Surgery 4th/409; Schwartz 10th/305]

- The clinically negative node (N0) is the most important indication for SNB.
- Presence of suspicious palpable axillary lymph nodes is contraindication for SLNB.
- Axillary lymph node dissection (ALND) may result in lymphedema. Sentinel lymph node biopsy (SLNB) is a less invasive method of assessing nodal involvement so chances of lymphedema are very less.

Sentinel Node Biopsy

◈ *L and B 27th/877*

- This technique has become the standard of care in ***the management of the axilla in patients with clinically node-negative disease.***
- The sentinel node is localised peroperatively by the injection of patent blue dye and radioisotope labelled albumin in the breast.
- The recommended site of injection is in the subdermal plexus around the nipple although some still inject on the axillary side of the cancer.

- ***Morbidity rates are substantially lower with sentinel node biopsy than with axillary dissection.*** Sentinel node biopsy is an outpatient procedure that does not require a drain, allows rapid return to full mobility, and permits return to work weeks sooner than after axillary dissection. ***Longer term morbidity, including lymphedema, numbness, and chronic pain, is greatly reduced***- *Sabiston 19th/854*
- The concept of SLNB is based on the notion that tumors drain in an orderly manner through the lymphatic system. Therefore, the SLN is the first to be affected by metastasis if the tumor has spread, and a tumor-free SLN makes it highly unlikely for other nodes to be affected. Sentinel lymph node biopsy has become the standard of care for primary treatment of early breast cancer and has replaced **axillary lymph node dissection (ALND)** to stage clinically node-negative patients, thus reducing ALND-associated morbidity.

Indications of SLNB

- ***The clinicall y negative node (N0) is the most important indication for SNB.*** Therefore, the candidates for SNB should be picked from the patients with N0.
- When no histological information is available, patients whose tumor is 20 mm or smaller are candidates for SNB.
- When histological information is available, the SNB indication extends to patients whose type of tumor has histologically good prognosis or a low probability of having nodal involvement, regardless of tumor size.

Contraindications of SLNB

- ***Presence of suspicious palpable axillary lymph nodes;***
- Ductal carcinoma in situ (DCIS) when mastectomy is not planned, therefore not requiring axillary node assessment;
- ***Pregnant patients if blue dye is used in the technique***
- Inflammatory breast cancer.
- **Multifocal breast cancer**- *Manipal Surgery 4th/409*

189. Ans. a. Generalized weakness, b. Iron deficiency anemia, e. Apple core lesion on radiography

[Ref: L and B 27th/1261-64; CSDT11th/ 719; Schwartz 9th/1041-50; Manipal Surgery 4th/711]

- Weakness occur due to anaemia

"Tumours of the left side of the colon which are far more common. It usually present with a change in bowel habit or rectal bleeding, while more **proximal lesions** typically present later with ***iron deficiency anaemia or a mass***"- *L and B 26th/1164*

Hematochezia is the passage of fresh blood through the anus, usually in or with stools (contrast with melena).It is commonly occur in rectal cancer. In carcinoma left colon, there may be gross blood in stool. In right colon carcinoma, there is occult blood(malena)"- *Manipal Surgery 4th/711*

Double contrast barium enema: *Show apple core deformity or napkin ring*- *Manipal Surgery 4th/714*

Table *(Manipal Surgery 4th/711; L and B 25th/ 1180)*: **Symptoms and signs of colorectal cancer**

Right-sided tumours: Iron deficiency anaemia, abdominal mass

Left-sided tumours: Rectal bleeding, alteration in bowel habit, tenesmus, obstruction

Metastatic disease: Jaundice, ascites, hepatomegaly; other symptoms and signs from rarer sites of metastasis

There may be considerable overlap between these symptoms

190. Ans. a. Full thickness is most common in adult, b. Mucosal prolapse is most common in children, c. Diarrhoea in children may be precipitating factor for mucosal prolapse, e. Rectal prolapse in adults is often associated with third-degree haemorrhoids

[Ref: L and B 27th/1321-24; Manipal Surgery 4th/788-89]

"Mucosal prolapse in children often commences after an attack of diarrhoea, or from loss of weight and consequent loss of fat in the ischiorectal fossae. It may also be associated with cystic fibrosis, neurological causes and maldevelopment of the pelvis"-*L and B 27th/1321*

"**Rectal prolapse** in adults is often associated with **third-degree haemorrhoids**"- *L and B 27th/1322*

Rectal Prolapse

◈ *L and B 27th/1322*

- It may be mucosal or full thickness
- If full thickness, the whole wall of the rectum is included
- It commences as a rectal intussusception
- In ***children, the prolapse is usually mucosal*** and should be treated conservatively
- In the ***adult, the prolapse is often full thickness*** and is frequently associated with incontinence
- Surgery is necessary for full-thickness rectal prolapse
- The operation is performed either via the perineum or via the abdomen

191. Ans. a. Up to 5 mm in width, d. Conservative management is done initially, e. In chronic and recurrent cases lateral internal sphincterotomy is helpful

[Ref: L and B 27th/1351-53; Sabiston 19th/1391; Manipal Surgery 4th/802-03; Schwartz 9th/1225]

- They are *mostly (85-90%)* ***located posteriorly in the midline*** *at 6'o clock position*
- ***Diagnosed by visually inspecting the anal verge*** *with gentle separation of gluteal cleft as patients are* ***often too tender for DRE, anoscopy orproctoscopy.***
- Combination of medical therapies may offer up to 98% cure rates.
- Surgical procedures are generally reserved for people with anal fissure who have tried medical therapy for at least one to three months and have not healed (recurrent and chronic cases). Lateral internal sphincterotomy (LIS) is the surgical procedure of choice for anal fissures due to its simplicity and its high success rate (95%).

Anal Fissure

◈ *L and B 27th/1352*

- Acute or chronic
- Ischaemic ulcer in the ***midline of the anal canal***

- Ectopic site suggests a more sinister cause
- Symptoms:
  - Pain on defaecation
  - Bright-red bleeding
  - Mucous discharge
  - Constipation

Treatment of an Anal Fissure

◈ *L and B 27th/1353*

- **Conservative initially,** consisting of stool-bulking agents and softeners, and chemical agents in the form of ointments designed to relax the anal sphincter and improve blood flow
- **Surgery if above fails**, consisting of lateral internal sphincterotomy or anal advancement flap

Anal Fissure

◈ *Sabiston 19th/1391*

- *The average anal fissure usually sizes up to 1 cm in length, up to 3-5 mm in width (basal) and about 2-3 mm in depth.*
- Anal fissures usually extend from the anal opening to dentate line. They are *mostl y (85-90%) located posteriorlv in the midline at 6'o clock position.* probably because of the relatively unsupported nature and poor perfusion of the anal wall in that location. About 10-15% occurring in the anterior (front) midline. A small number of patients may actually have fissures in both the front and the back locations
- Lateral internal sphincterotomy (LIS) is the surgical procedure of choice for anal fissures due to its simplicity and its high success rate (-95%).

192. Ans. b. Fever and abdominal pain are common presentation, c. High risk of mortality, d. Antibiotics may be given prior to bacterial culture report, e. Leukocytosis

[Ref: Harrison 20th/953-54; L and B 27th/1053; Sabiston 19th/1100-02; Schwartz 9th/124-25]

"When first described, the ***mortality rate exceeded 90%,*** *but it has been reduced to* ***approximately 20%*** *with early diagnosis & treatment"- L and B 27th/1053*

Spontaneous Bacterial Peritonitis

◈ *Sabiston 19th/1100-02*

- The diagnosis of SBP is made initially by demonstrating more than ***250 neutrophils/mm³*** of ascitic fluid in a clinical setting consistent with this diagnosis, that is, ***abdominal pain, fever, or leukocytosis*** in a patient with low-protein ascites
- ***Broad-spectrum antibiotics, such as a third-generation cephalosporin, are started immediately*** in patients suspected of having ascitic fluid infection. These agents cover about 95% of the flora most commonly associated with SBP. ***The spectrum of the antibiotic coverage may be narrowed once the results of antibiotic sensitivity tests are known.***
- The immediate mortality risk due to SBP is low, particularly if recognized and treated expeditiously. However, the development of other **complications** of hepatic failure, including gastrointestinal hemorrhage or hepatorenal syndrome, contributes to the death of many of these patients during the hospitalization in which SBP is detected.

Primary (Spontaneous) Bacterial Peritonitis

◈ *Harrison 20th/953-54*

- In adults, **primary bacterial peritonitis (PBP)** occurs most commonly in conjunction with ***cirrhosis of the liver*** (frequently the result of alcoholism).
- The presentation of PBP differs from that of secondary peritonitis.
- ***The most common manifestation is fever, which is reported in up to 80% of patients.***
- Ascites is found but virtually always predates infection.
- ***Abdominal pain***, an acute onset of symptoms, and peritoneal irritation during physical examination can be helpful diagnostically, but the absence of any of these findings does not exclude this often subtle diagnosis.
- ***The finding of >250 PMNs/μL is diagnostic for PBP***, according to Conn. This criterion does not apply to secondary peritonitis
- The **diagnosis of PBP** is not easy. It depends on the exclusion of a primary intraabdominal source of infection. Contrast-enhanced CT is useful in identifying an intraabdominal source for infection. It may be difficult to recover organisms from cultures of peritoneal fluid, presumably because the burden of organisms is low.
- Because bacteremia frequently accompanies PBP, blood should be cultured simultaneously.
- ***PBP has a high rate of recurrence. Up to 70% of patients experience a recurrence within 1 year.*** Antibiotic prophylaxis is recommended for patients with a history of PBP to reduce this rate to <20% and improve short-term survival rates.
- **Treatment for PBP** is directed at the isolate from blood or peritoneal fluid. Gram's staining of peritoneal fluid often gives negative results in PBP. ***Therefore, until culture results become available, therapy should cover gram-negative aerobic bacilli and gram-positive cocci.*** Third-generation cephalosporins such as cefotaxime (2 g q8h, administered IV) provide reasonable initial coverage in moderately ill patients

193. Ans. d. Hematesis

[Ref: Harrison 20th/1904; Robbins 9th/753;;Schwartz 10th/990-92]

- There is *progressive dysphagia for both solids and liquids.* Dysphagia is worsened by emotional stress and hurried eating.
- Other features may include ***regurgitation*** and pulmonary aspiration
- ***Esophagitis with ulceration*** may occur due to chronic retention of food.
- ***Loss of appetite & Weight loss*** *can occur if the condition become chronic.*

Achalasia Cardia

◈· *Harrison 20th/1904*

- Clinical manifestations may include ***dysphagia, regurgitation***, chest pain, and weight loss. Most patients report ***solid and liquid food dysphagia.***

- Regurgitation occurs when food, fluid, and secretions are retained in the dilated esophagus.
- Patients with advanced achalasia are at risk for bronchitis, pneumonia, or lung abscess from chronic regurgitation and aspiration.
- **Chest pain** is frequent early in the course of achalasia, thought to result from esophageal spasm. Patients describe a squeezing, pressure-like retrosternal pain, sometimes radiating to the neck, arms, jaw, and back.
- Paradoxically, some patients complain of heartburn that may be a chest pain equivalent. Treatment of achalasia is less effective in relieving chest pain than it is in relieving dysphagia or regurgitation.
- **Chest X-ray** shows absence of gastric air bubble, an air-fluid level in mediastinum in upright position.
- Barium swallow shows ***'Bird beak'*** or ***'rat tailed'*** *appearance.* There is *megaesophagus (diffuse esophageal dilatation or sigmoid esophagus).*
- Manometry is the diagnostic procedure of choice

194. Ans. a. Nonpulmonary visceral metastases

[Ref: www.ncbi.nlm.nih.gov; www.cancer.ca]

- Presence of Nonpulmonary visceral metastases is an intermediate prognostic factor. All other are good progsotic factors
- Any primary site and any level of tumor markers if present with no nonpulmonary visceral metastasis are considerd good prognostic factors.

The International Germ Cell Consensus Classification (IGCCC) Prognostic Criteria for Seminoma

Good-prognosis seminomia (90% of seminomas) 5-year survival 86% 5-year progression-free survival (PSF) 82%	Any primary site No nonpulmonary visceral metastases Normal AFT, any hCG, any LDH
Intermediate prognosis seminoma (10% of seminomas) 5-year survival 72%; 5 year PSF 67%	Any primary site Nonpulmonary visceral metastases Normal AFT, any hCG, any LDH
Poor	No seminoma patients are classified as poor prognosis

195. Ans. c. Herniation of Midgut, d. Goes back around 4 week after herniation, e. Goes back around 10 week of fetus age

[Ref: BDC 6th Vol. II/273; Embryology by Inderbir Singh 10th/198-200; radiopaedia.org Langman Embryology 9th/Chap 10]

"**Midgut** *is in the form of primary intestinal loop. At the apex of the loop it is connected to the yolk sac & grows very rapidly during 6th week, so much so that it protrudes into the umbilical cord. This is* ***called physiological hernia. After an interval of 4 week****, i. e* ***at 10 week*** *it returns back into the enlarged abdominal cavity. During this herniation & return the midgut loop rotates by 270 degree in a counter clockwise direction*" *(BDC 6th Vol. II/273)*

"Herniated coils of intestine return to the abdominal ***cavity at 3 months***"- Embryology by Inderbir Singh 10th/200

Physiological Gut Herniation

◈ *radiopaedia.org*

- It is a natural phenomenon that occurs in early pregnancy. It usually ***occurs from around 6-8 weeks up until 13 weeks in-utero, after which the bowel returns to the abdominal cavity.***
- It occurs as a result of the bowel (particularly ileum) growing faster than the abdominal cavity during the early gestational period. In the physiological situation, the intestine elongates and moves outside of the embryonic abdomen herniating into the base of the umbilical cord.
- This occurs at ~8 weeks gestational age and is due to a number of factors including rapid growth of the cranial end of the ***midgut*** (which will form the small intestine), and the large size of the developing liver and kidneys.
- While the bowel is within the umbilical cord, the midgut rotates 90 degrees counter-clockwise (facing the embryo).
- At approximately 10-11 weeks the abdomen enlarges and the intestines return to the abdominal cavity. The midgut then rotates an additional 180 degrees counter-clockwise fixing to the posterior retroperitoneum.

OBSTETRICS & GYNECOLOGY

196. Ans. a. Clear cell, b. Mixed mullerian, d. Serous

[Ref: Robbins 9th (SAE)/1014-17; Shaw's Gynac 17th/432-34; Dutta's Gynae 7th/293]

Endometrial carcinoma *are of* **two types** *based upon biological & histological behavior- DutaGynae 7th/293*

"Type I*: **endometrioid & mucinous***;* **Type II***: **serous, clear cell,*** *undifferentiated & carcinosarcoma"-Harshmohan 8th/771*

Type II (Serous) Carcinoma

◈ *Robbins 9th (SAE)/1017*

- These generally occur in women who are about 10 years older than those with type I carcinomas, and in contrast to type I carcinoma they usually arise in the setting of *endometrial atrophy*
- Type II tumors are by definition poorly differentiated (grade 3) tumors and account for approximately 15% of cases of endometrial carcinoma.
- The most common subtype is ***serous carcinoma***, referred to as such because of morphologic and biologic overlap with ovarian serous carcinoma.
- Several less common histologic subtypes (***clear cell carcinoma and malignant mixed müllerian tumor***) are also included within this category

Table: *(Robbins 9th (SAE)/1015; DutaGynae 7th/293)*: **Carcinoma Endometrial II Type and I Type of Characteristics**

Characteristics	Type I	Type II
Age	55–65 yr	65–75 yr

Contd...

Characteristics	Type I	Type II
Clinical setting	Unopposed estrogen Obesity Hypertension Diabetes	Atrophy Thin physique
Morphology	Endometrioid	Serous Clear cell Mixed mullerian tumor
Precursor	Hyperplasia	Serous endometrial intraepithelial carcinoma
Behavior	Indolent Spreads via lymphatics	Aggressive Intraperitonealand lymphatic spread

197. Ans. a. OCP

[Ref: Robbins 9th (SAE)/1014-17; Shaw's Gynae 17th/433; DutaGynae 7th/294]

*"Both ovarian & endometrial malignancies are **less common** among **regular users of OCP**"- Shaw's Gynae 17th/264*

Table: *(Shaw's Gynae 17th/433):* **Risk factors for endometrial cancer**

Risk factor	Relative risk
Long-term unopposed oestrogen	10–20
Lynch syndrome	6–20
Oestrogen-producing tumour	>5
Older age	2–3
Higher income and education	1.5–2
White race	2
Nulliparity	3
Menstrual irregularity	1.5
History of infertility	2–3
Late age at menopause	2–3
Early age at menarche	1.5–2
Tamoxifen	2–3
Obesity	2–5
History of type 2 diabetes mellitus (T2DM), hypertension (HTN) or thyroid disorder	1.3–3

198. Ans. a. ≤2.5 cm

[Ref: Duta Obs 9th/294-95; Obs by JB Sharma 1st/458]

Predictors of Preterm Labor

◈ *Duta Obs 9th/295 Obs by JB Sharma 1st/458*

- **Clinical Predictors** (i) History of prior preterm birth; (ii) Multiple pregnancy; (iii) Presence of genital tract infection; (iv) Symptoms of PTL
- **Biophysical predictors:** (i) Uterine contractions (UC) >4/hr; (ii) Bishop score >4; (iii) ***Cervical length (TVS) <25 mm.***
- **Biochemical predictors:** (i) Fetal fibronectin (fFN) in cervicovaginal discharge (>50 ng/mL); (ii) Others IL-6, IL-8, TNF-α

199. Ans. b. Follicular phase is constant, d. Ovulation occur after 14 day of menstruation

[Ref: Ganong 25th/402,399; Shaw's Gynae 17th/55; Duta Gynae 7th/75]

"The **luteal phase** i,e. Time between ovulation & menstruation, is ***fairly constant at 14 days*** in a menstrual cycle"- *Shaw's Gynae 17th/55*

"Ovulation occur approx. 10-12 hour after LH peak or 32-36 hours after the onset of LH surge"- *DutaGynae 7th/75*

"LH peak occurs about 24-36 hours before ovulation- *Shaw's Gynae 17th/55*

Table: *(DutaGynae 7th/75):* **Approx.time interval of events in menstrual cycle prior to ovulation**

Events	Hours
Onset of LH surge	34-36
LH peak	10-12
Progesterone rise	8
Estradiol rise	83
Estradiol peak	24-36

200. Ans. b. True gestational sac, c. Corpus luteum in ovary, d. Fetal pole, e. Yolk sac

[Ref: Duta Obs 9th/66; Obs by JB Sharma 1st/69,726]

"A **pseudogestational sac**, also known as a **pseudosac** or **intracavitary fluid**, is the concept that a small amount of intrauterine fluid in the setting of a positive pregnancy test and abdominal pain could be erroneously interpreted as a true gestational sac in ***ectopic pregnancy***"- radiopaedia.org

Ultrasonographic Finding of Intrauterine Pregnancy

◈ *Duta Obs 9th/66; Obs by JB Sharma 1st/726*

- *Intrauterine pregnancy is usually diagnosed by a positive pregnancy test and demonstration of a **gestational sac in the uterus.***
- *A transvaginal scan (more sensitive than a transabdominal scan) can detect an intrauterine **gestational sac** at 4 weeks, an embryo (yolk sac) at 5 weeks.*
- *A **fetal pole** with heart tone is typically seen by the completion of 7 menstrual weeks.*
- *In cases of ectopic pregnancy, a pseudo sac (due to decidual reaction in the endometrium) may give a false impression of an intrauterine pregnancy.*
- *In the first 8 weeks of pregnancy, the corpus luteum is often identified as a cystic mass measuring 1-3 cm in diameter.*

Table: *(Obs by JB Sharma 1st/69):* **Summary of Diagnosis of pregnancy**

Presumptive symptoms
• Amenorrhoea of varying period • Nausea, vomiting (morning sickness) • Frequency of micturition

Contd...

Presumptive signs
• Discoloration of vaginal mucosa • Breast changes • Skin changes • Fatigue • Quickening
Probable signs
• Changes in the size, shape and consistency of uterus • Softening of cervix • Various signs described in early pregnancy • Abdominal enlargement • Braxton Hicks contractions • External and internal ballotment
Absolute signs
• Auscultation of fetal heart sound • Palpation of fetal parts and perception of active fetal movements • Ultrasonography ***evidence of gestational sac and embryo in early pregnancy and fetal parts*** later

201. Ans. a. 46 XX, b. 46 XY

[Ref: Duta Obs 9th/180-87; Obs by JB Sharma 1st/143-49; Dutta Gynae 7th/298-300; William's Obs23rd/257-61]

"In general ***completes moles have a 46XX karyotype (85%),*** the molar chromosomes are derived entirely from the father. The ovum nucleus may be either absent (empty ova) or inactivated which have been fertilized by a haploid sperm. It then duplicates its own chromosomes after meosis. Infrequently, the chromosome pattern may be ***46XY or 45X"***- *Duta Obs 9th/181; C'‘s by JB Sharma 1st/143*

"**Partial mole**: 69XXX or 69XXY"- *Obs by JB Sharma 1st/143; Duta Obs 9th/186*

Table: *(COGDT; Duta Obs 9th/187):* **Comparison of Complete and Partial Hydatidiform Moles**

Features	Complete mole	Partial mole
Karyotype	Diploid (46, XX or 46, XY)	Triploid (90%) (69, XXX or 69, XXY); diploid (10%)
Embryo/fetus	Absent	Often present
Villi	Hydropic	Few hydropic
Trophoblasts	Diffuse hyperplasia	Mild focal hyperplasia
Implantation site trophoblast	Diffuse atypia	Focal atypia
Fetal RBCs	Absent	Present
β-hCG	High (> 50,000)	Slight elevation (< 50,000)
Frequency of classic clinical symptoms1	Common	Rare
Risk for persistent GTT	20–30%	< 5%

202. Ans. a. Loss of deep tendon reflex, b. Decreased respiratory rate, c. Decreased urine output

[Ref: Dutta's Obs 9th/222; William's Obs 23rd/737-39; Obs by J B Sharma 1st/437-39]

Box (*Duta Obs 9th/222*)**: Detection of magnesium toxicity**

- Loss of deep tendon reflex (Depression of patellar reflex is the earliest sign of patellar toxicity)
- Decreased respiratory rate (<12 per minute)
- Decreased Urine output (<30 mL/h)
- Chest pain, ***heart block***, pulmonary edema
- ***Cardiac arrest***
- O_2 saturation monitoring (PaO2 <95%)
- Double vision
- Slurred speech
- Nausea-vomiting
- Muscular weakness

203. Ans. a. Lower 1/3rd of vagina, e. Pelvis wall

[Ref: Shaw's Gynae 17th/425; DutaGynae 7th/282; obgyn.onlinelibrary.wiley.com]

Option a-e

Lower 1/3rd Vagina: Stage IIIA
Pelvic wall:Stage IIIB
Upper 2/3rd Vagina: Stage IIA
Parametrium involvement (Partial/complete): Stage IIB

Changes in Latest FIGO (2018) Staging (from Previous FIGO Staging)

◈ *obgyn.onlinelibrary.wiley.com*

- One of the major changes from the prior 2014 FIGO staging system is that stage ***IB disease now includes three sub-groups rather than two***
- Another major change in the current staging system is the incorporation of ***nodal status into stage III*** disease staging.
- Cases with lymph node metastasis are now specifically designated as stage **IIIC disease**, stage IIIC1 for pelvic lymph node metastasis only or stage IIIC2 for paraaortic lymph node metastasis. This new staging system clearly reflects the importance of lymph node metastasis as a major prognostic factor in cervical cancer

Revised FIGO Staging of Cervical Carcinoma (2018)

Stage I

The carcinoma is strictly confined to the cervix uteri (extension to the corpus should be disregarded)

- **IA** Invasive carcinoma that can be diagnosed only by microscopy, with maximum depth of invasion <5 mm[a]
  - **IA1** Measured stromal invasion <3 mm in depth
  - **IA2** Measured stromal invasion ≥3 mm and <5 mm in depth
- **IB** Invasive carcinoma with measured deepest invasion ≥5 mm (greater than stage IA), lesion limited to the cervix uteri[b]
  - **IB1** Invasive carcinoma ≥5 mm depth of stromal invasion and <2 cm in greatest dimension
  - **IB2** Invasive carcinoma ≥2 cm and <4 cm in greatest dimension
  - **IB3** Invasive carcinoma ≥4 cm in greatest dimension

Stage II

The carcinoma invades beyond the uterus, but has not extended onto the lower third of the vagina or to the pelvic wall

- **IIA** Involvement limited to the upper two-thirds of the vagina without parametrial involvement
  - **IIA1** Invasive carcinoma <4 cm in greatest dimension
  - **IIA2** Invasive carcinoma ≥4 cm in greatest dimension
- **IIB** With parametrial involvement but not up to the pelvic wall

Stage III

The carcinoma involves the lower third of the vagina and/or extends to the pelvic wall and/or causes hydronephrosis or non-functioning kidney and/or involves pelvic and/or paraaortic lymph nodesc

- **IIIA** Carcinoma involves the lower third of the vagina, with no extension to the pelvic wall
- **IIIB** Extension to the pelvic wall and/or hydronephrosis or non-functioning kidney (unless known to be due to another cause)
- **IIIC** Involvement of pelvic and/or paraaortic lymph nodes, irrespective of tumor size and extent (with r and p notations) c
  - **IIIC1** Pelvic lymph node metastasis only
  - **IIIC2** Paraaortic lymph node metastasis

Stage IV

The carcinoma has extended beyond the true pelvis or has involved (biopsy proven) the mucosa of the bladder or rectum. A bullous edema, as such, does not permit a case to be allotted to stage IV

- **IVA** Spread of the growth to adjacent organs
- **IVB** Spread to distant organs

- Adding notation of r (imaging) and p (pathology) to indicate the findings that are used to allocate the case to stage IIIC. For example, if imaging indicates pelvic lymph node metastasis, the stage allocation would be stage IIIC1r and, if confirmed by pathological findings, it would be Stage IIIc1p. The type of imaging modality or pathology technique used should always be documented. When in doubt, the lower staging should be assigned

204. Ans. b. Causes primary amenorrhoea

[Ref: Shaw's Gynae 17th/350; DutaGynae 7th/378]

Asherman's syndrome *cause* **secondary amenorrhoea**- *DutaGynae 7th/378*

Uterine Synechiae (Asherman's Syndrome)

◈ *DutaGynae 7th/378*

- There is formation of adhesions following post-abortal and puerperal curettage and also following diagnostic curettage in dysfunctional uterine bleeding.
- Rarely, it follows tubercular endometritis.
- Menstrual abnormalities include hypomenorrhea, oligomenorrhea or amenorrhea.
- Progesterone challenge test is negative
- Hysterosalpingography shows honeycomb appearance.
- Transvaginal sonography or saline infusion sonography is helpful to the diagnosis. But definitive diagnosis is made by hysteroscopy.
- Hysteroscopy reveals the extent of adhesions directly. It has got its therapeutic value also

205. Ans. a. Congenital anomalies are more common when the infection occurs during 12-20 weeks of gestation, c. Immunoglobulins can be given to the neonates whose mother had varicella 5 days before to 2 days after the delivery

[Ref: Duta Obs 9th/281; Park 25th/158; Obs by JB Sharma 1st/558]

If varicella develops in a mother **within 5 days** after delivery, the newborn is at risk of disseminated disease & should receive varicella-zoster immunoglobulin- *Park 25th/158*

"The risk of **congenital malformation** *is nearly* **absent** *when maternal infection* **occurs after 20 weeks**"- *Duta Obs 9th/281*

The **risk depends** upon the timing of pregnancy being 0.4% in first trimester, 2% from 13 to 20 weeks increasing to ***17 to 30% if onset of varicella in the mother is from 5 days before delivery to 2 days after delivery***. VZIG should be given within 72 hours of exposure to all pregnant women with significant exposure to VZV with no history of chickenpox to reduce morbidity in mother & newborn. VZIG should also be administered to the neonates within 5 days of delivery- *Obs by JB Sharma 1st/558*

"Use of **acyclovir** *in the first trimester does not increase birth defects & it should be the antiviral* **drug of choice in early pregnancy**"*-www.aafp.org*

*"**Women should not get vaccinated** during pregnancy or during the 30 days before becoming pregnant- www.ijdvl.com*

206. Ans. b. Rotterdam criteria decreases the prevalence in the population, c. More in Caucasian as compared to Asian

[Ref: www.ncbi.nlm.nih.gov; Shaw's Gynae 17th/314-16; DutaGynae 7th/378-82]

Option a (Correct): Prevalence of PCOS in Chinese population is >5% (~5.6%: table below)

Estimated prevalence of PCOS in unselected female populationwww.ncbi.nlm.nih.gov

Ethnicity	Estimated prevalence (%) of PCOS in general female population (with 95% CrI)		
	1990 NIH	2003 Rotterdam	2006 AES
White (Caucasian)	5.5 (4.8–6.3)	–	–
Black (African-American and Afro-Brazilian)	7.4 (6.3–8.7)	–	–
Chinese	–	5.6 (4.4–7.3)	–
Middle East (Iranian and Turkish)	6.1 (5.3–7.1)	16.0 (13.8–18.6)	12.6 (11.3–14.2)

Option b (Wrong): Rotterdam Criteria Increases the Prevalence

"For the same ethnicity, the prevalence of PCOS was estimated to be the highest for the 2003 Rotterdam and the lowest for the 1990 NIH with the prevalence under the 2006 AES lying in-between"-www.ncbi.nlm.nih.gov

Option c (Wrong): Less Incidence Among Caucausian

"In a community-based study in the United Kingdom (UK), it was found that polycystic ovaries (PCO) were particularly common among women of South Asian origin (52%), compared to the prevalence of PCO observed in a predominately Caucasian population (22%). The South Asian population, in general, also exhibit a higher prevalence of insulin resistance and type 2 diabetes, which may increase long term morbidity among those with PCOS. Recent research indicated higher insulin concentrations and lower insulin sensitivity in South Asian women with PCOS compared to Caucasian women with PCOS. This research also concluded that South Asians presenting with anovular PCOS were significantly younger, had ***more severe hirsuitism*** and a higher prevalence of acanthosis nigricans than their Caucasian counterparts"- www.ncbi.nlm.nih.gov

Option d (Correct): Prevalence of PCOS varies in different population due to use of different diagnostic criteria

The three major diagnostic criteria of PCOS widely followed are criteria raised by National Institutes of Health (NIH), 2003 Rotterdam Consensus raised by European Society of Human Reproduction and Embryology (ESHRE) and American Society for Reproductive Medicine (ASRM) and criteria raised by Androgen Excess Society (AES)

Option e (Correct)

*PCOS: Greater concordance has been reported in **monozygotic twins** versus dizygotic twins"-www.ncbi.nlm*

Current Criteria for the Definition of PCOS

◈ *academic.oup.com*

Study	Criteria
NIH, 1990 (5)	To include all of the following: • Hyperandrogenism and/or hyperandrogenemia • Oligoovulation • Exclusion of related disorders
ESHRE/ASRM (Rotterdam), 2003 (6, 7)	To include two of the following, in addition to exclusion of related disorders: • Oligo- or anovulation • Clinical and/or biochemical signs of hyperandrogenism • Polycystic ovaries

"While there are a number of definitions of PCOS, the ***Rotterdam consensus is the most widely accepted*** across Europe, Asia and Australia and was the definition used for the guideline"- www.racgp.org.au

207. Ans. b. Colposcopy & biopsy, e. Hysterectomy

[Ref: Shaw's Gynae 17th/409-15; DutaGynae 7th/266-68; Novak's Gynae 15th/588]

- **Hysterectomy** may be an option for those women who ***have completed their family***

HSIL *includes **CINII, CINIII and CIS**- Shaw's 16th/88*

High-Grade Squamous Intraepithelial Lesions

◈ *Novak's Gyae 15th/588*

- ***Any woman with a cytologic specimen suggesting the presence of HSIL should undergo colposcopy and directed biopsy***. This is because two-thirds of patients with this cytologic finding will have CIN 2 or greater.
- After colposcopically directed biopsy and determination of the distribution of the lesion, excisional or ablative therapy that addresses the entire transformation zone should be performed
- *"Since cytology alone does not give a clue to which abnormal cells progress to invasive cancer and aneuploidy which suggest the risk of progression is not routinely performed, it is necessary to submit all women with HSIL **cytology for colposcopic study and biopsy of suspicious lesions**"- Shaw's 16th/489*
- *"A single pap smear has a diagnostic sensitivity of about 60%. False negative results may be up to 25%. False negative rate of Pap smear after 3 consecutive negative tests is less than 1%. **Error in cytology could be reduced further by liquid-based thin layer slide preparation** and automated (computer) screening methods. **Abnormal cytology is an indication of colposcopic evaluation and directed biopsy**"-Dutta Gynae 6th/113*

208. Ans. a. LNG, b. CuT < 5 days of unprotected sex, c. Progesterone only pill, d. Progesterone and estrogen pill

[Ref: Shaw's Gynae 17th/269-70; Dutta Gynae 6th/493; Novak's Gynaecology 14th/283-85; William's Obstetrics 23rd/694]

*"In 2009, US FDA has approved the use of **progestin only emergency contraception** (called plan B) without a prscription **(over the counter)** to woman 17 years or older due to efficacy, safety & intent in preventing unwanted adolescent pregnancies" (Obs By JB Sharma 1st/698)*

*"**LNG alone**, 0.75 initially followed by another 0.75mg 12 hours apart, is more effective than the combination of Ethinyl estradiol (EE) & lower dose LNG & **clearly the emergency contraceptive method of choice at present. Alternately 2 tablets (1.5 mg) can be taken as a single dose**" (Novak's Gynaecology 14th/284 & Shaw's Gynaecology 16th/278)*

"The *progestin-only* method uses the progestin **levonorgestrel** in a dose of 1.5 mg, either as two 750 μg doses 12 hours apart, or ***more recently as a single dose within 72 hours of unprotected sex***" *(www.wikipedia.org)*

Table: Methods of Emergency Contraception

Regimen	Dose	Time period
Estrogen alone		
• Ethinyl estradiol (EE)	2.5 mg BD x 5 days	Within 72 hrs
• Conjugated estrogen	15 mg BD x 5 days	-do-
Progestogen alone		
• Levonorgestrel (LNG) (Method of choice)	0.75 mg stat then 0.75 mg after 12 hrs or 1.5 mg stat	-do-

Contd...

Regimen	Dose	Time period
Estrogen + Progestogen (Yuzpe method) • Oral (EE 50 mg + LNG 0.25 mg) • Low dose OCP's	2 tabs stat F/B 2 tabs after 12 hrs 4 tabs stat F/B 4 tabs after 12 hr	-do-
Copper IUD	–	Within 5-7 days
Mifepristone	50-600 mg single dose (Now 10 mg)	On day 27 of mens. Cycle

209. Ans. a. Increase in Middle cerebral artery Peak systolic velocity, b. By platting Lilly zone graph, c. Doppler flow velocity waveforms in umbilical artery, d. Disproportionate growth on USG

[Ref: Dutta's Obs 9th/311-17; Obs by JB Sharma 1st/579-81]

"**Rh Immunisation**: *Currently, MCA PSV is the mainstay of fetal surveillance in a case with red cell alloimmunization.* ***Middle cerebral artery Peak systolic velocity (MCA PSV)*** *>1.5 MoM (multiples of median) for the corresponding gestational age, predicts moderate to severe fetal anaemia"- Duta Obs 9th/316; Obs by JB Sharma 1st/583*

"Doppler flow velocity waveforms in umbilical artery is used to detect fetal anaemia & acidosis"- Duta Obs 9th/316

"Using spectrometer, the optical density 'deviation bulge' of the liquor is observed at 450nm wavelength for the severity of fetal hemolysis. The height of the deviation bulge falls within one of the three zones when plotted in ***Liley's graph*** *depending upon the gestation"- Obs by JB Sharma 1st/584*

Liley zone: Zone1 (low zone), zone 2 (mid zone) & zone 3 (high zone) - *Duta Obs 9th/316*

Doppler USG is useful to assess the fetal gestational age & also to detect the early onset of fetal hydrops*- Duta Obs 9th/316*

210. Ans. c. Immobilization of sperms

[Ref: KDT 8th/349-50; Shaw's 17th/264]

◈ *Immobilization of sperms is not mechanism of action*

Mechanism of Action of Progesterone

◈ *Shaw's 17th/264*

- Thick cervical mucous secretion hostile to sperm penetration is evoked by progestin action KDT 8th/350
- Atrophic changes in endometrium & prevents nidation

Table: *(KDT 8th/349):* **M/A of contraceptives**

				Oral pills	Injections
		Combined E +P	**Progestin-only P**	**Postcoital only P**	**Progestin-only**
1.	FSH inhibition	++	–	–	+
2.	LH inhibition	+++	+	+	+++
3.	Antiovulatory effect	+++	+	+,–	++
4.	Hostile cervical mucus	+++	+++	–	+++
5.	Endometrium	Hypersecretory	Out of phase	Unfavourable	Atrophic
6.	Failure rate (on perfect use)	0.3%	2–3%	2–4%	<0.5%
7.	Contraceptive efficacy	++++	+++	++	++++

211. Ans. a. A combination of hepatitis B immune globulin (HBIG) and hepatitis B vaccination should be initiated within 24 hours of delivery, b. HBIG can be given up to 72 hours after birth, e. 4 doses of vaccine should be given post natally

[Ref: Dutta's Obs 9th/272; O.P. Ghai 8th/217-18; Obs by JB Sharma 1st/533-34]

"In mothers with an unknown HBsAg positivity status at delivery the birth dose of hepatitis B vaccine should be given within 24 hours of birth & HBIG is administered as soon as possible if mother tests positive, ideally within 72 hours of delivery"-indianpaediatric.net

"In the case of **preterm babies** of HBsAg positive mothers, the ***birth dose is indicated even if the baby weighs less than 2 kilograms,*** but should be followed by a further three doses starting at six weeks of age. This is due to the reduced immunogenicity of hepatitis B vaccine in preterms weighing <2 kilograms in the first month of life"- indianpaediatric.net

Management of HBV During Pregnancy

◈ *Dutta's Obs 9th/272*

- HBV Infection can be prevented by vaccination and the recombinant vaccine is safe in pregnancy.
- Pregnant woman who is seronegative, should have HB immunoglobulin (HBIG), 0.06 mL/kg IM,Soon following exposure and a second dose after 1 month. Then she should be given recombinant DNA vaccine intramuscularly 1 mL, 3 doses at 0, 1 and 6 months.
- All infants born to HBsAg positive mothers should have HBIG 0.5 mL IM ***within 12 hours of birth.*** Active immunization with HB vaccine (0.5 mL) is also given IM at a separate site at the same time schedule. This is very effective (85-95%) to protect the infant from HBV infection.
- Breastfeeding is not contraindicated.
- Similar to HIV, perinatal transmission of HBV depends on maternal viral load.

- Tenofovir and HBIG are effective to reduce the transplacental transmission of HBV to the fetus. Tenofovir is given 300 mg/day from 34 weeks.

PAEDIATRICS

212. Ans. **a. Most common age group is 5-10 yr, d. Leaves children unware, e. Precipitated by hyperventilation**

[Ref: Harrison 20th/3051-52; CPDT 17th/749; O.P. Ghai 8th/555; Nelson 20th/2835-36]

Absence Seizures

◈ *Nelson 20th/2835-36*

- Simple (typical) absence (petit mal) seizures are characterized by a sudden cessation of motor activity or speech with a blank facial expression and flickering of the eyelids.
- ***Usually start at 5-8 yr of age*** are never associated with an aura, ***rarely persist longer than 30 sec***, and are ***not associated with a postictal state.*** These features tend to differentiate absence seizures from complex partial seizures.
- Children with absence seizures may experience countless seizures daily, whereas complex partial seizures are usually less frequent.
- Patients do not lose body tone, but their head may fall forward slightly.
- Immediately after the seizure, patients resume preseizure activity with ***no indication of postictal impairment.***
- Automatic behavior frequently accompanies simple absence seizures.
- ***Hyperventilation for 3–5 min routinely produces an absence seizure.***
- The **EEG** shows a ***typical 3 Hz spike and generalized wave discharge.***
- **Complex (atypical) absence** seizures have associated motor components consisting of myoclonic movement of the face, fingers, or extremities and, on occasion, loss of body tone. These seizures produce atypical EEG spike and wave discharges at 2–2.5/sec.

Childhood Absence Seizures

◈ *CPDT 17th/749*

- Incidence higher in girls than in boys
- Age at onset, 3–12 y (peak 6–7 years)
- 10–200 seizures per day
- 3/s spike–wave EEG
- Most remit at puberty

Typical Absence Seizures

◈ *Harrison 20th/3051-52*

- Typical absence seizures are characterized by ***sudden, brief lapses of consciousness without loss of postural control.***
- The seizure usually lasts for ***only seconds***, consciousness returns as suddenly as it was lost, and there is *no postictal confusion.*
- Although the brief loss of consciousness may be ***clinically inapparent*** or the sole manifestation of the seizure discharge, absence seizures are ***usually accompanied by subtle, bilateral motor signs*** such as rapid blinking of the eyelids, chewing movements, or small-amplitude, clonic movements of the hands.
- Typical absence seizures are associated with a group of genetically determined epilepsies with onset usually in childhood (***ages 4–10 years***) or ***early adolescence*** and are the main seizure type in 15–20% of children with epilepsy.
- The seizures can occur hundreds of times per day, but the child may be ***unaware of or unable to convey their existence.***
- ***Hyperventilation tends to provoke these electrographic discharges*** and even the seizures themselves and is routinely used when recording the EEG

213. Ans. **c. Anti-La (SS-B), d. Anti-Ro (SSA), e. Anti-U1RNP**

[Ref: O.P. Ghai 9th/625; emedicine.medscape.com Nelson 20th/1179, 3107; CPDT 17th/850]

"**Neonatal lupus erythematosus (NLE)** is related to the ***anti-Ro (SSA) antibody*** in *more than 90% of patients.* Occasionally, patients only have ***anti-La (SSB) or anti-U1RNP antibodies.*** These maternal autoantibodies cross the placenta and can react with various fetal tissues, causing an increased risk of acquiring NLE"- emedicine.medscape.com

"**Neonatal lupus erythematosus** (NLE): It is a clinical spectrum of cutaneous, cardiac, and systemic abnormalities observed in the newborn or infants whose mothers have ***autoantibodies against Ro/SSA and/or La/SSB.*** Congenital complete heart block is the most serious manifestation of NLE that can develop *in utero* or after birth"- *www.indianjrheumatol.com*

"Neonatal lupus: In most cases, it is the ***anti-Ro/SSA antibody, the anti-La/SSB antibody***, or both. In rare cases, the **skin rash associated** with neonatal lupus has been associated with another autoantibody that reacts against another type of ribonucleoprotein (the test is called ***anti-RNP***). Other symptoms such as congenital heart block are not thought to occur with anti-RNP but a few isolated cases have been recently published, the importance of which is not yet clear"-*rarediseases.org*

Table *(Harrison 19th/2126)*: **Autoantibodies in Systemic Lupus Erythematosus (SLE)**

Antibody	Pre valence %	Antigen Recognized	Clinical Utility
Antinuclear antibodies	98	Multiple nuclear	Best screening test; repeated negative tests make SLE unlikely
Anti-ds DNA	70	DNA (double-stranded)	High titers are SLE-specific and in some patients correlated with disease activity, nephritis, vasculitis

Contd...

Antibody	Pre valence %	Antigen Recognized	Clinical Utility
Anti-RNP	25	Protein complexed to 6 species of nuclear U1 RNA	Specific for SLE; no definite clinical correlation, most patients also have anti-RNP, more common in blacks and Asians than whites
Anti-RNP	40	Protein complexed to U1 RNA	No specific for SLE
Anti-Ro (SS-A)	30	Protein complexed to hY RNA, primarily 60 kDa and 52 kDa	Not specific for SLE
Anti-La (SS-B)	10	47-kDa protein complexed to hY RNA	Usually associated with anti-Ro, associated with decreased risk for nephritis
Antihistone	70	Histones associated with DNA (in nucleosome, chromatin)	More frequent in drug-induced lupus than in SLE
Antiphospholipid	50	Phospholipids, β_2 glycoprotein 1 cofactor prothrombin	Three tests available- ELSIAs for cardiolipin and β_2 G1 sensitive sensitive prothrombin time (DRVVT); predisposes to clotting, fetal loss, thrombocytopenia
Antierythrocyte	60	Erythrocyte membrane	Measured as direct Coombs test; a small proportion develops overt hemolysis
Antiplatelet	30	Surface and altered cytoplasmic antigens on platelets	Associated with thrombocytopenia but sensitivity and specificity are not good; this is not a useful clinical test
Antineuronal (includes anti-glutamate receptor)	60	Neuronal and lymphocyte surface antigens	In some series a positive test in CSF correlates with active CNS lupus.
Antiribosomal P	20	Protein in ribosomes	In some series a positive test in serum correlated with depression or psychosis due to CNS lupus

214. Ans. a. Modified Blalock–Taussig shunt, b. Waterston-Cooley shunt, c. Pott's shunt

[Ref: O.P. Ghai 9th/417-19; Nelson 20th/2214-15; CPDT 17th/590]

- Aortoplasty & Cutting & end to end anastomosis of aorta have no role in TOF

Tetralogy of Fallot

◈ *Hurst's The Heart 12th/Chap82*

- Palliation, when it is now performed, almost inevitably involves a ***modified Blalock-Taussig shunt*** that interposes a graft between the subclavian artery and the ipsilateral pulmonary artery, usually on the side opposite the aortic arch.
- The performance of some previous palliative operation (***Waterston or Pott's shunts***) but not a palliative Blalock-Taussig shunt was associated with higher mortality.

"A **Waterston shunt is a form of palliative surgery performed in patients with** tetralogy of Fallot prior to the ability to repair the defect. It consists of a shunt formed between the ascending aorta and the right pulmonary artery"-radiopaedia.org

"A **Pott shunt is a form of palliative surgery performed in patients with** tetralogy of Fallot prior to the ability to repair the defect. It consists of a shunt formed between the descending thoracic aorta **and the** left pulmonary artery"- radiopaedia.org

The ***modified Blalock-Taussig shunt*** is currently the most common aortopulmonary shunt procedure and consists of a Gore-Tex conduit anastomosed side to side from the subclavian artery to the homolateral branch of the pulmonary artery. Sometimes the shunt is brought directly from the ascending aorta to the main pulmonary artery and in this case is called a central shunt. The Blalock-Taussig operation can be successfully performed in the newborn period with shunts 3–4 mm in diameter and has also been used successfully in premature infants. *Nelson 20th/2214-15;* CPDT 17th/590

215. Ans. a. Preterm baby, c. Shoulder, d. Fetus

[Ref: Behl 10th/12; Nelson 20th/795; CPDT 17th/5; Avery Neonatology 6th/331]

"***Premature infants***: Fine, soft, immature hair, **lanugo**, frequently covers the ***scalp and brow*** and may also cover the **face** of **premature infants**. Lanugo has usually been lost or replaced by vellus hair in ***term infants***"-*Nelson 20th/795*

"**Lanugo**: Downy hair on the body of a fetus or newborn baby. Lanugo is the first hair to be produced by the fetal hair follicles, and it usually appears on the ***fetus at about 5 months of gestation***. ***Lanugo is very fine, soft, and usually unpigmented***. Although ***lanugo is normally shed before birth***, around 7 or 8 months of gestation, it is sometimes present at birth. This is ***not a cause for concern***: Lanugo disappears of its own accord within a few days or weeks"-www.medicinenet.com

"It is ***more common to see lanugo on preemies, but full-term newborns can be born with this soft***, downy hair covering, too. It can be found everywhere on a baby's body, ***except on the palms, lips, and soles of the feet (so shoulder also)***.It might be surprising to see, but it is ***normal***. Usually, there is no need to worry"- www.verywellfamily.com; *CPDT 17th/5*

216. Ans. a. Crouzon syndrome, b. Carpenter syndrome, c. Pfeiffer syndrome

[Ref: O.P. Ghai 9th/37; Nelson 20th/2817-19; CPDT 17th/769]

"Condtions associated with ***Craniosynostosis: Apert syndrome, Crouzon syndrome, Carpenter syndrome & Pfeiffer syndrome***"- *O.P.Ghai 9th/37*

Craniosynostosis is premature closure of cranial sutures. The most prevalent genetic disorders associated with craniosynostosis include *Crouzon, Apert, Carpenter, Chotzen, and Pfeiffer syndromes- Nelson 20th/2817*

TABLE: *(Nelson 20th/2817):* **Syndromic craniosynostosis**

Name of disorder	Cause
Antler-Bixler syndrome	Unknown
Apert syndrome	Usually one of two mutations in $FGFR_2$
Baere-Stevenson syndrome	Mutation in $GFGR_2$ or $FGFR_3$
Bailler-Gerold syndrome	Mutation in *TWIST*heterogenous
Carpenter syndrome	Unknown
Craniofrontonasal dysplasia	Unknown gene at Xp22
Crouzon syndrome	Numerous different mutations at *$FGFR_2$*
Crouzonomesodermoskeletal syndrome	Mutation in *$FGFR_3$*
Jackson-Weiss syndrome	Mutation in *$FGFR_2$*
Muenke syndrome	Mutation in *$FGFR_3$*
Pfeiffer syndrome	Mutation in *$FGFR_1$* or numerous mutation in *$FGFR_2$*
Saethre-Chotzen syndrome	Mutation in *TWIST*
Shprintzen-Goldberg syndrome	Mutation in *$FBEN_1$*

217. Ans. a. Associated with aniridia, b Mostly unilateral, c. Surrounded by pseudocapsule, e. Associated with palpable abdominal mass

[Ref: O.P. Ghai 9th/609-10; O.P. Ghai 8th/617-18; Nelson 20th/2464-68; CPDT 17th/931]

"Wilms tumor manifests as a solid intrarenal mass with a ***pseudocapsule*** and distortion of the renal parenchyma and collecting system"- pubs.rsna.org

Wilms Tumor

❖ *O.P. Ghai 8th/617-18*

- Most common malignant tumour of kidney, accounting for 6–7% of all childhood malignancy
- 80% of patients with Wilm's tumour present under age of 5 yr
- The peak age at diagnosis is 2–4 yr
- 6% patient have bilateral disease
- While a vast majority of tumour is sporadic, 1–2% may be familial
- Most patients present with an asymptomatic abdominal mass detected by parents or physician during routine examination
- Most patients presents with a asymptomatic abdominal mass
- *At diagnosis **30% presents with abdominal pain***
- Features of congenital syndrome may be present in 13–28% of patients
- ***Renal lump is ballottable****-Kundu 4th/255*
- Wilms tumor occurs in the setting of associated malformations or syndromes, including
- aniridia, hemihypertrophy, genitourinary malformations (eg, cryptorchidism, hypospadias, gonadal dysgenesis, pseudohermaphroditism, horseshoe kidney), Beckwith–Wiedemann syndrome, Denys–Drash syndrome, and WAGR syndrome (Wilms tumor, ***aniridia,*** ambiguous genitalia, mental retardation) - *CPDT 17th/931*

Wilms Tumor

❖ *Nelson 20th/2464-68*

- Familial predisposition to Wilms Tumor is inherited in an **autosomal dominant manner.**
- It may arise in one or both kidneys; the incidence of ***bilateral Wilms Tumor is 7%.***
- It ***usually occurs in children between 2–5 yr of age***, although it has also been encountered in neonates, adolescents, and adults.

Wilms Tumor

❖ *Robbins 9th/479-81*

- The peak incidence for Wilms Tumor is between 2 and 5 years of age, and 95% of tumors occur before the age of 10 years.
- ***Approximately 5% to 10% of Wilms tumors involve both kidneys***, either simultaneously *(synchronous)* or one after the other *(metachronous).s*

218. Ans. c. High positive end expiratory pressure (PEEP), d. Long inspiration time, e. Low tidal volume

[Ref: O.P. Ghai 9th/393; Nelson 20th/1990; CPDT 17th/380-83; www.cancertherapyadvisor.com]

CMV Guidelines for Paediatric ALI/ARDS as Adapted from NHLBI ARDS Network

❖ *www.cancertherapyadvisor.com*

- Set mode to volume assist-control, pressure regulated volume control or similar modes.
- Set initial ***tidal volume to 6-8 mL/kg ideal body weight***.
- Set the ***rate to approximate patients rate but not to exceed 35/min.***
- **Optimally, PEEP should be adjusted** to a level above the lower inflection point of the patients inspiratory pressure volume curve.
- Reduce tidal volume by 1 mL/kg every two hours or less until a tidal volume of 4-6 mL/kg is reached and pH and plateau pressure goals are reached.
- Goal plateau pressure 30 cm water or less.
- Check plateau pressure every 4 hours and after every adjustment of PEEP and oxygen.
- If the plateau pressure is greater than 30, the tidal volume is decreased by 1 mL/kg to a tidal volume of 4 mL/kg or a plateau pressure of less than 30 is reached.

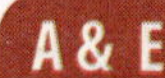

- ***FiO$_2$* less than 0.60** is desired to prevent additional lung toxicity.

Acute Respiratory Distress Syndrome (ARDS)

◈ *Nelson 20th/1990*

- A-aO_2 gradient >300
- The clinician must consider the potential adverse effects of therapeutic interventions such as oxygen, endotracheal intubation, and mechanical ventilation as part of the pathophysiologic consequences of ARDS.
- ***High concentrations of inspired oxygen*** have a risk of pulmonary capillary and epithelial cell injury;
- The mechanical ventilation strategy aimed at minimizing ventilator-induced lung injury in ARDS includes alveolar recruitment and maintenance of adequate FRC throughout the respiratory cycle with an ***optimum PEEP***, and ventilation with ***relatively low (6–8 mL/kg) tidal volume.***
- ***High PEEP or inverse ratio*** ventilation- *O.P. Ghai 9th/393*

"Inverse ratio ventilation (IRV) in ARDS: IRV **is a mode of ventilation which is designed to improve oxygenation at a given level of inspired oxygen. Conventional ventilation uses the times of inspiration and expiration in a ratio of 1:4 or 1:2, giving a longer time for expiration, which is generally a passive process.** Inverse ratio ventilation **reverses this ratio to give a longer inspiratory time** (1:1 or 2:1) by using rapid inspiratory flow rates and decelerating flow patterns during the inspiratory phase. The effect of inverse ratio ventilation **is to increase mean** airway pressures **and thus recruit alveoli in an effect similar to** PEEP"- www.sciencedirect.com

Ventilatory Support for ARDS

◈ *CPDT 17th/382-83*

- Current ventilatory management of ARDS is directed at the rerecruitment of areas of dependent alveolar collapse and the protection of noncollapsed areas from overdistention.
- Since an FiO_2 greater than 60% over 24 hours can cause additional injury to the lung, mean airway pressure should be increased to provide an adequate PaO_2 (> 55 mm Hg) at an ***FiO$_2$* of 60% or less.**
- In general, this can be accomplished by ***incremental increases in PEEP*** every 15–30 minutes until adequate oxygenation is achieved or until a limiting side effect of the PEEP is reached.
- Ventilation with ***high levels of PEEP*** acts by helping to prevent dependent collapse of edematous lung units. PEEP levels of 12–14 cm H_2O are not unusual, and levels as high as 20–25 cm H_2O have been used successfully in these patients.
- Before increasing PEEP significantly, the physician should optimize conditions by making sure that the patient's intravascular volume is appropriate, the endotracheal tube does not leak, and the patient is heavily sedated and paralyzed.
- Current practice for pediatric ARDS patients should consist of ventilation ***with tidal volumes in the 6–8 mL/kg range***, or at least with tidal volumes small enough to keep ***alveolar pressures below 30–35 cm H_2O***

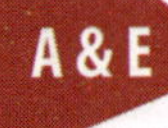

219. Ans. a. Fragile-X syndrome, b. Pierre-Robin syndrome, c. Turner syndrome, d. De-George syndrome, e. Choanal atresia

[Ref: Benumof Airway Management 2nd/277; www.ncbi.nlm]

"Difficult or failed ventilation and endotracheal intubation are amongst the situations that anesthesiologists fear most. Patients with **choanal atresia** are considered to be at high risk for experiencing difficulty with anesthesia."-www.ncbi, nim, nith, gov

Difficult Airway in Congenital Syndromes Based on Anatomical Site

Nasopharynx	• Mucopolysccharidoses (Hurler's/Hunter's syndrome)
Oral cavity/ oropharynx	• Trisomy 21 (Down syndrome) • Beckwith-Wiedemann syndrome • Mucopolysaccharidoses (Hurler's/Hunter's syndrome) • Crouzone syndrome • Pfeiffer syndrome • Freeman-Sheildon syndrome • Halleman-Streiff syndrome
Mandible/ maxilla	• Pierre Robin sequence • Treacher Collins syndrome • Goldenhar syndrome • Apert syndrome • Stickler syndrome • Cri-du-chat syndrome • Edward syndrome • Turner syndrome • De-George syndrome • Fragile-X syndrome
Pharynx/ Larynx	• Trisomy 21 (Down syndrome) • Cri-du-chat syndrome
Trachea	• Trisomy 21 (Down syndrome) • Mucopolysaccharidoses (Hurler's/Hunter's syndrome)
Cervial spine	• Trisomy 21 (Down syndrome) • Klippel-Feil syndrome • Goldenhar syndrome • Mucopolysaccharidoses (Hurler's/Hunter's syndrome) • Arthrogryposis • Fibrodysplasia ossificans progressiva

Acquired Causes of Difficult airway

Infections	Supraglottis Croup Abscess (introral, retropharygeal) Ludwig's angina
Arthritis	Rheumatoid arthritis Ankylosing spondylitis
Tumors	Cystic hygroma Lipoma adenoma, gotier
Truma	Facial injury Cervial spine injury Laryngeal/tracheal trauma
Others	Obesity Acromegaly Acute burns

220. Ans. a. Also k/a kinky hair disease, b. Hypotonia, c. Mental retardation, e. Trichorhexis nodosa

[Ref: Harrison 20th/2318; ghr.nlm.nih.gov]

"**Trichorrhexis nodosa** is a commonly occurring abnormality of the hair shaft. It is characterised by the presence of nodules in the hair strand that cause hair breakage and alopecia. Trichorrhexis nodosa is also observed along with many other syndromes and conditions like Netherton's syndrome, ***Menke's kinky hair*** syndrome, iron deficiency, ectodermal dysplasia (aberrant growth and development of hair, skin and nails) and also hyperthyroidism has been associated to this condition"- www.richfeel.com

Menkes Kinky Hair Syndrome

◈ *Harrison 20th/2318*

- It is an ***X-linked metabolic*** disturbance of copper metabolism characterized by ***mental retardation, hypocupremia, and decreased circulating ceruloplasmin.***
- This syndrome is caused by mutations in the copper-transporting ***ATP7A gene.***
- Children with this disease often die within 5 years because of dissecting aneurysms or cardiac rupture.

Menkes Kinky Hair Syndrome

◈ *ghr.nlm.nih.gov*

- Menkes syndrome is a disorder that affects copper levels in the body.
- It is characterized by ***sparse, kinky hair; failure to gain weight and grow at the expected rate (failure to thrive***); and deterioration of the nervous system.
- Additional signs and symptoms include ***weak muscle tone (hypotonia),*** sagging facial features, ***seizures,*** developmental delay, and ***intellectual disability***.
- Children with Menkes syndrome typically begin to develop symptoms during infancy and often do not live past age 3.
- Early treatment with copper may improve the prognosis in some affected individuals. In rare cases, symptoms begin later in childhood.
- **Occipital horn syndrome** (sometimes called X-linked cutis laxa) is a less severe form of Menkes syndrome that begins in early to middle childhood. It is characterized by wedge-shaped calcium deposits in a bone at the base of the skull (the occipital bone), coarse hair, and loose skin and joints.

ORTHOPAEDICS

221. Ans. b. Failed closed reduction, c. Non-union of old fracture, d. Displaced intra-articular fractures

[Ref: Maheshwari 6th/16,103]

Long bone fractures & Fracture of lateral condyle of humerus are not absolute indication for open reduction

Fracture of **Lateral condyle of humerus in children**: A displaced fracture is treated by ***open reduction & internal fixation*** using two K-wires. An undisplaced fracture (uncommon situation) needs support in an above-elbow plaster slabs for 2-3 weeks"- *Maheshwari 6th/103,58*

Table: *(Maheshwari 6th/16):* **Indications for open reduction**

Absolute
- ***Failure of closed reduction***
- ***Displaced intra-articular fractures***
- Some displaced epiphyseal injuries (types III and IV)
- Major avulsion fractures e.g., fracture of patella
- ***Non-union***

Relative
- Delayed union and malunion
- Multiple fractures
- Pathological fractures
- Where closed reduction is known to be ineffective e.g., fracture of the neck of the femur
- Fractures with vascular or neural injuries

222. Ans. a. Bone scan, b. Bone biopsy, c. CT scan, d. MRI scan

[Ref: Maheshwari 6th/239-41; Apley 9th/208]

It is a case of osteosarcoma

Osteosarcoma: *Investigations Maheshwari 6th/240-41; Apley 9th/208*

- Radiological examination: *Periosteal reaction, Codman's triangle, Sun-ray appearance*
- Serum alkaline phosphatase: Generally elevated, but is of no diagnostic significance
- Biopsy: A open biopsy is performed to confirm the diagnosis
- CT scan may be required in cases where the metastatic lesion is unclear on chest X-ray
- Methods used for precise evaluation of spread of the tumor locally: bone scan for finding the intra-medullary spread (skip lesions), CT & MRI scans for finding the soft tissue spread

Osteosarcoma

◈ *Maheshwari 6th/239*

- Primary osteosarcoma occurs in age group of 15-25 years.
- Secondary osteosarcoma occur in older age (45 years onward)
- Common sites of origin (in decreasing order of frequency): lower end of femur, upper end of the tibia, upper end of humerus

223. Ans. a. Sickle cell anaemia, c. Osteoblastic metastasis, d. Paget's disease of bone, e. Lymphoma

[Ref: Danhert Radiology 7th/192; Sumer Sethi 6th/93; radiopaedia.org]

Ivory Vertebrae: Lost from Chomp

◈ *Danhert Radiology Review Manual 7th/192*

= Increase in opacity of vertebral body retaining its size & contours

- Lymphoma
- Osteopetrosis
- Sickle cell disease
- Trauma, T.B, Spondylitis
- Fluorosis
- Renal osteodystrophy

- Osteoblastic metastasis
- Myelosclerosis
- Chronic sclerosing osteomyelitis, Chordoma
- Hemangioma
- Osteosarcoma
- Myeloma
- Pagets disease of bone

Ivory Vertebrae

◈ *Sumer Sethi 6th/93*

- Lymphoma
- Infection
- Metastasis
- Pagets disease

The **ivory vertebra sign refers to diffuse and homogeneous increase in opacity of a** vertebral body **that otherwise retains its size and contours, and with no change in the opacity and size of adjacent** intervertebral disks- *Danhert Radiology 7th/192*

224. Ans. a. Flexion at the knee, posterior subluxation & external rotation of tibia, e. Seen in TB

[Ref: curofy.com]

Triple Deformity of Knee

◈ *curofy.com*

- It includes
  - Flexion at the knee
  - Posterior subluxation of the tibia
  - External rotation of tibia (abduction)
- Can be seen in
  - Tuberculosis of knee joint
  - Rheumatoid arthritis
  - Rheumatic fever
  - Polio (less frequently)
- Treatment Bilateral knee atroplasty If failed, Bilateral knee replacement

Triple Deformity of Knee is seen in: "TRIPLE"

T - Tuberculosis (most common cause)
R - Rheumatoid arthritis
I - Iliotibial band contacture
P - Polio
L - Low clotting capacity
E - Excess bleeding/hemophilia

225. Ans. a. Subtalar joint, c. Calcaneocuboid joint, d. Talo-navicular joint

[Ref: Maheshwari 6th/216; emedicine.medscape.com; Adam's Ouline of orthopaedics 14th/Chap 26]

Triple Arthrodesis

◈ *Maheshwari 6th/216; emedicine.medscape.com*

- Operative method for CTEV
- This consists of fusion of **three joints of the foot** –***subtalar (talocalcaneal), calcaneo-cuboid &talo-navicular***
- Of the three, talo-navicular joint fusion is most difficult to achieve
- The primary goals of a triple arthrodesis are to relieve pain from arthritic, deformed, or unstable joints.
- Other important goals are the correction of deformity and the creation of a stable, balanced plantigrade foot for ambulation

226. Ans. a. Closed tibial fractures, b. Supracondylar fracture of humerus, c. Forearm bone fractures

[Ref: Maheshwari 6th/47; Apley 9th/295,713]

Compartment Syndrome

◈ *Maheshwari 6th/47*

- Rise in pressure in compartments (enclosed by bones, fascia & interosseous membrane) may jeopardize the blood supply to muscles & nerves within the compartment
- Injuries with high risk of developing compartment syndrome are as follows:
  - Supracondylar fracture of the humerus
  - Forearm bone fractures
  - Closed tibial fractures
  - Crush injuries to leg & forearm
- High risk injuries are fracture of elbow, forearm bones, proximal third of tibia & also multiple fracture of the hand or foot- Apley 9th/295
- Stretch test: Earliest sign of impending compartment syndrome
- Surgical decompression is necessary in established cases by: fasciotomy &fibulectomy

"Tibial fracture- both open & closed- are among the commonest causes of compartment syndrome in the leg"-*Apley 9th/902*

227. Ans. d. Highly radiosensitive tumour, e. Very aggressive tumor

[Ref: Maheshwari 6th/243,173; Apley 9th/212-13; Harrison 20th/656-57; Robbins 9th/1203; Harrison 19th/119e-4; Nelson 20th (SAE)/2473]

Ewing Sarcoma

◈ *Maheshwari 6th/243; Apley 9th/212-13; Harrison 20th/657*

- This is highly malignant tumour occurring b/w the age of ***10-20 years***, sometimes up to 30 years
- **Site:** The tumour may benign anywhere, but ***diaphysis of the long bone*** is the ***most common site***
- ***Often there is associated fever***, in which case it may be confused with osteomyelitis
- The classic cytogenetic abnormality associated with this disease is a reciprocal translocation of the long arms of chromosomes 11 and 22, t (11; 22), which creates a chimeric gene product of unknown function with components from the *fli-1* gene on chromosome 11 and *ewson* 22
- The presence of p30/32, the product of the *mic-2* gene, is a cell-surface marker for Ewing's sarcoma (and other members of the Ewing's family of tumors, previously also called PNETs).
- This ***disease is very aggressive,*** and it is therefore considered a systemic disease. Common sites of metastases are lung, bones, and bone marrow

- The plain radiograph may show a characteristic "onion peel" periosteal reaction with a generous soft tissue mass, which is better demonstrated by CT or MRI.
- This ***a highly radiosensitive tumour***, melts quickly but recurs.
- ***Systemic chemotherapy is the mainstay of therapy, often being used before surgery***. Doxorubicin, cyclophosphamide or ifosfamide, etoposide, vincristine, and dactinomycin are active drugs. Topotecan or irinotecan in combination with an alkylating agent is often used in relapsed patients. Targeted therapy with an anti-IGF-I receptor antibody in combination with an inhibitor of mammalian target of rapamycin (mTOR) has shown promising activity in refractory cases.
- Local treatment for the primary tumor includes surgical resection, usually with limb salvage or radiation therapy.

228. Ans. a. Periosteal reaction, b. New bone formation, e. Fever

[Ref: Maheshwari 6th/243,173; Apley 9th/212]

From chronic osteomyelitis, Ewing sarcoma can be differentiated by the following feature in the former *Maheshwari* 6th*/243*

- Sequestrum
- Located at metaphysis
- Well-defined cloacae & a rather smooth periosteal reaction

Ewing Sarcoma

◈ *Maheshwari* 6th*/243,173*

- Subperiosteal new bone formation
- Sunray appearance & Codman's triangle (Usually associated with osteosarcoma) may occur
- Fever
- Sometime pain & swelling
- Diaphysis

Chronic Osteomyelitis

◈ *Maheshwari* 6th*/172*

- New bone formation
- Pain & fever during acute exacerbations

Sunburst appearance is a ***type of periosteal reaction*** giving the appearance of a sunburst secondary to an aggressive periostitis. It is frequently associated with osteosarcoma but can also occur with other aggressive bony lesions such as an ***Ewing sarcoma*** or osteoblastic metastases (e.g. prostate, lung or breast cancer).- radiopaedia.org

229. Ans. b. Reactive arthritis

[Ref: Harrison 19th/836; Maheshwari 6th/178,286-88]

This is case of reactive arthritis (Reiter's syndrome). Points favouring this diagnosis

- Young patient
- Arthritis
- Conjunctivitis (erythema with pain) Keratoderma blenorrhagicum (yellowish brown keratotic papule)
- Urethritis (burning micturition & urethral discharge)

About other Options

- **Bechet disease:** It is characterized by a triad of recurrent oral ulcers, genital ulcers & uveitis
- **RA & psoriasis** can present with arthritis but there is no history of conjunctivitis & urethritis
- **Secondary syphilis** can present with similar rash. Rash is usually asymptomatic bilateral symmetrical macule or maculopapular which occurs on palm & soles. But arthritis is rare & there is no history of conjunctivitis & urethritis

Postinfectious or Reactive Arthritis (Reiter's Syndrome)

◈ *Harrison* 19th*/836*

- Reactive polyarthritis develops several weeks after ~1% of cases of nongonococcal urethritis and 2% of enteric infections, particularly those due to *Yersinia enterocolitica*, *Shigella flexneri*, *Campylobacter jejuni*, and *Salmonella* species.
- Only a minority of these patients have the other findings of ***classic reactive arthritis, including urethritis, conjunctivitis, uveitis, oral ulcers, and rash***.
- Studies have identified microbial Reactive arthritis is most common among young men (except after *Yersinia* infection) and has been linked to the HLA-B27 locus as a potential genetic predisposing factor.
- Patients report painful, asymmetric oligoarthritis that affects mainly the knees, ankles, and feet.
- Low-back pain is common, and radiographic evidence of sacroiliitis is found in patients with long-standing disease.
- Most patients recover within 6 months, but prolonged recurrent disease is more common in cases that follow chlamydial urethritis.
- **Age:** Reactive arthritis occurs most frequently in adults between the ***ages of 20 and 40***- www.mayoclinic.org
- **Sex:** Women and men are equally likely to develop reactive arthritis in response to foodborne infections. However, men are more likely than are women to develop reactive arthritis in response to sexually transmitted bacteria- www.mayoclinic.org

Symptoms of Reactive Arthritis

◈ *www.webmd.com*

- The first symptoms of reactive arthritis are painful urination and a discharge from the penis if there is inflammation of the urethra.
- Diarrhea may occur if the intestines are affected.
- This is then followed by arthritis four to 28 days later that usually affects the fingers, toes, ankles, hips, and knee joints. Typically, only one or a few of these joints may be affected at one time.
- Other symptoms include:
  - Mouth ulcers
  - Inflammation of the eye
  - ***Keratoderma blennorrhagica*** (patches of scaly skin on the palms, soles, trunk, or scalp)
  - Back pain from sacroiliac (SI) joint involvement
  - Pain from inflammation of the ligaments and tendons at the sites of their insertion into the bone (enthesitis)

ANESTHESIA

230. Ans. a. Epidural is contraindicated in HELLP syndrome, b. Risk of aspiration is increased as lower oesophageal sphincter tone is reduced due to progesterone, d. Dose of local anesthesia is decreased while giving epidural anesthesia for caesarean, e. General anesthesia is preferred only for emergency caesarean

[Ref: Ajay Yadav 6th/231-33; Morgan Anaesthesia 5th/825,843; Lee13th/657-65; Miller Anaesthesia 7th2207-10]

"The diagnosis of HELLP syndrome is a ***relative, if not absolute, contraindication to the use of epidural anaesthesia***. If the clinical history and examination is negative for evidence of abnormal haemostasis and both the platelet count and the bleeding times are within the normal range, then an ***epidural block may be offered***. Because the platelet count often continues to decrease postpartum and bleeding complications are common in patients with HELLP Syndrome, it is prudent to remove the epidural catheter as soon as possible after delivery."-link.springer.com

"Premedication should include H_2 blockers or sodium citrate to minimize the risk of aspiration as lower ***oesophageal sphincter tone is reduced due to circulating progesterone*** especially after 16 weeks of gestation"- *www.aeronline.org*

Pregnant patients display enhanced sensitivity to local anesthetics during regional anesthesia and analgesia, and neural blockade occurs at reduced concentrations of local anesthetics; dose requirements may be reduced as much as 30%- *Morgan Anaesthesia 5th/825*

In the United States most elective cesarean sections are performed under spinal anesthesia. Regional anesthesia has become the preferred technique because general anesthesia has been associated with a greater risk of maternal morbidity and mortality-*Morgan Anaesthesia 5th/855*

Anesthesia for Caesarean Section

- *Ajay Yadav 6th/231-33*
- Regional anesthesia is preferred over general anesthesia
- GA is usually given for fetal distress when there is no time to give spinal or if there is contraindication for spinal anesthesia
- **Advantage of Regional** (Epidural/spinal over general anesthesia)
  - Risk of pulmonary aspiration (which is 4 times more in obstetrics) can be avoided
  - The possibility of failed intubation (which is 8 times more in obstetrics) can be avoided
  - Because of pulmonary aspiration & failed intubation the mortality in obstetrics during GA is twice as compared to regional anesthesia
  - Effect of anesthetic drugs on fetus can be avoided
- **Disadvantage of Regional** (Epidural/spinal over general anesthesia)
  - Increase procedural time makes regional anesthesia unsuitable for emergency situations like severe fetal distress
  - Pregnant patients are more vulnerable for high spinal &postspinal headache after spinal & accidental dural puncture after epidural
- As pregnant patients are very vulnerable for high spinal, doses of local anesthetics should be reduced by 30-40%
- Left lateral tilt should be maintained to prevent supine hypotension syndrome

Caesarean section: Epidural is most commonly used for women who already have epidural analgesia in labour. Spinal is most popular technique for elective CS, although in some centers combined spinal epidural are preferred"-Oxford manual of Anesthesia 3rd/755

Continuous lumbar epidural analgesia is the most versatile and most commonly employed technique, because it can be used for pain relief for the first stage of labor as well as analgesia/anesthesia for subsequent vaginal delivery or cesarean section, if necessary- *Morgan Anaesthesia 5th/843*

231. Ans. c. For post-operative pain caudal block is used, d. Low dose of drug is required as compared to adult in regional anaesthesia, e. Abdominal surgeries preferred in general anaesthesia

[Ref: Ajay Yadav 6th/238-41,173,38; Morgan Anaesthesia 5th/891-95; Lee13th/625; Miller Anaesthesia 7th/Chap 81]

Regional anesthesia in paediatric patients: *Age is no bar for regional anesthesia; any block can be given at any age. Dose of local anesthetic reuired is less because drug can easily diffuse in the nerve due to lose sheath*

Child: Size & length of **ETT** is ***according to age***-*Ajay Yadav 6th/38-39*

The appropriate diameter inside the endotracheal tube can be estimated by a formula based on age:4 + Age/4 = Tube diameter (in mm) - *Morgan Anaesthesia 5th/891*

There is also a formula to estimate endotracheal length: *Morgan Anaesthesia 5th/892*

12 + Age/2 = Length of tube (in cm)

Caudal block (Epidural sacral block): *Used for analgesia in children-Ajay Yadav 6th/176*

Regional Anesthesia and Analgesia

- *Morgan Anaesthesia 5th/894*
- The primary uses of regional techniques in pediatric anesthesia have been to supplement and reduce general anesthetic requirements and to provide better postoperative pain relief
- ***Caudal blocks have proved useful*** following a variety of surgeries, including circumcision, inguinal herniorrhaphy, hypospadias repair, anal surgery, clubfoot repair, and other subumbilical procedures.
- "Single dose caudal anesthesia is well established for lower body surgery"-*Lee 13th/625*

Absolute Contraindications to Neuraxial Blocks

- *Miller Anaesthesia 7th/Chap 81*
- Seven medical conditions contraindicate neuraxial blocks in children:

- Severe coagulation disorders, which may be either constitutional (hemophilia), acquired (disseminated intravascular coagulation), or therapeutic
- Severe infection such as septicemia or meningitis
- Hydrocephaly and intracranial tumoral process
- True allergy to local anesthetics, a very rare condition even with aminoesters
- Certain chemotherapies (such as with cisplatin) prone to induce subclinical neurologic lesions that can be acutely aggravated by a block procedure
- Uncorrected hypovolemia; and
- Cutaneous or subcutaneous lesions, whatever their nature (infection, angioma, dystrophic or tumoral, tattoo) at the contemplated site of puncture.

Parental refusal is a nonmedical absolute contraindication.

232. Ans. b. Bronchodilator

[Ref: 268; Morgan Anaesthesia 5th/182-83]

Day care: *Propofol is agent of choice for induction. Desflurane is inhlational agent of choice. Mivacurium is preferred muscle relaxant. Remifentanyl is most preferred opiod"- Ajay Yadav 6th/268*

Ketamine

◈ *Ajay Yadav 6th/112-13*

- Increase ICT
- Causes tachycardia &Hypertention: So IV anesthesia of choice
- ***Potent bronchodilator**: Used in treatment of refractory status asthmaticus; Induction of agent of choice in asthmaticus*

Table: *(Morgan Anaesthesia 5th/182):* **Summary of nonvolatileanesthetic effects on organ systems**

	Cardiovascular		Respiratory		Cerebral		
Agent	**HR**	**MAP**	**Vent**	**B'dil**	**CBF**	**$CMRO_2$**	**ICP**
Barbiturates							
Thiopental	↑↑	↓↓	↓↓↓	↓	↓↓↓	↓↓↓	↓↓↓
Thiamylal	↑↑	↓↓	↓↓↓	↓	↓↓↓	↓↓↓	↓↓↓
Methohexital	↑↑	↓↓	↓↓↓	0	↓↓↓	↓↓↓	↓↓↓
Benzodiazepines							
Diazepam	0/↑	↓	↓↓	0	↓↓	↓↓	↓↓
Lorazepam	0/↑	↓	↓↓	0	↓↓	↓↓	↓↓
Midazolam	↑	↓↓	↓↓	0	↓↓	↓↓	↓↓
Ketamine	↑↑	↑↑	↓	↑↑↑	↑↑	↑	↑↑
Etomidate	0	↓	↓	0	↓↓↓	↓↓↓	↓↓↓
Propofol	0	↓↓	↓↓↓	0	↓↓↓	↓↓↓	↓↓↓

233. Ans. a. Bupivacinae 0.5%, e. Lidocaine 5%

[Ref: Ajay Yadav 6th/167; Morgan Anaesthesia 5th/956; Lee13th/490; Miller Anaesthesia 7th/]

Drug used for Spinal Anesthesia

◈ *Ajay Yadav 6th/167*

- Lidocaine concentration used is 5%
- Bupivacaine: Most commonly used drug for spinal. The concentration used is 0.5%

Bupivacaine: Low concentration (0.1-0.125%) is used for postoperative analgesia- *Lee13th/490*

Table: *(Morgan Anaesthesia 5th/956; Ajay Yadav 6th/167)* **Some spinal anaesthetic agents**

Agent
Bupivacaine
0.5% in 8.25% dextrose
0.5% plain
Lidocaine
2% plain
5% in 7.5% dextrose
Procaine
10% plain
2.5% in water
Tetracaine
0.5% in water
0.5%in D_5W

234. Ans. d. Atracurium

[Ref: Miller 7th/926; Morgan 4th/200-203; K. D. T 8th/406]

"Atracurim: Undergo spontaneous degradation in plasma called as Hoffman degradation. So can be safely used in hepatic failure"- Ajay Yadav 6th/135,129

"Halothane: About 20% of halothane that enters blood is metabolized in the liver, the rest is exhaled out"- K. D. T 8th/406

"Propofol: Mainly metabolized in liver but significant (30%) extrahepatic metabolism also occur in kidney"-Ajay Yadav 6th/109

"Metabolism of amides (including lidocaine) occur in liver, whereas aminoesters metabolise in plasma by pseudocholinesterase"-*Lee 13th/382*

SKIN

235. Ans. b. Caused by Herpes simplex virus 6 & 7, d. Deposition of IgG in dermis, e. Lesion common on flexure surfaces

[Ref: Neena Khanna 5th/89-91; Harriosn 20th/356,358-59]

Dermatitis herpetiformis, also known as DH and Duhring's disease, is a chronic skin condition caused by a reaction to gluten ingestion. The vast majority of patients with DH also have an ***associated gluten sensitive enteropathy (celiac disease)*** "- celiac.org

Dermatitis Herpetiformis (DH)

Harriosn 20th/358-59

- DH is an intensely pruritic, papulovesicular skin disease characterized by lesions symmetrically distributedover ***extensor surfaces*** (i.e., elbows, knees, buttocks, back, scalp, andposterior neck)
- Primary lesions in this disorder consistof ***papules, papulovesicles, or urticarial plaques***.
- Because pruritus isprominent, patients may present with excoriations and crusted papules but no observable primary lesions.
- Almost all DH patients have associated,usually subclinical, ***gluten-sensitive enteropathy*** and
- >90% express the HLA-B8/DRw3 and HLA-DQw2 haplotypes.
- DH may present at any age, including in childhood; onset in the second to fourth decades is most common. The disease is typically chronic.
- Biopsy of early lesional skin reveals neutrophil-rich infiltrates within dermal papillae. Neutrophils, fibrin, edema, and microvesicle formation at these sites are characteristic of early disease.
- Patients with DH have **granular deposits of IgA** in their epidermal basement membrane zone and should be distinguished from individuals with linear IgA deposits at this site
- As is true for patients with ***celiac disease,*** this gastrointestinal abnormality can be reversed by a gluten-free diet.
- As in patients with celiac disease, dietary gluten sensitivity in patients with DH is associated with IgA anti-endomysial autoantibodies that target tissue transglutaminase.
- Patients with DH also have an increased incidence of thyroid abnormalities, achlorhydria, atrophic gastritis, and autoantibodies to gastric parietal cells.
- The **mainstay of treatment of DH is dapsone,** a sulfone. Gluten restriction can control DH and lessen dapsone requirements; this diet must rigidly exclude gluten to be of maximal benefit.

Immunologically Mediated Blistering Dis

Disease	Clinical manifestations	Histology	Immunopathology	Autoantigensa
Dermatitis herpetiformis (Harriosn 20th/356)	Extremely pruritic small papules and vesicles on elbows, knees, buttocks, and posterior neck	Subepidermal blister with neutrophils in dermal papillae	Granular deposits of IgA in dermal papillae	Epidermal transglutaminase

236. Ans. a. Onycholysis, b. Oil drop discolouration, c. Subungual hyperkeratosis, d. Nail pitting

[Ref: Neena Khanna 5th/50-51; Harrison 19th/348; Roxburg 17th/129]

"***Pterygium*** *is diagnostic & is a manifestation of severe* ***lichen planus*** *of nails"- Neena Khanna 5th/65*

Nail Changes in Psoriasis

Neena Khanna 5th/50-51; Harrison 19th/348

- ***Punctate pitting***
- *Nail plate thickening*
- ***Subungual hyperkeratosis***
- ***Discolouration*** *& dystrophy of nail plate*
- *Onycholysis*
- Oilspots (*oil drop or salmon patch- www.dermnetnz.org*) -yellow red discolouration in center of nail

Nail Changes in Lichen Planus

Neena Khanna 5th/64-65

- *Thinning & distal splitting of nail plates*
- *Trachyonychia*
- *Tenting of nail plate: pup tent sign*
- *Pterygium*

PSYCHIATRY

237. Ans. a. Common in extradural hemorrhage, b. Period of sanity, d. Occur in mania

[Ref: Reddy 34th/243,499; Harrison 20th/3066; Niraj Ahuja 7th/26]

Epidural Hematomas: They are often accompanied by a **"lucid interval"** of several minutes to hours prior to neurological deterioration-Harrison 20th/3184

Extradural haemorrhage: ***Lucid interval*** of few hours (2 to 4) to a week. Lucid interval is seen only in 30-40% cases- Reddy 34th/243

Lucid Interval

- **Lucid interval** *is a* ***period occurring in insanity,*** *during which all symptoms are insanity disappear completely- Reddy 34th/449*
- *In* ***mania & melancholia*** *lucid intervals are common- Reddy 34th/449*
- Postictal psychosis is a rare phenomenon that typically occurs after a period of increased seizure frequency. There is usually a brief lucid interval lasting up to a week, followed

by days to weeks of agitated, psychotic behavior- Harrison 20th/3066

- **Lewy body dementia**: Lucid interval can be present in b/w fluctuations"- *Niraj Ahuja7th/26*
- **Acute Subdural Hematoma:** Up to one-third of patients have a **lucid interval** lasting minutes to hours before coma supervenes, but most are drowsy or comatose from the moment of injury- Harrison 20th/3184

238. Ans. a. Cyclophosphamide, b. Azathioprine

[Ref: Niraj Ahuja 7th/98; Kaplan and Sadock 11th/424-25; Harrison 20th/3268]

- Cyclophosphamide & Azathioprine are **anti-cancer drugs**- KDT 8th/916
- Anti-psychotic drugs are also used in refractory cases

Treatment of OCD

- *Niraj Ahuja 7th/98*
- **Antidepressant**: Clomipramine, ***SSRIs***
- **Antipsychotic in OCD**: These are occasionally used in low doses (e.g haloperidol, risperidone, olanzapine, aripiprazole, pimozide) in treatment of severe, disabling anxiety- *Niraj Ahuja 7th/98*
- **Buspirone**: *As adjunct for augmentation of SSRIs, in some patients*

Treatment of OCD

- *Kaplan and Sadock 11th/424-25; Harrison 20th/3268*
- Because OCD symptoms appear to be largely refractory to psychodynamic psychotherapy and psychoanalysis, pharmacological and behavioral treatments have become common
- The standard approach is to ***start treatment with an SSRI*** or clomipramine and then move to other pharmacological strategies if the serotonin-specific drugs are not effective
- **Selective Serotonin Reuptake Inhibitors**. Fluoxetine, fluvoxamine, paroxetine, sertraline, citalopram -has been approved by the US Food and Drug Adinistration (FDA) for the teatment of OCD.
- The best clinical outcomes occur when ***SSRs are used in combination with behavioral therapy***
- **Clomipramine**. Of all the tricyclic and tetracyclic drugs, clomipramine is the most selective for serotonin reuptake versus norepinephrine reuptake and is exceeded in this respect only by the SSRis.
- If treatment with clomipramine or an SSRI is unsuccessful, many therapists augment the frst drug by the addition of valproate, lithium, or carbamazepine.
- Other drugs that can be tied in the treatment of OCD are venlafaxine, pindolol, and the monoamine oxidase inhibitors (MAOis), especially phenelzine.
- Other pharmacological agents for the treatment of unresponsive patients include buspirone, 5-hydroxytryptamine (5-HT), L-tryptophan, and clonazepam.
- Adding an ***atypical antipsychotic such as risperidone*** (Risperdal) has helped in some cases.
- **Behavior Therapy**
  - Although few head-to-head comparisons have been made, ***behavior therapy is as effective as pharmacotherapies in OCD,*** and some data indicate that the beneficial effects are longer lasting with behavior therapy.
  - Many clinicians, therefore, consider behavior therapy the treatment of choice for OCD.
  - Behavior therapy can be conducted in both outpatient and inpatient settings.
  - The principal behavioral approaches in OCD are exposue and response prevention.
  - Desensitization, thought stopping, flooding, implosion therapy, and aversive conditioning have also been used in patients with OCD.
  - In behavior therapy, patients must be truly committed to improvement

239. Ans. c. Duloxetine, d. Venlafaxine, e. Desvenlafaxine

[Ref: KDT 8th/481; Harrison 20th/3264]

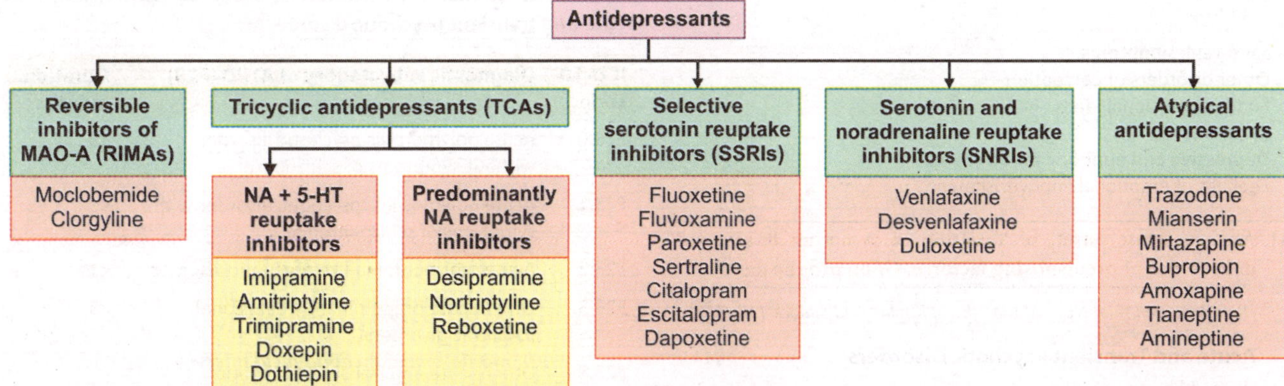

Table: *(Harrison 20th/3264):* **Mixed Norepinephrine/Serotonin Reuptake Inhibitors (SNRI) and Receptor Blockers**

Name		Side-effect	Comment
Venlafaxine (Effexor)	75–375	Nausea; dizziness; dry mouth; headaches; increased blood pressure; anxiety and insomnia	Bid-tid dosing (extended release available); lower potential for drug interactions than SSRIs; contraindicated with MAOIs
Desvenlafaxine (Pristiq)	50–400	Nausea, dizziness, insomnia	Primary metabolite of venlafaxine; no increased efficacy with higher dosing
Duloxetine (Cymbalta)	40–60	Nausea, dizziness, headache, insomnia, constipation	May have utility in treatment of neuropathic pain and stress incontinence
Mirtazapine (Remeron)	15–45	Somnolence, weight gain; neutropenia rare	Once-a-day dosing
Vilazodone (Viibryd)	40	Nausea, diarrhea, headache; dosage adjustment if given with CYP3A4 inhibitor/stimulator	Also 5-HT 1a receptor partial agonist
Vortioxetine (Brintellix)	5–20	Nausea, diarrhea, sweating, headache; low incidence of sedation or weight gain	No specific p450 effects; 5-HT3a and 5-HT7 receptor antagonist, 5-HT1b partial agonist, and 5-HT1a agonist
Levomilnacipran (Fetzima)	40–120	Nausea, constipation, sweating; rare increase in blood pressure/pulse	Most noradrenergic of SNRIs

240. Ans. d. Perplexity

[Ref: Niraj Ahuja 6th/55; Kaplan & Saddok's Synopsis of Psychiatry 10th/467-75]

- **Perplexity** *is Second-rank symptom. All other are first rank symptoms*

Table: *(Kaplan 10th/467-68):* **Kurt Schneider Criteria for Schizophrenia**

First-rank symptoms
- Audible thoughts
- Voices arguing or discussing or both
- Voices commenting
- Somatic passivity experiences
- Thought insertion
- Thought withdrawal and other experiences of influenced thought
- Thought broadcasting
- Delusional perceptions
- All other experiences involving volition made affects, and made impulses

Second-rank symptoms
- Other disorders of perception
- Sudden delusional ideas
- Perplexity
- **Depressive and euphoric mood changes**
- Feelings of emotional impoverishment

241. Ans. a. Acute onset, b. Variation in symptom & severity, d. Presence of predisposing factor, e. Good prognosis

[Ref: Park 25th/444; Niraj Ahuja 7th/76; Kaplan and Sadock 11th/339]

Acute and Transient Psychotic Disorders

◈ *oxfordmedicine.com*

- The heterogeneous group of acute and transient psychotic disorders are characterized by three typical features, listed below in descending order of priority:
  - ***Sudden/Acute/Abrupt onset*** (within 2 weeks or less);
  - **Presence of typical syndromes** with polymorphic (changing and variable) or schizophrenic symptoms;
  - ***Presence of associated acute stress*** (stressful events such as bereavement, job loss, psychological trauma, etc.).
- The onset of the disorder is manifested by an obvious change to an abnormal psychotic state. This is considered to be abrupt when it occurs within 48 h or less. Abrupt onset often indicates a better outcome.
- Full recovery occurs within 3 months and often in a shorter time (a few days or weeks). However, a small number of patients develop persistent and disabling states.
- Overall prognosis is good
- ICD-10 offers four specific and two non-specific subcategories of ATPD based on ***variability of clinical picture, presence of schizophrenic symptoms, and duration of the episode***

Table: **International Classification of Diseases nomenclature of acute and transient psychotic disorders**

ICD-10 code	Diagnostic subcategory of ATPD (F23)	Duration, months
F23.0	Acute polymorphic psychotic disorder without symptoms of schizophrenia	<3
F23.1	Acute polymorphic psychotic disorder with symptoms of schizophrenia	<1
F23.2	Acute schizophrenia-like psychotic disorder	<1
F23.3	Other acute predominantly delusional psychotic disorders	<3
F23.8	Other acute and transient psychotic disorders	<3
F23.9	Acute and transient psychotic disorders, unspecified	<3

242. Ans. **a. Acamprosate, c. Naltrexone, d. Disulfiram**

[Ref: Katzung 13th/564; NirajAhuja 7th/42,44,132; Pharmacology by Satoskar 24th/165]

*"**Acamprosate, naltrexone** & SSRIs (such as fluoxetine) are among the medications tried as **anti-craving agents** in alcohol dependence"- Niraj Ahuja 7th/42*

"The μ opioid receptor antagonist and partial agonist **naltrexone** is FDA-approved for indication in ***opioid and alcohol addiction***. Its effect is modest and may involve a modulation of endogenous opioid systems"- *Katzung 13th/564*

"Since its introduction, **naltrexone** has been tried for the treatment of a wide range of psychiatric disorders, including, among others, ***eating disorders, autism, self-injurious behavior, cocaine dependence, gambling, and alcoholism.*** Naltrexone was approved for the treatment of ***alcohol dependence*** in 1994"-*Kaplon and Sadock 11th/1004*

"Alcohol Dependence: **Opioid receptor antagonists are also used as adjuncts to cognitive-behavioral programs for treatment of alcohol dependence. Opioid receptor antagonists** *reduce alcohol craving and alcohol consumption,* **and they** *ameliorate the severity of relapses*"- ***Kaplon and Sadock 11th/1006***

Medications for Relapse Prevention of Alcohol Dependence

◈ *www.ncbi.nlm.nih.gov*

	US-FDA approved?	Grade of strength of evidence	Clinical recommendations
Disulfiram	Yes	B (Fair)	Not recommended for routine use in primary care
Naltrexone	Yes	A (Good)	FDA-approved option for treatment of alcohol dependence in conjunction with behavioral therapy
Acamprosate	Yes		
SSRI	No	I (insufficient)	Recommended for patients with comorbid depressive disorders
Ondansetron	No		Recommended to reduce drinking frequency and increase.
Topiramate	No		Abstinence

243. Ans. **b. Schizophrenia, c. Anxiety, d. Flash-back, e. Psychosis**

[Ref: Kaplan and Sadock 11th/646]

Cannabis (marijuana) *is obtained from the flowering tops & leaves of the Indian Hemp plant (cannabis sativa)*

"Those reporting high levels of cannabis use (more than 50 occasions) were at ***six-fold increased risk of schizophrenia*** compared with nonusers. The use of amphetamines, cocaine and similar drugs should raise particular concern because of their marked ability to increase psychotic symptoms"- *Kaplan and Sadock 11th/302*

"**Cannabis-induced anxiety disorder** is a common diagnosis for acute cannabis intoxication, which in many persons induces short-lived anxiety states often provoked by paranoid thoughts"- *Kaplan and Sadock 11th/646*

Cannabis Intoxication Delirium: The delirium associated with cannabis intoxication is characterized by marked impairment on cognition and performance tasks. Even modest doses of cannabis impair memory, reaction time, perception, motor coordination, and attention"- *Kaplan and Sadock 11th/646*

"**Flashbacks:** There are case reports of persons who have experienced-at times significantly-sensations related to cannabis intoxication after the short-term effects of the substance have disappeared"-*Kaplan and Sadock 11th/646*

244. Ans. **a. Attempted suicide is now decriminalized, b. More common in depression, c. Related to substance abuse, d. Elderly people are more predisposed**

[Ref: Park 25th/444; Niraj Ahuja 7th/222-24; Kaplan and Sadock 11th/766-70]

*"The **Section 309 of IPC** which deals with **attempted suicide was decriminalized** under the Mental Healthcare Act in May 2018"- www.newindianexpress.com*

Depression is a major risk factor for suicide- *Niraj Ahuja 7th/223*

Suicide

◈ *Park 25th/444*

- Majority of cases are below 29 yrs followed by 30-44 years of age group
- In India, an average 369 suicides take place every day, out of these 248 are committed by males & 121 by females
- Family problems & illness are main cause of suicide

Variables Enhancing Risk of Suicide Among Vulnerable Groups

◈ *Kaplan and Sadock 11th/768*

- Adolescence and late life
- Bisexual or homosexual gender identity
- Criminal behavior
- Cultural sanctions for suicide
- Delusions
- Disposition of personal property
- Divorced, separated, or single marital status
- Early loss or separation from parents
- Family history of suicide
- Hallucinations
- Homicide
- Hopelessness
- Hypochondriasis
- Impulsivity
- Increasing agitation
- Increasing stress
- Insomnia
- Lack of future plans
- Lack of sleep
- Lethality of previous attempt
- Living alone

- Low self-esteem
- Male sex
- Physical illness or impairment
- Previous attempts that could have resulted in death
- Protestant or nonreligious status
- Recent childbirth
- Recent loss
- Repression as a defense
- Secondary gain
- Severe family pathology
- Severe psychiatric illness
- Sexual abuse
- Signals of intent to die
- Suicide epidemics
- Unemployment
- White race

Table: *(Niraj Ahuja 7th/223):* **Risk factor for suicide**

The presence of following increase the risk of completed suicide:

- Age > 40 years
- Male gender
- Staying single
- Previous suicidal attempt (s)
- Depression (risk about 25 times more than usual)
    - Presence of guilt, self-accusation, agitation, nihilistic ideation, worthlessness, hypochondriacal delusions and/or severe insomnia.
    - Risk is usually higher at the beginning or towards the end of a depressive episode.
    - Risk can often be higher soon after response to treatment rather at the peak of depression; this applies to all forms of treatment but particularly so with antidepressant treatment.
    - There is a higher risk of suicide in the week after discharge from a psychiatric inpatient unit.
- Suicidal preoccupation (for example, a written 'suicide note' and/or detailed plans are made for committing suicide)
- ***Alcohol or drug dependence***
- Severe, disabling, painful or untreatable physical illness
- Recent serious loss or major stressful life event
- Social isolation
- Higher degree of impulsivity

Table: *(Niraj Ahuja 7th/223):* **Summary of Risks & protective factors for suicide**

Factors	Biological	Psychological	Social
Predisposing	Genetic Factors Male gender ***Older age***	Early childhood trauma ***Personality traits***	Poor social support Unemployment
Precipitating	Discontinuation of antidepressant Psychiatric diagnosis	Separation from spouse Hopelessness Worthlessness	Financial difficulties Easy availability of lethal means
Perpetuating	Alcohol and drug misuse	Poor self-esteem	Poor social support
Protective	Children: elderly parents: religious and moral values: good engagement with treatment		

RADIOLOGY

245. Ans. d. Pneumoperitoneum

[Ref: radiopaedia.org; Sumer Sethi 6th/122; Danhert Radiology Review Manual 7th/449; Radiology by S. Bhadury 2nd/24]

Supine film sign of Pneumoperitoneum*Sumer Sethi 6th/122; Danhert Radiology Review Manual 7th/772*

- ***Tell Tale Triangle sign***: Air b/w bowel loop
- Football sign
- Riglers sign
- Cupola sign: Large amount of gas under diaphragm

"The **telltale triangle sign**, also known as the **triangle sign** or **telltale triangle**, is a radiographic sign seen on plain abdominal radiograph that signifies presence of **pneumoperitoneum.** It describes the appearance of a radiolucent triangle of gas formed between three loops of bowel or between two loops of bowel and the abdominal wall"-radiopaedia.org

"**Pleural effusion**: Vanishing or pseudo tumor (loculated pleural effusion in interlobar fissure"- *Sumer Sethi 6th/49; Danhert Radiology Review Manual 7th/446*

Pneumomediastinum: Spinnaker sail sign & continuous diaphragm sign-*Danhert Radiology Review Manual 7th/449*

Pericardial effusion: Money bag or leather bottle or flask shaped heart- *Sumer Sethi 6th/76*

246. Ans. d. USG > e. Lateral decubitus

[Ref: Sumer Sethi 6th/49; Danhert Radiology Review Manual 7th/446; Radiology by S. Bhadury 2nd/19]

Pleural Effusion: Minimal Amount Required to be Detected (For X-ray)

Sumer Sethi 6th/49

- **Lateral decubitus:** <10 ml pleural fluid (25 ml-*Dánhert 7th/446)*
- Lateral view: 75 ml pleural fluid
- PA view 100-200 ml pleural fluid

- Lateral decubitus view of same side: best view to detect minimal fluid
- USG best investigation to detect minimal fluid

"Pleural fluid is detectable in the costophrenic recesses on lateral upright chest radiograph after 50mL has accumulated. On standard **posterior-anterior chest radiograph**, blunting of the costophrenic recesses and obliteration of the hemidiaphragm are seen when >200mL and >500mL of pleural fluid have accumulated, respectively"- www.ncbi.nlm.nih.gov

"**Pleural ultrasound** can detect physiologic amounts of pleural fluid (***5ml***),but a minimal volume of 20ml is more reliably detected, and ultrasound is 100% sensitive for effusions >100ml"- www.ncbi.nlm.nih.gov

While a minimum of 150 mL is required to detect effusion by radiography in the erect position, effusions as ***small as 5 mL can be detected ultrasonographically with 100% sensitivity***"- www.e-ultrasonography.org

247. Ans. a. Half-life 6 hr, b. Most commonly used radionuclide, c. Can detect ectopic gastric tissue, d. Generator originated nuclide

[Ref: Sumer Sethi 6th/27, 44; Danhert Radiology Review Manual 7th/1112; Radiology K. Thayalam 1st/285-87]

Tc-99m *is used in clinical medicine as* ***sodium pertechnetate-99m*** *which is used for imaging tissues e.g* ***thyroid, gastric mucosa*** *& salivary glands, due to similarity to iodine & chloride ions"- Radiology K. Thayalam 1st/286*

'Technetium 99m' (99mTc) Pertechnetate

◈ *Danhert 7th/1112; Sumer Sethi 6th/27, 44*

- Half life- 6 hrs
- *Administration: oral/IV*
- *Parent molecules: Molybdenum-99*
- *Decay:* ***By photon emission*** *of 140 keV*
- *Mode of production:* ***Radionuclide generator***
- *Uptake: thyroid, salivary glands, gastric mucosa, choroid plexus*
- *Excretion: Mostly in feces, some in urine*
- *Advantage: Low cost & reduced radiation exposure*
- **Gastric mucosa**: ***Active uptake by gastric mucosa.*** *Dectetion& localization of a Meckel's diverticulum containing heterotropic gastric mucosa- Danhert Radiology Review Manual 7th/1137, Sumer Sethi 6th/4*

'Technetium 99m

◈ *www.radioactivity.eu.com*

- **Tc- 99m**' is a long-lived *isomer* of technetium 99, widely used in nuclear medicine.
- The term 'isomer' refers to those nuclei that are able to survive in excited states for abnormally long periods of time. Excited nuclei normally return to their ground states after a fraction of a second, though in rare cases this transition can be inhibited and greatly slowed down. This is the case with technetium 99m, which exists for several hours before returning to the normal state of technetium.
- This excited state has a name (technetium 99m) that distinguishes it from ordinary technetium 99, as the 6-hour half-life of technetium 99m gives researchers enough time to put these nuclei to use.
- In order to leave the excited state, technetium-99m nuclei ***emits 140 keV characteristic gamma rays without accompanying beta rays.*** This property makes them highly desirable in medicine.
- Gamma rays are absorbed far from the examined organ, minimizing the danger posed to living matter.
- The technetium-99 precursor is molybdenum-99, a radioactive nuclei generally produced in reactors. The 66 hours molybdenum radioactive half-life give enough time to transport it to hospitals and to extract chemically technetium 99m.
- The radioisotople placed in a radiopharmaceutical serum is then injected into the patient, which allows gamma camera scans providing accurate pictures of the patient's body.
- ***Technetium 99m is the most commonly used radioisotope in the field of nuclear imaging being involved in 80% of scintigraphies***

248. Ans. b. Oxygen cylinder should not take inside of MRI room, e. MR scanner installation enclosed in Faraday cage

[Ref: Sumer Sethi 6th/14-18; Radiology K. Thayalam 1st/369-402]

No ionizing radiation (safe in pregnancy) - *Sumer Sethi 6th/19*

"The entire MR scanner installation is enclosed in a ***stainless or copper shield*** *known as* ***Faraday cage*** *that blocks out* ***radiofrequency signals*** *from local radio & TV stations that might influence the MR signals- Sumer Sethi 6th/15; Radiology K. Thayalam 1st/398*

Biosafety in MRI

◈ *Radiology K. Thayalam 1st/396-98*

- ***Hazards arise from static magnetic field, gradient field & RF field, cryogenic liquids, claustrophobia & noise***
- **Static magnetic field**: *Patients with implants, prosthesis, aneurysm clips, pacemakers, heart valves, etc should be away from MRI area. Pregnant patients should not be exposed to >2.5T*
- **Fringe field**: *Fringe field can affect watches, erase CD data & credit cards, distort video display & photo multiplier tubes (PMT)*
- **Projectile effect**: *Attraction of ferromagnetic objects varies with square of the magnetic field & inversely with cube of distance. Scissors, scalpel etc can become lethal projectile in MRI room. Oxygen cylinder, patient bed & the fire fitting apparatus have caused major injuries in past*

249. Ans. a. Double atrial shadow, c. Associated with mitral stenosis, d. Splaying of the carina, e. Posterior displacement of left upper lobe bronchus

[Ref: Sumer Sethi 6th/75; Danhert Radiology Review Manual 7th/597; P.J. Mehta 15th/160-61]

"Downward & outward extension of the apex is seen in left ventricle enlargement"*-Radiology by Samarjit Bhadury 2nd/38*

LAE: seen in ***mitral valve disease****- Sumer Sethi 6th/75*

Left Atrial Enlargement

◈ *Danhert Radiology Review Manual 7th/597*

PA View Chest X-ray

- ***Right retrocardiac double density***
- *>75⁰ splaying of carina* with horizontal orientation of distal left mainstream bronchus
- Enlargement of left atrial appendages

Lateral View

- Increased convexity of postero-superior cardiac margin
- ***Posterior displacement of left upper lobe bronchus***

Left Heart Enlargement

◈ *P.J. Mehta 15th/160*

- Double density seen through right upper border (AP view) (*i.e.,* ***double atrial shadow)***
- Esophagus curving around the dilated left atrium
- ***Straightened left border***
- ***Splaying of mainstem bronchi*** (*i.e.,* ↑ed carinal angle)
- Small aorta (due to decrease of forward cardiac output)
- Normal/Undersized LV

250. Ans. c. I 127

[Ref: Sumer Sethi 6th/38; Danhert Radiology Review Manual 7th/1112; Harrison 19th/263e-3; Dutta Gynaecology 5th/484, 4th/465; Merdith Radiation Physics & Nuclear Medicine/28]

"I-127 is stable isotope of iodine. Its radioactive isotope of medical importance is I-131" *(K.D.T 7th/256)*

Radiolabeling with Radioisotopes of Iodine

◈ *www.sciencedirect.com*

- Isotopes of iodine have been extensively used in clinical nuclear medicine imaging and radiation therapy. Out of the 37 known isotopes of iodine, 4—^{123}I, ^{124}I, ^{125}I, and ^{131}I—are suitable for SPECT or PET imaging.
- With a 60-day half-life, γ-emitter ^{125}I is useful for the long-term tracking and imaging of radiolabeled NPs.
- ^{131}I (half-life 8 days) is a strong γ-emitter, but due to its mode of β-decay, it is used for β-therapy, commonly in treating thyroid cancer.
- Dual-purpose theranostic radionuclides, for example, ^{131}I, or the pair ^{124}I/^{131}I can be used for imaging followed by therapy using the same radiolabeling procedure

Iodine Radio-isotopes

"I-125: *Used in cancer brachytherapy (prostate & brain"- Sumer Sethi 6th/38*

"I-131: *Widely used in treating thyroid cancer & in imaging the thyroid"- Sumer Sethi 6th/38*

"I-123: *Increasingly used for diagnosis of thyroid function"-Agent of choice for thyroid imaging- Danhert 7th/1112*

Iodine 125 (I125) *-It is used in gynaecological malignancies brachytherapy- Dutta gynaecology 5th/484 (Table)*

"I-131 emits β & γ rays" *(Harrison 19th/263e-3, 18th/1790)*

"I-131 *is* ***contraindicated during pregnancy. Foetal thyroid will be destroyed*** *resulting in cretinism, other abnormalities if given during first trimester" (K.D.T 7th/256)*

"For radioactive iodine scanning I-131 & I-123 are used. ***For treatment of hyperthyroidism & thyroid cancer I-131 is used"*** *(CMDT06/1127)*

MAY

2018

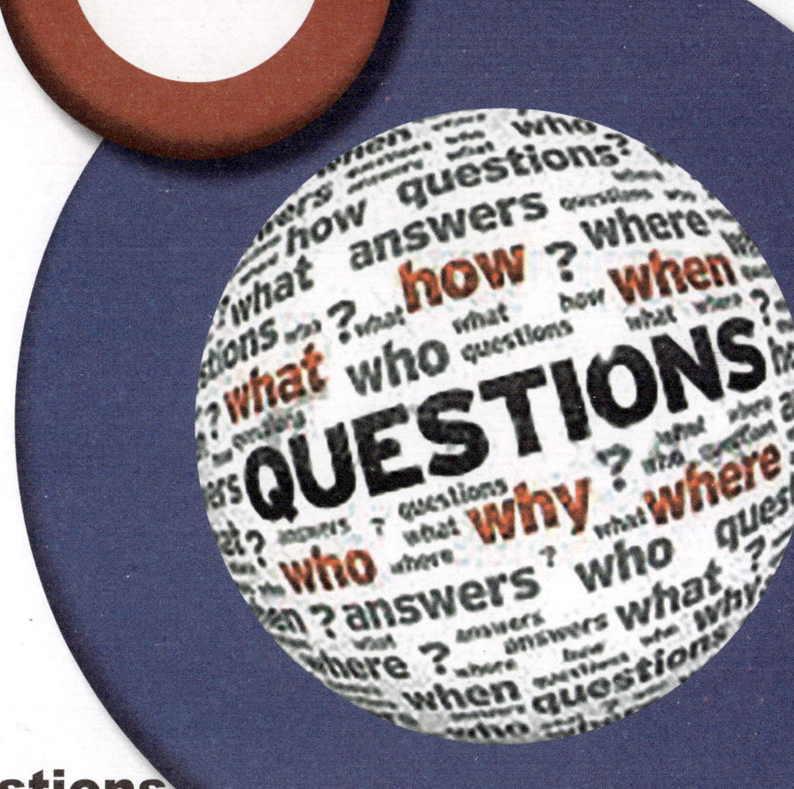

Multiple Choice Questions
Answers & Explanations

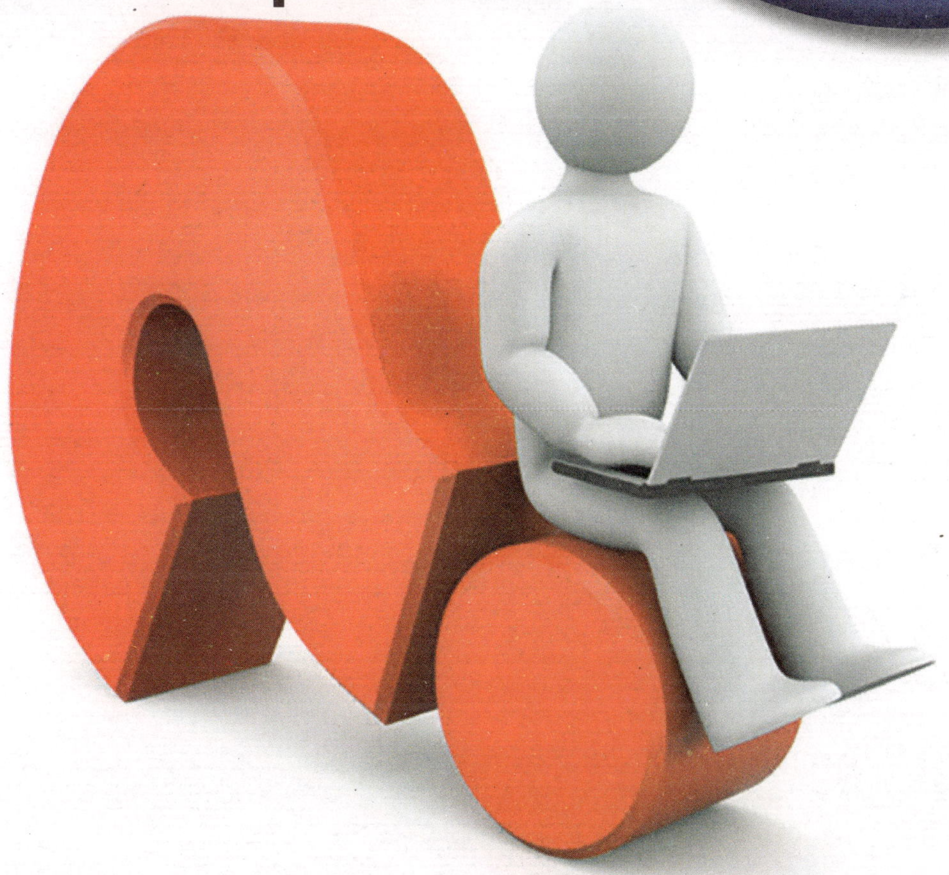

MAY 2018 MULTIPLE CHOICE QUESTIONS

ANATOMY

1. **Which of the following muscles is/are supplied by posterior interosseous nerve:**
   a. Extensor carpi ulnaris
   b. Extensor carpi radialis longus
   c. Extensor carpi radialis brevis
   d. Extensor digitorum communis
   e. Brachioradialis
2. **Which of the following is/are muscle form rotator cuff except:**
   a. Teres minor
   b. Teres major
   c. Subscapularis
   d. Supraspinatus
   e. Infraspinatus
3. **In the aortic opening of diaphragm, which of the following structures passes:**
   a. Azygous vein
   b. Thoracic duct
   c. Hemiazygos vein
   d. Esophagus
   e. Greater splanchnic nerve
4. **Which of following statement(s) is/are false about anatomy of genitourinary region:**
   a. Penile skin is supplied by superficial external pudendal artery
   b. Nerve supply of penile skin is from obturator nerve
   c. There are at least 5 urethral sphincters
   d. Penis receives three venous drainage systems
   e. Dorsal artery of penis is branch of bulbourethral artery
5. **Which of the following is/are true regarding anatomy of kidney:**
   a. Kidney extend b/w upper border of 1st lumbar vertebrae & lower border of 3rd lumbar vertebrae
   b. Long axis of the kidney is directed upward & laterally
   c. Anterior segmental artery is first & most constant branch of renal artery
   d. Supplied by preganglionic T8-T12 sympathetic fibers
   e. Papilla of renal pyramids terminates into minor calyx
6. **Component(s) of inner Waldeyer's ring:**
   a. Jugulo-digastric lymph nodes
   b. Jugulo-omohyoid lymph nodes
   c. Tubal tonsil
   d. Nasopharyngeal tonsil
   e. Lingual tonsil
7. **All are true about parotid except:**
   a. 2nd largest salivary gland
   b. Stenson's duct opens into the vestibule of the mouth opposite upper third molar
   c. Divided into superficial and deep lobe by facial nerve
   d. Majority of lymph nodes are embedded in deep lobe
   e. Deep lobe abscess can extend into parapharyngeal space
8. **Cavernous vein/sinus receives input from:**
   a. Cephalic vein
   b. Superior ophthalmic vein
   c. Superior petrosal sinus
   d. Inferior petrosal sinus
   e. Superficial middle cerebral vein
9. **Which of the following develop from 4th aortic arch:**
   a. Pulmonary artery
   b. Right umbilical artery
   c. Arch of aorta
   d. Left subclavian artery
   e. Right subclavian artery
10. **A case of pulmonary TB came to emergency department ith complaints of recurrent hemoptysis. In this case which of the following vessel(s) should be considered for angiographic evaluation:**
   a. Pulmonary artery
   b. Pulmonary vein
   c. Bronchial artery
   d. Bronchial vein
   e. Superior vena cava
11. **True statement about terminal bronchiole:**
   a. Most distal portion of the conducting zone
   b. Lined by columnar epithelium
   c. Composed of C-shaped hyaline cartilage rings
   d. Wall is composed of smooth muscle & glands
   e. Gaseous exchange takes places
12. **True about anatomy of heart:**
   a. SA node lies in left atrial appendages
   b. SA node is located at junction of left atrial appendages & superior vena cava
   c. AV node located in triangle of Koch
   d. AV node located at atrial & ventricular junction
   e. Bundle of His lies posteroinferiorly in ventricular septum
13. **External anal sphincter is supplied by:**
   a. S2, S3, S4
   b. S2, S3
   c. S1, S2
   d. L5, S1
   e. L2, L3

Answer

1.	a,c, d.	2.	b.	3.	a, b, c.	4.	b, c, e.	5.	e.	6.	c, d, e.	7.	a, b, d.
8.	b, e.	9.	c, e.	10.	a, c.	11.	a, b.	12.	c, e.	13.	a.		

14. **Not derived from ventral mesogastrium:**
    a. Falciform ligament
    b. Right coronary ligament
    c. Left coronary ligament
    d. Greater omentum
    e. Triangular ligament

PHYSIOLOGY

15. **Which of the following are true about HbA2**
    a. Constitutes around 2% of total haemoglobin
    b. Consists of 2 alpha and 2 beta chains
    c. Prevents polymerization of deoxy-sickle haemoglobin present in sickle cell disease
    d. Level is increased in β-thalassemia trait
    e. Decreased level is seen in iron deficiency anaemia
16. **Normal concentration of H^+ ions in blood is:**
    a. 35 mmol/L
    b. 40 mmol/L
    c. 45 mmol/L
    d. 50 mmol/L
    e. 55 mmol/L
17. **Which of the following is correctly matched sensory receptor and sensation:**
    a. Meissner corpuscle-slow adopting
    b. Merkel's disc-cold temperature
    c. Pacinian corpuscles- vibration
    d. Krause's end organs –pain
    e. Ruffini's end organ – pressure
18. **Hyperprolactinemia is/are associated with:**
    a. Inhibition of suppressing effect of dopamine on prolactin
    b. Pituitary apoplexy
    c. Pregnancy
    d. Pituitary adenoma
    e. Lactation
19. **Which of the following is/are causes of hypercalcemia with normal or increased parathormone levels:**
    a. Primary hyperparathyroidism
    b. Familial hypocalciuric hypercalcemia
    c. Vitamin D intoxication
    d. Milk-alkali syndrome
    e. Thiazide diuretic use
20. **True statement(s) regarding hypoxemia:**
    a. Decrease O_2 partial pressure in blood
    b. Decrease in O_2 delivery to tissues
    c. Decreased alveolar ventilation
    d. Inadequate utilization of oxygen by tissue despite normal delivery of oxygen
    e. All of the above
21. **True about functions of loop of Henle (LoH):**
    a. Thin ascending limb permeable to water
    b. Thick ascending limb actively absorb Cl^- ion
    c. Descending limb receive hypotonic fluid from PCT
    d. Descending limb permeable to water
    e. Thin ascending limb actively absorb sodium ion
22. **Which of the following are true with respect to red pulp of spleen:**
    a. It has B cell rich lymphoid tissues
    b. Composed of splenic cords and sinusoids
    c. It has T cell rich periarticular lymphatic sheath
    d. Perisinusoidal macrophages are present
    e. Removes senescent erythrocytes from circulation
23. **Which of these is/are true with respect to cardiac muscle:**
    a. Beta-1 stimulation increases intracellular calcium concentration
    b. Beta-1 stimulation increases cGMP level inside myocardium
    c. Sarcoplasmic reticulum regulates the release and reuptake of calcium inside the cell
    d. Titin protein connects the Z lines to the M lines
    e. Calcium attachment to troponin C causes initiation of contraction of muscle
24. **Regarding transpulmonary pressure, which of the following is/are true:**
    a. Alveolar pressure minus intrapleural pressure
    b. Intrapleural pressure minus alveolar pressure
    c. Under physiological conditions the transpulmonary pressure is always positive
    d. Lungs collapses if transpulmonary pressure become zero

BIOCHEMISTRY

25. **β-galactosidase deficiency is/are seen in:**
    a. Fabry's disease
    b. Krabbe's disease
    c. Metachromatic leukodystrophy
    d. Gaucher's disease
    e. Morquio syndrome
26. **Feature(s) of vitamin E deficiency:**
    a. Peripheral neuropathy
    b. Posterior column involvement
    c. Alopecia
    d. Hemolysis
    e. Thrombocytopenia
27. **Vitamin C deficiency may lead to:**
    a. Increase incidence of oxalate stones
    b. Diarrhoea
    c. Constipation
    d. Delayed wound healing
    e. Seizure

Answer

14. d.	15. a, c, d, e.	16. None.	17. c, e.	18. a, c, d, e.	19. a, b.	20. a.
21. b, c, d.	22. b, d, e.	23. a, c, d, e.	24. a, c, d.	25. b, e.	26. a, b, c, d.	27. b, d.

28. **Which of the following acts as antioxidant:**
    a. Vitamin A
    b. Vit E
    c. Vit C
    d. Glutathione reductase
    e. Zinc
29. **Pyridoxine acts as coenzyme for:**
    a. Deamination
    b. Transamination
    c. Carboxylation
    d. Decarboxylation
    e. Tryptophan metabolism
30. **True about phenylketonuria:**
    a. Mental retardation may be present
    b. Musty odour due to phenylalanine in sweat
    c. Autosomal recessive inheritance
    d. Deficiency of the hepatic enzyme phenylalanine hydroxylase
    e. Light coloured skin
31. **Which of the following is/are substrates for gluconeogenesis**
    a. Even chain fatty acids
    b. Glycerol
    c. Pyruvate
    d. Lysine
    e. Alanine
32. **Which of the following is/are uncoupler of oxidative phosphorylation:**
    a. Cyanide
    b. 2, 4-Dinitrophenol
    c. Thyroxine
    d. Thermogenin
    e. Hydrogen sulphide
33. **Which of the following is/are co-factor required in de novo synthesis of fatty acid in human:**
    a. Biotin
    b. Pyridoxine
    c. NADPH
    d. ATP
    e. ADP
34. **Which of the following is/are examples of chaperons except:**
    a. Hsp 40, 70 and 60
    b. Calreticulin
    c. Calbindin
    d. Calnexin
    e. Immunoglobulin binding protein (BiP)
35. **Enzyme not involved in Purine metabolism:**
    a. Ornithine transcarbamylase (OTC)
    b. Urtidylic acid decarboxylase
    c. Carbamoyl phosphate synthetase
    d. Hypoxanthine Guanine phosphoribosyl transferase (HGPRT)
    e. Phosphoribosylpyrophosphate (PRPP) synthetase
36. **Coenzyme used in transamination reactions:**
    a. Flavin adenine dinucleotide (FAD)
    b. Pyridoxine
    c. Nicotinamide adenine dinucleotide (NAD)
    d. Vit. B7 (Biotin)
    e. Thiamine
37. **Between E and F helices of hemoglobin, oxygen binds to which of the following amino acid:**
    a. Histidine
    b. Lysine
    c. Proline
    d. Tyrosine
    e. Glycine

IMMUNOGENETICS & MOLECULER BIOLOGY

38. **Which of the following size DNA fragment will be towards the negative end in electrophoresis:**
    a. 50 bp
    b. 150 bp
    c. 550 bp
    d. 5500 bp
    e. 50000 bp
39. **Which of the following is not true about mutation of p53:**
    a. Cell cycle will continue to multiply
    b. Neoplastic changes
    c. Cell cycle will be arrested
    d. DNA repair will be affected
    e. Cells will not get mutated because other tumor suppressor genes can still control the cell cycle at different check points
40. **All are true about Okazaki fragments except:**
    a. Present in leading strand
    b. Present in lagging strand
    c. Gap on these fragments are filled by DNA Polymerase enzyme
    d. Require RNA primer
    e. Helicase used for DNA unwinding
41. **Which of the following is used to study protein-protein interaction:**
    a. Fluorescence life imaging
    b. Bimolecular fluorescence complementation (BiFC)
    c. Fluorescence resonance energy transfer (FRET)
    d. Fluorescence polarization
    e. Fluorescence in situ hybridization (FISH)
42. **True statement regarding transfer RNA:**
    a. Act as adaptor molecules b/w mRNA and the amino acids coded by it
    b. Contain codon arm
    c. Have Anticodon arm
    d. Has unusal bases
    e. Have blunt ends

Answer

28. All (a,b,c,d,e.)	29. a, b, d, e.	30. a, c, d, e.	31. b, c, e.	32. b, c, d.	33. a, c, d.	34. c.
35. a, b, c.	36. b.	37. a.	38. e.	39. c, e.	40. a.	41. a, b, c, d.
42. a, c, d.						

43. Which of the following is not found in RNA:
a. Uracil
b. Thymine
c. Deoxyribose sugar
d. Adenine
e. Cytosine

44. All are true about satellite DNA except:
a. Highly repetitive DNA in tandem
b. Short sequences of DNA stretches in satellite DNA are unique
c. Transcriptionally it is very active
d. Present in centromere and telomeres
e. They are part of 'junk DNA'

45. Isothermal amplification technique include(s):
a. Nested PCR
b. Reverse PCR
c. Ligase chain reaction
d. Nucleic acid sequence-based amplification (NASBA)
e. Loop-mediated amplification (LAMP)

46. True about telomerase:
a. Reverse transcriptase enzyme
b. RNA dependent DNA polymerase
c. DNA dependent RNA polymerase
d. Activity high in stem cell and cancer cells
e. Telomerase increases the longevity of cells

PATHOLOGY

47. Which of the following is/are lower in anaemia of chronic diseases as compared to iron deficiency anaemia:
a. TIBC (Total iron binding capacity)
b. Serum ferritin
c. Serum iron
d. Transferrin saturation
e. Iron stores

48. Microcytosis on peripheral blood smear is/are seen in:
a. Iron deficiency anemia
b. Thalassaemia
c. Sideroblastic anemia
d. Vit. B12 deficiency
e. Folate deficiency

49. Karyotyping is/are not necessary in which of the following conditions:
a. Recurrent abortions
b. Child with multiple malformation
c. Pregnancy in advance maternal age with previous pregnancy with an abnormal chromosomal complement
d. Child with seizure
e. Down syndrome

50. In Down syndrome which is/correct
a. Most common cause of death is congenital heart disease
b. 95% have an extra 21st chromosome
c. Increased nuchal fold thickness on USG
d. Karyotyping is required in all cases for prenatal diagnosis
e. Advanced paternal age (>35 years) is a risk factor

51. Which of following dyads are correct:
a. Marfan syndrome: Autosomal recessive
b. Phenylketonuria: Autosomal dominant
c. Vit. D resistant rickets: Autosomal dominant
d. Alkaptonuria: Autosomal recessive
e. Duchene muscle dystrophy: X-linked recessive

52. Causes of unconjugated hyperbilirubinemia is/are:
a. Hemolysis due to ABO incompatibility
b. Criggler-Najar syndrome
c. Gilbert syndrome
d. Sepsis
e. Roter's syndrome

53. A patient presented with hemoptysis and hematuria. On renal biopsy, it show crescentic glomerulonephritis. Immunofluorescence microscopy shows linear IgG and C3 deposits. Which of the following is the most appropriate diagnosis:
a. Thin basement disease
b. Good pasture syndrome
c. Wegener granulomatosis
d. PSGN
e. Minimal change disease

54. In hereditary spherocytosis, which of the following is/are increased:
a. Haptoglobin
b. Spleen size
c. MCHC
d. MCV
e. LDH

55. All of the following are feature of waldenstorm macroglobulinemia except:
a. Hyperviscosity
b. Polycythemia
c. Treated with alkylating agents
d. Low grade lymphoplasmacytoid lymphoma
e. IgG paraprotein

56. Which of the following are feature of anaplasia:
a. Metaplasia
b. Pleomorphism
c. Loss of cell polarity
d. Abnormal nuclear morphology
e. Abnormal mitosis

57. Dysmorphic RBC's in urine is/are seen in:
a. Glomerulonephritis
b. Renal vascular injury
c. Renal stone
d. Pyelonephritis
e. Interstitial nephritis

Answer

43. b, c. 44. c. 45. d, e. 46. a, b, d, e. 47. a. 48. a, b, c. 49. d.
50. a, b, c. 51. d, e. 52. a, b, c, d. 53. b. 54. b, c, e. 55. b, e. 56. b, c, d, e.
57. a.

58. **Alcohol is a risk factor for which of the following cancers:**
   a. Liver b. Esophagus
   c. Gastric d. Cervical
   e. Breast

59. **Which of the following involved in leukocyte attachment and emigration during inflammation:**
   a. Complement C5a
   b. Integrin
   c. L-selectin
   d. Leukotriene B4
   e. Interleukin-8

60. **Acanthocytes are seen in:**
   a. Hallervorden-Spatz disease
   b. Abetalipoproteinemia
   c. Severe liver disease
   d. Ataxia telangiectasia
   e. McLeod syndrome

61. **Which of the infections is/are predisposes to cholangiocarcinoma:**
   a. Paragonimus westermani
   b. Fasiciola hepatica
   c. Schistosoma hematobium
   d. Opisthorchis viverrini
   e. Clonorchis sinensis

62. **When CSF is collected by lumbar puncture in 4 vials, regarding 1st vial which is correct:**
   a. Biochemical test like protein and glucose
   b. To count cells and differential count
   c. Bacterial culture and gram stain
   d. No use, discard the first vial
   e. Mycobacterial and fungal culture and staining

63. **True about liver haemangioma are all except:**
   a. Most common benign tumor of liver
   b. Pregnancy is risk factor
   c. Thrombocytopenia may occur
   d. Diagnosis by MRI and CT scan
   e. Need surgical removal in every case because chances of rupture is high

64. **Which of the following is/are features of acute hepatitis:**
   a. Interface hepatitis
   b. Mononuclear cell infiltration
   c. Apoptosis of hepatocyte
   d. Portal tracts Inflammation
   e. Bridging fibrous

65. **Which of the following are false about electron microscopy**
   a. High resolving power
   b. Can see both live and dead objects
   c. Vacuum is required
   d. Three-dimensional images can be obtained
   e. Coloured images are seen

66. **Microscopy which can be performed with minimum optical illumination:**
   a. Dark field
   b. Phase contrast
   c. Bright-field microscopy
   d. Fluorescent microscopy
   e. Inverted microscopy

67. **Increased prothrombin time (PT) is seen with**
   a. Vitamin K deficiency
   b. Factor V deficiency
   c. Factor VIII deficiency
   d. Factor IX deficiency
   e. Warfarin administration

PHARMACOLOGY

68. **Which of the following is/are adverse effect(s) of tricyclic antidepressants(TCA):**
   a. Tremor
   b. Hypertension
   c. Weight loss
   d. Diarrhoea
   e. Urinary retention

69. **Which inotropes act on both D receptor and alpha receptor:**
   a. Dopamine
   b. Epinephrine
   c. Isoprenaline
   d. Norepinephrine
   e. Phenylephrine

70. **First dose syncope occur with which of the following drug(s):**
   a. ACE inhibitor
   b. CCB
   c. Alpha blockers
   d. Beta blockers
   e. Thiazide diuretics

71. **Which of the following drug acts by inhibiting protein synthesis:**
   a. Penicillin
   b. Chloramphenicol
   c. Fluoroquinolones
   d. Vancomycin
   e. Aminoglycosides

72. **Which of the following is/are indications of use of antibiotics in diarrhoea:**
   a. Cholera
   b. Traveller's diarrhoea
   c. Diarrhoea caused by shiga toxin-producing E. coli
   d. Bacillary dysentery
   e. All of above

Answer

58. a, b, c, e. 59. b, c. 60. a, b, c, e. 61. d, e. 62. b. 63. e. 64. b, c, d.
65. b, e. 66. a. 67. a, b, e. 68. a, e. 69. a. 70. a, c. 71. b, e.
72. a, b, d

73. Which of the following drugs is/are used in treatment of mucormycosis:

a. Fluconazole
b. Amphotericin B
c. Voriconazole
d. Posaconazole
e. 5-flurocysteine

74. Which of the following anti-platelet drug acts through adenosine receptor antagonism:

a. Aspirin
b. Prasugrel
c. Cloipidogrel
d. Abciximab
e. Ticagrelor

75. Which of the following diuretics is/are carbonic anhydrase inhibitors:

a. Acetazolamide
b. Topiramate
c. Thiazide
d. Spironolactone
e. Bumetanide

76. Which of the following drug(s) is /are used for acute asthma

a. Terbutaline
b. Budesonide
c. Salbutamol
d. Formoterol
e. Ipratropium

77. Which of the following anti-viral drug is/are prodrug:

a. Acyclovir
b. Oseltemivir
c. Valganciclovir
d. Valaciclovir
e. Ganciclovir

78. Regarding 1st order drug kinetics, which of the following is true

a. Constant fraction of drug is eliminated per unit time
b. Rate of elimination has no correlation with concentration of drug
c. As concentration of drugs increases, rate of elimination increases
d. Elimination half-life is dose dependent
e. Clearance (CL) increases as drug concentration increases

79. Anti-androgenic drugs are:

a. Abiraterone
b. Anastrozole
c. Ketoconazole
d. Finasteride
e. Danazol

80. A tuberculosis patient was sputum positive even 5 months after treatment with isoniazid, rifampicin, kanamycin, moxifloxacin and streptomycin. He belongs to which drug resistance category:

a. Multidrug resistance (MDR-TB)
b. Poly-drug resistance TB
c. Extensively drug resistance (XDR-TB)
d. Pro-extensively drug resistance
e. Mono-resistance TB

81. WHO updated new treatment for MDR-T.B in 2016. It includes 4-6 month intensive phase and 5 month continuation phase for short regimen. Which of the following drugs are included in the intensive phase regimen apart from pyrizinamide+ ethambutol+kanamycin+moxifloxacin:

a. Delamanid
b. Bedaquiline
c. High dose isoniazid
d. Clofazimine
e. Linezolid

82. If dopamine is given at rate of 8μg/kg /min which of the following actions are seen:

a. Increased stroke volume
b. Decreased systemic vascular resistance
c. Increased systemic vascular resistance
d. Renal vasodilation
e. Increased heart rate

83. Which of the following drugs should not be used in myasthenia gravis:

a. Neostigmine
b. Paracetamol
c. Amikacin
d. Edrophonium
e. Atropine

84. Which of the following antiseizure drug(s) is/are sodium channel blocker:

a. Ethosuximide
b. Felbamate
c. Phenytoin
d. Levetiracetam
e. Ezogabine

MICROBIOLOGY

85. Which of the following is/are examples of type 3 hypersensitivity reaction(s):

a. Serum sickness
b. Arthus reaction
c. Erythroblastosis fetalis
d. Farmer's lung
e. Goodpasteur's syndrome

86. Which of the following organism(s) cannot be cultured in artificial media:

a. Mycobacterium leprae
b. Klebsiella rhinoscleromatis
c. Rhinosporidium *seeberi*
d. Pneumocystis jirovecii
e. Aeromonas hydrophila

87. Which of the following is/are vector borne disease:

a. Malaria
b. Dengue
c. Plague
d. Kyasanur forest disease
e. Tuberculosis

Answer

73. b, d. 74. b, c, e. 75. a, b. 76. a, c. 77. All (a,b,c,d,e.) 78. a, c. 79. a, c, d.
80. c. 81. c, d. 82. a, b, d, e. 83. c, e. 84. c. 85. a, b, d. 86. a, c, d.
87. a, b, c, d.

88. Which of the following is/are causes lymphatic filariasis:
a. Loa-Loa
b. Oncocerca volvulus
c. Wuchereria bancrofti
d. Brugia malayi
e. Brugia timori

89. Cell wall of gram negative bacteria contains:
a. Teichuronic acids
b. Peptidoglycan
c. Lipopolysaccharide
d. Teichoic acid
e. Lipoprotein

90. Which of the following has least risk of HIV transmission in case of contact with the infected source for the first time:
a. Anal intercourse: Receptive
b. Anal intercourse: Insertive
c. Penile Oral sex: Receptive
d. Penile Oral sex: Insertive
e. Vaginal intercourse: Female to male

91. Which of the following larva is/are found in stools:
a. *Strongyloides stercoralis*
b. Ankylostoma duodenale
c. Ascaris lumbricoides
d. Hymenolepis nana
e. Enterobius vermicularis

92. Common organism involved in community acquired-native valve infective endocarditis:
a. Staphylococcus aureus
b. Pseudomonas aerogenosa
c. Streptococcus viridans
d. Enterococcus
e. Candida

93. Which of the following is/are causes fever with rash:
a. Streptococcus pyogens
b. Staphylococcus aureus
c. Vibrio cholerae
d. Neisseria meningitidis
e. Salmonella typhi

94. Which of the following causes hemorrhagic fever:
a. Lassa fever
b. Yellow fever
c. Crimean-Congo fever
d. West Nile fever
e. Kyasanur forest disease

95. Which of the following halophilic vibrio:
a. V. alginolyticus
b. V. parahaemolyticus
c. V. cholerae
d. V. damsela
e. V. vulnificus

96. Category A bioterrorism agents is/are:
a. Anthrax
b. Cl. Botulinum toxin
c. Vibrio cholerae
d. Burkholderia pseudomallei
e. Yersinia pestis

97. Food poisoning caused due to preformed toxin of:
a. Bacillus cereus
b. Cl. botulinum
c. Shigella
d. Vibrio cholera
e. Staphylococcus aureus

98. Which of the following is/are the components of innate immune system:
a. NK cell
b. Beta defensins
c. T cell
d. B–cell
e. Dendritic cell

99. Class II MCH molecule are expressed on:
a. Dendritic cell
b. Basophils
c. Eosinophils
d. Activated T-cell
e. Macrophages

100. Which of the following immunoglobulins are commonly present in antigen binding site of B cell:
a. IgA
b. IgG
c. IgD
d. IgM
e. IgE

101. True about Severe Combined Immunodeficiency
a. Autosomal dominant transmission
b. Both B & T cell defect
c. Decreased lymphocyte count
d. More common in boys
e. Absent tonsils

102. Which of the following will give positive β-D-Glucan test:
a. Mucor
b. Candida
c. Pseudomonas aeruginosa
d. Aspergillus
e. Cryptococcus

FORENSIC MEDICINE

103. Which is/are false regarding post-mortem changes:
a. Fixation of cadaveric lividity occur in around 8 hr(range 6-12 hr)
b. Rigor mortis occur when ATP decreased to 85%of normal level
c. Cheery red colour occur due to CO poisoning
d. Rigor mortis delay & persists longer in cholera & typhoid
e. Livor mortis usually occur on dependent part

104. Punishment for insulting the modesty of a woman comes under:
a. IPC 375
b. IPC 376
c. IPC 354
d. IPC 509
e. IPC 506

Answer

88. c, d, e.	89. b, c, e.	90. d.	91. a.	92. a, c, d.	93. a, b, d, e.	94. a, b, c, e.
95. a, b, d, e.	96. a, b, e.	97. a, b, e.	98. a, b, e.	99. a, d, e.	100. c, d.	101. b, c, d, e.
102. b, c, d.	103. d.	104. c, d.				

105. Cephalic index in Indian population is:
a. 70-75
b. 75-80
c. 80-85
d. 85-90
e. 90-95

106. BAL used as an antidote in poisoning with:
a. Mercury
b. Arsenic
c. Iron
d. Cadmium
e. Lead

107. According to "Treatment of Terminally-Ill Patients Bill 2016", incompetent patient is below the age of:
a. 12 years
b. 14 years
c. 16 years
d. 21 years
e. 24 years

108. Bolam test deals with:
a. Identification
b. Age estimation
c. Negligence by patient
d. Named after John Bolam
e. Medical negligence

109. Which of the following is/are true regarding identification:
a. Most common pattern in dactylography is loop
b. In india, dactylography was first used by sir William herschel
c. Sex determination by pelvis is more accurate than skull
d. 10 year child has 14 temporary & 8 permanent teeth
e. In poroscopy, no of sebaceous gland pores are counted

110. A 15 year old child presented to emergency with altered sensorium, B.P-90/50, PR- 40/m RR-9/mm with gasping respiration. There is increased lacrimation, salivation & sweating. On examination meiosis is present. What is the drug/poisoning is most likely suspected-
a. Opioid
b. Organophosphorus
c. Phencyclidines
d. Barbiturates
e. Cocaine

111. Sin needle used to kill animals is made of:
a. Dhatura seeds
b. Ratti seeds
c. Lead peroxide
d. Arsenic
e. Strychnine

PSM

112. Primary prevention for Hypertension are all except:
a. Early diagnosis
b. Treatment with Anti-hypertensive drug
c. Low salt intake
d. Reduction in weight
e. Regular exercise

113. Screening tests should be:
a. More specific
b. Easy to perform
c. Expensive
d. Difficult to perform
e. Low sensitivity

114. True regarding Odd-ratio:
a. Calculated in case-control study
b. Calculated in cohort study
c. Closely related to relative risk
d. It is a cross-product ratio calculated by 2x2 table
e. Measure the strength of the association between risk factor and outcome

115. In ESI scheme which of the following benefits is/are given by cash:
a. Maternity benefit
b. Funeral benefit
c. Dependent benefit
d. Sickness benefit
e. Medical benefit

116. Regarding public health surveillance, which of the following is/are true is:
a. Done to evaluate the disease load in the society
b. Identify risk factors associated with health conditions
c. It can be both active and passive
d. It helps in framing new health programmes
e. Only done for rare disease

117. True about Elimination of disease:
a. This is a stage b/w control and eradication
b. It has an element of area association
c. Complete interruption of disease transmission
d. Incomplete interruption of disease transmission
e. Agent is absent but vector is present

118. All are true about vasectomy except:
a. Non-scalpel vasectomy has less complication than conventional method of vasectomy
b. Unprotected intercourse is allowed only after two consecutive semen analyses show absence of spermatozoa
c. Failure rate is 1 in 300
d. Increased risk of testicular cancer
e. Antibodies to sperm may formed

Answer

105. a.	106. a, b, e.	107. c.	108. d, e.	109. a, b, c.	110. b.	111. a, b.
112. a, b.	113. a, b.	114. a, c, d, e.	115. a, b, c, d.	116. a, b, c, d.	117. a, b, d.	118. c, d.

OPHTHALMOLOGY

119. Cause(s) of hypopyon include:
- a. Fungal corneal ulcer
- b. Episcleritis
- c. Rifabutin drug use
- d. Behcet's disease
- e. Retinitis pigmentosa

120. Which of the following is/are feature of superior oblique muscle lesion:
- a. Head tilt to opposite normal shoulder
- b. Chin liftto opposite side
- c. Hypertropia of the affected eye
- d. Diplopia
- e Blepharoptosis

121. With respect to tarsal plate which is/are true:
- a. Attached to lateral palpebral ligaments
- b. Meibomian gland is present here
- c. Upper lid tarsal plate is larger than lower lid tarsal plate
- d. Forms skeleton of eyelid
- e. Superior tarsal muscle associated with superior tarsal plate is innervated by the sympathetic nervous system

122. A person presented with lens subluxation. What will help in phacoemulsification:
- a. Capsular hooks
- b. Lid retractor
- c. Phacoemulsification is not done in subluxated lens
- d. Iris repositor
- e. High power settings phacoemulsification is used

123. In Iridocorneal endothelial (ICE) syndromes which is/are not present:
- a. Cataract
- b. Iris atrophy
- c. Iris nodules
- d. Corectopia
- e. Iris cyst

124. Risk factor for steroid induced glaucoma includes:
- a. Primary open angle glaucoma (POAG)
- b. Male sex
- c. Family history
- d. Hypermetropia
- e. TIGR gene presence

125. True about macular corneal dystrophy:
- a. Autosomal recessive inheritance
- b. Opacities are present throughout the cornea with clear paces in between
- c. Abnormal stromal deposit of mucopolysaccharide which stain positive with Alcian blue
- d. Recurs after corneal transplant
- e. Laser therapy can be done

126. Which of the following is/are associated with congenital cataract:
- a. Zellweger syndrome
- b. Neonatal hypoglycemia
- c. Canavan's syndrome
- d. Deposition of lipofuscin
- e. Reiger's syndrome

127. Procedures for thyroid related orbitopathy (TAO) includes:
- a. Lateral tarsorrhaphy
- b. Eyelid surgery with skin graft
- c. Extraocular muscle surgery
- d. Levator palpebrae superioris (LPS) muscle resection
- e. No role of orbital decompression

ENT

128. Clinical feature of Zygomatic fracture includes:
- a. Flattening of cheek
- b. Trismus
- c. Step deformity
- d. Hypoesthesia along distribution of infraorbital nerve
- e. CSF rhinorrhea

129. Tone decay test can be used to detect:
- a. Otosclerosis
- b. Meniere's disease
- c. Cochlear deafness
- d. SNHL
- e. Otitis media

130. True about rhinitis medicamentosa:
- a. Caused by excessive use of corticosteroid sprays
- b. Caused by long term use of α-adrenergic sprays
- c. Edema and redness of mucosa along with hypertrophy of turbinate may occur
- d. Regress by oral & nasal steroids
- e. Cocaine use may cause

131. True about Caldwell-Luc operation:
- a. Infraorbital nerve damage may occur as complication
- b. Opening of maxillary antrum through gingivobuccal incision
- c. Used for the treatment of chronic maxillary sinusitis & for obtaining biopsy for antral malignancy
- d. Sublabial approach leading to opening of mandibular antrum
- e. It may be done under local anaesthesia with nerve block

132. True about otosclerosis:
- a. Autosomal dominant mode of inheritance in hereditary cases
- b. More common in male
- c. Increases during pregnancy
- d. Commonly involve stapes which results in fixation & conductive deafness
- e. Reddish blushover promontory

Answer

119. a, c, d.	120. a, c, d.	121. a, b, c, d, e.	122. a.	123. a, e.	124. a, c, e.	125. a, c, d, e.
126. b, e.	127. a, b, c, d.	128. a, b, c, d.	129. b, c, d.	130. b, c, d, e.	131. a, b, c, e.	132. a, c, d, e.

133. False about Mondini dysplasia:
a. Inner ear malformation
b. Always occur as an isolated anomaly
c. Cochlear implants are used in treatment
d. Doesn't lead to sensorineural hearing loss
e. May be associated with Pendred syndrome & DiGeorge syndrome

134. Crouzon syndrome consists of:
a. Hypertelorism
b. Maxillary hypoplasia
c. Syndactyly
d. Hydrocephalus
e. Macrocephaly

135. True statement regarding use of head mirror & Bull lamp in ENT examination:
a. Distance between the doctor and the patient must be more than 10 inches
b. Applied on right eye
c. Right eye should be closed during examination
d. Both eye should be open while examining
e. Light from bull lamp is diffuse but strong

136. Facies leprosa is characterized by:
a. Collapse of nasal bridge
b. Loss of upper incisors teeth
c. Diffuse infiltration of face
d. Resorption of anterior nasal spine
e. Madarosis

137. True about anatomy of nasolacrimal duct & lacrimal apparatus:
a. Length of both upper and lower canaliculi is around 8-10 mm
b. In majority of population upper and lower canaliculi combines to form single common canaliculus
c. Nasolacrimal duct open in inferior meatus
d. Commonly injured in major facial fractures
e. Canalicus is lined by cilliary stratified columnar epithelium

MEDICINE

138. Which of the following cardiac manifestations is/are expected in stroke patients:
a. Mitral stenosis
b. Aortic regurgitation
c. Constrictive pericarditis
d. Recurrent atrial arrythmia
e. Patent foramen ovale

139. True about Emery-Dreifuss muscular dystrophy:
a. In X-linked form, female is most commonly affected
b. Facial muscle is always spared
c. Conduction defect may present
d. Cardiac involvement is rare
e. Contracture usually develops

140. True statement about infective endocarditis:
a. Janeway lesions are haemorrhagic lesion present on palm and sole
b. Janeway lesion are tender
c. Janeway lesions are non-tender
d. Osler nodes are present on pulp of finger & toes
e. Osler's nodes are non-tender

141. False statement(s) about porphyria:
a. In acute intermittent porphyria photosensitivity is seen
b. HMB-synthasedeficiency is seen in acute intermittent porphyria
c. Uroporphyrinogen synthase deficiency is seen in congenital erythropoietic porphyria
d. Beta carotene- decreases photosensitivity
e. Uroporphyrinogen decarboxylase is deficient in porphyria cutanea tarda

142. Diagnostic criteria for Guillain-Barré syndrome include(s):
a. CSF white cell > 10×10^6 cells/L
b. Progressive weakness of arms and legs with hyperreflexia
c. Absence of fever
d. Absence of an identified alternative diagnosis for weakness
e. Albuminocytological dissociation

143. Endocrine cause of weight gain include(s)
a. Hypothyroidism
b. Thyrotoxicosis
c. Addison's disease
d. Cushing syndrome
e. Insulinoma

144. Component of qSOFA score include(s)
a. Systolic blood pressure
b. Respiratory rate
c. Altered mental status
d. Pulse rate
e. Oxygen saturation

145. Which of the following is/are specific antibody for Systemic Lupus Erythematosus (SLE):
a. Anti-ds DNAantibody
b. Anti-histone antibody
c. Anti-Sm antibody
d. Antinuclear antibodies
e. Anti-RNP

146. Regarding scleroderma, which of the following is true:
a. Limited variants usually involves extremities and face
b. Majority of patient presents with Raynaud's phenomenon
c. Skin thickening is the hallmark
d. Pulmonary artery hypertension can also occur without lung fibrosis
e. ACE inhibitorscan precipitate sclerodermic renal crisis

147. Pulsus paradoxus is/are not present in:
a. Severe asthma
b. Constrictive pericarditis
c. Cardiac tamponade
d. Aortic regurgitation
e. Cor pulmonale

Answer

133. b, d. 134. a, b, d. 135. b, d, e. 136. b, d. 137. a, b, c, d. 138. a, d, e. 139. c, e.
140. a, c, d. 141. a. 142. c, d, e. 143. a, d, e. 144. a, b, c. 145. a, c. 146. a, b, c, d.
147. a, b, c.

148. Components of Cushing's triad includes:
a. Hypotention b. Hypertention
c. Bradycardia d. Tachycardia
e. Irregular respiration

149. Which of the following are true about diabetic ketoacidosis:
a. pH < 7.3
b. Bicarbonate <15 mEq/L
c. Blood glucose >300 mg/dL
d. Ketonemia
e. Absence of ketone bodies in urine

150. True about Clubbing:
a. The angle between the nail plate and the skin overlying the proximal part of the distal phalanx is >160 degree
b. Scramoth sign may present
c. Hypertrophic osteoarthropathy may be associated
d. Not found in cyanotic congenital heart disease

151. All are true about diabetic nephropathy except:
a. Screening for albuminuria should commence 5 years after the onset of type 1 DM
b. Microalbuminuria is the first clinical manifestation
c. Nephropathy is a risk factor for retinopathy
d. Persistent macroalbuminuria leads to renal impairment
e. Renal biopsy is always necessary for diagnosis

152. Which of the following are of importance in a patient of chronic kidney disease [CKD]:
a. Hypertensive control
b. Keep blood glucose in limit
c. Low salt intake
d. Peritoneal hemodialysis
e. Use of ACE inhibitors &ARB

153. Regarding Henoch-schonleinpurpura (HSP), which is/are true:
a. Leukocytoclastic vasculitis responds to corticosteroids
b. More commonly seen in adult and elderly
c. Palpebral purpura occurs
d. Thrombocytopenia due to immune cause
e. May progresses to chronic renal failure

154. True about 10% rule in pheochromocytoma:
a. 10% Bilateral b. 10% Malignant
c. 10% Familial d. 10% Extra-adrenal
e. 10% Benign

155. Which of the following are true about second heart sound(H2):
a. A_2-P_2 splitting increases with inspiration and decreases during expiration
b. A_2-P_2 splitting decreases with inspiration and increases during expiration
c. Wide fixed splitting in ASD
d. Narrow split in pulmonary arterial hypertension
e. A2 is delayed in LBBB & P2 is delayed in RBBB

156. Features of parkinsonism include all except:
a. Intention tremors b. Resting tremors
c. Mask face d. Rigidity
e. Flaccidity

SURGERY

157. True about elastic compression stockings in venous insufficiency:
a. Elastic compression stocking's cause dynamic sequential compression of leg veins
b. Improve venous circulation of leg
c. Compression occur maximum at calf
d. Worn in the morning and taken off at night before bedtime
e. Worn even after ulcer heals to prevent recurrence

158. Not true about frost bite:
a. Trench foot is a type of frostbite of foot
b. Initial treatment is rewarming
c. On face it is superficial & on extremities severe form occurs
d. Autoamputation may occur in severe cases
e. In First and second degree frostbite affected part show redness and edema

159. Cause of chronic empyema include(s):
a. Inadequate drainage of acute empyema
b. Inadequate needle aspiration of acute empyema
c. Inadequate antibiotic treatment of acute empyema
d. Drainage of plural effusion
e. Due to persistent foreign body in bronchioles

160. True about pyogenic liver abscess:
a. More common in left lobe
b. Can cause right pleural effusion
c. Surgical drainage is initial treatment of choice
d. Associated with polymicrobial flora
e. May arise from sepsis outside the hepatobiliary tree

161. True regarding deep partial thickness burn:
a. Involve subcutaneous fat & deeper tissue
b. May be associated with hypertrophic scarring and contractures
c. Painless
d. Epithelisation is completed in 10–14 days
e. Dry leathery skin

162. True about splenial hernia:
a. Protrude through linea alba
b. Occur where transversus abdominis muscle is defective
c. Arise from lateral aspect of rectus abdominis
d. Internal organs including small intestine may protrude
e. Usually occur at or above to accurate line

Answer

148. b, c, e.	149. a, b, c, d.	150. a, b, c.	151. e.	152. a, b, c, d, e.	153. a, c, e.	154. a, b, c, d.
155. a, c, d, e.	156. a, e.	157. a, b, d, e.	158. a, c.	159.All (a, b, c, d, e.)	160. b, d, e.	161. b, d.
162. b, c, d, e.						

163. Regarding phyllodes tumors which of the following is are true:
a. Associated with BRCA2
b. Second most benign tumor of breast
c. Reliable diagnosis by FNAC
d. Treatment by wide local excision or mastectomy
e. Around 90% cases are benign

164. Which of the following are true regarding ulcerative colitis:
a. Has malignant potential
b. Almost always involve rectum
c. Skip lesion
d. On abdominal radiographs gives thumbprinting pattern
e. Presents with pain and bloody diarrhoea

165. Which of the following is/are examples of contaminated wound:
a. Resection of intestinal fistula
b. Ruptured appendix surgery
c. Inguinal hernia repair surgery
d. Resection of unprepared bowel
e. Hysterectomy

166. True about Opsite wound dressing:
a. Wound can be visualized
b. Permeable to gases c. Permeable to water
d. Impermeable to bacteria
e. Increased chance of maceration

167. Indication of Hemorrhodectomy in haemorrhoids includes:
a. Large 1st and 2nd degree haemorrhoids
b. 3rd and 4th degree hemorhoids
c. If not able to differentiate prolapsed hemorhoids from low rectal prolapse
d. Strangulated hemorrhoid
e. Thrombosed external hemorrhoids

168. True about Chronic Pancreatitis:
a. Predispose to carcinoma of pancreas
b. Lipase and amylase will be always elevated
c. Can present with steatorrhoea & malabsorption
d. Present with epigastric pain radiating to back
e. Total pancreatectomy relieves pain in majority of patients

169. In a patient with ileal resection, ileocecal valve is spared. Which of the following is/are seen:
a. Steatorrhoea b. Constipation
c. Cholelithiasis
d. Small intestinal bacterial overgrowth
e. Renal oxalate stones

170. True about extradural haematoma:
a. On CT, extradural haematomas appear as a biconvex lentiform hyperdense appearance
b. More dangerous than acute subdural haematoma
c. Mainly arterial blood
d. Common after injury at pterion of skull
e. Located on lateral side of cerebral hemisphere

171. Feature of compartment syndromes include(s)
a. Swollen fingers b. Pallor
c. Paraesthesia d. Pain on passion flexion
e. Pain on active flexion

172. True statement about Urinary bladder cancer:
a. Intravesical BCG immunotherapy is helpful in recurrent cases
b. In muscle-invasive bladder cancer removal of visible lesion is sufficient
c. Smoking is a risk factor
d. Urothelial carcinomas is most common subtype
e. Schistosomiasis is not a risk factor

173. Poor prognosis of breast cancer is associated with:
a. Increased expression of Estrogen and Progesterone receptor
b. Over expression of HER-2/neu
c. Triple negative tumor
d. <5% cells in S-phase of mitosis
e. >20% of cells expressing Ki 67 marker

174. True about Luminal A breast cancer:
a. Low grade tumor
b. Her 2/neu amplification
c. Good prognosis
d. High grade tumor
e. Associated with cytokeratin 8 and 18

175. Regarding acute sialadenitis, which of the following is/are true:
a. Viral infection is common etiology
b. Transoral removal of stone by probing through oral route
c. Swollen gland
d. Most commonly involves the submandibular gland
e. Can present with stasis of saliva

176. Feature of 10-0 suture in comparison to 1-0 suture (made up of same material):
a. Smaller diameter
b. More tensile strength
c. More elasticity and plasticity
d. More chance of tissue reaction
e. Less chance of tissue reaction

177. In examination of acute abdomen which of the following signs is/are elicited in supine position:
a. Rovsing's sign b. Iliopsoas sign
c. Carnett's sign d. Obturator sign
e. Balance sign

178. True about esophageal squamous cell carcinoma:
a. Usually occur in middle 1/3rd of esophagus
b. Barret's esophagus is a risk factor
c. Staging is done by CECT
d. Chemoradiation has little role in inoperable cases
e. Stomach, jejunum or colon can be used for replacement after surgical removal

Answer

163. a, d, e. 164. a, b, d, e. 165. b, d. 166. a, b, d. 167. b, d. 168. a, c, d, e. 169. a, c, e.
170. a, c, d. 171. All (a, b, c, d, e.) 172. a, c, d. 173. b, c, e. 174. a, c, e. 175. a, b, c, e. 176. a, e.
177. a, b, c, d. 178. a, c, e.

179. True about lymphedema:
a. Milroy disease is hereditary
b. Filariasis is most common cause world wide
c. Meig syndrome occur in infancy
d. Not much responsive to diuretics
e. Can be complicated by cellulitis

180. True about hyperplastic gastric polyps:
a. More common in young adults
b. Chronic atrophic gastritis is a predisposing factor
c. Pre-malignant lesion with high malignant potential
d. Most common variety of gastric polyp
e. Surgery is done if they are symptomatic

181. Which of the following is /are true about Primary intestinal lymphoma:
a. Most common site is jejunum
b. Most of them are non-Hodgkin's lymphomas
c. May have T or B cell origin
d. May cause intestinal obstruction
e. Treatment may include surgical resection, chemotherapy & radiotherapy

182. Steps taken to prevent post-operative infection include(s):
a. Antibiotic is given at time of induction of anesthesia
b. Shaving hair is better than clipping
c. Preoperative skin preparation with alcohol-based solutions
d. Start antibiotic at least 1 day preoperatively
e. Prevent perioperative hypothermia

183. True statement(s) about colon carcinoma:
a. Right side colon carcinoma is associated with early obstruction
b. Left side colon carcinoma is associated change in bowel habit
c. Left side colon carcinoma is associated with early obstruction
d. Anaemia & melena are more common in right colon cancer
e. Colonoscopy is the gold standard for establishing the diagnosis of colon cancer

OBSTETRICS AND GYNECOLOGY

184. True statement(s) about $MgSO_4$ use in severe pre-eclampsia & eclampsia:
a. Used to treat hypertension
b. Seizure can be prevented by maintaining 4-7 mEq/Lconcentration
c. In $MgSO_4$ toxicity calcium gluconate is given
d. Initial dose cannot be given without checking patient's renal status
e. $MgSO_4$ can be given by continuous infusion or intermittent i.m injection

185. Which of the following is/are contraindication to pregnancy:
a. Severe pulmonary hypertension
b. Severe aortic stenosis
c. Moderate aortic regurgitation
d. Marfan's syndrome with dilated aortic root
e. Atrial septal defect(ASD)

186. Which of the following is/are true regarding estimation of gestational age:
a. Gestational sac diameter at 5–7 week
b. Crown rump length(CRL) at 7–10 week
c. CRL at 10–13 weeks
d. CRL at 14–18
e. BPD at 18–20 week

187. Regarding CIN & cervical carcinoma which of the following is/are true:
a. 50% cases of carcinoma cervix is associated with HPV-16
b. High-risk subtypes of HPV are 16 & 18
c. CIN-I is kept under observation with PAP smear or HPV DNA test
d. All cases of CIN-1 regresses in 2 year
e. Route of infection is usually through cervical columnar epithelium

188. Which of the following is/are cause(s) of primary amennorhoea:
a. Turner's syndrome
b. Kallmann syndrome
c. Meyer-Rokistansky Kauster Hauser (MRKH) syndrome
d. Sheehan's syndrome
e. PCOD

189. Which of the following is/are not effective in controlling hot flushes of menopause:
a. Hormone replacement therapy
b. Calcium
c. Tibolone
d. Vitamin E
e. Raloxifene

190. In shoulder dystocia, shoulder delivery is/are done by:
a. Suprapubic pressure
b. McRoberts Manoeuvre
c. Wood corkscrew method
d. Lovset manoeuvre
e. Pinnard manoeuvre

191. In antenatal screening for aneuploidy, which of the following is/are true:
a. Nuchal translucency is seen at 11-14 weeks
b. Quadruple test is done at 10-12 weeks
c. AFP is tested in Down syndrome
d. Fetal cell DNA from maternal blood is used
e. Anomaly scan is done at 12-16 week

Answer

179. a, b, d, e.	180. b, d, e.	181. b, c, d, e.	182. a, c, e.	183. b, c, d, e.	184. b, c, e.	185. a, b, d.
186. a, b, e.	187. a, b, c, e.	188. a, b, c, e.	189. b, e.	190. a, b, c.	191. a, c, d.	

192. A clinical case of abnormal uterine bleeding with endometrial hyperplasia and without atypia is diagnosed. Treatment of this condition includes:
  a. LNG- IUD insertion
  b. Medroxyprogesterone acetate for 3 cycles
  c. Medroxyprogesterone acetate for 6 cycles
  d. Medroxyprogesterone acetate for 3 months
  e. Medroxyprogesterone acetate for 6 months

193. According to recent WHO guideline for semen analysis, which of the following is true about normal semen analysis:
  a. Normal morphology >4%
  b. Sperm motility>25%
  c. Volume>1.5 ml
  d. PH <6.5
  e. Sperm count 1.5 million/mL

194. True about risk factor of pre-eclampsia:
  a. More in those who are exposed to chorionic villi for first time
  b. More in those who exposed to excess chorionic villi like twins
  c. Genetic predisposition
  d. Family history of hypertension
  e. Smoking

195. Which of the following important points needed to be informed to a pregnant woman when taking consent for vaginal birth after caesarean section (VBAC):
  a. Previous classical C.S is contraindication
  b. Chance of uterine rupture 4% after 1 LSCS
  c. Chance of fetal compromises are 15–25%
  d. Induction of labour with oxytocin is totally safe
  e. Increases risk of placenta accreta

196. Regarding fibroid which of the following is/are true:
  a. Sarcomatous changes in >1% of cases
  b. Calcareous degeneration occur in pregnancy
  c. Does not increase in size during pregnancy
  d. Anterior wall fibroid causes mostly hydro-ureter
  e. Broad ligament fibroid causes mainly menstrual irregularities

197. Marker raised in ovarian dysgerminoma include(s):
  a. AFP
  b. Lactate dehydrogenase (LDH)
  c. Placental alkaline phosphatise (PLAP)
  d. Inhibin
  e. β-hCG

198. In comparison of large loop excision of the transformation zone(LLETZ) with laser ablation therapy, which is/are true regarding management of carcinoma in situ(of cervix):
  a. A loop size of less than 2 cm gives a better cone than a larger one
  b. Cheaper than laser
  c. Takes longer time w.r.t. laser
  d. Costlier than laser
  e. Low voltage is used

199. Major diagnostic criteria of PCOD include(s):
  a. Insulin resistance
  b. Size of ovary >10 cm with single follicle
  c. Hirsutism
  d. Oligomenorrhoea
  e. Obesity

200. Moskowitz procedure is/are done for:
  a. Secondary vault prolapse
  b. Cystourethrocele
  c. Adenomyosis
  d. Chronic inversion of uterus
  e. Enterocele

201. Which of the following intervention is/are not used in active management of 3rd stage labour:
  a. Early cord clamping
  b. Manual removal of placenta
  c. Control cord traction
  d. Oxytocin drip infusion
  e. Normal saline infusion

202. After B/L salpingo-oophorectomy what is the chance of occurrence of peritoneal/ovarian/uterine cancer22.high risk patient undergoes prophylactic salpingo oophorectomy, wat are her future chances of getting malignancy
  a. 4%
  b. 6%
  c. 8%
  d. 10%
  e. 15%

203. Investigation(s) which are part of Pre-conceptional advice to diabetic mother:
  a. Check HbA1c level
  b. TSH estimation
  c. Frequent blood sugar estimation
  d. LH & FSH estimation
  e. All of above

PEDIATRICS

204. Features of hypoxic ischemic injury in newborn may include(s):
  a. Mortality in more than 30% cases in severe asphyxia
  b. Umbilical arterial blood pH <7.5
  c. Acute tubular necrosis
  d. Seizure
  e. Cerebral edema

205. Which of the following is true about breast milk:
  a. Contains all vitamins except vitamin A
  b. Breast milk contains factors for cell growth and differentiation of intestinal cells
  c. Contain antibacterial factors including Bifidus factor
  d. Breast milk is a suspension of Protein and Fats in Carbohydrate
  e. Main secretory Ig present is IgG

Answer

192. a, b, d.	193. a, c, e.	194. a, b, c, d.	195. a.	196. None	197. b, c, e.	198. a, b, e.
199. c, d.	200. e.	201. a, b.	202. a.	203. a, b, c.	204. a, c, d, e.	205. b, c.

206. Which of the following is/are true regarding infant leukemia except:
a. Ratio of ALL: AML is around 2:1
b. Most children have MLL nutation
c. CNS infiltration is commonly seen in AML
d. Overall good prognosis
e. Poor prognosis

207. Feature(s) of hypertrophic pyloric stenosis are all except:
a. Projectile vomiting
b. Bilous vomiting
c. Non-bilous vomiting
d. Non-projectile vomiting

ORTHOPEDICS

208. In posterior dislocation of hip, attitude of limb is/are all except:
a. Abduction
b. Adduction
c. Flexion
d. Extension
e. Internal rotation

209. A 30-years-old male met with fracture of femur bone. He develops fat embolism. Major feature of Gurd's criteria for fat embolism include(s):
a. CNS depression
b. Axillary or Conjunctival petechiae
c. Tachycardia
d. Pulmonary edema
e. Unexplained decreased platelet count

210. Feature(s) of Achondroplasia:
a. Autosomal recessive inheritance
b. Abnormal sexual development
c. Disproportionate body dwarfism
d. Trident hand
e. Subnormal intelligence

211. All are feature(s) of inflammatory arthritis except:
a. Pain during active movement of the joint
b. Pain decrease after walking
c. Morning stiffness of joint
d. No inflammatory cell in aspirated fluid of joint
e. Elevated ESR

212. Which of the following fracture is/are specific for child abuse:
a. Posterior rib fracture
b. Scapula fracture
c. Pelvic fracture
d. Multiple fractures at different stages of healing
e. Mandible dislocation

213. Risk factor for Legg-Calve-Perthes disease include(s):
a. Adult & elderly age group
b. Accelerated skeletal growth
c. Passive smoking
d. Positive family history
e. Hypercoagulation state

214. True about management of fracture in children:
a. Supracondylar fracture of humerus can be managed by closed reduction
b. Displaced lateral condylar fracture of humerus- Open reduction & internal fixation
c. Lateral condylar fracture of humerus is known as fracture of necessity
d. Undisplaced medial epicondyle fracture of humerus- open reduction & internal fixation
e. Forearm fracture in children can be managed by closed reduction & casting

215. In a patient with L4-5 disc prolapse of, which of the following nerve root is likely to be compressed:
a. L4
b. L5
c. S1
d. S2
e. S2-4

216. True statement(s) regarding osteogenesis imperfect:
a. Dual-Energy X-ray Absorptiometry (DEXA) scan will help to assess osteoporosis and osteopenia in children
b. Bisphosphonates can be given to children to prevent skeletal damage
c. Can present as lethal skeletal dysplasia
d. Always autosomal dominant inheritance

217. All are true about septic arthritis except:
a. Most common cause is E. coli
b. Staphylococcus aureus is the most common cause
c. Common in children
d. Affects growth plate
e. Aspiration of joint fluid is used for diagnosis

ANESTHESIA

218. Diagnostic criteria for blood stream infection from central venous catheter include all except:
a. Apparent source of blood stream infection present other than catheter
b. At least one positive peripheral blood culture
c. Blood culture from catheter shows colony formation at least 2 hours before the peripheral blood culture
d. Semi-quantitative catheter tip culture showing >15 CFU/catheter segment whereby the same organism (species and anti-biogram) is isolated from the catheter segment and peripheral blood culture
e. Colony count from catheter culture is 5 times more than peripheral blood culture

Answer

206. d.	207. b, d.	208. a, d.	209. a, b, d.	210. c, d.	211. a.	212. a, b, d.
213. c d, e.	214. a, b, c, e.	215. b.	216. a, b, c.	217. a.	218. a.	

219. Which of the following is/are true regarding Intra-jugular vein catheterization (IJV) and subclavian vein catheterization (SCV):
- a. SCV catheterisation is have lesser success rate in first attempt
- b. SCV catheterisation is a/w more line infection
- c. SCV catheterisation associated with more artery damage
- d. IJV catheterization is easy for inexperienced hand
- e. SCV catheterisation associated with more pneumothorax

220. Sterile zone of operation theater consists of:
- a. Scrub room
- b. Anesthesia Induction Room
- c. Preoperative room
- d. Sterile store
- e. Changing room

221. In Caesarean section operation, after 8 min of spinal anesthesia, female develop hypotension. Which of the following drug(s) is/are used for management of hypotension:
- a. Ephedrine
- b. Adrenaline
- c. Dopamine
- d. Phenylephrine
- e. Mephentermine

222. In renal disease, which of the following agents should not be used:
- a. Succinylcholine
- b. Methoxyflurane
- c. Pancuronium
- d. Atracurium
- b. Desflurane

223. True statement(s) about local anesthetics:
- a. Lidocaine is used for awake intubation
- b. Bupivacaine more cardiotoxic & longer acting than lidociane
- c. Intralipid is used for cardiotoxicity of bupivacaine
- d. Ropivacaine- used in peripheral nerve block
- e. Cocaine can produce hypotension

224. True about muscle relaxants:
- a. Succinylcholine is short acting muscle relaxant
- b. Succinylcholine is used for rapid-sequence induction in full stomach patients
- c. Recuronium is muscle relaxant of choice in paediatric patients
- d. Rocuronium can be used for rapid-sequence induction
- e. Pancuronium is used in day care surgery

225. Which of the following is/are false regarding gases used in anesthesia:
- a. Sevoflurane is the agent of choice for children & asthma patients
- b. In day care surgery, halothane is most commonly used inhalational agent
- c. Sevoflurane can be safely used in liver disease
- d. Desflurane should not be used for induction in children
- e. Sevoflurane fresh gas flow rates should be at least 2 L/min for exposures greater than 1 hour

226. Which of the following is/are correct about cardiac arrest management according 2015 American Heart association guidelines for cardiopulmonary resuscitation (CPR) & Emergency cardiovascular care (ECC):
- a. Ventricular fibrillation requires synchronized cardioversion
- b. Monophasic defibrillators are preferred over biphasic devices
- c. Epinephrine (1 mg) is the DOC for cardiac arrest
- d. Lidocaine may be considered as an alternative to amiodarone for unresponsive VF/pVT
- e. Vasopressin provides added advantage when combined with epinephrine

227. True about pre-anaesthesia checkup (PAC):
- a. Used for evaluation of vitals, co-morbid conditions & relevant investigation
- b. Decreases anxiety of patient
- c. In day care surgeries it is not required
- d. Help in planing anaesthetic technique
- e. Not needed in infants

DERMATOLOGY

228. Which of the following is/are not a subtype of lichen planus:
- a. Ulcerative lichen planus
- b. Lichen nitidus
- c. Hypertrophic lichen planus
- d. Lichen scrofulosorum
- e. Lichen planus pigmentosus

229. Nail changes in psoriasis is/are:
- a. Onycholysis
- b. Oil drop discolouration
- c. Subungual hyperkeratosis
- d. Nail pitting
- e. Pterygium formation

230. Scarring alopecia is seen in all except:
- a. Trichotillomania
- b. Lichen planus
- c. Tinea capitis
- d. DLE [discoid lupus erythematosus]
- e. Sarcoidosis

231. Which of the following is/are causes of painful ulcers:
- a. Herpes genitalis
- b. Chancroid
- c. Donovanosis
- d. Lymphogranuloma venereum (LGV)
- e. Primary syphilis

232. Langerhans cell is/are decreased/absent in:
- a. Langerhans cell histiocytosis
- b. Oral lichen planus
- c. Basal cell carcinoma
- d. Contact dermatitis
- e. Sarcoidosis

Answer

219. a, d, e. 220. a, b. 221. All (a,b,c,d,e.) 222. a, b, c. 223. a, b, c, d. 224. a, b, d. 225. b.

226. c, d. 227. a, b, d. 228. d. 229. a, b, c, d. 230. a, c. 231. a, b. 232. c, e.

233. Which of the following are true regarding leg ulcers & their locations:
- a. Tip of toes is more common location for arterial ulcers
- b. Arterial ulcers more common above medial malleolus
- c. Venous ulcers are more common above lateral malleolus than above medial malleolus
- d. Diabetic foot ulcers are more common in ball of greater toe & plantar surface of metatarsals head
- e. Pressure ulcer - common at heels

PSYCHIATRY

234. According to Diagnostic and Statistical Manual of Mental Disorders, fifth edition(DSM-5), which is/are not paraphilia:
- a. Exhibitionism
- b. Tribadism
- c. Frotteurism
- d. Adultery
- e. Masochism

235. Which of the following(s) is/are not feature of mania:
- a. Delusion of grandeur
- b. Delusion of guilt
- c. Delusion of persecution
- d. Delusion of infidelity
- e. Nihilistic delusion

236. Which of the following is/are true about suicide:
- a. More common in young males
- b. Genetic predisposition
- c. Suicide and parasuicide are same thing
- d. Loneliness increases chance
- e. Hopelessness is predisposing factor

237. Feature(s) of Antisocial personality disorder:
- a. Low concern for others feeling
- b. Inability to feel guilt
- c. Suicidal threats may present
- d. Low tolerance to frustration
- e. Disrupted self image

238. A patient with paranoid schizophrenia talks about 'omni micro', but he is unable to explain it in detail & reach a conclusion. He often repeats the last syllable of one word of the last sentence. This can be related to:
- a. Neologism
- b. Perseveration
- c. Circumstantiality
- d. Knight's move thinking
- e. Logoclonia

239. Defense mechanism in obsessive compulsive disorder is/are:
- a. Isolation of affect
- b. Conversion
- c. Reaction formation
- d. Undoing
- e. Projection

RADIOLOGY

240. Which of the following is/are present inside the nucleus of an atom:
- a. Electron
- b. Proton
- c. Neutron
- d. Photon
- e. None of above

241. Which of the following imaging modalities is/are used to see the lesion of white matter of brain:
- a. MR spectroscopy (MRS)
- b. Magnetic resonance imaging (MRI)
- c. Computed tomography (CT)
- d. Positron emission tomography (PET)
- e. Skull radiograph

242. Natural radioisotope are:
- a. Cobalt-60
- b. Radium- 226
- c. Iridium-192
- d. Strontium-90
- e. Cesium-137

243. Claw sign on x-ray is seen in:
- a. Ischemic colitis
- b. Intussusception
- c. Sigmoid volvulus
- d. Crohn's disease
- e. Iliocaecal tuberculosis

244. Which of the following ray(s) is/are used in tele-therapy:
- a. Gamma rays
- b. X-rays
- c. Alpha rays
- d. Beta rays
- e. Electron beam

245. Posterior urethral valve in neonate is diagnosed by:
- a. Micturating Cystourethrography (MCU)
- b. Prenatal USG
- c. PET scan
- d. Postnatal USG
- e. CT scan

246. Radiological features of neurofibromatosis-1 include(s):
- a. Posterior scalloping of vertebral bodies
- b. Sphenoid wing dysplasia
- c. Narrowing of neural foramina
- d. Scoliosis
- e. Microcephaly

247. Unit of radiation exposure /Radiation exposure in linear accelerator is measured in:
- a. Becquerel
- b. Rad/min
- c. Curie/sec
- d. Rad/sec
- e. Roentgen/min

248. Which of the following is/are true about hepatocellular carcinoma:
- a. USG is used for initial screening
- b. Contrast enhanced MRI - Enhancement in arterial phase & washout in venous phase
- c. Multidetector row CT with intravenous contrast shows hypervascular appearance
- d. PET-scan is better than CT scan & MRI scan
- e. AFP is invariably increased

Answer

233. a, d, e.	234. c, e.	235. b, d.	236. b, d, e.	237. a, b, c, d, e.	238. b, e.	239. a, c, d.
240. b, c.	241. a, b, c, d.	242. b, d, e.	243. b.	244. a, b, e.	245. a, b, d.	246. a, b, d.
247. b.	248. a, b, c.					

MAY 2018 ANSWERS & EXPLANATIONS

ANATOMY

1. Ans. a. Extensor carpi ulnaris; c. Extensor carpi radialis brevis; d. Extensor digitorum communis.

[Ref: BDC 7th/ Vol. I 181, 138-140; Moore Anatomy 7th/764; Gray's 40th/784; Anatomy by Kulkarni 8th/112]

Extensor Carpi Radialis Longus, Brachioradialis, Triceps & Anconeus *are directly supplied by radial nerve*

◈ *BDC 7th/ Vol. I 181(table)*

Radial nerve *has two terminal branch-superficial Anterior interosseous nerve (purely cutaneous branch) & deep Posterior interosseous nerve(motor)- Moore Anatomy 7th/764; BDC 7th/ Vol. I 115*

Table: Posterior interosseous nerve (Deep division of Radial nerve) *(BDC 7th/ Vol. I 181,138,140)*

	Cubital fossa	Back of forearm	Wrist
Muscular	• Extensor carpi radialis brevis • Supinator	• Abductor pollicis longus • Extensor pollicis brevis • Extensor pollicis longus • Extensor digitorum (Extensor digitorum communis) • Extensor indicis • Extensor digiti minimi • Extensor carpi ulnaris	–
Articular	–		To inferior radio-ulnar, wrist & intercarpal joints

Posterior Interosseous Nerve Palsy

◈ *Gray's 40th/784*

- Many causes include trauma and inflammatory swellings
- Pain is similar in nature to that of radial tunnel syndrome and is later accompanied by weakness and paralysis.
- There are no sensory disturbances,

2. Ans. b. Teres major

[Ref: BDC 7th/ Vol. I 72-74; Snell 9th/359; Campbell's 11th/2607; Gray's 40th/807]

- Teres major is not a part of rotator cuff

Musculotendinous Cuff or Rotator Cuff of Shoulder

◈ *BDC 7th/ Vol. I 72-74; Snell 9th/359*

- *Muscles are-* ***subscapularis, supraspinatus, infraspinatus & teres minor***
- *Cuff muscles arise from the scapula & inserted into the lesser & greater tubercles of the humerus*
- *It strengthens the capsule of shoulder joint except inferiorly- that is why dislocation of humerus occur commonly in an anteroinferior direction*
- *During injury to rotator cuff, tendons are affected, not the muscles. Supraspinatus tendon is affected most frequently*

Rotator Cuff Disorders

◈ *Apley's 9th/337; Gray's 40th/807*

- Supraspinatus impingement syndrome & *Tendinitis (including acute calcific tendinitis; Subacute tendinitis-painful arc syndrome)*
- *Tears/Ruptures*
- *Frozen shoulder (Adhesive capsulitis)*

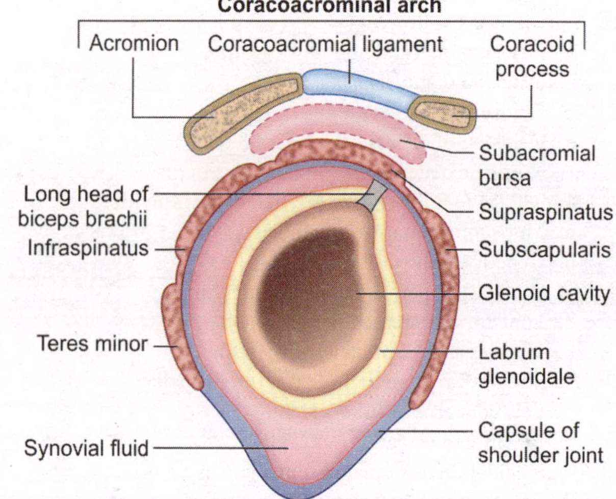

Fig: Rotator Cuff of shoulder (*BDC 7th/ Vol. I 72)*

3. Ans. a. Azygous vein; b. Thoracic duct; c. Hemiazygos vein

[Ref: BDC 7th/ Vol. I 202; Keith Moore 7th/308-09; Gray's 40th/1007-08]

- **Hemiazygos vein***: Pierces left crus of diaphragm & also sometimes passes through* ***aortic opening***

"The **aortic opening** ***transmits the aorta, thoracic duct, lymphatic trunks from the lower posterior thoracic wall and, sometimes, the azygos and hemiazygos veins***"*-Gray's 40th/1007*

The **aortic hiatus** transmits ***descending aorta, thoracic duct and sometimes the azygos and hemi-azygos veins***"*- Keith Moore 7th/309*

"**Hemiazygos vein** *pierces the left crus of the diaphragm, ascends on the left side of the vertebrae* ***overlapped by the aorta***"*- BDC 7th/ Vol. I 233*

Table: Large openings in thoracoabdominal diaphragm *(BDC 7th/ Vol. I 202)*

Opening	Situation	Shape	Structures passing	Effect on contraction
Vena cava	T8, junction of right and median leaflet of central tendon	Quadrilateral	IVC Right phrenic nerve Lymphatic of liver	Dilation
Oesophageal	T10, splitting of right crus	Elliptical	Oesophagus Both vagal trunks Left gastric vessels	Constriction
Aortic	T12, behind median arcuate ligament	Rounded	Aorta Thoracic duct Azygos vein	No change

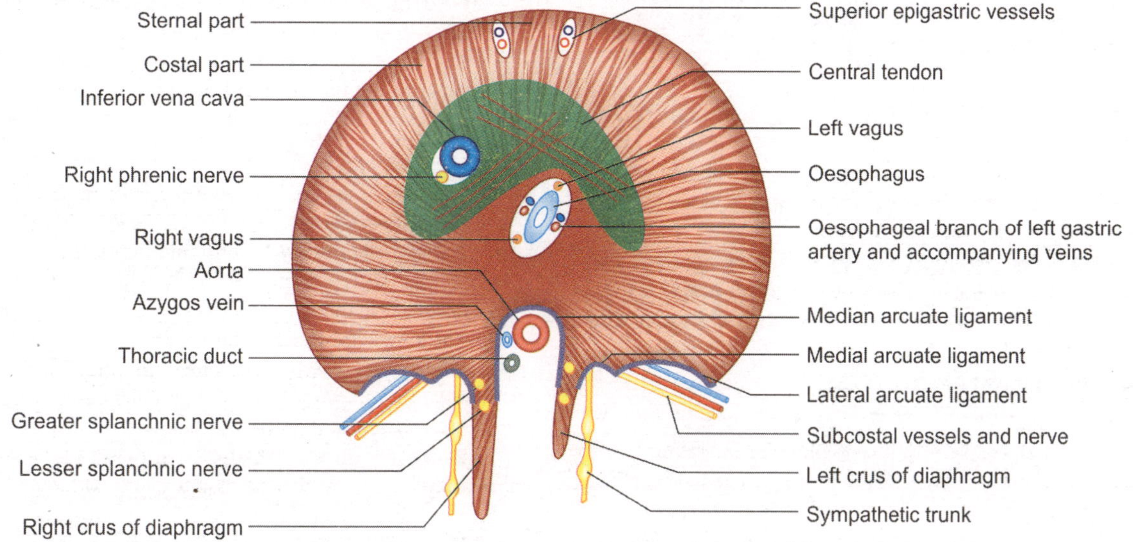

Fig: Structure passing through the diaphragm *(BDC 7th/ Vol. I 202)*

Apertures of Diaphragm

◈ *Gray's 40th/1007-08; Keith Moore 7th/309*

- A number of structures pass between the thorax and abdomen via apertures in the diaphragm. There are ***three large openings***, for the aorta, oesophagus and inferior vena cava and a number of smaller ones
- In addition to the three main apertures, there is a small opening, the **sternocostal triangle** (foramen). This triangle transmits lymphatic vessels from the diaphragmatic surface of the liver and the superior epigastric vessels
- There are **two small apertures** in each crus of the diaphragm; one transmits the greater splanchnic nerve and the other the lesser splanchnic nerve.

4. Ans. b. Nerve supply of penile skin is from obturator nerve; c. There are at least 5 urethral sphincters; e. Dorsal artery of penis is branch of bulbourethral artery

[Ref: BDC 7th/ Vol. II 242; Snell 9th/315-16; Gray's 40th/1093-94, 1274-75; Moore 7th/422, 712]

- ***Dorsal artery of penis** is branch of **internal pudendal artery; there are 2*** **urethral sphincters and obturator nerve does not supply penile skin**

The **urethral sphincter** is a muscular structure that regulates the outflow of urine from the bladder into the urethra. There are **2 urethral sphincters**, the ***external and internal urethral sphincters***. When these muscles contract, the urethra narrows and urination stops or slows. The urethral sphincter is critical for the maintenance of urinary continence"- *www.ncbi.nlm.nih.gov; BDC 7th/Vol. II 411-12*

*Obturator nerve supplies **adductor muscles** of medial compartment of thigh"- BDC 7th/ Vol. II 143*

Arteries of Penis

◈ *BDC 7th/ Vol. II 242*

- ***Superficial external pudendal artery** (Br. of femoral artery): **supplies skin & fascie of the penis***
- **Superficial** and **deep branches of the external pudendal arteries** supply the penile skin, anastomosing with branches of the internal pudendal arteries.
- *Deep artery of penis (Br. of internal pudendal artery)*
- ***Dorsal artery of penis** (Br. of **internal pudendal artery**): supplies glans penis, distal part of corpus spongiosum, prepuce & frenulum*
- *Artery of bulb of penis **Also k/a Bulbourethral artery** (Br. of internal pudendal artery): Supplies bulb & proximal half of corpus cavernosa*

Penis

◈ *Snell 9th/315-16*

- **Arterial supply**: Deep artery of penis (corpora cavernosa), artery of the bulb(corpus spongiosum) & dorsal artery of penis- all are branches of *internal pudendal artery*
- *Lymphatic drainage: superficial inguinal L.N (skin of penis) & internal iliac node (deep structures of penis)*

Nerve Supply of Penis

◈ *BDC 7th/ Vol. II 242; Snell 9th/316*

- *Sensory supply: dorsal nerve of penis & ilioinguinal nerve*
- *Muscular supply: perineal branch of the pudendal nerve*
- *Autonomic nerves: Derived from pelvic plexus via prostatic plexus*

Penis Venous System

◈ *urologicsurgery.wordpress.com*

- **The penis is drained by three venous systems: superficial, intermediate and deep.**
- **Superficial veins: contained in the dartos fascia on the dorsolateral aspects of the penis unite** at its base to form a single superficial dorsal vein.
- **Intermediate system contains the deep dorsal and circumflex veins, lying within and beneath Buck's fascia:**
- **DEEP drainage system consists of the crural and cavernosal veins.**

Venous Drainage of Penis

◈ *BDC 7th/ Vol. II 242*

- Superficial dorsal vein: drains prepuce & penile skin
- Deep dorsal vein: receives blood from glans penis & corpora cavernosa

5. Ans. e. Papilla of renal pyramids terminates into minor calyx

[Ref: BDC 7th/ Vol. II 341-46; Snell 9th/206-07; Gray's 40th/1225-33; A.K.Jain 6th/501-07]

- ***Posterior segmental artery is first & most constant branch of renal artery; supplied by postganglionic sympathetic (T10-L1) fibres; long axis of the kidney is directed downward & laterally & kidney extends up to upper border of twelth thoracic vertebra***

Kidney

◈ *BDC 7th/ Vol. II 341-46*

- *Vertically extend from* ***upper border of twelfth thoracic vertebra to the centre of the body of third lumbar vertebra***
- *Right kidney is slightly lower than the left & the left kidney is a little nearer to the median plane than the right*
- *The* **long axis** ***of the kidney is directed downwards & laterally****, so that the* ***upper poles are nearer to the median plane than the lower poles.*** *The* **transverse axis** *is directed laterally & backwards*
- ***Kidney is supplied by the renal plexus****, an off shoot of the celiac plexus. It contains* **sympathetic(T10-L1)** *fibres which are chiefly vasomotor. The afferent nerves of the kidney belong to segment T10 to T 12*
- The *renal plexus* is located around the renal artery and contains ***postganglionic fibers*** from the sympathetic nervous system (T10 to L2)-*www.urology-textbook.com*

Blood Supply: Kidney

◈ *urologicsurgery.wordpress.co*

- The renal artery splits into four or more branches, with five being the most common. These are the renal segmental arteries.
- Each segmental artery supplies a distinct portion of the kidney with no collateral circulation between them. Thus, occlusion or injury to a segmental branch will cause segmental renal infarction.
- Generally, the ***first and most constant branch is the posterior segmental branch***, which separates from the renal artery before it enters the renal hilum.
- There are typically **four anterior branches**, which from superior to inferior are apical, upper, middle and lower.

Kidney

◈ *Gray's 40th/1225*

- Superiorly they are level with the ***upper border of the 12th thoracic vertebra, inferiorly with the third lumbar vertebra.***
- The right is usually slightly inferior to the left, reflecting its relationship to the liver. The left is a little longer and narrower than the right and lies nearer the median plane
- The **long axis of each kidney** is ***directed inferolaterally and the transverse axis posteromedially***, which means that the anterior and posterior aspects usually described are in fact anterolateral and posteromedial.

Renal pyramids (or **malpighian pyramids** or **Malpighi's pyramids** are cone-shaped tissues of the kidney. In humans, the renal medulla is made up of 10 to 18 of these conical subdivisions. The broad base of each pyramid faces the renal cortex and **its apex, or papilla**, points internally towards the pelvis. The pyramids appear striped because they are formed by straight parallel segments of nephrons and collecting ducts. The ***base of each pyramid originates at the corticomedullary border and the apex terminates in a papilla, which lies within a minor calyx***, made of parallel bundles of urine collecting tubules.- *www.sciencedirect.com; wikipedia*

The **pyelocaliceal system** consists of the ***renal pelvis and calyces***. The urine from the collecting ducts (which cross the renal pyramids to open into the papillae) is collected in the small calyces (minor or secondary). At the renal level, there are 8–18 pyramids, but only 7–13 minor calyces, some of the latter having more than one papilla. These calyces converge to form the major calyces, which in turn open into the renal pelvis through the caliceal infundibula.

6. Ans. c. Tubal tonsil; d. Nasopharyngeal tonsil; e. Lingual tonsil.

[Ref: BDC 7th/ Vol. III 237; Snell 9th/639; Gray's 40th/567; Keith Moore 7th/1038]

Jugulo-digastric lymph nodes & Jugulo-omohyoid lymph nodes are deep group of H & N lymph nodes while Waldeyer's ring is deepest group of H & N lymph nodes- *BDC 7th/ Vol. III 162-64*

Waldeyer's Ring

◈ *Gray's 40th/567; Keith Moore 7th/1038; BDC 7th/ Vol. III 237*

- Waldeyer's ring is a circumpharyngeal ring of mucosa-associated lymphoid tissue which surrounds the openings into the digestive and respiratory tracts.
- It is made up anteroinferiorly by the ***lingual tonsil***, laterally by the ***palatine and tubal tonsils*** and posterosuperiorly by the ***nasopharyngeal tonsil*** and smaller collections of lymphoid tissue in the intertonsillar intervals

Waldeyer's Ring

◈ *www.juniordentist.com*

- Waldeyer's lymphatic ring is a collection of lymphoid tissue. It is also called as **Waldeyer's-Pirogov tonsillar ring**
- **It is divided into 2 types based on its location:**
    - Waldeyer's outer ring: present in the neck
    - Waldeyer's inner ring/Waldeyer's tonsillar ring: The lymphatic ring present around the pharynx
- **Waldeyer's outer ring**: It is composed of various lymph nodes in the neck – mostly cervical lymph nodes. **The component lymph nodes are:** Occipital, Postauricular, Preauricular, Parotid, Facial (superficial – upper, middle, lower; deep), Submandibular, Submental, Superficial cervical & Anterior cervical.

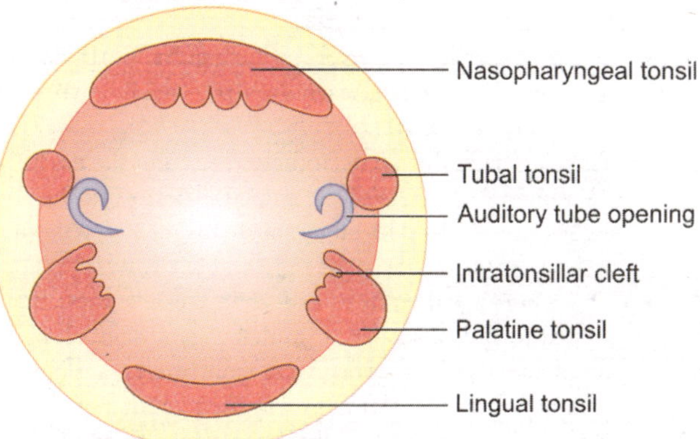

Fig: Waldeyer's lymphatic ring *(BDC 7th/ Vol. III 237)*

7. **Ans.** **a. 2nd largest salivary gland; b. Stenson's duct opens into the vestibule of the mouth opposite upper third molar; d. Majority of lymph nodes are embedded in deep lobe**

[Ref: BDC 7th/ Vol. III 108-13; Snell 9th/630-32; Essential Anatomy by Moore 2nd/954-55; Gray's 40th/495-97]

- ***The majority of lymph nodes lie in the superficial part of the gland***

"The **facial nerve** divides the gland into ***superficial and deep lobes***"- *Snell 9th/630*

"Facial layer is very thick superficially but very thin on the deep side of the parotid gland where ***parotid abscess can burst to form a parapharyngeal abscess*** and thence spread to the mediastinum"-*P.L.Dingra 6th/263*

Parotid Gland

◈ *BDC 7th/ Vol. III 108-13*

- It is the ***largest of salivary glands.***
- **Stenson's duct** opens into the vestibule of the mouth opposite the crown of the ***upper second molar teeth***
- "**Superficial surface of parotid** is covered with a ***few deep parotid lymph nodes embedded in the gland***"- *BDC 7th/ Vol. III 110*
- **Facial nerve** lies in relation to isthmus of the gland which ***separates large superficial part from small deep part of the gland.*** Facial nerve divides into two branches—temporofacial and cervicofacial nerve"- *BDC 7th/ Vol. III 111*

Parotid Gland

◈ *Gray's 40th/495-97*

- The paired parotid glands are ***the largest of the salivary glands.***
- Lymph nodes occur in the skin overlying the parotid gland (***preauricular nodes***) and in the substance of the gland.
- There are usually 10 lymph nodes present in the gland, ***the majority lie in the superficial part of the gland*** above the plane related to the facial nerve. Lymph from the parotid gland drains to the upper deep cervical lymph nodes.

"**Parotid:** The parotid lymph nodes are a small group of nodes ***located superficially to the parotid gland.*** They collect lymph from the nose, the nasal cavity, the external acoustic meatus, the tympanic cavity and the lateral borders of the orbit. There are also ***parotid lymph nodes deep to the parotid gland*** that drain the nasal cavities and the nasopharynx"- *teachmeanatomy.info*

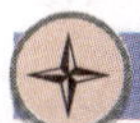

Also Know

"Gustatory sweating (Frey's syndrome or auriculotemporal syndrome): Gustatory sweating (auriculotemporal syndrome) commonly occurs following parotid surgery or other surgery or trauma that results in opening of the parotid capsule"
- Gray's 40th/495

8. **Ans.** **b. Superior ophthalmic vein; e. Superficial middle cerebral vein**

[Ref: BDC 7th/ Vol. III 200; Gray's 40th/429-30]

Tributaries or incoming channels of Cavernous Sinus

◈ *BDC 7th/ Vol. III 200*

I-From Orbit

- ***Superior ophthalmic vein***
- *Inferior ophthalmic vein branch or may vein itself*
- *Central vein of retina may drain*

II- From Brain

- ***Superficial middle cerebral vein***
- *Inferior cerebral vein from temporal lobe*

III- From meninges

- *Sphenoparietal sinus*
- *Frontal trunk of middle meningeal vein may drain*

Cavernous Sinus

◈ *Gray's 40th/429-30*

- Tributaries of the cavernous sinus are the ***superior ophthalmic vein, inferior ophthalmic vein (either a branch***

or the whole vessel), superficial middle cerebral vein, inferior cerebral veins and sphenoparietal sinus.

- Less frequently, the ***central retinal vein and frontal tributary of the middle meningeal vein drains into it***.
- The **cavernous sinus drains** to the transverse sinus via the superior petrosal sinus; to the internal jugular vein via the inferior petrosal sinus and a plexus of veins associated with the internal carotid artery; to the pterygoid plexus by veins traversing the emissary sphenoidal foramen, foramen ovale and foramen lacerum; and to the facial vein via the superior ophthalmic vein
- The **cavernous sinuses** are two large venous plexuses that lie on either side of the body of the sphenoid bone, extending from the superior orbital fissure to the apex of the petrous temporal bone, with an average length of 2 cm and width of 1 cm.

9. Ans. c. Arch of aorta; e. Right subclavian artery

[Ref: Embryology by I.B.Singh 11th/244-247; Gray's 40th/597]

Table: Adult derivatives of truncus arteriosus, aortic sac and aortic arches *(Embryology by I.B.Singh 11th/247)*

Adult Derivatives	Embryological Structures
Ascending aorta	Truncus arteriosus
Arch of aorta	Aortic sac, left horn of aortic sac and ***left 4th arch artery***
Descending aorta	Left dorsal aorta and fused dorsal aorta
Brachiocephalic artery	Right horn of aortic sac
Right subclavian artery	***Right 4th arch artery*** and 7th cervical intersegmental artery
Left subclavian artery	Left 7thr cervical intersegmental artery
Common carotid artery	Proximal part of 3rd arch artery
Internal carotid artery	Distal part of 3rd arch artery and cervical part of dorsal aorta
External carotid artery	As a bud from 3rd arch artery
Pulmonary trunk	Truncus arteriosus
Pulmonary artery	Part of 6th arch artery
Ductus arteriosus	Part of left 6th arch artery between lung bud and aorta

Table: Pharyngeal arch *(Gray's 40th/597)*

Arch No.	Ach name	Nerve	Artery
1	Mandibular	Trigeminal (V) Mandibular division	First aortic arch artery [transitory]
2	Hyoid	Facial (VII)	Stapedial artery [transitory]
3	Third	Glossopharyngeal (IX)	Common carotid artery, first part of internal carotid artery
4	Fourth	Vagus (X) Pharyngeal branch	Proximal part of subclavian artery on the right, Arch of aorta between origins of left common carotid and left subclavian arteries
6	Sixth	Vagus (X) Recurrent laryngeal branch	Part between the pulmonary trunk and dorsal aorta. Becomes ductus arteriosus on left, disappears on right

Contd...

Pharyngeal arch arteries & their fate

◈ *Embryology by I.B.Singh 11th/244-247*

- *The greater part of the first & second arch arteries disappears*
- *In adult life, the first arch is represented by the maxillary artery*
- *The fifth arch also disappears*
- *Aortic sac is connected only with the arteries of 3rd, 4th, & 6th arches*

Aortic Arches

◈ *Langman's Embryology 13th/ 202-04*

- When pharyngeal arches form during the fourth and fifth weeks of development, each arch receives its own cranial nerve and its own artery
- These arteries, the **aortic arches,** arise from the **aortic sac,** the mowst distal part of the truncus arteriosus. The aortic arches are embedded in mesenchyme of the pharyngeal arches and terminate in the right and left dorsal aortae.
- The **pharyngeal arches** and their vessels appear in a cranial to caudal sequence, so that they are not all present simultaneously. The aortic sac contributes a branch to each new arch as it forms, giving rise to a total of five pairs of arteries. (The fifth arch either never forms or forms incompletely and then regresses. Consequently the five arches are numbered I, II, III, IV and VI. During further development, this arterial pattern becomes modified and some vessels regress completely.
- The **fourth aortic arch** persists on both sides, but its ultimate fate is different on the right and left sides. **On the left** it forms part of the ***arch of the aorta***, between the left common carotid and the left subclavian arteries. **On the right** it forms the most proximal segment of the ***right subclavian artery***, the distal part of which is formed by a portion of the right dorsal aorta and the seventh intersegmental artery

"The **umbilical arteries, *initially paired ventral branches of the dorsal aorta,*** course to the placenta in close association with the allantois. During the fourth week, however, each artery acquires a secondary connection with the dorsal branch of the aorta, the common iliac artery and loses its earliest origin. After birth, the proximal portions of the umbilical arteries persist as the internal iliac and superior vesical arteries and the distal parts are obliterated to form the medial umbilical ligaments"- *Langman's Embryology 13th/ 202*

10. Ans. a. Pulmonary artery; c. Bronchial artery

[Ref: Harrison 19th/245-46,1108; Davidson 23rd/559-60www.ncbi.nlm.nih.go]

Cavitary TB: *Hemoptysis (source is usually a* ***Bronchial Artery****):* *Rasmussen aneurysm-Danhert Radiology 7th/549*

Hemoptysis

◈ *Harrison 19th/245*

- Pneumonias of any sort can cause hemoptysis. Tuberculous infection, which can lead to bronchiectasis or cavitary pneumonia, is a very common cause of hemoptysis worldwide. Patients may present with a chronic cough productive of blood-streaked sputum or with larger volume bleeding.
- *Rasmussen's aneurysm* (the ***dilation of a pulmonary artery*** in a cavity formed by previous tuberculous infection) ***remains a source of massive, life-threatening hemoptysis in the developing world***. Community-acquired pneumonia and lung abscess can also result in bleeding. Once again, if the infection results in cavitation, there is a greater likelihood of bleeding due to erosion into blood vessels.
- Infections with *Staphylococcus aureus* and gram-negative rods (e.g., *Klebsiella pneumoniae*) are especially likely to cause necrotizing lung infections and thus to be associated with hemoptysis

"Rasmussen's aneurysm, a very rare complication of active pulmonary tuberculosis (TB), is a *pulmonary artery aneurysm* adjacent to or within a tuberculous cavity. It may lead to rupture and life threatening massive hemoptysis, an uncommon but challenging medico-surgical emergency"- www.ncbi.nlm.nih.gov; radiopaedia.org

Massive Hemoptysis

◈ *Schwartz 10th/661-63*

- The lungs have two sources of blood supply: the ***pulmonary and bronchial arterial systems***.
- ***Most cases of massive hemoptysis involve bleeding from the bronchial artery circulation or from the pulmonary circulation***
- ***Aneurysms of the pulmonary artery (referred to as Rasmussen's aneurysm) can develop within pulmonary cavities and can result in massive bleeding.***
- Massive hemoptysis in patients with lung cancer is typically caused by malignant invasion of pulmonary artery vessels by large central tumors. Although rare, it is often a terminal event.
- **Recurrence after bronchial artery embolization** is less common in the setting of ***malignancy and active tuberculosis*** but does occur and can ultimately result in patient death

11. Ans. a. Most distal portion of the conducting zone; b. Lined by columnar epithelium

[Ref: BDC 7th/ Vol. I 252,254-55; Morgan Anesthesia 5th/489-500; Gray's 40th/999]

Terminal Bronchiole

◈ *BDC 7th/ Vol. I 252,254-55*

- *Less than 1 mm in diameter*
- *Lined by* ***columnar epithelium***
- *No smooth muscles & gland*
- They do not contain cartilage in their walls like bronchi. The epithelium is comprised of simple columnar ciliated cell- radiopaedia.org
- It is the most distal portion of the conducting zone that branches off the lesser bronchioles. Every single terminal bronchiole gets divided to form respiratory bronchioles that comprise a small number of alveoli- *www.britannica.com*
- It supplies oxygen to each pulmonary acini in the body. The main function of these tubular structures is conduction of gas and they are too thick to allow the exchange of air- www.britannica.com
- *Respiratory bronchiole: lined by cuboidal epithelium, wall made up of smooth muscle fibers & elastic fibers; gaseous exchanges takes place.*

Respiratory Passage

◈ *Harshmohan 7th/442*

- *Trachea, major bronchi & their branching possess cartilage, smooth muscle & mucous glands in their walls, while the* ***bronchioles*** *have smooth muscle but* ***lack cartilage as well as the mucous glands***
- *Bronchioles undergo 3 to 4 divisions leading to the* ***terminal bronchioles*** *which are less than 2 mm in diameter*
- *The part distal to a terminal bronchiole is called an acinus*
- *Acinus composed of 3-5 respiratory bronchioles, alveolar duct & alveoli*

"The **trachea** is a longer section of the respiratory tract, shaped like a tube and approximately 5 inches in length. It has several ***C-shaped hyalines cartilage rings*** which are lined with ***pseudostratified ciliated columnar epithelium***. These rings keep the trachea open for air all the time. They are C-shaped in order to allow the open end to face the esophagus. This allows the esophagus to expand into the area normally occupied by the trachea in order to permit larger chunks of food to pass through"- *adrenalfatiguesolution.com*

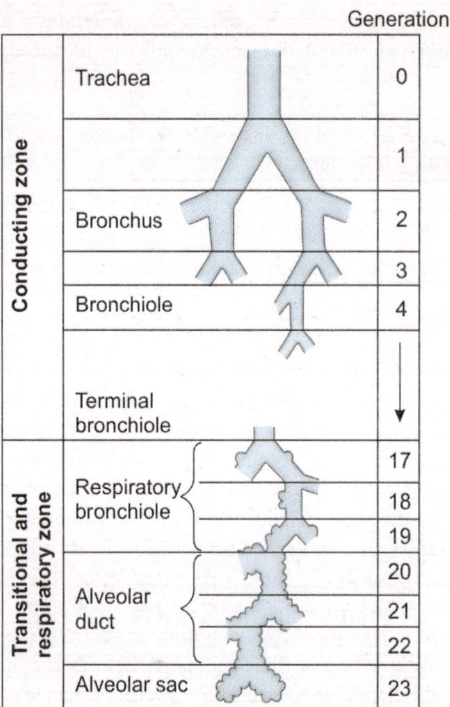

Fig: Dichotomous division of the airways *(Morgan Anesthesia 5th/489)*

12. Ans. c. AV node located in triangle of Koch; e. Bundle of His lies posteroinferiorly in ventricular septum

[Ref: BDC 7th/ Vol. I 277; Snell 9th/85; Gray's 40th/977; Davidson 23rd/445]

Conducting System

◈ *BDC 7th/ Vol. I 277*

- **SA node**: ***situated at atriocaval junction***
- The SA node is situated at ***the junction of the superior vena cava and RA***- *Davidson 23rd/445*
- **AV node**: *situated in the lower & dorsal part of the* ***atrial septum*** *just above the opening of the coronary sinus*
- **AV node**: The node, with its transitional zones, is located within the **atrial component of the muscular atrioventricular septum**. Its anatomical landmarks are the ***boundaries of the triangle of Koch*** (the attachment of the septal cusp of the tricuspid valve inferiorly, the ostium of the coronary sinus basally and the tendon of Todaro superiorly) *Gray's 40th/977*
- **AV bundle or bundle of His**: *It begins as AV node, crosses AV ring & decsends along the* ***posteroinferior border of the membranous part of the ventricular septum***
- **AV bundle** *descends behind the septal cusp of the tricuspid valve to reach the* ***inferior border of the membranous part of the ventricular septum****. At the upper border of muscular part of the septum, it divides into two branches, one for each ventricle- Snell 9th/85*

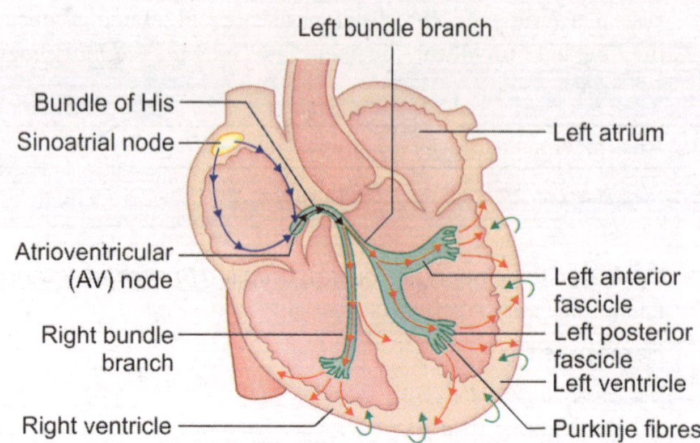

Fig: The cardiac conduction system *(Davidson 23rd/445)*

13. Ans. a. S2, S3, S4

[Ref: BDC 7th/ Vol. II451; Snell 9th/; Gray's 40th/1092, 1094]

"External sphincter is supplied by the ***inferior rectal nerve(S2,3,4)*** *& by the perineal branch of the* ***fourth sacral*** *nerve"- BDC 7th/ Vol. II 451*

The **external anal sphincter** is innervated mainly by the ***inferior rectal branch of the pudendal nerve (anterior divisions of the second, third and fourth sacral spinal nerves).*** It may also receive some direct supply via fibres which leave the ventral rami of these nerves as they exit the sacral foramina and run beneath the fascia over levator ani to reach the anorectal junction- *Gray's 40th/1159*

External Anal Sphincter

◈ *Gray's 40th/1094*

- The external anal sphincter is an oval tube of striated muscle which surrounds the lowest part of the anal canal. The uppermost (deepest) fibres blend with the lowest fibres of puborectalis; the two are seen to be continuous on endoanal ultrasound and magnetic resonance imaging.
- Anteriorly, some of these upper fibres decussate into the superficial transverse perineal muscles. Posteriorly, some fibres are attached to the anococcygeal raphe. The majority of the middle fibres of the external anal sphincter surround the lower part of the internal sphincter and are attached anteriorly to the perineal body and posteriorly to the coccyx via the anococcygeal ligament.

14. Ans. d. Greater omentum

[Ref: Gray's 40th/1206,1209; Embryology by I.B.Singh 11th/177-78; masterofmedicine.com]

The Derivatives of Dorsal and Ventral mesogastrium are

I.B.Singh 11th/177-78; masterofmedicine.com

Dorsal mesogastrium

- Greater omentum
- Gastrosplenic ligament
- Gastrophrenic ligament
- Lienorenal ligament

Ventral Mesogastrium

- Lesser omentum
- ***Falciform ligament***
- ***Coronary ligament***
- Right and left triangular ligament

PHYSIOLOGY

15. Ans. **a. Constitutes around 2%...; c. Prevents polymerization of deoxy-sickle...; d. Level is increased in β-thalassemia trait; e. Decreased level is seen in iron ...**

[Ref: Nelson 20th/2307-09; Ganong 25th/555; Wintrobe's Clinical Hematology 12th/Chap7; A K Jain 6th/61]

Hemoglobin A2 (α2δ2)

◈ *A K Jain 6th/61*

- "Approx. **2.5%** of the total haemoglobin"- *Ganong 25th/555; A K Jain 6th/61*
- Level: **2.3-3.5%** (*www.sickle-thal.nwlh.nhs.uk*)
- Hemoglobin A2 ***(alpha2delta2)***, which is present at low concentration ***(1-2%)*** in the circulating red cells of normal individuals- www.ncbi.nlm.nih.gov
- It produces no abnormality and is regarded as normal haemoglobin
- ***Iron deficiency anaemia- low level*** (www.ncbi.nlm.nih.gov)

Adult Hemoglobins

◈ *Nelson 20th/2308*

- ***At birth, <1.0% of Hb A_2 is seen, but by 12 moths of age the normal level of 2.0–3.4% is attained. Throughout life, the normal ratio of Hb A to A_2 is about 30:1.***
- The ***normal adult level of Hb A_2 (2.0–3.4%) is seldom*** *altered.*
- ***Levels of Hb A_2>3.4% are found in most persons with the β-thalassemia trait*** and in those with megaloblastic anemias secondary to vitamin B_{12} and folic acid deficiency. Decreased ***Hb A_2 levels are found in those with iron-deficiency anemia and α-thalassemia***- *Nelson 20th/2309*
- ***HbA2 is increased in people with thalassemia***-www.ijcrr.com

"HbA2, a tetramer of a- and d-globin chains, provides a diagnostic clue to the presence of β-thalassaemia trait. This minor haemoglobin, which forms about 2–3% of the total, has ***no known physiological role,*** but has the ***interesting property of preventing polymerization of deoxy-sickle haemoglobin.*** If it were possible to increase the level of HbA2 sufficiently it could have ***a benefit in sickle cell disease*** similar to that of foetal haemoglobin. Moreover, HbA2 is present in all erythrocytes, an advantage not found with foetal haemoglobin, which is heterocellularly expressed"-www.ijcrr.com/uploads

Table: **Normal Human Hemoglobins** *(Wintrobe's Clinical Hematology 12th/Chap 7)*

Name	Designation Molecular Structure	Proportion in	
		Adults	Newborns
Adult hemoglobin A	α2β2	97%	20%
Hemoglobin A2	α2δ2	2.5%	0.5%
Fetal hemoglobin F	α2γ2	<1%	80%
Portland	ζ2γ2	0	0
Gower I	ζ2∊2	0	0
Gower II	α2∊2	0	0

16. Ans. **None**

[Ref: A K Jain 6th/31; www.lakesidepress.com; medical-dictionary.thefreedictionary.com]

- ***Correct answer is 40 nmol/L*** *(not 40 mmol/L) - so none of the options*

A **pH of 7.4 represents a [H⁺] of 40 nmoles/L** (for univalent ions, mmoles/ L equal mEq/L). By definition pH does not have units-*www.lakesidepress.com*

Arterial blood pH (the most readily measured) varies inhealth within the range of ***7.36-7.44 or $[H^+]$ = 40 nmol.L^{-1}*** *-medical-dictionary.thefreedictionary.com*

Plasma (pH= 7.35 to 7.45, or $[H^+]$= **35 to 45 nmol/l**) "-*www.jfmed.uniba.sk*

The **hydrogen ion concentration of the blood** is normally controlled within narrow limits, in health rarely exceeding ***46 nmol/L or falling below 35 nmol/L***"- *www.sciencedirect.com*

The normal range of hydrogen ion concentration in the **extracellular fluid (ECF)** is between ***35 and 45 nmol/L,*** which translates to a pH of 7.35 to 7.45.- www.sciencedirect.com

pH and $[H^+]$

◈ *A K Jain 6th/31*

- Optimal pH range for blood at which human body functions properly is 7.35 to 7.45.
- Clinically, blood pH <7.35 is referred as acidosis and blood pH >7.45 as alkalosis

Table: **pH and $[H^+]$ of various body fluid** *(A K Jain 6th/31)*

	pH	[H+] nmol/L or nEq/L = 10^{-9}mol/L
8.00	(Maximum alkaline urine)	10
7.70	Of plasma (severe alkalosis)	20
7.41	(Arterial blood)	
7.40	(Plasma)	40 How? Plasma at pH 7.4 i.e. $[H^+]$ of 40 × 10^{-9} mol/L
7.38	(Mixed venous blood)	
7.30	(CSF)	50
7.20	(RBC)	
7.10	(ICF)	80

Contd...

	pH	[H+] nmol/L or nEq/L = 10^{-9}mol/L
7.00	(Pure water) 'neutral'	100; pH of water at 250°C, in which H^+ and OH– are present in equal numbers, $[H^+]= [OH^-]= 10^{-7}$ mol/L
6.9	Of plasma (severe acidosis)	126
6.0	(Normal urine)	1000
4.5	(Urine maximum acidity)	31600
1.0	(Pure gastric juice)	108

17. Ans c. Pacinian corpuscles- vibration; e. Ruffini's end organ – pressure

[Ref: Ganong 25th/160; Guyton (SEA) 13th/714-15; AK Jain 6th/864-65]

Cutaneous Receptors

◈ *AK Jain 6th/865*

- Cutaneous receptors respond to touch, pressure, pain and temperature- AK Jain 6th/864
- Meissner's corpuscles-light touch
- Merkle's corpuscles-touch
- Free terminal-pain
- Pacinian corpuscles-deep pressure
- Ruffini corpuscles-warmth

"Merkel's disks respond to light touch. Meissner's corpuscles respond to touch and low-frequency vibration. Ruffini endings detect stretch, deformation within joints and warmth. ***Pacinian corpuscles detect transient pressure and high-frequency vibration. Krause end bulbs detect cold***"- courses. lumenlearning.com

Receptors

◈ *Ganong 25th/160*

- Touch and pressure are sensed by four types of mechanoreceptors.
- **Meissner corpuscles** are dendrites encapsulated in connective tissue and respond to changes in texture and slow vibrations.
- **Merkel cells** are expanded dendritic endings and they respond to sustained pressure and touch.
- **Ruffini's corpuscles** are enlarged dendritic endings with elongated capsules and they respond to ***sustained pressure.***
- **Pacinian corpuscles** consist of unmyelinated dendritic endings of a sensory nerve fber, 2 μm in diameter, encapsulated by concentric lamellae of connective tissue that give the organ the appearance of a cocktail onion. These ***receptors respond to deep pressure and fast vibration.***

"**Merkel's discs and Meissner's corpuscles** *are tactile receptors. They are* ***rapidly adapting receptors****. This is why we do not feel our clothes once they are put on"-AK Jain 6th/864*

"**Pacinian corpuscles:** *They respond to deformation caused by firm pressure and are* ***quickly adapting****. This is why we do not feel seat pressure when sitting"- AK Jain 6th/864*

"**Joint receptors** *are mainly the pacinian corpuscles,* **Golgi tendon organs** *and Ruffini's end organs which are situated in the ligaments of the joint. They are* ***quickly adapting receptors****"- AK Jain 6th/865*

"The ***pacinian corpuscle adapts very rapidly,*** hair receptors adapt within a second or so and ***some joint capsule and muscle spindle receptors adapt slowly.*** Furthermore, some sensory receptors adapt to a far greater extent than others"-*Guyton 12th (SAE) /688*

Adaptation of Receptors–*Two types*

◈ *AK Jain 6th/870*

- **Tonic receptors***: They are poor,* ***slow and incompletely adapting receptors****, therefore, they can continue to transmit the information for many hours even if the intensity of stimulus remains absolutely constant over many days. E.g* ***Muscle spindle; Sensation of pain and cold; Baroreceptors and chemoreceptors***
- **Phasic (or rate) receptors:** *These are* ***rapidly adapting receptors*** *and transmits signals only when the stimulus strength is changed.e.g* ***touch, olfactory and pressure***

Classification of Receptor by Rate of Adaptation

◈ *wikipedia*

- **Slowly adapting:** Slowly adapting mechanoreceptors include Merkel and Ruffini corpuscle end-organs and some free nerve endings. Slowly adapting type I mechanoreceptors have multiple Merkel corpuscle end-organs. Slowly adapting type II mechanoreceptors have single Ruffini corpuscle end-organs.
- **Intermediate adapting**: Some free nerve endings are intermediate adapting.
- **Rapidly adapting**: Rapidly adapting mechanoreceptors include ***Meissner corpuscle end-organs, Pacinian corpuscle end-organs, hair follicle receptors and some free nerve endings.***
- Rapidly adapting type I mechanoreceptors have multiple Meissner corpuscle end-organs.
- Rapidly adapting type II mechanoreceptors (usually called Pacinian) have single Pacinian corpuscle endorgans

Table: Principle sensory modalities *(Ganong 25th/160)*

Sensory system	Modality	Stimulus	Receptor class	Receptor cell types
Somatosensory	Touch	Tap, flutter 5-40 Hz	Cutaneous mechanoreceptor	Meissner corpuscles
Somatosensory	Touchw	Motion	Cutaneous mechanoreceptor	Hair follicle receptors
Somatosensory	Touch	Deep pressure, vibration 60-300 Hz	Cutaneous mechanoreceptor	Pacinian corpuscles

Contd...

Sensory system	Modality	Stimulus	Receptor class	Receptor cell types
Somatosensory	Touch	Touch, pressure	Cutaneous mechanoreceptor	Merkel cells
Somatosensory	Touch	Sustained pressure	Cutaneous mechanoreceptor	Ruffin corpuscles
Somatosensory	Proprioception	Stretch	Mechanoreceptor	Muscle spindles
Somatosensory	Proprioception	Tension	Mechanoreceptor	Golgi tendon organ
Somatosensory	Temperature	Thermal	Thermoreceptor	Cold and warm receptors

18. Ans. a. Inhibition of suppressing effect of dopamine on prolactin; c. Pregnancy, d. Pituitary adenoma; e. Lactation

[Ref: Harrison 19th/2266; Ganong 25th/398; Guyton (SEA) 13th/694; A K Jain 6th/671]

Pituitary Apoplexy

Acute intrapituitary hemorrhagic vascular events can cause substantial damage to the pituitary and surrounding sellar structures. ***Pituitary apoplexy*** may occur spontaneously in a preexisting adenoma; postpartum (Sheehan's syndrome); or in association with diabetes, hypertension, sickle cell anemia, or acute shock. ***Hypopituitarism is common after apoplexy"***- *Harrison 19th/2266*

Hyperprolactinemia

◈ *Harrison 19th/2266*

- Hyperprolactinemia is the most common pituitary hormone hypersecretion syndrome in both men and women. PRL-secreting ***pituitary adenomas (prolactinomas) are the most common cause of PRL levels*** >200 μg/L
- ***Pregnancy*** and lactation are the important physiologic causes of hyperprolactinemia
- Drug-induced inhibition or disruption of dopaminergic receptor function is a common cause of hyperprolactinemia
- Prescription drug use is a common cause of hyperprolactinemia. ***Prolactin secretion in the pituitary is suppressed by the brain chemical dopamine. Use of drugs that block the effects of dopamine can cause the pituitary to secrete prolactin***- *Ganong 25th/398*

Table: Etiology of Hyperprolactinemia *(Harrison 19th/2266)*

- **Physiologic hypersecretion:** ***Pregnancy***, Lactation, Chest wall stimulation, Sleep, Stress
- **Hypothalamic–pituitary stalk damage**
- **Tumors:** Craniopharyngioma, Suprasellar pituitary mass, Meningioma, Dysgerminoma, Metastases
  - Empty sella
  - Lymphocytic hypophysitis
  - Adenoma with stalk compression
  - Granulomas
  - Rathke's cyst
  - Irradiation
  - Trauma: Pituitary stalk section, Suprasellar surgery
- **Pituitary hypersecretion**: Prolactinoma, Acromegaly
- **Systemic disorders**
  - Chronic renal failure
  - Hypothyroidism
  - Cirrhosis
  - Pseudocyesis
  - Epileptic seizures

Contd...

- **Drug-induced hypersecretion**
  - Dopamine receptor blockers
    - Atypical antipsychotics: risperidone
    - Phenothiazines: chlorpromazine, perphenazine
    - Butyrophenones: haloperidol
    - Thioxanthenes
    - Metoclopramide
  - Dopamine synthesis inhibitors
    - α-Methyldopa
  - Catecholamine depletors
    - Reserpine
  - Opiates
  - H_2 antagonists
    - Cimetidine, ranitidine
  - Imipramines
    - Amitriptyline, amoxapine
  - Serotonin reuptake inhibitors
    - Fluoxetine
  - Calcium channel blockers
    - Verapamil
    - Estrogens
    - TRH

19. Ans. a. Primary hyperparathyroidism; b. Familial hypocalciuric hypercalcemia

[Ref: Harrison 19th/2469-70;Ganong 25th/381-82; Davidson 23rd/662]

- ***Milk-alkali syndrome, Thiazide diuretic use and Vitamin D intoxication*** cause low **parathyroid hormone (PTH) level**-so excluded from answer

Table: Causes of hypercalcaemia *(Davidson 23rd/662)*

With normal or elevated PTH levels	With low PTH levels
• ***Primary or tertiary hyperparathyroidism*** • Lithium-induced hyperparathyroidism • ***Familial hypocalciuric hypercalcaemia***	• Malignancy (lung, breast, myeloma, renal, lymphoma, thyroid) • Elevated 1,25 (OH) 2 vitamin D (***vitamin D intoxication***, sarcoidosis, HIV, other granulomatous disease) • Thyrotoxicosis • Paget's disease with immobilisation • ***Milk-alkali syndrome*** • ***Thiazide diuretics*** • Glucocorticoid deficiency

Familial Hypocalciuric Hypercalcemia (Familial Benign Hypercalcemia)

- Patients with this disorder are usually asymptomatic and the hypercalcemia is identified by chance during routine investigation for other conditions. The parathyroid glands are normal, ***PTH levels are inappropriately normal***"- Nelson 18th/Chap 574
- FHH (also called *familial benign hypercalcemia*) is inherited as an autosomal dominant trait. Affected individuals are discovered because of asymptomatic hypercalcemia. Most cases of FHH (FHH1) are caused by an inactivating mutation in a single allele of the CaSR, leading to ***inappropriately normal or even increased secretion of PTH***"- *Harrison 19th/2475*

Evaluation of patients with hypercalcemia

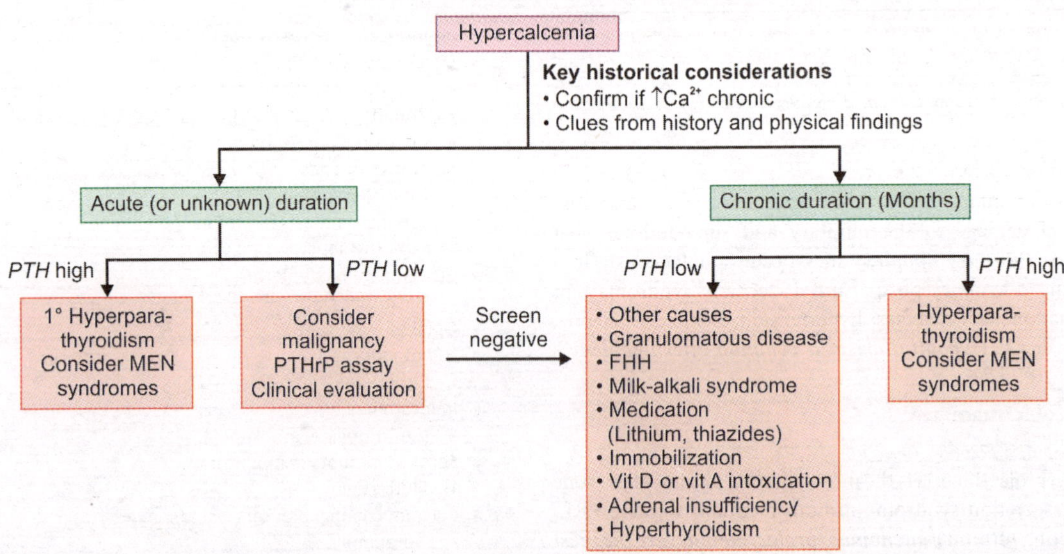

Fig: Algorithm for the evaluation of patients with hypercalcemia *(Harrison 19th/2479)*

Abbreviations: FHH, familial hypocalciuric hypercalcemia; MEN, multiple endocrine neoplasia; PTHrP, parathyroid hormone–related peptide

20. Ans. a. Decrease O_2 partial pressure in blood; c. Decreased alveolar ventilation

[Ref: Ganong 25th/647; Guyton (SEA) 13th/374; www.ncbi.nlm.nih.gov]
[Ref: Harrison 19th/2469-70; Ganong 25th/381-82; Davidson 23rd/662]

"By definition, hypoxemia is a condition of ***reduced arterial Po2***. Hypoxemia is a problem in normal individuals at high altitudes and is a complication of pneumonia and ***a variety of other diseases of the respiratory system***"- *Ganong 25th/647*

"**Hypoxia** is O_2 deficiency at the tissue level. It is a more correct term than **anoxia** (lack of O_2), since there is rarely no O_2 at all left in the tissues"-*Ganong 25th/646*

Hypoxemia and Hypoxia

◈ *www.ncbi.nlm.nih.gov*

- The term hypoxia and hypoxemia are not synonymous.
  - **Hypoxemia** is defined as a ***decrease in the partial pressure of oxygen in the blood*** whereas **hypoxia** is defined by ***reduced level of tissue oxygenation***. It can be due to ***either defective delivery or defective utilization of oxygen by the tissues.***
- Hypoxemia and hypoxia do not always coexist.
- Patients can develop hypoxemia without hypoxia if there is a compensatory increase in hemoglobin level and cardiac output (CO).
- Similarly, there can be hypoxia without hypoxemia.
- In cyanide poisoning, cells are unable to utilize oxygen despite having normal blood and tissue oxygen level.
- There are various mechanisms of hypoxemia. These are ***V/Q mismatch, right-to-left shunt, diffusion impairment, hypoventilation and low inspired PO_2***

Some of the Most Common Causes of Hypoxemia Include

◈ *my.clevelandclinic.org*

- Heart conditions, including heart defects
- Lung conditions such as asthma, emphysema and bronchitis
- Locations of high altitudes, where oxygen in the air is lower
- Strong pain medications or other problems that slow breathing
- Sleep apnea (impaired breathing during sleep)
- Inflammation or scarring of the lung tissue (as in pulmonary fibrosis)

What are the Symptoms of Hypoxemia

◈ *my.clevelandclinic.org*

- Headache
- Shortness of breath
- Fast heartbeat
- Coughing
- Wheezing
- Confusion
- Bluish color in skin, fingernails and lips

Table: Classification of hypoxia *(Guyton (SEA) 13th/374)*

- Hypoxic hypoxia:
  - Low atmospheric and alveolar oxygen content
  - Impairment of diffusion across the respiratory membrane
  - Venous-to-arterial shunts
  - Ventilation–perfusion mismatches
- Anemic hypoxia:
  - Anemia or abnormal hemoglobin
  - Poisoning by carbon monoxide
- Stagnant hypoxia:
  - General circulatory deficiency
  - Localized circulatory deficiency (peripheral, cerebral and coronary vessels)
- Histotoxic hypoxia:
  - Poisoning of cellular oxidation enzymes
  - Diminished cellular metabolic capacity for using oxygen because of toxicity, vitamin deficiency, or other factors

21. Ans. b. Thick ascending limb actively absorb Cl^- ion; c. Descending limb receive hypotonic fluid from PCT; d. Descending limb permeable to water

[Ref: Ganong 25th/683-84; Guyton (SEA) 13th/510-12; A K Jain 6th/521]

- Thin ascending limb actively passively sodium ion and thin ascending limb is impermeable to water

Tubular fluid remains isotonic in the proximal tubule (so fluid reaching **descending limb is also isotonic)** - *Guyton 13th (SAE) /509*

Loop of Henle

◈ *A K Jain 6th/521*

- **Thin descending segment**: ***highly permeable to water*** but relatively impermeable to solids (Specially NaCl)
- **Thin ascending segment**: impermeable to water but permeable to NaCl and urea; causes ***passive*** reabsorption of NaCl
- **Thick ascending segment**: impermeable to water and solute but ***actively reabsorbs NaCl*** by Na^+ –K^+ pump and Na^+ –$2Cl^-$ – and K^+ are reabsorbed (mostly in the thick ascending limb)

Loop of Henle

◈ *Ganong 25th/683-84*

- The **descending limb of the loop** of Henle is permeable to water, due to the presence of **aquaporin-1** in both the apical and basolateral membranes, but the ***ascending limb is impermeable to water***. Na^+, K^+ and Cl^- are cotransported out of the thick segment of the ascending limb.
- "The fluid in the ***descending limb of the loop of Henle becomes hypertonic*** as water moves out of the tubule into the hypertonic interstitium. ***In the ascending limb it becomes more dilute*** because of the movement of Na^+ and Cl^- out of the tubular lumen and ***when fluid reaches the top of the ascending limb (called the diluting segment) it is now hypotonic to plasma.***
- In the **thick ascending limb**, a carrier cotransports one Na^+, one K^+ and $2Cl^-$ from the tubular lumen into the tubular cells. This is another example of secondary active transport; the ***Na^+ is actively transported from the cells into the interstitium*** by Na, K ATPase in the basolateral membranes of the cells, keeping the intracellular Na^+ low

Table: Summary of tubule characteristics-urine concentration (Guyton 13th (SAE) /511)

		Permeability		
	Active NaCl Transport	**H_2O**	**NaCl**	**Urea**
Proximal tubule	++	++	+	+
Thin descending limb	0	++	+	+
Thin ascending limb	0	0	+	+
Thick ascending limb	++	0	0	0
Distal tubule	+	+ADH	0	0
Cortical collecting tubule	+	+ADH	0	0
Inner medullary collecting duct	+	+ADH	0	++ADH

0, minimal level of active transport or permeability; +, moderate level of active transport or permeability; ++, high level of active transport or permeability; +ADH, permeability to water or urea is increased by ADH

22. Ans. b. Composed of splenic cords and sinusoids; d. Perisinusoidal macrophages are present; e. Removes senescent erythrocytes from circulation

[Ref: BDC 7th/ Vol. II 325; Guyton 13th (SAE)/252; A.K.Jain 6th/116; Gray's 40th/1193; Harshmohan 7th/366-67; Schwartz 10th/1425–26]

- B and T cells (option a and c) are component of white pulp

"**White pulp**: *It consists of* ***lymphatic nodules arranged around an arteriole called malpighian corpuscle***"- *BDC 7th/ Vol. II 325*

Red pulp: *Formed by collection of cells in the interstices of reticulum, in b/w the* ***sinusoids****. It consists of* ***fixed and free macrophages***"*-BDC 7th/ Vol. II 325*

Spleen

◈ *Schwartz 10th/1425-26*

- The **red pulp** is comprised of large numbers of **venous sinuses (Sinusoids),** which ultimately drain into tributaries of the splenic vein. The sinuses are surrounded and separated by a fibrocellular network, called the reticulum, consisting of collagen fibers and fibroblasts. Within this network or mesh lie ***splenic macrophages***. These intersinusoidal regions appear as ***splenic cords***. The red pulp serves as a dynamic filtration system, enabling ***macrophages to remove microorganisms, cellular debris, antigen/antibody complexes and senescent erythrocytes from circulation.***
- **White pulp**: Around the terminal millimeters of splenic arterioles, a ***periarticular lymphatic sheath*** replaces the native adventitia of the vessel. The sheath is ***comprised of T lymphocytes and intermittent aggregations of B lymphocytes or lymphoid follicles***. When antigenically stimulated, the follicles, which are centers of lymphocyte proliferation, develop germinal centers.

- At the junction between the white and red pulp is the **marginal zone**, where lymphocytes are more loosely aggregated. Blood is delivered from this zone to the red pulp, where lymphocytes and locally produced immunoglobulins ultimately enter the systemic circulation.

Microstructure of Spleen

◈ *Gray's 40th/1193*

- The spleen is essentially concerned with phagocytosis and immune responses. In the fetus it is also an important site of haemopoiesis. Postnatally it may become haemopoietic in certain pathological conditions.
- Although important to the **defence of the body** it is not absolutely essential: if the spleen is removed, many of its functions can be assumed by the liver and by other lymphoid tissues.
- Microscopically, the parenchymal tissue of the spleen consists of **two major components**, ***white pulp and red pulp,*** named on the basis of their appearance when a fresh spleen is transected
- The ***white pulp is composed of lymphoid tissue in which B and T lymphocytes mature*** and proliferate under antigenic stimulation
- The **red pulp** is a unique filtration device that enables the spleen to clear particulate material from the blood as it perfuses the spleen. It is composed of a complex system of interconnected spaces populated by large ***numbers of phagocytic macrophages*** that ***remove effete red blood cells,*** microorganisms, cellular debris and other particulate matter from the circulation.

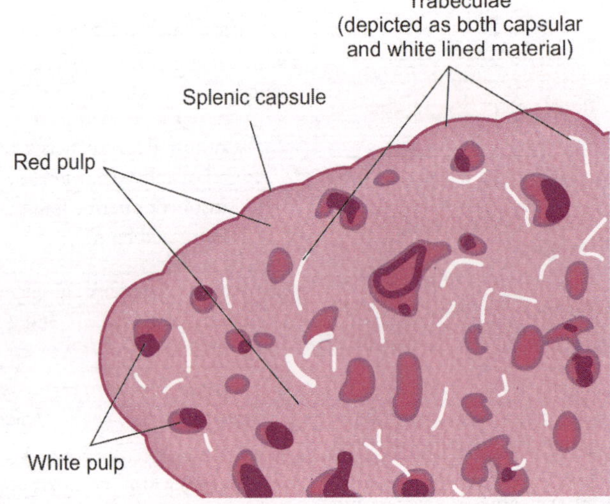

Fig: Splenic architecture *(Schwartz 10th/1426)*

23. Ans. **a. Beta-1 stimulation increases intracellular calcium concentration; c. Sarcoplasmic reticulum regulates the release and reuptake of calcium inside the cell; d. Titin protein connects the Z lines to the M lines; e. Calcium attachment to troponin C causes initiation of contraction of muscle**

[Ref: Ganong 25th/99-105; Guyton (SEA) 13th/87-93; A K Jain 6th/160-65; KDT 7th/133;Katzung 13th/135-36]

"Effector Pathway of β Receptor Activation: *cAMP↑, Ca^{2+} channel↑*"

◈ *KDT 8th/139*

Skeletal Muscle and Cardiac Muscle

◈ *Ganong 25th/101; A K Jain 6th/163*

- ***Light and electron microscopic feature of skeletal and cardiac muscles are same***- *A K Jain 6th/175*
- Each of the three troponin subunits has a unique function: Troponin T binds the troponin components to tropomyosin, troponin I inhibits the interaction of myosin with actin and ***troponin C contains the binding sites for the Ca2+ that helps initiate contraction***- *Ganong 25th/101*
- Some additional structural proteins that are important in skeletal muscle function include **actinin, titin** and **desmin.**
- Actinin binds actin to the Z lines.
- ***Titin, the largest known protein (with a molecular mass near 3,000,000 Da), connects the Z lines to the M lines and provides scaffolding for the sarcomere.***
- Desmin adds structure to the Z lines in part by binding the Z lines to the plasma membrane
- The **sarcoplasmic reticulum of cardiac muscle** is found to be much less extensive and less precisely arranged in relation to the cross-banded pattern of the myofibrils, than it is in skeletal - www.ahajournals.org

"Sarcoplasmic reticulum has a special organization that is extremely important in ***regulating calcium storage, release*** and reuptake and therefore muscle contraction"- *Guyton (SEA) 13th/93*

Beta Receptors

◈ *Katzung 13th/135-36*

- Activation of all three receptor subtypes (`1, `2 and `3) results in stimulation of ***adenylyl cyclase and increased conversion of adenosine triphosphate (ATP) to cAMP***
- Activation of the cyclase enzyme is mediated by the stimulatory coupling protein Gs. **Cyclic AMP** is the major second messenger of `-receptor activation. In the heart, `-receptor-activated cAMP synthesis ***increases the influx of calcium across the cell membrane and its sequestration inside the cell.***
- Beta adrenoceptors may activate voltage-sensitive calcium channels in the heart via Gs-mediated enhancement independently of changes in cAMP concentration. Under certain circumstances, `2 receptors may couple to Gq proteins. These receptors have been demonstrated to activate additional kinases, such as MAP kinases, by forming multi-subunit complexes within cells, which contain multiple signaling molecules

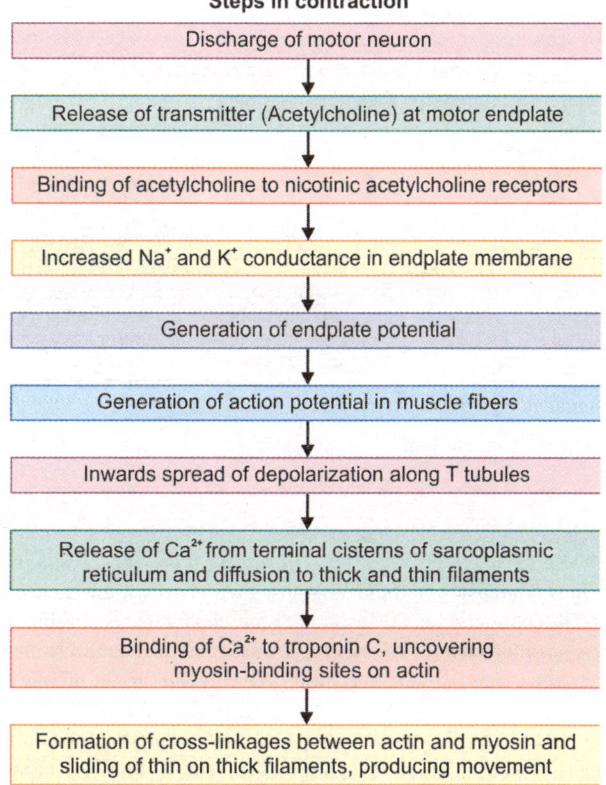

Fig: Steps in contraction *(Ganong 25th/105)*

24. Ans. **a. Alveolar pressure minus intrapleural pressure; c. Under physiological conditions the transpulmonary pressure is always positive; d. Lungs collapses if transpulmonary pressure become zero**

[Ref: Ganong 25th/628; Morgan Anesthesia 5th/494; Guyton (SEA) 13th/336; www.atsjournals.org; www.sciencedirect.com]

Transpulmonary Pressure

◈ *Guyton (SEA) 13th/336*

The ***difference between the alveolar pressure and the pleural pressure*** is called the *transpulmonary pressure.*

- It is the pressure difference between that in the alveoli and that on the outer surfaces of the lungs and it is a ***measure of the elastic forces in the lungs that tend to collapse the lungs*** at each instant of respiration, called the recoil pressure

Transpulmonary Pressure

◈ *www.atsjournals.org;www.sciencedirect.com*

- **Transpulmonary pressure** is the difference between the alveolar pressure and the intrapleural pressure in the pleural cavity. During human ventilation, air flows because of pressure gradients.
- $P_{tp} = P_{alv} - P_{ip}$. Where P_{tp} is transpulmonary pressure, P_{alv} is alveolar pressure and P_{ip} is intrapleural pressure.
- Since atmospheric pressure is relatively constant, pressure in the lungs must be higher or lower than atmospheric pressure for air to flow between the atmosphere and the alveoli.
- If **'transpulmonary pressure' = 0** (alveolar pressure = intrapleural pressure), such as when the lungs are removed from the chest cavity or air enters the intrapleural space (a pneumothorax), ***the lungs collapse as a result of their inherent elastic recoil.***

- ***Under physiological conditions the transpulmonary pressure is always positive; intrapleural pressure is always negative and relatively large***, while ***alveolar pressure moves from slightly negative to slightly positive as a person breathes.***
- For a given lung volume the transpulmonary pressure is equal and opposite to the elastic recoil pressure of the lung.
- Transpulmonary pressure can be measured by placing pressure transducers. The alveolar pressure is estimated by measuring the pressure in the airways while holding one's breath. The intrapleural pressure is estimated by measuring the pressure inside a balloon placed in the esophagus
- Measurement of transpulmonary pressure assists in spirometry in availing for calculation of static lung compliance.

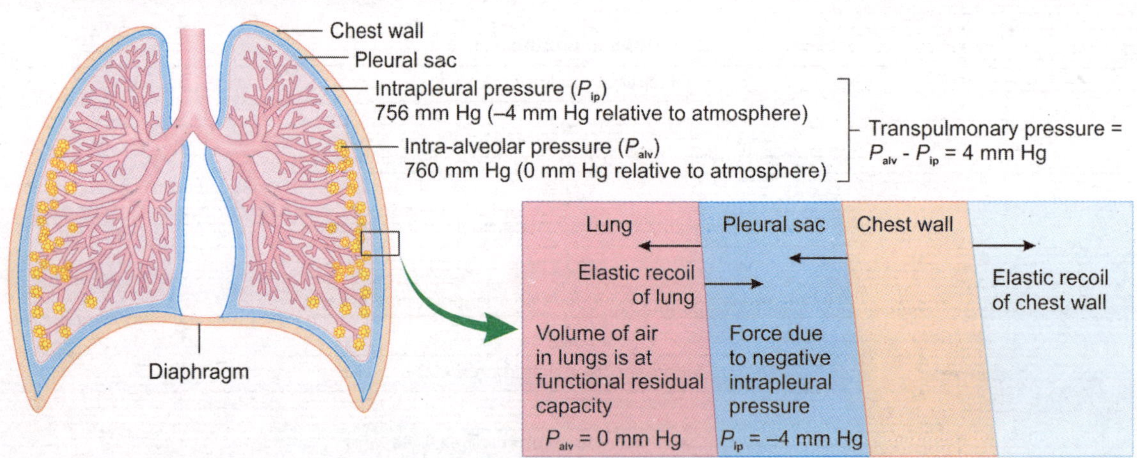

Figs A and B: Transpulmonary pressure

Inspiration and Expiration

◈ *Ganong 25th/628*

- The pressure in the "space" between the lungs and chest wall ***(intrapleural pressure) is subatmospheric***
- ***If the chest wall is opened, the lungs collapse;*** and if the lungs lose their elasticity, the chest expands and becomes barrel-shaped.
- Inspiration is an active process. The contraction of the inspiratory muscles increases intrathoracic volume. The **intrapleural pressure** at the base of the lungs, which is ***normally about –2.5 mm Hg*** (relative to atmospheric) at the start of inspiration, ***decreases to about –6 mm Hg***. The lungs are pulled into a more expanded position. The pressure in the airway becomes slightly negative and air flows into the lungs.
- At the end of inspiration, the lung recoil begins to pull the chest back to the expiratory position, where the recoil pressures of the lungs and chest wall balance pressure in the airway becomes slightly positive and air flows out of the lungs.
- ***Strong inspiratory efforts reduce intrapleural pressure to values as low as –30 mm Hg***, producing correspondingly greater degrees of lung inflation.

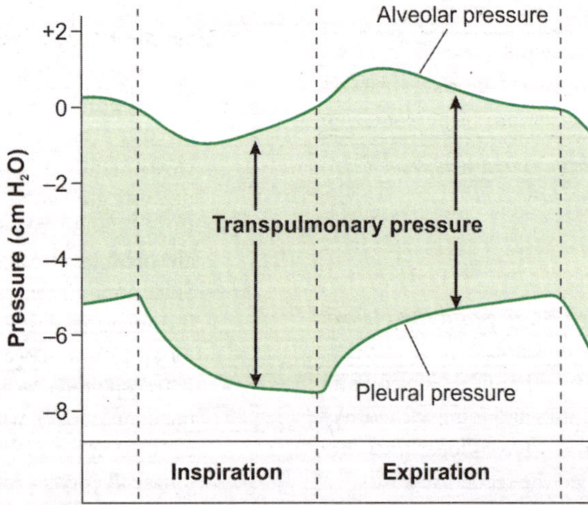

Fig: Changes in alveolar pressure, pleural pressure and transpulmonary pressure during normal breathing *(Guyton (SEA) 13th/335)*

BIOCHEMISTRY

25. Ans. b. Krabbe's disease, e. Morquio syndrome

[Ref: Harper 30th/ 251; Harrison 19th/432e-2; Satyanarayan 4th/ 309]

"Mucopolysaccharidosis IV B (Morquio): *β-Galactosidase Deficiency*"

◈ *Harrison 19th/432e-2*

"**Beta-galactosidase** is a lysosomal enzyme responsible for catalyzing the hydrolysis of gangliosides. The deficiency of this enzyme can lead to one of the following conditions: ***GM1 gangliosidosis, Morquio syndrome B and galactosialidosis***" -*www.mayomedicallaboratories.com*

Table: Examples of Sphingolipidoses *(Harper 30th/ 251; Satyanarayan 4th/ 309)*

Disease	Enzyme deficiency	Clinical symptoms
Tay-Sachs disease	Hexosaminidase A	Mental retardation, blindness, muscular weakness
Fabry's disease	α-Galactosidase	Skin rash, kidney failure (full symptoms only in males; X-linked recessive)
Metachromatic leukodystrophy	Arylsulfatase A	Mental retardation and psychologic disturbances in adults; demyelination
Krabbe' disease	***β-Galactosidase***	Ental retardation; myelin almost absent
Gaucher's disease	β-Glucosidase	Enlarged liver and spleen, erosion of long bones, mental retardation in infants
Niemann-Pick disease	Sphingomyelinase	Enlarged liver and spleen, mental retardation; fatal in early life
Farber's disease	Ceramidase	Hoarseness, dermatitis, skeletal deformation, mental retardation; fatal in early life

26. Ans. a. Peripheral neuropathy, b. Posterior column involvement, c. Alopecia, d. Hemolysis

[Ref: Harper 30th/553; Harrison 19th/96e-8; O.P.Ghai 8th/116; Davidson 23rd/713]

Vitamin E Deficiency

◈ *Harper 30th/553*

- In experimental animals, vitamin E. deficiency results in resorption of fetuses and testicular atrophy.
- The erythrocyte membranes are abnormally fragile as a result of lipid peroxidation, leading to ***hemolytic anemia***
- It is involved in the anti-inflammatory and immune systems- Davidson 23rd/713
- "***Vit. E also boosts immune response***- Vasudevan 5th/291

Vitamin E deficiency

◈ **Harrison** *19th/96e-8*

- Dietary deficiency of vitamin E does not exist. Vitamin E deficiency is seen only in severe and prolonged malabsorptive diseases, such as celiac disease, or after small-intestinal resection or bariatric surgery.
- Children with cystic fibrosis or prolonged cholestasis may develop vitamin E deficiency characterized by ***areflexia and hemolytic anemia***. Children with abetalipoproteinemia cannot absorb or transport vitamin E and become deficient quite rapidly.
- Vitamin E deficiency causes axonal degeneration of the large myelinated axons and ***results in posterior column and spinocerebellar symptoms***.
- ***Peripheral neuropathy*** is initially characterized by areflexia, with progression to an ataxic gait and by decreased vibration and position sensations.
- Ophthalmoplegia, skeletal myopathy and pigmented retinopathy may also be features of vitamin E deficiency.
- A deficiency of either vitamin E or selenium in the host has been shown to increase certain viral mutations and, therefore, virulence. The laboratory diagnosis of vitamin E deficiency is based on low blood levels of α-tocopherol

Table: Principal clinical findings of vitamin malnutrition *(Harrison 19th/96e-1)*

Nutrient	Clinical finding
Vitamin E	Peripheral neuropathy, spinocerebellar ataxia, skeletal muscle atrophy, retinopathy

27. Ans. b. Diarrhoea, d. Delayed wound healing

[Ref: Harper 30th/ 562; O.P.Ghai 8th/120; Harrison 19th/96e-1-5,1867]

"**Vitamin C supplements** are associated with an ***increased risk of calcium oxalate stone formation,*** possibly because of raised levels of oxalate in urine. Thus, ***calcium oxalate stone formers should be advised to avoid vitamin C supplements***. Although high doses of supplemental vitamin B_6 may be beneficial in selected patients with type 1 primary hyperoxaluria, the benefit of supplemental vitamin B_6 in other patients is uncertain"- Harrison 19th/1867

Vitamin C Deficiency

◈ *O.P.Ghai 8th/120*

- Prolonged vitamin C deficiency results in scurvy.
- It usually occurs in those who are deprived of citrus fruits, fresh vegetables or vitamins for some cultural or geographic reasons.
- In infancy, features of scurvy are ***anorexia, diarrhea, pallor, irritability and increased susceptibility to infections.***
- Subperiosteal hemorrhages and long bone tenderness (Pseudoparalysis of lower extremities) can occur; radiologic abnormalities are frequent.
- In older children, hemorrhagic signs predominate, with bleeding from gums, conjunctiva and intestinal tract.

Vitamin C deficiency causes scurvy: Signs of vitamin C deficiency include skin changes, fragility of blood capillaries, gum decay, tooth loss and bone fracture, many of which can be attributed to deficient collagen synthesis- *Harper 30th/ 562*

Vitamin C Deficiency

◈ *Harrison 19th/96e-5*

- Vitamin C deficiency causes scurvy.
- In addition to generalized fatigue, symptoms of scurvy primarily reflect impaired formation of mature connective tissue and include bleeding into the skin (***petechiae, ecchymoses, perifollicular hemorrhages***); inflamed and bleeding gums; and manifestations of bleeding into joints, the peritoneal cavity, the pericardium and the adrenal glands.
- In children, vitamin C deficiency may cause impaired bone growth.

Table: Principal clinical findings of vitamin malnutrition *(Harrison 19th/96e-1)*

Vitamin C deficiency	Scurvy: ***Petechiae, ecchymosis, coiled hairs, inflamed and bleeding gums, joint effusion, poor wound healing, fatigue***

28. Ans. a. Vitamin A, b. Vit E, c. Vit C, d. Glutathione reductase, e. Zinc

[Ref: Harper 30th/543,550; Lippincot 6th/148; Vasudevan 5th/ 357; Satyanarayan 4th/658-59]

"**Antioxidant nutrients- *zinc,*** copper, carotene and ***vitamins A (beta-carotenes) C and E***"- *Harper 30th/550*

Antioxidants

◈ *Vasudevan 5th/ 357*

- **Vitamin E** is the lipid phase antioxidant
- **Vitamin C** is the aqueous phase antioxidant
- Ceruloplasmin can act as an antioxidant in extracellular fluid
- Caffeine is another effective anti-oxidant
- Cysteine, ***glutathione*** and **vitamin A** are minor Antioxidants. **Beta carotene** can act as a chain breaking antioxidant, but is less effective than alpha tocopherol

Antioxidants used as Therapeutic Agents

◈ *Vasudevan 5th/ 357*

- **Vitamin E**
- **Vitamin C**
- Dimethyl thio urea
- Dimethyl sulfoxide
- Allopurinol

Commercial use of Antioxidants

◈ *Vasudevan 5th/ 357*

"Antioxidants are regularly used in food industry to increase the shelf-life of products. Commercially used food preservatives are Vitamin E, propyl gallate, butylted hydroxyl anisole (BHA) and butylated hydroxyl toluene (BHT). They prevent oxidative damage of oils, particularly those containing PUFA and prevent rancidity"

Antioxidants *in Biological System*

◈ *Satyanarayan 4th/658-59*

- Antioxidants in relation to lipid peroxidation
  - Preventive antioxidants that will block the initial production of free radicals e.g. catalase, ***glutathione peroxidase***
  - Chain breaking antioxidants that inhibit the propagative phase of lipid peroxidation e.g. superoxide dismutase, vitamin E, uric acid.
- Antioxidants according to their location
  - **Plasma antioxidants** e.g. β-carotene, ascorbic acid, bilirubin, uric acid, ceruloplasmin, transferrin
  - **Cell membrane antioxidants** e.g. α-tocopherol
  - **Intracellular antioxidants** e.g. superoxide dismutase, catalase, glutathione peroxidase
- Antioxidants according to their nature and action
  - **Enzymatic antioxidants** e.g. superoxide dismutase, catalase, glutathione peroxidase, ***glutathione reductase***
  - **Non-enzymatic antioxidants**
    - **Nutrient antioxidants** e.g. carotenoids (β-carotene), α-tocopherol, ascorbic acid, selenium
    - **Metabolic antioxidants** e.g. glutathione, ceruloplasmin, albumin, bilirubin, transferrin, ferritin, uric acid

29. Ans. a. Deamination, b. Transamination, d. Decarboxylation, e. Tryptophan metabolism

[Ref: Harper 30th/550; Shinde 7th/173-74; Lippincot 6th/378]

Pyridoxal Phosphate Role (as a Coenzyme)

◈ *Shinde 7th/173-74*

- *In **tryptophan metabolism**, pyridoxal-P acts as a coenzyme for the enzyme kynureninase. In Vit B6 deficiency, niacin synthesis from tryptophan does not take place*
- ***Intramitochondrial fatty acid synthesis:*** *Coenzyme for condensing enzyme*
- Co-enzyme for biosynthesis of arachidonic acid from linoleic acid

"**B6 (Pyridoxine, pyridoxal, pyridoxamine):** Coenzyme in ***transamination and decarboxylation of amino acids*** and glycogen phosphorylase; modulation of steroid hormone action"- *Harper 30th/550 (Table)*

Pyridoxine (Vitamin B6)

◈ *Lippincot 6th/378*

- Vitamin B6 is a collective term for ***pyridoxine, pyridoxal and pyridoxamine***, all derivatives of pyridine.
- They differ only in the nature of the functional group attached to the ring. Pyridoxine occurs primarily in plants, whereas pyridoxal and pyridoxamine are found in foods obtained from animals.
- All three compounds can serve as precursors of the biologically active coenzyme, pyridoxal phosphate. Pyridoxal phosphate functions as a coenzyme for a large number of enzymes, particularly those that catalyze reactions ***involving amino acids.***

Table: **Pyridoxal phosphate as a coenzyme**

Reaction type	Example
Transamination	Oxaloacetate + glutamate → aspartate + α-ketoglutarate
Deamination	Serine → pyruvate + NH_3
Decarboxylation	Histidine → histamine + CO_2
Condensation	Glycine + succinyl CoA → d-aminolevulinic acid

30. Ans. a. Mental retardation may be present, c. Autosomal recessive inheritance, d. Deficiency of the hepatic enzyme phenylalanine hydroxylase, e. Light coloured skin

[Ref: Harper 30th/304; Harrison 19th/434e-1; Lippincot 6th/270-71; Satyanarayan 4th/351]

- ***Musty odour due to phenylacetate accumulation***

Hyperphenylalaninemias

◈ *Harrison 19th/434e-1*

- The hyperphenylalaninemias result from impaired conversion of phenylalanine to tyrosine.
- The most common and clinically important is *phenylketonuria* (frequency 1:10,000), which is an ***autosomal recessive disorder*** characterized by an increased concentration of phenylalanine and its by-products in body fluids and by ***severe mental retardation*** if untreated in infancy. It results from reduced activity of ***phenylalanine hydroxylase***.
- Phenylalanine is a competitive inhibitor of tyrosinase, a key enzyme in the pathway of melanin synthesis and accounts for the ***hypopigmentation of hair and skin***.
- Untreated children with classic phenylketonuria are normal at birth but fail to attain early developmental milestones, develop microcephaly and demonstrate progressive impairment of cerebral function.
- ***Hyperactivity, seizures and severe intellectual disability are major clinical problems later in life. Electroencephalographic abnormalities; "mousy" odor of skin, hair and urine (due to phenylacetate accumulation); and a tendency to develop hypopigmentation and eczema*** complete the devastating clinical picture.

"Phenylketonuria (PKU), caused by a deficiency of the hepatic enzyme ***phenylalanine hydroxylase***, is the most common clinically encountered inborn error of amino acid metabolism"- *Lippincot 6th/270; Satyanarayan 4th/351*

Characteristics of Classic PKU

◈ *Lippincot 6th/271*

- **Elevated phenylalanine:** Phenylalanine is present in elevated concentrations in tissues, plasma and urine. ***Phenyllactate, phenylacetate and phenylpyruvate***, which are not normally produced in significant amounts in the presence of functional phenylalanine hydroxylase, are also elevated in PKU. These metabolites give urine a characteristic ***musty ("mousey") odor***. [Note: The disease acquired its name from the ***presence of a phenylketone (now known to be phenylpyruvate) in the urine***.]
- **CNS symptoms: *Mental retardation***, failure to walk or talk, seizures, hyperactivity, tremor, microcephaly and failure to grow are characteristic findings in PKU. The patient with untreated PKU typically shows symptoms of mental retardation by the age of 1 year and rarely achieves an IQ greater than 50. [Note: These clinical manifestations are now rarely seen as a result of neonatal screening programs.]
- **Hypopigmentation:** Patients with phenylketonuria often show a ***deficiency of pigmentation*** (fair hair, light skin color and blue eyes). The hydroxylation of tyrosine by tyrosinase, which is the first step in the formation of the pigment melanin, is competitively inhibited by the high levels of phenylalanine present in PKU

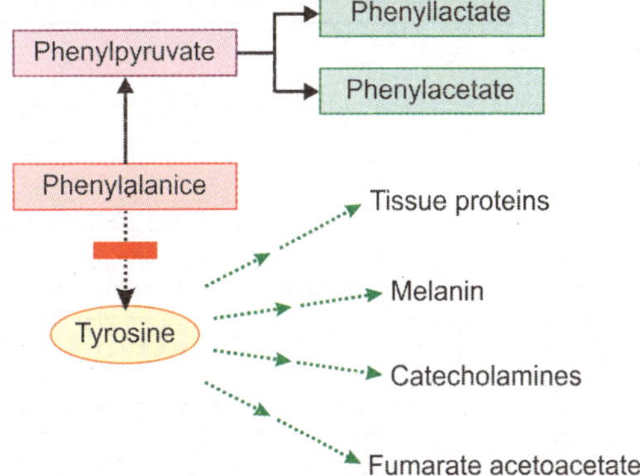

Fig: Pathways of phenylalanine metabolism in normal individuals and in patients with phenylketonuria *(Lippincott)*

31. Ans. b. Glycerol, c. Pyruvate, e. Alanine

[Ref: Harper 30th/185; Lippincot 6th/117-18; Vasudevan 5th/96; Satyanarayan 4th/258-59]

*"Propionyl CoA is formed from odd chain fatty acids and carbon skeleton of some amino acids. It is converted to succinyl CoA. It is a **minor source for glucose. Even chain fatty acids cannot be converted to glucose; they are not substrate for gluconeogenesis**"- Vasudevan 5th/96*

Substrate for Gluconeogenesis

◈ *Lippincot 6th/117; Shinde 7th/342*

- Lactate
- Pyruvate
- Glycerol
- Alpha-keto acids
- Propionic acid (important in ruminants) andpropionyl-CoA (Human beings)

Glycogenic and Ketogenic Amino Acids

◈ *Satyanarayan 4th/48-49*

- **Glycogenic amino acid:** These amino acids can serve as precursors for the formation of glucose or glycogen, e.g. ***alanine, aspartate, glycine, methionine*** etc
- **Ketogenic amino acids:** Fat can be synthesized from these amino acids. Two amino acids ***leucine and lysine*** are exclusively ketogenic

- **Glycogenic and ketogenic amino acids:** The four amino acids isoleucine, phenylalanine, tryptophan, tyrosine are precursors for synthesis of glucose as well as fat.

Gluconeogenesis

◈ *Harper 30th/185 Satyanarayan 4th/258-59*

- Gluconeogenesis is the process of synthesizing glucose or glycogen from noncarbohydrate precursors. The major substrates are the ***glucogenic amino acids, lactate, glycerol and propionate***.
- Liver and kidney are the major gluconeogenic tissues; the kidney may contribute up to 40% of total glucose synthesis in the fasting state and more in starvation.

32. Ans. b. 2, 4-Dinitrophenol, c. Thyroxine, d. Thermogenin

[Ref: Harper 30th/132-33; Lippincott 6th/79; Satyanarayan 4th/233-34; Chatterjea 7th/132-34]

Uncouplers

◈ *Satyanarayan 4th/233-34*

- The uncouplers allow oxidation of substrates without ATP formation
- *Uncouplers are:* **2,4-dinitrophenol (DNP),** *Dinitrocresol, Trifluoro carbonyl cyanide phenylhydrazone, Pentachlorophenol, Aspirin (in high dose)*
- *Physiological uncouplers: High concentration of* ***thermogenin, thyroxine****, long chain free fatty acids*
- Antibiotics- valinomycin, gramicidin A and nigercin

Many Poisons Inhibit the Respiratory Chain

◈ *Harper 30th/132*

- They may be classified as inhibitors of the ***respiratory chain, inhibitors of oxidative phosphorylation and uncouplers of oxidative phosphorylation.***
- **Barbiturates such as amobarbital** inhibit electron transport via Complex I by blocking the transfer from Fe-S to Q. At sufficient dosage, they are fatal in vivo.
- ***Antimycin A and dimercaprol*** inhibit the respiratory chain at Complex III.
- The classic poisons ***H_2S, carbon monoxide and cyanide*** inhibit Complex IV and can therefore totally arrest respiration.
- **Malonate** is a competitive inhibitor of Complex II.
- **Atractyloside** inhibits ***oxidative phosphorylation***
- The antibiotic **oligomycin** completely blocks oxidation and phosphorylation
- The uncoupler that has been used most frequently is **2, 4-dinitrophenol**, but other compounds act in a similar manner. **Thermogenin** (or the uncoupling protein) is a physiological uncoupler found in brown adipose tissue

Table: Inhibitors of ETC *(Chatterjea 7th/134)*

Site—I (Complex-I):
- **Rotenone:** A fish poison and also insecticide. Inhibits transfer of electrons through complex-I- NADH-Q- reductase.
- **Amobarbital (Amytal) and Secobarbital:** Inhibits electron transfer through NADH-Q reductase
- **Piericidin A:** An antibiotic. Blocks electron transfer by competing with CoQ.
- **Drugs:** Chlorpromazine and hypotensive drug like guanethidine

Site-II (Complex III): Blocks electron transfer from cyt b to C_1
- Antimycin A
- BAL (Dimer-Coprol)
- Hypoglycaemic drugs: like phenformin

Site-III (Complex IV): Inhibits terminal transfer of electrons molecular O_2
- Cyanide
- H_2S to
- Azide
- **CO (Carbon monoxide):** Inhibits cyt. Onydase by combining with O_2 binding site. It can be reversed by illumination with light

Complex II: Succinate dehydrogenase FAD: Specifically inhibit transfer of reducing equivalent from succinate dehydrogenase
- Carboxin
- TTFA
- **Malonate:** A competitive inhibitor of succinate dehydrogenase

33. Ans. a. Biotin, c. NADPH, d. ATP

[Ref: Harper 30th/232-33; Lippincot 6th/183; Vasudevan 5th/138-40; Satyanarayan 4th/297-98; Shinde 7th/174]

- Pyridoxine is used for chain elongation of fatty acid (not in de novo fatty acid synthesis)

The Main Pathway for de Novo Synthesis of Fatty Acids (Lipogenesis) Occurs in the Cytosol

◈ *Harper 30th/232-33; Satyanarayan 4th/297-98*

- This system is present in many tissues, including liver, kidney, brain, lung, mammary gland and adipose tissue.
- Its cofactor requirements include ***NADPH, ATP, Mn^{2+}, biotin and HCO_3^-*** (as a source of CO_2). **Acetyl-CoA** is the immediate substrate and **free palmitate** is the end product

"Intramitochondrial FA synthesis: Pyridoxal phosphate required as a coenzyme with condensing enzyme for chain elongation of F.A in intramitochondrial F.A. synthesis"-*Shinde 7th/174*

"Biosynthesis of F.A: ***Pantothenic acid*** is a constituent of a compound called as "Acyl-carrier protein" (ACP) and also a constituent of multienzyme complex" in mammals, which is used in the **extramitochondrial 'de Novo' fatty acid synthesis"**- *Shinde 7th/178*

34. Ans. c. **Calbindin**

[Ref: Harper 30th/608-09; Lippincot 6th/; Vasudevan 5th/434; Satyanarayan 4th/561]

"Synthesis of the intracellular calcium-binding protein, calbindin, required for calcium absorption, is induced by vitamin D"- *Harper 30th/541*

Chaperones are Proteins That Stabilize Unfolded or Partially Folded Proteins

◈ *Harper 30th/608-09*

- **Molecular chaperones** are proteins which **stabilize unfolded or partially folded intermediates,** allowing them time to fold properly and prevent inappropriate interactions, thus combating the formation of nonfunctional structures.
- Most chaperones exhibit **ATPase activity** and bind ADP and ATP.
- **Chaperonins** are the second major class of chaperones.
- The structure of the bacterial chaperonin **GroEL** has been studied in detail.
- The heat shock protein **Hsp60** is the equivalent of GroEL in eukaryotes.

"Two major chaperones groups: *1) Hsp 70 system:includes Hsp 70 and 40 and 2) Chaperonin system:* includes Hsp 60 and 10"- *Satyanarayan 4th/561*

Chaperones Faculty

◈ *washington.edu*

- General chaperones: ***GRP78/BiP (Immunoglobulin heavy chain binding protein)***, GRP94, GRP170.
- Lectin chaperones: ***calnexin and calreticulin***
- Non-classical molecular chaperones: HSP47 and ERp29
- Folding chaperones:Protein disulfide isomerase (PDI), *Peptidyl prolyl cis-trans-isomerase* (PPI) and ERp57

Tab *(Harper 30th/609)*: Some Properties of Chaperone Proteins

- Present in a wide range of species from bacteria to humans
- Many are so-called heat shock proteins (Hsp)
- Some are inducible by conditions that cause unfolding of newly synthesized proteins (eg, elevated temperature and various chemicals)
- They bind to predominantly hydrophobic regions of unfolded proteins and prevent their aggregation
- They act in part as a quality control or editing mechanism for detecting misfolded or otherwise defective proteins
- Most chaperones show associated ATPase activity, with ATP or ADP being involved in the protein-chaperone interaction
- Found in various cellular compartments such as cytosol, mitochondria and the lumen of the endoplasmic reticulum

35. Ans. a. **Ornithine transcarbamylase (OTC), b. Uridylic acid decarboxylase, c. Carbamoyl phosphate synthetase**

[Ref: Harper 30th/348-351, 356; Harrison 19th/431e-3]

- Ortidylic acid decarboxylase is enzyme of pyrimidine metabolism

"Urea cycle: Condensation of CO_2, ammonia and ATP to form **carbamoyl phosphate** is catalyzed by mitochondrial **carbamoyl phosphate synthase I. L-Ornithine transcarbamoylase** catalyzes transfer of the carbamoyl group of carbamoyl phosphate to ornithine, forming citrulline and orthophosphate"- *Harper 30th/293-94*

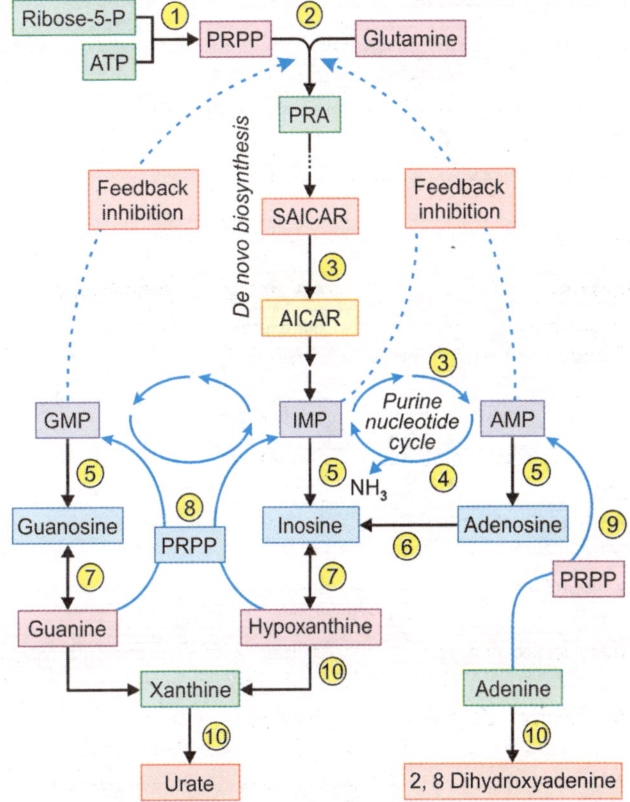

Fig: Abbreviated scheme of purine metabolism *(Harrison 19th/431e-3)*

Abbreviations: (1) Phosphoribosylpyrophosphate (PRPP) synthetase, (2) amidophosphoribosyltransferase (amidoPRT), (3) adenylosuccinate lyase, (4) (myo-) adenylate (AMP) deaminase, (5) 5′-nucleotidase, (6) adenosine deaminase, (7) purine nucleoside phosphorylase, (8) hypoxanthine phosphoribosyltransferase (HPRT), (9) adenine phosphoribosyltransferase (APRT) and (10) xanthine oxidase. PRA, phosphoribosylamine; SAICAR, succinylaminoimidazole carboxamide ribotide; AICAR, aminoimidazole carboxamide ribotide; GMP, guanylate; IMP, inosine monophosphate; ATP, adenosine triphosphate

Table: Metabolic disorders of purine and pyrimidine metabolism *(Harper 30th/356)*

Defective enzyme	Major signs and symptoms
Purine metabolism	
Hypoxanthine-guanine phosphoribosyltransferase	Lesch-Nyhan syndrome. Uncemia, self-mutilation
Prpp synthase	Gout gouty arthritis
Adenosine deaminase	Severely compromised immune system
Purine nucleoside phosphorylase	Autoimmune disorders; benign I and opportunistic infections
Pyrimidine metabolism	
Dihydropyrimidine dehydrogenase	Can develop toxicity to 5-fluorouracil, also a substrate for this dehydrogenase
Orotate phosphoribosyl transferase and oroticlytic acid decarboxyiase	Orotic acid aciduna type 1; megaloblastic anemia
Orotidylic acid decarboxylase	Orotic acid aciduna type 2

Table: Inborn error of purine metabolism *(Harrison 19th/431e-3)*

Enzyme	Activity	Inheritance	Clinical features	Laboratory features
Hypoxanthine phosphoribosyltransferase	Complete deficiency	X-linked	Self-mutilation, choreoathetosis, gout and uric acid lithiasis	Hyperuricemia, hyperuricosuria
	Partial deficiency	X-linked	Gout and uric acid lithiasis	Hyperuricemia, hyperuricosuria
Phosphoribosyl pyrophosphate synthetase	Overactivity	X-linked	Gout, uric acid lithiasis and deafness	Hyperuricemia, hyperuricosuria
Adenine phosphoribosyl transferase	Deficiency	Autosomal recessive	2, 8-Dihydroxyadenine lithiasis	—
Xanthine oxidase	Deficiency	Autosomal recessive	Xanthinuria and xanthine lithiasis	Hypouricemia, hypouricosuria
Adenylosuccinate lyase	Deficiency	Autosomal recessive	Autism and psychomotor retardation	—
Myoadenylate deaminase	Deficiency	Autosomal recessive	Myopathy with exercise intolerance or asymptomatic	—
Adenosine deaminase	Deficiency	Autosomal recessive	Severe combined immunodeficiency disease and chondro-osseous dysplasia	—
Purine nucleoside phosphorylase	Deficiency	Autosomal recessive	T cell—mediated immunodeficiency	—

36. Ans. b. Pyridoxine

[Ref: Harper 30th/550; Shinde 7th/173-74; Lippincott 6th/378]

"**B6 (Pyridoxine, pyridoxal, pyridoxamine):** Coenzyme in transamination and decarboxylation of amino acids and glycogen phosphorylase; modulation of steroid hormone action"- *Harper 30th/550 (Table)*

37. Ans. a. Histidine

[Ref: Harper 30th/52; biology.kenyon.edu]

Hemoglobin Protein Structure

◈ *biology.kenyon.edu*

- The hemoglobin molecule is made up of four polypeptide chains: two alpha chains of 141 amino acid residues each and two beta chains of 146 amino acid residues each.
- The alpha and beta chains have different sequences of amino acids, but fold up to form similar three-dimensional structures. The four chains are held together by noncovalent interactions.
- There are four binding sites for oxygen on the hemoglobin molecule, because each chain contains one heme group.
- In the **alpha chain**, the 87th residue is ***histidine F8*** and in the **beta chain** the ***92nd residue is histidine F8***. A heme group is attached to each of the four histidines.
- Each polypeptide chain is made up of ***eight or nine alpha-helical segments*** and an equal number of nonhelical ones placed at the corners between them and at the ends of the chain. ***The helices are named A-H***, starting from the amino acid terminus and the nonhelical segments that lie between

the helices are named AB, BC, CD, etc. The nonhelical segments at the ends of the chain are called NA at the amino terminus and HC at the carboxyl terminus.

- There are nine positions in the amino acid sequence that contain the same amino acid in all or nearly all species studied thus far. These conserved positions are especially important for the function of the hemoglobin molecule. Several of them, such as ***histidines F8 (His87) and E7 (His63),*** are directly involved in the oxygen-binding site
- Phenylalanine CD1 (Phe43) and leucine F4 (Leu83) are also in direct contact with the heme group.
- Tyrosine HC2 (Tyr140) stabilizes the molecule by forming a hydrogen bond between the H and F helices.
- Glycine B6 (Gly25) is conserved because of its small size: a side chain larger than a hydrogen atom would not allow the B and E helices to approach each other as closely as they do.
- Proline C2 (Pro37) is important because it terminates the C helix.
- Threonine C4 (Thr39) and lysine H10 (Lys127) are also conserved residues, but their roles are uncertain.

Histidines F8 and E7 Perform Unique Roles in Oxygen Binding

◈ *Harper 30th/52*

- The heme of myoglobin lies in a crevice between helices E and F oriented with its polar propionate groups facing the surface of the globin. The remainder resides in the nonpolar interior.
- The fifth coordination position of the iron is occupied by a nitrogen from the imidazole ring of the histidine, His F8. The distal histidine, His E7, lies on the side of the heme ring opposite to His F8

IMMUNOGENETICS & MOLECULER BIOLOGY

38. Ans. e. 50000 bp

[Ref: www.khanacademy.org;www.yourgenome.org]

- ***In Gel electrophoresis: DNA fragments move towards the positive electrode as they are negatively charged. As larger fragments move slowly w.r.t smaller fragments, it is more towards the negative ends, so the answer is e (Largest fragment)***

Gel Electrophoresis

◈ *www.khanacademy.org*

- **Gel electrophoresis** is a technique used to separate DNA fragments (or other macromolecules, such as RNA and proteins) according to their size.
- DNA samples are loaded into wells (indentations) at one end of a gel and an electric current is applied to pull them through the gel.
- ***DNA fragments are negatively charged, so they move towards the positive electrode.*** Because all DNA fragments have the same amount of charge per mass, small fragments move through the gel faster than large ones.
- When a gel is stained with a DNA-binding dye, the DNA fragments can be seen as **bands**, each representing a group of same-sized DNA fragments

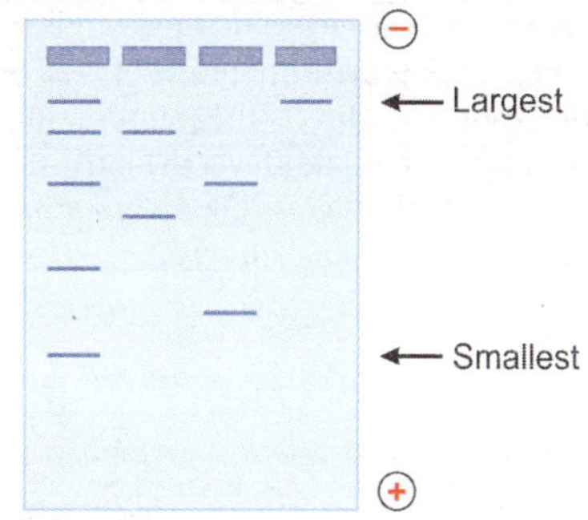

Fig: *www.khanacademy.org*

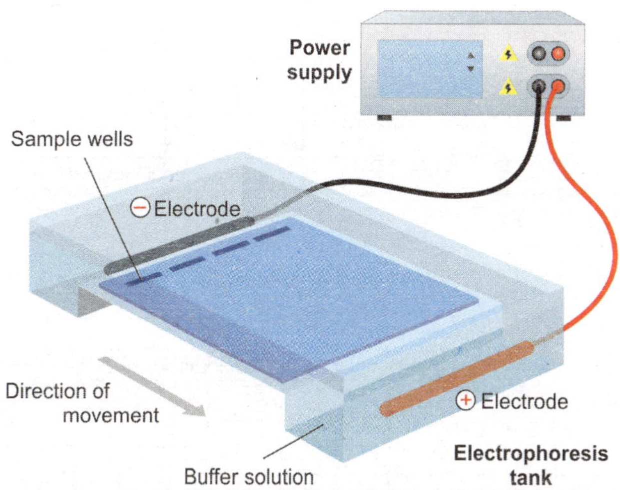

Fig: Electrophoresis setup *(www.yourgenome.org)*

39. Ans. c. Cell cycle will be arrested, e. Cells will not get mutated because other tumor suppressor genes can still control the cell cycle at different check points

[Ref: Robbins 9th/ 293-96; Harsh mohan 7th/206]

Tp53 (Guardian of the Genome)

◈ *Robbins 9th/293-95*

- ***TP53,*** a tumor suppressor gene that ***regulates cell cycle progression, DNA repair, cellular senescence and apoptosis,*** is the most frequently mutated gene in human cancers.
- **Loss-of-function mutations in *TP53*,** located on chromosome 17p13.1, are ***found in more than 50% of cancers.***
- Moreover, *TP53* mutations occur with some frequency in virtually every type of cancer, including carcinomas of the lung, colon and breast—the three leading causes of cancer death.
- **Once activated, p53 thwarts neoplastic transformation by inducing either transient cell cycle arrest, senescence (permanent cell cycle arrest), or programmed cell death (apoptosis).**

- The key target genes that execute the functions of p53 are not completely defined, but appear to fall into three major categories: (1) ***those that cause cell cycle arrest***; (2) ***those that cause apoptosis***; and (3) *those that enhance catabolic metabolism or inhibit anabolic metabolism.*
- The name is due to its molecular mass: it is in the 53 kilo dalton fraction of cell proteins
- **p53-induced apoptosis.** Apoptosis of cells with irreversible DNA damage is the ultimate protective mechanism against neoplastic transformation. p53 directs the transcription of several pro-apoptotic genes such as *BAX* and *PUMA*, which are believed to tip the balance in favor of cell death via the intrinsic (mitochondrial) pathway
- ***"P53 gene (TP53): Two major function of p53 in normal cell cycle are: (1) In blocking mitotic activity and (2) In promoting apoptosis"***- *Harsh mohan 7th/206*

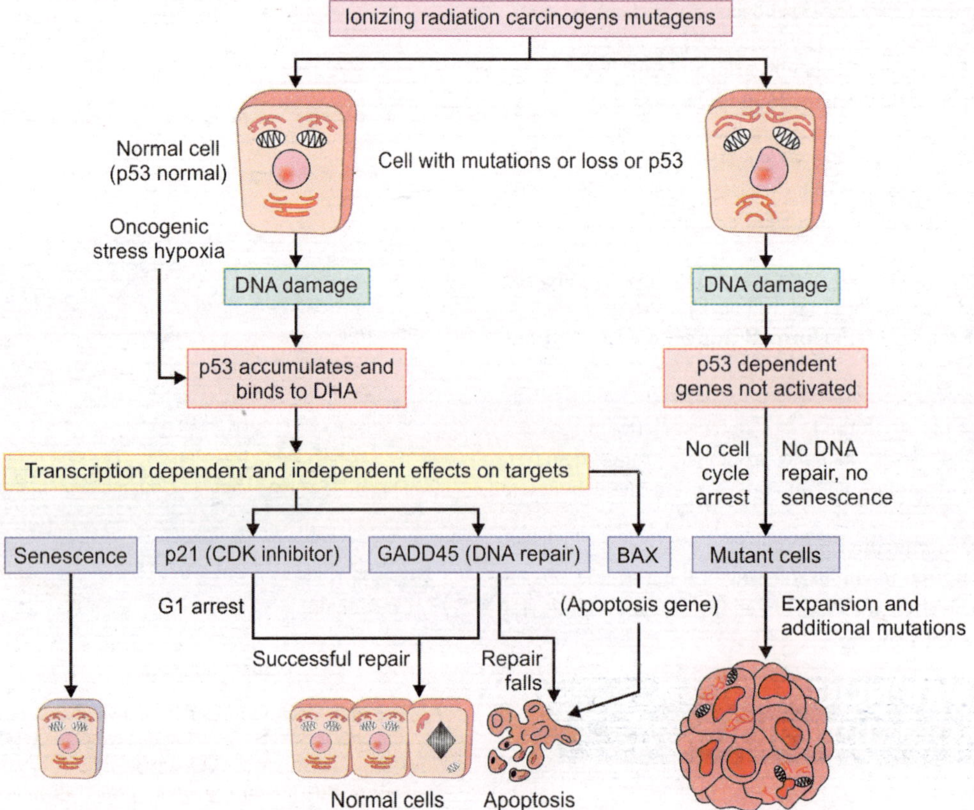

Fig: The role of p53 in maintaining the integrity of the genome *(Robbins 9th/295)*

40. Ans. a. Present in leading strand

[Ref: Lippincott 6th/402-03; Harper 30th/ 383,385]

Formation of Replication Fork

◈ *Harper 30th/ 383*

- DNA polymerases only synthesize DNA in the 5' to 3' direction and only one of the several different types of polymerases is involved at the replication fork. Because the DNA strands are antiparallel, the polymerase functions asymmetrically.
- On the leading (forward) strand, the DNA is synthesized continuously.
- On the lagging (retro-grade) strand, the DNA is synthesized in short (1-5 kb) fragments, the so-called Okazaki fragments.
- Several Okazaki fragments (up to a thousand) must be sequentially synthesized for each replication fork. To ensure that this happens, the helicase acts on the lagging strand to unwind dsDNA in a 5' to 3' direction.
- The helicase associates with the primase to afford the latter proper access to the template. This allows the RNA primer to be made and, in turn, the polymerase to begin replicating the DNA. This is an important reaction sequence since DNA polymerases cannot initiate DNA synthesis de novo. The mobile complex between helicase and primase has been called a primosome. As the synthesis of an Okazaki fragment is completed and the polymerase is released, a new primer has been synthesized. The same polymerase molecule remains associated with the replication fork and proceeds to synthesize the next Okazaki fragment

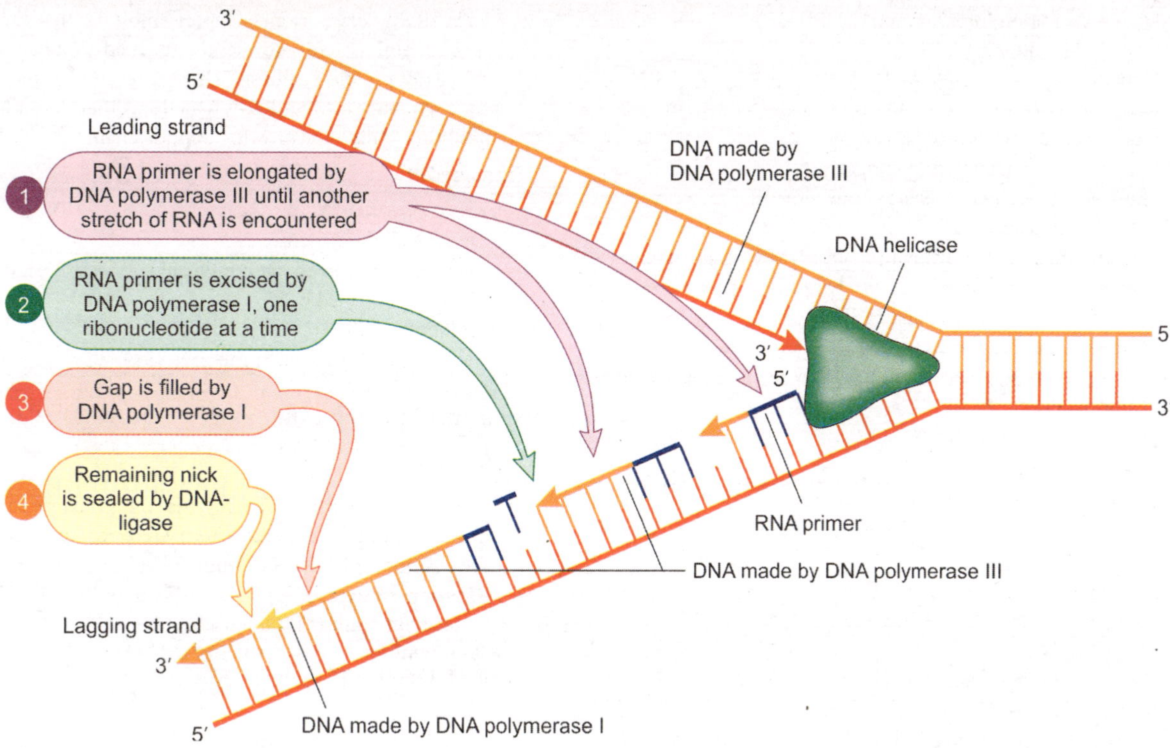

Fig: Removal of RNA primer and filling of the resulting "gaps" by DNA polymerase I on okazaki fragment *(Lippincott 6th/406)*

41. Ans. a. Fluorescence life imaging, b. Bimolecular fluorescence complementation (BiFC), c. Fluorescence resonance energy transfer (FRET), d. Fluorescence polarization

[Ref:www.hindawi.com; wikipedia]

"Fluorescence *in situ* hybridization (FISH) is a molecular cytogenetic technique that uses fluorescent probes that bind to only those parts of the chromosome with a high degree of sequence complementarity. It was developed by biomedical researchers in the early 1980sand is used to detect and localize the presence or absence of specific DNA sequences on chromosomes"-*www.nature.com*

In Vivo Techniques to Predict Protein-Protein Interactions

www.hindawi.com

- Y2H method is an in vivo method applied to the detection of PPIs
- Other widely used techniques, such as bioluminescence resonance energy transfer (BRET), fluorescence resonance energy transfers (FRET) and bimolecular fluorescence complementation (BiFC), require extensive instrumentation.

Protein-protein Interaction

◈ *www.hindawi.com*

- Protein-protein interaction plays key role in predicting the protein function of target protein and drug ability of molecules.
- The majority of genes and proteins realize resulting phenotype functions as a set of interactions.
- The in vitro and in vivo methods like affinity purification, Y2H (yeast 2 hybrid), TAP (tandem affinity purification) and so forth have their own limitations like cost, time and so forth and the resultant data sets are noisy and have more false positives to annotate the function of drug molecules.
- Thus, in silico methods which include sequence-based approaches, structure-based approaches, chromosome proximity, gene fusion, in silico 2 hybrid, phylogenetic tree, phylogenetic profile and gene expression-based approaches were developed.
- Protein-protein interactions (PPIs) handle a wide range of biological processes, including cell-to-cell interactions and metabolic and developmental control
- Protein-protein interaction is becoming one of the major objectives of system biology.
- The study of PPIs is also important to infer the protein function within the cell.
- PPIs can (i) modify the kinetic properties of enzymes; (ii) act as a general mechanism to allow for substrate channeling; (iii) construct a new binding site for small effector molecules; (iv) inactivate or suppress a protein; (v) change the specificity of a protein for its substrate through interaction with different binding partners; (vi) serve a regulatory role in either upstream or downstream level.

Methods to Investigate Protein–Protein Interactions

◈ *wikipedia.org*

Biophysical and Theoretical Methods

- Surface plasmon resonance (SPR)

- Dual polarisation interferometry (DPI)
- Static light scattering (SLS)
- Dynamic light scattering (DLS)
- Flow-induced dispersion analysis (FIDA)
- Fluorescence polarization/anisotropy
- Fluorescence correlation spectroscopy,
- Fluorescence resonance energy transfer (FRET)
- Bio-layer interferometry
- Protein activity determination by NMR multi-nuclear relaxation measurements
- Isothermal titration calorimetry (ITC)
- Microscalethermophoresis (MST)
- Rotating cellbased ligand binding assay using radioactivity or fluorescence
- Single colourreflectometry (SCORE)

Biochemical Methods

- Co-immunoprecipitation
- Bimolecular fluorescence complementation (BiFC)
- Affinity electrophoresis
- Pull-down
- Label transfer
- Phage display,
- Tandem affinity purification (TAP)
- Chemical cross-linking
- Chemical cross-linking followed by high mass MALDI mass spectrometry
- SPINE (Strepprotein interaction experiment)
- Quantitative immunoprecipitation combined with knock-down (QUICK)
- Proximity ligation assay (PLA)

Genetic Methods

- The yeast two-hybrid and bacterial two-hybrid screen

Computational Methods

- Protein–protein docking
- Network analysis

42. Ans. a. Act as adaptor molecules b/w mRNA and the amino acids coded by it, c. Have Anticodon arm, d. Has unusal bases

[Ref: Lippincott 6th/418; Vasudevan 5th/428-29; Horper 30th/411]

- tRNA have no codon arm
- DNA ends may be blunt or sticky

Transfer RNA

◈ *Lippincott 6th/418*

- tRNAs are the smallest (4S) of the three major types of RNA molecules.
- There is at least one specific type of tRNA molecule for each of the 20 amino acids commonly found in proteins.
- Together, tRNAs make up about 15% of the total RNA in the cell.
- The tRNAmolecules contain a high percentage of unusual bases (for example, dihydrouracil, pseudouridine, hypoxanthine) and have extensive intrachainbase-pairing (Figure) that leads to characteristic secondary and tertiary structure.
- Each tRNA serves as an "adaptor" moleculethat carries its specific amino acid—covalently attached to its 3'-end—to the site of protein synthesis. There it recognizes the genetic code sequence on an mRNA, which specifies the addition of its amino acid to the growing peptide chain

Transfer RNA

◈ *Vasudevan 5th/428-29*

- Clover leaf like structure
- The tRNA act as adaptor molecules b/w mRNA and the amino acids coded by it
- Contains 4 arm
- **Acceptor arm:** At 3' end. This area has 7 base pairs. The end sequence is CCA-3'
- **Anticodon arm:** It recognizethe triplet nucleotide codon present in mRNA. The specificity of tRNA resides in the anticodon site
- **DHU or D arm:** Named due to the presence of dihydrouridine in that area. It serves as recognition site for the enzyme which adds the amino acids
- **Pseudouridinearm:** It contains pseudouridine. It is involved in binding tRNA to ribosome

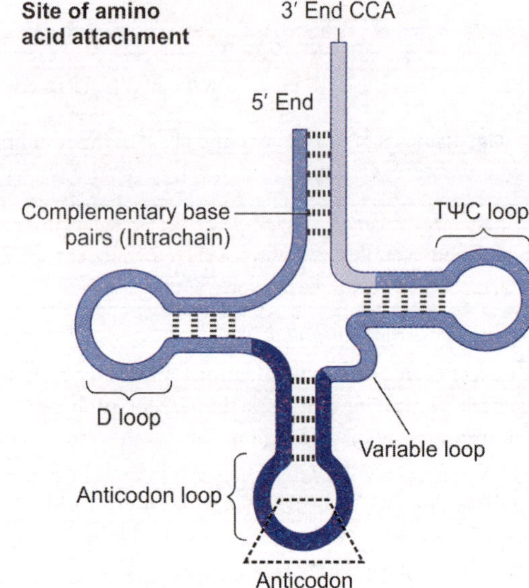

Fig: Characteristic tRNA secondary structure *(Lippincott 6th/418)*

43. Ans. b. Thymine, c. Deoxyribose sugar

[Ref: Lippincott 6th/417-18; Harper 30th/ 362-63; Davidson 22rd/43]

The Chemical Nature of RNA Differs from that of DNA

◈ *Harper 30th/ 362-63;Davidson;Lippincott 6th/417-1822rd/43*

- RNA is a polymer of purine and pyrimidine ribonucleotides linked together by 3′, 5′-phosphodiester bonds analogous to those in DNA
- Although sharing many features with DNA, **RNA possesses several specific differences:**
  - In RNA, the **sugar moiety** to which the phosphates and purine and pyrimidine bases are attached is riboserather than the **2′-deoxyribose of DNA**

- The pyrimidine components of RNA can differ from those of DNA. Although RNA contains the ribonucleotides of **adenine, guanine and cytosine**, it **does not possess thymine**. Instead of thymine, RNA contains the ribonucleotide of uracil.
- RNA typically exists as a **single strand**, whereas DNA exists as a double-stranded helical molecule.
- 4. Since the RNA molecule is a single strand complementary to only one of the two strands of a gene, its guanine content does not necessarily equal its cytosine content, nor does its adenine content necessarily equal its uracil content.
- RNA can be hydrolyzed by alkali to 2′, 3′ cyclic diesters of the mononucleotides, compounds that cannot be formed from alkali-treated DNA because of the absence of a 2′-hydroxyl group. The alkali lability of RNA is useful both diagnostically and analytically.

44. Ans. c. Transcriptionally it is very active

[Ref: Genetics by Thompson 8th/10; Reddy 34th/430; www.ncbi.nlm.nih.gov; Horper 30th/377-78]

"Satellite DNA: The *majority of these sequences are transcriptionally inactive* and some of these sequences play a structural role in the chromosome"-*Horper 30th/377*

Satellite DNA Consists of Arrays of Tandemly Repeating Sequences that Are Widely Present (>30%) in the Genome

◈ *Horper 30th/377-78;www.news-medical.net*

- Satellite DNA is mainly present in heterochromatin or the tightly packed regions of chromosomes in centromeres, telomeres and sometimes even in the euchromatin region (active region of the genome).
- Although conventionally satellite DNA has been known to be 'non-coding' (i.e. it does not encode protein), recent evidence suggests that some of the satellite DNA does undergo transcription.

Satellite DNA Structure

- Satellite DNA consists of arrays of ***tandem repeats*** or repeats arranged side-by-side. These repeats can be as small as 1–2 bp long or as long as 10–60 bps long. The short tandem repeats (1-2 bp long) are called microsatellite or simple sequence repeats (SSRs), while the longer tandem repeats (10-60bp long) are called minisatellites or variable number tandem repeats (VNTRs).
- The regions in between two simple sequence repeats or microsatellite are termed as 'inter simple sequence repeats' or ISSRs. Due to the presence of large number of repeats, the mutation rate is high in satellite DNA. It is speculated that as most of these sequences do not code for proteins, the detrimental consequences of high mutation rate is low. Thus, there is no selection pressure against it.

Functions of Satellite DNA

- **Although popularly satellite DNA is thought to be part of 'junk DNA' or 'selfish DNA'** which occupy the genome but have no effect on the fitness of an organism, recent studies show several distinct biological functions.
- They **reside in the centromeric and pericentrometric** regions and regulate centromere function.
- They are involved in the formation of heterochromatin.
- Transcripts of satellite RNA have been found in invertebrates, vertebrates and plants where they are transcribed at a particular developmental stage in certain cells and tissues.
- As the sequences of satellite DNA are highly diverse and variable, sequence-specific regulatory signals are speculated to be present in satellite DNA which fine tune gene expression

Applications

- The short sequences of DNA stretches in satellite DNA vary from individual to individual. These variations in the length and sequence of satellite DNA are **unique to each individual.**
- This uniqueness can be exploited to identify each individual based on their DNA map. This technique is called DNA fingerprinting and it is used to identify criminals, perform paternity tests and diagnose genetic disorders.

45. Ans. d. Nucleic acid sequence-based amplification (NASBA), e. Loop-mediated amplification (LAMP)

[Ref: Harrison 19th/1247; link.springer.com]

- *PCR and LCR are **thermal cycling procedures***

"The **NASBA technique** involves the ***isothermal amplification*** of a sequence within the gag region of HIV in the presence ofinternal standards and employs the production of multiple RNA copies through the action of T7-RNA polymerase"-*Harrison 19th/1247*

Loop-mediated amplification (LAMP): It is ***ani sothermal amplification technique***. It is a very sensitive, easy and time efficient method. The LAMP reaction proceeds at a constant temperature using a strand displacement reaction"-*www.premierbiosoft.com*

Isothermal Amplification Technique

◈ *pubs.rsc.org;www.ncbi.nlm.nih.go*

- This review highlights various methods that can be used for a sensitive detection of **nucleic acids without using thermal cycling procedures, as is done in PCR or LCR** (Ligase chain reaction)
- Topics included are **nucleic acid sequence-based amplification (NASBA)**, strand displacement amplification (SDA), **loop-mediated amplification (LAMP),** Invader assay, rolling circle amplification (RCA), signal mediated amplification of RNA technology (SMART), helicase-dependent amplification (HDA), recombinase polymerase amplification (RPA), nicking endonuclease signal amplification (NESA) and nicking endonuclease assisted nanoparticle activation (NENNA), exonuclease-aided target recycling, Junction or Y-probes, split DNAZyme and deoxyribozyme amplification strategies, template-directed chemical reactions that lead to amplified signals, non-covalent DNA catalytic reactions, hybridization chain reactions (HCR) and detection via the self-assembly of DNA probes to give supramolecular structures.

- The majority of these **isothermal amplification methods** can detect DNA or RNA in complex biological matrices and have great potential for use at point-of-care.
- Nucleic acid sequence-based amplification (NASBA) is an isothermal amplification method designed to detect RNA targets
- Loop-mediated amplification (LAMP) is an isothermal method that has been shown to display amplification levels that approach that of PCR

"The **Polymerase Chain Reaction (PCR)** is a well-known approach to amplify a specific DNA sequence. PCR involves the reiterative *cycling of a reaction cocktail between different temperatures* to achieve amplification. As routine as PCR is in the molecular biology and molecular diagnostic laboratory, there are other methods of sequence-specific DNA amplification. These alternative approaches often do not require changing the reaction temperature and are, therefore, often referred to as sequence-**specific isothermal amplification protocols"- www.neb.com**

46. Ans. a. Reverse transcriptase enzyme, b. RNA dependent DNA polymerase, d. Activity high in stem cell and cancer cells, e. Telomerase increases the longevity of cells

[Ref: Lippincott 6th/415,408;Harper 30th/ 374-75]

Telomeres and Telomerase

◈ *Harper 30th/ 374-75*

- The ends of each chromosome contain structures called **telomeres. Telomeres consist of short TG-rich repeats.** Human telomeres have a variable number of repeats of the sequence 5′-TTAGGG-3′, which can extend for several kilobases.
- **Telomerase,** a multisubunit RNA template-containing complex related to viral **RNA-dependent DNA polymerases (reverse transcriptases),** is the enzyme responsible for telomere synthesis and thus for **maintaining the length of the telomere.**
- Since **telomere shortening has been associated with both malignant transformation and aging,** this enzyme has become an attractive target for cancer chemotherapy and drug development

Telomerase

◈ *Lippincott 6th/408,415*

- This complex contains a protein that acts as a **reverse transcriptase** and a short piece of RNA that acts as a template.
- The CA-rich RNA template base-pairs with the GT-rich, single-stranded 3'-end of telomeric DNA. The **reverse transcriptase** uses the RNA template to synthesize DNA in the usual 5'→3' direction, extending the already longer 3'-end.
- Telomerase then translocates to the newly synthesized end and the process is repeated. Once the GT-rich strand has been lengthened, primase can use it as a template to synthesize an RNA primer. The **RNA primer is extended by DNA polymerase** and the primer is removed
- Telomeres may be viewed **as mitotic clocks** in that their length in most cells is inversely related to the number of times the cells have divided. The study of telomeres is providing insight intothe biology of aging and cancer
- **Telomeres** are stretches of **highly repetitive DNA** complexed with protein that **protect the ends of linear chromosomes.** As most cells divide and age, these sequences are shortened, contributing to senescence.
- In cells that do not senesce (for example, **germ line and cancer cells**), telomerase employs its enzyme component reverse transcriptase to extend the telomeres, using its **RNA as a template**

Telomeres

◈ *Lippincott 6th/407-08*

- **Telomeres are complexes of noncoding DNA plus proteins located at the ends of linear chromosomes.**
- They maintain the structural integrity of the chromosome, preventing attack by nucleases and allow repair systems to distinguish a true end from a break in dsDNA.
- **Telomere shortening:** Eukaryotic cells face a special problem in replicating the ends of their linear DNA molecules. Following removal of the RNA primer from the extreme 5'-end of the lagging strand, there is no way to fill in the remaining gap with DNA. Consequently, in most normal human somatic cells, telomeres shorten with each successive cell division.
- Once telomeres are shortened beyond some critical length, the cell is no longer able to divide and is said to be senescent.
- In **germ cells and other stem cells, as well as in cancer cells, telomeres do not shorten** and the cells do not senesce. This is a result of the presence of a ribonucleoprotein, telomerase, which maintains telomeric length in these cells

PATHOLOGY

47. Ans. a. TIBC (Total iron binding capacity)

[Ref: Harshmohan 7th/278; Harrison 19th/628-30; Davidson 23rd/942]

- **Transferrin saturation,** although decreased in **anemia of chronic disease** (ACD), but its level is greater than iron deficiency anaemia
- ACD-despite the ***presence of normal or increased iron store, there is inadequate iron delivery to the marrow***

Anemia of Chronic Inflammation/Infection *(AI Also k/a anemia of chronic disease) Harrison 19th/628-30*

- AI—which encompasses inflammation, infection, tissue injury and conditions (such as cancer) associated with the release of proinflammatory cytokines—is one of the most common forms of anemia seen clinically.
- It is the most important anemia in the differential diagnosis of iron deficiency, because many of the features of the anemia are brought about ***by inadequate iron delivery to the marrow,*** despite the presence of normal or increased iron stores. This is reflected by ***a low serum iron, increased red cell protoporphyrin, a hypoproliferative marrow,***

transferrin saturation in the range of 15–20% and a normal or increased serum ferritin.

- The **serum ferritin** values are often the ***most distinguishing features*** between true iron-deficiency anemia and the iron-restricted erythropoiesis associated with inflammation. Typically, ***serum ferritin values increase threefold over basal levels***
- The **distinction between true iron deficiency anemia and AI** is among the most common diagnostic problems encountered by clinicians.
- Usually, ***AI is normocytic and normochromic***. The iron values usually make the differential diagnosis clear, as the ***ferritin level is normal or increased*** and the ***percent transferrin saturation and TIBC are typically below normal***"-*Harrison 19th/628*

Table: Diagnosis of Hypoproliferative Anemias *(Harrison 19th/630)*

Tests	Iron Deficiency	Inflammation
Anemia	Mild to severe	Mild
MCV (fL)	60–90	80–90
Morphology	Normo-microcytic	Normocytic
SI (μg/dL)	<30	<50
TIBC (μg/dL)	>360	<300
Saturation (%)	<10	10–20
Serum ferritin (μg/dL)	<15	30–200
Iron stores	0	2–4+

Table: Diagnosis of microcytic anemia *(Harrison 19th/628)*

Tests	Iron deficiency	Inflammation	Thalassemia	Sideroblastic anemia
Smear	Micro/hypo	Normal micro/hypo	Micro/hypo with targeting	Variable
Serum iron (mg/dL)	<30	<50	Normal to high	Normal to high
TIBC (mg/dL)	>360	<300	Normal	Normal
Percent saturation	<10	10-20	30-80	30-80
Ferritin (mg/L)	<15	30-200	50-300	50-300
Hemoglobin pattern on electrophoresis	Normal	Normal	Abnormal with β thalassemia; can be normal with a thalassemia	Normal

Table: Investigations to differentiate anaemia of chronic disease from iron deficiency anaemia (*Davidson 23rd/942*)

Tests	Ferritin	Iron	TIBC	Transferrin saturation	Soluble transferrin receptor
Iron deficiency anaemia	↓	↓	↑	↓	↑
Anaemia of chronic disease	↑/Normal	↓	↓	↓	↓/Normal

Anaemia of Chronic Disease (ACD)

◈ *Davidson 22nd/1023*

- It occurs in the setting of chronic infection, chronic inflammation or neoplasia.
- ***The serum iron is low but iron stores are normal or increased, as indicated by the ferritin or stainable marrow iron.***
- It has recently become clear that the key regulatory protein that accounts for the findings characteristic of ACD is hepcidin, which is produced by the liver
- Inhibition or blockade of hepcidin is a potential target for treatment of this form of anaemia.

48. Ans. a. Iron deficiency anemia, b. Thalassaemia, c. Sideroblastic anemia

[Ref: Harrison 19th/ 394; Davidson 23rd/921; William's Haematology 7th/ Chap 40]

Table: *Davidson 23rd/921*

Microcytosis (reduced average cell size, MCV < 76 fL)
- Iron deficiency
- Sideroblastic anaemia
- Thaassaemia

Macrocytosis (increased average cell size, MCV > 100 fL)
- Vitamin B_{12} or folate deficiency
- Drugs (e.g. zidovudine, trimethoprim, phenytoin, methotrexate)
- Liver disease, alcohol
- Hypothyroidism

Table: Red blood cell indices *(Harrison 19th/ 394)*

Index	Normal Value
Mean cell volume (MCV) = (hematocrit x 10)/(red cell count x 106)	90 ± 8 fL
Mean cell hemoglobin (MCH) = (hemoglobin x 10)/(red cell count x 106)	30 ± 3 pg
Mean cell hemoglobin concentration = (hemoglobin x 10)/hematocrit, or MCI-1/MCV	33 ± 2%

Anemia

◈ *William's Haematology 7th/Chap 40*

- The forms of anemia that must be distinguished from iron-deficiency anemia most frequently include those of ***thalassemia minor, chronic inflammatory disease, malignancy, chronic liver disease, chronic renal disease, hemolytic anemia and aplastic anemia.***
- It is the microcytic anemias that are most likely to be confused with iron deficiency.

Table: Microcytic disorders *(William's Haematology 7th/Chap 40)*

Thalassemias and hemoglobinopathies
β-thalassemia major
β-thalassemia minor
αβ-thalassemia minor
α-thalassemia minor
Hemoglobin Lepore trait
Hemoglobin E trait
Homozygous hemoglobin E disease
Hemoglobin H disease
Combination of above (compound heterozygotes)
Blockade of heme synthesis caused by chemicals
Lead
Pyrazinamide
Isoniazid
Other disorders
Sideroblastic anemias
Hereditary sex-linked
Idiopathic acquired
Anemia of chronic disease

A & E

49. Ans. d. Child with seizure

[Ref: www.healthline.com; Robbins 9th/158-61;Harshmohan 7th/252-55; Obs by GB Sharma 1st/118]

"Investigation for **Recurrent miscarriage-*Karyotype***"-*Obs by G.B.Sharma 1st/118*

An unusual number of chromosomes, incorrectly arranged chromosomes, or malformed chromosomes can all be signs of a genetic condition. Genetic conditions vary greatly, but two examples are ***Down syndrome*** and Turner syndrome"-*www.healthline.com*

Karyotype

◈ *atlasgeneticsoncology.org*

- The karyotype is the study of the individual chromosomal complement through which one can detect chromosomal rearrangements constitutional or acquired on at least one band equivalent to 10^3 to 10^4 K bases; since the scale is not at the gene level the karyotpe is useless in monogenic diseases (except in research).
- 10% of children with a congenital defect would have a chromosomal anomaly
- Karyotype can be done on peripheral lymphocytes, tumour cells (bone marrow) fibroblasts, gametes, amniocytes or trophoblasts upon indications.

Indications of Karyotype

◈ *atlasgeneticsoncology.org*

- **During the perinatal period In a stillbirth:** Karyotype on fibroblasts (umbilical cord, lung, muscle) if the etiology in unknown or when one suspects a chromosomal disease (for instance in dysmorphic syndromes and /or visceral anomalies); a complete anatomo-pathological examination is indicated (foeto-pathology).

  During the neonatal period.
  - In ***any dysmorphic syndrome and/or malformation***(s) and/ or neurological deficit, unless a known etiology is likely involved (teratogenic embryopathy or monogenic disease).
  - In ambiguous genitalia: Pseudohermaphrodism, gonadal dysgenesis, true hermaphrodyte
- **During childhood and adolescence if**
  - Psycho motor retardation (fra X, Klinefelter)
  - Dysmorphism with visceral anomalies undetected during infancy
  - Unexplained short stature (Turner)
  - Hypogonadism (Klinefelter, Turner).
- **During adulthood**
  - Parents of a child with a chromosomal disorder
  - Sterility workup once gynaecological or endocrine causes have been ruled out (Klinefelter, Turner,Testicular feminization).
  - If more than two spontaneous miscarriages cytogenetic studies are indicated on the parents to rule out a translocation carrier; a foetal karyotype is recommended if at all possible.
- **During pregnancy**

  Tissues: amniotic fluid cells obtained by amniocentesis, chorionic villi, lymphocytes obtained by cordocentesis. Indications:

- Advanced maternal age
  - ***Previous pregnancy with an abnormal chromosomal complement***
- Previous stillbirth with an abnormal chromosomal complement
- Balanced chromosomal rearrangement (translocation, inversion,...) or not (marker, mosaicism, sexual aneuploidy) in one of the parents
- Abnormal maternal serological screening test
- Abnormal foetal ultrasound
- Risk of an unstable chromosomal syndrome
  - Confirmation of foetal mosaicism diagnosed earlier during the pregnancy

(This procedure has a 1% risk of miscarriage)

"Approximately 4% of patients with Down syndrome have a translocation and because recurrence risks are different for families of these individuals, ***all patients with clinically identified Down syndrome should have a karyotype to look for translocations***"- www.labtestsonline.org.au

Karyotyping: Stained Cells are Examined

◈ *www.healthline.com*

- Extra chromosomes
- Missing chromosomes
- Missing portions of a chromosome
- Extra portions of a chromosome
- Portions that have broken off of one chromosome and reattached to another

50. Ans. a. Most common cause of death is congenital heart disease, b. 95% have an extra 21st chromosome, c. Increased nuchal fold thickness on USG

[Ref: Robbins (SEA) 9th/ 161-63; O.P.Ghai 9th/635-37; Harrison 19th/83e1-4; Danhert 5th/925; Nelson 18th/508]

- ***Advanced maternal age is a risk factor***

"Parents who wish to get a prenatal diagnosis have a number of options- invasive test(fetal karyotype by chorionic villus sampling or amniocentesis) or non-invasive initial screening test like maternal serum markers and USG- O.P.Ghai 9th/637(so Karyotyping is not required in all cases for prenatal diagnosis-option d)

"Presence of heart disease is the chief factor in determining survival- *O.P.Ghai 9th/636*

"Cardiac problems are *responsible for the majority of the deaths in infancy and early childhood*"-*Robbins (SEA) 9th/ 163*

"Fetal USG in Down syndrome: ***Increased nuchal fold thickness****"- O.P.Ghai 9th/635*

Trisomy 21 (Down Syndrome)

◈ *O.P.Ghai 8th/637-38*

- *Chromosome no. 21 is present in triplicate, the origin of extra chromosome 21 being* ***either maternal or paternal***
- *In* ***most cases the extrachromosome from the mother***
- *Trisomy is found in 94% cases.*
- *Approx. 1% of cases are mosaic and* ***rest (5%) are due to trans-locations, most commonly involving chromosome 21 and 14***

Trisomy 21 (Down Syndrome)

◈ *Robbins (SEA) 9th/ 161*

- Down syndrome is the most common of the chromosomal disorders and is a major cause of mental retardation.
- **Approximately 95%** of affected ***individuals have trisomy 21***
- Maternal age has a strong influence on the incidence of trisomy 21. It occurs once in 1550 live births in women under age 20, in contrast to 1 in 25 live births for mothers older than age 45. The correlation with **maternal age** suggested that ***most cases the meiotic nondisjunction of chromosome 21 occurs in the ovum***.
- Indeed, studies in which DNA polymorphisms were used to trace the parental origin of chromosome 21 have revealed that in ***95% of the cases with trisomy 21 the extra chromosome is of maternal origin***.

Systemic Abnormalities in Down Syndrome

◈ *Nelson 18th/508*

- **GIT:** ***Duodenal, ileal and jejunal atresia***, tracheoesophogeal fistula, hirschsprung's disease, meckel's diverticulum, imperforate anus, omphalocele.
- **Eye:** Brushfield spot,↑ed risk of cataract, nystagmus and squint.
- **CVS:** Endocardial cushion defect (MC), VSD, Ostium primum ASD and AV valve malformation
- **Hearing defects:** Serous otitis media; conductive and/or ***sensorineural hearing loss*** (Nelson 18th/508)
- **Thyroid-dysfunction:** Hypothyroidism
- Atlanto-occipital dislocation/subluxation
- **Malignancy:** ↑ed risk of AML and ALLQ
- ***Early onset of Alzheimer disease***
- Abnormal immune response

51. Ans. d. Alkaptonuria: Autosomal recessive, e. Duchene muscle dystrophy: X-linked recessive

[Ref: Robbins (SAE) 9th/141-42]

Mendelian Disorders

◈ *Robbins 9th (SAE)/141-42,144*

- ***Duchene muscle dystrophy- X-linked recessive***
- ***Vit D resistant rickets- X-linked dominant***
- **Marfan syndrome: *Autosomal dominant*** (70% to 85% of cases)

Table: Autosomal recessive disorders *(Robbins 9th/141)*

System	Disorder
Metabolic	Cystic fibrosis
	Phenylketonuria
	Galactosemia
	Homocystinuria
	Lysosomal storage diseases
	a1-Antitrypsin deficiency
	Wilson disease
	Hemochromatosis
	Glycogen storage diseases
Hematopoietic	**Sickle cell anemia**
	Thalassemias
Endocrine	Congenital adrenal hyperplasia
Skeletal	Ehlers-Danlos syndrome (some variants)
	Alkaptonuria
Nervous	Neurogenic muscular atrophies
	Friedreich ataxia
	Spinal muscular atrophy

52. Ans. a. Hemolysis due to ABO incompatibility, b. Criggler-Najar syndrome, c. Gilbert syndrome, d. Sepsis

[Ref: Nelson 20th/1923; Robbins (SAE) 9th/854; O.P.Ghai 9th/169; Harrison 19th/282,2000-04; Davidson 23rd/860-61]

- Roter's syndrome causes conjugated hyperbilirubinemia
- **Sepsis** cause ***both conjugated and uncojugated hyperbilirubinemia***-*Harshmohan 7th/583*

Table: Causes of isolated hyperbilirubinemia *(Harrison 19th/282)*

Indirect hyperbilirubinemia
• Hemolytic disorders ▪ Inherited • Spherocytosis, elliptocytosis Glucose-6-phosphate dehydrogenase and pyruvate kinase deficiencies • Sickle cell anemia ▪ Acquired • Microangiopathic hemolytic anemias • Paroxysmal nocturnal hemoglobinuria • Spur cell anemia • ***Immune hemolysis (ABO*** and Rh incompatibility- O.P.Ghai 9th/169) • Parasitic infections ▪ Malaria ▪ Babesiosis • Ineffective erythropoiesis ▪ Cobalamin, folate, thalassemia and severe iron deficiencies • Drugs ▪ Rifampicin, probenecid, ribavirin • Inherited conditions ▪ ***Crigler-Najjar types I and II*** ▪ Gilbert's syndrome
Direct hyperbilirubinemia
• Inherited conditions ▪ Dubin-Johnson syndrome ▪ ***Rotor's syndrome***

53. Ans. b. Good pasture syndrome

[Ref: Robbins (SAE) 9th/ 910,92-26; Harrison 19th/1846; Davidson 23rd/404]

- ***Most appropriate diagnosis is Goodpasture syndrome (presence of all feature: Linear IgG and C3 deposit, hemoptysis, hematuria, crescent)***

Exclusion of other Options

- **Wegener granulomatosis:** ***no deposits***
- **Minimal change disease**: ***no deposit, no hemoptysis, no crescent***
- **Post-streptococcal GN**(Postinfectious glomerulonephritis): ***Granular IgG and C3 deposit, no hemoptysis, no crescent***
- **Thin basement membrane lesion** (Benign Familial Hematuria): ***thinned glomerular basement membrane, no deposit***

Rapidly Progressive (Crescentic) Glomerulonephritis

◈ *Robbins (SAE) 9th/ 912-13*

- *Causes:* **Type I Anti-GBM antibody-mediated disease** (e.g ***Goodpasture syndrome***), **Type III** (***Pauci-Immune, e.g Wegener granulomatosis***)
- *The most common histologic picture is the presence of crescents in most of the glomeruli (**crescentic glomerulonephritis**).*
- **Anti-GBM antibody-mediated disease**, *characterized by **linear deposits of IgG and, in many cases, C3** in the GBM.*
- **Pauci-immune RPGN**, *defined by the* ***lack of detectable anti-GBM antibodies or immune complexes by immunofluorescence*** *and electron microscopy.* Most patients with this type of RPGN have circulating *antineutrophil cytoplasmic antibodies* (ANCAs)

Immunological cause of hemoptysis- ***Goodpasture syndrome,*** Wegener granulomatosis and polyarteritis nodosa- P.J.M 20th/382

Pulmonary-renal Syndromes

◈ *Harrison 19th/1846*

- Several diseases can present with catastrophic hemoptysis and glomerulonephritis associated with varying degrees of renal failure. The usual causes include ***Goodpasture's syndrome, granulomatosis with polyangiitis (Wegener), microscopic polyangiitis, Churg-Strauss vasculitis and, rarely, Henoch-Schönlein purpura or cryoglobulinemia***.
- **Pulmonary bleeding** in this setting is life-threatening and often results in airway intubation and acute renal failure requires dialysis. Diagnosis is difficult initially because biopsies and serologic testing take time.

Table: Summary of major primary glomerulo *(Robbins (SAE) 9th/ 910)*

Disease	Most frequent clinical presentation	Pathogenesis	Glomerular pathology		
			Light microscopy	**Fluorescence microscopy**	**Electron microscopy**
Postinfectious Glomerulone-phritis	Nephritic syndrome	Immune complex mediated; circulating or planted antigen	Diffuse endocapillary proliferation; leukocytic infiltration	Granular IgG and C3 in GBM and mesangium; Granular igA. In some cases	Primarily subepithelial humps; subendothelial deposits in early disease stages.
Goodpasture syndrome	Rapidly progressive glomerulonephritis	Anti-GBM COL4-A3 antigen	Extracapillary proliferation with crescents; necrosis	Liner IgG and C3; fibrin in crescents	No deposits; GBM disruptions; fibrin
Minimal change disease	Nephrotic syndrome	Unknown; loss of glomerular polyanion; podocyte injury	Normal; lipid in tubules	Negative	Loss of foot process; no deposits
IgA nephropathy	Recurrent hematuria or proteinuria	Unknown	Focal mesangial proliferative glomerulonephritis; mesangial widening	IgA ± IgG, IgM and C3 in mesangium	Mesangial and paramesangialdense deposits

54. Ans. b. Spleen size, c. MCHC, e. LDH

[Ref: Robbins (SAE) 9th/633-34; Harrison 19th/649; Davidson 23rd/947-48]

In HS: ***MCV is usually normal or slightly decreased-*** *Harshmohan 7th/292*

Features Common to Most Patients with a Hemolytic Disorder (Including HS)

Harrison 19th/649

General examination	Jaundice, pallor
Other physical findings	Spleen may be enlarged; bossing of skull in severe congenital cases
Hemoglobin level	From normal to severely reduced
MCV, MCH	Usually increased
Reticulocytes	Increased
Bilirubin	Increased (mostly unconjugated)
LDH	Increased (up to 10 time normal with intravascular hemolysis)
Haptoglobin	Reduced to absent (if hemolysis in part intravascular)

Hereditary Spherocytosis (HS)

Harrison 19th/651-52

- The presence of *osmotic fragility* is the main diagnostic test for HS.
- The main clinical findings are jaundice, ***an enlarged spleen*** and often gallstones; indeed, it may be the finding of gallstones in a young person that triggers diagnostic investigations.
- An **increased mean corpuscular hemoglobin concentration (MCHC)** on an ordinary blood count report should raise the suspicion of HS, because HS is almost the only condition in which this abnormality occurs.

Hereditary Spherocytosis

Robbins (SAE) 9th/633-34

- **It is caused by intrinsic defects in the red cell membrane skeleton**
- The characteristic clinical features are *anemia, splenomegaly and jaundice.* The generally stable clinical course is sometimes punctuated by *aplastic crises,* usually triggered by an acute parvovirus infection.
- Gallstones, found in many patients, can also produce symptoms.
- Splenectomy treats the anemia and its complications, but brings with it an increased risk of sepsis, since the spleen acts as an important filter for blood borne bacteria.

55. Ans. b. Polycythemia, e. IgG paraprotein

[Ref: Robbins (SAE) 9th/; Harrison 19th/717-18; Davidson 23rd/966]

- In **waldenstorm macroglobulinemia: *Anaemia and IgM paraprotein***

Waldenström Macroglobulinaemia

Davidson 23rd/966

- This is a ***low grade lymphoplasmacytoid lymphoma*** associated with an ***IgM paraprotein***, causing clinical features of **hyperviscosity syndrome**.
- It is a rare tumour occurring in the elderly and affects males more commonly.
- Patients classically present with ***features of hyperviscosity***, such as nose bleeds, bruising, confusion and visual disturbance. However, presentation may be with ***anaemia***, systemic symptoms, splenomegaly or lymphadenopathy.
- Patients are found on investigation to have an ***IgM paraprotein*** associated with a raised plasma viscosity. The bone marrow has a characteristic appearance, with infltration of lymphoid cells and prominent mast cells.
- If patients show symptoms of hyperviscosity and anaemia, plasmapheresis is required to remove IgM and make blood transfusion possible. ***Chemotherapy with alkylating agents, such as chlorambucil***, has been the mainstay of treatment, controlling disease in over 50%. Fludarabine may be more effective but has more side effects. Rituximab can also be effective. The median survival is 5 years.

Waldenström's Macroglobulinemia

Harrison 19th/717-18

- Major clinical manifestation is ***hyperviscosity syndrome.***
- Like myeloma, the disease involves the bone marrow, but unlike myeloma, it does not cause bone lesions or hypercalcemia.
- Physical examination reveals adenopathy and hepatosplenomegaly and ophthalmoscopic examination may reveal vascular segmentation and dilation of the retinal veins characteristic of ***hyperviscosity states.***
- Patients may have a ***normocytic, normochromic anemia***, but rouleaux formation and a positive Coombs' test are much more common than in myeloma.
- Malignant lymphocytes are usually present in the peripheral blood.
- About 10% of macroglobulins are cryoglobulins. These are pure M components and are not the mixed cryoglobulins seen in rheumatoid arthritis and other autoimmune diseases.

56. Ans. b. Pleomorphism, c. Loss of cell polarity, d. Abnormal nuclear morphology, e. Abnormal mitosis

[Ref: Harshmohan 7th/189-90; Robbins (SAE) 9th/268-70]

Normal tissue → Metaplasia → Dysplasia → Carcinoma in situ → Invasive cancer *(Harshmohan 7th/40-41)*

Anaplasia

Harshmohan 7th/189-90

- It is ***lack of differentiation and is a characteristic feature of most malignant tumours***
- Depending upon the degree of differentiation, the extent of anaplasia is also variable i.e. poorly differentiated malignant tumours have high degree of anaplasia

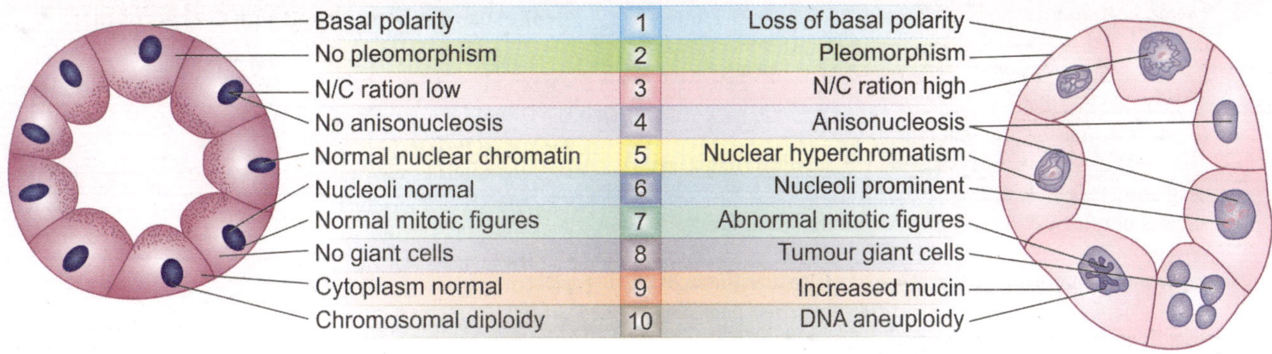

Fig: Anaplasia-changes *(Harshmohan 7th/189)*

Anaplasia and Differentiation

◈ *Robbins (SAE) 9th/268-70*

- **Differentiation refers to the extent to which neoplastic parenchymal cells resemble the corresponding normal parenchymal cells, both morphologically and functionally; lack of differentiation is called *anaplasia*.**
- Malignant neoplasms that are composed of poorly differentiated cells are said to be *anaplastic*. **Lack of differentiation, or anaplasia, is considered a hallmark of malignancy.**
- The term *anaplasia* means "to form backward," implying a reversal of differentiation to a more primitive level.
- **Lack of differentiation, or anaplasia, is often associated with many other morphologic changes.**

- **Pleomorphism**: Cancer cells often display pleomorphism—variation in size and shape
- **Abnormal nuclear morphology**. Characteristically, the nuclei are disproportionately large for the cell, with a nuclear-to-cytoplasm ratio that may approach 1: 1 instead of the normal 1: 4 or 1: 6.
- **Mitoses**. More important as a morphologic feature of malignancy are *atypical, bizarre mitotic figures*, sometimes with tripolar, quadripolar, or multipolar spindles
- Loss of polarity. In addition to the cytologic abnormalities, the orientation of anaplastic cells is markedly disturbed.

Table: Difference b/w metaplasia and dysplasia *(Harshmohan 7th/41)*

Feature	Metaplasia	Dysplasia
• Definition	Change of one type of epithelial or mesenchymal cell to another type of adult epithelial or mesenchymal cell	Disordered cellular development, may be accompanied with hyperplasia or metaplasia
• Types	Epithelial (squamous, columnar) and mesenchymal (osseous cartilaginous)	Epithelial only
• Tissues affected	Most commonly affects bronchial mucosa, uterine endocervix; others mesenchymal tissues (cartilage, arteries)	Uterine cervix, bronchial mucosa
• Cellular changes	Mature cellular development	Disordered cellular development (pleomorphism, nuclear hyperchromasia, mitosis, loss of polarity)
• Natural history	Reversible on withdrawal of stimulus	May regress on removal of inciting stimulus, or may progress to higher grades of dysplasia or carcinoma in situ

57. Ans. a. Glomerulonephritis

[Ref: Robbins (SAE) 9th/898; Harrison 19th/1805]

Urine Analysis

◈ *Harrison 19th/1805*

- ***Glomerulonephritis may lead to dysmorphic red blood cells or red blood cell casts.***
- ***Interstitial nephritis may lead to white blood cell casts.***

- **Urine eosinophils** have a limited role in differential diagnosis; they can be seen in interstitial nephritis, pyelonephritis, cystitis, atheroembolic disease, or glomerulonephritis.
- Crystalluria may be important diagnostically.
- The finding of oxalate crystals in AKI should prompt an evaluation for ethylene glycol toxicity.
- Abundant uric acid crystals may be seen in the tumor lysis syndrome

"**Microscopic hematuria** may also appear with the onset of benign prostatic hypertrophy, ***interstitial nephritis,*** papillary necrosis, hypercalciuria, ***renal stones,*** cystic kidney diseases, or renal vascular injury. However, when red blood cell casts or **dysmorphic red blood cells** are found in the sediment, ***glomerulonephritis is likely***"- *Harrison 19th/1834*

Urine microscopy	Casts or dysmorphic red cells suggest ***glomerulonephritis*** Leucocytes suggest infection/ ***interstitial nephritis*** Crystals may be observed in drug-induced or uric acid nephropathy

"*Nephritic syndrome* is a clinical entity caused by glomerular disease and is dominated by the acute onset of either grossly visible hematuria (red blood cells in urine) or microscopic hematuria with ***dysmorphic red cells*** and red cell casts on urinalysis, diminished GFR, mild to moderate proteinuria and hypertension. It is the classic presentation of **acute poststreptococcal glomerulonephritis**"-Robbins (SAE) 9th/898

"Two main types of red blood cells, **is omorphic and dysmorphic**, are found in the urine sediment, indicating ***nonglomerular and glomerular hematuria***, respectively. Occasionally, however, other types of red blood cells such as sickle cells, anisocytes, poikilocytes, elliptocytes and dacryocytes can be seen in the urine sediment of patients with hematuria"- *www.karger.com*

58. Ans. a. Liver, b. Esophagus, c. Gastric, e. Breast

[Ref: Harshmohan 7th/236; Robbins (SAE) 9th/ 277; Harrison 19th/ 477]

- *Association of alcohol with cervical cancer is less conclusive*

"Consuming **alcohol,** even frequently and in large quantities, is ***not a risk factor for developing cervical cancer***- It is based on analysis of the scientific research evidence, that is the conclusion of the American Cancer Society, the United States Centers for Disease Control and Prevention (CDC), the National Cancer Institute, the United Kingdom's National Health Service, the Canadian Cancer Society, Cancer Council Australia, the World Health Organization (WHO), the Mayo Clinic and other health agencies and organizations"-www.alcoholproblemsandsolutions.org

"**Alcohol consumption**: Alcohol abuse alone increases the risk of carcinomas of the ***oropharynx (excluding lip), larynx and esophagus and, by the development of alcoholic cirrhosis, hepatocellular carcinoma.*** Alcohol and tobacco together synergistically increase the risk of cancers in the upper airways and digestive tract"- *Robbins (SAE) 9th/ 277*

Alcohol use has been Linked with Cancers of the:

- *www.cancer.org (American cancer society)*
- Mouth
- Throat (pharynx)
- Voice box (larynx)
- ***Esophagus***
- ***Liver***
- Colon and rectum
- ***Breast***
- Alcohol may also increase the risk of cancers of the pancreas and ***stomach.***

"Heavy alcohol intake has been linked to increased risk of several cancers, including cancer of the colon, rectum, ***female breast***, oral cavity, pharynx, larynx, ***liver*** and ***esophagus;*** whereas light-to-moderate drinking (up to one drink per day for women and up to two drinks per day for men) is not appreciably associated with cancer risk and may be beneficial for cardiovascular disease"-*www.sciencedirect.com*

"Clear patterns have emerged between **alcohol consumption** and the development of the following types of cancer: ***Head and neck cancer, Esophageal cancer, Liver cancer: Breast cancer: Colorectal cancer.*** Evidence is accumulating that alcohol is associated with increased risks of melanoma and of prostate and pancreatic cancers . However, for cancers of the ovary, prostate, stomach, uterus and bladder, either no association with alcohol use has been found or the evidence for an association is inconsistent. Alcohol consumption has also been associated with decreased risks of kidney cancers and non-Hodgkin lymphoma in multiple studies"- *www.cancer.gov*

Table: Suspected carcinogens *(Harrison 19th/ 477)*

Carcinogensa	Associated cancer or neoplasm
Alkylating agents	Acute myeloid leukemia, bladder cancer
Androgens	Prostate cancer
Aromatic amines (dyes)	Bladder cancer
Arsenic	Cancer of the lung, skin
Asbestos	Cancer of the lung, pleura, peritoneum
Benzene	Acute myelocytic leukemia
Chromium	Lung cancer
Diethylstilbestrol (prenatal)	Vaginal cancer (clear cell)
Epstein-Barr virus	Burkitt's lymphoma, nasal T cell lymphoma
Estrogens	Cancer of the endometrium, liver, breast
Ethyl alcohol	Cancer of the ***liver, esophagus, head and neck***
Helicobacter pylori	Gastric cancer, gastric MALT lymphoma
Hepatitis B or C virus	Liver cancer
Human immunodeficiency virus	Non-Hodgkin's lymphoma, Kaposi's sarcoma, squamous cell carcinomas (especially of the urogenital tract)
Human papilloma virus	Cervix cancer, head and neck cancer

Contd...

Carcinogensa	Associated cancer or neoplasm
Human T cell lymphotropic virus type I (HTLV-I)	Adult T cell leukemia/lymphoma
Immunosuppressive agents (azathioprine, cyclosporine, glucocorticoids)	Non-Hodgkin's lymphoma
Ionizing radiation (therapeutic or diagnostic)	Breast, bladder, thyroid, soft tissue, bone, hematopoietic and many more
Nitrogen mustard gas	Cancer of the lung, head and neck, nasal sinuses
Nickel dust	Cancer of the lung, nasal sinuses
Phenacetin	Cancer of the renal pelvis and bladder
Polycyclic hydrocarbons	Cancer of the lung, skin (especially squamous cell carcinoma of scrotal skin)
Schistosomiasis	Bladder cancer (squamous cell)
Sunlight (ultraviolet)	Skin cancer (squamous cell and melanoma)
Tobacco (including smokeless)	Cancer of the upper aerodigestive tract, bladder
Vinyl chloride	Liver cancer (angiosarcoma)

59. Ans. b. Integrin, c. L-selectin

[Ref: Harshmohan 7th/120,125; Robbins (SAE) 9th/ 75-77]

- ***Complement C5a, Leukotriene B4 and Interleukin-8 are chemo-attractant (help in chemotaxis)***

Exudation of Leucocyte; Steps

◈ *Harshmohan 7th/120*

- Change in formed elements of blood
- Rolling and adhesion(Selectin, Integrin and immunoglobulin gene superfamily adhesion molecules)
- Emigration
- Chemotaxis (***Complement C5a, Leukotriene B4 and Interleukin-8)***

The journey of leukocytes from the vessel lumen to the tissue is a multistep process that is mediated and controlled by adhesion molecules and cytokines called chemokines. This process can be divided into sequential phases: *Robbins (SAE) 9th/ 75*

- In the lumen: *margination, rolling and adhesion to endothelium.* Vascular endothelium in its normal, unactivated state does not bind circulating cells or impede their passage. In inflammation, the endothelium is activated and can bind leukocytes as a prelude to their exit from the blood vessels.
- **Migration across the endothelium** and vessel wall
- **Migration in the tissues** toward a ***chemotactic stimulus***

Leukocyte Adhesion and Migration

◈ *Robbins (SAE) 9th/ 76*

The two major families of molecules involved in leukocyte adhesion and migration are the selectins and integrins and their ligands. They are expressed on leukocytes and endothelial cells.

- The **initial rolling interactions** are mediated by a family of proteins called *selectins.* There are three types of selectins: one expressed on leukocytes (**Lselectin**), one on endothelium (**Eselectin**) and one in platelets and on endothelium (**Pselectin**).
- The ligands for selectins are sialylated oligosaccharides bound to mucinlike glycoprotein backbones. The expression of selectins and their ligands is regulated by cytokines produced in response to infection and injury. Tissue macrophages, mast cells and endothelial cells that encounter microbes and dead tissues respond by secreting several cytokines, including ***tumor necrosis factor (TNF), IL1 and chemokines*** *(chemo**attractant cytokines**)*.
- **TNF and IL1** act on the endothelial cells of postcapillary venules adjacent to the infection and induce the coordinate expression of numerous adhesion molecules. Within 1 to 2 hours the endothelial cells begin to express ***Eselectin and the ligands for Lselectin***..
- Leukocytes express **Lselectin** at the tips of their microvilli and also express ligands for E and Pselectins, all of which bind to the complementary molecules on the endothelial cells. These are lowaffnity interactions with a fast offrate and they are easily disrupted by the flowing blood. As a result, the bound leukocytes bind, detach and bind again and thus begin to roll along the endothelial surface.
- These weak rolling interactions slow down the leukocytes and give them the opportunity to bind more firmly to the endothelium. Firm adhesion is mediated by a family of heterodimeric leukocyte surface proteins called *integrins.*
- TNF and IL1 induce endothelial expression of ligands for **integrins**, mainly vascular cell adhesion molecule 1 (VCAM1, the ligand for the b1 integrin VLA4) and intercellular adhesion molecule1 (ICAM1, the ligand for the b2 integrins LFA1 and Mac1). Leukocytes normally express integrins in a low affnity state.
- Chemokines that were produced at the site of injury bind to endothelial cell proteoglycans and are displayed at high concentrations on the endothelial surface. These chemokines bind to and activate the rolling leukocytes. One of the consequences of activation is the conversion of VLA4 and LFA1 ***integrins*** on the leukocytes to a high affinity state.

Table: Endothelial and leukocyte adhesion molecules *(Robbins (SAE) 9th/ 76)*

Family	Molecule	Distribution
Selection	L-selectin (CD62L)	Neutrophils, monocytes T cells (naive and central memory) B cells (naive)
	E-selectin (CD62E)	Endothelium activated by cytokines (TNF, IL-1)
	P-selectin (CD62P)	Endothelium activated by cytokines (INF, IL-1), histamine, or thrombin

Contd...

A & E

Family	Molecule	Distribution
Integrin	LFA-1 (C011aC018) MAC-1 (CD11bCD18) VLA-4 (CD49aCD29) α4b7 (C049DCD29)	Neutrophils, monocytes, T cells (naive, effector, memory) Monocytes, DCs Monocytes T cells (naive effector. memory) Monocytes T cells (gut homing naive effector, memory)
Ig	CD31	Endothelial cells, leukocytes

Chemotaxis of Leukocytes

◈ *Robbins (SAE) 9th/ 77; Harshmohan 7th/120*

- **After exiting the circulation, leukocytes move in the tissues toward the site of injury by a process called *chemotaxis,*** which is defined as locomotion along a chemical gradient. Both exogenous and endogenous substances can act as chemo attractants.
- The most common exogenous agents are *bacterial products*, including peptides that possess an Nformyl methionine terminal amino acid and some lipids.
- Endogenous chemoattractants include several chemical mediators: (1) *cytokines*, particularly those of the chemokine family (e.g., ***IL8***); (2) *components of the complement system, particularly C5a*; and (3) *arachidonic acid (AA) metabolites, mainly leukotriene B4 (LTB4)*.
- ***All these chemotactic agents bind to specific seven transmembrane G protein coupled receptors on the surface of leukocytes.***
- The net result is that leukocytes ***migrate toward the inflammatory stimulus in the direction of the locally produced chemoattractants.***

60. Ans. a. Hallervorden-Spatz disease, b. Abetalipoproteinemia, c. Severe liver disease, e. McLeod syndrome

[Ref: Harshmohan 7th/270; William's Haematology 7th/Chap 44; emedicine.medscape.com]

Acanthocytosis

◈ *William's Haematology 7th/Chap 44*

- Spiculated red cells are classified into two types: acanthocytes and echinocytes.
- *Acanthocytes* are contracted, dense cells with irregular projections from the red cell surface that vary in width and length.
- **Acanthocytes** are present on the blood films of patients with ***severe liver disease, abetalipoproteinemia*(Bassen-Kornzweig Syndrome), *certain inherited neurologic disorders without abetalipoproteinemia and in association with inheritance of certain red cell antigen polymorphisms such as the McLeod phenotype.***
- "The **McLeod syndrome** is an X-linked anomaly of the Kell blood group system characterized by mild compensated hemolytic anemia with variable ***acanthocytosis*** and, in some patients, late-onset myopathy or chorea"- *William's Haematology 7th/Chap 44*
- Smaller numbers of acanthocytes (<10%) may be seen in patients with ***myelodysplasia, hypothyroidism and anorexia nervosa.***

Acanthocytosis

◈ *William's Haematology 7th/Chap 44*

- **Inherited neuroacanthocytosis syndromes** other than chorea-acanthocytosis have been described.
- The syndromes include (1) a recessively inherited syndrome with acanthocytosis, tics, parkinsonism and occasional motor neuron disease; (2) mitochondrial myopathy with encephalopathy, lactic acidosis, strokelike symptoms and acanthocytosis; (3) **Hallervorden-Spatz disease** (progressive dementia, dystonia, spasticity, pallidal and retinal degeneration) with acanthocytosis; and (4) HARP syndrome (*h*ypoprebetalipoproteinemia, *a*canthocytosis, *r*etinitis pigmentosa and *p*allidal degeneration with iron deposition).

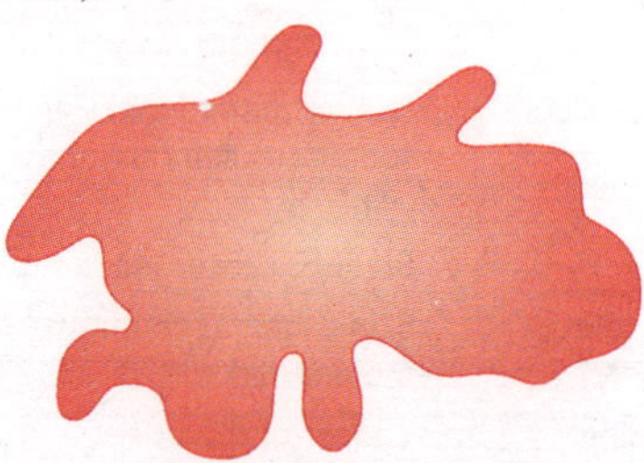

Fig: Acanthocyte *(Harshmohan 7th/270)*

Some of the Common Morphological Abnormalities of Red Cells

◈ *Harshmohan 7th/270*

- *Schistocytosis*: thalassaemia, hereditary elliptocytosis, megloblastic anaemia, iron deficiency anaemia, micro-angiopathic haemolytic anaemia and in severe burns.
- *Leptocytosis*is: severe iron deficiency and thalassaemia.
- *Target cell*: in iron deficiency, thalassaemia, chronic liver disease and after splenectomy.
- *Sickle cells or drepanocytes*: sickle cell disease
- *Acanthocytosis*: ***Splenectomised subjects, chronic liver disease.***
- *Burr cells:* uraemia
- *Stomatocytosis*is: Hereditary stomatocytosis and chronic alcoholism
- *Ovalocytosis or elliptocytosis*is: Hereditary ovalocytosis and elliptocytosis, megaloblastic anaemia and hypochromic anaemia

61. Ans. d. Opisthorchis viverrini, e. Clonorchis sinensis

[Ref: Harrison 19th/552; Davidson 23rd/907; Paniker 7th/144]

"**No association to hepatic malignancy** has been ascribed to fascioliasis (F. hepatica)"-Paniker 7th/153

Paragonimus westermani is lung fluke- *Paniker 7th/157*

Parasite Associated with Malignancy

◈ *Paniker 7th/144*

- *Clonorchis sinensis- Bile duct carcinoma*
- *Opisthorchis viverrini-Bile duct carcinoma*
- **Schistosoma hematobium**- ***bladder carcinoma***

Cholangiocarcinoma (CCC)

◈ *Harrison 19th/552*

- CCC typically refers to mucin-producing adenocarcinomas (different from HCC) that arise from the biliary tract and have features of cholangiocyte differentiation.
- Nodular tumors arising at the bifurcation of the common bile duct are called *Klatskin* tumors and are often associated with a collapsed gallbladder, a finding that mandates visualization of the entire biliary tree.
- **Predisposing diseases** include primary sclerosing cholangitis (10–20% of primary sclerosing cholangitis [PSC] patients), an autoimmune disease and liver fluke in Asians, especially ***Opisthorchis viverrini* and *Clonorchis sinensis***.
- CCC seems also to be associated with any cause of chronic biliary inflammation and injury, with alcoholic liver disease, choledocholithiasis, choledochal cysts (10%) and Caroli's disease (a rare inherited form of bile duct ectasia).
- **Cholangiocarcinoma:** In the Far East, particularly northern Thailand, chronic liver fluke infection (***Clonorchis sinensis***) is a major risk factor for the development of CCA in men-Davidson 23rd//907

62. Ans. b. To count cells and differential count

[Ref: www.med.uottawa.ca; emedicine.medscape.com]

Table: CSF sample collection *(www.med.uottawa.ca)*

Tube	Study
Tube 1	Cell count
Tube 2	Stat gram stain and culture (C+S) (2 cc.)
Tube 3	Glucose and protein
Tube 4	Cell count (for comparison to Tube 1)
Tube 5 (Optional)	Virology, mycology, cytology, etc.

Different institutions have different protocols for the studies performed on the various CSF tubes. **The classic approach is to send the 4 CSF tubes** for the following studies (*emedicine.medscape.com)*:

- ***Tube 1 - Cell count and differential***
- Tube 2 - Glucose and protein levels
- Tube 3 - Gram stain, culture and sensitivity (CandS)
- ***Tube 4 - Cell count and differential (for comparison to tube 1)***

At some institutions, only 3 tubes are sent for analysis and tube 4 is reserved for special studies when indicated. In this approach, the following studies are done (*emedicine.medscape.com*):

- Tube 1 - Protein and glucose levels
- Tube 2 - Gram stain, CandS
- Tube 3 - Cell count and differential

63. Ans. e. Need surgical removal in every case because chances of rupture is high

[Ref: Schwartz 10th/1289-90; Robbins 9th/867; Harrison 19th/553; CSDT 14th/559; Sabiston 19th/1452-53]

"**Pregnant women** and women using estrogen replacement therapy have a ***higher risk*** of developing a large ***hemangioma.*** This is because estrogen may contribute to the growth of liver hemangiomas. Most liver hemangiomas don't require treatment and only need monitoring. However, a hemangioma may need to be removed surgically if it's large and causing symptoms"- *www.mayoclinic.org*

Hemangioma

◈ *Schwartz 10th/1289-90*

- Hemangiomas (also referred to as *hemangiomata*) are the ***most common solid benign masses that occur in the liver***.
- They consist of large endothelial-lined vascular spaces and represent congenital vascular lesions that contain fibrous tissue and small blood vessels that eventually grow.
- They are ***predominantly seen in women*** and occur in 2% to 20% of the population.
- They can range from small (≤1 cm) to giant cavernous hemangiomas (10 to 25 cm). Most hemangiomas are discovered incidentally with little clinical consequence. However, large lesions can cause symptoms as a result of compression of adjacent organs or ***intermittent thrombosis***, which in turn results in further expansion of the lesion.
- **Spontaneous rupture (bleeding) is rare**, but surgical resection can be considered if the patient is symptomatic. Resection can be accomplished by enucleation or formal hepatic resection, depending on the location and involvement of intrahepatic vascular structures and hepatic ducts.
- The majority of hemangiomas can be diagnosed by liver imaging studies. On ***biphasic contrast CT scan***, large hemangiomas show asymmetrical nodular peripheral enhancement that is isodense with large vessels and exhibit progressive centripetal enhancement fill-in over time .
- On ***MRI, hemangiomas*** are hypointense on T1-weighted images and hyperintense on T2-weighted images.With gadolinium enhancement, hemangiomas show a pattern of peripheral nodular enhancement similar to that seen on contrast CT scans. Caution should be exercised in ordering a liver biopsy if the suspected diagnosis is hemangioma because of the risk of bleeding from the biopsy site, especially if the lesion is at the edge of the live

"Hemangiomas are the ***most common and are entirely benign.*** Treatment is unnecessary unless their expansion causes symptoms"- *Harrison 19th/553*

Hemangiomas

◈ *Sabiston 19th/1452-53*

- Rupture, change in size and development of the **Kasabach-Merritt syndrome** are indications for resection.
- In rare cases of diagnostic uncertainty, resection may be necessary to make a definitive diagnosis
- The natural history of liver hemangioma is generally benign and it appears that most of these tumors remain stable over long periods of time with a low risk for rupture or hemorrhage.
- Growth and development of symptoms do occur, ***however, occasionally requiring resection.***

- An asymptomatic patient with a secure diagnosis can therefore be simply observed.
- Symptomatic patients undergo a thorough evaluation, looking for alternative explanations for the symptoms, but are candidates for resection if no other cause is found.
- Rupture, change in size and development of the Kasabach-Merritt syndrome are indications for resection.

Hemangioma

- *CSDT 14th/559*
- ***Hemangioma is the most common benign hepatic tumor***
- **Cavernous hemangiomas, blood vessel tumors identical to those occurring elsewhere, are the most common benign liver tumors**- Robbins 9th/867
- Women are affected more often than men
- Kasabach–Merritt syndrome is usually seen in children and is associated with ***thrombocytopenia and a consumptive coagulopathy***; both of these complications are exceedingly uncommon.
- Fortunately, biopsy is very rarely indicated, since the diagnosis can be made with certainty in most cases by contrast-enhanced CT or MRI scans.
- ***Irrespective of their size, the only reasons to resect hemangiomata are for symptoms***, most commonly pain, or diagnostic uncertainty (rare). Symptomatic hemangiomas should be excised by lobectomy or enucleation. Even large lesions can be safely removed.

64. Ans. b. Mononuclear cell infiltration, c. Apoptosis of hepatocyte, d. Portal tracts Inflammation

[Ref: Robbins (SAE) 9th/ 837-38; Harshmohan 7th/595-97]

- ***Portal tracts Inflammation is less severe in acute hepatitis (scant mononuclear infiltrate)***

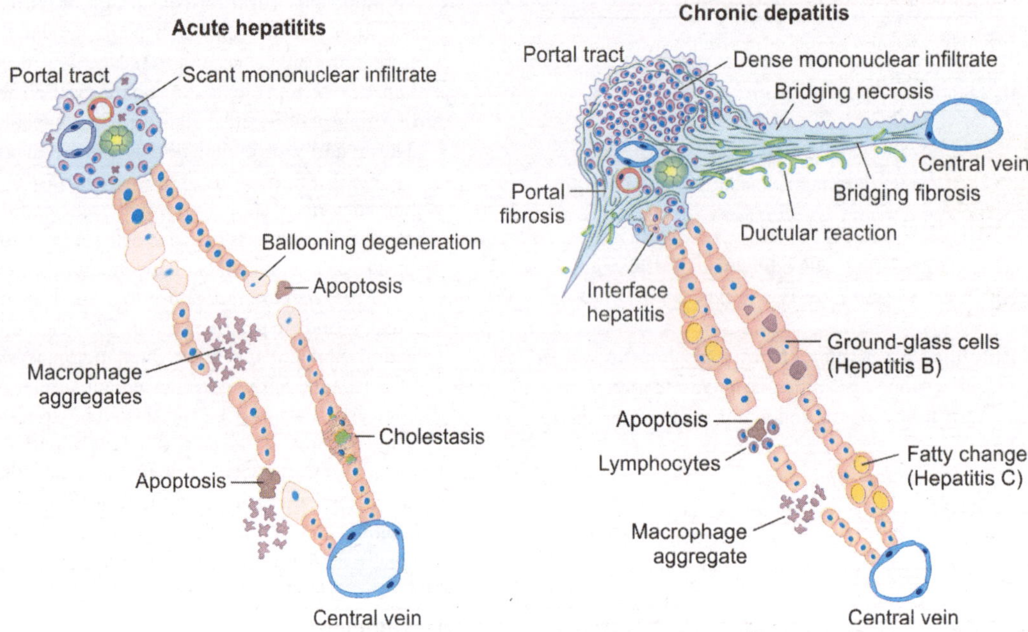

Fig: Morphological feature of acute and chronic hepatitis *Robbins (SAE) 9th/ 838:*

Table: Main morphologic features of acute and chronic viral hepatitis *(Robbins (Basic) 9th/ 613)*

I-acute hepatitis- parenchymal changes (microscopic)
• Hepatocyte injury: swelling (ballooning degeneration) Cholestasis: canalicular bile plugs HCV: mild fatty change of hepatocytes • Hepatocyte necrosis: isolated cells or clusters Cytolysis (rupture) or apoptosis (shrinkage) *If severe*: ***bridging necrosis*** (portal-portal, central-central, portal-central)

Contd...

- Lobular disarray: loss of normal architecture
- Regenerative changes: hepatocyte proliferation
- Sinusoidal cell reactive changes
  Accumulation of phagocytosed cellular debris in Kupffer cells
  Influx of mononuclear cells into sinusoids
- ***Portal tracts Inflammation: predominantly mononuclear***. Inflammatory spillover into adjacent parenchyma, with hepatocyte necrosis

II-Chronic Hepatitis

- Changes shared with acute hepatitis
  Hepatocyte injury, necrosis, apoptosis and regeneration
  Sinusoidal cell reactive changes
- Portal tracts
  - Inflammation Confined to portal tracts, *or* Spillover into adjacent parenchyma, with necrosis of hepatocytes ("***interface hepatitis***"), *or* ***Bridging inflammation and necrosis***
  - Fibrosis
    Portal deposition, *or* Portal and periportal deposition, *or*
    Formation of bridging fibrous septa
- HBV: Ground-glass hepatocytes (accumulation of HBsAg)
- HCV: Bile duct epithelial cell proliferation, lymphoid aggregate formation

Acute and Chronic Hepatitis

◈ *Robbins (Basic) 9th/ 611-13*

- Unlike most other organ systems in which the distinction between acute and chronic inflammation depends on the predominant type of inflammatory cell—neutrophilic in acute injury, mononuclear in chronic phases—***mononuclear infiltrate predominate in all phases of most hepatitic diseases*** because they all invoke T cell–mediated immunity.
- Thus, **the distinction between acute and chronic hepatitis is based on the pattern of cell injury and severity of inflammation, with acute hepatitis often showing less inflammation and more hepatocyte death than chronic hepatitis.**
- ***Portal inflammation in acute hepatitis is minimal or absent***; dense **mononuclear portal infiltrate** of variable prominence are the defining lesion of **chronic hepatitis**.
- There is often **interface hepatitis** as well, distinguished from lobular hepatitis by its location at the interface between hepatocellular parenchyma and portal stroma (or scars, when present). The hallmark of severe chronic liver damage is scarring.

65. Ans. b. Can see both live and dead objects, e. Coloured images are seen

[Ref: Ananthanarayan 10th/12; Jawetz 27th/12-13;Microbiology by Baveja 5th/10-11]

"Gas molecules scatters electrons and it is therefore ***necessary to examine the object in a vaccum.*** Hence, ***only dead and dried objects can be examined*** in the electron microscope"- Ananthanarayan 10th/12

"A major disadvantage is- ***inability to examine living cells.*** A method introduced to overcome this disadvantage is freeze-etching"- *Microbiology by Baveja 5th/11*

Electron Microscopes

◈ *www.jic.ac.uk/microscop*

- Transmission electron microscopes produce two-***dimensional, black and white images.***
- Because the SEM image ***relies on electron interactions at the surface rather than transmission it is able to image bulk samples and has a much greater depth of view*** and so can produce images that are a good representation of the ***3D structure of the sample.***
- SEM images are therefore considered to ***provide us with 3D, topographical information about the sample surface but will still always be only in black and white***

The Electron Microscope

◈ *Jawetz 27th/12-13*

- ***High resolving power***
- The superior resolution of the electron microscope is due to the fact that electrons have a much shorter wavelength than the photons of white light.
- There are two types of electron microscopes in general use: the **transmission electron microscope (TEM),** which has many features in common with the light microscope and the **scanning electron microscope (SEM).**
- The SEM generally has a lower resolving power than the TEM; however, it is ***particularly useful for providing three-dimensional images*** of the surface of microscopic objects.

Table: Electron microscope versus light microscope

Electron Microscope	Light Microscope
Only fixed specimens are studied	Both living and fixed specimens can be studied
It Is very large and complicated	Microscope is compact and handy
Illuminating source is beam of electrons	Illuminating source is light
The objects is ultrathin, 0.1 mm or below	The object is 5 mm or thicker
Only dehydrated specimens are used	The specimen need not be dehydrated
Vacuum is essential for its operation	A vacuum is not required

Contd...

Electron Microscope	Light Microscope
High voltage electric current is required (50,000 volts and above)	There is no need for high voltage electricity
Tungsten filament is used to produce electrons	A filament is not used
It has a cooling system to take out heat generated by high voltage electric current	There is no cooling system
There is risk of radiation leakage	Radiation risk is absent
It employs elecromagnets	Light microscope uses glass lenses
Image is seen only on a fluorescent screen	Image can be seen directly
Specimen is coated with heavy metals in order to reflect electrons	Specimen is stained by coloured dyes
Image black and white	Image is colored
Resolving power is 0.5-5-0 A°, though theoretically it can be 0.25 A°	Resolving power is 0.25 pm or 250 nm (2500A°)
Magnification is up to 300,000	Magnification is up to 4000
Electron microscope is used in the study of external surface (Scanning Electron Microscope SEM), ultra structure of cell and very small organism (Transmission Electron Microscope TEM)	It is used for the study of detailed gross internal structure

66. Ans. a. Dark field

[Ref: Jawetz 27th/11-13; Microbiology by Baveja 5th/10-11]

"In **darkfield microscopy** the condenser is designed to form a hollow cone of light , as apposed to **brightfield microscopy** ***that illuminates the sample with a full cone of light***. In darkfield microscopy, the objective lens sits in the dark hollow of this cone and ***light travels around the objective lens, but does not enter the cone shaped area.*** The entire field of view appears dark when there is no sample on the microscope stage. However, when a sample is placed on the stage it appears bright against a dark background. It is similar to back-lighting an object that may be the same color as the background it sits against - in order to make it stand out"- www.microscopeworld.com

"Inverted microscopes have both the ***light source and condenser set up high above the stage and pointing down toward the stage,*** while the objectives and objective turret are located beneath the stage pointing up. The two basic types of inverted microscopes include biological inverted microscopes and metallurgical inverted microscopes. Biological inverted microscopes are used to observe living cells or organisms at the bottom of a petri dish or tissue"- culture flask"- www.microscopeworld.com

The Light Microscope

◈ *Jawetz 27th/11-13*

- **Several types of light** microscopes are commonly used in microbiology:
  - **Bright-Field Microscope:** The bright-field microscope is most commonly used in microbiology courses and consists of two series of lenses **(objective** and **ocular lens),** which function together to resolve the image. With this microscope, specimens are rendered visible because of the differences in **contrast** between them and the surrounding medium.
  - **Phase Contrast Microscope:** The phase contrast microscope was developed to improve contrast differences between cells and the surrounding medium, ***making it possible to see living cells without staining them;*** with bright-field microscopes, killed and stained preparations must be used. ***The phase contrast microscope takes advantage of the fact that light waves passing through transparent objects, such as cells, emerge in different phases depending on the properties of the materials through which they pass.*** This effect is amplified by a special ring in the objective lens of a phase contrast microscope, leading to the formation of a ***dark image on a light background.***
  - **Dark-Field Microscope:** The dark-field microscope is a light microscope in which the ***lighting system has been modified to reach the specimen from the sides only.*** This is accomplished through the use of a special condenser that both blocks direct light rays and deflects light off a mirror on the side of the condenser at an oblique angle. ***This creates a "dark field" that contrasts against the highlighted edge of the specimens*** and results when the oblique rays are reflected from the edge of the specimen upward into the objective of the microscope. Resolution by dark-field microscopy is quite high. Thus, this technique has been particularly useful for observing organisms such as *Treponema pallidum*
  - **Fluorescence Microscope:** The fluorescence microscope is used to visualize specimens that **fluoresce,** which is the ability to absorb short wavelengths of light (ultraviolet) and give off light at a longer wavelength (visible).
  - Differential Interference Contrast (DIC) Microscope: **Differential interference contrast** microscopes employ a polarizer to produce polarized light.

67. Ans. a. Vitamin K deficiency, b. Factor V deficiency, e. Warfarin administration

[Ref: Robbins 9th/118; Harrison 19th/406]

"The ***prothrombin time*** **(PT) assay** assesses the function of the proteins in the extrinsic pathway (factors ***VII, X, V, II and fibrinogen***). In brief, tissue factor, phospholipids and calcium are added to plasma and the time for a fibrin clot to form is recorded"- Robbins 9th/118

Table: Hemostatic disorders and coagulation test abnormalities *(Harrison 19th/406)*

Prolonged Activated Partial Thromboplastin Time (aPTT)
No clinical bleeding—↓ factor XII, high-molecular-weight kininogen, prekallikrein
Variable, but usually mild, bleeding—↓ factor XI, mild ↓ factor VIII and factor IX
Frequent, severe bleeding—severe deficiencies of factors VIII and IX
Heparin and direct thrombin inhibitors

Contd...

Prolonged Prothrombin Time (PT)

Factor VII deficiency

Vitamin K deficiency—early

Warfarin anticoagulation

Direct Xa inhibitors (rivaroxaban, apixaban)

Prolonged aPTT and PT

Factor II, V, X, or fibrinogen deficiency

Vitamin K deficiency—late

Direct thrombin inhibitors

Prolonged Thrombin Time

Heparin or heparin-like inhibitors

Direct thrombin inhibitors (e.g., dabigatran, argatroban, bivalirudin)

Mild or no bleeding—dysfibrinogenemia

Frequent, severe bleeding—afibrinogenemia

Prolonged PT and/or aPTT Not Corrected with Mixing with Normal Plasma

Bleeding—specific factor inhibitor

No symptoms, or clotting and/or pregnancy loss—lupus anticoagulant

Disseminated intravascular coagulation

Heparin or direct thrombin inhibitor

Abnormal Clot Solubility

Factor XIII deficiency

Inhibitors or defective cross-linking

Rapid Clot Lysis

Deficiency of α2-antiplasmin or plasminogen activator inhibitor

Treatment with fibrinolytic therapy

PHARMACOLOGY

68. Ans. a. Tremor, e. Urinary retention

[Ref: K. D. T 8th/486-87; Katzung 13th/525;Satoskar Pharma 25th/214-15]

- ***TCA adverse effect(s) are- hypotension, weight gain and constipation***

Adverse Effects of TCAs

❖ *KDT 8th/486-87*

- **Anticholinergic:** Dry mouth, bad taste, ***constipation***, epigastric distress, ***urinary retention*** (especially in males with enlarged prostate), blurred vision, palpitation.
- Sedation, mental confusion and weakness, especially with amitriptyline and more sedative congeners.
- Increased appetite and ***weight gain*** is noted with most TCAs and trazodone, but not with SSRIs, SNRIs and bupropion.
- Some patients receiving any antidepressant may abruptly '*switch over*' to a dysphoric-agitated state or tom mania. Most likely, these are cases of bipolar depression, the other pole being unmasked by the antidepressant. Patients receiving higher doses, especially of TCAs, are at greater risk than those receiving lower doses and SSRIs or bupropion.
- Sweating (despite antimuscarinic action) and ***fine tremors*** are relatively common.
- Seizure threshold is lowered– fits may be precipitated, especially in children. Bupropion, clomipramine, amoxapine have greater propensity, while desipramine, SSRIs and SNRIs are safer in this regard
- ***Postural hypotension***, especially in older patients. It is less severe with desipramine- like drugs and insignificant with SSRIs/SNRIs.
- Sexual distress: especially delay or interference with erection, ejaculation and occasionally with orgasm.
- Cardiac arrhythmias
- Rashes and jaundice

"The primary adverse effects of TCAs: **Constipation**, urinary retention, blurred vision and confusion, ***orthostatic hypotension***, **weight gain** and sedation, arrhythmogenic at higher doses (TCAs are also class 1A antiarrhythmic agents)"- *Katzung 13th/525*

69. Ans. a. Dopamine

[Ref: K. D. T 8th/142,146-47;Satoskar Pharma 25th/276,269]

Dopamine: *It is **dopaminergic (D1 and D2) as well as adrenergic α** and β1(but not β2) agonist- K. D. T 8th/146*

KDT 8th/142

Adrenaline (Epinephrine): $\alpha_1 + \alpha_2 + \beta_1 + \beta_2$ and weak β_3 action

Noradrenaline (Norepinephrine): $\alpha_1 + \alpha_2 + \beta_1 + \beta_3$ but no β_2 action

Isoprenaline: $\beta_1 + \beta_2 + \beta_3$ but no α action

Phenylephrine: *It is a selective α_1 agonist with negligible β action- K. D. T 8th/148*

Dobutamine: *A derivative of DA, but a D1 or D2 receptor agonist. Act on both α and β (but relatively selective β1 agonist)- K. D. T 8th/147; Satoskar Pharma 25th/276*

70. Ans. a. ACE inhibitor, c. Alpha blockers

[Ref: K. D. T 8th/155;Davidson 23rd/182;Satoskar Pharma 25th/ 284]

Prazosin (*α blocker*): *Postural hypotension **occur in beginning** causing dizziness and fainting as **first dose effect**-K. D. T 8th/155*

Captopril (ACE inhibitors): *An **initial sharp fall in BP** occurs especially in diuretics treated and CHF patients- K. D. T 8th/531*

Propranolol (β blocker): *There is **little acute change in BP**- K. D. T 8th/159*

"Historically, the **"first dose effect"** with symptomatic orthostatic hypotension and possible syncope, accompanied by tachycardia and palpitations, is probably the most well-known adverse effect of alpha-blocking drugs"- *www.sciencedirect.com*

First-dose Syncope

❖ *en wikipedia.org*

- The **first-dose phenomenon** is a sudden and severe fall in blood pressure that can occur when changing from a lying to a standing position the first time that an ***alpha blocker*** drug is used or when resuming the drug after many months off.
- This postural hypotension usually happens shortly after the first dose is absorbed into the blood and can result in syncope (fainting).

- **Syncope** occurs in approximately 1% of patients given an initial dose of 2 **mg prazosin** or greater. This adverse effect is self-limiting and in most cases does not recur after the initial period of therapy or during subsequent dose titration
- For this reason, treatment with prazosin should always be initiated with a low dose and should be taken at bedtime to avoid standing position.
- The **alpha blocker prazosin** is most notorious for producing a first dose phenomenon. **Other drugs** of the same family, doxazosin and terazosin, can also cause this phenomenon, though less frequently.
- This effect is also observed after the administration of the first dose of drugs in the ***ACEi class (angiotensin-converting enzyme inhibitor).***
- The first dose phenomenon in ACEi is reduced and made safer by avoiding diuretics for 24 hours prior to first dose, taking first dose at night (so avoiding falls, etc) and starting on low doses and titrating upwards.

'First dose' Hypotension and Venodilatation

◈ *bpspubs.onlinelibrary.wiley.com*

- Profound falls in blood pressure may occur in some patients when commencing ***captopril or enalapril.***
- The patients at greatest risk of **'first dose' reactions** when commencing ACE inhibitors are now well recognised and include those with heart failure, hyponatraemia, salt depletion, high renin or aldosterone II levels, those with renovascular or severe hypertension and the elderly
- Similar 'first dose' reactions have been described with ***phentolamine, prazosin, ketanserin, renin inhibitors etc.***
- Although the underlying mechanism was originally assumed to be arterial vasodilatation, often enhanced by bradycardia, recent evidence suggests that venous dilatation may also be important.
- Furthermore, **classical 'first dose' hypotensive reactions*do not occur*** with 'pure' arterial vasodilators such as *nifedipine, felodipine or hydralazine*, in spite of occasionally marked reductions in systemic vascular resistance and blood pressure.

71. Ans. b. Chloramphenicol, e. Aminoglycosides

[Ref: K. D. T 8th/ 785, 7th/734,689-90]

Bacterial Protein Synthesis and Site of Action of Antibiotics

◈ *K. D. T 8th/785, 7th/734*

- **Aminoglycosides** bind to several sites at 30S and 50S subunits as well as to their interface–freeze initiation, interfere with polysome formation and cause misreading of mRNA code.
- **Tetracyclines** bind to 30S ribosome and inhibit aminoacyl tRNA attachment to the 'A' site
- **Chloramphenicol** binds to 50S subunit–interferes with peptide bond formation and transfer of peptide chain from 'P' site.
- **Erythromycin and clindamycin** also bind to 50S ribosome and hinder translocation of the elongated peptide chain back from 'A' site to 'P' site and the ribosome does not move along the mRNA to expose the next codon. Peptide synthesis may be prematurely terminated

Mechanism of Action of Drugs

◈ *KDT 7th/689-90; Katzung 12th/803*

- **Inhibit cell wall synthesis:** Penicillins, Cephalosporins, Cycloserine, Vancomycin, Bacitracin.
- **Cause leakage from cell membranes:** Polypeptides Polymyxins, Colistin, Bacitracin. Polyenes-Amphotericin B, Nystatin, Hamycin.
- **Inhibit protein synthesis:** Tetracyclines, Chloramphenicol, Erythromycin, Clindamycin, Linezolid.
- **Cause misreading of m-RNA code and affect permeability: Aminoglycosides**-Streptomycin, Gentamicin, etc.
- **Inhibit DNA gyrase:** Fluoroquinolones-Ciprofloxacin and others.
- **Interfere with DNA function:** Rifampin.
- **Interfere with DNA synthesis:** Acyclovir, Zidovudine.
- **Interfere with intermediary metabolism:** Sulfonamides, Sulfones, PAS, Trimethoprim, Pyrimethamine, Metronidazole

72. Ans. a. Cholera, b. Traveller's diarrhoea, d. Bacillary dysentery

[Ref: OP Ghai 8th/296; Satoskar Pharma 25th/607]

"**Antibiotics** *are not recommended for routine treatment of acute diarrhea in children. In acute diarrhea antimicrobial are indicated in* ***bacillary dysentery, cholera, amoebiasis and giardiasis****. Escherichia coli are normal gut flora and their growth on stool culture is not an indication for antibiotics" -O.P. Ghai 8th/296*

"If the patient's clinical presentation suggests the possibility of **Shiga toxin–producing *E. coli*** (e.g., bloody diarrhea, history of eating seed sprouts or rare ground beef, proximity to an outbreak), ***antibiotic use should be avoided*** because it may increase the risk of hemolytic uremic syndrome"-*www.aafp.org*

"The bacteria causing **bacillary dysentery** *are-shigella species, Enterotoxigenic and Enterohemorrhagic E. Coli, salmonella and Campylobacter jejuni"- OP Ghai 8th/297*

Traveller's diarrhea *can be either simple diarrhea or dysentery- Satoskar Pharma 25th/608*

Traveller's diarrhea: *Enterotoxigenic E. Coli* *causes traveller's diarrhea-Ananthanarayan 10th/285*

Enterohemorrhagic E. Coli *produces two potent toxins, verocytotoxin (VT) or* ***Shiga-like toxin (SLT)****. They can give rise to diarrhea ranging in severity from mild diarrhea to fatal hemorrhagic colitis and hemorrhagic uremic syndrome (HUS)-Ananthanarayan 10th/286*

Antibiotic Therapy

◈ *www.aafp.org*

- Because acute diarrhea is most often self-limited and caused by viruses, routine antibiotic use is not recommended for most adults with non severe, watery diarrhea.
- Additionally, the **overuse of antibiotics** can lead to resistance (e.g., *Campylobacter*), harmful eradication of normal flora, prolongation of illness (e.g., super infection

with *C. difficile*), prolongation of carrier state (e.g., delayed excretion of *Salmonella*), induction of Shiga toxins (e.g., from Shiga toxin–producing *E. coli*) and increased cost

- However, when used appropriately, **antibiotics are effective** for ***shigellosis, campylobacteriosis, C. difficile, traveler's diarrhea and protozoal infections.***
- **Antibiotic treatment of traveler's diarrhea** (usually a quinolone) is associated with decreased severity of illness and a two-or three-day reduction in duration of illness.
- Conservative management without antibiotic treatment is less successful for diarrhea lasting more than 10 to 14 days and testing and treatment for protozoal infections should be considered.

73. Ans. b. Amphotericin B, d. Posaconazole

[Ref: Harrison 19th/1350-54; K. D. T 8th/841; Şatoskar Pharma 25th/716]

Fluconazole *is* ***not active*** *against mucormycosis-Satoskar Pharma 25th/716*

Mucormycosis

- Fungi of the order Mucorales belong to seven medically relevant families, all of which can cause mucormycosis. Among the Mucorales, *Rhizopusoryzae* (in the family Mucoraceae) is by far the most common cause of infection in the Western Hemisphere- Harrison 19th/1353
- **Fluconazole is not effective** for the treatment of aspergillosis, ***mucormycosis***, or *scedosporium apiospermum ear infections*- Harrison 19th/1330
- **Amphotericin B** (AmB) deoxycholate remains the ***only licensed antifungal agent for the treatment of mucormycosis.*** However, lipid formulations of AmB are significantly less nephrotoxic, can be administered at higher doses and are probably more effective than AmB deoxycholate for this purpose- Harrison 19th/1352
- ***Posaconazole is the only FDA-approved azole with in vitro activity against the Mucorales.***

Table: Choice of drugs for systemic mycoses *(KDT 8th/841)*

Disease	Drugs	
	1st Choice	2nd choice
• Candidiasis oral/vaginal/ cutaneous deep/invasive	FLU/NYS/CLO AMB/VORI	ITR FLU/CAS/POSA
• Cryptococcosis	AMB ± 5-FC	FLU
• Histoplasmosis	ITR/AMB	FLU
• Coccidioidomycosis	AMB/FLU	ITR
• Blastomycosis	ITR/AMB	FLU
• Sporotrichosis (disseminated)	AMB	ITR
• Paracoccidiodomycosis	ITR	AMB
• Aspergillosis	VORI/AMB	ITR/CAS/POSA
• Mucormycosis	AMB	POSA
• Chromomycosis	ITR	TER/POSA

Abbreviation: AMB–Amphotericin, B; 5-FC–Flucytosine; KTZ–Ketoconazole; FLU–Fluconazole; ITR– Itraconazole; NYS–Nystatin; CLO– Clotrimazole; VORI–Voriconazole; CAS–Caspofungin; POSA–Posaconazole; TER–Terbinafine

74. Ans. b. Prasugrel, c. Cloipidogrel, e. Ticagrelor

[Ref: K. D. T 8th/677-79; Satoskar Pharma 25th/486]

ADP receptor (P_2Y_{12}) antagonistsprevents activation of platelets, their recruitment to the site of injury and aggregation- *Satoskar Pharma 25th/486*

Antiplatelet Agents Classification

◈ *K. D. T 8th/677; Satoskar Pharma 25th/486;www.drugbank.ca*

- **Prostacyclin PGI_2**
- **Inhibitors of TXA_2 formation,** e.g. aspirin
- **ADP receptor (P_2Y_{12}) antagonists,** e.g. clopidogrel, prasugrel, ticagrelor, Ticlopidine, Cangrelor
- **Phosphodiesterase inhibitors,** e.g. dipyridamole
- **Glycoprotein IIb/IIIa antagonists,** e.g. abciximab
- **Protease activated receptor (PAR-1) antagonist,** e.g. vorapaxar

"Cangrelor is an intravenous, direct-acting, reversible P2Y12 inhibitor for patients undergoing percutaneous coronary intervention (PCI) who have not been yet treated by oral P2Y12 inhibitors. An advantage Cangrelor provides **over oral P2Y12 inhibitors** (such as ***prasugrel, ticagrelor and clopidogrel)*** is that it is an active drug not requiring metabolic conversion therefore providing a rapid onset and offset of action. Cangrelor was approved by the FDA in June 2015 for intravenous application"- *www.drugbank.ca*

75. Ans. a. Acetazolamide, b. Topiramate

[Ref: K. D. T 8th/624; Satoskar Pharma 25th/560]

"Topiramate: weak **carbonic anhydrase inhibitor** with antiepileptic property"-*K. D. T 8th/624; Satoskar Pharma 25th/560*

Classification of Diuretics

◈ *K. D. T 8th/624, 7th/579*

- High efficacy diuretics (Inhibitors of Na^+- K^+-$2Cl^-$ Cotransport): Furosemide, ***Bumetanide***, Torasemide
- Medium efficacy diuretics (Inhibitors of Na^+-Cl^-symport)
  - Benzothiadiazines (**thiazides**): Hydrochlorothiazide, Benzthiazide, Hydroflumethiazide, Bendroflumethiazide
  - Thiazide like (related heterocyclics): Chlorthalidone, Metolazone, Xipamide, Indapamide, Clopamide
- Weak or adjunctive diuretics
  - **Carbonic anhydrase inhibitors**: ***Acetazolamide***
  - Potassium sparing diuretics
    - *Aldosterone antagonist:* ***Spironolactone***, Eplerenone
    - *Inhibitors of renal epithelial Na+ channel:* Triamterene, Amiloride.
  - *Osmotic diuretics*: Mannitol, Isosorbide, glycerol

Carbonic Anhydrase Inhibitors (Antiglaucoma)

◈ *reference.medscape.com*

- *acetazolamide*
- *Azopt*
- *brinzolamide*
- *Diamox Sequels*
- *dorzolamide*

- *methazolamide*
- *Neptazane*
- *Trusopt*

76. Ans. a. Terbutaline, c. Salbutamol

[Ref: K. D. T 8th/242-43, 7th/222; Harrison 19th/1676-79; Satoskar Pharma 25th/ 374-75]

Ipratropium bromide: *It is **not recommended for acute attack**. It has slow onset of action (30 min) and lower efficacy than $\beta_2$agonists in the management of acute attack- Satoskar Pharma 25th/ 376*

Drug therapy During an Acute Attack

◈ *Satoskar Pharma 25th/ 374-75*

- ***Salbutamol***
- Levosalbutamol
- ***Terbutaline***, fenoterol, bitolterol

Drugs for prevention of acute attack (Maintenance therapy) *Satoskar Pharma 25th/ 377-78*

- *Inhaled long-acting B agonist e.g, salmeterol, **formoterol***
- *Inhaled glucocorticoids (beclomethasone, **budesonide** and fluticasone)*
- Oral theophylline
- Oral leukotriene modifier

"**Theophylline** is the most effective bronchodilator and it has been shown repeatedly both to relieve airflow obstruction in **acute asthma** and to reduce the severity of symptoms and time lost from work or school in patients with chronic asthma"- Katzung 11th/346

77. Ans. a. Acyclovir, b. Oseltemavir, c. Valganciclovir, d. Valaciclovir, e. Ganciclovir

[Ref: K. D. T 7th/800; Satoskar Pharma 25th/809]

Acyclovir-*Prodrug*

◈ *K. D. T 7th/23*

Valacyclovir: Ester ***prodrug of acyclovir***- *K. D. T 7th/800*

Valganciclovir-*prodrug* - *K. D. T 7th/801*

Valganciclovir is an orally bioavailable ***prodrug*** that is rapidly metabolized to ganciclovir in intestinal tissues and the liver- Harrison 19th/1193;*Satoskar Pharma 25th/810*

Oseltamivir-prodrug *of oseltamivir carboxylate- Satoskar Pharma 25th/811*

Oseltamivir phosphate is an ethyl ester ***prodrug*** that is converted to oseltamivir carboxylate by esterases in the liver- Harrison 19th/215e-1

Ganciclovir is activated intracellularly- K. D. T 7th/801

Ganciclovir (GCV) is a guanosine analog ***used as a prodrug*** to obtain a suicide effect in cells transfected with the herpes virus thymidine kinase gene (HSV-tk). Ganciclovir is approved by the FDA for the treatment of cytomegalovirus (CMV) infections"- www.invivogen.com

Famciclovir-prodrug of penciclovir-*Satoskar Pharma 25th/809*

A & E

78. Ans. a. Constant fraction of drug is eliminated per unit time, c. As concentration of drugs increases, rate of elimination increases

[Ref: K. D. T 8th/38-39, 7th/30-31; Satoskar Pharma 24th/22-23]

First Order Kinetic

◈ *K. D. T 8th/38-40, 7th/30-31*

- The **rate of elimination** is ***directly proportional to the drug concentration, CL (clearance) remain constant;*** or a ***constant fraction of the drug present in the body is-eliminated in unit time***
- This ***applied to majority of drugs*** which do not saturate the elimination processes (transporters, enzymes, blood flow etc.) over the therapeutic concentration range
- However, if the dose is high enough, elimination pathways of all drugs will get saturated
- ***T1/2 remain constant*** because V (volume of distribution) and ***CL (clearance) do not change with dose***

Zero Order Kinetic

◈ *K. D. T 8th/38-39, 7th/31*

- ***Few drugs*** normally saturate eliminating mechanisms and handled by zero order kinetics
- The ***rate of elimination remain constant irrespective of the drug concentration***, CL decreases with increase in concentration; or a *constant amount is eliminated in unit time*

79. Ans. a. Abiraterone, c. Ketoconazole, d. Finasteride

Antiandrogens

◈ *Satoskar Pharma 25th/978*

- Any compound which antagonizes or interferes with the action of androgens at the tissue level is referred to as an antiandrogen. **Estrogens** and **potent progestins** such as medroxyprogesterone block the synthesis of androgens by their central gonadotropin inhibiting action and thus act as antiandrogen.
- Drugs which act as antiandrogens are:
- **Steroid synthesis inhibitors: *Ketoconazol***e; relatively toxic in the doses needed and hence not used
- **5-Alpha-reductase inhibitors: *Finasteride***
- **Noncompetitive androgen receptor antagonists:** Cyptoterone
- **Competitive androgen receptor antagonists:** Flutamide and spironolactone

"**Abiraterone acetate** is converted in vivo to abiraterone, an ***androgen biosynthesis inhibitor***, that inhibits 17 a-hydroxylase/ C17,20-lyase (CYP17). This enzyme is expressed in testicular, adrenal and prostatic tumor tissues and is required for androgen biosynthesis"-www.centerwatch.com; Katzung 13th/ 720

"**Danazol,** an isoxazole derivative of ethisterone with weak progestational a***ndrogenic*** and glucocorticoid activities, is used to suppress ovarian function. Danazol inhibits the midcycle surge of LH and FSH. Danazol binds to androgen, progesterone and glucocorticoid receptors and can translocate the androgen receptor into the nucleus to initiate androgen-specific RNA synthesis"- Katzung 13th/ 720

Anastrozole, a selective nonsteroidal ***inhibitor of aromatase*** (the enzyme required for estrogen synthesis, is effective in some women whose breast tumors have become resistant to tamoxifen- *Katzung 13th/ 720*

80. Ans. c. Extensively drug resistance (XDR-TB)

[Ref: Park 24th/189;Suryakantha Community Medicine 4th/389;K. D. T 8th/824, 7th/775-76]

- ***This patient is resistance to: 3 first line drug, 1 fluoroquinoloneand one of three second-line injectable drugs. So he belongs to Extensively drug resistance (XDR-TB) category***

TB Resistance Category

◈ *Park 24th/189; K. D. T 8th/824*

- **Monoresistance:** Resistance to one first-line anti-TB drug but not R-resistant
- **Polydrug resistance:** Resistance to more than one first-line anti-TB drug (other than both isoniazid and rifampicin)
- **Multidrug resistance (MDR-TB):** Resistance to ***at least both isoniazid and rifampicin***
- **Extensive drug resistance (XDR-TB):** ***Resistance to any fluoroquinolone and at least one of three second-line injectable drugs (capreomycin, kanamycin and amikacin), in addition to multidrug resistance***
- **Rifampicin resistance:** Resistance to rifampicin detected using phenotypic or genotypic methods, with or without resistance to other anti-TB drugs. It includes any resistance to rifampicin, whether monoresistance, multidrug resistance, polydrug resistance or extensive drug resistance
  - These categories are not all mutually exclusive. When enumerating rifampicin-resistant TB (RR-TB), for instance, multidrug-resistant TB (MDR-TB) and extensively drug-resistant TB (XDR-TB) are also included.
  - While it has been the practice until now to limit the definitions of monoresistance and polydrug resistance to first-line drugs only, future drug regimens may make it important to classify patients by their strain resistance patterns to fluoroquinolones, second-line injectable agents and any other anti-TB drug for which reliable DST becomes available

81. Ans. c. High dose isoniazid, d. Clofazimine

[Ref: http:apps.who.int; Park 24th/199-200; Suryakantha Community Medicine 4th/390]

In 2016, WHO published two regimen- ***short (9-12 month)*** *and* ***long (conventional)*** *regimen for MDR-TB. The* ***question is asking for drugs of intensive phase of short regimen***

"2016 WHO guidelines: The shorter MDR-TB regimen recommended by the WHO consists of a **4–6-month intensive phase** with ***kanamycin, moxifloxacin, ethionamide, clofazimine, pyrazinamide, high-dose isoniazid, ethambutol*** and a 5-month continuation phase with moxifloxacin, clofazimine, pyrazinamide and ethambutol"-*www.ncbi.nlm.nih.gov*

2016 WHO Guidelines for MDR TB

◈ *apps.who.int*

- **Shorter MDR-TB regimen for adults and children** In patients with RR-TB or MDR-TB who were not previously treated with second-line drugs and in whom resistance to fluoroquinolones and second-line injectable agents was excluded or is considered highly unlikely, **a *shorter MDR-TB regimen of 9–12 months*** may be used ***instead of the longer regimens*** (conditional recommendation, very low certainty in the evidence).
- **Longer MDR-TB regimens for adults and children** (2a) In **patients with RR-TB or MDR-TB**, a regimen with at least five effective TB medicines during the intensive phase is recommended, including pyrazinamide and four core second-line TB medicines – one chosen from Group A, one from Group B and at least two from Group C2 (conditional recommendation, very low certainty in the evidence). If the minimum number of effective TB medicines cannot be composed as given above, an agent from Group D2 (***bedaquiline, delamanid***) and other agents from Group D3 may be added to bring the total to five **(2b) Inpatients with RR-TB or MDR-TB,** it is recommended that the regimen be further strengthened with high-dose isoniazid and/or ethambutol (conditional recommendation, very low certainty in the evidence). It is recommended that any patient – child or adult – with RR-TB in whom isoniazid resistance is absent or unknown be treated with a recommended MDR-TB regimen. It could either be a shorter MDR-TB regimen, or a longer MDR-TB regimen to which isoniazid is added. As a result of the update, the grouping of medicines used in the treatment of MDR/RR-TB has been revised from the one used in the last guidance to reflect the updated evidence on the efficacy and safety of the different agents. This reclassification of medicines has a bearing on the choice of medicines when users design longer, individualized regimens for patients withdrug-resistant TB. There is no change in the recommended use of bedaquiline and delamanid from those defined by the WHO interim guidance. These two new medicines now occupy a unique subgroup within the add-on agents used to treat MDR/RR-TB.
- **Surgical interventions in patients with MDR-TB**: In patients with RR-TB or MDR-TB patients, elective partial lung resection (lobectomy or wedge resection) may be used alongside a recommended MDR-TB regimen (conditional recommendation, very low certainty in the evidence).

Group A = levofloxacin, moxifloxacin, gatifloxacin;

Group B = amikacin, capreomycin, kanamycin, (streptomycin);

Group C = ethionamide (or prothionamide), cycloserine (or terizidone), linezolid, clofazimine; in children with nonsevere disease Group B medicines may be excluded (see guidelines text for how disease severity was assessed).

Group D = Pyrazinamide, ethambutol, high dose INH

Group D2 = bedaquiline, delamanid;

Group D3 = p-aminosalicylic acid, imipenem–cilastatin, meropenem, amoxicillin clavulanate, (thioacetazone). Bedaquiline is only recommended for adults; delamanid may also be used in patients aged 6–17 years.

Main changes to the who policy recommendations for the treatment of drug-resistant TB

The main changes in the 2016 recommendations are as follows:

- A shorter MDR-TB treatment regimen is recommended under specific conditions.
- Medicines used in the design of longer MDR-TB treatment regimens are now regrouped differently based upon current evidence on their effectiveness and safety. Clofazimine and linezolid are now recommended as core second-line medicines in the MDR-TB regimen while p-aminosalicylic acid is an add-on agent.
- MDR-TB treatment is recommended for all patients with RR-TB, regardless of confirmation of isoniazid resistance.
- Specific recommendations are made on the treatment of children with RR-TB or MDR-TB.
- Clarithromycin and other macrolides are no longer included among the medicines to be used for the treatment of MDR/RR-TB.
- Evidence-informed recommendations on the role of surgery are now included.

(**Bedaquiline and delamanid** have now been assigned to **a *specific subgroup of add-on agents.*** In October 2016, WHO published its new policy on delamanid. Delamanid may now also be used alongside longer MDR-TB regimens in patients aged 6–17 years. Bedaquiline is still only recommended for adults)

82. Ans. **a. Increased stroke volume, b. Decreased systemic vascular resistance, d. Renal vasodilation, e. Increased heart rate**

[Ref: K. D. T 7th/134; Satoskar Pharma 25th/276; Morgan 5th/247]

- **Increased systemic vascular resistance** occurs with high dose((**10-20 μg/kg /min), *when α_1 effect become prominent***

At large dose (10-20 μg/kg /min), α_1 effect become prominent causing ***increase in peripheral vascular resistance-*** *Morgan 5th/247*

Table: Pharmacological Effects of Dopamine *(Satoskar Pharma 25th/276; Morgan 5th/247)*

Dose (by infusion mcg/kg/min)	Effects
2-5 (Dopaminergic range)	Renal, mesenteric and cerebral vasodilation by action on dopamine (D_1) receptors
5-10 (Dopaminergic + β_1 range)	Same as above plus increase in myocardial contractility with ***increase in heart rate and cardiac output***, by action on dopamine and b_1 receptors. This is of advantage in the treatment of shock. ***The peripheral resistance is lowered or unchanged.***
11-20 (β_1 range)	Predominantly cardiac action
More than 20 (α_1 range)	***Vasoconstriction***, decrease in renal blood flow and urine output and sometimes aggravation of heart failure, by action on α_1 adrenergic receptors

Dopamine (DA)

◈ *K. D. T 8th/146,7th/134*

- It is a dopaminergic (D1 and D2) as well as adrenergic α and b_1 (but not b_2) agonist.
- The D1 receptors in renal and mesenteric blood vessels are the most sensitive: IV infusion of **low dose of DA** dilates these vessels (by raising intracellular cAMP). This increases g.f.r. in addition DA exerts natriuretic effect by D1 receptors on proximal tubular cells.
- **Moderately high doses** produce a positive inotropic (direct b_1 and D1 action + that due to NA release), but little chronotropic effect on heart.
- ***Vasoconstriction (α_1 action)*** occurs only when **large doses** are infused.
- At doses normally employed, it raises cardiac output and systolic BP with little effect on diastolic BP. It has practically no effect on nonvascular α and β receptors; does not penetrate blood-brain barrier– no CNS effects
- Dopamine is used in patients of cardiogenic or septic shock and severe CHF wherein it increases BP and urine outflow.
- It is administered by IV infusion (0.2–1 mg/min) which is regulated by monitoring BP and rate of urine formation

83. Ans. **c. Amikacin, e. Atropine**

[Ref: K. D. T 8th/ 120-22; Harrison 19th/2702-06; Satoskar Pharma 25th/298]

"Myasthenia Gravis (MG): Aminoglycosides (amikacin, gentamicin, kanamycin, ***neomycin,*** streptomycin, tobramycin) should be avoided because they can cause neuromuscular weakness"-*www.myastheniagravis.org*

"Atropine is contra-indicated in myasthenia gravis (except to reduce muscarinic side-effects of anticholinesterases)"-*www.medicines.org.uk*

Anticholinesterase Medications for MG

◈ *Harrison 19th/2704; K. D. T 8th/ 120*

- Pyridostigmine and ***Neostigmine*** areused
- In some patients, muscarinic side effects of the anti-cholinesterase drugs medication (diarrhea, abdominal cramps, salivation, nausea) may limit the dose tolerated.
- Atropine/diphenoxylateor loperamide is useful for the treatment of GI symptoms.

Anticholinesterase Test

◈ *Harrison 19th/2702*

- Drugs that inhibit the enzyme AChE allow ACh to interact repeatedly with the limited number of AChRs in MG, producing improvement in muscle strength.
- **Edrophonium** is used most commonly for diagnostic testing
- An initial IV dose of 2 mg of edrophonium is given. If definite improvement occurs, the test is considered positive and is terminated.

Drugs to Avoid in Myasthenic Patients

◈ *Harrison 19th/2706*

- Many drugs have been reported to exacerbate weakness in patients with MG, but not all patients react adversely to all of these.

- Conversely, not all "safe" drugs can be used with impunity in patients with MG. As a rule, the listed drugs should be avoided *whenever possible* and myasthenic patients should be followed closely when *any new drug* is introduced.

Table: Drugs with Interactions in Myasthenia Gravis (MG) *(Harrison 19th/2706)*

I-Drugs that May Exacerbate MG
Antibiotics
• Aminoglycosides: e.g., streptomycin, tobramycin, kanamycin
• Quinolones: e.g., ciprofloxacin, levofloxacin, ofloxacin, gatifloxacin
• Macrolides: e.g., erythromycin, azithromycin
Nondepolarizing Muscle Relaxants for Surgery
• d-Tubocurarine (curare), pancuronium, vecuronium, atracurium
Beta-blocking Agents
• Propranolol, atenolol, metoprolol
Local Anesthetics and Related Agents
• Procaine, Xylocaine in large amounts
• Procainamide (for arrhythmias)
Botulinum Toxin
• Botox exacerbates weakness
Quinine Derivatives
• Quinine, quinidine, chloroquine, mefloquine (Lariam)
Magnesium
• Decreases acetylcholine release
Penicillamine
• May cause MG
II_Drugs with Important Interactions in MG
Cyclosporine
• Broad range of drug interactions, which may raise or lower cyclosporine levels.
Azathioprine
• Avoid allopurinol—combination may result in myelosuppression.

84. Ans. c. Phenytoin

[Ref: K. D. T 7th/414; Harrison 19th/2548; Satoskar Pharma 25th/133]

Mechanisms of Action of Antiepileptic Drugs

◈ *Harrison 19th/2548*

- Antiepileptic drugs appear to act primarily by blocking the initiation or spread of seizures. This occurs through a variety of mechanisms that modify the activity of ion channels or neurotransmitters and in most cases, the drugs have pleiotropic effects.
- The mechanisms include inhibition of **Na^+-dependent action potentials** in a frequency-dependent manner (e.g., ***phenytoin, carbamazepine, lamotrigine, topiramate, zonisamide, lacosamide, rufinamide***), **inhibition of voltage-gated Ca^{2+} channels** (phenytoin, gabapentin, pregabalin), **facilitating the opening of potassium channels** (***ezogabine***), **attenuation of glutamate activity** (lamotrigine, topiramate, **felbamate**), **potentiation of GABA receptor function** (*benzodiazepines and barbiturates*), **increase in the availability of GABA** (valproic acid, gabapentin, tiagabine) **and modulation of release of synaptic vesicles** (***levetiracetam***).
- The two most effective drugs for absence seizures, ***ethosuximide*** and valproic acid, probably act by inhibiting T-type Ca^{2+} channels in thalamic neurons

Table: Major mechanisms of anticonvulsant action *(K. D. T 7th/414)*

Prolongation of Na^+ channel inactivation	Facilitation of GABA mediated Cl^- channel opening	Inhibition of 'T' type Ca^{2+} current
Phenytoin	Barbiturate	Ethosuximide
Carbamazepine	Benzodiazepine	Valproate
Valproate	Vigabatrin	Zonisamide
Lamotrigine	Valproate	
Topiramate	Gabapentin	
Zonisamide	Tiagabine	
Lacosamide		

Classification of AEDs according to their mechanism of action (*Satoskar Pharma 25th/133)*

- **Decrease in the neuronal excitability by delaying the recovery of inactivated Na^+ channels:** ***Phenytoin***, carbamazepine, lamotrigine, topiramate
- **Decrease in the low threshold calcium currents (T-current) in the thalamic neurons:** Ethosuximide
- **Action similar to both phenytoin and ethosuximide as mentioned earlier:** Sodium valproate, zonisamide
- Enhancement of inhibition through GABA:
  - Acting through GABA-related receptors: Barbiturates and benzodiazepines
  - By releasing GABA from neuronal endings: Gabapentin
  - By inhibiting GABA transaminase: Sodium valproate and vigabatrin
  - By inhibiting neuronal reuptake of GABA: Tiagabine
- **Decrease release of excitatory neurotransmitter glutamate:** Lamotrigine
- **Miscellaneous:** Levetiracetam and acetazolamide

Note: A given drug may act through multiple mechanisms

MICROBIOLOGY

85. Ans. a. Serum sickness; b. Arthus reaction; d. Farmer's lung

[Ref: Ananthanarayan 9th/162-67; Robbins 9th/201; Jawetz 27th/145-46; Greenwood 16th/144]

Farmer's lung is a type of arthus reaction*- Ananthanarayan 10th/168*

***Erythroblastosis fetalis** (Hemolytic anaemia) & **Goodpasteur's syndrome** are type II **Hypersensitivity Reactions**- Davidson 22nd/88*

Type 3 Hypersensitivity Reaction (Immune-Complex Disease)

◈ *Ananthanarayan 9th/162*

- *It is two types-**arthus reaction & serum sickness***
- *Here the damage is caused by antigen-antibody complexes.*

These may precipitate in & around small blood vessels causing damage to cells secondarily, or on membranes, interfering with their function

Table: Mechanism of Hypersensitivity Reactions *(Robbins 9th/201)*

Type	Immune Mechanisms	Histopathological Lesions	Prototypical Disorders
Immediate (type I) hypersensitivity	Production of IgE → antibody immediate release of vasoactive amines and other mediators from mast cells; later recruitment of inflammatory cells	Vascular dilation, edema, smooth muscle contraction, mucus production, tissue injury, inflammation	Anaphylaxis: allergies; bronchial asthma (atopic forms)
Antibody-mediated type (II) hypersensitivity	Production of IgG, IgM → binds to antigen on target cell or tissue → phagocytosis or lysis of target cell by activated complement or Fc receptors; recruitment of leukocytes	Phagocytosis and lysis of cells: Inflammation; in some diseases, functional derangements without cell or tissue injury	Autoimmune hemolytic anemia; Good pasture syndrome
Immune complex-mediated (type III) hypersensitivity	Deposition of antigen-antibody complexes → complement activation → recruitment of leukocytes by complement products and Fc receptors → release of enzymes and other toxic molecules	Inflammation, necrotizing vasculitis (fibrinoid necrosis)	Systemic lupus erythematosus; some forms of glomerulonephritis; serum sickness; Arthus reaction
Cell-mediated (type IV) hypersensitivity	Activated T lymphocytes → (1) release of cytokines, inflammation and macrophage activation: (2) T: cell-mediated cytotoxicity	Perivascular cellular infiltrates: edema: granuloma formation: cell destruction	Contact dermatitis: multiple sclerosis: type 1 diabetes tuberculosis

Type I Hypersensitivity (IgE)	Type II hypersensitivity (IgG&IgM) Cytotoxic, complement medicated lysis
Includes: • Local: Eczema, Hay fever, Asthma (Atopy) • Systemic: Anaphylaxis	**Includes:** • Complement mediated lysis • Antibody dependent cell mediated toxicity (formerly classified as type I) • Changes in cellular function (former type V) • Increased function: Grave's disease. • Decreased function: M. Gravis. • Phagocytosis.

Contd...

• **Examples** • Theoblad Smith Phenomenon: This is anaphylaxis in guinea pigs. • PK reaction (Prusnitz Kunster) • Demonstrate that IgE is	• **Examples Includes:** • Those with Ag on RBC. • Blood transfusion reaction. • Hemolytic aneamia e.g. with I.M. and mycoplasma • Those with Ag on Neutrophils: • Agranulocytosis
• homocytotropici.g. specific. • Casoni's test: Immediate type (IgE) H.S	• Those with Ag on platelets: e.g. ITP. • T-hose with Ag on basement membrane: Good pasture's
Type III Immune complex (IgG)	**Type IV Delayed hypersensitivity (cellular immunity)**
Includes: • Local Arthus reaction • Systemic: serum sickness. • Examples: • Shick's test. • Post streptococcal G.N. • Detected by RAJI Assay.	**Includes:** • Tuberculin test • Lepromin test • Contact dermatitis • Jones-Mote reaction (cutaneous basophilic hypersensitivity). • Graft rejection (Chronic).

86. Ans. a. Mycobacterium leprae; c. Rhinosporidium seeberi; d. Pneumocystis jirovecii

[Ref: Ananthanarayan 10th/352;Dhingra 7th/178; Baveja 5th/284;Jawetz 27th/319]

M. leprae: *non-cultivable in vitro*

◈ *Ananthanarayan 10th/352*

M. leprae ***has not be cultivated*** *on non-living bacteriological media"-Jawetz 27th/319*

Mycobacterium leprae has never been cultured in vitro- *Ballenger's Otorhinolaryngology 16th/646*

"**Rhinosporidium seeberi** has ***not been cultivated in artificial culture media***"- *Ananthanarayan 10th/352*

Rhinosporidium seeberi has ***not been possible to culture*** *or transfer the disease to experimental animals- Dhingra 7th/178*

"**Pneumocystis jirovecii-** ***It can not be cultured***"- *Ananthanarayan 10th/618*

"**Rhinoscleroma:** Causative organism **Klebsiella rhinoscleromatis** or Frisch bacillus ***can be cultured*** from the biopsy material"- *Dhingra 7th/175*

Aeromonas hydrophila*: It grow well on nutrient agar, blood agar, MacConky agar, DCA& TCBS agar- Baveja 5th/284*

87. Ans. a. Malaria; b. Dengue; c. Plague; d. Kyasanur forest disease

[Ref: Ananthanarayan 10th/74;Park 24th/102,805]

Table: Arthropod-borne disease *(Park 24th/805)*

Arthropod	Diseases transmitted
1. Mosquito	***Malaria***, filaria, viral encephalitis (e.g., Japanese encephalitis), viral fevers (e.g., ***dengue***, West Nile, viral haemorrhagic fevers (e.g., yellow fever, dengue haemorrhagic fever)
2. Housefly	Typhoid and paratyphoid fever, diarrhea, dysentery, cholera, gastroenteritis, amoebiasis, helminthic infestations, poliomyelitis, conjunctivitis, trachoma, anthrax, yaws, etc
3. Sandfly	Kala-azar, oriental sore, sandfly fever, oraya fever
4. Tsetse fly	Sleeping sickness
5. Louse	Epidemic typhus, relapsing fever, trench fever, pediculosis
6. Rat flea	***Bubonic plague***, endemic typhus, chiggerosis, hymenolepisdiminuta
7. Blackfly	Onchocerciasis
8. Reduviid bug	Chagas disease
9. Hard tick	Tick typhus, viral encephalitis, viral fevers, viral haemorrhagic fever, (e.g., ***Kyasanur forest disease***), tularemia, tick paralysis, human babesiosis.
10. Soft tick	Q fever, relapsing fever
11. Trombiculid mite	Scrub typhus, Rickettsial-pox
12. Itch-mite	Scabies
13. Cyclops	Guinea-worm disease, fish tapeworm (D. latus)
14. Cockroaches	Enteric pathogens

Epidemiological Classification of Vector-borne Disease

◈ *Park 24th/103*

- By vector
  - Invertebrate type: Arthropod vectors fall into seven orders largely
    - Diptera– flies and mosquitoes
    - Siphonaptera– fleas
    - Orthoptera– cockroaches
    - Anoplura– sucking lice
    - Hemiptera– bugs, including kissing bugs
    - Acarina– ricks and mites
    - Copepoda– Cyclops
  - Vertebrate type–Mice, rodents, bats

- By transmission chain: Vector-borne diseases are classified under heterogeneous infection chain and involve three principal patterns:
  - Man and a non-vertebrate host
    - Man–arthropod–man (malaria)
    - Man–snail–man (schistosomiasis)
  - Man, another vertebrate host and a non-vertebrate host
    - Mammal–arthropod–man (plaque)
    - Bird–arthropod–man (encephalitis)
  - Man and 2 intermediate hosts
    - Man–Cyclops-fish-man (fish tape worm)
    - Man-snail-fish-man (Clonorchis sinensis)
    - Man–snail–crab–man (Paragonimiasis)
- By methods in which vectors transmit agent
  - Biting
  - Regurgitation
  - Scratching-in of infective faeces
  - Contamination of host with body fluids of vectors
- By methods in which vectors are involved in the transmission and propagation of parasites

88. Ans. **c. Wuchereria bancrofti; d. Brugia malayi; e. Brugia timori**

[Ref: Harrison 19th/1417-18;Park 24th/287]

Lymphatic filariasis is caused by ***W. bancrofti, B. malayi, or B.*** timori. The thread like adult parasites reside in lymphatic channels or lymph nodes, where they may remain viable for more than two decades"- *Harrison 19th/1417*

Table: Characteristics of the Filariae *(Harrison 19th/1418)*

Organism	Periodicity	Vector	Location of Adult	Microfilarial Location	Sheath
Wuchereria bancrofti	Nocturnal	*Culex, Anopheles* (mosquitoes)	*Lymphatic tissue*	Blood	+
	Subperiodic	*Aedes* (mosquitoes)	*Lymphatic tissue*	Blood	+
Brugia malayi	Nocturnal	*Mansonia, Anopheles* (mosquitoes)	*Lymphatic tissue*	Blood	+
	Subperiodic	*Coquillettidia, Mansonia* (mosquitoes)	*Lymphatic tissue*	Blood	+
B. timori	Nocturnal	*Anopheles* (mosquitoes)	*Lymphatic tissue*	Blood	+
Loa loa	Diurnal	*Chrysops* (deerflies)	Subcutaneous tissue	Blood	+
Onchocerca volvulus	None	*Simulium* (blackflies)	Subcutaneous tissue	Skin, eye	–
Mansonella ozzardi	None	*Culicoides* (midges)	Undetermined site	Blood	–
		Simulium (blackflies)			
M. perstans	None	*Culicoides* (midges)	Body cavities, mesentery, perirenal tissue	Blood	–
M. streptocerca	None	*Culicoides* (midges)	Subcutaneous tissue	Skin	–

89. Ans. **b. Peptidoglycan; c. Lipopolysaccharide; e. Lipoprotein**

[Ref: Ananthanarayan 10th/16; Jawetz 27th/23-29]

"Lipopolysaccharides (LPS): *Present on cell wall of gram-negative bacteria* account for their endotoxic activity"- *Ananthanarayan 10th/16*

Cell Wall of Gram-negative Bacteria

◈ *Ananthanarayan 10th/16*

- ***Lipopolysaccharides (LPS)***
- Outer membrane proteins
- ***Lipoprotein***
- ***Peptidoglycan***

"Special Components of Gram-Negative Cell Walls: Gram-negative cell walls contain three components that lie outside of the peptidoglycan layer: ***lipoprotein, outer membrane and lipopolysaccharide***"- *Jawetz 27th/26-29*

Special Components of Gram-Positive Cell Walls: Most gram-positive cell walls contain considerable amounts of **teichoic** and **teichuronic acids**. In addition, some gram-positive walls may contain polysaccharide molecules"-*Jawetz 27th/25*

Table: Comparison of cell walls of Gram-positive and gram-negative bacteria *(Ananthanarayan 10th/16)*

	Gram-positive	Gram-negative
Thickness (***peptidoglycan***)	Thicker	Thinner
Variety of amino acids	Few	Several
Aromatic and sulphur containing amino acids	Absent	Present
LPS and outer membrane	Absent	Present
Teichoic acid	Present	Absent

A & E

90. Ans. d. Penile Oral sex: Insertive

[Ref: Harrison 19th/1220-21; www.cdc.gov]

- *In above options- **oral sex(d>c)** has least chance of HIV transmission(**Anal>Vaginal>oral**)*

"Oral sex is a ***much less efficient mode of transmission* of HIV *than is anal intercourse or vaginal intercourse*"**- *Harrison 19th/1221*

Table: Estimated per-act probability of acquiring HIV from an infected source, by exposure act *(Harrison 19th/1220; www.cdc.gov)*

Type of Exposure	Risk per 10,000 Exposures
Parenteral	
Blood Transfusion	9,250
Needle-Sharing During Injection Drug Use	63
Percutaneous (Needle-Stick)	23
Sexual	
Receptive Anal Intercourse	138
Insertive Anal Intercourse	11
Receptive Penile-Vaginal Intercourse	8
Insertive Penile-Vaginal Intercourse	4
Receptive Oral Intercourse	Low
Insertive Oral Intercourse	Low
Other[a]	
Biting	Negligible
Spitting	Negligible
Throwing Body Fluids (Including Semen or Saliva)	Negligible
Sharing Sex Toys	Negligible

*a*HIV transmission through these exposure routes is technically possible but unlikely and not well documented

Penile-Oral Sex

◈ *www.poz.com*

- The risk of penile-oral sex causes the greatest amount of confusion in terms of risk—and it raises the greatest number of questions. But most experts agree that fellatio (blow jobs) is not an efficient route of HIV transmission.
- Because unprotected fellatio allows body fluids from one person to come into contact with the mucosal tissues or open cuts, sores or breaks in the skin of another person, there is a "theoretical risk" of HIV transmission, meaning that passing an infection from one person to another is considered possible. But the likelihood of it happening is rare, as there are only a few documented cases. These instances all involved MSM(men who have sex with men)—***men who were the receptive partners (the person doing the sucking) during unprotected oral sex with an HIV-positive man.***
- There haven't been any instances of HIV transmission among female receptive partners during unprotected oral sex. And ***there hasn't been a single documented case of HIV transmission to an insertive partner*** (the person being sucked) during unprotected oral sex, either among MSM or heterosexuals.

Oral-Vaginal Sex

◈ *www.poz.com*

- Like fellatio, this is also considered a low-risk activity. Reports document one case of female-to-female transmission of HIV via cunnilingus and another case of female-to-male transmission of HIV via cunnilingus. Both of these cases involved transmission from receptive partner (the one receiving oral sex) to the insertive partner (the one performing oral sex).
- There haven't been any documented cases of HIV transmission from the insertive partner to the receptive partner.

91. Ans. a. Strongyloides stercoralis

[Ref: Panikar Parasitology 7th/6-7; Chatterjee Parasitology 13th/263-65]

*"The larvae are found in the feces in **Strongyloides stercoralis** infection"- Panikar Parasitology 7th/7*

In **ankylostoma duodenale: *Eggs are passed in stool & are not infective.*** Rhabditiform & filariform larva(infective form) develops in soil- *Panikar Parasitology 7th/184*

Table: Parasites and Their Developmental Stages found in stool *(Panikar 7th/6)*

Cysts/Trophozoites	Eggs		Larvae	Adult worms
Entamoeba histolytica	CESTODES	Gastrodiscoides horminis	Strangyloides stercoralis	Taeniasolium
Giardia lamblia	Taenia spp.	Heterophyes heterophyes		Taeniasaginata
Balantidium coli	Hymenolepis nana	Metagonimus yokogawai		Diphyllobothrium latum
Sarcocystis spp	Hymenolepis diminuta	Opisthorchis spp.		Ascaris lumbricoides
Isospora belli	Dipylidium caninum	**NEMATODES**		Enterobius vermicularis
Cyclospora cayetanensis	Diphyllobothrim latum	Trichuris trichiura		Trichinella spiralis
Cryptosporidium parvum	**TREMATODES**	Enterobius vermicularis		
	Schistosoma spp.	Ascaris lumbricoides		

Contd...

Cysts/Trophozoites	Eggs		Larvae	Adult worms
	Fasciolopsis buski	Ancyclostoma duodenale		
	Fasciola hepatica	Necator americanus		
	Fasciola gigantica	Trichostrongylus orientalis		
	Clonorchis sinensis			

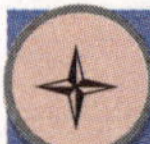

Also Know

Parasites found in urine *Panikar Parasitology 7th/7*

- Schistosoma haemtobium
- Wuchereria bancrofti
- Trichomonas vaginalis

Parasites found in peripheral Blood film *panikar parasitology 7th/7*

Gram-positive	Gram-negative
• Plasmodium spp. • Babesia spp. • Tryponosoma spp. • Leishmania spp.	• Wuchereriabancrofti • Brugiamalayi • Loa loa • Mansonella spp.

92. Ans. a. **Staphylococcus aureus; c. Streptococcus viridans; d. Enterococcus**

[Ref: Harrison 19th/816-17;Davidson 23rd/528;Robbins 9th/559-60]

Table: Organisms Causing Major Clinical Forms of Endocarditis *(Harrison 19th/817)*

Organism	Native Valve Endocarditis		Prosthetic Valve Endocarditis at Indicated Time of Onset (Months) after Valve Surgery		
	Community-Acquired (n =1718)	Health Care–Associated (n =1110)	<2 (n = 144)	2–12 (n = 31)	>12 (n = 194)
Streptococci[a]	40	13	1	9	31
Pneumococci	2	—	—	—	—
Enterococci[b]	9	16	8	12	11
Staphylococcus aureus	28	52[c]	22	12	18
Coagulase-negative staphylococci	5	11	33	32	11
Fastidious gram-negative coccobacilli (HACEK group)[d]	3	—	—	—	6
Gram-negative bacilli	1	1	13	3	6
Candida spp.	<1	1	8	12	1
Polymicrobial/miscellaneous	3	3	3	6	5
Diphtheroids	—	<1	6	—	3
Culture-negative	9	3	5	6	8

[a]Includes viridans streptococci; *Streptococcus gallolyticus*; other non–group A, groupable streptococci; and *Abiotrophia* and *Granulicatella* spp. (nutritionally variant, pyridoxal-requiring streptococci). [b]Primarily E. *faecalis* or nonspeciated isolates; occasionally *E. faecium* or other, less likely species. [c]Methicillin resistance is common among these S. *aureus* strains. [d]Includes *Haemophilus* spp., *Aggregatibacter aphrophilus*, *Aggregatibacter actinomycetemcomitans*, *Cardiobacterium hominis*, *Eikenella* spp. and *Kingella* spp

Table: Microbiology of infective endocarditis *(Davidson 23rd/528)*

			Of prosthetic valve	
Pathogen	**Of native valve (n = 280)**	**In IV drug users (n = 87)**	**Early (n = 15)**	**Late (n = 72)**
Staphylococci	124 (44%)	60 (69%)	10 (67%)	33 (46%)
Staph. aureus	106 (38%)	60 (69%)	3 (20%)	15 (21%)
Coagulase-negative	18 (8%)	0	7 (47%)	18 (25%)
Streptococci	86 (31%)	7 (8%)	0	25 (35%)
Oral	59 (21%)	3 (3%)	0	19 (26%)
Others (non-enterococcal)	27 (10%)	4 (5%)	0	6 (8%)
Enterococcus spp.	21 (8%)	2 (2%)	1 (7%)	5(7%)
HACEK group (see text)	12 (4%)	0	0	1 (1%)
Polymicrobial	6 (2%)	8 (9%)	0	1 (1%)
Other bacteria	12(4%)	4(5%)	0	2(3%)
Fungi 3 (1%)	2 (2%)	0	0	
Negative blood culture	16 (6%)	4 (5%)	4(27%)	5 (7%)

"Over three-quarters of cases are caused by streptococci or staphylococci. Staph. aureus has now overtaken streptococci as the most common cause of acute endocarditis"- *Davidson 23rd/528*

"Yeasts and fungi, such as *Candida* and *Aspergillus*, may attack previously normal or prosthetic valves, particularly in immunocompromised patients or those with in-dwelling intravenous catheters"-*Davidson 23rd/528*

Infective Endocarditis: Etiology

◈ *Harrison 19th/816*

- **Health care–associated native valve endocarditis (NVE),** most commonly caused by **Staphylococcus aureus, coagulase-negative staphylococci (CoNS) and enterococci**, may have either a nosocomial onset (55%) or a ***community onset*** (45%); community-onset cases develop in patients who have had extensive contact with the health care system over the preceding 90 days.
- **Prosthetic valve endocarditis (PVE)** arising within 2 months of valve surgery is generally nosocomial, the result of intraoperative contamination of the prosthesis or a bacteremic postoperative complication.
- This nosocomial origin is reflected in the primary microbial causes: *S. aureus*, CoNS, facultative gram-negative bacilli, diphtheroids and fungi. The portals of entry and organisms causing cases beginning >12 months after surgery are similar to those in community-acquired NVE.
- **Injection drug use**–associated endocarditis, especially that involving the tricuspid valve, is commonly caused by *S. aureus*, which in many cases is resistant to methicillin. Left-sided valve infections in addicts have a more varied etiology.

Infective Endocarditis

◈ *Robbins 9th/559-60*

- The causal organisms differ among the major high-risk groups.
- **Endocarditis of native** but previously damaged or otherwise abnormal valves is caused most commonly (50% to 60% of cases) by *Streptococcus viridans*, a normal component of the oral cavity flora.
- In contrast, more virulent *S. aureus* organisms commonly found on the skin can infect either ***healthy or deformed valves*** and are responsible for 20% to 30% of cases overall; notably, *S. aureus* is the major offender in IE among intravenous drug abusers.
- Other bacterial causes include enterococci and the so-called HACEK group (*Haemophilus, Actinobacillus, Cardiobacterium, Eikenella* and *Kingella*), all commensals in the oral cavity.
- **Prosthetic valve endocarditis** is caused most commonly by coagulase-negative staphylococci (e.g., *S. epidermidis*).
- Other agents causing endocarditis include gram-negative bacilli and fungi. In about 10% of all cases of endocarditis, no organism can be isolated from the blood ("culture negative" endocarditis); reasons include prior antibiotic therapy, difficulties in isolating the offending agent, or because deeply embedded organisms within the enlarging vegetation are not released into the blood.

93. Ans. a. Streptococcus pyogens; b. Staphylococcus aureus; d. Neisseria meningitides; e. Salmonella typhi

[Ref: Harrison 19th/127-34]

"**Fever and Rash:** Diseases with fever and rash may be **classified by type of eruption:** *centrally distributed maculopapular,* *peripheral, confluent desquamative erythematous, vesiculobullous, urticaria-like, nodular, purpuric, ulcerated, or with eschars"- Harrison 19th/127*

"Typhoid fever **(Salmonella typhi***)* Transient, blanchable ***erythematous macules and papules,*** 2–4 mm, usually on trunk **(rose spots)"**- *Harrison 19th/129*

Table: Diseases Associated with Fever and Rash(Summarized) *(Harrison 19th/128-34)*

Disease	Etiology	Description
Rubeola (measles, first disease)	Paramyxovirus	Discrete lesions that become confluent as rash spreads from hairline downward, sparing palms and soles; Koplik's spots
Rubella (German measles, third disease)	Togavirus	Spreads from hairline downward, clearing as it spreads; Forchheimer spots
Erythema infectiosum (fifth disease)	Human parvovirus B19	Brightred "slapped-cheeks" appearance followed by lacy reticular rash
Exanthem subitum (roseola, sixth disease)	Human herpesvirus 6	Diffuse maculopapular eruption over trunk and neck; resolves within 2 days
Epidemic typhus	*Rickettsia prowazekii*	Maculopapular eruption appearing in axillae, spreading to trunk and later to extremities; usually spares face, palms, soles
Endemic (murine) typhus	*Rickettsia typhi*	Maculopapular eruption, usually sparing palms, soles
Scrub typhus	*Orientia tsutsugamushi*	Diffuse macular rash starting on trunk; eschar at site of mite bite
Relapsing fever	*Borrelia* species	Central rash at end of febrile episode; petechiae in some cases
Rocky Mountain spotted fever	*Rickettsia rickettsii*	Rash beginning on wrists and ankles
Scarlet fever (second disease)	***Group AStreptococcus*** (pyrogenic exotoxins A, B, C)	Diffuse blanchable erythema beginning on face and spreading to trunk and extremities
Staphylococcal toxic shock syndrome	***S. aureus*** (toxic shock syndrome toxin 1, enterotoxin B or C)	Diffuse erythema involving palms; pronounced erythema of mucosal surfaces; conjunctivitis; desquamation 7–10 days into illness
Staphylococcal scaldedskin syndrome	***S. aureus***, phage group II	Diffuse tender erythema, often with bullae and desquamation; Nikolsky's sign
Disseminated *Vibrio vulnificus* infection	*V. vulnificus*	Erythematous lesions evolving into hemorrhagic bullae and then into necrotic ulcers
Acute meningococcemia	***Neisseria meningitidis***	Initially pink maculopapular lesions evolving into petechiae; petechiae rapidly becoming numerous, sometimes enlarging and becoming vesicular
Purpura fulminans	Severe disseminated intravascular coagulation	Large ecchymoses with sharply irregular shapes evolving into hemorrhagic bullae and then into black necrotic lesions
Disseminated gonococcal infection	*Neisseria gonorrhoeae*	Papules (1–5 mm) evolving over 1–2 days into hemorrhagic pustules with gray necrotic centers;

94. Ans. **a. Lassa fever; b. Yellow fever; c. Crimean-Congo fever; e. Kyasanur forest disease**

[Ref: Ananthanarayan 10th/524; Davidson 23rd/245]

West Nile fever- belongs to ***febrile group*** (fever with/without rash)- *Ananthanarayan 10th/524; www.cdc.gov*

Hemorrhagic Fever

- *Ananthanarayan 10th/524*
- Chikungunya
- Dengue type 1-4
- ***Yellow fever***
- ***Kyasanur forest disease***
- Omsk hemorrhagic fever
- ***Crimean Congo fever***

Roden-Borne Hemorrhagic Fever

- *Ananthanarayan 10th/524*
- Hanta virus pulmonary syndrome
- ***Lasaa fever***
- Hemorrhagic fever with Renal syndrome

Table: Viral haemorrhagic fevers *(Davidson 23rd/245)*

Disease	Reservoir	Mortality rate	Clinical features of severe disease
Lassa fever	Multimammate rats (Masto mysnatalensis)	15%	Haemorrhage, shock, encephalopathy, ARDS (responds to ribavirin);Deafness in survivors
Ebola fever	Undefined (?Bats)	25-90%	Hemorrhage, hepatic and renal failure
Marburg fever	Undefined	25-90%	Haemorrhage, diarrhea, encephalopathy, orchitis
Yellow fever	Monkeys	~15%	Hepatic failure, renal failure, haemorrhage
Dengue	Humans	<10%	Haemorrhage, shock
Crimean congo haemorrhagic fever	Small vertebrates Domestic and wild animals	30%	Encephalopathy, haemorrhage, hepatic or renal failure, ARDS
Rift Valley fever	Domestic Livestock	1%	Haemorrhage, bilindess, menin goencephalitis (complications only in a minority)
Kyasanur fever	Monkeys	5-10%	Haemorrhage, pulmonary Oedema, neurological features, iridokeratitis in survivors

95. Ans. a. V. alginolyticus; b. V. parahaemolyticus; d. V.damsela; e. V.vulnificus

[Ref: Ananthanarayan 10th/317; Microbiology by Baveja 5th/276-77; Harrison 19th/1065]

Halophilic Vibrios

◈ *Ananthanarayan 10th/317; Microbiology by Baveja 5th/277*

- Vibrios that have a high requirement of sodium chloride are known as halophilicvibrios. Their natural habitat is sea water and marine life.
- Some halophilicvibrios have been known to cause human disease–***V.parahaemolyticus,*** ***v.alginolyticus and V. vulnificus***

V. cholerae is halotolerant (*unlike V.parahaemolyticus which is halophilic* *& needs higher concentration of NaCl)- Ananthanarayan 10th/310*

"A halophilic gram-negative bacillus, *P. damsela* was initially described as ***V. damsela,*** later classified as *L. damsela* and was recently reclassified as P. damsela on the basis of phenotypic data. Strains of P. damsela are commonly found in marine fish and it is a pathogen that is found in both fish and humans. Generally, *P. damsela* is considered to be less virulent than *Vibrio vulnificus*, which is regarded as the most virulent bacillus in the genus"- *academic.oup.com*

V.mimicus *is a non-haophilic vibrio- Microbiology by Baveja 5th/277*

Table: Features of Selected Noncholera Vibrioses *(Harrison 19th/1065])*

Organism	Vehicle or Activity	Syndrome
V. parahaemolyticus	Shellfish, seawater	Gastroenteritis
	Seawater	Wound infection
Non-O1/O139 V. *cholerae*	Shellfish, travel	Gastroenteritis
	Seawater	Wound infection, otitis media
V. vulnificus	Shellfish	Sepsis, secondary cellulitis
	Seawater	Wound infection, cellulitis
V. alginolyticus	Seawater	Wound infection, cellulitis, otitis
	Seawater	Sepsis

96. Ans. a. Anthrax; b. Cl. Botulinum toxin; e. Yersinia pestis

[Ref: Harrison 19th/261e-1; Ananthanarayan 10th/662]

Table: CDC Category A, B and C Agents *(Harrison 19th/261e-1)*

Category A
Anthrax (***Bacillus anthracis***) Botulism (***Clostridium botulinum*** toxin) Plague (***Yersinia pestis***) Smallpox (*Variola major*) Tularemia (*Francisella tularensis*) Viral hemorrhagic fevers Arenaviruses: Lassa, New World (Machupo, Junin, Guanarito and Sabia) Bunyaviridae: Crimean-Congo, Rift Valley Filoviridae: Ebola, Marburg

Contd...

Category B
Brucellosis (*Brucella* spp.)
Epsilon toxin of *Clostridium perfringens*
Food safety threats (e.g., *Salmonella* spp., *Escherichia coli* 0157:H7, *Shigella*)
Glanders (*Burkholderia mallei*)
Melioidosis (*B. pseudomallei*)
Psittacosis (*Chlamydophila psittaci*)
Q fever (*Coxiella burnetii*)
Ricin toxin from *Ricinus communis* (castor beans)
Staphylococcal enterotoxin B
Typhus fever (*Rickettsia prowazekii*)
Viral encephalitis [alphaviruses (e.g., Venezuelan, eastern and western equine encephalitis)]
Water safety threats (e.g., *Vibrio cholerae, Cryptosporidium parvum*)
Category C
Emerging infectious diseases threats such as Nipah, hantavirus, SARS or MERS coronavirus and pandemic influenza.

Abbreviations: MERS, Middle East respiratory syndrome; SARS, severe acute respiratory syndrome

Microbial Bioterrorism

Harrison 19th/261e-1

- The U.S. Centers for Disease Control and Prevention (CDC) classifies potential biologic threats into three categories: ***A, B and C***
- **Category A agents** are the *highest-priority pathogens.* They pose the greatest risk to national security because they (1) can be easily disseminated or transmitted from person to person, (2) result in high mortality rates and have the potential for major public health impact, (3) might cause public panic and social disruption and (4) require special action for public health preparedness.
- **Category B agents** are the *second highest priority* pathogens and include those that are moderately easy to disseminate, result in moderate morbidity rates and low mortality rates and require specifically enhanced diagnostic capacity.
- **Category C agents** are the *third highest priority.* These include certain emerging pathogens to which the general population lacks immunity; that could be engineered for mass dissemination in the future because of availability, ease of production and ease of dissemination; and that have a major public health impact and the potential for high morbidity and mortality rates.
- It should be pointed out, however, that these A B and C designations are empirical and, depending on evolving circumstances such as intelligence-based threat assessments, the priority rating of any given microbe or toxin could change. The CDC classification system also largely reflects the severity of illness produced by a given agent, rather than its accessibility to potential terrorists.

97. Ans. a. Bacillus cereus; b. Cl. Botulinum; e. Staphylococcus aureus

[Ref: Harrison 19th/856; Microbiology by Baveja 5th/233;Park 24th/253-54]

"Incubation period for Bacterial Gastroenteritis 1-7 days for common agents (e.g., *Campylobacter, E. coli, Shigella, Salmonella);* a few hours for **bacteria producing preformed toxins** (e.g., ***Staphylococcus aureus, Bacillus cereus***)"- *Harrison 19th/1287*

"**Cl. botulinum is** non-invasive and its pathogenicity is due to the ***action of preformed toxin,*** the manifestations of which are called botulism. Botulism is of three types—foodborne, infant and wound botulism"-*Microbiology by Baveja 5th/ 233*

Table: Association between Pathobiology of Causative Agents and Clinical Features in Acute Infectious Diarrhea *(Harrison 19th/266)*

Pathobiology/Agents	Incubation Period
Toxin producers	
Preformed toxin	
Bacillus cereus, Staphylococcus aureus,	1–8 h
Clostridium perfringens	8–24 h
Enterotoxin	
Vibrio cholerae, enterotoxigenic *Escherichia coli, Klebsiella pneumoniae, Aeromonas* species	8–72 h
Enteroadherent	
Enteropathogenic and enteroadherent *E. coli, Giardia* organisms, cryptosporidiosis, helminths	1–8 d
Cytotoxin producers	
C. difficile	1–3 d
Hemorrhagic *E. coli*	12–72 h
Invasive organisms	
Minimal inflammation	
Rotavirus and norovirus	1–3 d
Variable inflammation	
Salmonella, Campylobacter and *Aeromonas* species, *Vibrio parahaemolyticus, Yersinia*	12 h–11 d
Severe inflammation	
Shigella species, enteroinvasive *E. coli, Entamoeba histolytica*	12 h–8 d

98. Ans. a. NK cell; b. Beta defensins; e. Dendritic cell

[Ref: Robbins 9th/186-88, 7th/194-96; Harrison 19th/372e1-7]

Innate & Adaptive Immunity

Robbins 9th/186-88, 7th/194

- **Innate immunity** (also called ***natural, or native, immunity***) refers to defense mechanisms that are present even before infection and have evolved to specifically ***recognize microbes and protect multicellular organisms against infections.***

- **Adaptive immunity** (also called ***acquired, or specific, immunity***) consists of mechanisms that are stimulated by (adapt to) microbes and are capable of also recognizing nonmicrobial substances, called antigens.
- ***Innate immunity is the first line of defence, because it is always ready***

"*There are* **two main types of adaptive immunity**—*cell-mediated (or cellular) immunity, which is responsible for defense against intracellular microbes and humoral immunity, which protects against extracellular microbes and their toxins.***Cellular immunity** *is mediated by* ***T (thymus-derived) lymphocytes*** *and* **humoral immunity** *is mediated by* ***B (bone marrowderived) lymphocytes*** *and their secreted products" (Robbins 9th/189)*

Table: Major Components of the Innate Immune System *(Harrison 19th/372e-2, 17th/2021)*

Pattern recognition receptors (PRR)	C type lectins, leucine-rich proteins, scavenger receptors, pentraxins, lipid transferases, *integrins*
Antimicrobial peptides	α-Defensins, β-defensins, cathelin, protegrin, granulsyin, histatin, secretory leukoprotease inhibitor and probiotics
Cells	***Macrophages***, dendritic cells, NK cells, NK-T cells, neutrophils, eosinophils, mast cells, basophils and epithelial cells
Complement components	***Classic and alternative complement pathway*** and proteins that bind complement components
Cytokines	Autocrine, paracrine, endocrine cytokines that mediate host defense and inflammation, as well as recruit, direct, and regulate adaptive immune responses

Table: Cells of the Innate Immune System *(Harrison 19th/372 e-5, 17th/2021)*

Cell Type	Major Role in Innate Immunity
Macrophages	Phagocytose and kill bacteria; produce antimicrobial peptides; bind (LPS); produce inflammatory cytokines
Plasmacytoid dendritic cells (DCs) of lymphoid lineage	Produce large amounts of interferon-α (IFN-α) which has antitumor and antiviral activity and are found in T cell zones of lymphoid organs; they circulate in blood
Myeloid dendritic cells are of two types; interstitial and Langerhans derived	Interstitial DCs are strong producers of IL-12 and IL-10 and are located in T cell zones of lymphoid organs, circulate in blood and are present in the interstices of the lung, heart and kidney; Langerhans DCs are strong producers of IL-12; are located in T cell zones of lymph nodes, skin epithelia and the thymic medulla; and circulate in blood
Natural killer (NK) cells	Kill foreign and host cells that have low levels of MHC+ self peptides. Express NK receptors that inhibit NK function in the presence of high expression of self-MHC.
NK-T cells	Lymphocytes with both T cell and NK surface markers that recognize lipid antigens of intracellular bacteria such as M. tuberculosis by CD1 molecules and kill host cells infected with intracellular bacteria.
Neutrophils	Phagocytose and kill bacteria, produce antimicrobial peptides
Eosinophils	Kill invading parasites
Mast cells and basophils	Release TNF-α, IL-6, IFN-γ in response to a variety of bacterial PAMPs
Epithelial cells	Produce anti-microbial peptides; tissue specific epithelia produce mediator of local innate immunity, e.g., lung epithelial cells produce surfactant proteins (proteins within the collectin family) that bind and promote clearance of lung invading microbes

Contd...

99. Ans. a. Dendritic cell; d. Activated T-cell; e. Macrophages

[Ref: Robbins 9th/ 194-95; Harrison 19th/373e-1; Anathanarayan 10th/ 142;Jawetz 27th/132]

HLA class II antigens are found on: ***Macrophages, dendritic cells, activated T cells & particularly on B cell***- Anathanarayan 10th/ 142

"In contrast to class I molecules, **class II MHC molecules** are mainly expressed on cells that present ingested antigens and respond to T-cell help (***macrophages, B lymphocytes and dendritic cells***)"- *Robbins 9th/ 195*

Class I MHC molecules are expressed on ***all nucleated cells and platelets***- *Robbins 9th/ 194*

Table: Important Features of Some Human MHC Gene Products *(Jawetz 27th/132)*

	Class I	Class II
Genetic loci (partial list)	HLA-A, -B and -C	HLA-DP, -DQ and -DR
Cell distribution	All nucleated somatic cells, except cells of brain & retina	***Antigen-presenting cells (macrophages, B cells, etc), activated human T cells***
Present peptide antigens to	CD8 T cells	CD4 T cells

100. Ans. c. IgD; d. IgM

[Ref: Harrison 19th/379e19-20; Anathanarayan 10th/135,138; Jawetz 27th/135]

"B cells display immunoglobulin molecules (10^5/cell) on their surface. These immunoglobulins serve as receptors for a specific antigen, so that each B cell can respond to only one antigen or a closely related group of antigens. All immature B cells carry ***IgM immunoglobulins on their surface and most also carry IgD***. B cells also have surface receptors for the Fc portion of immunoglobulins and for several complement components"- *Jawetz 27th/135*

"**Membrane-bound immunoglobulins** are associated non-covalently with two accessory peptides, forming the ***B-cell antigen receptor complex.*** The first antigen receptors expressed by B cells are IgM and IgD"- www.thermofisher.com

"The ***first Ig class to be appear on the B cell surface is monomeric IgM. Subsequently other classes(IgG, IgA or IgE) may be present along with IgD.*** T cells do not have surface Ig"- Anathanarayan *10th/135*

"The light chains combine with the μ chains, replacing the surrogate light chains, to form four-chain ***IgM molecules*** (each with two μ chains and two light chains). These molecules then insert into the plasma membrane, where they function as receptors for antigen. At this point, the cell is called an immature naïve B cell. After leaving the bone marrow, the cell starts to produce cell-surface ***IgD molecules*** as well, with the same antigen-binding site as the IgM molecules. It is now called a mature naïve B cell. It is this cell that can respond to foreign antigen in peripheral lymphoid organs"-*wikipedia*

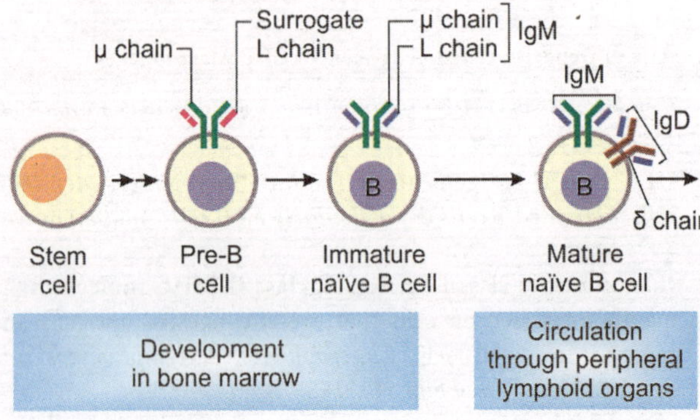

Fig: The main stages in B cell development (*www.ncbi.nlm.nih.gov*)

101. Ans. b. Both B & T cell defect, c. Decreased lymphocyte count, d. More common in boys, e. Absent tonsils

[Ref: Robbins 9th/239- 40; Harrison 19th/2107-08; Ananthanarayan 9th/ 174-76]

Severe Combined Immunodeficiency (SCID)

◈ *Harrison 19th/2107-08*

- Diagnosis of SCID can be suspected based on the patient's clinical history and, possibly, a family history of deaths in very young children (suggestive of ***either X-linked or recessive inheritance***).
- ***Lymphocytopenia*** is strongly suggestive of SCID in more than 90% of cases.
- The ***absence of a thymic shadow*** on a chest x-ray can also be suggestive of SCID. An accurate diagnosis relies on precise determination of the number of circulating T, B and NK lymphocytes and their subsets.
- Although counts are usually low (<500/μL of blood), higher maternal T cell counts may, under some circumstances, initially mask the presence of SCID.
- **Severe combined immunodeficiency caused by a cytokine-signaling deficiency**: The most frequent SCID phenotype (accounting for 40–50% of all cases) is the absence of both T and NK cells
- **Severe combined immunodeficiency (SCID, Bubble boy disease, Glanzmann Riniker syndrome, Alymphocytosis):** Lymph nodes and tonsils may be absent"- www.amboss.com
- *"SCID: **Absent tonsils and absent thymus are key clinical markers** that may point to the diagnosis"- indianpediatrics. net*

Severe Combined Immunodeficiency

◈ *Robbins 9th/239-40; Ananthanarayan 9th/174-75*

- The SCID syndrome is characterized by gross functional impairment of both *humoral and cell-mediated immunity*
- Persons with SCID are extremely susceptible to recurrent, severe infections by a wide range of pathogens, including *Candida albicans, Pneumocystis jiroveci, Pseudomonas*, cytomegalovirus, varicella and a whole host of bacteria.
- Without HSC transplantation, *death occurs within the first year of life.*
- The most common form, accounting for 50% to 60% of cases, is ***X-linked*** and hence SCID is ***more common in boys than in girls***. The genetic defect in the X-linked form is a **mutation in the common γ-chain (γc) subunit of cytokine receptors**
- **Autosomal recessive SCID:** The remaining forms of SCID are autosomal recessive disorders. The most common cause of autosomal recessive SCID is a deficiency of the enzyme adenosine deaminase (ADA). Other is Mutations of an intracellular kinaseJak3 & Mutations in recombinase activating genes (RAG)
- Although the mechanisms by which ADA deficiency causes SCID are not entirely clear, it has been proposed that deficiency of ADA leads to accumulation of deoxyadenosine and its derivatives (*e.g.*, deoxy-ATP), which are toxic to rapidly dividing immature lymphocytes, especially those of the T-cell lineage. Hence there may be a greater reduction in the number of T lymphocytes than of B lymphocytes.
- *Currently, HSC transplantation is the mainstay of treatment*, but X-linked SCID is the first human disease in which gene therapy has been successful.
- The syndrome has been associated with mutations in one of several genes whose products are necessary for the normal differentiation of ***T, B and, sometimes, NK cells***

Table: **Disorder of specific immunity** *(Ananthanarayan 9th/174; 8th/156)*

Humoral immunodeficiency (B cell defect)	Cellular immunodeficiency (T cell defect)	Combined immune deficiency (B and T cell defect
X-linked Agammaglobulinemia Common Variable Immunodeficiency Selective Ig deficiency	DiGeorge Syndrome Chronic Mucocutaneous Candidiasis	Nezelof Syndrome Ataxia-Telangiectasia Wiskott-Aldrich syndrome Severe combined immunodeficiency (SCID

102. Ans. **b. Candida; c. Pseudomonas aeruginosa; d. Aspergillus**

[Ref: www.ncbi.nlm.nih.gov; academic.oup.com]

β-D-Glucan

- Detection of fungal antigens in body fluids, including cryptococcus capsular polysaccharide, histoplasma antigen, galactomannan and β-D-glucan, is viewed as being clinically useful for at least the presumptive diagnosis of invasive fungal infections. **β-D-Glucan** is an attractive antigen in that it is found in a broad range of fungal agents, including the commonly encountered agents ***Candida* spp., *Aspergillus* spp. and *Pneumocystis jirovecii*.**- *www.ncbi.nlm.nih.gov*
- An abundant cell wall polysaccharide, (1-3)-β-D-glucan (BDG) is found in most fungi, with the notable **exception of the cryptococci, the zygomycetes and *Blastomyces dermatitidis***, which either lack the glucan entirely or produce it at minimal levels- www.ncbi.nlm.nih.gov
- While the cell wall of yeast has been suggested to contain less glucan than filamentous molds, glucans are a major constituent of the cell wall of saprophytic and pathogenic fungi with the ***exception of* Mucor, Rhizopus, Blastomyces dermatitidis *and* Cryptococcus *species*** -*academic.oup.com*
- **False positives** test can also occur with contamination of clinical specimens with the bacteria *Streptococcus pneumoniae*, ***Pseudomonas aeruginosa*** and *Alcaligenes faecalis*, which also ***produce (1→3)β-D-glucan***. This test can aid in the detection of ***Aspergillus, Candida and Pneumocystis jirovecii.*** This test **cannot** be used to detect ***Mucor or Rhizopus***, the fungi responsible for mucormycosis, as they do not produce (1,3)-beta-D-glucan

FORENSIC MEDICINE

103. Ans. **d. Rigor mortis delay & persists longer in cholera & typhoid**

[Ref: Parikh 7th/144-150; Reddy 34th/150-55]

Hypostasis (Livor Mortis, PM staining, ***Cadaveric lividity***) usually well developed within 4 hours & reaches a maximum ***b/w 6 to 12 hours***. It occurs on a dependable part. It becomes fixed when blood leaks into the surrounding soft tissue due to haemolysis & breakdown of blood vessels-Reddy 34th/148,150

*"**Cadaveric lividity**is **fully developed & fixed in about 6-8 hours**"-Parikh 7th/144*

"**Rigor mortis:** *When the ATP is reduced to a **critical level(85% of the normal),** it causes hardness & rigidity of muscle rigor. The rigidity of the muscle is at its maximum, when the level of ATP is reduced to 15% & lactic acid level is 0.3%- Reddy 34th/152*

"In carbon monoxide poisoning, the colour is cherry-red-*Reddy 34th/151*

" The onset of **rigor is early & duration is short in** deaths from diseases causing great exhaustion & wasting e.g., ***cholera, typhoid***, tuberculosis, cancer etc"- *Reddy 34th/153-54*

104. Ans. **c. IPC 354; d. IPC 509**

[Ref: Parikh 7th/713-16; Reddy 34th/384-86; indiankanoon.org]

- **S. 354 IPC: Assault or criminal force to woman with intent to outrage her modesty.**—Whoever assaults or uses criminal force to any woman, intending to outrage or knowing it to be likely that he will thereby outrage her modesty, shall be punished with imprisonment of either description for a term which may extend to two years, or with fine, or with both(*indiankanoon.org*); 1year may extend to 5 years (*Reddy 34th/384 Parikh 7th/713)*
- **S. 509 IPC: Word, gesture or act intended to insult the modesty of a woman.**—Whoever, intending to insult the modesty of any woman, utters any word, makes any sound or gesture, or exhibits any object, intending that such word or sound shall be heard, or that such gesture or object shall be seen, by such woman, or intrudes upon the privacy of such woman, shall be punished with simple imprisonment for a term which may ***extend to one year, or with fine, or with both(indiankanoon.org);*** simple imprisonment up to ***3 years & also fine****(Reddy 34th/386)*
- **S.375 IPC**: *Definition of rape- Reddy 34th/384*
- **S.376 IPC**: *Punishment for rape- Reddy 34th/384*
- **S.504 IPC**: Intentional insult with intent to provoke breach of the peace.—Whoever intentionally insults and thereby gives provocation to any person, intending or knowing it to be likely that such provocation will cause him to break the public peace, or to commit any other offence, shall be punished with imprisonment of either description for a term which may extend to two years, or with fine, or with both- *indiankanoon.org*

105. Ans. **a. 70-75**

[Ref: Parikh 7th/78; Reddy 34th/57; Pillay Forensic 18th/70; pgblazer.com]

- ***Cephalic index in Indian population is 70-75 (Aryans)***

*"The **skull of Aryans, aborigines & black is dolichocephalic**, that of Europeans & Chinese mesaticephalic& that of the Mongolian race brachycephalic"- Parikh 7th/78*

Table: Cephalic index *Pillay Forensic 18th/ 70; Reddy 34th/57*

Cephalic index	Type of skull	Race
80-85	Brachycephalic (Short-headed)	Mongolian
75-80	Mesati-cephalic (Medium headed)	Europeans and Chinese
70-75	**Dolico-cephalic (Long-headed)**	**Pure Aryans**, Aborigines and Negroes

106. Ans. **a. Mercury; b. Arsenic; e. Lead**

[Ref: KDT 8th964-65; Parikh 7th/518; Reddy 34th/481-82]

- "**BAL is contraindicated** *in* ***iron & cadmium*** *poisoning because the dimercaprol-Fe &dimercaprol-Cd complex is itself toxic"- KDT 8th965*
- **BAL (British anti-lewisite; dimercaptopropanol; dimercaprol)**: *Used as physiological antidote in* ***arsenic, lead, bismuth, copper, mercury,gold, thallium & antimony***"-*Reddy 34th/482*

A & E

107. Ans. c. 16 years

[Ref: www.insightsonindia.com;www.iasparliament.com]

The Treatment of Terminally Ill Patients Bill, 2016-Key facts:*www.insightsonindia.com;www.iasparliament.com*

- According to the Bill, "every competent patient, ***including minors aged above 16 years***, has a right to take a decision and express the desire to the medical practitioner attending on her or him."
- The Bill goes on to say that **such a decision will be binding on the medical practitioner**. He or she has to inform the spouse, parents or any other close relative of the patient and desist from carrying out the decision for a period of three days after informing them.
- The Bill provides **protection to patients and doctors from any liability** for withholding or withdrawing medical treatment and states that palliative care (pain management) can continue.
- The **Medical Council of India has been given the authority to formulate guidelines** from time to time for the guidance of medical practitioners and might review and modify the guidelines periodically.
- In case any patient is not competent enough to take a decision then his or her next of kin, including spouse, parents or sibling, **can approach the High Court**, which will have to take a decision **within a period of one month**.

The Treatment of Terminally Ill Patients Bill, 2016*http://www.prsindia.org*

- This Act may be called the Treatment of Terminally-ill Patients Act, 2016.
- It shall come into force on such date as the Central Government may, by notification in the Official Gazette, appoint. In this Act, unless the context otherwise requires,—
  - "Adult"means an individual who is of eighteen years of age or more;
  - "Advance medical directive" (called living will) means a directive given by a person that he shall or shall not be given medical treatment in future when he becomes terminally-ill;
  - "Attending medical practitioner" means a physician who has primary responsibility for care of the patient and treatment of the patient's terminal disease;
  - "Competent patient" means a patient who is not an incompetent patient;
  - "**Incompetent patient**" means a patient who is a ***minor below the age of sixteen years*** or a person of unsound mind or a patient who is unable to—
    - Understand the information relevant to an informed decision about his medical treatment;
    - Retain that information;
    - Use or weigh that information as part of the process of making his informed decision;
    - Make an informed decision because of impairment of or a disturbance in the functioning of his mind or brain; or (v) communicate his informed decision (whether by speech, language or any other mode) as to medical treatment

108. Ans. d. Named after John Bolam; e. Medical negligence

[Ref: medical-dictionary.thefreedictionary.com; www.lawteacher.net;www.gponline.com]

Bolam Test

◈ *medical-dictionary.the freedictionary.com*

- A test that arose from English tort law, which is used to assess ***medical negligence***.
- Bolam holds that law imposes a duty of care between a doctor and his patient, but the standard of that care is a matter of medical judgement.
- Under Bolam, the plaintiff seeking to prove medical negligence needs to (1) show that there was a duty of care between the doctor or nurse and the patient, which is usually a straight forward exercise and (2) that the act or omission of the doctor or nurse breached the duty of care.
- In Bolam v Friern Hospital Management Committee [1957], the court held that there is no breach of standard of care if a responsible body of similar professionals support the practice that caused the injury, even if the practice was not the standard of care. The ruling meant that the accused doctor need only to find an expert who would testify to having done the same thing. Thus, Bolam was criticised for its overreliance on medical testimony and personal judgement of experts chosen by the defendant.
- Bolam has been subsequently modified by the Bolitho test

Bolam Case

◈ *www.gponline.com*

- In 1954, John Bolam was admitted to Friern Hospital with relapse of depression. In accordance with the hospital's usual practice of not administering a relaxant or applying manual restraint, the psychiatrist Dr Allfrey gave him electro convulsive therapy (ECT). Nurses were present on either side to prevent him from falling off the couch, but Bolam suffered acetabular fracture of both hips.
- He sued, alleging that the hospital was negligent in (a) not giving muscle relaxant (b) failing to provide manual restraint during convulsions and (c) failing to warn him of the risks. At the trial, the expert witnesses said that a large body of medical opinion was not in favour of using relaxant drugs. Some experts felt that more restraint meant more likelihood of fracture.

109. Ans. a. Most common pattern in dactylography is loop; b. In India, dactylography was first used by Sir William Herschel; c. Sex determination by pelvis is more accurate than skull

[Ref: Parikh 7th/67; Reddy 34th/82-83; Pillay Forensic 18th/75]

Dactylography (Fingerprints, Dermatoglyphics, Galton System, Galton-Henry system)

◈ *Patterns Parikh 7th/67; Reddy 34th/82*

- ***Loops(60-70%)-Most common***
- *Whorls(20-35%)*
- *Arches(6-7%)*
- *Composite(1-2%)*

A & E

- *This system was first used in India in 1858 by Sir William Herschel in Bengal*

"According to Krogman, when the entire skeleton is available, sex can be determined with 100% certainty, ***from pelvis alone 95%, from skull alone 90%****, from both skull & pelvis 98% & from long bones it can be done with 80% certainty"- Pillay Forensic 18th/75*

Poroscopy

◈ *Reddy 34th/83; Parikh 7th/69*

- *Pores are formed by* ***subepidermal sweat glands***
- *Useful when only fragments of fingerprints are available*
- *These pores are permanent & unchanged during life*

Teeth

◈ *Reddy 34th/63-64*

- *Between 7 to 12 years, 24 teeth are present*
- *At age 10yr: 16 permanent teeth(8 incisors, 4 premolars,4 molars) & 8 deciduous teeth(4 molars & 4 cannines)*
- *At age 9 yr: 12 permanent teeth& 12 deciduous teeth*

---

110. Ans. b. Organophosphorus

[Ref: Reddy 34th/485; A.K.Khurana 6th/504;K. D. T 7th/400; SatoskarPharma 25th/154-55]

Points in Favor of Organophosphorus as Compared to Other Options in the Question

- **Increased lacrimation, salivation & sweating**-Reddy 34th/485 **(opioid-** ***reduced secretion of saliva, increased sweating****: Satoskar Pharmacology 25th/154,155)*
- **Miosis (Barbiturate-** ***alternate contraction & dilation of pupil*****)**
- **Organophosphorus poisoning** *Reddy 34th/484-86*
- These compounds are **irreversible inhibitors of enzyme cholinesterase**, an enzyme which hydrolyzes acetylcholine. Thus organophosphates inhibit cholinesterase and protect acetylcholine from hydrolysis. This results in increased concentration of acetylcholine and excessive cholinergic activity.
- **They inhibit cholinesterase by phosphorylating the catalytic site of enzyme.** ***Less than 50% of cholinesterase activity in indicative of poisoning.***

Clinical Features

- Clinical features of poisoning are due to excessive cholinergic activity
- Local muscarinic manifestations at the site of exposure (skin, eye, GIT) occur immediately and are followed by complex, systemic effects due to muscarinic, nicotinic and central actions. They are:
  - **Lacrimation,** ***salivation, sweating, miosis*** **(*pinpoint pupil*)** breathlessness, **bronchospasm with** asthma like symptoms, involuntary defecation and urination
  - **There is pulmonary edema**
  - Fall in BP, **bradycardia or tachycardia,** cardiac arrhythmias
  - **Muscular fasciculation,** ***weakness,*** **respiratory paralysis**
  - Excitement, **tremor**, ataxia, convulsions, coma and death
  - Death is due to respiratory failure
  - ***Chromolacryorrhea*****:** Shedding of red color tear due to abnormal porphyria metabolism
- Chronic exposure to certain organophosphates, e.g. triorthocresyl phosphate (addictive in lubricating oil) may cause:
  - ***Delayed neuropathy*** (1-2 weeks after exposure) associated with ***demyelination of axons***. It is not caused by cholinesterase inhibition but rather by ***neuropathy target esterase (NTE)*** inhibition
  - ***Intermediate syndrome*** (after 1-4 days) caused by cholinesterase inhibition. There is **muscle weakness,** motor cranial nerve palsies and respiratory paralysis may occur. ***It does not respond to oximes or atropine***

Morphine/ Heroin Poisoning has Three Stages

- **Stage of excitement**- Hallucination, euphoria, maniacal features
- **Stage of stupor**-Headache, nausea, vomiting, incapacity for exertion, a sense of weight in limbs, giddiness, drowsiness, stupor
- **Stage of coma**-Abolished reflex, ***Pin point non reacting pupil****, All secretions are suspended except sweat,* **hypotension** hypothermia, cyanosis, bradycardia, slow and shallow breathing, *respiratory depression* and paralysis.
  - **They may be white froth from mouth, in PM examination**

Barbiturate Poisoning

- Manifestations are due to excessive CNS depression-patient is flabby and comatose with shallow and failing respiration **cyanosis, fall in BP** and cardiovascular collapse, renal shut down, pulmonary complications, bullous eruption ***(barbiturate blisters)*** and **hypothermia**. Finally there is **coma**
- Important **specific features** are (i) **constricted pupil (*there may be alternate constriction and dilatation, i.e. hippus reaction)*** and (ii) **liquid gold urine.**

Opium poisoning

The odour of breath, slow pulse and moist perspiring skin are prominent. The triad of coma, pinpoint, immobile pupils and respiratory depression are diagnostic- Reddy 34th/544

Barbiturate poisoning

Shallow respiration, deep coma, no response to painful stimuli, deep reflexes re depressed, subnormal temperature, low blood pressure, thread pulse, ***dilated pupils***- Reddy 34th/544

Poisoning	Clinical presentation
Phencylidine *(Reddy 34th/553)*	Miosis, tachycardia, hypertension
Cocaine *(Parikh Forensic 7th/680)*	Stimulant, dilated pupil, rapid pulse
Barbiturates *(Parikh Forensic 7th/677)*	Cerebral depressant, drowsiness, deep sleep, shallow breathing, fall of blood pressure, alternate contraction & dilation of pupils, cardiorespiratory failure Pupil (Reddy 34th/547)- Usually slightly contracted but react to light; they may dilate during terminal asphyxia
Morphine *(Parikh Forensic 7th/686)*	Start with excitement , later drowsiness & deep coma, pin point pupil, fall of BP, Low respiratory rate(2-4/min) Pupil dilate before death Pupil (Reddy 34th/544)- during stage of coma pupil contracted to pin point size & do not react to light but dilate during the agonal asphyxia phase caused by respiratory depression & ultimate paralysis
Organophosphorus *(Parikh Forensic 7th/687)*	Contracted pupil

111. Ans. a. Dhatura seeds; b. Ratti seeds

[Ref: Reddy 34th/516-17; Parikh 7th/566-67]

"**Suis (sin needle)** are fine needles prepared by decorticating the ***Abrus precatorius(Rati,*** Gunchi) seeds & powdering them, followed by mixing the powder with ***opium, onion, dhatura & spirit or water*** to make into a paste & then paste shaped into small sharp needles, which are allowed to harden by drying. Suis are used to kill cattle either to produce cheap hides or for revenge"- *Reddy 34th/516-17; Parikh 7th/566-67*

PSM

112. Ans. a. Early diagnosis; b. Treatment with Anti-hypertensive drug

[Ref: Park 24th/394-95; Community Medicine by Piyush Gupta 1st/490; Community Medicine with Recent Advances by Suryakantha 4th/ 566]

- Early diagnosis & treatment with Anti-hypertensive drug **comes under secondary prevention**

Primary prevention

◈ *Park 24th/394*

- Defined as: **all measures to reduce the incidence of disease** in a population by reducing the risk of onset
- In connection with primary prevention terms such as **population strategy & High-risk strategy** have become established. WHO has recommended these approaches in the prevention of hypertension. Both the approaches are complementary

Table: Lifestyle modifications to mange hypertension (HTN) *(Park 24th/395)*

Modification	Recommendation (Reduction, Range)	Approximate systolic BP
Weight reduction	Maintain normal body weight (BMI, 18.5–24.9)	5–20mm Hg/10 kg weight loss
Adopt DASH (Dietary approaches to stop HTN) eating plan	Consume a diet rich in fruits, vegetables and low-fat dairy products with a reduced content of saturated fat and total fat	8–14 mm Hg
Dietary sodium reduction	Reduce dietary sodium intake to no more than 100 mEq/d (2.4 g sodium or 6 g sodium chloride)	2–8 mm Hg
Physical activity	Engage in regular aerobic physical activity such as brisk walking (at least 30 minutes per day, most days of the week)	4–9 mm Hg
Moderation of alcohol consumption	Limit consumption to no more than two drinks per day (1 oz or 30 m ethanol eg. 24 oz beer, 10 oz wine, or 3 oz 80-proof whisky) in most men and no more than one drink per day in women and lighter-weight persons	2–4 mm Hg

Box 1: Strategies for prevention of Hypertension *(Piyush Gupta 1st/490)*

- *Primordial prevention:* Preventing hypertension by measures aimed at reducing the blood pressure levels in the population as a whole
- *Primary prevention:* Early identification and effective management of individuals who are 'at risk' of hypertension (e.g., individuals with obesity, genetic predisposition, or stressful life styles).
- *Secondary prevention:* ***Identification and management of hypertensive individuals,*** with/without manifestation of end organ disease, to reduce the morbidity and mortality

Secondary prevention

◈ *Suryakantha 4th/ 566*

- **Early diagnosis** (Identification of hypertensive individual)
- Instituting nonpharmacological management of HTN in all
- ***Use of appropriate drugs to control the blood pressure***
- Regular follow-up to ensure control of BP & compliance of management

113. Ans. a. More specific; b. Easy to perform

[Ref: Park 24th/ 149;Community Medicine by Piyush Gupta 1st/591-93; Community Medicine with Recent Advances by Suryakantha 4th/305-06]

Screening Test: Criteria to be Fulfilled

◈ *Suryakantha 4th/306*

- ***Simple, cheap, safe & rapidly applied***
- *"The disease sought to be screened should be a public health problem"- Piyush Gupta 1st/593*
- Acceptable by people
- Reliable(reproducible or repeatable)
- Valid (accurate). Validity has 2 component- **sensitivity & specificity**
- **"An ideal screening test should be both 100% sensitive & 100% specific. Practically, this is never the case"- Piyush Gupta 1st/593**

Table: Screening and diagnostic test contrasted *(Park 24th/ 145)*

Screening test	Diagnostic test
• Done on apparently healthy	Done on those with indications or sick
• Applied to groups	Applied to single patients, all diseases are considered
• Test results are arbitrary and final	Diagnosis is not final but modified in light of new evidence, diagnosis is the sum of all evidence
• Based on one criterion or cut-off point	Based on evaluation of a number of symptoms, signs (e.g., diabetes) and laboratory findings
• ***Less accurate***	More accurate
• Less expensive	More expensive
• Not a basis for treatment	Used as a basis for treatment
• The initiative comes from the investigator or agency providing care	The initiative comes from a patient with a complaint

114. Ans. a. Calculated in case-control study; c. Closely related to relative risk; d. It is a cross-product ratio calculated by 2x2 table; e. Measure the strength of the association between risk factor and outcome

[Ref: Park 24th/78; Community Medicine by Piyush Gupta 1st/586; Community Medicine with recent Advances by Suryakantha 4th/261]

Odds Ratio (Cross-product Ratio)

◈ *Park 24th/78*

- From a case control study, we can derive what is known as odds Ratio (OR) which is a measure of the **strength of the association between risk factor and outcome.**
- *Odds ratio is **closely related to relative risk.***
- "Case control study: **Generally yields only estimate of relative risk(odd ratio)- *Park 24th/84***
- The derivation of odds ratio is based on three assumptions: **(a) the disease being investigated must be relatively rare; (b) the cases must be representative of those with the disease and (c) the controls must be representative of those without the disease.**
- The odds ratio is the cross product of the entries in Table which is reproduced below:

Table: Case control study- A 2x2 table for computing odds ratio
Piyush Gupta 1st/586, Park 24th/78

	Diseases	
	Yes	No
Exposed	a	b
Not exposed	c	d
Odds radio = ad/bc		

Odds Ratio: Overview

◈ *lifeinthefastlane.com*

- An odds ratio (OR) is a measure of **association between an exposure and an outcome.**
- The OR represents the odds that an outcome will occur given a particular exposure, compared to the odds of the outcome occurring in the absence of that exposure.
- Odds are different to probability — odds is the ratio of the probability that the event of interest occurs to the probability that it does not
- Don't confuse odds with probability and don't confuse odds with odds ratio!
- Odds ratio is not as intuitive as relative risk
- Must be used in case-control studies rather than relative risk (RR) as there is no information on the numbers of all exposed and non-exposed
- Used in logstic regression

Interpretation

- OR is not equivalent to risk
- ***OR is approximately the same as the relative risk (RR) when the outcome is rare (approx <10%)***
- OR <1 tends to underestimate RR, OR >1 tends to overestimate RR; degree of mis-estimation increases at higher base event rates
- OR of 1 means no association
- If OR is reported with a CI which includes 1 then the OR is not significant

115. Ans. a. Maternity benefit; b. Funeral benefit; c. Dependent benefit d. Sickness benefit

[Ref: Park 24th/853-54; Community Medicine by Piyush Gupta 1st/754; Community Medicine with recent Advances by Suryakantha 4th/ 241]

- In medical benefit, **no cash is given (only full medical care provided)**

ESI: Benefit to employees *(First 5 benefits in cash & 6th one in kind)* *Suryakantha 4th/ 241; Park 24th/853-54*

1. ***Sickness benefit**: Periodic **cash payment** (91 days or 309 days)*
2. ***Maternity benefit:** Payable in **cash** to insured woman*
3. ***Disablement benefit**: **Cash payment**, besides free medical treatment*
4. ***Dependent benefit**: **Periodic payment***
5. ***Funeral benefit**: **Cash payment** upto 10,000 (w.e.f 1.4.11)*
6. *Medical benefit: Full medical care(through ESI hospital, dispensaries & panel of private hospital)*
7. *Rehabilitation benefit: continue to get medical treatment after permanent disablement or retirement*

Cost of medical benefit: Steadily increasing. In 2001-02, Rs 905 per capita- *Park 24th/854*

116. Ans. a. Done to evaluate the disease load in the society; b. Identify risk factors associated with health conditions; c. It can be both active and passive; d. It helps in framing new health programmes

[Ref: Park 24th/99,135; Community Medicine by Piyush Gupta 1st/594-97; Cummunity Medicine with recent Advances by Suryakantha 4th/274-78]

- ***Statement (e) is false***

"**Surveillance** is the systematic and continuous collection, analysis and interpretation of data, closely integrated with the timely and coherent dissemination of the results and assessment to those who have the right to know so that action can be taken. The final phase in the surveillance chain is the *application of information to health promotion and to disease prevention and control.* A surveillance system includes a functional capacity for data collection, analysis and ***dissemination lined to public health programs.***"- *Piyush Gupta 1st/594*

Mode of Data Collection Community

◈ *Medicine by Piyush Gupta 1st/595*

- Passive surveillance: Involves routine reporting through the normal channel. No specific efforts are made to make sure all cases are reported. E.g. Surveillance of acute flaccid paralysis
- Active surveillance would be when the public health staff actively seeks cases from the community or healthcare facilities. E.g HIV sentinel Surveillance

Table: Uses of surveillance data *(Piyush Gupta 1st/595)*

- ***Estimate burden of disease and health conditions** to **define public health priorities***
- ***Estimate the burden of risk factors for health conditions***
- Monitor trends in prevalence, incidence of disease and/or risk factors, geographic distribution and risk group distribution
- Detect outbreaks
- Generate hypotheses during outbreaks
- Identify new syndromes
- Identify risk factors associated with health conditions
- Generate hypotheses for subsequent epidemiological investigation
- ***Provide health information to design rational intervention programs***
- Evaluate the effectiveness of health intervention strategies such as vaccines, health education/behavioral programs, legislation, etc.
- Ascertain cases for epidemiological studies
- Detect changes in health practice
- Allocate resources for prevention and control programs
- Project future healthcare needs

Methods of Surveillance (Data Collecting Procedures)

◈ *Suryakantha 4th/276-77*

- ***Active & passive surveillance***
- *Reporting of notifiable diseases*
- *Laboratory based surveillance*
- *Volunteer providers*
- *Registries*
- *Surveys*
- *Information systems*
- *Sentinel events*
- *Record linkages*
- *Combinations of surveillance methods*

117. Ans. a. This is a stage b/w control and eradication; b. It has an element of area association; d. Incomplete interruption of disease transmission

[Ref: Park 24th/ 99; Community Medicine by Piyush Gupta 1st/179]

"**Control → elimination → eradication**" *Piyush Gupta 1st/179*

*The term **elimination** is sometimes used to **describe eradication of disease from a large geographic region** or political jurisdiction- Park 24th/ 99*

Eradication

***Termination of all transmission of infection by extermination of the infectious agent** through surveillance & containment- Park 24th/ 99*

Elimination

◈ *Piyush Gupta 1st/179*

- The reduction of **disease incidence to zero within a defined geographical area** is called elimination.
- In disease control and elimination phases, continued intervention efforts are required to prevent the reemergence of infection.
- Certain disease elimination programs have defined the term in a different manner, i.e. 'reduction of case transmission to a predetermined very low level'. For example, leprosy elimination was defined as a reduction in the prevalence of leprosy cases to less than 1/10000 under the national leprosy Eradication Program of India. Similarly, neonatal tetanus elimination is said to be achieved when the new cases is less than 1 per 1000 live births in every district of a country
- Some disease related programs are aimed at "eliminating a disease as a public health threat," and this is interpreted to imply reducing incidence to an arbitrarily defined "acceptable" level but not necessarily to zero.

Eradication

◈ *Piyush Gupta 1st/179*

- The term denotes the **certified total absence of human cases**, the **absence of reservoir for the organism in nature** and **absolute containment of any infectious source**.
- Continued intervention efforts are either no longer required or markedly reduced.
- Smallpox has been eradicated.
- There are no levels of eradication. It is **either eradicated or not eradicated.**

118. Ans. c. Failure rate is 1 in 300; d. Increased risk of testicular cancer

[Ref: Park 24th/543; Community Medicine by Piyush Gupta 1st/637-38; Community Medicine with recent Advances by Suryakantha 4th/686; Shaw's Gynae 16th/280; Dutta Gynae 7th/406-07]

"Non-scalpel **vasectomy (NSV):** *There is **no increase in testicular cancer** or heart disease. Risk of prostate cancer is considered to have no causal association*"- *Dutta Gynae 7th/407*

Two semen analysis reports *must confirm the absence of sperms before the man can be declared sterile-Shaw's Gynae 16th/280*

"Semen should be examined either by one test after 16 weeks or by two tests at 12 & 16 weeks after vasectomy & if the **two consecutive semen analyses** ***show absence of spermatozoa****, the man is declared as sterile"- Dutta Gynae 7th/407*

Vasectomy

◈ *Park 24th/543*

- It is a permanent sterilization operation done in the male where a ***segment of vas deferens*** of both the sides are resected & the cut ends are ligated
- It is a simple, cheap, safe, very effective, permanent & quick surgical method of family planning
- **Failure rate** is generally low, ***0.15 pregnancies per 100 persons*** in the first year after the procedure- *Park 24th/543; Dutta Gynae 7th/406*
- **Failure rate is 0.15-1/HWY**- *Piyush Gupta 1st/637*
- ***Additional contraceptive protection is needed for about 2-3 months or at least 20-30 ejaculation***(whichever comes first) following operations, i.e. till the semen becomes free of sperm
- It is ***not castration, it does not affect the testes & it does not affect sexual ability***. Some men may complain of diminution of sexual vigour, impotence, headache, fatigue etc. Such adverse psychological effects are seen in men who have undergone vasectomy under emotional pressure
- Autoimmune response: ***Normally, 2% of fertile men have circulating antibodies against their own sperm***. In men who have had vasectomies, the figure can be as ***high as 54%.*** There is no reason to believe that such antibodies are harmful to physical health
- The ***incidence of recanalization is 0-6% after procedure***
- In no-scalpel vasectomy(NSV): In this instead of incision, small puncture is made & require no suturing of punctured site, just a small bandage is sufficient
- NSV- It is an improvement on the conventional vasectomy with shorter duration,less painful & bruising, shorter recovery time & ***practically no side effects or complication***- *Piyush Gupta 1st/637; Suryakantha 4th/686*

OPHTHALMOLOGY

119. Ans. **a. Fungal corneal ulcer; c. Rifabutin drug use; d. Behcet's disease**

[Ref: A.K.Khurana 6th/ 102-03; Parson 22nd/ 196; Oxford Handbook of Ophthalmology 3rd/892]

Mycotic Corneal Ulcer

Usually a big hypopyon is present even if the ulcer is very small- A.K.Khurana 6th/ 106

"Cause of hypopyon: *Behcet's disease*, endophthalmitis, panuveitis/panophthalmitis and ***adverse reactions to some drugs*** (such as ***rifabutin***)**"**-*en.wikipedia.org;www.sciencedirect.com*

The **differential diagnosis of hypopyon:** *www.djo.harvard.edu*

- Infectious etiologies include hypopyon associated with corneal ulcers or endophthalmitis.
- Severe acute iridocyclitis can also present as hypopyon uveitis.
- Certain systemic drugs (e.g. ***rifabutin***)
- Retained intraocular foreign bodies, including toxic lens syndrome &after trauma.
- Surgical causes:refractive surgery, pars plana vitrectomy with silicone oil injection.
- Necrosis of intraocular tumors or metastases (e.g. leukemia, non-Hodgkins lymphoma and retinoblastoma)

Hypopyon: Causes

◈ *www.actforlibraries.org*

Hypopyon is the collection of pus in the bottom of the anterior chamber of the eye. It can be clearly visualized as a fluid level and the sedimentation is governed by the gravity. The composition of the pus would be only white cells or leucocytes without any pathogens of bacterial, fungal or even viral origin

Infections of the iris and the uvea can be caused by both systemic as well as local conditions. Some of them are,

a. **Corneal ulcers**
b. **Tuberculosis**
c. **Herpes Simplex and Herpes Zoster:** These viruses that are causative organisms for the herpes infection and chicken pox are culprits in creating a form of hypopyon.
d. **Lyme disease and toxocariasis:**Both of these infections are systemic infections that can manifest as a hypopyon.
e. **Multiple sclerosis and Psoriatic arthritis:** The conditions are being driven by an autoimmune process and it has been found to cause pus formation in the eye without a underlying infection.

Causative Organisms

Many pyogenic organisms (staphylococci, streptococci, gonococci, Moraxella) may produce hypopyon, but by far the most dangerous are *pseudomonas pyocyanea* **and** *pneumococcus*"- *A.K.Khurana 6th/ 102-03; Parson 22nd/ 196*

About Other Options

- **Episcleritis** is an inflammatory disorder involving the episcleral tissue that lies superficial to the sclera, just beneath Tenon's capsule. Episcleritis is usually mild, characterized by slight conjunctival injection and the presence of a foreign body sensation. The episodes often resolve without treatment, but can recur-*A.K.Khurana 6th/ 141*
- **Retinitis pigmentosa**: This retinal dystrophy is a hereditary disorder predominantly affecting the rods more than the cones.

120. Ans. **a. Head tilt to opposite normal shoulder; c. Hypertropia of the affected eye; d. Diplopia**

[Ref: A.K.Khurana 6th/ 337-39; Parson 22nd/ 441-42]

"Blepharoptosis is an abnormal low-lying upper eyelid margin with the eye in primary gaze. Neurogenic blepharoptosis may result from ***third nerve palsy***"- eyewiki.aao.org

Paralysis of the Superior Oblique

◈ *Parson 22nd/ 441-42*

- There is ***hypertropia of the affected eye*** with limitation of movement downwards and towards the sound side; the face is turned downwards and towards the sound side with a ***slight tilt of the head towards the shoulder of the sound or the normal side.***
- ***Homonymous diplopia*** occurs on looking down; the false image is lower and its upper end is tilted towards the true image (the image is intorted because the eye is extorted when the superior oblique is paralysed). The distance between the images increases on looking down and towards the sound side and the inclination of the false image increases on looking down to the *paralysed* side.
- A congenital left superior oblique palsy produces a compensatory ***head tilt to the right with chin depression and slight face turn to the right***. Thus, binocular vision is maintained in the primary position.
- When the head is forcibly tilted to the left, reflex intorsion is excited. This can now only be undertaken by the left superior rectus which is stimulated to overact. The result is an unopposed overelevation of the left eye (Bielschowsky head tilt test).
- Bilateral superior oblique palsy may follow head trauma and give rise to a form of **diplopia** which is often unrecognized because it is due to ***excyclotropia.***

"Hypertropia is an ocular disorder characterized by either constant or intermittent upwards deviation of one eye in comparison to the other eye. On the other hand, hypotropia involves downward deviation of one eye compared to the other. Hypertropia can also be referred to as vertical strabismus. The most common type of vertical strabismus is a ***trochlear nerve palsy.***1 The fourth cranial nerve, aka trochlear nerve, innervates the superior oblique muscle"-eyewiki.aao.org

"Among the diagnostic features distinguishing bilateral from unilateral paralysis were a right hypertropia in left gaze and left hypertropia in right gaze and a positive Bielschowsky test on tilting the head toward either shoulder. However, absence of either sign did not exclude bilateral paralysis. Large excyclotropia and a V-pattern esotropia are suggestive of but not diagnostic for bilateral paralysis. Complaints about cyclotropia are limited to acquired paralysis. Cyclotropia in the normal eye, head tilt toward the involved side, or absence of any abnormal head posture limits the diagnostic value of these associated signs. jamanetwork.com

Superior Oblique Palsy

◈ *Review of Ophthalmology by William B. Trattler 2nd/149*

- ***Findings:*** diplopia (vertical, horizontal, or torsional). In long-standing cases of SO palsy, comitance develops and the deviation becomes more difficult to localize (hypertropia can be present in all fields of gaze)
- ***Bilateral:*** objective torsion is often >10° of excyclotorsion(measure with double Maddox rod), often have inferior oblique overaction with V-pattern ET and chin-down head posture, alternate hypertropia with head tilt
- ***Diagnosis:*** Parks-Bielschowsky 3-step test (i.e. ***right superior oblique palsy produces right hypertropia in*** *primary gaze*, **worsens in left gaze and in right head tilt)**

"Superior oblique palsy may cause double vision because of misalignment of the eyes (the brain perceives an image from two different directions). The double vision may be vertical (one image on top of the other), diagonal (vertically and horizontally separated) and less often torsional (rotated or twisted). The torsional phenomenon occurs more frequently with acquired cases of superior oblique palsy"-***aapos.org***

"Diplopia chart for a case with paralysis of the **right superior oblique**: The r***ight eye is hypertropic***, extorted and esotropicas the superior oblique is a depressor, intortor and abductor. The diplopia is thus homonymous and the false image belonging to the right eye is lower and intorted"- ***Parson 22nd/ 442***

121. Ans. a. Attached to lateral palpebral ligaments; b. Meibomian gland is present here; c. Upper lid tarsal plate is larger than lower lidtarsal plate; d. Forms skeleton of eyelid; e. Superior tarsal muscle associated with superior tarsal plate is innervated by the sympathetic nervous system

[Ref: Gray's Anatomy 40th/670-71;A.K.Khurana 6th/ 363; Parson 22nd/449-50]

Tarsal Plates

◈ *Gray's Anatomy 40th/670-71*

- The two tarsal plates are thin, elongated, ***crescent-shaped*** plates of firm, dense fibrous tissue approximately 2.5 cm long. There is one in each eyelid to provide support and determine eyelid form. Each is convex and conforms to the configuration of the anterior surface of the eye.
- The free ciliary border is straight and adjacent to the eyelash follicles. The orbital border is convex and attached to the orbital septum.
- The **superior tarsus**, the ***larger of the two***, is semi-oval, approximately 10 mm in height centrally. Its inferior edge is parallel to and approximately 2 mm from, the lid margin.
- The **smaller inferior tarsus** is ***narrower*** and approximately 4 mm in vertical height.
- The tarsal plates are connected to the margins of the orbit by the orbital septum and by the medial and ***lateral palpebral (canthal) ligaments.***
- The **medial palpebral ligament** passes from the medial ends of the two tarsal plates to the anterior lacrimal crest and the frontal process of the maxilla. It splits at its insertion into the tarsal plates to surround the lacrimal canaliculi and lies in front of the nasolacrimal sac and the orbital septum.
- The **lateral palpebral ligament** is relatively poorly developed. It passes from the lateral ends of the tarsal plates to a small tubercle on the zygomatic bone within the orbital margin and is more deeply situated than the medial palpebral ligament.
- It lies beneath the orbital septum and the lateral palpebral raphe of orbicularis oculi. The ***deepest fibres of the aponeuros is of levator palpebrae superioris are attached to the anterior surface of the superior tarsus.*** The superior and inferior tarsal plates are also associated with a thin

lamina of smooth muscle forming the **superior and inferior tarsalmuscles** respectively.

- Opposite the equator of the eye the **superior tarsal muscle** passes from the inferior face of levator palpebrae superioris to a fibrous extension which projects to the upper margin of the superior tarsus. The ***muscle is innervated by the sympathetic nervous system*** and on contraction, elevates the eyelid. Although it may be regarded as supplementing the action of the levator muscle, its full role is not clear. (The mild ptosis that is a characteristic feature of Horner's syndrome is the result of an interruption to the ***sympathetic supply to the superior tarsal muscle.***)
- **Tarsal (Meibomian) glands** are modified sebaceous glands embedded in the tarsal plates
- *Tarsal plates:* There are two plates of dense connective tissue, one for each lid, which give shape and firmness to the lids. The upper and lower tarsal plates join with each other at medial and lateral canthi; and are attached to the orbital margins through medial and lateral palpebral ligaments. In the substance of the tarsal plates lie ***meibomian glands in parallel rows***- *A.K.Khurana 6th/ 363*

122. Ans. **a. Capsular hooks**

[Ref: A.K.Khurana 6th/203-04; Parson 22nd/278-82;www.ascrs.org;www.touchophthalmology.com]

- *Low power settings phacoemulsification is used*

"Iris repository: Two limbed instrument ***used to remove the iris during posterior chamber maneuvers***"- *en.wikipedia.org*

Ophthalmology instrument

Iris repositor

- **Iris hook**: Straight shaft, blunt curved hook. Flat handle. Overall length: 125mm- www.accutome.com
- **Desmarres Lid Retractor** is a handheld ophthalmologic retractor used for ***retaining primarily the upper eyelid and eyelashes.*** It may be used to pull down the lower lid as well. The curved, saddle style blade contours to the round shape of the eye as well as the curvature of the eyelid created when it is retracted- *www.sklarcorp.com; A.K.Khurunu 6th/596*
- **Phacoemulsification** should be performed with ***minimal pressure*** exerted on the zonules. Whichever technique is chosen, ***lowering all of the settings is advisable.*** This is carried out to avoid exerting undue pressure on the capsule and zonules. Besides the direct hydrostatic forces on the capsule and zonules, the zonular laxity allows for transudation of the fluid into the vitreous, with resultant vitreous hydration causing increased positive posterior pressure with possible vitreous loss. A technique described by Osher as **'slow motion phacoemulsification,'** uses a bottle height between 35–50 cm, aspiration rate around 12 cc per minute, vacuum below 30 mmHg and ***low ultrasound power.*** This was shown to produce only very minor intraocular pressure fluctuations during phacoemulsification, protecting against AC shallowing"-www.touchophthalmology.com

Iris Hooks

◈ *www.touchophthalmology.com*

- Iris hooks have been used to fixate and support the anterior capsule following capsulorrhexis.[39,40] Also available are hooks designed specifically for the capsule. As is the case for iris retraction, four equidistant stab incisions are made for insertion of the hooks. The hooks engage the edge of the capsulorrhexis and are carefully retracted to provide evenly distributed support to the capsule. Hydrodissection and the remaining steps are performed as described above and the hooks are removed after the lens is inserted.
- One proposed benefit of the iris hooks compared with a CTR is that the hooks offer protection against anteroposterior movement, since with a CTR the whole bag can still move along with the zonules.[39] They also do not trap cortex beneath them as can occur with a CTR inserted early in the case. Hooks can also be combined with CTR in cases of dialysis from 3 to 6 clock hours.[19] Given the smaller profile of the hooks, one possibility is inserting the hooks just after completing capsulorrhexis so that the CTR does not have to be inserted with the nucleus still in place.

The surgical approach to phacoemulsification of the subluxated crystalline lens differs depending on the degree of zonulopathy and the underlying pathophysiologic origin. In cases in which the zonular abnormality is less than 3 contiguous clock hours, attentive surgical technique may suffice for a successful surgical outcome, although ***capsule retractors*** may provide additional support- *www.ascrs.org*

Management of Subluxated Cataracts

◈ *crstodayeurope.com*

- Surgical management of ectopialentis is one of the major challenges faced by cataract surgeons today.Ectopialentis signifies a displacement or malposition of the crystalline lens, irrespective of cause. It may occur congenitally or as part of developmental anomalies or result from blunt external trauma or iatrogenic zonular dehiscence during complicated cataract surgery.
- In eyes with ectopialentis, the **phacoemulsification technique** used depends on the degree of zonulopathy and its underlying pathophysiologic origin.
- When the zonular abnormality is less than 3 contiguous clock hours, slow and careful surgery may be sufficient for a successful surgical outcome, with adjunctive support from ***capsule retractors.***
- When the area of zonular dialysis is small, with otherwise strong zonular attachment elsewhere, as in trauma, a ***capsular tension ring (CTR)*** may not be routinely required.
- On the other hand, the use of a CTR is mandatory even in mild cases of zonular laxity that have a progressive pathologic nature, as in PXF, Weill-Marchesani syndrome, Marfan syndrome, or retinitis pigmentosa. These are cases in which the zonular pathology worsens with time and the CTR can be helpful for secondary fixation of the bag if necessary. It is wise to implant a CTR in every case in which zonular disturbance is suspected.

- In younger patients with such risk factors, ***bag fixation to the sclera*** with a capsular tension segment (CTS) is advisable from the beginning. The operating surgeon is the ultimate judge, but he or she should remain flexible in these cases and be prepared to handle a greater degree of difficulty than anticipated during the preoperative assessment.
- **Five pearls for challenging surgery of sublaxated lens are:**
  - **Incision:** The modern cataract surgeon is likely accustomed to using a clear corneal temporal incision. The dictum in eyes with lens subluxation is that the main incision should not lie directly over the area of zonulopathy when possible. The paracentesis wound for a second instrument should be more corneal to prevent injury to the rhexis margin, which tends to be slightly anteriorly tented after fixation of iris hooks.
  - **Capsulorrhexis:**
    - The capsulorrhexis is the most challenging step of cataract surgery in eyes with ectopialentis because capsulorrhexis completion and bag preservation are mandatory for successful phacoemulsification.
    - The first capsular puncture can be made with a standard cystotome or a straight 25-gauge needle
    - In most unstable lenses, microforceps or a hook may be used to provide countertraction during the continuous tear of the capsule. This second instrument should be placed at least 2 to 3 clock hours from the leading edge of the capsulorrhexis to avoid runaway
    - Countertraction with a ***Kuglen hook*** during capsulorrhexis creation (A) and countertraction with an iris hook and centration of a subluxated lens
  - **Stabilization of the Capsular Bag:**
    - If zonular dysfunction involves a large area, for instance in the range of 3 to 6 clock hours, then the capsule must be supported during surgery. This can be done using flexible iris retractors strategically placed through limbal stab incisions to hook the capsulorrhexis edge and support the bag
    - The disadvantage of this approach is that the hook ends can inadvertently tear the rhexis edge. They also tend to bring the capsular bag into a more anterior plane and sometimes in extreme subluxation the lens itself can be in the anterior chamber. Capsular hooks, therefore, are a better alternative, as they support the bag by its equator and keep it distended, reducing the risk of aspiration of the bag equator
    - The capsular bag can be stabilized with an Ahmed CTS by hooking the fixation eyelet with an iris retractor. In patients with deep anterior chambers, a capsular hook may be placed through a prelimbal stab incision to reduce the chance of the hook slipping
    - The best way to stabilize a compromised capsular bag is to place a CTR. Segmental designs with eyelets, such as the Cionni or Ahmed CTS, can be sutured to the sclera to stabilize focal defects. Alternatively, the CTS can be fixed by passing an iris hook through an eyelet.
  - **Phacoemulsification:**
    - The next important phase of surgery is phacoemulsification of the cataractous lens. Zonulopathy makes the situation more difficult, as mobilization of the nucleus in the bag is nearly impossible due to a lack of countertraction.
    - The risk of damaging the bag can be reduced with meticulous and repeated hydrodissection and viscodissection, crucial steps in this procedure. Slow-motion phacoemulsifcation with low parameters is mandatory.
  - **Long-term Bag Fixation:** Available tools for bag fixation include standard CTRs, the Cionni ring and the Ahmed CTS. The process of selecting which tool to use is ruled by the degree of zonular damage and its chance of progression.

123. Ans. a. Cataract; e. Iris cyst

[Ref: A.K.Khurana 6th/ 253; Parson 22nd/254]

Glaucomas Associated with Iridocorneal Endothelial Syndromes *A.K.Khurana 6th/ 253*

- Iridocorneal endothelial (ICE) syndromes include three clinical entities:*Progressive iris atrophy, Chandler's syndrome andCogan-Reese syndrome.*
- ***Pathogenesis.*** The common feature of the ICE syndromes is the presence of abnormal corneal endothelial cells which proliferate to form an endothelial membrane in the angle of anterior chamber. Glaucoma is caused by secondary synechial angle-closure as a result of contraction of this endothelial membrane.
- The ICE syndromes typically affect middle-aged women. The raised IOP is associated with characteristic features of the causative condition.
- In *'progressive iris atrophy'*, iris features predominate with marked ***corectopia, atrophy and hole formation.***
- While in *Chandler's syndrome,* changes in iris are mild to absent and the corneal oedema even at normal IOP predominates (corneal edema can be microcystic-http://eyewiki.aao.org)
- Hallmark of *Cogan-Reese syndrome* is ***nodular or diffuse pigmented lesions of the iris*** (therefore also called as *iris naevus syndrome*) which may or may not be associated with corneal changes

Essential (Progressive) Atrophy of the Iris

Parson 22nd/254

- This disease of unknown aetiology is characterized by a slowly progressive atrophic change in the tissues of the iris, which leads to the complete disappearance of large portions of this tissue. It forms part of the iridocornealendothelial (ICE) syndromes.
- The disease usually starts insidiously in early adult life by the development of large areas of atrophy which coalesce and progress to form lacunae. Vision is eventually lost by the gradual onset of glaucoma due to downgrowth of an endothelial membrane over the tissues at the angle of the anterior chamber.

- Contraction of the membrane produces ***synechiae, corectopia, iris atrophy from ischaemia, ectropionuveae, dyscoria*** (abnormal shape of the pupil), polycoria (more than one pupil due to secondary holes in the iris) and ***nodules in the iris***. The prognosis is poor, but fortunately the disease is usually unilateral

"An iris cyst is an epithelial-lined space that involves a layer of the iris. A primary iris cyst does not have a recognizable etiology. A secondary iris cyst has a recognizable etiology, such as surgical or nonsurgical trauma"-eyewiki.aao.org

124. Ans. a. Primary open angle glaucoma (POAG); c. Family history; e. TIGR gene presence

[Ref: Shields Textbook of Glaucoma 6th/346; pdfs.semanticscholar.org; A.K.Khurana 6th/251; Parson 22nd/ 294,302]

Higher than Average Risk for Steroid Glaucoma is Found in Patients with

◈ *Shields Textbook of Glaucoma 6th/346*

- ***Primary open angle glaucoma (POAG)***
- A first degree relative with POAG(a personal or ***family history of glaucoma***-*www.saeyeinstitute.com*)
- A history of previous steroid induced intraocular pressure (IOP) elevation
- Type 1 Diabetes Mellitus
- Very young age (age less than six years old) or an older age
- Connective tissue disease
- Penetrating keratoplasty, especially in eyes with Fuchs endothelial dystrophy or keratoconus
- High myopia
- ***No gender*** & racial predilection exists for Steriod induced glaucoma-pdfs.semanticscholar.org
- Glucocorticoids may exert their effect by increased expression of MYOC [***Trabecular meshwork-induced glucocorticoid response (TIGR)***] gene at locus GLC1A-*pdfs.semanticscholar.org*

Risk Factorsfor Steroid Induced Glaucoma

The possibility of high response is greater in the following cases: patients with primary open-angle glaucoma ***(POAG)*** or glaucoma suspects, ***first-degree relatives with POAG***, old age or age less than 6 years, connective tissue disease, especially rheumatoid arthritis in men, ***high myopia***, type 1 diabetes mellitus and angle recession glaucoma. Patients with predisposing risk factors should be monitored more diligently when receiving corticosteroids"-*www.karger.com*

Steroid-Induced Glaucoma

◈ *A.K.Khurana 6th/251*

- It is a type of ***secondary open-angle glaucoma*** which develops following topical and sometimes systemic steroid therapy.
- ***Etiopathogenesis.*** It has been postulated that the response of IOP to steroids is genetically determined. Following theories have been put forward: *Glycosaminoglycans (GAG) theory, Endothelial cell theory &Prostaglandin theory.*
- ***Clinical features.*** Steroid-induced glaucoma typically resembles POAG
- ***Management.*** It can be *prevented* by a judicious use of steroids and a regular monitoring of IOP when steroid therapy is a must.

125. Ans. a. Autosomal recessive inheritance; c. Abnormal stromal deposit of mucopolysaccharide which stain positive with Alcian blue; d. Recurs after corneal transplant; e. Laser therapy can be done

[Ref: A.K.Khurana 6th/129; Parson 22nd/ 213]

- *Opacities are present throughout the cornea with **no clear spaces between***

Macular Corneal Dystrophy (Groenouw type-II or Fehr Spotted Dystrophy)

◈ *A.K. Khurana 6th/129*

- It is an ***autosomal recessive*** dystrophy characterized by appearance of dense grey opacity in the central cornea.
- Genetic locus is 16q22
- The condition results due to ***accumulation of mucopolysaccharides*** owing to a local enzyme deficiency.
- It occurs in childhood (5 to 10 years) and leads to marked defective vision in early life, which usually requires penetrating keratoplasty

"Accumulation of glycosaminoglycans in the cornea (stroma, Descemet's, endothelium) which stain with colloidal iron or ***Alcian blue***"- *eyewiki.aao.org*

"A macular form of **corneal dystrophy** has a recessive heredity and in it the visual acuity tends to be affected at an early age. The ***opacities are present throughout the cornea with no clear spaces between.*** Histopathological examination of the cornea by ***special stains*** after keratoplastydemonstrates the nature of the material deposited. Intracellularly and extracellularly in the corneal stroma, endothelium and Descemet's membrane"-*Parson 22nd/ 213*

"Macular corneal dystrophy: Since the condition affects the entire corneal stroma, Descemet membrane and corneal endothelium, lamellar keratoplasty does not excise all damaged tissue. ***Corneal transplantation*** may therefore be needed. Vision can be restored by corneal grafting but ***opacities may recur in the graft after many years***"- *rarediseases.info.nih.gov*

"Substantial corneal erosions and a slight reduction in visual acuity can be treated with Phototherapeutic keratectomy (PTK) using an excimer laser. PTK usually only works well for very superficial opacities. A severe reduction in visual acuity or large and deep opacities usually necessitate a corneal transplant. ***Even after a corneal transplant the corneal deposits can come back after time***"-*www.mastereyeassociates.com*

126. Ans. b. Neonatal hypoglycaemia; e. Reiger's syndrome

[Ref: A.K.Khurana 6th/182-83; Parson 22nd/264;Nelson Paediatrics 18th/Chap 627]

- ***Neonatal hypoglycemia & Reiger's syndrome*** causes **cataract** (*Nelson table*)
- **Zellweger syndrome (Hepato-cerebral renal syndrome)** is associated with ***developmental glaucoma***-*A.K.Khurana 6th/228*

- **Rieger syndrome**: Ocular malformations, called Rieger eye malformations, include underdeveloped iris, a small cornea (microcornea), an opaque ring around the outer edge of the cornea, adhesions (abnormal union of surfaces normally separate) in the front of the eye and/or displacement of the pupil of the eye so that it is not centered. **Glaucoma** (increased pressure within the eyeball) may result from the ocular malformations associated with Rieger syndrome"- www.encyclopedia.com; *A.K.Khurana 6th/228*
- "**Canavan disease** is a progressive, fatal neurological disorder that begins in infancy. It is caused by an inherited genetic abnormality: the lack of an essential enzyme causes deterioration of the white matter (myelin) in the brain, thereby preventing the proper transmission of nerve signals. Symptoms of Canavan disease vary, but generally include rapidly increasing head circumference, lack of head control, reduced visual responsiveness and abnormal muscle tone such as stiffness or floppiness"- www.canavanfoundation.org

Congenital Cataracts Often Occur as Part of the following Birth Defects

◈ *medlineplus.gov*

- Chondrodysplasia syndrome
- Congenital rubella
- Conradi-Hünermann syndrome
- Down syndrome (trisomy 21)
- Ectodermal dysplasia syndrome
- Familial congenital cataracts
- Galactosemia
- Hallermann-Streiff syndrome
- Lowe syndrome
- Marinesco-Sjögren syndrome
- Pierre-Robin syndrome
- Trisomy 13

Table: Differential Diagnosis of Cataracts *(Nelson Paediatrics 18th/ Chap 627)*

Genetic Disorders
Multisystem Genetic Disorders
Alport syndrome (hearing loss, renal disease)
Alström syndrome (nerve deafness, diabetes mellitus)
Apert disease (craniosynostosis, syndactyly)
Cockayne syndrome (premature senility, skin photosensitivity)
Conradi disease (chondrodysplasiapunctata)
Crouzon disease (dysostosis craniofacialis)
Hallermann-Streiff syndrome (microphthalmia, small pinched nose, skin atrophy and hypotrichosis)
Hypohidrotic ectodermal dysplasia (anomalous dentition, hypohidrosis, hypotrichosis)
Ichthyosis (keratinizing disorder with thick, scaly skin)
Incontinentia pigmenti (dental anomalies, mental retardation, cutaneous lesions)

Contd...

Genetic Disorders
Lowe syndrome (oculocerebrorenal syndrome: hypotonia, renal disease)
Marfan syndrome
Meckel-Gruber syndrome (renal dysplasia, encephalocele)
Myotonic dystrophy
Nail-patella syndrome (renal dysfunction, dysplastic nails, hypoplastic patella)
Marinesco-Sjögren syndrome (cerebellar ataxia, hypotonia)
Nevoid basal cell carcinoma syndrome (autosomal dominant, basal cell carcinoma erupts in childhood)
Peters anomaly (corneal opacifications with iris-corneal dysgenesis)
Reiger syndrome (iris dysplasia, myotonic dystrophy)
Rothmund-Thomson syndrome (poikiloderma: skin atrophy)
Rubinstein-Taybi syndrome (broad great toe, mental retardation)
Smith-Lemli-Opitz syndrome (toe syndactyly, hypospadias, mental retardation)
Sotos syndrome (cerebral gigantism)
Spondyloepiphyseal dysplasia (dwarfism, short trunk)
Werner syndrome (premature aging in 2nd decade of life)
Inborn Errors of Metabolism
Abetalipoproteinemia (absent chylomicrons, retinal degeneration)
Fabry disease (α-galactosidase A deficiency)
Galactokinase deficiency
Galactosemia (galactose-1-phosphate uridyltransferase deficiency)
Homocystinemia (subluxation of lens, mental retardation)
Mannosidosis (acid α-mannosidase deficiency)
Niemann-Pick disease (sphingomyelinase deficiency)
Refsum disease (phytanic acid α-hydrolase deficiency)
Wilson disease (accumulation of copper leads to cirrhosis and neurologic symptoms)
Endocrinopathies
Hypocalcemia (hypoparathyroidism)
Hypoglycemia
Diabetes mellitus
IDIOPATHIC

Congenital and Developmental Cataracts

◈ *A.K. Khurana 6th/ 182-83*

- These occur due to some disturbance in the normal growth of the lens. When the disturbance occurs before birth, the child is born with a *congenital cataract.* Therefore, in congenital cataract the opacity is limited to either embryonic or foetal nucleus.
- *Developmental cataract* may occur from infancy to adolescence. Therefore, such opacities may involve infantile or adult nucleus, deeper parts of cortex or capsule.

- **Etiology**-*Metabolic disorders* of the foetus or infant such as galactosemia, galactokinase deficiency and ***neonatal hypoglycemia***.

127. Ans. a. Lateral tarsorrhaphy; b. Eyelid surgery with skin graft; c. Extraocular muscle surgery; d. Levator palpebrae superioris (LPS) muscle resection

[Ref: A.K.Khurana 6th/414-16;Ophthalmology by Myron Yanoff 3rd/233]

"**Acquired myogenic ptosis**: Occur due acquired disorder of levator palpebrae superioris muscle (LPS). It may occur **in *muscle thyrotoxicosis.*** Treatment includes ***LPS muscle resection***"-*A.K.Khurana 6th/380-81*

Non-pharmacologic Treatment

◈ *Ophthalmology by Myron Yanoff 3rd/233*

- Prism, patches, tape, eye exercises
- ***Sequence of Surgical Interventions***
  - ***Orbital decompression***
  - Ocular muscle surgery
  - Adjustment of eyelid margin
  - Blepharoplasty
  - Retrobulbar radiation therapy (up to 2000 cGy).

"Surgery involves moving the eyelids into a more normal position. In the upper eyelids this is usually performed by removing or stretching the scarred muscles. In the ***lower eyelids, a graft is often needed to help push the eyelid upward***"-*www.gdatf.org*

"Eyelid surgery may involve recession of the upper eyelid retractors, recession of the lower eyelid retractors ***with or without a spacer graft and conservative blepharoplasty***"-www.ijo.in/article.asp

Tarsorrhaphy

◈ *www.ncbi.nlm.nih.go*

- It may be- lateral, medial, or central; total or partial; temporary or permanent
- A temporary central tarsorrhaphy with a drawstring that allows it to be repeatedly opened and closed for examining the eye.
- A permanent lateral tarsorrhaphy that leaves the central lids open, allowing the patient to see and the eye to be examined.
- Tarsorrhaphy is most commonly performed to protect the cornea from exposure caused by inadequate eyelid coverage, as may occur in ***Graves disease*** or facial nerve (CN VII) dysfunctions such as Bell palsy"-*www.aao.org*

Management of Graves' Ophthalmopathy

◈ *A.K.Khurana 6th/414-16*

- *Topical artificial tear drops*
- *Guanethidine 5% eyedrops*may decrease the lid retraction caused by overaction of Muller's muscle.
- *Systemic steroids*
- *Radiotherapy (2000 rads given over 10 daysperiod).*
- ***Lateral tarsorrhaphy*** should be performed in patients with exposure keratopathy (with mild to moderate proptosis) not responding to topical artificial tears.
- *Extraocular muscle surgery*. It should be carried out for left-out diplopia in primary gaze
- *Surgical orbital decompression.* It should be performed in patients with marked proptosis associated with severe exposure keratopathy and/or optic neuropathy with imminent danger of permanent visual loss.
- *Cosmetic surgery for persistent lid retraction.* ***It consists of levator and Muller's muscle recession***. Recently, implantation of scleral grafts has become a popular technique.
- *Blepharoplasty.* It may be performed by removal of excess fatty tissue and redundant skin from around the eyelids

Thyroid-associated Orbitopathy (TAO)

◈ *emedicine.medscape.com*

- TAO, frequently termed Graves ophthalmopathy, is part of an autoimmune process that can affect the orbital and periorbital tissue, the thyroid gland and rarely, the pretibial skin or digits (thyroid acropachy)
- Approximately 5% of patients with thyroid-associated orbitopathy (TAO) may require surgical intervention..
- The timing of surgery is important.
- The **sequence of surgery** is also important. If the patient has marked proptosis, strabismus and lid deformity, perform surgery in the following order:
  - *Orbital decompression*
  - *Strabismus surgery*
  - *Lid-lengthening surgery*
  - *Blepharoplasty*

ENT

128. Ans. a. Flattening of cheek, b. Trismus, c. Step deformity, d. Hypoesthesia along distribution of infraorbital nerve

[Ref: Dhingra 7th/205-06; Logan and Turner 10th /90-91]

- CSF rhinorrhea is feature of maxilla fracture

Zygoma/Zygomatic Fracture (Tripod Fracture): *Features*

◈ *Dhingra 7th/205-06*

- After nasal bone, zygoma is the second most frequently fractured bone
- ***Flattening of malar prominence***
- ***Step deformity*** of infraorbital margin
- ***Anesthesia in distribution of infraorbital nerve***
- ***Trismus***
- Diplopia, restricted ocular movements

Zygomatic Complex Fracture

◈ *Logan and Turner 10th /90-91*

- Patient may complain of diplopia, pain on mouth opening/ ***trismus,*** or ***reduced projection of the cheek*** (due to zygoma depression, a late sign caused by swelling).
- There is usually lateral subconjuctival haemorrhage and if the zygomaticotemporal or zygomaticobuccal branches of the ***infraorbital nerve*** are involved, there will be ***paraesthesia of the overlying skin.***
- Examination should look directly at the area for bony deficiency or displacement, as well as those structures that can be indirectly involved – the eye and brain.

Fractures of Maxilla–They are *classified into* three types:

◈ *Dhingra 7th/207*

- **Le Fort I (transverse), Le Fort II (pyramidal) & Le Fort III** (craniofacial disjunction).
- ***Malocclusion of teeth*** with anterior open bite
- Elongation of midface
- Mobility in the maxilla
- ***CSF rhinorrhea.***

129. Ans. b. Meniere's disease, c. Cochlear deafness, d. SNHL

[Ref: Dhingra 7th/28, 511; ENT by Hazarika3rd/65]

- ***Tone decay test mainly used to identify retrocochlear type of SNHL(Marked tone decay indicates Retro-Cochlear Pathology).*** *But it may be used in cochlear lesion(mild tone decay)-see below references*
- ***Meniere's diseases causes cochlear SNHL.*** **Otosclerosis & otitis media** causes ***conductive deafness***

SNHL: *Cochlear (Sensory) & Neural*

◈ *(peripheral-8th CN & central)-Dhingra 7th/31*

Tone decay test: It is a Measure of Nerve Fatigue and is used to *Detect Retrocochlear Lesion*

◈ *Dhingra 7th/28*

Tone Decay Test -

◈ *ENT by Hazarika3rd/65*

- It is a measure of nerve fatigue and is used to ***detect retrocochlear lesion.***
- This test may be performed with standard audiometry and is believed to be useful in ***distinguishing lesions from cochlea from those in other areas of auditory pathway.***
- Threshold is established for a selected frequency (say 1000 Hz) and the tone allowed to persist unchanged in intensity until the patient indicates it can no longer be heard. The intensity is then raised again until it is heard and until it decays and so no, intensity being charted against time.
- Normally the threshold tone is perceived for longer than half a minute and should not 'decay' during this time by more than 5 dB. Normal person can hear a tone continuously for 60 seconds. In nerve fatigue he stops hearing earlier.

"TDT: A *decay of between 15 and 20 decibels is indicative of cochlear* hearing loss and the *decay more than 25 decibels is indicative of damage to the vestibulocochlear nerve*"-*www.denochearing.com*

Tone Decay Test (TDT)

◈ *www.denochearing.com*

- The tone decay test (also known as the threshold tone decay test or TTDT) is used to detect and measure auditory fatigue.
- In people with normal hearing, a tone whose intensity is only slightly above their absolute threshold of hearing can be heard continuously for 60 seconds. The tone decay test produces a measure of the "decibels of decay", i.e. the number of decibels above the patient's absolute threshold of hearing that are required for the tone to be heard for 60 seconds.
- Normal value is 0-15 dB. A ***decay of between 15 and 20 decibels is indicative of cochlear*** hearing loss and the ***decay more than 25 decibels is indicative of damage to the vestibulocochlear nerve***-*Dhingra 7th/113(table)*

TDT: (Tone Decay Test): TDT is the most commonly used tests because the test can be reliably carried out on any pure tone audiometer and helps in diagnosing ***neural lesions like acoustic neuroma***- **www.bhj.org.in**

130. Ans. b. Caused by long term use of α-adrenergic sprays, c. Edema and redness of mucosa along with hypertrophy of turbinate may occur, d. Regress by oral & nasal steroids, e. Cocaine use may cause

[Ref: Dhingra 7th/191; Logan and Turner 10th /73-74; ENT by Hazarika3rd/298-99; Ballenger H & N Surgery 16th/788,764]

Rhinitis Medicamentosa (Rebound Rhinitis)

◈ *Dhingra 7th/191, emedicine.medscape.com www.ncbi.nlm.nih.govwww.jacionline.org*

- It is triggered by the overuse of topical vasoconstrictive medications, most notably intranasal decongestants; recreational use of ***intranasal cocaine*** may also cause a similar condition
- Intranasal decongestants are best reserved for patients in whom nasal congestion is so severe that it precludes the use of other topical preparations such as intranasal corticosteroids
- **Sympathomimetic amines** mimic the actions of the sympathetic nervous system, ultimately stimulating the α ***receptors*** and resulting in vasoconstriction. They also are mild β receptor agonists and cause rebound nasal dilatation after the α effect has waned. The imidazolines (e.g, **oxymetazoline, xylometazoline, naphazoline, clonidine**) are **primary α_2-agonists**, causing vasoconstriction. The decongestive effect of these medications initially lasts approximately 7 to 9 hours but decreases with prolonged use.
- **Benzalkonium chloride**, used as a preservative in some nasal sprays, has also been incriminated in causing nasal mucosa swelling.
- **Rhinitis medicamentosa** can lead to chronic rhinosinusitis, atrophic rhinitis, ***turbinate hyperplasia,*** psychological dependence and an abstinence syndrome upon intranasal decongestant withdrawal that may include headaches, sleep disturbances, restlessness, irritability and anxiety
- Clinical rhinoscopic examination is non-specific, showing areas of ***red, thickened mucosa*** and dull zones-www.sciencedirect.com
- The first goal in the treatment of rhinitis medicamentosa is the *immediate discontinuation of topical nasal decongestants*
- **Nasal glucocorticosteroids *decrease nasal edema, inflammation and congestion associated with rhinitis medicamentosa***
- If a treatment program is not effective, treat the patient with oral prednisone, 15 mg 3 times a day for 5 days
- Turbinate surgery has a major place in the management of nasal congestion induced by mucosal oedema. Various technical modalities (turbinoplasties, radiofrequency, laser,

microresection) can be proposed as a complement to the alternative treatments

131. Ans. **a. Infraorbital nerve damage may occur as complication, b. Opening of maxillary antrum through gingivobuccal incision, c. Used for the treatment of chronic maxillary sinusitis & for obtaining biopsy for antral malignancy, e. It may be done under local anaesthesia with nerve block**

[Ref: Dhingra 7th/469-70; ENT by Hazarika3rd/406-07,332]

- Sublabial approach leading to opening of maxillary antrum

"Caldwell-Luc Operation: It is Process of *Opening the Maxillary Antrum* Through Canine Fossa by *Sublabial Approach* & Dealing with *Pathology Inside Antrum*. Operation is also Called Anterior Antrostomy"- *Dhingra 7th/469*

Complication: *Anaesthesia of the cheek due to stretching of **infraorbital Nerve.** It may last for a few weeks or months- Dhingra 7th/469*

Caldwell-Luc Operation: Indications

◈ *ENT by Hazarika3rd/407;Dhingra 7th/469*

- ***Chronic maxillary sinusitis*** with irreversible mucosal changes which is refractory to other modalities of treatment.
- Recurrent antro-choanal polyp if the patient is more than 18 years old (after eruption of the second molar tooth).
- Removal of benign tumors/dentigerous cyst.
- As an approach for Vidian neurectomy
- As an approach for maxillary artery ligation.
- Invasive fungal sinusitis of the maxillary sinus
- Hemoantrum
- Blow-out fracture of the orbit

Caldwell-LUC Operation

◈ *Ballenger H & N Surgery 16th/779-80*

- This procedure may be performed under ***general anesthesia or locoregional anesthesia via blocks of the infraorbital, sphenopalatine and posterosuperior alveolar nerve.*** Topical 4%cocaine can be placed intranasally in the region of the anterior ethmoid nerve and the medial wall ofthe maxillary sinus.
- Technique.
    - The procedure begins with a ***gingivobuccal incision***, made from the second molar tothe ipsilateral canine tooth . The incisionshould be made just above the apex of the buccogingival sulcus to preserve an inferior flap of soft tissue that will facilitate closure.
    - Dissection proceeds sharply through the submucosal tissue and the ***maxillary periostium*** down to bone. A periostial elevatoris used to raise the periosteum and overlying soft tissue superiorly to the level of the infraorbital foramen, being careful not to injure the neurovascular bundle. Medially, the periosteum is elevated to thepyriform aperture. Once adequate exposure is achieved, the ***maxillary sinus*** in entered through its anterior wall using an osteotome or cutting bur.
    - ***The antrum is entered superior to the roots of the canine and premolar teeth.*** A sphenoid punch and a Kerrison Rongeur are used to remove additional bone and enhance exposure. Bone can be removed superiorly,medial and lateral to the infraorbital nerve, ***preserving the infraorbital foramen itself.***
    - The approach gives good visualization of allportions of the maxillary sinus and allows complete removal of infectious material and masses that would not be easily reached through a middle meatal antrostomy.
    - Furthermore, creation of an inferior meatus antrostomy, which is typically performed in conjunction with the Caldwell-Lucprocedure, is nonphysiologic in terms of mucociliaryclearance patterns and may result in recirculation of purulent material.
    - At the conclusion of the maxillary sinus procedure, the ***gingivobuccal incision***is closed with either interrupted or running absorbable suture.
- ***Complications: The most common complication of the Caldwell-Luc approach is paresthesia or anesthesia of the cheek, teeth and gingiva secondaryto traction on the infraorbital nerve.*** Fortunately, this is self-limited in the majority of cases and resolves in less than 6 months. However, as many as 30% of patients will report some degree of persistent dysesthesia in the infraorbital nerve distribution.Other complications include hematoma formation, maxillary tooth root injury and superior alveolar nerve damage.

132. Ans. **a. Autosomal dominant mode of inheritance in hereditary cases, c. Increases during pregnancy, d. Commonly involve stapes which results in fixation & conductive deafness, e. Reddish blushover promontory**

[Ref: Dhingra 7th/95-99; Logan and Turner 10th /433-441; Current D & T in Otolaryngology 3rd/689-90]

Otosclerosis

◈ *Dhingra 7th/95-99*

- Hereditary: About 50% have positive family history. Genetic study reveal that it is an ***autosomal dominant*** trait
- Family history: Up to two-thirds of patients have a positive family history- *Logan and Turner 10th /435*
- Sex: ***Females are affected twice*** as often as males but in India, otosclerosis seems to predominate in males
- Hearing loss due to otosclerosis may be initiated or ***made worse by pregnancy***
- ***Stapedial otosclerosis causing stapes fixation & conductive deafness*** is the most common variety (other two subtypes are: cochlear otosclerosis & histological otosclerosis.
- ***Reddish hue may be seen on the promontory*** through the tympanic membrane (Schwartze sign). This is indicative of active focus with increased vascularity

Otosclerosis

◈ *Current D & T in Otolaryngology 3rd/689-90*

- In practice, otosclerosis is ***seen more oftenin women*** than in men by the ratio of approximately **2:1.** However, it has been proposed that the incidence may bethe same in both sexes and that ***hormonal influences during pregnancy*** might cause a more rapid progression in women, bringing them to clinical attention.

- In most cases, the disease is inherited as a simple ***autosomal dominant*** trait with incomplete penetrance and variable expressivity
- While otosclerosis may potentially involve any part of the bony labyrinth, it carries a distinct predilection for the region near the anterior border of the oval window (fissula ante fenestram). When disease involves the annular ligament of the oval window and ***stapesfootplate***, a ***conductive hearing loss*** (CHL) invariablyoccurs.
- The most common location of the otosclerotic focus is the region of the otic capsule anterior to the stapes footplate (the region of the fissula ante fenestram).
- In active disease, the astute clinician may appreciate a ***reddish blush*** (**Schwartze sign**) over both the ***promontory and the oval window niche*** owing to the prominent vascularity associated with an otospongiotic focus.

133. Ans. **b. Always occur as an isolated anomaly, d. Doesn't lead to sensorineural hearing loss**

[Ref: Dhingra 7th/129;rarediseases.info.nih.gov;emedicine.medscape.com]

Mondini Dysplasia

◈ *arediseases.info.nih.gov;emedicine.medscape.com*

- It is a type of ***inner ear*** malformation that is present at birth (congenital).
- Individuals with Mondini dysplasia have one and a half coils of the cochlea instead of the normal two coils.
- It may occur in one ear (unilateral) or both ears (bilateral) and can cause ***varying degrees of sensorineural hearing loss***, although most individuals have profound hearing loss.
- The condition can also predispose affected individuals to recurrent meningitis
- It is caused by disruption in the embryonic development of the inner ear during the seventh week of gestation.
- The **condition may be isolated** (occurring with no other conditions or malformations) or may occur with other ear malformations or a number of syndromes.
- Syndromes that have been associated with MD include Klippel Feil syndrome, ***Pendred syndrome, DiGeorge syndrome*** and some chromosomal trisomies.
- Treatment options may include surgical repair of the defect to prevent recurrent meningitis; amplification aids for those with residual hearing; and ***cochlear implantation***

134. Ans. **a. Hypertelorism, b. Maxillary hypoplasia, d. Hydrocephalus**

[Ref: Dhingra 7th/130; Logan and Turner 10th /591; Ballenger's Otorhinolaryngology 16th/34]

Crouzon Syndrome (Craniofacial Dystosis)

◈ *Dhingra 7th/130*

- ***Hypertelorism***
- *Mandibular prognathism*
- *Frog eye(Exophthalmos with divergent squint)*
- *Parrot-beak nose*
- *Premature closure of cranial sutures with mental retardation*
- *Conductive or mixed hearing loss*
- *Autosomal dominant inheritance*

Crouzon Syndrome

◈ *rarediseases.org*

- In most individuals with Crouzon syndrome, early sutural fusion causes the head to appear unusually short and broad (brachycephaly). In other cases, the head may appear long and narrow (scaphocephaly) or triangular (trigonocephaly). Rarely, premature closure of multiple sutures (known as Kleeblattschadel type craniosynostosis) causes the skull to be abnormally divided into three lobes (cloverleaf skull deformity).
- Eyes are spaced apart wider than usual (***hypertelorism***)
- Crouzon syndrome is associated with additional craniofacial abnormalities. Affected individuals often have a prominent forehead (frontal bossing); a curved nose; unusually flat or underdeveloped mid-facial regions (midface hypoplasia); and a short upper lip.
- In addition, a small, underdeveloped upper jaw (***hypoplastic maxilla***) with protrusion of the lower jaw (relative ***mandibular prognathism***) may also occur.
- Clefting of the lip and/or palate (incomplete closure of the palate or an abnormal groove in the upper lip) can occur rarely. Typical dental problems include a highly arched narrow palate with crowded teeth and upper and lower teeth that don't meet when biting (malocclusion).
- Approximately 30% of individuals with Crouzon syndrome develop ***hydrocephalus***.
- Some affected individuals have hearing impairment due to an inability to transmit sound impulses to the brain (*sensorineural hearing loss*). In some infants, breathing problems may occur in infancy due to various abnormalities of the face and upper airway. In severe instances, this can lead to life-threatening breathing complications

Table: Important genetic syndromes associated with childhood deafness *(Logan and Turner 10th /591)*

Syndrome	Inheritance	Important manifestations
Pendred syndrome	AR	Sensorineural loss and thyroid goitre +/- enlarged vestibular aqueduct
Usher syndrome	AR	Sensorineural loss and retinitis pigmentosa
Jervell Lange-Nielson syndrome	AR	Sensorineural loss and prolonged Q-T interval on electrocardiogram
Waardenburg syndrome	AD	Sensorineural loss, heterochromiairidis, white forelock
Crouzon syndrome	AD	Conductive loss and external ear anomalies. Craniosynostosis and exophthalmos

Contd...

Syndrome	Inheritance	Important manifestations
Apert syndrome	AD (majority sporadic)	Conductive loss due to fixation of stapes. Craniosynostosis and ***syndactyly***
Alport syndrome	X-linked or AR	Glomerulonephritis and sensorineural loss
Down syndrome	Sporadic	Increased risk of senorineural loss and glue ear. Increased risk of middle ear anomalies
CHARGE syndrome	Sporadic	Coloboma, heart defects, atresia of choana, retardation of growth, genital anomalies, ear anomalies—abnormal pinna, ossicular anomalies, malformed cochlea (Mondini dysplasia)
Cleft palate	Variable	Almost universal glue ear due to poor Eustachian tube function

Cause of Syndactyly

◈ **Danhert Radiology** *6th/Chap1*

= osseous ± cutaneous fusion of digits

- Apert syndrome
- Carpenter syndrome
- Down syndrome
- Neurofibromatosis
- Poland syndrome
- Others

135. Ans. **b. Applied on right eye, d. Both eye should be open while examining, e. Light from bull lamp is diffuse but strong**

[Ref: www.drbalu.com;ENT by Hazarika3rd/841-42]

Illumination used in Otolaryngologcial Examination

◈ *www.drbalu.com*

- Two types of illumination is used in otolaryngologcial examination: *www.drtbalu.co.in*
  - Semi mobile illumination like the Bull's lamp
  - Mobile illumination like the Clair's head light, or cold light based head bands.
  - **Bull's lamp**: is a semi mobile source of illumination. It has a 100 watts milk white bulb which provide the source of illumination. This light is focused with the plano-convex lens placed in front of the bulb. Ideally the ***Bulls lamp is placed 6 inches above and behind the left shoulder of the patient***, at the level of left ear of the patient.
- A bright lamp is positioned adjacent to patient's head, pointing toward the physician's face- *wiki*
- The examiner and the patient must be conveniently seated on adjustable stools. While using a Bull's lamp the examiner must focus the light using a head mirror to illuminate the patient.
- The head mirror is a concave mirror. It has a hole in the centre. The ***approximate focal length of the mirror is about 10 inches***. It has a plastic head band with a lever with 2 ball and socket joints. The joints are at right angles to each other.

Focusing the Light with Head Mirror

- The art of focusing the light to the desired spot comes only with practice. But there are certain **basic** steps which must be followed.
  - The patient sitting on the stool must be at **the** same level as the doctor.
  - The patient's legs must be placed to one side of the examiner.
  - The ***distance between the doctor and the patient must not be more than 8 inches*** (i.e. the focal length of the head mirror).
  - The ***mirror is fixed over the right eye in such a way part of the mirror touches the nose.***
  - The mirror is adjusted in such a way that the ***right eye sees through the hole in the mirror***. The mirror is ***adjusted while keeping the left eye closed and the right eye is* kept *open. Then both eyes are opened.***
- Clair's head light provides mobile illumination. The source of light is from a small 9 volt bulb. It is placed in front of a adjustable concave mirror. The mirror and the bulb are held via a plastic adjustable head band. The power supply to the bulb is from a 9 volt transformer. The major advantage of this illumination is that it is freely mobile and the patient may be examined in various positions. This illumination is highly useful while performing operative procedures inside the theatre.

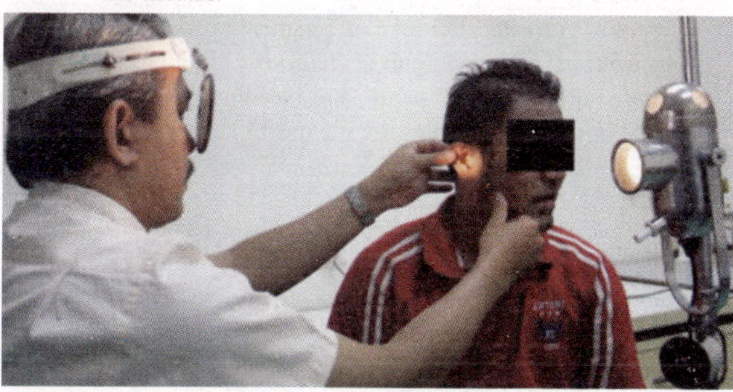

136. Ans. **b. Loss of upper incisors teeth, d. Resorption of anterior nasal spine**

[Ref: Dhingra 7th/176; Logan and Turner 10th /47; ENT by Hazarika3rd/307]

- *Other options in Q are also feature of leprosy, but not included in feature of* ***Faciesleprosa***

New Criteria for the Characterization of Facies Leprosa

◈ *www.researchgate.ne*

Facies leprosa is characterized by a combination of nasal change and ***resorption of nasal bone, anterior nasal spine,*** *supra-incisive alveolar region and anterior alveolar process of the maxilae,* ***associated with the loss of upper incisors teeth,*** according to the criteria of radiographic interpretation.

"**Facies leprosa** is characterized by a combination of ***nasal change and resorption of nasal bone, anterior nasal spine,***

supraincisive alveolar region and anterior alveolar process of the maxillae, associated with the loss of upper incisors teeth, *according to the criteria of radiographic interpretation.* The clinical aspect of faciesleprosa is termed Bergen Syndrome I (nasal leprosy) and Bergen Syndrome II (the leprogenic changes of the alveolar process of the maxilla)"- pdfs.semanticscholar.org

Table: Deformities occurring in leprosy *(Park 24th/345)*

Face	Mask face, ***facies leonine***, sagging face, ***lagophthalmos***, loss of eyebrows (superciliary madarosis) and eyelashes, (ciliarymadarosis), corneal ulcer and opacities, perforated nose, depressed nose, ear deformities, e.g. nodules on the ear and elongated lobules
Hands	Claw hand, wrist-drop, ulcers, absorption of digits thumb-web contracture, hollowing of the interosseous spaces and swollen hand.
Feet	Plantar ulcers, foot-drop, inversion of the foot, clawing of the toes, absorption of the toes, collapsed foot, swollen foot and callosities.
Other deformities	Gynaecomastia and perforation of the palate

"The nose is by far the most frequently involved site in the upper aerodigestive tract. Approximately 95% of patients with lepromatous leprosy have nasal involvement. Lesions begin as a pale, nodular, plaque-like thickening of the nasal mucosa. Untreated lesions can progress to ***ulceration, septal perforation and saddle-nose deformity***. Symptoms include rhinitis, obstruction, crusting and bleeding. The anterior end of the inferior turbinate is the site most likely to give a positive biopsy"-*Ballenger's Otorhinolaryngology 16th/646*

137. Ans. a. Length of both upper and lower canaliculi is around 8-10 mm, b. In majority of population upper and lower canaliculi combines to form single common canaliculus, c. Nasolacrimal duct open in inferior meatus, d. Commonly injured in major facial fractures

[Ref: Kanski 4th/369-372;A.K.Khurana 6th/386-87;Review of ophthalmology by William B. Trattler 2nd/166]

The nasolacrimal duct is approximately 18 mm long and descends from the lacrimal sac to ***open anteriorly in the inferior meatus*** of the nose at an expanded orifice- *Gray's 40th/674*

"Injuries to nasolacrimal system: Isolated nasoethmoid-orbital injuries are common. The most frequent causes are ***high-energy traumas, such as motor vehicle accidents,*** by an impact force applied to the upper portion of the bridge of nose. The patient with nasolacrimal injuries may present with significant concurrent ***facial wounds*** and multiple system injuries"

Lacrimal Apparatus

◈ *A.K.Khurana 6th/386-87*

- The lacrimal apparatus comprises (1) Main lacrimalgl and, (2) Accessory lacrimal glands and (3) Lacrimal passages, which include: puncta, canaliculi, lacrimal sac and nasolacrimal duct (NLD)
- Nasolacrimal duct (NLD)
  - It extends from neck of the lacrimal sac to inferior meatus of the nose. It is about 15-18 mm long and lies in a bony canal formed by the maxilla and the inferior turbinate. Direction of the NLD is downwards, backwards and laterally. Externally its location is represented by a line joining inner canthus to the ala of nose. The upper end of the NLD is the narrowest part
  - There are numerous membranous valves in the NLD, the most important is the *valve of Hasner*, which is present at the lower end of the duct and prevents reflux from the nose
- Lacrimal canaliculi
  - These join the puncta to the lacrimal sac. Each canaliculus has two parts: vertical (1-2 mm) and horizontal (6-8 mm) which lie at right angle to each other. The horizontal part converges towards inner canthus to open in the sac. The two canaliculi may open separately or may join to form common canaliculus which opens immediately into the outer wall of lacrimal sac. A fold of mucosa at this point forms the *valve of Rosenmuller* which prevents reflux of tears.
  - "The ***superior and inferior lacrimal canaliculi are lined with stratified squamous epithelium*** that is non-keratinized and non-mucin-producing. The **common canaliculus** is also lined with ***stratified squamous epithelium***, but its lumen is much narrower than the lumen of the superior and inferior canaliculi. The common canaliculus opens into an ample space called the vestibule, where the epithelium changes to *high pseudostratified columnar* and then low pseudostratified columnar"-www.ncbi.nlm.nih.go

Canaliculi

◈ *Review of ophthalmology by William B. Trattler, 2nd/166*

- ***10 mm long*** (2 mm vertical segment [ampulla] and 8 mm horizontal portion parallel to lid margin)
- Combine to form single common canaliculus in 90% ofindividuals
- Valve of Rosenmüller prevents reflux from lacrimal sacinto canaliculi

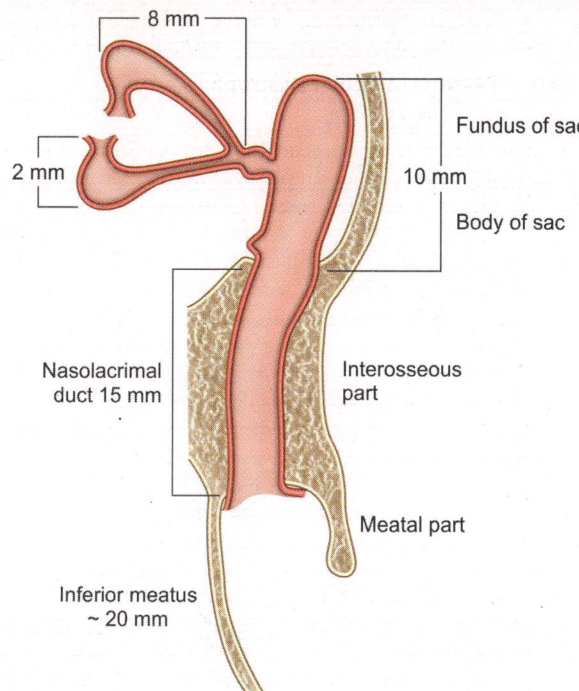

Fig: Lacrimal Apparatus *(Review of ophthalmology by William B. Trattler, 2nd/166)*

MEDICINE

138. Ans. a. Mitral stenosis, d. Recurrent atrial arrythmia, e. Patent foramen ovale

[Ref: Robbins 9th/1264-65; Harrison 19th/2563-65; Davidson 23rd/1153]

Table: Causes of Ischemic Stroke *(Harrison 19th/2565)*

Common Causes	Uncommon Causes
• Thrombosis ▪ Lacunar stroke (small vessel) ▪ Large vessel thrombosis ▪ Dehydration • Embolic occlusion ▪ ***Artery-to-artery*** ◆ Carotid bifurcation ◆ Aortic arch ◆ Arterial dissection • Cardioembolic ▪ Atrial fibrillation ▪ Mural thrombus ▪ Myocardial infarction ▪ Dilated cardiomyopathy	• Hypercoagulable disorders • Protein C deficiency • Protein S deficiency • Antithrombin III deficiency • Antiphospholipid syndrome • Factor V Leiden mutation • Prothrombin G20210 mutationa • Homocysteinemia • Thrombotic thrombocytopenic purpura • Disseminated intravascular coagulation • Dysproteinemia • Nephrotic syndrome • Inflammatory bowel disease • Oral contraceptives • Venous sinus thrombosis • Fibromuscular dysplasia • Vasculitis
• Valvular lesions ▪ ***Mitral stenosis*** ▪ Mechanical valve ▪ Bacterial endocarditis • Paradoxical embolus ▪ Atrial septal defect ▪ ***Patent foramen ovale*** • Atrial septal aneurysm • Spontaneous echo contrast	▪ Systemic vasculitis [PAN, granulomatosis with polyangiitis (Wegener's), Takayasu's, giant cell arteritis] ▪ Primary CNS vasculitis ▪ Meningitis (syphilis, tuberculosis, fungal, bacterial, zoster) • Cardiogenic ▪ Mitral valve calcification ▪ Atrial myxoma ▪ Intracardiac tumor ▪ Marantic endocarditis ▪ Libman-Sacks endocarditis • Subarachnoid hemorrhage vasospasm • Drugs: cocaine, amphetamine • Moyamoya disease • Eclampsia

Contd...

Cardioembolic Stroke

◈ *Harrison 19th/2563-64*

- Cardioembolism is responsible for ~20% of all ischemic strokes. Stroke caused by heart disease is primarily due to embolism of thrombotic material forming on the atrial or ventricular wall or the left heart valves.
- These thrombi then detach and embolize into the arterial circulation. The thrombus may fragment or lyse quickly, producing only a TIA. Alternatively, the arterial occlusion may last longer, producing stroke.
- Emboli from the heart most often lodge in the intracranial internal carotid artery, the MCA, the posterior cerebral artery (PCA), or one of their branches; infrequently, the anterior cerebral artery (ACA) is involved.
- The most significant causes of cardioembolic stroke in most of the world are ***nonrheumatic (often called nonvalvular) atrial fibrillation, MI, prosthetic valves, rheumatic heart disease and ischemic cardiomyopathy***.
- ***Nonrheumatic atrial fibrillation*** is the most common cause of cerebral embolism overall.
- Rheumatic heart disease usually causes ischemic stroke when there is ***prominent mitral stenosis*** or atrial fibrillation. Recent MI may be a source of emboli, especially when transmural and involving the anteroapical ventricular wall and prophylactic anticoagulation following MI has been shown to reduce stroke risk.
- Mitral valve prolapse is not usually a source of emboli unless the prolapse is severe.
- Paradoxical embolization occurs when venous thrombi migrate to the arterial circulation, usually via a ***patent foramen ovale or atrial septal defect.***

Mitral Valve Prolapse is Associated with a Variety of Typically Benign Arrhythmias, Atypical Chest Pain and a Very *Small Risk of Embolic Stroke or TIA*-*Davidson 23rd/520*

Cardiac Risk Factor for Stroke: *Atrial fibrillation, Congestive Cardiac Failure & Infective Endocarditis, Myocardiac Infaraction (Previous Episode)*-*Davidson 23rd/1153 (Table)*

139. Ans c. Conduction defect may present, e. Contracture usually develops

[Ref: Robbins 9th/1244; Harrison 19th/462e-5,e-9; Davidson 23rd/1143]

- Facial muscle may be involved (though less common) & cardiac involvement is common

Emery-Dreifuss Muscular Dystrophye

◈ *medicine.medscape.com*

- ***Face, thigh and hand weakness*** *(uncommon, may occur late)*
- ***Cardiac disease (nearly universal)***
- EDMD1 is caused by mutations in the *EMD* gene on the X chromosome
- EDMD2/EDMD3 is due to mutations (autosomal dominant and autosomal recessive, respectively) in the *LMNA* gene that codes for lamins A and C
- ***Males are affected in X-linked EDMD.*** About 10-20% of female carriers have ***cardiac conduction defects***, weakness, or both and they can die from ***sudden cardiac death.***
- In autosomal dominant EDMD, males and females are affected in equal numbers.
- The ***major cause of mortality and morbidity in EDMD is cardiac disease, which is consistently present.***
- Early onset of ***contractures*** (often before weakness has developed) is common in EDMD.
- The following **triad of symptoms** strongly suggests EDMD:
    - Slowly progressive muscle weakness and wasting in a scapulohumeroperoneal distribution
    - ***Early contractures*** of the elbow, ankle and posterior neck
    - ***Cardiac conduction defects, cardiomyopathy***, or both

Emery-Dreifuss Muscular Dystrophy

◈ *Harrison 19th/462e-9*

- There are at least five genetically distinct forms of Emery-Dreifuss muscular dystrophy (EDMD). Emerin mutations are the most common cause of ***X-linked*** EDMD, although mutations in *FHL1* may also be associated with a similar phenotype, which is X-linked as well.
- Mutations involving the gene for lamin A/C are the most common cause of ***autosomal dominant*** EDMD (also known as LGMD1B) and are also a common cause of hereditary cardiomyopathy.
- Less commonly, autosomal dominant EDMD has been reported with mutations in nesprin-1, nesprin-2 and *TMEM43*.
- ***Prominent contractures*** can be recognized in early childhood and teenage years, often preceding muscle weakness. The contractures persist throughout the course of the disease and are present at the ***elbows, ankles and neck.***
- Muscle weakness affects humeral and peroneal muscles at first and later spreads to a limb-girdle distribution.
- The cardiomyopathy is potentially life threatening and may result in sudden death. ***A spectrum of atrial rhythm and conduction defects includes atrial fibrillation and paralysis and atrioventricular heart block.*** Some patients have a ***dilated cardiomyopathy.***
- Female carriers of the X-linked variant may have cardiac manifestations that become clinically significant.

Table: Progressive Muscular Dystrophies *(Harrison 19th/462e-5; Davidson 23rd/1143)*

Type	Inheritance	Defective Gene/Protein	Onset Age	Clinical Features	Other Organ Systems Involved
Emery-Dreifuss	XR/AD	Emerin/Lamins A/C Nesprin-1, Nesprin 2, TMEM43	Childhood to adult	Elbow contractures, humeral and peroneal weakness	Cardiomyopathy

140. Ans. a. Janeway lesions are haemorrhagic lesion present on palm and sole, c. Janeway lesions are non tender, d. Osler nodes are present on pulp of finger & toes

[Ref: Robbins 9th/561; Harrison 19th/818; Davidson 23rd/528-30]

- "Complications of IE: ***erythematous or hemorrhagic nontender lesions on the palms or soles (Janeway lesions),subcutaneous nodules in the pulp of the digits (Osler nodes) a***nd retinal hemorrhages in the eyes (Roth spots)"- *Robbins 9th/561*
- **Janeway lesions** are one of the stigmata of infectious endocarditis. They are irregular, ***erythematous***, flat, ***painless*** macules on the ***palms, soles, thenar and hypothenar eminences of the hands, tips of the fingers and plantar surfaces of the toes;*** they rarely present as a diffuse rash and are very rare in clinical practice"-*www.ncbi.nlm.nih.gov*
- "Osler nodes are red-purple, slightly raised, tender lumps, often with a pale centre. ***Pain*** often precedes the development of the visible lesion by up to 24 hours. They are typically found on the ***fingers and/or toes***"- *www. dermnetnz.org*
- "Janeway lesions: On toe and plantar surface of the foot in subacute *Neisseria mucosa* endocarditis"- *Harrison 19th/818*
- *"Subacute endocarditis:* ***Osler's nodes are painful tender swellings at the fingertips*** *that are probably the product of vasculitis; they are rare"-Davidson 23rd/528*

141. Ans. a. In acute intermittent porphyria photosensitivity is seen

[Ref: Davidson 23rd/378-80,1263-64;Harrison 19th/ 2521-30, CMDT 2016/1655-56; Nelson 18th/645-46]

Erythropoietic Protoporphyria (EPP)

Oral β-carotene (120–180 mg/dL) may improve tolerance to sunlight in some patients. *The beneficial effects of β-carotene may involve quenching of singlet oxygen or free radicals.Mildskin discoloration due to carotenemia is the only significant side effect"- Harrison 19th/2533*

- "In contrast to other forms of porphyria, ***cutaneous photosensitivity is absent in AIP***"- *CMDT 2016/165*
- "AIP: This hepatic porphyria is an autosomal dominant condition resulting from the half-normal level of ***HMB synthase*** activity"- *Harrison 19th/2526*

AIP: Due to Deficiency of Enzyme *PBG (Porphobilinogen) Deaminase* or *UPG (Uroporphyrinogen)-1 Synthase"*

◈ *Vasudevan 5th/264*

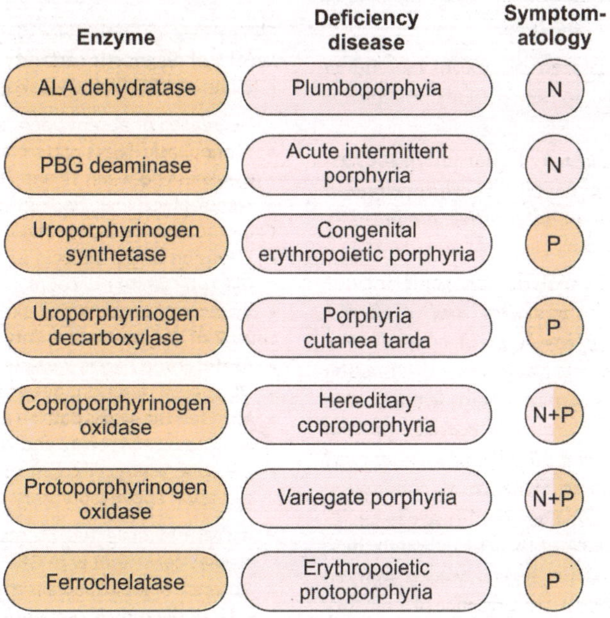

Enzyme	Deficiency disease	Symptomatology
ALA dehydratase	Plumboporphyia	N
PBG deaminase	Acute intermittent porphyria	N
Uroporphyrinogen synthetase	Congenital erythropoietic porphyria	P
Uroporphyrinogen decarboxylase	Porphyria cutanea tarda	P
Coproporphyrinogen oxidase	Hereditary coproporphyria	N+P
Protoporphyrinogen oxidase	Variegate porphyria	N+P
Ferrochelatase	Erythropoietic protoporphyria	P

Fig: Enzyme defects responsible for the porphyrias
Abbreviations: N, neurovisceral; P, photosensitive *(Davidson 23rd/378)*

Table: Human Porphyrias-major clinical and laboratory features *(Harrison 19TH/2522)*

Porphyria	Deficient Enzyme	Inheritance	Principal Symptoms NV or CP	Enzyme Activity% of Normal	Increased porphyrin precursors and/or Porphyrins		
					Erythrocytes	Urine	Stool
Hepatic Porphyrias							
5-ALA dehydratase deficient porphyria (ADP)	ALA-dehydratase	AR	NV	~S	Zn-protoporphyrin	ALA, Coproporphyrin III	–
Acute intermittent porphyria (AIP)	***HMB-synthase***	***AD***	NV	~50	–	ALA, ***PBG***, Uroporphyrin	–
Porphyria cutanea tarda (PCT)	URO-decarboxylase	AD	CP	~20	–	Uroporphyrin, 7-crboxylate porphyrin	Isocoproporphyrin
Hereditary coproporphyria (HCP)	COPRO-oxidase	AD	NV & CP	~50	–	ALA, PBG, Coproporphyrin III	Coproporphyrin III
Variegate porphyria (VP)	PROTO-oxidase	AD	NV & CP	~50	–	ALA, PBG, Coproporphyrin III	Coproporphyrin III Protoporphyrin
Erythropoietic Porphyrias							
Congenital erythropoietic porphyria (CEP)	URO-synthase	AR	CP	1-5	Uroporphyrin I Coproporphyrin I	Uroporphyrin I Coproporphyrin I	Coproporphyrin I
Erythropoietic protoporphyria (EPP)	Ferrochelatase	AD[a]	CP	~20-30	Proto-porphyrin	–	Protoporphyrin

Abbreviations: *AD, autosomal dominant; ALA, 5'-aminolevulinic acid; AR, autosomal recessive; CP, cutaneous photosensitivity; COPRO, coproporphyrinogen; HMB, hydroxymethylbilane; ISOCOPRO, isocoproporphyrin; NV, neurovisceral; PBG, porphobilinogen; PROTO, protoporphyrinogen; URO, uroporphyrinogen*

142. Ans. c. Absence of fever, d. Absence of an identified alternative diagnosis for weakness, e. Albuminocytological dissociation

[Ref: Harrison 19th/2694-98;Davidson 23rd/1140]

- "**Hyporeflexia or areflexia** is seen in 70% of patients at presentation and eventually in all patients"-*emedicine. medscape.com*
- ***"The CSF protein is raised, but may be normal in the first 10 days. There is usually no increase in CSF white cell count (> 10 × 10^6 cells/L suggests an alternative diagnosis)"***- *Davidson 23rd/1140*
- **Diagnostic criteria** for Guillain-Barré syndrome include the presence of ***progressive weakness and areflexia***, relative symmetry, mild sensory involvement, ***cranial nerve involvement***, at least partial recovery, autonomic dysfunction and ***absence of fever.*** Cerebrospinal fluid features that strongly support the diagnosis are an ***increase in protein beyond the first week, cell count < 10 (albuminocytological dissociation).*** Electrophysiologic evidence of conduction slowing, block, prolonged distal latency or F-wave latencies are also strongly supportive (80% of the case), though these abnormalities may be delayed for several weeks. Marked persistent asymmetry of weakness, the presence of a sensory level, bowel/bladder involvement at onset and a prominent pleocytosis, often cast doubt on the diagnosis, so is the presence of another cause for the neuropathy"- *emedicine. medscape.com*

Diagnosis of GBS

◈ *Harrison 19th/2697*

- Acute inflammatory demyelinating polyneuropathy(AIDP), the most common and best-studied type of GBS; ***the concept extends to all of the subtypes of GBS***
- The **diagnosis of AIDP** is made by recognizing the pattern of ***rapidly evolving paralysis with areflexia, absence of fever or other systemic symptoms*** and characteristic antecedent events.
- In 2011, the **Brighton** Collaboration developed a new set of case definitions for GBS in response to needs of epidemiologic studies of vaccination and assessing risks of GBS. These criteria have subsequently been validated.
- Laboratory tests are helpful primarily to exclude mimics of GBS. EDX features may be minimal and the ***CSF protein level may not rise until the end of the first week.*** If the diagnosis is strongly suspected, treatment should be initiated without waiting for evolution of the characteristic EDX and CSF findings to occur. GBS patients with risk factors for HIV or with ***CSF pleocytosis should have a serologic test for HIV***

Table: Brighton Criteria for Diagnosis of Guillain-Barré Syndrome (GBS) *(Harrison 19th/2698)*

Clinical case definitions for diagnosis of GBS

Level 1 of diagnostic certainty
- Bilateral AND flaccid weakness of the limbs
- Decreased or absent deep tendon reflexes in weak limbs
- Monophasic illness pattern and interval between onset and nadir of weakness between 12 and 28 days and subsequent clinical plateau
- Electrophysiologic findings consistent with GBS

Cytoalbuminologic dissociation
- Elevation of CSF protein level above laboratory normal value and CSF total white cell count <50 cells/µL
- *Absence of an identified alternative diagnosis for weakness*

Level 2 of diagnostic certainty
- Bilateral and flaccid weakness of the limbs
- Decreased or absent deep tendon reflexes in weak limbs
- Monophasic illness pattern and interval between onset and nadir of weakness between 12 and 28 days and subsequent clinical plateau
- CSF total white cell count <50 cells/µL (with or without CSF protein elevation above laboratory normal value) or
- If CSF not collected or results not available, electrophysiologic studies consistent with GBS
- Absence of identified alternative diagnosis for weakness

Level 3 of diagnostic certainty
- Bilateral and flaccid weakness of the limbs
- Decreased or absent deep tendon reflexes in weak limbs
- Monophasic illness pattern and interval between onset and nadir of weakness between 12 and 28 days and subsequent clinical plateau
- Absence of identified alternative diagnosis for weakness

Table: Key diagnostic criteria and Brighton case definitions for Guillain-Barré syndrome *(academic.oup.com)*

	Level of diagnostic certainty			
Diagnostic criteria	**1**	**2**	**3**	**4**
Bilateral and flaccid weakness of limbs	+	+	+	+/–
Decreased or absent deep tendon reflexes in weak limbs	+	+	+	+/–
Monophasic course and time between onset-nadir 12 hours to 28 days	+	+	+	+/–
CSF cell count <50/µl	+	+[a]	–	+/–
CSF protein concentration > normal value	+	+/–[a]	–	+/–
NCS findings consistent with one of the subtypes of GBS	+	+/–	–	+/–
Absence of alternative diagnosis for weakness	+	+	+	+

+ = present; – = absent; +/– = present or absent; NCS = nerve conduction studies; [a] If CSF is not collected or results not available, nerve electrophysiology results must be consistent with the diagnosis Guillain-Barré syndrome.

143. Ans. a. Hypothyroidism, d. Cushing syndrome, e. Insulinoma

[Ref: Davidson 23rd/700, 786;Harrison 19th/415e-4]

Table: Potentially reversible cause of weight gain *(Davidson 23rd/700)*

Endocrine factors	Drug treatments
• ***Hypothyroidism*** • ***Cushing's syndrome*** • ***Insulinoma*** • Hypothalamic tumours or injury	• Atypical antipsychotics (e.g. olanzapine) • Sulphonylureas, thiazolidinediones, insulin • Pizotifen • Corticosteroids • Sodium valproate • β-blockers

Specific Syndromes Associated with Obesity

◈ *Harrison 19th/415e-4*

- Patients with **insulinoma** often gain weight as a result of overeating to avoid hypoglycemic symptoms
- Much of the weight gain that occurs in **hypothyroidism** is due to myxedema
- Although obese patients commonly have central obesity, hypertension and glucose intolerance, they lack other specific stigmata of Cushing's syndrome
- *Craniopharyngioma and other disorders involving the hypothalamus:* Whether through tumors, trauma, or inflammation, hypothalamic dysfunction of systems controlling satiety, hunger and energy expenditurecan cause varying degrees of obesity

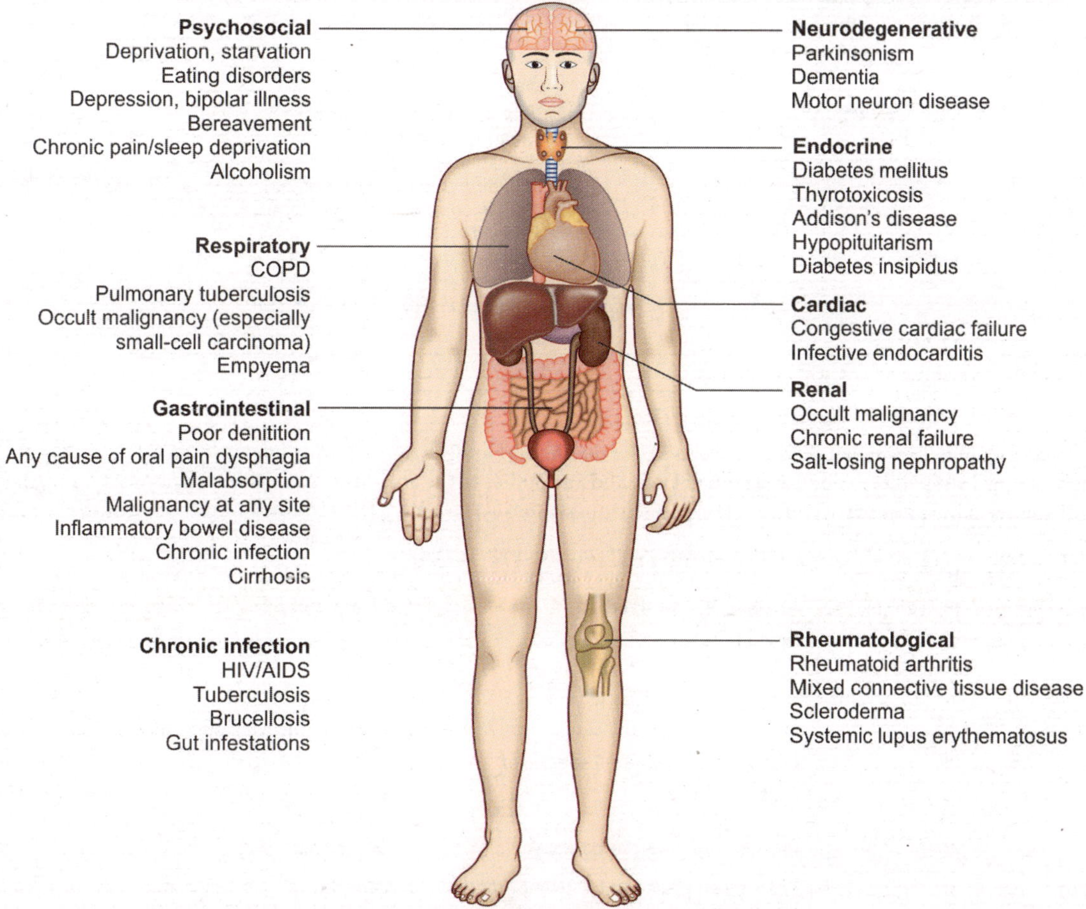

Fig: Some important causes of weight loss *(Davidson 23rd/786)*

144. Ans. a. Systolic blood pressure, b. Respiratory rate, c. Altered mental status

[Ref: www.qsofa.org/what.php; Paul Marino ICU book 3rd/1001]

- "Patients with suspected infection who are likely to have a **prolonged ICU stay** or to die in the hospital can be promptly identified at the bedside with **qSOFA**, i.e, ***alteration in mental status, systolic blood pressure ≤100 mm Hg, or respiratory rate ≥22/min***"- *jamanetwork.com/journal*

qSOFA	CURB65
Criteria • Abnormal mental status • RR >22 • SBP < 100	• Confusion • RR > 30 • SBP <90 or diastolic BP < 60 mm • BUN > 19 mg/dL • Age > 65 YO
Interpretation • > 1: sepsis (mortality ~10%)	**Interpretation** • 0: 0.6% mortality • 1: 2.7% mortality • 2: 6.8% mortality • 3: 14% mortality • 4-5: 28% mortality

Contd...

Table: Quick sequential organ failure assessment (SOFA) score

qSOFS (Quick SOFA) Criteria	Points
Respiratory rate >22/min	1
Change in mental status	1
Systolic blood pressure <100 mm Hg	1

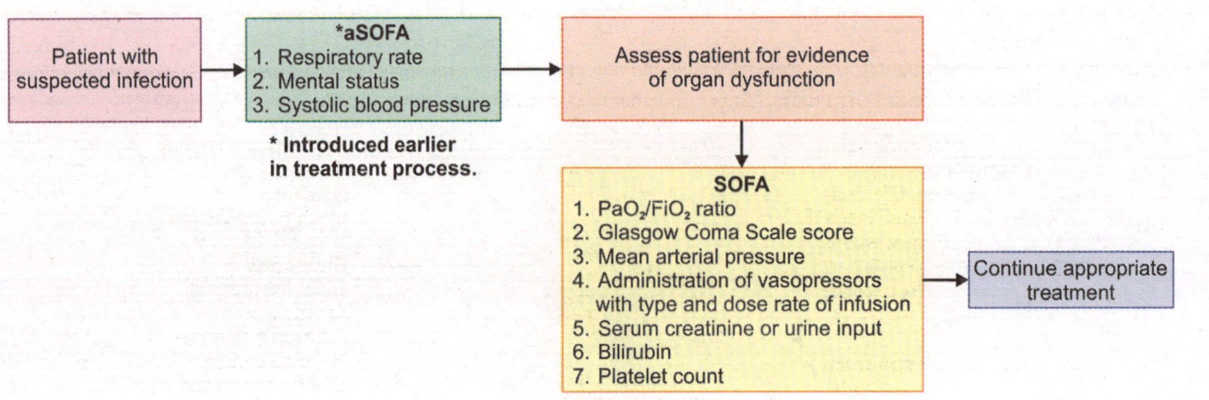

Fig: aSOFA vs SOFA

145. Ans. a. Anti-ds DNA antibody, c. Anti-Sm antibody

[Ref: Robbins 9th/219; Harrison 19th/2126; Davidson 23rd/1036]

- *"Antibodies to **double-stranded DNA and the so-called Smith (Sm) antigen** are **virtually diagnostic** of SLE"-Robbins 9th/219*
- "High-titer IgG antibodies to **double-stranded DNA and antibodies to the Sm antigen** are ***both specific for SLE*** and, therefore, favor the diagnosis in the presence of compatible clinical manifestations"- *Harrison 19th/2126*

Table: Autoantibodies in systemic lupus erythematosus (SLE) *(Harrison 19th/2126)*

Antibody	Prevalence, %	Antigen Recognized	Clinical Utility
Antinuclear antibodies	98	Multiple nuclear	Best screening test; repeated negative tests make SLE unlikely
Anti-dsDNA	70	DNA (double-stranded)	High titers are SLE-specific and in some patients correlate with disease activity, nephritis, vasculitis
Anti-Sm	25	Protein complexed to 6 species of nuclear U1 RNA	Specific for SLE; no definite clinical correlations; most patients also have anti-RNP; more common in blacks and Asians than whites
Anti-RNP	40	Protein complexed to U1 RNA	Not specific for SLE;
Anti-Ro (SS-A)	30	Protein complexed to hY RNA, primarily 60 kDa and 52 kDa	Not specific for SLE; associated with sicca syndrome,
Anti-La (SS-B)	10	47-kDa protein complexed to hY RNA	Usually associated with anti-Ro; associated with decreased risk for nephritis

Contd...

Antibody	Prevalence, %	Antigen Recognized	Clinical Utility
Antihistone	70	Histones associated with DNA (in nucleosome, chromatin)	More frequent in drug-induced lupus than in SLE
Antiphospholipid	50	Phospholipids, β_2 glycoprotein 1 cofactor, prothrombin	Three tests available—ELISAs for cardiolipin and β_2G1, sensitive prothrombin time (DRVVT); predisposes to clotting, fetal loss, thrombocytopenia
Antierythrocyte	60	Erythrocyte membrane	Measured as direct Coombs test; a small proportion develops overt hemolysis
Antiplatelet	30	Surface and altered cytoplasmic antigens on platelets	Associated with thrombocytopenia but sensitivity and specificity are not good; this is not a useful clinical test
Antineuronal (includes anti-glutamate receptor)	60	Neuronal and lymphocyte surface antigens	In some series a positive test in CSF correlates with active CNS lupus.
Antiribosomal P	20	Protein in ribosomes	In some series a positive test in serum correlates with depression or psychosis due to CNS lupus

Abbreviations: CNS, central nervous system; CSF, cerebrospinal fluid; DRVVT, dilute Russell viper venom time; ELISA, enzyme-linked immunosorbent assay.

146. Ans. a. Limited variants usually involves extremities and face, b. Majority of patient presents with Raynaud's phenomenon, c. Skin thickening is the hallmark, d. Pulmonary artery hypertension can also occur without lung fibrosis

[Ref: Harrison 19th/2154-55;Davidson 23rd/1037-38]

- "**Raynaud's phenomenon**, the ***most frequent extracutaneous complication of system sclerosis (SSc)***, is characterized by episodes of reversible vasoconstriction in the fingers and toes"-*Harrison 19th/2159*
- "While early-stage SSc is associated with edematous skin changes, ***skin thickening is the hallmark*** that distinguishes SSc from other connective tissue diseases. The distribution of skin thickening is invariably symmetric and bilateral"-*Harrison 19th/2159*
- ***"Skin involvement restricted to sites distal to the elbow or knee (apart from the face) is classified as 'limited disease' or CREST syndrome*** (Calcinosis, Raynaud's, Esophageal involvement, Sclerodactyly and Telangiectasia).. ***Involvement proximal to the knee and elbow and on the trunk is classified as 'diffuse disease'***-*Davidson 23rd/1037*
- "**Pulmonary Arterial Hypertension (PAH)**, develops in approximately 15% of patients with SScand can occur in ***association with ILD or as an isolated abnormality***"-*Harrison 19th/2161*
- "Patients presenting with **scleroderma renal crisis** should be immediately hospitalized. Once other causes of renal disease are excluded, treatment should be started promptly with ***titration of short-acting ACE inhibitors***, with the goal of achieving rapid normalization of the blood pressure. In patients with hypertension persisting despite ACE inhibitor therapy, addition of angiotensin II receptor blockers, calcium channel blockers and direct renin inhibitors should be considered"- *Harrison 19th/2164*

Table: Subsets of Systemic Sclerosis (SSc): Limited Cutaneous SSc versus Diffuse Cutaneous SSc *(Harrison 19th/2155)*

Features	Limited Cutaneous SSc	Diffuse Cutaneous SSc
Skin involvement	Indolent onset. Limited to ***fingers, distal to elbows, face; slow*** progression	Rapid onset. Diffuse: fingers, extremities, face, trunk; rapid progression
Raynaud's phenomenon	***Precedes skin involvement;*** Sometimes by years; may be associated with critical ischemia in the digits	Onset coincident with skin involvement; critical ischemia less common
Musculo-skeletal	Early arthralgia	Severe arthralgia, carpal tunnel syndrome, tendon friction rubs
Interstitial lung disease	Slowly progressive, generally mild	Frequent, early onset & progression; can be severe
Pulmonary arterial hypertension	***Frequent, late, may occur as isolated complication***	Often occur in association with Interstitial lung disease
Scleroderma renal crisis	Very rare	Occurs in 15%; generally early(<4 years from disease onset)
Calcinosis cutis	Frequent, prominent	Less common, mild
Chara-cteristic auto-antibodies	Anticentromere	Antitopoisomerase I (Scl-70), anti-RNA polymerase III

Table: Internal Organ Involvement: Limited Cutaneous and Diffuse Cutaneous Forms of Systemic Sclerosis (*Harrison 19th/2158)*

Features	Limited Cutaneous SSc (%)	Diffuse Cutaneous SSc (%)
Skin involvement	90*	100
Raynaud's phenomenon	99	98
Esophageal involvement	90	80
Pulmonary fibrosis	35	65
Pulmonary arterial hypertension	15	15
Myopathy	11	23
Cardiac involvement	9	12
Scleroderma renal crisis	2	15

*10% of LCSSc patients have SSc sine scleroderma.

147. Ans. a. Severe asthma, b. Constrictive pericarditis, c. Cardiac tamponade

[Ref: Harrison 19th/1450;PJM 20th/40-42;www.jpgmonline.com]

Table: Features that distinguish cardiac tamponade from constrictive pericarditis and similar clinical disorders (Partial) *(Harrison 19th/1473)*

Character istic	Tam ponade	Con strictive Pericar ditis	Restrictive Cardiomy opathy	RVMI	Effusive constrictive Pericarditis
Pulsus paradoxus	+++	+	+	+	+++

- **"Absent pulsus paradoxus in cardiac tamponade[Aortic regurgitation (AR)]:** In the presence of AR, the left ventricle can fill from the aorta during inspiration. Therefore, if aortic dissection produces both AR and tamponade, ***pulsus paradoxus may be absent***"-*www.jpgmonline.com*
- "Disease states in which **cardiac tamponade may occur without pulsus paradoxus** include the following:Co-existing disease that significantly increases left or right ventricular diastolic pressure such severe systemic hypertension, ***aortic stenosis***, or ***corpulmonale***- *www.ncbi.nlm.nih.gov*
- "**Pericardial tamponade** *can be diagnosed with a sensitivity of 98%, a specificity of 83% and a positive likelihood ratio of 5.9 by a* ***pulsu sparadoxus*** *that exceeds 12 mmHg in a patient with a large pericardial effusion*"- *Harrison 19th/1450*

Pulsus Paradoxus

◈ *Harrison 19th/1444-45*

- *It refers to a fall in systolic pressure >10 mm Hg with* inspiration that is seen in patients with ***pericardial tamponade*** but also is described in those with *massive pulmonary embolism, hemorrhagic shock, severe obstructive lung disease and tension pneumothorax*
- It can be difficult to measure pulsus paradoxus in patients with tachycardia, atrial fibrillation, or tachypnea.
- A pulsus paradoxus may be palpable at the brachial artery or femoral artery level when the pressure difference exceeds 15 mmHg. This inspiratory fall in systolic pressure is an exaggerated consequence of interventricular dependence.
- **Reversed pulsus paradoxus**, a rise in systolic blood pressure during inspiration, was first described by Massumi et al in patients with idiopathic hypertrophic subaortic stenosis, isorhythmic ventricular rhythm and patients of left ventricular failure on positive pressure ventilation. A rise in peak systolic pressure on inspiration by more than 15 mm Hg is considered significant. A reverse pulsus paradoxus in mechanically ventilated patients is a sensitive indicator of hypovolaemia- *www.jpgmonline.com*

Causes of Pulsusparadoxus

◈ *www.jpgmonline.com*

Cardiac causes

- ***Cardiac tamponade***
- Pericardial effusion
- ***Constrictive pericarditis***
- Restrictive cardiomyopathy
- Pulmonary embolism
- Acute myocardial infarction
- Cardiogenic shock

Extracardiac pulmonary causes

- ***Bronchial asthma***
- Tension pneumothorax

Extracardiac non-pulmonary causes

- Anaphylactic shock (during urokinase administration)
- Volvulus of the stomach
- Diaphragmatic hernia
- Superior vena cava obstruction
- Extreme obesity

148. Ans. b. Hypertention, c. Bradycardia, e. Irregular respiration

[Ref: Guyton 11th/213;CSDT 11th/890; Harrison 19th/1778-79;Manipal Surgery 4th/1038]

- "**Cushing triad of increased ICP**: ***Bradycardia, hypertension & irregular respiration***" *(Manipal Surgery 4th/1038)* "**Blood pressure elevation** accompanied by ***bradycardia and respiratory slowing*** classically results from raised intracranial pressure. This "Cushing response," however, usually appears only when intracranial hypertension is severe"-*(CSDT 11th/890)*

Features of Increased ICT

- Loss of the normal autoregulation of blood pressure and pulse, called the ***Cushing's reflex, is a hallmark of severe brain injury or imminent crisis***. This generally results in a *sudden rise in blood pressure and a slowing of the pulse.*
- Signs of increased ICP include ***decreasing level of consciousness***, paralysis or weakness on one side of the body and ***a blown pupil, one that fails to constrict in response to light or is slow to do so.***
- **Cushing's triad,** a slow heart rate with high blood pressure and respiratory depression is a classic manifestation of significantly raised ICP.

- Anisocoria, unequal pupil size, is another sign of serious traumatic brain injury

149. Ans. a. pH < 7.3, b. Bicarbonate <15 mEq/L, c. Blood glucose >300mg/dL, d. Ketonemia

[Ref: Harrison 19th/ 2417-18; Davidson 22nd /812-13; Lippincott 6th/339, 345]

- "**Ketones,** *an indicator of* **diabetic ketoacidosis**, *should be measured in individuals with type* ***1 DM when the plasma glucose is >16.7 mmol/L (300 mg/dL)***, *during a concurrent illness, or with symptoms such as nausea, vomiting, or abdominal pain. Blood measurement of β-hydroxybutyrate is preferred over urine testing with nitroprusside-based assays that measure only acetoacetate and acetone. DKA and HHS exist along a continuum of hyperglycemia, with or without ketosis"- Harrison 19th/ 2417*

Diabetic Ketoacidosis

Harrison 19th/ 2418

- In DKA, the ketone body, β-hydroxybutyrate, is synthesized at a threefold greater rate than acetoacetate; however, acetoacetate is preferentially detected by a commonly used ketosis detection reagent (nitroprusside).
- ***Serum ketones*** *are present at significant levels (usually positive at serum dilution of ≥1:8).*
- *The timely diagnosis of DKA is crucial and allows for prompt initiation of therapy.*
- *DKA is characterized by* ***hyperglycemia, ketosis and metabolic acidosis*** *(increased anion gap) along with a number of secondary metabolic derangements.*
- *Occasionally, the serum glucose is only minimally elevated. Serum bicarbonate is frequently <10 mmol/L and* ***arterial pH ranges between 6.8 and 7.3,*** *depending on the severity of the acidosis.*

All are Useful in Diagnosis of Diabetic Ketoacidosis (DKA)

Davidson 22nd /812–1 3

- *Venous blood*: for urea and electrolytes, ***glucose and bicarbonate*** (severe acidosis is indicated by a venous plasma bicarbonate < 12 mmol/L).
- ***Urine or blood analysis for ketones***
- *ECG.*
- *Infection screen*: full blood count, blood and urine culture, C-reactive protein, chest X-ray. Although leukocytosis invariably occurs in DKA, this represents a stress response and does not necessarily indicate infection.

Table: Laboratory values in diabetic ketoacidosis (DKA) and Hyperglycemic Hyperosmolar state (HHS) (Representative Ranges at presentation) *(Harrison 19th/2417)*

	DKA	HHS
Chloride	Normal	Normal
Phosphate	Normal	Normal
Creatinine	Slightly ↑	Moderately ↑
Osmolality (mOsm/mL)	300–320	330-380
Plasma ketones	++++	+/–
Serum bicarbonate, mEq/L	<15 mEq/L	Normal to slightly ↓
Arterial pH	6.8–7.3	>7.3
Glucose, mmol/L	13.9–33.3	33.3–66.6
Sodium, mEq/L	125–135	135–145
Potassium	Normal to ↑	Normal
Magnesium	Normal	Normal
Arterial PCO_2, mmHg	20-30	Normal
Anion gap [Na–(Cl + HCO_3)]	↑	Normal to slightly ↑
Glucose (mg/dl)	250-600	600-1200

Contd...

150. Ans. a. The angle between the nail plate and the skin overlying the proximal part of the distal phalanx is >160 degree, b. Scramoth sign may present, c. Hypertrophic osteoarthropathy may be associated

[Ref: Harrison 19th/250; www.medscape.com]

Clubbing

Harrison 19th/250

- The selective bulbous enlargement of the distal segments of the fingers and toes due to proliferation of connective tissue, particularly on the dorsal surface, is termed *clubbing*; there is also increased sponginess of the soft tissue at the base of the clubbed nail.
- Clubbing may be hereditary, idiopathic, or acquired and **associated** with a variety of disorders, including ***cyanotic congenital heart disease***, *infective endocarditis and a variety of pulmonary conditions (among them primary and metastatic lung cancer, bronchiectasis, asbestosis, sarcoidosis, lung abscess, cystic fibrosis, tuberculosis and mesothelioma), as well as with some gastrointestinal diseases (including inflammatory bowel disease and hepatic cirrhosis)*. In some instances, it is occupational, e.g., in jackhammer operators.
- Clubbing in patients with primary and metastatic lung cancer, mesothelioma, bronchiectasis, or hepatic cirrhosis may be associated with ***hypertrophic osteoarthropathy***. In this condition, the subperiosteal formation of new bone in the distal diaphysis of the long bones of the extremities causes pain and symmetric arthritis-like changes in the shoulders, knees, ankles, wrists and elbows.
- The diagnosis of ***hypertrophic osteoarthropathy*** may be confirmed by bone radiograph or magnetic resonance imaging (MRI).
- Although the mechanism of clubbing is unclear, it appears to be secondary to humoral substances that cause dilation of the vessels of the distal digits as well as growth factors released from platelet precursors in the digital circulation. In certain circumstances, clubbing is reversible, such as following lung transplantation for cystic fibrosis.

Clubbing

◈ *www.medscape.com*

- Normally, the angle between the nail plate and the skin overlying the proximal part of the distal phalanx is about 160 degrees or less. ***With clubbing, proliferation of tissue under the nail plate causes this angle to increase to more than 160 degrees***. In fact, the angle may be entirely lost and the nail plate and skin lie in a straight line (180-degree angle). ***As clubbing progresses, the angle exceeds 180 degrees***. Eventually, the profile of the fingertip becomes bulbous.
- "*Obliteration in clubbed fingers of the diamond-shaped window* normally produced when the dorsal surfaces of the corresponding finger of each hand are opposed (**Schamroth sign**) may useful for the ***identification of clubbing***"
- "Two signs are characteristic of early clubbing: the "floating nail" sign and the "profile" sign.
- *Hypertrophic osteoarthropathy* is an advanced stage of clubbing.
- Conditions which are commonly associated with clubbing include: Lung cancer, bronchiectasis, interstitial lung disease such as idiopathic pulmonary fibrosis, empyema, pulmonary tuberculosis and cystic fibrosis; Congenital heart disease, Gastrointestinal conditions (celiac sprue, cirrhosis, Crohn's disease and ulcerative colitis), Endocrine problems(Hyperthyroidism, especially Grave's disease)"

151. Ans. **e. Renal biopsy is always necessary for diagnosis**

[Ref: Harrison 19th/1817,1820-21; Davidson 23rd/757; CMDT 2016/930-31]

Diabetic Nephropathy

- "**Screening for albuminuria** should commence ***5 years after the onset of type 1 DM*** and at the *time of diagnosis of type 2 DM*"- *Harrison 19th/2425*
- Although the appearance of microalbuminuria in type 1 DM is an important risk factor for progression to macroalbuminuria, only ~50% of individuals progress to macroalbuminuria over the next 10 years. In some individuals with type 1 diabetes and microalbuminuria of short duration, the microalbuminuria regresses. ***Microalbuminuria*** is alsoa risk factor for CVD-*Harrison 19th/2425*
- ***Once macroalbuminuria is present, there is a steady decline in GFR and ~50% of individuals reach ESRD in 7-10years.*** Once macroalbuminuria develops, blood pressure rises slightly and the pathologic changes are likely irreversible-*Harrison 19th/2425*
- Duration of DM and degree of glycemic control are the best predictors of the **development of retinopathy**; hypertension and ***nephropathy are also risk factors***-*Harrison 19th/2424*
- ***Diabetic nephropathy presents in its earliest stage with low levels of albumin (microalbuminuria) in the urine***-*www.aafp.org*

Diabetic Nephropathy

◈ *CMDT 2016/930-31*

- Type 1 diabetes mellitus carries a 30–40% risk of nephropathy after20 years, whereas type 2 has a 15–20% risk after 20 years.ESRD is much more likely to develop in persons with type 1diabetes mellitus, in part due to fewer comorbidities and deaths before ESRD ensues. Diabetic nephropathy
- High GFR (hyperfiltration) → microalbuminuria → frank proteinuria → decline in GFR"- CMDT 2016/919
- The first stage of diabetic nephropathy is hyperfiltration with an increase in GFR, followed by the development of microalbuminuria (30–300 mg/day).
- ***Kidney biopsy is not required in most patients***, though, unless atypical findings are present, such as sudden onset of proteinuria, nephritic spectrum features (see above), massive proteinuria (>10 g/d), urinary white cell casts, or rapid decline in GFR.

152. Ans. **a. Hypertensive control, b. Keep blood glucose in limit, c. Low salt intake, d. Peritoneal hemodialysis, e. Use of ACE inhibitors & ARB**

[Ref: Harrison 19th/1817,1820-21; Davidson 23rd/757-58]

- "**CKD**: Uremia (asterixis, pericardial rub or effusion, encephalopathy, uremic bleeding) leads to disturbances in the function of virtually every organ system. ***Chronic dialysis (peritoneal Dialysis***, hemodialysis, hemofiltration and other hybrid procedures) can reduce the incidence and severity of many of these disturbances, so that the overt and florid manifestations of uremia have largely disappeared in the modern health setting. However, even optimal dialysis therapy is not completely effective as renal replacement therapy, because some disturbances resulting from impaired kidney function fail to respond to dialysis"-*Harrison 19th/1814,1810*

Management of Hypertension in CKD

◈ *Harrison 19th/1817*

- The overarching goal of hypertension therapy in CKD is to ***prevent the extrarenal complications*** of high blood pressure, such as cardiovascular disease and stroke.
- In CKD patients with diabetes or proteinuria >1 g per 24 h, ***blood pressure should be reduced to 130/80 mmHg***, if achievable without prohibitive adverse effects.
- ***Salt restriction*** should be the first line of therapy. When volume management alone is not sufficient, the choice of antihypertensive agent is similar to that in the general population.
- ***ACE inhibitors and ARBs appear*** to ***slow the rate of decline of kidney function*** in a manner that extends beyond reduction of systemic arterial pressure and that involves correction of the intraglomerular hyperfiltration and hypertension involved in progression of CKD described above.

"The optimal therapy for diabetic nephropathy(an important cause of CKD) is prevention by control of glycemia. Interventions effective in slowing progression of albuminuria include **(1) *improved glycemic control*, (2) *strict blood pressure control* and (3) *administration of an ACE inhibitor or ARB.*** Dyslipidemia should also be treated"-*Harrison 19th/2425;Davidson 23rd/757-58*

153. Ans. a. Leukocytoclastic vasculitis responds to corticosteroids, c. Palpebral purpura occurs, e. May progresses to chronic renal failure

[Ref: Robbins 9th/926; Harrison 19th/2190; Davidson 23rd/1043]

- **Cutaneous leukocytoclastic angiitis**: It is not one specific disease but a manifestation that can be seen in a variety of settings.***Glucocorticoids are often used*** in the treatment of idiopathic cutaneous vasculitis. In cases that prove refractory to glucocorticoids, a trial of a cytotoxic agent may be indicated"-*Harrison 19th/2192*
- *"**Henoch–Schönlein purpura**:* This condition ***most commonly occurs in children*** but can also be observed in adults. The prognosis is good, with spontaneous resolution, but ***some, particularly adults, progress to develop ESRD***"-*Davidson 23rd/1043*

IgA vasculitis (Henoch-Schönlein)

◈ *Harrison 19th/2190*

- It is a ***small-vessel vasculitis*** characterized by ***palpable purpura*** (most commonly distributed over the buttocks and lower extremities), arthralgias, gastrointestinal signs and symptoms and glomerulonephritis.
- It is ***usually seen in children***; most patients range in age from 4 to 7 years; however, the disease may also be ***seen in infants and adults***. The male-to-female ratio is 1.5:1.
- A seasonal variation with a peak incidence in spring has been noted
- The presumptive pathogenic mechanism is immune-complex deposition.
- In pediatric patients, palpable purpura is seen in virtually all patients; most patients develop polyarthralgias in the absence of frank arthritis.
- Gastrointestinal involvement, which is seen in almost 70% of pediatric patients, is characterized by colicky abdominal pain usually associated with nausea, vomiting, diarrhea, or constipation and is frequently accompanied by the passage of blood and mucus per rectum; bowel intussusception may occur.
- **Renal involvement** occurs in 10–50% of patients and is usually characterized by mild glomerulonephritis leading to proteinuria and microscopic hematuria, with red blood cell casts in the majority of patients; ***it usually resolves spontaneously without therapy***. Rarely, a progressive glomerulonephritis will develop.
- Laboratory studies generally show a mild leukocytosis, ***a normal platelet count*** and occasionally eosinophilia. Serum complement components are normal and IgA levels are elevated in about one-half of patients.
- The complete blood count may reveal a normal or elevated white blood cell count and possible eosinophilia. Sedimentation rate and ***platelet count may be elevated***"-*www.aafp.org*
- The diagnosis of IgA vasculitis (Henoch-Schönlein) is based on clinical signs and symptoms. Skin biopsy specimen can be useful in confirming ***leukocytoclastic vasculitis with IgA and C3 deposition by immunofluorescence***. Renal biopsy is rarely needed for diagnosis but may provide prognostic information in some patients.
- The prognosis is excellent. Mortality is exceedingly rare and ***1–5% of children progress to endstage renal disease.***

154. Ans. a. 10% Bilateral, b. 10% Malignant, c. 10% Familial, d. 10% Extra-adrenal

[Ref: Robbins 9th/1134-36; Harrison 19th/2329-32; Davidson 23rd/675]

The classic "rule of tens" for pheochromocytomas states that ***~10% are bilateral, 10% are extra-adrenal and 10% are malignant***"- *Harrison 19th/2329*

- **Pheochromocytoma:** *Review of facts*
  - It is catecholamine producing tumour of sympathetic or Parasympathetic nervous system
  - Pheochromocytomas usually subscribe to a convenient "**rule of 10**" (*Robbins, Harrison & CMDT*)
  - *10% are bilateral*
  - *10% are malignant*
  - ***10% are extra adrenal***
  - *10% are associated with familial syndrome*
  - *10% arise in childhood*
  - *Approximately 10% are in thorax*
  - *Most are < 10 cm in diameter*
  - *10% not associated with Hypertension*
  - *About 10% tumour involves both adrenal gland*
  - *10% extra-adrenal tumour are extra abdominal*

155. Ans. a. A2-P2 splitting increases with inspiration and decreases during expiration, c. Wide fixed splitting in ASD, d. Narrow split in pulmonary arterial hypertension, e. A2 is delayed in LBBB& P2 is delayed in RBBB

[Ref: Harrison 19th/1447; Davidson 23rd/459]

Heart sound

◈ *Harrison 19th/1447*

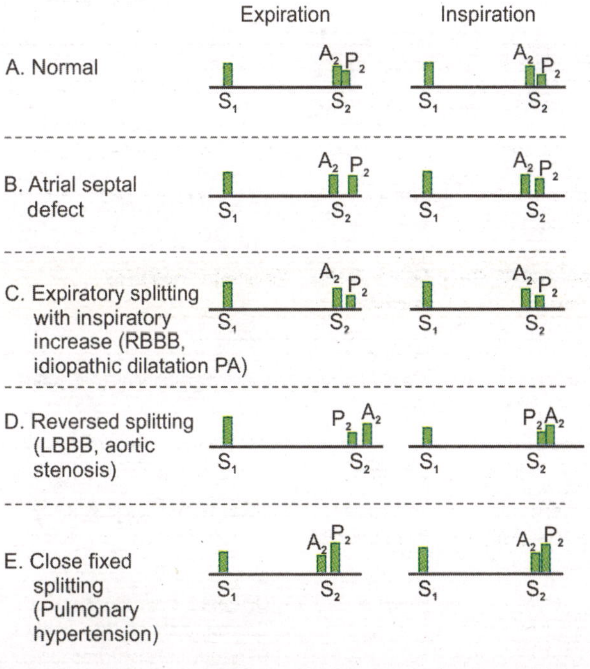

Fig: Heart sounds. A. Normal. S1, first heart sound; S2, second heart sound; A2, aortic component of the second heart sound; P2, pulmonic component of the second heart sound. B.Atrial septal defect with fixed splitting of S2.*C.*Physiologic but wide splitting of S2 with right bundle branch block (RBBB). PA, pulmonary artery.D. Reversed or paradoxical splitting of S2 with left bundle branch block (LBBB). E. ***Narrow splitting of S 2 with pulmonary hypertension***. (Harrison 19th/1447)

- *Aortic and pulmonic valve closure constitutes the second heart sound (S2). With normal or physiologic splitting, the* ***A2–P2interval increases with inspiration and narrows during expiration****. This physiologic interval will* ***widen with right bundle branch block*** *because of the further delay in pulmonic valve closure and in patients with severe MR because of the premature closure of the aortic valve.*
- *An* ***unusually narrowly split or even a singular S2 is a feature of pulmonary arterial hypertension****.*
- **Fixed splitting of S2**, *in which the A2–P2 interval is wide and does not change during the respiratory cycle, occurs in patients with a* ***secundum atrial septal defect.***
- **Reversed or paradoxical splitting** *refers to a pathologic delay in aortic valve closure, such as that which occurs in patients with* ***left bundle branch block****, right ventricular pacing, severe AS, HOCM and acute myocardial ischemia.*
- *With* **reversed or paradoxical splitting**, *the individual components of S2 are audible at end expiration and their interval narrows with inspiration, the opposite of what would be expected under normal physiologic conditions. P2 is considered loud when its intensity exceeds that of A2 at the base, when it can be palpated in the area of the proximal main pulmonary* artery (second left interspace), or when both components of S2 can be appreciated at the lower left sternal border or apex. The intensity of A2 and P 2decreases with aortic and ***pulmonic stenosis***, respectively. In these conditions, a single S2may result

Table: Normal and abnormal heart sounds *(Davidson 23rd/459)*

Sound	Timing	Characteristics	Mechanisms	Variable features
First heart sound (S1)	Onset of systole	Usually single or narrowly split	Closure of mitral and tricuspid valves	Loud: hyperdynamic circulation (anaemia, pregnancy, thyrotoxicosis); mitral stenosis Soft: heart failure; mitral regurgitation
Second heart sound (S2)	End of systole	Split on inspiration single on expiration	Closure of aortic and pulmonary valve A_2 first P_2 second	Fixed wide splitting with atrial septal defect Wide but variable splitting with delayed right heart emptying (e.g. right bundle branch block) Reversed splitting due to delayed left heart emptying (e.g. left bundle branch block)
Third heart sound (S3)	Early in diastole, just after S2	Low pitch, often heard as 'gallop'	From ventricular wall due to abrupt cessation of rapid filling	**Physiological:** Young people, pregnancy **Pathological:** Heart failure, mitral regurgitation
Fourth heart sound (S4)	End of diastole just before S1	Low pitch	Ventricular origin (stiff ventricle and augmented atrial contraction) related to atrial filling	Absent in atrial fibrillation A feature of severe left ventricular hypertrophy (e.g. hypertrophic cardiomyopathy)

156. Ans. a. Intention tremors, e. Flaccidity

[Ref: Harrison 19th/2609-11; CMDT 2015/988]

"Intention tremor occur in *cerebellar lesion*"-A.K.Jain 6th/971

Table: Clinical feature Parkinson's disease (PD) *(Harrison 19th/2609)*

Cardinal Motor Features	Other Motor features	Nonmotor Features
Bradykinesia	Micrographia	Anosmia
Rest tremor	Masked facies (hypomimia)	Sensory distubances (e.g. pain)
Rigidity	Reduced eye blinking	Mood disorders (e.g. depression)
Gait disturbance/ postural instability	Soft voice (hypophonia)	Sleep disturbances (e.g. RBD)
	Dysphagia Freezing	Autonomic disturbances • Orthostatic hypotension • Gastrointestinal disturbances • Genitourinal disturbances • Sexual dysfunction Cognitive impairment (MCI/ dementia)

SURGERY

157. Ans. a. Elastic compression stocking's cause dynamic sequential compression of leg veins, b. Improve venous circulation of leg, d. Worn in the morning and taken off at night before bedtime, e. Worn even after ulcer heals to prevent recurrence

[Ref: Manipal Surgery 4th/134; CSDT 14th/835; L and B 27th/984-85, 977; Schwartz 10th/931-32]

"The Compression Stockings are Worn all Day to Diminish Venous Distention During Standing and are Removed at night"—

- *CSDT 14th/835*
- The ***stockings work by exerting the greatest degree of compression at the ankle***, with the level of compression gradually decreasing up the garment. The ***pressure gradient ensures that blood flows upward toward the heart*** instead of refluxing downward to the foot or laterally into the superficial veins. The application of adequate graduated compression reduces the diameter of major veins, which increases the velocity and volume of blood flow. **Graduation compression** can reverse venous hypertension, augment skeletal-muscle pump, facilitate venous return and improve lymphatic drainage"- www.ncbi.nlm.nih.gov

- "There is evidence that high-compression (30–40 mm Hg) stockings are more effective than medium- and low-compression stockings in ***promoting venous ulcer healing and preventing recurrence***"- www.ncbi.nlm.nih.gov
- Compression stockings squeeze legs to compress veins and keep blood moving in the right direction. The squeeze is ***generally tighter at the ankle and gradually lessens farther up the leg***. The strength of compression stockings is measured in millimeters of mercury or mmHg. This is represented in a range (i.e. 20-30mmHg) from lowest compression to the highest compression. 20-30mmHg is the most commonly prescribed strength of stocking for its effective compression and ease of use. ***After varicose vein treatment, it is important to wear compression stockings to ensure treatment efficacy***"-www.ivein.com

Elastic Compression Stockings

◈. *Manipal Surgery 4th/ 134*

- Elastic compression bandage and elevation of leg: It forms the fundamental steps in treating varicose veins. This can be advised in asymptomatic cases of varicose veins and in secondary varicose veins.
    - Usually 20–30 mmHg stockings are sufficient.
    - It should be worn from *ankle to below knee.*
    - It should be ***worn during working hours (entire day).***
    - Should be ***removed while lying down*** but legs should be kept elevated.
    - Above knee stockings should never be prescribed as they are difficult to put on and tend to roll down.
- Unna boot: It is a three-layered dressing.
- Pneumatic compression devices not commonly used.

Compression Therapy

◈ *Schwartz 10th/931-32*

- *Compression therapy is the mainstay of CVI management. Compression can be achieved using a variety of techniques, including **elastic compression stockings**, paste gauze boots (Unna's boots), multilayer elastic wraps or dressings and pneumatic compression devices.*
- ***Nonelastic compression bandages generally achieve higher and more prolonged degrees of compression than elastic compression bandages.***
- *The exact mechanism by which compression therapy can improve CVI remains uncertain. **An improvement in skin and subcutaneous tissue microcirculatory hemodynamics as well as a direct effect on subcutaneous pressure have been hypothesized as the mechanisms of efficacy of compression therapy.***
- *Additionally, compression therapy has demonstrated quantifiable differences in **ulcer healing** with decreases in matrix metalloproteins and inflammatory cytokines. Clinically, routine use of elastic and nonelastic bandages reduces lower extremity edema in patients with CVI. In addition, supine perimalleolar subcutaneous pressure has been demonstrated to increase with elastic compression.*
- ***With edema reduction**, cutaneous metabolism may improve due to enhanced diffusion of oxygen and other nutrients to the cellular elements of skin and subcutaneous tissues.*
- Compression therapy is most commonly achieved with **graduated elastic compression stockings**. Elastic compression stockings are available in various compositions, strengths and lengths and can be customized for a particular patient. The benefits of **elastic compression stocking therapy** for the treatment of ***CVI and healing of ulcerations*** have been well documented. The rate of ulcer recurrence was lower in patients who were compliant with their compression therapy.
- *In addition to promoting ulcer healing*, elastic compression therapy can also improve quality of life in patients with CVI. Patient compliance with compression therapy is crucial in treating CVI and especially ***venous leg ulcers***.

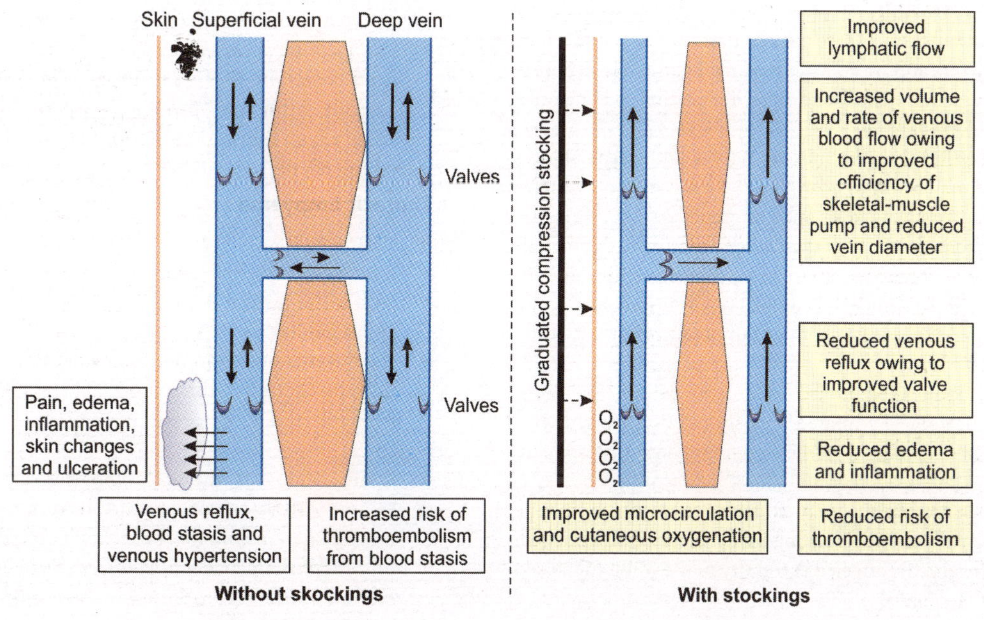

Fig: The mechanisms of action of graduated compression stockings (www.ncbi.nlm.nih.gov)

158. Ans. a. Trench foot is a type of frostbite of foot, c. On face it is superficial & on extremities severe form occurs

[Ref: L and B 27th/422; Park 24th/785; Reddy 34th/295; Manipal Surgery 4th/94; Harrison 19th/1650; Schwartz 10th/480]

- "Peripheral cold injuries include both ***freezing (Frostbite)*** and ***nonfreezing injuries*** to tissue. The two most common nonfreezing peripheral cold injuries are *chilblain (pernio)* and ***immersion (trench) foot***"- *Harrison 19th/478e-4*
- "Immersion injury is a cold injury which does ***not involve actual freezing of the tissue*** and is commonly caused by prolonged ***immersion in cold water*** (hence '**trench foot**')"- *L and B 27th/422*
- **"Trench foot,** also known as immersion foot syndrome, is a type of ***non-freezing cold injury***. It is a condition that develops when feet are cold and wet for a long time and affects the skin"- *www.medicalnewstoday.com*

Tissue loss and ***autoamputation are potential consequences of frostbite.*** Frostbite usually affects the hands, feet, nose, cheeks and ears. **Superficial frostbite** *injures the skin and tissues just beneath the skin, but usually does not permanently injure tissue.* **Deep frostbite,** which also affects *muscle, nerves and blood vessels*, may result in tissue death, a condition known as gangrene"- *pennstatehershey.adam.com* ***(severity depend on degree of frostbite, not site involved)***

- "Frostbite is infarction of peripheral digits with edema, redness and later necrosis"- Reddy 34th/295

Frostbite

◈ *Harrison 19th/1650*

- Tissue injury results from both freezing and vasoconstriction.
- Frostbite usually affects the distal aspects of the extremities or exposed parts of the face, such as the ears, nose, chin and cheeks.
- **Two type**- Superficial frostbite (first or second degree) or deep frostbite (third or fourth degree) *www.dermnetnz. org*
- **Superficial frostbite** involves the skin and subcutaneous tissue. Patients experience pain or paresthesia and the skin appears white and waxy. After rewarming, there is cyanosis and erythema, wheal-and-flare formation, edema and superficial blisters.
- **Deep frostbite** involves muscle, nerves and deeper blood vessels. It may result in edema of the hand or foot, vesicles and bullae, tissue necrosis and gangrene
- ***Initial treatment is rewarming***, performed in an environment where re-exposure to freezing conditions will not occur. Rewarming is accomplished by immersion of the affected part in a water bath at temperatures of 40°–44°C (104°–111°F).
- Massage, application of ice water and extreme heat are contraindicated. The injured area should be cleansed with soap or antiseptic and sterile dressings should be applied. Analgesics are often required during rewarming.
- Antibiotics are used if there is evidence of infection. The efficacy sympathetic blocking drugs is not established. After recovery, the affected extremity may exhibit increased sensitivity to cold.
- Treatment includes rapid rewarming to 40 to 42°C, analgesia, debridement of blisters, hydrotherapy, elevation, topical antimicrobials, topical antithromboxanes (aloe vera) and systemic antiprostaglandins (aspirin)-Schwartz 10th/480

Degree of Frostbite

◈ *www.dermnetnz.org; wikipedia*

- In **first-degree frostbite**, hyperemia and edema are evident.
- **Second-degree frostbite is** characterized ***by hyperemia and edema, with large, clear blisters*** that may extend the entire length of the involved limb, digit, or facial feature. The blisters can be quite large and interfere with function, especially if they involve the digits of the hand or the soles the feet.
- **Third-degree frostbite is** characterized by hyperemia, edema, and vesicles filled with hemorrhagic fluid that are usually smaller than those of second-degree frostbite and do not extend to the tip of the involved digit. The hemorrhagic component of the blisters is a sign of underlying deeper tissue injury.

159. Ans. a. Inadequate drainage of acute empyema, b. Inadequate needle aspiration of acute empyema, c. Inadequate antibiotic treatment of acute empyema, d. Drainage of plural effusion, e. Due to persistent foreign body in bronchioles

[Ref: S.Das Textbook of Surgery 5th/751-53;CSDT 14th/345-48; L and B 27th/922; Sabiston 19th/1597-98; Schwartz 10th/ 684-85]

Chronic Empyemas

◈ *S.Das Textbook of Surgery 5th/751-53*

- *Majority of chronic empyemas are due to* ***mismanagement of acute or subacute empyema****. Some are due to failure of diagnosis in the acute or subacute stage.*
- *A few cases are due to chronic pathology in the lung(e.g* ***bronchiectasis****, neoplasm etc), in pleura (foreign bodies or actinomycosis) or in the chest wall(osteomyelitis)*
- *Main feature of chronic empyema is the absence of toxicity & acute condition. There is no dypnoea or fever or anemia*

"An **occult bronchial foreign body** can lead to chronic respiratory symptoms, complicating to ***bronchiectasis,*** recurrent infections(pneumonia), lobar collapse"-*www.ncbi.nlm.nih.gov*

Thoracic Empyema

◈ *CSDT 14th/345*

- Pyothorax (empyema thoracis) is the accumulation of pus within the pleural cavity. The pus is usually thick, creamy and malodorous.
- If empyema occurs in the setting of underlying suppurative lung disease (ie, pneumonia, lung abscess, or ***bronchiectasis***), it is referred to as a parapneumonic empyema (60% of cases).
- Other causes of thoracic empyema are surgery (20%), trauma (10%), esophageal rupture, other chest wall or mediastinal infections, bronchopleural fistula, ***extension of a subphrenic or hepatic abscess, instrumentation of the pleural space*** (***thoracentesis, chest tube placement***, etc)

and, rarely, hematogenous seeding from a distant site of infection.

- Empyemas are divided into three phases based on their natural history: *acute exudative, fibrinopurulent and* ***chronic organizing***

"Options for treatment include *repeated thoracentesis, closed tube thoracostomy***,** rib resection and open drainage, decortication and empyemectomy, thoracoplasty and muscle flap closure. Adjunctive maneuvers reported to aid in the disruption and drainage of loculated empyemas include instillation of fibrinolytic enzymes (such as tPA) and video assisted thoracoscopic debridement"- *CSDT 14th/346*

"***Antibiotics*** are an important adjunct in the treatment of empyemas, but it must be emphasized that ***drainage is the primary treatment modality.*** Although antibiotic therapy is always instituted early in the course of therapy when signs of systemic infection generally are present, they need not be continued once effective drainage is established. In fact, overuse of antibiotics may lead to the generation of resistant bacteria and therefore compromise the success of any subsequent procedures designed to obliterate residual intrathoracic space"- *CSDT 14th/348*

Table: Conditions that predispose to empyema formation *(L and B 27th/922)*

Pulmonary infection	Unresolved pneumonia Bronchiectasis Tuberculosis Fungal infections Lung abscess
Aspiration of pleural effusion	Any aetiology
Trauma	Penetrating injury Surgery Oesophageal perforation
Extrapulmonary sources	Subphrenic abscess
Bone infections	Osteomyelitis of ribs or vertebrae

Pathogenesis of Empyema

◈ *Schwartz 10th/ 685*

- **I-Contamination from a source contiguous to the pleural space**(50%–60%)
- Lung, Mediastinum, Deep cervical area, Chest wall and pine & Subphrenic area
- **II-Direct inoculation of the pleural space (30%–40%)** Minor thoracic interventions, Postoperative infections, Penetrating chest injuries
- III-**Hematogenous infection of the pleural space from a distant** site (<1%)

160. Ans. b. Can cause right pleural effusion, d. Associated with polymicrobial flora, e. May arise from sepsis outside the hepatobiliary tree

[Ref: Manipal Surgery 4th/517-18;CSDT 14th/579; L and B 27th/1168; Schwartz 10th/1284; Sabiston 19th1440-44]

Pyogenic Liver Abscess

◈ *Manipal Surgery 4th/517-18*

- *In majority of cases, it is* ***polymicrobial infection***
- Majority of the infective bacteria are derived from gastro-ntestinal tract
- In ***most cases, the organism is of enteric origin***- *CSDT 14th/579*
- Pyogenic liver abscesses are generally treated with b***oth IV antibiotics and percutaneous drainage of the abscess. Some patients may require surgical drainage***- www.amboss.com

Pyogenic Liver Abscess

◈ *L and B 27th/1168*

- ***Mixed growths are common.***
- ***Treatment is with antibiotics and ultrasound-guided aspiration.*** Often, repeated aspirations may be necessary.
- Percutaneous drainage without ultrasound guidance should be avoided as an empyema may follow drainage through the pleural space.
- ***A source for the liver abscess should be sought, particularly from the colon.*** Atypical clinical or radiological findings should raise the possibility of a necrotic neoplasm.

Pyogenic Liver Abscess

◈ *Schwartz 10th/1284*

- They may be single or multiple and are more frequently found in the ***right lobe of the liver***
- Approximately 40% of abscesses are monomicrobial, an ***additional 40% are polymicrobial*** and 20% are culture-negative.
- The current cornerstones of treatment include correction of the ***underlying cause and IV antibiotic therapy***. Empiric antibiotic therapy should cover gram-negative and anaerobic organisms; ***percutaneous needle aspiration*** and culture of the aspirate may be useful in guiding subsequent antibiotic therapy. IV antibiotic therapy should be continued for at least 8 weeks and can be expected to be effective in 80% to 90% of patients.
- ***Placement of a percutaneous drainage catheter is beneficial only for a minority of patients, as most pyogenic abscesses are quite viscous and catheter drainage is often ineffective.***
- ***Surgical drainage either via the laparoscopic or open approach may become necessary if initial therapies fail***

Complications of Pyogenic Liver Abscess

◈ *www.amboss.com*

- Rupture
    - Into the abdomen → peritonitis
    - Into the chest → empyema
    - Into the retroperitoneum → retroperitoneal abscess
- Sepsis
    - Pneumonia
    - Pleural effusion

Table: Features of Amoebic Versus Pyogenic Liver Abscess *(Sabiston 19th/1443)*

Clinical Features	Amoebic Abscess	Pyogenic Abscess
Age (yr)	20-40	>50
Male-to-female ratio	≥10: 1	1.5: 1
Solitary vs. multiple	Solitary 80%[*]	Solitary 50%
Location	Usually right liver	Usually right liver
Travel in endemic area	Yes	No
Diabetes	Uncommon (~2%)	More common (~27%)
Alcohol use	Common	Common
Jaundice	Uncommon	Common
Elevated bilirubin	Uncommon	Common
Elevated alkaline phosphatase	Common	Common
Positive blood culture	No	Common
Positive amebic serology	Yes	No

* In acute amebic abscess, 50% are solitary

161. Ans b. May be associated with hypertrophic scarring and contractures, d. Epithelisation is completed in 10-14 days

[Ref: L and B 27th/622 ; CSDT 14th/227-28; Manipal Surgery 4th/187; CSDT 14th/227-28; Schwartz10th/229-30]

- "**Deep partial-thickness**: These burns usually ***heal with minimal scarring in 10-14 days*** unless they become infected"- *CSDT 14th/228*
- "**Deep partial-thickness**: Spontaneous healing may require up to six weeks and is ***often associated with hypertrophic scarring and joint contractures***"- *www.ebmedicine.net*
- "**Second-degree or partial-thickness** (2 subtype superficial & deep) burns are deeper, ***involving all of the epidermis and some of the corium or dermis***. Superficial partial-thickness burns usually heal with ***minimal scarring in 10-14 days*** unless they become infected. **Deep partial-thickness** burns heal over a period of ***4-8 weeks*** with only a ***fragile epithelial*** covering developing that arises from the residual uninjured epithelium of the deep dermal sweat glands and hair follicles. ***Severe hypertrophic scarring occurs when such an injury heals***; the resulting epithelial covering is prone to blistering and breakdown"-*CSDT 14th/228*

Deep Partial-thickness Burn

◈ *L and B 27th/622*

- These burns involve damage to the ***deeper parts of the reticular dermis***. Clinically, the ***epidermis is usually lost.*** The exposed dermis is not as moist as that in a superficial burn. There is often abundant fixed capillary staining, especially if examined after 48 hours.
- The colour does not blanch with pressure under the examiner's finger. Sensation is reduced and the patient is unable to distinguish sharp from blunt pressure when examined with a needle.
- ***Deep dermal burns take 3 or more weeks to heal without surgery*** and usually lead to ***hypertrophic scarring***

Table: Burn depth classification *(www.ebmedicine.net)*

Depth	Histology	Appearance	Sensation	Healing
First-degree:	Epidermis only	Erythema; blanches with pressure	Intact; mild to moderate pain	3-6 days without scarring
Second degree:				
Superficial	Epidermis and superficial dermis; skin appendages intact	Erythema, blisters, moist, elastic; blanches with pressure	Intact; severe pain	1-3 weeks; scarring unusual
Deep	Epidermis and most dermis; most skin appendages destroyed	White ap pearing with erythema tous areas, dry, waxy, less elastic; reduced blanching to pressure	Decreased; may be less painful	>3 weeks; often with scarring and contractures
Third-degree	Epidermis and all of dermis; destruction of all skin appendages	White, charred, tan, thrombosed vessels; dry and leathery; does not blanch	Anesthetic; not painful (although surrounding areas of second-degree burns are painful)	Does not heal; severe scarring and contractures

Burn Classification

◈ *CSDT 14th/227-28*

- Traditionally, burns have been classified as ***first-, second- and third-degree***, but the current emphasis on burn healing has led to classification as **partial-thickness burns**, which can heal spontaneously and **full-thickness burns**, which require skin grafting, although deep partial-thickness burns are usually excised and grafted as well.
- A **first-degree burn** involves only the epidermis and is characterized by ***erythema and minor microscopic changes; tissue damage is minimal, protective functions of the skin are intact, skin edema is minimal and systemic effects are rare***. Pain, the chief symptom, usually resolves in 48-72 hours and healing takes place uneventfully. In 5-10 days, the damaged epithelium peels off in small scales, leaving no residual scarring.
- **Second-degree or partial-thickness (Superficial and deep)** burns are deeper, involving ***all of the epidermis*** and

some of the corium or dermis. The systemic severity of the burn and the quality of subsequent healing are directly related to the amount of undamaged dermis.

- **Superficial burns** ***are often characterized by blister formation***, while ***deeper partial-thickness burns have a reddish appearance or a layer of whitish, nonviable dermis firmly adherent to the remaining viable tissue. Complications from superficial second degree burns are mainly severe pain related.*** These burns usually heal with minimal scarring in 10-14 days unless they become infected.
- **Deep dermal burns**
- **Full-thickness (third-degree) burns** have a characteristic white, dry, waxy appearance and may appear to the untrained eye as unburned skin. Burns caused by prolonged exposure to heat, with ***involvement of fat and underlying tissue***, may be brown, dark red, or black. ***The diagnostic findings of full-thickness burns are lack of sensation in the burned skin, lack of capillary refill and a leathery texture that is unlike normal skin. All dermal epithelial elements are destroyed, leaving no potential for reepithelialization.***

Superficial Partial-thickness Burns

◈ *L and B 27th/622*

- The damage in these burns goes no deeper than the papillary dermis.
- The clinical features are ***blistering and/or loss of the epidermis.***

Deep Partial-thickness Burn

◈ *L and B 27th/622*

- These burns involve damage to the deeper parts of the reticular dermis. Clinically, the epidermis is usually lost.
- Sensation is reduced and the patient is unable to distinguish sharp from blunt pressure when examined with a needle.

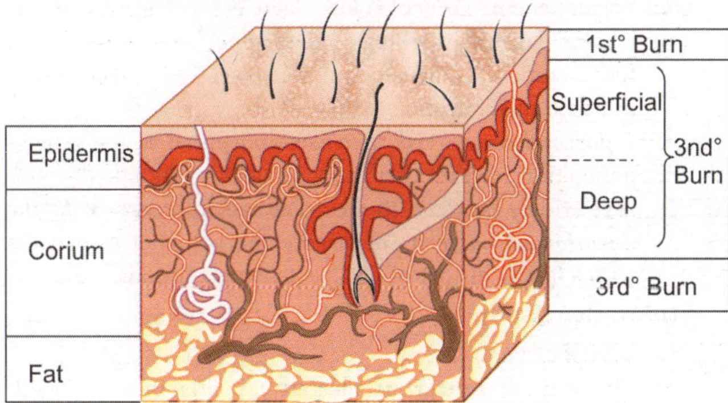

Fig: Layers of the skin showing depth of first-degree, second-degree (Partial thickness) and third-degree burns. *(CSDT 14th/228)*

162. Ans. b. Occur where transversus abdominis.., c. Arise from lateral aspect..., d. Internal organs including small..., e. Usually occur at or above to accurate...

[Ref: L and B 27th/1041-42; Manipal Surgery 4th/871; Schwartz 10th/1455;Sabiston 19th/1135]

- **Epigastric hernia** - Small lumps along the ***linea alba*** reflecting openings through which preperitoneal fat can protrude; may be adjacent to the umbilicus (umbilical hernia) or more cephalad (ventral hernia [epiplocele]) *Schwartz 10th/1455; emedicine.medscape.com(It is epigastric hernia* ***not splengial hernia that protrude through linea alba****)*
- "***Splenial hernia:*** The most common sac content is ***omentum but intestine, appendix, gall bladder, stomach or ovary*** have been reported"- *www.ncbi.nlm.nih.gov*
- "In most cases, the hernial sac contains the ***omentum*** and in some cases may also contain a segment of ***small intestine or colon*** that may cause intestinal obstruction. Several cases of congenital **Spigelian hernia** with *undescended testis* also have been reported"- *www.sciencedirect.com*
- "**Spigelian hernia**: *Located typically at the* ***junction of the arcuate line & lateral border of rectus abdominis****- Manipal Surgery 4th/871*

Spigelian Hernia

◈ *L and B 27th/1041-42*

- These hernias are uncommon although are probably underdiagnosed.
- They affect men and women equally and can occur at any age, but are most common in the elderly.
- They arise through a defect in the Spigelian fascia which is the ***aponeurosis of the transversus abdominis muscle.***
- Often these hernias advance through the internal oblique as well and spread out deep to the external oblique aponeurosis. The Spigelian fascia ***extends between the transversus muscle and the lateral border of the rectus sheath*** from the costal margin to the groin where it blends into the conjoint tendon.
- Most Spigelian hernias appear below the level of the umbilicus near the edge of the rectus sheath but they can be found anywhere along the 'Spigelian line'.
- There is a ***common misconception*** that they protrude below the arcuate line owing to deficiency of the posterior rectus sheath at that level, ***but in fact the defect*** is ***almost always above the arcuate line.***
- In young patients they usually contain extraperitoneal fat only but in older patients there is often a peritoneal sac and they can become very large indeed.
- Young patients usually present with ***intermittent pain,*** due to pinching of the fat, similar to an epigastric hernia.
- Older patients generally present with a reducible swelling at the edge of the rectus sheath and may have symptoms of ***intermittent obstruction.***
- Surgery is recommended as the narrow and fibrous neck predisposes to strangulation. Surgery can be open or laparoscopic.

Spigelian Hernias

◈ *Sabiston 19th/1135*

- *Spigelian* hernias can occur anywhere along the length of the Spigelian line or zone—an aponeurotic band of variable width at the ***lateral border of the rectus abdominis.***
- However, the most frequent location of these rare hernias is ***at or slightly above the level of the arcuate line.***

- These are not always clinically evident as a bulge and may come to medical attention because of pain or incarceration.

163. Ans. **a. Associated with BRCA2, d. Treatment by wide local excision or mastectomy, e. Around 90% cases are benign**

[Ref: L and B 27th/870 ; CSDT 14th/300; Manipal Surgery 4th/382-83 ; Schwartz 10th/555;Robbins 9th/1069;Sabiston 19th/845]

"Phyllodes Tumors: Account for Less than 1% of all Breast Neoplasm

◈ *Manipal Surgery 4th/382*

- "The value of **FNAC** in diagnosis of phyllodes tumour ***remains controversial***, but core needle biopsy has high sensitivity and negative predictive value"- *www.ncbi.nlm.nih.gov*
- "**Core needle biopsy** is preferred, although it is difficult to classify phyllodes tumours with benign or intermediate malignant potential based on a limited sampling. Thus, the ***final diagnosis is best made by excisional biopsy, followed by careful pathological review***- *Sabiston 19th/845*
- "Reports have suggested, however, that about ***85-90% of phyllodes tumors are benign*** and that approximately 10-15% are malignant"- *emedicine.medscape.com*
- "Most Phyllodes tumors are benign, but ***10 percent are malignant*** (cancerous)"- www.hopkinsmedicine.org "***About 1 in 10 are cancerous***"- *rarediseases.info.nih.gov*
- "**Phyllodes tumors**: The most frequently detected **genetic alteration** occurred in the *TERT* promoter region (70.6%), followed by *MED12* (64.7%). *EGFR* amplification and *TP53* alteration were detected in four MPTs without genetic alterations in *MED12* and *TERT* promoter regions. Genetic alterations of *RARA* and *ZNF703* were repeatedly found in PTs with local recurrence and genetic alterations of *SETD2*, ***BRCA2***, and *TSC1* were detected in PTs with distant metastasis. Especially, MPT harboring *PTEN* and *RB1* copy number deletion showed rapid disease progression"- *www.ncbi.nlm.nih.gov*
- The majority of phyllodes tumors have been described as benign (35% to 64%), with the remainder divided between the borderline and malignant subtypes.

Phyllodes Tumour (Previously Sometimes Known as *Serocystic Disease of Brodie or Cystosarcoma Phyllodes*)

◈ *L and B 27th/870*

- Usually occur in women over the age of 40 years but can appear in younger women.
- Treatment for the benign type is enucleation in young women or ***wide local excision***. Massive tumours, recurrent tumours and those of the malignant type will require mastectomy
- The treatment of malignant phyllodes tumor is more controversial, but ***complete removal of the tumor with a rim of normal tissue avoids recurrence***. Because these tumors may be large, ***simple mastectomy is sometimes necessary***. Lymph node dissection is not performed, since the sarcomatous portion of the tumor metastasizes to the lungs and not the lymph nodes- *CSDT 14th/300; Schwartz 10th/555*

164. Ans. **a. Has malignant potential, b. Almost always involve rectum, d. On abdominal radiographs gives thumbprinting pattern, e. Presents with pain and bloody diarrhoea**

[Ref: L and B 27th/1267-71; CSDT 14th/723-27; Manipal Surgery 4th/677;Harrison 19th/1956]

- "**Thumbprinting** is a radiographic sign of large bowel wall thickening, usually caused by oedema, related to an infective or inflammatory process (colitis). The normal haustra become thickened at regular intervals appearing like thumbprints projecting into the aerated lumen. It may be seen in: ***inflammatory bowel disease*** (Crohn disease & ***ulcerative colitis***), infection (i.e. pseudomembranous colitis), ischaemic bowel, diverticulitis, typhlitis etc"- radiopaedia.org
- "Earlier features of **intestinal ischemia** seen on abdominal radiographs include bowel-wall edema, known as "***thumbprinting***"-*Harrison 19th/1979*
- "UC: The ***disease always start in the rectum***- *Manipal Surgery 4th/677*
- "**Cancer risk in UC**: *Overall incidence is* ***3%****(when disease has been present for 15 years) &* ***20%****(at the end of 25 yr)"- Manipal Surgery 4th/679*

Ulcerative Colitis

◈ *CSDT 14th/723-27*

- UC is a diffuse but contiguous mucosal inflammatory disease.
- UC classically starts at the rectum and extends proximally ***without skip lesions***. The disease is confined to the rectum (proctitis) or up to the rectosigmoid region (proctosigmoiditis) in at least half of patients.
- Patients commonly report frequent, ***small volume watery stools mixed with blood***, pus and mucus accompanied by tenesmus, rectal urgency and even fecal incontinence
- Barium enema x-ray of colon. There is shortening of colon, loss of haustral markings (***"lead pipe" appearance***) and fine serrations at the edges of the bowel wall that represent multiple small ulcers
- ***Colorectal cancer risk increases*** above that of the general population 10 years after the onset of UC, although the rates vary widely between studies. The ***risk increases with the duration and severity of disease*** and is higher in patients with a family history of CRC, extensive colitis and PSC

Ulcerative Colitis

◈ *L and B 27th/1267-71*

- The **risk of cancer** in ulcerative colitis increases with duration of disease. At ten years from diagnosis, it is around 1 per cent. This increases to 10–15 per cent at 20 years and may be as high as 20 per cent at 30 years.
- Clinical presentation depends in large part on the extent of disease and the presence or otherwise of complications. ***If confined to the rectum (proctitis),*** there is usually no systemic upset and extra alimentary manifestations are rare. The main symptoms will be rectal bleeding, tenesmus and mucous discharge. ***The disease remains confined to the rectum in 90 per cent of cases but proctitis may spread proximally over time.***

- **Colitis** is almost always associated with ***bloody diarrhoea and urgency*** that can be incapacitating.
- Pain is unusual.
- The more extensive the disease, the more likely ***extraintestinal manifestations*** are to occur. Extensive colitis is also associated with systemic illness, characterized by malaise, loss of appetite and fever.
- ***Diarrhoea may be profuse and bloody***, resulting in anaemia, hypoproteinaemia and electrolyte disturbance.
- Approximately 30 per cent of patients have inflammation extending to the sigmoid colon and spread proximal to the splenic flexure occurs in 20 per cent.

Table: Different Clinical, Endoscopic and Radiographic Features *(Harrison 19th/1956)*

	Ulcerative Colitis	Crohn's Disease
Clinical		
Gross blood in stool	Yes	Occasionally
Mucus	Yes	Occasionally
Systemic symptoms	Occasionally	Frequently
Pain	Occasionally	Frequently
Abdominal mass	Rarely	Yes
Significant perineal disease	No	Frequently
Fistulas	No	Yes
Small intestinal obstruction	No	Frequently
Colonic obstruction	Rarely	Frequently
Response to antibiotics	No	Yes
Recurrence after surgery	No	Yes
ANCA-positive	Frequently	Rarely
ASCA-positive	Rarely	Frequently
Endoscopic		
Rectal sparing	Rarely	Frequently
Continuous disease	Yes	Occasionally
"Cobblestoning"	No	Yes
Granuloma on biopsy	No	Occasionally
Radiographic		
Small bowel significantly abnormal	No	Yes
Abnormal terminal ileum	No	Yes
Segmental colitis	No	Yes
Asymmetric colitis	No	Yes
Stricture	Occasionally	Frequently

165. Ans. b. Ruptured appendix surgery, d. Resection of unprepared bowel

[Ref: L and B 27th/53; CSDT 14th/86;Manipal Surgery 4th/10]

- Hysterectomy- Clean contaminated; Resection of intestinal fistula-dirty; Inguinal hernia repair surgery-clean

Table: Classification of surgical wounds: *Manipal Surgery 4th/10; www.bcbst.com*

Wounds class	Definition	Examples of typical procedures	Wound infection rate (%)
Clean	• Nontraumatic • Elective surgery • Gastrointestinal, respiratory or genitourinary tract not entered.	• Mastectomy • Vascular procedures • Thyroidectomy • Herniorrhaphy (All types)	2
Clean contami nated	• Respiratory, genitourinary or gastrointestinal tracts entered but minimal contamination	• Gastrectomy • ***Hysterectomy*** • Cholecystectomy	< 10
Contami nated	• Open, fresh, traumatic wounds • Uncontrolled spillage from an • Unprepared viscus • Minor break in sterile technique	• **Ruptured appendix** • **Resection of unprepared bowel** •	20
Dirty	• Open, traumatic dirty wounds • Traumatic perforated viscus • Pus in the operative field	• Resection of gangrene • ***Bowel resection (with fistula/*** perforation/ peritonitis)	30–70

Table: Wound classification *(CSDT 14th/86; www.researchgate.net)*

Clean	*These are uninfected operative wounds in which no inflammation is encountered and the respiratory, alimentary, genital, or uninfected urinary tracts are not entered*
Clean/ contaminated	*These are operative wounds in which the respiratory, alimentary, genital, or urinary tract is entered under controlled conditions and without unusual contamination*
Contaminated	*These include open, fresh, accidental wounds, operations with major breaks in sterile technique or gross spillage from the gastrointestinal tract and incisions in which acute, nonpurulent inflammation is encountered*
Dirty-Infected	Old traumatic wounds with retained devitalized tissue and those that involve existing clinical infection or perforated viscera. This definition suggests that the organisms causing postoperative infection were present in the operative field before the operation.

166. Ans. a. Wound can be visualized, b. Permeable to gases, d. Impermeable to bacteria

[Ref: L and B 27th/41,60 ; Sabiston 19th/171;]

- Opsite wound dressing are waterproof

Skin Adhesive Strips

◈ *L and B 27th/41*

- For the skin, self-adhesive tapes or steristrips may be used where there is no tension and not too much moisture, such as after a wide excision of a breast lump. They may also be used to minimise 'spreading' of a scar.
- Other adhesive polyurethane films, such as **Opsite**, Tegaderm or Bioclusive, may provide a similar benefit, while such transparent dressings also allow ***wound inspection and may protect against cross-infection.***

Table: Type of dressing *(partial) (Sabiston 19th/171)*

Category	Composition & characteristic	Function	Examples	Comment
Occlusive Films	Clear polyurethane membranes with acrylic adhesive on one side	Insulation, moisture retention, ***protective barrier acts against bacteria***	Tegaderm, mefilm, carrafilm, bioclusive, transeal, **opsite**	***Waterproof; permeable to oxygen, carbon dioxide and water vapor***; do not interfere with patient function; allow visualization of wound; ***nonabsorptive***, can leak; require intact skin around wound area; wound contraction may be slowed, removal may disrupt new epithelium

Benefits Of Opsite Post-Op Dressing

◈ *www.healthproductsforyou.com*

- **Waterproof:** Opsite Post-Op Waterproof Dressing is impermeable to water and body fluids, allowing the patient to shower without changing dressings.
- **Bacterial Barrier: Opsite** Post-Op film provides a bacterial barrier, helping to reduce the risk of secondary infection.
- **High MVTR** (Moisture Vapour Transmission Rate)**:** It has a unique molecular structure that switches on in the presence of moisture, preventing accumulation of moisture underneath the dressing, which ***reduces bacterial growth and the risk of maceration.***
- **Transparent Film:** The clear film allows the user to monitor the level of fluid and check for infection without removing the dressing, thus increasing wear time.
- **Absorbent, Low-adherent Pad:** The thick pad is highly absorbent, minimizing the number of dressing changes whilst protecting the wound from further injury. The low-adherent wound contact layer leaves the wound site clean and comfortable, reducing pain when changing the dressing.
- **Conformable:** Opsite Post-Op **Transparent Dressing** is highly conformable, even over the most awkward body contours. Its extensibility does not restrict movement, ensuring that it is comfortable for the patient. The unique dressing carrier keeps the film firm, allowing easy application.

167. Ans. b. 3rd and 4th degree hemorhoids, d. Strangulated hemorrhoid

[Ref: Manipal Surgery 4th/793-95;CSDT 14th/744; L and B 27th/1354-61; Schwartz 10th/1233;Sabiston 19th/1388-89]

Table: Treatment of haemorrhoids (Summarized from text) *(Schwartz 10th/1233)*

Medical therapy	• Bleeding from 1st & 2nd degree hemorrhoids often improve with dietary fibers, stool softeners & other diet regulations
Rubber band ligation	• It is the simplest, most effective and most widely used method • Done for 1st, 2nd & selective 3rd degree hemorrhoids
Infrared photocoagulation	• For 1st and 2nd degree hemorrhoids
Sclerotherapy	• Done for 1st, 2nd & selective 3rd degree hemorrhoids
Elliptical Excision	• Done for ***thrombosed external hemorrhoids***
Operative hemorrhoidectomy (excisional hemorrhoidectomy)	• Surgical method is the method of choice for: ▪ ***3rd & 4th degree hemorrhoids*** ▪ *Other degrees not cures by conservative methods* ▪ Mixed (combined internal/external) hemorrhoids ▪ *Hemorrhoids complicated by strangulations* or associated pathology, such as ulceration, fissure or fistula

The Indications for Haemorrhoidectomy Include

◈ *L and B 27th/1357*

- ***Third- and fourth-degree haemorrhoids***
- Second-degree haemorrhoids that have not been cured by non-operative treatments
- Fibrosed haemorrhoids

- Intero-external haemorrhoids when the external haemorrhoid is well defined.

"Hemorrhoidectomy is the best means of curing hemorrhoidal disease and should be considered whenever patients fail to respond satisfactorily to repeated attempts at conservative measures; hemorrhoids are severely prolapsed and require manual reduction; hemorrhoids are complicated by ***strangulation or associated pathology, such as ulceration, fissure, fistula; or hemorrhoids are associated with symptomatic external hemorrhoids or large anal tags.* For *simple thrombosed external hemorrhoids, excision in the office is best performed early*** in the course of the disease, during the period of maximum pain. To remove complex internal or external hemorrhoids, an open or closed hemorrhoidectomy can be performed as an outpatient procedure"-*Sabiston 19th/1389*

Table: Internal Hemorrhoids: Grading and Management *(Sabiston 19th/1388; L and B 27th/1355)*

Grade	Symptoms and Signs	Management
First degree	Bleeding; no prolapse	Dietary modifications[*]
Second degree	Prolapse with spontaneous reduction	Rubber band ligation
	Bleeding, seepage	Coagulation
		Dietary modifications
Third degree	Prolapse requiring digital reduction	Surgical hemorrhoidectomy
	Bleeding, seepage	Rubber band ligation
		Dietary modifications
Fourth degree	Prolapsed, cannot be reduced	Surgical hemorrhoidectomy
	Strangulated	Urgent hemorrhoidectomy
		Dietary modifications

Technique of Haemorrhoidectomy

◈ *L and B 27th/1357.*

- Haemorrhoidectomy can be performed using an ***open or a closed technique.***
- The open technique is known as the Milligan–Morgan operation
- Both involve ligation and excision of the haemorrhoid, but in the open technique the anal mucosa and skin are left open to heal
- ***If a patient with a thrombosed external hemorrhoid is seen within 3 days of the onset of symptoms then excision of the clot may be beneficial.***

"Rectal prolapse describes a condition in which the entire layer of the rectal wall protrudes through the anal canal. A common pitfall in the diagnosis of **rectal prolapse** is the potential for confusion with ***prolapsed incarcerated internal hemorrhoids.*** These conditions may be distinguished by close inspection of the direction of the prolapsed tissue folds. ***In the case of rectal prolapse, the folds are always concentric,*** whereas *hemorrhoidal tissue develops radial invaginations defining the hemorrhoidal cushions.* Prolapsed, incarcerated hemorrhoids produce extreme pain and can be accompanied by fever and urinary retention. ***Unless incarcerated, rectal prolapse is easily reducible and painless***"-Sabiston 19th/1367

168. Ans. a. Predispose to carcinoma of pancreas, c. Can present with steatorrhoea & malabsorption, d. Present with epigastric pain radiating to back, e. Total pancreatectomy relieves pain in majority of patients.

[Ref: CSDT 14th/621-22; L and B 27th/1230-32; Schwartz 10th/1370-76; Sabiston 19th/1520-28]

- "**Adenocarcinoma of the pancreas** occurs with greater frequency in patients with familial chronic pancreatitis than in the general population"- *CSDT 14th/622*
- ***"Patients with intractable pain and diffuse disease may plead for a total pancreatectomy in the expectation that removing the offending organ will relieve their pain"***- *L and B 27th/1231-32*
- ***"Longitudinal pancreaticojejunostomy relieves pain in about 80% of patients with a dilated duct.*** The results of pancreaticoduodenectomy are good in 80% of patients, but removal of the distal pancreas is less successful. ***Total pancreatectomy, which is principally reserved for failures of other operations, gives satisfying relief in 30%-90% of patients depending on the series.*** The reasons for these widely differing results are not known"- *CSDT 14th/623*

Chronic Pancreatitis

◈ *Schwartz 10th/1370-76*

- "**Pain** is the most common symptom of chronic pancreatitis. It is usually ***midepigastric in location*** but may localize or involve either the left or right upper quadrant of the abdomen. Occasionally, it is perceived in the lower midabdomen but is frequently described as ***penetrating through to the back***"- *Schwartz 10th/1371*
- Nausea or vomiting may accompany the pain, but anorexia is the most common associated symptom.
- The **surgical relief of pain** due to obstructive pancreatopathy may be dependent on the degree of underlying fibrosis rather than the presence of ductal obstruction
- **Malabsorption and Weight Loss:** When pancreatic exocrine capacity falls below 10% of normal, ***diarrhea and steatorrhea develop.***
- **Lipase deficiency** tends to manifest itself before trypsin deficiency, so the presence of steatorrhea may be the first functional sign of pancreatic insufficiency.
- The direct measurement of pancreatic enzymes (e.g., **lipase and amylase**) by blood test is highly sensitive and fairly specific in acute pancreatitis but is ***seldom helpful in the diagnosis of chronic pancreatitis.*** The pancreatic endocrine product that correlates most strongly with chronic pancreatitis is the **PP response** to a test meal

- "**Amylase**—In acute exacerbations, serum and urinary amylase levels may be elevated, but most often they are not, perhaps because pancreatic fibrosis has destroyed so much of the enzyme-forming capacity of the parenchyma. Elevated bilirubin or alkaline phosphatase levels may result from fibrotic entrapment of the lower end of the bile duct"- *CSDT 14th/622*
- The **incidence of carcinoma** in patients with chronic pancreatitis ranges from ***1.5% to 6%,*** which is at least 10-fold greater than that of patients of similar age seen in a hospital setting- *Schwartz 10th/1375*

169. Ans. a. Steatorrhoea, c. Cholelithiasis, e. Renal oxalate stones

[Ref: Manipal Surgery 4th/694-95;CSDT 14th/676-77; L and B 27th/ 283,1256; Schwartz 10th/1171]

- "**Small intestinal bacterial overgrowth (SIBO)** is defined as the presence of an abnormally high number of ***coliform bacteria in the small bowel.*** It is associated with a broad range of predisposing small intestinal motility disorders and with surgical procedures that result in bowel stasis. The most common symptoms associated with SIBO include *diarrhea, flatulence, abdominal pain and bloating.* There are several endogenous **defence mechanisms** for preventing bacterial overgrowth: gastric acid secretion, intestinal motility, ***intact ileocaecal valve***, immunoglobulins within intestinal secretion and bacteriostatic properties of pancreatic and biliary secretion.
- **An intact ileocaecal valve *inhibits retrograde translocation of bacteria from the colon to the small bowel***"-www.ncbi.nlm.nih.gov
- "An **intact ileocecal valve** is believed to be associated with ***decreased malabsorption***. The *ileocecal valve delays transit of chyme from the small intestine into the colon,* thereby prolonging the contact time between nutrients and the small-intestinal absorptive mucosa"-*Schwartz 10th/1171; CSDT 14th/676*
- "With an **ileal resection** greater than 100 cm, there is a gradual loss in the total bile salt pool, eventually leading to impairment in fat absorption and the onset of ***steatorrhea***. Ileal resections are also associated with ***lithogenic bile,*** such that ***gallstone formation*** is seen in approximately 30% of patients who have undergone such surgery. ***Calcium oxalate urinary tract calculi form in 7%-10% of patients who have extensive ileal resection*** and an intact colon, due to excessive absorption of oxalate from the colon"- *CSDT 14th/677*
- "**Complications of short bowel syndrome** include peptic ulceration related to gastric hypersecretion, ***cholelithiasis*** and ***hyper oxaluria as a result of the increased absorption of oxalate in the colon predisposing to renal stones***"-*L and B 27th/ 283*

Ileum

◈ *L and B 27th/ 283*

- ***The ileum is the only site of absorption of vitamin B12 and bile salts.*** Bile salts are essential for the absorption of fats and fat-soluble vitamins.
- ***Depletion of the bile salt pool results in fat malabsorption.***
- In addition, loss of bile salts into the colon affects colonic mucosa, ***causing a reduction in salt and water absorption, which increases stool losses***
- Following ileal resection, the colon receives a much larger volume of fluid and electrolytes and it also receives bile salts, which reduce its ability to absorb salt and water, resulting in **diarrhoea**.
- Even the loss of 100 cm of ileum causes **steatorrhoea**, which may necessitate the administration of oral cholestyramine to bind bile salts. With larger resections (>100 cm) dietary fat restriction may be necessary. Regular parenteral vitamin B12 is required.

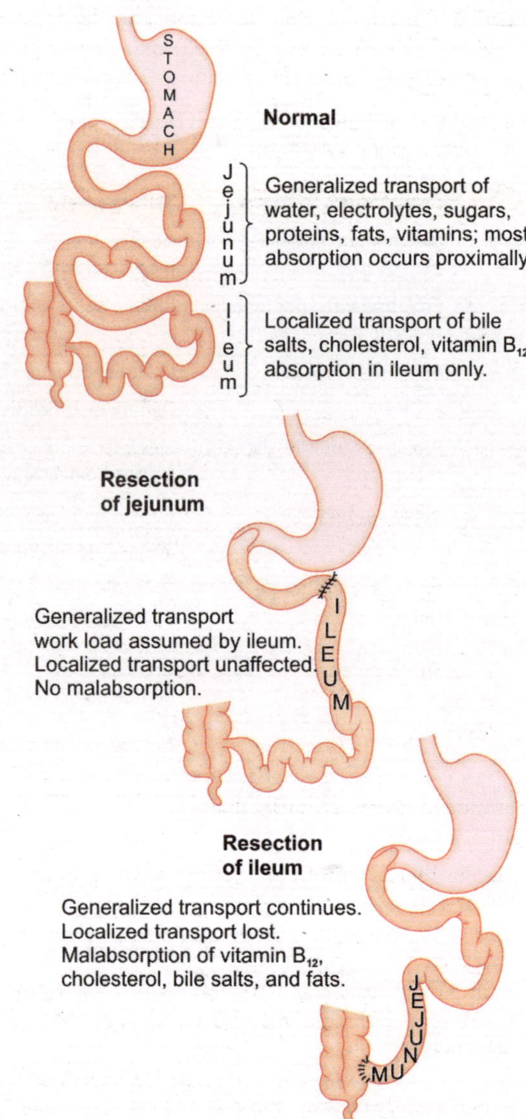

Fig: The consequences of complete resection of jejunum or ileum are predictable in part from the loss of regionally localized transport processes *(CSDT 14th/677)*

170. Ans. **a. On CT, extradural haematomas appear ..., c. Mainly arterial blood, d. Common after injury...**

[Ref: Harrison 19th/457e-3;Danhert Radiology 7th/289-90;CSDT 14th/867-68; Schwartz 10th/174,1719;Chandrasoma Taylor 3rd/924,438; Sumer Sethi 6th/144; Manipal 4th/1037]

Option B: Not True (See below)

- "Because the primary injury in an isolated **epidural hematoma** ***does not involve the brain***, *the neurological outcome is excellent if the diagnosis and treatment are prompt*"*-CSDT 14th/867*
- "**Epidural Hematoma**: These usually e***volve more rapidly than subdural hematomas and are correspondingly more treacherous***"*-Harrison 19th/457e-3*
- **"Subdural haemorrhage**: Relatively severe trauma. 50 per cent mortality"*- L and B 26th/316*
- "Due to associated parenchymal injury, subdural hematomas have a much worse prognosis than epidural collections"*-Schwartz 10th/174*
- "The prognosis for functional recovery is significantly worse for acute SDH than EDH because it is associated with greater primary injury to brain parenchyma from high-energy impacts"*-Schwartz 10th/1719*
- **"Acute Subdural Hematomas (ASDH):** Focal bruising of the brain is often present beneath the subdural hematoma. Outcomes are often poor, with a mortality of 50%-90%. Survivors often have significant disabilities"*-CSDT 14th/868*

"**Extradural haematoma Location**: ***In 66% temporoparietal*** *(most often from laceration of middle meningeal artery); in 29% at frontal lobe, parietooccipital region, b/w occipital lobes, posterior fossa(most often from laceration of dural sinuses by fracture)"- Danhert Radiology 7th/290*

Pterion is a point of clinical significance – the skull is very thin at this point. In addition to being structurally weak due to being the point of union between several bones, it also lies over the **anterior division of the middle meningeal artery.** Fracture of the skull at this point can therefore disrupt the middle meningeal artery, leading to an extradural (epidural) haematoma-*anatomyzone.com*

"Convex, lens-shaped hyperdensity that may cross the midline. **An epidural hematoma is a neurosurgical emergency!** Since bleeding is under arterial pressure, the hematoma may expand rapidly. Prompt drainage is almost always necessary. 5%-10% mortality if treated within the first few hours. Mortality is largely due to increased intra-cranial pressure and herniation"*-casemed.case.edu*

Extradural Hematoma	Subdural Hematoma
• Biconvex or lenticular • Temporal or temporoparietal • Middle meningeal artery • 0.5% of all head injured pts • "Lucid" Interval classically • Outcome related to status prior to surgery	• Diffuse and concave • Entire surface of brain • Tearing of bridging veins • 30% of severe head injuries • Underlying brain damage more severe • Prognosis is worse than extradural

Extradural Haematoma

◈ *L and B 27th/333-34*

- Extradural haematoma is a neurosurgical emergency. It results from rupture of ***an artery, vein or venous sinus,*** in association with a skull fracture.
- ***Typically, it is damage to the middle meningeal artery under the thin temporal bone.***
- On CT, extradural haematomas appear as a ***lentiform (lens shaped or biconvex)*** hyperdense lesion between skull and brain.
- Overall mortality is around 10–20 per cent, but is considerably lower in isolated extradural haematoma.

171. Ans. **a. Swollen fingers, b. Pallor, c. Paraesthesia, d. Pain on passion flexion, e. Pain on active flexion**

[Ref: Ebnezar 4th/33-34; Current Diagnosis and Treatment in Orthopedics 2006/Chap3; Campbell's Operative Orthopaedics, 11th/Chap 71; CSDT 14th/1062]

"Hand compartment syndrome: Consider the diagnosis when nonspecific aching of the hand, increased pain, loss of digital motion and ***continued swelling are present.*** A tight, ***swollen hand*** in an intrinsic minus position—with the digits in metacarpophalangeal (MCP) extension and proximal interphalangeal (PIP) flexion—is highly indicative. Pain with certain movements, particularly ***passive stretching of the muscles,*** is the earliest clinical indicator of compartment syndrome. A patient may report ***pain with active flexion***"-**emedicine.medscape.co**

Forearm Compartment Syndrome Campbell's Operative Orthopaedics

◈ *11th/Chap 71*

- A crush injury or fracture of the forearm or elbow, especially in the supracondylar area of the humerus, should raise suspicion that a **forearm compartment syndrome** may develop.
- Pain is the most consistent symptom, although it may not be discovered in a comatose patient. ***Passive extension of the fingers increases the pain.***
- The ***forearm is tender and tense with swelling*** and sensibility of the fingertips may be diminished.
- The radial pulse may or may not be palpable.
- The diagnosis of a compartment syndrome of an individual interosseous muscle can be difficult. The hand is swollen and tense and the ***fingers are held almost rigid in a partially flexed position with the wrist in neutral.***
- ***Any passive movement of the fingers that causes metacarpophalangeal joint extension usually causes considerable pain.*** The adductor compartment of the thumb can be tested by pulling the thumb into palmar abduction and stretching the adductor muscle. The thenar muscles rarely are involved

"Forearm compartment syndrome: physical examination-pain with passive stretch of fingers (most sensitive finding); palpable swelling"-*www.orthobullets.com*

Compartment Syndrome

◈ *Current Diagnosis and Treatment in Orthopedics 2006/Chap3*

- The term **compartment syndrome** refers to pathologic developments in a closed space in the body caused by buildup of pressure.
- Most commonly, such compartments are circumscribed by fascia and incorporate one or more bones.
- The **five P's** (***pulselessness, paresthesia, paresis, pain and pressure***) ***characteristic of compartment syndrome*** are helpful, but not diagnostic, for the experienced clinician.
- Pulses are poor indicators of compartment syndrome as they generally remain intact until late.
- **Paresthesias** occur only when the syndrome is significantly advanced.
- **Pain with passive stretching** of involved muscles is also a subjective finding and must be differentiated from pain arising from the original injury. To the experienced clinician, pain with passive stretching is a reliable clinical sign.
- Pressure is a key component of compartment syndrome, but palpation of a soft compartment does not rule out the diagnosis of compartment syndrome.

Compartment Syndrome

◈ *CSDT 14th/1062*

- Although, it most commonly occurs in ***the forearm and leg, it can occur in the foot, thigh and arm.*** Compartment syndrome typically presents as a ***painful, swollen, tense extremity.***
- ***Pain with passive range of motion of the digits and pain out of proportion are considered to be the most reliable early indicators of compartment syndrome.***
- Clinical signs of compartment syndrome include the ***5 Ps: pain, poikilothermia, pallor, paresthesias and finally pulselessness.***

172. Ans. a. Intravesical BCG immunotherapy is helpful in recurrent cases, c. Smoking is a risk factor, d. Urothelial carcinomas is most common subtype

[Ref: CSDT 14th/1000-03; L and B 27th/1446-52; Campbell-Walsh Urology, 9th/Chap 77]

Bladder Cancer Type

- Transitional(Urothelial) cell cancer: 90%
- Squamous cell cancer: 5-10%
- Adenocarcinoma:2%

"**Muscle-invasive bladder cancer**: ***Radical cystoprostatectomy*** in the male patient and ***anterior exenteration in the female patient,*** coupled with en bloc pelvic lymphadenectomy, remain the standard surgical approaches to muscle-invasive bladder carcinoma in the absence of metastatic disease"- *Campbell-Walsh Urology, 9th/Chap 77*

Non Muscle-invasive bladder cancer: TUR of bladder tumor (TURBT) under regional or general anesthesia is the initial ***treatment for visible lesions*** and is performed both to remove all visible tumors and to provide specimens for pathologic examination to determine stage and grade. After all visible tumor is resected, an additional pass of the cutting loop or a cold cup biopsy can be obtained to send to pathology separately to determine the presence of muscle invasion of the tumor base"- *Campbell-Walsh Urology, 9th/Chap 76*

"***Schistosoma haematobium*** cystitis appears to be causally related to the ***development of bladder cancer***—often SCC. In Egypt, where schistosomiasis is endemic among males, ***SCC of the bladder*** (bilharzial bladder cancer) is the most common malignancy. However, there is also an ***increased incidence of TCCs*** in males with schistosomiasis"- *Campbell-Walsh Urology, 9th/Chap 75*

Urinary Bladder Cancer

◈ *CSDT 14th/1000-03*

- Men are affected twice as often as women.
- ***More than 90% of tumors are urothelial carcinomas***, while a few are squamous cell carcinomas (associated with chronic inflammation, as in ***bilharziasis***) or adenocarcinomas (often seen at the dome of the bladder in patients with a urachal remnant).
- ***Most urothelial carcinomas (70%-80%) are nonmuscle invasive (not invasive into the bladder detrusor musculature) when recognized.*** Only 10%-15% of recurrent tumors become invasive
- The cause of urothelial carcinoma is unknown; ***there is a strong association with chronic cigarette smoking*** and exposure to chemicals prevalent in dye, rubber, leather, paint and other chemical industries

Intravesical Therapy

◈ *CSDT 14th/1002-03*

- A variety of chemotherapeutic agents have been used in patients with recurrent low-grade, low-stage tumors. Immunotherapeutic drugs, which include BCG, are effective in prophylaxis (60%) of ***recurrent papillary tumors*** and curative (70%) in carcinoma *in situ*, a highly malignant lesion less responsive to the cytotoxic agents described earlier. ***Intravesical BCG is the gold-standard first line therapy for carcinoma in situ of the bladder.***
- The combination of BCG and interferon alpha has shown nearly 50% response rates and is occasionally used in patients who have failed BCG.

Urothelial Cell Carcinoma of the Bladder

◈ *L and B 27th/1446*

- Strongly associated with **Schistosoma haematobium infection (bilharzial bladder cancer)** in regions where the parasite is endemic
- **Muscle-invasive bladder cancer: Radical primary treatment** options include ***radical cystectomy, urinary diversion and thorough lymph node dissection which tends to be offered as first line, or radical external beam radiotherapy***- *L and B 27th/1448*
- **Non-muscle-invasive bladder cancer (NMIBC):** The **incidence of recurrence** of this disease can be reduced by **intravesical chemotherapy and immunotherapy**. High-risk superficial disease (any grade 3 disease) is best managed by BCG immunotherapy followed by radical treatment if disease persists- *L and B 27th/1447*

Table: Treatment and prognosis of tumors related to stage of disease *(CSDT 14th/1001)*

Conventional state	TNM stage	Tumor involvement	Treatment	Five-Year survival (%)
0	Ta	Mucosa only	Transurethral resection	85-90
A	T1	Submucosal invasion (lamina propria)	Transurethral resection and intravesical chemoimmunotherapy	60-80
B1	T2a	Superficial muscle invasion	Total cystectomy and pelvic lymphadenectomy	50-55
B2	T2b	Deep muscle invasion		30-50
C	T3	Perivesical fat invasion		30-40
D1	T3-4N+	Regional lymph node invasion	Systemic chemo-therapy	6-35
D2	T3-4M1	Distant metastases		0-10

173. Ans. **b. Over expression of HER-2/neu, c. Triple negative tumor, e. >20% of cells expressing Ki 67 marker**

[Ref: Manipal Surgery 4th/404-05; L and B 27th/875; Harshmohan 7th/757-58; Schwartz 10th/514-19]

"**Favourable Prognosis:** *ER-PR Positive, HER2/Neu Under Expression*"- *Harshmohan 7th/757*

Table: Summary of prognostic markers and predictive factors for invasive breast cancer *(Internet, Harshmohan 7th/758)*

Prognostic factors	Favourable, low recurrence	Unfavourable, high recurrence
Lymph node status	Negative	Positive
Size	T0T1	T2T3
Histological grade	Low	High
Histological type	Tubular, colloid, papillary	Invasive ductal Ca (of NST)
Necrosis	Absent	Present
Hormone receptors (ER, PR)	Positive	**Negative**
DNA flow cytometry	Diploid	Aneuploid
Proliferative ability by ***S phase*** fraction	Low (<5%)	**High (>5%)**
Lymphatic or vascular invasion	Absent	Present
Her-2/neu oncogene	Low	**High**
Cathepsin-D	Low	High
Epidermal growth factor receptor		
PCNA & ***Ki-67 expression***	Negative	**Positive**

Contd...

Ki67

- *Manipal Surgery 4th/404*
- Also known as MK167
- ***Higher value suggests aggressive tumor***
- A ***cut off value of <14%*** is generally used to ***denote low & high values***

Triple-negative

- *www.breastcancer.org*
- Breast cancer cells tested negative for estrogen receptors (ER-), progesterone receptors (PR-) and HER2 (HER2-). Testing negative for all three means the cancer is **triple-negative** [negative for estrogen receptors (ER-), progesterone receptors (PR-) and HER2 (HER2-)]
- Triple-negative breast cancer does not respond to hormonal therapy (such as tamoxifen or aromatase inhibitors) or therapies that target HER2 receptors, such as Herceptin (chemical name: trastuzumab). However, other medicines can be used to treat triple-negative breast cancer.
- About 10-20% of breast cancers — more than one out of every 10 — are found to be triple-negative
- Triple negative breast cancer ***can be more aggressive and difficult to treat***. Also, the cancer is ***more likely to spread and recur***- *www.nationalbreastcancer.org*

174. Ans. **a. Low grade tumor, c. Good prognosis, e. Associated with cytokeratin 8 and 18**

[Ref: Schwartz 10th/536; ww5.komen.org; www.breastcancer.org]

Luminal A

- *ww5.komen.org*
- Luminal tumor cells look the most like cells of breast cancers that start in the inner (luminal) cells lining the mammary ducts.
- Luminal A tumors tend to be: Estrogen receptor-positive (ER-positive), ***HER2 receptor-negative*** (HER2-negative) & ***Tumor grade 1 or 2***
- About 30-70 percent of breast cancers are luminal A tumors
- Of the **4 subtypes, luminal A** tumors tend to have the ***best prognosis***, with fairly ***high survival rates and fairly low recurrence rate***

"**Luminal A** breast cancer is hormone-receptor positive (estrogen-receptor and/or progesterone-receptor positive), ***HER2 negative*** and has low ***levels of the protein Ki-67***, which helps control how fast cancer cells grow. Luminal A cancers are low-grade, tend to grow slowly and have the best prognosis"- *www.breastcancer.org*

"basal-like **(CK5+ER-)**, ***luminal (CK8/18+ER+)*** and **ERBB2+ (HER2+)**"- *onlinelibrary.wiley.com*

"CK8/18 is another marker which can be called ***luminal marker*** as it represents nor-mal luminal epithelial differentiation"- *www.researchgate.net*

Four Main Intrinsic or Molecular Subtypes of Breast Cancer

◈ *www.mayoclinic.org*

- **Group 1 (luminal A).** This group includes tumors that are ER positive and PR positive, but negative for HER2. Luminal A breast cancers are likely to benefit from hormone therapy and may also benefit from chemotherapy.
- **Group 2 (luminal B).** This type includes tumors that are ER positive, PR negative and HER2 positive. Luminal B breast cancers are likely to benefit from chemotherapy and may benefit from hormone therapy and treatment targeted to HER2.
- **Group 3 (HER2 positive).** This type includes tumors that are ER negative and PR negative, but HER2 positive. HER2 breast cancers are likely to benefit from chemotherapy and treatment targeted to HER2.
- **Group 4 (basal-like).** This type, which is also called triple-negative breast cancer, includes tumors that are ER negative, PR negative and HER2 negative. Basal-like breast cancers are likely to benefit from chemotherapy.

Table: Molecular subtype of breast cancer

	Luminal A	Luminal B	Her-2/neu	Basal-like
		Luminal B tends to be higher histological grade than luminal A	**TP53 mutation common** More likely to be high grade and node positive	TP 53 mutation common; **BRCA-1 dysfunction** (germline sporadic)
Histological correlation	Tubular carcinoma Cribriform carcinoma Low grade IDC (NOS) lobular carcinoma	IDC (NOS) Micropapillary carcinoma	High grade IDC (NOS)	High grade IDC (NOS) Metaplastic carcinoma Medullary carcinoma
Treatment	Respond to endocrine therapy	Respond to endocrine therapy (tamoxifen& aromatase inhibitors)	Respond to trastuzumab	No response to Endocrine therapy and trastuzumab
Response to chemotherapy	Variable	Variable (> in luminal A)	Good (anthracycline based chemotherapy)	Good (platinum-based chemotherapy
Prognosis	Good prognosis	Prognosis not as good as for luminal A	Generally poor prognosis	Generally poor prognosis

175. Ans. a. Viral infection is common etiology, b. Transoral removal of stone by probing through oral route, c. Swollen gland, e. Can present with stasis of saliva

[Ref: Manipal Surgery 4th/303-05;P.L.Dhingra 7th/260-61; Sabiston 19th/811-12; CSDT 14th/ 256; L and B 27th/ 780-81,786; L & T 11th/248]

- There is some confusion regarding most commonly gland involvement- Majority of references favor parotid gland

"Sialadenitis is ***most common in the parotid gland.*** The most common causative organism is Staphylococcus aureus; others include streptococci, coliforms and various anaerobic bacteria"- www.msdmanuals.com

Sialadenitis

◈ *teachmesurgery.com*

- It most ***commonly affects the parotid gland***
- **Viruses are much more common** than bacteria as pathogens causing sialadenitis. Of viral causes, mumps is the most common, affecting either the parotid (more common) or the submandibular gland, yet other viral causes include coxsackie, parainfluenza and HIV
- Patients will commonly report **painful swelling and tenderness of the gland**. Pyrexia, lymphadenopathy and erythema of the affected gland can all also develop
- *"**Acute sialadenitis** is rarely aspirated because it is usually diagnosed clinically as a postoperative complication, **viral** or fungal infection, or secondary bacterial infection resulting from an obstruction such as sialolithiasis. **Most cases affect the parotid gland**"- www.sciencedirect.com*

Acute Sialadenitis

◈ *radiopaedia.org*

- **Sialadenitis** can occur in various forms ranging from acute bacterial sialadenitis (acute suppurative sialadenitis) to acute viral sialadenitis to chronic sialadenitis.
- Acute sialadenitis is most commonly caused by an ascending bacterial infection, with *Staphylococcus aureus* or *Streptococcus viridans* being the most common organisms.
- Sialolithiasis is often present (causing obstructive sialadenitis) and stones are found in ***~85% of submandibular ducts and ~15% of parotid duct***
- Due to calculi being a dominant aetiological factor, the distribution of sialadenitis follows that of sialolithiasis and therefore the ***submandibular glands are the most commonly affected.***
- Sialography is contraindicated in acute sialadenitis because it can worsen the infection
- In acute sialadenitis, the ***affected gland appears enlarged,*** hypoechoic and hyperaemiac on ultrasound
- Acute sialadenitis: CT: ***enlarged intra- or extra-glandular lymph nodes*** may also be seen but this is non-specific and can occur in other conditions such as malignancy

Acute Sialadenitis

◈ *www.aafp.org*

- Patients with acute sialadenitis typically present with acute onset of pain and ***swelling of the affected gland.*** Physical examination may reveal induration, edema and extreme localized tenderness.
- Massage of the gland may express pus from the respective intraoral orifice
- Management involves treating the infection and reversing the underlying medical condition and predisposing factors.
- This includes stimulation of salivary flow by application of warm compresses, administration of sialagogues such as lemon drops or vitamin C lozenges, hydration, salivary gland massage, oral hygiene & Empiric antimicrobial therapy
- Rarely, acute suppurative sialadenitis can lead to **abscess formation**; surgical drainage is indicated in these cases.

Sialadenitis and Sialoiithiasis

◈ *CSDT 14th/ 256*

- Infection of the salivary glands may be either viral or bacterial in etiology.
- **Viral sialadenitis**is most commonly secondary to mumps, which presents with a flu-like prodrome followed by ***parotid gland swelling.***
- Bacterial sialadenitis may be acute or chronic. ***The parotid gland is affected in the majority of cases secondary to the diminished bacteriostatic activity of its serous saliva.***
- ***Salivary stasis***, ductal obstruction and decreased saliva production appear to be predisposing conditions to acute sialadenitis. Patients usually present with fever, systemic toxicity and ***tender swelling and enlargement of the affected glands.***

Sialadenitis

◈ *rarediseases.info.nih.gov*

- Sialadenitis usually occurs after ***decreased flow of saliva*** (hyposecretion) or duct obstruction, but may develop without an obvious cause.
- Signs and symptoms of sialadenitis may include fever, chills and ***unilateral pain and swelling in the affected area.***
- The affected gland may be ***firm and tender,*** with redness of the overlying skin. Pus may drain through the gland into the mouth
- Sialadenitis is most commonly due to bacterial infections caused by Staphylococcus aureus. Other bacteria which can cause the infections include streptococci, coliforms and various anaerobic bacteria.
- Although less common than bacteria, several viruses have also been implicated in sialadenitis. These include the mumps virus, HIV, coxsackievirus, parainfluenza types I and II, influenza A and herpes

Sialolithiasis

◈ *P.L.Dhingra 7th/260-61*

- ***90% stones are seen in the submandibular gland but only 10% in the parotid***
- *Calculi are formed by deposition of calcium phosphate on the organic matrix of mucin or cellular debris*
- *The presenting feature is **intermittent swelling of the involved gland** & the pain due to **obstruction to outflow of saliva***
- ***Stones in the peripheral part of submandibular or parotid ducts can be removed intraorally**, while those a hilum or in parenchyma require excision of the gland*

176. Ans. **a. Smaller diameter, e. Less chance of tissue reaction**

[Ref: Instruments by Vinod Pusdekar 1st/144-45; Manipal Surgery 4th/1140; L and B 27th/ 89-90; Sabiston 19th/233]

- "The **diameter of the suture** will affect its **handling properties** and **tensile strength**. The larger the size ascribed to the suture, the smaller the diameter is, for example a 7-0 suture is smaller than a 4-0 suture"-*teachmesurgery.com*

Number of Suture Material

◈ *Vinod Pusdekar 1st/145*

- Number of suture material, indicates thickness of the suture
- Depending on the thickness of the suture, the No may be 2, 1, 0, 1–0, 2–0, 3–0, 4–0, etc.
- Higher the number, thicker the suture, like No 2 is thicker than 1
- ***But, if '0' is prefixed by the higher numbers, then the sutures become finer or less thick,*** like 3–0 is finer and thinner than 2–0 suture.

Gauge: Size of Suture

◈ *coreem.net/core*

- ***Strength of suture*** proportional to ***square of the diameter*** of the thread
- Usually best to select smallest suture that provides adequate tensile strength as ***more material increases tissue reaction***
- Standardized by United States Pharmacopedia
  - Scale runs from 11-0 (smallest) to 7 (largest)
  - Sizes are a number or a zero
    - #2>#1>0>2-0 (00)
  - Zero sizes are pronounced with the number of zeros first
  - E.g. 7-0 is pronounced "seven-oh"
- Metric system used in other parts of the world
  - Sized in tenths of a millimeter
  - Eg. 5-0 is 0.1mm in diameter and size 1 metric

Background: Suture Characteristics

◈ *fpnotebook.com*

- Tensile Strength
  - ***Related to Suture size***
  - Related to weight required to break a Suture
- Knot strength
  - Force required for a knot to slip
- Configuration
  - Monofilament (less risk of infection)
  - Braided multifilament (easier to handle and tie)
- Elasticity
  - Degree Suture stretches and return to original length
- Memory or Suture stiffness

- High memory: Suture stiff, difficult handling, unties
- Tissue reactivity (inflammatory response to Suture)
  - Reaction peaks in first 2 to 7 days

Table: List of common thread sizes, as indicated in the United States Pharmacopoeia (USP) and European Pharmacopoeia (EP) *(www.researchgate.net)*

USP size code	EP size code (mm)	Diameter range (mm)
12/10	0.01	0.001-0.009
11/0	0.1	0.010-0.019
10.0	0.2	0.020-0.029
9/0	0.3	0.030-0.039
8/0	0.4	0.040-0.049
7/0	0.5	0.050-0.069
6/0	0.7	0.070-0.099
5/0	1.0	0.100-0. 149
4/0	1.5	0. 150-0. 199
3/0	2.0	0. 200-0. 249
2/0	2.5	0. 250-0. 299
1/0	3.0	0. 300-0. 349
0	3.5	0.350-0.399
1	4.0	0.400-0.499
2	5.0	0.500-0.599
3	6.0	0.600-0.699
5	7.0	0.700-0.799
6	8.0	0.800-0.899
7	9.0	0.900-0.999

Table: Size of suture material *(L and B 27th /90)*

Metric (EurPh)	Range of diameter (mm)	USP ('old')
1	0. 100-0. 149	5-0
1.5	0. 150-0. 199	4-0
2	0. 200-0. 249	3-0
3	0. 300-0. 349	2-0
3.5	0. 350-0. 399	0
4	0. 400-0. 499	1
5	0. 500-0. 599	2

Suture

◈ *emedicine.medscape.com*

- Understanding the various characteristics of available suture materials is important to make an educated selection. No one suture possesses all desirable characteristics. The ***optimal suture should be easy to handle and have high tensile strength and knot security***. Any ***tissue reaction should be minimal*** and the material should resist infection and ***have good elasticity and plasticity to accommodate wound swelling***. A low cost is preferred. Although some of the newer materials available have many of these properties, no one material is ideal and compromises must be made.
- The physical characteristics of a suture material determine its utility; these characteristics include ***configuration, diameter, capillarity and fluid absorption, tensile strength, knot strength, elasticity, plasticity and memory.***
- **Sizes**: United States Pharmacopeia (USP) sizes are standardized and related to a specific diameter range (in millimeters) that is necessary to produce a certain tensile strength. These diameter ranges vary with the different categories of suture material. These categories include natural materials, synthetic absorbable materials and synthetic nonabsorbable materials. Sizes are expressed with zeroes, such as 3-0, 4-0, 5-0 and 6-0; more zeroes indicate a smaller size.
- The **tensile strength** of a material is the maximal stress that it can withstand before breaking. The rate at which a suture loses its tensile strength over time is not the same as its absorption and varies among suture materials. The implantation and tying of a suture decrease its tensile strength. Dry, unused, absorbable suture loses 4-13% of its initial strength after being soaked in sodium chloride solution for 24 hours. Knotted sutures have two-thirds the strength of unknotted sutures. In selecting suture material, the tensile strength of a suture does not need to exceed that of the tissue it is securing.
- **Plasticity and elasticity**: Plasticity is the ability of the suture to retain its new form and length after stretching. Plasticity allows a suture to accommodate wound swelling, thereby decreasing the risk of strangulated tissue and crosshatch marks. As swelling subsides, however, the suture retains its new size and may not continue to adequately approximate the wound edges. Elasticity is the ability of a suture to regain its original form and length after stretching. After the swelling of a wound recedes, the suture returns to its original length and keeps the wound well approximated. *Most sutures are elastic; few are plastic.*
- **Memory** is the ability of a suture to return to its original shape after deformation by tying. Memory is related to plasticity and elasticity. Sutures with a high degree of memory, particularly monofilament sutures, are stiff and difficult to handle and may be more prone to knot loosening and untying.
- **Tissue reaction:** Different suture materials produce varying degrees of tissue reaction, specifically inflammation. Significant inflammation reduces the resistance to infection and delays the onset of wound healing. The ***type of material and size of the suture are thought to be the major factors contributing to this reaction***. *Natural materials are absorbed by proteolysis, which causes a prominent inflammatory response, while synthetic materials are absorbed by hydrolysis, which produces a minimal reaction.*

Suture Material: Desired Characteristics

◈ *(L and B 27th/ 89)*

- Easy to handle
- Predictable behaviour in tissues
- Predictable tensile strength
- Sterile
- Glides through tissues easily
- Secure knotting ability
- Inexpensive

- Minimal tissue reaction
- Non-capillary
- Non-allergenic
- Non-carcinogenic
- Non-electrolytic
- Non-shrinkage

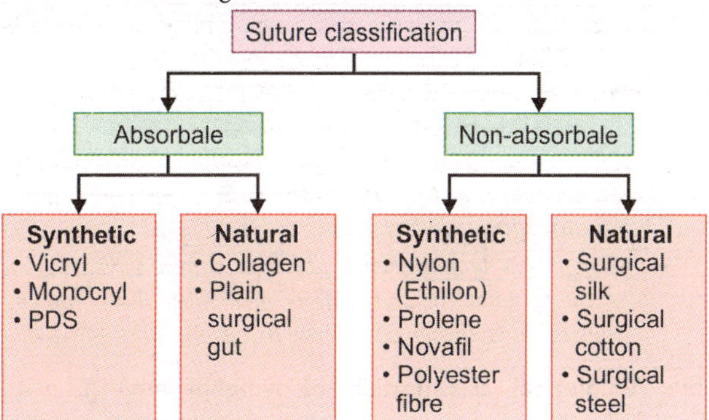

177. Ans. a. Rovsing's sign, b. Iliopsoas sign, c. Carnett's sign, d. Obturator sign

[Ref: Harrison 19th/1987; Manipal Surgery 4th/828-29; L and B 27th/1303; Schwartz 10th/1244]

- **Ballance's sign**: *medical-dictionary* "dull percussion resonance sound heard on the right flank of a patient lying in the ***left decubitus position***, an indication of a ruptured spleen. The sound is caused by an accumulation of liquid blood on the right side and coagulated blood on the left"
- ***"Obturator test:*** *Passive internal rotation of flexed right thigh with the patient in* ***supine position*** *with elicit pain. This positive obturator sign is diagnostic of pelvic appendicitis"-S. Das Textbook5th/1027*

Carnett's Sign

◈ *fpnotebook.com*

- Patient lies ***supine***
- Clinician identifies maximal point of abdominal tenderness
- Intra-Abdominal Pain source (Negative Carnett's Sign)
- Abdominal Muscle Wall Pain (Positive Carnett's Sign)

"Supine Position: The patient is ***lying flat on the back*** with the arms at the sides or above the head. This position facilitates examination of the chest, heart, abdomen and extremities. The head and neck can be examined in this position as well as certain neurologic reflex testing"- study.com/academ

Table: Classic signs of appendicitis in patients with abdominal *(Harrison 19th/1987; L and B 27th/1303)*

Pain (all three sign examined in supine position)

Maneuver	Findings
Rovsing's sign	Palpating in the left lower quadrant causes pain in the right lower quadrant
Obturator sign	Internal rotation of the hip causes pain, suggesting the possibility of an inflamed appendix located in the pelvis
Iliopsoas sign	Extending the right hip causes pain along posterolateral back and hip, suggesting retrocecal appendicitis

178. Ans. a. Usually occur in middle 1/3rd of esophagus, c. Staging is done by CECT, e. Stomach, jejunum or colon can be used for replacement ...

[Ref: Robbins 9th/758-59;Harrison 19th/532-33; CSDT 14th/473-75; L and B 27th/1085-92; Schwartz 10th/1003-04; Sabiston 19th/1049-52]

- "***Esophageal adenocarcinoma usually occurs in the distal third of the esophagus*** and may invade the adjacent gastric cardia In contrast to adenocarcinoma, ***half of squamous cell carcino-mas occur in the middle third of the esophagus***"-Robbins 9th/758-59
- "Tumors that arise within the ***middle third of the esophagus are squamous carcinomas*** most commonly"- *Schwartz 10th/1005*
- "**Squamous cell carcinoma** generally affects the ***upper two-thirds*** of the oesophagus and adenocarcinoma the lower one-third"-*L and B 27th/1085-86*
- "Endoscopy is the first-line investigation for most patients. **Computed tomography scanning with intravenous contrast** (contrast CT scan) is the modality most used to ***identify haematogenous metastases***"- *L and B 27th/1088,1090*
- "**Computed tomographic (CT) scanning** of the chest, abdomen and pelvis provides information on local invasion of the primary cancer, LN involvement, or disseminated disease. In summary, esophageal cancer is diagnosed
- With endoscopic biopsy and is ***staged with CT scanning of the chest and abdomen***, EUS and PET scan for all patients with CT or EUS evidence of advanced disease (T2 or greater, N1-2 or NX)"-*Schwartz 10th/1005*

Treatment of Carcinoma of the Oesophagus

◈ *L and B 27th/1092*

- Radical oesophagectomy is the most important aspect of curative treatment
- Neoadjuvant treatments before surgery may improve survival in a proportion of patients
- ***Chemoradiotherapy alone may cure selected patients, particularly those with squamous cell cancers***
- Useful palliation may be achieved by chemo/radiotherapy or endoscopic treatments

"Dysphagia as a result of esophageal cancer can be graded from Grade I, eating normally, to grade VI, unable to swallow saliva. Grades I–III often can be managed with radiation therapy, usually in combination with chemotherapy. When surgical resection is not anticipated in the future, this is termed definitive ***chemoradiation therapy*** and usually is palliative"-Schwartz *10th/1008*

"In Western countries, **esophageal reconstruction** by ***colonic interposition*** is preferred, even in the patients who are capable to undergo reconstruction with the ***gastric tube*** in order to avoid gastroesophageal reflux, which appears to be beneficial for preventing the development of Barrett's esophagus and adenocarcinoma"-*medical-clinical-reviews.imedpub.com*

"Re-establishment of **gastrointestinal continuity** is a critical determinant of quality of life following esophagectomy. Current options for esophageal replacement include the ***stomach, the right and left colon and the jejunum***"-*www.ncbi.nlm.nih.gov*

"**Barrett's oesophagus:** When intestinal metaplasia occurs, there is an increased risk of ***adenocarcinoma* of the oesophagus,** which is about 25 times that of the general population"-*L and B 27th/1082*

Some Etiologic Factors Associated with Squamous Cell Cancer of the Esophagus

◈ *Harrison 19th/532*

- Excess alcohol consumption
- Cigarette smoking
- Other ingested carcinogens
- Nitrates (converted to nitrites)
- Smoked opiates
- Fungal toxins in pickled vegetables
- Mucosal damage from physical agents
- Hot tea
- Lye ingestion
- Radiation-induced strictures
- Chronic achalasia
- Host susceptibility
- Esophageal web with glossitis and iron deficiency (i.e., Plummer-Vinson or
- Paterson-Kelly syndrome)
- Congenital hyperkeratosis and pitting of the palms and soles (i.e., tylosis
- palmaris et plantaris)
- ? Dietary deficiencies of selenium, molybdenum, zinc and vitamin A

Some Etiologic Factors Associated with Adenocarcinoma of the Esophagus

◈ *Harrison 19th/533*

- Chronic gastroesophageal reflux
- Obesity
- ***Barrett's esophagus***
- Male sex
- Cigarette smoking

179. Ans. a. Milroy disease is hereditary, b. Filariasis is most common cause world wide, d. Not much responsive to diuretics, e. Can be complicated by cellulitis

[Ref: Manipal Surgery 4th/;CSDT 14th/848-49; L and B 27th/997-1011; Schwartz 10th/ 934-36]

- "***Meige's disease** is similar to Milroy's disease, except that the lymphoedema generally develops between puberty and middle age (50 years)"-L and B 27th/1004*
- "**Filariasis**: *This is the **most common cause of lymphoedema worldwide**, affecting up to 100 million individuals. It is particularly prevalent in Africa, India and South America where 5–10 percent of the population may be affected"-L and B 27th/1003*
- ***Diuretics are of no value in pure lymphedema**-L and B 27th/1011*
- "***Diuretics can be useful for acute exacerbation of edema secondary to infection or for coexisting venous stasis disease, but these agents are not recommended for long-term use in lymphedema.*** The mainstay of treatment is external compression and meticulous skin care"-*CSDT 14th/849*
- "**Antibiotic Therapy:** *Patients with lymphedema are at **increased risk of developing cellulitis** in the affected extremity due to microscopic breakdown in the skin barrier either secondary to swelling or unrecognized and untreated tinea pedis. Recurrent infection can damage the lymphatics, aggravating the edema and increasing the risk for subsequent infection. Staphylococcus and β-hemolyticStreptococcus are the most common organisms causing soft tis-sue infection. Aggressive antibiotic therapy and elevation with compression are recommended at the earliest signs or symptoms of cellulitis"- Schwartz 10th/ 935*
- *"Congenital lymph-edema develops before 1 year of age, is usually bilateral and affects men more than women; **if familial, it is known as Milroy disease**"-CSDT 14th/848*

Table: Aetiological classification of lymphoedema *(L and B 27th/998)*

• **I-Primary lymphedema** (thought to be caused by 'congenital lymphatic dysplasia')	• **II-Secondary lymphedema** (clear underlying cause)
Congenital (onset <2 years old): sporadic; familial (***Nonne–Milroy's disease***) • Praecox (onset 2–35 years old): sporadic; familial (***Letessier–Meige's disease***) • Tarda (onset after 35 years old)	▪ Parasitic infection ***(filariasis)*** ▪ Fungal infection (tinea pedis) ▪ Exposure to foreign body material (silica particles) ▪ Primary lymphatic malignancy ▪ Metastatic spread to lymph nodes ▪ Radiotherapy to lymph nodes ▪ Surgical excision of lymph nodes ▪ Trauma (particularly degloving injuries) ▪ Superficial thrombophlebitis ▪ Deep venous thrombosis

180. Ans. b. Chronic atrophic gastritis is a predisposing factor, d. Most common variety of gastric polyp, e. Surgery is done if they are symptomatic

[Ref: Robbins 9th/770;Sabiston 19th/1206; L and B 26th/1045; Schwartz 10th/1076-77]

- ***Hyperplastic polyps are most common in individuals b/w 50 & 60 yr of age & usually develop in association with chronic gastritis. Up to 75% of all gastric polyps are inflammatory or hyperplastic polyps**- Robbins 9th/770*
- "***Hyperplastic polyps are among the most frequently observed polyps and compose 28% to 75% of all gastric polyps.*** The lesions are typically less than 1.5 cm in size and arise in a setting of chronic atrophic gastritis 40% to 75% of the time. Most commonly, the ***chronic atrophic gastritis*** is secondary to *H. pylori* infection, the treatment of which

may result in polyp regression. ***Although the hyperplastic polyp itself is non-neoplastic, dysplastic changes may occasionally develop in the polyp***. Frank adenocarcinoma is detected in 2% of hyperplastic polyps. When detected, endoscopic polypectomy is indicated for histologic examination"- *Sabiston 19th/1206*

Polyps

◈ *Chwartz 10th/1076-77*

- Benign gastric polyps are classified as neoplastic (adenoma and fundic gland polyps) or ***nonneoplastic (hyperplastic polyp***, inflammatory polyp, hamartomatous polyp).
- In general, inflammatory and hamartomatous polyps have little or no malignant potential.
- Fundic gland polyps, commonly seen in patients on long term proton pump inhibitor therapy, are not premalignant but in patients with familial adenomatous polyposis, dysplasia in these lesions is not uncommon.
- ***Hyperplastic polyps usually occur in the setting of chronic inflammation***. Large hyperplastic polyps may harbor dysplasia or carcinoma in situ and gastric cancer may develop remote from the hyperplastic polyp in an area of associated chronic inflammation.

181. Ans. b. Most of them are non-Hodgkin's lymphomas, c. May have T or B cell origin, d. May cause intestinal obstruction, e. Treatment may include surgical resection, chemotherapy & radiotherapy

[Ref: Harrison 19th/537; Manipal Surgery 4th/693;CSDT 14th/680; L and B 27th/1251; Schwartz 10th/ 1159-60]

Intestinal Lymphoma

◈ *Harrison 19th/537*

- Primary intestinal lymphoma accounts for ~20% of malignancies of the small bowel. ***These neoplasms are non-Hodgkin's lymphomas***; they usually have a diffuse, large-cell histology and are of ***T cell origin***.
- ***Intestinal lymphoma involves the ileum, jejunum and duodenum, in decreasing frequency***—a pattern that mirrors the relative amount of normal lymphoid cells in these anatomic areas.
- ***Resection of the tumor constitutes the initial treatment modality.*** While postoperative radiation therapy has been given to some patients following a total resection, most authorities favor short-term (three cycles) systemic treatment with combination chemotherapy.

"**Treatment** of small bowel *lymphoma* ***requires conservative resections*** with para-aortic and mesenteric lymph node sampling, liver biopsy and bone marrow biopsy performed for staging. ***Low-grade localized lesions are treated with resection alone,*** while for intermediate and high-grade lesions resection and chemotherapy is recommended. Radiation is used only for palliation in poor performance patients. This modality is associated with significant side effects, such as bowel necrosis, bleeding and perforation and is offered for palliation only to patients unfit for surgery or chemotherapy"- *CSDT 14th/684*

- **Intestinal lymphoma** is very rare. Lymphomas are classified as either Hodgkin or non-Hodgkin lymphoma according to its characteristics, but ***intestinal lymphoma is usually non-Hodgkin lymphoma originated in the B or T-cells***"- lymphomanewstoday.com
- "Lymphoma of Small Intestine can either be a B-cell lymphoma or a T-cell lymphoma. B-cell lymphomas are far more common than T-cell lymphomas"- www.dovemed.com
- "Lymphoma may involve the small intestine primarily or as a manifestation of disseminated systemic disease. ***Primary small-intestinal lymphomas are most commonly located in the ileum***, which contains the highest concentration of lymphoid tissue in the intestine. Although ***partial small bowel obstruction is the most common mode of presentation***, 10% of patients with small-intestinal lymphoma present with bowel perforation"-*Schwartz 10th/ 1160*

Table: Features of small-intestinal malignancies *(Schwartz 10th/ 1159)*

Tumor type	Cell of origin	Frequency	Predominant site
Adenocarcinoma	Epithelial cell	35%–50%	Duodenum
Carcinoid	Enterochromaffin cell	20%–40%	Ileum
Lymphoma	Lymphocyte	10%–15%	Ileum
GIST	?Interstitial cell of Cajal	10%–15%	—

Lymphoma

◈ *L and B 27th/1251*

- Small bowel lymphoma may be primary, or more commonly secondary to systemic lymphoma.
- ***Most western-type lymphomas are non-Hodgkin's B-cell lymphomas.***
- They present with anaemia, bleeding, perforation, anorexia and weight loss.
- T-cell lymphoma develops in patients with coeliac disease.
- Worsening of the patient's diarrhoea, with pyrexia of unknown origin together with ***local obstructive symptoms***, are the usual features
- ***The mainstay of treatment for these conditions is chemotherapy, however surgery may be required for obstruction, perforation or bleeding***

182. Ans. a. Antibiotic is given at time of induction of anesthesia, c. Preoperative skin preparation with alcohol-based solutions, e. Prevent perioperative hypothermia

[Ref: L and B 27th/52-56 ; CSDT 14th/88]

- Avoiding hair removal; ***clipping instead of shaving***, if necessary- *CSDT 14th/88*

Table: Potential measures to prevent surgical site infections. *(CSDT 14th/88)*

- Optimizing the patient's nutritional status
- Appropriate perioperative antibiotic prophylaxis (choice, dosing and timing)
- Adequate glucose level control in diabetic patients

A & E

- Maintenance of perioperative normoglycemia in all patients
- Maintenance of strict asepsis
- ***Preoperative skin preparation with alcohol-based solutions***
- Gentle skin handling and minimization of cautery-related tissue damage
- Improving ventilation and laminar air flow in the OR
- ***Maintenance of perioperative normothermia***
- ***Avoiding hair removal; clipping instead of shaving, if necessary***
- Perioperative oxygen supplementation
- ***Preoperative antibacterial soap showers***
- Antibacterial coated sutures
- Antibacterial irrigation solutions
- Operative wound barriers
- Antibacterial dressing

"Antiseptic baths (usually chlorhexidine) are popular in Europe, but there is no hard evidence for their value in reducing wound infections. ***Preoperative skin shaving*** should be undertaken in the operating theatre ***immediately before surgery*** as the SSI rate after clean wound surgery may be doubled if it is performed the night before; minor skin injury enhances superficial bacterial colonisation. Cream depilation is messy and ***hair clipping is best***, with the lowest rate of infection"- *L and B 27th/52*

Avoiding Surgical Site Infections

◈ *L and B 26th/62*

- Staff should always wash their hands between patients
- Length of patient stay should be kept to a minimum
- ***Preoperative shaving should be done immediately before surgery***
- Antiseptic skin preparation should be standardised
- Attention to theatre technique and discipline
- ***Avoid hypothermia perioperatively*** and ensure supplemental oxygenation in recovery

Prophylactic Antibiotics

◈ *L and B 27th/53*

- If antibiotics are given to prevent infection after surgery or instrumentation, they should be used when local wound defences are not established (the decisive period). Ideally, maximal blood and tissue levels should be present at the time at which the first incision is made and before contamination occurs.
- ***Intravenous administration at induction of anaesthesia is optimal.*** In long operations or when there is excessive blood loss or when unexpected contamination occurs, ***antibiotics may be repeated at 4-hourly intervals during the surgery***, as tissue antibiotic levels often fall faster than serum levels.
- There is no evidence that further doses of antibiotics after surgery are of any value in prophylaxis against infection and the practice can only encourage the development of antibiotic resistance.

Choice of Antibiotics for Prophylaxis

◈ *L and B 27th/53*

- Not required in clean surgery unless a prosthetic is implanted
- Use antibiotics that are effective against expected pathogens with local hospital guidelines
- ***Plan for single-shot intravenous administration at induction of anaesthesia***
- Repeat only during long operations or if there is excessive blood loss

183. Ans. b. Left side colon carcinoma is associated change in bowel habit, c. Left side colon carcinoma is associated with early obstruction, d. Anaemia & melena are more common in right colon cancer, e. Colonoscopy is the gold standard for establishing the diagnosis of colon cancer

[Ref: CSDT 14th/702; L and B 27th/1262; Schwartz 10th/1209;Sabiston 19th/1350-51]

- "Because of the caliber of the bowel and the consistency of the stool, **left-sided tumors** are ***more likely to cause obstruction*** than are right-sided tumors *Schwartz 10th/1209*

Colorectal Cancers

◈ *Sabiston 19th/1350-51*

- Cancers located in the **left colon** are often constrictive in nature. Patients with left-sided colon cancers may notice a ***change in bowel habit***, most often reported as ***increasing constipation***.
- Cancers in the **right colon** more often present with ***melena, fatigue associated with anemia***, or, if the tumor is advanced, abdominal pain. Although ***obstructive symptoms are more commonly associated with cancers of the left colon***, any advanced colorectal cancer can cause a change in bowel habits and intestinal obstruction
- ***Colonoscopy is the gold standard for establishing the diagnosis of colon cancer.*** It permits biopsy of the tumor to verify the diagnosis while allowing inspection of the entire colon to exclude metachronous polyps or cancers (the incidence of a synchronous cancer is about 3%). Colonoscopy is generally performed even after a cancer is detected by barium enema to obtain a biopsy and to detect (and remove) small polyps that may be missed by the contrast study

Colon Cancer

◈ *CSDT 14th/702*

- Compared with the left colon, tumors of the **right colon** may reach a more advanced stage before they cause symptoms. ***Obstruction is rare because the right colon is larger*** in diameter and has liquid stool. If these tumors bleed, melena, or more commonly occult blood, will be present in the stool. There may be associated vague abdominal pain. Ten percent of patients present with a palpable abdominal mass.
- In contrast, the **left colon and rectum** has a smaller diameter and semisolid feces. Tumors here can cause luminal narrowing and ***obstruction resulting*** in narrowing of the stool, constipation and ***increased frequency of bowel movements***.

Carcinoma of the Colon

◈ *L and B 27th/1262*

- Carcinoma of the colon typically occurs in patients over 50 years of age and is most common in the eighth decade of life.

- Twenty per cent of cases present as an emergency with intestinal obstruction or peritonitis.
- Those with first-degree relatives who have developed colorectal cancer at the age of 45 years or below are at higher risk and may be part of one of the colorectal cancer familial syndromes.
- Tumours of the **left side** of the colon which are far more common usually present with a **change in bowel habit or rectal bleeding**, while **more proximal lesions** typically present later with ***iron deficiency anaemia or a mass.***

OBSTETRICS AND GYNECOLOGY

184. Ans. b. Seizure can be prevented by maintaining 4-7 meq/ Lconcentration, c. In $MgSO_4$ toxicity calcium gluconate is given, e. MgSO4 can be given by continuous infusion or intermittent i.m injection

[Ref: DuttaObs 9th/ 221-22,625; William's Obs 23rd/737-38; Obs by JB Sharma 1st/437-39]

- ***The initial standard dose of magnesium sulfate can be safely administered without knowledge of renal function***

Magnesium Sulphate

◈ *DuttaObs 9th/ 221-22,625; J B Sharma 1st/437-39*

- Magnesium sulphate is drug of choice as ***anticonvulsant in eclampsia***
- It ***does not control hypertension***
- The ***therapeutic level of serum magnesium is 4-7 mEq/L***
- ***Various regimens: Pritchard (IV+IM), Sibai (IV), Zuspan(IV) and Dhaka regimen (IV+IM).***
- ***In India, most hospital use Pritchard regimen (magnesiumsulphate 4 g is given IV slowly over 3-4 min immediately followed by 5 g in each buttock IM) as it is safer***
- Serum magnesium level may be monitored in selected cases (***renal insufficiency***, absent deep tendon reflex)
- Magnesium toxicity and serum magnesium level is seen in (a) loss of deep tendon reflex > 7 mEq/L (b) respiratory depression more than 10 mEq/L and (c) cardiac arrest more than 25 mEq/L
- For magnesium toxicity: Inj calcium gluconate 10 mL(10% solution), IV slowly

Magnesium Sulfate to Control Convulsions

◈ *William's Obs 23rd/737-38*

- In more severe cases of preeclampsia, as well as eclampsia, magnesium sulfate administered parenterally is an **effective anticonvulsant agent**
- It may be given ***intravenously by continuous infusion or intramuscularly by intermittent injection***
- The dosage schedule for severe preeclampsia is the same as for eclampsia.
- **Magnesium sulfate is not given to treat hypertension.**
- **Because magnesium is cleared almost exclusively by renal excretion, plasma magnesium concentration, using the doses described previously, is excessive if glomerular filtration is decreased substantively.**
- ***The initial standard dose of magnesium sulfate can be safely administered without knowledge of renal function.*** Renal function is thereafter estimated by measuring plasma creatinine and whenever it is 1.3 mg/dL or higher, only half of the maintenance intramuscular magnesium sulfate dose is given.
- When magnesium sulfate is being given intravenously by continuous infusion, serum magnesium levels are used to adjust the infusion rate. **With either method, when there is renal insufficiency, plasma magnesium levels must be checked periodically.**
- **Treatment with calcium gluconate, 1 g intravenously, along with withholding further magnesium sulfate usually reverses mild to moderate respiratory depression**
- Magnesium sulfate is discontinued 24 hr after delivery
- Measure serum magnesium level at 4–6 hr and adjust infusion to maintain levels between 4–7 mEq/L (4.8–8.4 m/ dL).

185. Ans. a. Severe pulmonary hypertension, b. Severe aortic stenosis, d. Marfan's syndrome with dilated aortic root

[Ref: DuttaObs 9th/ 257-261; William's Obs 23rd/962-78; Obs by JB Sharma 1st/498-500; Normal and Problem Pregnancy by Gabbe 6th/832-41]

- ***In Atrial septal defect(ASD), pregnancy is well tolerated***

Absolute Contraindications of Pregnancy (Indications of MTP) in Heart Disease

◈ *Obs by JB Sharma 1st/499*

- Eisenmenger's syndrome
- ***Primary pulmonary hypertension***
- Single ventricle
- Pulmonary veno-occlusive disease
- ***Marfan's syndrome with dilated aortic root*** (> 4cm on echocardiography)
- Dilated cardiomyopathy (Peripartum cardiomyopathy) with residual left ventricular function impairment.
- Bicuspid aortic valve with aortic root > 5 cm.

Relative Contraindications of Pregnancy (Relative Indications for MTP) in Heart Disease

◈ *Obs by JB Sharma 1st/499*

- Severe obstructive lesion. Left ventricular ejection fraction < 30%.
- Parous woman with grade III or IV lesion
- Past history of cardiac failure with heart disease MTP should be done using suction and evacuation before 12 weeks of pregnancy (preferably before 8 weeks).

Clinically significant **aortic stenosis** is uncommonly encountered during pregnancy. Although mild to moderate degrees of stenosis are well tolerated, ***severe disease is life threatening.*** The principal underlying hemodynamic **problem** is the fixed cardiac output associated with severe stenosis. During pregnancy, a number of factors commonly decrease preload further and thus aggravate the fixed cardiac output. Because of these considerations, ***severe aortic stenosis may be extremely dangerous during pregnancy"***- *William's Obs 23rd/967*

"Aortic insufficiency is ***generally well tolerated during pregnancy***. Symptoms necessitate therapy for heart failure, including bed rest, sodium restriction and diuretics"- *William's Obs 23rd/967*

- **"Atrial Septal Defects**: ***Most are asymptomatic*** until the third or fourth decade. Pregnancy is well tolerated unless pulmonary hypertension has developed, but this is rare because pulmonary artery pressures are usually low"- *William's Obs 23rd/968*
- "Although ***pregnancy is contraindicated with severe disease***, milder degrees of **secondary pulmonary hypertension** probably go unnoticed"- *William's Obs 23rd/971*
- *"Women with* **pulmonary hypertension** *& right ventriculay dysfunction should be strongly discouraged from being pregnant"- Gabbe 6th/844*
- **"Marfan Syndrome:** Progressive aortic dilatation causes aortic valve insufficiency and there may be infective endocarditis and mitral valve prolapse with insufficiency. ***Aortic dilatation and dissecting aneurysm are the most serious abnormalities, aortic dilatation of more than 40 mm or mitral valve dysfunction are high-risk factors for life-threatening cardiovascular complications during pregnancy***. Conversely, women with minimal or no dilatation and those with normal cardiac function by echocardiography, are counseled regarding the small but serious potential risk of aortic dissection. Elkayam and colleagues (1995) also concluded that *pregnancy was safer in women* with Marfan syndrome who had no cardiovascular manifestations or ***aortic arch dilatation***"- *William's Obs 23rd/977*

Table: : Risks for Maternal Mortality Caused by Various Types of Heart Disease (*William's Obs 22nd*)

Cardiac Disorder	Mortality
Group 1—Minimal Risk	0–1%
Atrial septal defect	
Ventricular septal defect	
Patent ductus arteriosus	
Pulmonic or tricuspid disease	
Fallot tetralogy, corrected	
Mitral stenosis, NYHA class I and II	
Group 2—Moderate Risk	5–15%
2A:	
Mitral stenosis, NYHA class III and IV	
Aortic stenosis	
Aortic coarctation without valvular involvement	
Fallot tetralogy, uncorrected	
Previous myocardial infarction	
Marfan syndrome, normal aorta	
2B:	
Mitral stenosis with atrial fibrillation	
Artificial valve	
Group 3--Major Risk	25–50%
Pulmonary hypertension	
Aortic coarctation with valvular involvement	
Marfan syndrome with aortic involvement	

186. Ans. a. Gestational sac diameter at 5-7 week, b. Crown rump length (CRL) at 7-10 week, e. BPD at 18-20 week

[Ref: DuttaObs 9th/ 67; William's Obs 23rd/350-52; Obs by JB Sharma 1st/70; Normal and Problem Pregnancy by Gabbe 6th/184]

Estimation of Gestational Age: USG Findings

◈ *DuttaObs 9th/ 67*

- ***Gestational sac- at 5 weeks***
- ***Measurement of crown rump length (CRL) detected at 7 weeks,*** *aprrox. 10mm; at* ***10 weeks-34 mm****(CRL in cm + 6.5= week of pregnancy)*
- ***First trimester- CRL is most accurate***
- *Second trimester by* ***BPD****, HC, AC & FL measurement. Most accurate when done* ***b/w 12 & 20*** *weeks(variation ± 8 days)*
- *Third trimester-less reliable, variation ±16 days*

"B/w 14-26 week a combination of BPD or HC & FL is used"*- Obs by JB Sharma 1st/70*

Determining Gestational Age

◈ *William's Obs 23rd/352*

- ***For determining gestational age in the first trimester, the crown-rump length is most accurate***(variation of only 3 to 5 days)
- ***Between 14 and 26 weeks, the biparietal diameter (BPD) is usually the most accurate parameter***, with a variation of 7 to 10 days.
- The head circumference (HC) also is measured. If the head shape is flattened (*dolichocephaly*) or rounded (*brachycephaly*), this measurement is more reliable than the BPD.
- The femur length (FL) correlates well with both BPD and gestational age(variation of 7 to 11 days in the second trimester.)
- The abdominal circumference (AC) is the parameter with the widest variation of 2 to 3 weeks.
- By the third trimester, all individual measurements become less accurate. Estimates are improved by taking an average of the various parameters—the BPD, HC, AC and FL.

187. Ans. a. 50% cases of carcinoma cervix is associated with HPV-16, b. High-risk subtypes of HPV are 16 & 18, c. CIN-I is kept under observation with PAP smear or HPV DNA test, e. Route of infection is usually through cervical columnar epithelium

[Ref: Shaw's Gynae 16th/485-86; Dutta Gynae 7th/262-66, 280-86; Novak's Gynae 15th/574-80; Harrison 19th/1197-98]

- ***CIN-I persists in 10-20% cases and progress in 1-4% cases***
- "There are 14 high-risk HPV subtype: **two of high-risk subtypes, 16 & 18,** are fund in 62% of cervical carcinoma"- Novak 15th/1305
- "HPV is **epitheliotropic.** ***Cervical epithelium*** → Infection (latent/active with virus replication) → Oncogenic-

Contd...

HPV-DNA integration to human genome → Neoplastic transformation" -*DuttaGynae* 7th/265

- "**CIN I:** *Women with CIN I, confirmed on biopsy, is* ***kept under observation with pap smear follow up at 6 months or HPV DNA tests*** *at 12 months. If both tests are negative routine recall (screening) is done*" (*DuttaGynae. 6th/326; Shaw's 16th/491*)

Cervical Intraepithelial Neoplasia (CIN)

◈ *Novak's Gynae 15th/574-80*

- CIN most often arises in an area of metaplasia in the transformation zone at the advancing squamocolumnarjunction (SCJ). Metaplasia advances from the original SCJ inward, toward the external os and over the columnar villi, to establish the transformation zone.
- The ***spontaneous regression rate of biopsy-proven CIN 1 is 60% to 85% in prospective studies***. The ***regressions typically occur within a 2-year follow-up*** with cytology and colposcopy.
- The cervix is composed of columnar epithelium, which lines the endocervical canal and squamous epithelium, which covers the exocervix. The point at which they meet is called the squamocolumnar junction (SCJ)
- **Type 16** is the most common HPV found in invasive cancer and in CIN 2 and CIN 3 and it is ***found in 47% of women*** with cancer in all stages. It is the most common HPV type found in women with normal cytology.
- HPV-18 is more specific than HPV-16 for invasive tumors.

"The causative virus appear to be transmitted to susceptible women during intercourse"- *DuttaGynae* 7th/265

Table: *Shaw's Gynae 16th/486*

	Regression	Persistence	Progresses	Age
CIN I	80–90%	10–20%	1–4%	<30 years
CIN II	30–40%	40%	20%	30–35 years
CIN III	20–30%	50–60%	Almost all	35–45 years

HPV

◈ *Harrison 19th/1197-98*

- More than 125 HPV types have been identified and are numerically designated according to a unique L1 gene sequence.
- The International Agency for Research on Cancer concludes that HPV types 16, 18, 31, 33, 35, 39, 45, 51, 52, 56, 58 and 59 are carcinogenic in the uterine cervix.
- ***HPV-16 is particularly virulent and causes 50% of cervical cancers.***
- ***Worldwide, HPV-16 and HPV-18 cause 70% of cervical squamous cell carcinomas and 85% of cervical adenocarcinomas.*** Oncogenic types other than HPV-16 and HPV-18 cause the remaining 30% of cervical cancers.
- HPV-16 and HPV-18 also cause nearly 90% of anal cancers worldwide
- In addition to cervical and anal cancer, other HPV-associated cancers include vulvar and vaginal cancer, which are associated with HPV in 50–70% of cases; penile cancer, which is caused by HPV in 50% of cases; and oropharyngeal squamous cell carcinoma (OPSCC)

188. Ans. a. Turner's syndrome, b. Kallmann syndrome, c. Meyer-Rokistansky Kauster Hauser (MRKH) syndrome, e. PCOD

[*Ref: Shaw's Gynae 16th/322-23, 326-27; Dutta Gynae 7th/371-72,377*]

- **Sheehan's syndrome** *causes* ***secondary amenorrhoea****-Shaw's Gynae 16th/326-27*
- **PCOD** causes both ***primary & secondary amenorrhoea****-Shaw's Gynae 16th/322, 326*

Primary Amenorrhoea

◈ *Shaw's Gynae 16th/322*

- The spectrum of diagnosis presenting clinically as primary amenorrhoea can be conventionally **classified** according to the status of her serum FSH levels into ***hypergonadotropic (FSH>40 mIU/mL), eugonadotropic or hypogonadotropic***
- "**Kallmann's syndrome**-*inadequate GnRH pulse secretion* ***reduced FSH & LH***" (*DuttaGynae 6th/450-54*)

Table: Classification of primary amenorrhea as per serum FSH level

Hypergonadotropic primary Amenorrhoea(Show's)	Eugonadotropic primary amenorrhoea (Show's)
• Gonadal dysgenesis: 45 OX (Turner's syndrome mosaics, abnormal X.)	**A. Absence of Mullerian development**
• 46 XX pure gonadal dysgenesis	• Androgen insensitivity syndrome (testicular feminization)
• 46 XY gonadal dysgenesis–Swyer syndrome, testicular feminizing syndrome	• Mullerian agenesis– absence of uterus/vagina. Rokitansky-kuster-hauser syndrome
• Gonadotropin-resistant ovary syndrome-Savage syndrome	**B. Norma mullerian development**
	• Female or true intersex
	• Polycystic ovary syndrome
	• Adrenal or thyroid diseases
	C. Cryptomenorrhoea-imperforate hymen, vaginal septum cervical atresia.
	D. Tubercularendometritis
	E. Constitutional delay-nutrition

Hypogonadotropic Primary Amenorrhoea (Shaw's)
A. Hypothalamic causes:
• Delayed menarche and puberty
• Hypothalamic hypogonadism (***Kallmann syndrome***). GnRh deficiency syndrome
• Psychogenic causes, weight loss. Stress anorexia nervosa and malnutrition

Contd...

Hypogonadotropic Primary Amenorrhoea (Shaw's)

B. Pituitary causes:

- Pituitarism causes short stature, obesity genital dystrophy, mental retardation, polydactyly and retinitis pigmentosa.
- Neoplasma-prolactinomas, craniopharyngiomas, adenomas and empty sellaturcica
- Hypopituitary states-Simmond's disease, Chiari-frommel syndrome, Forbes-Albright syndrome and pineal gland tumour

C. Severe systemic disease like tuberculosis, syphilis.

D. Other endocrinal disorders-thyroid or adrenal gland.

189. Ans. b. Calcium, e. Raloxifene

[Ref: Shaw's Gynae 16th/67-71; DuttaGynae 7th/48-52; Novak's Gynae 15th/ 1235-38]

"raloxifene does not improve hot flush or urogenital atrophy" *-DuttaGynae 7th/50*

"Vitamin d3 & calcium reduces osteoporosis & fracture" *-DuttaGynae 7th/49*

Raloxifene side effect-hot flush" *-Shaw's Gynae 16th/73*

"Tibolone: relieves vasomotor symptoms(hot flush)"*-Shaw's Gynae 16th/73*

"Benefit of hormone replacement therapy: improvement of vasomotor symptoms" *-DuttaGynae 7th/50; Shaw's Gynae 16th/71*

"Vitamin e reduces hot flush"*-DuttaGynae 7th/50*

Options for Treatment of Vasomotor Symptoms

Novak's Gynae 15th/1238

Hormone Therapy

- Estrogen therapy
- Progestin therapy$
- Combination estrogen/progestin therapy

Nonhormonal Prescription Medications

- Clonidine
- Selective serotonin and norepinephrine reuptake inhibitors: Paroxetine & Venlafaxine
- Gabapentin

Nonprescription Medications

- ***Isoflavone supplements***
- Soy products
- Black cohosh
- ***Vitamin E***

Lifestyle Changes

- Reducing body temperature
- Maintaining a healthy weight
- Smoking cessation
- Relaxation response techniques
- Acupuncture
- *$-Not US FDA –approved for vasomotor symptoms*

190. Ans. a. Suprapubic pressure, b. McRoberts Manoeuvre, c. Wood corkscrew method

[Ref: Dutta Obs 9th/381; William's Obs 23rd/962-63; Obs by JB Sharma 1st/317-18]

- ***Pinnard maneuver & lovset's maneuver are used for management of complicated breech***

"Management of complicated breech: *Pinnard maneuver & lovset's maneuver*" *- DuttaObs 9th/361-62*

Management of Shoulder Dystocia

JB Sharma 1st/317-18; DuttaObs 9th/ 381

I. First Line Maneuvers

- Large episiotomy
- Avoid fundal pressure
- ***McRoberts maneuver & Suprapubic pressure***

II. Second Line Maneuvers

- *Delivery of posterior shoulder*
- ***Wood's corkscrew manoeuvre***
- *Rubin's maneuver*
- *Gaskin position*

III. Third Line Maneuvers

- *Cleidotomy*
- Zanelli manoever
- Symphysiotomy

191. Ans. a. Nuchal translucency is seen at 11-14 weeks, c. AFP is tested in Down syndrome, d. Fetal cell DNA from maternal blood is used

[Ref: Dutta Obs 9th/ 102-07; William's Obs 23rd/292-302; Obs by JB Sharma 1st/153-56]

Quadruple (Quad) Screening: Done at **15-20 week**- DuttaObs 9th/104 (table)

Cell-free Fetal DNA *is tested for trisomy & single gene disorders after 10 weeks- DuttaObs 9th/ 104 (table)*

Anomaly Scan (Ultrasound Level II)/Mid-pregnancy or 20-Week Scan/Morphology Scan

www.pregnancybirthbaby.org.au

- The only reason this mid-pregnancy scan is sometimes called an anomaly scan, is because the sonographer will be looking for any ***fetal abnormalities*** at this time
- During the scan sonographer examines each part of the fetal body, determine the position of the placenta, assess the amount of amniotic fluid and measure fetal growth. Special attention is paid to the brain, face, spine, heart, stomach, bowel, kidneys and limbs.

First Trimester Screening

J B Sharma 1st/155; DuttaObs 8th/128

- It uses *PAPP-A* ***(lower in Down syndrome) and free β-hCG(higher in Down's syndrome)*** b/w 11 and 14 weeks
- It can detects 62% Down's syndrome pregnancies with a 5%false-positive rate

Second Trimester Screening

J B Sharma 1st/155

- Double test (MSAFP is lower while total hCG or free β-hCGis raised in Down's syndrome

- Triple test- MSAFP, hCG and uE3 (unconjugated estriol)
- Quadruple test- MSAFP, hCG, uE3 and inhibin-A
- Penta screen- AFP, hCG, uE3, diametric inhibin-A and hyperglycosylated hCG

Screening for Down's Syndrome

◈ *(Davidson 22nd/63)*

- Antenatal screening in the first and second trimesters identifies fetuses at risk of Down's syndrome. Tests which currently have sensitivity > 60% and specificity > 95% include:
- *First trimester* (***11–14 weeks***): ***nuchal translucency***; or nuchal translucency, human chorionic gonadotrophin (hCG) and pregnancy-associated plasma protein-A (PAPP-A)
- *Second trimester* (13–20 weeks): triple test (hCG, α-fetoprotein, unconjugated oestriol, uE3)
- Other combinations are available for use from 11 to 20 weeks.

Box : Procedures for early detection of fetal: (i) Genetic, (II) Chromosomal and (III) structural abnormalities *(DuttaObs 9th/ 103)*

- Triple test (combined test): MSAFP, unconjugated estriol (uE3) and hCG
- Quadruple test: (MSAFP, uE3, hCG, inhibin A)
- Integrated test: NT, PAPP-A + hCG
- ***Cell-free fetal DNA from maternal plasma/blood***
- Maternal serum alpha fetoprotein (MSAFP)
- Chorionic villus biopsy
- Cordocentesis
- Amniocentesis
- ***Fetal cell isolation from maternal blood***–(from isolated fetal nucleated red blood cells or trophoblast cells)
- High resolution ultrasonography (for (nuchal thickening, nasal bone)
- Peri-implantation genetic diagnosis
- 3D or 4D ultrasound with increased resolution
- Fetoscopy

192. Ans. a. LNG- IUD insertion, b. Medroxyprogesterone acetate for 3 cycles, d. Medroxyprogesterone acetate for 3 months

[Ref: Shaw's Gynae 16th/343-44; DuttaGynae 7th/157-58;Novak 15th/409]

Endometrial Hyperplasia

◈ *Shaw's Gynae 16th/347, innovativegyn.com*

- *Endometrial hyperplasia* typically causes ***abnormal uterine bleeding*** and most commonly occurs in post-menopausal women. Long-term unopposed estrogen production causes overgrowth of the uterine lining and results in endometrial hyperplasia.
- **Simple without atypia**: One percent risk of uterine cancer
- ***Progesterone therapy can be used to treat endometrial hyperplasia without atypia.*** Oral progesterone, Depo Provera (injection) or IUD (***Intrauterine device***) are all possible treatment options
- **LNG-IUS** *is recommended as a first line therapy for a women with heavy menstrual bleeding, in the absence of any structural or histological abnormality"- Dutta Gynae 7th/158*

Medical Management of DUB

◈ *DuttaGynae 7th/157*

- While isolated progestins therapy is highly effective in anovular DUB, in ovular DUB combined preparations of progestogen and estrogen (combined oral pills) are effective.
- **The preparations are used:**
  - Cyclic therapy
  - Continuous therapy
- To stop bleeding and regulate the cycle: Norethisterone preparations (5 mg tab) are used thrice daily till bleeding stops, which it usually does by 3–7 days.
- Cyclic therapy
  - 5th–25th day course
  - 15th–25th day course.
- **5th to 25th day course:**
  - In ovular bleeding: Any low dose combined oral pills are effective when given from 5th to 25th day of cycle for ***3 consecutive cycles.*** It causes endometrial atrophy. It is more effective compared to progesterone therapy as it suppress the hypothalamo-pituitary axis more effectively. Normal menstruation is expected to resume with restoration of normally functioning pituitary-ovarian-endometrial axis. It reduces menstrual blood loss by 50%. It serves as a contraceptive as well.
  - In **anovular bleeding**: Cyclic progestogen preparation of medroxyprogesterone acetate (MPA) 10 mg or norethisterone 5 mg is used from 5th to 25th day of cycle ***for 3 cycles.***
- 15th-25th day course: less effective than 5th-25th day course
- *Continuous progestin*: **Medroxyprogesterone acetate** *10 mg thrice daily is given & treatment is usually continued for at* ***least 90 days****- DuttaGynae 7th/158*

Table: Medical management of DUB *(DuttaGynae 7th/157)*

A. Prostaglandin synthetase inhibitors (PSI): Fenamates (Mefenamic acid)

B. Antifibrinolytic agents: Tranexamic acid (TA)

C. Hormones

- Norelhindone acetate
- Medroxyprogesterone acetate
- Progestin releasing IUCD: LNG–IUS
- Dydrogesterone
- Equine conjugated estrogen
- Combined estrogen and progestogen (contraceptive pills)
- 19 Norsteroid derivative (gestrinone)
- Danazol (17 a-ethinyl testosterone)
- Mifepristone (RU 486)
- GnRH analogs
- Desmopressin

193. Ans. a. Normal morphology >4%, c. Volume>1.5 ml, e. Sperm count 1.5 million/mL

[Ref: Shaw's Gynae 16th/243; DuttaGynae 7th/ 190]

In 1980, the WHO recruited a team of physicians and scientists to publish a manual describing in detail what the **normal semen parameters** of a fertile man should be and how to analyse semen in the laboratory. Since then, they have updated the manual four times, with the ***latest being in 2010***

Semen analysis (WHO-2010)(*DuttaGynae 7th/190; Shaw's Gynae 16th/243***)**

Semen analysis	Normal reference value	Lower reference limit
Volume	2.0 mL or more	1.5 mL
pH	7.2–7.8	
Viscosity	< 3 (scale 0–4)	
Sperm concentration	20 million/mL	15 million/mL
Total sperm count	> 40 million/ejaculate	39 million/ejaculate
Motility	> 50% progressive forward motility	Progressive motility = 32%
Morphology	> 14% normal form	4%
Viability	75% or more living	58%
Leukocytes	Less than 1 million/ mL	
Round cells	< 5 million/mL	
Sperm agglutination	< 10% spermatozoa with adherent particles	

Table: Lower reference limits (5th centiles and their 95% confidence intervals) for semen characteristics *(apps.who.int)*

Parameter	Lower reference limit
Semen volume (ml)	1.5 (1.4–1.7)
Total sperm number (106 per ejaculate)	39 (33–46)
Sperm concentration (106 per ml)	15 (12–16)
Total motility (PR+NP, %)	40 (38–42)
Progressive motility (PR, %)	32 (32–34)
Vitality (live spermatozoa, %)	58 (55–63)
Sperm morphology (normal forms, %)	4 (3.0–4.0)
Other consensus threshold values	
pH	≥7.2
Peroxidase-positive leukocytes (106 per ml)	<1.0
Mar test (motile spermatozoa with bound particles, %)	<50
Immunobead test (motile spermatozoa with bound beads, %)	<50
Seminal zinc (mmol/ejaculate)	≥2.4
Seminal fructose (mmol/ejaculate)	≥13
Seminal neutral glucosidase (mU/ejaculate)	≥20

194. Ans. a. More in those who are exposed to chorionic villi for first time, b. More in those who exposed to excess chorionic villi like twins, c. Genetic predisposition, d. Family history of hypertension

[Ref: DuttaObs 9th/208-09; William's Obs 23rd/962-63; Obs by JB Sharma 1st/422-24]

- ***Smoking reduces risk of pre-eclampsia****-Obs by JB Sharma 1st/424*

Abnormal Trophoblastic Invasion and Placental Ischemia Theory

◈ *Obs by JB Sharma 1st/422-23*

- According to abnormal trophoblastic invasion and placental ischemia theory, pre-eclampsia is a ***two-stage placental disease.***
- In the **first stage**, there is incomplete ***trophoblastic invasion*** of spiral arteries with failure of secondary wave and deficient blood supply to the placenta.
- The **second stage** includes the effects for ***placental ischemia*** on both the mother and the fetus.
- There is also increased micro deportation of syncytiontrophoblast microvillous membrane particles and glycogen accumulation in syncytiontrophoblasts in patients with pre-eclampsia.
- **"Genetic imprinting:** Pre-eclampsia and eclampsia may develop based on a single recessive gene or a dominant gene which explains its higher prevalence in daughters of pre-eclamptic women than their daughters-in-law"-*Obs by JB Sharma 1st/422-23*

Table: Causes of pre-eclampsia -*(DuttaObs 9th/208)*

Risk factors for pre-eclampsia	Etiopathological factors for pre-eclampsia
• Primigravida: Young or elderly (first time exposure to chorionic villi)	• Failure of trophoblast invasion (abnormal placentation)
• Family history: Hypertension, pre-eclampsia	• Vascular endothelial damage
• Placental abnormalities: ▪ Hyperplacentosis: ***Excessive exposure to chorionic villi***—(molar pregnancy, ***twins,*** diabetes) ▪ Placental ischemia	• Inflammatory mediators (cytokines)
• **Obesity**: BMI > 35 kg/m2, insulin resistance	• Immunological intolerance between maternal and fetal tissues: Coagulation abnormalities

Contd...

Risk factors for pre-eclampsia	Etiopathological factors for pre-eclampsia
• **Pre-existing vascular disease**	• Increased oxygen-free radicals
• **New paternity, pregnancy following ART**	• Imbalance of angiogenic and antiangiogenic proteins
• **Thrombophilias** [antiphospholipid syndrome, protein C, S deficiency, factor V Leiden	• ***Genetic predisposition*** (polygenic disorder)
	• Dietary deficiency or excess

195. Ans. a. **Previous classical C.S is contraindication**

[Ref: DuttaObs 9th/309-10; William's Obs 23rd/962-63; Obs by JB Sharma 1st/595; Normal and Problem Pregnancy by Gabbe 6th/462]

"Contraindication for TOLAC (Indication for Cesarean delivery): Previous classical or inverted T-shaped uterine incision, ***previous two or more lower segment CS***"- *DuttaObs 9th/310*

- VBAC- ***Risk of uterine rupture (1%)***- *Obs by JB Sharma 1st/595*
- "Although the risk of **uterine rupture** was higher among women undergoing a trial of labor, the absolute risk was small—***only 7 per 1000***. Not surprisingly, rates of stillbirth and hypoxic ischemic encephalopathy were significantly greater in the trial of labor arm"-*William's Obs 23rd/962*
- "**Oxytocin** for augmentation of labour may be used selectively & judiciously. Augmentation of labour ***increases the risk of uterine scar rupture*** & the risk of C.S"- *DuttaObs 9th/309*

What is a Trial of Labor After Caesarean Delivery (TOLAC)

◈ *www.mayoclinic.org*

- A TOLAC is the attempt to have a VBAC. If it is successful, TOLAC results in a vaginal birth. If it is not successful, there is need of another caesarean delivery
- In fact, research on women who attempt a trial of labor after cesarean (TOLAC) shows that about 60 to 80 percent have a successful vaginal delivery
- "**VBAC**: The baby is less likely to have respiratory (breathing) problems following the birth, so it less likely that you and your baby will be separated. 6 in 100 (***6%)*** babies have respiratory problems after a caesarean birth, compared to 3 in 100 (3%) following a vaginal birth"- www.cyh.com
- "VBAC-2(Vaginal birth after two caesarean sections) success rate was 71.1%, uterine rupture rate 1.36%, hysterectomy rate 0.55%, blood transfusion 2.01%, neonatal unit admission rate 7.78% and ***perinatal asphyxial injury/ death 0.09%***"-*www.ncbi.nlm.nih.gov*

Benefits and Risks of Planning a VBAC Compared to Planning an Elective Repeat

◈ *Cesareanwww.vbac.com/201*

- Mothers who have a ***VBAC will avoid the risk of hysterectomy,*** bowel or bladder injury, blood transfusion, infection and ***placental complications such as placenta previa*** and ***accreta***.
- Induction or **augmentation of labor** remains an option for women who want to labor after a prior cesarean, but the ***risk of uterine rupture is higher.***
- The ***risk of uterine rupture with a low-transverse uterine incision is 05-0.9% with one prior cesarean***. The risk is similar for women with one low vertical uterine scar. ACOG states that the risk of rupture reported in the literature is between ***.09% to 3.7% with more than one prior cesarean.***
- "While there are risks to TOLAC, most are related to complications, such as hemorrhage, that may arise from cesarean section in the setting of an unsuccessful trial of labor. However, TOLAC is still offered to patients as an option due to the significant risks associated with **multiple repeat cesarean deliveries**. Risks of ***placenta accreta***, cystotomy, bowel injury, ureteral injury and ileus, the need for postoperative ventilation, intensive care unit admission, hysterectomy and blood transfusion requiring 4 or more units and the duration of operative time and hospital stay significantly increase with increasing number of cesarean deliveries. In the NICHD MFMU study (Obstetrics and Gynecology 2006), ***Placenta accreta was present in 0.24%*** (1st cesarean sections [CS]) 0.31% (2nd CS), 0.57% (3rd CS), 2.13% (4th CS), 2.33% (5th CS), 6.74% (6 or more CS). Hysterectomy was required in 0.65% (1st CS) 0.42% (2nd CS) (0.90% (3rd CS) 2.41% (4th CS) 3.49% (5th CS) and 8.99% (6 or more CS). In 723 women who had previa in this study, risk for placenta accreta was 3% (1st CS), 11% (2nd CS), 40% (3rd CS) 61% (4th CS) and 67% (5 or more CS)"- *www.obgproject.com*

Table: Benefits and the risks of TOLAC *(DuttaObs 9th/310)*

Benefits of VBAC	Risks of elective repeat cesarean delivery	Complications of unsuccessful TOLAC
• Decreased maternal morbidity (infection and others) • Reduced length of hospital stay • Decreased need for blood transfusion • Decreased risk of abnormal placentation and need for successive cesarean delivery in next pregnancy	• Increased maternal morbidity • Increased length of hospital stay • Increased risk of hemorrhage and need for blood transfusion • Increased risk of abnormal placentation, hemorrhage and successive cesarean delivery in the next pregnancy	**Maternal** • Uterine wound dehiscence • *Uterine rupture (0.5–1%)* • Increased blood transfusion • Increased risks of hysterectomy due to uterine rupture • Infections, increased maternal morbidity **Perinatal:** Low Apgar score, admission to NICU, hypoxic ischemic encephalopathy (HIE), neonatal death, rarely stillbirth

Contd...

Risk for uterine rupture with trial of labor after cesarean (*Gabbe 6th/462*)	
Prior incision type	**Rupture rate (%)**
Low transverse	0.5–1.0
Low-vertical	0.8–1.1
Classical	4–9

Perinatal outcomes after uterine rupture term pregnancies (*Gabbe 6th/463*)	
Outcome	**Term pregnancies with uterine rupture (N = 114)**
Intrapartum stillbirth	0
Hypoxic-ischemic encephalopathy	7 (6.2)
Neonatal death	2 (1.8)
Admission to the neonatal intensive care unit	46 (40.4)
5-minute Apgar score <5	16 (14.0)
Umbilical artery blood pH <7.0	23 (33.3)

Table: Complication of TOLAC in woman with a previous CS (*William's Obs 23rd/566*)

Complication	**Trial of Labor group n = 17, 898 No. (%)**	**Elective Repeat Cesarean Group n = 15,801 No. (%)**
Uterine rupture	124 (0.7)	0
Uterine dehiscence	119 (0.7)	76 (0.5)
Hysterectomy	41 (0.2)	47 (0.3)
Thromboembolic disease	7 (0.04)	10 (0.1)
Transfusion	304 (1.7)	158 (1.0)
Uterine infection	517 (2.9)	285 (1.8)
Maternal death	3 (0.02)	7 (0.04)
Antepartum stillbirth[a]		
37-38 weeks	18 (0.4)	8 (0.1)
≥ 39 weeks	16 (0.2)	5 (0.1)
Intrapartum stillbirth[a]	2	0
Term HIE[a]	12 (0.08)	0
Term neonatal death[a]	13 (0.08)	7 (0.05)

Table: Types of Prior Uterine Incisions and Estimated Risks for Uterine Rupture (*William's Obs 23rd/569, 24th*)

Prior incision	**Estimated Rupture Rate (%)**
Classical	2–9
T-shaped	4–9
Low-vertical	1–7
One low-transverse	0.2–0.9
Multiple low-transverse	0.9–1.8
Prior preterm cesarean delivery	"increased"
Prior uterine rupture	
Lower segment	2–6
Upper uterus	9–32

196. Ans. None

[Ref: Shaw's Gynae 16th/391-400; DuttaGynae 7th/221-28]

- *Myomas are known to* ***increase in size during pregnancy &*** *with oral contraceptives & shrink after delivery- Shaw's Gynae 16th/392;DuttaGynae 7th/222*
- ***Sarcomatous change not more than 0.5%****- Shaw's Gynae 16th/395; less than 0.1%- DuttaGynae 7th/224*
- **Broad ligament fibroid** *can cause* ***hydroureter & hydronephrosis*** *which is reversible following surgery- Shaw's Gynae 16th/397*
- *Subserous,* **broad ligament** *or cervical fibroids are* ***usually unassociated*** *with* ***menstrual abnormalities****- DuttaGynae 7th/225*
- ***Calcareous degenerations usually occur in postmenopausal women****/old patient with long lasting myoma- DuttaGynae 7th/224; Shaw's Gynae 16th/395*

- **Pressure symptoms are rare in body fibroids.** The **fibroids in the posterior wall** may be impacted in the pelvis producing constipation, dysuria or even retention of urine. A **broad ligament fibroid** may produce ureteric compression → hydroureteric and hydronephrotic changes → infection → pyelitis" *-DuttaGynae 7th/225*

197. Ans. b. Lactate dehydrogenase (LDH), c. Placental alkaline phosphatise (PLAP), e. β-hCG

[Ref: Shaw's Gynae 16th/441; DuttaGynae 7th/ 314; Novak's Gynae 15th/1394,1397]

- "**Dysgerminomas:** The tumour is neutral & does not secrete either male or female sex hormones but ***placental alkaline phosphatise (PLAP), lactate dehydrogenase (LDH) & β-hCG****- Shaw's Gynae 16th/441*
- "In **dysgerminomas**, diagnosis is usually confirmed by positive immunohistochemical staining for ***LDH, CA-125, β-hCG, PALP, NSE, cytokeratin 18 and S-100 protein***"- *www.cancerjournal.net*
- **"Germ cell tumors**: Some of these tumors produce elevated levels of human chorionic gonadotropin (hCG), which can lead to isosexual precocious puberty. As with testicular tumors, some of these tumors tend to produce ***AFP (yolk sac tumors)*** or ***hCG*** (embryonal carcinoma, choriocarcinomas and some ***dysgerminomas***) that are reliable tumor markers"- *Harrison 19th/594*

Dysgerminoma: Immunohistochemistry

◈ *www.sciencedirect.com*

- Dysgerminoma cells contain abundant intracytoplasmic glycogen that can be highlighted by PAS that disappears with diastase digestion.
- The cells typically show strong cytoplasmic membrane staining for ***PLAP***. Recently, *c-kit (CD117) and OCT4 positivity* has been reported in up to 92% and 100% of dysgerminomas respectively.
- Tumor cells are frequently positive for vimentin, LDH and neuron-specific enolase (NSE).
- Approximately 30% of dysgerminomas contain scattered cells positive for cytokeratin. They are negative for EMA, CEA, S-100 protein, leukocyte common antigen (LCA) and AFP. Syncytiotrophoblast cells stain for β-hCG.
- LDH is a nonspecific tumor marker and is reported to be elevated in up to 95% of cases β-hCG may be produced in low levels (<200 IU/L).

Table: Tumor markers that may be elevated in the presence of germ cell neoplasms *(CDTOG 10th/Chap 52)*

Neoplasm	AFP	hCG
Dysgerminoma	*	+/–
Endoderal sinus tumor	+	–
Immature teratoma	+/–	–
Mixed germ cell tumor	+/–	+/–
Choriocarcinoma	–	+
Embryonal carcinoma	+/–	+

AFP, α-fetoprotein; hCG, human chorionic gonadotropin.
– = negative (not elevated);
+ = positive (elevated above normal level);
* = borderline (<16 ng/mL) elevations in case reports.

198. Ans. a. A loop size of less than 2 cm gives a better cone than a larger one, b. Cheaper than laser, e. Low voltage is used

[Ref: Shaw's Gynae 16th/492-93; DuttaGynae 7th/269-70; Novak's Gynae 15th/603-04]

- "LEEP uses a ***low-voltage electrified wire*** to remove abnormal tissue that has been identified in a colposcopy, which provides a magnified view of the cervix. ***LEEP can also remove abnormal tissue higher in the cervix*** not visible with colposcopy. LEEP is preferred in these instances over conization"*-cancer.coloradowomenshealth.com*
- "Laser surgery may be used to destroy abnormal cells in the cervix. This procedure directs a very strong, hot beam of light at the abnormal cells to burn them away. The procedure takes about 10–15 minutes"*-canceraustralia.gov.au*
- LLETZ/LEEP: A ***loop(2-3cm)*** of very thin stainless-steel wire is used for excision of transformation zone. Blended current(cutting & coagulation) of ***low voltage*** is used"- *DuttaGynae 7th/269*

Comparison of Different Methods of Treatment of Dysplasia and CIN

◈ *Shaw's Gynae 16th/493*

- **Large loop excision of the transformation zone (LLETZ)** uses ***low-voltage diathermy*** under local anaesthesia. The loop is advanced into the cervix lateral to the lesion until the required depth is reached. It is then taken across to the opposite side and a cone of tissue removed. ***A loop size of less than 2 cm gives a better cone than a larger one. The low cost of the equipment and harmless effects on personnel***

A & E

makes LLETZ more popular than laser. Besides, it takes ***shorter time to perform*** with similar success and recurrence as that of laser.

- *Loop electrosurgical excision procedure (LEEP)* is even simpler than LLETZ, LEEP is applicable anywhere in the lower genital tract; whereas, ***LLETZ is applicable only to the cervix.***
- With the availability of LEEP, a simple and effective method, laser seems to have taken a backseat
- **Laser ablation** boils, steams and explodes the cells. The laser is very expensive and can be harmful to the personnel (burn injury to the skin and eyes). It destroys the tissue up to 5 mm deep.
- *However, laser ablation is useful when* the CIN extends up to the vaginal vault.
- Laser causes minimal bleeding, no infection, no post-laser scar formation and no deeper excision. It is an OPD procedure done under local anaesthesia and under colposcopic guidance.
- More importantly, laser does not cause indrawal of squamocolumnar junction and therefore, repeat laser is possible for residual lesion unlike cautery or cryosurgery. Recurrence of 2-8% is reported.
- **Excisional and cone biopsy** *provide tissue for histopathological study and can be therapeutic.*
- **Punch biopsy** under colposcopic view can remove the entire lesion, if small and can be performed under sedation or local anaesthesia.

Treatment Options for CIN-II & CIN-III

◈ *Shaw's 16th/491*

- **Local destructive methods:** Cryosurgery, fulgration/ electrocoagulation & laser abalation
- **Excision of abnormal tissue:** Cold-knife conization, laser conization, LLETZ, LEEP & NETZ
- **Surgery:** Therapeutic conization, hysterectomy, hysterectomy with removal of vaginal cuff if carcinoma in situ extends to the vaginal vault
- Follow up with coloposcopy &/or cytology

Flow chart 1: Management of CIN *(Shaw's 16th/494)*

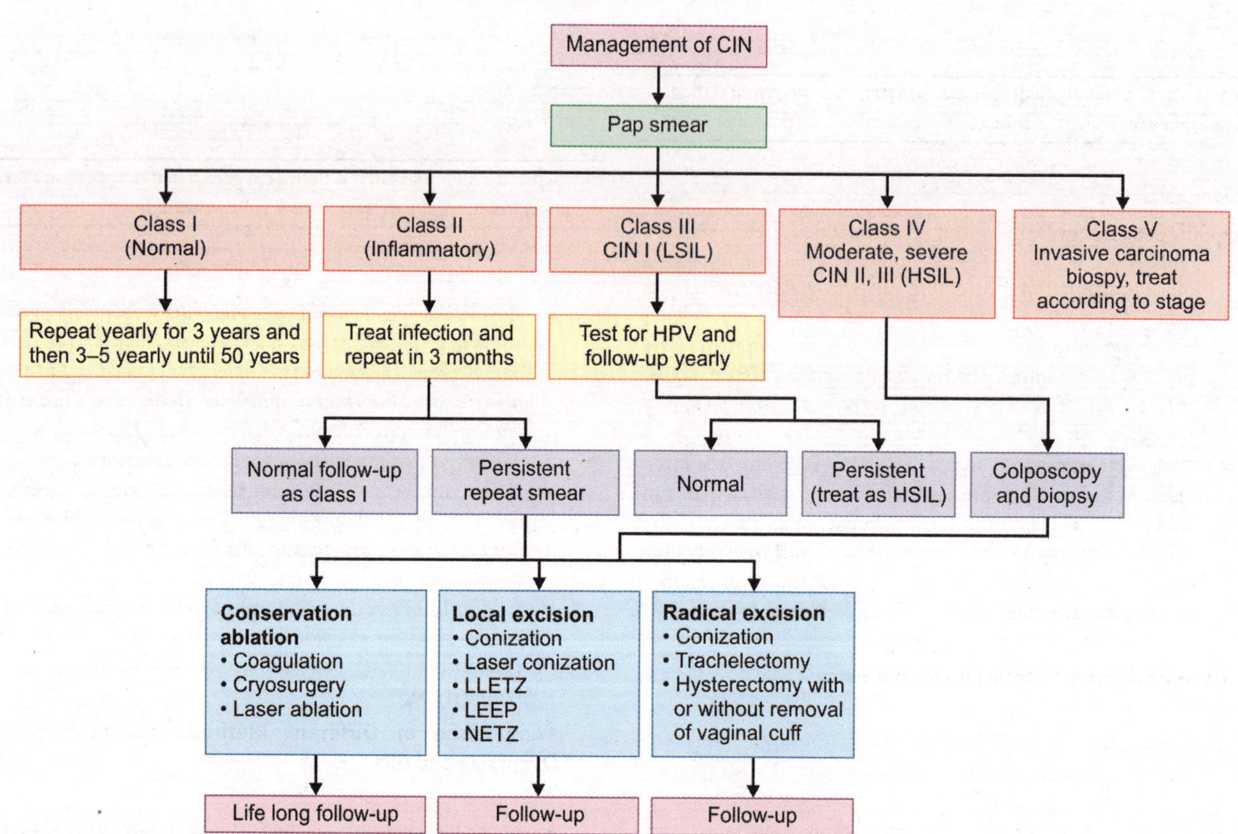

Table: Comparison of different methods of treatment of dysplasia and CIN *(Shaw's 16th/492)*

Characteristics	Laser ablation	Laser conization	LEEP	LLETZ
Place	OPD	OPD/OT	OPD	OPD
Anesthesia	Nil analgesia	Local	Local	Local
Instrument cost	Expensive	Expensive, Not portable	Cheap, Portable	Cheap,Portable
Risk of equipment	Yes	Yes	Nil	Nil
Complication during surgery	Personnel	Personnel	Nil	Nil
Depth of destruction	7 mm	-	-	-
Pain	Slight	Slight	Slight	Nil
Bleeding	Nil	Slight		Slight
Sepsis	Nil	Nil	Slight	Slight
Healing	4 weeks	4 weeks	4-6 weeks	4-6 week
Cure rate	90-97%	90-95%	90-95%	90-95%
Postoperative transformation zone	Seen			

199. Ans. c. **Hirsutism, d. Oligomenorrhoea**

[Ref: Shaw's Gynae 16th/430-34; DuttaGynae 7th/ 378-81; Novak's Gynae 15th/1076]

PCOD: Diagnosis is Based Upon the Presence of any two of the following three Criteria (ASRM/ESHRE 2003 Criteria)

◈ *DuttaGynae 7th/ 378*
- Oligomenorrhoea &/or anovulation
- Hyperandrogenism (Clinical &/or biochemical)
- Polycystic ovaries

PCOD: Diagnosis is Based Upon the Presence of any two of the following three Criteria (ASRM/ESHRE 2003 Criteria)

◈ *Shaw's Gynae 16th/432*
- Oligo/amenorrhoea, anovulation, infertility
- Hirsutism-acne
- Ultrasound finding-***enlarged ovary***, multiple follicles, ruled out ovarian tumour, endometrial hyperplasia(if present)

Table: Diagnostic criteria for Rotterdam diagnosis of polycystic ovary syndrome *(Novak's Gynae 15th/1076, www.racgp.org.au)*

- While there are a number of definitions of PCOS, the Rotterdam consensus is the most widely accepted across Europe, Asia and Australia and was the definition used for the guideline.
- It encompasses the National Institutes of Health definition, which generally describes women with a more severe form of PCOS and requires the presence of both hyperandrogenism and oligo/anovulation.
- The Rotterdam Criteria require the presence of two of the following: oligo/anovulation, hyperandrogenism or polycystic ovaries on ultrasound
- Two of the following **three criteria** are required:
  - ***oligo/anovulation***
  - ***hyperandrogenism: clinical (hirsutism or less commonly male pattern alopecia) or biochemical (raised FAI or free testosterone)***
  - ***polycystic ovaries on ultrasound***

- **Oligo/anovulation** is usually seen in women with menstrual cycles greater than 35 days apart or, conversely, with short cycles of less than 21 days. It is important to remember that even women with regular cycles may be anovulatory. For these women a measure of luteal progesterone (day 21 in a 28 day cycle) will determine ovulatory status
- **Hyperandrogenism**: Hirsutism is difficult to assess as most women treat this so it is not obvious on examination. Hyperandrogenaemia is best measured with free testosterone; either calculated free testosterone, free androgen index (FAI) or bioavailable testosterone. Most laboratories will offer at least one of these. Hormonal contraceptive use will affect free testosterone measures. If appropriate, assess after 3 months cessation; alternative contraception should be discussed for this time.[4] If free testosterone is significantly raised or there is evidence of rapid virilisation, further investigations are required to exclude late onset congenital adrenal hyperplasia and virilising tumours
- **Polycystic ovaries** on ultrasound are diagnosed when ***10 small antral follicles are seen in each ovary***. A unilateral polycystic ovary is rare but still clinically significant.

Contd...

- Other aetiologies must be excluded such as congenital adrenal hyperplasia androgen secreting tumours, Cushing syndrome, thyroid dysfunction and hyperprolactinaemia
- All other frequently encountered manifestations offer less consistent findings and therefore qualify only as minor diagnostic criteria for PCOS. They include elevated LH-to- FSH (follicle-stimulating hormone) ratio, insulin resistance, perimenarchal onset of hirsutism and obesity.

PCOS

◈ *Shaws 16th/431-34*

- PCOS includes chronic nonovulation, hyper-androgenismassociated with normal or raised oestradiol level (E2), raised LH & low FSH/LH ratio
- Patients are mostly 15-25 years of age. The disease has genetic & familial tendency & may be autosomal dominant inherited
- **HAIR-AN Syndrome**: In patients with PCOS, this syndrome is characterized by ***hyperandrogenism, insulin resistance & acanthosis nigricans***

Table: Presentations of PCOD *(Shaws 16th/430)*

Clinical features	Hormonal	Sequelae
• Young woman	• ↑ E2 level	Diabetes (15%)
• Central obesity	• FSH normal; ↑ LH > 10 IU/ml	CVS disorder
BMI > 30 kg/cm2	• ↓ FSH/LH ratio	Lipidaemia
Waist line >88 cm (35")	• ↑ Androgens	Hypertension
• Oligomenorrhoea, amenorrhoea	• ↑Testosterone, epiandrostenedione,	Endometrial cancer
• Infertility (20%)	• ↑ dehydroepiandrosterone	Breast cancer
• Hirsutism	• 17-alpha-hydroxy progesterone > 300 ng/dl	Premature ovarian failure following surgery
• Acanthosis nigra due to insulin resistance. Thick pigmented skin over the nape of neck, inner thigh and axilla. • Most androgen from ovary • Fasting insulin >10mIU/L	• Testosterone > 2 ng/ml • Most androgens from ovary • Prolactin ↑ • Sex hormone binding globulin (SHBG) ↓ • ↓ E2/oestrone (E1) ratio • F.blood glucose/fasting insulin ratio < 4.5	

200. Ans. e. Enterocele

[Ref: Shaw's Gynae 16th/361; DuttaGynae 7th/174, 177; Novak's Gynae 15th/]

"Abdominal repair of enterocele is done by obliterating the pouch of douglas to prevent herniation of bowel. This is known as *moskowitz procedure*"-*DuttaGynae 7th/177; Shaw's Gynae 16th/361*

Vault prolapse: primary (enterocele) & secondary (following vaginal & abdominal hysterectomy)-*DuttaGynae 7th/168*

"Failure to recognize & repair the enterocele can lead to vault prolapsed later"- *Shaw's Gynae 16th/361*

"Adenomyosis: localized excision/hysterectomy"- *Shaw's Gynae 16th/422*

Chronic inversion of uterus: spinelli's operation/vaginal hysterectomy/abdominal hysterectomy-*Shaw's Gynae 16th/369*

Table: Type of prolapse and the common surgical repair procedures *(DuttaGynae 7th/174)*

Organ descent	Clinical condition	Type of operation
Vaginal wall		
Anterior (Upper 2/3) or whole	Cystocele/cystourethrocele Paravaginal defect	• Anterior colporrhaphy • Paravaginal defect repair
Posterior (Lower 2/3)	Rectocele	• Colpoperineorrhaphy
Posterior (Upper 1/3)	Enterocele	• Vaginal repair of enterocele with PFR • McCall culdoplasty • Moskowitz procedure
Combined anterior and posterior	Cystocele and rectocele	• PFR (combined procedure)
Uterovaginal		
Uterus along with vaginal walls	Uterovaginal prolapse	• Vaginal hysterectomy with PFR (Elderly woman, family completed) • Fothergill's operation (Preservation of uterus)
Vaginal wall Following hysterectomy (Vaginal or abdominal)	Vault prolapse (secondary)	**Vaginal**: i. Repair of vaginal vault along with PFR ii. Sacrospinouscolpopexy iii. Colpocleisis (Le fort) **Abdominal**: i. Sacral colpopexy
Uterus (Without vaginal walls)	Congenital or nulliparous prolapse (Young women)	Cervicopexy or sling (Purandare's) operation
Pelvic organ prolapse (POP)	POP with stress in continence	• Vaginal: TOT operation • **Abdominal**: Burch operation

Abbreviations: PFR Pelvic floor repair; TOT, Transobturator tape procedure

201. Ans. **a. Early cord clamping, b. Manual removal of placenta**

[Ref: DuttaObs 9th/133-34; William's Obs 23rd/397-98; Obs by JB Sharma 1st/217-18]

In active management of 3rd stage labour, delayed cord clamping is done. Manual cord removal is drawback of active management of 3rd stage labour

Drawback of active management of 3rd stage labour: slight increased incidence of retained placenta (1–2%) & consequent increased incidence of manual removal"-*DuttaObs 9th/134,Obs by JB Sharma 1st/218*

"Oxytocin is given in 500 ml normal saline infusion in management of third stage labour" *William's Obs 23rd/399*

Management of the third Stage of Labor and Prevention of Postpartum Hemorrhage

◈ *www.obtsguidelines.org (Updated on 10/2/2017)*

- The 2012 WHO guidelines for active management of the third stage of labor recognize the need to balance hemorrhage prevention and the benefits of delayed cord clamping, which ACOG has also acknowledged in the Practice Bulletin on postpartum hemorrhage.
- Based on review of the WHO guidelines, ACOG Practice Bulletin and recent literature, the following is recommended for deliveries in GHS hospitals.
- **Delayed cord clamping** should be practiced for most deliveries, allowing at least 30 to 60 seconds topass before clamping. The cord should be clamped immediately if the newborn requires immediate resuscitation or if stabilization of the mother needs to take precedence.
- At vaginal delivery, administer **oxytocin** 30 units in 500mL of normal saline given IV at the time of cord clamping. This should be run in over 30 minutes.
- If IV access is not available, oxytocin 20 units IM may be given as an alternative, also given at the time of cord clamping. Misoprostol 600 mcg PO is an alternative if oxytocin is unavailable.
- For cesarean deliveries, oxytocin 40 units in 1000 mL to be started at cord clamping and infused over 30-60 minutes.
- In both cases, the full dose should be given.
- At vaginal delivery, controlled cord traction may be used to facilitate delivery of the placenta. Uterine massage prior to placental delivery is not recommended, but should be performed following placental delivery.

- If a patient's risk of postpartum hemorrhage is high, additional prophylactic oxytocin may be given in the first postpartum hours.
- If active hemorrhage occurs, initiate the postpartum hemorrhage plan while continuing oxytocin administration.

WHO Recommendations for Active Management of the Third Stage of Labour (AMTSL), 2012

apps.who.int

- The use of uterotonics for the prevention of postpartum haemorrhage (PPH) during the third stage of labour is recommended for all births. Oxytocin (10 IU, IV/IM) is the recommended uterotonic drug for the prevention of PPH.
- In settings where skilled birth attendants are available, controlled cord traction (CCT) is recommended for vaginal births if the care provider and the parturient woman regard a small reduction in blood loss and a small reduction in the duration of the third stage of labour as important. In settings where skilled birth attendants are unavailable, CCT is not recommended.
- ***Sustained uterine massage is not recommended as an intervention to prevent PPH in women who have received prophylactic oxytocin.*** Postpartum abdominal uterine tonus assessment for early identification of uterine atony is recommended for all women.
- Postpartum vigilance: Immediately assess uterine tone to ensure a contracted uterus; continue to check every 15 minutes for 2 hours. If there is uterine atony, perform fundal massage and monitor more frequently
- CCT is the recommended method for removal of the placenta in caesarean section.

Flow chart: Scheme of management of third stage of labour *(Dutta Obs 9th/132)*

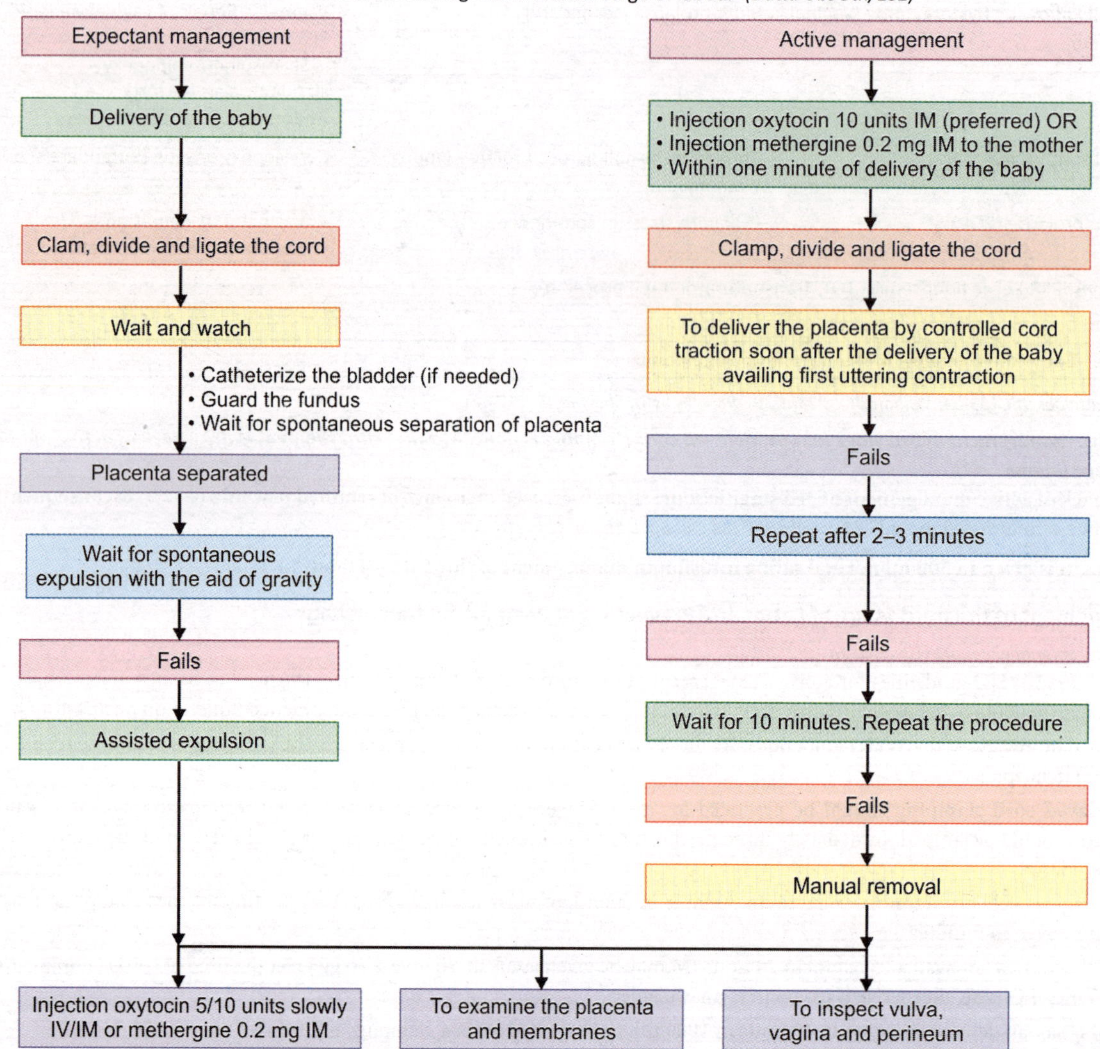

Components of Active Management of third Stage

◈ *Obs by JB Sharma 1st/218*

- Use of oxytocic
- Delivery of placenta by ***controlled cord traction (CCT)***
- ***Uterine massage***
  - Some include delayed cord clamping as part of active management of the third stage.
  - Latest WHO guideline recommends only oxytocin use for active management of third stage. It does not recommend sustained uterine massage if the women has already received prophylactic oxytocin. However, postpartum abdominal uterine tone assessment for early identification of uterine atony is recommended for all births.
  - Controlled cord traction is only recommended if skilled birth attendant is available. In absence of skilled birth attendant, CCT is not recommended.

202. Ans. **a. 4% (Most probably)**

[Ref: Shaw's Gynae 16th/451; DuttaGynae 7th/244; Novak's Gynae 15th/1364,807 Johns Hopkins Manual of Gynecology and Obstetrics 3rd/ Chap 44]

- "The performance of a **prophylactic salpingo-oophorectomy** significantly reduces, but does not totally eliminate, the risk of non-uterine pelvic cancers; because the entire peritoneum is at risk, peritoneal carcinomas can occur in ***2% to 3%*** of women even after prophylactic bilateral salpingo-oophorectomy"-*Novak's Gynae 15th/ 1360*
- "**Prophylactic oophorectomy** may also be employed for the prevention of ovarian and breast cancers among high-risk women. A prospective cohort study evaluating the outcomes of *BRCA* mutation carriers demonstrated a statistically significant association between prophylactic oophorectomy and a reduced incidence of ovarian or primary peritoneal cancer (36% relative risk reduction, or a ***4.5% absolute difference).*** Studies of prophylactic oophorectomy for prevention of breast cancer in women with genetic mutations have shown relative risk reductions of approximately 50%; the risk reduction may be greatest for women having the procedure at younger (i.e., <50 years) ages.All of the evidence concerning the use of prophylactic mastectomy and oophorectomy for prevention of breast and ovarian cancer in high-risk women has been observational in nature; such studies are prone to a variety of biases, including case selection bias, family relationships between patients and controls and inadequate information about hormone use. Thus, they may give an overestimate of the magnitude of benefit"- *Harrison 19th/479*
- **"Prophylactic Salpingo-oophorectomy**: Bilateral salpingo-oophorectomy can reduce the risk of developing ovarian and fallopian tube cancers by over 90% and breast cancer by 50%. Tubal ligation by reduce the risk of ovarian cancer by 30-60%"-*jgh.ca/upload*

Prophylactic Salpingo-oophorectomy in High-Risk Women

◈ *Novak's Gynae 15th/ 1364*

- The value of prophylactic salpingo-oophorectomy in these patients is documented
- The protection against ovarian cancer is excellent: the performance of a prophylactic salpingo-oophorectomy reduced the risk of BRCA-related gynecologic cancer by 96%
- Although the risk of ovarian cancer is significantly diminished, there remains the small risk of peritoneal carcinoma, a tumor for which women who have mutations in BRCA1 and BRCA2 may have a higher predisposition. In these series, the subsequent development of peritoneal carcinoma was ***0.8% and 1%, respectively***. The risk of developing subsequent breast cancer was reduced by 50% to 80%.

Risk-reducing Bilateral Salpingo-oophorectomy (rrBSO)

◈ *www.uptodate.com*

- Risk-reducing bilateral salpingo-oophorectomy (rrBSO) is an important option for decreasing the risk of epithelial ovarian and fallopian tubal cancer in women who have the highest likelihood of developing this malignancy. Other preventive measures and surveillance measures are available, but are of limited efficacy in reducing the high rates of cancer mortality.
- Emerging data suggest that some apparent ovarian cancers, particularly in women with *BRCA* gene mutations, are initiated in the fallopian tubes, thus, risk-reducing surgery must include bilateral removal of the tubes as well as the ovaries
- In addition, women with a hereditary ovarian cancer syndrome may also be at risk for other malignancies, including breast and peritoneal cancer in *BRCA* gene mutation carriers and endometrial or colon cancer in those with Lynch syndrome (hereditary nonpolyposis colorectal cancer). Decisions regarding various cancer risk reduction must take into account prevention or surveillance of these other tumors
- "Prophylactic Bilateral Salpingo-Oophorectomy. Women over age 45 who are undergoing any pelvic surgery may consider prophylactic removal of the ovaries. A bilateral salpingo-oophorectomy will essentially eliminate her risk for developing ovarian cancer (although the risk of primary peritoneal cancer still exists after removal of both ovaries). The potential for surgical menopause must be weighed against the potential benefit of averting ovarian malignancy. Women at high risk of ovarian cancer (Lynch syndrome, BRCA mutations) should consider a prophylactic bilateral salpingo-oophorectomy"- Johns Hopkins Manual of Gynecology and Obstetrics 3rd/Chap 44

203. Ans. **a. Check HbA1c level, b. TSH estimation, c. Frequent blood sugar estimation**

[Ref: DuttaObs 9th/266; William's Obs 23rd/176; Obs by JB Sharma 1st/512; care.diabetesjournals.org]

Preconception Care of Women With Diabetes: Laboratory evaluation

◈ *care.diabetesjournals.org*

The evaluation should focus on assessment of metabolic control and detection of diabetic complications that may affect or be affected by pregnancy:

- A1C test
- ***Frequent blood sugar estimation***- *www.arhp.org*
- Serum creatinine and urinary excretion of total protein and/or albumin (albumin-to-creatinine ratio or 24-h excretion rate).
- Measurement of **serum thyroid stimulating hormone** and/or free thyroxine level in women with type 1 diabetes because of the 5–10% coincidence of hyper- or hypothyroidism
- Other tests as indicated by physical exam or history

Table: American Diabetes Association Recommendations for the Preconceptional Care of Women with Diabetes *(William's Obs 23rd/176)*

Medical and Obstetrical History

- Duration and type of diabetes
- Acute complications, including history of infections, ketoacidosis and hypoglycemia
- Chronic complications, including retinopathy, nephropathy, hypertension, atherosclerotic vascular disease and neuropathy
- Diabetes management, including insulin regimen, use of glucose lowering agents, self-glucose monitoring regimens and results, nutrition and physical activity
- Concomitant medical conditions
- Menstrual and pregnancy history, contraceptive use
- Support systems

Physical Examination

- Blood pressure, including testing for orthostatic changes
- Retinal examination with pupillary dilatation
- Cardiovascular examination for evidence of cardiac or peripheral vascular disease—if present, screen for evidence of coronary artery disease
- Neurological examination

Laboratory Evaluation

- ***Hemoglobin A1c***
- *Serum creatinine*
- **Urine protein:** Protein excretion >190 mg/24 hours may increase the risk for hypertensive disorders during pregnancy; protein excretion >400 mg/24 hours may increase the risk for fetal-growth restriction
- ***Thyroid function tests***: 5- to 10-percent coincidence of type 1 diabetes and thyroid dysfunction

Initial Management Plan

- Counseling
  - Risk and prevention of congenital anomalies
  - Fetal and neonatal complications of maternal diabetes
  - Effects of pregnancy on maternal diabetic complications
  - Risks of obstetrical complications that occur with increased frequency in diabetic pregnancies
  - Need for effective contraception until glycemia is well controlled
- Insulin regimen selected to achieve the following goals:
  - Capillary plasma glucose before meals 80–110 mg/dL
  - Capillary plasma glucose 2 hours after meals less than 155 mg/dL[a]
- Monitor hemoglobin A1c levels at 1- to 2-month intervals until stable with the goal to achieve a concentration less than 1 percent above the normal range

Note: [a]There are no data to suggest that postmeal glucose monitoring has a specific role in preconception diabetes care beyond what is needed to achieve the target hemoglobin A1c. Thus, a focus on preprandial monitoring is recommended initially to assist patients in self-selection of insulin doses.

PEDIATRICS

204. Ans. a. Mortality in more than 30% cases in severe asphyxia, c. Acute tubular necrosis, d. Seizure, e. Cerebral edema

[Ref: O.P.Ghai 9th/ 162-64; Nelson 20th/ 838-42,2850;CPDT 17th/29-30]

Hypoxic-ischemic Encephalopathy (HIE)

Nelson 20th/ 838-42

- HIE is an important cause of permanent damage to CNS tissues that may result in neonatal death or manifest later as cerebral palsy or developmental delay.
- ***Fifteen to 20-30% of infants with hypoxic-ischemic encephalopathy (HIE) die in the neonatal period*** and ~33–50% of survivors are left with permanent neurodevelopmental abnormalities (cerebral palsy, mental retardation). The greatest risk of adverse outcome is seen in infants with severe fetal acidosis (pH <6.7) (***90% death/impairment***) & a base deficit > 25 mmol/L (72% mortality).
- In stage 3 HIE, half of neonates die & remaining half tend to have poor neurodevelopment outcomes. In stage 2 HIE adverse neurological outcome is present in 20% of babies
- Perinatal asphyxia: The single best predictor of outcome is the severity of clinical hypoxic-ischemic encephalopathy (severe symptomatology including coma carries a 75% chance of death and a 100% rate of neurologic sequelae among survivors)-*CPDT 17th/30*
- Perinatal asphyxia: low cord pH of < 7.00- *CPDT 17th/30*

Table: Essential criteria for perinatal asphyxia *(O.P.Ghai 9th/163)*

- Prolonged metabolic or mixed academia (pH <7.0) on an umbilical arterial blood sample
- Persistence of Apgar score of 0–3 for >5 minutes
- Neurological manifestations, e.g. seizures, coma, hypotonia or hypoxic ischemic encephalopathy (HIE) in the immediate neonatal period
- Evidence of multiorgan dysfunction in the immediate neonatal period

Table: Multiorgan Systemic Effects of Asphyxia *(Nelson 20th/838)*

System	Effect
Central nervous system	Hypoxic-ischemic encephalopathy, infarction, intracranial hemorrhage, seizures, ***cerebral edema***, hypotonia, hypertonia
Cardiovascular	Myocardial ischemia, poor contractility, cardiac stun, tricuspid insufficiency, hypotension
Pulmonary	Pulmonary hypertension, pulmonary hemorrhage, respiratory distress syndrome

System	Effect
Renal	Acute tubular or cortical necrosis
Adrenal	Adrenal hemorrhage
Gastrointestinal	Perforation, ulceration with hemorrhage, necrosis
Metabolic	Inappropriate secretion of antidiuretic hormone, hyponatremia, hypoglycemia, hypocalcemia, myoglobinuria
Integument	Subcutaneous fat necrosis
Hematology	Disseminated intravascular coagulation

205. Ans. b. Breast milk mcontains factors for cell growth and differentiation of intestinal cells, c. Contain antibacterial factors including Bifidus factor

[Ref: O.P.Ghai 9th/ 145;CSDT 17th/302; Guyton(SEA) 13th/696]

"Milk is a source of all vitamins except vitamin C"-*Park 24th/668*

Breast Milk

◈ *O.P.Ghai 9th/ 145*

- *It contains a number of protective factors which include immunoglobulin-mainly* ***secretary IgA****, macrophages, lymphocytes, lactoferrin, lysozyme,* ***bifidus factor*** *& interferon among others. Breastfeed babies are less likely to develop infection*
- "Immunoglobulins, present in particularly high concentrations early in lactation, are found in breast milk as secretory IgA (SIgA), the most predominant form, followed by SIgG. These provide immunological protection to the infant, whilst its own immune system matures"- www.researchgate.net
- *Breast milk contains a number of growth factor, enzymes & hormones. The epidermal growth factor in breast milk enhances maturation of the intestinal cells & reduces the risk of allergy in later life*
- *Vitamins & minerals- The quantity & bioavailability of vitamins & minerals is sufficient to the needs of the baby in the first 6 months of life*
- Human breast milk contains adequate amounts of most vitamins to support normal infant growth, except for vitamins D and K-*www.ncbi.nlm.nih.gov*
- ***"Milk (all type) is a good source of all vitamins except vitamin C***- *Park 24th/668*

Regarding Option D (Breast Milk is a Suspension of Protein and Fats in Carbohydrate)-Not True (see Explanation)

- An ***emulsion is a suspension of droplets of one liquid into another liquid. Milk is an emulsion of fat in water***- www4.ncsu.edu
- A colloidal solution is when matter exists in a state of division in between a true solution, which is sugar in water and a suspension, which is chalk in water. The characteristics of a colloid are small particle size, electrical charge and affinity of the particles for water molecules.
- In milk, the whey proteins are in colloidal solution. The casein proteins are in colloidal suspension www4.ncsu.edu
- Technically, milk is an ***emulsion of fat globules in a plasma phase*** (skim milk), which itself contains casein micelles (protein particles) in a colloidal suspension in a serum phase (whey)-blogs.commons.georgetown.edu
- The particles in suspensions are larger than those found in solutions. Components of a suspension can be evenly distributed by a mechanical means, like by shaking the contents, but the components will settle out. Example: Oil and Water- www.thoughtco.com

Antibodies and other Anti-infectious Agents in Milk

◈ *Guyton(SEA) 13th/696*

- Not only does milk provide the newborn baby with needed nutrients, but it also provides important protection against infection. For instance, multiple types of *antibodies* and other anti-infectious agents are secreted in milk along with the nutrients.
- Also, several different types of white blood cells are secreted, including both *neutrophils* and *macrophages*, some of which are especially lethal to bacteria that could cause deadly infections in newborn babies. Particularly important are antibodies and macrophages that destroy *Escherichia coli* bacteria, which often cause lethal diarrhea in newborns.
- When cow's milk is used to supply nutrition for the baby in place of mother's milk, the protective agents in it are usually of little value because they are normally destroyed within minutes in the internal environment of the human being.

Table: The composition of milk (per 100 kcal) *(CSDT 17th/302)*

Nutrient (unit)	Minimal Level Recommended	Mature Human Milk	Typical commercial Formula	Cow's Milk (Mean)
Protein (g)	1.8	1.3–1.6	2.3	5.1
Fat (g)	3.3	5	5.3	5.7
Carbohydrate (g)	–	10.3	10.8	7.3
Linoleic acid (mg)	300	560	2300	125
Vitamin A (IU)	250	250	300	216
Vitamin D (IU)	40	3	63	3
Vitamin E (IU)	0.7/g linoleic acid	0.3	2	0.1

Contd...

Nutrient (unit)	Minimal Level Recommended	Mature Human Milk	Typical commercial Formula	Cow's Milk (Mean)
Vitamin K (mg)	4	2	9	5
Vitamin C (mg)	8	7.8	8.1	2.3
Thiamin (mg)	40	25	80	59
Riboflavin (mg)	60	60	100	252
Niacin (mg)	250	250	1200	131
Vitamin B_6 (mg)	15 mg of protein	15	63	66
Folic acid (mg)	4	4	10	8
Pantothenic acid (mg)	300	300	450	489
Vitamin B_{12} (mg)	0.15	0.15	0.25	0.56
Biotin (mg)	1.5	1	2.5	3.1

206. Ans. d. Overall good prognosis

[Ref: Nelson 20th/2444-45; www.ncbi.nlm.nih.gov]

Infant Leukemia

◈ *Nelson 20th/2444-45*

- About 2% of cases of leukemia during childhood occur before the age of 1 yr. In contrast to older children, the ratio of ***ALL to AML is 2: 1.***
- Some cases may be due to maternal exposure to naturally occurring DNA topoisomerase II inhibitors.
- Several unique biologic features and a ***particularly poor prognosis*** are characteristic of ALL during infancy.
- **More than two thirds** of the cases demonstrate rearrangements of the **MLL gene**, found at the site of the 11q23 band translocation; this subset of patients largely accounts for the very high relapse rate. These patients often present with hyperleukocytosis and extensive tissue infiltration producing organomegaly, including CNS disease.
- Subcutaneous nodules, known as **leukemia cutis** and tachypnea due to diffuse pulmonary infiltration by leukemic cells are observed more often in infants than in older children. The leukemic cell morphology is usually that of large irregular lymphoblasts (FAB L2), with a phenotype negative for the CD10 (cALLa) marker.
- Very intensive chemotherapy programs including stem cell transplantation are being explored in infants with rearrangement of MLL in band 11q23, but none has yet proved satisfactory.
- Infants with leukemia who lack the 11q23 rearrangements have a prognosis similar to that of older children with ALL.
- ***Infants with AML often present with CNS or skin involvement*** and have the FAB M4 subtype, which is commonly known as **acute myelomonocytic leukemia.**
- The treatment may be the same as that for older children with AML. Meticulous supportive care is necessary because of the young age and aggressive therapy needed in these patients.

Infant Leukemias

◈ *www.ncbi.nlm.nih.gov*

- The term "infant leukemia" generally refers to acute lymphoblastic leukemia (ALL) or acute myeloid leukemia (AML) diagnosed in a child before 1 year of age.
- The incidence of ALL in infants is significantly lower than in children aged 1 to 14 years old and approximately the same as adolescents. In contrast, the incidence of AML in infants is approximately twice that of older children and adolescents.
- Interestingly, females have a higher risk of developing infant leukemia than males but a lower risk of developing leukemia beyond the first birthday.[1]
- ***MLL*** gene translocations occur in up to 80% of cases of ALL, in up to 50% of cases of AML in infants and in 80% of monoblastic variants of AML in infants and young children
- Compared with older children, infants with acute leukemia tend to present with ***more aggressive features,*** including high WBC counts, hepatosplenomegaly, CNS involvement and leukemia cutis (skin infiltration)
- Perhaps most importantly, the eventual outcomes for infants with leukemia in terms of relapse-free survival are poor compared with leukemia in older children despite the use of maximally intensified standard therapies (chemotherapy with or without hematopoietic stem cell transplantation [HSCT]).

207. Ans. b. Bilous vomiting, d. Non-projectile vomiting

[Ref: Robbins 9th/751; Nelson 18th/1555-57]

Congenital Hypertrophic Pyloric Stenosis (CHPS)

◈ *Robbins 9th/751*

- It generally presents between the third and sixth weeks of life as new onset regurgitation, ***projectile, nonbilious vomiting*** after feeding and frequent demands for re-feeding.
- Physical examination reveals a firm, ovoid, 1 to 2 cm abdominal mass. In some cases abnormal left to right hyperperistalsis is evident during feeding and immediately before vomiting. This constellation of findings stems from hyperplasia of the pyloric muscularis propria, which obstructs the gastric outflow tract. Edema and inflammatory changes in the mucosa and submucosa may aggravate the narrowing.
- Surgical splitting of the muscularis (myotomy) is curative.

ORTHOPEDICS

208. Ans. a. Abduction, d. Extension

[Ref: Maheswari 5th/131-32; Apley 9th/ 843]

Posterior Dislocation of Hip

- *Maheswari 5th/131-32*
- *Deformity seen: Flexion, adduction & internal rotation*
- *Shortening of leg*
- *Reduction is an emergency, since longer the head remains out, more the chances of it becoming avascular*
- *There are three types of dislocation of hip-posterior(commonest), anterior & central fracture dislocation*
- *Also k/a dashboard injury*

"**Posterior dislocation of hip:** In straightforward case the diagnosis is easy; the leg is short & lies adducted, internally rotated & slightly flexed. However, if long bone (like femur) is fractured, limb can adopt any position"- *Apley 9th/ 843*

Hip Condition	Deformity
Synovitis	Flexion, abduction, external rotation, apparent lengthening
Arthritis	Flexion, adduction, internal rotation, true shortening
Anterior dislocation	Flexion, abduction, external rotation, true lengthening
Femoral neck fracture	External rotation, later adduction & flexion
Intertrochanteric fracture	Marked external rotation, later adduction & flexion

209. Ans. a. CNS depression, b. Axillary or Conjunctival petechiae, d. Pulmonary edema

[Ref: Barash 6th/1388; academic.oup.com; Maheswari 5th/43; Apley 9th/681]

Table: Gurd's criteria for diagnosis of fat embolus syndrome[a] *(Barash 6th/1388)*

MAJOR
• Axillary/subconjunctival petechiae
• Hypoxemia (PaO_2 <60 mm Hg; FiO_2 <0.4)
• Central nervous system depression (disproportionate to hypoxemia)
• Pulmonary edema
Minor
• Tachycardia (>110 beats/min)
• Hyperthermia
• Retinal fat emboli
• Urinary fat globules
• Decreased platelets/hematocrit (unexplained)
• Increased erythrocyte sedimentation rate
• Fat globules in sputum

[a]Diagnosis of fat embolus syndrome requires at least one sign from the major and four signs from the minor criteria categories

Table: Lindeques criteria *academic.oup.com*

Sustained PaO_2<8 kPa
Sustained PCO_2 of >7.3 kPa or a pH <7.3
Sustained respiratory rate >35 breaths min^{-1}, despite sedation
Increased work of breathing: dyspnea, accessory muscle use, tachycardia and anxiety

Table: Schonfeld's criteria *academic.oup.com/bjaed*

Petechiae
Chest X-ray changes (diffuse alveolar infiltrates)
Hypoxaemia (Pa_{a2}<9.3 kPa)
Fever (>38°C)
Tachycardia (>120 beats min^{-1})
Tachycardia (>30 bpm)
Cumulative score >5 required for diagnosis

Fat Embolus Syndrome

- *Barash 6th/1388*
- Fat embolus syndrome (FES) is associated with multiple traumatic injuries and surgery involving long-bone fractures.
- Risk factors include male gender, age (20 to 30 years), hypo-volemic shock, intramedullary instrumentation, rheumatoid arthritis, total hip arthroplasty using the technique of cementing femoral stems designed for press-fit application and bilateral total knee surgery.
- The incidence of FES in isolated long-bone fractures is 3 to 4% and the mortality rate associated with this condition is significant, ranging from 10 to 20%.
- Clinical and laboratory signs of FES have been classified by ***Gurd as major or minor***, with a diagnosis requiring at least one major and four minor criteria, as well as the exclusion of other posttraumatic causes of hypoxemia.
- Symptoms usually occur 12 to 40 hours after the injury and can range from mild dyspnea to frank coma. Decreased arterial oxygen tension is the most consistent abnormal laboratory value.
- Fulminant episodes can occur within hours of the traumatic injury, causing severe hypoxemia, respiratory failure and severe neurologic impairment.
- Disseminated intravascular coagulation can also occur in conjunction with FES.

210. Ans. c. Disproportionate body dwarfism, d. Trident hand

[Ref: Maheswari 5th/316; Apley 9th/ 163-64; Robbins 9th/1184; Adam's Ouline of orthopaedics 14th/61]

Achondroplasia

- *Apley 9th/ 163-64; Adam's Outline of orthopaedics 14th/61*
- *Disproportionately short limb (rhizomelic shortening)*
- *The fingers appear stubby & somewhat splayed (**trident hands**)*

- ***AD transmission***
- A trident hand is a description where the hands are short with stubby fingers, with a separation between the middle and ring fingers.
- trident hand = separation of 2nd + 3rd digit and inability to approximate 3rd + 4th finger- *Danhert Radiology 6th/Chap1*
- There is no mental impairment

Achondroplasia

Maheswari 5th/316

- ***Dwarfism is disproportionate***; the limbs being out of proportion with the trunk. Shortening is especially marked in the proximal segments of the limbs.
- ***Intelligence is normal.***
- Typically, the patient has a large skull with a bulging vault and forehead, a flat nose, short limbs, ***short and stubby fingers*** and increased lumbar lordosis.
- These patients lead a near normal life, except for a few who develop spinal canal stenosis

Achondroplasia

Robbins 9th/1184

- **Achondroplasia is the most common skeletal dysplasia and a major cause of dwarfism.** ***It is an autosomal dominant disorder*** resulting in retarded cartilage growth.
- Affected individuals have shortened proximal extremities, a trunk of relatively normal length and an enlarged head with bulging forehead and conspicuous depression of the root of the nose.
- The skeletal abnormalities are usually not associated with ***changes in longevity, intelligence, or reproductive status.***

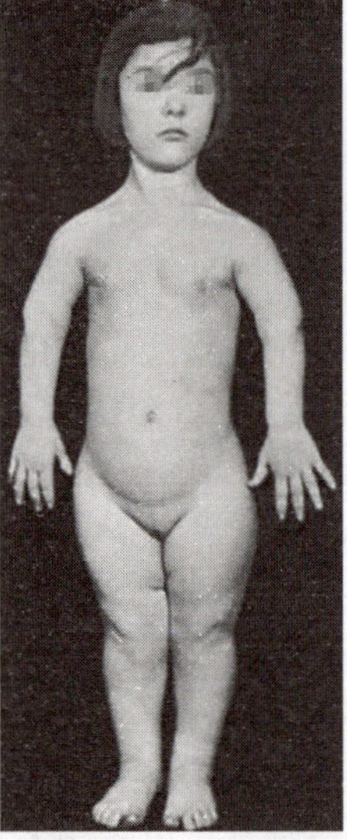

Fig: Achondroplasia, showing the typical features in a child. The dwarfing is due to shortness of the limbs, especially in their proximal segments; development of the trunk is but little impaired. Note the ***'trident' hands.*** (*Adam's Outline of orthopaedics 14th/61*)

211. Ans. a. Pain during active movement of the joint

[Ref: Harrison 19th/2216; Maheswari 5th/177]

Inflammatory Versus Noninflammatory Arthritis

Harrison 19th/2216

- Inflammatory disorders may be infectious (*Neisseria gonorrhoeae* or *Mycobacterium tuberculosis*), crystal-induced (gout, pseudogout), immune-related (rheumatoid arthritis [RA], systemic lupus erythematosus [SLE]), reactive (rheumatic fever, reactive arthritis), or idiopathic.
- Inflammatory disorders may be identified by any of the four cardinal signs of inflammation (***erythema, warmth, pain, or swelling***), systemic symptoms (***fatigue, fever, rash, weight loss***), or laboratory evidence of inflammation (elevated erythrocyte sedimentation rate [ESR] or C-reactive protein [CRP], thrombocytosis, anemia of chronic disease, or hypoalbuminemia).
- ***Articular stiffness commonly accompanies chronic musculo-skeletal disorders. The duration of stiffness may be prolonged (hours) with inflammatory disorders (such as RA or polymyalgia rheumatica) and may improve with activity.***
- By contrast, ***intermittent stiffness (also known as gel phenomenon) is typical of noninflammatory conditions (such as osteoarthritis [OA]), shorter in duration (<60 min) and exacerbated by activity.***
- **Noninflammatory disorders** are often characterized by *pain without synovial swelling or warmth, absence of inflammatory or systemic features, daytime gel phenomena rather than morning stiffness and normal (for age) or negative laboratory investigations.*

What are the Results of Joint Inflammation

www.webmd.com

- Increased blood flow and release of these chemicals attract white blood cells to the sites of inflammation.
- The ***increased number of cells and inflammatory substances*** within the joint can cause irritation, wearing down of cartilage (cushions at the end of bones) and swelling of the joint lining (synovium)

Symptoms of Inflammation

www.webmd.com

- Redness
- Joint swelling
- Joint pain
- Joint stiffness
- Loss of joint function

Often, only a few of these symptoms are present.

Inflammation may also be Associated with General "Flu"-Like Symptoms Including

www.webmd.com

- Fever
- Chills
- Fatigue/loss of energy
- Headaches
- Loss of appetite
- Muscle stiffness

Table: **Synovial fluid examination** (*Maheswari 5th/177)*

Points	Normal	Non-inflammatory	Inflammatory	Septic
Gross examination				
• Volume (ml)	Often < 3.5 ml	Often > 3.5 ml	Often > 3.5 ml	>3.5 ml.
• Viscosity	High	High	Low	Variable
• Colour	Colourless	Straw yellow	Yellow	Variable
• Clarity	Transparent	Transparent	Translucent	Opaque
Examination in lab.				
• WBC count	< 200	200-2000	2000-7500	> 10000
• PMN leucocytes	< 25%	< 25%	> 50%	> 75%
• Culture	–	–	–	+
• Mucin clot	Firm	Firm	Friable	Friable
• Glucose level	Equal to blood glucose	Nearly equal to blood glucose	< 25 mg% of blood glucose	> 25 mg% of blood glucose
Crystal examination:	Positive in Gout–Sodium biurate,		Positive in Pseudogout–Ca pyrophosphate	

212. Ans. a. Posterior rib fracture, b. Scapula fracture, d. Multiple fractures at different stages of healing

[Ref: Reddy 34th/417-18; www.aafp.org]

Table: **Fracture Types and Their Association with Child Abuse** *(www.aafp.org)*

Likelihood of Nonaccidental Trauma		
Low	**Moderate**	**High**
Clavicular fracture	Multiple fractures, especially bilateral	Metaphyseal lesion
Long-bone shaft fracture	Fractures of different ages Posterior rib fracture	
Linear skull fracture	Vertebral body fracture/subluxation	Scapular fracture
	Digital fracture	Spinous process fracture
	Complex skull fracture	Sternal fracture
	Epiphyseal separation	

When Is a Fracture Suspicious for Child Abuse

◈ *pediatrics.aappublications.org*

- No history of injury
- History of injury not plausible—mechanism described not consistent with the type of fracture, the energy load needed to cause the fracture, or the severity of the injury
- Inconsistent histories or changing histories provided by caregiver
- Fracture in a nonambulatory child
- Fracture of high specificity for child abuse (e.g., rib fractures)
- Multiple fractures
- Fractures of different ages
- Other injuries suspicious for child abuse
- Delay in seeking care for an injury

Battered baby syndrome or Caffey's syndrome or child abuse

◈ *Injuries: Reddy 34th/417-18*

- Skull fractures are common in occipitoparietal area, The fractures are multiple, depressed and wide. Large periosteal haematomas are common because periosteum is readily stripped in infants. Bleeding under the periosteum causes calcification, which is seen on X-ray as an extra line of opacity running alongside the affected length of bone.
- The violent forces applied to the limbs involve pulling and twisting, both capable of producing epiphyseal separation and periosteal shearing. Transverse and spiral fractures of long bones result from compression, bending and direct forcible blows.
- Anteroposterior compression of the chest causes ***fractures of ribs in midaxillary line***. Violent squeezing of the chest from side to side causes fractures at the ***costochondral junctions***.
- ***Multiple rib fractures also occur along the posterior angles of the ribs.*** After one to two weeks, callus is formed and on X-ray" a string of beads" appearance is seen in the paravertebral gutter (NOBBING FRACTURES). Avulsion of the metaphysis or chipping of the edges of the metaphyses or epiphyses may occur, with small fragments seen isolated on X-ray
- *Before autopsy, a whole body X-ray should be taken to detect* ***old fractures & especially metaphyseal & epiphyseal injuries in various stages of healing***

213. Ans. c. Passive smoking, d. Positive family history, e. Hypercoagulation state

[Ref: Maheswari 5th/318; Apley 9th/511-14; www.dovemed.com]

Legg-Calvé-Perthes disease (LCP, Perthes disease) CDTO 4th/Chap 11;

◈ *Apley 9th/511-14*

- It is a serious but self-limited pediatric hip disorder. Although its cause is unknown, the disease is thought to be related to avascular necrosis of the hip.

- It affects children between 4 and 10 years of age and is somewhat more common in boys.
- Children with the disease are ***often small for their age and have retarded bone age***. The disease is generally unilateral.
- Newer investigations suggest that some cases of LCP might be related to a variety of transient or permanent ***hypercoagulation states***. This research is not yet been confirmed in multiple centers. Surprisingly, trauma is not considered a causative factor in LCP

Table: Risk Factors for Perthes disease *online.epocrates.com/diseases*

Strong	Weak
Male sex	Urban population
Age 4 to 8 years	Eskimos, Japanese, some central European races
Socioeconomic deprivation	Transient hip synovitis
Hypercoagulable states	Hip joint effusion
	Passive smoking
	Skeletal dysplasia
	Congenital anomalies
	Trisomy 21
	Behavior disorders
	Endocrinopathy

LCPD (Legg-Calve Perthes Disease)

◈ *www.dovemed.com*

- It is a rare, but painful condition that develops in childhood, when blood supply to the ball portion of the hip joint (the femoral head) is temporarily disrupted
- Without sufficient supply of blood, the hip joint dies causing severe irritation and inflammation
- Perthes Disease may occur in children of any gender, race and ethnic group. However, Caucasian, Asian and Eskimo children are at a higher risk
- Boys, between the ages of 4 and 10 years, have the highest rate of incidence
- Common risk factors associated with Perthes Disease include:
  - Children between the ages of 4-8 years old
  - Boys are more likely to develop this condition, than girls, in a 5:1 ratio
  - Family history of Perthes Disease
- It is important to note that having a risk factor does not mean that one will get the condition. A risk factor increases ones chances of getting a condition compared to an individual without the risk factors. Some risk factors are more important than others.
- Also, not having a risk factor does not mean that an individual will not get the condition. It is always important to discuss the effect of risk factors with your healthcare provider.
- Signs and symptoms of Perthes Disease include:
  - Pain within the hip, knee
  - Pain in the thigh and groin
  - Disproportionate leg length
  - Reduced range of motion within the hip, difficulty walking
  - Stiffness of the hip

214. Ans. a. Supracondylar fracture of humerus can be managed by closed reduction, b. Displaced lateral condylar fracture of humerus-Open reduction & internal fixation, c. Lateral condylar fracture of humerus is known as fracture of necessity, e. Forearm fracture in children can be managed by closed reduction & casting

[Ref: Maheswari 5th/109, 97-99; Apley 9th/ 763]

Medial Epicondyle Fracture of Humerus

◈ *Maheswari 5th/105; Apley 9th/ 764*

- Treatment is generally conservative, by immobilisation in an above-elbow slab
- If displaced into the joint, it may require open reduction & internal fixation

"Fracture of **lateral condyle of humerus** in paediatric age group is notorious for non union. Attempts to treat these fractures usually lead to displacement and requiring open reduction and internal fixation. Hence these fractures are called "Fracture of necessity"- http:jorjournal.com/wp-content

Supracondylar Fracture of Humerus

◈ *Maheswari 5th/97-99*

- Undisplaced fracture: Immobilisation in an above-elbow plaster slab
- Displaced fracture (1) Closed reduction & percutaneous K-wire fixation, (2) Open reduction & K-wire fixation

Lateral Condylar Fracture of Humerus

◈ *Maheswari 5th/103; Apley 9th/ 763*

- *Undisplaced fracture:* Immobilisation in an above-elbow plaster slab for 2-3 week
- *Displaced fracture: Open reduction & internal fixation using two K-wires*

Fracture of Forearm Bones

◈ *Maheswari 5th/109*

- There may be fracture of either radius or ulna or both
- In children, these fractures are often undisplaced or minimally displaced, but in adults they are notoriously prone to severe displacement
- Conservative treatment is sufficient in most cases. This consists of closed reduction by manipulation under GA & immobilisation in an above-elbow plaster cast
- For adults with displaced fractures, operative treatment is often required

215. Ans. b. L5

[Ref: Maheswari 5th/255; Apley 9th/821-23; Campbell's Operative Orthopaedics, 11th/Chap 39]

- These 3 references & many websites advocates that in L4-L5 disc prolapse, ***only L5 nerve root is compressed***
- "***Fifth lumbar nerve*** is impinged upon by a prolapse b/w L4 & L5"-Adam's Outline of Orthopaedics 14th/236

Table: ***Neurological deficit in disc prolapse*** *(Maheswari 5th/255)*

Level	Nerve root affected	Motor weakness	Sensory loss	Reflexes
L_3-S_1	S1 root	Weakness of plantar flexors of the foot	Over lateral side of the foot	Ankle jerk sluggish or absent
L_4-L_5	L5 root	Weakness of EHL* and dorsiflexors of the foot	Over dorsum of foot and lateral side of the leg	Ankle jerk normal
L_3-L_4	L4 root	Weakness of extensors of the knee	Over great toe and medial side of the leg	Knee jerk sluggish or absent

*EHL: *extensor halluces longus*

"***Unilateral disc herniation between L4 and L5 results in compression of the L5 root.*** L5 root radiculopathy should produce pain in the dermatomal pattern. Numbness, when present, follows the L5 dermatome along the anterolateral aspect of the leg and the dorsum of the foot, including the great toe. The autonomous zone for this nerve is the dorsal first web of the foot and the dorsum of the third toe. Weakness may involve the extensor hallucis longus (L5), gluteus medius (L5), or extensor digitorum longus and brevis (L5). Reflex change usually is not found. A diminished posterior tibial reflex is possible, but difficult to elicit"- Campbell's Operative Orthopaedics, 11th/Chap 39

L5 Root Compression

◈ *(Campbell's Operative Orthopaedics, 11th/Chap 39)*

- Sensory Deficit
  - Anterolateral leg, dorsum of the foot and great toe
- Motor Weakness
  - Extensor hallucis longus
  - Gluteus medius
  - Extensor digitorum longus and brevis
- Reflex Change
  - Usually none
  - Posterior tibial (difficult to elicit)

216. Ans. a. Dual-Energy X-ray Absorptiometry (DEXA) scan will help to assess osteoporosis and osteopenia in children; b. Bisphosphonates can be given to children to prevent skeletal damage, c. Can present as lethal skeletal dysplasia

[Ref: Maheswari 5th/316; Apley 9th/ 172-74; Robbins 9th/1185;Harrison 19th/2509]

"Children with severe OI may be treated medically with cyclical bisphosphonates to increase bone mineral density & reduce the tendency to fracture"-*Apley 9th/ 172*

Bisphosphonates show Promise for Decreasing the Incidence of Fractures"

◈ *CPDT 17th/813*

"Radiographs reveal cortical bone thinning and excessive trabecular bone transparency. This finding, however, is subjective and may be difficult to assess with conventional radiography and its detection requires a significant reduction (about 30 to 50%) in calcified bone mass. Bone densitometry by dual-energy X-ray absorptiometry (DEXA) is currently the optimal method to detect decreased bone mineral density, but in children, accurate interpretation of the results requires a good knowledge of the potential pitfalls related to age, sex, pubertal stage and skeletal maturation. Decreased bone mineral density is not specific for OI; it may be encountered in metabolic disorders (hypogonadism, growth hormone deficiency, hyperthyroidism, juvenile diabetes mellitus, calcium and vitamin D deficiency, etc.). However, when such causes have been excluded, DEXA may help to establish the diagnosis of OI and to monitor the response to bisphosphonates-*www.ncbi.nlm.nih.gov*

Table: **Characteristics of Osteogenesis Imperfecta** *(pediatrics.aappublications.org)*

Fragile bones with few, some, or many of the following findings:
• Poor linear growth
• Macrocephaly
• Triangular-shaped face
• Blue sclerae
• Hearing impairment as a result of otosclerosis
• Hypoplastic, translucent, carious, late-erupting, or discolored teeth
• Easy bruisability
• Inguinal and/or umbilical hernias
• Limb deformities
• Hyperextensible joints
• Scoliosis and/or kyphosis
• Wormian bones of the skull
• Demineralized bones

Diagnosis

◈ *Harrison 19th/2509-10*

- OI is usually diagnosed on the basis of clinical criteria. The presence of fractures together with blue sclerae, dentinogenesis imperfecta, or family history of the disease is usually sufficient to make the diagnosis.
- X-rays usually reveal a ***decrease in bone density that can be verified by photon or x-ray absorptiometry***. Bone microscopy can be helpful in the diagnosis.
- The diagnosis, as in other genetic disorders, is now routinely determined using targeted candidate gene sequencing and exome sequencing, but whole-genome sequencing may be used in the future
- About half of children have a substantial increase in growth when given growth hormone.
- ***Treatment with bisphosphonates to decrease bone loss has been introduced for moderate to severe forms of OI***. Improvements in bone mineral density are consistently seen in patients. Some clinical trials observed improvements in bone pain and fracture incidence;

however, there are still unresolved questions about the best delivery protocols and the risks associated with long-term use in OI patients.

- For these reasons, the current consensus is that bisphosphonate therapy should be restricted to moderate to severe OI, where the possible benefits outweigh risks. Also, a clinical trial was performed in which patients were treated by intravenous infusion of cells from bone marrow referred to as mesenchymal stem cells, or multipotential stromal cell

Osteogenesis Imperffecta

◈ *(Fragilitas ossium, Vroliks disease) Maheswari 5th/316*

- This is a condition characterized by tendency for *frequent fractures* because of *weak and brittle* bones. It results from defective collagen synthesis and thus affects other collagen containing soft tissues such as the skin, sclera, teeth, ligaments etc., as well.
- The disease is ***commonly inherited as an autosomal dominant*** disorder, but a ***severe variant is known to occur where the inheritance is autosomal recessive.***
- Typically, the patient has a tendency for frequent fractures, usually with minimal trauma. Associated features are blue sclera, joint laxity and otosclerosis in adulthood.
- Patients with the ***severe type do not survive beyond a few years***, but those with the milder disease live their full life interrupted by frequent fractures.
- The fractures unite normally but deformities secondary to malunion or fracture often reduces with age.

Osteogenesis Imperfecta

◈ *Robbins 9th/1185*

- *Osteogenesis imperfecta (OI), also known as "brittle bone disease," is actually a group of genetic disorders caused by defective synthesis of type I collagen.* Because type I collagen is a major component of extracellular matrix in other parts of the body, there are also numerous extraskeletal manifestations (affecting skin, joints, teeth and eyes, for example).
- The mutations underlying OI characteristically involve the coding sequences for α1 or α2 chains of type I collagen. Because collagen synthesis and extracellular export require formation of a complete and intact triple helix, any primary defect in a collagen chain tends to disrupt the entire structure and results in its premature degradation (an example of a *dominant negative mutation*). As a consequence, ***most defects manifest as autosomal dominant disorders*** and may be associated with severe malformations. There is, however, a broad spectrum of severity and mutations that result in qualitatively normal collagen but at only reduced levels generally have milder manifestations.
- *The fundamental abnormality in all forms of OI is too little bone,* resulting in extreme skeletal fragility. Four major subtypes are recognized. The type II variant is uniformly fatal in utero or immediately postpartum as a consequence of multiple fractures that occur before birth. By contrast, patients with type I OI have a normal lifespan, with only a modestly increased proclivity for fractures during childhood (decreasing in frequency after puberty). The classic finding of *blue sclerae* in type I OI is attributable to decreased scleral collagen content; this deficit causes a relative transparency that allows the underlying choroid to be seen.
- *Hearing loss* can be related to conduction defects in the middle and inner ear bones and *small misshapen teeth* are a result of dentin deficiency.

Table: Imperfecta osteogenesis of subtypes *(Robbins 9th/1185)*

Subtype	Inheritance	Major clinical features	Prognosis
I	Autosomal dominant	Postnatal fractures, blue sclera Normal stature; Skeletal fragility Dentinogenesis imperfecta Hearing impairment Joint laxity Blue sclerae	Compatible with survival
II	Most autosomal recessive some autosomal dominant new mutations	Death in utero or within days of birth skeletal deformity with excessive fragility and multiple fractures blue sclera Blue sclera	Perinatal lethal
III	Autosomal dominant (75%) Autosomal recessive (25%)	Compatible with survival Growth retardation Multiple fractures Progressive kyphoscoliosis Blue sclera at birth that become white Heating impairment dentinogenesis imperfecta	Progressive deforming

217. Ans. a. Most common cause is E. coli

[Ref: Apley 9th/43-45; Maheshwari 5th/175-78; Harrison 19th/833-34]

Septic Arthritis

◈ *Maheshwari 5th/175*

- ***Staphylococcus aureus is the commonest causative organism.*** Other organisms are streptococcus pneumococcus & gonococcus
- It is ***more common in children*** & males are more susceptible
- Knee is the commonest joint affected
- ***Joint aspiration is the quickest & the best method of diagnosing septic arthritis***

Infectious Arthritis

◈ *Harrison 19th/833-34*

- Although *Staphylococcus aureus*, *Neisseria gonorrhoeae* and other bacteria are the most common causes of infectious arthritis, various mycobacteria, spirochetes, fungi and viruses also infect joints

- Since acute bacterial infection can destroy articular cartilage rapidly, all inflamed joints must be evaluated without delay to exclude noninfectious processes and determine appropriate antimicrobial therapy and drainage procedures.
- Aspiration of synovial fluid—an essential element in the evaluation of potentially infected joints—can be performed without difficulty in most cases by the insertion of a large-bore needle into the site of maximal fluctuance or tenderness or by the route of easiest access. Ultrasonography or fluoroscopy may be used to guide aspiration of difficult-to-localize effusions of the hip and, occasionally, the shoulder and other joints.
- The usual presentation consists of moderate to severe pain that is uniform around the joint, effusion, muscle spasm and decreased range of motion.
- Plain radiographs show evidence of soft-tissue swelling, joint space widening and displacement of tissue planes by the distended capsule. Narrowing of the joint space and bony erosions indicate advanced infection and a poor prognosis.
- Ultrasound is useful for detecting effusions in the hip and CT or MRI can demonstrate infections of the sacroiliac joint, the sternoclavicular joint and the spine very well.

ANESTHESIA

218. Ans. a. Apparent source of blood stream infection present other than catheter

[Ref: www.ncbi.nlm.nih.gov; www.idsociety.org; academic.oup.com]

Catheter-related Bloodstream Infection (CRBSI, also Called Catheter-related sepsis)

- CRBSI is defined as the presence of bacteraemia originating from an i.v. catheter. It is one of the most frequent, lethal and costly complications of central venous catheterization.
- It is also the most common cause of nosocomial bacteraemia. Although the use of central venous catheters (CVC) is increasing, there is evidence that the problem of CRBSI can be reduced
- CRBSI is unlikely in the first 3–4 days of catheterization; thereafter it is likely that the risk incidence (risk per catheter per day) is constant, although the cumulative incidence increases over time.
- Majority of CRBSIs are associated with CVCs and in prospective studies, the relative risk for CRBSI is up to 64 times greater with CVCs than with peripheral venous catheters.
- Detection of CRBSI includes both clinical as well as laboratory examination.
- The diagnosis of CRBSI is often suspected clinically in a patient using a CVC who presents with fever or chills, unexplained hypotension and no other localizing sign.

Laboratory Diagnosis of Catheter Related Bloodstream Infections

- The diagnosis of CRBSI requires a positive culture of blood from a peripheral vein and clear evidence that the catheter is the source.
- CRBSI means a patient with an intravascular catheter has at least one positive blood culture obtained from a peripheral vein, clinical manifestations of infections (i.e., fever, chills and/or hypotension) and ***no apparent source for the BSI, except the catheter.***
- In addition, one of the following is also present: A positive semi-quantitative (>15 CFU/catheter segment) or quantitative (>10^3CFU/catheter segment) catheter tip culture also, the same organism (species and anti-biogram) is isolated from the catheter segment and peripheral blood culture.
- ***Simultaneous quantitative paired blood cultures with a >5:1 ratio CVC versus peripheral, or differential time to positivity, whereby a non-quantitative blood culture drawn from the CVC that becomes positive at least 2 hr earlier than the peripheral blood culture, is a new method for the diagnosis of CRBSI without removing the catheter***

Quantitative Paired Blood Culture

- CRBSI is defined as a ***quantitative blood culture ratio of >5:1 (CVC versus peripheral***) with proven identity of isolates from positive peripheral and CVC blood cultures confirmed by pulsed-field gel electrophoresis.
- CRBSI can be diagnosed when colony counts are at least 3-fold higher in cultures of blood obtained via the CVC than in cultures of blood taken from a peripheral vein. The fold difference between the CVC and peripheral blood varies in the literature with suggested cuts offs from 3-fold to 10-fold.
- To diagnose CRBSI with the CVC *in situ*, most experts recommend comparative blood cultures obtained via the CVC and a peripheral vein prior to initiating antibiotics. Cultures should be obtained from all lumens of the CVC, it is the most specific method of diagnosing CRBSI. If a blood sample cannot be drawn from a peripheral vein, it is recommended that 2 blood samples should be drawn through different catheter lumens and the colony count for the blood sample drawn through one lumen is at least 3-fold greater than the colony count for the blood sample obtained from the second lumen should be considered to indicate possible CRBSI.

Differential Time to Positivity

- CRBSI is suggested when blood from the ***CVC demonstrates microbial growth at least 2 h earlier than growth is detected in blood collected*** simultaneously from a peripheral vein. Most currently used automated blood culture systems can readily provide this information and it is likely that this will become a standard diagnostic test.

Short-term Catheters, Including Arterial Catheters

- For short-term catheter tip cultures, the roll plate technique is recommended for routine clinical microbiological analysis. For suspected pulmonary artery catheter infection, the introducer tip is cultured.

Long-term Catheters

- Semi-quantitative growth of 15 cfu/catheter segment of the same microbe from both the insertion site culture and the catheter hub culture strongly suggests that the catheter is the source of a bloodstream infection. A venous access subcutaneous port is removed for suspected CRBSI and the port is sent to the microbiology laboratory for qualitative culture of the port reservoir contents, in addition to the catheter tip

219. Ans. **a. SCV catheterisation is have lesser success rate in first attempt; d. IJV catheterization is easy for inexperienced hand; e. SCV catheterisation associated with more pneumothorax**

[Ref: Morgan Anaesthesia 5th/100; Lee13th/ 231-32; Miller Anaesthesia 7th/Chap40]

Techniques & Complications

◈ *Morgan 5th/100*

- Central venous cannulation involves introducing a catheter into a vein so that the catheter's tip lies with the venous system within the thorax. Generally, the optimal location of the catheter tip is just superior to or at the junction of the superior vena cava and the right atrium. When the catheter tip is located within the thorax, inspiration will increase or decrease CVP, depending on whether ventilation is controlled or spontaneous. Measurement of CVP is made with a water column (cm H2O), or, preferably, an electronic transducer (mm Hg). The pressure should be measured during end expiration.
- Various sites can be used for cannulation.
- All cannulation sites have an increased risk of line-related infections the longer the catheter remains in place.
- Compared with other sites, the ***subclavian vein is associated with a greater risk of pneumothorax during insertion, but a reduced risk of other complications during prolonged cannulations*** (e.g., in critically ill patients).
- The **right internal jugular vein** provides a ***combination of accessibility and safety.***
- **Left-sided internal jugular vein** catheterization has an ***increased risk of pleural effusion and chylothorax***

Table: Relative rating of central venous access* *(Morgan 5th/101)*

	Basilic	External Jugular	Internal Jugular	Subclavian	Femoral
Ease of cannulation	1	3	2	5	3
Long-term use	4	3	2	1	5
Success rate (pulmonary artery catheter placement)	4	5	1	2	3
Complications (technique-related)	1	2	4	5	3

***In each category, 1=best, 5=worst**

Subclavian Vein

◈ *Miller Anaesthesia 7th/Chap40*

- The subclavian vein is an important site for central venous cannulation and is particularly popular among surgeons and other physicians who place central venous catheters for emergency volume resuscitation and long-term intravenous therapy or dialysis rather than for shorter-term monitoring purposes.
- Advantages of subclavian venous cannulation include a ***lower risk of infection than with internal jugular or femoral sites, ease of insertion in trauma patients who may be immobilized in a cervical collar and increased patient comfort, especially for long-term intravenous therapy such as hyperalimentation and chemotherapy.***
- Of greatest importance, however, the clinician should resist the temptation to make multiple needle passes if the subclavian vein is not punctured on the second or third attempt. It is clear that complications from this procedure, particularly the incidence of pneumothorax and subclavian artery puncture, are directly related to the number of attempts.
- Bilateral attempts at subclavian venipuncture are highly discouraged because of the serious morbidity of ***bilateral pneumothorax and the difficulty detecting and treating injury to the subclavian artery. Perhaps to an even greater degree than with internal jugular vein cannulation, the safety of subclavian venous line placement rests in the experience of the operator.*** In more practiced hands, the incidence of complications should be low, with pneumothorax developing in less than 2% and arterial puncture in less than 5% of cases

"The internal jugular vein is often the access site of choice for central venous cannulation. **Advantages** include a *superficial location, easy ultrasonic visualization and a straight course to the superior vena cava (on the right).* Internal jugular cannulation avoids the subclavian "pinch-off syndrome". Furthermore, for renal failure patients, it avoids potential subclavian vein stenosis which would preclude use of the extremity for hemodialysis access via arteriovenous shunt/fistula"- *www.ncbi.nlm.nih.gov*

"The **subclavian vein,** long favored by surgeons, offers an alternative to the internal jugular vein for central venous access. It may be associated with ***fewer infectious complications than the internal jugular vein*** and will remain accessible after localized thrombosis of the internal jugular vein. Well-designed studies comparing the internal jugular and subclavian approaches are sparse. Review of multiple nonrandomized studies suggests the ***arterial puncture is more frequent with the internal jugular approach,*** catheter malposition is more frequent with the subclavian approach and the incidences of pneumothorax, hemothorax and thrombosis are equivalent"- *www.ncbi.nlm.nih.gov*

"The **subclavian vein** access has been the standard recommended approach for central venous catheterization both for short and long term use. The advantages are attributed to its large size, patient comfort and lowest rate of catheter related infections. It also carries a lower risk of thrombosis when compared to femoral or internal jugular vein cannulation"- *www.apicareonline.com*

220. Ans. **a. Scrub room; b. Anesthesia Induction Room**

[Ref: www.peerlesshospital.com/services/ot.html]

Zones of Operation Theatre

◈ *www.peerlesshospital.com/services/ot.html*

- For an unbreachable sterile OT compound, it has been segregated in various zones which are area of varying degrees of cleanliness in which the bacteriological count progressively diminishes from the outer to the inner zones (operating area) and is maintained by a differential decreasing positive pressure ventilation gradient from the inner zone to the outer zone. They are of following types.
- ***Protective Zone: Areas included in this zone are:***
  - Reception
  - Waiting area
  - Trolley bay
  - Changing room
- ***Clean Zone: Areas included in this zone are:***
  - Pre-op room
  - Recovery room
  - Plaster room
  - Staff room
  - Store
- ***Sterile Zone: Areas included in this zone are:***
  - Operating Suite
  - Scrub Room
  - Anesthesia Induction Room
  - Set up Room
- ***Disposal Zone: Areas included in this zone are:***
  - Dirty Utility
  - Disposal corridor

Criteria for Zoning

◈ *www.shareyouressays.com/115980/zoning*

The aim of zoning is that when staff members, patients or supplies enter the OT suite, the risk factors of carrying the chances of infection with them get lesser and lesser, as they pass from the protective through clean to aseptic zone.

- **Sterile Zone:** The OT suite organisation revolves around the central aseptic work area, i.e. the actual operating rooms. Activities take place in these zones that require full aseptic conditions, such as exposure of living tissues and handling sterile instruments. Here, the highest level of cleanliness and aseptic condition are maintained.
- **Clean Zone:** The clean zone is designed around the aseptic zone. This zone is only accessible to staff having changed their outer clothing in the protective zone and prepared patients transferred from the ward trolley to OT stretcher and clean supplies. 'Patient holding and preparation area' is earmarked in the clean zone.
- **Protective zone:** Outside the clean zone is the protective zone forming a barrier between the clean area of the suite and the less clean rest of the hospital area. This zone contains the administration" elements including theatre nurse supervisor's office, where stores are received and personnel enter the department, where locker and change rooms are located, patients are received and held.
- **Disposal zone:** Disposal zone is the corridor from where used instruments and used linen and operating room debris is taken out. This zone must have an independent access to the outside corridor. Disposal zone has only one-way traffic, viz. from inside the operating room to the outside and never vice versa

221. Ans. a. Ephedrine; b. Adrenaline c. Dopamine; d. Phenylephrine; e. Mephentermine

[Ref: Ajay Yadav 6th/170; Morgan Anaesthesia 5th/946;Lee13th/510; Miller Anaesthesia 7th/1617]

Four Most Commonly used Sympathomimetics in Hypotension During Central Neuraxial Blockade

◈ *Lee13th/510*

- ***Epinephrine(adrenaline)***
- ***Phenylephrine***
- *Metaraminol*
- ***Ephedrine***

Treatment of Hypotension During Spinal Anesthesia

◈ *Ajay Yadav 6th/170*

- *Ephedrine is most preferred vasopressor for treatment of spinal anesthesia. However, mephentermine is more frequently used in India*
- *Other vasopressor which can be used are methoxamine, phenylephrine, metaraminol & ephinephrine as vasopressor of last resort*
- **Inotropes (dopamine, dobutamine): The inotropes only benefit by improving the cardiac output therefore are hardly ever used**

Ephedrine is the drug most commonly used to treat hypotension. Dopamine, in low-to-moderate doses, has also been shown to correct the hemodynamic changes induced by central neuraxial block. Dopamine may be preferable to ephedrine for long-term infusion because tachyphylaxis can develop to repeated ephedrine boluses. Pure α-adrenergic agonists, most commonly **phenylephrine**, are also used to correct hypotension during spinal anesthesia."-*Barash Anesthesia 6th/Chap 37*

222. Ans. a. Succinylcholine; b. Methoxyflurane; c. Pancuronium

[Ref: KDT 7th/353; Ajay Yadav 6th/203; Morgan Anaesthesia 5th/659; Lee13th/ 802; Miller Anaesthesia 7th/Chap 65]

- "**Renal disease:** ***Desflurane is the inhalational agent of choice*** *because it does not produce fluoride"- Ajay Yadav 6th/203*
- "**Renal disease**: *As these patients exhibit hyperkalemia,* ***succinylcholine should not be used****"- Ajay Yadav 6th/203*
- "**Cisatracurium and atracurium** are degraded by plasma ester hydrolysis and nonenzymatic Hofmann elimination. These agents are often the ***drugs of choice for muscle relaxation in patients with kidney failure***, especially in clinical situations where neuromuscular function monitoring is difficult or impossible"- *Morgan Anaesthesia 5th/659*
- "**Pancuronium** is primarily dependent on renal excretion (60–90%). Although pancuronium is metabolized by the liver into less active intermediates, its elimination half-life is still primarily dependent on renal excretion (60–80%).

Neuromuscular function should be ***closely monitored if these agents are used in patients with abnormal renal function***"- *Morgan Anaesthesia 5th/660*

Approximately 40% to 50% of **pancuronium** is excreted in urine. A portion of this excretion occurs after biotransformation to the less active metabolite 3-hydroxypancuronium. Pancuronium has a prolonged terminal elimination half-life in patients with reduced renal function, so it should be ***administered cautiously, particularly when several doses are required***-*Miller Anaesthesia 7th/Chap 65*

- **Anesthetic Agents in Renal Failure**: With the exception ***of methoxyflurane and possibly enflurane***, anesthetic agents do not directly cause renal dysfunction or interfere with the normal compensatory mechanisms activated by the stress response. The nephrotoxicity of methoxyflurane appears to be due to its metabolism, which results in release of the ***fluoride ions*** believed responsible for the renal injury"- Barash 6th/Chap 52

"Muscle relaxants are the most likely group of drugs used in anesthetic practice to produce prolonged effects in ESRD because of their dependence on renal excretion. ***Only succinylcholine, atracurium, cis-atracurium and mivacurium appear to have minimal renal excretion of the unchanged parent compound***"- *Miller Anaesthesia 7th/Chap 65*

- **Succinylcholine** can be safely used in patients with kidney failure in the absence of hyperkalemia at the time of induction. When serum potassium is known to be increased or is in doubt, a nondepolarsing muscle relaxant should be substituted"-*Morgan 5th/659*

223. Ans. **a. Lidocaine is used for awake intubation; b. Bupivacaine-more cardiotoxic & longer acting than lidociane; c. Intralipid is used for cardiotoxicity of bupivacaine; d. Ropivacaine- used in peripheral nerve block;**

[Ref: Ajay Yadav 6th/151-56; Morgan Anaesthesia 5th/274;Lee13th/ 381; KDT 8th/391]

- "**Bupivacaine**- ***long acting(2-3hr),*** lidocaine-medium acting (30-90 min)- *Lee13th/ 381; Morgan Anaesthesia 5th/272*
- ***Bupivacaine is far more cardiotoxic than lignocaine***- *Ajay Yadav 6th/156*
- "**Bupivacainecardiotoxicity**: ***Intralipid is used****. Intralipid binds the active form of bupivacaine"- Ajay Yadav 6th/157*
- ***Cocaine cause Hypertension***-*KDT 8th/391*
- **Ropivacaine** is used for spinal, epidural, infiltration , ***peripheral nerve block***"-*Morgan Anaesthesia 5th/272*

What Nerve Blocks Could be Helpful During Awake Intubation?

◈ *Morgan Anaesthesia 5th/338*

- The lingual and some pharyngeal branches of the glossopharyngeal nerve that provide sensation to the posterior third of the tongue and oropharynx are easily blocked by ***bilateral injection of 2 mL of local anesthetic*** into the base of the palatoglossal arch (also known as the anterior tonsillar pillar) with a 25-gauge spinal needle.
- Bilateral **superior laryngeal nerve blocks** and a transtracheal block would anesthetize the airway below the epiglottis. The hyoid bone is located and ***3 mL of 2% lidocaine*** is infiltrated 1 cm below each greater cornu, where the internal branch of the superior laryngeal nerves penetrates the thyrohyoid membrane.
- A transtracheal block is performed by identifying and penetrating the CTM while the neck is extended. After confirmation of an intratracheal position by aspiration of air, ***4 mL of 4% lidocaine*** is injected into the trachea at end expiration. A deep inhalation and cough immediately following injection distribute the anesthetic throughout the trachea.
- Although these blocks may ***allow the awake patient to tolerate intubation better***, they also obtund protective cough reflexes, depress the swallowing reflex and may lead to aspiration. Topical anesthesia of the pharynx may induce a transient obstruction from the loss of reflex regulation of airway caliber at the level of the glottis

Cardiovascular Toxicity

◈ *Morgan Anaesthesia 5th/274*

- Unintentional intravascular injection of ***bupivacaine during regional anesthesia may produce severe cardiovascular toxicity***
- Multiple studies have demonstrated that bupivacaine is associated with more pronounced changes in conduction and a greater risk of terminal arrhythmias than comparable doses of lidocaine.
- Recent reports suggest that bolus administration of ***nutritional lipid solutions*** at 1.5 mL/kg can resuscitate bupivacaine-intoxicated patients who do not respond to standard therapy.

Table: Comparative features of commonly used local anesthetics *(KDT 8th/392)*

Drug	Relative potency	Onset	Duration (Min)	Cardio toxicity
Lidocaine	1	Fast	60-120	+
Bupivacaine	4-5	Inter-mediate	120-360	+++
Ropivacaine	3-4	Slow	120-300	++

224. Ans. **a. Succinylcholine is short acting muscle relaxant; b. Succinylcholine is used for rapid-sequence induction in full stomach patients; d. Rocuronium can be used for rapid-sequence induction**

[Ref: Ajay Yadav 6th/124,268; Morgan Anaesthesia 5th/200]

- "**Succinylcholine** is the ideal muscle relaxant for intubation however due to the side effects its use is only restricted to ***rapid sequence*** or difficult airway management situations"- *Ajay Yadav 6th/124*
- "Rocuronium (0.9–1.2 mg/kg) has an onset of action that approaches succinylcholine(60–90s), making it a suitable alternative for ***rapid-sequence inductions***, but at the cost of a much longer duration of action "-*Morgan Anaesthesia 5th/200*

- "**Rapid sequence induction (RSI)** is a method of achieving rapid control of the airway whilst minimising the risk of regurgitation and aspiration of gastric contents. Intravenous induction of anaesthesia, with the application of cricoid pressure, is swiftly followed by the placement of an endotracheal tube (ETT). For many decades, ***suxamethonium (succinylcholine) has been the standard of care for RSI***. Rocuronium is an alternative agent"- *http: anaesthesiology.gr*
- "**Day care surgeries:** Short duration of action(10 min) makes mivacurium as preferred muscle relaxant for day-care surgery. Succinylcholine, in spite of having short duration, is usually not preferred due to high incidence of postoperative myalgia"- *Ajay Yadav 6th/268*
- **Pancuronium** is ***long acting muscle relaxant*** (duration 60-120 min: KDT 8th/378; 30-40 min: *Ajay Yadav 6th/128*), ***so not used for day care surgery***
- **Muscle relaxant in paediatric patients**: *Atracurium & cis-atracurium are relaxant of choice as they are not dependent on hepatic & renal functions. Succinylcholine should be avoided in children*"- *Ajay Yadav 6th/239*

Table: A summary of the pharmacology of non-depolarizing muscle relaxants *(Morgan 5th/211)*

Relaxant	Metabolism	Primary Excretion	Onset[2]	Duration[3]	Histamine Release[2]	Vagal Blockade[3]
Atracurium	+++	Insignificant	++	++	+	0
Cisatracurium	+++	Insignificant	++	++	0	0
Pancuronium	+	Renal	++	+++	0	++
Vecuronium	+	Biliary	++	++	0	0
Rocuronium	Insignificant	Biliary	+++	++	0	+
Gantacurium	+++	Insignificant	+++	+	+	0

[1]Onset; +, slow; ++, moderately rapid; +++, rapid
[2]Duration: +, short; ++, intermediate; +++, long
[3]Histamine release: 0, no effect; +, slight effect; ++, moderate effect; +++, marked effect
[4]Vagal blockade: 0, no effect; +, slight effect; ++, moderate effect

225. Ans. b. In day care surgery, halothane is most commonly used inhalational agent

[Ref: Ajay Yadav 6th/99; Morgan Anaesthesia 5th/172]

Nonpungency and rapid increases in alveolar anesthetic concentration make sevoflurane an ***excellent choice for smooth and rapid inhalation inductions in pediatric*** and adult patients- *Morgan 5th/171*

"Faster, pleasant & smooth induction with no significant systemic toxicity ***makes sevoflurane as the agent of choice for induction in children, however due to high cost, halothane is still very commonly used agent for induction in India.*** *Isoflurane & desflurane have irritating induction & can produce severe laryngospasm therefore, must not be used for induction. But anesthesia is best maintained with desflurane "- Ajay Yadav 6th/239,99*

"Sevoflurane depresses respiration and ***reverses bronchospasm*** to an extent similar to that of isoflurane"- *Morgan Anaesthesia 5th/172*

"Because of bronchodialtion **Sevoflurane** *is the inhalational agent of choice for asthmatics in present day practice" Ajay Yadav 6th/99*

"Sevoflurane *is inhalational* ***agent of choice for hepatic patients***"- *Ajay Yadav 6th/99*

"Desflurane *has earliest induction & recovery, therefore, is the inhalational agent of choice for day-care patients. In case of non-availability of desflurane, sevoflurane serves as an excellent alternative"- Ajay Yadav 6th/268*

"Irritation during **desflurane** induction can be manifested by salivation, breath-holding, coughing and laryngospasm. ***Airway resistance may increase in children with reactive airway susceptibility.*** These problems make desflurane a poor choice for inhalation induction"- *Morgan's clinical aneasthesia 5th/170*

"United States Food and Drug Administration recommends the use of sevoflurane with fresh gas flow rates at least 1 L/min for exposures up to 1 hour and at least 2 L/min for exposures greater than 1 hour. The FDA was concerned that sevoflurane may cause adverse renal effects at low flows because it is degraded by the strong bases in CO^2 absorbents to fluoromethyl-2,2-difluoro-1-(trifluoromethyl) vinyl ether (compound A)"- *www. ncbi.nlm.nih.gov; Ajay Yadav 6th/100; Morgan Anaesthesia 5th/172*

226. Ans. c. Epinephrine (1 mg) is the DOC for cardiac arrest; d. Lidocaine may be considered as an alternative to amiodarone for unresponsive VF/pVT

[Ref: circ.ahajournals.org/]

- ***Unsynchronized cardioversion is used in ventricular fibrill-ation***

Synchronized Cardioversion

◈ *acls-algorithms.com*

- It is a LOW ENERGY SHOCK that uses a sensor to deliver electricity that is synchronized with the peak of the QRS complex (the highest point of the R-wave). When the "sync" option is engaged on a defibrillator and the shock button pushed, there will be a delay in the shock. During this delay, the machine reads and synchronizes with the patients ECG rhythm. This occurs so that the shock can be delivered with or just after the peak of the R-wave in the patients QRS complex

- The most common **indications** for synchronized cardioversion are unstable ***atrial fibrillation, atrial flutter, atrial tachycardia and supraventricular tachycardias***. If medications fail in the stable patient with the before mentioned arrhythmias, synchronized cardioversion will most likely be indicated.

Unsynchronized Cardioversion (Defibrillation)

◈ *acls-algorithms.com*

- It is a HIGH ENERGY shock which is delivered as soon as the shock button is pushed on a defibrillator. This means that the shock may fall randomly anywhere within the cardiac cycle (QRS complex).
- Unsynchronized cardioversion (defibrillation) is used when there is no coordinated intrinsic electrical activity in the heart (***pulseless VT/VF)*** or the defibrillator fails to synchronize in an unstable patient

Synchronized Cardioversion Versus Defibrillation

◈ *Acls.com/free resources*

- Both defibrillation and cardioversion impose a therapeutic dose of electrical energy on the myocardium. Defibrillation is used to treat certain types of arrhythmias (ventricular fibrillation and pulseless ventricular tachycardia) while cardioversion is used to treat others (i.e. unstable narrow and wide complex tachyarrhythmias such as atrial fibrillation, atrial flutter and ventricular tachycardia), but there is a very important distinction between the two.
- Defibrillation involves the use of a high energy shock which in *unsynchronized*; that is, the shock is delivered as soon as the shock button is pushed. As mentioned above, it is used to treat conditions such as pulseless monomorphic ventricle tachycardia and ventricular fibrillation.
- A synchronized shock is different because it is timed to be delivered at a specific period of time during the cardiac cycle. It is used to treat cardiac arrhythmias such as atrial flutter and atrial fibrillation when medications have failed to convert the rhythm, or when the patient is unstable and the rhythm must be immediately terminated.
- Success rates may vary for patients who undergo synchronized cardioversion. According to the National Heart, Lung and Blood Institute, the success rates of cardioversion are 75 percent or greater.
- The combined use of vasopressin and epinephrine offers no advantage to using standard-dose epinephrine in cardiac arrest.
- Also, vasopressin does not offer an advantage over the use of epinephrine alone. Therefore, to simplify the algorithm, vasopressin has been removed from the Adult Cardiac Arrest Algorithm–2015

2015 AHA BLS and ACLS Guidelines

◈ *alliedhealth.ceconnection.com*

- Based on their greater success in dysrhythmia termination, defibrillators using ***biphasic waveforms*** (biphasic truncated exponential or rectilinear biphasic) are ***preferred to monophasic defibrillators.***
- The recommended energy dose for **biphasic defibrillators** is 120 to 200 joules (J); if the manufacturer's recommended energy dose is unknown, using the maximum energy dose available should be considered. Subsequent defibrillation energy doses should be equivalent or higher.
- The shock energy dose for a **monophasic defibrillator** is 360 J.
- Perform CPR for 2 minutes after defibrillation and obtain I.V. or I.O. access if not already established. If VF/pVT persists with a rhythm check during the compressor role change at 2 minutes, defibrillate again. Biphasic doses can be equivalent to the first shock administered (120 to 200 J) or higher. Monophasic doses remain at 360 J. If the defibrillator unit is capable of escalating energies, it's reasonable to use them for the second and third shock.
- After the second defibrillation attempt, continue CPR for 2 minutes and administer ***I.V./I.O. epinephrine 1 mg.*** This dose may be repeated every 3 to 5 minutes. Epinephrine's vasoconstrictor effects, which increase coronary and cerebral perfusion pressure during CPR, are beneficial in cardiac arrest
- A **single dose of I.V./I.O. vasopressin** was an option to consider in pVT/VF, pulseless electrical activity (PEA) and asystole to replace either the first or second dose of I.V./I.O. epinephrine in the 2010 guidelines. However, ***one notable change in the 2015 guidelines is the removal of vasopressin from the adult cardiac arrest algorithm***. Studies indicate that vasopressin has no advantage over epinephrine and has been removed to simplify the cardiac arrest algorithm.1
- If pVT/VF persists, another shock is administered after 2 minutes of CPR. At this time, an anti arrhythmic agent may be considered. Recommendations include I.V./I.O. amiodarone; I.V./I.O. ***lidocaine may be considered as an alternative to amiodarone for pVT/VF unresponsive to CPR***, defibrillation and vasopressor therapy

227. Ans. a. Used for evaluation of vitals, co-morbid conditions & relevant investigation; b. Decreases anxiety of patient; d. Help in planing anaesthetic technique

[Ref: Ajay Yadav 5th/53,194,225; Morgan Anaesthesia 5th/ 296-97; Lee13th/3; Miller Anaesthesia 7th/1001-10]

- ***PAC is equally necessary in infant & children (in fact, even more than adult).***

*"**Infants are at much greater risk of anesthetic morbidity & mortality** than older children; risk is generally inversely proportional to age. In addition, pediatric patients are prone to medical illness that require unique surgical & anesthetic strategies"-Morgan Anesthesia 5th/878*

"Prior assessment of a patient for day-care surgery should be done"-*Ajay Yadav 6th/267*

Pre-anaesthetic Checkup (PAC): Goals

◈ Ajay Yadav 5th/53
- *To* ***reduce anxiety & educate the patient about anaesthesia***
- *To obtain information about patient's medical history*
- *To perform physical examination*
- *To* ***determine which test are required***
- ***To plan anaesthetic technique***
- To obtain informed consent
- To give any preoperative instructions

"Based on preoperative assessment, the patients are classified ***into six categories*** **by American Society of** Anesthesiologist **(IVI)**" *(Ajay Yadav 5th/53)*

Table: Preanaesthetic checkup (PAC) or preoperative evaluation: *(Miller Anaesthesia 7th/1001- Miller Anaesthesia 7th/1001)*

1.	The **anesthesia preoperative evaluation** is the clinical foundation and framework of ***perioperative patient management and can potentially reduce operative morbidity and enhance patient outcome***s.
2.	The fundamental purpose of preoperative evaluation is to obtain pertinent information regarding the patient's current and past medical history and to formulate an assessment of the patient's intraoperative risk and requisite clinical optimization.
3.	***Basic and complex medical diseases and syndrome***s that can potentially affect anesthesia perioperative management require the anesthesiologist to be clinically knowledgeable and current in many aspects of internal medicine.
4.	***Patients require preoperative diagnostic and laboratory studie***s that are consistent with their medical history, the proposed surgical procedure and the potential for intraoperative blood loss. Routine preoperative testing cannot be justified and is costly and clinically inappropriate.
5.	Preoperative patient education and individual discussion ***can significantly reduce patient anxiety and fears of the perioperative anesthesia process***.
6.	**Under the clinical directorship of an anesthesiologis**t, the anesthesia preoperative evaluation clinic can enhance operating room efficiency, decrease day-of-surgery cancellations and delays, reduce hospital costs and enhance the quality of patient care.
7.	New and updated preoperative evaluation consensus and evidence-based guidelines published by multiple medical specialties have led to evaluation protocols for ***preparing patients for anesthesia and surgery***.
8.	Increasing regulatory and reporting requirements involving preoperative issues by agencies such as the Joint Commission on Accreditation of Healthcare Organizations require awareness and compliance by anesthesiologists.
9.	Information technology and decision support systems in preoperative evaluation can ***enhance the quality of patient care and clinical managemen***t through electronic integration and standardization of patient data.
10.	The anesthesiologist is the perioperative medical specialist and th***e only preoperative evaluation physician who can truly evaluate the risks associated with anesthesia, discuss these risks with the patient and manage them intraoperativel***y

DERMATOLOGY

228. Ans. d. Lichen scrofulosorum

[Ref: Neena Khanna 5th/62-65; Harrison 19th/ 349; Roxburg 17th/145-46]

- ***There is Controversy Regarding Lichen Nitidus***

"The controversy regarding the etiology of lichen nitidus and its possible relationship to lichen planus is still unresolved. ***Some authors suggest that lichen nitidus represents a variant of lichen planus***"- *www.ncbi.nlm.nih.gov*

"Links between lichen nitidus and other diseases aren't well-understood, but they may include: **Lichen planus, Atopic dermatitis (eczema), Crohn's disease, Juvenile rheumatoid arthritis & Tuberculosis**"- *www.mayoclinic.org*

Lichen Planus (LP): Variant

◈ *Neena Khanna 5th/62; Roxburg 17th/145-46*
- *Annular LP*
- *Actinic LP*
- *Linear LP*
- *Follicular LP (Lichen planopilaris)*
- ***Hypertrophic LP (Commonest)***
- *Bullous LP*
- ***LP pigmentosus***
- ***Lichen nitidus: It is a rare variant of LP in which numerous tiny, pink, flat topped papule develop***- *Roxburg 17th/146*
- Ulcerative lichen planus-*wikipedia*

Cutaneous Tuberculosis: 4 Important Variant

◈ *Neena Khanna 5th/268*
- *Lupus vulgaris*
- *Scrofuloderma*
- *Tuberculosis verrucosa cutis*
- *Tuberculides:* ***lichen scrofulosorum*** *& papulonecrotic tuberculide*

Clinical Variants of Lichen Planus

◈ *onlinelibrary.wiley.com*
- *Annular lichen planus, Hypertrophic lichen planus, Atrophic lichen planus, Ulcerative lichen planus, Bullous lichen planus, Lichen planus pemphigoides, Lichen planus pigmentosus, Erythrodermic lichen planus, Inverse lichen planus, Linear lichen planus, Follicular lichen planus, Lichen planus follicularis decalvans & Actinic lichen planus*
- The classification presented takes morphology of the lesions, peculiarities of the topographic distribution and in individual cases the etiology into consideration.

229. Ans. a. Onycholysis; b. Oil drop discolouration; c. Subungual hyperkeratosis; d. Nail pitting

[Ref: Neena Khanna 5th/50-51; Harrison 19th/348; Roxburg 17th/129]

"**Pterygium** *is diagnostic & is a manifestation of severe* **lichen planus** *of nails*"- *Neena Khanna 5th/65*

Nail Changes in Psoriasis

- *Neena Khanna 5th/50-51; Harrison 19th/348*
- ***Punctate pitting***
- *Nail plate thickening*
- ***Subungual hyperkeratosis***
- ***Discolouration** & dystrophy of nail plate*
- *Onycholysis*
- Oilspots (*oil drop or salmon patch- www.dermnetnz.org*)- yellow red discolouration in center of nail

Nail changes in Lichen Planus

- *Neena Khanna 5th/64-65*
- *Thinning & distal splitting of nail plates*
- *Trachyonychia*
- *Tenting of nail plate: pup tent sign*
- *Pterygium*

230. Ans. **a. Trichotillomania; c. Tinea capitis.**

[Ref: Neena Khanna 5th/141; Harrison 19th/ 354-55]

Alopecia

- *Harrison 19th/ 354-55*
- The two major forms of alopecia are scarring and nonscarring.
- ***Scarring alopecia*** is associated with fibrosis, inflammation and loss of hair follicles. A smooth scalp with a decreased number of follicular openings is usually observed clinically, but in some patients, the changes are seen only in biopsy specimens from affected areas.
- In ***nonscarring alopecia***, the hair shafts are absent or miniaturized, but the hair follicles are preserved, explaining the reversible nature of nonscarring alopecia
- Scarring alopecia is more frequently the result of a primary cutaneous disorder such as *lichen planus, folliculitis decalvans, chronic cutaneous (discoid) lupus*, or *linear scleroderma (morphea)* than it is a sign of systemic disease. Although the scarring lesions of *discoid lupus* can be seen in patients with systemic lupus, in the majority of patients, the disease process is limited to the skin. Less common causes of scarring alopecia include *sarcoidosis* and *cutaneous metastases Harrison 19th/ 354*
- Scattered, poorly circumscribed patches of alopecia with a "moth-eaten" appearance are a manifestation of the secondary stage of syphilis

Table: Causes of Alopecia *(Harrison 19th/ 355)*

I. Nonscarring alopecia
A. Primary cutaneous disorders
▪ Telogen effluvium
▪ Androgenetic alopecia
▪ Alopecia areata
▪ Tinea capitis
▪ Traumatic alopecia[a]
B. Drugs
C. Systemic diseases
▪ Systemic lupus erythematosus
▪ Secondary syphilis
▪ Hypothyroidism
▪ Hyperthyroidism
▪ Hypopituitarism
▪ Deficiencies of protein, iron, biotin and zinc
II. Scarring alopecia
A. Primary cutaneous disorders
▪ Cutaneous lupus (chronic discoid lesions)
▪ Lichen planus
▪ Central centrifugal cicatricial alopecia
▪ Folliculitis decalvans
▪ Linear scleroderma (morphea)
B. Systemic diseases
▪ Discoid lesions in the setting of systemic lupus erythematosus
▪ Sarcoidosis
▪ Cutaneous metastases

[a] **Most patients with *trichotillomania*, pressure-induced alopecia, early stages of traction alopecia.**

231. Ans. **a. Herpes genitalis; b. Chancroid**

[Ref: Neena Khanna 5th/321; Harrison 19th/880; Khopkar 6th/232]

- **Primary syphilis (Hunterian chancre):** Single, clean, ***painless*** & indurated ulcer- *Neena Khanna 5th/321*
- **Primary Syphilis**: The typical primary chancre usually begins as a single painless papule that rapidly becomes eroded and usually becomes indurated -*Harrison 19th/1134*
- ***"Donovanosis (Granuloma inguinale):*** Begin as ***painless papule***, which leads to slowly progressive, autoinoculable ulcer"-*Ananthanarayan 10th/404*
- "Lymphogranuloma venereum: The primary lesion is a small, painless, papulovesicular lesion"-*Ananthanarayan 10th/404*
- ***LGV begins as a small painless papule*** that tends to ulcerate at the site of inoculation, often escaping attention- *Harrison 19th/1169*

Table: Clinical features of genital ulcers *(Harrison 19th/880)*

Feature	Syphilis	Herpes	Chancroid	Lymphogranuloma Venereum	Donovanosis
Incubation period	9-90 days	2-7 days	1-14 days	3 days-6 weeks	1-4 weeks (up to 6 months)
Early primary lesions	Papule	Vesicle	Pustule	Papule, pustule, or vesicle	Papule
No. of lesions	Usually one	Multiple	Usually multiple, may coalesce	Usually one; often not detected, despite lymphadenopathy	Variable

Contd...

Feature	Syphilis	Herpes	Chancroid	Lymphogranuloma Venereum	Donovanosis
Diameter	5-15 mm	1-2 mm	Variable	2-10	Variable
Edges	Sharply demarcated, elevated, round, or oval	Erythematous	Undermined, ragged, irregular	Elevated, round, or oval	Elevated, irregular
Depth	Superficial or deep	Superficial	Excavated	Superficial or deep	Elevated
Base	Smooth, nonpurulent, relatively nonvascular	Serous, erythematous, nonvascular	Purulent, bleeds easily	Variable, nonvascular	Red and velvety, bleeds readily
Induration	Firm	None	Soft	Occasionally firm	Firm
Pain	Uncommon	Frequently tender	Usually very tender	Variable	Uncommon
Lymphadenopathy	Firm, nontender, bilateral	Firm, tender, often bilateral with initial episode	Tender, may suppurate, loculated, usually unilateral	Tender, may suppurate, loculated, usually unilateral	None; pseudobuboes

232. Ans. **c. Basal cell carcinoma; e. Sarcoidosis**

[Ref: exp-oncology.com.ua; www.ncbi.nlm.nih.gov; jamanetwork.com]

"The **number of LCs** over ***basal cell carcinoma,*** squamous cell carcinoma and malignant melanoma was ***significantly lower than*** in normal skin and seborrheic keratosis"- *jamanetwork.com*

Oral lichen planus (OLP) is considered to be a mucocutaneous disease caused due to a cell-mediated immune reaction. Light and electron microscopic studies suggested that an ***intraepithelial accumulation of LCs*** takes place during the early stages. In OLP, changes in the local immune regulation may result in changes in the LCs. In a study it was suggested that the antigen presenting capability of LCs was increased in lichen planus"- www.ncbi.nlm.nih.gov

LCs are considered necessary to induce contact hypersensitivity as the phenomenon is taking place in the epidermis. The phenomenon of contact hypersensitivity has two phases: sensitization and elicitation of response. Sensitization of LCs takes place about 10 - 14 days and their number increased in the epidermis at 24 - 48 hrs. It was also found that ***LCs increased significantly*** in the connective tissue at the site of nickel application."- *www.ncbi.nlm.nih.gov*

Table: Difference between reduce and increased langerhans cells

Reduced Lngerhans cells *(ncbi.nlm.gov)*	**Increased Langerhans cells**
• Ageing	• Gingivitis and periodontitis
• ***Basal cell carcinoma of skin***	• ***Oral Lichen planus***
• Squamous cell carcinoma skin	• *Contact hypersensitivity*
• ***Sarcoidosis***	• Recurrent aphthous stomatitis
• HIV/AIDs	• Behcet's disease
• HPV infection	• Oral cancers
• Lichenoid drug eruptions	• ***Langerhans cell histiocytosis*** (LCH)

233. Ans. **a. Tip of toes is more common location for arterial ulcers; d. Diabetic foot ulcers are more common in ball of greater toe & plantar surface of metatarsals head; e. Pressure ulcer - common at heels**

[Ref: Roxburg 17th/173; Neena Khanna 5th/179; L and B 27th/984; Manipal Surgery 4th/ 60]

- **Venous ulcer**- *Medial malleolus commonly & ankle nearby- Roxburg 17th/173*
- ***Decubitus ulcer***- *Sacrum ischial region, heels, scapular region, back of head, elbows- Roxburg 17th/173*
- **Neuropathic ulcer** *(e.g diabetes & leprosy)- Site: soles of feet particularly- Roxburg 17th/173*

Location of Ulcer

- *Manipal Surgery 4th/ 60*
- *Arterial ulcer: Tip of the toes, dorsum of feet*
- *Long saphenous varicosity with ulcer: Medial side of leg*
- *Short saphenous varicosity with ulcer: Lateral side of the leg above the lateral malleolus*
- *Diabetes:* ***Pressure sore over plantar surface of the head of the metatarsals****- Manipal Surgery 4th/ 67*

Neuropathic ulcer or Neurogenic ulcer or trophic ulcer *(e.g diabetes, leprosy, nerve injuries etc): Ulcer develops on the pressure points such as beneath heel,* ***beneath the first & fifth metatarsals*** *& gluteal region (decubitus ulcer)"- Manipal Surgery 4th/ 65*

The **venous ulcer of the leg** characteristically develops in the skin of the gaiter region, the area between the muscles of the calf and the ankle. This is the region where many of the Cockett perforators join the posterior tibial vein to the surface vein, known as the posterior arch vein. The ***majority of ulcers develop on the medial side of the calf*** but ulcers associated with lesser saphenous incompetence may develop on the lateral side of the leg. Ulcers can develop on any part of the calf skin in patients with post-thrombotic legs; however, venous ulcers rarely extend onto the foot or into the upper calf and, if there is ulceration at these sites, other diagnoses should be seriously considered. *L and B 27th/984*

Table: Differential Diagnosis of leg ulcers *(Neena Khanna 5th/179)*

Aetiology	Location	Pain	Temperature of foot	Morphology of ulcers
Venous	Medial aspect of ankles	Painless or minimally painful	Warm	• Irregular • May be large in diameter & of varying depth floor of unhealthy granulation tissue • Floor of unhealthy granulation tissue • Surrounding pigmentation & lipodermatosclerosis
Arterial	Toes, heels & dorsae of feet	Severe pain	Cold with absent peripheral pulses	• Irregular (polycyclic) • May be deep • Floor black/grey with no granulation tissue. Islands of normal looking skin may be present
Vasculitic	Anywhere on legs	Painful	Warm	• Begin as palpable purpura • Punched out, shallow ulcers
Trophic	Pressure points, e.g. ***metatarsal arch & heels***	Painless	Warm	• Deep ulcers • Surrounded by hyperkeratotic thick callus • May be secondarily infected • Anaesthetic area. Loss of hair in surrounding area (evidence of trophic change)
Malignant	Any site	Generally painless	Warm	• Everted edges • Indurated • Regional lymphadenopathy

PSYCHIATRY

234. Ans. **c. Frotteurism, e. Masochism**

[Ref: Synopsis of Psychiatry by Kaplan & Saddock 11th/593-97; Reddy 34th/384, 401-404; Neeraj Ahuja 7th/124-26; Parikh 7th/ 411-12]

Tribadism ***is also k/a lesbianism or sapphism or*** *female homosexuality- Reddy 34th/401*

Classifications of Sexual Offences

◈ *Reddy 34th/384*

I. Natural offences:
   1. Rape
   2. Incest
   3. Adultery

II. Unnatural offences:
   1. Sodomy
   2. Tribadism
   3. Bestiality
   4. Buccal coitus

III. Sexual paraphilias
   1. Sadism
   2. Masochism
   3. Necrophilia
   4. Fetichism
   5. Transvestism
   6. Exhibitionism
   7. Masturbation
   8. Frotteurism
   9. Undinism, etc.

IV. Sex-linked offences:
   1. Stalking
   2. Voyeurism
   3. Sexual harassment
   4. Trafficking
   5. Indecent assault

Paraphilic Disorders

◈ *Kaplan&Saddock 11th/593-97*

- Paraphilias or perversions are sexual stimuli or acts that are deviations from normal sexual behaviors, but are necessary for some persons to experience arousal and orgasm.
- According to the **Diagnostic and Statistical Manual of Mental Disorders, fifth edition (DSM-5),** the term paraphilic disorder is reserved for those cases in which a sexually deviant fantasy or impulse has been expressed behaviorally.
- Individuals with paraphilic interests can experience sexual pleasure, but they are inhibited from responding to stimuli that are normally considered erotic. The paraphiliac person's sexuality is mainly restricted to specific deviant stimuli or acts.
- Persons that occasionally experiment with paraphilic behavior (e.g., infrequent episode of bondage or dressing in costumes), but are capable of responding to more typical erotic stimuli, are not seen as having paraphilic disorders.
- DSM-5 lists ***pedophilia, frotteurism, voyeurism, exhibitionism, sexual sadism, sexual masochism, fetishism and transvestism*** with explicit diagnostic criteria because of their threat to others and/or because they are **relatively common paraphilias**. There are ***many other paraphilias that may be diagnosed***
- In **DSM-5,** the criteria for paraphilic disorder requires the patient to have experienced intense and recurrent arousal

from their deviant fantasy for ***at least 6 months*** and to have acted on the paraphilic impulse.

- **Special Note:** Homosexuality (gay and lesbianism) was previously listed as a paraphilia in the DSM-I and DSM-II, but this was declassified from DSM-III, DSM-IV & DSM-V, consistent with the change of attitude among psychiatrists and psychologists. ***Homosexuality is no longer considered a paraphilia.***
- **Section-497- Adultery:**"Whoever has sexual intercourse with a person who is and whom he knows or has reason to believe to be the wife of another man, without the consent or connivance of that man, such sexual intercourse not amounting to the offence of rape, is guilty of the offence of adultery and shall be punished with imprisonment of either description for a term which may extend to five years, or with fine, or with both. In such case, the wife shall not be punishable as an abettor"- *Reddy 34th/399*

235. Ans. b. Delusion of guilt; d. Delusion of infidelity

[Ref: Niraj Ahuja 7th/70-71,83; Kaplan and Sadock 11th/333-34; Harrison 19th/2717]

Manic Episode

◈ *Niraj Ahuja 7th/70-71*

- *There can be **delusions of grandeur (grandiosity)**, with marked inflated self-esteem*
- ***Delusion of persecution** may sometime develop secondary to the delusions of grandeur (e.g. I am so great that people are against me)*
- *Delusion of control, may be present in some cases*

Depressive Episode

◈ *Niraj Ahuja 7th/72*

- *Mood congruent features- **nihilistic delusions, delusion of guilt,** delusion of poverty*
- *Mood incongruent features- delusion of control*

"**Othello syndrome:** The **delusion** of infidelity of a spouse or partner. The Othello syndrome affects males and, less often, females. It is characterized by recurrent accusations of infidelity, searches for evidence, repeated interrogation of the partner, tests of their partner's fidelity and sometime stalking. The syndrome may appear by itself or in the course of paranoid schizophrenia, alcoholism, or cocaine addiction. As in *Othello*, the play by Shakespeare, the syndrome can be highly dangerous and result in disruption of a marriage, homicide and suicide"- *www.medicinenet.com*

"**Nihilistic delusions** are associated with delusions of enormity when the patient believes that he can produce a catastrophe by some action, e.g. refuse to pass water because he will flood the world"-*saminkie.blogspot.com*

236. Ans. b. Genetic predisposition; d. Loneliness increases chance; e. Hopelessness is predisposing factor.

[Ref: Niraj Ahuja 7th/22-23; Kaplan and Sadock 11th/ 763-69]

"**Parasuicidal Behavior:** Parasuicide is a term introduced to describe patients who in jure themselves by self -mutilation (e.g., cutting the skin), but ***who usually do not wish to die.*** Studies show that about 4 percent of all patients in psychiatric hospitals have cut themselves; the ***female-to-male ratio is almost 3 to 1.*** Self-injury is found in about 30 percent of all abusers of oral substances and 10 percent of all intra venous users admitted to substance-treatment units"-*Kaplan and Sadock 11th/ 768*

"**Age:** For all groups, suicide is rare before puberty. Suicide rates increase with age and underscore the significance of the midlife crisis. ***Among men, suicides peak after age 45;*** among women, the ***greatest number of completed suicides occurs after age 55***"-*Kaplan and Sadock 11th/ 763*

Genetic Factors: Suicidal behavior, as with other psychiatric disorders, tends to run in families. In psychiatric patients, a family history of suicide increases the risk of attempted suicide and that of completed suicide in most diagnostic groups. In medicine, the strongest evidence for involvement of genetic factors comes from twin and adoption studies and from molecular genetics- *Kaplan and Sadock 11th/ 767*

Table: An Example of Summary of Risks and Protective Factors for Suicide *(Niraj Ahuja 7th/223)*

Factors	Biological	Psychological	Social
Predisposing	Genetic factors Male gender Older age	Early childhood trauma Personality traits	Poor social support Unemployment
Precipitating	Discontinuation of antidepressant Psychiatric diagnosis	Separation from spouse ***Hopelessness*** Worthlessness	Financial difficulties Easy availability of lethal means
Perpetuating	Alcohol and drug misuse	Poor self-esteem	Poor social support
Protective	Children; elderly parents; religious and moral values; good engagement with treatment		

Variables Enhancing Risk of Suicide Among Vulnerable Groups

◈ *Kaplan and Sadock 11th/ 768*

- Adolescence and late life
- Bisexual or homosexual gender identity
- Criminal behavior
- Cultural sanctions for suicide
- Delusions
- Disposition of personal property
- Divorced, separated, or single marital status
- Early loss or separation from parents
- Family history of suicide
- Hallucinations
- Homicide

Hopelessness

- Hypochondriasis
- Impulsivity
- Increasing agitation
- Increasing stress
- Insomnia
- Lack of future plans
- Lack of sleep
- Lethality of previous attempt

Living Alone

- Low self-esteem
- Male sex
- Physical illness or impairment
- Previous attempts that could have resulted in death
- Protestant or nonreligious status
- Recent childbirth
- Recent loss
- Repression as a defense
- Secondary gain
- Severe family pathology
- Severe psychiatric illness
- Sexual abuse
- Signals of intent to die
- Suicide epidemics
- Unemployment
- White race

237. Ans. a. Low concern for others feeling; b. Inability to feel guilt; c. Suicidal threats may present; d. Low tolerance to frustration, e. Disrupted self-image

[Ref: Niraj Ahuja 7th/115; Kaplan and Sadock 11th/748-49]

Borderline Personality Disorder

◈ *Niraj Ahuja 7th/117*

- ***Unstable & intense interpersonal relationship patterns***
- ***Significant & persistent disturbances of identity of self, 'who am I'. There is marked uncertainty about major issue in life***
- *Deliberate self-harm is common in the form of self-mutilation, suicidal gestures, or accident proneness*

Antisocial Personality Disorder: Traits are

◈ *Niraj Ahuja 7th/115*

- ***Callous unconcern for the feelings of others***
- Gross and persistent attitude of irresponsibility and disregard for social norms, rules and obligations,
- Incapacity to maintain enduring relationships,
- ***Very low tolerance to frustration*** and a low threshold for discharge of aggression,
- ***Incapacity to experience guilt*** and to profit from experience, particularly punishment and
- Marked proneness to blame others

DSM-5 Diagnostic Criteria for Antisocial Personality Disorder

◈ *Kaplan and Sadock 11th/748*

- **A pervasive pattern of disregard for and violation of the rights of others, occurring since age 1 5 years, as indicated by three (or more) of the following:**
  - Failure to conform to social norms with respect to lawful behaviors, as indicated by repeatedly performing acts that are grounds for arrest.
  - Deceitfulness, as indicated by repeated lying, use of liases, or conning others for personal profit or pleasure.
  - Impulsivity or failure to plan ahead.
  - Irritability and aggressiveness, as indicated by repeated physical fights or assaults.
  - Reckless disregard for safety of self or others.
  - Consistent irresponsibility, as indicated by repeated failure to sustain consistent work behavior or honor financial obligations.
  - Lack of remorse, as indicated by being indifferent to or rationalizing having hurt, mistreated, or stolen from another.
- **The individual is at least age 18 years.**
- There is evidence of conduct disorder with onset before age 15 years.
- The occurrence of antisocial behavior is not exclusively during the course of schizophrenia or bipolar disorder

Antisocial Personality Disorder: Clinical Features

◈ *Kaplan and Sadock 11th/748-49*

- Patients with antisocial personality disorder can often seem to be normal and even charming and ingratiating. Their histories, however, reveal many areas of disordered life functioning.
- Lying, truancy, running away from home, thefts, fights, substance abuse and illegal activities are typical experiences that patients report as beginning in childhood. These patients often impress opposite-sex clinicians with the colorful, seductive aspects of their personalities, but same-sex clinicians may regard them as manipulative and demanding.
- Patients with antisocial personality disorder exhibit no anxiety or depression, a lack that may seem grossly incongruous with their situations, although ***suicide threats and somatic preoccupations may be common***.
- Their own explanations of their antisocial behaviour make it seem mindless, but their mental content reveals the complete absence of delusions and other signs of irrational thinking. In fact, they frequently have a heightened sense of reality testing and often impress observers as having good verbal intelligence.
- Persons with antisocial personality disorder are highly representative of so-called con men. They are extremely manipulative and can frequently talk others into participating in schemes for easy ways to make money or to achieve fame or notoriety. These schemes may eventually lead the unwary to financial ruin or social embarrassment or both.
- Those with this disorder do not tell the truth and cannot be trusted to carry out any task or adhere to any conventional standard of morality. Promiscuity, spousal abuse, child abuse and drunk driving are common events in their lives. A notable finding is a ***lack of remorse for these actions;*** that is, they appear to lack a conscience.

238. Ans. b. **Perseveration; e. Logoclonia**

[Ref: Niraj Ahuja 7th/56-58; Kaplan and Sadock 11th/202,313]

Perseveration: Types

◈ *Revision Notes in Psychiatry By Basant Puri, Annie Hall, Roger Ho 3rd/4*

- **Palilalia:** The person repeats a word with increasing frequency
- **Logoclonia:** The person repeats the last syllable of the last word
  - ***Logoclonia:*** A nearextinct term for a variation of palilalia in which there is a meaningless repetition of the last syllables of a word or phrase and formerly regarded by some authors as typical of presenile and senile dementias, general paresis and other neurological diseases"- *medical-dictionary*
  - ***Feature of schizophrenia:*** Perseveration (persistent repetition of words beyond their relevance), echolalia (repetition or echoing by the patient of words or phrases of examiner) etc.- *Niraj Ahuja 7th/56*

Table: Formal thought disorders *(Kaplan and Sadock 11th/202)*

- **Circumstantiality:** Overinclusion of trivial or irrelevant details that impede the sense of getting to the point.
- **Clang associations:** Thoughts are associated by the sound of words rather than by their meaning (e.g., through rhyming or assonance).
- **Derailment:** (Synonymous with loose associations.) A breakdown in both the logical connection between ideas and the overall sense of goal-directedness. The words make sentences, but the sentences do not make sense.
- **Flight of ideas:** A succession of multiple associations so that thoughts seem to move abruptly from idea to idea; often (but not invariably) expressed through rapid, pressured speech.
- **Neologism.** The invention of new words or phrases or the use of conventional words in idiosyncratic ways.
- **Perseveration.** Repetition of out of context of words, phrases, or ideas.
- **Tangentiality.** In response to a question, the patient gives a reply that is appropriate to the general topic without actually answering the question.
- **Thought blocking.** A sudden disruption of thought or a break in the flow of ideas.

"Perseveration is the tendency to focus on a specific idea or content without the ability to move on to other topics. The perseverative patient will repeatedly come back to the same topic despite the interviewer's attempts to change the subject"- *Kaplan and Sadock 11th/202*

"**Neologism:** New word or phrase whose derivation cannot be understood; ***often seen in schizophrenia***" *(Kaplan & Sadock's Synopsis of Psychiatry 11th/1415)*

Knight's move thinking *Mastering Psychiatry: A Core Textbook for Undergraduates By Melvyn WB Zhang Chap/3*

Schizophrenia patient changes from one topic to another b/w abruptly & there is no logical link b/w thoughts. The train of thought is similar to the knight's movement in chess

239. Ans. a. **Isolation of affect; c. Reaction formation; d. Undoing**

[Ref: Ahuja 7th/208-10,97; Kaplon & Saddock 11th/161-62]

- ***Conversion is seen in conversion disorder (Hysteria)****- Ahuja 7th/208*
- ***Projection is seen in persecutory delusions & hallucinations****- Ahuja 7th/208*

Defense Mechanism in Obsessive Compulsive Disorder (OCD)

◈ *Ahuja 7th/208-10,97*

- ***Reaction formation***
- ***Displacement***
- ***Undoing***
- ***Isolation of affect***
- ***Inhibition***

RADIOLOGY

240. Ans.. b. **Proton; c. Neutron**

[Ref: Radiology & Imaging by K. Thayalam 1st/10-11; Harrison 19th/103e-4; Sumer Sethi 6th/162]

Atomic Structure Radiology & Imaging by

◈ *K. Thayalam 1st/10-11*

- Every atom has central core, k/a nucleus
- ***Nucleus consists of two particle- protons & neutrons***, collectively k/a nucleons
- **Proton:** positively charged
- **Neutron:** no charge
- Electron circulate around nucleus
- **Electron:** Negatively charged
- Number of electrons in an atom = number of protons
- Mass number of atom = total number of protons & neutrons in the nucleus
- Atomic number of atom = number of proton = number of electrons

Photon

◈ *www.zmescience.com*

- A photon is the smallest discrete amount or quantum of electromagnetic radiation. It is the basic unit of all light
- Photons are always in motion and, in a vacuum, travel at a constant speed to all observers of 2.998×10^8 m/s. This is commonly referred to as the speed of light, denoted by the letter *c*.
- The basic properties of photons are:
  - They have zero mass and rest energy. They only exist as moving particles.
  - They are elementary particles despite lacking rest mass.
  - They have no electric charge.
  - They are stable.
  - They are spin-1 particles which makes them bosons.
  - They carry energy and momentum which are dependent on the frequency.

- They can have interactions with other particles such as electrons, such as the Compton effect.
- They can be destroyed or created by many natural processes, for instance when radiation is absorbed or emitted.
- When in empty space, they travel at the speed of light

241. Ans. a. MR spectroscopy (MRS); b. Magnetic resonance imaging (MRI); c. Computed tomography (CT); d. Positron emission tomography (PET)

[Ref: Sumer Sethi 6th/149; Radiology & Imaging by K. Thayalam 1st/377; Harrison 19th/440e-1; Davidson 23rd/1072-73]

White matter disorders- mri is the most sensitive modality- *Sumer Sethi 6th/149*

"Plain skull X-rays *now have a very limited role in neurological disease.* CT or MRI is needed for intracranial imaging"- *Davidson 23rd/1073*

Neuroimaging in Neurologic Disorders

◈ *Harrison 19th/440e-1-4*

- The clinician caring for patients with neurologic symptoms is faced with myriad imaging options, including computed tomography (CT), CT angiography (CTA), perfusion CT (pCT), magnetic resonance (MR) imaging (MRI), MR angiography (MRA), functional MRI (fMRI), MR spectroscopy (MRS), MR neurography (MRN), diffusion and diffusion tensor imaging, susceptibility-weighted MR imaging
- (SWI), arterial spin label MRI (ASL) and perfusion MRI (pMRI).
- In general, ***MRI is more sensitive than CT*** for the detection of lesions affecting the central nervous system (CNS), particularly those of the spinal cord, cranial nerves and posterior fossa structures.
- CT is the primary study of choice in the evaluation of an acute change in mental status, focal neurologic findings, acute trauma to the brain and spine, suspected subarachnoid hemorrhage and conductive hear-ing loss- *Harrison 19th/440e-2*
- FLAIR images are more sensitive than standard spin echo images for any water-containing lesions or edema-*Harrison 19th/440e-4*

"White matter diseases include a wide spectrum of disorders that have in common impairment of normal myelination, either by secondary destruction of previously myelinated structures (demyelinating processes) or by primary abnormalities of myelin formation (dysmyelinating processes). Demyelinating disorders can be further divided into autoimmune, infectious, vascular and toxic-metabolic processes"- pubs.rsna.org

Neurological Imaging

◈ *Davidson 23rd/1072-73*

- Neurological imaging has traditionally allowed only ssessment of structure but advances are allowing much more sophistication.
- Imaging modalities can use X-rays (plain X-rays, computed tomography (CT), CT angiography, myelography and angiography), magnetic resonance (MR imaging (MRI), MR angiography (MRA)), ultrasound (Doppler imaging of blood vessels) and nuclear medicine techniques (single photon emission computed tomography (SPECT) and positron emission tomography (PET).
- Specialist MR techniques, such as functional MRI (fMRI), MR spectroscopy or diffusion tensor imaging (DTI), can be used to assess brain metabolism and chemical compositions. This may be dynamic and can provide 'maps' of cortical function to help plan lesionectomy and epilepsy surgery.
- Similarly, **MR spectroscopy** can outline the chemical composition of specific regions, providing notions of whether lesions are ischaemic, neoplastic or inflammatory
- Some degenerative neurological conditions cause functional rather than structural abnormalities that make metabolic and neurochemical assessment increasingly useful. **PET scanning** can display glucose metabolism in dementia and epilepsy. **SPECT scanning** uses the lipid-soluble properties of radioactive tracers to mark cerebral blood flow at the time of injection to help in investigating seizures. Dopaminergic pathway tracers can assess the integrity of the nigrostriatal pathway in patients with possible parkinsonism.
- **Magnetic Resonance (MR) spectroscopy** is a noninvasive diagnostic test for measuring biochemical changes in the brain, especially the ***presence of tumors.*** While magnetic resonance imaging (MRI) identifies the anatomical location of a tumor, MR spectroscopy compares the chemical composition of normal brain tissue with abnormal tumor tissue. This test can also be used to detect tissue changes in stroke and epilepsy"- *www.mayfieldclinic.com*
- **Magnetic Resonance (MR) spectroscopy: Useful to identify metabolic disorders, infections & treatment evaluation**-*Radiology & Imaging by K. Thayalam 1st/393*

PET

◈ *scan www.healthline.com Radiology & Imaging by K. Thayalam 1st/296-98*

- **Glucose** is the main fuel of the brain. During PET scans, tracers "attach" to compounds such as glucose. By attaching to glucose, the PET scan is able to detect which areas of the brain are utilizing glucose at the highest rates.
- PET scans are used to help diagnose and manage many central nervous system (CNS) disorders, including: Alzheimer's disease, depression, epilepsy, head trauma, Parkinson's disease etc
- Used to evaluate brain abnormalities, such as tumors, memory disorders, seizures and other central nervous system disorders- www.radiologyinfo.org

Table: Guidelines for the Use of CT, Ultrasound and MRI *(Harrison 19th/440e-1)*

Condition	Recommended Technique
Hemorrhage	
Acute parenchymal	CT, MR
Subacute/chronic	MRI
Subarachnoid hemorrhage	CT, CTA, lumbar puncture → aniogrphy
Aneurysm	Angiography > CTA, MRA
Ischemic infarction	
Hemorrhagic infarction	CT or MRI
Bland infarction	MRI with diffusion > CT, CTA, angiography
Carotid or vertebral dissection	MRI/MRA
Vertebral basilar insufficiency	CTA, MRI/MRA
Carotid stenosis	CTA, MRA > US
Suspected mass lesion	
Neoplasm, primary or metastatic	MRI + contrast
Infection/abscess	MRI + contrast
Immunosuppressed with focal findings	MRI + contrast
Vascular malformation	MRI ± angiography
White matter disorders	***MRI***
Demyelinating disease	MRI ± contrast
Dementia	MRI > CT
Trauma	
Acute trauma	CT
Shear injury/chronic hemorrhage	MRI + susceptibility-weighted imaging
Headache/migraine	CT / MRI
Seizure	
First time, no focal neurologic deficits	MRI > CT
Partial complex/refractory	MRI
Cranial neuropathy	MRI with contrast
Meningeal disease	MRI with contrast

Contd...

Abbreviations: CT, computed tomography; CTA, CT angiography; MRA, magnetic resonance angiography; MRI, magnetic resonance imaging

Table: Imaging techniques for the nervous system *(Davidson 23rd/1072)*

Technique	Applications	Advantages	Disadvantages	Comments
X-ray/CT	Plain X-rays, CT, CTA Radiculography Myelography Intra-arterial angiography	Widely available Relatively cheap Relatively quick	Ionising radiation Contrast reactions Invasive (myelography and angiography)	X-rays: used for fractures or foreign bodies CT: First line for stroke intra-arterial angiography: gold standard for vascular lesions
MRI	Structural imaging MRA Functional MRI MR spectroscopy	High-quality soft tissue images, useful for posterior fossa and temporal lobes No ionizing radiation No-invasive	Expensive Less widely available MRA images blood flow, not vessel anatomy Claustrophobic Pacemakers are a contraindication contrast (gadolinium) reactions	Functional MR and spectroscopy: mainly research tools
Ultrasound	Doppler Duplex scans	Cheap Quick Non-invasive	Operator-dependent Poor anatomical definition	Screening tool to assess need for carotid endarterectomy
Radioisotope	Isotope brain scan spect pet	In vivo imaging of functional anatomy (ligand binding, blood flow)	Poor spatial resolution Ionising radiation Expensive Not widely available	**Isotope Scans:** Obsolete **Spect:** Usuful In Movment Disorders, Epilepsy And Dementias **PET:** Mainly research tool

242. Ans. **b. Radium- 226; d. Strontium-90; e. Cesium-137.**

[Ref: Sumer Sethi 6th/38-40,163-64; Dutta Gynae7th/419; Radiology & Imaging by K. Thayalam 1st/307; Harrison 19th/263e-1]

"Cobalt-60, is a ***synthetic radioactive isotope of cobalt*** with a half-life of 5.2714 years. It is produced artificially in nuclear reactors"-*www.britannica.com*

"Unlike more stable isotopes iridium-191 and 193, ***iridium-192 does not occur in nature***"- www.theguardian.com

***"Iridium-192 does not typically occur naturally.* Instead,** scientists must put iridium-191 in a nuclear reactor and bombard it with neutrons. The iridium-191 then takes up an extra neutron to become iridium-192-*www.livescience.com*

"Important naturally occurring radioisotapes are hydrogen (H-3), beryllium (Be-10), carbon (C-14), ***radium (Ra-226), radon (Rn-222), cesium (Cs-37)***, sodium (Na-22), silicon (Si-32), chlorine (Cl-36), argon (Ar-39), krypton (Kr-81, Kr-78), iodine (I-129, I-131), potassium (K-40), ***strontium (Sr 90),*** calcium (Ca-48), germanium (Ge-76), zirconium- (Zr-96), samarium, (Sm-147, 148) selenium (Se-82), rubidium (Ru-87), molybdenum (Mo-100), cadmium (Cd-113, Cd-116), xenon (Xe-136), barium (Ba-130), gadolinium (Gd-152), tungsten (Tn-180), platinum (Pt-190), bismuth (Bi-209), thorium (Th-232, Th-230) and uranium (U-235, 236, 237, 238)"-*britanica.com*

Natural Background Exposure

◈ *Radiology & Imaging by K. Thayalam 1st/307*

- Natural background exposure includes (1) radon & thoron (2) cosmic rays (3)terrestrial (4) internal sources
- Cosmic rays: protons & C-14
- Terrestrial-Mainly U-238,Th-232 & their decay products & K-40
- Internal exposure- U-238,Th-232 & K-40

Natural isotopes must be either stable, have a half-life exceeding about 7×10^7 years (there are 34 isotopes in this category, see stable isotope for more details) or are generated in large amounts cosmogenically (e.g. ^{14}C, which has a half life of only 6000 years but is made by cosmic rays colliding with ^{14}N)-wiki

243. Ans. b. Intussusception

[Ref: Sumer Sethi 6th/123; Manipal Surgery 4th/752; Danhert Radiology Review Manual 7th/862]

Intussusception:

◈ *Radiological signs Sumer Sethi 6th/123*

- ***Claw sign***
- ***Coiled spring appearance***
- ***Empty right iliac fossa***
- ***Double target appearance***

Radiological Signs

- *Sigmoid volvulus:* Bird of prey sign, Liver overlap sign & left flank overlap sign- *Sumer Sethi 6th/124*
- *Ischemic colitis:* Thumb printing- *Sumer Sethi 6th/124*
- *Pneumoperitoneum:* Football sign, Cupola sign & triangle sign- *Sumer Sethi 6th/122*
- Crohn's Disease:String sign of kantor, Halo sign on CT, Cobblestone appearance- *Sumer Sethi 6th/120-21*
- **Ulcerative colitis:** Pipe stem colon(ahaustral), pseudopolyps- *Sumer Sethi 6th/120*
- *Ileocaecal kochs:* String sign, sterlein sign, purse string sign, Fleishner or inverted umbrella sign- *Sumer Sethi 6th/119*

244. Ans. a. Gamma rays; b. X-rays; e. Electron beam.

[Ref: Sumer Sethi 6th/175; Harrison 19th/103e-4;Dutta Gynae 7th/418-19]

Teletherapy (External beam Therapy)

◈ *Sumer Sethi 6th/175*

- *Three main type of radiation are used in radiation therapy-gamma rays, X-rays & electron beams*
- *Linear accelerators or Co-60 machines are used commonly for external beam radiation therapy*
- *Electron beam therapy- choice for skin & shallow targets*
- *Gamma rays & X-rays: choice for deeper target*

Radiotherapy

◈ *Dutta Gynae 7th/418-19*

- Ionizing radiation used for therapy- Electromagnetic radiation & particulate radiation
- *Electromagnetic radiation are of two types-* ***X-ray & gamma rays***
- ***X-ray & gamma rays are collectively called photons***
- Particulate radiation: This consists of atomic subparticles such as ***electrons, protons & neutrons***. Only ***electrons (βrays*** are used in radiotherapy)

Beta decay: *The process of radioactive decay, in which an electron or positron is ejected is called the beta decay. The electron emission is denoted by β-(beta minus decay) & the positron emission is denoted by β+"- Radiology & Imaging by K. Thayalam 1st/276*

Therapeutic Radiation

◈ *Harrison 19th/103e 4*

- *Therapeutic radiation is delivered in three ways: (1) teletherapy, with focused beams of radiation generated at a distance and aimed at the tumor within the patient; (2) brachytherapy, with encapsulated sources of radiation implanted directly into or adjacent to tumor tissues; and (3) systemic therapy, with radionuclides administered, for example, intravenously but targeted by some means to a tumor site.*
- ***Teletherapy with x-ray or gamma-ray photons is the most commonly used form of radiation therapy. Particulate forms of radiation are also used in certain circumstances, such as the use of proton beams.***
- *The difference between photons and protons relates to the volume in which the greatest delivery of energy occurs. Typically protons have a much narrower range of energy deposition, theoretically resulting in more precise delivery of radiation with improvement in the degree to which adjacent structures may be affected, in comparison to photons.*
- ***Electron beams*** *are a particulate form of radiation that, in contrast to photons and protons, have a very low tissue penetrance and are* ***used to treat cutaneous tumors***.
- *Apart from sparing adjacent structures, particulate forms of radiation are in most applications not superior to x-rays or gamma rays in clinical studies reported thus far, but this is an active area of investigation.*

245. Ans. a. Micturating Cystourethrography (MCU); b. Prenatal USG; d. Postnatal USG.

[Ref: O.P.Ghai 8th/470; Nelson 20th/2573-75 Paediatric Nephrology 3rd/94]

"**Posterior urethral valve:** The diagnosis is established with a VCUG or by perineal ultrasonography"- *Nelson 20th/2573*

"Because congenital urologic abnormalities increase the risk of UTI, radiologic evaluation of first UTI has been routinely recommended. These recommendations usually include routine ***ultrasound of the kidneys and voiding cystourethrogram (VCUG).*** Boys with first UTI should be studied to detect posterior urethral valves, an important congenital abnormality that requires surgery"-*CPDT 18th/731*

Radiographic Investigations for Posterior Urethral Valves (PUVs)

- *Paediatric Nephrology 3rd/94*

1. ***Micturating cystourethrogram (MCU)***
2. ***Ultrasound***

   A. *Antenatal ultrasound*
   - Marked distention and hypertrophy of the bladder
   - Hydronephrosis and hydroureter
   - In severe cases oligohydrarnnios and renal
   - Keyhole sign

   B. *Postnatal ultrasound*
   - Bladder is typically thick-walled and trabeculated with an elongated and dilated posterior urethra (keyhole sign)
   - Hydronephrosis
   - Kidneys may also be hyperechoic with loss of the normal corticomedullary differentiation, a manifestation of renal dysplasia
   - Examination of the posterior urethra can be performed longitudinally through the perineum during micturition at which. Time the proximal urethra can be seen to dilate. Diameter of more than 6 mm is considered abnormal and is highly specific and sensitive to the diagnosis.

Micturating Cystourethrogram (MCU)

- *O.P.Ghai 8th/470*
- ***MCU*** is necessary for studying the lower urinary tract.
- A sterile catheter is introduced into the bladder, which is filled with contrast medium; films are taken during and end-micturition.
- MCU provides precise details of the anatomy of the bladder and urethra, presence of vesicoureteric reflux and obstruction in the lower urinary tract (e.g. ***posterior urethral valves***, urethral stenosis).

Posterior Urethral Valves

- *Neonatology by Buonocore (2012)/1075*
- PUVs is a congenital disease of high mortality and morbidity, starting in the uterus and leading to progressive renal dysfunction.
- PUVs are recognized as the most common cause of bladder outlet obstruction in boys
- Commonly, PUVs consist of two folds arising from the urethra at the level of the veru montanum and fusing anteriorly in the midline. A much rarer form is a diaphragm extending across the lumen of the urethra just beyond the veru montanum.
- The degree of obstruction can vary from minimal with associated symptoms of dysfunctional voiding to severe with dilated posterior urethra, trabeculated bladder and severely hydronephrotic kidneys.
- Antenatal Diagnosis: The antenatal diagnosis is made on the finding of dilated upper tracts associated with a thick-walled bladder and oligohydramnios. A detailed sonographic evaluation of the fetus is carried out to exclude extrarenal abnormalities. MRI is reported of benefit when used in addition to US if the resolution of US is impaired by oligohydramnios
- PUVs are diagnosed by VCUG or cystoscopy revealing an obstruction at the urethral level in males. VCUG can reveal the presence, grade and position of the VUR. In addition, ***dynamic radioisotope renography MAG3*** can provide information about the flow of urine. Drainage from a very-dilated upper tract might be slower than normal even if there is no anatomical obstruction"- *Neonatology by Buonocore (2012)/1082*

"**Anterior urethral valves:** The diagnosis is suspected on physical examination and is confirmed by the VCUG"- *Nelson 20th/2575*

246. Ans. a. Posterior scalloping of vertebral bodies; b. Sphenoid wing dysplasia; d. Scoliosis

[Ref: Harrison 19th/603; Davidson 22nd/1216; Maheswari 5th/317; Danhert Radiology Review Manual 7th/320]

Skeletal manifestations of NF-1

- *Danhert Radiology Review Manual 7th/320*
- *Seen in 25-40%*
- ***Scoliosis***
- ***Macrocranium + macroencephaly***
- **Posterior scalloping of vertebral bodies due to dural ectasia**
- **Partial absence of lesser & greater wing of sphenoid**
- **Sphenoid dysplasia** is a characteristic defect of the posterosuperior orbital wall that is attributed to mesodermal dysplasia, although a review suggests that the dysplasia may be secondary to interactions with plexiform neurofibromas early in life. Findings include hypoplasia of the greater and lesser sphenoid wings along with enlargement of the middle cranial fossa-*www.ajronline.org*
- **Enlargment of neural foramina**
- Rib penciling is caused by underlying mesodermal dysplasia and bony remodeling from adjacent neurofibroma. Rib penciling is present when rib width is narrower than the narrowest portion of the second rib- *www.ajronline.org*

"**Neurofibromatosis:** A generalized variety of neurofibromatosis (von Recklinghausen's disease) may have skeletal disturbances like scoliosis, solitary bone lesions, pseudarthrosis of the tibia, compressive myelopathy, local gigantism, limb length inequality etc. In addition, other soft tissue manifestations of the disease may be present"- *Maheswari 5th/317*

Table: Neurofibromatosis 1 and Neurofibromatosis 2: Clinical Feature *(Davidson 22nd/1216)*

Neurofibromatosis 1	Neurofibromatosis 2
Skin Cutaneous/subcutaneous neurofibromas Angiomas Café au lait patches (> 6) Axillary/groin freckling Hypopigmented patches	Much less commonly affected then NF1 Café au lait patches (usually <6) Cutaneous schwannomas: plaque lesions Subcutaneous schwannomas
Eyes Lisch nodules (Iris fibromas) Glaucoma Congenital ptosis	**Cataracts** Retinal hamartoma ***Optic nerve meningioma***
Nervous system Plexiformneurofibromas Malignant peripheral nerve sheath tumours Aqueduct stenosis Slight tonsillar descent Cognitive impairment Epilepsy	Vestibular schwannomas Cranial nerve schwannomas (not 1 and 2) Spinal schwannomas Peripheral nerve schwannomas Cranial meningiomas Spinal meningiomas Spinal/brainstem ependymomas Spinal/cranial astrocytoma
Bone Scoliosis Osteoporosis Pseudoarthrosis	
Cardiorespiratory systems Pulmonary stenosis Hypertension Renal artery stenosis Compression from neurofibroma causing restrictive lung defect	
Gastrointestinal system Gastrointestinal stromal tumour Dysplasia Duodenal carcinoid tumour	

247. Ans. b. Rad/min

[Ref: Sumer Sethi 6th/170-71; Radiology & Imaging by K. Thayalam 1st/108-09; Radiology by S. Bhadury 2nd/197; Harrison 19th/363e-4]

"**Dose rate in telethrapy:** measured in Monitor unit or rad per minute"- *Innovations in Radiation Oncology by H. Rodney 1st/100*

Monitor Units

- *Ozradonc.wikidot.com*
- A monitor unit is a measurement of ionisation occurring in a treatment beam within the treatment head. One monitor unit is typically equal to a specific dose of radiation, at a specific depth in a water phantom, for a beam of a particular energy, with a particular field size and at a certain distance from the target. Monitor units are used to measure the output of the machine to deliver accurate dose.
- For teletherapy machines, treatment time is used instead of monitor units. The treatment time is based on similar measurements to monitor units, but uses the known output of the radioactive source to calculate the time required to leave the source in the 'on' position
- Factors influencing calculation of Monitor Units
    - Beam Energy
    - Source Surface Distance
    - Tissue-Phantom Ratio / Tissue-Maximum Ratio (TPR)
    - Percentage Depth Dose (PDD)
    - Output Factor (OF)
    - Wedge Factor (WF).
    - Calibration Factor (CF)

Radiation Units Radiology & Imaging by

- *K. Thayalam 1st/ 108-09*
- Exposure is a source related term
- Unit of exposure is- Roentgen(R)
- Activity (disintegration rate) = Curie & Becquerel (SI unit)
- Absorbed dose = Gray/Rad
- Equivalent dose = Sievert (Sv) & Rem

Table: *Sumer Sethi 6th/171*

Unit	Quantity Measured	Definition
Roentgen (R)	Exposure	Amount of X-rays or gamma rays that produces a specific amount of ionization in a given volume of air
Rad	Dose	100 ergs deposited per gram of tissue
Gray (Gy)	Dose	SI unit of dose; equals 100 rad
Rem	Dose equivalence	Unit that reflects the biologic response. It is used to compare various types of radiation
Sievert (Sv)	Dose equivalence For X-rays: 1 Gy = 1 Sv.	SI unit of dose equivalence; equals 100 rem

248. Ans. a. USG is used for initial screening; b. Contrast enhanced MRI - Enhancement in arterial phase & washout in venous phase; c. Multidetector row CT with intravenous contrast shows hypervascular appearance

[Ref: Davidson 23rd/890-91;Harrison 19th/547; Danhert Radiology Review Manual 7th/739-40]

Contrast enhanced MRI scan Danhert

- *Radiology Review Manual 7th/740*
- **Arterial Phase**
    - *Intense homogenous enhancement for tumor <2 cm*
    - *Heterogenous enhancement for lesion >2 cm*
- *Portal venous & equilibrium phase*
    - *Rapid loss of enhancement becoming isointense/ hypointense (= venous washout)*

Hepatocellular Carcinoma

◈ *Radiology Harrison 19th/547*

- ***An ultrasound examination of the liver is an excellent screening tool.*** The two characteristic vascular abnormalities are hyper-vascularity of the tumor mass (neovascularization or abnormal tumor-feeding arterial vessels) and thrombosis by tumor invasion of otherwise normal portal veins.
- To determine tumor size and extent and the presence of portal vein invasion accurately, a **helical/triphasic CT scan** of the abdomen and pelvis, with fast-contrast bolus technique, should be performed to detect the vascular lesions typical of HCC.
- **Magnetic resonance imaging (MRI)** can also provide detailed information, especially with the newer contrast agents
- A prospective comparison of ***triphasic CT, gadolinium-enhanced MRI, ultrasound and fluorodeoxyglucose positron emission tomography (FDG-PET) showed similar results for CT, MRI and ultrasound;*** PET imaging appears to be positive in only a subset of HCC patients.
- MRI requires a longer examination and ascites can cause artifacts, but MRI is better able to distinguish dysplastic or regenerative nodules from HCC.
- **Imaging criteria** have been developed for HCC that do not require biopsy proof, as they have >90% specificity.
- The altered tumor vascularity that is a consequence of molecularly targeted therapies is the basis for newer imaging techniques including contrast-enhanced ultrasound (CEUS) and dynamic MRI

"Screening for HCC, by ***ultrasound scanning and AFP measurements at 6-month intervals, is indicated in high-risk patients,*** such as those with cirrhosis due to hepati-tis B and C, haemochromatosis, alcohol, NASH and α1 -antitrypsin deficiency"- *Davidson 23rd/891*

Serologic Assays

◈ *Harrison 19th/547*

- **AFP** is a serum tumor marker for HCC; however, it is only ***increased in approximately one-half*** of U. S. patients.
- γ-Glutamyl transpeptidase and alkaline phosphatase may be particularly important in the 50% of HCC patients who have low AFP levels.
- ***Alpha-fetoprotein (AFP) is produced by 60% of HCCs.*** Levels increase with the size of the tumour and are often normal or only minimally elevated in small tumours detected by ultrasound screening- *Davidson 23rd/890-91*

Imaging in HCC

◈ *Davidson 23rd/891*

- Ultrasound will detect focal liver lesions as small as 2–3 cm. The use of ultrasound contrast agents has increased sensitivity and specificity, but is highly user-dependent. Ultrasound may also show evidence of portal vein involvement and features of coexistent cirrhosis.
- **Multidetector row CT**, following intravenous contrast, identifies HCC by its classical hypervascular appearance. Small lesions of less than 2 cm can be difficult to differentiate from hyperplastic nodules in cirrhosis. MRI can be used instead of CT.
- Angiography is now seldom performed and has been superseded by the above techniques.
- Combination of imaging modalities more accurately diagnoses and stages the extent of disease and using at least two modalities (typically, ***CT or MRI following initial screening ultra-sound identification of a mass lesion***) is recommended

"Rising or elevated levels of *serum α-fetoprotein* are found in 50% of persons with advanced HCC. However, it is insensitive as a screening test for premalignant or early lesions as these usually do not produce particularly high levels of the protein"-*Robbins 9th/873*

ANSWER SHEET

1 – 50		51 – 100		101 – 150		151 – 200		201 – 250	
1	A B C D E	51	A B C D E	101	A B C D E	151	A B C D E	201	A B C D E
2	A B C D E	52	A B C D E	102	A B C D E	152	A B C D E	202	A B C D E
3	A B C D E	53	A B C D E	103	A B C D E	153	A B C D E	203	A B C D E
4	A B C D E	54	A B C D E	104	A B C D E	154	A B C D E	204	A B C D E
5	A B C D E	55	A B C D E	105	A B C D E	155	A B C D E	205	A B C D E
6	A B C D E	56	A B C D E	106	A B C D E	156	A B C D E	206	A B C D E
7	A B C D E	57	A B C D E	107	A B C D E	157	A B C D E	207	A B C D E
8	A B C D E	58	A B C D E	108	A B C D E	158	A B C D E	208	A B C D E
9	A B C D E	59	A B C D E	109	A B C D E	159	A B C D E	209	A B C D E
10	A B C D E	60	A B C D E	110	A B C D E	160	A B C D E	210	A B C D E
11	A B C D E	61	A B C D E	111	A B C D E	161	A B C D E	211	A B C D E
12	A B C D E	62	A B C D E	112	A B C D E	162	A B C D E	212	A B C D E
13	A B C D E	63	A B C D E	113	A B C D E	163	A B C D E	213	A B C D E
14	A B C D E	64	A B C D E	114	A B C D E	164	A B C D E	214	A B C D E
15	A B C D E	65	A B C D E	115	A B C D E	165	A B C D E	215	A B C D E
16	A B C D E	66	A B C D E	116	A B C D E	166	A B C D E	216	A B C D E
17	A B C D E	67	A B C D E	117	A B C D E	167	A B C D E	217	A B C D E
18	A B C D E	68	A B C D E	118	A B C D E	168	A B C D E	218	A B C D E
19	A B C D E	69	A B C D E	119	A B C D E	169	A B C D E	219	A B C D E
20	A B C D E	70	A B C D E	120	A B C D E	170	A B C D E	220	A B C D E
21	A B C D E	71	A B C D E	121	A B C D E	171	A B C D E	221	A B C D E
22	A B C D E	72	A B C D E	122	A B C D E	172	A B C D E	222	A B C D E
23	A B C D E	73	A B C D E	123	A B C D E	173	A B C D E	223	A B C D E
24	A B C D E	74	A B C D E	124	A B C D E	174	A B C D E	224	A B C D E
25	A B C D E	75	A B C D E	125	A B C D E	175	A B C D E	225	A B C D E
26	A B C D E	76	A B C D E	126	A B C D E	176	A B C D E	226	A B C D E
27	A B C D E	77	A B C D E	127	A B C D E	177	A B C D E	227	A B C D E
28	A B C D E	78	A B C D E	128	A B C D E	178	A B C D E	228	A B C D E
29	A B C D E	79	A B C D E	129	A B C D E	179	A B C D E	229	A B C D E
30	A B C D E	80	A B C D E	130	A B C D E	180	A B C D E	230	A B C D E
31	A B C D E	81	A B C D E	131	A B C D E	181	A B C D E	231	A B C D E
32	A B C D E	82	A B C D E	132	A B C D E	182	A B C D E	232	A B C D E
33	A B C D E	83	A B C D E	133	A B C D E	183	A B C D E	233	A B C D E
34	A B C D E	84	A B C D E	134	A B C D E	184	A B C D E	234	A B C D E
35	A B C D E	85	A B C D E	135	A B C D E	185	A B C D E	235	A B C D E
36	A B C D E	86	A B C D E	136	A B C D E	186	A B C D E	236	A B C D E
37	A B C D E	87	A B C D E	137	A B C D E	187	A B C D E	237	A B C D E
38	A B C D E	88	A B C D E	138	A B C D E	188	A B C D E	238	A B C D E
39	A B C D E	89	A B C D E	139	A B C D E	189	A B C D E	239	A B C D E
40	A B C D E	90	A B C D E	140	A B C D E	190	A B C D E	240	A B C D E
41	A B C D E	91	A B C D E	141	A B C D E	191	A B C D E	241	A B C D E
42	A B C D E	92	A B C D E	142	A B C D E	192	A B C D E	242	A B C D E
43	A B C D E	93	A B C D E	143	A B C D E	193	A B C D E	243	A B C D E
44	A B C D E	94	A B C D E	144	A B C D E	194	A B C D E	244	A B C D E
45	A B C D E	95	A B C D E	145	A B C D E	195	A B C D E	245	A B C D E
46	A B C D E	96	A B C D E	146	A B C D E	196	A B C D E	246	A B C D E
47	A B C D E	97	A B C D E	147	A B C D E	197	A B C D E	247	A B C D E
48	A B C D E	98	A B C D E	148	A B C D E	198	A B C D E	248	A B C D E
49	A B C D E	99	A B C D E	149	A B C D E	199	A B C D E	249	A B C D E
50	A B C D E	100	A B C D E	150	A B C D E	200	A B C D E	250	A B C D E

NAME OF THE CANDIDATE	ROLL NO.	CENTRE NO.	QUESTION BOOKLET NO.	BOOKLET CODE
CATEGORY SC ○ ST ○ OBC ○ GEN ○ CW ○ PH ○	0 0 0 0 0 1 1 1 1 1 2 2 2 2 2 3 3 3 3 3 4 4 4 4 4 5 5 5 5 5 6 6 6 6 6 7 7 7 7 7 8 8 8 8 8 9 9 9 9 9	0 0 1 1 2 2 3 3 4 4 5 5 6 6 7 7 8 8 9 9	0 0 0 0 0 1 1 1 1 1 2 2 2 2 2 3 3 3 3 3 4 4 4 4 4 5 5 5 5 5 6 6 6 6 6 7 7 7 7 7 8 8 8 8 8 9 9 9 9 9	A B C D

INSTRUCTIONS FOR FILLING THE SHEET

1. This sheet should not be folded or crushed.
2. Use only blue/black ball pen to fill the circles.
3. Use of pencil is strictly prohibited.
4. Circles should be darkened properly and completely.
5. Cutting & erasing on this sheet is not allowed.
6. Do not use any stray marks on the sheet.
7. Do not use marker, white fluid or any other device to hide the shading already done.

WRONG METHOD

CORRECT METHOD

CANDIDATE'S SIGNATURE
(in ball - point pen)

INVIGILATOR'S SIGNATURE
(in ball - point pen)

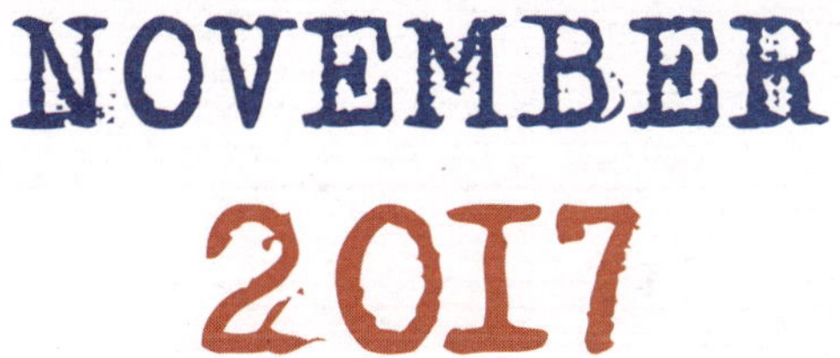

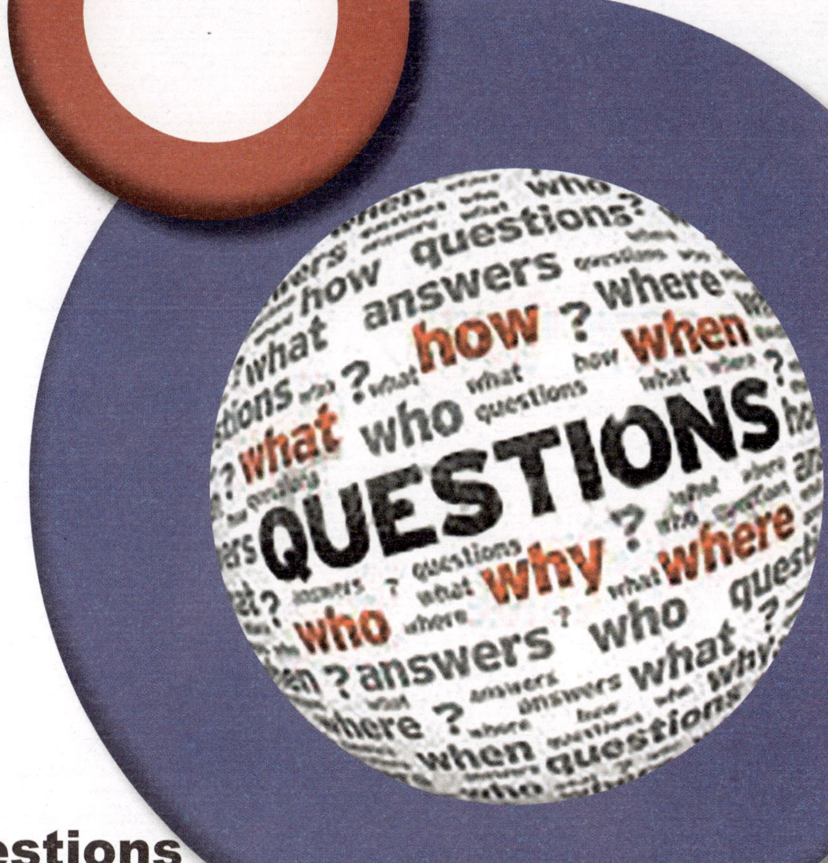

Multiple Choice Questions
Answers & Explanations

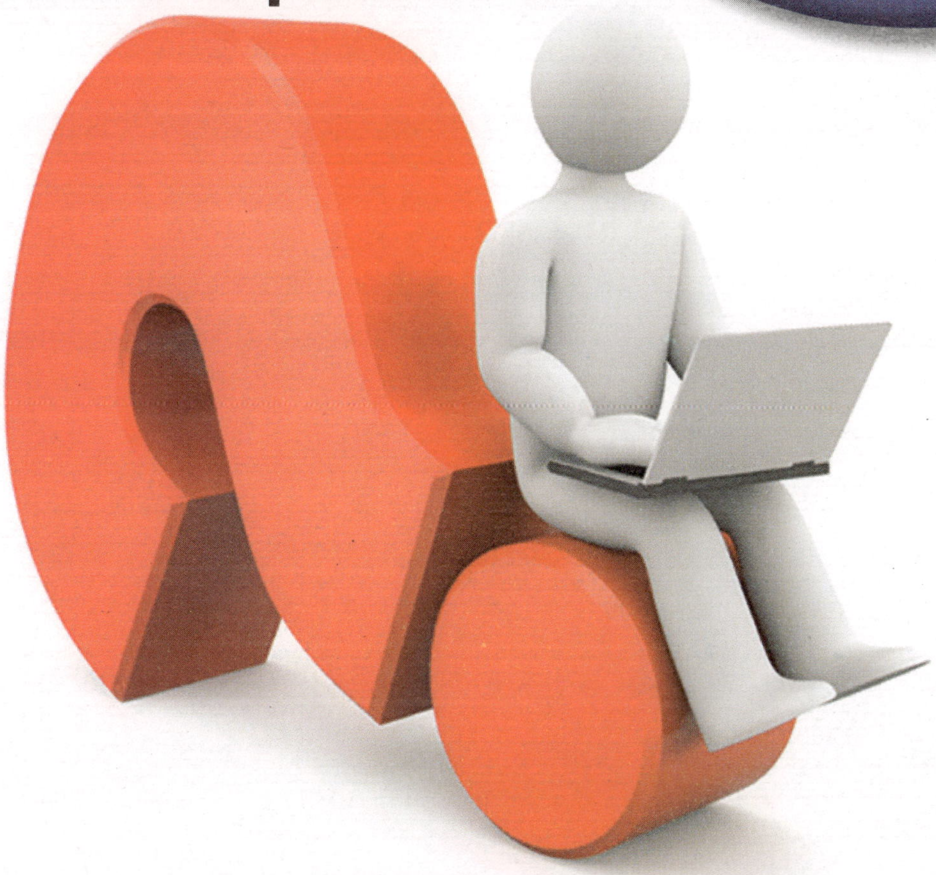

NOVEMBER 2017 MULTIPLE CHOICE QUESTIONS

ANATOMY

1. **Muscle(s) of anterior compartment of leg is/are:**
   a. Peroneus tertius
   b. Peroneus brevis
   c. Peroneus longus
   d. Flexor digitorum longus
   e. Extensor hallucis longus
2. **True about epiglottis:**
   a. Contains serous gland
   b. Contains mucous secreting glands
   c. It is oval shaped
   d. Made up of elastic cartilage
   e. Has bilateral lymphatic supply
3. **Which of the following is/are true about perineal membrane of urogenital diaphragm:**
   a. Posterior border is attached medially to perineal body
   b. Triangular in shape
   c. Carry pudendal nerve and internal pudendal artery
   d. Perforated by ureter and vaginal
   e. Supports pelvic floor
4. **Blood supply of ureter is/are from all, except:**
   a. Middle rectal artery
   b. Internal pudendal artery
   c. Gonadal vessel
   d. Common Iliac artery
   e. Vesical artery
5. **Tributaries of coronary sinus are all except:**
   a. Great cardiac vein
   b. Anterior cardiac vein
   c. Oblique vein of the left atrium
   d. Middle cardiac vein
   e. Small cardiac vein
6. **True about Trochlear nerve:**
   a. Cranial nerve with longest intracranial course
   b. Smallest cranial nerve
   c. It terminates on the superior oblique muscle on the same of the nucleus of origin
   d. Only cranial nerve which arises anteriorly
   e. It passes b/w the anterior and middle cerebral artery
7. **Trigeminal nerve lesion may lead to:**
   a. No weakness in jaw opening
   b. Weakness in jaw closing
   c. Loss of corneal reflex
   d. Sensory loss of face
   e. Paralysis of temporalis and masseter muscle
8. **Which of the following structure(s) traverse parotid gland:**
   a. External carotid artery
   b. Cervicofacial trunk of facial nerve
   c. Retromandibular vein
   d. Lingual nerve
   e. Facial artery
9. **True about Thyroid gland:**
   a. Thyroid lies in between 2 layers of deep cervical fascia
   b. Berry ligament derived from deep cervical fascia
   c. Left recurrent laryngeal nerve is larger than right recurrent laryngeal nerve
   d. Superior thyroid artery runs in close relation with superior laryngeal nerve
   e. The superior parathyroid glands are usually located ventral to the recurrent laryngeal nerve
10. **True statement (s) about events in Prophase of Meiosis I:**
    a. Sister chromatids duplicates
    b. Sister chromatids separate
    c. Homologous chromosomes separate
    d. Homologous chromosomes duplicates
    e. Haploid daughter cells
11. **Correct statement(s) regarding the anatomy of vertebrae is/are:**
    a. T_7 has vertically oriented articular process
    b. C_6 has prominent lateral mass
    c. T_3 has smallest spinous process
    d. T_{12} has large costal facet
    e. C_7 has no foramen transversarium

PHYSIOLOGY

12. **True regarding Rennin-angiotensin system:**
    a. Renin is secreted by modified smooth muscle cells of efferent arteriole
    b. Macula densa is a part of renin-angiotensin system
    c. Renin converts angiotensinogen to angiotensin-I
    d. Angiotensin-converting enzyme is present in endothelium of the lung vessels
    e. Angiotensin-II stimulates release of aldosterone from zona glomerulosa
13. **True about function Loop of Henle:**
    a. Fluid reaching descending limb from proximal convoluted tubule is hypotonic
    b. Descending limb reabsorbs water
    c. Thin ascending limb actively absorbs sodium chloride
    d. Thick ascending limb permeable to water
    e. Descending limb imperable to water
14. **Main features of Brown-Séquard syndrome:**
    a. Ipsilateral loss of pain and temperature sense
    b. Contralateral posterior column involvement
    c. Ipsilateral posterior column involvement
    d. Ipsilateral extensive weakness of lower limbs
    e. Contralateral extensive weakness of lower limbs

Answer

1. a, e.	2. b,d,e.	3. a,b,e.	4. b.	5. b.	6. a,b.	7. b,c,d,e.
8. a,b,c.	9. a,b,c.	10. c.	11. a.	12. b,c,d,e.	13. b.	14. c. d.

15. Solute diuresis is/are seen in:
a. Diabetes mellitus
b. Central diabetes insipidus
c. Nephrogenic diabetes insipidus
d. Diuretic overuse

16. Vitamin K is/are involved in synthesis of which of the clotting factors:
a. Factor 9
b. Factor 13
c. Factor 10
d. Factor 11
e. Factor 12

17. ACTH convert progesterone into:
a. Deoxycorticosterone
b. Cortisol
c. DHEA
d. Aldosterone
e. Androstenedione

18. Which of the following tests is/are useful for assessment of anterior pituitary gland function:
a. Serum prolactin level estimation
b. Serum growth hormone level after oral glucose ingestion
c. Serum oxytocin level
d. Water deprivation test
e. ACTH stimulation test

19. Which of the following statements are true regarding diffusion of gas in lung:
a. CO_2 diffuses 20 times faster than O_2
b. PO_2 gradient is low between alveoli & blood vessel in case of restrictive lung disease
c. Diffusion of oxygen is perfusion limited
d. Diffusion of gas is decreased in emphysema
e. Diffusion capacity of O_2 is 25

20. True statement(s) about nerve muscle physiology :
a. Contraction is mainly because of extracellular calcium
b. Action potential traverses along T tubules
c. Rynadine receptors sense the action potiential
d. Actin pulls the myosin
e. ATP binds to myosin

BIOCHEMISTRY

21. Which of the following urea cycle enzymes is/are found in cytosol:
a. Carbamoyl phosphate synthetase I
b. Ornithine transcarbomylase
c. Arginosuccinate synthetase
d. Arginosuccinate lyase
e. Arginase

22. Which of the following is/are feature(s) of homocystinuria:
a. Cystine stone formation in kidney
b. Mental retardation
c. Autosomal dominant inheritance
d. Ectopia lentis

23. True about mucopolysaccharidoses:
a. It is a type of lysosomal storage disorder
b. All are autosomal recessive except Morquio syndrome
c. Skeletal defect is manifested as dystosis multiplex
d. Research is going on to develop give therapy for Morquio syndrome

24. Which of the following are omega-6 fatty acid except:
a. Palmitic acid
b. Alpha-linolenic acid
c. Linoleic acid
d. Gamma linolenic acid
e. Arachidonic acid

25. Which of the following statement(s) is/are true regarding vitamin B12 deficiency:
a. ↓Erythocyte transketolase level
b. Muscle weakness may occur
c. Peripheral sensory nerve involvement is usually present
d. Neuronal symptom improves with Vit B12 therapy

26. True statement(s) about vitamin A:
a. 1600 U retinol is used for treatment of xerophthalmia
b. >1% prevalence of night-blindness is the criteria for determining the xerophthalmia problem in the population at risk (6m-6yr)
c. Retinol is not present in milk
d. Chronic vitamin A intoxication causes papilledema

27. Glycolysis is/are regulated by:
a. Hexokinase
b. Pyruvate kinase
c. Phosphofructokinase
d. Glucose 1,6 bisphosphatase
e. Pyruvate dehydrogenase

28. Which of the following is/are non-reducing sugar(s):
a. Glucose
b. Isomaltose
c. Sucrose
d. Galactose
e. Trehalose

29. Apolipoproteins present in HDL cholesterol is/are:
a. Apo I
b. Apo II
c. Apo B-48
d. Apo 100
e. Apo D

30. Uridine diphosphoglucose (UDPG) help in:
a. Galactose synthesis
b. Glycogen synthesis
c. Bilirubin metabolism
d. Ganglioside synthesis
e. Heaprin synthesis

31. True about copper metabolism:
a. Copper excretion mainly occurs in urine
b. 95% bond to albumin in the serum
c. Ceruloplosmin contains 6 atoms of copper
d. Failure to synthesize ceruloplasmin causes Wilson's disease
e. Intestinal absorption occurs in duodenum

Answer

15. a, d.	16. a, c.	17. a, b, e.	18. a, b, e.	19. a, c, d, e.	20. b, c, e.	21. c, d, e.
22. b, d.	23. a, c, d.	24. a, b.	25. b, c, d.	26. b, d.	27. a, b, c	28. c, e.
29. a, b, e.	30. a, b, c, d, e.	31. c, d, e.				

32. Poor wound healing is vitamin 'C' deficiency is/are due to:
a. Defective collagen synthesis
b. Inhibition of collagen synthesis
c. Defective post-translational modification of collagen
d. Defective hydroxylation
e. Defect in antioxidant system

IMMUNOGENETICS & MOLECULAR BIOLOGY

33. Which of the following DNA polymerase used in PCR has proofreading activity:
a. Pfu polymerase
b. Taq polymerase
c. Bestaq DNA Polymerase
d. Pwo polymerase
e. Tth polymerase

34. Which of the following motif is/are involved in specific protein-DNA interactions:
a. Helix-turn-helix
b. Zinc finger
c. Helix-loop-helix
d. Leucine zipper

35. Which of the following protein(s) is/are required for DNA strand separation:
a. DNA Helicase
b. Single-stranded DNA-binding (SSB) proteins
c. Ligase
d. DNA polymerase
e. DnaA protein

36. Component(s) involved in RNA-induced silencing complex (RISC):
a. miRNa
b. Drosha
c. Dicer
d. Pasha
e. Slicer

37. In which of the following autosomal non-disjunction is/are seen:
a. Patau syndrome
b. Edward syndrome
c. Klinefelter syndrome
d. Cri-du-chat syndrome
e. William syndrome

38. Microsatellite instability disorder(s) is/are:
a. Myotonic dystrophy
b. Huntington chorea
c. Ataxia telangiectasia
d. Spinocerebellar ataxia
e. Xeroderma pigmentosa

39. Which of the following is/are part of 30S initiation complex:
a. ATP
b. GTP
c. Initiation factor
d. Elongation factor
e. mRNA

40. Single mutation in DNA of somatic cell of multicellular organism results in:
a. No effect on organism
b. Every cell in the entire organism will be affected
c. May result in 100 abnormal cells
d. Can be transmitted to progeny

41. 30S ribosome interacts with all except:
a. GTP
b. ATP
c. mRNA
d. Elongation factor
e. Initiation factor

42. Enzymes required for mRNA synthesis is/are:
a. RNA polymerase I
b. RNA polymerase II
c. Primase
d. Topoisomerase
e. Ligase

43. Complementary DNA differs from genomic DNA in:
a. Has coded segments
b. Has introns
c. Has only exons
d. Uses reverse transcriptase
e. Larger

PATHOLOGY

44. Feature(s) of DiGeorge syndrome is/are all except:
a. Results from failure of development of the third and fourth pharyngeal pouches
b. Absent thyroid
c. Absent parathyroid glands
d. B cell defect
e. Enhanced susceptibility of bacterial infection

45. Which of the following is not associated with prolonged prothrombin time:
a. Haemophilia A
b. Von-Willebrand disease
c. Factor VII deficiency
d. Disseminated intravascular coagulation (DIC)
e. Liver disease

46. Primary extranodal neoplasms is/are:
a. Burkitt lymphoma
b. Waldeyer's ring lymphoma
c. Gastric lymphoma
d. Thyroid lymphoma
e. Mycosis fungoides

47. Pathological feature(s) of rheumatic heart disease is/are:
a. Widened mitral annulus
b. McCallum plaques
c. Rupture of papillary muscle
d. Aschoff nodules
e. Aortic valve thickening

Answer

32. a, c, d, e. 33. a, c, d. 34. a, b, c, d. 35. a, b, e. 36. a, c, e. 37. a, b. 38. a, b, d
39. b, c, e. 40. c. 41. b, d. 42. b. 43. a, c, d. 44. d. 45. a, b
46. b, c, d, e 47. a, b, d, e

48. Which of the following Dyads are correctly matched:
a. RB1-retinoblastoma
b. PTEN- Melanoma
c. BRCA2-Breast cancer
d. N-MYC-Neuroblastoma
e. WT1 = Wilm's tumor

49. Paraneoplastic syndrome(s) associated with lymphoma:
a. SIADH
b. Hypercalcemia
c. Cushing's syndrome
d. Acanthosis nigricans

50. Dystrophic calcification is/are found in:
a. Monckeberg's medial sclerosis
b. Papilary carcinoma thyroid
c. Hyperparathyroidism
d. Meningioma
e. Vitamin D intoxication

51. Features of irreversible cell injury is/are:
a. Lysosomal rupture
b. Pyknosis
c. Bleb formation on membrane
d. Severe mitochondrial dysfunction

52. Which of the following is/are released from dense granules of platelets:
a. Serotonin
b. Histamine
c. PDGF
d. ATP
e. Lysosome

53. Which of the cell derived chemical mediators of inflammation is/are preformed in secretory granules:
a. Histamine
b. Lysosomal enzymes
c. Leukotrienes
d. Prostaglandins
e. Serotonin

54. CD markers for natural killer cells is/are:
a. CD 16
b. CD 117
c. CD 56
d. CD 1
e. CD 4

55. Combined B and T cell immunodeficiency is/are seen in:
a. Severe Combined Immunodeficiency
b. Adenosine deaminase deficiency
c. Wiskott-Aldrich syndrome
d. Ataxia telangiectasia
e. DiGeorge syndrome

56. Which of the following dyads are correctly matched regarding urinary casts and associated condition:
a. Hyaline casts- may be normally present in healthy person
b. Muddy brown casts-acute tubular necrosis
c. WBC cast - pyelonephritis
d. Epithelial cast – acute glomerulonephritis
e. Myogolobin cast - Rhabdomyolysis

57. Which of the following statement(s) is/are true about primary sclerosing cholangitis:
a. May be complicated by bacterial infection
b. Rarely progress to biliary cirrhosis
c. Involve only intrahepatic bile duct not extrahepatic bile ducts
d. Associated with Inflammatory bowel disease
e. Narrowing of bile duct

58. About autoimmune hepatitis, which of the following is true:
a. More common in female
b. Anti–liver kidney microsome-1 (anti-LKM-1) antibody is found in type I subtype only
c. Oral corticosteroids are given in severe cases
d. Associated with other autoimmune disease
e. Rarely lead to cirrhosis

59. Which of the following is/are not feature of Turner syndrome:
a. Tall stature
b. Associated with celiac disease
c. 45XO karyotype
d. 45XO/46XY karyotype
e. Hypertension

60. True about morphological feature(s) of alcoholic steatosis:
a. Fat droplet in hepatocyte
b. Mallory body may be seen
c. May cause hepatic necrosis
d. Perivenular fibrosis may be seen
e. Macro-nodule formation

61. On which cell cycle checkpoints BRCA-2 acts:
a. G2-M
b. G1-M
c. M phase
d. G1 phase
e. S phase

62. Vascular changes of malingnant hypertension is/are:
a. Necrotizing arteriolitis
b. Hyaline arteriosclerosis
c. Hyperplastic arterioscleroesis
d. Aortic dissection
e. Onion skinning

PHARMACOLOGY

63. Resistance to which of the following drugs is included in definition of Extensively drug resistance-TB (XDR-TB):
a. Amikacin
b. Fluroquinolones
c. Ethambutol
d. Pyrazinamide
e. Streptomycin

64. Which of the following drug(s) can cause Diarrhea as side-effect?
a. Proton pump inhibitors (PPI)
b. Calcium channel blockers
c. NSAIDS
d. Aluminium hydroxide
e. Magnesium hydroxide

65. Which of the following statement(s) is/are true about salicylate poisoning and its treatment except:
a. Alkaline diuresis is used for increased excretion of drug
b. Activated charcoal has no role
c. Hemodialysis for removal of absorbed drug
d. Liver toxicity may occur
e. Tinnitus is seen

Answer

48. a, c, d, e.	49. a, b.	50. a, b, d.	51. a, b, d.	52. a, b, d.	53. a, b, e.	54. a, c.
55. a, b, c, d.	56. a, b, c, e.	57. a, b, d, e.	58. a, c, d, e.	59. a.	60 a, d.	61. a, e.
62. a, c, d, e.	63. a, b.	64. a, e.	65. b.			

66. IFN-alpha is/are used in:
a. Chronic hepatitis B
b. Chronic hepatitis C
c. Hairy cell leukaemia
d. Mycosis fungoides
e. Multiple sclerosis

67. Which drug(s) do/does not cause significant bone marrow depression:
a. Vinblastine
b. Vincristine
c. Cyclophosphamide
d. Clorambucil Cisplatin
e. 5-Fluorouracil

68. True about Bedaquilline:
a. It is a bactericidal drug of newer class diarlyquinolone
b. It works by blocking the enzyme ATP synthase in mycobacterium and affects energy supply
c. Causes liver and cardiac damage
d. Always should be used in combination with other drugs
e. Can be used up to 12 months

69. Which of the following causes pink/red discoloration of urine:
a. Drug such as Rifampicin and phenazopyridine
b. Ingestion of beetroot
c. Phenol poisoning
d. Aniline dyes ingestion
e. Alkaptonuria

70. True about first order kinetics of drug elimination:
a. Elimination half-life is dose dependent
b. Clearance (CL) remains constant
c. Constant fraction of drug is eliminated
d. Constant amount of drug is eliminated
e. Rate of drug elimination is inversely proportional to the drug concentration

71. True statement(s) about competitive antagonist in relation to drug response curve (DRC) of agonist:
a. Antagonism can be overcome by increasing dose of agonist
b. Decrease potency of agonist
c. Parallel rightward shift of agonist DRC
d. Decrease efficacy of agonists
e. Parallel leftward shift of agonist DRC

72. Which are direct-acting cholinomimetic drugs:
a. Neostigmine
b. Donepezil
c. Bethanechol
d. Methacholine
e. Pilocarpine

73. Which of the following dyads of oral hypoglycaemic drug-mechanism of action is/are true:
a. Canagliflozin- Inhibitors of Sodium Glucose Transport-2
b. Acarbose: α-glucosidase inhibitor
c. Exenatide: Dipeptidyl dipeptidase-4 inhibitor
d. Repaglinide: K+ ATP channel blocker
e. Sitagliptin: Glucagon Like peptide (GLP-1) agonist

74. According to the latest guideline, chemotherapy for Glioblastoma Multiforme include(s):
a. Methotrexate
b. Dacarbazine
c. Temozolomide
d. Thiotepa
e. Cyclophosphamide

75. Management of monomorphic/acute ventricular tachycardia includes:
a. Amiodarone
b. Propanolol
c. Diltiazem
d. Lidocaine
e. Procainamide

76. True about treatment of leprosy:
a. Multibacillaryleprosy is treated by 3 drugs
b. Paucibacillary leprosy is treated by 1 drug
c. Paucibacillary leprosy is treated for 1 year
d. Post-treatment surveillance for multibacillary leprosy is for 5 years
e. Clofazimine is first line drug

77. Alternative to rifampicin based treatment of leprosy in patient with hepatitis:
a. Clofazimine
b. Ofloxacin
c. Minocycline
d. Clarithromycin
e. Moxifloxacin

78. Physiological antagonism is found in:
a. Salbutamol and leukotrienes
b. Isoprenaline and adrenaline
c. Isoprenaline and propranolol
d. Adrenaline and histamine
e. Isoprenaline and salbutamol

79. A patient has platelet count<1 lakh, hemoglobin 8gm. Which of the following anticancer drug can be used:
a. Cisplatin
b. Methotrexate
c. Vincristine
d. Vinblastin
e. Bleomycin

80. Primaqunie sensitivity is seen in anemia with following enzyme deficiency except:
a. Pyruvate dehydrogenase
b. Hexokinase
c. Glucose-6-phosphate dehydrogenase
d. Glucose 6 phosphate

MICROBIOLOGY

81. Non-gonococcal urethritis is/are caused by:
a. Mycoplasma hominis
b. Mycoplasma genitalium
c. Chlamydia trachomatis
d. Treponema pallidum
e. None of above

Answer

66. a, b, c, d. 67. a. 68. a, b, c, d. 69. a, b, d. 70. b, c. 71. a, b, c. 72. c, d, e.
73. a, b, d. 74. c. 75. a, b, c, d. 76. a, d, e. 77. a, b, d, e. 78 a, d. 79. c, e.
80. a, b, d. 81. a, b, c.

82. Which of the following disease is/are not caused by family Spirochetes?
- a. Lyme's disease
- b. Yaws
- c. Syphilis
- d. Pinta
- e. Leptospira

83. True about Human papillomavirus (HPV):
- a. ssDNA containing virus
- b. Icosahedral symmetry
- c. HPV type 16 and 18 causes cervical cancer
- d. Recently nine valent vaccine passed phase 3 clinical trial
- e. 5 genera of HPV identified

84. True about Ebola virus:
- a. Flavivirus
- b. Icosahedral symmetry
- c. Predominantly found in Africa
- d. Spreads by direct contact with the blood or body fluids
- e. Currently there is no specific treatment for this disease

85. True statement about genital ulcer:
- a. Donovanosis- Painful and multiple lesion
- b. Granuloma inguinale causes donovanosis
- c. Haemophilus ducrei causes chancroid
- d. Systemic feature common in primary syphilis and H.ducrei infection
- e. Primary syphilis-Painful and indurated papule

86. A patient is presenting with multiple painful ulcers and discharging inguinal lymphadenopathy. Which of the following finding is suggestive of this disease:
- a. Demonstration of school of fish appearance of bacilli
- b. Culture of H. ducreyi from an aspirate of suppurative lymph nodes
- c. Microscopic identification of Donovan bodies in tissue smear
- d. Evidence of Treponema pallidum infection by dark-field examination of ulcer exudate
- e. Herpes simplex virus in the ulcer exudate

87. Which of the following is/are feature of streptococcus agalactiae rather than staphylococcus aureus?
- a. Catalase positive
- b. Bacitracin resistant
- c. Coagulase negative
- d. α hemolysis
- e. β hemolysis

88. True about tapeworm:
- a. Taenia solium is more prevalent
- b. Taenia saginata is beef tapeworm
- c. Infection is acquired by ingestion of cysticercus in raw beef
- d. Infectious form to animal is egg

89. True regarding erysipelas:
- a. Caused by streptococcus pyogenes
- b. Superficial skin lesion
- c. More seen on face than trunk
- d. Has history of recent sore throat infection

90. Not true about candida albicans.
- a. Forms pseudohyphae
- b. Yeast like fungus
- c. Reynolds-Braude phenomenon
- d. Forms true hyphae
- e. Dimorphic fungus

91. True about aspergillus infection:
- a. Causes subcutaneous infections
- b. Branched at 90°
- c. Nonseptate
- d. Septate
- e. Forms hyphae

92. Which of the following Nanoparticle(s) inhibit both E coli and staph aureus:
- a. Zinc oxide
- b. Silver nanoparticle (SNP)
- c. Iron oxide
- d. Aluminum oxide
- e. Copper oxide

FORENSIC MEDICINE

93. Magnan's symptom is seen in poisoning with:
- a. Cocaine
- b. Lead
- c. Cannabis
- d. Mercury

94. True about Gustafson's method:
- a. Useful in dead person
- b. Useful in living person
- c. Transparency of root is most reliable component
- d. Used for identification of sex
- e. Used for age estimation

95. Which of the following bone/joint epiphysis ossification is used for age estimation in age group 21-25 year:
- a. Ankle
- b. Knee
- c. Wrist
- d. Inner end of clavicle
- e. Fusion of ischial tuberosity

96. Which of the following statement(s) is/are true regarding rape, after October 11, 2017 verdict of supreme court:
- a. Sex with wife age < 15 year is rape
- b. Sex with wife age < 15 year is not rape
- c. Sex with wife of age group 15-18 years is rape
- d. Age of consent for wife >16 year
- e. Exception 2 of S. 375 IPC is validated

97. Section of IPC related to sodomy:
- a. Section 321 IPC
- b. Section 322 IPC
- c. Section 323 IPC
- d. Section 324 IPC
- e. Section 377 IPC

Answer

82. e.	83. b, c, d, e.	84. c, d, e.	85. b, c.	86. a, b.	87. c.	88. b, c, d.
89. a, b, c, d.	90. None.	91. d,e.	92. a, e.	93. a.	94 a, c, e.	95. d, e.
96. a, c.	97. e.					

98. **Which of the following combination(s) is/are correct:**
   a. Castor seed - not poisonous when consumed unbroken with cover
   b. Neem- excessive use can cause renal failure
   c. Dhatura-neurotoxic
   d. Cannabis- CNS depressant

PREVENTIVE & SOCIAL MEDICINE

99. **Post exposure prophylaxis is/are given in:**
   a. Hepatitis A infection
   b. Hepatitis B infection
   c. Hepatitis C infection
   d. Rabies
   e. Varicella zoster virus infection

100. **True statement(s) about epidemiological studies:**
   a. Cross sectional study: concept of causativity can be deducted
   b. Case control study: Suitable for study of rare disease
   c. Cohort study help in assessing concept of causativity
   d. In cohort study groups are allocated by randomization
   e. Case control study-estimates only odd ratio

101. **Which of the following statement(s) is/are true:**
   a. Sensitivity and specificity of test-depend on prevalence of disease
   b. Predictive value reflects the diagnostic power of the test
   c. Positive predictive value -depend on prevalence of disease
   d. Sensitivity and specificity of test- characteristics of the test

102. **Which of the following statement(s) is/are true about Dengue:**
   a. According to WHO, dengu is classified only in 2 category- DF and DHF
   b. Subsequent infection with different strain produces severe form of dengu
   c. Most infection with dengu virus is asymptomatic
   d. Vector is Aedes mosquito

103. **Which of following is/are component vaccine:**
   a. DaPT vaccine
   b. Pneumococcal (PCV-7) vaccine
   c. Hepatitis B vaccine
   d. OPV vaccine
   e. MMR vaccine

104. **True statement about iodine deficiency disorder:**
   a. Exclusively found in Himalayan goiter belt
   b. Goiter prevalence of 10% is cut-off value for endemicity
   c. Strabismus is also a manifestation
   d. Only monitored by blood thyroid test

105. **According to biomedical waste rule 2016, incineration/deep burial/plasma pylorysis is done for bag having colour code:**
   a. Blue
   b. Red
   c. Yellow
   d. White
   e. None

106. **True statement(s) regarding National programme for control of blindness (NPCB):**
   a. Launched in 1962
   b. Dr Rajendra Prasad Center for Ophthalmic Sciences , AIIMS is apex body for implementation of NPCB
   c. Promotion of eye camp and mobile unit
   d. Intra ocular lens implantation better than convention conventional surgery
   e. NGOs are sidelined in this programme

107. **90:90:90 target in National Health Policy 2017 stand for:**
   a. 90% of all people living with HIV know their HIV status
   b. 90% of all people diagnosed with HIV infection receive sustained antiretroviral therapy
   c. 90% of all people living with HIV and TB know their HIV status
   d. 90% of all people diagnosed with HIV infection and TB receive sustained antiretroviral therapy and ATT
   e. 90% of all people receiving antiretroviral therapy will have viral suppression

108. **Which of the following is/are true about Six-Sigma:**
   a. Developed by Motorola
   b. Only practiced in Motorola company
   c. Represents an ideology that focuses on statistical improvements to a business process
   d. It is a quality-control program

109. **Which of the following vaccine may be used as candidate vaccine in Leprosy:**
   a. BCG vaccine
   b. Killed M.leprae + BCG vaccine
   c. Vaccination with M. indicus pranii
   d. BCG vaccine + M. vaccae

110. **Which of the following is/are true about sewage disposal:**
   a. Biochemical oxygen demand (BOD) is indicator of the organic content of sewage
   b. BOD is amount of oxygen absorbed by a sample of sewage
   c. Undergo both aerobic and anaerobic reaction in sewage purification
   d. Untreated sewage is thrown into rivers

111. **High risk group for influenza is/are:**
   a. Morbid obese
   b. Young adult
   c. Children
   d. Pregnant women
   e. Elderly person

OPHTHALMOLOGY

112. **Feature of fungal corneal ulcer is/are all except:**
   a. Mucopurulent discharge may be present
   b. Satellite lesion may be present around the ulcer
   c. Flat and mobile hypopyon
   d. Fungi can penetrate into the anterior chamber without perforation
   e. Wesseley ring may present

Answer

98. a, b, c.	99. a, b, d, e.	100. b, c, e.	101. b, c, d.	102. b, c, d.	103. b, c.	104. b, c.
105. c.	106. b, c, d.	107. a, b, e.	108. a, c, d.	109. a, b, c, d.	110. a, b, c.	111. a, b, c, d, e.
112. c						

113. True about adenovirus conjunctivitis:
a. Virus has ssDNA
b. Incubation period is 6-10 days
c. Ganciclovir only modality available for treatment
d. True membrane lining lower fornix and palpebral conjunctiva may be present

114. Upper eyelid consists of:
a. Levator palpebrae superioris muscle (LPS)
b. Skin
c. Muller muscle
d. Fat
e. Orbicularis oris muscle

115. True about blood supply of optic pathway:
a. Optic nerve is supplied by pial network of vessels
b. Optic tract is supplied by anterior choroidal artery
c. Cilioretinal artery arise from central retinal artery
d. Lateral geniculate body is supplied by choroidal arteries
e. Optic radiation is supplied by middle cerebral arteries

116. Branches of ophthalmic artery is/are:
a. Central retinal artery
b. Anterior choroidal artery
c. Anterior ciliary artery
d. Short posterior ciliary artery

117. Which of the following not causes lens dislocation:
a. Ehlers-Danlos syndrome
b. Marfan's syndrome
c. Sulphite oxidase deficiency
d. Diabetes mellitus

118. In which of the following condition there is decreased corneal sensitivity:
a. Viral keratitis
b. Herpes simplex keratitis
c. Acanthamoeba keratitis
d. Keratoplasty fully restores the corneal sensitivity

119. Unilateral mydriasis is/are seen in:
a. Adie's tonic pupil
b. Marcus gunn pupil
c. Argyll Robertson pupil
d. Horner syndrome

ENT

120. Which of the following statement(s) is/are true about neck dissection in H and N surgery:
a. Submandibular nodes belong to level 2A
b. Posterior triangle group nodes belong to level 4
c. Level I to V nodes are removed in radical neck dissection
d. Internal jugular vein is preserved in modified radical neck dissection
e. Hypoglossal nerve is removed in radical neck dissection

121. Which of the following is true regarding vestibular system:
a. Semicircular canal responds to linear acceleration
b. Utricle responds to linear acceleration
c. Otolith organs responds to angular acceleration
d. Saccule responds to rotational acceleration
e. Saccule responds to linear acceleration

122. True statement about Schwartz sign:
a. Contraindication to surgery
b. Can be seen in early disease
c. More common during pregnancy
d. Reddish hue over the promontory
e. Indicate active lesion

123. Which of the following is/are feature(s) of tongue tie:
a. Usually lead to severe respiratory difficulty
b. Predisposes to dental caries
c. Difficulty in articulation of speech
d. Difficult breast-feeding
e. Significant tongue tie need surgical release

124. True abut Auditory Brainstem Implant (ABI):
a. Restores hearing when hearing loss is due to the destruction of the auditory nerve
b. Indicated in profoundly deaf person
c. Indicated in bilateral acoustic neuromas after surgery
d. Cochlear nerve agenesis is contraindication
e. Electrode is placed on the surface of the Brainstem

125. Cochlear implant is contraindicated in:
a. Michel aplasia
b. Enlarged vestibular aqueduct syndrome
c. Absent cochlear nerve
d. Mild intracochlear ossification
e. Persistent otitis media and mastoiditis without eradication of the disease

126. True about development of Cochléa:
a. Cochlea start develop by 5th week of gestation
b. Vestibular labyrinth develop later than cochlea
c. Cochlea development completes by 8 week of gestation
d. Cochlea development completes at 20th week of gestation
e. Cochlea develops from endoderm

127. Premalignant lesion of tongue includes:
a. Erythroplakia
b. Lichen planus
c. Psoriasis
d. Aphthous ulcer
e. Fordyce's spot

128. True about allergic fungal sinusitis:
a. Allergic mucin containing scattered fungal hyphae is pathological hallmark
b. Invasion of the sinus mucosa with fungus
c. Allergic reaction to fungus
d. Antifungal agents are main drug used for treatment
e. In severe cases corticosteroids are used for treatment

129. Which of the following is/are true about the T-stage of maxillary sinus carcinoma:
a. Stage T4a- Frontal sinus involvement
b. Stage T3-Ethmoid sinus involvement
c. Stage T2-Sphenoid sinus involvement
d. Stage T2- bone of the posterior wall of maxillary sinus

Answer

113. b.	114. a, b, c, d.	115. a, b, d, e.	116. a, c, d.	117. d.	118. a, b, c.	119. a, b.
120. c, d.	121. b, e.	122. b, c, d, e.	123. b, c, d, e.	124. a, b, c, e.	125 a, c, e.	126. a, d.
127. a, b.	128. a, c, e	129. a, b.				

MEDICINE

130. Features of milk alkali syndrome:

a. Hypercalcemia
b. Hypervolumeia
c. Hyperparathyroidism
d. Nephrocalcinosis
e. Diarrhea

131. True statement(s) about adrenocortical carcinoma are all except:

a. Part of Li-Fraumeni syndrome
b. Surgery is the treatment of choice for solitary tumor
c. Resection of tumors with metastasis is also useful
d. In big size functioning tumor debulking is also useful
e. There is no role of chemotherapy and radiotherapy

132. Ventilator-Induced lung injuries occur due to:

a. Subtracheal stenosis
b. Barotrauma
c. Biotrauma
d. Atelectrauma
e. Altectasis

133. Malignancies associated with AIDS:

a. Non hodgkin lymphoma
b. Cervical cancer
c. Kaposi sarcoma
d. Ovarian cancer
e. Anal cancer

134. Criteria of febrile neutropenia include(s):

a. Axillary temperature >39°C
b. One oral temperature ≥38.5°C
c. A sustained oral temperature >38°C for more than 1 hour
d. Absolute neutrophil count $<0.5 \times 10^9$/L
e. Absolute neutrophil count $<1.0 \times 10^9$/L with a predictable decline to $\leq 0.5 \times 10^9$/l in 24–48 h

135. Which of the following may be present in patent ductus arteriosus

a. Continuous murmur
b. Aortic ejection systolic murmur
c. Loud P2
d. Mitral opening snap
e. Mid diastolic murmur at apex

136. Which of the following findings are seen in atrial septal defect except:

a. Wide and fixed splitting of 2nd heart sound
b. Soft 1st heart second
c. An apical holosystolic murmur indicates associated mitral or tricuspid regurgitation or a ventricular septal defect
d. Pulmonary ejection systolic murmur
e. Mid diastolic murmur at the lower left sternal border

137. True about atrial premature beats:

a. Associated with abnormal P wave
b. All P waves are normal in morphology
c. Each P wave is followed by QRS complex
d. Each P wave is not always followed by QRS complex
e. Shows saw-tooth pattern in lead II

138. Partial Pressure of Oxygen in aortic blood (PaO_2) is/are decreased in all except:

a. Pulmonary edema
b. Pulmonary Fibrosis
c. Polycythemia
d. Cor pulmonale
e. Pulmonary atelectasis

139. In comparison to obstructive lung disease, restrictive lung disease, on pulmonary function test, shows decrease of

a. FEV1
b. Forced residual capacity (FRC)
c. FEV1/FVC
d. Total lung capacity (TLC)
e. Residual volume

140. Which of the following is/are true about management of Non-ST segment elevation myocardial infarction except:

a. Management includes aspirin, clopidegrel and LMWH
b. Increase serum troponin level
c. Fibrinolytic therapy is not useful
d. Thrombolysis should be done within 48 hour
e. Low risk patient may be evaluated by angiography after 48-72 hour

141. Liver transplantation is contraindicated in all except:

a. MELD score >15
b. Hepatocellular carcinoma
c. Active alcoholic abuser
d. Active drug user
e. Child–Pugh grade C

142. Which of the following is/are true about Kaposi's sarcoma:

a. African form mainly occurs in older men
b. European form found in all age group
c. IFN-alpha is used for treatment
d. HIV associated Kaposi's sarcoma regresses with antiretroviral therapy
e. Caused by HHV-8

143. True statement(s) about management of acute pancreatitis except:

a. Aggressive fluid resuscitation
b. Early enteric feeding within 2-3 days
c. Prophylactic antibiotic is not necessary
d. Pancreatic pseudocysts can be treated by drainage into the stomach, duodenum or jejunum
e. Only conservative management should be done for pancreatic necrosis

144. Cause(s) of fever following blood transfusion:

a. Transfusion-related acute lung injury (TRALI)
b. Septicemia
c. Transfusion related CMV infection
d. Acute Hemolytic Transfusion Reactions

145. Which of the following is increased in Iron deficiency anemia:

a. Serum iron
b. Total Iron-Binding Capacity
c. Transferrin saturation
d. Serum ferritin
e. Red blood cell distribution width (RDW) index

Answer

130. a, d	131. e.	132. a, b, c, d.	133. a, b, c, e.	134. b, c, d, e.	135. a, b, c, d , e.	136. b.
137. a, d.	138. c.	139. b, d, e.	140. d.	141. a, b, e.	142 c, d, e.	143. .e
144. a, b, c, d.	145. b, e					

146. In contrast to Iron deficiency anaemia, which of the following are decreased in anemia of chronic disease:

a. Mobilization of iron stores
b. Total Iron-Binding Capacity
c. Transferrin saturation
d. Serum Ferritin
e. Iron store

147. Diagnostic Criteria for Severe aplastic anemia include(s)

a. Absolute neutrophil count <500/μL
b. Platelet count <20,000/μL
c. Hemoglobin < 8g/dL
d. Bone marrow cellularity <25%
e. Absolute reticulocyte count <60,000/μL

148. All of the following shows rise in reticulocyte count except:

a. Acute severe haemorrhage
b. Congenital Dyserythropoietic anemia
c. Aplastic anemia
d. Hereditary spherocytosis
e. Treatment of megaloblastic anemia with vitamin B12

149. A cancer patient who is ambulatory and about more than 50% is waking hours .He not able to perform work activities but able to perform his daily activities for self-care without assistance. Which of the following performance scale/index, he belongs:

a. ECOG Grade 1
b. ECOG Grade 2
c. ECOG Grade 3
d. Karnofsky Performance Index 60
e. Karnofsky Performance Index 70

150. Continuous murmur is seen is:

a. Ventricular septal defect
b. Tetrology of fallot
c. Pregnancy
d. Coarctation of aorta
e. Patent ductus arteriosus

SURGERY

151. Which is true regarding frostbite injury:

a. In First and second degree frostbite affected part show redness and edema
b. Spontaneous recovery without any treatment is rule
c. Extensive involvement in frostbite is called chilbain
d. Initial treatment is rewarming
e. Autoamputation may occur in severe cases

152. True about Small bowel diarrhea:

a. Loperamide should not be given because it causes drug dependence
b. Causes watery diarrhea
c. Pain relieves after defaecation
d. Cause malabsorption of vitamins
e. Pain usually occur in periumbilical area

153. True about small bowel resection:

a. If jejunum is cut, ileum can compensate jejunal function
b. If Ileum is cut, jejunum can compensate ileum function
c. Ileum resection is generally better tolerated, as jejunal shows better capacity to compensate
d. Bile acid malabsorption lead to diarrhea

154. True statement about splenosis:

a. Occur after traumatic rupture of the spleen
b. Function as normal spleen
c. Multiple small implants of splenic tissue on the peritoneal surfaces
d. Peritoneal nodules of metastatic carcinoma
e. Benign tumor of spleen

155. True statement(s) regarding tubercular peritonitis and ascites:

a. SAAG <1.1 g/dL in ascitic fluid
b. Elevated adenosine deaminase level
c. Protein < 25–30 g/L
d. The diagnosis can be made by laparoscopy with directed biopsy of the peritoneum

156. All are true about arteriovenous-fistula except:

a. Trauma is most common cause of acquired fistula
b. Congenital fistula is easier to repair by surgery than acquired fistula
c. Artificial fistula is surgically created fistulas for hemodialysis access
d. High blood pressure from artery results in arterialization of vein
e. Large A-V fistula may casue thrombocytopenia

157. Proximally obliterated processus vaginalis is/are seen in:

a. Vaginal hydrocele
b. Congenital hydrocele
c. Infantile hydrocele
d. Encysted hydrocele of cord
e. Inguino-scrotal hydrocele

158. True about gastric bezoar:

a. After gastrectomy- it does not occurs
b. Caused by ingestion of fruits, vegetable fibers and hairs
c. In Rapunzel syndrome, bezoar has a tail-like extension into the small bowel
d. Surgery is always indicated
e. It increases chance of gastric ulceration

159. True about abdominal compartment syndrome:

a. Normal intra-abdominal pressure is 0-5 mm Hg
b. Intra-abdominal hypertension is measured by bladder pressure
c. Earliest sign-kidney failure
d. Management of choice is abdominal opening
e. Multi-organ failure may occur

160. Which of the following suture(s) is/are not degraded by proteolytic enzymes:

a. Catgut
b. Polyglyconate
c. Polyglactin
d. Monofilament Nylon

Answer

146. a, b. 147. a, b, d, e. 148. b. 149. b, e. 150. c, d, e. 151. a, d, e. 152. b, c, d, e.
153. a, b, d. 154. a, b, c. 155. a, b, d. 156. b. 157. a, c, d, e. 158. b, c, e. 159. a, b, d, e.
160. b, c, d

161. One French (F) size of angiographic catheter corresponds to:
a. 0.33 mm
b. 1.67 mm
c. 0.133 inch
d. 0.013 inch
e. 0.057 inch

162. Clinical feature of acute arterial embolism is/are:
a. Pulselessness
b. Pain
c. Erythema of distal part
d. Numbness
e. Sensory loss

163. Which of the following is/are commonly present in middle mediastinum:
a. Schwannoma b. Thymoma
c. Bronchogenic cyst d. Teratoma
e. Substernal thyroid

164. True regarding axillary lymph node dissection in breast cancer:
a. Axillary dissection can be carried out through the incision for a mastectomy
b. Level I,II and III nodes are removed in modified radical mastectomy
c. In Halsted radical mastectomy all breast tissue and skin, the nipple-areola complex, the pectoralis major and pectoralis minor muscles and the level I, II and III axillary lymph nodes are removed
d. Arm is kept abducted at 900 during axillary dissection
e. Halsted radical mastectomy preserves pectoralis major and the lateral pectoral nerve

165. True about acute ischemic colitis:
a. Most common site involved are sigmoid colon and splenic flexure
b. Most commonly occur in young female
c. Abdominal radiographs show thumb print sign
d. Commonly presents as pain in abdomen with bloody dirrhoea
e. Acute thrombotic mesenteric occlusion is also k/a intestinal angina

166. True about esophageal perforation:
a. Morbidity is mainly d/t mediastinal infection
b. Partial tear involving mucosa should be managed conservatively
c. Simple exploration and end to end anastomosis is done as soon as possible in all cases
d. Spontaneous perforation most commonly occur in midthoracic esophagus
e. Serum amylase levels may be high as a result of absorption of amylase from the pleural cavity

167. True about transurethral resection of the prostate (TURP):
a. More morbidity than retropubic prostatectomy
b. Can causes retrograde ejaculation
c. Open prostatectomy is preferred in larger obstructive mass
d. There is less risk of bleeding in transurethral laser vaporization than in TURP
e. Resectoscope is passed through the urethra and prostate is resected into multiple pieces and removed

168. Risk factors for gastric cancer includes:
a. Chronic atrophic gastritis b. Obesity
c. Smoking d. H.pylori infection
e. Menetriers disease

169. All are true about pilonidal sinus except:
a. More common in young female
b. It may occur d/t combination of buttock friction and shearing forces in affected area
c. Direction of the sinuses are cephaloid
d. May l/t recurrent abscess formation
e. Recurrence is common even after surgery

170. True about chest wall tumor:
a. Fibrous dysplasia is the most common malignant soft tissue tumor
b. Lipomas are the most common benign tumors
c. Desmoid is low-grade sarcomas of soft tissue of chest wall
d. Lung metastasis with direct chest wall extension should be treated with radical en bloc resection of the chest wall and underlying lung
e. Rhabdomyosarcoma is the second most common chest wall tumor in children

171. Regarding lipoma which of the statement(s) is/are true:
a. Lipoma is the most common benign soft tissue tumor in adult
b. 25% of all lipomas are multiple (Dercum disease)
c. Intramuscular lipoma are ill defined and difficult to palpate than subcutaneous lipoma
d. Usually progress to liposarcoma

172. True about low velocity ballistic injury:
a. Abdominal injury usually requires full exploratory laparotomy
b. Spinal cord and brain injury may require bullet fragment removal if compressive symptoms present
c. Injuries are typically associated with a low infection rate
d. Conservative management in superficial abdominal injury
e. Prophylactic antibiotic has no role

173. Unlike cellulitis, erysipelas has feature(s) of:
a. Clearly demarcated margin
b. Elevated edge
c. More deeper skin involvement
d. More generalized spread
e. More abrupt onset

Answer

161. a, d.	162. a, b, d, e.	163. c.	164. a, b, c, d.	165. a, c, d, e.	166. a, b, e.	167. b, c, d, e.
168. a, b, c, d, e.	169. a.	170. b, c, d, e.	171. a, c.	172. a, b, c, d.	173 a, b, e.	

174. Which of the following is/are true except:
- a. Surgical blade direction should be downward and away from surgeon
- b. During bowel anastomosis, hemostatic forceps are used to grasp intestine
- c. Needle holding forceps damage sutures as it is crushing in nature
- d. Toothed forceps is used of bone to grasp skin, subcuatneous tissue, muscles and sheath
- e. Handle of Surgical blade is hold with thumb and middle finger

175. Reverse Trendelenburg position is/are not used for:
- a. Prophylaxis against thromboembolism
- b. High intracranial tension
- c. Thyroid surgery
- d. Hyperparathyroid surgery

OBSTETRICS & GYNECOLOGY

176. Most common cause of secondary postpartum hemorrhage:
- a. Trauma
- b. Atonic uterus
- c. Bleeding disorders
- d. Retained products of conception
- e. Coagulopathy

177. Management of postmenopausal women with stress urinary incontinence include(s):
- a. Kegel pelvic floor exercise
- b. Retropubic cystourethropexy
- c. Intermittent self catheterization
- d. Anticholinergic drugs
- e. Retopubic midurethral sling procedures

178. Absolute contraindication of medical abortion:
- a. Previous LSCS
- b. Previous myomectomy
- c. Suspected ectopic pregnancy
- d. Prostaglandin hypersensitivity
- e. Severe rheumatic heart disease

179. Which of the following contraceptive will be effective when used alone after 15 day of menstrual cycle:
- a. Levonorgestrel IUCD
- b. Progesterone only pill
- c. Combined oral contraceptives (COC)
- d. CuT IUCD
- e. LNG emergency pill

180. A women forget to take 3 Combined oral contraceptive (COC) active pills. What should she do now:
- a. Take all missing piles at a time and continue rest pills as usual
- b. For 2–3 day use barrier method and continue rest pills as usual
- c. Immediately switch to non hormonal contraceptives (e.g. CuT-IUD) and discontinue COC
- d. If she exposed to recent intercourse, use emergency contraceptive
- e. Use another method of contraception like barrier method for remaining period and start next COC pack without break

181. Which of the following is/are true regarding haemodynamic changes in pregnancy:
- a. Maximum cardiac changes occurs at 8 weeks of gestation
- b. Venocaval compression begins at about 16 weeks of gestation
- c. There is midtrimester fall in blood pressure
- d. Systolic murmur may occur normally
- e. Cardiac output return to pregnant level by 20 days after delivery

182. Screening test(s) for aneuploidy in 1st trimester:
- a. PAPP-A and β-hCG estimation
- b. Quadruple test
- c. Chorionic villus Sampling
- d. Amniocentesis
- e. Triple test

183. Double test in 2nd trimester for screening of Down syndrome includes:
- a. PAPP and AFP
- b. MSAFP and hCG
- c. MSAFP and uE3
- d. MSAFP and inhibin-A

184. True about adenomyosis:
- a. Capsulated lesion
- b. Associated with dysmenorrhea and menorrhagia
- c. Total hysterectomy is the treatment of choice
- d. Asymmetrically enlarged and tender uterus
- e. Tenderness of uterus may be seen before and during menses

185. A lady with secondary amenorrhea is negative for progesterone challenge test but positive for combined estrogen and progesterone challenge test. What is the probable cause(s):
- a. Hypothalamic and pituitary cause
- b. Ovarian failure
- c. PCOD
- d. Asherman syndrome
- e. Pregnancy

186. True about chronic hypertension in pregnancy:
- a. Hypertension before pregnancy, elevation of blood pressure during the first half of pregnancy, or high blood prêssure that lasts for longer than 12 weeks after delivery
- b. Fetal complication may occur
- c. Incidence is about 50%
- d. High blood pressure may require antihypertensive medications

187. Which of the following are true about Breech presentation:
- a. Frank breech is most common breech presentation
- b. Complete breech is more common in multiparae
- c. Frank breach is more common in primigravida
- d. Chance of cord prolapse in footling presentation is 5–6%
- e. Chance of cord prolapse in complete breech is 5%

Answer

174. b.	175. a.	176. d.	177. a, b, e.	178. c, d, e.	179. d.	180. d, e.
181. b, c, d, e.	182. a, c.	183. b.	184. b, c, e.	185. a, b.	186 a, b, d.	187. a, b, c, e.

188. True about benign gestational trophoblastic disease:
a. Occur due to proliferation of placenta
b. No risk of carcinoma
c. Fetus may be absent
d. Karyotype 69XXY may result from fertilization of 1 ovum and 2 sperm
e. Snowstorm appearance on USG

189. Pap smear of a patient with condyloma accuminita shows what kind of smear:
a. Inflammatory
b. High-Grade Squamous Intraepithelial Lesion (HSIL)
c. Squamous cell carcinoma
d. Low-Grade Squamous Intraepithelial Lesion (LSIL)
e. Normal

190. High-grade squamous intraepithelial lesions (HSIL) are found in pap smear. Next step(s) of management:
a. HPV DNA Testing
b. Liquid based cytology
c. Colposcopy study and biopsy of suspicious lesion
d. Hysterectomy
e. Radiotherapy

191. Indication(s) of postoperative radiotherapy in vulval carcinoma is/are all except:
a. Lymphovascular space permeation
b. Positive margins
c. Margin < 8-10 mm
d. Single metastatic nodule with capsular involvement
e. Only one microscopically positive lymph node

192. A female with IUCD develops pelvic inflammatory disease. Which of the following should be done?
a. Keep the IUCD, give antibiotic, follow up for antibiotic response and then take decision regarding IUCD removal
b. Start antibiotics and then remove IUCD
c. Remove IUCD and then start antibiotics
d. Wait till next menstrual cycle for any intervention
e. Do nothing

193. Mutation involved in serous ovarian carcinoma:
a. KRAS
b. WT1
c. TP53
d. PTEN
e. ARID1A

PEDIATRICS

194. All are true about Attention deficit hyperactivity disorder except:
a. In Two-third cases symptoms may continue in adulthood
b. For making the diagnosis, the behavioral changes must begin before 5 year of age
c. May associated with mood disorder
d. Amphetamine and busiprone may be used for treatment
e. More prevalent in boys

195. Preferred diagnostic test used for HIV detection in neonate born by caesarean section whose mother is HIV positive:
a. HIV DNA PCR
b. ELISA
c. Viral culture
d. HIV P24 antigen assay
e. HIV RNA PCR

196. Most common route of TB infection in neonate born by caesarean section:
a. Hematogenously spread
b. Through Skin contact
c. Inhalational of aerosol
d. Tansplacental
e. By aspiration of infected amniotic fluid

197. True about febrile seizure:
a. Most common cause of seizure in childhood
b. May persist beyond 5 years if associated with atypical feature
c. Family h/o is a risk factor
d. Febrile seizure is always associated with neurologically abnormal child

198. Causes of macrocephaly includes:
a. *Galactosemia*
b. Weaver syndrome
c. Rett syndrome
d. Sostos syndrome
e. Morquio syndrome

199. Feature(s) of Rett's syndrome:
a. Developmental delay starts from birth
b. Loss of purposeful learned hand movements
c. Incoordinated gait
d. Expressive speech defect
e. Normal head circumference at birth

ORTHOPEDICS

200. Which of the following is/are true about Kienbock disease:
a. Osteochondritis of scaphoid bone
b. Osteochondritis of lunate bone
c. Painful flexion and extension of wrist
d. Passive dorsiflexion of middle finger produces pain
e. Positive ulnar variance is a predisposing factor

201. Feature(s) of Hangman's fracture:
a. Fracture of C2 vertebrae
b. Neural arch disturbed
c. Traumatic spondylolisthesis of C2 on C3
d. C2-3 intervertebral disc may be torn
e. C2-3 intervertebral disc is always preserved

Answer

188. a, c, d, e.	189. d.	190. a, b ,c.	191. e.	192. a.	193. a, c, d.	194. b.
195. a, e.	196. c.	197. a, b, c.	198. a, d, e.	199. b, c, d, e.	200 b, c, d.	201. a, b, c, d.

202. Which of the following condition affects primarily the metaphysis:

a. Osteomyelitis
b. Osteosarcoma
c. Giant cell tumor
d. Osteoclastoma

203. True about osteoarthritis:

a. Knee is the most commonly affected joint in Indian population
b. Hip osteoarthritis is more common than knee osteoarthritis in India
c. Causes movement restriction and instability of the joint
d. Synovial thickening occur early
e. Heberden's nodes occur more commonly in female

204. A 28 yr old lady came with nausea, vomiting and abdominal pain. On X-ray, lytic eccentric lesion and cortex thinning seen in wrist joint. What will be the next step(s) in management:

a. Bone biopsy
b. Bone curettage alone
c. Bone curettage and adjuvant treatment with phenol only
d. Bone curettage, adjuvant treatment with phenol and bone cementing
e. PTH and serum calcium level measurement

205. A Child presented with tenderness and crepitus on lateral condyle of humerus with flexion deformity of elbow, following fall on extended hand. Long term complication of this fracture include(s):

a. Malunion
b. Nonunion
c. Volkmann's ischemic contracture
d. Ulnar nerve palsy
e. Recurrent dislocation

206. Which of the following is/are feature(s) of compound palmer Ganglion:

a. Swelling is hour glassed shaped but fluctuation can not be elicited
b. Complete excision is the best treatment
c. Present both above and below the flexor retinaculum
d. A very painful swelling

207. Cause of recurrent dislocation of patella include(s):

a. Underdeveloped medial femoral condyle
b. Excessive ligamental laxity
c. Vastus medialis agenesis
d. High oblique insertion of the vastus medialis
e. Flattening of the intercondylar groove

208. Feature(s) of pyogenic osteomyelitis:

a. Most common causal organism is staphylococcus aureus
b. Most commonly affects diaphysis of long bones
c. Involucrum is piece of dead bone
d. Cloacae are holes in involucrum
e. Sequestrum is dense sclerotic bone overlying lesion site

ANESTHESIA

209. Which of the following may be used in management of Post-dural puncture headache (PDPH):

a. Caffeine
b. Clonidine
c. Epidural blood patch
d. Synthetic ACTH in refractory cases
e. NSAIDS

210. Child came to emergency room with respiratory depression, shock and fever. Endotracheal intubation is planned. Which of the following drug(s) should be avoided in this child:

a. Ketamine
b. Thiopentone
c. Etomidate
d. Fentanyl
e. Propofol

211. True statement(s) about sugammadex:

a. Antisuccinylcholine in action
b. Selectively binds to rocuronium
c. Used along with rocuronium for rapid induction Anesthesia
d. Discovered to reverse the effects of atracurium
e. Specific for depolarizing neuromuscular blocking agents

212. Metabolism of atracurium is/are by:

a. Hofmann Elimination
b. Non-specific esterase
c. Acetylcholinesterase
d. Pseudocholinesterase
e. Ester hydrolysis

213. Which of the following is/are use of capnography:

a. For confirmation of intubation
b. For diagnosing pulmonary edema
c. For assessing pulmonary embolism
d. To check adequate ventilation

214. Which of the following statement(s) is/are correct regarding perfluorocarbon emulsions used as blood substitute:

a. Chemically combine with oxygen
b. Low capacity for carrying oxygen at physiological pO_2 levels
c. Transported oxygen is more completely offloaded than blood-transported oxygen
d. Sigmoid shaped oxygen dissociation curve
e. All oxygen carried by the perfluorocarbon is in the dissolved state

215. Pre-anaesthetic medication is given to:

a. Reduction of secretion of saliva
b. Reduce anxiety and fear
c. To produce amnesia
d. To prevent undesirable reflexes
e. Prevent vomiting

Answer

202. a, b.	203. a, c, d, e.	204. a, d, e.	205. a, b, d, e.	206. b, c.	207. b, c, d, e.	208. a, d.
209. a, c, d, e.	210. b, c, d, e.	211. b.	212. a, b, e.	213. a, c, d.	214 b, c, e.	215. All (a,b,c,d,e).

216. Methods of regional anaesthesia is/are:

a. Spinal anaesthesia
b. Bier's block
c. Rapid sequence induction
d. Conscious sedation
e. Surface anaesthesia

DERMATOLOGY

217. Which of the following play(s) a role in pathogenesis of Rosacea:

a. Demodex folliculorum
b. Propionobacterium acne
c. H.pylori
d. Malassezia furfur

218. Treatment for genital warts include (s):

a. 10–30% Tricholoroacetic acid
b. 50–70%Tricholoroacetic acid
c. 10-25% Podophyllin resin
d. Clindamycin
e. Imiquimod (5% cream)

219. Sporotrichoid pattern is/are seen in:

a. Sporotrichosis
b. Lichen nitidus
c. Lichen planus
d. Fish tank granuloma
e. Lupus vulgaris

220. Agent (s) associated with allergic contact dermatitis:

a. Poison ivy
b. Nickel
c. Gold
d. Paraphenylene diamine
e. Rubber

221. Which of the following is/are vascular malformation:

a. Campbell de Morgan spots
b. Hutchinson freckle
c. Angiokeratoma
d. Keratoacanthoma
e. Pyogenic granuloma

222. Spongiosis involves which part of skin:

a. Epidermis
b. Dermis
c. Stratum spinosum
d. Stratum corneum
e. Prickle cell layer

223. Koebner's phenomenon is seen in-

a. Pemphigus vulgaris   b. DLE
c. Lichen planus   d. Acne rosae
e. Genital warts

PSYCHIATRY

224. Which of the following is/are true regarding cannabis use and schizophrenia:

a. Increased incidence of schizophrenia in genetically susceptible person with long term use of cannabis
b. Stopping cannabis prevent development of schizophrenia
c. Cannabis is most common cause of substance abuse psychosis
d. Schizophrenic persons are more prone to cannabis use
e. There is no association of schizophrenia with cannabis use

225. All are somatoform disorder(s) except:

a. Somatisation disorder
b. Illness anxiety disorder
c. Persistent somatoform pain disorder
d. Somatic passivity disorders
e. Hypochondriacal disorders

226. Which is/are selective serotonin and noradrenaline reuptake inhibitors (SNRIs):

a. Duloxetine   b. Venlafaxine
c. Milnacipran   d. Dapoxetine
e. Paroxetine

227. Side effects of Clozapine include(s):

a. Seizures   b. Sedation
c. Dry mouth   d. Hypothermia
e. Constipation

228. Treatment of mania includes:

a. ECT
b. Mood stabilizer
c. Antidepressant drugs
d. Antipsychotic drugs

229. Psychiatric illness included in criminal responsibility of insane person:

a. Delusion   b. Hallucination
c. Illusion   d. OCD
e. Mania

230. Feature(s) of catatonic schizophrenia:

a. Waxy flexibility   b. Automatic obedience
c. Somatic passivity   d. Rigidity
e. Mutism

RADIOLOGY

231. Unit of absorbed radiation is/are:

a. Rem
b. Gray
c. Curie
d. Rad
e. Becquerel

Answer

216. a, b, e.   217. a, c.   218. b, c, e.   219. a, d, e.   220. a, b, d, e.   221. a, c, e.   222. a, c, e.
223. b, c, e.   224. a, d.   225. b, d.   226. a, b, c.   227. a, b, e.   228 a, b, d.   229. a, b.
230. All (a,b,c,d,e). 231. b, d

232. Which of the following radio-diagnostic tests should be done in a traumatic patient:

a. Cervical X-ray A-P view
b. Chest X-ray A–P view
c. Focused assessment with sonography for trauma(FAST)
d. X-ray of visible injury site
e. X-ray pelvis AP view

233. Which of the following statement(s) is/are true regarding X-ray abdomen:

a. Gas under diaghragm- seen in perforated gastric ulcer
b. Rigler sign-seen in acute peritonistis with pneumoperitoneum
c. Differentiation of small and large bowel obstruction can be done by location of distended bowel loop
d. Large intestine- shows taenia coli and haustration
e. Valvulae conniventes are circular folds reach around the whole circumference of the large intestine

234. Which of the following may not lead to infertility/sterility:

a. Whole body radiation
b. I-131 therapy
c. Strontium-89
d. Pelvic radiation
e. High dose alkylating agent

235. X-ray findings of Tetralogy of Fallot include(s):

a. Pulmonary plethora
b. Decreased pulmonary vascularity
c. Left ventricular hypertrophy
d. Coeur en sabot
e. Left atrial hypertrophy

236. On CT scan, Hilar lymph node calcification seen in:

a. Asbestosis
b. Silicosis
c. Amyloidosis
d. Berylysosis
e. Coal worker pneumoconiosis

237. Advantage of MRI is/are:

a. Images can be readily produced in axial, sagittal or coronal without changing position of the patient
b. Uses less ionizing radiation
c. Blood vessel can be seen without contrast
d. Lung pathology is better visualized than CT scan

238. Egg-shell calcification is/are seen in:

a. Silicosis
b. Sarcoidosis
c. Lymphoma after treatment
d. Aspergilloma
e. TB

239. Isotope(s) used for brachytherapy is/are-

a. Radon-222
b. Radium-226
c. Iodine-125
d. Cobalt-60
e. Cesium-137

240. Isotope(s) used for metastatic bone pain is/are-

a. Selenium
b. Samarium-153
c. Phosphorus-32
d. Thallium
e. Strontium-89

241. Drug(s) used for radiation protection is/are:

a. Amifostine
b. Metronidazole
c. Actinomycin-D
d. Pentoxiphylline
e. Hydroxyurea

Answer

232. a, b, c, d, e. 233. a, b, c, d. 234. c. 235. b, d. 236. b, d, e. 237. a, c. 238. a, b, c, e.
239. All (a,b,c,d,e). 240. b, c, e. 241. a, d.

NOVEMBER 2017 ANSWERS & EXPLANATIONS

ANATOMY

1. Ans. a. Peroneus tertius, e. Extensor hallucis longus

[Ref: BDC 7th/Vol. II 101-02; Essential Anatomy by Moore 2nd/360-63]

"The four muscles in the **anterior compartment** of the leg are- ***tibialis anterior, extensor digitorum longus, extensor hallucis longus and fibularis (Peroneus) tertius***"- *Moore 2nd/360*

Muscle of posterior compartment of leg: Superficial- Gastrocnemius, soleus and plantaris; **Deep-*Flexor digitorum longus***, popliteus, flexor halluces longus and tibialis posterior- BDC 7th/Vol. II 118

Table: *(Essential Anatomy by Moore 2nd/360-63)*: **Muscles of anterior and lateral compartment of leg**

Muscle	Proximal attachment	Distal attachment	Innervation	Main action (s)
Anterior compartment				
Tibialis anterior	Lateral condyle and superior half of lateral surface of tibia and interosseous membrane	Medial and inferior surfaces of medial cuneiform and base of 1st metatarsal	Deep fibular (peroneal) nerve (L4 and L5)	Dorsiflex ankle and inverts foot
Extensor hallucis longus	Middle part of anterior surface of fibula and interosseous membrane	Dorsal aspect of base of distal phalanx of great toe (hallux)	Deep fibular (peroneal) nerve (L5 and S1)	Extends great toe and dorsiflexes ankle
Extensor digitorum longus	Lateral condyle of tibia and superior three fourths of anterior surface of interosseous membrane	Middle and distal phalanges of lateral four digits	Deep fibular (peroneal) nerve (L5 and S1)	Extends lateral four digits and dorsiflexes ankle
Fibularis ***(Peroneus) Tertius***	Inferior third of anterior surface of fibula and interosseous membrane	Dorsum of base of 5th metatarsal	Deep fibular (peroneal) nerve (L5 and 51)	Dorsiflexes ankle and aids in eversion of foot
Lateral compartment				
Fibularis ***(peroneus) longus***	Head and superior two thirds of lateral surface of fibula	Base of 1st metatarsal and medial cuneiform	Superficial fibular (peroneal) nerve (L5, S1 and S2)	Evert foot and weakly plantar flex ankle
Fibularis ***(peroneus) brevis***	Inferior two thirds of lateral surface of fibula	Dorsal surface of tuberosity on lateral side of base of 5th metatarsal	Superficial fibular (peroneal) nerve (L5, S1 and S2)	Evert foot and weakly plantar flex ankle

2. Ans. b. Contains mucous secreting glands, d. Made up of elastic cartilage, e. Has bilateral lymphatic supply

[Ref: BDC 7th/Vol. III 264; Snell's 8th/802; Moore 2nd/628; Gray's 40th/577-78, 588; Dhingra 6th/283-85; H and N Cancer by L B Harrison 3rd/368; H and N Surgery by Satalof 1st/693]

Epiglottis/Epiglottic Cartilage

◈ *BDC 7th/Vol. III 264*

- The epiglottis is a ***leaf-shaped structure.***
- It is a flap that is made of ***elastic cartilage tissue*** covered with a mucous membrane, attached to the entrance of the larynx
- The epiglottis is one of **nine cartilaginous** structures that make up the larynx (voice box). While one is breathing, it lies completely within the pharynx. When one is swallowing it serves as part of the anterior of the larynx.
- The epiglottis has two surfaces, a lingual and a laryngeal surface, related to the oral cavity and the larynx respectively
- The entire lingual surface and the apical portion of the laryngeal surface (since it is vulnerable to abrasion due to its relation to the digestive tract) are covered by a *stratified squamous non-keratinized epithelium.*
- The rest of the laryngeal surface on the other hand, which is in relation to the respiratory system, has respiratory epithelium: pseudostratified, ciliated columnar cells and ***mucus secreting Goblet cells.***

Lymphatic Drainage

◈ *Gray's 40th/588; Moore 2nd/628*

- The vocal cords, with their firmly bound mucosa and paucity of lymphatics, provide a clear demarcation between the upper and lower areas of the larynx.
- **Above the vocal cords**, the lymph vessels draining the supraglottic part of the larynx accompany the superior laryngeal artery, pierce the thyrohyoid membrane and end in the upper deep cervical lymph nodes, ***often bilaterally.*** The supraglottic lymphatics also communicate with those at the base of the tongue. (Note: Epiglottis is supraglottic part of larynx- *Dhingra 6th/283)*
- Below the vocal cords, some of the lymph vessels pass through the conus elasticus to reach the prelaryngeal (Delphian) and/or pretracheal and paratracheal lymph nodes, while others accompany the inferior laryngeal artery and join the lower deep cervical nodes.

- "The supraglottis has ***extensive bilateral network of lymphatics*** that result in frequent regional metastases"-L B Harrison 3rd/368
- "Unlike the other two anatomic sites (glottis and subglottis) of the larynx, the supraglottis is formed without midline union and consequently has ***bilateral lymphatic drainage***"-R Satalof 1st /693

3. **Ans. a. Posterior border is attached medially to perineal body, b. Triangular in shape; e. Supports pelvic floor**

[Ref: BDC 7th/Vol.II388-89; Snell's 9th/314-15; Gray's 40th/1094]

"Perineal membrane: a layer of tough fascia, which is perforated by the ***urethra (and also the vagina in the female).*** The role of the membrane is to provide attachment for the muscles of the external genitalia"- *teachmeanatomy.info*

"Contents of the superficial perineal space: The **branches** of the **internal pudendal vessels** and the **pudendal nerves."** *download.videohelp.com (so not pass through* **perineal membrane)**

Perineal Membrane (Previously the Inferior Fascia of the Urogenital Diaphragm)

◈ *Gray's 40th/1094*

- The perineal membrane is a ***triangular membrane,*** which stretches almost horizontally across the deep perineal pouch.
- It is attached **laterally** to the periosteum of the ischiopubic rami and its apex is attached to the arcuate ligament of the pubis. It is particularly thick in this area and is here referred to as the transverse perineal ligament.
- The **posterior border** is fused with the ***deep part of the perineal body*** and is continuous with the fascia over the deep transverse perinei.
- In the **male**, the perineal membrane is crossed by the urethra, 2–3 cm behind the inferior border of the symphysis pubis; the *vessels and nerves to the bulb of the penis*; the ducts of the bulbourethral glands, posterolateral to the urethral orifice; the *deep dorsal vessels and dorsal nerves of the penis*, behind the pubic arch in the midline; and the *posterior scrotal vessels and nerves,* anterior to the transverse perinei.
- In the **female,** the perineal membrane is less well defined than in the male. It is divided almost into two halves by the ***vagina and urethra*** such that it forms a triangle on each side of these structures; the pubourethral ligament (the female equivalent of the transverse perineal ligament in males) links the two sides anteriorly behind the pubic arch. It is crossed by the urethra, 2–3 cm behind the inferior border of the symphysis pubis; the vagina, centrally; the ducts of Bartholin's glands, posterolateral to the urethral orifice; the *deep dorsal vessels and dorsal* nerves of the clitoris, behind the pubic arch in the midline; the posterior labial vessels and nerves, anterior to the transverse perinei.
- "**Urogenital diaphragm:** There is a triangular sheet of dense musculofascial tissue that ***spans the anterior half of the pelvic outlet***. Rather than forming an uninterrupted sheet in the female, as it does in the male, the ***urogenital diaphragm attaches the vagina and perineal body to the anterior bony outlet. The medial attachments of the urogenital diaphragm are to the walls of the vagina and to the perineal body.*** Within the substance of the urogenital diaphragm, there is skeletal muscle, called the deep transversus perineus"- *www.glowm.com*
- "The **primary function of the urogenital diaphragm** in relation to obstetrics has to do with its attachment to the vagina and perineal body. By attaching these structures to the pelvic bones, ***their descent is limited during the great downward pressure*** that is exerted on the vagina and perineum during the second stage of labor. If these attachments remain intact after parturition, they will contribute to the normal support of the vaginal outlet. If torn or detached from the vagina and perineal body, then the ***pelvic floor sags and the introitus gapes***"- *www.glowm.com*
- "The **pudendal nerve and vessels:** They leave the pelvis through the greater sciatic foramen by hooking around the ischial spine and sacrospinous ligament to enter the pudendal (Alcock's) canal through the lesser sciatic foramen. In passing around the sacrospinous ligament, the nerve and vessels enter the pudendal canal on the inner aspect of the obturator internus muscle in the ischiorectal fossa. As the vessels ***reach the posterior border of the urogenital diaphragm***, they bend forward to supply the structures of the perineum"- *www.glowm.com*

Perineal Membrane

◈ *BDC 7th/Vol.II388*

Perineal membrane is almost ***triangular membrane***

- Laterally attached to periosteum of ischiopubic rami
- Apex attached to arcuate ligament of pubis, where the membrane is attached to this arcuate ligament of pubis, it is particularly thick and is called *transverse perineal ligament*
- **Posterior border** is fused to deep parts of perineal body and is continuous with the fascia over deep transversus perinei

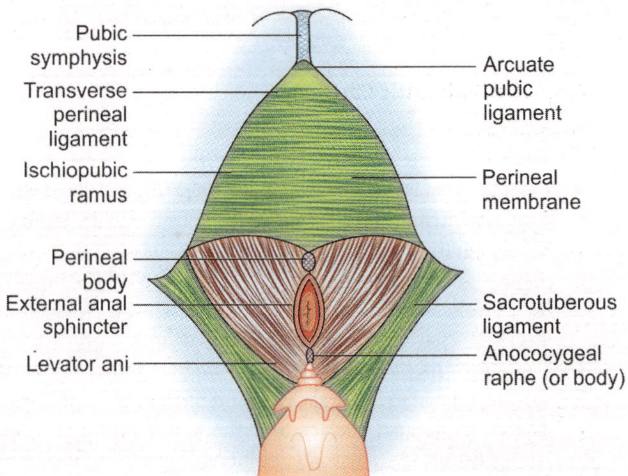

Fig: *(aibolita.com/sundries)*: Perineal membrane

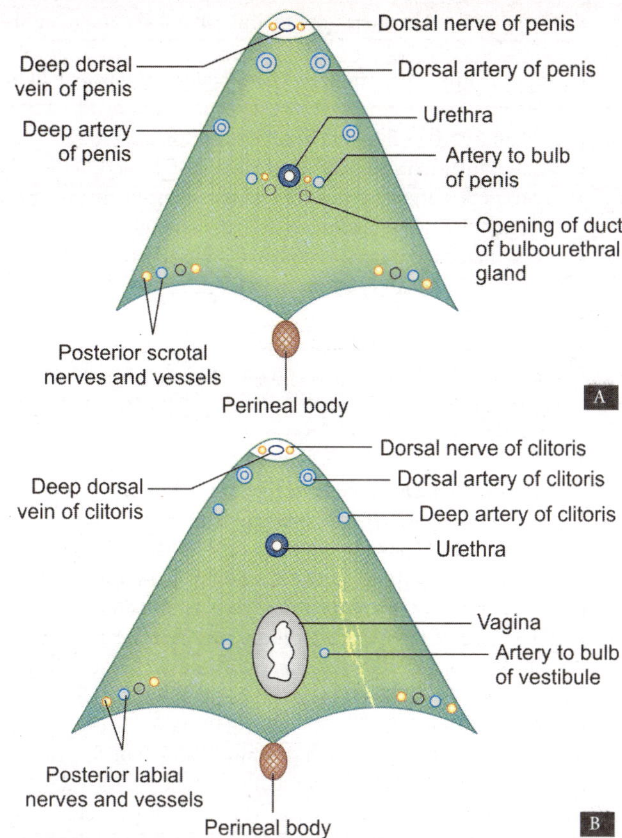

Fig: *(BDC 7th/Vol. II 388; aibolita.com/sundries)*: Structures piercing the perineal membrane: (A) Male; (B) Female

4. Ans. b. Internal pudendal artery

[Ref: BDC 7th/Vol.II352; Gray's 40th/1241]

Arteries Supplying Ureter

◈ *Gray's 40th/1241*

- The ureter is supplied by branches from the ***renal, gonadal, common iliac, internal iliac, vesical and uterine arteries and the abdominal aorta***
- The pattern of distribution is subject to much variation.
- The abdominal ureter is supplied from vessels originating medial to the ureter, while the pelvic ureter is supplied by vessels lateral to the ureter.
- There is a good longitudinal anastomosis between these branches on the wall of the ureter, which means that the ureter can be safely transected at any level intraoperatively and a uretero-ureterostomy performed, without compromising its viability. The branches from the inferior vesical artery are constant in their occurrence and supply the lower part of the ureter as well as a large part of the trigone of the bladder. The branch from the renal artery is also constant and is preserved whenever possible in renal transplantation to ensure good vascularity of the ureter.

Arteries Supplying Ureter-*BDC 7th/Vol.II 352*

Part of ureter	Arteries supplying
Upper part	Renal artery. Also by- gonadal or colic vessel
Middle part	Branches from aorta. Also by-gonadal or iliac vessel
Pelvic part	Vesical, middle rectal or uterine vessels

"The **internal pudendal** artery is a branch of the anterior division of the internal iliac artery and is the primary supply of the perineum. It is a larger vessel in males than in females. It **branches include:** inferior rectal artery, deep artery of the penis/clitoris, dorsal artery of the penis/clitoris, perineal artery, posterior scrotal artery, transverse perineal artery, urethral artery and artery to the bulb. *It* **supplies:** perineum, genitalia, anal region, erectile tissues"- BDC 7th/Vol.II456; *radiopaedia.org*

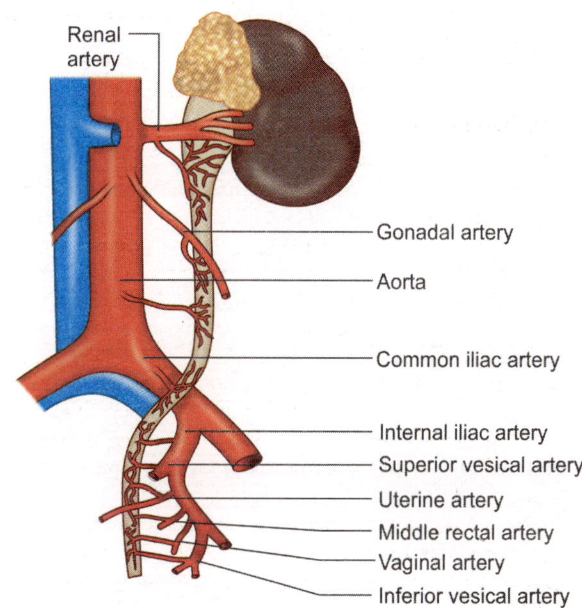

Fig: *(Gray's 40th/1241)*: Arterial supply of the left ureter. The proximal part takes its blood supply medially and the distal part is supplied laterally

5. Ans. b. Anterior cardiac vein

[Ref: BDC 7th/Vol.I 281-82; Snell's 9th/89; Gray's 40th/981-82]

Anterior cardiac vein: ***Open directly into the right atrium*** through its anterior wall- BDC 7th/Vol.I 282

Coronary Sinus

◈ *BDC 7th/Vol.I 281-82; Gray's 40th/981-82*

- It is the largest vein of the heart
- It is 2 or 3 cm long, lying in the posterior atrioventricular groove between the left atrium and ventricle. The sinus opens into the right atrium between the opening of the inferior vena cava and the right atrioventricular orifice; the opening is guarded by an endocardial fold (semilunar valve of the coronary sinus)

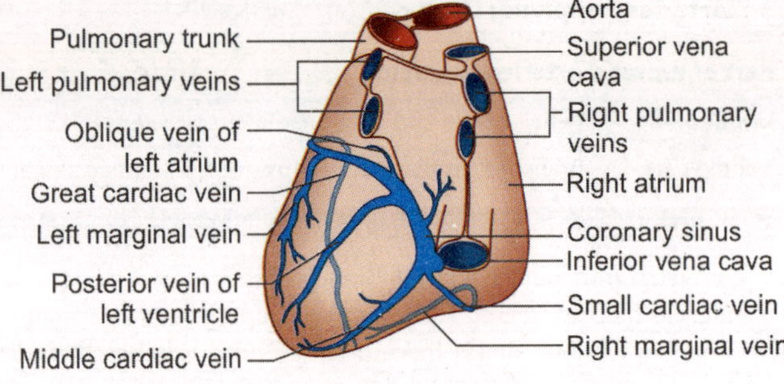

Fig: *(Gray's 40th/982)*: The principal veins of the heart

- Its **tributaries** are the ***great, small and middle cardiac veins, the posterior vein of the left ventricle and the oblique vein of the left atrium***; all except the last have valves at their orifices.

6. Ans. a. Cranial nerve with longest intracranial course, b. Smallest cranial nerve

[Ref: BDC 7th/Vol.IV 63-64; Snell's 9th/607; Gray's 40th/666]

Trochlear Nerve

◈ *BDC 7th/Vol.IV 63-64*

- *Only nerve which emerges from **dorsal aspects** of the brainstem- BDC 7th/Vol.IV 64*
- *It is only cranial nerve whose fibers **emerge posteriorly**-PJM 20th/308*
- *It passes b/w the **posterior cerebral and superior cerebellar arteries** to appear ventrally b/w the temporal lobe and upper border of pons- BDC 7th/Vol.IV 64*
- *It **terminates on the superior oblique muscle on the side opposite to the nucleus of origin**- PJM 20th/308*

It is the *smallest cranial nerve (by number of axons)*, yet has the *longest intracranial course*. It has a purely somatic motor function- *teachmeanatomy.info*

It is the **only cranial nerve to emerge from the dorsal surface** of the brain stem, passing from the midbrain onto the lateral surface of the crus of the cerebral peduncle- *Gray's 40th/666*

The trochlear nerves lie between the posterior cerebral and superior cerebellar arteries- *Gray's 40th/288*

Important facts and points about Cranial Nerves: *www.juniordentist.com; mympsc.com*

- Trigeminal nerve is the largest cranial nerve
- Trochlear nerve is the smallest cranial nerve
- Olfactory nerve is the shortest cranial nerve
- Vagus nerve is with Vague or Extensive Distribution
- Trochlear nerve shows largest intracranial course
- Smallest branch of Trigeminal nerve is the Ophthalmic branch
- Largest branch of Trigeminal nerve is Mandibular branch

7. Ans. b. Weakness in jaw closing, c. Loss of corneal reflex, d. Sensory loss of face e. Paralysis of temporalis and masseter muscle

[Ref: BDC 7th/Vol.IV 68-69; P.J.M 20th/312-15; Snells' Anatomy 9th /608-10]

Trigeminal Nerve Injury

◈ *BDC 7th/Vol.IV 68-69*

- It comprises 3 branches-ophthalmic, maxillary and mandibular
- Ophthalmic nerve injury: There is ***loss of corneal blink reflex***
- Maxillary nerve injury: There is loss of sneeze reflex
- Mandibular nerve injury: There is loss of jaw jerk reflex
- ***Flaccid paralysis of muscles of mastication*** in injury to mandibular nerve leading to decrease strength for bitting
- Hypoacusis i.e., partial deafness to low pitched sound due to paralysis of tensor tympani muscle
- ***Sensory loss of face***
- The patient is asked to open the mouth. Normally the jaw is central. If there is paralysis on one side, the jaw will deviate to that side being pushed by the healthy lateral pterygoid muscle- *P.J.M 20th/313*
- *The patient is asked to clench the teeth. Normally the masseters and temporalis on the both sides stand out with equal prominence. If there is paralysis on one side, the muscles on that side do not become prominent- P.J.M 20th/313*

Lesions at or proximal to the Gasserian ganglion *results in **ipsilateral sensory loss of the whole face**- P.J.M 20th/313*

"The ***paired temporalis and masseter muscles function in jaw closure and the medial pterygoid muscle closes the jaw and moves it from side-to-side*** (grinding motion). The **lateral pterygoid muscles** (along with some of the upper neck muscles) open the jaw in concert with a downward and opposing inward motion. When one lateral pterygoid is weak, the jaw deviates toward the weak side on opening, with the inward vector of the opposite pterygoid being unopposed"- *www.dartmouth.edu*

The motor component of the **mandibular division (V3) of the trigeminal nerve** controls the movement of ***eight muscles***, includingthe four muscles of mastication: ***the masseter, the temporalis and the medial and lateral pterygoids***. The other four muscles are the tensor veli palatini, the mylohyoid, the anterior belly of the digastric and the tensor tympani"- *BDC 7th/Vol.III 129; en.wikipedia.org*

The trigeminal nerve is responsible for transmitting sensations to the mouth, teeth, face and nasal cavity *www.healthline.com*

Lesions of the Trigeminal Nerve

◈ *www.derangedphysiology.com*

- Absent corneal reflex
- Absent sensation in the sensory distribution
- ***Weakness/wasting of the muscles of mastication (masseter and temporalis)***

Causes of a Unilateral Lesion of the Trigeminal Nerve

◈ *www.derangedphysiology.com*

- A higher central lesion (e.g. cerebral or thalamic) will have to be *contralateral* to the clinical findings.
- Brainstem lesions would be *ipsilateral*.

8. Ans. a. External carotid artery, b. Cervicofacial trunk of facial nerve, c. Retromandibular vein

[Ref: BDC 7th/Vol.III 111; Gray's 40th/496]

Structures Within the Parotid Gland

◈ *Gray's 40th/496*

- ***The external carotid artery, retromandibular vein and facial nerve, either in part or in whole, traverse the gland and branch within it.***
- The **external carotid artery** enters the posteromedial surface and divides into the maxillary artery, which emerges from the anteromedial surface and the superficial temporal artery, which gives off its ***transverse facial branch*** in the ***gland*** and ascends to leave its upper limit. The posterior auricular artery may also branch from the external carotid artery within the gland, leaving by its posteromedial surface.
- The **retromandibular** is superficial to the external carotid artery. It descends in the parotid gland and emerges behind the apex of the gland

Structures within the Parotid Gland

◈ *BDC 7th/Vol.III 111*

From medial to the lateral side, these are as follows.

- **Arteries:** The ***external carotid artery*** enters the gland through its posteromedial surface. The ***maxillary artery*** leaves the gland through its anteromedial surface. The ***superficial temporal artery*** gives ***transverse facial artery*** and emerges at the anterior part of the superior surface
- ***Veins:*** The ***retromandibular vein*** is formed within the gland by the union of the superficial temporal and vein divides into anterior and posterior divisions which emerge close to the apex (lower pole) of the gland
- ***The facial nerve*** exits from cranial cavity through stylomastoid foramen and enters the gland through the upper part of its posteromedial surface and divides into its terminal branches within the gland. The branches leave the gland through its anteromedial surface and appear on the surface at the anterior border.

Facial nerve lies in relation to isthmus of the gland which separates large superficial part from small deep part of the gland. Facial nerve divides into two branches:

- *Temporofacial*: Divides into temporal and zygomatic branches
- *Cervicofacial*: Divides into buccal, marginal mandibular and cervical branches.

The various branches (5–6) of facial nerve radiate like a goose-foot from the curved anterior border of the parotid gland to supply the respective muscles of facial expression.

"The **facial artery** arises in the carotid triangle from the external carotid artery a little above the lingual artery and, sheltered by the ramus of the mandible, passes obliquely up beneath the digastric and stylohyoid muscles, over which it arches to enter a groove on the ***posterior surface of the submandibular gland***"-*BDC 7th/Vol. III 71*

The **lingual nerve** is a branch of the ***mandibular division of the trigeminal nerve***"- *BDC 7th/Vol.III 129*

9. **Ans. a. Thyroid lies in between 2 layers of deep cervical fascia, b. Berry ligament derived from deep cervical fascia, c. Left recurrent laryngeal nerve is larger than right recurrent laryngeal nerve**

[Ref: L and B 26th/742; Schwartz 10th/1523]

Thyroid Gland

◈ *Schwartz 10th/1523-25*

- The thyroid gland is enveloped by a loosely connecting fascia that is formed from the partition of the deep cervical fascia into anterior and posterior divisions (false capsule)
- The true capsule of the thyroid is a thin, densely adherent fibrous layer that sends out septa that invaginate into the gland, forming pseudolobules.
- The thyroid capsule is condensed into the posterior suspensory or **Berry's ligament** near the cricoid cartilage and upper tracheal rings.
- "The false capsule is derived from the pretracheal layer of the deep cervical fascia. It is thin along the posterior border of the lobes, but thick on the inner surface of the gland where it forms a **suspensory ligament (of berry)**, which connects the lobe to the cricoid cartilage"- *BDC 7th/Vol III 145*

"The course of the **recurrent laryngeal nerves** on the right and left sides is different. The left RLN is longer than the right, because it crosses under the arch of the aorta at the ligamentum arteriosum. The lower origin and consequently, a longer course of the left RLN makes it more vulnerable to injury than the right RLN."- emedicine.medscape.com;– *BDC 7th/Vol IV 83*

"Superior thyroid artery: It runs downwards and forwards in intimate relation to external laryngeal nerve"- *BDC 7th/Vol III 147*

"About 85% of individuals have four parathyroid glands that can be found within 1 cm of the junction of the inferior thyroid artery and the RLN. The superior glands are usually located dorsal to the RLN, whereas the inferior glands are usually found ventral to the RLN" -*Schwartz 10th/1523*

10. **Ans. c. Homologous chromosomes separate**

[Ref: Gray's 40th/22-23;I B Singh 10th/13-15; Langman's Medical Embryology 9th/6-7

During diplotene stage of prophase I, pairs of homologous chromosome separates

Prophase of Meiosis I-Contains 5 Steps

◈ *Gray's 40th/22-23; I B Singh 10th/13-15*

- **During leptotene,** homologous chromosomes (maternal and paternal copies of the same chromosome), which were replicated in a preceding S phase and each ***consist of sister chromatids joined at the centromere***, locate one another within the nucleus and the process of ***genetic recombination is initiated.*** Cytologically, chromosomes begin to condense, appearing as individual threads that are attached via their telomeres to the nuclear membrane.
- **Zygotene stage:** During zygotene, the homologous chromosomes initiate a process known as **synapsis**, during which they become intimately associated with one another. The pairs of synapsed homologues, also known as bivalents, are linked together by a highly structured fibrillar band, the synaptonemal complex.
- **Pachytene stage:** When synapsis is complete for all chromosomes, the cell is said to be in pachytene. Each bivalent looks like a single structure, but is actually ***two pairs of sister chromatids held together by the synaptonemal complex. Genetic recombination is completed at this point***, with sites where it has occurred (usually one per

chromosome arm) appearing as nodules in the center of the synaptonemal complex.

- **Diplotene stage:** During diplotene, the synaptonemal complex disassembles and ***pairs of homologous chromosomes, now much shortened, separate except where crossing over has occurred*** (chiasmata). At least one chiasma forms between each homologous pair, exchanging maternal and paternal sequences and up to five have been observed.
- **Diakinesis:** Diakinesis is the prometaphase of the first meiotic division.

Meiosis I (All other Steps Except Prophase) and Meiosis II

◈ *Gray's 40th/22-23; I B Singh 10th/13-15*

- Meiosis consists of 2 successive division called first and second meiotic division
- Meiosis I consists of-Prophase I (Leptotene, Zygotene, **Pachytene,** Diplotene and Diakinesis), metaphase I, **Anaphase I and telophase I**
- Metaphase I resembles mitotic metaphase, except that the bodies attaching to the spindle microtubules are ***bivalents, not single chromosomes***. These become arranged so that the homologous pairs occupy theequatorial plane of the spindle.
- Anaphase I of meiosis begins with the ***release of cohesion between the arms of sister chromatids, much as it does during mitosis***. In meiosis, this 'unties' the topological knots of the chiasmata and ***allows homologous chromosomes to separate and migrate to opposite spindle poles***. As positioning of bivalent pairs is random, assortment of maternal and paternal chromosomes in each telophase nucleus is also random. ***Critically, sister centromeres and thus chromatids, do not separate during anaphase I.***
- In Telophase I, two daughter nuclei are formed. The division of nucleus is followed by division of the cytoplasm
- During meiosis I, cytoplasmic division occurs by specialized mechanisms. In females, the division is highly asymmetric, producing one egg and ***one tiny cell known as a polar body***. In males, the process does not go to full completion, resulting in ***production of spermatocytes*** that remain joined by small cytoplasmic bridges.
- "Meiosis II is similar to mitosis. However, because of crossing over that has occurred during the meiosis I, the daughter cells are not identical in genetic content"- *I B Singh 10th/15*
- Meiosis II commences after only a short interval during which no DNA synthesis occurs. The centromeres of sister chromatids remain paired, but rotate so that each one can face an opposite spindle pole. Onset of anaphase II is triggered by loss of cohesion between the centromeres, as it is in mitosis. This ***second division is more like mitosis, in that chromatids separate during anaphase***, but, unlike mitosis, ***the separating chromatids are genetically different*** (the result of genetic recombination). ***Cytoplasmic division also occurs and thus, in the male, four haploid cells result from meiosis I and II.***

11. Ans. a. T_7 has vertically oriented articular process

[Ref: BDC 7th/Vol. I 213-15; Gray's 40th/716-23;Textbook of Skeletal Anatomy /716]

Thoracic Vertebrae (Regarding Options a, c & d)

- There are 12 thoracic vertebrae. T_2-T_9 are typical thoracic vertebrae & T_1, T_{10}, T_{11} & T_{12} are atypical thoracic vertebrae
- Thoracic vertebrae (including T_3) have long spinous process, Small spinous processes are seen in cervical vertebrae (except for C_7).
- T_{11}& T_{12} do not have costal facets
- Articular process(of typical T vertebrae): Vertically placed & interlocked; so that dislocation can only occur if they are fractured

Cervical Vertebrae (Regarding Option b & e)

- Lateral mass is seen in C_1 (not in C_6)
- There are 7 cervical vertebrae of which 3-6 are typical and 1st, 2nd and 7th are atypical.
- Characteristic features of typical cervical vertebra are:-
  - Foramen transversarium is present in the transverse process. Foramina transversaria of C_1 to C_6 vertebrae transmit vertebral artery, vertebral vein and sympathetic plexus and that of C_7 transmits only vertebral veins.
  - Body is small and broad transversely (side to side)
  - Spinous process is small and bified.
  - Vertebral foramen is large and triangular.
- Atypical vertebrae: Important features
  - First cervical vertebra (atlas) is ring like bone having lateral mass on each side connected by a smaller anterior arch and a larger posterior arch.
  - Second cervical vertebra (axis) is characterized by presence of *odontoid process or dens*
  - Seventh cervical vertebra is called as vertebra prominens because it has most promenentspinous process which is not *bifid*. Foramen transversarium transmits only vertebral vein, not vertebral artery.

Features of Typical Vertebrae

Feature	Cervical vertebra	Thoracic vertebra	Lumbar vertebra
Vertebral foramen	Large and triangular	Small and circular	Trinagular
Body	*Small and broad from side to side*	Medium size and heart shaped	Large and kidney shaped
Spinous process	Small and bifid	Long and inclined downwards	Short, flat and projected backwards
Transverse process	*Have foramen transversarium* for passage of vertebral artery	Posses costal facets (not on T_{11} and T_{12})	Long and slender

Contd...

Features of Typical Vertebrae			
Feature	**Cervical vertebra**	**Thoracic vertebra**	**Lumbar vertebra**
Superior articular facets face	*Backwards and upwards*	Backwards and laterally	Medially
Inferior articular facets face (opposite of superior)	Downwards and forwards	Forwards and medially	Laterally

PHYSIOLOGY

12. Ans. b. Macula densa is a part of renin-angiotensin system; c. Renin converts angiotensinogen to angiotensin-I; d. Angiotensin-converting enzyme is present in endothelium of the lung vessels; e. Angiotensin-II stimulates release of aldosterone from zona glomerulosa

[Ref: Ganong 25th/699-706; Guyton 13th (SAE)/272-74; A K Jain 6th/506]

Angiotensin-converting enzyme is present in the *endothelium of the lung vessels*- *Guyton 13th (SAE)/273*

"**Angiotensin II**: *It stimulates zona glomerulosa of adrenal cortex to increase aldosterone secretion- A K Jain 6th/506*

"Renin is synthesized and stored in an inactive form called *prorenin* **in the** *juxtaglomerular cells* **(JG cells) of the kidneys. The JG cells are modified smooth muscle cells located** *in the walls of the* ***afferent arterioles*** *immediately proximal to the glomeruli.* **When the arterial pressure falls, intrinsic reactions in the kidneys themselves cause many of the *prorenin molecules in the JG cells to split and release renin.* Most of the renin enters the renal blood and then passes out of the kidneys to circulate throughout the entire body. However, small amounts of the renin do remain in the local fluids of the kidney and initiate several intrarenal functions"**- *Guyton 13th (SAE)/273*

The juxtaglomerular apparatus (JGA) consists of three types of cells: *A K Jain 6th/504-05*

- **Macula densa**, a part of the distal convoluted tubule of the same nephron: They function as chemoreceptors. They are stimulated by a decreased sodium ion load ***thereby causing increased renin release***
- **Juxtaglomerular cells**, (also known as granular cells) which ***secrete renin***
- **Mesangial cells or lacis cell:** supporting cell. Play a role in the regulation of glomerulation filtration. They show granulation to secrete renin in conditions of extreme hyperactivity

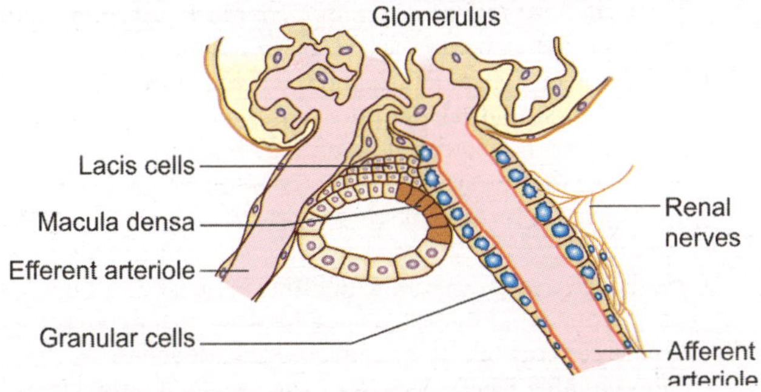

Fig: *(Ganong 25th/703)*: Diagram of glomerulus, showing the juxtaglomerular apparatus

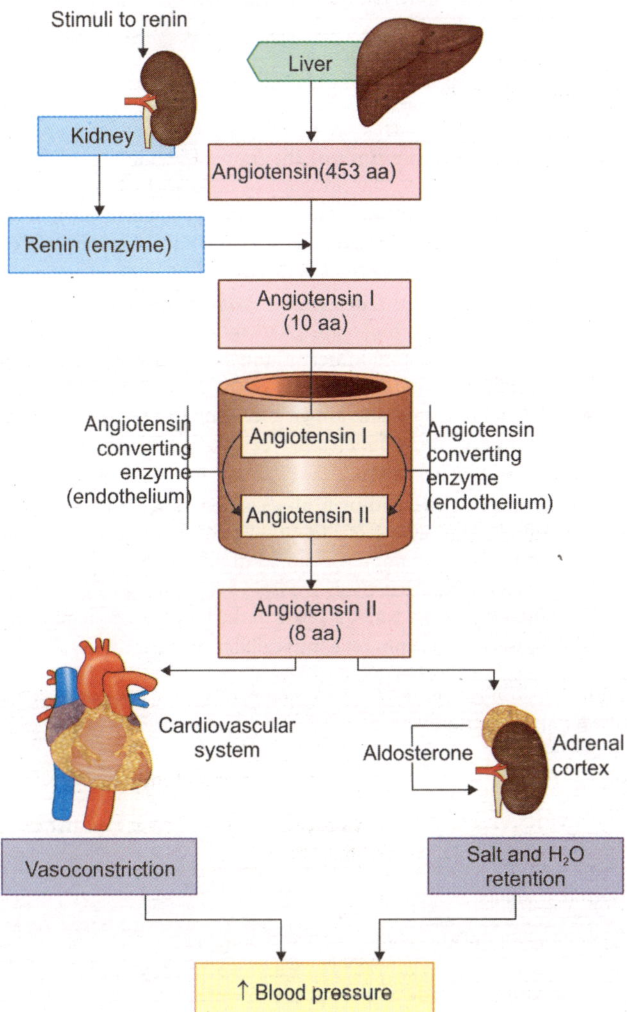

Fig: *(Ganong 25th/699)*: Summary of the renin-angiotensin system and the stimulation of aldosterone secretion by angiotensin II. The plasma concentration of renin is the rate-limiting step in the renin-angiotensin system; therefore, it is the major determinant of plasma angiotensin II concentration

13. Ans. b. Descending limb reabsorbs water

[Ref: Ganong 25th/683-84; Guyton 13th (SAE)/510-12; A K Jain 6th/521]

Tubular fluid remains isotonic in the proximal tubule (so fluid reaching **descending limb is also isotonic)**- *Guyton 13th (SAE)/509*

Loop of Henle

◈ *A K Jain 6th/521*

- **Thin descending segment**: highly permeable to water but relatively impermeable to solids (Specially NaCl)
- **Thin ascending segment**: impermeable to water but permeable to NaCl and urea; causes ***passive*** resbsorption of NaCl
- **Thick ascending segment**: impermeable to water and solute but ***actively reabsorbs NaCl*** by Na^+ –K^+ pump and Na^+ –$2Cl^-$ – and K^+ are reabsorbed (mostly in the thick ascending limb)

Loop of Henle

◈ *Ganong 25th/683-84*

- The **descending limb of the loop** of Henle is permeable to water, due to the presence of **aquaporin-1** in both the apical and basolateral membranes, but the ***ascending limb is impermeable to water***. Na+, K^+ and Cl^- are cotransported out of the thick segment of the ascending limb.
- "The fluid in the ***descending limb of the loop of Henle becomes hypertonic*** as water moves out of the tubule into the hypertonic interstitium. ***In the ascending limb it becomes more dilute*** because of the movement of Na^+ and Cl^- out of the tubular lumen and ***when fluid reaches the top of the ascending limb (called the diluting segment) it is now hypotonic to plasma***.
- In the **thick ascending limb**, a carrier cotransports one Na^+, one K^+ and $2Cl^-$ from the tubular lumen into the tubular cells. This is another example of secondary active transport; the ***Na^+ is actively transported from the cells into the interstitium*** by Na, K ATPase in the basolateral membranes of the cells, keeping the intracellular Na^+ low.

Table: *Guyton 13th (SAE)/511*: **Summary of Tubule Characteristics-Urine Concentration**

		Permeability		
	Active NaCl Transport	H_2O	NaCl	Urea
Proximal tubule	++	++	+	+
Thin descending limb	0	++	+	+
Thin ascending limb	0	0	+	+
Thick ascending limb	++	0	0	0
Distal tubule	+	+ADH	0	0
Cortical collecting tubule	+	+ADH	0	0
Inner medullary collecting duct	+	+ADH	0	++ADH

0, minimal level of active transport or permeability; +, moderate level of active transport or permeability; ++, high level of active transport or permeability; +ADH, permeability to water or urea is increased by ADH.

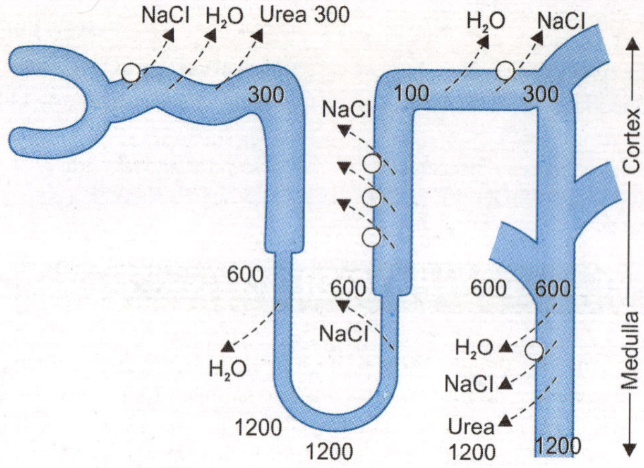

Fig: *(Guyton 13th (SAE)/512)*: Formation of a concentrated urine when antidiuretic hormone (ADH) levels are high

14. Ans. c. Ipsilateral posterior column involvement, ... d. Ipsilateral extensive weakness of lower limbs

[Ref: Ganong 25th/172; Harrison 19th/2652; A K Jain 6th/934-35]

Brown-Sequard Hemicord Syndrome **This consists of *ipsilateral weakness (corticospinal tract) and loss of joint position and vibratory sense (posterior column)*, with *contralateral loss of pain and temperature sense (spinothalamic tract)* one or two levels below the lesion. Segmental signs, such as radicular pain, muscle atrophy, or loss of a deep tendon reflex, are unilateral. Partial forms are more common than the fully developed syndrome"**- *Harrison 19th/2652*

Brown-Sequard Syndrome: Below the level of the lesion, on the ***same side, there is extensive motor loss*** but little sensory loss; while on the ***opposite side there is extensive sensory loss but little motor loss***"- A K Jain 6th/935

Brown-Séquard Syndrome

◈ *Ganong 25th/172*

- A functional hemisection of the spinal cord causes a characteristic and easily recognized clinical picture that reflects damage to ascending sensory (dorsal column pathway, ventrolateral spinothalamic tract) and descending motor (corticospinal tract) pathways, which is called the Brown-Séquard syndrome.
- The lesion to fasciculus gracilus or fasciculus cuneatus leads to ***ipsilateral loss of discriminative touch, vibration and proprioception*** below the level of the lesion.
- The loss of the spinothalamic tract leads to ***contralateral loss of pain and temperature sensation*** beginning one or two segments below the lesion.
- Damage to the corticospinal tract produces ***weakness and spasticity in certain muscle groups on the same side of the body.***
- Although a precise spinal hemisection is rare, the syndrome is fairly common because it can be caused by a spinal cord tumor, spinal cord trauma, degenerative disk disease and ischemia.

Pyramidal tract includes **corticospinal tract and corticobulbar tract**

15. Ans. a. Diabetes mellitus; d. Diuretic overuse

[Ref: Harrison 19th/294-95; Davidson 22nd/435]

Polyuria

❖ *Harrison 19th/2*

- Poorly controlled ***diabetes mellitus with glucosuria is the most common cause of a solute diuresis,*** leading to volume depletion and serum hypertonicity.
- Since the urine sodium concentration is less than that of blood, more water than sodium is lost, causing hypernatremia and hypertonicity.
- **Common iatrogenic solute diuresis** occurs in association with ***mannitol administration, radiocontrast media and high-protein feedings (enteral or parenteral),*** leading to increased urea production and excretion.

Abnormalities of Urine Volume: Polyuria

❖ *Harrison 19th/294-95*

- Polyuria results from two potential mechanisms: (1) excretion of ***nonabsorbable solutes*** (such as ***glucose***) or (2) excretion of water (usually from a defect in ADH production or renal responsiveness).

Flowchart: *(Harrison 19th/294):* Approach to the patient with polyuria

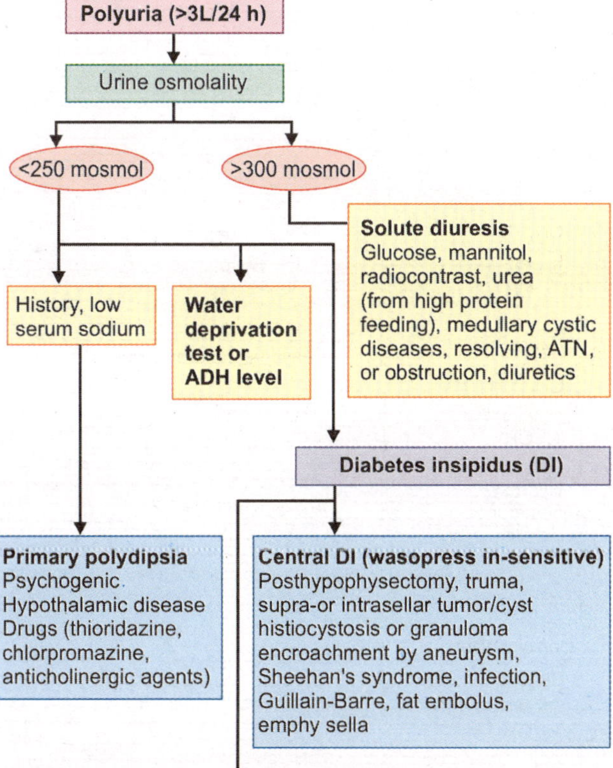

- The average person excretes between 600 and 800 mosmol of solutes per day, primarily as urea and electrolytes.
- If the urine output is >3 L/d and the urine is dilute (<250 mosmol/L), total mosmol excretion is normal and a ***water diuresis*** is present. This circumstance could arise from polydipsia, inadequate secretion of vasopressin (*central diabetes insipidus*), or failure of renal tubules to respond to vasopressin (*nephrogenic diabetes insipidus*).
- If the urine volume is >3 L/d and urine osmolality is >300 mosmol/L, a ***solute diuresis*** is clearly present and a search for the responsible solute (s) is mandatory.

16. Ans. a. Factor 9; c. Factor 10

[Ref: A K Jain 6th/102; O.P.Ghai 8th/116]

"**Vit. K** *carboxylates glutamic acids of translation products of vitamin K-dependent proteins, to produce ϒ-carboxyglutamate.* ***Factor II, VII, IX and X*** *are procoagulant proenzymes whereas proteins C and S are anticoagulant proenzymes" (O. P. Ghai 8th/116)*

"Vit. K is required for synthesis of prothrombin ***(factor II) and factors VII, IX and X*** *in the liver"- A K Jain 6th/102*

The vitamin K–dependent proteins can be divided into two classes: Procoagulant (factors II, VII, IX and X; and anticoagulant (protein C, protein S and protein Z. The vitamin K–dependent proteins are part of a family of serine proteinases (except for protein S and protein Z) related to the trypsin/chymotrypsin superfamily- Wintrobe's Clinical Hematology 12th/Chap 20

17. Ans. a. Deoxycorticosterone, b. Cortisol; e. Androstenedione

[Ref: Ganong 25th/357-58; Guyton 13th(SAE)/641; A K Jain 6th/718]

Not very sure about answer. Please explore yourself.

"ACTH is ***not concerned with aldosterone synthesis*** *(it is regulated by renin angiotensin system)"- A K Jain 6th/718*

"Aldosterone is secreted from the zona glomerulosa under the control of three principal secretagogues, angiotensin II, potassium and to a *lesser extent ACTH*"- *Williams Textbook of Endocrinology 11th/Chap14*

ACTH Receptor and ACTH Effects on the Adrenal

❖ *Williams Textbook of Endocrinology 11th/Chap14*

- ***The effects of ACTH on the adrenal include both immediate and chronic effects; the end result is the stimulation of adrenal steroidogenesis*** and growth.
- Acutely, steroidogenesis is stimulated through a StAR-mediated increase in cholesterol delivery to the CYP11A1 enzyme in the inner mitochondrial membrane
- Chronically (within 24 to 26 hours of exposure), ***ACTH acts to increase the synthesis of all steroidogenic CYP enzymes (CYP11A1, CYP17, CYP21A2, CYP11B1) in addition to adrenodoxin,*** effects which are mediated at the transcriptional level.

"In vivo conversion of *progesterone to deoxycorticosterone (DOC) by peripheral 21 hydroxylation* was studied in normal men and women. The technique used was to infuse labeled progesterone under steady state conditions and isolate the precursor and product from blood by multiple chromatography steps. Acute ACTH increases both progesterone and DOC and almost all of the DOC in plasma is from direct secretion"-*www.ncbi. nlm. nih. gov*

Flowchart (Ganong 25th/358): Hormone Synthesis in the Zona Glomerulosa The zona glomerulosa lacks 17α-hydroxylase activity and only the zona glomerulosa can convert corticosterone to aldosterone because it is the only zone that normally contains aldosterone synthase. ANG II, angiotensin II.

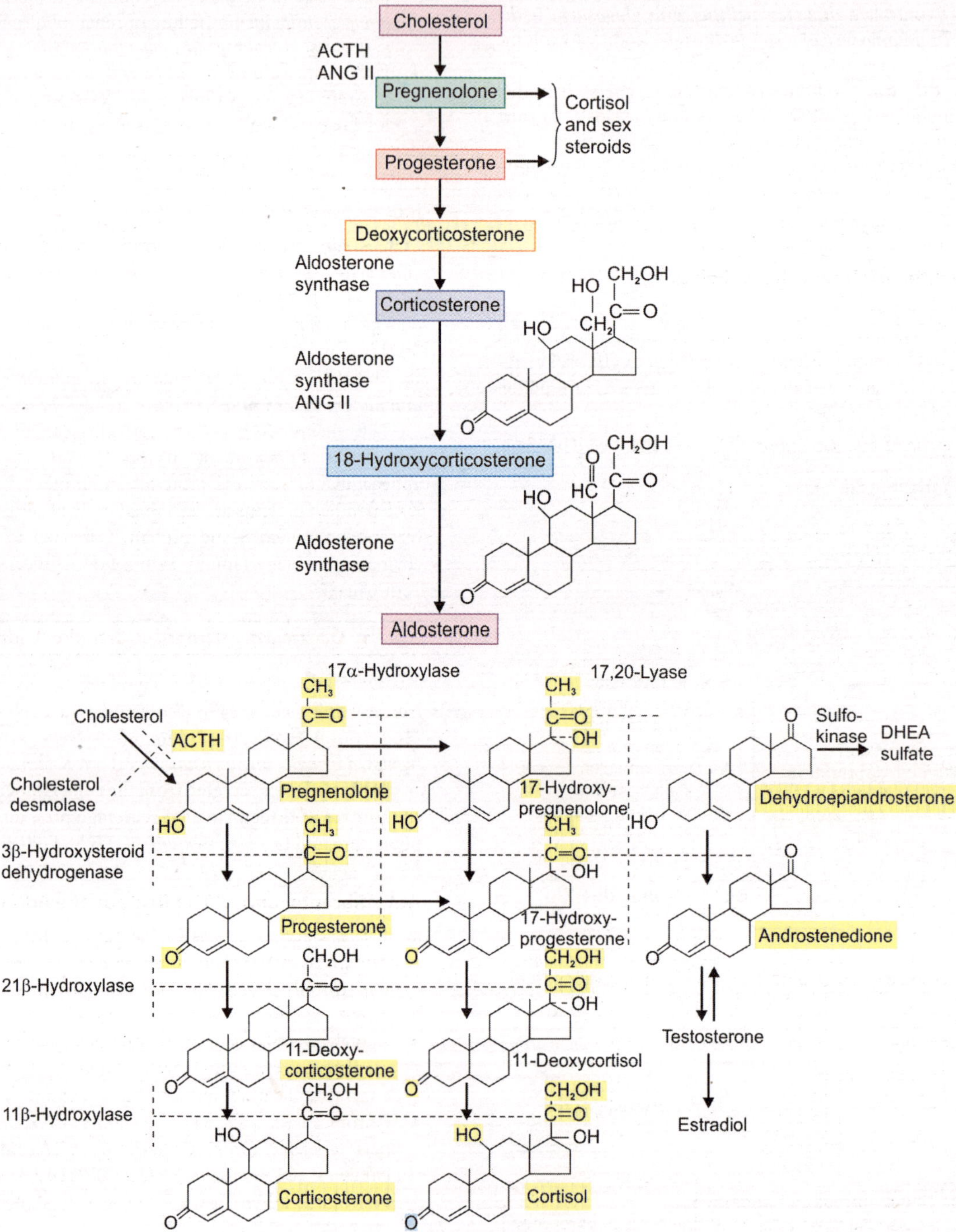

Fig: *(Ganong 25th/357):* Outline of hormone biosynthesis in the zona fasciculata and zona reticularis of the adrenal cortex. The major secretory products are underlined. The enzymes for the reactions are shown on the left and at the top of the chart. When a particular enzyme is deficient, hormone production is blocked at the points indicated by the shaded bars

Flowchart *(Williams Textbook of Endocrinology 11th/Chap14)*: Adrenal Steroidogenesis. After the steroidogenic acute regulatory (StAR) protein-mediated uptake of cholesterol into mitochondria within adrenocortical cells, aldosterone, cortisol and adrenal androgens are synthesized through the coordinated action of a series of steroidogenic enzymes in a zone-specific fashion. A'Dione androstenedione; DHEA, dehydroepiandrosterone; Doc, deoxycorticosterone.

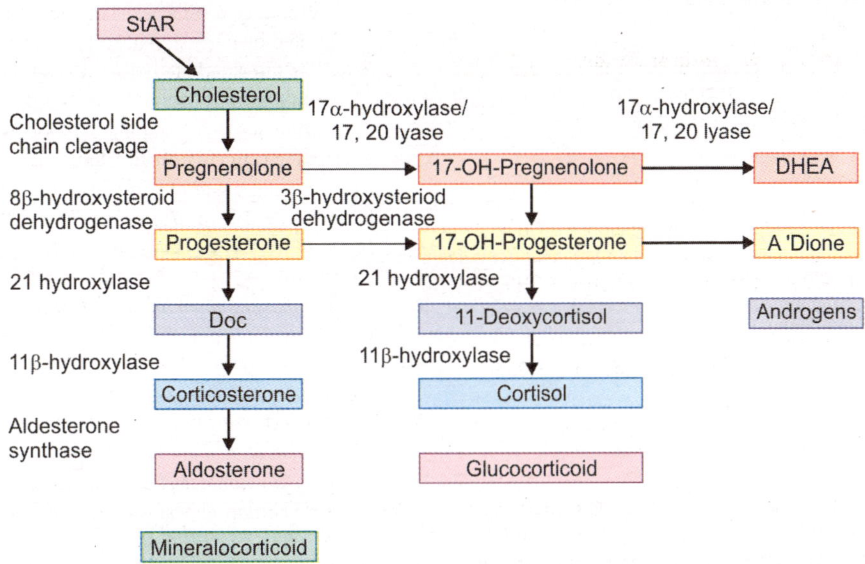

18. Ans. a. Serum prolactin level estimation; b. Serum growth hormone level after oral glucose ingestion; e. ACTH stimulation test

[Ref: Harrison 19th/2257-58; Guyton 13th(SAE)/588]

ADH clinical tests: ***water deprivation test*** *and water load test"- Guyton 13th (SAE)/588*

Oxytocin is secreted by posterior pituitary gland

Prolactin Test

www.healthcommunities.com

- To ***diagnose and monitor pituitary tumors***
- To evaluate patients with amenorrhea (absence of menstruation) or galactorrhea (abnormal secretion of milk)
- To determine the cause of headaches and visual disturbances
- To diagnose erectile dysfunction
- To diagnose infertility
- To diagnose, monitor the treatment of or detect recurrence of prolactinomas

"Growth hormone (GH), as its name implies, plays a central role in regulating the body's growth. If a blood test indicates an elevated level of GH, a ***GH suppression test,*** **which** ***measures GH levels in response to glucose*** (a sugar that normally suppresses GH secretion) is done to confirm the finding. If the blood level of GH is low, a ***GH stimulation test*** is performed to measure GH levels in response to substances that normally stimulate GH secretion (such as the hormone insulin, the amino acid arginine, or growth hormone-releasing hormone, or GHRH)"- *www.healthcommunities.com*

GH suppression test: Blood samples are drawn between 6 AM and 8 AM using venipuncture to record pre-test GH levels. Person is asked to **drink a glucose solution**. Additional blood samples are drawn at several intervals over the next 2 hours so that they can be analyzed for GH levels in response to the glucose"-*www.healthcommunities.com*

ACTH, or corticotropin, is a pituitary hormone that stimulates the adrenal gland to release cortisol and other hormones. ***Measuring ACTH levels*** in the blood can aid in the diagnosis of adrenal gland abnormalities, such as Cushing's syndrome (overproduction of cortisol) and Addison's disease (a form of adrenal insufficiency marked by underproduction of cortisol). To help diagnose Cushing's syndrome, the **dexamethasone suppression test** may be performed to measure the effect that dexamethasone, a drug similar to cortisol, has on cortisl levels. Alternatively, to evaluate adrenal insufficiency the **ACTH stimulation test** is used to measure the adrenal response to ACTH administration"- *www.healthcommunities.com*

Laboratory Investigation

Harrison 19th/2257

- Biochemical diagnosis of **pituitary insufficiency** is made by demonstrating ***low levels of respective pituitary trophic hormones*** in the setting of low levels of target hormones.
- Provocative tests may be required to assess pituitary reserve. GH responses to insulin-induced hypoglycemia, arginine, L-dopa, growth hormone–releasing hormone (GHRH), or growth hormone–releasing peptides (GHRPs) can be used to assess GH reserve.
- Corticotropin releasing hormone (CRH) administration induces **ACTH release** and administration of synthetic ACTH (cosyntropin) evokes adrenal cortisol release as an indirect indicator of pituitary ACTH reserve. ACTH reserve is most reliably assessed by measuring **ACTH and cortisol levels** during insulin-induced hypoglycemia. However,

this test should be performed cautiously in patients with suspected adrenal insufficiency because of enhanced susceptibility to hypoglycemia and hypotension.

Table: *(Harrison 19th/2258)*: **Tests of pituitary sufficiency**

Hormone	Test	Interpretation
Growth hormone (GH)	Insulin tolerance test: Regular insulin (0. 05-0. 15 U/Kg IV)	Glucose <40 mg/dL; GH should be >3 mg/L
	GHRH test: 1 mg/kg IV	Normal response is GH >3 mg/L
	L-Arginine test: 30 g IV over 3 min	Normal response is GH >3 mg/L
	L-Dopa test: 200-500mg IV	Normal response is GH >3 mg/L
Prolactin	TRH test: 200-500 mg IV	Normal prolactin Is >2 mg/L and Increase >200%0 baseline
ACTH	Insulin tolerance test: regular insulin (0. 05-0. 15 U/kg IV)	Glucose <40 mg/dL
	CRH test: 1 mg/kg ovine CRH IV at 8 am.	Cortisol should increase by >7 mg/dL or to >20 mg /dL
	Standard ACTH stimulation test: ACTH 1–24 (cosyntropin), 0. 25 mg IM or IV	Normal response is cortisol >21 g/dL and aldosterone response of >4 ng/dL above baseline

19. Ans. a. CO_2 diffuses 20 times faster than O_2; c. Diffusion of oxygen is perfusion limited; d. Diffusion of gas is decreased in emphysema; e. Diffusion capacity of O_2 is 25.

[Ref: Ganong 25th/634-35; Guyton 13th/368; Textbook of Respiratory Physiology 3rd/913]

Diffusion of Gas is Decreased In Emphysema (Due to Decreased Surface Area of Respiratory Membrane)

◈ *Guyton 13th/368*

PO_2 gradient, i.e PAO_2-PaO_2 (Theoretical Alveolar oxygen- Actual arterial oxygen) is increased in case of restrictive lung disease (diffusion defect)-*Textbook of Respiratory Physiology 3rd/913*

Diffusion Across The Alveolocapillary Membrane

◈ *Ganong 25th/634*

- Gases diffuse from the alveoli to the blood in the pulmonary capillaries or vice versa across the thin alveolocapillary membrane made up of the pulmonary epithelium, the capillary endothelium and their fused basement membranes
- Whether or not substances passing from the alveoli to the capillary blood reach equilibrium in the 0.75 s that blood takes to traverse the pulmonary capillaries at rest depends on their reaction with substances in the blood. Thus, for example, the anesthetic gas nitrous oxide (N_2O) does not react and reaches equilibrium in about 0.1 s
- In this situation, the amount of **N_2O** taken up is not limited by diffusion but by the amount of blood flowing through the pulmonary capillaries; that is, it is **flow-limited.**
- On the other hand, **carbon monoxide (CO)** is taken up by hemoglobin in the red blood cells at such a high rate that the partial pressure of CO in the capillaries stays very low and equilibrium is not reached in the 0.75 s the blood is in the pulmonary capillaries. Therefore, the transfer of CO is not limited by perfusion at rest and instead is diffusion-limited.
- **O_2** is intermediate between **N_2O** and CO; it is taken up by hemoglobin, but much less avidly than CO and it reaches equilibrium with capillary blood in about 0.3 s. Thus, its uptake is **perfusion-limited.**

"The normal value of diffusing capacity for CO (Dlco) at rest is about 25 mL/min/mm Hg. The ***diffusing capacity for O_2, like that for CO at rest, is about 25 mL/min/mm Hg***"-Ganong 25th/635

"The diffusing capacity for carbon-dioxide at rest is slightly more than 20 times of that of oxygen (about 400-450 mL/min/mm Hg)"-*Guyton 13th/368*

Calculation of the A-a gradient helps to distinguish basic patghogenic cause of hypoxia

- **Increased** A-a gradient is seen in:-
  - *Diffusion defect **(e.g. restrictive lung diseases)***
  - *Ventilation perfusion defect*
  - *Right to left shunt*
- **Normal** A-a gradient is seen in
  - *Hypoventilation*
  - *High altitude*

20. Ans. b. Action potential traverses...; c. Rynadine receptors sense the action potiential; e. ATP binds to myosin

[Ref: Ganong 25th/101-06; Guyton 13th/91-96; A.K.Jain 6th/165]

- *Myosin pulls actin by powerstroke*
- *It is **intracellular calcium**, which is responsible for contraction(not extracellular)*

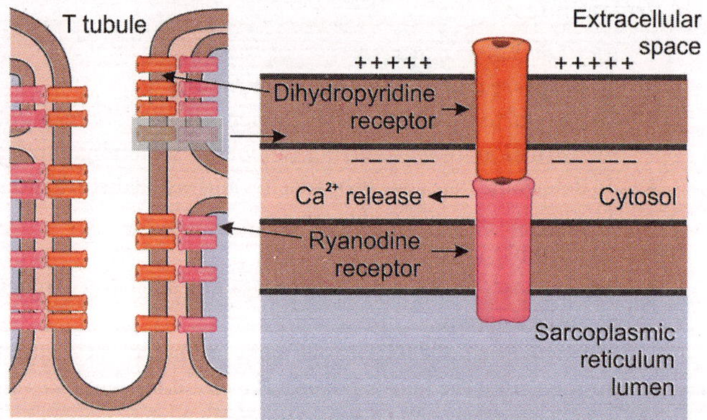

Fig: (Ganong 25th/106): Relation of the T tubule to the sarcoplasmic reticulum in Ca^{2+} transport. In skeletal muscle, the voltage-gated dihydropyridine receptor in the T tubule triggers Ca^{2+} release from the sarcoplasmic reticulum (SR) via the ryanodine receptor (RyR). Upon sensing a voltage change, there is a physical interaction between the sarcolemmal-bound DHPR and the SR-bound RyR. This interaction gates the RyR and allows for Ca^{2+} release from the SR.

Steps in contraction[a]

↓

Discharge of motor neuron

↓

Release of transmitter (acetylcholine) at motor endplate

↓

Binding of acetylcholine to nicotinic acetylocholine receptors

↓

Increased Na^+ and K^+ conductance in endplate membrane

↓

Generation of endplate potenital

↓

Generation of action potenital in muscle fibers

↓

Inward spread of depolarization along T tubules

↓

Release of Ca^{2+} from terminal cisterns of sarcoplasmic reticulum and diffusion to thick and thin flaments

↓

Binding of Ca^{2+} to troponin C, uncovering myosin-binding sites on actin

↓

Formation of cross-linkages between actin and myosin and slinding of thin on thick filaments, producing moverment

Fig *(Ganong 25th/105)*: Flow of information that leads to muscle contraction

21. Ans. c. Arginosuccinate synthetase, d. Arginosuccinate lyase, e. Arginase

[Ref: Harper 30th/293; Lippincott 6th/252-54; Vasudevan 5th/180-81; Satyanarayan 4th/337]

"Urea synthesis is a five step cyclic process, with five distinct enzyme. The first two reactions (Catalyzed by Carbamoyl phosphate synthetase I and ornithine transcarbomylase) leading to the synthesis of urea occur in the mitochondria, whereas the **remaining cycle enzymes (reaction 3-5; *Arginosuccinate synthetase, Arginosuccinate lyase and arginase*) are *located in the cytosol*"**- *Lippincott 6th/252-54; Harper 30th/293*

High yielding facts

- Carbomyl phosphate synthetase I reaction is rate limiting step in urea formation- *Vasudevan 5th/180*
- Urea cycle is also k/a Krebs-Henseleit cycle or ornithine cycle- *Satyanarayan 4th/337; Vasudevan 5th/180*
- *Urea has two amino groups, one derived from NH_3 and the other from aspartate. Carbon atom is supplied by CO_2- Satyanarayan 4th/337*
- *Urea is synthesized in liver*

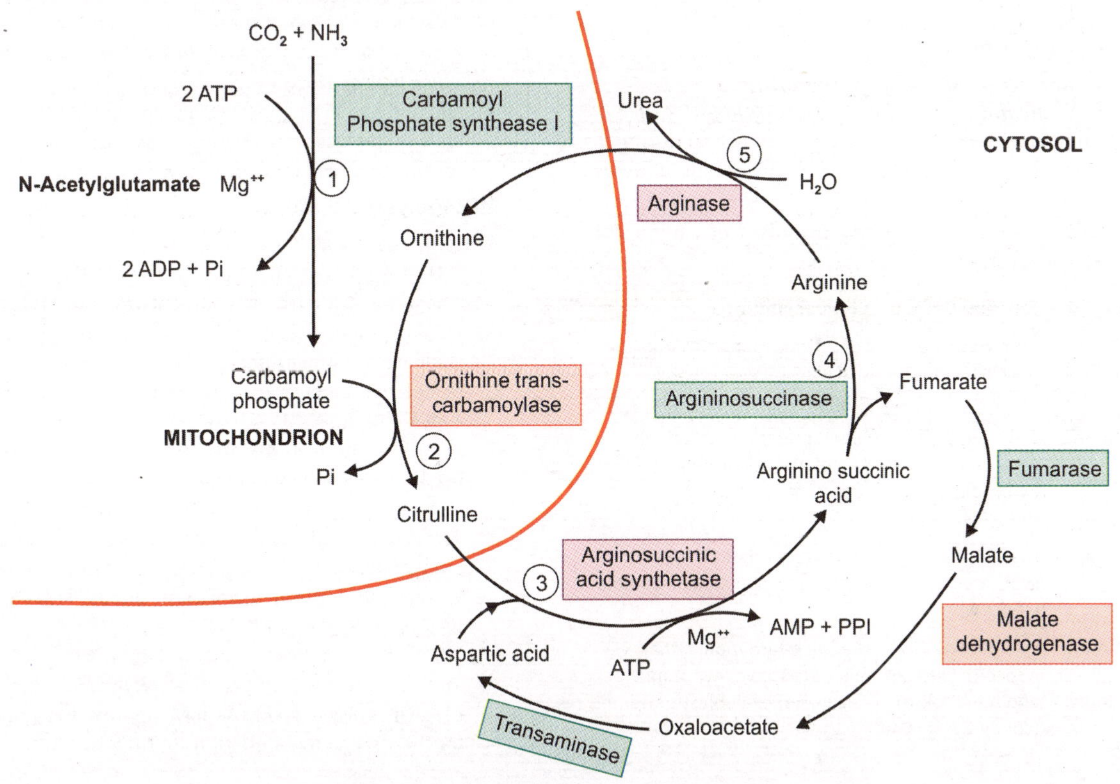

Fig: Biosynthesis of urea or ornithine – urea cycle

22. Ans. b. Mental retardation; d. Ectopia lentis

[Ref: Harper 30th/316; Lippincott 6th/273,269; Shinde 7th/477-78; Vasudevan 5th/194; Satyanarayan 4th/362]

Cystine kidney stones are due to cystinuria, an inherited (genetic) disorder of the transport of an amino acid (a building block of protein) called cystine that results in an excess of cystine in the urine (cystinuria) and the formation **of *cystine stones***- *Lippincott 6th/249; healthline.com*

Homocystinuria

◈ *Lippincott 6th/273,269*

- The homocystinurias are a group of disorders involving defects in the metabolism of homocysteine.
- The diseases are inherited as autosomal recessive illnesses, characterized by ***high plasma and urinary levels of homocysteine and methionine and low levels of cysteine.***
- The most common cause of homocystinuria is a defect in the enzyme cystathionine β-synthase, which converts homocysteine to cystathionine
- Individuals who are homozygous for cystathionine β-synthase deficiency exhibit ***ectopia lentis (displacement of the lens of the eye), skeletal abnormalities, a tendency to form thrombi (blood clots), osteoporosis and neurological deficits.***
- ***Mental retardation***- *Satyanarayan 4th/362*
- Treatment includes restriction of methionine intake and supplementation with vitamins B6, B12 and folate.

Homocystinurias (Hyperhomocysteinemias)

◈ *Harrison 19th/434e1-4*

- Most patients present between 3 and 5 years of age ***with dislocated optic lenses and intellectual disability (in about half of cases)***. Some patients develop a ***marfanoid habitus and radiologic evidence of osteoporosis.***
- ***Life-threatening vascular complications (affecting coronary, renal and cerebral arteries)*** can occur during the first decade of life and are the major cause of morbidity and mortality.

Table: *(Harrison 19th/434e-2)*: **Inherited Disorders of Amino Acid Metabolism (Partial list)**

Condition	Enzyme Defect	Clinical Findings
Homocystinuria	Cystathionine β-synthase	Lens dislocation, thrombotic vascular disease, mental retardation, osteoporosis
Homocystinuria	5, 10 - Methylenetetra-hydrofolate reductase	Mental retardation, gait and psychiatric abnormalities, recurrent strokes
Homocystinuria	Methionine synthase (cblE, -G)	Mental retardation, hypotonia, seizures, megaloblastic anemia
Homocystinuria and methylmalonic acidemia	Vitamin B12 lysosomal efflux and metabolism (cbl C, -D, -F)	Mental retardation, lethargy, failure to thrive, hypotonia, seizures, megaloblastic anemia

23. Ans. a. It is a type of lysosomal storage disorder; c. Skeletal defect is manifested as dystosis multiplex; d. Research is going on to develop give therapy for Morquio syndrome

[Ref: Harper 30th/638-39; O.P.Ghai 8th/661; Nelson 20th/741,706; Lippincott 6th/163-64; Satyanarayan 4th/281-82; Harrison 19th/432e-1-6]

Mucopolysaccharidoses

◈ *Lippincott 6th/163-64*

- The mucopolysaccharidoses are hereditary diseases caused by a ***deficiency of any one of the lysosomal hydrolases*** normally involved in the degradation of heparan sulfate and/or dermatan sulfate. They are progressive disorders characterized by accumulation of glycosaminoglycans in various tissues, causing a range of symptoms, such as ***skeletal and extracellular matrix deformities*** and ***mental retardation***.
- ***All are autosomal recessive diseases except Hunter syndrom***e, which is X-linked.
- Bone marrow and cord blood transplants have been used to treat **Hurler and Hunter syndromes**. ***Enzyme replacement therapy (ERT) is currently available for both syndromes.***

Mucopolysaccharidos

◈ *O.P.Ghai 8th/661*

- Skeletal changes observed include thickening of the skull, marked deformity of sella turcica, brad spatula like ribs, beak shaped vertebrae (around L1 vertebrae) and proximal tapering of metacarpals; these abnormalities are referred to as ***dystosis multiplex***
- ***Enzyme replacement therapy is available for type I,II and type VI but the cost is prohibitive. Trial are underway for other type of MPS***
- In 2014, the FDA approved a recombinant human GALNS enzyme replacement therapy (elosulfase alfa, or Vimizim) for the treatment of MPS IVA- *rarediseases.org*

Mucopolysaccharidose

◈ *Harrison 19th/432e-1-6*

- It is a type of lysosomal storage diseases (LSDs).
- There are two current treatments for the MPS I diseases. Hematopoietic stem cell transplantation (HSCT) is the standard treatment for patients presenting at <2 years of age who appear to have or are at risk for neurologic degeneration.
- A combination of **enzyme therapy and HSCT** has been used, with enzyme therapy initiated prior to transplantation in an attempt to reduce the disease burden.
- The experience with this approach is not well documented, but it appears to have advantages over HSCT alone. Enzyme therapy for ***Maroteaux-Lamy disease (MPS VI)*** has received U.S. FDA approval.
- HSCT has not been successful in treating CNS disease associated with MPS II. The FDA and the European Medicines Agency (EMA) have approved enzyme therapy for the visceral manifestations of MPS II.

How is Mucopolysaccharidosis Type IV Treated?

◈ *www.dovemed.com*

The treatment measures may include:

- **Enzyme replacement therapy**: *Replacement of the missing enzyme to help in the breakdown of glycosoaminoglycans*
- Other organ specific treatments as specified by the healthcare provider including:
  - Orthopedic surgery for correcting bone and joint abnormalities
  - Surgical correction for spinal cord and vertebral defects
  - Hernia repair for inguinal and umbilical hernia
  - Corneal transplant for vision abnormalities
  - Tonsillectomy for frequent ear and throat infections
  - Correction of hearing defects
- For improving motor skills, special therapeutic treatment (by physical and occupational therapists) and supportive care is required
- **Bone marrow transplant**: Presently, this is not found to be a very effective treatment option
- ***Research is being currently undertaken to treat Mucopolysaccharidosis Type IV using gene therapy***

Table: *(Harper 30th/639):* **The Mucopolysaccharidoses**

Disease Name	Abbreviation	Symptoms
Hurler-, Scheie-Hurler-Scheie syndrome	MPS I	Mental retardation, coarse facial features, hepatosplenomegaly, cloudy cornea
Hunter syndrome	MPS II	Mental retardation
Sanfilippo syndrome A	MPS IIIA	Delay in development, motor dysfunction
Sanfilippo syndrome B	MPS IIIB	As MPS IIIA
Sanfilippo syndrome C	MPS IIIC	As MPS IIIA
Sanfilippo syndrome D	MPS IIID	As MPS IIIA
Morquio syndrome A	MPS IVA	Skeletal dysplasia, short stature
Morquio syndrome B	MPS IVB	As MPS IVA
Maroteaux-Lamy syndrome	MPS VI	Curvature of the spine, short stature, skeletal dysplasia, cardiac defects
Sly syndrome	MPS VII	Skeletal dysplasia, short stature, hepatomegaly, cloudy cornea
Natowicz syndrome	MPS IX	Joint pain, short stature

24. Ans. a. Palmitic acid; b. Alpha-linolenic acid

[Ref: Harper 30th/214; Lippincott 6th/182]

Palmitic acid is a saturated fatty acid

Table: *(Harper 30th/214):* **Unsaturated Fatty Acids of Physiologic and Nutritional Significance**

Number of C Atoms and No. and Position of Common Double Bonds	Family	Common Name	Systematic Name	Occurrence
Monoenoic acids (one double bond)				
16:1; 9	ω7	Palmitoleic	cis-9-Hexadecenoic	In nearly all fats
18:1; 9	ω9	Oleic	cis-9-Octadecenoic	Possibly the most common fatty acid in natural fats; particularly high in olive oil
18:1; 9	ω9	Elaidic	trans-9-Octadecenoic	Hydrogenated and ruminant fats
Dienoic acids (two double bonds)				
18:2; 9,12	ω6	Linoleic	all-cis-9,12-Octadecadienoic	Corn, peanut, cottonseed, soy bean and many plant oils
Trienoic acids (three double bonds)				
18:3; 6,9,12	ω6	γ-Linolenic	all-cis-6,9,12-Octadecatrienoic	Some plants, e.g., oil of evening primrose, borage oil; minor fatty acid in animals
18:3; 9,12,15	w3	α-Linolenic	all-cis-9,12,15-Octadecatrienoic	Frequently found with linoleic acid but particularly in linseed oil
Tetraenoic acids (four double bonds)				
20:4; 5,8,11,14	ω6	Arachidonic	all-cis-5,8,11,14-Eicosatetraenoic	Found in animal fats; important component of phospholipids in animals
Pentaenoic acids (five double bonds)				
20:5; 5,8,11,14,17	w3	Timnodonic	all-cis-5,8,11,14,17-Eicosapentaenoic	Important component of fish oils, e.g., cod liver, mackerel, menhaden, salmon oils
Hexaenoic acids (six double bonds)				
22:6; 4,7,10,13,16,19	w3	Cervonic	all-cis-4,7,10,13,16,19-Docosahexaenoic	Fish oils, algal oils, phospholipids in brain

Table: *(Lippincott 6th/364):* **Effects of dietary fats**

Type of Fat	Metabolic Effects	Effects on Disease Prevention
Trans fatty acid	↑LDL ↓ HDL	↑ Incidence of coronary heart disease
Saturated fatty acid	↑LDL Little effect on HDL	↑ Incidence of coronary heart disease; may increase risk of prostate, colon cancer
Monounsaturated fatty acid	↓ LDL ↓ HDL	↓ Incidence of coronary heart disease
Polyunsaturated fatty acids ω-6	↓ LDL ↓ HDL Provide arachidonic acid which is an important precursor of prostaglandins and leukotrienes	↓ Incidence of coronary heart disease
Polyunsaturated fatty acids ω-3	Little effect on LDL and HDL Suppress cardiac arrhythmias, reduce serum triacylglycerols, decrease the tendency for thrombosis, lower blood pressure	↓ Incidence of coronary heart disease ↓ Risk of sudden cardiac death

25. Ans. b. Muscle weakness may occur; c. Peripheral sensory nerve involvement is usually present; d. Neuronal symptom improves with Vit B12 therapy

[Ref: Harrison 19th/96e-3; Davidson 22nd/1024-26]

Neurological Findings in B12 Deficiency

◈ *Davidson 22nd/1024*

Peripheral nerves
- Glove and stocking paraesthesiae
- Loss of ankle reflexes

Spinal cord
- Subacute combined degeneration of the cord
  Posterior columns: |diminished vibration sensation and proprioception
  Corticospinal tracts: upper motor neuron signs

Cerebrum
- Dementia
- Optic atrophy

Autonomic Neuropathy

Megaloblastic Anemia not due to Cobalamin or Folate Deficiency or Altered Metabolism: In thiamine-responsive megaloblastic anemia, there is a genetic defect in the high-affinity thiamine transport (SLC19A2) gene. This causes defective RNA ribose synthesis through ***impaired activity of transketolase, a thiamine-dependent enzyme*** in the pentose cycle. This leads to reduced nucleic acid production"- *Harrison 19th/649*

"Blood and urine assays for thiamine are not reliable for diagnosis of deficiency. **Erythrocyte transketolase activity** and the percentage increase in activity (in vitro) following the addition of thiamine pyrophosphate (TPP) may be more accurate and reliable"- *Harrison 19th/2690*

Cobalamin (Vitamin B12)

◈ *Harrison 19th/2690,643*

- Cobalamin deficiency may cause a ***bilateral peripheral neuropathy or degeneration (demyelination) of the posterior and pyramidal tracts of the spinal cord and, less frequently, optic atrophy or cerebral symptoms.*** The patient, more frequently male, p***resents with paresthesias, muscle weakness,*** or difficulty in walking and sometimes dementia, psychotic disturbances, or visual impairment.
- EDx shows an ***axonal sensorimotor neuropathy.*** CNS involvement produces abnormal somatosensory and visual evoked potential latencies.
- The **diagnosis is confirmed** by finding reduced serum cobalamin levels. In up to 40% of patients, anemia and macrocytosis are lacking. Serum methylmalonic acid and homocysteine, the metabolites that accumulate when cobalamin-dependent reactions are blocked, are elevated. Antibodies to intrinsic factor are present in approximately 60% and antiparietal cell antibodies in about 90%, of individuals with pernicious anemia.
- *Treatment for cobalamin deficiency usually does not completely reverse the clinical manifestations and at least 50% of patients exhibit some permanent neurologic deficit.*
- "Vitamin B12 deficiency is treated with hydroxycobalamin 1000 µg IM for 6 doses 2 or 3 days apart, followed by maintenance therapy of 1000 µg every 3 months for life. The reticulocyte count will peak by the 5th–10th day after starting replacement therapy. ***A sensory neuropathy may take 6–12 months to correct; long-standing neurological damage may not improve***"- *Davidson 22nd/1026*
- **Megaloblastic anaemia:** Vitamin B12 deficiency, but not folate deficiency, is associated with neurological disease in up to 40% of cases, although advanced neurological disease due to B12 deficiency is now uncommon in the developed world- *Davidson 22nd/1024*

26. Ans. b. 1% prevalence of night-blindness is the criteria for determining the xerophthalmia problem...; d. Chronic vitamin A intoxication causes papilledema

[Ref: Park 24th/653-54; Harrison 19th/96e5-6; Suryakanth Recent Advances in Community Medicine 4th/161-62; Harper 30th/547, 551; Lippincott 6th/381-83; Shinde 7th /152-56]

Vitamin A

◈ *Harrison 19th/96e5-6*

- *Vitamin A*, in the strictest sense, refers to retinol. However, the oxidized metabolites retinaldehyde and retinoic acid are also biologically active compounds. The term *retinoids* includes all molecules (including synthetic molecules) that are chemically related to retinol.

- Retinaldehyde (11-*cis*) is the essential form of vitamin A that is required for normal vision, whereas retinoic acid is necessary for normal morphogenesis, growth and cell differentiation. Retinoic acid does not function in vision and, in contrast to retinol, is not involved in reproduction.
- As judged by deficient serum retinol (<0.70 μmol/L [20 μg/dL]), vitamin A deficiency worldwide is present in >90 million preschool-age children, among whom >4 million have an ocular manifestation of deficiency termed ***xerophthalmia.***
- This condition includes milder stages of ***night blindness*** and conjunctival *xerosis* (dryness) with *Bitot's spots* (white patches of keratinized epithelium appearing on the sclera) as well as rare, potentially blinding corneal ulceration and necrosis.
- Any stage of xerophthalmia should be treated with ***60 mg*** (or RAE) of vitamin A in oily solution, usually contained in a soft-gel capsule.
- WHO is according high priority to prevention in communities where xerophthalmia occurs, giving single prophylactic oral doses of ***60 mg retinyl palmitate (providing 200 000 U retinol)*** to pre-school children. This also reduces mortality from gastroenteritis and respiratory infections"- *Davidson 22nd/127*
- **Chronic vitamin A intoxication**: Manifestations include dry skin, cheilosis, glossitis, vomiting, alopecia, bone demineralization and pain, hypercalcemia, lymph node enlargement, hyperlipidemia, amenorrhea and features of pseudotumor cerebri with increased intracranial pressure and ***papilledema***

"Vit. A is found in animal as preformed Vit. A (retinol) and in plant as provitamins (carotenes). Animal foods rich in retinol are liver, eggs, butter, cheese, ***whole milk***, fish and meat. Fish liver oils are the richest natural sources of retinol"- *Park 24th/653*

Toxicity of Vit. A: Nausea, vomiting, anorexia and sleep disorders followed by skin desquamation and then an enlarged liver and ***papillar edema***"- Park 24th/654

Table: *(Park 24th/654)*: **Prevalence criteria for determining the xerophthalmia problem**

Criteria	Prevalence in the population at risk (6m-6yr)
Night blindness	More than 1%
Bitot's spots	More than 0.5%
Corneal xerosis/corneal ulceration/Keratomalacia	More than 0.01%
Corneal ulcer	More than 0.05%
Serum retinol (<10 mcg/dl)	More than 5%

1 μg retinol = 3.3IU of Vit A=12μg of –carotene-O.P.Ghai 8th/110

Table: Daily intake of vitamin A recommended by ICMR (2010)

	Group	Retinol (μg) Or β-carotene (μg)*	
Adults	Man	600	4,800
	Woman	600	4,800
	Pregnancy	800	6,400
	Lactation	950	7,600
Infants	0 to 6 months	350	–
	6 to 12 months	350	2800
Children	1 to 6 years	400	3,200
	7 to 9 years	600	4,800
Adolescents	10 to 17 years	600	4,800

* A Conversion ratio of 1: 8 is used

27. Ans. a. Hexokinase; b. Pyruvate kinase; c. Phosphofructokinase

[Ref: Harper 30th/172; Lippincott 6th/96-98; Vasudevan 5th/89]

Glycolysis is Regulated at three Steps Involving Nonequilibrium Reactions

Harper 30th/172; Vasudevan 5th/89

- Although most of the reactions of glycolysis are freely reversible, three are markedly exergonic and must therefore be considered to be physiologically irreversible.
- These reactions, catalyzed by **hexokinase** (and glucokinase), **phosphofructokinase** and **pyruvate kinase,** are the major sites of regulation of glycolysis.

"Citric acid cycle-*Pyruvate dehydrogenase*"- *Harper 30th/169*

28. Ans. c. Sucrose; e. Trehalose

[Ref: Lippincott 6th/84-85; Vasudevan 5th/107; Satyanarayan 4th/18]

- **Non-reducing disaccharides**: *no free aldehydes or keto group e.g.* ***sucrose, trehalose****"- Satyanarayan 4th/18*
- **Reducing disaccharides**: *free aldehydes or keto group e.g.* ***maltose, isomaltose,lactose****"- Satyanarayan 4th/18*

Reducing Sugars

Lippincott 6th/84-85,90

- The sugar can act as a reducing agent and is termed a reducing sugar. Such sugars can react with chromogenic agents (for example, Benedict's reagent or Fehling's solution) causing the reagent to be reduced and colored, with the aldehyde group of the acyclic sugar becoming oxidized. [Note: Only the state of the oxygen in the aldehyde group determines if the sugar is reducing or nonreducing.]
- **Reducing substances: Reducing sugars (*glucose, fructose, galactose, xylulose, lactose*)**, amino acids, ascorbic acid and certain drugs and drug metabolites.
- ***Sucrose is not a reducing sugar***

Table: *(Vasudevan 5th/107)*: **Reducing substances in urine**

Sugars	Non-carbohydrates
Glucose *Fructose* *Lactose* *Galactose* *Pentoses*	*Homogentisic acid* *Salicylates* *Ascorbic acid* *Glucuronides of drugs*

29. Ans. a. Apo I; b. Apo II; e. Apo D

[Ref: Harper 30th/255; Lippincott 6th/229-30; Satyanarayan 4th/318]

"Apolipoproteins in HDL- *AI, AII, CI, CII, CIII, D and E*"- *Satyanarayan 4th/318*

The Distribution of Apolipoproteins Characterizes the Lipoprotein *Harper 30th/255*

- ***Some apolipoproteins are integral and cannot be removed (e.g., apo B)***, whereas ***others are bound to the surface and are free to transfer to other lipoproteins, eg, apos C and E).***
- The ***major apolipoproteins of HDL*** **(α-lipoprotein)** ***are apoAs***
- The main **apolipoprotein of LDL** (β-lipoprotein) is apo B (B-100), which is found also in VLDL. Chylomicrons contain a truncated form of apo B (B-48) that is synthesized in the intestine, while B-100 is synthesized in the liver.
- Apo E, found in VLDL, HDL, chylomicrons and chylomicron remnants, is also freely transferable; it accounts for 5% to 10% of total VLDL apolipoproteins in normal subjects.
- Apolipoproteins carry out several roles: (1) they ***can form part of the structure of the lipoprotein***, for ***example, apo B***; (2) they are ***enzyme cofactors***, for example, C-II for ***lipoprotein lipase,*** A-I for ***lecithin:cholesterol acyltransferase***, or **enzyme inhibitors**, for example, apo A-II and apo C-III for lipoprotein lipase, apo C-I for cholesteryl ester transfer protein; and (3) they act as ligands for interaction with lipoprotein receptors in tissues, for example, apo B-100 and apo E for the LDL receptor, apo E for the LDL-receptor-related protein-1 (LRP-1), which has been identified as the remnant receptor and apo A-I for the HDL receptor.

Table: *(nopr.niscari.res.in/bitstream)*: **Major apolipoproteins**

Apolipoprotein	Functional activity	Lipoprotein carrier(s)
Apo A-I	Cofactor LCAT	Chylomicron, HDL
Apo A-II	Not known	HDL
Apo A-IV	Activation of LCAT Secretion of triglyceride from liver binding protein to LDL receptor	Chylomicron, HDL
Apo B-48	Secretion of triglyceride from intestine	Chylomicron
Apo B-100	Cholesterol transport from liver	LDL
Apo C-I	Activation of LCAT (?)	Chylomiron, VLDL, HDL
Apo C-II	Cofactor of LPL	Chylomiron, VLDL, HDL
Apo C-III	Inhibition of apo CIII, activation of LPL	Chylomiron, VLDL, HDL
Apo D	Unknown	HDL
Apo E	Facilitation of uptake of chylomicron remnant and LDL	Chylomiron, VLDL, HDL
Apo (a)	Unknown	Lp (a)

Contd...

30. Ans. a. Galactose synthesis; b. Glycogen synthesis; c. Bilirubin metabolism; d. Ganglioside synthesis; e. Heaprin synthesis

[Ref: Harper 30th/187; Lippincott 6th/126-27,141-42; Shinde 7th/210]

Uridine Nucleotides

◈ *Shinde 7th/210*

- UTP reacts with Glucose-1-P to from **uridine diphosphoglucose (UDPG)**, in presence of the enzyme *UDPG-Pyrophosphorylase.*
- UDPG can donate glucose to a "Primer" molecule of glycogen and is involved in ***glycogen synthesis.***
- UDPG is also required for UDP-Glucose-Galactose *epimerase* for the interconversion of glucose and ***galactose in the liver***
- Galactose-1-P and UTP similarly can form uridinediphospho-galactose (UDPGal). Both UDPG and UDP-Gal can be oxidized to ***UDP-glucuronic acid*** and UDP-Galacturonic acid respectively by NAD^+ -dependant dehydrogenase

UDP-Glucuronic Acid is used for

- ***Conjugation and detoxication of bilirubin, benzoic acid, sterols, estrogens and drugs***
- Also used in the ***biosynthesis of hyaluronic acid, heparin and several other MPS.***

UDP–Galacturonic acid and UDP–L-iduronic acids are used for the biosynthesis of chondroitin–SO_4.

"Glycogen synthesis involves a different pathway via ***uridine diphosphate glucose*** **and glycogen synthase"**- *Harper 30th/187*

Uridine Diphosphoglucose

◈ *Functions en.wikipedia.org*

- It is used in nucleotide sugars metabolism as an activated form of glucose as a substrate for enzymes called glucosyltransferases.
- It is a precursor of glycogen and can be converted into **UDP-galactose** ***and*** **UDP-glucuronic acid,** which can then be

used as substrates by the enzymes that make polysaccharides containing galactose and glucuronic acid.

- UDP-glucose can also be used as a precursor of sucrose lipopolysaccharides and glycosphingolipids.
- UDP-Glucose is the Substrate for Sucrose Synthesis in Plants-www.bioinfo.org.cn/book

"Uridine diphosphate glucose is a key intermediate in carbohydrate metabolism. Serves as a precursor of glycogen, can be metabolized into UDPgalactose and UDPglucuronic acid which can then be incorporated into polysaccharides as galactose and glucuronic acid. **Also serves as a precursor of *sucrose lipopolysaccharides and glycosphingolipids*"**-*www.hmdb.ca*

"Glycosphingolipids include: Cerebrosides, Gangliosides and Globosides"-*wiki*

31. Ans. c. Ceruloplosmin contains 6 atoms of copper; d. Failure to synthesize ceruloplasmin causes Wilson's disease; e. Intestinal absorption occurs in duodenum

[Ref: Shinde 7th/584-86;Harrison 20th/2318; O.P.Ghai 9th/122; Satyanarayan 4th/417]

"Copper(Cu): Primarily Absorbed from the Duodenum)"

◈ *Shinde 7th/584*

Copper is Present in Serum in two Distinct forms

◈ *Shinde 7th/585*

- Direct reacting Cu which is loosely bound to albumin. Approx. 4% present in this form
- Bound form, which remain bound to α-globulin fraction of serum called ceruloplasmin (about 96%)

"Excretion: Under normal conditions, 85 to 99% of the ingested Cu is excreted in the faeces via the bile & remaining 1 to 15% in the urine"- *Shinde 7th/585*

"Wilson disease: Mainly two defects. First is, defect in incorporation of Cu into newly synthesized apo-ceruloplasmin to form ceruloplasmin. Second is, impaird ability of the liver to excrete Cu into bile"- *Shinde 7th/586*

"Ceruloplasmin: It contains about 0.34% copper(6-8 atoms of Cu per molecules, half in cuprous & half in cupric state)"- *Satyanarayan 4th/417*

Ceruloplasmin: It has eight sites for binding copper-contains about eight atoms of copper per molecule"-*Shinde 7th/96*

32. Ans. a. Defective collagen synthesis; c. Defective post-translational modification of collagen; d. Defective hydroxylation; e. Defect in antioxidant system;

[Ref: Shinde 7th/164;Harper 31st/539; Harrison 20th/2313; Satyanarayan 4th/132-33]

Vitamin C

◈ *Shinde 7th/164; Harper 31st/539*

- Asorbic acid (Vit. C) is also called antiscorbutic factor.
- It is very heat labile, especially in basic medium.
- Maximum amount of vitamin C is found in adrenal cortex.
- Amla is the richest source
- Vitamin C deficiency causes scurvy.
- Ascorbic acid functions as a reducing agent and scavenger of free radicals (antioxidant).
- Its major functions are following:
  - In collagen synthesis: Vitamin C is required for post-translational modification by hydroxylation of proline and lysine residues converting them into hydroxyproline and hydroxylysine. Thus vitamin C is essential for the conversion of procollagen to collagen, which is rich in hydroxyproline and hydroxylysine. Though collagen synthesis, it plays a role in formation of matrix of bone, cartilage, dentine and connective tissue.
  - Synthesis of norepinephrine from dopamine by dopamine-β-monoxygenase (dopamine- β hydroxylase) requires Vitamin C.
  - Carnittine synthesis
  - Bile acid synthesis:- 7-α-hydroxylase requires vitamin C.
  - Absorption of iron is stimulated by ascorbic acid by conversion of ferric to ferrous ions.
  - During adrenal steroid synthesis, ascorbic acid is required during hydroxylation reactions.
  - Tyrosine metabolism:- Oxidation of P-hydroxy-phenylpyruvate to homogentisate.
  - Folate metabolism:- Folic acid is converted to its active form tetrahydrofolate by help of Vitamin C.

IMMUNOGENETICS & MOLECULAR BIOLOGY

33. Ans. a. Pfu polymerase; c. Bestaq DNA Polymerase; d. Pwo polymerase

[Ref: Lippincott 6th/482; Vasudevan 5th/458]

"Taq polymerase remains to be the most ubiquitously used polymerase for PCR. This enzyme has a high rate of dNTP incorporation but does **not have any proof-reading activity.** This means that Taq is prone to introducing base-pair errors during PCR amplification. If the PCR product is to be used for functional protein analysis, then this can be problematic"-*www.sciencedirect.com*

Alternative Polymerases and PCR Modifications

- Since the introduction of *Taq* polymerase, a variety of other thermostable polymerases from other thermophilic organisms have also been used in PCR.
- ***Pfu* polymerase** from *Pyrococcus furiosus* is used when increased accuracy is desired because ***it possesses proofreading ability***—unlike *Taq* polymerase.

Tli* polymerase** isolated from Thermococcus litoralis (Vent™ DNA polymerase) also has 3′ to 5′ ***proofreading exonuclease activity to create accurate copies- www.sciencedirect.com

*"Both **Bestaq DNA Polymerase** and Kodaq DNA Polymerase have excellent **proofreading ability** and processivity, with a*

processing speed of 3-4kb and 1kb per minute, respectively"-www.abmgood.com

"Tth polymerase is derived from Thermus thermophilus, a thermophilic thermal vent bacterium (25). Tth DNA polymerase functions optimally at 75°C with high processivity, but ***lacks proofreading 3'-5' exonuclease activity***"-*www.abmgood.com*

"Pwo DNA polymerase is derived from the ultra-thermophilic archaeon Pyrococcus woesei found in deep marine environments (24). Pwo polymerase functions optimally at 100-103°C and displays ***high proofreading 3'-5' exonuclease activity*, giving it 18-fold higher fidelity than Taq polymerase**"-*www.abmgood.com*

KOD DNA polymerase is a recombinant form of DNA polymerase derived from the thermophilic solfatara bacterium Thermococcus kodakaraensis KOD1 type strain. KOD DNA polymerase functions optimally at 85°C and displays 3'-5' ***exonuclease proofreading activity*,** producing blunt-ended DNA products- *www.abmgood.com*

"Bacillus stearothermophilus is a thermophilic species of bacteria common to soil, hot spring and ocean sediment environments. **Bst DNA polymerase** isolated from this species displays helicase-like activity to unwind DNA strands in addition to its polymerase activity. While Bst polymerase has 5'-3' exonuclease activity, it **cannot proofread as** it lacks 3'-5' exonuclease activity"- *www.abmgood.com*

"Bsu DNA polymerase is isolated from the mesophilic soil bacterium Bacillus subtilis. Bsu DNA polymerase operates optimally at 25-30° and denatures at 75°C, making it unsuitable for PCR. Bsu polymerase **cannot proofread as it** lacks 3'-5' exonuclease activity"- *www.abmgood.com*

DNA Polymerase in PCR

◈ *www.bioline.com*

- *VELOCITY DNA- have proofreading 3'–5' exonuclease activity*
- *RANGER DNA- have proofreading 3'–5' exonuclease activity*
- *VELOCITY DNA- proofreading 3'–5' exonuclease activity*

34. Ans. a. Helix-turn-helix; b. Zinc finger; c. Helix-loop-helix; d. Leucine zipper

[Ref: Harper 30th/444-45;Satyanarayan 4th/573-74]

Several Motifs Compose the DNA Binding Domains of Regulatory Transcription

◈ *Harper 30th/444-45; Satyanarayan 4th/573-74*

- The specificity involved in the control of transcription requires that regulatory proteins bind with high affinity and specificity to the correct region of DNA.
- Four unique motifs—the **helix-turn-helix,** the **zinc finger,** ***Helix-loop-helix motif*** and the **leucine zipper**— account for many of these specific protein-DNA interactions.
- The first motif described was the **helix-turn-helix.**

Table: *(Harper 30th/444)*: **Examples of Transcription Factors That Contain Various DNA Binding Motifs**

Binding Motif	Organism	Regulatory Protein
Helix-turn-helix	E coli Phage Mammals	lac repressor, CAP Icl, cro and 434 repressors Homeobox proteins Pit-1, Oct1, Oct2
Zinc finger	E coli Yeast Drosophila Xenopus Mammals	Gene 32 protein Gal4 Serendipity, hunchback TFIIIA Steroid receptor family, Sp1
Leucine zipper	Yeast Mammals	GCN4 C/EBP, fos, Jun, Fra-1, CRE binding protein (CREB), c-myc, n-myc, l-myc

35. Ans. a. DNA Helicase; b. Single-stranded DNA-binding (SSB) proteins; e. DnaA protein

[Ref: Harper 30th/453; Lippincott 6th/399-400;Satyanarayan 4th/525]

Formation of the Replication Fork

◈ *Lippincott 6th/399-400*

- **Proteins required for DNA strand separation:** Initiation of DNA replication requires the recognition of the origin of replication by a group of proteins that form the prepriming complex. These proteins are responsible for maintaining the separation of the parental strands and for unwinding the double helix ahead of the advancing replication fork. These proteins include the following:
  - **DnaA protein:** DnaA protein binds to specific nucleotide sequences at the origin of replication, causing short, tandemly arranged (one after the other) AT-rich regions in the origin to melt. Melting is ATP-dependent and results in ***strand separation*** with the formation of localized regions of ssDNA.
  - **DNA helicases:** These enzymes bind to ssDNA near the replication fork and then move into the neighboring double-stranded region, ***forcing the strands apart—in effect, unwinding the double helix.*** Helicases require energy provided by ATP [Note: DnaB is the principal helicase of replication in E. coli. Its binding to DNA requires DnaC.]
  - **Single-stranded DNA-binding (SSB) proteins:** These proteins bind to the ssDNA generated by helicases . They bind cooperatively—that is, the binding of one molecule of SSB protein makes it easier for additional molecules of SSB protein to bind tightly to the DNA strand. The SSB proteins are not enzymes, but rather serve to shift the equilibrium between dsDNA and ssDNA in the direction of the single-stranded forms. These proteins not only keep the ***two strands of DNA separated in the area of the replication origin***, thus providing the single stranded

template required by polymerases, but also protect the DNA from nucleases that degrade ssDNA.

- **Solving the problem of supercoils:** To solve this problem, there is a group of enzymes called DNA topoisomerases, which are responsible for removing supercoils in the helix.
  - **Type I DNA topoisomerases:** These enzymes reversibly cut one strand of the double helix. They have both nuclease (strand-cutting) and ligase (strand-resealing) activities.
  - **Type II DNA topoisomerases:** These enzymes bind tightly to the DNA double helix and make transient breaks in both strands. Type II DNA topoisomerases are also required in both prokaryotes and eukaryotes for the separation of interlocked molecules of DNA following chromosomal replication. **DNA gyrase, a Type II topoisomerase** found in bacteria and plants, has the unusual property of being able to ***introduce negative supercoils*** into relaxed circular DNA using energy from the hydrolysis of ATP.

Table: *(Harper 30th/453)*: **Some of the Enzymes Used in Recombinant DNA Research**

Enzyme	Reaction	Primary Use
DNA ligase	Catalyzes bonds between DNA molecules	Joining of DNA molecules
DNA polymerase I	Synthesizes double-stranded DNA from single-stranded DNA	Synthesis of double-stranded cDNA; nick translation; generation of blunt ends from sticky ends
Thermostable DNA polymerases	Synthesize DNA at elevated temperatures (60°-C-80°C)	Polymerase chain reaction (DNA synthesis)
DNase I	Under appropriate conditions, produces single-stranded nicks in DNA	Nick translation; mapping of hypersensitive sites; mapping protein-DNA interactions
Reverse transcriptase	Synthesizes DNA from RNA template	Synthesis of cDNA from mRNA; RNA (5′ end) mapping studies
RNAse H	Degrades the RNA portion of a DNA-RNA hybrid	Synthesis of cDNA from mRNA
Terminal transferase	Adds nucleotides to the 3′ ends of DNA	Homopolymer tailing
CRISPER-Cas9	RNA-targeted DNA-directed nuclease	Genome editing and modulation of gene expression

36. Ans. a. miRNa; c. Dicer; e. Slicer

[Ref: Harper 30th/409-10; Lippincott 6th/459]

"Degradation of homologous RNA in RNA interference is carried out by functional **RNA-induced silencing complex (RISC). RISC contains *Dicer, Argonaute protein, siRNA and other components*"- www.ncbi.nlm.nih.gov**

"The Argonaute family of proteins, specifically **Argonaute 2** (also known as Ago2, eIF2C2 or ***Slicer***) are essential **components of RISC**, which are involved in mRNA cleavage"- *www.abcam.com*

"MicroRNAs (miRNAs) associate with Argonaute (Ago), GW182 and FXR1 proteins to form RNA-induced silencing complexes (RISCs). RISCs represent a critical checkpoint in the regulation and bioavailability of miRNAs"-www.jneurosci.org

"The **RNA-induced silencing complex,** or **RISC,** is a multiprotein complex, specifically a ribonucleoprotein, which incorporates ***one strand of a single-stranded RNA (ssRNA) fragment, such as microRNA (miRNA), or double stranded small interfering RNA (siRNA).*** The single strand acts as a template for RISC to recognize complementary messenger RNA (mRNA) transcript. Once found, one of the proteins in RISC, called ***Argonaute***, activates and cleaves the mRNA. This process is called RNA interference (RNAi) and it is found in **many eukaryotes; it is a key process in gene silencing and defense against viral infections"**-*wiki*

"The cytoplasmic **RNA-induced silencing complex (RISC)** contains dsRNA binding proteins, including ***protein kinase RNA activator (PACT), transactivation response RNA binding protein (TRBP) and Dicer,*** that process pre-microRNAs into mature microRNAs (miRNAs) that target specific mRNA species for regulation. There is increasing evidence for important functional interactions between the miRNA and nuclear receptor (NR) signaling networks, with recent data showing that estrogen, acting through the estrogen receptor, can modulate initial aspects of nuclear miRNA processing. Here, we show that the ***cytoplasmic RISC proteins PACT, TRBP and Dicer*** are steroid receptor RNA activator (SRA) binding NR coregulators that target steroid-responsive promoters and regulate NR activity and downstream gene expression. Furthermore, ***each of the RISC proteins, together with Argonaute 2,*** associates with SRA and specific pre-microRNAs in both the nucleus and cytoplasm, providing evidence for links between NR-mediated transcription and some of the factors involved in miRNA processing"-www.ncbi. nlm. nih.gov

"**DGCR8/Pasha** is an essential cofactor for Drosha, a nuclear RNase III that cleaves the local hairpin structures embedded in long primary microRNA transcripts (pri-miRNAs) in eukaryotes. DsRNA-binding proteins that contain dsRNA-binding domains (dsRBDs) serve diverse roles during RNA metabolism. A recently emerging theme in RNA silencing pathways is that multidomain RNase III proteins, such as ***Drosha and Dicer,*** necessitate dsRNA-binding proteins for ***miRNA processing and/or RISC formation***. For example, Dcr-1 in Drosophila interacts with Loquacious/R3D1 that contains three dsRBDs and is required for miRNA processing and possibly also for RISC assembly"- www.ncbi. nlm. nih. gov

The **Microprocessor complex** is a protein complex involved in the early stages of processing microRNA (miRNA) in animal cells. The complex is minimally composed of the ribonuclease enzyme ***Drosha*** and the RNA-binding protein DGCR8 (also known as ***Pasha***) and cleaves primary miRNA substrates to pre-miRNA in the cell nucleus-wikipedia

Micro-RNAs Are Derived from Large Primary Transcripts Through Specific Nucleolytic Processing *Harper 30th/409*

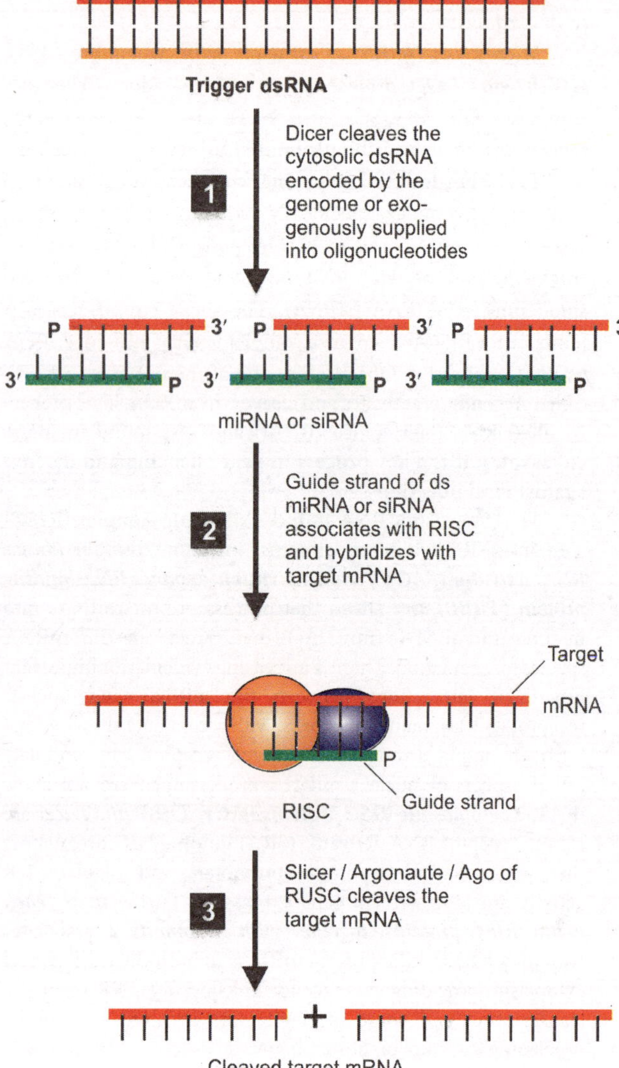

Fig *(Lippincott 6th/459)*: RNA interference or RNAi by cleavage of target mRNA. [Note: RNAi can also result from inhibition of target mRNA translation.]

- The majority of miRNAs are transcribed by RNA pol II into **primary transcripts** termed **pri-miRNAs**. pri-miRNAs are 5′-capped and 3′-polyadenylated. pri-miRNAs are synthesized from transcription units encoding one or several distinct miRNAs; these transcription units are either located independently in the genome or within the intronic DNA of other genes. Given this organization miRNA-encoding genes must therefore minimally possess a distinct promoter, coding region and polyadenylation/termination signals. pri-miRNAs have extensive 2° structure and this intramolecular structure is maintained following processing by the **Drosha-DGCR8 nuclease**; the portion containing the RNA hairpin is preserved, transported through the nuclear pore via the action of exportin 5 and once in the cytoplasm, further processed by the heterodimeric **dicer nuclease-TRBP complex** to a **21 or 22-mer**.
- Ultimately, one of the two strands is selected for loading into the **RNA-induced silencing complex** (**RISC**), which is composed of one of four **Argonaute proteins (Ago 1→4)**, to form a mature, functional 21-22 nt single stranded miRNA. siRNAs are produced similarly. Once in the **RISC complex**, ***miRNAs*** can modulate mRNA function by one of three mechanisms: (a) promoting mRNA degradation directly; (b) stimulating CCR4/NOT complex- mediated poly A tail degradation; or (c) inhibition of translation by targeting the 5′-methyl cap binding translation factor eIF4 or the ribosome directly. Recent data suggest that regulatory miRNA-encoding genes may be linked and hence co-evolve with their target genes.

37. Ans. a. Patau syndrome; b. Edward syndrome

[Ref: Robbins 9th (SAE)/100,163,165; Harrison 19th/439,83e-6,2350]

- *Klinefelter syndrome involves sex chromosome* ***non-disjunction*** *(so not autosomal)*

Williams syndrome and Cri-du-chat syndrome are chromosome deletion syndromes

"Nondisjunction is the ***failure of homologous chromosomes or sister chromatids to separate*** properly during cell division. There are **three forms of nondisjunction:** *failure of a pair of homologous chromosomes to separate in meiosis I, failure of sister chromatids to separate during meiosis II and failure of sister chromatids to separate during mitosis.* Nondisjunction results in daughter cells with abnormal chromosome numbers (aneuploidy)"-*www.medicinenet.com*

Consequences Nondisjunction

◈ *www.angelfire.com,wiki; Robbins 9th (SAE)/100,163,165;Harrison 19th/439, 83e-6, 2350*

- Monosomy-***Turner syndrome (X monosomy) (45, X0)***
- Autosomal trisomy: Down syndrome (trisomy 21), ***Edwards syndrome (trisomy 18) and Patau syndrome*** (trisomy 13)
- **Sex chromosome aneuploidy**: ***Klinefelter syndrome (47, XXY)***, XYY Male (47, XYY) and Trisomy X (47, XXX)
- Uniparental disomy (Prader-Willi syndrome and Angelman syndrome)
- Mosaicism syndromes (Pallister-Killian syndrome and Hypomelanosis of Ito)
- Mosaicism in malignant transformation (Human retinoblastoma)

"**Klinefelter syndrome:** The classic form of KS (47, XXY) occurs after meiotic ***nondisjunction of the sex chromosomes*** during gametogenesis (40% during spermatogenesis, 60% during oogenesis)"- *Harrison 19th/2350*

"Humans have 22 homologous pairs of autosomes and one pair of sex chromosomes. The **main difference** between autosomes and sex chromosomes is that **autosomes are involved in determining the somatic characters of an individual and sex chromosomes are involved in determining the sex and the sex-related hormonal traits"-www.pediaa.com**

"The first **chromosome deletion syndromes** were diagnosed clinically and were subsequently demonstrated to be caused by a chromosome deletion on cytogenetic analysis. Examples of these disorders include the Wolf-Hirschhorn syndrome, which is associated with deletions of a small region of the short arm of chromosome 4 (4p); the **cri-du-chat syndrome,** associated with ***deletion of a small region of the short arm of chromosome 5 (5p)***; **Williams syndrome,** which is associated with ***interstitial deletions of the long arm of chromosome 7*** (7q11. 23); and the DiGeorge/velocardiofacial syndromes, associated with interstitial deletions of the long arm of chromosome 22 (22q11. 2)"- *Harrison 19th/83e-6*

38. Ans. a. Myotonic dystrophy; b. Huntington chorea; d. Spinocerebellar ataxia

[Ref: Harrison 19th/440; Harper 30th/378; Lippincott 6th/]

"**Trinucleotide sequences** that increase in number (microsatellite instability) can cause disease. The unstable (CGG)n repeat sequence is associated with the **fragile X syndrome.** Other trinucleotide repeats that undergo dynamic mutation (usually an increase) are associated with ***Huntington's chorea (CAG), myotonic dystrophy (CTG), spinobulbar muscular atrophy (CAG) and Kennedy disease (CAG)***"- *Harper 30th/378*

Nucleotide Repeat Expansion Disorders

◈ *Harrison 19th/440*

- Several diseases are associated with an increase in the number of nucleotide repeats above a certain threshold
- The repeats are sometimes located within the coding region of the genes, as in ***Huntington's disease or the X-linked form of spinal and bulbar muscular atrophy (SBMA; Kennedy's syndrome).*** In other instances, the repeats probably alter gene regulatory sequences.
- If an expansion is present, the DNA fragment is unstable and tends to expand further during cell division. The length of the nucleotide repeat often correlates with the severity of the disease. When repeat length increases from one generation to the next, disease manifestations may worsen or be observed at an earlier age; this phenomenon is referred to as *anticipation.*

Table: *(Harriosn 19th/440)*: **Selected Trinucleotide Repeat Disorders**

Disease	Repeat	Inheritance	Gene Product
X-chromosomal spinobulbar muscular atrophy (SBMA)	CAG	XR	Androgen receptor
Fragile X-syndrome (FRAXA)	CGG	XR	FMR-1 protein
Fragile X-syndrome (FRAXE)	GCC	XR	FMR-2 protein
Dystrophia myotonica (DM)	CTG	AD, variable penetrance	Myotonin protein kinase
Huntington's disease (HD)	CAG	AD	Huntingtin
Spinocerebellar ataxia type 1 (SCA1)	CAG	AD	Ataxin 1
Spinocerebellar ataxia type 2 (SCA2)	CAG	AD	Ataxin 2
Spinocerebellar ataxia type 3 (SCA3); Machado-Joseph disease (MD)	CAG	AD	Ataxin 3
Spinocerebellar ataxia type 6 (SCA6, CACNAIA)	CAG	AD	Alpha 1A voltage-dependent L-type calcium chan-nel
Spinocerebellar ataxia type 7 (SCA7)	CAG	AD	Ataxin 7
Spinocerebellar ataxia type 12 (SCA12)	CAG	AD	Protein phosphatase 2A
Dentorubral pallidoluysian atrophy (DRPLA)	CAG	AD	Atrophin 1
Friedreich ataxia (FRDA1)	GAA	AR	Frataxin

Contd...

"Roughly 100 syndromes of familial cancer have been reported, although many are rare. The majority are inherited as autosomal dominant traits, although some of those associated with **DNA repair abnormalities *(xeroderma pigmentosum,*** Fanconi's anemia, ***ataxia telangiectasia***) are autosomal recessive"-*Harrison 19th/101e-4*

39. Ans. b. GTP; c. Initiation factor; e. mRNA

[Ref: Satyanarayan 4th/557]

"30S initiation complex (30SIC) contains ***mRNA, fMet-tRNA^{fMet} and initiation factors IF1 and GTP-bound IF2***"-**www.nature.com**

"In bacteria, during the initiation phase of protein synthesis three initiation factors (IFs: IF1, IF2 and IF3), the messenger RNA (mRNA) and initiator tRNA (fMet–tRNA) assemble in a ***30S pre-initiation complex*** (preIC) in which proper codon–anticodon base pairing has not yet taken place"-*academic. oup. com*

Initiation of translation in prokaryotes

◈ *Satyanarayan 4th/557*

- The 30S ribosomal subunit is bound to ***initiation factor 3 (IF-3) and attached to ternary complex of IF-2, formyl met-tRNA and GTP***
- Another initiation factor namely IF-1 also participates in the formation of preinitiation complex
- A 50S ribosome unit is now bound with the 30S unit to produce 70S initiation complex

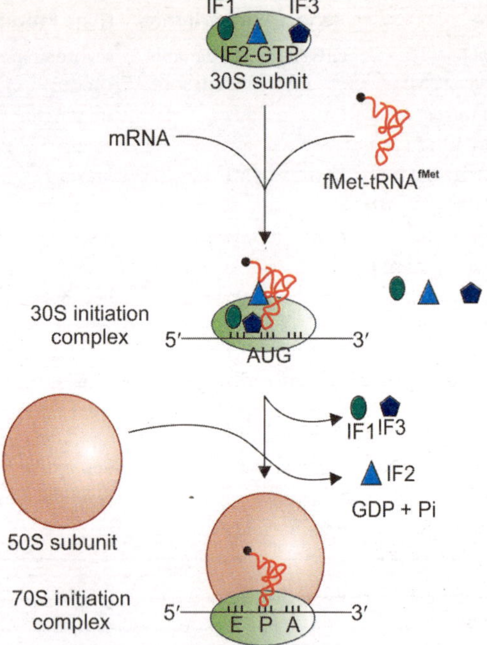

Fig: Initiation complex formation in bacteria

40. Ans. c. May result in 100 abnormal cells

[Ref: Harrison 19th/432; ib.bioninja.com.au]

- ***As tissue (collection of cells) can be formed from mutant somatic cells, so option c (100 abnormal cells) may be true***

In multicellular organisms, mutations can be classed as either somatic or germline: *ib. bioninja.com.au*

- **Somatic mutations**: ***occur in a single body cell and cannot be inherited (only tissues derived from mutated cell are affected)***
- *Germline mutations*: occur in gametes and can be passed onto offspring (every cell in the entire organism will be affected)

Mutation

◈ *Harrison 19th/432*

- Some mutations may be lethal, others are less deleterious and some may confer an evolutionary advantage.
- Mutations can occur in the **germline** (sperm or oocytes); these can be ***transmitted to progeny***. Alternatively, mutations can occur during embryogenesis or in ***somatic tissues.***
- Mutations that occur **during development** lead to *mosaicism*, a situation in which tissues are composed of cells with different genetic constitutions.
- If the germline is mosaic, a mutation can be transmitted to some progeny but not others, which sometimes leads to confusion in assessing the pattern of inheritance.
- **Somatic mutations** that do not affect cell survival can sometimes be detected because of ***variable phenotypic effects in tissues*** (e.g., pigmented lesions in McCune-Albright syndrome).
- Other somatic mutations are ***associated with neoplasia*** because they confer a growth advantage to cells. Epigenetic events may also influence gene expression or facilitate genetic damage. With the exception of triplet nucleotide repeats, which can expand, mutations are usually stable.

Mutations and Evolution

◈ *www.thoughtco.com*

Sometimes, during replication, mistakes can be made and these mutations can change the DNA in the cells of the body. ***However, if there is a mutation in a somatic cell, it most likely will not contribute to the evolution of the species.***

Since **somatic cells** are in no way involved in the process of sexual reproduction, ***any changes in the DNA of somatic cells will not get passed down to the offspring*** of the mutated parent.

Since the offspring will not receive the changed DNA and any new traits the parent may have will not be passed down, ***mutations in the DNA of somatic cells will not cause evolution.***

If there happens to be a **mutation in a gamete**, that ***can drive evolution***. Mistakes can happen during meiosis that can either change the DNA in the haploid cells, or create a chromosome mutation which can add or delete portions of DNA on various chromosomes. If one of the offspring is created from a gamete that has a mutation in it, then that offspring will have different traits that may or may not be favorable for the environment

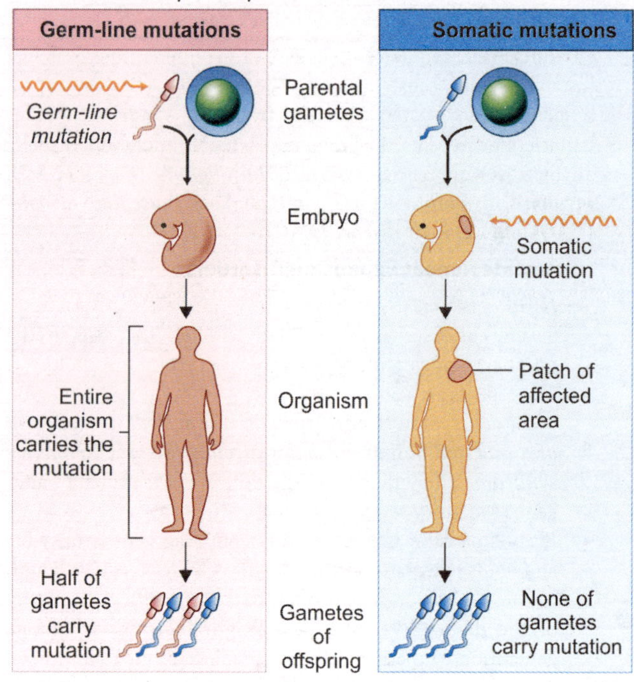

41. Ans. b. ATP; d. Elongation factor

[Ref: Lippincott 6th/438-42; Dinesh Puri 3rd/482-83]

Question is asked about interaction of 30S ribosome (of 0prokaryotes). Interaction of 30S occur in initiation step only (in elongation & termination stage, interaction occurs with 70S subunit)

Functionally Competent Ribosomes

◈ *Lippincott 6th/435*

- The prokaryotic 50S and 30S ribosomal subunits together form a 70S ribosome.
- The eukaryotic 60S and 40S subunits form an 80S ribosome

Steps In Protein Synthesis

◈ *Lippincott 6th/438-42*

A. Initiation

- Initiation of protein synthesis involves the assembly of the components of the translation system before peptide bond formation occurs. These components include the two ribosomal subunits, the ***mRNA to be translated, the aminoacyl-tRNA specified by the first codon in the message, GTP*** (which provides energy for the process) and initiation factors that facilitate the assembly of this initiation complex.
- [Note: In prokaryotes, three initiation factors are known ***(IF-1, IF-2 and IF-3)***, whereas in eukaryotes, there are over ten (designated eIF to indicate eukaryotic origin). ***Eukaryotes also require ATP for initiation.]***
- There are two mechanisms by which the ribosome recognizes the nucleotide sequence (AUG) that initiates translation:
    - Shine-Dalgarno sequence &
    - Initiation codon
- There is formation of 70S initiation complex by joining 50S & 30S subunits

B. Elongation

- It requires 70S complex, aminoacyl t-RNA & elongation factors

C. Termination

- Termination occurs when one of the three termination codons moves into the A site.
- These codons are recognized in E. coli by release factors: RF-1, which recognizes the termination codons UAA and UAG and RF-2, which recognizes UGA and UAA

42. Ans. b RNA polymerase I

[Ref: Lippincott 6th/422;Harper 31st/378;363]

Table: *(Harper 31st/378):* **Nomenclature and properties of Mammalian Nuclear DNA-Dependent RNA polymerases**

Form of RNA polymerase	Sensitivity to α-amanitin	Major products
I	Insensitive	rRNA
II	High sensitivity	mRNA, IncRNA, miRNA, SnRNA
III	Intermediate sensitivity	tRNA, 5s rRNA

Table *(Harper 31st/363)*: **Classes of proteins Involved in DNA replication**

Protein	Function
DNA polymerases	Deoxynucleotide polymerization
Helicases	ATP-driven processive unwindin of DNA
Topoisomerases	Relieve torsional strain that results from helicase-induced unwinding
DNA primase	Initiates synthesis of RNA primers
Single-strand binding proteins (SSBs)	Prevent premature reannealing of dsDNA
DNA ligase	Seals the single strand nick between the nascent chain and okazaki fragments on lagging strand

43. Ans. a. Has coded segments; c. Has only exons; d. Uses reverse transcriptase;

[Ref: Shinde 7th/265;Lehninger 5th/940-60]

Gene library Shinde

◈ *7th/265;Lehninger 5th/940-60*

- It is cloned (recombinant) DNA fragments is called DNA library or shotgun collection
- It is of two types-Genomic library & Complementary DNA (cDNA) library

Table: Difference between genomic library & complementary DNA (cDNA) library

cDNA library	Genomic library
Only *exons* are represented	Entire genome (***exon+intron***) represented
Smaller	***Larger***
Uses ***reverse transcriptase*** (for preparation of cDNA from mRNA)	Uses ***restriction enzymes*** for partial digestion of total DNA
cDNA has only ***coding sequences*** therefore can be directly expressed in prokaryotic system	Expression of genes takes from genomic library is difficult in prokaryotic system like bacteria due to absence of splicing mechanism
Plasmids are the ideal & preferred vector	Phage vectors are ideal & preferred

PATHOLOGY

44. Ans. d. B cell defect

[Ref: Robbins 9th/241,163-64; Harrison 19th/2483; Ananthanarayan 10th/175; Davidson 22nd/80]

DiGeorge Syndrome (Thymic Hypoplasia)

◈ *Robbins 9th/241*

- **DiGeorge syndrome is a T-cell deficiency that results from failure of development of the third and fourth pharyngeal pouches**. The latter give rise to the thymus, the parathyroids, some of the C cells of the thyroid and the ultimobranchial body. Thus, individuals with this syndrome have a ***variable loss of T cell–mediated immunity*** (***resulting from hypoplasia or lack of the thymus***), tetany (resulting from ***lack of the parathyroids***) and congenital defects of the heart and great vessels.
- Absence of cell-mediated immunity is caused by ***low numbers of T lymphocytes in the blood*** and lymphoid tissues and ***poor defense against certain fungal and viral infections.***
- The T-cell zones of lymphoid organs—paracortical areas of the lymph nodes and the periarteriolar sheaths of the spleen—are depleted. Ig levels may be normal or reduced, depending on the severity of the T-cell deficiency.
- "Patients who survives the neonatal period show ***enhanced susceptibility to viral, fungal and bacterial infections,*** which ultimately prove fatal"- *Ananthanarayan 10th/175*

- Patients with DGS may have poor T-cell production compared to their peers and as a result, have an increased susceptibility to ***viral, fungal and bacterial infections***- primaryimmune.org

DiGeorge Syndrome

◈ *Harrison 19th/2483*

- A form of hypoparathyroidism associated with defective development of both the thymus and the parathyroid glands is termed the *DiGeorge syndrome*, or the ***velocardiofacial syndrome.***
- Congenital cardiovascular, facial and other developmental defects are present and patients may die in early childhood with ***severe infections***, hypocalcemia and seizures, or cardiovascular complications.
- Most cases are sporadic, but an autosomal dominant form involving microdeletions of chromosome 22q11.2 has been described.

45. Ans. a. Haemophilia A; b. Von-Willebrand disease

[Ref: Robbins 9th/119; Harrison 19th/733; Harshmohan 7th/307-08]

Prothrombin time assay assesses the function of the proteins in the extrinsic and common pathways (factor VII, X, V, II and fibrinogen) *(Robbins 9th/119)*

Table: *(Harshmohan 7th/307)*

Prothrombin time (Normal value- 10 to 14 second)	Evaluation of extrinsic and common pathway (deficiency of factor I, II, V, VII and X)	Increased in —***oral anticoagulant therapy, DIC and liver disease, Vit K deficiency***

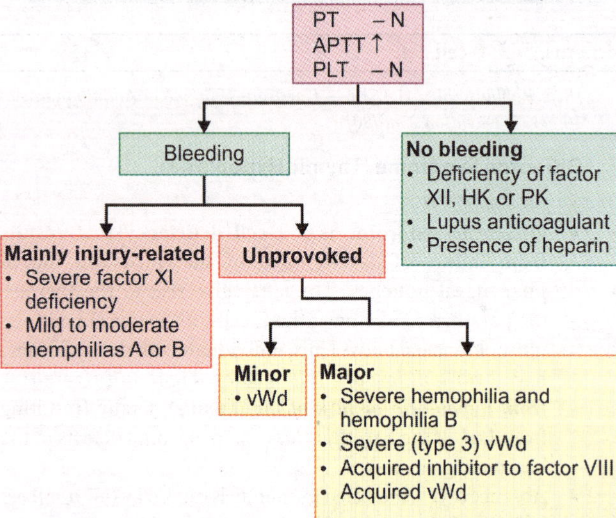

Fig: *(William Hematology 7th/Chap 109): APTT, activated partial thromboplastin time; HK, high molecular weight kininogen; N, normal; PK, prekallikrein; PLT, platelets; PT, prothrombin time; vWd, von Willebrand disease*

46. Ans. b. Waldeyer's ring lymphoma; c. Gastric lymphoma; d. Thyroid lymphoma; e. Mycosis fungoides

[Ref: Robbins 9th/588,605-06; Harshmohan 7th/359,357]

Burkitt Lymphoma is predominantly nodal neoplasms

Table: *(slideplayer.com):* **Extranodal Lymphoma**

Waldeyer's Ring Lymphomas	Primary Muscle Lymphoma
Sinus Lymphomas	Bone Lymphoma
Salivery Gland Lymphoma	Pancreatic Lymphoma
Thyroid Lymphomas	Cardiac Lymphomas
Nasal and nasopharyngeal Lymphomas	Testicular Lymphoma
Adnexal lymphomas	Uterine and Cervical Lymph
Ocular Lymphomas	Pulmonary Lymphomas
Central Nervous Lymphomas	Prostatic Lymphoma
Gastric Lymphoma	Small Bowel Lymphomas
Large Bowel and Anorectal Lymphomas	Bladder Lymphoma
Hepatic Lymphomas	Breast Lymphomas
Splenic Lymphoma	Renal Lymphomas

Table: *(William's Hematology 7th/Chap95)*: **WHO Classification of Lymphoid Neoplasms**

B Cell Neoplasms
• Precursor B cell neoplasm
• Precursor B lymphoblastic leukemia/lymphoma
• Mature B cell neoplasms
• Predominantly disseminated/leukemic neoplasms
• Chronic lymphocytic leukemia/small lymphocytic lymphoma
• B cell prolymphocytic leukemia
• Lymphoplasmacytic lymphoma/Waldenström macroglobulinemia
• Splenic marginal zone lymphoma
• Hairy cell leukemia
• Plasma cell neoplasms
• Plasma cell myeloma
• Plasmacytoma
• Monoclonal immunoglobulin deposition disease
• Heavy chain diseases
Primary extranodal neoplasm
• Extranodal marginal zone B cell lymphoma ***(MALT lymphoma)***
• Mediastinal (thymic) large B cell lymphoma
• Intravascular large B cell lymphoma
• Primary effusion lymphoma
• Lymphomatoid granulomatosis
• Predominantly nodal neoplasms
• Nodal marginal zone B cell lymphoma
• Follicular lymphoma

Contd...

- Mantle cell lymphoma
- Diffuse large B cell lymphoma
- Burkitt lymphoma/leukemia

T Cell Neoplasms

- Precursor T cell neoplasm
- Precursor T lymphoblastic leukemia/lymphoma
- Mature T cell neoplasms
- Predominantly disseminated/leukemic neoplasms
- T cell prolymphocytic leukemia
- T cell large granular lymphocytic leukemia
- Aggressive NK cell leukemia
- Adult T cell leukemia/lymphoma

Primary extranodal neoplasms

- Extranodal NK/T cell lymphoma, nasal type
- Enteropathy-type T cell lymphoma
- Hepatosplenic T cell lymphoma
- Subcutaneous panniculitis-like T cell lymphoma
- Blastic NK cell lymphoma
- Mycosis fungoides/Sézary syndrome
- Primary cutaneous CD-30 positive T cell lymphoproliferative disorders

Predominantly nodal neoplasms

- Angioimmunoblastic T cell lymphoma
- Peripheral T cell lymphoma, unspecified
- Anaplastic large cell lymphoma

Extranodal non-Hodgkin lymphoma (NHL) in head and neck region is ***most commonly seen in the*** Waldeyer's ring. Waldeyer's ring is a unique subtype of mucosa associated lymphoid tissue (MALT), which shows rarity of low-grade or MALT-type lymphomas and a high incidence of diffuse large B cell lymphoma (DLBCL) - www.ncbi.nlm.nih.gov

47. Ans. a. Widened mitral annulus; b. McCallum plaques; d. Aschoff nodules; e. Aortic valve thickening

[Ref: Robbins 9th/557-59; Harrison 19th/2149-54; Harshmohan 7th/420-22]

"The papillary muscles are muscles located in the ventricles of the heart. They attach to the cusps of the atrioventricular valves (also known as the mitral and tricuspid valves) via the chordae tendineae and contract to prevent inversion or prolapse of these valves on systole (or ventricular contraction). Papillary muscle rupture can be caused by a myocardial infarct and dysfunction can be caused by ischemia. Both complications may lead to worsening of mitral regurgitation"-mvpresource.com; Robbins 9th/554

"Chronically, rheumatic fever leads to commissural fusion, valve thickening and calcification. The appearance of the mitral valve with shortened, fused chordae and scarred commissures has been likened to the mouth of a catfish (fish-mouth deformity). There is also diffuse scarring of the aortic valve, with commissural fibrosis and thickening of the leaflets"-emedicine.medscape.com

The widening of the mitral annulus can happen when the left ventricle of the heart becomes enlarged, usually because of rheumatic heart disease (a complication of rheumatic fever) or cardiomyopathy, which is an inherited disease of the heart muscle-www.your.md

Morphology

◈ *Robbins 9th/558-59*

- During acute RF, focal inflammatory lesions are found in various tissues. Distinctive lesions occur in the heart, called **Aschoff bodies**, consisting of foci of T lymphocytes, occasional plasma cells and plump activated macrophages called **Anitschkow cells** (pathognomonic for RF).
- During acute RF, diffuse inflammation and **Aschoff bodies** may be found in any of the three layers of the heart, resulting in pericarditis, myocarditis, or endocarditis (**pancarditis**) .
- Subendocardial lesions, perhaps exacerbated by regurgitant jets, can induce irregular thickenings called **MacCallum plaques**, usually in the left atrium.
- The cardinal anatomic changes of the **mitral valve** in chronic RHD are **leaflet thickening, commissural fusion and shortening and thickening and fusion of the tendinous cords**
- In ***chronic disease the mitral valve*** is virtually always involved. The mitral valve is affected in isolation in roughly two thirds of RHD and along with the **aortic valve** in another 25% of cases. Tricuspid valve involvement is infrequent and the pulmonary valve is only rarely affected.
- In **rheumatic mitral stenosis,** calcification and fibrous bridging across the ***valvular commissures create "fish mouth" or "buttonhole" stenoses.*** With tight mitral stenosis, the left atrium progressively dilates and may harbor mural thrombi that can embolize.
- Microscopically, valves show organization of the acute inflammation, with post-inflammatory neovascularization and transmural fibrosis that obliterate the leaflet architecture.
- ***Aschoff bodies are rarely seen in surgical specimens or autopsy tissue from patients with chronic RHD***, as a result of the long intervals between the initial insult and the development of the chronic deformity.

Chronic Rheumatic Heart Disease

◈ *www.histopathology-india.net*

- In chronic recurrent rheumatic heart disease the **valve involvement**, which was of little clinical significance during the acute attack, becomes the major problem. For example the **mitral valve** which is most frequently and severely involved valve, shows ***conspicuous, irregular thickening and calcification of its leaflets, often with fusion of its***

A & E

commissures and thickening and fusion of the chordae tendineae. As a result the valve is often severely stenotic and when viewed from the atrial aspect has a narrowed orifice described as having a "fish mouth" appearance.

- The **aortic valve**, the second most commonly involved valve, shows ***typical fusion of the commissures and later pronounced thickening and calcification of the cusps, with resulting stenosis or insufficiency.***
- The **tricuspid valve** is similarly involved, although less frequently than the aortic and mitral valves and the pulmonary valve is the least frequently involved.
- The ***subendocardial collections of Aschoff nodules***, usually in the left atrium, induce thickenings called ***MacCallum plaques (patch)***

Papillary muscle function

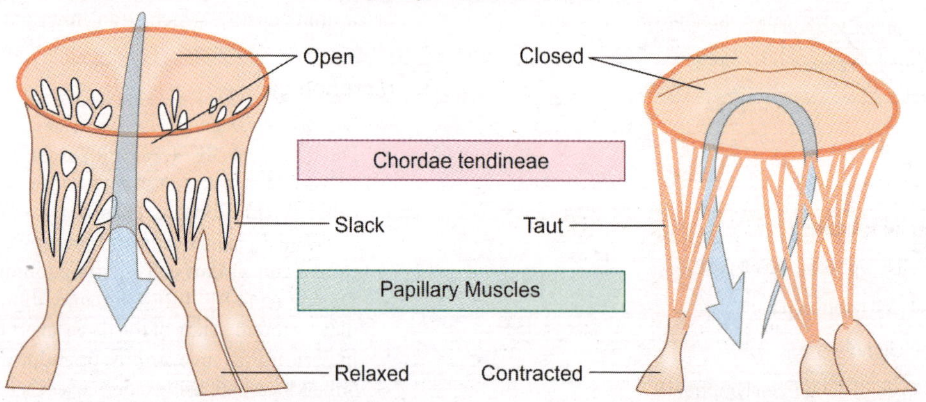

48. Ans. a. RB1-retinoblastoma; c. BRCA2-Breast cancer; d. N-MYC-Neuroblastoma; e. WT1 = Wilm's tumor

[Ref: Robbins 9th/284,291; Harrison 19th/494; Harshmohan 7th/420-21]

Table: *(Robbins 9th/291)*: **Selected tumor suppressor genes and associated familial**

Syndromes and Cancers (Partial list)

Gene	Familial Syndromes	Sporadic Cancers
PTEN	Cowden syndrome (variety of benign skin, GI and CNS growths; breast, endometrial, and thyroid carcinoma)	Diverse cancers, particularly carcinomas and lymphoid tumors
RB	Familial retinoblastoma syndrome (retinoblastoma, osteosarcoma, other sarcomas)	Retinoblastoma; osteosarcoma carcinomas of breast, colon, lung
WT1	Familial Wilms tumor	Wilms tumor, certain leukemias
BRCA1, BRCA2	Familial breast and ovarian carcinoma; carcinomas of male breast; chronic lymphocytic leukemia (BRCA2)	Rare
APC	Familial colonic polyps and carcinomas	Carcinomas of stomach, colon, pancreas; melanoma
CDKN2A	Familial melanoma	Pancreatic, breast and esophageal carcinoma, melanoma, certain leukemias

"The **retinoblastoma tumor-suppressor gene (*Rb1*)** mutational inactivation of both *Rb1* alleles is the primary molecular alteration causing the pediatric cancer ***retinoblastoma***" - www.nature.com

Table: *(Harrison 19th/101e-2)*: **Common oncogenes altered in human cancers**

Oncogene	Neoplasm
AKT1	Stomach
AKT2	Ovarian, breast, pancreatic
BRAF	Melanoma, lung, colorectal
CTNNB1	Colon, prostate, melanoma, skin, others
FOS	Osteosarcomas
ERBB2	Breast, ovary, stomach, neuroblastoma
JUN	Lung
MET	Osteocarcinoma, kidney, glioma
MYB	AML, CML, colorectal, melanoma
C-MYC	Breast, colon, gastric, lung
L-MYC	Lung, bladder
N-MYC	Neuroblastoma, lung
HRAS	Colon, lung, pancreas
KRAS	Melanoma, colorectal, AML
NRAS	Various carcinomas, melanoma
REL	Lymphomas
WNT1	Retinoblastoma

Melanoma: Genetic Susceptibility

◈ *Harrison 19th/494*

- Approximately 20–40% of cases of hereditary melanoma (0.2–2% of all melanomas) are due to germline mutations in the cell cycle regulatory gene ***cyclindependent kinase inhibitor 2A (CDKN2A).***
- In fact, 70% of all cutaneous melanomas have mutations or deletions affecting the CDKN2A locus on chromosome 9p21. This locus encodes two distinct tumor suppressor proteins from alternate reading frames: **p16 and ARF** (p14ARF).
- The p16 protein inhibits CDK4/6-mediated phosphorylation and inactivation of the **retinoblastoma (RB)** protein, whereas ***ARF inhibits MDM2 ubiquitin-mediated degradation of p53***. The end result of the loss of CDKN2A is inactivation of ***two critical tumor-suppressor pathways, RB and p53***, which control entry of cells into the cell cycle.
- Germline mutations in the melanoma lineage specific oncogene microphthalmia-associated transcription factor (***MITF***) predispose to both familial and sporadic melanomas.
- **The melanocortin-1 receptor** (***MC1R***) gene is a moderate-risk inherited melanoma susceptibility factor.

49. Ans. a. SIADH; b. Hypercalcemia

[Ref: Robbins 9th/331; Harrison 19th/609; Williams Textbook of Endocrinology 11th/Chap 43]

"**SIADH** also occurs occasionally in a wide range of carcinomas, including as many as 2% of squamous carcinomas of the head and neck, adenocarcinoma of the colon, ***Hodgkin's disease, non-Hodgkin's lymphomas*** and several varieties of brain tumors"- *Williams Textbook of Endocrinology 11th/Chap 43*

Most extrapancreatic tumors that cause **hypoglycemia** do so by secreting IGF-II. Fibrosarcomas, rhabdomyosarcomas, leiomyosarcomas, mesotheliomas and hemangiopericytomas account for more than 50% of cases. Hepatocellular carcinomas (hepatomas), carcinoid tumors and adrenocortical carcinomas account for about 25% of cases and the remainder are made up of various carcinomas, ***leukemias and lymphomas***- *Williams Textbook of Endocrinology 11th/Chap 43*

Table: *(Harrison 19th/609)*: **Paraneoplastic Syndromes Caused by Ectopic Hormone Production**

Paraneoplastic Syndrome	Ectopic Hormone	Typical Tumor Types
Common		
Hypercalcemia of malignancy	Parathyroid hormone-related protein (PTHrP)	Squamous cell (head and neck, lung, skin), breast, genitourinary, gastrointestinal
	1,25 dihydroxyvitamin D	Lymphomas
	Parathyroid hormone (PTH) (rare)	Lung, ovary
	Prostaglandin E2 (PGE2) (rare)	Renal, lung
Syndrome of inappropriate antidiuretic hormone secretion (SIADH)	Vasopressin	Lung (squamous, small cell), gastrointestinal, genitourinary, ovary
Cushing's syndrome	Adrenocorticotropic hormone (ACTH)	Lung (small cell, bronchial carcinoid, adenocarcinoma, squamous), thymus, pancreatic islet, medullary thyroid carcinoma
	Corticotropin-releasing hormone (CRH) (rare)	Pancreatic islet, carcinoid, lung, prostate
	Ectopic expression of gastric inhibitory peptide (GIP), luteinizing hormone (LH) / human chorionic gonadotropin (hCG), other G protein–coupled receptors (rare)	Macronodular adrenal hyperplasia
Less Common		
Non-islet cell hypoglycemia	Insulin-like growth factor (IGF-II)	Mesenchymal tumors, sarcomas, adrenal, hepatic, gastrointestinal, kidney, prostate
	Insulin (rare)	Cervix (small cell carcinoma)
Male feminization	hCGb	Testis (embryonal, seminomas), germinomas, choriocarcinoma, lung, hepatic, pancreatic islet
Diarrhea or intestinal hypermotility	Calcitoninc	Lung, colon, breast, medullary thyroid carcinoma
	Vasoactive intestinal peptide (VIP)	Pancreas, pheochromocytoma, esophagus
Rare		
Oncogenic osteomalacia	Phosphatonin [fibroblast growth factor 23 (FGF23)]	Hemangiopericytomas, osteoblastomas, fibromas, sarcomas, giant cell tumors, prostate, lung
Acromegaly	Growth hormone–releasing hormone (GHRH)	Pancreatic islet, bronchial and other carcinoids
	Growth hormone (GH)	Lung, pancreatic islet
Hyperthyroidism	Thyroid-stimulating hormone (TSH)	Hydatidiform mole, embryonal tumors, struma ovarii
Hypertension	Renin	Juxtaglomerular tumors, kidney, lung, pancreas, ovary

Table: *(Robbins 9th/331):* **Paraneoplastic Syndromes**

Clinical Syndromes	Major Forms of Underlying Cancer	Causal Mechanism
Endocrinopathies		
Cushing syndrome	Small cell carcinoma of lung	ACTH or ACTH-like substance
	Pancreatic carcinoma	
	Neural tumors	
Syndrome of inappropriate antidiuretic hormone secretion	Small cell carcinoma of lung; intracranial neoplasms	Antidiuretic hormone or atrial natriuretic hormones
Hypercalcemia	Squamous cell carcinoma of lung	Parathyroid hormone-related protein (PTHRP), TGF-α, TNF, IL-1
	Breast carcinoma	
	Renal carcinoma	
	Adult T-cell leukemia/lymphoma	
	Ovarian carcinoma	
Hypoglycemia	Fibrosarcoma	Insulin or insulin-like substance
	Other mesenchymal sarcomas	
	Hepatocellular carcinoma	
Carcinoid syndrome	Bronchial adenoma (carcinoid)	Serotonin, bradykinin
	Pancreatic carcinoma	
	Gastric carcinoma	
Polycythemia	Renal carcinoma	Erythropoietin
	Cerebellar hemangioma	
	Hepatocellular carcinoma	
Nerve and Muscle Syndromes		
Myasthenia	Bronchogenic carcinoma	Immunologic
Disorders of the central and peripheral nervous systems	Breast carcinoma	
Dermatologic disorders		
Acanthosis nigricans	Gastric carcinoma	Immunologic; secretion of epidermal growth factor
	Lung carcinoma	
	Uterine carcinoma	
Dermatomyositis	Bronchogenic, breast carcinoma	Immunologic
Osseous, Articular and Soft Tissue Changes		
Hypertrophic osteoarthropathy and clubbing of the fingers	Bronchogenic carcinoma	Unknown
Vascular and Hematologic Changes		
Venous thrombosis (Trousseau phenomenon)	Pancreatic carcinoma	Tumor products (mucins that activate clotting)
	Bronchogenic carcinoma	
	Other cancers	
Nonbacterial thrombotic endocarditis	Advanced cancers	Hypercoagulability
Anemia	Thymic neoplasms	Unknown
Others		
Nephrotic syndrome	Various cancers	Tumor antigens, immune complexes

Abbreviations: ACTH, adrenocorticotropic hormone; TGF, transforming growth factor; TNF, tumor necrosis factor; IL, interleukin.

50. Ans. a. Monckeberg's medial sclerosis; b. Papilary carcinoma thyroid; d. Meningioma

[Ref: Robbins 9th/65-66; Harshmohan 7th/34-36]

"Mönckeberg's arteriosclerosis, or Mönckeberg's sclerosis, also called **medial calcific sclerosis** or **Mönckeberg medial sclerosis,** is a form of arteriosclerosis or vessel hardening, where calcium deposits are found in the muscular middle layer of the walls of arteries (the tunica media) . It is an example of dystrophic calcification- *Harshmohan 7th/35,* **wiki**

"**Dystrophic calcification**: ***Psammoma bodies*** *or calcospherites such as in* ***meningioma, papillary serous cystadenocarcinoma of the ovary and papillary carcinoma of the thyroid***"- *Harshmohan 7th/35*

Pathologic Calcification

◈ *Robbins 9th/65-66*

- **Pathologic calcification is the abnormal tissue deposition of calcium salts, together with smaller amounts of iron, magnesium and other mineral salts.**
- There are two forms of pathologic calcification. When the deposition occurs locally in dying tissues it is known as ***dystrophic calcification***; it occurs despite normal serum levels of calcium and in the absence of derangements in calcium metabolism.
- In contrast, the deposition of calcium salts in otherwise normal tissues is known as ***metastatic calcification*** and it almost always results from hypercalcemia secondary to some disturbance in calcium metabolism.

Dystrophic Calcification

◈ *Robbins 9th/65*

- **Dystrophic calcification is encountered in areas of necrosis,** whether they are of coagulative, caseous, or liquefactive type and in foci of enzymatic necrosis of fat.
- Calcification is almost always present in the ***atheromas of advanced atherosclerosis***. Sometimes a tuberculous lymph node is virtually converted to stone.
- **Histologically:** In the course of time, **heterotopic** bone may be formed in the focus of calcification. The progressive acquisition of outer layers may create lamellated configurations, called **psammoma bodies** because of their resemblance to grains of sand. Some types of **papillary cancers** (e.g., thyroid) are apt to develop psammoma bodies.

Metastatic Calcification

◈ *Robbins 9th/65*

- Metastatic calcification can occur in normal tissues whenever there is **hypercalcemia**. The major causes of hypercalcemia are (1) *increased secretion of parathyroid hormone,* due to either primary parathyroid tumors or production of ***parathyroid hormone***–related protein by other malignant tumors; (2) *destruction of bone* due to the effects of accelerated turnover (e.g., ***Paget disease***), immobilization, or tumors (increased bone catabolism associated with multiple myeloma, leukemia, or diffuse skeletal metastases); (3) *vitamin D-related disorders* including ***vitamin D intoxication*** and *sarcoidosis* (in which macrophages activate a vitamin D precursor); and (4) *renal failure,* in which phosphate retention leads to *secondary hyperparathyroidism.*

51. Ans. a. Lysosomal rupture; b. Pyknosis; d. Severe mitochondrial dysfunction

[Ref: Robbins 9th/40; Harshmohan 7th/12-13]

Table: *(Harshmohan 7th/12)*: **Summarized from figure**

Organelles	Reversible cell injury	Irreversible cell injury
Membrane	***Bleb****, cell swelling, myelin figure, intramembranous particles*	Disruptions, Myelin figure
Mitochondria	Swelling, amorphous densities	Swollen with vacuoles, large densities
Lysosomes	Autophagy	*Swollen,* ***ruptured***
Cytoskeleton	Aggregated	Disrupted
Nucleus	Clumped chromatin	***Pyknosis****, Karyorrhexis, Karyolysis*
RER and ribosomes	RER-Swelling Ribosomes- dispersed	RER-Lysed Ribosomes- dispersed

EXTRA EDGE

Table *(Robbins 9th/40)*: **Features of Necrosis and Apoptosis**

Feature	Necrosis	Apoptosis
Cell size	Enlarged (swelling)	Reduced (shrinkage)
Nucleus	Pyknosis → karyorrhexis → kaiyolysis	Fragmentation into nucleosome-size fragments
Plasma membrane	Disrupted	Intact: altered structure, especially orientation of lipids
Cellular contents	Enzymatic digestion: may leak out of cell	Intact: may be released in apoptotic bodies
Adjacent inflammation	Frequent	No
Physiologic or pathologic role	Invariably pathologic (culmination of irreversible cell injury)	Often physiologic, means of eliminating unwanted cells: may be pathologic after some forms of cell injury, especially DNA damage

52. Ans. a. Serotonin; b. Histamine; d. ATP

[Ref: Ganong 25th/79-81; Robbins 9th/19-20; Harshmohan 7th/101; Wintrobe's Clinical Hematology 12th/Chap 19]

Platelets

◈ *Harshmohan 7th/101*

- **Dense bodies:** ***ADP, ionic calcium, serotonin, histamine*** *and epinephrine*
- **Alpha granules:** *Fibrogen, fibronectin,* ***platelet-derived growth factor (PDGF),*** *platelet factor 4 (an antiheparin) and thrombospondin*

Dense Bodies

◈ *Wintrobe's Clinical Hematology 12th/Chap 19*

- Dense bodies, numbering approximately five per platelet, are exceptionally electron-dense and easily appreciated by electron microscopy because of their distinctive "bull's-eye" appearance
- With an approximate diameter of 250 nm, these granules contain a ***large reservoir of ADP***, a critical agonist for platelet activation that amplifies the effect of other stimuli.
- In addition to this nonmetabolic pool of **ADP**, the dense bodies are **rich in ATP**, ***pyrophosphate, calcium and serotonin (5-hydroxytryptamine), with lesser amounts of guanosine triphosphate (GTP), guanosine diphosphate (GDP) and magnesium.***
- There is ***more ADP than ATP in dense bodies*** and both can lead to adenosine monophosphate (AMP). In turn, AMP can be dephosphorylated to adenosine or cyclized to produce cyclic AMP, an inhibitor of the platelet-stimulatory response.
- The dense granule membrane ***contains P-selectin and granulophysin***

Platelets

◈ *Ganong 25th/79-81*

- Their cytoplasm contains actin, myosin, glycogen, ***lysosomes*** and two types of granules: (1) **dense granules,** which contain the nonprotein substances that are secreted in response to platelet activation, including ***serotonin, ADP and other adenine nucleotides***; and
- α-granules, which contain secreted proteins. These proteins include clotting factors and **platelet-derived growth factor (PDGF).**

53. Ans. a. Histamine; b. Lysosomal enzymes; e. Serotonin

[Ref: Robbins 9th/83; Robbins Basic 9th/45; Harshmohan 7th/122-23]

"Histamine **and** ***serotonin***: They are ***stored as preformed molecules in cells*** and are therefore among the first mediators to be released during inflammation"- *Robbins 9th/83*

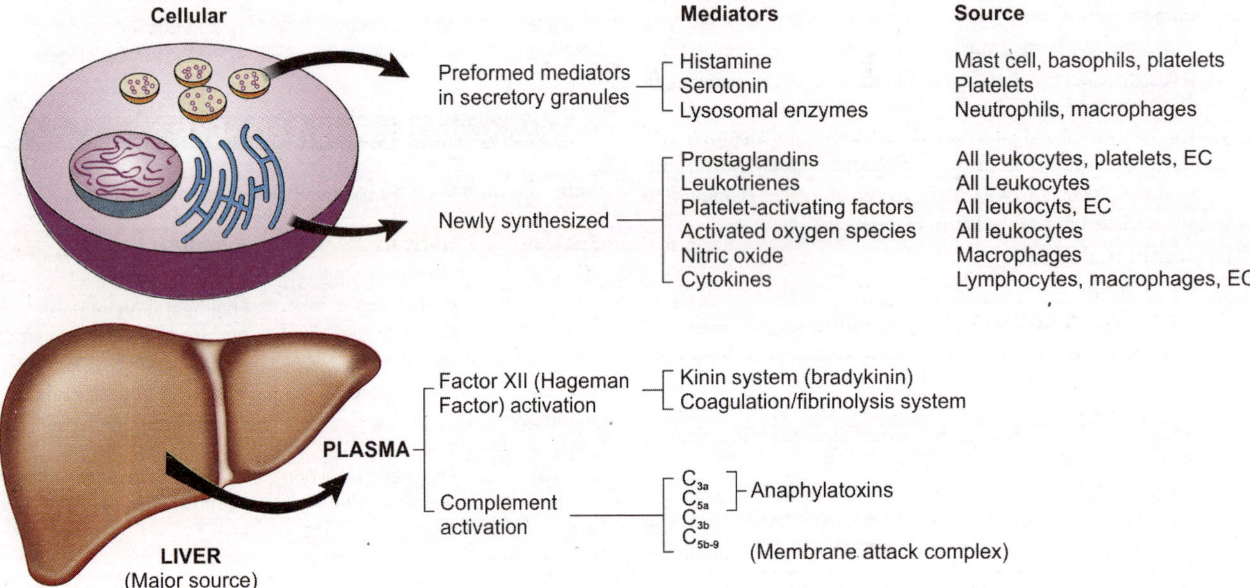

Fig: *(Robbins Basic 9th/45)*: Mediators of inflammation. The principal cell-derived and plasma protein mediators are shown. *EC, endothelial cells*

"Mediators are either secreted by cells or generated from plasma proteins. *Cell-derived mediators* are normally sequestered in intracellular granules and can be rapidly secreted by granule exocytosis (e.g., histamine in mast cell granules) or are **synthesized de novo** (e.g., ***prostaglandins and leukotrienes, cytokines)*** in response to a stimulus"-*Robbins 9th/83*

"Lysosomal Enzymes and Other Lysosomal Proteins: Neutrophils and monocytes contain lysosomal granules that contribute to microbial killing and, when released, may contribute to tissue damage. Neutrophils have two main types of granules. The smaller specific (or secondary) ***granules contain lysozyme***, collagenase, gelatinase, lactoferrin, plasminogen activator, histaminase and alkaline phosphatase. The larger azurophil (or primary) granules contain myeloperoxidase, bactericidal factors (***lysozyme***, defensins), acid hydrolases and a variety of neutral proteases (elastase, cathepsin G, nonspecific collagenases, proteinase 3). Both types of granules can fuse with phagocytic vacuoles containing engulfed material, or the granule contents can be released into the extracellular space"- *Robbins 9th/80*

Lysosomal Enzymes *are cell derived mediators of inflammation- Harshmohan 7th/123*

54. Ans. a. CD 16; c. CD 56

[Ref: Robbins 9th/590; Harrison 19th/372e6-7; Harshmohan 7th/46]

Mast/stem cell growth factor receptor (SCFR), also known as **proto-oncogene c-Kit** or **tyrosine-protein kinase Kit** or **CD117**, is a receptor tyrosine kinase protein that in humans is encoded by the ***KIT***gene

*"**NK cell** carry surface molecules of CD2, **CD16 and CD56** but negative for T cell marker CD3"- Harshmohan 7th/46*

Large Granular Lymphocytes/Natural Killer Cells

Harrison 19th/372e6-7

- NKs cells express surface receptors for the ***Fc portion of IgG (CD16) and for NCAM-I (CD56)***
- NK cells express some T lineage markers, **particularly CD8** and proliferate in response to IL-2.
- NK cells arise in both bone marrow and thymic microenvironments.
- Functionally, NK cells share features with both monocytes-macrophages and neutrophils in that *they mediate both antibody-dependent cellular cytotoxicity (ADCC) and NK cell activity.*
- NK cell activity may play an *important role in immune surveillance and destruction of malignant and virally infected host cells*

Table: *(Robbins 9th/590):* **Some Immune Cell Antigens Detected by Monoclonal Antibodies**

Antigen Designation	Normal Cellular Distribution
Primarily T-Cell Associated	
CD1	Cortical thymocytes and Langerhans histiocytes
CD3	Thymocytes, peripheral T cells
CD4	Helper subset of peripheral T cells, single positive medullary thymocytes and CD4/CD8 double positive thymocytes
CD5	T cells and a small subset of B cells
CD8	Cytotoxic subset of peripheral T cells, single positive medullary thymocytes, double positive cortical thymocytes and ***some NK cells***
Primarily B-Cell Associated	
CD10	Marrow pre-B cells and germinal center B cells; also called CALLA
CD19	Marrow pre-B cells and mature B cells but not plasma cells
CD20	Marrow pre-B cells after CD19 and mature B cells but not plasma cells
CD21	EBV receptor; present on mature B cells and follicular dendritic cells
CD23	Activated mature B cells
CD79a	Marrow pre-B cells and mature B cells.
Primarily Monocyte or Macrophage Associated	
CD11c	Granulocytes, monocytes and macrophages; also expressed by hairy cell leukemias
CD13	Immature and mature monocytes and granulocytes
CD14	Monocytes
CD15	Granulocytes; also expressed by Reed-Sternberg cells and variants in classical Hodgkin lymphoma
CD33	Myeloid progenitors and monocytes
CD64	Mature myeloid cells
Primarily NK-Cell Associated	
CD16	NK cells and granulocytes
CD56	NK cells and a subset of T cells
Primarily Stem Cell and Progenitor Cell Associated	
CD34	Pluripotent hematopoietic stem cells and progenitor cells of many lineages
Activation Markers	
CD30	Activated B cells, T cells and monocytes; also expressed by Reed-Sternberg cells and variants in classical Hodgkin lymphoma
Present on All Leukocytes	
CD45	All leukocytes; also known as leukocyte common antigen (LCA)

Abbreviations: CD, cluster designation; NK, natural killer; CALLA, common acute lymphoblastic leukemia antigen; EBV, Epstein-Barr virus.

55. **Ans. a. Severe Combined Immunodeficiency; b. Adenosine deaminase deficiency; c. Wiskott-Aldrich syndrome; d. Ataxia telangiectasia**

[Ref: Ananthanarayan 10th/174; Robbins 9th/239-43; Harshmohan 7th/51]

Table 10 *(Ananthanarayan 10th/174)*: **Classification of primary immunodeficiency syndrome**

A. Disorders of specific Immunity

I. Humoral immunodeficiencies (B ceil defects)

a) X.linked agammaglobulinemia
b) Transient hypogammaglobullnernia of Infancy
c) Common variable immunodeficiency (late onset hypogammaglobulinemia)
d) Selective immunoglobulin deficiencies (IpA IgM or IgG subclasses)
e) Immunodeficiency with hyper-IgM
f) Transcobalamin II deficiency

II. Cellular immunodeficiencies (T all defects)

a) Thymic hypoplasia (DiGeorge syndrome)
b) Chronic mucocutaneous candidosis
c) Purine nucleoside phosphorylase (PNP) deficiency

III. Combined immunodeficiencies (B and T cell defects)

a) Cellular Immunodeficiency with abnormal immunoglobulin synthesis (Nezelof syndrome)
b) *Ataxia telangiectasia*
c) *Wiskott-Aldrich syndrome*
d) Immunodeficiency with thymoma
e) Immunodeficiency with short-limbed dwarfism
f) Episodic lymphopenla with lymphocytotoxin

Contd...

d) Selective immunoglobulin deficiencies (IpA IgM or IgG subclasses)
e) Immunodeficiency with hyper-IgM
f) Transcobalamin II deficiency

B. Disorders of complement
a) Complement component deficiencies
b) Complement inhibitor deficiencies

C. Disorders of phagocytosis
a) Chronic granulomatous disease
b) Myeloperoxidase deficiency
c) Chediak-Higashi syndrome
d) Leukocyte GOPD deficiency
e) Job's syndrome
f) Tuftsin deficiency
g) Lazy leukocyte syndrome
h) Hyper-IgE syndrome
i) Actin binding protein deficiency
j) Shwachman's disease

56. Ans. a. Hyaline casts- may be normally present in healthy person; b. Muddy brown casts-acute tubular necrosis; c. WBC cast – pyelonephritis; e. Myogolobin cast – Rhabdomyolysis

[Ref: Robbins 9th/929; Harrison 19th/294; CMDT 2015/891]

- "**Hyaline casts** can be seen ***even in healthy patients***. They may be seen in increased numbers during dehydration, exercise or diuretic medicine"-*laboratoryinfo.com/types*
- "**Renal Tubular Epithelial Cell Cast**: These casts are composed of renal epithelial cells. These casts are seen in conditions such as ***renal tubular necrosis***, viral disease (such as CMV nephritis) and kidney transplant rejection"-laboratoryinfo.com/types

"The "**muddy brown cast**" seen in acute tubular necrosis is a type of granular cast"-wikipedia

"**Rhabdomyolysis: myoglobin cast**"-watermark.silverchair.com; www.scielo.br; www.humanpathol.com

Casts in CRD

◈ *Harrison 19th/294*
- In chronic renal disease, degenerated cellular casts called waxy casts can be seen in urine.
- Broad casts are thought to be arise in the dilated tubules of enlarged nephrons that have undergone compensatory hypertrophy in response to reduced renal mass (i.e., *chronic renal failure*)
- **WBC cast are seen in -** ***Pyelonephritis****, interstitial nephritis,* SLE and transplant rejection.
- RBC cast are seen in - *Acute glomerulonephritis*

Table: *(CMDT 2015/891)*: **Significance of specific urinary casts**

Type	Significance
Hyaline casts	Concentrated urine, febrile disease, after strenuous exercise, in the course of diuretic therapy (***not indicative of renal disease***)
Red cell casts	Glomerulonephritis
White cell casts	***Pyelonephritis***, interstitial nephritis (indicative of infection or inflammation)
Renal tubular cell casts	Acute tubular necrosis, interstitial nephritis
Coarse, granular casts	Nonspecific; can represent acute tubular necrosis
Broad, waxy casts	Chronic renal failure (indicative of stasis in enlarged collecting tubules)

Contd...

57. Ans. a. May be complicated by bacterial infection; b. Rarely progress to biliary cirrhosis; d. Associated with Inflammatory bowel disease; e. Narrowing of bile duct

[Ref: Robbins 9th/859-60; Harrison 19th/2061; Davidson 22nd/965-66; Harshmohan 7th/611]

"Patients with primary sclerosing cholangitis (PSC) are at increased risk for **bacterial cholangitis** because of biliary strictures and bile stasis. A subset of PSC patients suffer from repeated episodes of ***bacterial cholangitis***, which can lead to frequent hospitalizations and impaired quality of life"- www.ncbi.nlm.nih.gov

In addition to ***bacterial infections common for PSC, fungal infections*** are becoming an increasingly recognized complication associated with a poor prognosis"- *link.springer.com*

"Broad-spectrum antibiotics (e.g. ciprofloxacin) should be given for ***acute attacks of cholangitis*** but have no proven value in preventing attacks"-*Davidson 22nd/966*

Primary Sclerosing Cholangitis

◈ *Harrison 19th/2061*
- PSC is a chronic cholestatic syndrome that is characterized by diffuse inflammation and fibrosis involving the ***entire biliary tree***, resulting in chronic cholestasis. This pathologic process ultimately results in ***obliteration of both the intra- and extrahepatic biliary tree***, leading to ***biliary cirrhosis,*** portal hypertension and liver failure.
- Pathologic changes that can occur in PSC show ***bile duct proliferation as well as ductopenia and fibrous cholangitis (pericholangitis)*** . Often, liver biopsy changes in PSC are not pathognomonic and establishing the diagnosis of PSC must involve imaging of the biliary tree.
- ***Periductal fibrosis*** is occasionally seen on biopsy specimens and can be quite helpful in making the diagnosis.
- ***As the disease progresses, biliary cirrhosis is the final, end-stage manifestation of PSC.***
- The usual clinical features of PSC are those found in cholestatic liver disease, with fatigue, pruritus, steatorrhea, deficiencies of fat-soluble vitamins and the associated consequences.
- Most patients have at least a twofold increase in ALP and may have elevated aminotransferases as well. Albumin levels may be decreased and prothrombin times are prolonged in a substantial proportion of patients at the time of diagnosis.

- ***Over 50% of patients with PSC also have ulcerative colitis (UC)***

Primary Sclerosing Cholangitis

◈ *Robbins 9th/859-60*

- **PSC is characterized by inflammation and obliterative fibrosis of intrahepatic and extrahepatic bile ducts with dilation of preserved segments.**
- Characteristic "beading" on radiographs of the intrahepatic and extrahepatic biliary tree is attributable to these irregular, biliary strictures and dilations
- ***Inflammatory bowel disease, particularly ulcerative colitis,*** *coexists in approximately 70% of individuals with PSC.*
- **Large duct inflammation** is similar to that seen in ulcerative colitis: acute, neutrophilic infiltration of the epithelium superimposed on a chronic inflammatory background. Inflamed areas ***develop strictures*** because edema and ***inflammation narrows the lumen or because of subsequent scarring.***
- The **smaller ducts,** however, often have little inflammation and show a striking **circumferential "onion skin" fibrosis** around an increasingly atrophic duct lumen, eventually ***leading to obliteration*** by a "tombstone" scar.
- As the disease progresses the liver becomes ***markedly cholestatic, culminating in biliary cirrhosis*** much like that seen with chronic obstruction and primary biliary cirrhosis.
- Biliary intraepithelial neoplasia may develop and cholangiocarcinoma appears usually with a fatal outcomes.

58. Ans. a. More common in female; c. Oral corticosteroids are given in severe cases; d. Associated with other autoimmune disease; e. Rarely lead to cirrhosis

[Ref: Robbins 9th/839-40; Harrison 19th/2049-51; Davidson 22nd/962-63]

Autoimmune Hepatitis

◈ *Robbins 9th/839-40*

- **Autoimmune hepatitis is a chronic, progressive hepatitis with all the features of autoimmune diseases in general:** *genetic predisposition,* ***association with other autoimmune diseases,*** *presence of autoantibodies and therapeutic response to immunosuppression.*
- Strong HLA-associations for autoimmune hepatitis support a genetic predisposition.
- There is a ***female predominance*** (78%).
- *Autoimmune hepatitis is classified into types 1 and 2, based on the patterns of circulating antibodies.* **Type 1**, more common in middle-aged to older individuals, is characterized by the presence of antinuclear (ANA), anti–smooth muscle actin (SMA), anti–soluble liver antigen/liver-pancreas antigen (anti-SLA/LP) antibodies and less commonly, anti-mitochondrial (AMA) antibodies.
- In **type 2**, usually seen in children and teenagers, the main serologic markers are ***anti–liver kidney microsome-1 (anti-LKM-1) antibodies,*** which are mostly directed against CYP2D6 and anti– liver cytosol-1 (ACL-1) antibodies
- An acute appearance of clinical illness is common (40%) and a fulminant presentation with hepatic encephalopathy within 8 weeks of disease onset may also occur. The mortality of patients with severe untreated autoimmune hepatitis is approximately 40% within 6 months of diagnosis and **cirrhosis develops** in at least 40% of survivors.
- The **mainstay of management in autoimmune hepatitis is glucocorticoid therapy**-*Harrison 19th/2051*

Management of Autoimmune Hepatitis

◈ *Davidson 22nd/962-63*

- ***Treatment with corticosteroids is life-saving in autoimmune hepatitis, particularly during exacerbations of active and symptomatic disease.*** Initially, prednisolone 40 mg/day is given orally; the dose is then gradually reduced as the patient and LFTs improve.
- Azathioprine can also be used as the sole maintenance immunosuppressive agent in patients with low-activity disease.
- Newer agents such as mycophenolate mofetil (MMF) are increasingly being used but formal evidence to inform practice in this area is lacking. Patients should be monitored for acute exacerbations (LFT and IgG screening with patients alerted to the possible symptoms) and such exacerbations should be treated with corticosteroids.

Type II autoimmune hepatitis, is associated not with ANA but with anti-LKM 1. This is the same anti-LKM seen in some patients with chronic hepatitis C. Anti-LKM2 is seen in drug-induced hepatitis and anti-LKM3 (directed against uridine diphosphate glucuronyl transferases) is seen in patients with chronic hepatitis D. More controversial is whether or not a third category of autoimmune hepatitis exists, type III autoimmune hepatitis. These patients lack ANA and anti-LKM1 but have circulating antibodies to soluble liver antigen. Type III autoimmune hepatitis does not appear to represent a distinct category but, instead, is part of the spectrum of type I autoimmune hepatitis; this subcategory has not been adopted by a consensus of international experts"-Harrison 19th/2050

Microsomal antibody	Antigen	Disease
anti-LKM 1	Cytochrome P450 2D6	Autoimmune hepatitis type II and chronic hepatitis C (10%)
anti-LKM 2	Cytochrome P450 2C9	Drug-induced hepatitis (tienilic acid–induced)
anti-LKM 3	Cytochrome P450 1A2	Chronic active hepatitis in association with autoimmune polyendocrine syndrome type 1; hepatitis D

59. Ans. a. Tall stature

[Ref: Robbins 9th/839-40; Harrison 19th/2049-51; Davidson 22nd/962-63]

"**Celiac disease** is also associated with diabetes mellitus type 1, IgA deficiency, Down syndrome and **Turner's syndrome**"-Harrison 19th/1942

"**Turner's syndrome** affects around 1 in 2500 females. It is classically associated with a **45XO karyotype** but other cytogenetic abnormalities may be responsible, including mosaic forms (e.g. **45XO/46XX or 45XO/46XY**) and partial deletions of an X chromosome"-*Davidson 22nd/765*

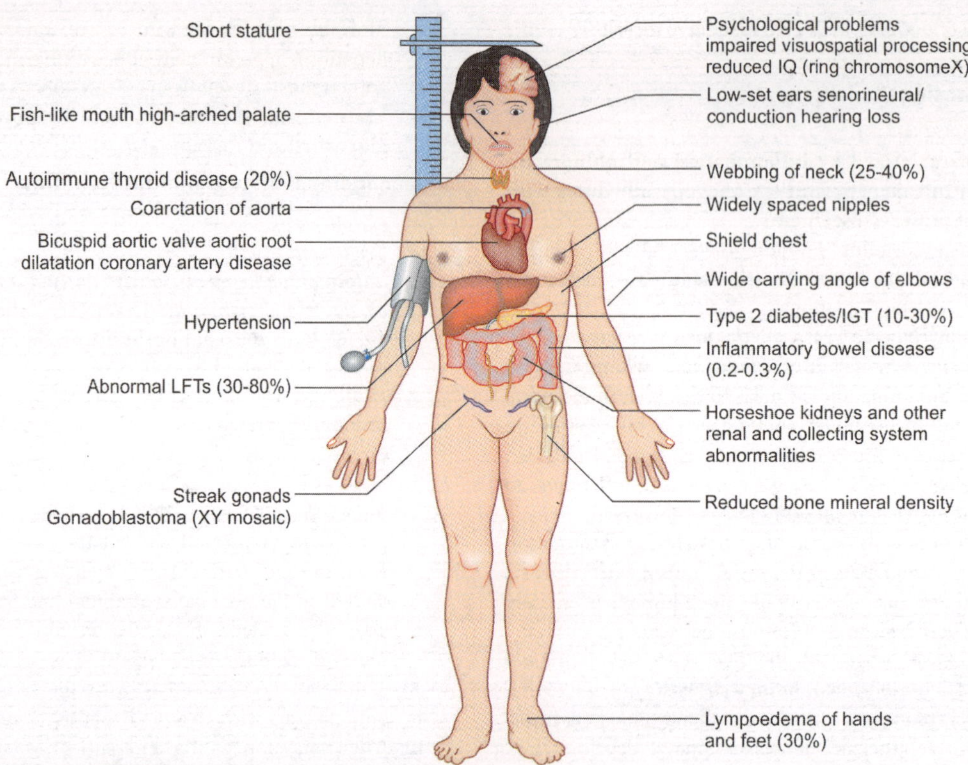

Fig: *(Davidson 22nd/765)*: Clinical features of Turner's syndrome (45XO) (IGT = impaired glucose tolerance)

60. Ans. a. Fat droplet in hepatocyte; d. Perivenular fibrosis may be seen

[Ref: Robbins 9th/842-44; Harrison 19th/2053; Davidson 22nd/958; Harshmohan 7th/19-20,606-07]

Perivenular fibrosis may be seen in both alcoholic steatosis and alcoholic hepatitis

ALCOHOLIC STEATOSIS (Fatty liver): Grossly, the liver is enlarged, yellow, greasy and firm with a smooth and glistening capsule. ***Microscopically***, the features consist of initial ***microvesicular large droplets*** of fat displacing the nucleus to the periphery. ***Fat cysts*** may develop due to coalescence and rupture of fat-containing hepatocytes. Less often, lipogranulomas consisting of collection of lymphocytes, macrophages and some multinucleate giant cells may be found"- Harshmohan 7th/606

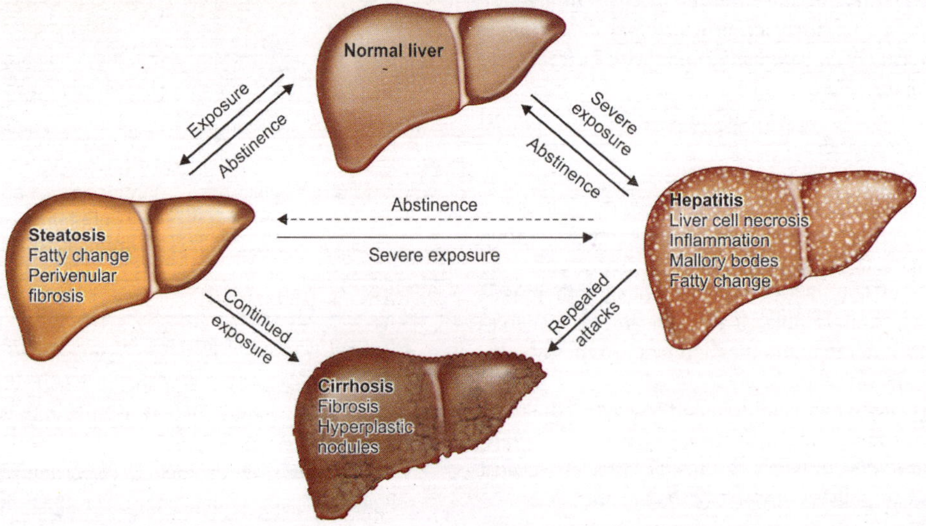

Fig: *(Robbins 9th/842)*: Alcoholic liver disease. The interrelationships among hepatic steatosis, alcoholic hepatitis and alcoholic cirrhosis are shown, along with depictions of key morphologic features. It should be noted that steatosis, alcoholic hepatitis and steatofibrosis may also develop independently. In particular some patients present initially with cirrhosis without any of the other forms of alcoholic liver disease

Alcoholic Liver Disease

◈ *Robbins 9th/842*

- There are three distinctive, albeit overlapping forms of alcoholic liver injury: (1) hepatocellular steatosis or fatty change, (2) alcoholic (or steato-) hepatitis and (3) steatofibrosis (patterns of scarring typical for all fatty liver diseases including alcohol) up to and including cirrhosis in the late stages of disease.

Hepatocellular Steatosis

◈ *Robbins 9th/842*

- It may cause hepatomegaly, with mild elevation of serum bilirubin and alkaline phosphatase levels. Severe hepatic dysfunction is unusual. Alcohol withdrawal and the provision of an adequate diet are sufficient treatment.
- All changes in alcoholic liver disease begin in acinus zone 3 and extend outward toward the portal tracts with increasing severity of injury.
- **Hepatic Steatosis (Fatty Liver).** After even moderate intake of alcohol, ***lipid droplets accumulate*** in hepatocytes increasing with amount and chronicity of alcohol intake. The ***lipid begins as small droplets that coalesce into large droplets which distend the hepatocyte and push the nucleus aside***

Alcoholic (Steato-)-*Hepatitis Robbins 9th/843*

Alcoholic hepatitis is characterized by:

- **Hepatocyte swelling and necrosis:** Single or scattered foci of cells undergo swelling (ballooning) and necrosis. The swelling results from the accumulation of fat and water, as well as proteins that are normally exported.
- **Mallory-Denk bodies**: These are usually present as clumped, amorphous, eosinophilic material in ballooned hepatocytes. They are made up of tangled skeins of intermediate filaments such as keratins 8 and 18 in complex with other proteins such as ubiquitin.
- **Neutrophilic reaction:** Neutrophils permeate the hepatic lobule and accumulate around degenerating hepatocytes, particularly those having ***Mallory-Denk bodies***. They may be more or less admixed with mononuclear cells

Alcoholic Steatofibrosis

◈ *Robbins 9th/843*

- Alcoholic hepatitis is often accompanied by prominent activation of sinusoidal stellate cells and portal fibroblasts, giving rise to fibrosis.
- Fibrosis begins with sclerosis of central veins. Perisinusoidal scar then accumulates in the space of Disse of the centrilobular region, spreading outward, encircling individual or small clusters of hepatocytes in a **chicken wire fence pattern**.
- With developing ***nodularity***, cirrhosis becomes established.
- When alcohol use continues without interruption over the long term, the continual subdivision of established nodules by new webs of, perisinusoidal scarring leads to a ***classic micronodular*** or **Laennec cirrhosis** first described for end-stage alcoholic liver disease

Alcoholic Liver Disease: Pathology

◈ *Harrison 19th/2053*

- The liver has a limited repertoire in response to injury. **Fatty liver** is the initial and most common histologic response to hepatotoxic stimuli, including excessive alcohol ingestion. The ***accumulation of fat within the perivenular hepatocytes*** coincides with the location of alcohol dehydrogenase, the major enzyme responsible for alcohol metabolism. Continuing alcohol ingestion results in ***fat accumulation throughout the entire hepatic lobule***. Despite extensive fatty change and distortion of the hepatocytes with **macrovesicular fat**, the cessation of drinking results in normalization of hepatic architecture and fat content. **Alcoholic fatty liver** has traditionally been regarded as entirely benign, but similar to the spectrum of nonalcoholic fatty liver disease, the ***appearance of steatohepatitis and certain pathologic features such as giant mitochondria, perivenular fibrosis and macrovesicular fat may be associated with progressive liver injury.***
- The transition between fatty liver and the development of alcoholic hepatitis is blurred. The **hallmark of alcoholic hepatitis** is hepatocyte injury characterized by ***ballooning degeneration, spotty necrosis, polymorphonuclear infiltrate and fibrosis in the perivenular and perisinusoidal space of Disse***. **Mallory-Denk bodies** are often present in florid cases but are neither specific nor necessary to establish the diagnosis.

---

61. Ans. a. G2-M; e. S phase

[Ref: Robbins 9th/289,1054-55; Harshmohan 7th/751]

BRCA1 is known to be required for **S and G2/M transitions** and is involved in the cellular response to DNA damage. **BRCA2** is believed to be involved in homologous recombination and regulating the S-***phase checkpoint*** and mutations of deficiencies in BRCA2 are strongly linked to tumorigenesis.-wiki

"It remains unclear whether BRCA2 participates directly in cell cycle regulation or checkpoint functions. Available evidence suggests that **BRCA2** mediates ***G2/M-phase control*** by interacting with a novel protein, BRCA2-associated factor 35 (BRAF35), which binds to branched DNA structures"-onlinelibrary.wiley.com

"Several requirements for **BRCA2** outside of homologous recombination have been suggested by protein interaction and cell culture studies, but these functions are far less understood. Most notably, **BRCA2** has been implicated in ***two S-phase checkpoints: the intra-S phase checkpoint and the replication checkpoint"***-journals.plos.org

"Mounting evidence indicates that BRCA1 is involved in all phases of the cell cycle and regulates orderly events during cell cycle progression. **BRCA1 deficiency**, consequently causes abnormalities in the ***S-phase checkpoint, the G2/M checkpoint***, the spindle checkpoint and centrosome duplication"- www.ncbi.nlm.nih.gov

Interaction of BRCT repeats of BRCA1 with CHK1 and Polo-like kinase (PLK1) regulates the G2/M and G1/S checkpoints and control apoptosis-Devita 8th/Chap 43

Cell-Cycle Checkpoints

- The cell cycle has its own internal controls, called ***checkpoints***. There are **two main checkpoints**, one at the ***G_1/S transition and another at G_2/M.***
- The S phase is the point of no return in the cell cycle and before a cell makes the final commitment to replicate, the G_1/S checkpoint checks for DNA damage.
- *Defect in cell-cycle checkpoint components is a major cause of genetic instability in cancer cells.*

Table: *(Robbins 9th/289; 8th/chap7):* **Main Cell-Cycle Components and Their Inhibitors**

Cell-Cycle Component	Main Function
Checkpoint Components	
• p53	Tumor suppressor altered in the majority of cancers; causes cell-cycle arrest and apoptosis. Acts mainly through p21 to cause cell-cycle arrest. Causes apoptosis by inducing the transcription of pro-apoptotic genes such as *BAX*. Levels of p53 are negatively regulated by MDM2 through a feedback loop. ***p53 is required for the G_1/S checkpoint and is a main component of the G_2/M checkpoint.s***
• Ataxia-telangiectasia mutated (*ATM*)	Activated by mechanisms that sense double stranded DNA breaks. Transmits signals to arrest the cell cycle after DNA damage. Acts through p53 in the G_1/S checkpoint. At the G_2/M checkpoint, it acts both through p53-dependent mechanisms and through the inactivation of CDC25 phosphatase, which disrupts the cyclin B-CDK1 complex. Component of a network of genes that include ***BRCA1* and *BRCA2***, which link DNA damage with cell-cycle arrest and apoptosis.

62. Ans. a. Necrotizing arteriolitis; c. Hyperplastic arterioscleroesis; d. Aortic dissection; e. Onion skinning;

[Ref: Robbins 9th/490;Harshmohan 8th/722]

Hypertension is Associated with two forms of Small Blood Vessels disease

◈ *Robbins 9th/490*

- Hyperplastic arteriosclerosis:
  - It is characteristic or **malignant hypertension**. There is concentrentic, laminated thickening of arteriolar wall → **onion skinning**. There is **mucinous intimal thickening** and **fibrous intimal thickening**.
  - There may be accompanied fibrinoid deposits with necrosis of the vessels wall →**fibrinoid necrosis** (or **necrotizing arteriolitis**).
- **Favoured sites for hyperplastic arteriosclerosis are kidney, small intestine, gall bladder, peripancreatic fat and periadrenal fat.**
- **Hyaline arteriolosclerosis**
  - There is homogenous, pink, hyaline thickening of arteriolar wall. The lumen becomes narrow. It is characteristic or **benign hypertension.**
  - It may also occur in **diabetes and aging**
- Beside these hypertension also causes:
  - **Atherosclerosis** in large arteries.
  - Degenerative changes in the walls of large and medium arteries that potentiate both aortic dissection and cerebrovascular hemorrhage.

PHARMACOLOGY

63. Ans. a. Amikacin; b.Fluroquinolones

[Ref: KDT 7th/776; Community Medicine by Suryakantha 4th/389; Community Medicine by Piyush Gupta 1st/202]

*"Multidrug resistance-TB (MDR-TB): resistance to **at least both isoniazid and rifampicin**" (Park 24th/189)*

"Extensively drug resistance (XDR-TB): resistance to any fluroquinolones and at least one of the three second-line injectable drugs (capreomycin, kanamycin andamikacin), in addition to multidrug resis7tance" -Community Medicine by Piyush Gupta 1st/202, Park 24th/189, Community Medicine by Suryakantha 4th/389; www.who.int

"Extensively drug resistance (XDR-TB): The bacilli are resistant to at least 4 most effective cidal drugs viz. H, R, FQ and one of Km/Am/Cm"-KDT 7th/776

"Multidrug resistance-TB (MDR-TB): *MDR-TB is defined as resistance to **both isoniazid and rifampicin and may (with or without) be any number of other 1st line drug (s)**"*- KDT *7th/775; Satoshkar Pharmacology 25th/761*

64. Ans. a. Proton pump inhibitors (PPI); e. Magnesium hydroxide

[Ref: Harrison 14th/427; KDT 7th/653; Satoskar 25th/626,613]

"Adverse Effect of Protein Pump Inhibitors (PPI): Loose stool"-KDT 7TH/653

Verapamil (Calcium channel blocker): ***Causes constipation***"-KDT 7th/548

Table: (Satoskar 25th/613): **Drugs Causing Diarrhea**

- ***Magnesium antacids***
- Antibiotics; Erythromycin, ampicillin, tetracyclines
- GI prokinetic drugs, e.g. cisapride
- Quinidine
- Prostaglandin analogues
- Anticholinesterases
- Colchicine
- Emetine
- Cytotoxic drugs
- Lithium

Table: *(Harrison 14th/427, not given in newer editions)*: **Drug causing Diarrhea or Colitis**

- Antibiotics (broad-spectrum)
- Clindamycin
- Cocaine
- Colchicine
- Digitalis
- Guanethidine
- Lactose excipients
- Lincomycin

Contd...

- ***Magnesium in antacids***
- Methyldopa
- Misoprostol
- Oral contraceptives
- Purgatives
- Reserpine
- Ticlopidine

Table: (Satoskar 25th/626): **Drugs Causing Constipation**

- Drugs with antimuscarinic action (atropine and its derivative; antihistaminics, antiparkinsonian agents, tricyclic antidepressants and phenothiazines)
- Prostaglandin inhibitors (NSAIDs)
- Opioids
- Calcium carbonate and ***aluminium hydroxide*** used as antacids
- Sympathomimetic amines
- Antidiarrheal agents
- Miscellaneous: Clonidine, iron, MAO inhibitors, verapamil and phenytoin

65. Ans. b. Activated charcoal has no role

[Ref: KDT 7th/197; Satoskar 25th/172-75]

- **Salicylate:** *Large doses particularly in children, can cause **hepatic damage and even necrosis**-Satoskar 25th/172*
- ***Salicylism:*** *Characterized by headache,dizziness, vertigo, **tinnitus,** difficulty in hearing, diminished vision, lethargy, mental confusion etc.- Satoskar 25th/174*

Acute Salicylate Poisoning

◈ *KDT 7th/197*

- It is more common in children. Fatal dose in adults is estimated to be 15-30g, but is considerably lower in children. Serious toxicity is seen at serum salicylate levels > 50 mg/dl.
- **Manifestations are:** Vomiting, dehydration, electrolyte imbalance, acidotic, breathing, hyper/hypoglycemia, petechial haemorrhages, restlessness, delirium, hallucinations, hyperpyrexia, convulsions, coma and death due to respiratory failure + cardiovascular collapse.
- **Treatment** is symptomatic and supportive. Most important is external cooling and i.v. fluid with Na^+, K^+, HCO^-_3 and glucose: according to need determined by repeated monitoring. ***Gastric lavage to remove unabsorbed drug; alkaline diuresis or haemodialysis*** to remove absorbed drug is indicated in severe cases. Blood transfusion and vit K should be given if bleeding occurs.

Table: (Satoskar 25th/175): **Principles of Management of Salicylate Poisoning**

- Hospitalization
- ***Activated charcoal 50 g orally***
- Correct hyperthermia, dehydration (5% dextrose), hypokalaemia, acid–base disturbances, ketosis
- ***Increase elimination by alkalinization, peritoneal dialysis or haemoperfusion***
- Vitamin K, blood transfusion
- Exchange transfusion in very small children

66. Ans. a. Chronic hepatitis B; b. Chronic hepatitis C; c. Hairy cell leukaemia; d. Mycosis fungoides

[Ref: KDT 7th/804-05; Satoskar 25th/813; Harrison 19th/2667]

In multiple sclerosis, IFN-β is used (not IFN-α)

Interferon-α: Use

◈ *KDT 7th/804-05; Satoskar 25th/813*

- ***Chronic hepatitis B***
- ***Chronic hepatitis C***
- Chronic hepatitis D
- Condyloma acuminata
- AIDS-related Kaposi sarcoma
- H.simplex, H.zoster and CMV
- **Hairy cell leukaemia** (IFN-aplha 2a and 2b)
- Melanoma (Peginterferon-alpha 2b)
- Multiple myeloma, ***cutaneous T-cell lymphoma***, follicular lymphoma, chronic myeloid leukaemia

Mycosis fungoides is the ***commonest form of cutaneous T cell lymphoma*** *-Neena Khanna 5th/404*

"DISEASE-MODIFYING THERAPIES FOR RELAPSING FORMS OF **Multiple sclerosis**: Ten such agents are approved by the U.S. FDA:

- ***IFN-β-1a (Avonex)***
- ***IFN-β-1a (Rebif)***
- ***IFN-β-1b*** (Betaseron or Extavia)
- Glatiramer acetate (Copaxone)
- Natalizumab (Tysabri)
- Fingolimod (Gilenya)
- Dimethylfumarate (Tecfidera)
- Teriflunomide (Aubagio)
- Mitoxantrone (Novantrone) and
- Alemtuzumab (Lemtrada)"- *Harrison 19th/2667; Satoskar 25th/241*

67. Ans. a. Vinblastine

[Ref: KDT 7th/865; Katzung 13th/932-33; Satoskar 25th/829,834; GandG 11th/1325-26]

Vincristine- *BM Depression is Minimal. Vinblastine- BM Depression is more Prominent-*

◈ *KDT 7th/865*

"Most alkylating agents, including nitrogen mustard, melphalan, ***chlorambucil, cyclophosphamide*** and ifosfamide, cause acute myelosuppression, with a nadir of the peripheral blood granulocyte count at 6–10 days and recovery in 14–21 days. Cyclophosphamide has lesser effects on peripheral blood platelet counts than do the other agents. **Busulfan** suppresses all blood elements, particularly stem cells and may produce a prolonged and cumulative myelosuppression lasting months or even years.

For this reason, it is used in preparation for allogeneic bone marrow transplantation"- *GandG 11th/1325-26*

*The major toxic effects of bolus-dose regimens result from the **myelosuppressive** action of **5-FU.** The nadir of leukopenia usually is between days 9 and 14 after the first injection of drug. Thrombocytopenia and anemia also may occur- GandG 11th/1344*

*"Although **less common than with vinblastine,** leukopenia may occur with vincristine and thrombocytopenia, anemia,*

polyuria, dysuria, fever and GI symptoms have been reported occasionally"-GandG 11th/1352

Vinorelbine: *Its primary toxicity is granulocytopenia, with only modest thrombocytopenia and less neurotoxicity than other vinca alkaloids. GandG 11th/1352*

Cisplatin causes ***mild-to-moderate myelosuppression****, with transient leukopenia and thrombocytopenia- GandG 11th/1334*

BM depression *results in agranulocytosis, granulocytopenia, thrombocytopenia, apasticanaemia. This is the most serious side effect of anti-cancer drug-KDT 7th/859*

Supportive Care During Cancer Treatment: Myelosuppression

◈ *Harrison 19th/103e-23*

- The common cytotoxic chemotherapeutic agents almost invariably affect bone marrow function.
- The normal kinetics of blood cell turnover influences the sequence and sensitivity of each of the formed elements. Polymorphonuclear leukocytes (PMNs; $t1/2$ = 6–8 h), platelets ($t1/2$ = 5–7 days) and red blood cells (RBCs; $t1/2$ = 120 days) have most, less and least susceptibility, respectively, to usually administered cytotoxic agents. The nadir count of each cell type in response to classes of agents is characteristic.
- Maximal neutropenia occurs 6–14 days after conventional doses ***of anthracyclines, antifolates and antimetabolites***. Alkylating agents differ from each other in the timing of cytopenias. ***Nitrosoureas, DTIC and procarbazine*** can display delayed marrow toxicity, first appearing 6 weeks after dosing.

68. Ans. a. It is a bactericidal drug of newer class diarlyquinolone; b. It works by blocking the enzyme ATP synthase in mycobacterium and affects energy supply; c. Causes liver and cardiac damage; d. Always should be used in combination with other drugs

[Ref: Park 24th/197; Katzung 13th/21; Satoskar 25th/757]

It is ***always administered with more than three drugs in MDR TB****-Satoskar 25th/757*

Take with a multidrug regimen consisting of ***at least 4 other drugs that the MDR-TB is likely susceptible for the entire 24 week duration***- *reference.medscape.com*

Bedaquiline should be given for a ***maximum of six months*** on top of the WHO recommended combination treatment regimen. The manufacturer recommends 400 mg daily (4 tablets) for 2 weeks followed by 200 mg 3 times per week for the remaining 22 weeks- www.who.int/tb/challenge; tbdrugmonographs.co.uk

Bedaquiline (BDQ)

◈ *Park 24th/197*

- BDQ is a ***new class of drug diarylquinoline***, that specifically ***targets mycobacterial ATP synthase***, an enzyme essential to ***supply of energy*** to *mycobacterium.*
- It is a ***bactericidal drug*** with high volume of tissue distribution, highly bound to plasma proteins and hepatically metabolized.
- The drug has extended half-life, which means that it is still present in the plasma up to 5.5 months post stopping BDQ.
- The basic criteria for patient selection is: (1) age of the patient should be ≥ 18 years having MDR—TB; (2) Pregnancy is a contraindication for BDQ therapy and the patient should be using non-hormonal based birth control measure throughout the treatment period or have been post-menopausal for past 2 years; and (3) Cardiac arrhythmia is a contraindication for BDQ treatment
- The most common side-effects reported with bedaquiline therapy are nausea (30%), arthralgia (26%), headache (22%), hemoptysis (14%), chest pain (9%), anorexia (7%) and rash (6%).

Important **cardiovascular adverse effect** is QT prolongation. Concurrent use of other QT-prolonging drugs causes additive QT prolongation. Other important adverse effect is elevation of ***hepatic transaminases***, which is moderate and reversible on discontinuation of therapy- *www.ncbi.nlm.nih.gov*

Bedaquiline has been reported to disturb the function of the heart and liver in particular- *www.who.int/tb/challenge*

Bedaquiline can also cause hepatotoxicity. Conditions and medications associated with hepatotoxicity could pose additional hepatotoxic risks- *www.ncbi.nlm.nih.go*

Liver function monitoring. Because a high incidence of liver toxicity have been seen in patients on bedaquiline, liver enzymes should be monitored monthly. If aminotransferase elevations are accompanied by total bilirubin elevation >2x upper limit of normal (ULN), or aminotransferase elevations are >5x the upper limit of normal, bedaquiline needs to be discontinued- *www.ncbi.nlm.nih.go*

69. Ans. a. Drug such as Rifampicin and phenazopyridine; b. Ingestion of beetroot; d. Aniline dyes ingestion

[Ref: Harrison 19th/434e-4; Reddy 34th/497; Henry's Clinical Diagnosis and Management by Laboratory Methods 22nd/446-47; emedicine. medscape.com; CMDT 2014/866]

"Myoglobinuria may give a red or brown colour in the urine. Other substances causing **red urine** include ***beetroot, blackberries, phenolphthalein*** in purgatives (if the urine is alkaline) and ***certain aniline dyes in sweets***"-French's Index of Differential Diagnosis An A-Z 16th/721; CMDT 2014/866

"Red or pink urine: Medications-Rifampin, ***phenazopyridine*** and laxatives containing senna"- www. mayoclinic.org

"Numerous medications can cause **red urine discoloration**. Most commonly, ***rifampin or phenazopyridine*** is the culprit, with tears and other bodily fluids generally also discolored. Others include chlorpromazine, thioridazine, senna and laxatives with a phenolphthalein component. Both ***mercury and lead poisoning*** have also been implicated in red urine discoloration. Other more benign causes of red urine discoloration are related to the ingestion of certain pigment-containing foods. Consumption of a large amount of **beets** can result in red urine with no observable erythrocytes on microscopy or heme on dipstick testing. Heavy consumption of rhubarb or carrots can also cause red urine"- emedicine. medscape.com

"Orange urine can result from: Medications that can turn urine orange include the anti-inflammatory drug sulfasalazine (Azulfidine); ***phenazopyridine*** (Pyridium); some laxatives; and certain chemotherapy drugs"- www.mayoclinic.org

"**Phenol**: Urine may be colourless or slightly ***green at first, but turns green or even black on exposure to air***"-Reddy 34th/497

Alkaptonuria: The diagnosis should be suspected in a patient whose urine darkens to blackness-Harrison 19th/434e-4

Alkaptonuria, also called **black urine disease**- emedicine. medscape.com

Table: (Henry's 22nd/446): **Appearance and color of urine**

Colour	Cause
Red	Hemoglobin Erythrocytes Myoglobin Porphyrin Fuscin, ***aniline dye*** ***Beets*** Menstrual contamination
Red-purple	Porphyrins
Red-brown	Erythrocytes Hemoglobin on standing Methemoglobin Myoglobin Bilifuscin (dipyrrole)
Brown-black	Methemoglobin ***Homogentisic acid***

Table: (Henry's 22nd/447): **Urine Color Changes with Commonly Used Drugs**

Drug	Color
Alcohol, ethyl	Pale, diuresis
Anthraquinone laxatives (senna, cascara)	Reddish, alkaline; yellow-brown, acid
Chlorzoxazone	Red
Deferoxamine mesylate	Red
Ethoxazene	Orange, red
Fluorescein sodium	Yellow
Furazolidone	Brown
Indigo carmine dye	Blue
Iron sorbitol	Brown on standing
Levodopa	Red then brown, alkaline
Methyldopa	Darkens; if oxidizing agents present, red to brown
Methylene blue	Blue, blue-green
Metronidazole	Darkening, reddish brown
Nitrofurantoin	Brown-yellow
Phenazopyridine	Orange-red, acid pH
Phenol poisoning	Brown; oxidized to quinones (green)
Phenolphthalein (purgative)	Red-purple, alkaline pH
Phenolsulfonphthalein	Pink-red, alkaline pH
Rifampin	Bright orange-red
Riboflavin	Bright yellow
Sulfasalazine	Orange-yellow, alkaline pH

70. Ans. b. Clearance (CL) remains constant; c. Constant fraction of drug is eliminated

[Ref: KDT 7th/30-31; Katzung 13th/45; Satoskar 25th/24-25; G and G 11th/12]

First Order Kinetics

◈ *Satoskar 25th/24-25; KDT 7th/30-31*

- ***Rate of drug elimination is directly proportional to the drug concentration***
- A ***constant fraction*** of the drug present in the body is eliminated in unit time
- ***Clearance (CL) remains constant***
- Applies to majority of drugs which do not saturate the elimination processes over the therapeutic concentration range
- The ***elimination half-life is independent of the dose***, the route of administration and the plasma concentration. It depends on Vd as well as on the metabolism and the renal excretion ($t1/2 = 0.693 \times Vd/C$

Zero Order Kinetics

◈ *Satoskar 25th/26*

- The increase in dose can cause an increase in the biological half-life
- A constant amount of the drug is eliminated in unit time
- Clearance (CL) decreases with increase in concentration

71. Ans. a. Antagonism can be overcome by increasing dose of agonist; b. Decrease potency of agonist; c. Parallel rightward shift of agonist DRC

[Ref: KDT 7th/58-59; Katzung 13th/23; Satoskar 25th/41; Ramg and Dale 8th/10-11]

*"Competitive antagonism: The **maximal response to agonist is**, however, **not impaired**"- Satoskar 25th/41*

The upper limit of DRC is the index of drug efficacy and refers to the maximal response that can be elicited by the drug- *KDT 7th/58*

Competitive (equilibrium type) KDT 7th/59	Noncompetitive
1. Antagonist binds with the same receptor as the agonist	Binds to another site of receptor
2. Antagonist resembles chemically with the agonist	Does not resemble
3. ***Parallel rightward shift of agonist DRC***	Flattening of agonist DRC
4. The ***same maximal response*** can be attained by increasing dose of agonist (surmountable antagonism)	Maximal response is suppressed (unsurmountable antagonism)

Contd...

Competitive (equilibrium type) KDT 7th/59	Noncompetitive
5. Intensity of response depends on the concentration of both agonist and antagonist	Maximal response depends only on the concentration of antagonist
6. Examples: Ach– Atropine Morphine–Naloxone	Diazepam– Bicuculline

Competitive and Irreversible Antagonists

◈ *Katzung 13th/23*

- In the presence of a fixed concentration of agonist, increasing concentrations of a reversible **competitive antagonist** ***progressively inhibit the agonist response; high antagonist concentrations prevent response completely.***
- Conversely, sufficiently high concentrations of agonist can surmount the effect of a given concentration of the antagonist; that is, the ***Emax*** *(It is the maximal response that can be produced by the drug)* ***for the agonist remains the same for any fixed concentration of antagonist***
- Because the **antagonism is competitive,** the presence of antagonist increases the agonist concentration required for a given degree of response and so The concentration (C') of an agonist required to produce a given effect in the presence of a fixed concentration ([I]) of competitive antagonist is greater than the agonist concentration (C) required to produce the same effect in the absence of the antagonist.

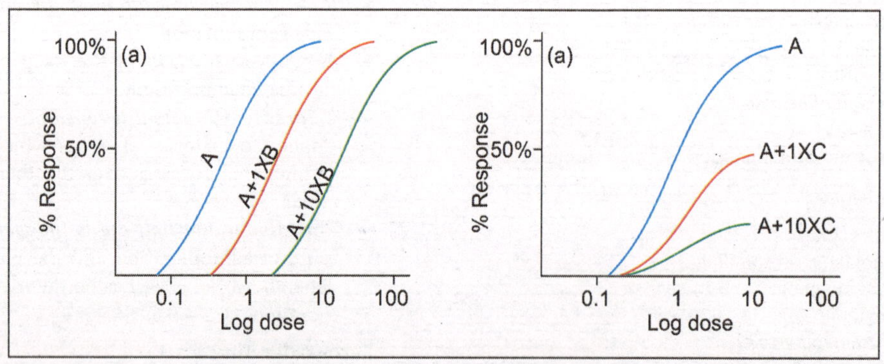

Fig: *(KDT 7th/59)*: Dose response curve showing competitive (a) and non-competitive (b) antagonism; A-agonist, B-competitive antagonist, C-Non-competitive antagonists

"**Potency** is the relationship between the dose of a drug and the therapeutic effect. It refers to the ***drug's strength***. A drug is considered potent when a small amount of the drug achieves the intended effect. Efficacy is the ability of a drug to produce the ***desired therapeutic*** effect. Efficacy means that the drug is effective. When comparing two drugs that work equally, the one with the lower dose has a higher potency. They have equal efficacy"- healthyliving.azcentral.com

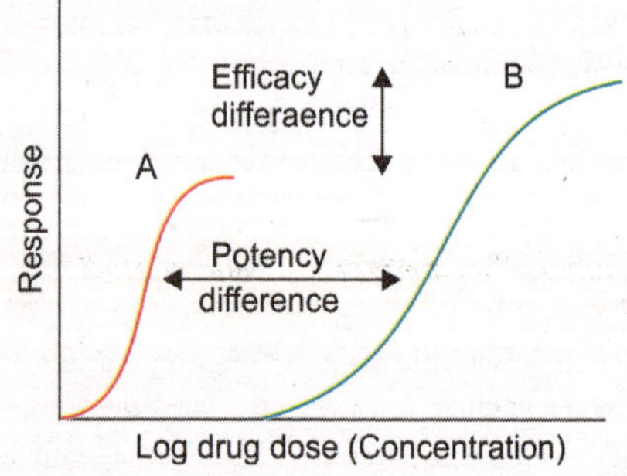

72. Ans. c. Bethanechol; d. Methacholine; e. Pilocarpine

[Ref: KDT 7th/102,105; Katzung 13th/120; Satoskar 25th/290-95]

The **direct-acting cholinomimetic drugs** can be divided on the basis of chemical structure into esters of choline (including acetylcholine) and alkaloids (such as muscarine and nicotine).

Anticholinesterase drugs are indirect acting drugs

Cholinergic Agonists

◈ *KDT 7th/102*

Choline esters	Alkaloids
Acetylcholine	Muscarine
Methacholine	Pilocarpine
Carbachol	Arecoline
Bethanechol	

Anticholinesterase-Reversible

◈ *KDT 7th/105*

Carbamates	Acridine
Physostigmine (Eserine)	Tacrine
Neostigmine	
Pyridostigmine	
Edrophonium	
Rivastigmine, ***Donepezil***	
Galantamine	

Anticholinesterase-Irreversible

◈ *KDT 7th/105*

Organophosphates	Carbamates
Dyflos (DFP)	Carbaryl* (SEVIN)
Echothiophate	Propoxur* (BAYGON)
Malathion*	*Insecticides
Diazinon* (TIK-20)	£Nerve gases for chemical warfare
Tabun£, Sarin£, Soman£	

73. Ans. a. Canagliflozin-Inhibitors of Sodium Glucose Transport-2; b. Acarbose- a-glucosidase inhibitor; d. Repaglinide -K+ ATP channel blocker

[Ref: KDT 7th/270; Satoskar 25th/895]

Classification of Oral Hypoglycemic Drugs

◈ *Satoskar 25th/895; KDT 7th/273*

- **Oral:**
  - **Stimulators of insulin release by beta cells (K^+_{ATP} channel modulators/blocker)** e.g., Sulfonylureas, Meglitinides (Repaglinide, Nateglinide)
  - **Inhibitors of hepatic gluconeogenesis, (AMPK activators)** e.g, Biguanides. (Metformin)
  - **Inhibitors of intestinal α-glucosidases, (α-glucosidases inhibitors)** e.g., Acarbose, Miglitol.
  - **Drugs which reduce insulin resistance, (PPAR activators)** e.g., Glitazones
    Inhibitors of dipeptidyl dipeptidase-4 (DPP-4) e.g. Sitagliptin, Linagliptin
  - **Inhibitors of Sodium Glucose Transport-2 (SGLT2)** e.g., Dapagliflozin, Canagliflozin
- **Parenteral:**
  - **Amylinomimetics,** e.g., Pramlinitide
  - **Glucagon Like peptide (GLP-1) agonists,** e.g., Exenatide, Liraglutide

74. Ans. c. Temozolomide

[Ref: CMDT 2017/1005; Harrison 19th/600; Davidson 22nd/1215; Satoskar 25th/830]

"Standard care for WHO grade IV **glioblastoma multiforme** is now combination radiotherapy with oral ***temozolomide chemotherapy***"-Davidson 22nd/1215

Grade IV Astrocytoma (Glioblastoma/GBM)

◈ *Harrison 19th/600*

- Glioblastoma accounts for the majority of high-grade astrocytomas.
- They are the most common malignant primary brain tumor
- Treatment involves maximal surgical resection followed by partial-field external-beam RT with concomitant ***temozolomide***, followed by 6–12 months of adjuvant ***temozolomide***.
- Implantation of biodegradable polymers containing the chemotherapeutic agent **carmustine** into the tumor bed after resection of the tumor also produces a modest improvement in survival.
- Treatment options for recurrent disease may include re-operation, **carmustine** wafers and alternate chemotherapeutic regimens. Reirradiation is rarely helpful. **Bevacizumab**, has activity in recurrent glioblastoma

Glioblastoma Multiforme

◈ *emedicine.medscape.com*

- **Temozolomide** is an orally active alkylating agent that is used for persons newly diagnosed with glioblastoma multiforme
- Carmustine (BCNU) and *cis* -platinum (cisplatin) have been the primary chemotherapeutic agents used against malignant gliomas.
- Genotyping of brain tumors may have applications in stratifying patients for clinical trials of various novel therapies.
- When used with ***irinotecan, bevacizumab*** improved 6-month survival in recurrent glioma patients to 46% compared with 21% in patients treated with ***temozolomide.***
- A small proportion of glioblastomas responds to ***gefitinib or erlotinib*** (tyrosine kinase inhibitors).

75. Ans. (All) a. Amiodarone; b. Propanolol; c. Diltiazem; d. Lidocaine; e. Procainamide

[Ref: KDT 7th/537-38; Satoskar 25th/406; Harrison 19th/473e-13; G and G 11th/907]

Ventricular Tachycardia

◈ *Pharmacotherapy by A. CHISHOLM-BURNS 2008/126-27*

- In the majority of patients with VT, the shape and appearance of the QRS complexes are consistent and similar and is referred to as **monomorphic VT**. However, some patients experience **polymorphic VT**, in which the shape and appearance of the QRS complexes vary.
- **Amiodarone** is considered the preferred first-line antiarrhythmic agent for management of VT, regardless of the patient's underlying LV function.
- In patients with normal LV function who do not respond to amiodarone, IV **procainamide** may be administered
- Data suggest superior efficacy of procainamide compared with that of **lidocaine**. However, in patients with HF due to LV dysfunction, procainamide should be avoided

Chronic Ventricular Tachycardia

◈ *KDT 7th/538*

- *Nonsustained VT- Suppression (oral **propranolol/ amiodarone**)*
- *Sustained VT- Abolition (i.v amiodarone ± propranolol or cardioversion or **propafenone/idocaine** (i.v)*
- *Sustained VT- Maintenance therapy (**amiodarone/sotalol,** implantable debrillator)*

Table: *(A.CHISHOLM-BURNS 2008/126)*: **Drugs for Termination of Ventricular Tachycardia**

Drug	Loading Dose	Maintenance Dose
Procainamide	12-17 mg/kg IV, no faster than 20 mg/minute	1-4 mg/minute continuous infusion
Lidocaine	0.5-0.75 mg/kg IV bolus Repeat every 5-10 minutes to a total of 3 mg/kg	1-4 mg/minute continuous infusion
Amiodarone	150 mg IV over 10 minutes	1 mg/minute continuous infusion for 6 hours, 0.5 mg/ minute for 18 hours

In patients who have experienced VT and are at risk for sudden cardiac death, implantation of an ***implantable cardioverter defibrillator*** *(ICD) is the treatment of choice.* ICDs have been found to be significantly more effective than antiarrhythmic agents such as ***amiodarone or sotalol*** for reducing the risk of sudden cardiac death; therefore, ICDs are preferred therapy. Combined pharmacotherapy with amiodarone and **a** β-blocker is more effective than monotherapy with sotalol or β-blockers for reduction in the frequency of ICD shocks"- *Pharmacotherapy by A. CHISHOLM-BURNS 2008/126*

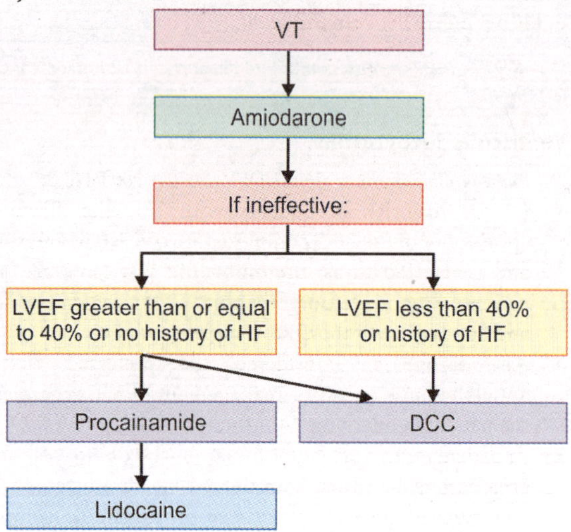

Fig: (Pharmacotherapy by A. CHISHOLM-BURNS 2008/127): Decision algorithm for termination of hemodynamically stable ventricular tachycardia. DCC, direct current cardioversion

"Hypertonic sodium bicarbonate (or hypertonic saline) for cardiac conduction delays and monomorphic ventricular tachycardia; ***lidocaine for monomorphic ventricular tachycardia*** (except when due to class Ib antiarrhythmics); ***magnesium, isoproterenol and overdrive pacing for polymorphic ventricular tachycardia;*** physostigmine for anticholinergic effects; naloxone for opioid effects; extracorporeal removal for some agents"-Harrison 19th/473e-13

"In stable patients with ***monomorphic VT*** and normal LV function, restoration of sinus rhythm is typically achieved with ***intravenous (IV) procainamide, amiodarone, or sotalol. Lidocaine*** may also be used, but this agent may have common and limiting side effects and, consequently, increase the overall mortality risk. A 12-lead electrocardiogram (ECG) is obtained before conversion"- emedicine.medscape.com

Outflow Tract Tachycardias

◈ *Braunwald's Heart Disease 8th/Chap 35*

- **Idiopathic VTs with monomorphic contours** can be divided into at least three types. Two types, ***paroxysmal VT and repetitive monomorphic VT***, appear to originate from the region of the right ventricular outflow tract.
- Vagal maneuvers, including adenosine, terminate the VT, whereas exercise, stress, isoproterenol infusion and rapid or premature stimulation can initiate or perpetuate the tachycardia. ***Beta blockers and verapamil*** can suppress this tachycardia as well.

Repetitive Monomorphic Ventricular Tachycardia

◈ *Hurst's The Heart 12th/Chap 39,43*

- Repetitive monomorphic ventricular tachycardia (RMVT), also referred to as right ventricular outflow tract VT is characterized by repetitive salvos of monomorphic nonsustained VT.
- ***β-Adrenergic receptor blockers and calcium channel antagonists*** are usually the first choice for the treatment of symptomatic VT, but their efficacy in preventing arrhythmia recurrence is modest.
- Verapamil was found to eliminate exercise-induced RMVT in 56 percent of patients who had RMVT induced during stress testing. In general, ***βblockers*** are effective in approximately 25 to 50 percent of patients, whereas ***calcium channel blockers*** are effective in approximately 25 to 30 percent
- Diltiazem is a ***calcium channel blocker****-KDT*
- **Propanolol-** ***βblockers***

76. Ans. a. Multibacillaryleprosy is treated by 3 drugs; d. Post-treatment surveillance for multibacillary leprosy is for 5 years; e. Clofazimine is first line drug;

[Ref: Harrison 20th/1264-65; Neena Khanna 5th/272-85; Park 25th/354]

Surveillance

◈ *Park 25th/354*

Paucibacillary: *Examined clinically at least once a year for a minimum of 2 years after completion of treatment*
Multibacillary: *Examined clinically at least once a year for a* ***minimum of 5 years after completion of treatment***

Duration of Treatment

◈ *Park 25th/351*

Multibacillary: MB blisterpacks for 12 months within 18 months
Paucibacillary: *PB blisterpacks for 6 months, within 9 months*

Table: *(Harrison 20th/1264)*: **Antimicrobial Regimens Recommended for the Treatment of Leprosy in Adults**

Form of Leprosy	More intensive regimen	WHO Recommended regimen (1982)
Tuberculoid (Paucibacillary)	Dapsone (100 mg/d) for 5 years	Dapsone (100 mg/d, unsupervised) plus rifampin (600 mg/month, supervised) for 6 months
Lepromatous (multibacillary)	Rifampin (600 mg/d) for 3 years plus dapsone (100 mg/d) indefinitely	Dapsone (100 mg/d) plus clofazimine (50 mg/d), unsupervised; and rifampin (600 mg) plus clofazimine (300 mg) monthly (supervised) for 1-2 years)

Leprosy Treatment

Harrison 20th/1264

- For treatment purposes, the WHO originally classified patients with few bacteria in the dermis (BI <2) as paucibacillary and those with many bacteria (BI >2) as multibacillary.
- The WHO recommended that **paucibacillary leprosy** in adults be treated with 100 mg of dapsone daily and 600 mg of rifampin monthly (supervised) for 6 months
- As an alternative for patients with single lesion paucibacillary leprosy, the WHO recommended a single dose of rifampin (600 mg), ofloxacin (400 mg) and minocycline (100 mg).
- The recommendation for **multibacillary leprosy** in adults was 100 mg of dapsone plus 50 mg of clofazimine daily (unsupervised) and with 600 mg of rifampin plus 300 mg of clofazimine monthly (supervised). Originally, the WHO recommended that lepromatous patients be treated for 2 years or until smears became negative (generally in ~5 years).
- In subsequent years, the WHO mandated several modifications to their original multidrug-treatment recommendation, primarily related to leprosy classification criteria and treatment duration

77. **Ans.** **a. Clofazimine; b. Ofloxacin d. Clarithromycin e. Moxifloxacin**

[Ref: KDT 8th/836-37 Park 24th/340-41; Goodman and Gilman's 11th/1204; Satoskar Pharma 24th/771-72; Rang and Dale 8th/640]

All above mentioned drug can be used in leprosy patients alternative to rifampin, but minocycline can cause hepatitis(Harrison), so excluded from answer

Alternative Regimens

KDT 8th/836-37

Many alternative regimens incorporating newer antileprotic drugs have been investigated. However, these are used only in case of ***rifampin-resistance*** or when it is impossible/inadvisable to employ the standard MDT regimen. Some of these are:

- **Intermittent ROM:** Rifampin 600 mg + ofloxacin 400 mg + minocycline 100 mg are given once a month for 3–6 month for PBL and for 12 or 24 month for MBL cases, without any drug in between
- **Single dose ROM:** A single dose of rifampin + ofloxacin + minocycline was given for single lesion PBL, but this has been discontinued.
- ***Cloflazimine*** 50 mg + any two of ofloxacin 400 mg/ minocycline 100 mg/clarithromycin 500 mg daily for 6 month, followed by clofazimine 50 mg daily for additional 18 months.
- **Four durg regimen** of rifampin 600 mg + sparfloxacin 200 mg + clarithromycin 500 mg + minocycline 100 mg daily for 12 weeks has yielded equivalent clinical improvement in MBL cases to standard 12 month MDT.
- **In case of refusal to accept clofazimine:** ofloxacin 400 mg or minocycline 100 mg daily can be substituted for it in the standard MDT. Use of ethionamide as a substitute is not recommended.
- **Intermittent RMMx: Moxifloxacin** 400 mg + minocycline 200 mg + rifampin 600 mg is administered once a month: 6 doses given for PBL and 12 doses given for MBL cases have produced rapid and marked clinical response.

Table: *(Goodman and Gilman's 11th/1204)*

Mycobacterial Species	First-Line Therapy	Alternative Agents
M. leprae	Dapsone + rifampin +/-clofazimine	Minocycline; moxifloxacin or gatifloxacin; clofazimine clarithromycin; ethionamide

"Other antimicrobial agents active against M. leprae in animal models and at the usual daily doses used in clinical trials include ***ethionamide/prothionamide;*** the aminoglycosides streptomycin, kanamycin and amikacin (but not gentamicin or tobramycin); ***minocycline; clarithromycin***; and several fluoroquinolones, particularly ofloxacin. Next to rifampin, ***minocycline, clarithromycin and ofloxacin*** appear to be most bactericidal for M. leprae, but these drugs have not been used extensively in leprosy control programs. Most recently, ***rifapentine and moxifloxacin*** have been found to be especially potent against M. leprae in mice. In a clinical trial in lepromatous leprosy, moxifloxacin was profoundly bactericidal, matched in potency only by rifampin"- ***Harrison 19th/1126***

In Case the Reference Laboratory Reports that the Patient is Harbouring rifampicin Resistant M. leprae the following Treatment Should be given

www.leprosy-ila.org/sit

- Administration of 50 mg of clofazimine, together with 400 mg of ofloxacin and 100 mg of minocycline, daily for six months;

- Administration of 50 mg of clofazimine, together with 100 mg of minocycline or 400 mg of ofloxacin daily for at least an additional 18 months.
- The above-mentioned treatment regimen is also to be used for patients reported to be harbouring both rifampicin and dapsone resistant M. leprae

Drug-causing Hepatitis

◈ *(Harrison 20th/2370-Table)*

- Halothane, fluothane
- Flutamide
- Isoniazid, rifampicin, nitrofurantoin, telithromycin, *minocycline*, pyrazinamide,
- trovafloxacine
- Phenytoin, carbamazepine, valproic acid, phenobarbital
- Iproniazid, amitriptyline, trazodone, venlafaxine, fluoxetine, paroxetine, duloxetine,
- sertraline, nefazodonee
- Ketoconazole, fluconazole, itraconazole
- Methyldopa, captopril, enalapril, lisinopril, losartan
- Ibuprofen, indomethacin, diclofenac, sulindac, bromfenac
- Risperidone
- Zidovudine, didanosine, stavudine, nevirapine, ritonavir, indinavir, tipranavir, zalcitabine
- Nifedipine, verapamil, diltiazem
- Tacrine
- Chlorothiazide
- Oxyphenisatinc
- Atomoxetine
- Troglitazone, acarbose

Mixed Hepatitis/Cholestatic

◈ *Harrison 20th/2370-Table*

- Amoxicillin-clavulanic acid, trimethoprim-sulfamethoxazole
- Clindamycin
- Terbinafine
- Cyproheptadine
- Azathioprine
- Nicotinic acid, lovastatin, ezetimibe

78. Ans. a. Salbutamol and leukotrienes; d. Adrenaline and histamine

[Ref: KDT 8th/68; Satoskar 25th/42]

Physiological Antagonists

- Physiological antagonists are those that produce opposite action by acting on different receptors. Example
  - Histamine causes bronchoconstriction viaH1 receptors and this action is antagonized by adrenaline which cause bronchodilodation through β2 receptors
  - Leukotrienescause bronchoconstriction via cystinyl leukotriene receptors and this action is antagonized by salbutamol which causes bronchodilatation through β2 receptors.

Receptor Antagonists (Pharmalogical Antagonists)

- Receptor antagonists are those drugs that blocks the action of agonist by acting on same receptors
- For example Isoprenaline is β1 and β2 receptor agonist while propranolol has antagonistic action on β1 and β2 receptors

About option a and b

◈ *KDT 8th/141*

Adrenaline ($\alpha_1 + \alpha_2 + \beta_1 + \beta_2$ +weak β_3 agonist), isoprenaline ($\beta_1 + \beta_2 + \beta_3$ agonist) and salbutamol (β_2 agonist) → all three are sympathomimetic drugs (not antagonists)

79. Ans. c. Vincristine; e. Bleomycin;

[Ref: KDT 8th/924;Katzung13th/926,928,933; Satoskar 25th/834]

"Vincristine Bone marrow depression is minimal"*KDT 8th/924*

"Bleomycin Bone marrow depression is minimal"-*Satoskar 25th/834*

"Cisplatin: Dose-related mylosuppression can occur"- *Satoskar 25th/834*

"**Vinblastine:** Bone marrow depression is more prominent"- *KDT 8th/924*

Methotrexate: It exerts major toxicity on bone marrow- low dose given repeatedly cause megaloblastic anaemia, but high dose produce pancytopenia"- *KDT 8th/921*

80. Ans. a. Pyruvate dehydrogenase; b. Hexokinase; d. Glucose 6 phosphate;

[Ref: KDT 8th/885; Satoskar 25th/781]

"Primaquine: The most important toxic potential is dose related hemolysis, methaemoglobinaemia, tachypnea and cyanosis. These are due to oxidant property of primaquine. **Those with G-6-PD**(Glucose-6-phosphate dehydrogenase) **deficiency are highly sensitive and hemolytic anemia can occur. Therefore it should be avoided in pregnancy as fetus with G6PD deficiency may develop hemolytic anemia**"- *KDT 8th/885*

MICROBIOLOGY

81. Ans. a. Mycoplasma hominis, b. Mycoplasma genitalium, c. Chlamydia trachomatis

[Ref: Ananthanarayan 10th/393; Harrison 19th/870-71; Greenwood 16th/385-86; Jawetz 27th/792; Microbiolgy by Baveja 5th/601]

Non-gonococcal urethritis (NGU): ***Chlamydia trachomatis (Type D-K), Mycoplasma genitalium and M.hominis***"- *Microbiology by Baveja 5th/601*

"**Urethritis in males:** *Neisseria gonorrhoeae,* ***Chlamydia trachomatis, Mycoplasma genitalium, Ureaplasma urealyticum*** **(subspecies** ***urealyticum*****),** ***Trichomonas vaginalis,*** **HSV and** *adenovirus."- Harrison 19th/870*

"**Cystitis/urethritis in female:** ***C. trachomatis, N. gonorrhoeae,*** **HSV**"- *Harrison 19th/870*

Nongonococcal Urethritis (NGU)

◈ *www.ashasexualhealth.org*

NGU is an infection of the urethra caused by pathogens (germs) other than gonorrhea. Several kinds of pathogens can cause NGU, including:

- *Chlamydia trachomatis*
- *Ureaplasma urealyticum*

A & E

- *Trichomonas vaginalis (rare)*
- *Herpes simplex virus (rare)*
- *Adenovirus*
- *Haemophilus vaginalis*
- *Mycoplasm genitalium*

Ureaplasma urealyticum causes non-gonococcal urethritis *and M.hominis and M.genitalium causes genital tract infections- Ananthanarayan 10th/393*

*"**M.genitalium has been strongly implicated as a cause of acute and chronic NGU**, but there is no evidence that this or other mycoplasma are a cause of acute or chronic prostatitis"- Greenwood 16th/386*

82. Ans. e. Leptospira

[Ref: Ananthanarayan 10th/376; Harrison 19th/1132]

Order* spirochetales** contain two family- ***Spirochaetaceae (spirochaetes/spirochetes) and Leptospiraceae

Spirochetes

◈ *Ananthanarayan 10th/376*

- Elongated, motile, flexible bacteria twisted spirally along the long axis are termed ***spirochetes*** (from speira, meaning coil and chaite, meaning hair)
- **Spirochetes** belong to the order spirochetales, comprising 2 families- ***Spirochaetaceae and leptospiraceae***
- Spirochaetaceae contains genera ***spirochaeta, cristispira, treponema and borrelia***
- Leptospiraceae containing the genus ***leptospira, leptonema and turneriella***
- The Spirochaetales include four genera that are pathogenic for humans and for a variety of other animals: ***Leptospira species, which cause leptospirosis; Borrelia species, which cause relapsing fever and Lyme disease; Brachyspira species, which cause intestinal infections; and Treponema species, which cause the diseases known collectively as treponematoses***- *Harrison 19th/1132*
- The *Treponema* species include *T. pallidum* subspecies *pallidum*, which causes venereal syphilis; *T. pallidum* subspecies *pertenue*, which ***causes yaws***; *T. pallidum* subspecies *endemicum*, which causes ***endemic syphilis or bejel***; and *T. carateum*, which causes ***pinta***- *Harrison 19th/1132*

83. Ans. b. Icosahedral symmetry; c. HPV type 16 and 18 causes cervical cancer; d. Recently nine valent vaccine passed phase 3 clinical trial; e. 5 genera of HPV identified

[Ref: Ananthanarayan 10th/557; Harrison 19th/1197-98; Baveja 5th/523-24]

Human papillomavirus (HPV)

◈ *Harrison 19th/1197-98*

- HPV is an ***icosahedral, nonenveloped, double-stranded DNA*** virus
- HPV capsid is non-enveloped, having a T = 7 ***icosahedral symmetry*** formed"- www.ncbi.nlm.nih.gov
- ***More than 125 HPV types*** have been identified and are numerically designated according to a unique L1 gene sequence.
- Approximately 40 HPV types are regularly found in the anogenital tract and are subdivided into high-risk and low-risk categories on the basis of the associated risk of cervical cancer. For example, HPV-6 and HPV-11 cause genital warts and ~10% of low-grade cervical lesions and are thus designated low risk. ***HPV-16 and HPV-18 cause dysplastic lesions and invasive cancers of the cervix*** and are considered high risk.
- HPV types 16, 18, 31, 33, 35, 39, 45, 51, 52, 56, 58 and 59 are carcinogenic in the uterine cervix. HPV-16 is particularly virulent and causes 50% of ***cervical cancers. Worldwide, HPV-16 and HPV-18 cause 70% of cervical squamous cell carcinomas*** and 85% of cervical adenocarcinomas. Oncogenic types other than HPV-16 and HPV-18 cause the remaining 30% of cervical cancers.
- Over **170 human papillomavirus types** have been completely sequenced. They have been **divided into 5 genera**: ***Alpha-papillomavirus, Betapapillomavirus, Gammapapillomavirus, Mupapillomavirus and Nupapillomavirus***-en.wikipedia.org
- *Family papovaviridae contain two genera- polyomavirus and papillomavirus. Papillomavirus contains several genera, **five of which cause human infection**- Ananthanarayan 10th/557*
- The 9-valent HPV vaccine, which protects against HPV ***types 6, 11, 16, 18, 31, 33, 45, 52 and 58***, is safe and effective and will further reduce the incidence of HPV infection, as well as HPV-related cancers- *www.ncbi.nlm.nih.gov*

Clinical trial of 9-Valent Human Papillomavirus Vaccine

◈ *www.ncbi.nlm.nih.go*

A Randomized, Double-Blind, **Phase III Study** of the Immunogenicity and Safety of a 9-Valent Human Papillomavirus L1 Virus-Like Particle Vaccine (V503) Versus Gardasil® in 9-15-Year-Old Girls:

- **RESULTS**- 2015 Sep
- The HPV 6/11/16/18 immune responses elicited by the 9vHPV vaccine were comparable with those elicited by the qHPV vaccine. All participants (except 1 for HPV 45) receiving the 9vHPV vaccine seroconverted for HPV 31/33/45/52/58. The 9vHPV and qHPV vaccines showed comparable safety profiles, although the incidence of injection-site swelling was higher in the 9vHPV vaccine group.

Phase IV prospective study measuring the immunogenicity (neutralizing antibody titles against each HPV vaccine genotype) of the 9-valent vaccine against HPV (Gardasil9®Merck, three doses at 0, 2 and 6 months) in HIV-positive women aged 15-40 years with fully suppressed HIV viremia on combined antiretroviral therapy. The safety of the vaccination (local or systemic reaction and impact on HIV viral control and immunodeficiency level) will be assessed. The cellular immune response will be assessed in a subgroup of patients.

Anticipated study start date	January 8, 2018
Estimated primary completion date	January 8, 2020
Estimated study completion date	January 8, 2021

84. Ans. c. Predominantly found in Africa; d. Spreads by direct contact with the blood or body fluids; e. Currently there is no specific treatment for this disease

[Ref: Jawetz 27th/559; Community Medicine by Piyush Gupta 1st/337-38; Park 24th/374; Ananthanarayan 10th/562-63; Harrison 19th/1323-29]

Ebola virus has helical symmetry and belong to filovirus

Flavivirus and cause widespread morbidity and mortality throughout the world. Some of the mosquitoes-transmitted viruses include: **Yellow Fever, Dengue Fever, Japanese encephalitis, West Nile viruses and Zika virus**"- www.cdc.gov

Ebola Virus

◈ *Harrison 19th/1323-28*

- The family **Filoviridae** comprises two antigenically and genetically distinct genera: *Marburgvirus* and *Ebolavirus.*
- Typical filovirus particles contain a ***single linear, negative-sense, single-stranded RNA*** arranged in a ***helical nucleocapsid.***
- After an **incubation period** of ***~7–10 days*** (range, ***3–16days***), the patient abruptly develops fever, severe headache, malaise, myalgia, nausea and vomiting. Continued fever joined by diarrhea (often severe), chest pain (accompanied by cough), prostration and depressed mentation.
- From 1976 (The first Ebola case), ***there have been around 20 Ebola epidemics which have mostly confined its boundaries to sub-saharan Africa***"- *Piyush Gupta 1st/337*
- **African Hemorrhagic Fevers (Marburg and Ebola Viruses)**: The large filovirus genome is ***single-stranded, nonsegmented, negative-sense RNA*** - *Jawetz 27th/559*

Ebola Virus

◈ *Park 24th/374*

- Incubation period is 2-21 days and is not infective during this period
- Case fatality rate may be as high as 70%
- The virus is transmitted through ***direct contact with blood, organs, body secretions or other body fluids*** of infected animals like chimpanzees, gorillas, monkeys, fruit bats etc.
- Human to human transmission is through blood or body fluids of an infected symptomatic person or through exposure to objects (such as needle) that have been contaminated with infected secretions
- It is ***not transmitted through air, water, or food***
- The illness is characterized by sudden onset of fever, intense weakness, muscle pain, headache, sorethroat, vomiting, diarrhea, rash, impaired kidney and liver function and in some both internal and external bleeding
- Currently there is ***no specific treatment for this disease***
- There is ***no vaccine against ebola***
- "Human infections typically occur through ***direct exposure of skin lesions or mucosal surfaces to contaminated bodily fluids or material or by parenteral inoculation (e.g., via accidental needle sticks or reuse of needles in poorly equipped hospitals)***" (Harrison 19th/1326-27)
- "Treatment of ebola is ***entirely supportive because no accepted/approved, efficacious, specific antiviral agents or vaccines are yet available. Pain management and administration of antipyretics and antiemetics should always be considered***" (Harrison 19th/1328)

85. Ans. b. Granuloma inguinale causes donovanosis; c. Haemophilus Ducrei causes chancroid

[Ref: Ananthanarayan 10th/404; Harrison 19th/880, 1012-13; Jawetz 27th/761]

Table: *(Harrison 19th/880)*: **Clinical Features of Genital Ulcer**

Feature	Syphilis	Herpes	Chancroid	Lymphogranuloma Venereum	Donovanosis
Incubation period	9-90 day	2-7 days	1-14 days	3 day-6 weeks	1-4 weeks (up to months)
Early primary lesion	Papule	Vesicle	Pustule	Papule, pustule, or vesicle	Papule
No. of lesion	Usually one	Multiple	Usually multiple, may coalesce	Usually one; often not detected, despite lymphadenopathy	Variable
Diameter	5-15 mm	1-2 mm	Variable	2-10 mm	Variable
Edges	Sharply demarcated, elevated, round, or oval	Erythematous	Undermined, ragged, irregular	Elevated, round or oval	Elevated irregular
Depth	Superficial or deep	Superficial	Excavated	Superficial or deep	Elevated
Base	Smooth, non-purulent, relatively nonvascular	Serous, erythematous nonvascular	Purulent, bleeds easily	Variable, nonvascular	Red and velvety bleeds readily
Induration	Firm	None	Soft	Occasionally firm	Firm
Pain	Uncommon	Frequent tender	Usually very tender	Variable	Uncommon
Lymphadenopathy	Firm, nontender, bilateral	Firm, tender, often bilateral with initial episode	Tender, may suppurate, loculated, usually unilateral	Tender, may suppurate, loculated, usually unilateral	None; pseudobuboes

Granuloma Inguinale (also known as Donovanosis) Calymmatobacterium Granulomatis)

◈ *Ananthanarayan 10th/404; Harrison 19th/880*

- It is a bacterial disease caused by Klebsiella granulomatis (formerly known as Calymmatobacterium granulomatis)
- It begin as ***painless papule*** on genitalia- *Ananthanarayan 10th/404*
- *Presents as one or more **painless granulomatous lesions**-Lippincott Microbiology 3rd/127*
- **Extragenital lesions** occur in 6% of cases and may involve the lip, gums, cheek, palate, pharynx, larynx and chest. Hematogenous spread with involvement of liver and bone has been reported. During pregnancy, lesions tend to develop more quickly and respond more slowly to treatment. Polyarthritis and osteomyelitis are rare complications. In newborn infants, donovanosis may present with ear infection.

Haemophilus Ducreyi

◈ *Harrison 19th/198e-1*

- *Haemophilus ducreyi* is the etiologic agent of ***chancroid (soft chancre)*** a sexually transmitted disease characterized by genital ulceration and inguinal adenitis.
- In addition to being a cause of morbidity in itself, chancroid is associated with HIV infection because of the role played by genital ulceration in HIV transmission. Chancroid increases the efficiency of transmission of and the degree of susceptibility to HIV infection.
- The ulcers are ***painful and bleed easily***; little or no inflammation of the surrounding skin is evident.
- Approximately half of patients develop enlarged, ***tender inguinal lymph nodes***, which frequently become fluctuant and ***spontaneously rupture***. Patients usually seek medical care after 1–3 weeks of painful symptoms
- The ***infection remain localized***- *Baveja 5th/315*
- *The infection remains localized, spreading only to the regional **lymph nodes which are enlarged and painful**-Ananthanarayan 10th/337*

Primary Syphilis

◈ *Harrison 19th/1134*

- The typical primary chancre usually begins as a ***single painless papule*** that rapidly becomes eroded and usually becomes ***indurated***, with a characteristic cartilaginous consistency on palpation of the edge and base of the ulcer. Multiple primary lesions are seen in a minority of patients.
- ***Regional (usually inguinal) lymphadenopathy*** accompanies the primary syphilitic lesion, appearing within 1 week of lesion onset. The nodes are firm, nonsuppurative and ***painless***.

Secondary Syphilis

◈ *Harrison 19th/1134-35*

- ***Constitutional signs and symptoms*** that may accompany or precede secondary syphilis include sore throat (15–30%), fever (5–8%), weight loss (2–20%), malaise (25%), anorexia (2–10%), headache (10%) and meningismus (5%).
- *Acute meningitis* occurs in only 1–2% of cases
- Less common complications of secondary syphilis include hepatitis, nephropathy, gastrointestinal involvement (hypertrophic gastritis, patchy proctitis, or a rectosigmoid mass), arthritis and periostitis.

86. Ans. a. Demonstration of school of fish appearance of bacilli; b. Culture of H. ducreyi from an aspirate of suppurative lymph nodes

[Ref: Ananthanarayan 10th/337; Harrison 19th/1013]

Patient is presenting feature of chancroid

A clinical diagnosis of **donovanosis** made by an experienced practitioner on the basis of the lesion's appearance usually has a high positive predictive value. The diagnosis is confirmed by microscopic identification of ***Donovan bodies*** in tissue smears-*Harrison 19th/198e-1*

Haemophilus Ducreyi

◈ *Ananthanarayan 10th/337*

- **Chancroid or soft sore** *is a venereal disease characterized by **tender non-indurated irregular ulcers on the genitalia***
- *The bacilli may be arranged in small groups or whorls or in parallel chains, giving a **'school of fish' or 'rail road track' appearance***
- *The infection remains localized, spreading only to the regional **lymph nodes which are enlarged and painful***

Haemophilus Ducreyi

◈ *Harrison 19th/1012-13*

- Infection is acquired as the result of a break in the epithelium during sexual contact with an infected individual.
- ***After an incubation period of 4–7 days***, the initial lesion-a papule with surrounding erythema, appears. In 2 or 3 days, the papule evolves into a pustule, which spontaneously ruptures and forms a sharply circumscribed ulcer that generally is not indurated
- The ***ulcers are painful and bleed easily***; little or no inflammation of the surrounding skin is evident.
- Approximately half of patients develop ***enlarged, tender inguinal lymph nodes***, which frequently become fluctuant and spontaneously rupture.
- Patients usually seek medical care after 1–3 weeks of painful symptoms.
- Multiple ulcers can coalesce to ***form giant ulcers***. Ulcers can appear and then resolve, with inguinal adenitis and suppuration following 1–3 weeks later; this clinical picture can be *confused with that of lymphogranuloma venereum*
- *Clinical diagnosis of chancroid is often inaccurate and* laboratory confirmation should be attempted in suspected cases.
- An **accurate diagnosis** of chancroid relies on ***culture of H. ducreyi*** from the lesion or from an aspirate of suppurative lymph nodes.

Diagnosis of Chancroid

◈ *Harrison 19th/1013*

- Clinical diagnosis of chancroid is often inaccurate and laboratory confirmation should be attempted in suspected cases. An accurate diagnosis of chancroid relies on culture of

H. ducreyi from the lesion or from an aspirate of suppurative lymph nodes. Since the organism can be difficult to grow, the use of selective and supplemented media is necessary. No polymerase chain reaction assay for *H. ducreyi* is commercially available; such tests can be performed by Clinical Laboratory Improvement Amendment (CLIA)–certified clinical laboratories that have developed their own assays.

- A **probable diagnosis of chancroid** can be made when the following criteria are met: ***(1) one or more painful genital ulcers; (2) no evidence of Treponema pallidum infection by dark-field examination of ulcer exudate or by a negative serologic test for syphilis performed at least 7 days after ulcer onset; (3) a typical clinical presentation for chancroid; and (4) a negative test for herpes simplex virus in the ulcer exudate.***

87. Ans. c. Coagulase negative

[Ref: Ananthanarayan 10th/210-13; Harrison 19th/964; Jawetz 27th/214]

β ***hemolysis and bacitracin resistance occur in both***

Staphylococcus Aureus

- ***Coagulase Positive****: Ananthanarayan 10th/210*
- ***Beta type of hemolyisis*** *on blood agar-Microbiology by Baveja 5th/175*

"Streptococci- ***coagulase negative****" Ananthanarayan 10th/218*

"Lancefield group B consists of a single species, **S. agalactiae,** which is definitively identified with specific antiserum to the group B cell wall–associated carbohydrate antigen. A streptococcal isolate can be classified presumptively as GBS on the basis of biochemical tests, including hydrolysis of ***sodium hippurate*** (in which 99% of isolates are positive), ***hydrolysis of bile esculin*** (in which 99–100% are negative), bacitracin susceptibility (in ***which 92% are resistant***) and ***production of CAMP factor*** (in which 98–100% are positive). CAMP factor is a phospholipase produced by GBS that causes ***synergistic hemolysis with β lysin produced by certain strains of S. aureus***"-*Harrison 19th/969*

Staphylococci produce ***catalase***, which converts hydrogen peroxide into water and oxygen. The catalase test differentiates the staphylococci, which are positive, from the ***streptococci, which are negative***- *Jawetz 27th/205*

Table: *Ananthanarayan 10th/210*

Species or common name	Lancefield group	Hemolysis	Laboratory test
S. pyogenes	A	Beta	Bacitracin-sensitive, PYR test-positive; Ribose not fermnted
S. agalactiae	B	Beta	CAMP test, Hippurate hydrolysis

Bacitracin Test *microbeonline.com*

- Positive: *Streptococcus pyogenes*
- Negative: *Streptococcus agalactiae*

The **bacitracin test** is useful for ***differentiating β-hemolytic Group A streptococci from β-hemolytic non-Group A streptococci. This is important because most streptococcal*** diseases are caused by Group A streptococci. The bacitracin test can also be used to differentiate the ***bacitracin-resistant Staphylococcus*** from the bacitracin-**susceptible** *Micrococcus*"-*www.austincc.edu.*

88. Ans. b. Taenia saginata is beef tapeworm; c. Infection is acquired by ingestion of cysticercus in raw beef; d. Infectious form to animal is egg;

[Ref:Paniker 7th/120-26;Chatterjee 13th/151-52]

Taenia Saginata & Taenia Solium

◈ *Paniker 7th/120-26; Chatterjee 13th/151-52*

- Taenia saginata: The beef tapeworm.
- Taenia solium: The pork tapeworm.
- Taenia saginata (beef tapeworm) is much more prevalent than Taenia Solium (Pork tapeworm).
- Habitat is small intestine (upper jejunum).
- **Definitive host is man**
- **Intermediate host** is cattle (cow or buffalo) for T saginata and Pig for T solium.
- **Mode of infection of tapeworms**
  a. T. saginata→Under cooked beef containg cysticercus bovis.
  b. ***T. solium→ Undercooked pork*** containg cysticercus cellulosae & rarely by ingestion of egg (autoinfection)
    - Occasionally man gets infected in the same way as pig, by ingestion of eggs (either by drinking contaminated water or by eating uncooked vegetables infected with eggs). In this cycle man acts both as definitive as well as intermediate host.

89. Ans. a. Caused by streptococcus pyogenes; b. Superficial skin lesion; c. True regarding erysipelas; d. True regarding erysipelas:

[Ref: Manipal Surgery 4th/24; Neena Khanna 5th/266-67;Roxburg 17th/44]

Erysipelas

◈ *Manipal Surgery 4th/24; Roxburg 17th/44*

- It is caused mostly by **streptococcus pyogenes** (group A Beta hemolytic streptococcus).
- **Erysipelas** is a ***superficial skin infection*** affecting upper dermis and extends into the superficial lymphatic.
- Symptoms and signs of erysipelas are usually abrupt in onset and often accompanied by fevers, chills and shivering.
- Erysipelas predominantly affects the skin of the lower limbs, but when it involves the face it can have a characteristic butterfly distribution on the cheeks and across the bridge of the nose.
- **Facial erysipelas, if untreated may prove fatal**- Neena Khanna 5th/267
- **The individual may report having sore throat (pharyngitis) or prior injuries to skin**
- The affected skin has a very sharp, raised border.

- It is bright red, firm and swollen. It may be finely dimpled (like an orange skin).
- It may be blisthered and in severe cases may become necrotic.
- Bleeding into the skin may cause purpura.

90. Ans. None (all options are correct)

[Ref: Ananthanarayan 10th/615-16;Harrison 20th/1529-30]

Candida Albican

◈ *Ananthanarayan 10th/615-16*
- Yeast like fungus
- It is Dimorphic
- Forms true hyphae
- It forms germ tubes within 2 hours when incubated on human serum at 37 degree centigrade ***(Reynold-Braude phenomenon)***
- Candida is a small, thin-walled, ovoid yeast that measures 4–6 μm in diameter and reproduces by budding. Organisms of this genus occur in three forms in tissue: blastospores, pseudohyphae and hyphae- *Harrison 20th/1529*
- A change from the blastospore stage to the pseudohyphal and hyphal stages is generally considered integral to *Candida's* penetration into tissue.- *Harrison 20th/1529*

91. Ans. d. Septate; e. Forms hyphae.

[Ref: Ananthanarayan 10th/612-13;Harrison 20th/1532-33;Baveja Microbiology 5th/559]

"Subcutaneous mycosis are caused by: mycetoma, chromoblastomycosis, sporotrichosis & rhinosporidiosis" *Baveja Microbiology 5th/547*

Aspergillosis

◈ *Ananthanarayan 10th/612-13*
- Cause Opportunistic mycosis
- A. niger is main pathogen
- Non-pigmented septate hyphae with characteristic dichomatous branching(at an angle of approx. 45 degree)- *Baveja Microbiology 5th/559*
- This hyaline (nonpigmented), septate, branching mold produces vast numbers of conidia (spores) on stalks above the surface of mycelial growth- *Harrison 20th/1532*
- 3 clinical form of systemic aspergillosis: respiratory disease, invasive aspergillosis & superficial infection

92. Ans. a. Zinc oxide; e. Copper oxide;

[Ref: www.ncbi.nlm.nih.gov]

Chemistry	Organisms	Proposed mechanism
ZnO	**Staphylococcus, Escherrichia coli**	ROS inhibition, membrane disruption
ZnO ions	*Pseudomonas aeruginosa, S aureus Candida albleris*	ROS inhibition
SNP	*E. coli, vibrio cholera, salmonella lyphi, P. aeruginosa*	Membrane disruption Ag ion interference with DNA replication
SNP	HIV-I	Binds to gp 120, inhibits binding to target cell
SNP	TB strains, *Candida sp*	Membrane disruption, ROS inhibition
SNP	Leishmania sp., Microfilria sp.	ROS inhibition
Cu	E. coli bacillus subtilis	Protein inactivation
CuO	**S aureus, MRSA, P. aeruginosa**	Membrane disruption
Fe_3O_4	*S. aureus. staphylococcus Epidermitis*	ROS inhibition, membrane disruption
Al_2O_3	*E. coli, B. subtilis, pseudomonas fluarrences*	ROS inhibition, Cell penetration, flocculation
TiO_2	*E. coli*	Membrane disruption
Chitosan	E. coli, S aureus, Interococcus sp. P. aeruginosa C. albious	Flocculation, membrane disruption chelation, enzyme dysfunction

FORENSIC MEDICINE

93. Ans a. Cocaine

[Ref: Reddy 34th/561; Parikh 7th/669]

Cocaine Habit/Chronic Cocaine Poisoning

◈ *Parikh 7th/669; Reddy 34th/561*
- ***Magnan's symptom*** or ***cocaine bugs*** is characteristic.
- In this there is feeling as if grains of sand are lying under the skin or some small insects are creeping on the skin giving rise to itching sensation (formication, tactile hallucination) with resultant excoriation, leading to irregular scratches and ulcers.

94. Ans. a. Useful in dead person; c. Transparency of root is most reliable component; e. Used for age estimation

[Ref: Reddy 34th/67; Parikh 7th/60; V V Pillay 18th/87; Principles of Forensic Medicine and Toxicology By Rajesh Bardale 1st/64-65]

Disadvantage of gustafson's method: cannot be used in living person"- *www.ijahs.net*

Advantage of Gustafson's Method

◈ *Rajesh Bardale 1st/64*
- Useful in adult population
- Fairly reliable method

Disadvantage of Gustafson's Method

Rajesh Bardale 1st/64-65

- ***It can not be used in living person, only in dead when extraction of a tooth is allowed***
- Too many age related changes needed to be considered making the method time-consuming
- The assessment of the scores is the result of a subjective evaluation of the changes

Gustafson's Method

Parikh 7th/60, Reddy 34th/67

- ***Age estimation of adult over 21 years*** depends on the physiological age changes in each of the dental tissues
- **Components includes**
  1. Attrition (A)
  2. Periodontosis (P)
  3. Secondary dentine (S)
  4. Cementum apposition (C)
  5. Root resorption (R)
  6. Transparency of the root (T)

Total score= A+P+S+C+R+T (a ranking scale 0–3 is given to each criteria)

Estimated age (years) = 11.43 + 4.56 × (Total score)

The transparency of root and secondary dentine have the highest correlation with age- *V V Pillay 18th/87*

The ***transparency of root is most reliable of all criteria***- *Reddy 34th/69*

If the eruption order of teeth could help determine the age up to 25 years, Gustafson's method is helpful in determining the ages beyond 25 years- www.doctoralerts.com, *V V Pillay 18th/87*

Gustafson's Method

gradestack.com

The AGE estimation of adult over 21 years depends on the physiological age changes in each of the dental tissue.

The various criteria used in Gustafson's method is:

- **Secondary dentine**: It develops within the pulp cavity and decrease the size of the cavity, start from base and reach the apex, finally obliterates the cavity.
- **Cementum opposition**: Near the end of root, increase cementum increases thickness, it is deposited throughout life and forms incremental lines.
- **Root resorption**: Because of cementum and dentine, absorption of root starts at the base and extends upwards.
- **Attrition**: Due to wear and tear upper surface of the teeth destroys gradually, first involving the enamel then dentine then pulp.
- **Paraodontosis**: Regression of gums and periodontal tissue surrounding the teeth, exposing the neck and adjacent part of root. Estimated before tooth extraction.
- **Transparency of the root**: Most RELIABLE criteria of Gustafson's. Seen after 30 years of age.

Canal in the dentine at first widens, increases with age because of deposition of minerals. They become invisible and dentine becomes transparent. It is a microscopic study. ***It is a method used for dead***. Anterior teeth are more reliable then posterior so merit of this method decrease from incisors to premolars.

"The present study concludes that regressive alterations of teeth can be used for estimation of age which ***helps in identification of the corpses; mutilated bodies; and is of importance for social, emotional and medicolegal aspects***. We also conclude that Gustafson's method is a reliable method for age estimation with some proposed modification"-www.ncbi.nlm.nih.gov

Boyde's method: Cross striation develop in the enamel of teeth, till the complete formation of enamel. They represent daily incremental lines. The age of an individual can be calculated in terms of days by counting the number of lines from the neonatal line onwards. It is useful to ***estimate the age of a dead infant***-gradestack.com

Stack's method: It is a method to know the age of infants from the weight and height of the erupting teeth of the infant. This method can be used on both deciduous and permanent teeth during their erupting phase -*gradestack.com*

Boyde's method and stack's method: other methods of age estimation from teeth- *Reddy 34th/69*

95. Ans. d. Inner end of clavicle; e. Fusion of ischial tuberosity

[Ref: Reddy 34th/78-79; Parikh 7th/61-63]

By the age of 18 years, bone age ***cannot be computed from hand and wrist radiographs***, therefore the medial end of the clavicle is used for bone age calculation in individuals aged 18—22 years"- *www.ncbi.nlm.nih.gov*

For Estimation of Age:

Reddy 34th/79

(A for appearance)

- **6-12 years :** *Take X-ray of* Elbow joint and Wrist joint
  - **6 years:**- center for lower end of ulna (A); medial epicondyle of the humerus (A)
  - **9 years:** *Olecranon (A)*
  - **9 to 11 years**: *Trochela of humerus (A)*
  - **10th to 11th year**: *Pisiform (A)*
  - **11th year**: *Lateral epicondyle of humerus (A)*
- **13 to 16 years:** *X-ray of elbow joint andpelvis*
  - **13th yr**–*separate centers in triradiate cartilage of acetabulum (A)*
  - **12 to 14 years:** *Lesser trochanter of femur (A)*
  - **14th year:** *Crest of ilium (A), fusion of medial epicondyle of humerus, lateral epicondyle with trochlea*
  - **15th year**: *fusion of triradiate cartilage of acetabulum*
  - **16th year**: Ischial tuberosity (A), Fusion of lower end of humerus; Olecranon of ulna and upper end of radius

Fusion of Bones/Joints in Male

Reddy 34th/79

- *16 years: elbow joint*
- ***16 to 17 years: Ankle joint***
- *17 to 18 years: Hip joint*
- *18 to 19 years: **Knee**, shoulder and wrist joint*
- *20 to 21 years: **Fusion of iliac crest, ischial tuberosity and inner end of clavicle***

In females fusion of bones occurs one year earlier than in males

*The opinion about the age should be given based on the findings of **physical, dental and radiological examination**. Multiple criteria of skeletal age should be used*

Region (Parikh 7th/62)	Girls	Boys
Elbow	13-14	15-17
Wrist	16-17	18-19
Shoulder	17-18	19-20
Crest of ilium	18-19	20-21
Ischial tuberosity	21-22	23-24
Inner end of clavicle	21-22	23-24

Ossification of Bone

◈ *Parikh 7th/61-62*

- Between 18 and 20 years, ***all the epiphyses at the wrist, knee, crest of ilium and lateral end of the clavicle should be united***. The acromion process should be united to the scapula.
- Soon after the 20th year, the articular facets of the ribs should be united.
- By 21-22 years, the ***ischial tuberosity should be fused in the females.***
- By 22 years, the ***inner (secondary) epiphysis of the clavicle fuses.***
- Between 18 and 22 years, the basiocciput should be fused with the basisphenoid.
- By 23 years, sacral vertebrae should be united with one another from below upwards.
- The four middle pieces of the sternum fuse with one another from below upwards between 14 and 25 years of ages.
- If ***all the epiphyses are united, the person is above 25 years of age***.
- From these data, it is seen that the probable age can be determined within a year or so before puberty and within a range of two years thereafter until the consolidation of the skeleton at 22 to 25 years.

96. Ans. a. Sex with wife age < 15 year is rape; c. Sex with wife of age group 15-18 years is rape

[Ref: Reddy 34th/384; Parikh 7th/389-90; www.livemint.com; www.thehindu.com]

October 11, 2017 verdict of supreme court on rape**: Age limit for wife raised to 18 year from 15 year and **Exception 2 of S. 375 IPC is now invalid

***"Exception 2 of S. 375 IPC- Sexual intercourse or sexual acts by a man with his own wife, the wife not being under fifteen years of age, is not rape"**- Reddy 34th/384*

October 11, 2017 Verdict of Supreme Court on Rape

◈ *www.livemint.com*

- In a landmark judgment, the Supreme Court on Wednesday ruled that a ***man who has sex with his minor wife is guilty of rape.***
- The move is expected to go a long way in discouraging the practice of child marriage in India.
- It is also likely to have a bearing on the criminality of marital rape, an issue which has been widely debated both by Parliament and the courts.
- "The **exception 2 carved out under section 375** (which defines rape) exempting marital rape for minors is ***artificial and contrary*** of Article 21 (right to life) of the Constitution of India," said justice Madan B. Lokur, while pronouncing the judgment.
- In a concurring judgment, passed by justices Lokur and Deepak Gupta, the court read down the provision of the Indian Penal Code (IPC), 1860 which exempted marital rape in case of minors.
- The purposive reading down was done to bring it in line with the Protection of Children from Sexual Offences Act (POCSO), 2012, in the spirit of other pro-child legislation and the human rights of a married girl child.
- ***The earlier age of 15 years has now been modified to 18 years for claiming exemption under the amended rape provisions.***
- Accordingly, the exemption clause now reads—"***sexual intercourse or sexual acts by a man with his own wife, the wife not being under eighteen years of age, is not rape***."
- It was also clarified that the court had not gone into the issue of **marital rape** since it did not form the subject matter of the case before it. Rights advocates welcomed the ruling.
- The court was ruling on a public interest litigation (PIL) by an NGO, Independent Thought, challenging the exception made out under provisions of the Indian Penal Code, which ***exempted marital rape of girls between 15 and 18 years of age by their husbands on the pretext of marriage.***
- ***The apex court ruling took into consideration the discrimination under the prevailing law where if a man had sex with a girl under 15 years of age, it was termed as rape—irrespective of consent. However, if she was below 18 years of age but more than 15 years and married, then there was no offence of rape.***

The exception had remained an anomaly because Section 375 itself mandated that sex with a girl below 18 years of age, with or without her consent, was statutory rape. An unmarried girl child can prosecute her rapist, but a married girl child aged between 15 and 18 could not even do that, Justice Lokur said, pointing out the injustice. The court, however, refrained from dealing with the issue of marital rape of a woman aged above 18. With this judgment, considered by experts as trigger to declaring child marriage void ab initio, the court ended the decades-old disparity between Exception 2 to Section 375 IPC and other child protection laws.

97. Ans. e. Section 377 IPC

[Ref: Reddy 34th/384;399,275; Parikh 7th/407]

Unnatural sex offences (S. 377, I.P.C): It is defined as sexual intercourse against the order of nature with any man or woman or animal. It includes sodomy, tribadism, bestiality, buccal coitus"- *Parikh 7th/407, Reddy 34th/399, 384*

I. P. C Related to Injury

◈ *Reddy 34th/275*

- *S.321, I. P. C: voluntarily causing hurt*
- *S.322, I. P. C: voluntarily causing grievous hurt*
- *S.323, I. P. C: Punishment for voluntarily causing hurt: imprisonment up to one year, or fine up to Rs 1000 or both*
- *S.324, I. P. C: voluntarily causing hurt by dangerous weapons or means (3 year imprisonment)*

- S.325, I. P. C: *Punishment for voluntarily causing grievous hurt: Imprisonment for a term extending to seven years and also fine.*
- S.326, I. P. C: Voluntarily causing grievous hurt by dangerous weapons or meAns. Imprisonment up to ten years and also fine

98. Ans. a. Castor seed - not poisonous when consumed unbroken with cover; b. Neem- excessive use can cause renal failure; c. Dhatura-neurotoxic

[Ref: Reddy 34th/515; Parikh 7th/565,633-34]

Ricinus Communis (Castor)

◈ *Parikh 7th/565, Reddy 34th/515*

- The entire plant is poisonous
- Castor seeds are poisonous when eaten in the raw state but ***harmless when swallowed entire*** (unbroken) or after cooking
- ***Castor oil does not contain ricin and therefore not poisonous***

Dhatura

◈ *Parikh 7th/633-34; Reddy 34th/556*

- *Contain alkaloid atropine, hyoscyamine and hyoscine*
- ***Anticholinergic effect***
- *First stimulate the **higher centers of brain**, then motor centers and finally cause depression and paralysis, especially of the vital centers in the medulla*

Neem *(Azadirachta indica)*: Liver and Kidney Damage

◈ *www.stylecraze.com*

- One of the serious side effects.
- Due to the natural antioxidant properties of neem, it is known to be beneficial for kidneys and several other bodily organs. ***When consumed in excess, neem is known to affect the organs thereby even damaging them***

Cannabis Sativa or Indica

◈ *Reddy 34th/558*

- It is a ***CNS stimulant***
- Psychoactive drug

PREVENTIVE AND SOCIAL MEDICINE

99. Ans. a. Hepatitis A infection; b. Hepatitis B infection; d. Rabies; e. Varicella zoster virus infection

[Ref: Park 24th/113, 226-33; Community Medicine by Piyush Gupta 1st/219, 212; Community Medicine with Recent Advances by Suryakantha 4th/296, 288]

Post-exposure Prophylaxis-*Rabies*- *Suryakantha 4th/296*

- ***Varicella-zoster virus infection** (chickenpox)- Piyush Gupta 1st/212*
- ***Hepatitis B**- Temporary immunity may be obtained by administering hepatitis B immunoglobulin (HBIG) for post-exposure prophylaxis- Piyush Gupta 1st/312*
- *Use of **hepatitis A** vaccine rather than passive prophylaxis with immune globulin should be considered for pre-exposure prophylaxis (e.g., travelers) and **post-exposure prophylaxis** (e.g., for close contacts of acute cases of hepatitis A)- Park 24th/227*
- ***Human immunoglobulin (Ig) against HAV infection**- Prophylaxis is achieved within hours of injection and is 80-90% effective when administered before or no later than 14 days after exposure- Park 24th/227*
- ***There is no PEP for hepatitis C**-www.hepch.ch*

"***Insufficient supporting data*** exist to endorse the use of directly acting anti-HCV antiviral (DAA) for PEP after HCV occupational exposures; additional studies examining efficacy, duration and cost-effectiveness are needed. Development of more oral drugs possessing a high barrier of resistance and equal activity against all HCV genotypes is anticipated"- *www.ncbi.nlm.nih.gov*

Post-exposure prophylaxis, also known as **post-exposure prevention (PEP)**, is any treatment started after exposure to a pathogen (such as a disease-causing virus), in order to prevent the infection from occurring.

100. Ans. b. Case control study: Suitable for study of rare disease; c. Cohort study help in assessing concept of causative; e. Case control study-estimates only odd ratio

[Ref: Park 24th/74, 88; Community Medicine by Piyush Gupta 1st/588]

Randomization is heart of control trial (e.g RCT)*. The essential difference b/w randomized control trial (RCT) and an analytic study (e.g., cohort, case-control, cross-sectional, ecological study) is that in the latter, there is **no randomization** because a differentiation into diseased and non-diseased (exposed or non-exposed) groups has already taken place. The only option left to ensure comparability in analytical studies is by matching"- Park 24th/88*

Cross-sectional Studies (Also k/a Prevalence Study)

◈ *Park 24th/74*

- **Cross-sectional studies** *is **single examination (so no follow up)** of a cross-section of population at one point in time- the results of which can be projected on the whole population*
- *Although it provides information about disease prevalence, it provides very little information about natural history of disease or about the rate of occurrence of new cases (incidence)*
- *The time sequence which is essential to the **concept of causativity cannot be deducted from cross-sectional data***

Case Control Study

◈ *Park 24th/84*

- ***Case control studies, often called retrospective studies**: No attrition problems, because case control studies **do not require follow-up** of individual into the future*
- *Generally yields only **estimate of relative risk (odd ratio)***
- ***Suitable for study of rare disease***

Cohort Study

◈ *Park 24th/80*

- ***Cohort*** (Known by a variety of names- ***prospective study, longitudinal study***, incidence study and forward looking study) is ***follow up study*** with individual as unit of study
- *Indicated when exposure is rare but incidence of disease high among exposed*
- *The basic approach is to work from cause to effect*
- *Yields incidence rate, Relative risk and attributable risk*
- As cohort studies measure potential causes before the outcome has occurred the study can demonstrate that these "**causes**" preceded the outcome, thereby avoiding the debate as to which is cause and which is effect
- Cohort studies provide the best information ***about the causation of disease***, because you follow persons from exposure to the occurrence of the disease. With data from cohort studies you can calculate cumulative incidences, which are the most direct measurement of the risk of developing disease-*www.theanalysisfactor.com*

101. Ans. b. Predictive value reflects the diagnostic power of the test; c. Positive predictive value -depend on prevalence of disease; d. Sensitivity and specificity of test- characteristics of the test

[Ref: Park 24th/149-50; Community Medicine by Piyush Gupta 1st/593;Biostatistics by Rao 2nd/70-71, 418; onlinecourses. science; wikipedia]

"Sensitivity and specificity are characteristics of the test. The population does not affect the results"-onlinecourses.science

"Positive and negative predictive values are influenced by the ***prevalence* of disease in the population** that is being tested. If we test in a high prevalence setting, it is more likely that persons who test positive truly have disease than if the test is performed in a population with low prevalence"-*onlinecourses. science*

"Using the same test in a population with higher prevalence, increases positive predictive value. Conversely, increased prevalence results in decreased negative predictive value. When considering predictive values of diagnostic or screening tests, recognize the influence of the prevalence of disease"-onlinecourses.science

"Neither sensitivity nor specificity are not influenced by the disease prevalence, meaning that results from one study could easily be transferred to some other setting with a different prevalence of the disease in the population. Nonetheless, sensitivity and specificity can vary greatly depending on the spectrum of the disease in the studied group"- *www.ncbi.nlm. nih.gov*

Predictive Accuracy

◈ *Park 24th/150*

- In addition to sensitivity and specificity, the performance of a screening test is measured by its "predictive value" which ***reflects the diagnostic power of the test.***
- The predictive accuracy ***depends upon sensitivity, specificity and disease prevalence.***
- The "predictive value of a positive test" indicates the probability that a patient with a positive test result has, in fact, the disease in question. The more prevalent a disease is in a given population, the more accurate will be the predictive value of a positive screening test.
- The ***predictive value of a positive result falls as disease prevalence declines.***

Sensitivity

◈ *Park 24th/149*

- The term **sensitivity** was introduced by Yerushalmy in 1940s as a statistical index of diagnostic accuracy. It has been defined as the ability of a test to identify correctly all those who have the disease, that is "true-positive".
- A 90 per cent of the diseased people screened by the test will give a "true-positive" result and the remaining 10 per cent a "false-negative" result.

Specificity

◈ *Park 24th/149*

- It is defined as the ability of a test to identify correctly those who do not have the disease, that is, "true-negatives".
- A 90 per cent specificity means that 90 per cent of the non-diseased persons will give "true-negative" result, 10 per cent of non-diseased people screened by the test will be wrongly classified as "diseased" when they are not.

"The positive and negative predictive values (PPV and NPV respectively) are the proportions of positive and negative results in statistics and diagnostic tests that are true positive and true negative results. The PPV and NPV describe the performance of a diagnostic test or other statistical measure. A high result can be interpreted as indicating the accuracy of such a statistic. ***The PPV and NPV are not intrinsic to the test; they depend also on the prevalence.*** The PPV can be derived using Bayes' theorem- *wikipedia*

Table: *(Park 24th/149)*: **Screening test result by diagnosis**

Screening Test Result	Diagnosis		Total
	Disease	Not disease	
Positive	A (true positive)	B (False positive)	A+B
Negative	C (False Negative)	D (True negative)	C+D
Total	A+C B+D		A+B+C+D

- *Sensitivity = A/(A+C) X 100*
- *Specificity = D/(B+D) X 100*
- *Predictive value of positive test = A/(A+B) X 100*
- *Predictive value of negative test = D/(C+D) X 100*
- *Percentage of false negative = C/(A+C) X 100*
- *Percentage of false positive = B/(B+D) X 100*

102. Ans. b. Subsequent infection with different strain produces severe form of dengu; c. Most infection with dengu virus is asymptomatic; d. Vector is aedes mosquito

[Ref: Park 24th/261-67; Community Medicine by Piyush Gupta 1st/263-67; Community Medicine with Recent Advances by Suryakantha 4th/471-73; Harrison 19th/1318- 19; Jawetz 27th/552-54]

Dengu

◈ *Park 24th/261*

- There are four virus serotypes which are designated as DENV-1, DENV-2, DENV-3 and DENV-4.

A & E

- All the 4 serotypes i.e dengu 1, 2, 3 and 4 have been isolated in India but at ***present DENV-1 and DENV-2 serotypes are widespread***
- Vector- ***Aedes aegypti and Aedes albopictus*** are the ***two most important vectors of dengu***
- Belong to ***genus flavivirus*** with positive sense RNA *(Harrison 19th 214e-1 table)*
- Infection with any one serotype confers lifelong immunity to that virus serotype
- Although all four serotypes are antigenically similar, they are different enough to elicit cross protection for only a few months after infection by any one of them. ***Secondary infection with dengue serotype 2 or multiple infection with different serotypes lead to severe form dengue DHF/DSS.***
- The first infection probably sensitizes the patient, while the second infection with different serotype appears to produce immunological catastrophy

"Three quarters of the people infected with dengue don't show any symptoms—and yet they are more likely to spread the disease than those who do"- *www.asianscientist.com/2015*

"Asymptomatic Infection: As ***many as one half of all dengue*** *infected individuals are asymptomatic, that is, they have no clinical signs or symptoms of disease"-www.cdc.gov*

"*Approximately, three-quarters of the dengue infections are asymptomatic.* Asymptomatic infection is therefore a major part of dengue burden and should be emphasized. In addition, asymptomatic cases may have a role in dengue transmission"- *www.sciencedirect.com*

"The first dengue vaccine, Dengvaxia (CYD-TDV) by Sanofi Pasteur, was first licensed in December, 2015, in Mexico. It has been registered for use in individuals 9-45 years of age living in endemic areas"-*www.who.int*

The **2009 WHO criteria classify dengue** according to levels of severity: ***dengue without warning signs; dengue with warning signs*** (abdominal pain, persistent vomiting, fluid accumulation, mucosal bleeding, lethargy, liver enlargement, increasing haematocrit with decreasing platelets); and ***severe dengue*** (dengue with severe plasma leakage, severe bleeding, or organ failure)"-*www.ncbi.nlm.nih.gov*

The **1997 guidelines classified dengue** into ***DF, DHF (Grades 1 and 2) and DSS (DHF Grades 3 and 4)***"-*www.ncbi.nlm.nih.gov*

Table: Classification of Dengue

Old WHO Classification	New WHO Classification
Classical dengue fever	Probable dengue (group A - OPD management)
Dengue Fever with hemorrhagic manifestations	Dengue with warning signs (Group B - inward observation and management) (patients are admitted for social reasons and when they are in high risk category)
DHF grade one	
DHF grade two	
DHF grade three	
DHF grade four DHF with unusual manifestations	Severe Dengue (Group C-resuscitation and management) 1. With compensated shock 2. With hypotensive shock 3. With severe organ impairment

Table: *(Park 24th/267)*: **WHO classification and grading of the severity of dengue infection**

DF/DHF	Grade	Symptoms/signs	Laboratory findings
DF		Fever with two or more of following Headache Retro-orbital pain Myalgia Arthralgia Rash Haemarrhagic manifestations No evidence of plasma leakage	Leucopenia (WBC < 5000 cells/cu. mm) Thrombocytopenia (platelet count < 150.000 cells /cu.mm) Rising haematocrit (5-10 per cent)
DHF	I	Above criteria for DF and haemorrhagic manifestation plus positive tourniquet test, evidence of plasma leakage	**Thrombocytopenia:** Platelet count < 100, 000/cu.mm. Haematorcit rise 20% or more
DHF	II	Above signs and symptoms plus some evidence of spontaneous bleeding in skin or other organs (black tarry stools, epistaxis, bleeding from gums, etc) and abdominal pain	Thrombocytopenia platelet count < 100, 000/cu.mm Haematocrit rise 20% or more
DHF	III	Above signs and symptoms plus circulating failure (weak rapid pulse, pule pressure < 20 mm Hg or high diastolic pressure, hypotension with the presence of cold clammy skin and restlessness)	Thrombocytopenia: Platelet count < 100, 000/cu.mm. Haematocrit rise more than 20%
DHF	IV	Signs as grade III plus profound shock with un-detectable blood pressure or pulse	Thrombocytopenia: Platelet count <100, 000/cu.mm. Haemotocrit rise more than 20%
DHF III and IV are dengue shock syndrome			

103. Ans. b. (Pneumococcal..) & c (Hepatitis..)

[Ref: Davidson 23rd/148-49;Park 25th/111-13; Piyush Gupta 1st/428; Suryakantha 4th/287; www.omicsonline.org]

- Correction from previous edition (on basis of Davidson)
- According to Davidson, Hepatitis B & pneumococcal vaccine are component vaccines

- Option a (DaPT vaccine): Mix or combined vaccine; option d (OPV vaccine): live attenuated vaccine & option e (MMR vaccine): mix or combination vaccine- Park 25th/111-13

Types of Vaccine

◈ *Davidson 23rd/148-49*

- Whole cell vaccines consist of live or inactivated (killed) microorganisms; component vaccines contain only extracted or synthesised components of microorganisms (e.g. polysaccharides or proteins).
- Live vaccines contain organisms with attenuated (reduced) virulence, which induce T-lymphocyte and humoral responses and are therefore more immunogenic than inactivated whole cell vaccines.
- Component vaccines consisting only of polysaccharides, such as the pneumococcal polysaccharide vaccine (PPV), are poor activators of T-lymphocytes and produce a short-lived antibody response without long-lasting memory. Conjugation of polysaccharide to a protein, as in the Haemophilus influenzae type B (Hib) vaccine, activates T lymphocytes, which results in a sustained response and immunological memory.
- Toxoids are bacterial toxins that have been modifed to reduce toxicity but maintain antigenicity.
- Vaccine response can be improved by co-administration with mildly proinflammatory adjuvants, such as aluminium hydroxide

Table: *(Davidson 23rd/149)*: **Vaccines in current clinical use**

Live attenuated vaccines

- *Measles, mumps, rubella (MMR)*
- *Oral poliomyelitis (**OPV**, not used in UK)*
- *Tuberculosis (bacille Calmette–Guérin, BCG)*
- *Typhoid (oral typhoid vaccine)*
- *Varicella zoster virus*
- *Rotavirus*

Inactivated (killed) whole-cell vaccines

- *Cholera*
- *Hepatitis A*
- *Influenza*
- *Poliomyelitis (inactivated polio virus, IPV)*
- *Rabies*

Component vaccines

- *Anthrax (adsorbed extracted antigens)*
- *Diphtheria (adsorbed toxoid)*
- *Hepatitis B (adsorbed recombinant HBsAg)*
- *Haemophilus influenzae type B (conjugated capsular polysaccharide)*
- *Human papillomavirus (recombinant capsid proteins)*
- *Meningococcal, quadrivalent A, C, Y, W135 (conjugated capsular polysaccharide)*

Contd...

- *Meningococcal, serogroup C (conjugated capsular polysaccharide)*
- *Pertussis (adsorbed extracted antigens)*
- ***Pneumococcal conjugate** (PCV; conjugated capsular polysaccharide, 13 serotypes)*
- ***Pneumococcal polysaccharide** (PPV; purifed capsular polysaccharide, 23 serotypes)*
- *Tetanus (adsorbed toxoid)*
- *Typhoid (purifed Vi capsular polysaccharide)*

*"PCV-7: It is a **Pneumococcal conjugate** vaccine"- cdc.gov*.

Component Vaccines: Vaccines that are employed in combination therapy for certain diseases can be termed as component vaccines. These are clinical vaccines discovered and employed for *combination therapies*. www.omicsonline.org **(In earlier edition(8th), I given this definition only)**

104. Ans. b. Goiter prevalence of 10% is cut-off value for endemicity; c. Strabismus is also a manifestation

[Ref: Park 24th/680-82, 662-63; Community Medicine by Piyush Gupta 1st/160-62; Community Medicine with Recent Advances by Suryakantha 4th/199-200]

Strabismus and nystagmus are manifestation of Iodine deficiency disorders- *Park 24th/662*

*"Result of annual sample survey (2009-10, Mohfw) conducted in 325 districts covering all the states/UT have revealed that 263 districts are **endemic** where the prevalence of IDD is **more than 10%**"- Park 24th/681*

The Problem of Iodine Deficiency

◈ *Park 24th/681*

- It has always been thought in India that goiter and cretinism were ***only found to a significant extent in the "Himalaya goiter belt"*** which is the world's biggest goiter belt. It stretches from Kashmir to the Naga Hills in the east, extending about 2, 400 km and affecting the northern States of Jammu and Kashmir, Himachal Pradesh, Punjab, Haryana, Delhi, Uttar Pradesh, Bihar, West Bengal, Sikkim, Assam, Arunachal Pradesh, Nagaland, Mizoram, Meghalaya, Tripura and Manipur.
- In recent years renewed surveys outside the conventional goiter belt have identified ***endemic foci of iodine deficiency and the associated IDD*** in parts of *Madhya Pradesh, Gujarat, Maharashtra andhra Pradesh, Kerala, Karnataka and Tamil Nadu.* More and more new areas are being identified.
- Even areas near the sea coast like Bharuch district in Gujarat and Ernakulam district in Kerala are found goiter-affected.
- ***In short, no State in India can be said to be entirely free from goiter***

Epidemiological Assessment of Iodine Deficiency

◈ *Park 24th/662-63*

- This is necessary before initiating an iodization programme and for surveillance of goiter control programmes. The following indicators are useful in this regard
  - Prevalence of goiter
  - Prevalence of cretinism
  - Urinary iodine excretion

- Measurement of thyroid function by determination of serum level of thyroxine (T_4) and pituitary thyrotropic hormone (TSH); and
- Prevalence of neonatal hypothyroidism

- Since the objective of goiter control programme is to increase iodine intake, indices of urinary excretion are particularly recommended for use in surveillance. Neonatal hypothyroidism has been found to be a sensitive indicator of environmental iodine deficiency. Serum T_4 level is a more sensitive indicator of thyroid insufficiency than T_3

"The **prevalence of goiter** in India is 7.3% of the total population. Endemic goiter is said to be present and considered as significant public health problems, when the prevalence of goiter (total goiter rate) ***exceeds 10% among school children aged 6 to 11 years***"- *Suryakantha 4th/199*

Table: *(Suryakantha 4th/200)*: **Endemicity of goiter**

Goiter prevalence rate	Grade of endemicity
<10%	Not significant
10-20%	Mild endemicity
20-30%	Moderate endemicity
>30%	Severe endemicity

105. Ans. c. Yellow

[Ref: http:cpcb.nic.in]

Table: Biomedical waste rule 2016 guideline

Cat.	Type of Bag/ Container used	Type of Waste	Treatment /Disposal options
Yellow	non-chlorinated plastic bags Separate collection system leading to effluent treatment system	a) Human anatomical waste b) Animal anatomical waste c) Soiled waste d) Expired or discarded medicines e) Chemical waste f) Micro, Bio-t and other clinical lab waste g) Chemical liquid waste	Incineration or Plasma Pyrolysis or deep burial
Red	non-chlorinated plastic bags or containers	Contaminated Waste (Recyclable) tubing, bottles, intravenous tubes and sets, catheters, urine bags, syringes (without needles) and gloves.	Auto/Micro/ Hydro and then sent for recycling. not be sent to landfill.
White	(Translucent) Puncture, Leak, tamper proof containers	Waste sharps including Metals	Auto or Dry Heat sterilization followed by shredding or mutilation or encapsulation
Blue	Cardboard boxes with blue colored marking	Glassware	Disinfection or auto/Micro/ hydro and then sent for recycling.

106. Ans. b. Dr Rajendra Prasad Center for Ophthalmic Sciences, AIIMS is apex body for implementation of NPCB; c. Promotion of eye camp and mobile unit; d. Intraocular Lens implantation better than convention conventional surgery

[Ref: Park 24th/458-60; Khurana 6th/480-86; Community Medicine by Piyush Gupta 1st/830]

National Programme for Control of Blindness

- *It was launched in the year 1976 and incorporates the earlier trachoma control programme started in the year 1968*
- *"For implementation of NPCB, an apex body, National Institute of Ophthalmology (**Dr Rajendra Prasad Center for Ophthalmic Sciences**) was established for manpower development, research and referral servces"- Piyush Gupta 1st/831*
- Government of India has adopted 'Vision 2020: Right to Sight' under National Programme for Control of Blindness. The initiative 'Vision 2020' has been launched with the objective to eliminate avoidable blindness by the year 2020- *Khurana 6th/480*
- **Eye camp approach** is of great help in reducing the backlog of cataract by mass surgeries. Recent emphasis is on reach-in-approach- *Khurana 6th/486*
- Development of Mobile Ophthalmic Units with Teleophthalmology Network and some fixed tele-models to cover difficult hilly terrains and difficult areas.
- **IOL surgery** for >80% by the year 2005 and for all by the year 2010- *Khurana 6th/483*
- **NPCB:** Recent surveys have confirmed ***higher success rates following cataract surgery with Intra Ocular Lens implantation*** as compared to conventional surgery- *www.ncbi.nlm.nih.gov*

Objectives of NPCB (2011-2017) *Piyush Gupta 1st/830*

1. To reduce the backlog of blindness through identification and treatment of blind at primary, secondary and tertiary levels based on assessment of the overall burden of visual impairment in the country.
2. Develop and strengthen the strategy of NPCB for "Eye Health and prevention of visual impairment; through provision of comprehensive eye care services and quality service delivery.
3. ***Strengthening and upgradation of Regional Institutes of Ophthalmology (RIOs) to become center of excellence in various sub-specialties of ophthalmology***
4. Strengthening the existing and developing additional human resources and infrastructure facilities for providing high quality comprehensive Eye Care in all Districts of the country;
5. To enhance community awareness on eye care and lay stress on preventive measures;
6. Increase and expand research for prevention of blindness and visual impairment
7. ***To secure participation of Voluntary Organizations/Private Practitioners in eye Care***

Strategies of Government of India to Control Blindness (Under NPCB)

Piyush Gupta 1st/831

- Comprehensive eye care services addressing major blinding causes: cataract, refractive errors and low vision, childhood blindness, corneal blindness, glaucoma, diabetic retinopathy.

- Development of eye care services and improvement in quality of eye care by training of personnel, supply of high tech equipment, strengthening follow up services and monitoring of services
- Decentralized implementation of the schemes through State and district health societies
- Reduction in backlog of blind persons active screening of population over 50 years, organizing screening camps and transporting operable cases to eye care facilities
- ***Involvement of voluntary organization in various NPCB activities***
- Participation of community and Panchayati raj institutions in organizing services in the rural area
- Screening of school going children for identification and treatment or refractive errors, with special attention to underserved areas
- Promoting eye donation, processing and utilization of donated eyes for treatment of corneal blindness
- Special focus of illiterate women in rural areas, convergence with ongoing schemes for development of Women and children
- Free treatment to poor patients through qualified government and ***non-governmental organizations***
- Public awareness about prevention and timely treatment of eye ailments
- "***Multipurpose district mobile ophthalmic units for better coverage***"- *Park 24th/459*

107. Ans. a. 90% of all people living with HIV know their HIV status; b. 90% of all people diagnosed with HIV infection receive sustained antiretroviral therapy; e. 90% of all people receiving antiretroviral therapy will have viral suppression

[Ref: pib.nic.in/newsite;vikaspedia.in/health/nrhm/national-health-policy-2017]

"National Health Policy 2017: *Achieve the global 2020 HIV target (also termed 90:90:90; 90 per cent of all people living with HIV know their HIV status, 90 per cent of all people diagnosed with HIV infection receive sustained antiretroviral therapy and 90 per cent of all people receiving antiretroviral therapy will have viral suppression)"*- pib.nic.in

National Health Policy 2017

◈ *pib.nic.in/newsite;indianexpress.com*

Key Highlights:

- The government aims in shifting focus from "sick-care" to "wellness", by promoting prevention and well-being.
- It intends on gradually increasing public health expenditure to 2.5% of the GDP.
- To strengthen health systems by ensuring everyone has access to quality services and technology despite financial barriers. The policy proposes increasing access, improving quality and reducing costs. It proposes free drugs, free diagnostics and free emergency and essential healthcare services in public hospitals.
- To focus on primary health care: The policy advocates allocating two-thirds (or more) of resources to primary care. It proposes two beds per 1, 000 of the population to enable access within the golden hour (the first 60 minutes after a traumatic injury).
- To reduce morbidity and preventable mortality of non-communicable diseases (NCDs) by advocating pre-screening.
- To promote Prime Minister 'Make in India' initiative by using drugs and devices manufactured in the country.
- It highlights AYUSH (Ayurveda, Yoga and Naturopathy, Unani, Siddha and Homeopathy) as a tool for effective prevention and therapy that is safe and cost-effective. It proposes introducing Yoga in more schools and offices to promote good health.
- Reforming medical education.
- The policy also lists quantitative targets regarding life expectancy, mortality and reduction of disease prevalence in line with the objectives of the policy.

Key Targets:

- Increase Life Expectancy at birth from 67.5 to 70 by 2025.
- Reduce infant mortality rate to 28 by 2019.
- Reduce Under Five Mortality to 23 by 2025.
- To reduce premature mortality from cardiovascular diseases, cancer, diabetes or chronic respiratory diseases by 25 per cent by 2025.

108. Ans. a. Developed by Motorola; c. Represents an ideology that focuses on statistical improvements to a business process; d. It is a quality-control program

[Ref: www.investopedia.com/terms/s/six-sigma.asp; www.simplilearn.com]

What is 'Six Sigma'

◈ *www.investopedia.com/terms/s/six-sigma.asp*

- Six Sigma is a ***quality-control program developed in 1986 by Motorola*** that emphasizes cycle-time improvement and the ***reduction of manufacturing defects*** to a level of no more than 3.4 per million.

As of 2016, Six Sigma has evolved into a more general business-management philosophy ***focused on meeting customer requirements, improving customer retention and improving and sustaining business products and services.***

Six Sigma is ***applicable to all industries and a number of vendors, including Motorola itself,*** offer Six Sigma training; special certifications include yellow belt, green belt and black belt.

Breaking Down 'Six Sigma'

Six Sigma represents an ideology that focuses on statistical improvements to a business process. Six Sigma advocates for qualitative measurements of success over qualitative markers. Therefore, practitioners of Six Sigma are those business people who use statistics, financial analysis and project management to achieve improved business functionality.

Six Sigma has evolved to define numerous ideas within business and is sometimes confusing. First, it's a statistical benchmark. Any business process that produces less than 3.4 defects per1 million chances is considered efficient; defects are considered anything that's produced outside of consumer satisfaction. Second, it's a training program and certification that teaches the core principles of Six Sigma. Practitioners can achieve Six Sigma belt levels, ranging from white belt to black belt. Finally, it's a philosophy that promotes the idea that all business processes can be measured and optimized.

Six Sigma DMAIC

◈ *searchcio.techtarget.com*

Here is a step-by-step breakdown of Six Sigma DMAIC:

- *Define: Identify the project goals and all customer deliverables.*
- *Measure: Understand current performance.*
- *Analyze: Determine root causes of any defects.*
- *Improve: Establish ways to eliminate defects and correct the process.*
- *Control: Manage future process performance.*

Sigma Level	Defects per Million	Yield
6	3.4	99.99966%
5	230	99.977%
4	6, 210	99.38%
3	66, 800	93.32%
2	308, 000	69.15%
1	690, 000	30.85%

109. Ans. a. BCG vaccine; b. Killed M.leprae + BCG vaccine; c. Vaccination with M. indicus pranii; d. BCG vaccine+ M. vaccae

[Ref: Park 24th/344; Community Medicine by Piyush Gupta 1st/283; Community Medicine with Recent Advances by Suryakantha 4th/548]

Leprosy Vaccine (Immunoprophylaxis)

◈ *Park 24th/344; Suryakantha 4th/548*

- *Trial in different population groups with BCG vaccine either alone or in combination with other vaccine (from killed M.lepae or atypical mycobacteria), have shown protective efficacy ranging b/w 28% and 60%*
- *High BCG coverage remains an important contribution to reducing the disease burden due to leprosy*

Table: *(Suryakantha 4th/548)*: **Candidate Vaccines against Leprosy**

Category I (Based on M. leprae)
Killed M. leprae
Killed M. leprae + BCG
Acetoacetylated M. leprae
Category II (Based on cultivable mycobacteriae)
BCG
BCG + M. vaccae
Killed M. vaccae
Killed ICRC bacilli
M. phlei
M. gordanae
M. habana
ICRC + BCG

Variants of Vaccination

◈ *www.news-medical.net*

- Adding killed ***M. leprae*** to BCG: Various modifications have been suggested, such as the addition of killed *M. leprae* to BCG. While it has not been conclusively proved to increase the protection rate, some studies have suggested that it almost doubles the vaccine efficacy in some populations. It fails, however, to increase the protection rate for patients below 15 years.
- Vaccination with ***M. indicus pranii:*** Earlier known as *Mycobacterium W*, this strain has been proved in one study to provide protection for up to nine years in both contacts and index cases. Unfortunately the immunity wanes with time and is higher for contacts than for cases.
- Indian cancer research center (ICRC) bacilli: ICRC bacilli are thought to belong to the *M. avium intracellulare* group and in one trial, they induced lepromin conversion in lepromatous leprosy patients and in lepromin-negative leprosy-free individuals. Its efficacy was reported to be 65.5 percent
- **M. vaccae**: This soil-dwelling mycobacterial species has been combined with BCG to provide greater protection, but a Vietnamese trial showed no such effect.
- **M. habana**: This organism induced lepromin positivity in monkeys and protected mice against the development of leprosy. It has been reported to induce lepromin conversion when used in a live vaccine.
- However, none of these organisms has replaced the BCG vaccine in common use.

110. Ans. a. Biochemical oxygen demand (BOD) is indicator of the organic content of sewage; b. BOD is amount of oxygen absorbed by a sample of sewage; c. Undergo both aerobic and anaerobic reaction in sewage purification

[Ref: Park 24th/799-800; Community Medicine by Piyush Gupta 1st/89-94]

Sewage

◈ *Park 24th/799-800*

- *Sewage is waste water from a community containing solid and liquid excreta, derived from houses, street and yard washing, factories and industries*
- *Sewage contains 99.9% water*
- *A standard test which is indicator of the organic content of sewage is **Biochemical oxygen demand***

Biochemical oxygen demand: It is defined as the amount of oxygen absorbed by a sample of sewage during a specified period, generally 5 days at a specified temperature usually 20 C for aerobic digestion. ***This is the most important test carried out on sewage***- *Piyush Gupta 1st/89-91*

Sewage purification: *The aim of sewage treatment is to convert an offensive and potentially dangerous mixture into an inoffensive effluent and sludge which can be **disposed of safely and without causing nuisance into rivers, sea or land**. The conversion of the complex organic matter in the sewage to simpler substances takes place by **both aerobic and anaerobic**- Piyush Gupta 1st/91*

111. Ans. (All) a. Morbid obese; b. Young adult; c. Children; d. Pregnant women; e. Elderly person

[Ref: Park 24th/167; Community Medicine by Piyush Gupta 1st/345-46; Community Medicine with Recent Advances by Suryakantha 4th/341]

Persons at Higher Risk for Complications of Influenza or for Influenza-Related Visits to Health Care Facilities

◈ *Harrison 19th/1211*

- All children from birth to <5 years, especially <2 years
- ***All persons ≥50 years old***
- ***Pregnant women***
- Adults and children who have chronic pulmonary (including asthma) or cardiovascular (except isolated hypertension), renal, hepatic, neurologic, hematologic, or metabolic disorders (including diabetes mellitus)
- Persons who have immunosuppression (including that caused by medications or by HIV infection)
- Children and adolescents (6 months to 18 years old) who are receiving long term aspirin therapy and who might be at risk for Reye's syndrome after influenza virus infection
- Residents of nursing homes and other long-term care facilities
- Native Americans/Alaska Natives
- Persons who are ***morbidly obese*** (body mass index ≥40 kg/m^2)

  In avian influenza H5N1 and in the pandemic influenza 2009
- "**H1N1:** The disease is more common ***among young adult***"- *Suryakantha 4th/341*

Seasonal Influenza

◈ *CMDT 2016/1387-88*

- Seasonal influenza viruses of types A and B produce clinically indistinguishable infections, whereas type C usually causes a minor illness.
- The main circulating seasonal influenza viruses that are the target of current vaccines are the A/California/7/2009 (H1N1) pandemic (pdm) 09-like virus, the A/Texas/50/2012 (H3N2)-like virus, the B/Massachusetts/2/2012-like virus and a B/Brisbane/60/2008-like virus.
- Attack rates with this pandemic strain are highest in children and young adults, particularly Hispanics, blacks and Native Americans, with relative sparing of ***adults older than 60 years*** of age presumably due to previous exposure with related strains (conferring some degree of crossprotection).
- High-risk groups include patients with ***severe obesity, asthma, immunosuppression, or neurologic disorders and especially pregnant and postpartum women.***
- ***Infection during pregnancy increases the risk for hospitalization and may be associated with severe illness,*** sepsis, pneumothorax and respiratory failure, spontaneous abortion, preterm labor and fetal distress.
- Overall case fatality rate is < 0.5% with 90% of deaths in those under 65 years of age and higher mortality recognized among men and patients with liver disease or a cancer diagnosis within the last year.

112. Ans. c. Flat and mobile hypopyon

[Ref: Khurana 6th/106-07; Parson 22nd/199-201]

The hypopyon, if present, is thick and immobile and may even have a convex upper surface- *Parson 22nd/199*

"Common symptoms of a patient with a **fungal keratitis** may include pain, photophobia, conjunctival injection, tearing, ***discharge (usually mucopurulent) and foreign-body sensation***"- *www.healio.com*

Mycotic Corneal Ulcer

◈ *Khurana 6th/106-07*

- The incidence of suppurative corneal ulcers caused by fungi has increased in the recent years due to injudicious use of antibiotics and steroids.
- The fungi more commonly responsible for mycotic corneal ulcers are Aspergillus (most common), Candida and Fusarium
- ***Symptoms*** are similar to the central bacterial corneal ulcer, but in general they are less marked than the equal-sized bacterial ulcer and the overall course is slow and torpid.
- ***Signs:*** A typical fungal corneal ulcer has following salient features
  - Corneal ulcer is ***dry-looking,*** greyish white, with ***elevated rolled out margins***
  - Delicate *feathery finger-like extensions* are present into the surrounding stroma under the intact epithelium.
  - A ***sterile immune ring*** (yellow line of demarcation) may be present where fungal antigen and host antibodies meet
  - Multiple, small ***satellite lesions*** may be present around the ulcer.
  - Usually a ***big hypopyon*** is present even if the ulcer is very small. Unlike bacterial ulcer, the hypopyon may not be sterile as the ***fungi can penetrate into the anterior chamber without perforation.***
  - *Perforation* in mycotic ulcer is rare but can occur.
  - *Corneal vascularization* is conspicuously absent.

Fungal Corneal Ulcer

◈ *Parson 22nd/201*

- Symptoms are much milder than the clinical signs would suggest. The ***slough in these ulcers is dry*** in appearance with feathery borders, surrounded by a yellow line of demarcation which gradually deepens into a ***gutter and there may also be a hypopyon***
- An **immune ring** (***Wesseley***) may be visible due to deposition of immune complexes and inflammatory cells around the ulcer. ***Satellite lesions may also be seen.***
- There is marked ciliary and conjunctival congestion, but ***symptoms of pain, watering and photophobia are disproportionately less as compared to those in cases of bacterial corneal ulcers.***
- **Bacterial corneal ulcer: *accumulation of purulent exudate on the cornea***- *Khurana 6th/100*

113. Ans. b. Incubation period is 6-10 days

[Ref: Khurana 6th/74-75; Ananthanarayan 10th/486-88; Harrison 19th/1208; Jawetz 27th/451-53]

Epidemic Keratoconjunctivitis

◈ *Khurana 6th/74-75*

- ***Mostly caused by adenovirus type 8 and 19***
- ***Incubation period after infection is about 8 day***
- ***Pseudomembrane*** *lining lower fornix and palpebral conjunctiva may formed in severe inflammation*
- ***Treatment***- It is usually supportive. Antiviral drugs are ineffective. Recently, promising results are reported with adenine ***arabinoside (Ara-A) and cidofovir***. Corticosteroids should not be used during active stage.

Adenovirus

◈ *Harrison 19th/1208*

- "G***enome is a linear double-stranded DNA***, no lipid envelop"- *Harrison 19th/214e-2(table)*
- Adenoviruses, particularly types 3 and 7, cause ***pharyngo-conjunctival fever***, a characteristic acute febrile illness of children that occurs in outbreaks, most often in summer camps. The syndrome is marked by ***bilateral conjunctivitis*** in which the bulbar and palpebral conjunctivae have a granular appearance.
- Only symptom-based treatment and supportive therapy are available for adenovirus infections and clinically useful antiviral therapy has not been established.
- ***Ribavirin and cidofovir*** are active in vitro against certain adenoviruses. Retrospective studies and anecdotes describe the use of these agents in disseminated adenovirus infections, but definitive efficacy data from controlled studies are not available. An oral liposomal form of ***cidofovir*** is being evaluated for adenovirus infections in immunosuppressed patients.

"Currently there are no drugs that are FDA approved for use in the management of *adenoviral* conjunctivitis. The use of topical **ganciclovir** is currently being investigated, but the adenoviral structural characteristics may prove too hardy for this anti-viral agent- *modernmedicine.com*

"After an ***incubation period of about 5 to 12 days***, conjunctival hyperemia, watery discharge and ocular irritation usually begin in one eye and spread rapidly to the other. Follicles may be present on the palpebral conjunctiva. Chemosis may be present. ***Pseudomembranes of fibrin*** and inflammatory cells on the tarsal conjunctiva, focal corneal inflammation, or both may blur vision."-*www.msdmanuals.com*

114. Ans. a. Levator palpebrae superioris muscle (LPS); b. Skin; c. Muller muscle; d. Fat

[Ref: Khurana 6th/363; Parson 22nd/449-50]

- ***Orbicularis oris muscle is a complex of muscles in the lips that encircles the mouth***

"Structures that must be considered in a description of ***lid anatomy*** are the skin and subcutaneous tissue; the orbicularis oculi muscle; the submuscular areolar tissue; the fibrous layer, consisting of the tarsi and the orbital septum; the lidretractors of the upper and lower eyelids; ***the retroseptal fat pads***; and the conjunctiva"- emedicine.medscape.com

- ***Eyelid:*** Underneath the skin, along with the subcutaneous tissue is a ***thin layer of fat***. However, the ***amount of fat is negligible when compared to other parts of the body***"- *www.eyeplastics.com*

Each eyelid consists (from anterior to posterior) of the following layers *Khurana 6th/363*

- ***The skin.*** It is elastic having a fine texture and is the thinnest in the body.

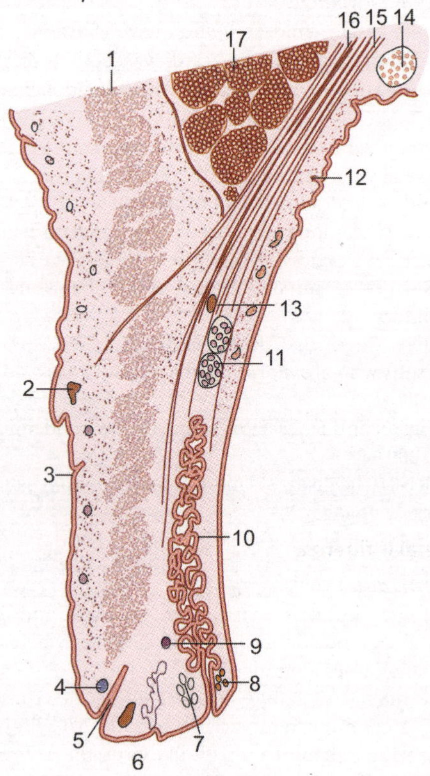

Fig: *(Parson 22nd/450)*: Section through the upper lid. 1, orbicularis muscle; 2, sweat gland; 3, hair follicle; 4, gland of Zeis; 5, cilium; 6, gland of Moll; 7, pars marginalis of orbicularis muscle; 8, pars subtarsalis of orbicularis muscle; 9, inferior arterial arcade; 10, meibomian gland; 11, gland of Wolfring; 12, conjunctival crypts; 13, superior arterial arcade; 14, gland of Krause; 15, Muller muscle; 16, levator palpebrae superioris; 17, fat.

- ***The subcutaneous areolar tissue.*** It is very loose and ***contains no fat.***
- ***The layer of striated muscle.*** It consists of ***orbicularis oculi muscle*** which forms an oval sheet across the eyelids. It comprises three portions: the *orbital, palpebral* and *lacrimal.* In addition, ***the upper lid also contains levator palpebrae superioris muscle (LPS).***
- ***Submuscular areolar tissue.*** It is a layer of loose connective tissue. The nerves and vessels lie in this layer.
- ***Fibrous layer.*** It is the framework of the lids and consists of two parts: the central tarsal plate and the peripheral septum orbitale

- ***Layer of non-striated muscle fibres.*** It consists of the palpebral muscle of Muller which lies deep to the septum orbitale in both the lids.
- ***Conjunctiva:*** The part which lines the lids is called *palpebral conjunctiva.* It consists of three parts: marginal, tarsal and orbital.

115. Ans. a. Optic nerve is supplied by pial network of vessels; b. Optic tract is supplied by anterior choroidal artery; d. Lateral geniculate body is supplied by choroidal arteries; e. Optic radiation is supplied by middle cerebral arteries

[Ref: Khurana 6th/311-12; Parson 22nd/11-12; Ophthalmology by Kaiser, Peter 2nd/49-52]

The cilioretinal arteries belong to the posterior ciliary artery system. They ***usually arise from the peripapillary choroid or directly from one of the short posterior ciliary arteries****- link. springer.com*

Blood Supply of Optic Pathway

◈ *Ophthalmology by Kaiser, Peter 2nd/49-52*

- Optic nerve → chiasm → optic tract → lateral geniculate body → optic radiation → occipital lobe

Optic Nerve: Blood supply

- **Orbital Portion:** Ophthalmic artery with meningeal anastomoses
- **Intracanalicular Portion:** ***pial branches from ophthalmic artery***; possibly internal carotid artery (ICA)
- **Intracranial Portion:** Small vessels from ICA, anterior cerebral and anterior communicating arteries
  - **Chiasm Blood supply:** ICA; occasionally by anterior cerebral and anterior communicating arteries
  - **Optic tract Blood supply:** Anterior choroidal artery; branches from posterior communicating artery
  - **Lateral geniculate body:** BLOOD SUPPLY-anterior communicating artery and choroidal arteries

Optic radiation Blood supply-***middle cerebral arteries***

Primary visual cortex (striate cortex, V1, Brodmann's area 17): ***Blood supply:*** middle and posterior cerebral arteries

Blood supply of the visual pathway *Khurana* 6th/311-12

- The visual pathway is ***mainly supplied by pial network of vessels*** except the orbital part of optic nerve which is also supplied by an axial system derived from the central artery of retina.
- ***Blood supply of the optic nerve head***
  - The *surface layer* of the optic disc is supplied by capillaries derived from the retinal arterioles.
  - *The prelaminar region* is mainly supplied by centripetal branches of the peripapillary choroid with some contribution from the vessels of lamina cribrosa.
  - The *lamina cribrosa* is supplied by branches from the posterior ciliary arteries and arterial circle of Zinn.
  - The *retrolaminar part* of the optic nerve is supplied by centrifugal branches from central retinal artery and centripetal branches from pial plexus formed by branches from the choroidal arteries, circle of Zinn, central retinal artery and ophthalmic artery.

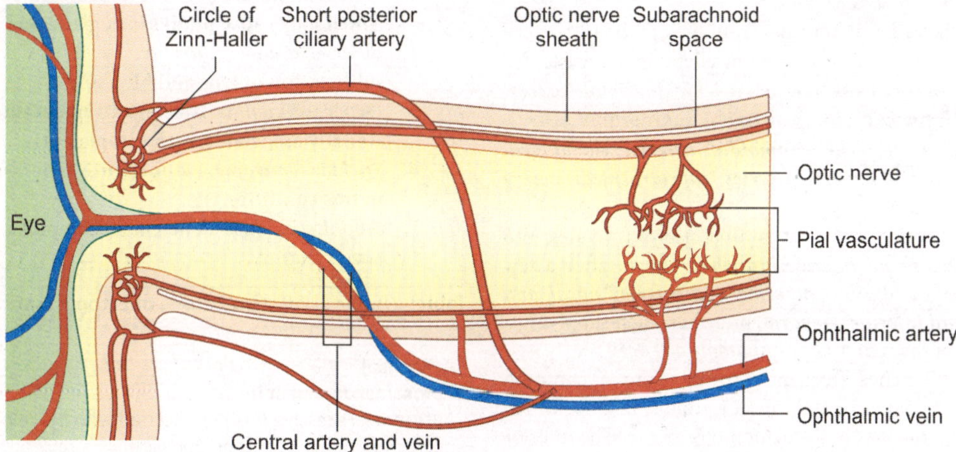

Fig: *(Ophthalmology by Kaiser, Peter 2nd/51):* Anterior optic nerve.
The sheath and the vascular supply to the intraocular and intraorbital portions are shown

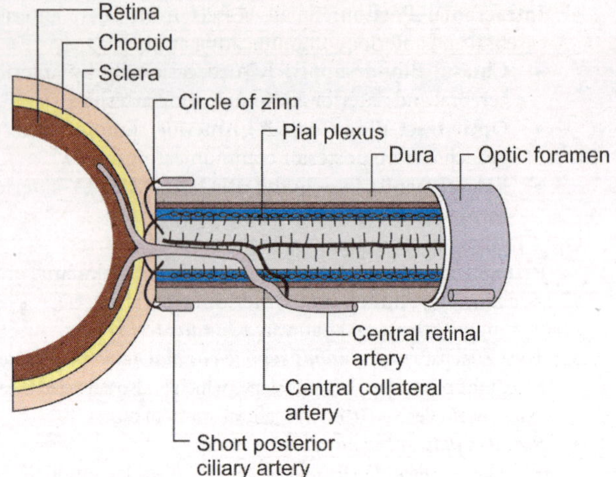

Fig: *(Khurana 6th/312)*: Blood supply of the optic nerve

116. Ans. a. Central retinal artery; c. Anterior ciliary artery; d. Short posterior ciliary artery

[Ref: Khurana 6th/5; Gray's Anatomy 40th/665-66]

"Internal carotid artery branch: Ophthalmic, ***anterior choroidal,*** anterior cerebral, middle cerebral and posterior communicating artery"- *www.meddean.luc.edu*

Ophthalmic Artery

◈ *Gray's Anatomy 40th/665-66*

- Although the order of branches from the ophthalmic artery is quite variable, a number may be identified consistently, including ***the central retinal artery, lacrimal artery, muscular branches, ciliary arteries, supraorbital artery, anterior and posterior ethmoidal arteries, meningeal branch, medial palpebral arteries, supratrochlear artery and dorsal nasal artery***.
- The central retinal artery at lamina cribrosa divides into equal ***superior and inferior branches***, which, after a few millimetres, divide into ***superior and inferior nasal and superior and inferior temporal***, branches, each supplying a 'quadrant' of the retina-*Gray's Anatomy 40th/693*
- **Muscular branches** frequently spring from a common trunk to form superior and inferior groups, most of which accompany branches of the oculomotor nerve. The inferior branch contains most of the ***anterior ciliary arteries***. Other muscular vessels branch from the lacrimal and supraorbital arteries or from the trunk of the ophthalmic artery.
- The ciliary arteries are distributed ***in long and short posterior and anterior groups.***

Ophthalmic Artery Branches

◈ *wikipedia*

Because of the obvious importance of the ocular globe, branches of the ophthalmic artery often are subdivided into two groups: those that supply the eyeball (ocular group) and those that supply non-ocular orbital structures (orbital group)

A. **Orbital group,** distributing vessels to the orbit and surrounding parts, includes:
   - Lacrimal artery
   - Supraorbital artery
   - Posterior ethmoidal artery
   - Anterior ethmoidal artery
   - Medial palpebral artery
   - Frontal artery, also called the Supratrochlear artery
   - Dorsal nasal artery

B. **Ocular group,** distributing vessels to the eye and its muscles, includes:
   - Long posterior ciliary arteries
   - ***Short posterior ciliary arteries***
   - ***Anterior ciliary artery***
   - ***Central retinal artery***
   - Superior muscular artery
   - Inferior muscular artery

117. Ans. d. Diabetes mellitus

[Ref: Khurana 6th/215-16; Parson 22nd/275; Ophthalmology by Kaiser, Peter 2nd/281]

Ectopia Lentis with Systemic Anomalies

◈ *Khurana 6th/215-16*

1. ***Marfan's syndrome:*** **In this condition lens is displaced upwards and temporally (bilaterally symmetrical)**
2. ***Homocystinuria:*** **In it the lens is usually subluxated downwards and nasally.**
3. ***Weil-Marchesani syndrome:*** **forward subluxation of lens which may cause pupil block glaucoma.**
4. ***Ehlers-Danlos syndrome.*** **In it the** *ocular features* **are subluxation of lens and blue sclera.**
5. ***Hyperlysinaemia***: **It is an extremely rare condition occasionally associated with ectopialentis.**
6. ***Stickler syndrome.*** **Ectopialentis is occasionally associated in this condition**
7. ***Sulphite oxidase deficiency:*** **Ectopialentis is a universal** ***ocular feature.***

Table: *(Parson 22nd/275)*: **Causes of Ectopia lentis**

A. Familial Autosomal dominant form Autosomal recessive form (associated with iris coloboma, aniridia, microspherophakia, ectopiapupillae)
B. Other systemic diseases Marfan, Ehlers-Danlos, Weil-Marchesani, Homocystinuria, Sulphite oxidase deficiency, Hyperlysinaemia
C. Secondary to eye diseases Uveitis, hypermature cataract, pseudoexfoliation syndrome, ciliary body tumour
D. Secondary to trauma (May or may not be associated with underlying defective zonules due to syphilis)

118. Ans. a. Viral keratitis; b. Herpes simplex keratitis; c. Acanthamoeba keratitis

[Ref: Khurana 6th/534; Parson 22nd/198, 205-07]

"Causes of decreased corneal sensations: *Viral keratitis,* neuro-paralytic keratitis, diabetic neuropathy and leprosy"- *Khurana 6th/534*

Stromal keratitis (Herpes simplex): ***Corneal sensations are diminished***- *Khurana 6th/109*

Causes of Decreased Corneal Sensation

◈ *medifactsonline.blogspot*

- Herpes simplex keratitis
- Neuroparalytic keratitis
- Leprosy
- Acoustic neuroma
- Absolute glaucoma

Corneal Hypoesthesia Differential Diagnosis

◈ *eyewiki.aao.org*

- Herpes simplex keratitis
- Herpes zoster ophthalmicus
- Surgical trauma (PK, LASIK, large limbal incisions, ablation of the trigeminal ganglion)
- Topical medications (anesthetics, NSAIDs, ß-blockers and carbonic anhydrase inhibitors)
- Cocaine abuse
- Cerebrovascular events
- Aneurysms
- Tumors (acoustic neuroma, neurofibroma, or angioma)
- Multiple sclerosis
- Hansen disease (leprosy)
- Hereditary causes - Familial dysautonomia (Riley-Day syndrome)

"***Decreased corneal sensation*** has contributed to the misdiagnosis of **Acanthamoeba** as herpes simplex keratitis. Misdiagnosis results in delayed treatment and worse outcome. The authors found that significantly decreased corneal sensation is a frequent finding in early Acanthamoeba keratitis. Therefore, physicians should consider Acanthamoeba keratitis as an alternative diagnosis in patients with presumed herpes simplex keratitis with ***decreased corneal sensation***"- *www.ncbi.nlm.nih.go*

Acanthamoeba keratitis- *mild pain to severe pain(out of proportion to degree of inflammation)- Khurana 6th/113*

Dendritic Ulcer

◈ *Khurana 6th/108*

- Dendritic ulcer is a typical lesion of recurrent epithelial keratitis.
- The ulcer is of an irregular, zigzag linear branching shape. The branches are generally knobbed at the ends
- ***Floor of the ulcer stains with fluoresce in*** and the ***virus-laden cells at the margin take up rose bengal.***
- There is ***an associated marked diminution of corneal sensations.***

Regarding Option (d)

"**Corneal sensitivity** is decreased in Fuchs dystrophy **compared** to normal and remains subnormal even at 3 years after endothelial keratoplasty. Decreased sensitivity is likely to be related to loss of subbasal nerves and abnormal nerve morphology, ***which persist after endothelial keratoplasty***"- *www.ncbi.nlm.nih.go*

"**Penetrating keratoplasty** is the procedure of choice to ***restore vision*** in those with significant corneal scarring due to recurrent HSV keratitis. However, serious consideration must be given to the possibility of recurrence and rejection especially when the fellow eye may be normal. In parts of the world where donor corneas are in short supply penetrating keratoplasty for HSK cannot be seen as a priority. PK is also performed to re-establish the integrity of the globe after ulceration and perforation. This procedure also reduces the viral load in the cornea responsible for repeated episodes of immune-mediated keratitis. The prognostic factors for corneal grafting in HSK are the presence of an inflamed eye and corneal vascularization. Patients with active disease, an inflamed eye and vascularization have poor graft survival"- *www.ijo.in/article.asp; Parson 22nd/207*

"There are two main types of cornea transplants: traditional, full thickness cornea transplant (also known as penetrating keratoplasty, or PK) and back layer cornea transplant (also known as endothelial keratoplasty, or EK)"- *www.allaboutvision.com*

119. Ans. a. Adie's tonic pupil; b. Marcus gunn pupil

[Ref: Khurana 6th/317, 504; Parson 22nd/32]

"***The Adie's tonic pupil.*** In this condition reaction to light is absent and to near reflex is very slow and tonic. The affected pupil is larger (anisocoria)"- Khurana 6th/317

"***Argyll Robertson pupil (ARP). Here the pupil is slightly small in*** size and reaction to near reflex is present but light reflex is absent, i.e., there is light near dissociation (to remember, the acronym ARP may stand for 'accommodation reflex present'). Both pupils are involved and dilate poorly with mydriatics. It is caused by a lesion (usually neurosyphilis) in the region of tectum"- Khurana 6th/317

"***Marcus Gunn pupil.*** It is the paradoxical response of a pupil of light in the presence of a relative afferent pathway defect (RAPD). It is tested by swinging flash light test. Normally, both pupils constrict equally and the pupil to which light is transferred remains tightly constricted. In the presence of relative afferent pathway defect in one eye, the ***affected pupil will dilate*** when the flash light is moved from the normal eye to the abnormal eye. This response is called '*Marcus Gunn pupil*' or a relative afferent pupillary defect (RAPD)"- *Khurana 6th/316,524*

Anisocoria

◈ *Khurana 6th/317*

- *Difference b/w the size of two pupil is called anisocoria*
- *Pathological anisocoria is usually due to a differenece of 2 mm or more and may either be due to abnormal miosis or mydriasis of one pupil*

Pupil

◈ *Khurana 6th/504*

- Normal pupil size varies from 3 to 4 mm depending upon the illumination. But it may be abnormally small (*miosis*) or large (*mydriasis*).

Causes of Miosis

- Effect of local miotic drugs (parasympathomimetic drugs).
- Effect of systemic morphine.
- Iridocyclitis (narrow, irregular, non-reacting pupil).
- ***Horner's syndrome.***
- Head injury (pontine hemorrhage).
- Senile rigid miotic pupil.
- Due to effect of strong light
- During sleep pupil is pinpoint.

Causes of Mydriasis

- Effect of topical sympathomimetic drugs (e.g., adrenaline and phenylephrine).
- Effect of topical parasympatholytic drugs (e.g., atopine, homatropine, tropicamide and cyclopentolate).
- Acute congestive glaucoma (vertically oval large immobile pupil).
- Absolute glaucoma.
- Optic atrophy.
- Retinal detachment.
- Internal ophthalmoplegia.
- 3rd nerve paralysis.
- Belladonna poisoning.

ENT

120. Ans. c. Level I to V nodes are removed in radical neck dissection; d. Internal jugular vein is preserved in modified radical neck dissection

[Ref: Dhingra 7th/442; L and B 26th/705; ENT by Hazarika 3rd/750-53; CSDT11th/1301]

Table (Dhingra 7th/441)	Division of Neck Nodes According to Levels
Level I	Submental (IA) Submandibular (IB)
Level II	**Upper jugular** Anterior to CNXI (IIA) Posterior to CNXI (IIB)
Level III	Mid jugular
Level IV	Lower jugular
Level V	**Posterior triangle group** (spinal accessory and transverse cervical chains) Above the level of intermediate tendon of omohyoid (VA) Below the level of intermediate tendon of omohyoid (VA)
Level VI	Prelaryngeal Pretracheal Paratracheal
Level VII	Nodes of upper mediastinum

Classical Radical Neck Dissection

◈ *Dhingra 7th/442; L and B 26th/705*

Structures removed are:

Lymph node of submental, submandibular, upper, middle and lower jugular and lateral (posterior) triangle regions, i.e., level I to V along with its fibrofatty tissue

- *Internal jugular vein*
- *Spinal accessory nerve*
- *Submandibular salivary gland*
- *Sternomastiod muscle*
- *Tail of parotid*
- Omohyoid muscle

Structure saved are:

Carotid artery

Brachial plexus, phrenic nerve, vagus nerve, cervical sympathetic chain, marginal mandibular br. of facial, lingual and ***hypoglossal nerves***

"RND does not removes nodes of postauricular, suboccipital, parotid (except those in tail), facial, retropharyngeal and pretracheal regions"- Dhingra 7th/442

Modified Radial Neck Dissection *L and B 26th/705; Dhingra 7th/442*

This is defined as a surgical procedure for a metastatic cervical node with radical clearance of the all the disease (nodes level 1 to 5) without sacrificing some of the lymph bearing structures that is resected in the radical neck dissection, with an intent to preserve their function

Structures preserved are one or more of the followings–

- *Spinal accessory nerve*
- *Sternocleidomastiod muscle*
- ***Internal jugular vein***

Classification of Neck Dissection

◈ *Dhingra 7th/442*

- Radical neck dissection
- Modified radical neck dissection
  - Type I–Preserves CN XI
  - Type II–Preserves CN XI and internal jugular vein
  - Type III– Preserves CN XI, internal jugular vein and sternocleidomastoid muscle
- **Selective neck dissection**
  - Supraomohyoid (or anterolateral) (removes level I to III)
  - Lateral (removes nodes in level II, III, IV)
  - Posterolateral (removes level II to V suboccipital and postauricular nodes)
  - Anterior compartment (removes level VI nodes)
- Extended neck dissection (vide infra)

121. Ans. b. Utricle responds to linear acceleration; e. Saccule responds to linear acceleration

[Ref: Dhingra 7th/19-20; Logan and Turner 11th/372-73; ENT by Hazarika 3rd/37-39]

Vestibular System

◈ *Dhingra 7th/19-20*

- *Consists of semicircular canals and otolith organs (utricle and saccule)*

- **Semicircular canals**: *They respond to* ***angular acceleration and deceleration***
- **Utricle** *is stimulated by* ***linear acceleration and deceleration*** *or gravitational pull during the head tilts*
- *The function of* **saccule** *is similar to that of utricle as the structure of maculae in the two organs is similar but experimentally, the saccule is also seen to respond to sound vibrations*
- **Macula of the saccule** *is at right angle to the macula of the utricle and may serve* ***linear acceleration****- Hazarika 3rd/37*
- ***Otolith for linear acceleration and semicircular canal for angular acceleration****- Logan and Turner 11th/373; Hazarika 3rd/37*

The saccule and utricle together make the otolith organs. The ***utricle is sensitive to a change in horizontal movement and the saccule gives information about vertical acceleration*** (such as when in an elevator)-www.ncbi.nlm.nih.gov

122. Ans. b. Can be seen in early disease; c. More common during pregnancy; d. Reddish hue over the promontory; e. Indicate active lesion

[Ref: Dhingra 7th/96,510; ENT by Hazarika 3rd/179; Ballenger's Otorhinolaryngology 16th/318]

"**Schwartz sign** is a pink reflex, seen through intact tympanic membrane, in the area of oval window. It indicates active otosclerosis usually during pregnancy"- Dhingra 7th/510

"**Schwartz sign**, a ***reddish hue over the promontory*** caused by increased vascularity of the bone immediately under the periosteum, may be seen in the early stages of the disease but is not present in all patients"- *Ballenger's Otorhinolaryngology 16th/318*

Schwartz Sign

◈ *wiki*

- **It** also known as Flemingo's pink sign, is a ***diagnostic indicator for otosclerosis***, a disease of the bones of the middle or inner ear.
- In clinical examination of the ear drum, ***increased vascularity of the promontory*** may be seen through the ear drum. This sign is ***known as Flemingo's flush sign or Schwartz's sign***. This ***indicates otospongiosis (active otosclerosis).***
- In about 10% of cases of otosclerosis, there is a redness of the promontory of the cochlea seen through the tympanic membrane due to ***prominent vascularity*** associated with an otospongiotic focus

◈ *www.ncbi.nlm.nih.gov*

- Otosclerosis is an ***otic capsule disorder*** that leads to progressive conductive and/or sensorineural hearing loss due to stapes footplate fixation and cochlear bone involvement.
- The disorder is bilateral in 70% of patients and it usually starts between the third and fifth decade. One of its characteristic clinical findings is **Schwartze sign** which refers to a reddish discoloration over the promontory seen beyond the intact tympanic membrane.
- **Schwartze sign, also known as Flemingo's flush sign or Rising sun sign** is believed to be associated with otospongiosis which is the ***active phase of the disease***.
- The prevalence of **Schwartze sign** is estimated to be 10%. The prevalence of bilateral sign has not been reported, but it is presumed to be too low.
- It seems that the ***surgery remains a therapeutic option, when the active phase of the disease is stabilized even following a short course of pharmacologic therapy***.

"Clinical examination: The ear drum in these patients is normal (mint condition). Rarely during active phase of the disease the *increased vascularity of the promontory* may be seen through the ear drum. This sign is known as Flemingo's flush sign or Schwartz's sign. This indicates otospongiosis (active otosclerosis)"- *www.drtbalu.co.in*

"Otosclerosis is a hereditary localised disease of the bone derived from the otic capsule characterised by alternating phases of bone resorption and new bone formation. The mature lamellar bone is removed by osteoclasis and replaced by woven bone of greater thickness, cellularity and *vascularity*. The redness of the outer wall of the cochlea in this patient is associated with a hypervascular bone of otosclerosis, termed Schwartze's sign. Otosclerosis only affects the endochondral bone of the inner ear, called the otic capsule"-journals.lww.com

123. Ans. b. Predisposes to dental caries; c. Difficulty in articulation of speech; d. Difficult breast-feeding; e. Significant tongue tie need surgical release

[Ref: Dhingra 7th/248; Embryology by Inderbir Singh 11th/170]

Ankyloglossia (Tongue Tie)

◈ *Dhingra 7th/248*

- True tongue tie which produces symptoms is uncommon. If tongue can be protruded beyond the lower incisors, it is unlikely to cause ***speech defects.***
- ***It interferes with speech****- Inderbir Singh 11th/170*
- A mobile tongue is important to maintain **orodental hygiene**-to clean the debris and prevent formation of ***dental plaques.***
- ***Treatment of any significant tongue tie is transverse release and vertical closure. Thin mucosal folds can be simply incised.***
- "A fold of tissue, the lingual frenulum, extends onto the inferior surface of the tongue from near the base of the tongue. It occasionally extends across the floor of the mouth to be attached onto the mandibular alveolus, known colloquially as a '**tongue tie**'; historically, this has been ***removed to aid speech***, but the evidence for this is scanty"- *Gray's 40th/501*

"Breastfeeding problems: To breastfeed successfully, the baby needs to latch on to both the breast tissue and nipple and their tongue needs to cover the lower gum so the nipple is protected from damage. *Babies with tongue-tie aren't able to open their mouths wide enough to latch on to the breast properly"- www.nhs.uk/conditions*

- "Tongue tie lead to poor oral and dental hygiene because of limitations in lingual mobility or habitual incorrect tongue posture usually accompany messy eating habits, with food debris remaining on teeth and lips and ***causing dental caries***"- *tonguetie.net/consequences*
- Treatment isn't necessary if your baby has tongue-tie but can feed without any problems. ***If their feeding is affected, treatment involves a simple procedure called tongue-tie division***"-*www.nhs.uk/conditions*

"Tongue-tie (ankyloglossia) is a condition present at birth that restricts the tongue's range of motion.

With tongue-tie, an unusually short, thick or tight band of tissue (lingual frenulum) tethers the bottom of the tongue's tip to the floor of the mouth. A person who has tongue-tie might have ***difficulty sticking out his or her tongue.*** Tongue-tie can also affect the way a ***child eats, speaks and swallows, as well as interfere with breast-feeding.***

Sometimes tongue-tie may not cause problems. Some cases may require a simple surgical procedure for correction"- *www.mayoclinic.org*

124. Ans. a. Restores hearing when hearing loss is due to the destruction of the auditory nerve; b. Indicated in profoundly deaf person; c. Indicated in bilateral acoustic neuromas after surgery; e. Electrode is placed on the surface of the Brainstem

[Ref: Dhingra 7th/141; Current Diagnosis and Treatment in Otolaryngology 3rd/804]

Auditory Brainstem Implant

◈ *Current Diagnosis and Treatment in Otolaryngology 3rd/804*

- An auditory brainstem implant is a method of restoring hearing ***when hearing loss is due to the destruction of the auditory nerve.***
- It is an ***alternate treatment option for the profoundly deaf because*** cochlear implants cannot be used in this patient population.
- The implantation of an auditory brainstem implant can be carried out at the same time as tumor removal. During surgery, the visualization of the cochlear nucleus complex is necessary, with a recommendation for intraoperative monitoring of the facial and glossopharyngeal nerves.

Auditory Brainstem Implant (ABI)

◈ *Dhingra 7th/141*

- This implant is designed to stimulate the cochlear nuclear complex in the brainstem directly by placing the implant in the lateral recess of the fourth ventricle. ***Such an implant is needed when CN VIII has been severed in surgery of vestibular schwannoma.*** In these cases, *cochlear* implants are obviously of no use.
- In unilateral acoustic neuroma, ABI is not necessary as hearing is possible from the contralateral side but in ***bilateral acoustic neuromas as in NF_2, rehabilitation is required by ABI.***

Auditory Brain Stem Implant (ABI)

◈ *academic.oup.com*

- This development from cochlear implant technology is ***indicated for totally deaf individuals*** who have ***no auditory nerves and who are thus not candidates for a cochlear implant.***
- In practice, this patient group comprises almost exclusively sufferers from ***neurofibromatosis type 2 (NF2)*** who have been deafened as a result of ***bilateral vestibular schwannomas*** (acoustic neuromas) or from the surgery to remove them.
- Other possible indications may emerge such as ***cochlear nerve agenesis*** or the ***unimplantable cochlea from excessive ossification***.

Auditory Brain Stem Implant (ABI)

◈ *hearnet.org.au*

Auditory Brainstem Implants are a small surgically implanted device connected to the brain stem of recipients with ***severe auditory nerve damage or profound Sensorineural Hearing Loss*** that results in an absence of any hearing ability.

Severely auditory nerve damage means the Cochlea – the organ that senses sound – cannot relay sound information to the Brainstem and then the rest of the brain. *As a result, Hearing Aids or Cochlear Implants are unable to help individuals with severe auditory nerve damage.*

One condition where an Auditory Brainstem Implant may be used is when a certain kind of tumor known as Neurofibromatosis Type 2 (NF2) occurs on the auditory nerve.

Unlike Cochlear Implants, ***the electrode is placed on the surface of the Brainstem rather than being inserted into the Cochlea.***

A person with an Auditory Brainstem Implant cannot usually distinguish between different sounds but instead that have an ability to know when sound is present or absent, which can assist with lip reading

125. Ans. a. Michel aplasia; c. Absent cochlear nerve; e. Persistent otitis media and mastoiditis without eradication of the disease

[Ref: Dhingra 7th/139;Ballenger's Otorhinolaryngology 16th/476-83; Logan and Turner 10th /327; ENT by Hazarika 3rd/89]

"Congenital inner ear abnormality is the most common cause of neurosensory hearing loss and **Michel aplasia** is characterized by a ***total absence of inner ear.*** Diagnosis is established based on cross-sectional imaging findings. There is ***no place for cochlear implantation in treatment***"-*www.ncbi.nlm.nih.gov*

Enlarged Vestibular Aqueducts

◈ *vestibular.org*

- When a vestibular aqueduct is larger than normal (>1.0-1.5 mm), it is known as a large vestibular aqueduct (LVA) or by the term used here, enlarged vestibular aqueduct (EVA).
- Hearing loss or balance symptoms associated with an EVA can occur when the endolymphatic duct and sac expand to fill the larger space. When EVA is associated with such symptoms, it is referred to as ***EVA syndrome (EVA).***
- Amplification in the form of hearing aids can be helpful. In the case of fluctuating or progressive hearing loss, hearing aids with flexible programming options are necessary. ***Cochlear implants have also proven to be beneficial in some patients with EVA*** (this will depend on the existence of any co-morbid inner ear anomalies

- "Children with **enlarged vestibular aqueducts (EVA),** will benefit from learning other forms of communication, such as sign language or cued speech, or using assistive devices, such as a hearing aid or ***cochlear implant***"- *www.nidcd.nih.go*

Table: *(www.researchgate. net)* **Contraindications for the cochlear implantation**

Absolute	Relative
Agenesia of Cochlea	Inappropriate medical conditions (e.g. pulmonary, cardiac, hematologic)
Agenesia of Cochlear Nerve	Uncontrolled epilepsy
Severe mental disease	Not being available for postoperative rehabilitation
Acute/chronic otitis media and mastoiditis without eradication of the disease	
Mental retardation to cooperate with speech training	

Contraindications

◈ *emedicine.medscape.com*

- Contraindications to cochlear implantation may include ***deafness due to lesions of the eighth cranial nerve or brain stem***.
- In addition, ***chronic infections of the middle ear and mastoid cavity or tympanic membrane perforation can be contraindications***.
- The ***absence of cochlear development as demonstrated on CT scans remains an absolute contraindication***.
- Certain medical conditions that preclude cochlear implant surgery (e.g., specific hematologic, pulmonary and cardiac conditions) also may be contraindications.
- The lack of realistic expectations regarding the benefits of cochlear implantation and/or a lack of strong desire to develop enhanced oral communication skills poses a strong contraindication for implant surgery.

Cochlear Implantation

◈ *Ballenger's Otorhinolaryngology 16th/476-83*

- ***Intracochlear ossification is not a contraindication to cochlear implantation*** but can limit the type and insertion depth of the electrode array that can be introduced into the cochlea.
- ***Congenital malformations of the cochlea are likewise not contraindications to cochlear implantation.***
- When an effusion occurs in an ear with a cochlear implant, no treatment is required as long as the effusion remains uninfected.
- ***Chronic otitis media, with or without cholesteatoma, must be resolved before implantation***; this is accomplished with conventional otologic treatments.
- **Prior ear surgery** that has resulted in a mastoid cavity ***does not contraindicate cochlear implantation***, but this situation may require mastoid obliteration with closure of the external auditory canal or reconstruction of the posterior bony ear canal

126. Ans. a. Cochlea start develop by 5th week of gestation; d. Cochlea development completes at 20th week of gestation

[Ref: Dhingra 6th/12; Logan and Turner 10th /410; Dhingra 7th/13-14;Gray's 40th/651,633- 34; Current Diagnosis and Treatment in Otolaryngology 3rd/604]

"Development of inner ear starts in the 3rd week of fetal life and is complete by the 16th week. **Ectoderm** in the region of hindbrain thickens to form an *auditory placode*, which is invaginated to form auditory vesicle or the *otocyst*. The latter then differentiates into the endolymphatic duct and sac; the utricle, the semicircular ducts; and saccule and the cochlea. ***Development of phylogenetically older part of labyrinth—pars superior (semicircular canals and utricle) takes place earlier than pars inferior (saccule and cochlea)***"-*Dhingra 7th/13-14*

Cochlea: ***Development begins at 3rd week and complete by 20th week***- *Dhingra 7th/12*

"*6 week:* The cochlea and semicircular canals start forming"- I.B.Singh Embryology 10th/374

"***Cochlea fully formed by the eleventh week***"- *Logan and Turner 10th /410*

Development the Inner Ear

◈ *Current Diagnosis and Treatment in Otolaryngology 3rd/604*

- Development The ***inner ear begins at 3 weeks*** gestation as a thickening of the ectoderm on the side of the embryo. This otic placode invaginates to form the otic pit. It then pinches off and begins to enlarge, forming the otocyst.
- Beginning in **weeks 5–6**, the otocyst elongates and partitions itself into what will become six different sensory structures (three semicircular canals, two otolithic organs and one cochlea) and the endolymphatic duct and sac.
- By 12 weeks, the formation of the membranous labyrinth is complete and the sensory cells have differentiated.
- By 16 weeks, cartilage has formed around the membranous labyrinth.
- By 23 weeks, this has undergone complete endochondral ossification to form the adult-size otic capsule.
- By 26 weeks, the human inner ear is sending auditory information to the brain.

Embryology

◈ *emedicine.medscape.com*

- ***During week 4 of embryonic development***, the human inner ear develops from the auditory placode, a ***thickening of the ectoderm*** that gives rise to the bipolar neurons of the cochlear and vestibular ganglions.
- As the auditory placode invaginates towards the embryonic mesoderm, it forms the auditory vesicle or otocysts.
- The auditory vesicle gives rise to the utricular and saccular components of the membranous labyrinth. They contain the sensory hair cells and otoliths of the macula of utricle and of the saccule, respectively
- Beginning in the **fifth week of development,** the auditory vesicle also gives rise to the ***cochlear duct, which contains the***

spiral organ of Corti and the endolymph that accumulates in the membranous labyrinth.

Table: *(Dhingra 7th/14)*: **Timing of development of ear in the week of gestation**

Development	Middle ear	Vestibular labyrinth	Cochlea
Begins	3rd	3rd	3rd
Complete	30th	20th	20th

127. Ans. a. Erythroplakia; b. Lichen planus

[Ref: Dhingra 7th/253-54,255; Logan and Turner 11th/228,270-71; L and B 26th/707; Logan and Turner 10th /126; ENT by Hazarika 3rd/502; Neena Khanna 5th/387]

Fordyce Spots

◈ *Dhingra 7th/248*

- They are aberrant sebaceous glands present under the buccal or labial mucosa and shine through it as ***yellowish or yellow-brown spots***.
- They are seen with equal frequency in both males and females and are ***considered normal.***

Premalignant Lesion for Oral Cavity Cancer

◈ *Dhingra 7th/253-54; Hazarika 3rd/502*

- ***Leukoplakia*** ("white patch") is induced by the same factors (tobacco, alcohol) that cause carcinomas. The ***malignant potential of leukoplakia corresponds to the degree of cellular dysplasia seen on biopsy***.
- ***Erythroplakia*** ("red patch") usually shows severe cellular dysplasia and carries a ***50% risk of malignant degeneration***
- ***Melanosis and mucosal hyperpigmentation:*** *May transform into malignant melanoma*
- ***Submucous fibrosis***
- Oral lichen planus –*Harshmohan 7th/507*

"Oral lichen planus is one of the potentially malignant disorders that may be seen in six different subtypes including papular, reticular, plaque-like, atrophic, erosive and bullous type, clinically. Atrophic and erosive subtypes have the greater increased malignant transformation risk compared to another subtypes"- *www.ncbi.nlm.nih.gov*

Aphthous ulcers are one of the most common problems that occur in the mouth. About 20% of the population (1 in 5 people) have aphthous ulcers at any given time. Aphthous ulcers typically last for 10-14 days and they heal without leaving a scar. There are many possible causes of aphthous ulcers. Often the cause is unknown"- *www.medicinenet.com;* Harshmohan 7th/507

"Behchets *syndrome (Oculo-oro-genital syndrome)*: *It is characterized by a triad of aphthous-like ulcer in oral cavity, genital ulceration and uveitis"-Dhingra 7th/246*

"The major signs and symptoms presented in the oral environment of a **psoriasis patient may include *geographic tongue, fissure tongue, gingival and/or mucosal lesions***"-*www.ncbi.nlm.nih.gov*

128. Ans. a. Allergic mucin containing scattered fungal hyphae is pathological hallmark; c. Allergic reaction to fungus; e. In severe cases corticosteroids are used for treatment

[Ref: Dhingra 7th/220; Logan and Turner 11th/56;Logan Turner 10th/51-52; Ballenger's Otorhinolaryngology 16th/764, 770]

Allergic Fungal Sinusitis

◈ *Dhingra 7th/220*

- It is an ***allergic reaction*** to the causative fungus and presents with sinunasal polyposis and mucin. The latter contains eosinophils, Charcot-Leyden crystals and fungal hyphae
- There is ***no invasion of the sinus mucosa with fungus***
- Usually more than one sinus are involved on one or both sides
- CT scan shows *mucosal thickening with hyperdense areas*
- There may be expansion of the sinus or bone erosion due to pressure, *but no fungal invasion*
- Treatment is endoscopic surgical clearance of the sinuses with provision of drainage and ventilation. This is combined with pre and postoperative systemic steroids

◈ *Ballenger's Otorhinolaryngology 16th/764, 770*

- Most patients with AFS are immunocompetent and present with features of refractory sinusitis and nasal polyposis. *Many also have a history of atopy or asthma.*
- The pathogenesis is incompletely understood, but evidence supports a Gell and Coombs *type I (IgE-mediated) immune response to fungal antigens. Type III and IV immune responses may also be involved.*
- The ***pathologic hallmark of AFS is "allergic mucin,*** consisting of eosinophils, Charcot-Leyden crystals and ***scattered fungal hyphae***. Although AFS is not thought to be invasive, bony erosion is seen on computed tomographic (CT) scans in 20% of reported cases.
- The *diagnosis of AFS is confirmed by demonstration of allergic mucin and culture of the fungus.*
- It is ***treated by surgical débridement*** and aeration of the involved sinus followed by the ***use of systemic and topical intranasal corticosteroids.***
- **Specific immunotherapy** with multiple relevant fungal and nonfungal antigens has reduced the necessity for ***corticosteroid therapy***, while preventing recurrence of the disease and the need for repeat surgery

Allergic Fungal Rhinosinusitis (AFS)

◈ *Current Diagnosis and Treatment in Otolaryngology 3rd /295*

- Allergic fungal sinusitis is characterized by the presence of **allergic mucin**, which is thick inspissated mucus with eosinophils and ***fungal hyphae.***
- Treatment is ***primarily surgical with postoperative topical and systemic steroids.*** Immunotherapy, systemic steroids and postoperative management by an allergist may be necessary to reduce recurrence.

Four Different Varieties of Fungal Infection of Sinuses are Seen *Dhingra 7th/220*

- *Fungal ball*
- *Allergic fungal sinusitis*

- *Chronic invasive sinusitis*
- *Fulminant fungal sinusitis*

"Invasive fungal sinusitis: The treatment consists of (1) debriding all involved structures, (2) *aggressive intravenous antifungal therapy* and (3) normalizing the underlying immuno-compromised state (usually neutropenia or uncontrolled diabetes)"- *Current Diagnosis and Treatment in Otolaryngology* 3rd /295

129. Ans. a. Stage T4a- Frontal sinus involvement; b. Stage T3- Ethmoid sinus involvement

[Ref: Dhingra 7th/234; Current Diagnosis and Treatment in Otolaryngology 3rd /312; Logan and Turner 10th /210; ENT by Hazarika 3rd/375]

Table: *(Dhingra 7th/234)*: **TNM classification and staging system of cancer of maxillary sinus**

Maxillary Sinus	
T_1	Tumour limited to maxillary sinus mucosa with no erosion or destruction of bone.
T_2	Tumour causing bone erosion or destruction including extension into the hard palate and/or middle nasal meatus, except extension to posterior wall of maxillary sinus and pterygoid plates
T_3	Tumour invades any of the following: ***bone of the posterior wall of maxillary sinus***, subcutaneous tissues, floor or medial wall of orbit, pterygoid fossa and ***ethmoid sinuses.***
T_{4a}	Tumour invades anterior orbital contents, skin of cheek, pterygoid plates, infratemporal fossa, cribriform plate, ***sphenoid or frontal sinuses.***
T_{4b}	Tumour invades any of the following: orbital apex, dura, brain, middle cranial fossa, cranial nerves other than maxillary division of trigeminal nerve (V_2), nasopharynx or clivus.

Maxillary Sinus Primary Tumor (T)

◈ *American Joint Committee on Cancer Atlas 2006/55-56*

- **TX** Primary tumor cannot be assessed
- **T0** No evidence of primary tumor
- **Tis** Carcinoma *in situ*
- **T1** Tumor limited to the maxillary sinus mucosa with no erosion or destruction of bone
- **T2** Tumor causing bone erosion or destruction including extension into the hard palate and/or middle nasal meatus, except extension to posterior wall of maxillary sinus and pterygoid plates
- **T3** Tumor invades any of the following: bone of the posterior wall of maxillary sinus, subcutaneous tissues, floor or medial wall of orbit, pterygoid fossa, ethmoid sinuses
- **T4a** Tumor invades anterior orbital contents, skin of cheek, pterygoid plates, infratemporal fossa, cribriform plate, sphenoid or frontal sinuses
- **T4b** Tumor invades any of the following: orbital apex, dura, brain, middle cranial fossa, cranial nerves other than maxillary division of trigeminal nerve V2, nasopharynx, or clivus

130. Ans. a. Hypercalcemia; d. Nephrocalcinosis

[Ref: Harrison 19th/2479; Davidson 22nd/130,767; Robbins 9th (SAE)/937]

***In* milk-alkali syndrome there is *suppression of endogenous PTH (not hyperparathyroidism)* and *some depletion of total-body water (*not hypervolemia)**

Hypervolemia, or **fluid overload,** is the medical condition where there is too much fluid in the blood- *www.healthline.com*

"Too much calcium can lead to **constipation** and toxicity has been observed in '**milk-alkali syndrome**"-Davidson 22nd/130

"**Hypercalcemia and Nephrocalcinosis** Disorders associated with hypercalcemia, such as hyperparathyroidism, or excess calcium intake (milk-alkali syndrome), may induce the formation of calcium stones and deposition of calcium in the kidney (**nephrocalcinosis**). Extensive degrees of calcinosis, under certain conditions, may lead to chronic tubulointerstitial disease and renal insufficiency"- *Robbins 9th (SAE)/937*

Milk-Alkali Syndrome

◈ *Harriosn 19th/2479*

- The milk-alkali syndrome is due to excessive ingestion of calcium and absorbable antacids such as milk or calcium carbonate. It is much less frequent since proton pump inhibitors and other treatments became available for peptic ulcer disease. For a time, the increased use of calcium carbonate in the management of secondary hyperparathyroidism led to reappearance of the syndrome.
- Several clinical presentations—acute, subacute and chronic—have been described, all of which feature ***hypercalcemia***, alkalosis and renal failure. The chronic form of the disease, termed *Burnett's syndrome*, is associated with irreversible renal damage. The acute syndromes reverse if the excess calcium and absorbable alkali are stopped.
- Development of hypercalcemia causes increased sodium excretion and ***some depletion of total-body water.*** These phenomena and perhaps some ***suppression of endogenous PTH secretion*** due to mild hypercalcemia lead to increased bicarbonate resorption and to alkalosis in the face of continued calcium carbonate ingestion.
- Calcium carbonate and sodium bicarbonate are potent antacids with varying levels of potential problems. The long-term use of calcium carbonate (converts to calcium chloride in the stomach) can lead to milk-alkali syndrome (***hypercalcemia, hyperphosphatemia with possible renal calcinosis*** and progression to renal insufficiency). Sodium bicarbonate may induce systemic alkalosis- Harriosn 19th/1920
- ***Parathyroid suppression***- seen in Milk-alkali syndrome- *Harriosn 19th/2461*
- In severe cases, ***treatment involves giving fluids*** through the vein (by IV). Otherwise, treatment involves drinking fluids along with reducing or stopping calcium supplements and antacids that contain calcium-*www.huronregional.org*

Milk-Alkali Syndrome Symptoms

◈ *www.huronregional.org*

In the beginning, the condition usually has no symptoms (asymptomatic). When symptoms do occur, they can include:

- Back, middle of the body and low back pain in the kidney area (related to ***kidney stones***)
- Confusion, strange behavior
- ***Constipation***
- Depression
- ***Excessive urination***
- Fatigue
- Irregular heartbeat (arrhythmia)
- Nausea or vomiting
- Other problems that can result from kidney failure

131. Ans. e. There is no role of chemotherapy and radiotherapy

[Ref: Harrison 19th/2321-23; L and B 26th/782]

Adrenocortical Carcinoma

◈ *Harrison 19th/2321-23*

- ACC is generally considereda highly malignant tumor; however, it presents with broad inter individual variability with regard to biologic characteristics and clinical behavior.
- Somatic mutations in the tumor-suppressor gene TP53 are found in 25% of apparently sporadic ACC. Germline TP53 mutations are the cause of the Li-Fraumeni syndrome associated with multiple solid organ cancers including ACC and are found in 25% of pediatric ACC cases
- FNA is not indicated in suspected ACC
- Metastasis in ACC most frequently occurs to liver and lung.
- ***Cure of ACC can only be achieved by early detection and complete surgical removal.*** Capsule violation during primary surgery, metastasis at diagnosis and primary treatment in a nonspecialist center are major determinants of poor survival. If the primary tumor invades adjacent organs, en bloc removal of kidney and spleen should be considered to reduce the risk of recurrence.
- ***Surgery can also be considered in a patient with metastases if there is severe tumor-related hormone excess.*** This indication needs to be carefully weighed against surgical risk, including thromboembolic complications and the resulting delay in the introduction of other therapeutic options.
- Patients with confirmed ACC and successful removal of the primary tumor should receive adjuvant treatment with **mitotane**
- **Single metastases** can be ***addressed surgically or with radiofrequency ablation as appropriate.*** If the tumor recurs or progresses during mitotane treatment, chemotherapy should be considered; the established first-line chemotherapy regimen is the combination of cisplatin, etoposide and doxorubicin plus continuing mitotane.
- ***Painful bone metastasis responds to irradiation.*** Overall survival in ACC is still poor, with 5-year survival rates of 30–40% and a median survival of 15 months in metastatic ACC

Adrenocortical Carcinoma

◈ *Treatment L and B 26th/782*

- ***Complete tumor resection (R0) is associated with favourable survival and should be attempted whenever possible.***
- In order to prevent tumor spillage and implantation metastases, the capsule must not be damaged. *En bloc* resection with removal of locally involved organs is often required and in case of tumor thrombus in the vena cava thrombectomy is needed. Laparoscopic adrenalectomyis associated with a high incidence of local recurrence and cannot be recommended.
- ***Tumor debulking plays a role in functioning tumors to control hormone excess.***
- ***Adjuvant radiotherapy may reduce the rate of local recurrence.***

132. Ans. a. Subtracheal stenosis; b. Barotrauma; c. Biotrauma; d. Atelectrauma

[Ref: ICU Book by Paul Marino 3rd/427,462; Harrison 19th/1741-43; Davidson 22nd/195; Morgan 5th/1289]

Ventilator-Induced Lung Injury

◈ *ICU Book by Paul Marino 3rd/462*

- Because inflation volumes are distributed preferentially to regions of normal lung function, inflation volumes tend to over distend the normal regions of diseased lungs. This tendency to over distend normal lung regions is exaggerated when large inflation volumes are used.
- The **hyperinflation of normal lung regions during mechanical ventilation can produce stress fractures at the alveolar-capillary interface.**
- These fractures may be the result of excessive alveolar pressures (*barotrauma*) or excessive alveolar volumes (*volutrauma*)
- Alveolar rupture can have three adverse consequences. The first is accumulation of alveolar gas in the pulmonary parenchyma (pulmonary interstitial emphysema), mediastinum (pneumomediastinum), or pleural cavity (pneumothorax). The second adverse consequence is a condition of inflammatory lung injury that is indistinguishable from ARDS. The third and possibly worst consequence is multiorgan injury from release of inflammatory mediators into the bloodstream. This latter process is known as ***biotrauma.***

Complications of Mechanical Ventilation

◈ *Harrison 19th/1743*

- Endotracheal intubation and mechanical ventilation have direct and indirect effects on the lung and upper airways, the cardiovascular system and the gastrointestinal system.
- Pulmonary complications include ***barotrauma, nosocomial pneumonia, oxygen toxicity, tracheal stenosis and deconditioning of respiratory muscles.***
- ***Barotrauma and volutrauma over distend and disrupt lung tissue***; may be clinically manifest by ***interstitial emphysema,***

pneumomediastinum, subcutaneous emphysema, or pneumothorax; and can result in the liberation of cytokines from over distended tissues, further promoting tissue injury. Clinically significant pneumothorax requires tube thoracostomy.

Ventilator Associated Lung Injury (VALI) can occur due to: *lifeinthefastlane.com*

- *volutramua*
- *barotrauma*
- *biotrauma*
- *recruitment/derecruitment injury (atelectotrauma)*
- *shearing injury*
- *oxygen toxicity*

"**Atelectotrauma** Injury to the lung caused by shearing forces as alveoli that are next to each other collapse and re-expand during mechanicalventilation. The condition may be prevented by applying enough positive end-expiratory pressure to limit alveolar collapse at end expiration"- *medical-dictionary*

133. Ans. a. Non hodgkin lymphoma; b. Cervical cancer; c. Kaposi sarcoma; e. Anal cancer

[Ref: Harrison 19th/1268; CMDT 2016/1322; Ananthanarayan 9th/576-77; Lippincott Microbiology 3rd/302; Davidson 22nd/405]

Neoplastic Diseases

◈ *Harrison 19th/1268*

- The neoplastic diseases considered to be AIDS defining conditions are ***Kaposi's sarcoma, non-Hodgkin's lymphoma and invasive cervical carcinoma.***
- In addition, there is also an increase in the incidence of a variety of **non-AIDS-defining malignancies** including ***Hodgkin's disease; multiple myeloma; leukemia; melanoma;, brain, testicular, oral, lung, gastric, liver, renal and anal cancers.***

"Four cancers are currently included in the CDC classification of AIDS *Kaposi sarcoma, non-Hodgkin lymphoma, primary lymphoma of the brain and invasive cervical carcinoma*"-*CMDT 2016/1322*

"HIV-related cancers The AIDS-defining cancers are ***Kaposi's sarcoma, cervical cancer and non-Hodgkin lymphoma***"-*Davidson 22nd/405*

134. Ans. b. One oral temperature ≥38.5°C; c. A sustained oral temperature >38°C for more than 1 hour; d. Absolute neutrophil count <0.5 × 10^9/L; e. Absolute neutrophil count <1.0 × 10^9/L with a predictable decline to ≤0.5 × 10^9/l in 24–48 h

[Ref: Harrison 19th/; Davidson 22nd/274]

Febrile Neutropenia

◈ *Harrison 19th/103e-23*

- Febrile neutropenia refers to the clinical presentation of fever (one temperature ≥38.5°C or three readings ≥38°C but ≤38.5°C per 24 h) in a neutropenic patient with an uncontrolled neoplasm involving the bone marrow or, more usually, in a patient undergoing treatment with cytotoxic agents.
- Mortality from uncontrolled infection varies inversely with the neutrophil count. If the nadir neutrophil count is >1000/μL, there is little risk; if<500/μL, risk of death is markedly increased.
- "Neutropenic fever is defined as a ***pyrexia of 38°C for over1 hour*** in a patient with a ***neutrophil count <1.0 × 10^9/L***"-*Davidson 22nd/274*

Febrile neutropaenia (or neutropaenic fever) is defined as *lifeinthefastlane.com*

- ***a single temperature measurement >38.5°C, or a sustained temperature >38C*** for more than 1 hour
- In a patient with a decreased absolute neutrophil count (ANC) of either **<0.5 x 10^9/L, or <1 x 10^9/L** with a predicted nadir of **<0.5 x 10^9/L** over the subsequent 48h

"Neutropenic fever is ***a single oral temperature of 38.3°C (101°F) or a temperature of greater than 38.0° C (100.4°F) sustained for more than 1 hour in a patient with neutropenia***"-emedicine.medscape.com

"Febrile neutropenia is defined as single oral temperature of *38.3°C (101.4°F) or 38.0°C (101°F) over 1 hour with less than 500 neutrophils/mm3 or less than 1,000 neutrophils/mm³ with a predicted decline to 500/mm3 over the next 48 hours.* In some situations, where fever may not be there but obvious infection is present and absolute neutrophil count (ANC) is low, it may be treated as FN. The single most important determinant of neutropenic fever is the ANC less than 100 and the duration of neutropenia (>14 days)" -*www.apiindia.org*

"Febrile neutropenia is defined as an **oral or tympanic membrane temperature** of ≥38°C on two occasions, at least one hour apart within a 12 h period or a single temperature of >38.5°C with ***an absolute neutrophil count of ≤0.5 × 10^9/l or ≤1.0 × 10^9/l with a predictable decline to ≤0.5 × 10^9/l in 24–48 h***"- *www.sciencedirect.com*

135. Ans. a. Continuous murmur; b. Aortic ejection systolic murmur; c. Loud P2; d. Mitral opening snap; e. Mid diastolic murmur at apex

[Ref: Harrison 19th/1523; Davidson 22nd/632; Hurst's The Heart 12th/Chap 82; O.P.Ghai 8th/417-18]

PDA

◈ O.P.Ghai 8th/417-18

- S1- accentuated (loud M1)
- ***P2 is louder than normal***
- It is difficult to evaluate the S2 because masking by continuous murmur
- Shunt murmur- ***continuous (machinery)***
- Flow murmurs- ***mitral delayed diastolic and aortic ejection systolic murmur***
- S3 with large shunt

Patent Ductus Arteriosus

◈ *Nelson 20th/2197*

- The apical impulse is prominent and, with cardiac enlargement, is heaving. A thrill, maximal in the 2nd left interspace, is often present and may radiate toward the left clavicle, down the left sternal border, or toward the apex. It is usually systolic but may also be palpated throughout the cardiac cycle.

- The **classic continuous murmur** is described as being ***like machinery or rolling thunder in quality***. It begins soon after onset of the 1st sound, reaches maximal intensity at the end of systole and wanes in late diastole. It may be localized to the 2nd left intercostal space or radiate down the left sternal border or to the left clavicle.
- When pulmonary vascular resistance is increased, the diastolic component of the murmur may be less prominent or absent. In patients with a large left-to-right shunt, a low-pitched ***mitral mid-diastolic murmur may be audible at the apex*** as a result of the increased volume of blood flow across the mitral valve.

Physical Examination

◈ *Hurst's The Heart 12th/Chap 82*

- The apical impulse may be increased or displaced in those with large shunts. The right ventricular impulse is increased in a premature infant with respiratory distress and in infants and children with significant pulmonary hypertension.
- The **typical murmur is a continuous or "machinery" murmur** best heard at the left upper sternal border and below the left clavicle. It is usually a rough murmur with eddy sounds, which are helpful in making the diagnosis and it peaks at or near the second heart sound.
- In patients with at least a **moderate shunt**, there is a ***middiastolic rumble at the apex as a result of relative mitral stenosis*** from increased flow across the mitral valve.
- The **second heart sound may be difficult to hear** because of the continuous murmur, but it is usually normal. The pulmonary component is accentuated in those with pulmonary hypertension.

"PDA In most adults with this anomaly, pulmonary pressures are normal and a gradient and shunt from aorta to pulmonary artery persist throughout the cardiac cycle, resulting in a characteristic thrill and a **continuous "machinery" murmur** with ***late systolic accentuation at the upper left sternal edge***"- *Harrison 19th/1523*

"**A continuous 'machinery' murmur is** heard with ***late systolic accentuation,*** maximal in the second left intercostal space below the clavicle"- *Davidson 22nd/632*

A mitral opening snap may be caused by *www.gpnotebook.co.uk*

- Mitral stenosis with a mobile valve
- Rapid mitral flow causes a soft snap e.g. ***left to right shunts such as a VSD or PDA***. Also may occur in severe mitral regurgitation

136. Ans. b. Soft 1st heart second

[Ref: Harrison 19th/1521; Davidson 22nd/633; O.P.Ghai 8th/413-14; Nelson (SAE) 20th/2189-91,2246-47]

Atrial Septal Defect (ASD)

◈ *O.P.Ghai 8th/413-14*

- ***S2 Wide fixed split, P2++***
- ***S1 Accentuated –loud T1***
- "An increased flow through the tricuspid valve may result in a ***soft delayed diastolic rumble at the lower left sternal border***"
- Shunt murmur-absent
- Flow murmur- Delayed diastolic (Tricupid), Ejection systolic (Pulmonary)

Atrial Septal Defect (ASD) Physical Examination

◈ *Harrison 19th/1521*

- Examination usually reveals a prominent RV impulse and palpable pulmonary artery pulsation. ***The first heart sound is normal or split***, with accentuation of the tricuspid valve closure sound.
- Increased flow across the pulmonic valve is responsible for a ***midsystolic pulmonary outflow murmur.*** The ***second heart sound is widely split and is fixed in relation to respiration.***
- A mid-diastolic rumbling murmur, loudest at the fourth intercostal space and along the left sternal border, Ref:lects increased flow across the tricuspid valve.
- In ostium primum ASD, an **apical holosystolic murmur** indicates associated mitral or tricuspid regurgitation or a ventricular septal defect (VSD).

ASD Clinical Features and Investigations

◈ *Davidson 22nd/633*

The characteristic physical signs are the result of the volume overload of the RV:

- **Wide, fixed splitting of the second heart sound** wide because of delay in right ventricular ejection (increased stroke volume and right bundle branch block) and fixed because the septal defect equalizes left and right atrial pressures throughout the respiratory cycle
- A **systolic flow murmur** over the pulmonary valve.
- In children with a large shunt, there may be a ***diastolic flow murmur over the tricuspid valve***. Unlike a mitral flow murmur, this is usually high-pitched.

Atrial Septal Defect

◈ *Nelson (SAE) 20th/2189-91*

- An ***ostium secundum defect in the region of the fossa ovalis is the most common form of ASD*** and is associated with structurally normal atrioventricular (AV) valves
- Examination of the chest may reveal a ***mild left precordial bulge. A right ventricular systolic lift is generally palpable at the left sternal border.***
- ***A loud 1st heart sound*** and sometimes a pulmonic ejection click can be heard. In most patients, the **2nd heart sound** is characteristically ***widely split and fixed in its splitting*** in all phases of respiration.
- A ***systolic ejection murmur is heard.***
- A ***short, rumbling mid-diastolic murmur***

137. Ans. a. Associated with abnormal P wave; d. Each P wave is not always followed by QRS complex

[Ref: A.K.Jain 6th/301; ECG Made Easy 8th/63; Davidson 22nd/564]

Atrial Extrasystoles

◈ *ECG Made Easy 8th/63,109; A.K.Jain 6th/301*

- ***Abnormal P waves*** followed by long PR interval because extrasystolic excitation impulse takes abnormal sinus path to reach AVN
- ***Normal QRS complex***
- There is pause b/w extrasystole and the next normal beat, therefore TP interval is more than its normal value of 0.2 sec

Atrial ectopic beats (extrasystoles, premature beats) *Davidson 22nd/564*

- These usually cause no symptoms but can give the sensation of a missed beat or an abnormally strong beat.
- The ECG shows a premature but **otherwise normal QRS complex**; ***if visible, the preceding P wave has a different morphology because the atria activate from an abnormal site.***
- In most cases, these are of no consequence, although very frequent atrial ectopic beats may herald the onset of atrial fibrillation. Treatment is rarely necessary but β-blockers can be used if symptoms are intrusive.

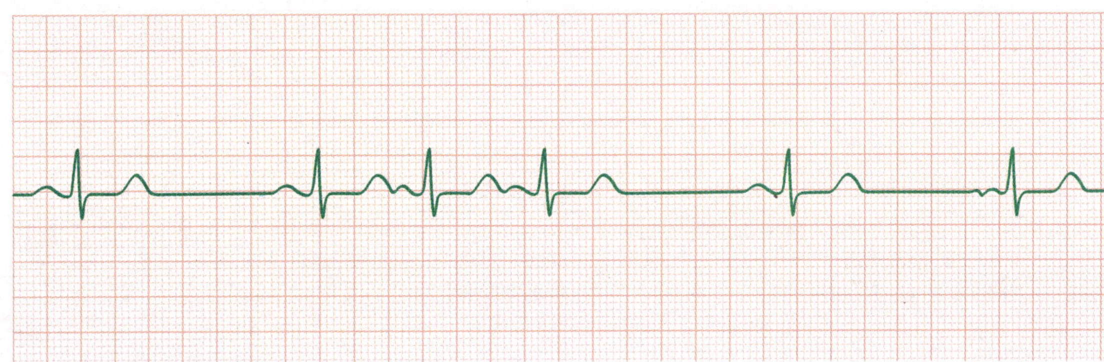

Fig: *(Davidson 22nd/564):* Atrial ectopic beats. The first, second and fifth complexes are normal sinus beats. The third, fourth and sixth complexes are atrial ectopic beats with ***identical QRS complexes and abnormal (sometimes barely visible) P waves.***

"**Atrial flutter** Most easily seen in Lead II. Atrial rate is greater than 250/min (b/w 200-350bpm). ECG shows ***saw-tooth pattern***"- *A.K.Jain 6th/301; ECG Made Easy 8th/68*

138. Ans. c. Polycythemia

[Ref: Harrison 19th/1731-32; Davidson 22nd/663-65]

- PaO_2 = measures oxygen in the blood (80-100 mm Hg)
- SaO_2 = measures tissue perfusion (pulse ox 95-100%)

PaO_2 (Partial Pressure of Oxygen in Arterial Blood)

◈ *webapp1.dlib.indiana.ed*

It reflects the amount of oxygen gas dissolved in the blood. It primarily measures the effectiveness of the lungs in pulling oxygen into the blood stream from the atmosphere.

Elevated pO_2 levels are associated with:

- Increased oxygen levels in the inhaled air
- ***Polycythemia***

Decreased PO_2 levels are associated with:

- *Decreased oxygen levels in the inhaled air*
- *Anemia*
- ***Heart decompensation***
- *Chronic obstructive pulmonary disease*
- *Restrictive pulmonary disease*
- *Hypoventilation*

"Cor pulmonale is a condition that causes the right side of the heart to fail. Long-term high blood pressure in the arteries of the lung and right ventricle of the heart can lead to cor pulmonale"- medlineplus.gov

Type II Respiratory Failure

◈ *Harrison 19th/1732*

- This type of respiratory failure is a consequence of **alveolar hypoventilation** and results from the inability to eliminate carbon dioxide effectively.
- Mechanisms are categorized by impaired central nervous system (CNS) drive to breathe, impaired strength with failure of neuromuscular function in the respiratory system and increased load(s) on the respiratory system.
- Reasons for diminished CNS drive to breathe include ***drug overdose, brainstem injury, sleep-disordered breathing and severe hypothyroidism.***
- Reduced strength can be due to impaired neuromuscular transmission (e.g., ***myasthenia gravis, Guillain Barre syndrome, amyotrophic lateral sclerosis) or respiratory muscle weakness (e.g., myopathy, electrolyte derangements, fatigue).***

Type I Acute Hypoxemic Respiratory Failure

◈ *Harrison 19th/1731*

- This type of respiratory failure occurs with alveolar flooding and subsequent intrapulmonary shunt physiology. Alveolar flooding may be a consequence of ***pulmonary edema, pneumonia, or alveolar hemorrhage.***
- Pulmonary edema can be further categorized as occurring due to elevated pulmonary microvascular pressures, as seen in heart failure and intravascular volume overload or ARDS ("low-pressure pulmonary edema,". This syndrome is defined by acute onset (≤1 week) of bilateral opacities

on chest imaging that are not fully explained by cardiac failure or fluid overload and of shunt physiology requiring positive end-expiratory pressure (PEEP).

- Type I respiratory failure occurs in clinical settings such as ***sepsis, gastric aspiration, pneumonia, near-drowning, multiple blood transfusions and pancreatitis.***
- The mortality rate among patients with ARDS was traditionally very high (50–70%), although changes in patient care have led to mortality rates closer to 30% (see below)

Table: *(Davidson 22nd/664)*: **How to interpret blood gas abnormalities in respiratory failure**

	Type I		**Type II**	
	Hypoxia (PaO_2 <8.0kPa (60 mmHg) Normal or low $PaCO_2$ (<6.6 kPa (50 mmHg)		Hypoxia (PaO_2 <8.0 kPa (60 mmHg) Raised $PaCO_2$ (> 6.6 kPa (50 mmHg)	
	Acute	Chronic	Acute	Chronic
H+	→	→	↑	→ or ↑
Bicarbonate	→	→	→	↑
Causes	Acute asthma Pulmonary edema Pneumonia Lobar collapse Pneumothorax Pulmonary embolus ARDS	COPD Lung fibrosis Lymphangitis Carcinomatosa Right-to-left shunts	Acute severe asthma Acute exacerbation of COPD Upper airway obstruction Acute neuropathies/paralysis Narcotic drugs Primary alveolar hypoventilation Flail chest injury	COPD Sleep apnea Kyphoscoliosis Myopathies/muscular dystrophy Ankylosing spondylitis

139. Ans. b. Forced residual capacity (FRC); d. Total lung capacity (TLC); e. Residual volume

[Ref: Harrison 19th/1662, Chap306e; Davidson 22nd/652 : Robbins 9th (SAE)/674; CMDT 2015/257- 58; http: //www. ncbi. nlm. nih. gov/ pubmed/19349398]

FEV1 decreases less in restrictive lung disease vis-à-vis obstructive lung disease

Table: Difference b/w obstructive and Restrictive lung diseases

	Obstructive lung disease (e.g emphysema)	**Restrictive lung disease**
Residual volume	Increase	Decrease
FRC	Increase	Decrease
Total lung capacity	Normal to increase	Decrease
Diffusion capacity	Normal (Except emphysema)	Decreased
Vital capacity	Decrease	Decrease
FEF 25-75%	Decrease	Normal
FEV1/FVC	Decrease	Normal to increase

"In individuas with **diffuse obstructive disorders**, pulmonary function tests show decreased maximal airflow rates during forced expiration, usually expressed as the ***forced expiratory volume at 1 second (FEV1) over the forced ventilatory capacity (FVC). An FEV1/FVC*** ratio of less than 0.7 generally indicates airway obstruction. Expiratory airflow obstruction may be caused by a variety of conditions that are ideally distinguished by distinct pathologic changes and different mechanisms of airflow obstruction. As discussed later, however, such neat distinctions are not always possible. In contrast, ***restrictive diseases are associated with proportionate decreases in both total lung capacity and FEV1, leading to normal FEV1/FVC ratio***"- Robbins 9th (SAE)/674

"The conventional FEV (1)/FVC test is the "gold standard" to quantitate airway obstruction, but elderly subjects or patients with severe respiratory diseases quite frequently cannot make such an effort. Many studies have investigated the usefulness of **FEV (1)/forced expired volume in 6 s (FEV 6)** measurements as an alternative for FEV (1)/FVC for ***diagnosis of airway obstruction***. FEV (1)/FEV (6) is a sensitive and specific test for the ***diagnosis of airway obstruction.*** FEV (1)/FEV (6) can be used as a valid alternative for FEV (1)/FVC in the diagnosis of airway obstruction"-www. ncbi. nlm. nih. gov/ pubmed/19349398

*"The data from the current study indicate that FEV1/FEV6, 73% and FEV6, 82% predicted can be used as a valid alternative for the FEV1/FVC, 70% and FVC, 80% pred cut-off points for the **detection of obstruction and restriction, respectively**" (erj. ersjournals. com/content/27/2/378. full. pdf)*

Measurement of Airway Obstruction

◈ *Davidson 22nd/652*

- Airway narrowing is assessed by asking patients to blow out as hard and as fast as they can into a peak flow meter or a spirometer. Peak flow meters are cheap and convenient for home monitoring of **peak expiratory flow (PEF)** in the detection and monitoring of asthma, but results are effort-dependent. More accurate and reproducible measures are obtained by inhaling fully, then exhaling at maximum effort into a spirometer.
- The forced expired volume in 1 second (FEV1) is the volume exhaled in the first second and the forced vital

capacity (FVC) is the total volume exhaled. ***FEV1 is disproportionately reduced in airflow obstruction***, resulting in FEV1/FVC ratios of less than 70%.

Table: *(Harrison)*: **Common abnormalities of pulmonary function. Pulmonary function values are expressed as a percentage of normal predicted values**

	Restriction due to Increased lung elastic recoil (pulmonary fibrosis)	Restriction due to chest wall abnormality (moderate obesity)	Restriction due to respiratory muscle weakness (myasthenia gravis)	Obstruction due to airway narrowing (acute asthma)	Obstruction due to decreased elastic recoil (severe emphysema)
TLC	60%	95%	75%	100%	130%
FRC	60%	65%	100%	104%	220%
RV	60%	100%	120%	120%	310%
FVC	60%	92%	60%	90%	60%
FEV1	75%	92%	60%	35% pre-b. d., 75% post-b. d	35% pre-b. d., 38% post-b. d.
Raw	1. 0	1.0	1.0	2.5	1.5
DLCO	60%	95%	80%	120%	40%

140. Ans. d. Thrombolysis should be done within 48 hour

[Ref: Harrison 19th/1595-98; Davidson 22nd/; CMDT 2016/363-65]

Acute Coronary Syndromes Without St-Segment Elevation

◈ *CMDT 2016/363*

- Distinction in acute coronary syndrome between patients with and without ST-segment elevation at presentation is ***essential to determine need for reperfusion therapy.***
- ***Fibrinolytic therapy is harmful in acute coronary syndrome without ST-segment elevation***, unlike with ST-segment elevation, where acute reperfusion saves lives.
- ***Antiplatelet and anticoagulation therapies and coronary intervention are mainstays of treatment.***

Reperfusion Therapy

◈ *CMDT 2016/370*

- The current recommendation is to treat patients with **STEMI** who seek medical attention within 12 hours of the onset of symptoms with reperfusion therapy, either primary PCI or thrombolytic therapy.
- Patients **without ST-segment elevation** (previously labeled "non-Q wave" infarctions) ***do not benefit and may derive harm, from thrombolysis.***

Non-ST segment Elevation MI and Unstable Angina Medical Treatment

◈ *Harrison 19th/1595-98*

- Patients should be placed at bed rest with continuous ECG monitoring for ST-segment deviation and cardiac arrhythmias. Ambulation is permitted if the patient shows no recurrence of ischemia (symptoms or ECG changes) and ***does not develop an elevation of a biomarker of necrosis for 12–24 h.***
- Medical therapy involves ***simultaneous anti-ischemic and antithrombotic treatments and consideration of coronary revascularization.***
- **Anti-Ischemic Treatment:** To provide relief and prevention of recurrence of chest pain, initial treatment should include bed rest, nitrates, beta adrenergic blockers and inhaled oxygen in the presence of hypoxemia.
- **Antithrombotic Therapy:** This is the second major cornerstone of treatment. There are two components of antithrombotic therapy antiplatelet drugs (aspirin And clopidogrel) and anticoagulants (unfractionated heparin -UFH, low-molecular-weight heparin-LMWH, bivalirudin and fondaparinux)

NSTEMI and Unstable Angina

◈ *ecgwaves.com*

- ***Most patients undergo coronary angiography within 48 hours or earlier if the patient is at high risk of death or other complications.***
- Low-risk patients may be evaluated by ***angiography*** after 48–72 hours
- Guidelines do not recommend acute angiography in patients with NSTEMI or unstable angina
- Because the coronary occlusion in NSTEMI and unstable angina is partial, there is some residual perfusion in the ischemic zone. Therefore, revascularization (PCI) is less urgent and can generally be delayed without worsening the prognosis.
- Symptoms, hemodynamic status, ECG changes, ***troponin levels*** and comorbidities dictates whether angiography should be performed promptly.
- Interestingly, acute angiography (which is routine in STEMI) has never proven to reduce mortality or morbidity in NSTEMI or unstable angina.
- Elevated troponins (with a pattern consistent with myocardial necrosis; refer to Diagnosis of Acute Myocardial ***Infarction is evidence for myocardial infarction (i.e NSTEMI), whereas normal troponins rule out myocardial infarction (i.e. unstable angina).***

141. Ans. a. MELD score >15; b. Hepatocellular carcinoma; e. Child–Pugh grade C

[Ref: Harrison 19th/2068-69; Davidson 22nd/978; Manipal Surgery 4th/1109-10]

"**Hepatocellular carcinoma** Theoretically liver transplant should offer the best chance of cure in HCC but there is always the risk of recurrence of HCC following transplant. Many transplant centres follow "Milan criteria" to decide the feasibility of liver transplant in HCC, which says that ***liver transplant can be considered in HCC when–there is a single nodule of < 5 cm or there are fewer than 3 nodules,*** the largest of which is measuring <3 cm. Those who follow the **"Milan criteria"** believe that the recurrence of HCC is very low if the criteria are strictly adhered to"- *Manipal Surgery 4th/1109*

C/I of Liver transplantation - ***Inability to abstain from alcohol when liver transplantation is being contemplated for alcoholic liver disease***- *Manipal Surgery 4th/1109*

"In the waiting list, candidate with ***higher MELD*** score come first. MELD score is nowadays preferred to Child-Pugh's score for being more objective"- Manipal Surgery 4th/1110

Table: *(Harrison 19th/2069):* **Contraindications to Liver Transplantation**

Absolute	Relative
Uncontrolled extrahepatobiliary infection	Age >70
Active, untreated sepsis	Prior extensive hepatobiliary surgery
Uncorrectable, life-limiting congenital anomalies	Portal vein thrombosis
Active substance or alcohol abuse	Renal failure not attributable to liver disease
Advanced cardiopulmonary disease	Previous extrahepatic malignancy (not including nonmelanoma skin cancer)
Extrahepatobiliary malignancy (not including nonmelanoma skin cancer)	Severe obesity
Metastatic malignancy to the liver	Severe malnutrition/wasting
Cholangiocarcinoma	Medical noncompliance
AIDS	HIV seropositivity with failure to control HIV viremia or CD4 <100/μL
Life-threatening systemic diseases	Intrahepatic sepsis Severe hypoxemia secondary to right-to-left intrapulmonary shunts (PO2<50 mmHg) Severe pulmonary hypertension (mean pulmonary artery pressure >35 mmHg) Uncontrolled psychiatric disorder

Indications for Liver Transplant Assessment for Cirrhosis

◈ *Davidson 22nd/978*

Complications

- First episode of bacterial peritonitis
- Diuretic-resistant ascites
- Recurrent variceal haemorrhage
- Hepatocellular carcinoma < 5 cm
- ***Persistent hepatic encephalopathy***

Poor Liver Function

- Bilirubin > 100 μmol/L (5.8 mg/dL) in primary biliary cirrhosis
- MELD score > 12
- ***Child–Pugh grade C***

"The main contraindications to transplantation are ***sepsis, extrahepatic malignancy, active alcohol or other substance misuse and marked cardiorespiratory dysfunction***"-*Davidson 22nd/978*

Liver Transplantation

◈ *CMDT 2016/692*

- Liver transplantation is **indicated in selected cases of irreversible, progressive chronic liver disease, acute liver failure and certain metabolic diseases in which the metabolic defect is in the liver.**
- ***Absolute contraindications include malignancy (except relatively small hepatocellular carcinomas in a cirrhotic liver), advanced cardiopulmonary disease (except hepatopulmonary syndrome) and sepsis.***
- ***Relative contraindications include age over 70 years, morbid obesity, portal and mesenteric vein thrombosis, active alcohol or drug abuse, severe malnutrition and lack of patient understanding.***

142. Ans. c. IFN-alpha is used for treatment; d. HIV associated Kaposi's sarcoma regresses with antiretroviral therapy; e. Caused by HHV-8

[Ref: Harrison 19th/1242, 1268-70; : Robbins 9th (SAE)/518; CMDT 2016/147]

Pathogenesis of Kaposi's Sarcoma

◈ *Harrison 19th/1242*

- There are at least four distinct epidemiologic forms of KS (1) the classic form that occurs in ***older men*** of predominantly Mediterranean or eastern **European Jewish** backgrounds with no recognized contributing factors; (2) the equatorial **African form** that occurs in ***all ages,*** also without any recognized precipitating factors; (3) the form associated with **organ transplantation** and its attendant iatrogenic immunosuppressed state; and (4) the form associated with **HIV-1 infection.**
- In HIV disease the development of KS is dependent on the interplay of a variety of factors including HIV-1 itself, human herpes virus 8 (HHV-8), immune activation and cytokine secretion.
- A number of epidemiologic and virologic studies have clearly linked HHV-8, which is also referred to as Kaposi's sarcoma– associated herpesvirus (KSHV), to KS not only in HIV infected individuals but also in individuals with the other forms of KS.

- In the majority of cases, effective cART will go a long way in achieving control. ***Antiretroviral therapy*** has been associated with the spontaneous regression of KS lesions- *Harrison 19th/1269*
- The use of systemic therapy, **either IFN-α or chemotherapy**, should be considered in patients with a large number of lesions or in patients with visceral involvement. The **response rate to IFN-α** for patients with CD4+ T cell counts >600/μL is ~80%, while the response rate for patients with counts <150/μL is <10%.
- In contrast to the other systemic therapies, ***IFN-α provides an added advantage of having antiretroviral activity; thus, it may be the appropriate first choice for single-agent systemic therapy for early patients with disseminated disease***-Harrison 19th/1270

Management of AIDS-Associate d Kaposi's Sarcoma

◈ *(Harrison 19th/1270)*

- Observation and optimization of antiretroviral therapy
- Single or limited number of lesions
- Radiation
- Intralesional vinblastine
- Cryotherapy

Extensive Disease

- Initial therapy
- Interferon α (if CD4-1- T cells >150/μL)
- Liposomal daunorubicin
- Subsequent therapy
- Liposomal doxorubicin
- Paclitaxel
- Combination chemotherapy with low-dose doxorubicin, bleomycin and vinblastine (ABV)
- Targeted radiation

Kaposi Sarcoma

◈ *Robbins 9th (SAE)/518*

- *Kaposi sarcoma (KS) is a vascular neoplasm caused by Kaposi sarcoma herpesvirus* (KSHV, also known as human herpesvirus- 8, or ***HHV-8***). Although it occurs in a number of contexts, *it is by far most common in patients with AIDS*; indeed, its presence is used as a criterion for the diagnosis.
- Four forms of KS, based on population demographics and risks, are recognized
- ***Classic KS* is a disorder of older men** of Mediterranean, Middle Eastern, or Eastern European descent (especially Ashkenazic Jews)
- ***Endemic African KS typically occurs in younger (under age 40) HIV-seronegative persons*** and can follow an indolent or aggressive course; it involves lymph nodes much more frequently than in the classic variant.
- *Transplantation-associated KS* occurs in solid organ transplant recipients in the setting of T cell immunosuppression.

Treatment

◈ *CMDT 2016/147*

- For Kaposi sarcoma in the elderly, palliative local therapy with intralesional chemotherapy or radiation is usually all that is required. In the setting of iatrogenic immunosuppression, the treatment of Kaposi sarcoma is primarily reduction of doses of immunosuppressive medications. In AIDS-associated Kaposi sarcoma, the patient should first be given ART.
- Other therapeutic options include cryotherapy or intralesional vinblastine (0.1–0.5 mg/mL) for cosmetically objectionable lesions; radiation therapy for accessible and space-occupying lesions; and laser surgery for certain intraoral and pharyngeal lesions.
- ***Systemic therapy is indicated in patients with rapidly progressive skin disease*** (more than 10 new lesions per month), with edema or pain and with symptomatic visceral disease or pulmonary disease. ART plus chemotherapy appears to be more effective than ART alone.
- Liposomal doxorubicin is highly effective in severe cases and may be used alone or in combination with bleomycin and vincristine. **Alpha-interferon** may also be used. Paclitaxel and other taxanes can be effective even in patients who do not respond to anthracycline treatment.

143. Ans. e. Only conservative management should be done for pancreatic necrosis

[Ref: Harrison 19th/2095-96; L and B 26th/1129-32; Davidson 22nd/892]

Early Management of Severe Acute Pancreatitis

◈ *(L and B 26th/1130)*

- Admission to HDU/ICU
- Analgesia
- ***Aggressive fluid rehydration***
- Oxygenation
- Invasive monitoring of vital signs, central venous pressure, urine output, blood gases
- Frequent monitoring of haematological and biochemical parameters (including liver and renal function, clotting, serum calcium, blood glucose)
- Nasogastric drainage
- ***Antibiotic prophylaxis can be considered*** (imipenem, cefuroxime)
- CT scan essential if organ failure, clinical deterioration or signs of sepsis develop
- ERCP within 72 hours for severe gallstone pancreatitis or signs of cholangitis
- Supportive therapy for organ failure if it develops (inotropes, ventilatory support, haemofiltration, etc.)
- If nutritional support is required, consider ***enteral (nasogastric) feeding***

Acute Pancreatitis Management

◈ *Harrison 19th/2095-96*

- It is important to note that ***85–90% of cases of acute pancreatitis are self-limited*** and subside spontaneously, usually within 3–7 days after initiation of treatment and do not exhibit organ failure or local complications.
- The management of acute pancreatitis begins in the emergency ward. After a diagnosis has been confirmed, ***aggressive fluid resuscitation is initiated***, intravenous

analgesics are administered, severity is assessed and a search for etiologies that may impact acute care is begun.

- Patients who do not respond to **aggressive fluid resuscitation** in the emergency ward should be considered for admission to a step-down or intensive care ***unit for aggressive fluid resuscitation, hemodynamic monitoring and management of necrosis or organ failure.***
- The most important treatment intervention for acute pancreatitis is safe, aggressive **intravenous fluid resuscitation.** The patient is made NPO to rest the pancreas
- **Nutritional Therapy** - ***A low-fat solid diet*** can be administered to subjects with mild acute pancreatitis after the abdominal pain has resolved. ***Enteral nutrition should be considered 2–3 days after admission in subjects with more severe pancreatitis instead of total parenteral nutrition (TPN).***
- Patients exhibiting signs of clinical deterioration despite aggressive fluid resuscitation and hemodynamic monitoring should be assessed for ***local complications, which may include necrosis, pseudocyst formation, pancreas duct disruption, peripancreatic vascular complications and extrapancreatic infections.***

Necrosis

◈ *Harrison 19th/2095-96*

- The management of necrosis requires a multidisciplinary team approach. ***Percutaneous aspiration of necrosis with Gram stain and culture should be performed*** if there are ongoing signs of possible pancreatic infection such as sustained leukocytosis, fever, or organ failure.
- There is ***currently no role for prophylactic antibiotics in necrotizing pancreatitis.*** It is reasonable to ***start broad-spectrum antibiotics in a patient who appears septic while awaiting the results of Gram stain and cultures.*** If cultures are negative, the antibiotics should be discontinued to minimize the risk of developing opportunistic or fungal superinfection.
- Repeated fine-needle aspiration and Gram stain with culture of pancreatic necrosis may be done every 5–7 days in the presence of persistent fever.
- In general, ***sterile necrosis* is most often managed conservatively unless complications arise**. Once a diagnosis of *infected necrosis* is established and an organism identified, ***targeted antibiotics should be instituted.***
- Pancreatic debridement (necrosectomy) should be considered for definitive management of *infected necrosis*, but clinical decisions are generally influenced by response to antibiotic treatment and overall clinical condition.

Management Comprises Several Related Steps

◈ *Davidson 22nd/892*

- Nasogastric aspiration is only required if paralytic ileus is present.
- **Enteral feeding**, if tolerated, ***should be started at an early stage in patients with severe pancreatitis because they are in a severely catabolic state and need nutritional support*** .
- Enteral feeding decreases endotoxaemia and so may reduce systemic complications. Nasogastric feeding is just as effective as the nasojejunal route.
- ***The use of prophylactic, broad-spectrum intravenous antibiotics, such as imipenem or cefuroxime, to prevent infection of pancreatic necrosis is of unproven benefit but they are often given empirically.***
- Patients with necrotizing pancreatitis or pancreatic abscess require urgent endoscopic or minimally invasive retroperitoneal pancreatic (MIRP) necrosectomy to debride all cavities of necrotic material.
- ***Pancreatic pseudocysts can be treated by drainage into the stomach, duodenum or jejunum.*** This is usually performed after an interval of at least 6 weeks, once a pseudocapsule has matured, by surgical or endoscopic cystogastrostomy

Acute Fluid Collection

◈ *L and B 26th/1131*

- No intervention is necessary unless a large collection causes symptoms or pressure effects, in which case it can be percutaneously aspirated under ultrasound or CT guidance.
- Transgastric drainage under EUS guidance is another option. An acute fluid collection that does not resolve can evolve into a ***pseudocyst or an abscess*** if it becomes infected.
- There is ***some evidence to support the use of prophylactic antibiotics in patients with severe acute pancreatitis***, but there is no consensus. The rationale is to prevent local and other septic complications. The regimens used include intravenous cefuroxime, or imipenem, or ciprofloxacin plus metronidazole.
- The ***duration of antibiotic prophylaxis should not exceed 14 days.*** Additional antibiotic use should be guided by microbiological cultures-*L and B 26th/1130*

144. Ans. a. Transfusion-related acute lung injury (TRALI); b. Septicaemia; c. Transfusion related CMV infection; d. Acute Hemolytic Transfusion Reactions

[Ref: Harrison 19th/138e3-5; Wintrobe's Clinical Hematology 12th/Chap 23; Willaim's Hematology 7th/131]

Febrile Reactions

◈ *Willaim's Hematology 7th/131*

- A febrile response associated with the administration of blood may be the result of a **hemolytic reaction, *sensitivity to leukocytes or platelets, bacterial pyrogens, or unidentifiable causes.*** Febrile reactions resulting from bacterial pyrogens have become uncommon with the introduction of commercially manufactured disposable transfusion equipment.
- A frequent cause of a **nonhemolytic febrile reaction** is sensitization to white cell or platelet antigens. ***Clinically there is a temperature rise*** during the administration of blood or shortly thereafter.
- **Transfusion-Related Lung Injury (TRALI;** Noncardiogenic Pulmonary Edema): Incompatibility to leukocyte antigens may also produce pulmonary edema of noncardiac origin, with acute respiratory distress, **chills, fever** and tachycardia usually occurring within 4 hours of transfusion
- **Bacterial Contamination** Blood may be contaminated by cold-growing organisms (*Pseudomonas* or colon-aerogenes

group). The infusion of large numbers of gram-negative microorganisms results in a serious reaction, endotoxin shock, **characterized by fever**, marked hypotension, abdominal pain, vomiting, diarrhea and the development of profound shock.

Acute Hemolytic Transfusion Reactions: Immune-mediated hemolysis occurs when the recipient has preformed antibodies that lyse donor erythrocytes. The ABO isoagglutinins are responsible for the majority of these reactions. Acute hemolytic reactions may present with hypotension, tachypnea, tachycardia, fever, chills, hemoglobinemia, hemoglobinuria, chest and/or flank pain and discomfort at the infusion site-Harrison 19th/138e3

Febrile Nonhemolytic Transfusion Reaction: The most frequent reaction associated with the transfusion of cellular blood components is a febrile nonhemolytic transfusion reaction (FNHTR). These reactions are characterized by ***chills and rigors and a ≥1°C rise in temperature****-Harrison 19th/138e4*

"Transfusion-related acute lung injury (TRALI) most commonly presents as severe respiratory distress of sudden onset, caused by a syndrome of noncardiogenic pulmonary edema resembling the adult respiratory distress syndrome. Chills, **fever,** chest pain, hypotension and cyanosis, as well as the usual manifestations of pulmonary edema, may be seen"-*Wintrobe's Clinical Hematology 12th/Chap 23*

Graft-versus-Host Disease: When transfused into immunoincompetent recipients, donor lymphocytes may proliferate in the patient and lead to the clinical syndrome of transfusion-associated graft-versus-host disease. **Fever is the most common symptom**, followed by a typical erythematous, maculopapular skin rash"- *Wintrobe's Clinical Hematology 12th/Chap 23*

Cytomegalovirus: The occurrence of CMV infection after transfusion was first noted in the 1960s as a postpump syndrome after open-heart surgery. Patients who received large quantities of fresh blood developed a syndrome of **fever,** rash, lymphadenopathy and splenomegaly, associated with an atypical lymphocytosis 8 to 12 weeks after surgery. It was later confirmed that this syndrome was associated with serologic ***evidence of CMV infection that had been transmitted by transfusion***"- Wintrobe's Clinical Hematology 12th/Chap 23

"Symptoms in recipients of **bacterially contaminated products** range from none to symptoms indistinguishable from those of a nonhemolytic febrile reaction, to **acute sepsis with fever**, hypotension and death"-Wintrobe's Clinical Hematology 12th/Chap 23

145. Ans. b. Total Iron-Binding Capacity; e. Red blood cell distribution width (RDW) index

[Ref: Robbins 9th/652; Harrison 19th/628]

Laboratory Iron Studies

- *Harrison 19th/627-28*
- The **serum iron** level represents the amount of circulating iron bound to transferrin. The normal range for the serum iron is 50–150 µg/dL
- **Total Iron-Binding Capacity** (TIBC) is an indirect measure of the circulating transferrin.; the normal range for TIBC is 300–360 µg/dL.
- **Transferrin saturation**, which is normally 25–50%, is obtained by the following formula serum iron × 100 ÷ TIBC. Iron deficiency states are associated with saturation levels below 20%.
- **Serum Ferritin**: Adult males have serum ferritin values averaging 100 µg/L, while adult females have levels averaging 30 µg/L. ***As iron stores are depleted, the serum ferritin falls to <15 µg/L. Such levels are diagnostic of absent body iron stores.***
- **Red blood cell distribution width (RDW) index** is generally normal in thalassemia and ***elevated in iron deficiency.***

Table: *(Harrison 19th/628)*: **Diagnosis of Microcytic Anemia**

Tests	Iron Deficiency	Inflammation	Thalassemia	Sideroblastic Anemia
Smear	Micro/hypo	Normal micro/hypo	Micro/hypo with targeting	Variable
Serum iron (µg/dL)	<30	<50	Normal to high	Normal to high
TIBC (µg/dL)	>360	<300	Normal	Normal
Percent saturation	<10	10–20	30–80	30–80
Ferritin (µg/dL)	<15	30–200	50–300	50–300
Hemoglobin pattern on electrophoresis	Normal	Normal	Abnormal with β thalassemia; can be normal with α thalassemia	Normal

146. Ans. a. Mobilization of iron stores; b. Total Iron-Binding Capacity

[Ref: Robbins 9th/653; Harrison 19th/630; Harshmohan 7th/278-79]

- **Transferrin saturation**, although decreased in **anemia of chronic disease** (ACD), but its level is greater than iron deficiency anaemia
- ACD-despite the ***presence of normal or increased iron stores there is inadequate iron delivery to the marrow***

Anemia of Acute and Chronic Inflammation/Infection

- *(AI Also k/a anemia of chronic disease)*
- AI—which encompasses inflammation, infection, tissue injury and conditions (such as cancer) associated with the release of proinflammatory cytokines—is one of the most common forms of anemia seen clinically.
- It is the most important anemia in the differential diagnosis of iron deficiency, because many of the features of the anemia are brought about ***by inadequate iron delivery to***

the marrow, despite the presence of normal or increased iron stores. This is reflected by ***a low serum iron, increased red cell protoporphyrin, a hypoproliferative marrow, transferrin saturation in the range of 15–20% and a normal or increased serum ferritin.***

- The **serum ferritin** values are often the ***most distinguishing features*** between true iron-deficiency anemia and the iron-restricted erythropoiesis associated with inflammation. Typically, ***serum ferritin values increase threefold over basal levels***
- The **distinction between true iron deficiency anemia and AI** is among the most common diagnostic problems encountered by cliniciAns. Usually, ***AI is normocytic and normochromic***. The iron values usually make the differential diagnosis clear, as the ***ferritin level is normal or increased*** and the ***percent transferrin saturation and TIBC are typically below normal***"-*Harrison 19th/628*

Table: *(Harrison 19th/630)*: **Diagnosis of Hypoproliferative Anemias**

Tests	Iron Deficiency	Inflammation	Renal Disease	Hypometabolic States
Anemia	Mild to severe	Mild	Mild to severe	Mild
MCV (fL)	60–90	80–90	90	90
Morphology	Normo-microcytic	Normocytic	Normocytic	Normocytic
SI (μg/dL)	<30	<50	Normal	Normal
TIBC (μg/dL)	>360	<300	Normal	Normal
Saturation (%)	<10	10–20	Normal	Normal
Serum ferritin (μg/dL)	<15	30–200	115–150	Normal
Iron stores	0	2–4+	1–4+	Normal

Table: *(Harshmohan 7th/278)*: **Laboratory diagnosis of hypochromic anaemias**

Test		Iron Deficiency	Chronic Disorders
1.	MCV, MCH, MCHC	Reduced	Low normal-to-reduced
2.	Serum iron	Reduced	Reduced
3.	TIBC	Raised	Low-to-normal
4.	Serum ferritin	Reduced	Raised
5.	Marrow-iron stores	Absent	Present
6.	Iron in normoblasts	Absent	Absent
7.	Hb electrophoresis	Normal	Normal

147. Ans. a. Absolute neutrophil count <500/μL; b. Platelet count <20,000/μL; d. Bone marrow cellularity <25%; e. Absolute reticulocyte count <60,000/μL

[Ref: Wintrobe's Clinical Hematology 12th/Chap 42; Robbins 9th/653-55; Harrison 19th/666; Harshmohan 7th/302-03]

Table: *(Wintrobe's)*: **Classification of Aplastic Anemia Based on Severity of Pancytopenia**

Severe aplastic anemia (SAA)
- Bone marrow cellularity <25%
- Two of three peripheral blood criteria:
- Absolute neutrophil count <500/mm^3
- Platelet count <20,000/mm^3
- Reticulocyte count <60,000/mm^3 or <1% corrected reticulocyte count

Very severe aplastic anemia (VSAA)
- Same as SAA with absolute neutrophil count <200/mm^3

Nonsevere (moderate) aplastic anemia
- Bone marrow cellularity <25%
- Peripheral blood cytopenias do not fulfill criteria for SAA

Severe Aplastic Anemia Prognosis

◈ *Harrison 19th/666*

- The natural history of severe aplastic anemia is rapid deterioration and death.
- The major prognostic determinant is the blood count. Severe disease has been defined by the presence of two of three parameters ***absolute neutrophil count <500/μL, platelet count <20,000/μL*** and corrected **reticulocyte count** <1% (or ***absolute reticulocyte count <60,000/μL***).
- In the era of effective immunosuppressive therapies, absolute numbers of reticulocytes (>25,000/μL) and lymphocytes (>1000/μL) may be better predictors of response to treatment and long-term outcome

Aplastic Anemia

◈ *Williams Hematology 7th/Chap 33*

- Anemia is associated with a low reticulocyte index. The reticulocyte count usually is less than 1.0 percent and may be zero despite the high levels of erythropoietin.

- ***An absolute neutrophil count less than 500 x 10^6/liter and a platelet count less than 20,000 x 10^6/liter are indicative of severe disease.***
- A neutrophil count ***less than 200 x 10^6/liter indicates very severe disease.***
- In severe aplastic anemia as defined by the International Aplastic Anemia Study Group, ***less than 25 percent cellularity or less than 50 percent cellularity with less than 30 percent hematopoietic cells is seen in the marrow.***

148. Ans. b. Congenital Dyserythropoietic anemia

[Ref: Robbins 9th/631; Harshmohan 7th/285]

"Normal Reticulocyte Count (%): 0.5-1.5"

◈ *Robbins 9th/631*

"**Acute Blood Loss** Initially, red cells appear normal in size and color (normocytic, normochromic). However, as marrow production increases there is a striking increase in the reticulocyte count ***(reticulocytosis)***, which reaches ***10% to 15% after 7 days.*** Reticulocytes are larger in size than normal red cells (macrocytes) and have a blue-red polychromatophilic cytoplasm."-*Robbins 9th/631*

"In **sickle cell anemia**, the peripheral blood demonstrates variable numbers of irreversibly sickled cells, **reticulocytosis** and target cells, which result from red cell dehydration. **Howell-Jolly bodies** (small nuclear remnants) are also present in some red cells due to the asplenia"-*Robbins 9th/636*

"**Treatment of megaloblastic anaemia by Vit B12 and folic acid *Reticulocytosis appears within 4-5*** *days after therapy is started and peaks at day 7"-Harshmohan 7th/285*

Although prompt hematologic ***response heralded by reticulocytosis*** follows the administration of folic acid, it should be remembered that the hematologic symptoms of vitamin B12 deficiency anemia also respond to folate therapy. As already mentioned, folate does not prevent (and may even exacerbate) the neurologic deficits seen in vitamin B12 deficiency states. It is thus essential to exclude vitamin B12 deficiency in megaloblastic anemia before initiating therapy with folate *Robbins 9th/649*

"***Hereditary spherocytosis*** The most specific morphologic finding is spherocytosis, apparent on smears as small, dark-staining (hyperchromic) red cells lacking the central zone of pallor. Other features are common to all hemolytic anemias. These include **reticulocytosis, marrow erythroid hyperplasia, hemosiderosis and mild jaundice**"-*Robbins 9th/633*

"**Diagnosis of Congenital Dyserythropoietic Anemia** CDA should be suspected in any individual with a chronic anemia that is largely due to ***ineffective erythropoiesis,*** as well as in individuals with unexplained iron overload. The presence of ineffective erythropoiesis would be indicated by a low absolute reticulocyte count for the degree of anemia despite erythroid hyperplasia in the marrow"- Wintrobe's Clinical Hematology 12th/Chap 44

Congenital dyserythropoietic anemia: **low reticulocyte counts,** the marrow features and findings of ***ineffective erythropoiesis***- *Williams Hematology 7th/Chap 37*

149. Ans. b. ECOG Grade 2; e. Karnofsky Performance Index 70

[Ref: Harrison 19th/470-72; Schwartz 10th/1947]

"In addition to tumor burden, a second major determinant of treatment outcome is the **physiologic reserve** of the patient. Physiologic reserve is a determinant of how a patient is likely to cope with the physiologic stresses imposed by the cancer and its treatment. This factor is difficult to assess directly. Instead, surrogate markers for physiologic reserve are used, such as the patient's age or **Karnofsky performance status or Eastern Cooperative Oncology Group (ECOG) performance status. *Older patients and those with a Karnofsky performance status <70 or ECOG performance status ≥3 have a poor prognosis*** unless the poor performance is a reversible consequence of the tumor"- *Harrison 19th/470-71*

Table: *(Harrison 19th/472)*: **The Eastern Cooperative Oncology Group (ECOG) Performance Scale**

ECOG Grade 0: Fully active, able to carry on all predisease performance without restriction

ECOG Grade 1: Restricted in physically strenuous activity but ambulatory and able to carry out work of a light or sedentary nature, e.g., light housework, office work

ECOG Grade 2: Ambulatory and capable of all self-care but unable to carry out any work activities. Up and about more than 50% of waking hours

ECOG Grade 3: Capable of only limited self-care, confined to bed or chair more than 50% of waking hours

ECOG Grade 4: Completely disabled. Cannot carry on any self-care. Totally confined to bed or chair

ECOG Grade 5: Dead

Table *(Harrison 19th/472)*: **Karnofsky Performance Index**

Performance Status	Functional Capability of the Patient
100	Normal; no complaints; no evidence of disease
90	Able to carry on normal activity; minor signs or symptoms of disease
80	Normal activity with effort; some signs or symptoms of disease
70	Cares for self; unable to carry on normal activity or do active work
60	Requires occasional assistance but is able to care for most needs
50	Requires considerable assistance and frequent medical care
40	Disabled; requires special care and assistance

Contd...

Performance Status	Functional Capability of the Patient
30	Severely disabled; hospitalization is indicated although death is not imminent
20	Very sick; hospitalization necessary; active supportive treatment is necessary
10	Moribund, fatal processes progressing rapidly
0	Dead

Prognostic Tool in Advanced Illness

◈ *Schwartz 10th/1947*

- Alternatively, the ***Karnofsky Performance Scale is a scale of functional status ranging from 100 (high level of function) to 0 (death).*** It is commonly used in palliative care to roughly assess patient anticipated needs as well as prognosis.
- The **Palliative Performance Scale** is a validated expansion of the *Karnofsky Performance Scale* that includes five palliative-focused domains, including a***mbulation, activity level, self-care, intake and level of consciousness,*** in addition to evidence of disease.
- The **Missoula- Vitas Quality of Life Index** is a 25-question scale specifically for palliative care and hospice patients that scores symptoms, function, interpersonal relationships, well-being and spirituality. Updates and Spanish versions are available

150. Ans. c. Pregnancy; d. Coarctation of aorta; e. Patent ductus arteriosus;

[Ref: Essentials of Medicine CECIL 3rd/712;Harrison 20th/1674]

Continuous Murmur

◈ *Harrison 20th/1674*

- A continuous murmur is predicated on a pressure gradient that persists between two cardiac chambers or blood vessels across systole and diastole. The murmurs typically begin in systole, envelop the second heart sound (S2) and continue through some portion of diastole.
- The classic example of a continuous murmur is that associated with a ***PDA***
- Other causes of a continuous murmur include a ruptured sinus of Valsalva aneurysm
- With creation of an aortic–right atrial or right ventricular fistula, a coronary or great vessel arteriovenous fistula and an arteriovenous fistula constructed to provide dialysis access.
- There are two types of benign continuous murmurs: cervical venous hum, heard in children or
- Adolescents & ***mammary soufflé of pregnancy.***

Physiological Classification of Continuous Murmur

Continuous murmurs due to rapid blood flow	Continuous mumurs due to high to low pressure shunts	Continuous murmur secondary to localized arterial obstruction
• Mammary soufflé (Pregnancy)	**Systemic artery to pulmonary artery**	• Branch pulmonary stenosis
• Hyper thryroidism	• Patent ductusareriosu	• ***Coarctation of the Aorta***
• Anaemia	• Aorto-pulmonary window	• Carotid occlusion
• Hyperemia of neoplasm	• Truncus arteriosus	• Celiac mesenteric occlusion
• Venous hum	• Pulmonary arteriosus	• Renal occlusion
	• Anomalous left coronary artery	• Femoral occlusion
	Systemic Artery to right heart	• Coronary occlusion
	• Ruptured sinus of valsalva	
	• Coronary artery fistula	
	Left to right atrial shunting.	
	• Lutembacher'ssyndrome	
	• Mitral atresia plus atrial septal defect.	
	Venovenous shunts	
	• Anomalous pulmonary veins	
	• Portosystemic shunts	
	Arteriovenous fistula	
	• Systemic	
	• Pulmonary	

Contd...

SURGERY

151. Ans. a. In First and second degree frostbite affected part show redness and edema; d. Initial treatment is rewarming; e. Autoamputation may occur in severe cases

[Ref: L and B 26th/400; Park 24th/785; Reddy 34th/295; Manipal Surgery 4th/94; Harrison 19th/1650; Schwartz 10th/480]

*"Frostbite is infarction of peripheral digits with **edema, redness** and later necrosis"- Reddy 34th/295*

Frostbite

◈ *Harrison 19th/1650*

- Tissue injury results from both ***freezing and vasoconstriction***.
- Frostbite usually affects the distal aspects of the extremities or exposed parts of the face, such as the ears, nose, chin and cheeks.

- Two type- Superficial frostbite (first or second degree) or deep frostbite (third or fourth degree)- *www.dermnetnz.org*
- **Superficial frostbite** involves the skin and subcutaneous tissue. Patients experience pain or paresthesia and the ***skin appears white and waxy***. After rewarming, there is ***cyanosis and erythema***, wheal-and-flare ***formation, edema and superficial blisters***.
- Deep frostbite involves muscle, nerves and deeper blood vessels. It may result in ***edema of the hand or foot, vesicles and bullae, tissue necrosis and gangrene***
- **Initial treatment is rewarming,** performed in an environment where reexposure to freezing conditions will not occur. Rewarming is accomplished by immersion of the affected part in a water bath at temperatures of 40°–44°C (104°–111°F).
- Massage, application of ice water and extreme heat are contraindicated. The injured area should be cleansed with soap or antiseptic and sterile dressings should be applied. Analgesics are often required during rewarming.
- Antibiotics are used if there is evidence of infection. The efficacy of sympathetic blocking drugs is not established. After recovery, the affected extremity may exhibit increased sensitivity to cold.
- Treatment includes rapid rewarming to 40 to 42°C, analgesia, debridement of blisters, hydrotherapy, elevation, topical antimicrobials, topical antithromboxanes (aloe vera) and systemic antiprostaglandins (aspirin)- *Schwartz 10th/480*

Degree of Frostbite

◈ *www.dermnetnz.org; wikipedia*

- In **first-degree frostbite**, ***hyperemia and edema are*** evident.
- **Second-degree frostbite** is characterized by ***hyperemia and edema,*** with large, clear blisters that may extend the entire length of the involved limb, digit, or facial feature. The blisters can be quite large and interfere with function, especially if they involve the digits of the hand or the soles of the feet.
- **Third-degree frostbite** is characterized by ***hyperemia, edema and vesicles filled*** with hemorrhagic fluid that are usually smaller than those of second-degree frostbite and do not extend to the tip of the involved digit. The hemorrhagic component of the blisters is a sign of underlying deeper tissue injury.
- **Fourth-degree frostbite,** the most severe type, involves complete necrosis, with gangrene and loss of the affected part. The amount of permanent damage can take one month or more to determine. *Autoamputation* ***can occur after two months.***

Frostbite

◈ *emedicine.medscape.com*

- Peripheral cold injury occurs on a spectrum from frost nip to varying depths of frostbite
- Once cold injury is identified and the affected parts rewarmed, it is vital to avoid refreezing; if refreezing occurs, the subsequent tissue damage will be catastrophic
- Simple management measures include rewarming, analgesia, blister débridement, the use of nonsteroidal anti-inflammatory drugs (NSAIDs) and aloe vera application
- It is difficult to predict the depth and severity of frostbite injury in the acute setting; it is best to allow the tissue to slowly demarcate over time (often 60-90 days) prior to the patient undergoing any form of surgical débridement

"The two most common **nonfreezing peripheral cold injuries** are *chilblain (pernio) and immersion (trench) foot.* **Chilblain** results from neuronal and endothelial damage induced by repetitive exposure to dry cold. Young females, particularly those with a history of Raynaud's phenomenon, are at greatest risk. Persistent vasospasticity and vasculitis can cause ***erythema, mild edema and pruritus***. Eventually plaques, blue nodules and ulcerations develop. These lesions typically involve the dorsa of the hands and feet"- *Harrison 19th/478e-4*

"There are milder conditions related to frostbite, including frostnip, ***chilblains*** and trench foot"- *www.emedicinehealth.com*

---

152. Ans. b. Causes watery diarrhea; c. Pain relieves after defaecation; d. Cause malabsorption of vitamins; e. Pain usually occur in periumbilical area

---

[Ref: Harrison 19th/1899; Schwartz 10th/1145-46; Katzung 13th/1065]

"Patients with ***colonic symptoms and findings*** such as ***bloody diarrhea, tenesmus, fever, or leukocytes in stool*** generally undergo sigmoidoscopy or colonoscopy to assess for colitis. Conversely, patients with symptoms and findings suggesting **small-bowel disease,** ***such as large volume watery stools, substantial weight loss and malabsorption of iron, calcium, or fat,*** may undergo upper endoscopy with duodenal aspirates for assessment of bacterial overgrowth and biopsies for assessment of mucosal diseases, such as celiac sprue"- *Harrison 19th/1899*

"Loperamide is a nonprescription opioid agonist that does not cross the blood-brain barrier and has ***no analgesic properties or potential for addiction. Tolerance to long-term use has not been reported.*** It is typically administered in doses of 2 mg taken one to four times daily"- *Katzung 13th/1065*

"Loperamide: This medication is ***used to treat sudden*** diarrhea (including traveler's diarrhea). It works by slowing down the movement of the gut. This decreases the number of bowel movements and ***makes the stool less watery***. It is also used to treat on-going diarrhea in people with inflammatory bowel disease.Loperamide treats only the symptoms, not the cause of the diarrhea (e.g., infection)"- *www.webmd.com/drug*

"Morning diarrhea is a term used to describe loose, watery stool and an urgent need to have a bowel movement upon waking. In some people, the need to pass stool may disturb sleep within the early hours of the morning. **Morning diarrhea**

is not a specific symptom that clearly indicates a definite cause. It is frequently seen in most gastrointestinal disorders where diarrhea is a feature. However, it tends to be more common in a ***person suffering with bowel disorders such as irritable bowel syndrome (IBS) and inflammatory bowel disease (IBD).*** This most likely indicates a psychosomatic element as both these disorders are aggravated with stress and anxiety"-*www.healthhype.com*

Table: Large bowel versus small bowel diarrhea

Clinical Sign	Small Intestine	Large Intestine
Frequency of defecation	Normal or slightly increased	Very frequent
Fecal volume	Large quantity of bulky or watery feces	Small quantities often
Urgency	Absent	Usually present
Tenesmus	Absent	Usually present
Mucus in feces	Usually absent	Frequent
Blood in feces	Dark black (melena)	Red (fresh)
Weight loss	May be present	Rare

Table: Differentiation between small bowel and large bowel diarrhea

Features	Small bowel	Large bowel
Volume	Large	Small
Blood	No	Usually present
Rectal symptoms	No	Yes
Steatorrhea (greasy stools)	Yes	No
Excessive flatulence (due to carbohydrate malabsorption)	Yes	No
Protein malabsorption	Pedal edema	Usually absent
Pain (if any)	***Periumbilical***, ↓ after stool	Hypogastric, ↓ after stool
Color of stool	Pale	Normal
Smell of stool	Unusually offensive	Normal
Vitamin deficiency	Frequent	Infrequent

153. Ans. a. If jejunum is cut, ileum can compensate jejunal function; b. If Ileum is cut, jejunum can compensate ileum function; d. Bile acid malabsorption lead to diarrhea

[Ref: L and B 26th/1144; A.K.Jain 6th/247; Schwartz 10th/1145-46]

*"**Capacity of jejunum to adopt is less than that of ileum. Removal of short segment of small intestine** (jejunum or ileum) leads to compensatory hypertrophy and hyperplasia of remaining mucosa with gradual return of the absorption function towards normal, called **intestinal adaptation**"-A.K.Jain 6th/247*

"**Distal small bowel resection (ileal resection)** *produces greater degree of malabsorption than removal of complete length of proximal small intestine (jejunum) because **resection of ileum prevents absorption of bile salts** causing **decreased fat absorption and unabsorbed bile salts** to enter the colon. **This inhibits Na+ and water reabsorption producing diarrhea**"-A.K.Jain 6th/247*

Intestinal Adaptation

◈ *Schwartz 10th/1145-46*

- Within a ***few hours after bowel resection, the remnant small intestine displays evidence of epithelial cellular hyperplasia.***
- ***Jejunal resection is generally better tolerated, as ileum shows better capacity to compensate.*** However, the magnitude of this response is limited. If enough small intestine is resected, a devastating condition known as the **short bowel syndrome results.**

Small Intestine

◈ *L and B 26th/1144*

- The jejunum is the principal site for digestion and absorption of fluid, electrolytes, iron, folate, fat, protein and carbohydrate, but the ***absorption of bile salts and vitamin B12 occurs in the terminal ileum where there are specific transporters.***
- ***If the jejunum is resected, the ileum can assume all the required absorptive functions, but resection of the terminal ileum will result in a diminished bile salt pool, B12 deficiency and may lead to deficiency of the fat-soluble vitamins A, D and K.***
- ***The clinical hallmarks of short bowel syndrome include diarrhea, fluid and electrolyte deficiency and malnutrition***-Sabiston
- Although there is considerable individual variation, ***resection of up to 70% of the small bowel usually can be tolerated if the terminal ileum and ileocecal valve are preserved.***

154. Ans. a. Occur after traumatic rupture of the spleen; b. Function as normal spleen; c. Multiple small implants of splenic tissue on the peritoneal surfaces

[Ref: CSDT 14th/647; Harrison 19th/413; www.ncbi.nlm.nih.gov]

Splenosis (Splenic Autotransplantation)

◈ *CSDT 14th/647*

- In splenosis, ***multiple small implants of splenic tissue grow in scattered areas on the peritoneal surfaces throughout the abdomen.***
- They arise from dissemination and autotransplantation of splenic fragments following ***traumatic rupture of the spleen.***
- Splenic implants or intentional autotransplants are capable of cell culling and ***some immunologic function*** appears to be exhibited in cases of intentional autotransplantation.

- Aggressive attempts at surgical excision are not warranted.
- Splenosis is usually an incidental finding discovered much later during laparotomy for an unrelated problem. However, the implants stimulate formation of adhesions and may be a cause of intestinal obstruction.
- They must be ***distinguished from peritoneal nodules of metastatic carcinoma*** *and from* ***accessory spleens.*** Histologically, they differ from accessory spleens by the absence of elastic or smooth muscle fibers in the delicate capsule.

"In a fraction of patients with splenic rupture, **peritoneal seeding of splenic fragments can lead to *splenosis***—the presence of multiple rests of spleen tissue not connected to the portal circulation. This ectopic spleen tissue may cause pain or gastrointestinal obstruction, as in endometriosis"-Harrison 19th/413

"Splenosis is the autotransplantation of splenic tissue that usually follows ***traumatic rupture of the spleen.*** Generally, the splenic implants are numerous and are located within the peritoneal cavity; however, ***extra-abdominal splenosis does occur. Splenic implants retain their ability to function and recurrence of a hematologic disease*** for which the spleen was previously removed should alter the clinician to the possibility of splenosis. The **differential diagnosis** includes ***accessory spleens, endometriosis, hemangiomas and metastatic cancer***"- www.ncbi.nlm.nih.gov

Splenosis

◈ *radiopaedia.org/articles*

Splenosis is one type of *ectopic splenic tissue* (the other being accessory spleen).

Abdominal splenosis is seen after ***abdominal trauma or surgery*** (e.g. splenectomy). They result from seeding of the peritoneal cavity with splenic tissue which recruits local blood supply.

They are typically small, sessile (as they grow on serosal/ peritoneal surfaces) and multiple. They may grow overtime to become quite sizeable. If located isolated ***intrahepatically***, they can cause serious diagnostic problems.

Similar process occurring in the thorax is called *thoracic splenosis.*

They are ***benign,*** their greatest importance being the need to distinguish them from more sinister pathology.

155. Ans. a. SAAG <1.1 g/dL in ascitic fluid; b. Elevated adenosine deaminase level; d. The diagnosis can be made by laparoscopy with directed biopsy of the peritoneum

[Ref: PJM 20th/70; Harrison 19th/287; L and B 26th/976; Davidson 22nd/691; Sabiston 19th/1101-02]

"The SAAG is calculated by subtracting the ascitic albumin concentration from the serum albumin level and does not change with diuresis. A SAAG ≥1.1 g/dL reflects the presence of portal hypertension and indicates that the ascites is due to increased pressure in the hepatic sinusoids. ***A SAAG <1.1 g/dL indicates that the ascites is not related to portal hypertension, as in tuberculous peritonitis***, peritoneal carcinomatosis, or pancreatic ascites"- Harrison 19th/287

"**Tuberculous peritonitis** is typically associated with ascitic fluid lymphocytosis but can be difficult to diagnose by paracentesis. A smear for acid-fast bacilli has a diagnostic sensitivity of only 0 to 3%; a culture increases the sensitivity to 35–50%. In patients without cirrhosis, an ***elevated ascitic adenosine deaminase level*** has a sensitivity of >90% when a cut-off value of 30–45 U/L is used. When the cause of ascites remains uncertain, ***laparotomy or laparoscopy with peritoneal biopsies for histology and culture remains the gold standard***"- *Harrison 19th/288*

Tuberculous Peritonitis

◈ *L and B 26th/976*

- ***Clinical or subclinical ascites is reported in virtually all patients with TB peritonitis*** and is frequently a presenting feature.
- Diagnosis is via abdominal ultrasound or CT to detect ascites and lymphadenopathy ± diffuse thickening of the peritoneum, mesentery and/or omentum
- Ascitic fluid is typically a ***straw-coloured exudate*** (***protein >25–30 g/***L) with white cells >500 mm3 and lymphocytes >40 per cent.
- ***Laparoscopy and peritoneal biopsy*** may thus be helpful to couple typical appearances with histology.

"**Tuberculous peritonitis:** The ascitic fluid is exudative and cellular, with a predominance of lymphocytes. ***Laparoscopy reveals multiple white 'tubercles' over the peritoneal and omental surfaces***"- Davidson 22nd/691

Tuberculous Peritonitis

◈ *Sabiston 19th/1101-02*

- The ***ascitic fluid SAAG is less than 1.1 g/dL, consistent with a high protein concentration*** within the ascitic fluid. Microscopic examination of the ascites shows erythrocytes and an increased number of leukocytes, most of which are lymphocytes.
- ***The diagnosis is made by laparoscopy with directed biopsy of the peritoneum. In more than 90% of cases, laparoscopy demonstrates multiple whitish nodules (<5 mm) scattered over the visceral and parietal peritoneum; histologic examination of these nodules demonstrates caseating granulomas.***

Table: *(PJM 20th/70)*: **Transudate and Exudate (of Ascites)**

	Transudate	Exudate
Process	Passive	Active
Serous structures	Others	Only local
Appearance	Clear	Clear/turbid
Specific Gravity	< 1.015	> 1.015
Proteins	< 3 gm/dL	> 3 gm/dL
Cells	Few mesothelial cells	Polymorphs or Lymphocytes

Contd...

	Transudate	Exudate
Clot formation	Nil	Present
SAAG	> 1.1 g/dL	< 1.1 g/dL
Example	Portal hypertension	Tuberculosis

156. Ans. b. Congenital fistula is easier to repair by surgery than acquired fistula

[Ref: Manipal Surgery 4th/259-62; L and B 26th/899; CSDT 14th/830]

Arteriovenous Fistulas

◈ *Manipal Surgery 4th/259-62*

- *Type- **congenital, acquired or iatrogenic***
- The most common etiology for ***acquired AVFs is penetrating trauma***- emedicine.medscape.com
- *High blood pressure from artery results in **arterialization of vein** that ultimately results in secondary varicose vein*
- *Therapeutic embolization is the treatment of choice for A-V fistula, in congenital cases*
- ***Acquired lesion need to be observed or treated by quadruple ligation***

"Extremely large AVFs or arteriovenous malformations (AVMs) may present with ***low platelet count (due to turbulence and trapping of platelets)*** and occasionally, with laboratory findings of consumptive coagulopathy, such as ***low platelets,*** elevated prothrombin time (PT) and partial thromboplastin time (PTT), increased bleeding time, low fibrinogen and elevated euglobulin clot lysis time (signs of fibrinolysis)"- emedicine.medscape.com

Arteriovenous Fistulas

◈ *CSDT 14th/830*

- Arteriovenous fistulas may be congenital, often called "malformations," or acquired. Abnormal communications between arteries and veins occur in many diseases and affect vessels of all sizes and in many locations.
- In **congenital fistulas**, the systemic effect is often not great, because although the communications may be multiple, they are small. When a limb is involved, extensive arteriovenous communications may exist with increased flow and increased muscle mass and bone length. ***Surgical correction is rarely successful because of the numerous A-V connections***. Massive swelling can be treated with ablation therapy but it also is rarely curative.
- ***Acquired fistulas are usually the result of trauma***, violent, or iatrogenic. These communications can have considerable ***flow and high-output heart failure*** can occur.
- The **third class of fistulas (artificial)** is ***surgically created fistulas for hemodialysis access.***
- ***Penetrating injuries either from trauma or iatrogenic ones from arterial punctures are the most common causes of acquired fistulas***. When large vessels are involved, the presentation may be dramatic. For example, if an aortic aneurysm ruptures into the inferior vena cava, the fistula enlarges rapidly and can result in *cardiac dilation and failure.*

◈ *L and B 26th/899*

- Communication between an artery and a vein (or veins) may be either a congenital malformation or the result of trauma.
- Arteriovenous fistulae for hemodialysis access are also created surgically. All arteriovenous communications have a structural and a physiological effect. The structural effect of arterial blood flow on the veins is characteristic; they ***become dilated, tortuous and thick walled (arterialized).***
- The physiological effect, if the fistula is big enough, is an increase in **cardiac output.**
- A thrill is detected on palpation and auscultation reveals a buzzing continuous bruit (**'machinery murmur'**). Dilated veins may be seen, in which there is rapid blood flow. Pressure on the artery proximal to the fistula reduces the swelling and the thrill and bruit cease.
- Treatment is by embolization. Excisional surgery can be advocated only rarely, perhaps for severe deformity or recurrent haemorrhage; the assistance of a plastic surgeon is wise.
- It is important to realize that ligation of a 'feeding' artery on its own is of no lasting value and is actually detrimental as it may preclude treatment by embolization.

Treatment

◈ *www.merckmanuals.com*

- For ***congenital fistula, endovascular treatment***
- For ***acquired fistulas, surgery***
- Congenital arteriovenous fistulas usually need treatment only if they cause symptoms. When necessary, doctors usually do an **endovascular procedure** to block the abnormal connection between the artery and vein. Arteriovenous fistulas near the eye, brain, or other major structures can be especially difficult to treat.
- ***Acquired arteriovenous fistulas usually have a single, large connection that can be corrected by a surgeon as soon as possible after diagnosis***. The surgeon cuts the connection and then sews shut the holes in the artery and vein.

157. Ans. a. Vaginal hydrocele; c. Infantile hydrocele; d. Encysted hydrocele of cord; e. Inguino-scrotal hydrocele

[Ref: Manipal Surgery 4th/988-89; L and B 26th/1382]

- **Processus vaginalis** is a pouch of peritoneum that is carried into the scrotum by the descent of the testicle and which in the scrotum forms the tunica vaginalis. But in some cases, it obliterated proximally, which results in hydrocele
- ***In congenital hydrocele, processus vaginalis remain patent (not closed)***

Processus Vaginalis

◈ *CSDT 14th/1255-56*

- The processus vaginalis may be ***obliterated at any location proximal to the testis or labium.***
- A hydrocele is fluid within the remnant processus vaginalis. It is characteristically long, non-tender soft mass.
- It may be around the testicle only (***testicular hydrocele***), extend up from the testicle into the inguinal region

(***inguinoscrotal hydrocele***), or be contained within a segment of the processus adjacent to the spermatic cord (***hydrocele of the cord***) or communicated with the ***peritoneal cavity (communicating hydrocele).***

- ***With a noncommunicating hydrocele (the first three hydroceles described above), the processus vaginalis has closed proximally***. The normal spermatic cord can usually be palpated above the level of the hydrocele.
- By connection with the peritoneal cavity via a ***patent processus vaginalis*** (***congenital***)- *L and B 26th/1382*

Encysted hydrocele of the cord: *In this condition the* ***sac is obliterated above*** *(inguinal canal) and* ***below*** *(scrotum) but patent at the root of the scrotum around spermatic cord- Manipal Surgery 4th/989*

Encysted hydrocele of the cord: *Localised oval swelling situated in scrotal region, inguinoscrotal region or in inguinal region-Textbook of Surgery by S.Das 5th/1309*

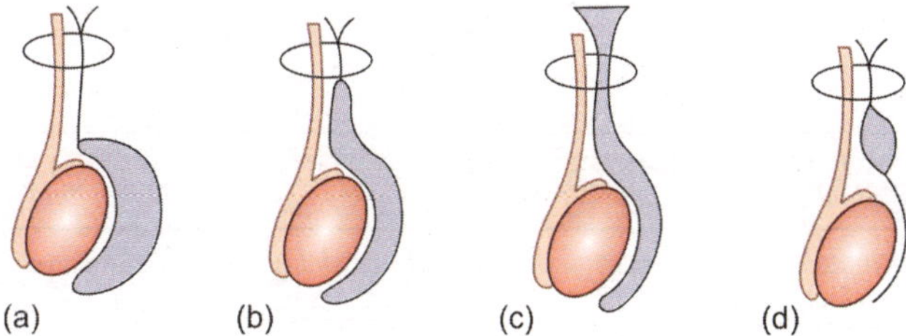

Fig: (L and B 26th/1382): (a) Vaginal hydrocele (very common); (b) 'infantile' hydrocele; (c) congenital hydrocele; (d) hydrocele of the cord.

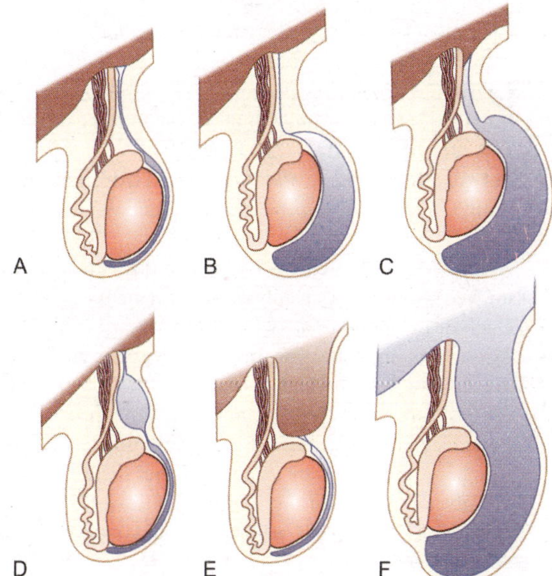

Fig: *(CSDT 14th/1255):* Spectrum of inguinoscrotal disorders. A: Normal anatomy. The processus vaginalis is obliterated and there is a small remnant, the tunica vaginalis, adjacent to the posterior surface of the testis. B: Scrotal hydrocele. C: Communicating hydrocele. Note the *proximal patency of the processus vaginalis.* D: Hydrocele of the spermatic cord. E: Inguinal hernia. F: Inguinoscrotal hernia

158. Ans. b. Caused by ingestion of fruits, vegetable fibers and hairs; c. In Rapunzel syndrome, bezoar has a tail-like extension into the small bowel; e. It increases chance of gastric ulceration

[Ref: CSDT 14th/538-39; L and B 26th/1056; Schwartz 10th/1089]

BEZOAR

◈ *CSDT 14th/538-39*

- Bezoars are concretions formed in the stomach. ***Trichobezoars are composed of hair*** and are usually found in young girls who pick at their hair and swallow it.
- ***Phytobezoars consist of agglomerated vegetable fibers.***
- Pressure by the mass can create a **gastric ulcer** that is prone to bleed or perforate.
- The ***postgastrectomy state predisposes to bezoar formation*** because pepsin and acid secretion are reduced and the triturating function of the antrum is gone.
- ***Orange segments or other fruits that contain a large amount of cellulose have been implicated in most cases.***
- Patients with symptomatic gastric bezoars may complain of abdominal pain. ***Ulceration and bleeding are associated with a death rate of 20%.***
- **Nearly all gastric bezoars** can be *broken up and dispersed by endoscopy*. Neglected lesions with complications (ie, bleeding or perforation) require **gastrectomy.**

Rapunzel syndrome is the term for a trichobezoar (gastric 'hair ball') which has a ***tail-like extension into the small bowel through the pylorus causing gastric outlet obstruction-*** *radiopaedia.org*

Trichobezoar and Phytobezoar

◈ *L and B 26th/1056*

- Trichobezoar (hair balls) are unusual and are virtually exclusively found in female psychiatric patients, often young. It is caused by the pathological ingestion of hair, which remains undigested in the stomach. The hair ball can lead to ***ulceration and gastrointestinal bleeding,*** perforation or obstruction.
- The diagnosis is made easily at endoscopy or, indeed, from a plain radiograph.
- ***Treatment consists of removal of the bezoar, which may require open surgical treatment.*** Phytobezoars are made of vegetable matter and found principally in patients who have gastric stasis. Often this follows gastric surgery.
- ***Treatment options include enzyme therapy (papain, cellulase, or acetylcysteine), endoscopic disruption and removal, or surgical removal***- *Schwartz 10th/1089*

159. Ans. a. Normal intra-abdominal pressure is 0-5 mm Hg; b. Intra-abdominal hypertension is measured by bladder pressure; d. Management of choice is abdominal opening; e. Multi-organ failure may occur

[Ref: Manipal Surgery 4th/645; L and B 26th/969; Schwartz 10th/217-18; CSDT 14th/58; Sabiston 19th/471-73, 309-11]

Normal IAP is 0-5 mm Hg *showing phasing variation with respiration- Manipal Surgery 4th/645*

Abdominal Compartment Syndrome Final effect *Manipal Surgery 4th/645*

- The major system affected in decreasing frequency of incidence and morbidity are: pulmonary, cardiovascular, renal, splanchnic, central nervous system
- ***End result can be***
  - ***Intractable hypoxia, hypercarbia, ARDS***
  - ***Cardiac insufficiency and cardiac arrest***
  - ***Oliguria, anuria, acute renal failure***
  - ***Cerebral edema and anoxia***

Abdominal Compartment Syndrome

◈ *L and B 26th/969*

- Surgeons are increasingly aware of the harmful effect of high intra-abdominal pressures which can occur in severe intraabdominal sepsis, such as pancreatitis and also aortic aneurysm rupture.
- High pressure leads to reduced blood flow and tissue ischaemia which contributes to **multiorgan failure**. While the abdominal wall has elasticity, if intra-abdominal volume increases due to fluid, gas, pus, tissue edema, etc., then maximal capacity may be reached and pressure rises to a critical level.
- ***Tension releasing incisions, equivalent to a fasciotomy, have been suggested although this is not widely practised.***
- In some cases, after surgery for severe intraperitoneal sepsis, the surgeon cannot close the abdomen and may leave the incision ***wide open, covering abdominal contents with mesh or a saline-soaked dressing, planning to return at a future date to close the defect. This is called a laparostomy.***

◈ *CSDT 14th/58*

- Aggressive resuscitation of patients, particularly those involved in trauma or requiring an emergent celiotomy, may result in increased abdominal pressure.
- **Intra-abdominal hypertension, as measured by bladder pressure**, is generally self-limiting; however, ***it can become dangerous when pressures exceed 30 mm Hg***. In this scenario ***venous outflow from the bowel and kidney may become compromised***.
- Furthermore, respiratory complications may ensue as the pressure exerted upon the diaphragm may decrease tidal volume and result in respiratory acidosis. ***In this situation, the abdominal compartment must be rapidly decompressed, usually by opening the abdomen, in order to reestablish flow from the viscera.***
- Similar to compartment syndrome of the extremities, the fascia resists stretch exerted by the muscle and other tissue after injury and resuscitation. ***However, a high index of suspicion, rapid diagnosis and expeditious treatment result in restoration of flow and prevention of morbidity in both scenarios.***

◈ *Schwartz 10th/217-18*

- ***Organ failure can occur over a wide range of recorded bladder pressures. Generally, no specific bladder pressure prompts therapeutic intervention, except when the pressure is >35 mm Hg.***
- Rather, emergent decompression is carried out when intra-abdominal hypertension reaches a level at which ***end-organ dysfunction occurs***.
- *Mortality is directly affected by the* ***timing of decompression****, with 60% mortality in patients undergoing presumptive decompression*, 70% mortality in patients with a delay in decompression and nearly uniform mortality in those not undergoing decompression.

Table: *(Schwartz 10th/217)*: **Abdominal compartment syndrome grading system**

Grade	Bladder Pressure	
	mmHg	cm H_2O
I	10–15	3–20
II	16–25	21–35
III	26–35	36–47
IV	>35	>48

160. Ans. b. Polyglyconate; c. Polyglactin; d. Monofilament Nylon

[Ref: Manipal Surgery 4th/1140-41; L and B 26th/37-38; Sabiston 19th/233-34]

- ***Sutures that lose the majority of their tensile strength within 60 days are considered absorbable.*** They are ***degraded by tissue enzymes or hydrolysis***- *www.dermnetnz.org*
- **Plain Catgut:** Phagocytosis and ***enzymatic degradation*** within 7–10 days- *L and B 26th/38*
- **Chromic Catgut**: Phagocytosis and ***enzymatic degradation*** within 90 days- *L and B 26th/38*
- **Catgut** also loses strength rapidly and unpredictably in the intestine and in infected wounds as a consequence of acid and ***enzyme hydrolysis***-CSDT 14th/70
- **Polyglactin** (*Braided Multifilament*): Hydrolysis minimal until 5–6 weeks. Complete absorption 60–90 day- *L and B 26th/38*
- **Nylon (Monofilament** or braided multifilament, Dyed or undyed) (raw material-**Polyamide polymer**):
- Degrades at approximately 15–20% per year *L and B 26th/37*
- "As a protein, **silk fibroin** is susceptible to biological degradation by ***proteolytic enzymes*** such as chymotrypsin, actinase and carboxylase"- www.ncbi.nlm.nih.gov
- **Polyglyconate:** Hydrolysis minimal until 8–9 weeks. Complete absorption by 180 days- *L and B 26th/38*
- Polyglycolic acid: Hydrolysis minimal at 2 weeks, significant at 4 weeks. Complete absorption 60–90 days- *L and B 26th/38*
- **Polydioxanone (PDS):** Hydrolysis minimal at 90 days. Complete absorption at 180 days- *L and B 26th/38*
- **Silk:** Fibrous encapsulation in body at 2–3 weeks. Absorbed slowly over 1–2 years- *L and B 26th/37*

Absorbable Suturs

◈ *omnisurge.co.za*

- Absorbable sutures are *naturally biodegradable in the body*, which makes it ideal for internal use. These sutures hold the body tissues together long enough to allow healing and then they disintegrate on their own, without requiring further procedures or manual removal.

Dissolvable sutures can be made of either ***natural or synthetic materials***.

Biological sutures are identified as foreign proteins and then naturally ***degraded by the body's*** proteolytic enzymes – the ***enzymes that digest proteins***.

However, the majority of absorbable sutures are now industrially produced from synthetic polymer fibers that can still be broken down successfully by the enzymes in the human body.

Synthetic absorbable sutures are industrially produced from polyglycolide, polylactide, polydioxanone and caprolactone. The chemical structures of these materials are similar to sugars and acids and they are therefore easily eliminated. ***Absorption takes place by hydrolysis***, which is the chemical breakdown of the compound due to its reaction with water or moisture.

Table: *(Sabiston 19th/233)*: **Comparison of Nonabsorbable Sutures**

Suture	Types	Tensile Strength Retention In Vivo
Silk Suture	Braided	Progressive degradation of fiber
Nylon Suture	Monofilament Braided	Progressive hydrolysis may result in gradual loss of tensile strength over time.
Polyester Fiber Suture	Braided Monofilament	No significant change known to occur in vivo.
Polyester Fiber Suture	Braided	No significant change known to occur in vivo.
Polypropylene Suture	Monofilament	Not subject to degradation or weakening by action of tissue enzymes.
Poly (hexa fluoropropylene -VDF Suture)	Monofilament	Not subject to degradation or weakening by action of tissue enzymes.

161. Ans. a. 0.33 mm; d. 0.013 inch

[Ref: Braunwald's Heart Disease 8th/Chap 19]

Catheters and Associated Equipment

◈ *Braunwald's Heart Disease 8th/Chap 19*

- Catheters used for ***cardiac catheterization*** are available in various lengths, sizes and shapes. Typical catheter lengths vary between 50 and 125 cm, with 100 cm being the most commonly used length for adult left-heart catheterization by the femoral approach.
- The outer diameter of the catheter is specified using French units; ***1 French unit (F) = 0.33 mm***. The inner diameter of the catheter is smaller than the outside diameter because of the thickness of the catheter material.
- ***0.33 mm equivalent to 0.013 inch***

The **French scale** or **French gauge** system is commonly used to measure the size of a catheter. It is most often abbreviated as Fr, but can often be seen abbreviated as Fg, Ga, FR or F. The ***French size is three times the diameter in millimeters***. A round catheter of 1 French has an external diameter of 1⁄3 mm and therefore the diameter of a round catheter in millimetres can be determined by dividing the French size by 3: D (mm) = Fr/3 or Fr = D (mm) * 3"-wikipedia

162. Ans. a. Pulselessness; b. Pain; d. Numbness; e. Sensory loss

[Ref: Manipal Surgery 4th/89; CSDT 14th/807; L and B 26th/888-89]

Acute Arterial Occlusion (Emboli)

◈ *Manipal Surgery 4th/89*

- Pain
- Pallor
- Paresis
- Pulselessness
- Paresthesia

Acute Lower Extremity Occlusive Disease

Clinical Findings CSDT 14th/807

- The Five Ps: ***Pain, Pallor, Pulselessness, Paresthesias and Paralysis***
- **Severe sudden pain** is present in 80% of patients and its onset usually indicates the time of vessel occlusion. Pain is absent in some patients because of prompt onset of anesthesia and paralysis and portends a poor prognosis.
- On examination, the key finding is a **lack of palpable pulses** in a diffusely painful extremity. It is important to determine if sensitivity to light touch is maintained. These fibers are highly susceptible to ischemia and their dysfunction heralds the beginning of irreversible ischemic changes.
- The *onset of motor paralysis implies impending gangrene*.
- Early intervention is critical.
- Swelling with acute tenderness of a muscle belly—usually in the calf following acute femoral artery occlusion—generally denotes irreversible muscle infarction.
- Skin and subcutaneous tissues have greater resistance to hypoxia than nerves and muscles, which may demonstrate irreversible histological changes after 3 hours or less of ischemia.

Acute Arterial Occlusion

◈ *L and B 26th/888-89*

- Sudden occlusion of an artery is usually caused by an embolus. It may also happen when thrombosis occurs on an atherosclerotic plaque
- Emboli may lodge in any organ and cause ischemic symptoms.
  - **Arm and leg**-***Pain, pallor, paralysis, pulselessness and paraesthesia***. Acute arterial occlusion due to an embolus differs from occlusion due to thrombosis on preexisting atheroma; in the latter case, a collateral circulation has often built up over time. It is essential to differentiate between the two as they require different management.
  - **Mesenteric vessels**-Possible gangrene of the corresponding loop of intestine.

163. Ans. c. Bronchogenic cyst

[Ref: Manipal Surgery 4th/1020; L and B 26th/868-69; Harrison 19th/1720; Schwartz 10th/673]

Neurilemmoma ***(schwannomas)*- posterior mediastinum; *substernal goiter*- anterior mediastinum**- *Manipal Surgery 4th/1020*

Schwannoma-Usually occur in ***posterior mediastinum***, asymptomatic - *www.pathologyoutlines.com*

"Bronchogenic cysts result from abnormal ventral budding or branching of the tracheobronchial tree during embryologic development. They are lined with pseudostratified columnar respiratory epithelium and their walls usually contain cartilage, smooth muscle and mucous gland tissue. They may be filled with clear, serous fluid or thick, mucoid material. They may occur in any part of the mediastinum, but *most are near the tracheal carina in the middle or posterior mediastinum.* Less often, they may occur within the lung parenchyma, pleura, or diaphragm"-pubs.rsna.org

Mediastinal Mass

◈ *CSDT 14th/358*

- An **anterior mediastinal mass** can indicate the following: thymoma (the most common), thymic hyperplasia, thymolipoma, thymic cyst, thymic carcinoid, thymic carcinoma, germ cell tumor (teratoma, seminoma and nonseminomatous germ cell tumor), lymphoma, parathyroid adenoma, ***substernal thyroid*** and lymphangioma.
- A **middle mediastinal mass** can include lymphoma, pericardial cyst, ***bronchogenic cyst***, aneurysm and lymphadenopathy.
- A **posterior mediastinal mass** can include neurogenic tumor, enteric cyst, bronchogenic cyst, meningocele, diaphragmatic or hiatus hernia and paravertebral abscess. The most common mediastinal masses in children are neurogenic tumors (50%-60%). In young children (< 4 years of age), they are invariably malignant (neuroblastomas).

Table: *(Harrison 19th/1720)*: **The Three compartment of the mediastinum**

	Anterior compartment	**Middle compartment**	**Posterior Compartment**
Contents	Thymus gland, anterior mediastinal lymph nodes, internal mammary arteries and veins	Pericardium, heart, ascending and transverse arch of aorta, superior and inferior vena Cavae, brachiocephalic arteries and veins, phrenic nerves, trachea and main bronchi and their contiguous lymph nodes, pulmonary arteries and veins	Descending thoracic aorta, esophagus, thoracic duct, azygos and hemiazygos veins, sympathetic chains and the posterior group of mediastinal lymph nodes
Common abnormalities	Thymoma, lymphomas, teratomatous neoplasms, thyroid masses, parathyroid masses, mesenchymal tumors, giant lymph node hyperplasia, hernia through foramen of Morgagni	Metastatic lymph node enlargement, granulomatous lymph node enlargement, pleuropericardial cysts, ***bronchogenic cysts***, masses of vascular origin	Neurogenic tumors, meningocele, meningomyelocele, gastroenteric cysts, esophgeal diverticula, hernia through foramen of Bochdalek, extramedullary hematopoiesis

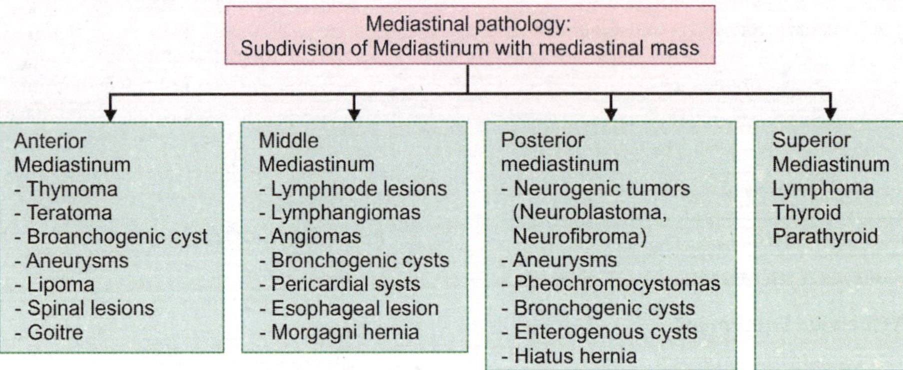

164. Ans. a. Axillary dissection can be carried out through the incision for a mastectomy; b. Level I,II and III nodes are removed in modified radical mastectomy; c. In Halsted radical mastectomy all breast tissue and skin, the nipple-areola complex, the pectoralis major and pectoralis minor muscles and the level I, II and III axillary lymph nodes are removed; d. Arm is kept abducted at 900 during axillary dissection

[Ref: CSDT 14TH/316; Manipal Surgery 4th/406-07; L and B 26th/813-14; Schwartz 10th/547-49]

A & E

Axillary Dissection

◈ *emedicine.medscape.com*

- Axillary dissection removes all the nodes and fat from axillary space.
- Clearance can be anatomically divided into **three levels** based on the relationship of the tissue to the pectoralis minor muscle.
- Patients are ***positioned lying supine, with the arm abducted*** and placed on an ***arm board at 90 degrees to the chest wall.***
- The ***head end is raised to 30 degrees***. The shoulder can be flexed to facilitate dissection of axillary level III nodes

- ***Axillary dissection can be carried out through the incision for a mastectomy. Patients having lumpectomy usually require a separate incision in the axilla.***
- **Simple and Modified Radical Mastectomy** *Sabiston 19th/852-53*
- **Simple or total mastectomy** refers to complete removal of the mammary gland, including the nipple and areola.
- Sentinel node biopsy may be added for axillary staging and may be performed through the ***mastectomy incision or through a separate axillary incision.***
- *Modified radical mastectomy* refers to removal of the mammary gland, nipple and areola with the ***addition of axillary dissection***

Mastectomy and Axillary Dissection

◈ *Schwartz 10th/547*

- An **extended simple mastectomy** removes all breast tissue, the nipple-areola complex, skin and the level I axillary lymph nodes.
- A **modified radical ('Patey') mastectomy** removes all breast tissue, the nipple-areola complex, skin and the ***levels I, II and III axillary lymph nodes***
- The **Halsted radical mastectomy** removes all breast tissue and skin, the nipple-areola complex, ***the pectoralis major and pectoralis minor muscles*** and the ***level I, II and III axillary lymph nodes.***

Modified Radical Mastectomy

◈ *Schwartz 10th/548-49*

- A modified radical mastectomy preserves the ***pectoralis major muscle*** with ***removal of level I, II and III (apical) axillary lymph*** nodes.

Conservative Breast Cancer Surgery

◈ *L and B 26th/813-14*

- This is aimed at removing the tumor plus a rim of at least 1 cm of normal breast tissue. This is commonly referred to as a wide local excision.
- Quadrantectomy and lumpectomy are usually combined with ***axillary surgery, usually via a separate incision in the axilla.***
- There are various options that can be used to deal with the axilla, ***including sentinel node biopsy, sampling, removal of the nodes behind and lateral to the pectoralis minor (level II) or a full axillary dissection (level III). Sentinel node biopsy is a reasonable alternative to axillary dissection in selected patients with invasive cancer-*** CDST 14TH/316

165. Ans. a. Most common site involved are sigmoid colon and splenic flexure; c. Abdominal radiographs show thumb print sign; d. Commonly presents as pain in abdomen with bloody dirrhoea; e. Acute thrombotic mesenteric occlusion is also k/a intestinal angina

[Ref: CSDT 14th/733-34; Sumer Sethi 6th/124; L and B 26th/1174; Schwartz 10th/1221-22]

Ischemic Colitis- Thumb Printing (Due to Marked Mucosal Edema)

◈ *Sumer Sethi 6th/124*

"The most common location is the sigmoid colon (40%) followed by the transverse colon (17%), splenic flexure (11%), ascending colon (12%) and the rectum (6%)"- CSDT 14th/734

Patients with **acute thrombotic mesenteric occlusion** also present with severe abdominal pain, but it is usually chronic postprandial abdominal pain ***(intestinal angina)*** accompanied by weight loss-*CSDT 14th/675; L and B 26th/886*

Nonocclusive mesenteric ischemia, also known as "***intestinal angina,***" is generally more insidious and most often seen in the aging population affected by atherosclerotic disease-*Harrison 19th/1979*

Ischaemic Colitis

◈ *L and B 26th/1174*

- Ischemia of the colon typically results from ***thrombosis or embolism.***
- Sudden embolic events present with ***severe pain out of proportion to the degree of peritonism, bloody diarrhea,*** severe hemodynamic instability and acidosis.
- Resuscitation and laparotomy are required with resection of gangrenous bowel and exteriorization of the bowel. Mortality is extremely high.
- Abdominal ***radiographs may show 'thumb printing'*** and endoscopy may demonstrate haemorrhagic edema. The ***left colon and, in particular, the splenic flexure are usually the worst affected.***

Intestinal Ischemia

◈ *Schwartz 10th/1221-22*

- Intestinal ischemia occurs ***most commonly in the colon.***
- ***Although the splenic flexure is the most common site of ischemic colitis***, any segment of the colon may be affected. The ***rectum is relatively spared*** because of its rich collateral circulation.

Ischemic colitis is a form of mesenteric ischemia limited to the colon. It is caused by a low flow state, usually affects the elderly and is likely due to the shunting of blood away from the mucosa. It often develops insidiously and many a times, no specific cause can be found. It manifests with ***lower abdominal pain, rectal bleeding and in later cases patients may develop symptoms of peritonitis***-www.clinicaladvisor.com

Ischemic Colitis

◈ *CSDT 14th/733-34*

- Ischemic colitis refers to colonic inflammation caused by inadequate perfusion.
- It is more common in **elderly patients** and has a mortality of 13%. It occurs as a result of an occlusive or non-occlusive insult. Examples of occlusive ischemic colitis include ***embolism, thrombosis (arterial or venous), atherosclerosis, trauma and postsurgical causes*** such as patients with loss of ***inferior mesenteric blood supply*** after aortic aneurysm

repair and those with inadequate perfusion to colonic anastomoses.

- Patients with ischemic colitis present with ***diarrhea (90%), hematochezia (65%) and abdominal pain (58%).***

Ischemic Bowel Disease

◈ *Robbins 9th/779-80*

- ***Intestinal segments at the end of their respective arterial supplies are particularly susceptible to ischemia. These watershed zones include the splenic flexure,*** where the superior and inferior mesenteric arterial circulations terminate and to a lesser extent, the sigmoid colon and rectum where inferior mesenteric, pudendal and iliac arterial circulations end.
- Although the ***colon is the most common site of gastrointestinal ischemia***, mucosal and mural infarction may involve any level of the gut from stomach to anus.

166. Ans. a. Morbidity is mainly d/t mediastinal infection; b. Partial tear involving mucosa should be managed conservatively; e. Serum amylase levels may be high as a result of absorption of amylase from the pleural cavity

[Ref: Harrison 19th/1910; CSDT 14th/476-77; Manipal Surgery 4th/452-53; L and B 26th/992-94; Schwartz 10th/1018]

Morbidity resulting from esophageal perforation is principally due to infection- *CSDT 14th/476*

Spontaneous rupture usually occurs into the left pleural cavity or just above the GEJ- Schwartz 10th/1018

Thoracentesis will reveal cloudy or purulent fluid, depending on how much time has passed since the time of perforation. The ***amylase content of the fluid is elevated and serum amylase levels may also be high as a result of*** absorption of amylase from the pleural cavity- CSDT 14th/477

Perforation of the esophagus: The key to optimum management is early diagnosis. The ***most favorable outcome is obtained following primary closure of the perforation*** within 24 hours, resulting in 80% to 90% survival- Schwartz 10th/1018

Spontaneous (Postemetic) Perforation (Boerhaave Syndrome)

◈ *CSDT 14th/476*

- Most cases follow a bout of heavy eating and drinking. ***The perforation most frequently occurs in the left posterolateral wall, 3-5 cm above the gastroesophageal junction.***
- The tear results from excessive intraluminal pressure, usually caused by violent retching and vomiting. Some cases have also been associated with childbirth, defecation, convulsions, heavy lifting and forceful swallowing. ***The overlying pleura are also torn, so both the mediastinum and the pleural cavity are contaminated with esophageal contents. The second-most common site of perforation is at the midthoracic esophagus,*** *on the right side at the level of the azygous vein.*

Esophageal Perforation

◈ *Harrison 19th/1910*

- ***Most cases of esophageal perforation are from instrumentation of the esophagus or trauma.*** Alternatively, ***forceful vomiting or retching can lead to spontaneous rupture at the gastroesophageal junction*** (Boerhaave's syndrome).
- Esophageal perforation causes pleuritic retrosternal pain that can be associated with pneumomediastinum and subcutaneous emphysema.
- ***Mediastinitis is a major complication of esophageal perforation*** and prompt recognition is key to optimizing outcome.
- CT of the chest is most sensitive in detecting mediastinal air. Esophageal perforation is confirmed by a contrast swallow, usually Gastrografin followed by thin barium.
- Treatment includes nasogastric suction and parenteral broad-spectrum antibiotics with prompt surgical drainage and repair in noncontained leaks. Conservative therapy with NPO status and antibiotics without surgery may be appropriate in cases of contained perforation that are detected early.
- ***Endoscopic clipping or stent placement may be indicated in nonoperated iatrogenic perforations*** or nonoperable cases such as perforated tumors.
- "Medical instrumentation is the most common cause of esophageal perforation (diagnostic or therapeutic endoscopy).Instrumental perforations are ***most likely to occur in the cervical esophagus.***The cricopharyngeal area is the most common site of injury"- CSDT 14th/476

Perforation

◈ *L and B 26th/992-94*

- Perforation of the esophagus is usually iatrogenic (at therapeutic endoscopy) or due to 'barotrauma' (spontaneous perforation).
- ***Many instrumental perforations can be managed conservatively, but spontaneous perforation is often a life-threatening condition that regularly requires surgical intervention***
- **Barotrauma (spontaneous perforation, Boerhaave syndrome):** This occurs classically when a person vomits against a closed glottis. The pressure in the esophagus increases rapidly and the esophagus bursts at its ***weakest point in the lower third, sending a stream of material into the mediastinum and often the pleural cavity as well.*** Boerhaave syndrome is the ***most serious type of perforation*** because of the large volume of material that is released under pressure. This causes rapid chemical irritation in the mediastinum and pleura followed by **infection if untreated**. Barotrauma has also been described in relation to other pressure events when the patient strains against a closed glottis (e.g. defaecation, labour, weight-lifting).
- Perforation of the esophagus usually leads to **mediastinitis.**

167. Ans. b. Can causes retrograde ejaculation; c. Open prostatectomy is preferred in larger obstructive mass; d. There is less risk of bleeding in transurethral laser vaporization than in TURP; e. Resectoscope is passed through the urethra and prostate is resected into multiple pieces and removed

[Ref: Manipal Surgery 4th/974-75; CSDT 14TH/976-77; L and B 26th/1348-49; Schwartz 10th/1665]

A resectoscope is passed through the urethra and prostate is resected into multiple pieces and removed- *Manipal Surgery 4th/974*

Open Prostatectomy Versus TURP Campbell

◈ *Walsh Urology, 9th/Chap 89*

- **Two approaches to open prostatectomy** are ***retropubic and suprapubic***
- Open prostatectomy should be considered when the obstructive tissue is estimated to weigh more than 75 g or sizable bladder diverticula or calculi exist.
- Before performing an open prostatectomy, the presence of prostate cancer should be excluded.
- **Potential risks of open prostatectomy** include *urinary incontinence, erectile dysfunction, retrograde ejaculation, urinary tract infection, bladder neck contracture, urethral stricture, deep vein thrombosis, pulmonary embolus and the need for blood transfusion.*
- Advantages of **open prostatectomy over TURP** are ***a lower retreatment rate, more complete removal of the prostatic adenoma under direct vision and no risk of TURP syndrome.***
- **Disadvantages of open prostatectomy over TURP** are a lower midline incision, longer hospitalization and increased ***potential for perioperative hemorrhage.***
- **Suprapubic prostatectomy** is ideal for men with a large median lobe, clinically significant bladder diverticulum, or large bladder calculi.

Prostatectomy

◈ *CSDT 14TH/976-77*

- There are two common approaches used in surgery for BPH: transurethral and transabdominal (open vs. minimally invasive).
- The **transurethral route** is by far the most common and preferred in patients with glands weighing less than 100 g because morbidity rates are lower and the hospital stay is shorter. With new technology, even larger glands can be managed with the transurethral approach.
- ***Larger glands, however, may require open surgery (suprapubic or retropubic enucleation)***, depending on the preference and experience of the urologist.
- ***Open surgery for BPH is the exception rather than the rule because of increased morbidity.***
- ***Transurethral approaches are the least invasive and require the shortest hospital stay*** (typically ambulatory or one night).
- The gold standard is the monopolar transurethral resection of the prostate (TURP), by which a ***resectoscope with a monopolar loop electrode is utilized to remove the obstructing BPH tissue***. Hypotonic irrigation solution is required and hyponatremia due to excess systemic absorption ("TURP Syndrome") is a unique complication of this approach.
- ***Additional complications of TURP include hematuria, UTI, stress incontinence, impotence, retrograde ejaculation***, urethral stricture and bladder neck contracture. ***Incontinence and impotence are rare complications in the hands of experienced surgeons (< 5%).***
- ***Transurethral laser vaporization of the prostate with holmium or KTP (potassium titanyl phosphate) laser technology has demonstrated similar efficacy to TURP in well selected patients with smaller glands.***
- ***The major advantage of the laser approaches is less risk of bleeding and even the ability to perform the procedure while patients remain on anticoagulation.***
- **Holmium-laser enucleation of the prostate (HOLEP)** utilizes laser energy to enucleate the prostate adenoma (rather than vaporize the tissue). The tissue must then be more cellated to be removed via the resectoscope.
- HOLEP has similar efficacy to TURP and laser vaporization but may be more technically challenging.

168. Ans. (All) a. Chronic atrophic gastritis; b. Obesity; c. Smoking; d. H.pylori infection; e. Menetriers disease

[Ref: CSDT 14th/534; Manipal Surgery 4th/488; Harrison 19th/534; L and B 26th/1045-48; Schwartz 9th/926-33; Sabiston 19th/1204-09]

Incidence of **proximal gastric carcinoma** *is increased- may be due to* ***obesity and rich in socioeconomic status patients***- *Manipal Surgery 4th/488*

"H. pylori is known to be a cause of ***chronic atrophic gastritis***, which in turn is a ***recognized precursor of gastric adenocarcinoma***. Epidemiologic studies have linked gastric H pylori infection with a 3.6-fold to 18-fold (all patients vs. women) increase in the risk of developing carcinoma of the body or antrum (not the cardia) and the risk is proportionate to serum levels of H pylori antibodies"- CSDT 14th/534

"Carcinoma is associated with ***cigarette smoking*** and dust ingestion from a variety of industrial processes. The ingestion of substances such as spirits may induce gastritis and, in the long term, cancer. The aetiology of proximal gastric cancer remains an enigma. It is not associated with Helicobacter but is associated with obesity and higher socioeconomic status"-L and B 26th/1046

Table: *(Schwartz 9th/928)*: **Factors increasing or decreasing the risk of gastric cancer**

Increase risk
Family history
Diet (high in nitrates, salt, fat)
Familial polyposis
Gastric adenomas
Hereditary nonpolyposis colorectal cancer
Helicobacter pylori infection: Atrophic gastritis, ***intestinal metaplasia***, dysplasia
Previous gastrectomy or gastrojejunostomy (>10 yr ago)
Tobacco use
Menetrier's disease
Decrease risk
Aspirin
Diet (high fresh fruit and vegetable intake)
Vitamin C

Risk Factors for Gastric Cancer

◈ *Davidson 22nd/877*

- ***H. pylori***

- ***Smoking***
- ***Alcohol***
- Dietary associations (see text)
- Autoimmune gastritis (pernicious anaemia)
- Adenomatous gastric polyps
- Previous partial gastrectomy (> 20 yrs)
- Ménétrier's disease
- Hereditary diffuse gastric cancer families (*HDC-1* mutations)
- Familial adenomatous polyposis

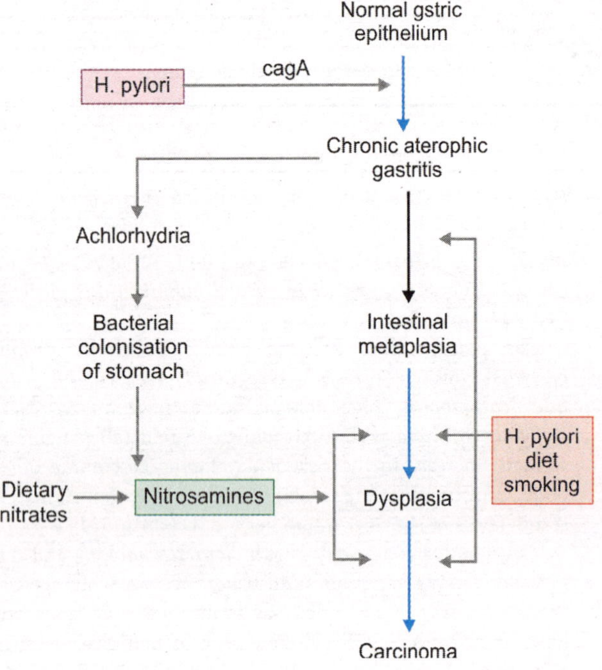

Fig: *(Davidson 22nd/877)*: Gastric carcinogenesis: a possible mechanism

169. Ans. a. More common in young female

[Ref: Manipal Surgery 4th/804-05; L and B 26th/1244]

Pilonidal Sinus

◈ *Manipal Surgery 4th/804-05*

- ***Common in hairy men** (20-30yr)*
- *In **spite of adequate surgical procedures, recurrence is common***
- ***Recurrent abscesses which rupture are common***
- *The **direction of the sinuses are cephaloid***
- *External opening of the **sinus seen just above the anal verge in the midline over the coccyx***

Pilonidal Sinus

◈ *L and B 26th/1244*

- The term 'pilonidal sinus' describes a condition found in the ***natal cleft overlying the coccyx***, consisting of one or more, usually non-infected, ***midline openings***, which communicate with a fibrous track lined by granulation tissue and containing hair lying loosely within the lumen. A common affliction among the military, it has been referred to as **'jeep disease'**.
- ***The disease mostly affects men, in particular hairy men.***
- ***Recurrence is common, even though adequate excision of the track is carried out.***
- ***It is thought that the combination of buttock friction and shearing forces in that area allows shed hair or broken hairs which have collected there to drill through the midline skin,*** or that infection in relation to a hair follicle allows hair to enter the skin by the suction created by movement of the buttocks, so creating a subcutaneous, chronically infected, midline track.
- Usually, but not invariably (when diagnosis may be confused with anal fistula or hidradenitis suppurativa), the sinus ***runs cephalad.***
- Carcinoma arising in chronic pilonidal disease has been described, but is exceedingly rare.
- ***The condition is seen much more frequently in men than in women, usually after puberty and before the fourth decade of life*** and is characteristically seen in dark-haired individuals rather than those with softer blond hair
- ***There is often a history of repeated abscesses*** that have burst spontaneously or which have been incised, usually ***away from the midline***. The primary sinus may have one or many openings, ***all of which are strictly in the midline between the level of the sacrococcygeal joint and the tip of the coccyx.***
- *Treatment of an acute exacerbation (abscess):* If rest, baths, local antiseptic dressings and the administration of a broad-spectrum antibiotic fail to bring about resolution, the abscess should be drained

170. Ans. b. Lipomas are the most common benign tumorsc; c. Desmoid is low-grade sarcomas of soft tissue of chest wall; d. Lung metastasis with direct chest wall extension should be treated with radical en bloc resection of the chest wall and underlying lung; e. Rhabdomyosarcoma is the second most common chest wall tumor in children

[Ref: CSDT 14th/341-43; Manipal Surgery 4th/; L and B 26th/871; Schwartz 10th/666-67]

"Lipomas—*Lipomas are the most common benign tumors of the chest wall*"- *CSDT 14th/341*

"Fibrous dysplasia (bone cyst, osteofibroma, fibrous osteoma and fibrosis ossificans) accounts for a ***third or more of benign skeletal tumors of the chest wall***"- CSDT 14th/341

Tumors of the chest wall*:* These can be tumors of any component of the chest wall, i.e. bone, cartilage and soft tissue. They are treated similarly to those that occur in other sites and require specialist surgical input only if major resection and chest wall reconstruction are contemplated"- *L and B 26th/871*

Malignant Soft Tissue Tumors

◈ *CSDT 14th/341*

- ***Roughly 50% of all chest wall masses are sarcomas***, yet overall they represent only a small percentage (5%) of all malignant soft tissue sarcomas. The development of metastasis greatly reduces the chances of survival. There are many histologic subtypes of soft tissue sarcoma. Typically, ***low-grade sarcomas include desmoids or liposarcomas with low-grade features.***

- **Desmoid tumors**-Soft tissue neoplasms arising from fascial or musculoaponeurotic structures, desmoid tumors consist of proliferations of ***benign-appearing fibroblastic cells***, abundant collagen and few mitoses. ***Surgical incisions (abdominal and thorax) have been the site of desmoid development,*** *either in or near the scar"- Schwartz 10th/666*
- Next most frequently seen are ***malignant fibrosarcoma, rhabdomyosarcoma and malignant fibrous histiocytoma***, which are usually high grade lesions.
- Individual histologic subtype is *not* by itself a significant prognostic variable, but histologic grade *is* significant. Metastases—either synchronous or metachronous—are ***most commonly to the lungs (75%)*** and should be resected if negative margins can be achieved and adequate lung function
- **Rhabdomyosarcoma—*Rhabdomyosarcoma is an uncommon tumor in adults but is the second most common chest wall tumor in children***-*CSDT 14th/341*

Metastatic Chest Wall Tumors

◈ *CSDT 14th/343*

- Metastases to bones of the thorax are often multiple and are usually from tumors of the kidney, thyroid, lung, breast, prostate, stomach, uterus, or colon. Renal cell and thyroid malignancies have a high propensity for metastasizing to the sternum.
- Involvement by direct extension occurs in carcinoma of the breast and lung.
- ***Lung metastasis with direct chest wall extension should be treated with radical en bloc resection of the chest wall and underlying lung.***

Tumors of Chest Wall

◈ *CSDT 14th/341-42*

- **Fibrosarcomas—*Fibrosarcoma is the most common primary soft tissue cancer of the chest wall***. It occurs most frequently in young adults..
- **Malignant fibrous histiocytoma/high-grade pleomorphic sarcoma**—Malignant fibrous histiocytoma has a bimodal distribution, with peaks between 20 and 30 years of age and between 50 and 60. ***Although they are the most common soft tissue sarcoma of adults***, they rarely rise from the chest wall.
- **Liposarcomas**—These tumors account for approximately one-third of all primary cancers of the chest wall.

171. Ans. a. Lipoma is the most common benign soft tissue tumor in adult; c. Intramuscular lipoma are ill defined and difficult to palpate than subcutaneous lipoma

[Ref: S.Das Textbook of Surgery 5th/92-93; Manipal Surgery 4th/214-15; Robbins 9th (SAE)/1220; Schwartz 10th/486]

Lipoma, a benign tumor of fat, is the most common soft tissue tumor of adulthood- *Robbins 9th (SAE)/1220*

Infrequently, ***lipomas are large, intramuscular and poorly circumscribed****- Robbins 9th (SAE)/1220*

Lipoma

◈ *Devita Oncology 8th/1751-52*

- ***Lipomas are the most common benign soft tissue neoplasm and usually arise in the subcutaneous tissue***. The trunk and proximal limbs are the most frequent sites. Although deep-seated benign lipomas do occur in the mediastinum or retroperitoneum, seemingly mature fatty neoplasms in the retroperitoneum should be regarded with suspicion because most are well-differentiated liposarcoma.
- Most lipomas are solitary, soft and painless and grow slowly; however, ***2% to 3% of patients have multiple lesions*** that are occasionally seen in a familial pattern.
- ***Lipomatosis is a term applied to a poorly circumscribed overgrowth of mature adipose tissue*** that grows in an infiltrating pattern.
- Solitary lipomas are well-circumscribed, lobulated lesions composed of fat cells but are demarcated from surrounding fat by a thin, fibrous capsule.
- ***Intramuscular lipomas differ from their more superficial counterparts by usually being poorly circumscribed and infiltrative***. These typically present in mid-adult life as slow-growing, deep-seated masses most often located in the thigh or trunk.
- Approximately 10% of intramuscular lipomas are noninfiltrative and well circumscribed. In a patient with a deep-seated fatty tumor, it is important to exclude an atypical lipomatous tumor (i.e. Liposarcoma), which tends to be more common than an intramuscular lipoma.
- ***"Lipomas are the most common subcutaneous neoplasm and have no malignant potential***.Surgical excision can be considered for symptomatic or large lesions that compromise musculoskeletal function"- *Schwartz 10th/486*

Lipoma

◈ *S.Das Textbook of Surgery 5th/92-93*

- A ***lipoma is one of the commonest and most benign of all tumors***
- **Lipomatosis (Multiple lipoma)** is not uncommon. ***Dercum's disease (adiposis dolorosa)*** is a variety of this condition in which there are tender lipomatous swellings particularly affecting the trunk

172. Ans. a. Abdominal injury usually requires full exploratory laparotomy; b. Spinal cord and brain injury may require bullet fragment removal if compressive symptoms present; c. Injuries are typically associated with a low infection rate; d. Conservative management in superficial abdominal injury

[Ref: Manipal Surgery 4th/; L and B 26th/293; Schwartz 10th/174,180]

Gunshot Wounds

◈ *CSDT 14th/168-69*

- Generally, fractures associated with low-velocity gunshot wounds are usually stable when a handgun is the weapon. ***These injuries are typically associated with a low infection rate*** and can be ***prophylactically treated with broad-spectrum antibiotics for 48 hours.***

- Any present neural injury, is usually secondary to "blast effect," in which the energy of the bullet is absorbed and transferred to the soft tissues. ***As a result, decompression is usually not indicated. An exception to this rule is if the bullet** fragment is found in the spinal canal between levels T12* ***and L5. Steroids after gunshot wounds to the spine are not*** *recommended.*
- Projectiles tend to be classified as ***low-velocity (<300 hm/second) or high-velocity (>300 hm/second).***
- Abdominal injuries are associated with a high incidence of internal injury. ***All but the most superficial penetrating wound of the abdomen require full exploratory laparotomy*** *-patient.info/doctor*
- When a neurologic deficit is present that correlates with radiographic findings of **neurologic compression, a retained bullet fragment within the spinal canal** in patients with incomplete motor deficits is a ***relative indication for surgical excision of fragment-*** *www.orthobullets.com*
- **Non-operative local wound care indications**- low velocity gun shot injury with no bone involvement and clean wound edges: local wound care, tetanus +/- ***short course of oral antibiotics*** *-www.orthobullets.com*
- The diagnostic approach differs for penetrating trauma and blunt abdominal trauma. ***As a rule, minimal evaluation is required before laparotomy for gunshot or shotgun wounds that penetrate the peritoneal cavity, because over 90% of patients have significant internal injuries.***
- ***Laparoscopy is another option to assess peritoneal penetration for tangential wounds. If there is doubt, however, it is always safer to explore the abdomen.***
- ***Gunshot wounds to the back or flank are more difficult to evaluate because of the retroperitoneal location of the injured abdominal organs.*** Triple-contrast CT scan can delineate the trajectory of the bullet and identify peritoneal violation or retroperitoneal entry, but may not identify the specific injuries-*Schwartz 10th/180*

173. Ans. a. Clearly demarcated margin; b. Elevated edge; e. More abrupt onset

[Ref: Manipal Surgery 4th /24/; L and B 26th/582-83; Harrison 19th/830]

"**Erysipelas** is a type of infection which is very near to the surface of skin and it's **more superficial than cellulitis infection**"- *www.cellutitis.org*

Primary Differences Between Erysipelas and Cellulitis

◈ *articles.mercola.com*

- In ***cellulitis, the infection is mostly found in the deep underlying tissues of skin***, including the deeper dermis and subcutaneous fat. ***Erysipelas affects the upper layers of the skin, or the upper dermis and superficial lymphatics.***
- Another factor that distinguishes these two conditions is the **age group** that acquires them. Erysipelas occurs in young children and older adults. On the other hand, cellulitis is found to occur more frequently among middle-aged individuals and older adults (although children may also be at risk for it).
- Although both of these conditions can occur in any area of your body, ***cellulitis more commonly manifests in the lower legs, while true erysipelas likely appears in the legs and face*** — these are parts of the body where there is very little subcutaneous tissue

Erysipelas *(articles.mercola.com)*	**Cellulitis**
An ***abrupt onset*** of fever accompanied by chills	You may experience a low-grade fever with a ***less abrupt onset***
Dark-skinned people may have brownish-grey skin, while Caucasians may have bright red skin	The skin appears brownish-black in dark skinned individuals and dull red in Caucasians
The infected area is hot, tender and spreads; the surface is shiny but vesicles and bullae (fluid- or air-filled sacs or lesions)	The ***border of the infected area is less well defined*** and fades into the surrounding skin; you will not see any blisters or lesions
Pain and swelling commonly occur	Pain and swelling commonly occur

Erysipelas

◈ *L and B 26th/582*

- Erysipelas is a ***sharply demarcated*** streptococcal infection of the ***superficial lymphatic vessels***, usually associated with broken skin on the ***face***. The area affected is erythematous and edematous.
- The patient may be febrile and have a leukocytosis.
- Prompt administration of broad-spectrum antibiotics after swabbing the area for culture and sensitivity is usually all that is necessary.

Cellulitis/lymphangitis

◈ *L and B 26th/582-83*

- This is a bacterial infection of the skin and subcutaneous tissue that is ***more generalized than erysipelas***. It is usually associated with broken skin or pre-existing ulceration.
- Cellulitis is characterised by an ***expanding area*** of erythematous edematous tissue that is painful and associated with a fever, malaise and leukocytosis.
- ***No edge****- Manipal Surgery 4th/16*
- Erythema tracking along lymphatics may be visible (***lymphangitis***).
- The most common causative organism is streptococcus. Blood and skin cultures for sensitivity should be taken before prompt administration of broad-spectrum intravenous antibiotics and elevation of the affected extremity.

Erysipelas

◈ *Harrison 19th/830*

- Erysipelas is due to *S. pyogenes* and is characterized by an abrupt onset of fiery-red swelling of the face or extremities.
- The distinctive features of erysipelas are ***well-defined indurated margins, particularly along the nasolabial fold; rapid progression; and intense pain.***
- Flaccid bullae may develop during the second or third day of illness, but extension to deeper soft tissues is rare.

- Treatment with penicillin is effective; swelling may progress despite appropriate treatment, although fever, pain and the intense red color diminish.

Cellulitis

◈ *Harrison 19th/830*

- Cellulitis is an acute inflammatory condition of the skin that is characterized by ***localized pain, erythema, swelling and heat.***
- It may be caused by indigenous flora colonizing the skin and appendages (e.g., *S. aureus* and *S. pyogenes*) or by a wide variety of exogenous bacteria.

174. Ans. b. During bowel anastomosis, hemostatic forceps are used to grasp intestine

[Ref: Manipal Surgery 4th/1129; L and B 26th/33; Surgical Instruments by V.Pusdekar 1st/11-13]

"*While doing* **intestinal resection and anastomosis,** ***mesenteric vessels*** *of the adjacent diseased intestine are held b/w the* ***hemostatic forceps*** *before resecting the segment of diseased intestine"- Surgical Instruments by V.Pusdekar 1st/21*

"BABCOCK intestinal forceps: It is used to hold ***tubular organs;*** the orifices in the blades accommodate some part of the tissue and reduce the intraluminal pressure, which protects the organs from getting damaged"-surgicalunits.com

"Skin incisions should be made with a scalpel with the ***blade being pressed firmly down*** at right angles to the skin and then drawn gently across the skin in the desired direction. The incision is facilitated by tension being applied across the line of the incision by the fingers of the non-dominant hand, but ***the surgeon must ensure that at no time is the scalpel blade directed at their own fingers as any slip may result in a self-inflicted injury"***-L and B 26th/33

"Care should be taken to avoid damage to the **suture material** when handling. ***Avoid the crushing or crimping application of surgical instruments, such as needle holders and forceps,*** to the strand except when grasping the free end of the suture during an instrument tie"- www.ruralareavet.org

"Mechanical trauma to the suture by surgical instruments can also result in suture failure. ***Compression of sutures between the needle holder jaws with teeth produced morphologic changes in sutures that resulted in a marked reduction in the suture*** breaking strength. Similarly, the sharp edges of needle holder jaws without teeth can even crush the suture and, thereby, decrease its strength"-www.covidien.com

"Toothed forceps are ***used for handling skin, subcuatneous tissue, muscles, sheath.*** NOT TO BE used when handling bowel or blood vessels"-www.themastersurgeon.com

Adson's toothed forceps: Fine dissectors with teeth for gripping fine but tougher tissues. Often used in plastic surgery and useful for grasping ***fascia, subcuatenous fast and tendons"***-www.surgicalexam.com

Bonney's toothed forceps: Heavy toothed forceps used for grasping larger tough tissue and handling heavy needles. Typically used on fascia such as when closing a laparotomy wound"-www.surgicalexam.com

Artery forceps (Haemostatic forceps): It is used to control bleeding, not only from arteries but also from veins and capillaries- They are also ***used to catch and pull the tip of needle*** by assistant during suturing . They are also ***used to hold the thread during stitching***- Manipal Surgery 4th/1129; Obs by J B Sharma 1st/736

The most important things to notice: medical-diagonosis. wonderhowto.com

- The ***scalpel is held between the thumb and the middle finger*** *(they hold both sides of the scalpel near the blade).*
- The ***index finger supports the axis blade from above.***
- This holding technique gives you better control over the scalpel.

175. Ans. a. Prophylaxis against thromboembolism

[Ref: L and B 26th/318]

"Prophylaxis against thromboembolism: Venous stasis induced by the ***reverse Trendelenburg position*** during laparoscopic surgery may be a particular risk factor for deep vein thrombosis, as is a lengthy operation and the obesity of many patients"- L and B 26th/97

"Initial measures for **raised intracranial pressure** include positioning the head up 20–30° ***(reverse Trendelenburg*** positioning by tilt of the whole bed if the spine has not been cleared)"-

"Thyroid surgery: The patient is supine on the operating table with the table tilted up 15° at the head end to reduce venous engorgement ***(reverse Trendelenburg)***"-L and B 26th/760

"Hyperparathyroid surgery: The patient is positioned in ***reverse Trendelenburg"-L and B 26th/774***

OBSTETRICS & GYNECOLOGY

176. Ans. d. Retained products of conception

[Ref: Dutta Obs 8th/483; William's Obs 24th/1395-96; Obs by JB Sharma 1st/341-42; Normal and Problem Pregnancy by Gabbe 6th/426]

Secondary Postpartum Hemorrhage

◈ *Dutta Obs 8th/483; Obs by JB Sharma 1st/341-42*

- *The bleeding usually occurs b/w 8th and 14th day of delivery*
- ***Retained bits of cotyledon or membranes*** *(most common)*
- ***Endometritis and subinvolution of placental site***
- ***Secondary hemorrhage from CS wound***
- *Withdrawl bleeding following estrogen therapy for suppression of lactation*
- *Infection and separation of slough over a deep cervicovaginal laceration*
- *Other rare cause- chorionepithelioma, carcinoma cervix, placental polyp, infected fibroid polyp, puerperal inversion of uterus*
- *Coagulopathy- Gabbe 6th/426 (Table)*

Late Postpartum Hemorrhage

◈ *William's Obs 24th/1395-96*

- The American College of Obstetricians and Gynecologists (2013) defines *secondary postpartum hemorrhage* as bleeding 24 hours to 12 weeks after delivery.

- Clinically worrisome uterine hemorrhage develops within 1 to 2 weeks in perhaps 1 percent of women. ***Such bleeding most often is the result of abnormal involution of the placental site.*** It ***occasionally is caused by retention of a placental fragment or by a uterine artery pseudoaneurysm.***
- Usually, retained products undergo necrosis with fibrin deposition and may eventually form a so-called *placental polyp*. As the eschar of the polyp detaches from the myometrium, hemorrhage may be brisk.
- Delayed postpartum hemorrhage may also be caused by von Willebrand disease or other inherited coagulopathies

"**Retained products of conception** (namely placental tissue and amniotic membrane) complicate 1 in 100-200 deliveries"- Gabbe 6th/435

"***Uterine inversion*** is a rare event, complicating about 1 2000 to 1in 23000 deliveries"- Gabbe 6th/437

Primary postpartum hemorrhage: Atonic uterus (80%) is the commonest cause- Dutta Obs 8th/475

177. Ans. a. Kegel pelvic floor exercise; b. Retropubic cystourethropexy; e. Retopubic midurethral sling procedures

[Ref: Shaw's Gynae 16th/229-32; Dutta Gynae 7th/331-32; Novak's 15th/882-900]

Management of Stress Incontinence

◈ *Dutta Gynae 7th/331-32*
- *Sympathomimetic drugs (α-adrenergic drugs)-Imipramine*
- ***Retropubic cystourethropexy*** *(colposuspension)*
- *Retopubic midurethral sling procedures*

Genuine Stress Incontinence (GSI)

◈ *Shaw's Gynae 16th/225*
- *Age:* ***Old postmenopausal women*** *with loss of pelvic muscle tone are liable to develop (estrogen deficiency)*
- ***GSI is the only kind which can be cured by surgical procedures****, hence the importance of making a correct diagnosis prior to planning any surgical repair*
- *GSI require to be differentiated from urge incontinence, DI and a neurological bladder*
- Lifestyle interventions can decrease stress urinary incontinence in many women
- Vaginal devices (pessaries) and ***urethral inserts*** are available for treating stress urinary incontinence. *Novak's 15th/885*
- Urethral inserts are sterile inserts placed into the urethra by the patient and removed before a void, after which a new sterile insert is placed. Such inserts are appropriate for women with relatively pure stress incontinence, no history of recurrent urinary tract infections and no serious contraindications to bacteriuria (e.g., artificial heart valves)- *Novak's 15th/885-86*

"**Anticholinergic Agents:** These agents represent first-line medicinal therapy in women with **urge incontinence**. These agents are useful in treating urinary incontinence associated with urinary frequency, urgency and nocturnal enuresis"- emedicine.medscape.com; Novak's 15th/887

Anticholinergic Agents are useful in Detrusor Instability-

◈ *Shaw's Gynae 16th/233; Novak's 15th/887*

"The mainstay in the treatment of **voiding difficulty** is clean, ***intermittent self catheterization.*** The most important protection against urinary tract infection is frequent and complete bladder emptying rather than avoiding the introduction of a foreign body into the bladder. Voiding difficulty may be caused by neurologic diseases, such as multiple sclerosis, medications (such as antihistamines and anticholinergic agents), infections (in particular, herpes simplex virus and urinary tract infections), obstruction (following bladder neck surgery, or in women with advanced pelvic organ prolapse), overdistension, severe constipation (particularly in the elderly) and, rarely, psychogenic factors"- Novak's 15th/900

Table: *(Shaw's Gynae 16th/230)*: **Management of stress incontinence**

Conservative	Drugs	Surgery
1st line of treatment • Young woman • Frail, old woman • Postpartum, previous failed surgery	• Oestrogen cream in menopausal woman • Venlafaxine 75 mg daily • Imipramine 10–20 mg BD	1. If others fail • Vaginal (Kelly) • Abdominal 2. Marshall–Marchetti–Krantz and Pereyra Burch • Combined vaginal and abdominal suspension • Slings • Tension –free sling • Transobturator type 3. Laparoscopic suspension of bladder neck
1. ***Kegel pelvic floor exercises*** × 4–6 months 2. Electric/magnetic stimulation for nerve damage, magnetic stimulation 3. Artificial urinary sphincter in neurological condition 4. Vaginal cones		

178. Ans. c. Suspected ectopic pregnancy; d. Prostaglandin hypersensitivity; e. Severe rheumatic heart disease

[Ref: Dutta Obs 8th/204,206; J B Sharma 1st/126; William's Obs 23rd/232; Novak's Gyae 15th/256-57; Robert Shaw Gynae 4th/435]

Absolute C/I of medical abortion: *Suspected ectopic pregnancy or undiagnosed adnexal mass; Allergy to any drug*"-*J B Sharma 1st/126*

Table: *(Robert Shaw Gynae 4th/435)*: **Contraindication of medical abortion**

Absolute contraindications
- Adrenal insufficiency
- Ectopic pregnancy
- Asthma
- ***Cardiac disease***
- Heavy smoker
- Older than 35 years
- On anticoagulants or bleeding disorder

Relative contraindications
- Heavy smoker
- >35 years
- Obesity
- Hypertension (diastolic > 100 mmHg)

Contraindications to Medical Abortion

◈ *Novak's Gyae 15th/256-57*

- Contraindications to medical abortion with mifepristone/ misoprostol include ***ectopic pregnancy; an IUD in place (remove IUD first); chronic adrenal failure; concurrent long-term corticosteroid therapy; history of allergy to mifepristone, misoprostol, or other prostaglandin; and the inherited porphyrias***.
- The mifepristone–misoprostol combination was studied for gestations at 9 to 13 weeks; although it is almost as effective as earlier in pregnancy, a larger proportion of patients will experience heavy bleeding and require vacuum curettage

Contraindications to Medical Abortion

◈ *William's Obs 23rd/232*

- In addition to specific allergies to the medicines, they have included an in situ intrauterine device, ***severe anemia, coagulopathy or anticoagulant use and significant medical conditions, such as active liver disease, cardiovascular disease and uncontrolled seizure disorders***.
- Additionally, because misoprostol can lower glucocorticoid activity, women with adrenal disease or with disorders requiring glucocorticoid therapy should be excluded.

179. Ans. d. CuT IUCD

[Ref: Shaw's Gynae 16th/275; Dutta Gynae 7th/270; Dutta Obs 8th/629-30]

*Answer should be those method which prevent present risk of pregnancy and provide medium and long term method of contraception. From above options, **CuT (>LNG-IUCD) is single best answer. CuT prevent implantation of even fertilized egg.** LNG-IUCD act through prevents penetration of sperm, endometrial atrophy and prevention of ovulation*

"Intercourse b/w 11th and 17th day may result in a pregnancy"- Shaw's Gynae 16th/265

Emergency Contraception (EC)

◈ *Dutta Obs 8th/629-30*

- *LNG (0.75 stat and after 12 hour)*
- ***Cu IUCD (gold standard):** Introduction within maximum period of 5 days can prevent conception following accidental unprotected exposure. **This prevent implantation. It is gold standard method to be offered to all women for EC***

IUD- CuT and LNG-IUS. It can be used as postcoital contraceptive- *Dutta Obs 8th/615-16*

COC: Simple regime of 3 week on and 1 week off is to be followed. New users should normally ***start their pills packet on day 1 of their cycle"***- Dutta Obs 8th/623

POP: *It has to be **taken daily from the 1st day of the cycle**- Dutta Obs 8th/627*

Minipill/Progestogen-*only pill: The tablet is **taken daily without break**. The bill should be started within 5-7 days of the menstruation and taken at same time with a leeway of 3 hr on either side of fixed time each day. If this regime is nt observed any day, the women continues with POP but observes extra precaution for 48 h"- Shaw's Gynae 16th/275*

IUD (Interval): ***It is preferable to insert 2-3 days after the period is over. But can be inserted any time during the cycle even during menstrual phase which has certain advantage***- *Dutta Obs 8th/616*

"It is advisable to insert IUCD during or soon after menstruation and after abortion or MTP. Lately, immediate postpartum insertion within 10 min of placental expulsion or within 24 hr of delivery is practical and is found effective"- *Shaw's Gynae 16th/270*

180. Ans. d. If she exposed to recent intercourse, use emergency contraceptive; e. Use another method of contraception like barrier method for remaining period and start next COC pack without break

[Ref: Dutta Obs 8th/624; Dutta Gynae 7th/400]

Missed Combined oral contraceptive (COCs): Management

◈ *Dutta Gynae 7th/400*

- When a woman forgets to take **one pill** (late up to 24 hours), she should take the missed pill at once and continue the rest as schedule. There is nothing to worry.
- When she **misses two pills** in the first week (days 1-7), she should take 2 pills on each of the next 2 days and then continue the rest as schedule. ***Extra precaution has to be taken for next 7 days either by using a condom or by avoiding sex.***
- If 2 pills are missed in the third week (days 15-21) or **if more than two active pills are missed at any time, *another form of contraception should be used as back up for next 7 days*** as mentioned above. ***She should start the next pack without a break.*** If she misses any of the **7 inactive pills** (in a 28-day pack only) she should throw away the missed pills. She should take the remaining pills one a day and start the new pack as usual.

"If she forgets to take a tablet, she should take two tablets the following day. ***If she forgets to take tablet more than once in a cycle, she is no longer adequately protected and must use a barrier method during that cycle"***- Shaw's Gynae 16th/273

Emergency contraceptive: *It should be used mainly as back-up methods. It is **used in misplaced IUCD and missed pills**"- Shaw's Gynae 16th/279*

181. Ans. b. Venocaval compression begins at about 16 weeks of gestation; c. There is midtrimester fall in blood pressure; d. Systolic murmur may occur normally; e. Cardiac output return to pregnant level by 20 days after delivery

[Ref: Dutta Obs 8th/60-61; Obs by JB Sharma 1st/49-52; Normal and Problem Pregnancy by Gabbe 6th/46-50]

Cardiovascular System in Pregnancy

◈ *Dutta Obs 8th/60-61*

- *Cardiac output starts to increase from 5th week of pregnancy and **reaches its peak 40-50% at about 30-34 weeks**.* CO increases further during labor (+50%) and immediately following delivery (+70%) over the pre-labor values
- *CO return to pre-labor values by 1 hr following delivery and to the **pre-pregnant level by another 4 weeks, time***
- ***Blood pressure unaffected or mid-pregnancy drop of diastolic pressure by 5-10 mm Hg***

- ***A systolic murmur may be audible in the apical or pulmonary area***
- *A continuous hissing murmur may be audible over the tricuspid area in the left second and third intercostal spaces called the mammary murmur*

Cardiovascular System in Pregnancy

◈ *Obs by JB Sharma 1st/49-51*

- An increase in cardiac output begins early in pregnancy (6 weeks) and reach peak at 32-34 week
- ***Changes in cardiac function become apparent during the first 8 weeks of pregnancy. Cardiac output is increased as early as the fifth week*** and reflects a reduced systemic vascular resistance and an increased heart rate- *William's Obs 23rd*
- *Cardiac output returns to normal by about 2 weeks following delivery*
- *Maternal BP decreases during pregnancy to reach the lowest peak at 24-26 weeks and increases thereafter to reach pre-pregnancy level at term. There is more fall in diastolic and mean arterial pressure (5-10 mm Hg) as compared with systolic BP.* ***The mid trimester fall in BP*** *may be absent in women with pre-eclamsia*
- **Systolic ejection murmur** *(d/t increased flow across pulmonary and aortic valve) can be heard in 90% cases of normal pregnancy. These physiological murmurs are mostly midsystolic and less than grade 3*
- *A* ***soft, diastolic murmur*** *may be hard transiently in 20% women*
- *A* ***continuing mammary murmur*** *may be heard in 10% women*

Cardiac changes in pregnancy *Normal and Problem Pregnancy by Gabbe 6th/49*

- CO- return to normal in 2-4 postpartum week
- By 5th week, CO has already risen by more than 10%

Supine hypotensive syndrome is caused when the inferior vena cava is compressed by the weight of a pregnant female's uterus, fetus, placenta and amniotic fluids while lying in the supine position This condition can develop as *early as the second trimester but is maximal during the third trimester, 36 to 38 weeks*- jacobburton.wordpress.com

"Vena cava compression *begins as early as 13 to 16 week's gestation* and nearly complete at term"- *Bonica's Management of Pain by Scott M. Fishman* 4th*/795*

182. Ans. a. PAPP-A and β-hCG estimation; c. Chorionic villus Sampling

[Ref: Dutta Obs 8th/128-130; William's Obs 23rd/292-93; Fernando Arias 3rd/44-45]

CVS is done for First Trimester Prenatal Diagnosis b/w 10-14 week-

◈ *B Sharma 1st/160*

First Trimester Screening *J B Sharma 1st/155; Dutta Obs 8th/128*

- It uses ***PAPP-A (lower in Down syndrome) and free β-hCG (higher in Down's syndrome)*** b/w 11 and 14 weeks
- It can detects 62% Down's syndrome pregnancies with a 5% false-positive rate

Second Trimester Screening

◈ *J B Sharma 1st/155*

- **Double test** (MSAFP is lower while total hCG or free β-hCG is raised in Down's syndrome
- **Triple test**- MSAFP, hCG and uE3 (unconjugated estriol)
- **Quadruple test**- MSAFP, hCG, uE3 and inhibin-A
- **Penta screen:** AFP, hCG, uE3, diameric inhibin-A and hyperglycosylated hCG

Table: *(Dutta Obs 8th/130)*: **Prentatal Diagnosis- CVS, Amniocentesis and Cordocentesis**

	Chorionic villus Sampling	Amniocentesis	Cordocentesis
Time	Transcervical 10–13 weeks Transabdominal 10 weeks to term	After 15 weeks (early 12-14 weeks)	18–20 weeks
Materials for study	Trophoblast cells	Fetal fibroblasts Fluid for biochemical study (see p. 741)	Fetal white blood cells (others–infection and biochemical study)
Karyotype result	Direct preparation: 24–48 hours Culture: 10–14 days	Culture: 3–4 weeks	Culture: 24–48 hours
Fetal loss	0.5–1%	0.5%	1–2%
Accuracy	Accurate; may need amniocentesis for confirmation	Highly accurate	Highly accurate
Termination of pregnancy when indicated	1st trimester–safe	2nd trimester–risky	2nd trimester–risky

183. Ans. b. MSAFP and hCG

[Ref: Dutta Obs 8th/128,132; J B Sharma 1st/155]

See Explanation of above Question

Screening Methods: First Trimester

◈ *Dutta Obs 8th/128-29*

Screening Parameters are:

- ***Biophysical:*** *(i) ultrasound measurement of nuchal transluceny (NT), (ii) nasal bone*
- ***Biochemical:*** *(i) free β –hCG, (ii) PAPP-A (Pregnancy associated plasma protein-A)*
- **Time of test: *b/w 11 weeks and 14 weeks***
- **Values:** *PAPP-A- reduced; β –hCG- increased; NT-measurement increased in trisomy 21*

Note:

- *NT is the fluid-filled space (detected by USG) b/w the fetal skin and the underlying soft tissue at the region of fetal neck. NT ≥ mm is abnormal. Combined tests can detect trisomy 21 in 92% cases with a false-positive rate of 5%*
- First trimester screening is either equal or even superior to second trimester screening

Screening Methods: Second Trimester

◈ *Dutta Obs 8th/129*

- *It is done b/w 15 weeks and 22 weeks*
- *MSAFP: Low level are found in down syndrome*
- ***Triple test:*** *It is a combine test which includes MSAFP, hCG and uE3 (unconjugated estriol). It is used for detection of down syndrome. In an affected pregnancy, levels of MSAFP and uE3 tend to low while that of hCG is high*
- ***Quadruple (Quad) screening include four biochemical analytes:*** *MSAFP, hCG, uE3 and dimeric inhibin-A. It can detect trisomy 21 in 85% cases. Level of serum analytes in cases with trisomy 21: MSAFP-reduced, hCG-increased, uE3-reduced and dimeric inhibin-A- elevated*
- ***Note:*** *Best screening procedure is combined first and second trimester procedures*

184. Ans. b. Associated with dysmenorrhea and menorrhagia; c. Total hysterectomy is the treatment of choice; e. Tenderness of uterus may be seen before and during menses

[Ref: Shaw's Gynae 16th/420-22; Dutta Gynae 7th/256-58; Novak's Gynae 15th/484-85; Robbins 9th/1012]

Adenomyosis

◈ *Shaw's Gynae 16th/420-22*

- Grossly, the uterus appears ***symmetrically enlarged*** to not more than 14 weeks size
- Unlike fibroid- ***there is no capsule surrounding the lesion-*** *Dutta Gynae 7th/257*
- Some are aymptomatic, others present with ***menorrhagia and progressively increasing dysmenorrhea,*** pelvic discomfort, backache and dyspareunia
- If a patient gives a history of ***menorrhagia with accompanying dysmenorrhea***, one should always consider the possibility of adenomyosis
- Uterus is tender
- NSAIDS are commonly used to control pain and bleeding. Treatment with progestins or cyclic estrogen and progestins have got little benefit. LNG-IUD is found to improve the menorrhagia and dysmenorrhea- *Dutta Gynae 7th/257*
- Since most women are elderly and past the age of age of childbearing, ***total hysterectomy is the treatment***

Adenomyosis

◈ *Novak's Gynae 15th/484-85*

- **Adenomyosis is defined as presence of endometrial stroma and glands within the myometrium, at least one low-power field from the basis of the endometrium, whereas endometriosis is characterized by ectopic endometrium appearing within the peritoneal cavity.**
- Although occasionally noted in women in their younger reproductive years, the average age of ***symptomatic women is usually older than 40 years.*** Increasing parity, early menarche and shorter menstrual cycles may all be risk factors according to one study
- Symptoms typically associated with ***adenomyosis include excessively heavy or prolonged menstrual bleeding, dyspareunia and dysmenorrhea. Symptoms often begin up to 2 weeks before the onset of a menstrual flow and may not resolve until after the cessation of menses.***
- The uterus is typically ***diffusely enlarged,*** although usually less than 14 cm in size and is often ***soft and tender, particularly at the time of menses.***
- The uterus is usually tender and slightly softened under bimanual examination performed premenstrually (Halban's sign)- *COGDT 2006/Chap 39*
- **Adenomyosis is a clinical diagnosis.**
- Imaging studies including pelvic ultrasound or MRI, although helpful, are not definitive
- The **management of adenomyosis** depends on the patient's age and desire for future fertility. Relief of secondary dysmenorrhea caused by adenomyosis can be ensured after ***hysterectomy***, but ***less invasive approaches can be tried initially.***
- NSAIDs, hormonal contraceptives and menstrual suppression using oral, intrauterine, or injected progestins or gonadotropin-releasing hormone agonists are all useful. Treatment follows the same protocol as treatment for endometriosis. Uterine artery embolization can be effective

185. Ans. a. Hypothalamic and pituitary cause; b. Ovarian failure

[Ref: Shaw's Gynae 16th/330-32; Dutta Gynae 7th/387, 441-43]

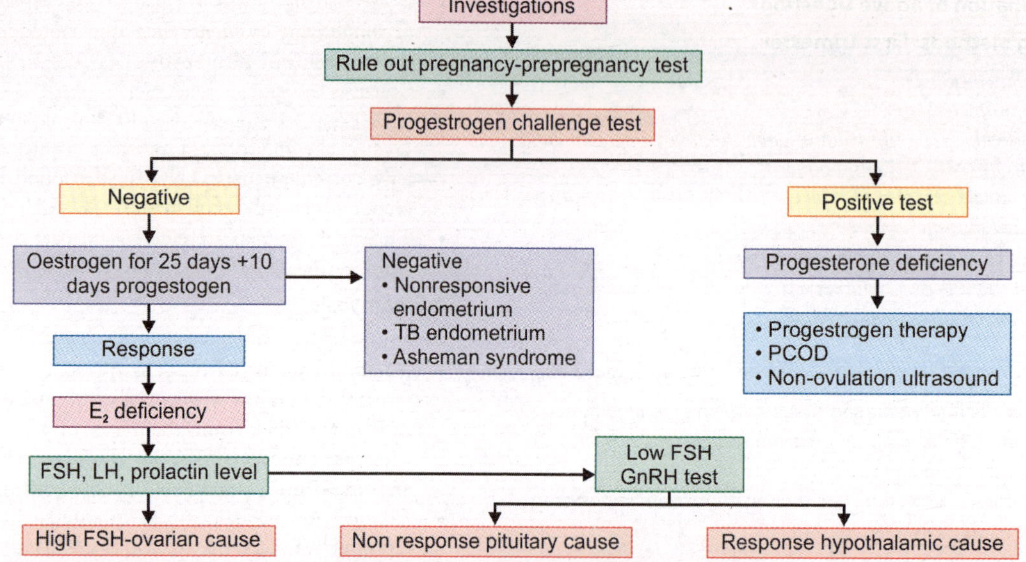

Fig: *(Shaw's Gynae 16th/332)*: Secondary amenorrhea

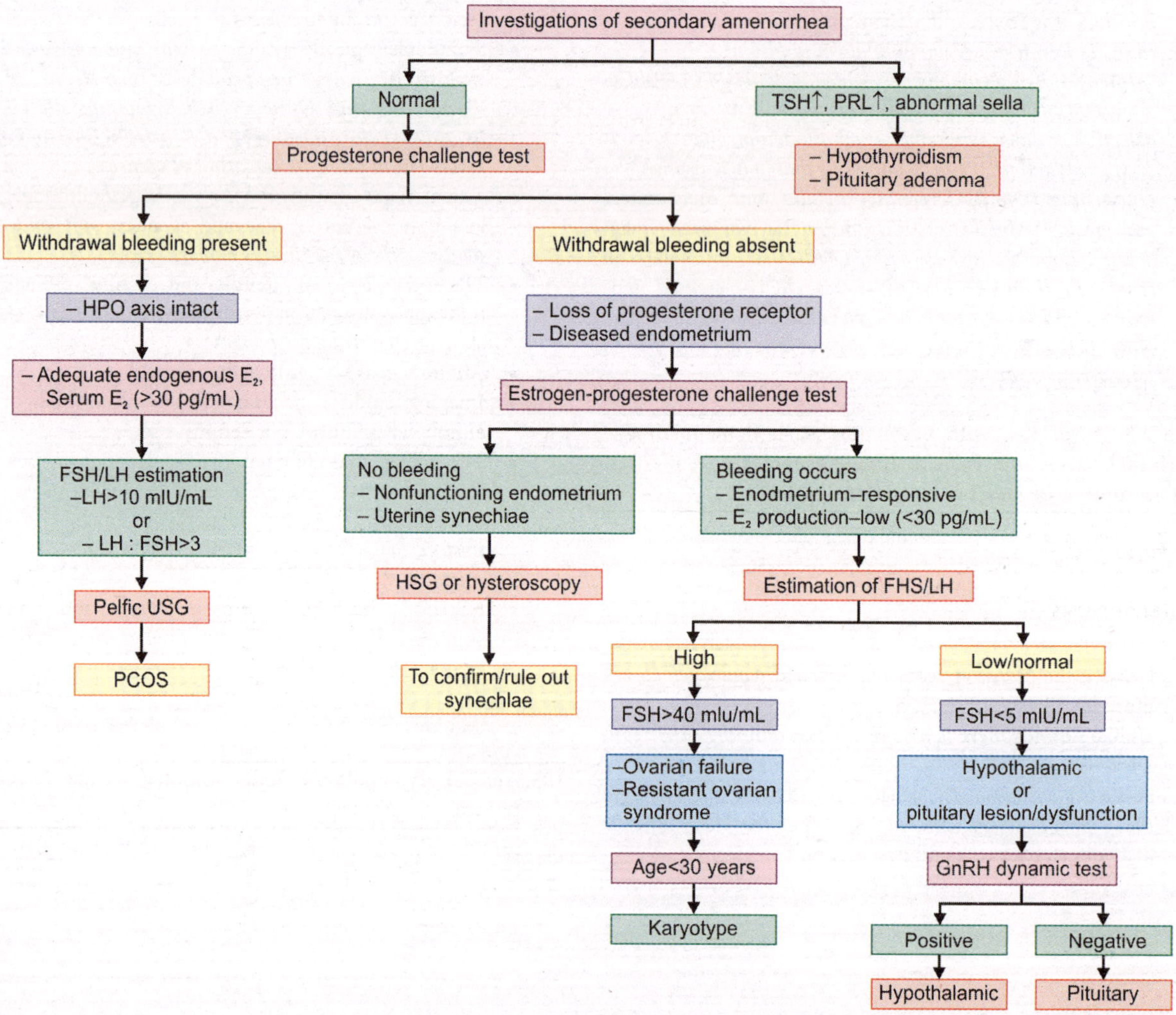

Investigations of secondary amenorrhea

Normal

TSH↑, PRL↑, abnormal sella

– Hypothyroidism
– Pituitary adenoma

Progesterone challenge test

Withdrawal bleeding present

– HPO axis intact

– Adequate endogenous E_2, Serum E_2 (>30 pg/mL)

FSH/LH estimation
–LH>10 mIU/mL
or
– LH : FSH>3

Pelfic USG

PCOS

Withdrawal bleeding absent

– Loss of progesterone receptor
– Diseased endometrium

Estrogen-progesterone challenge test

No bleeding
– Nonfunctioning endometrium
– Uterine synechiae

HSG or hysteroscopy

To confirm/rule out synechlae

Bleeding occurs
– Enodmetrium–responsive
– E_2 production–low (<30 pg/mL)

Estimation of FHS/LH

High

FSH>40 mlu/mL

–Ovarian failure
–Resistant ovarian syndrome

Age<30 years

Karyotype

Low/normal

FSH<5 mIU/mL

Hypothalamic
or
pituitary lesion/dysfunction

GnRH dynamic test

Positive

Hypothalamic

Negative

Pituitary

Fig: *(Dutta Gynae 7th/387)*: Secondary amenorrhea

A & E

186. Ans. a. Hypertension before pregnancy, elevation of blood pressure during the first half of pregnancy, or high blood pressure that lasts for longer than 12 weeks after delivery; b. Fetal complication may occur; d. High blood pressure may require antihypertensive medications

[Ref: Dutta Obs 8th/277; William's Obs 23rd/709; Obs by JB Sharma 1st/441-43; Normal and Problem Pregnancy by Gabbe 6th/781]

Chronic Hypertension in Pregnancy

◈ *Dutta Obs 8th/277*

- **Chronic hypertensive disease (CHD) is defined as the presence of hypertension of any cause antedating or before the 20th week of pregnancy and its presence beyond the 12 weeks after delivery.**
- The condition poses a difficult problem as regards the diagnosis and management when seen for the first time, beyond the 20th week of pregnancy.
- ***Overall incidence is 2-4% of which 90% are due to essential hypertension.***
- **The high risk factors for CHD are:** (i) Age (> 40 years), (ii) Duration of hypertension (>15 years), (iii) Level of BP (>160/110 mm of Hg), (iv) Presence of any medical disorder (renovascular) and (v) Presence of thrombophilias.
- Majority of women with CHD are low risk and have satisfactory maternal and fetal outcome without any antihypertensive therapy

Fetal complication of chronic hypertension of pregnancy
Obs by JB Sharma 1st/441

- *Abortions*
- *Fetal growth restriction (FGR)*
- *Intrauterine death*
- *Increased neonatal complications*
- *Prematurity*

Chronic Hypertension

◈ *COGDT 2006/Chap 19*

- Chronic hypertension ***complicates as many as 5% of pregnancies.***
- It is characterized by a history of ***high blood pressure before pregnancy, elevation of blood pressure during the first half of pregnancy, or high blood pressure that lasts for longer than 12 weeks after delivery.***
- After evaluating the possible causes of chronic hypertension, further assessment is directed at end-organs and systems most likely to be affected by hypertension, including the eyes, heart, kidneys, uteroplacental circulation and the fetus.
- Pregnancies complicated by chronic hypertension, regardless of the cause, are at ***increased risk for poor fetal growth.*** An initial ultrasound examination should be performed as early as possible to confirm the due date and to ensure that no obvious fetal anomalies are present. Thereafter, fetal growth may be assessed by ultrasound as needed, usually no more frequently than every 2–4 weeks. Antepartum fetal monitoring usually is started by 32–34 weeks.
- Pregnancy outcome usually is good in patients with mild chronic hypertension and no other serious medical conditions. ***Fetal growth restriction, superimposed preeclampsia, placental abruption and preterm delivery are the most common complications.***
- In pregnant women with mild hypertension and no evidence of renal disease, serious medical complications are rare.
- Women with sustained blood pressure ≥180/110 mm Hg or those with evidence of renal disease may be at higher risk for serious complications, such as heart attack, stroke, or progression of renal disease and are candidates for ***antihypertensive medication.***

187. Ans. a. Frank breech is most common breech presentation; b. Complete breech is more common in multiparae; c. Frank breech is more common in primigravida; e. Chance of cord prolapse in complete breech is 5%

[Ref: Dutta Obs 8th/435-36; William's Obs 23rd/527-35; Obs by JB Sharma 1st/302-03; Normal and Problem Pregnancy by Gabbe 6th/396]

Breech Presentation

◈ *Obs by JB Sharma 1st/302-03; Dutta Obs 8th/435-36*

- **Complete** (Flexed breech): It is ***commonly present in multiparae (10%)***
- Incomplete breech: 3 types (Frank, footling and Knee)
- Breech with extended leg (**Frank breech**): It is ***commonly present in primigravidae, about 70%***
- Footling presentation: 25% (10-30%)
- Knee presentation-rare
- ***Cord prolapse chance in Complete (Flexed breech): 4-6%***
- ***Cord prolapse chance in footling presentation: 12%***
- Cord prolapse chance in extended leg (Frank breech): 0.5%

Table: *(Gabbe 6th/396)*: **Breech categories**

Type	Overall % of breech	Risk (%) of prolapse	Premature
Frank	48-73	0.5	38
Complete	4.6-11.5	4-6	12
Footling	12-38	15-18	50

188. Ans. a. Occur due to proliferation of placenta; c. Fetus may be absent; d. Karyotype 69XXY may result from fertilization of 1 ovum and 2 sperm; e. Snowstorm appearance on USG

[Ref: Dutta Obs 8th/221-31; Dutta Gynae 7th/298-300; William's Obs 23rd/257-61; Obs by JB Sharma 1st/143-49]

"The development of ***choriocarcinoma following hydatidiform mole ranges b/w 2-10%"****- Dutta Obs 8th/226*

Gestational Trophoblastic Disease

◈ *Dutta Gynae 7th/298-300*

- It is a spectrum of abnormal growth and proliferation of the trophoblasts of the placenta that continue even beyond the end of pregnancy of the placenta
- **Benign GTD includes:** ***Hydatidiform mole-complete and partial***

- **GTN encompasses**: *persistent hydatiform mole, invasive mole, choriocarcinoma and a rare entity of placental site trophoblastic tumour*

H. mole:

◈ *(Short Review) Dutta Obs 8th/221-31*

- *It is prevalent among teenaged and elderly patients with high parity*
- It is best regarded as a benign neoplasia of chorion with malignant potential
- In general ***completes moles have a 45XX karyotype (85%),*** the molar chromosomes are derived entirely from the father. The ovum nucleus may be either absent (empty ova) or inactivated which have been fertilized by a haploid sperm. It then duplicates its own chromosomes after meosis. Infrequently, the chromosome pattern may be 46Xy or 45X
- The higher the ratio of paternal: maternal chromosomes, the greater is the molar change. ***Complete moles show 2: 0 paternal/maternal ratio whereas partial mole shows 2: 1 ratio***
- ***Symptoms***
  - Vaginal bleeding (Commonest, in 90%, "***white currant in red currant juice")***.
  - Varying degrees of lower abdominal pain
  - Constitutional symptoms like excessive vomiting, breathlessness, thyrotoxicosis, features of tremors or tachycardia
  - ***Expulsion of grape like vesicles per vaginum is diagnostic of vesicular mole***
  - History of quickenig is absent.
- ***Signs***
  - Ill looking patient, prominent pallor
  - ***Features of pre-eclampsia*** (hypertension, oedema and or proteinuria).
  - ***The size of the uterus is more than that expected for the period of amenorrhea***
  - Doughy, firm elastic feel of the uterus
  - ***Fetal parts are neither felt nor fetal movements***
  - ***Absence of Fetal Heart Sound***
  - ***High hCG in urine*** (positive pregnancy test) diluted up to 1: 200 to 1: 500 beyond 100 days of gestation is very much suggestive. Rapidly increasing value of serum hCG > 100, 000 mIU/ml, are usual with molar pregnancy. Normal pregnancy values are below 60, 0000 mIU/ml. *(there is no mention of doubling time)*
- **Sonography: *Characteristic snowstorm appearance***

Table: *(COGDT)*: **Comparison of Complete and Partial Hydatididiform Moles**

	Complete	Partial
Karyotype	Diploid (46,XX or 46,XY)	Triploid (69,XXX or 69,XXY)
Embryo/fetus	Absent	Often present
Villi	Hydropic	Few hydropic
Trophoblasts	Diffuse hyperplasia	Mild focal hyperplasia
Implantation-site trophoblast	Diffuse atypia	Focal atypia
Fetal RBCs	Absent	Present
β-hCG	High (> 50,000)	Slight elevation (< 50,000)
Frequency of classic clinical symptoms[1]	Common	Rare
Risk for persistent GTT	20–30%	< 5%

Contd...

[1]Hyperemesis, hyperthyroidism, excessive uterine enlargement, anemia and preeclampsia

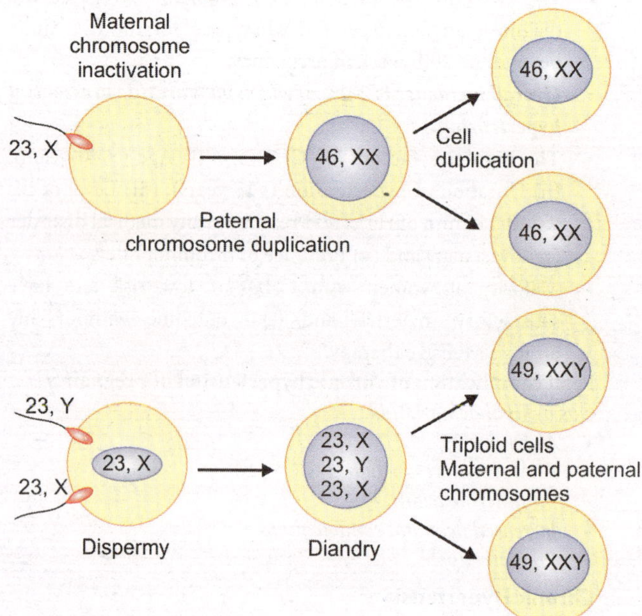

Fig: *(William's Obs):* Typical pathogenesis of complete and partial moles. A. A 46,XX complete mole may be formed if a 23,X-bearing haploid sperm penetrates a 23,X-containing haploid egg whose genes have been "inactivated." Paternal chromosomes then duplicate to create a 46,XX diploid complement solely of paternal origin. B. A partial mole may be formed if two sperm—either 23,X- or 23,Ybearing— both fertilize (***dispermy***) a 23,X-containing haploid egg whose genes have not been inactivated. The resulting fertilized egg is triploid with two chromosome sets being donated by the father (***diandry***)

189. Ans. d. Low-Grade Squamous Intraepithelial Lesion (LSIL)

[Ref: Shaw's Gynae 16th/157,88-89; Dutta Gynae 7th/90,128; Neena Khanna 5th/339-40; Gynae by Robert Shaw 4th/969]

"Condyloma acuminatum-Subcategory of LSIL" *pathologyoutlines.com*

What is Condyloma Acuminatum of Uterine Cervix

◈ *www.dovemed.com*

- Condyloma Acuminatum of Uterine Cervix is strongly associated with HPV type 6 and HPV type 11. The infection typically manifests as a benign wart on the mucous membrane of the cervix

- Treatment of the condition is necessary, since Condyloma Acuminatum of Uterine Cervix is termed as a variant of ***low-grade squamous intraepithelial lesion (SIL).*** Low-grade SIL is an early indicator for future 'invasive carcinoma' development
- The prognosis of Condyloma Acuminatum of Cervix depends upon 2 key factors, namely the type of HPV involved and the ***grade of the premalignant lesion present (whether low-grade or high-grade SIL)***
- Informing and educating the infected individuals on the importance of safe sex is essential to prevent the spread of HPV infection and thus of Cervical Condyloma Acuminatum

How is Condyloma Acuminatum of Uterine Cervix Diagnosed

◈ *www.dovemed.com*

- **Pap smear:** Cells are collected from the tip of the cervix and examined under the microscope for any associated precancerous or cancerous lesions. Pap smear results may indicate abnormalities such as low-grade squamous intraepithelial lesion
- Cervical Condyloma Acuminata is a variant of ***low-grade squamous intraepithelial lesion (SIL),*** which are asymptomatic lesions, but present a low risk for future cancer

Table: *(Shaw's Gynae 16th/88)*: **Comparison of different classification**

Pap Smear (1943)	CIN (WHO 1975)	SIL Bethesda (1988)
I	Normal	Normal
II	Inflammatory	Inflammatory – HPV – ASCUS
III	CIN I	Low SIL
IV	CIN II, CIN III, CIS	High SIL
V	SCC	SCC

ASCUS: atypical squamous cell of undetermined significance: CIN: Cervical intraepithelial neoplasia; CIS: carcinoma in situ; SIL: squamous intraepithelial lesion and SCC: squamous cell carcinoma

190. Ans. a. HPV DNA Testing; b. Liquid based cytology; c. Colposcopy study and biopsy of suspicious lesion

[Ref: Shaw's 16th/88-90; Dutta Gynae 6th/111-15, 323-28; Novak's Gyae 15th/588]

HSIL *includes* ***CINII, CINIII and CIS***- *Shaw's 16th/88*

High-Grade Squamous Intraepithelial Lesions

◈ *Novak's Gyae 15th/588*

- ***Any woman with a cytologic specimen suggesting the presence of HSIL should undergo colposcopy and directed biopsy***. This is because two-thirds of patients with this cytologic finding will have CIN 2 or greater.
- After colposcopically directed biopsy and determination of the distribution of the lesion, excisional or ablative therapy that addresses the entire transformation zone should be performed

"Since cytology alone does not give a clue to which abnormal cells progress to invasive cancer and aneuploidy which suggest the risk of progression is not routinely performed, it is necessary to submit all women with HSIL ***cytology for colposcopic study and biopsy of suspicious lesions****"- Shaw's 16th/489*

"A ***combined HPV testing and pap smear yields 96% sensitivity*** *as compared to only 60-70% with* ***pap smear*** *alone. PCR, southern blot or hybrid capture detects HPV DNA"-Shaw's 16th/491*

"A single pap smear has a diagnostic sensitivity of about 60%. False negative results may be upto 25%. False negative rate of Pap smear after 3 consecutive negative tests is less than 1%. *Error in cytology could be reduced further by liquid-based thin layer slide preparation* ***and automated (computer) screening methods.*** *Abnormal cytology is an indication of colposcopic evaluation and directed biopsy"-Dutta Gynae 6th/113*

"In 2003, the FDA approved *HPV DNA testing combined with cervical cytology* ***as a screening technique for women older than age 30. When the results of both tests are negative, the woman does not have to be retested for 3 years. The negative predictive value of a double negative*** test exceeds 99% . Because most HPV infections are transient, clear spontaneously and do not lead to real cancer precursors (especially in young women), it should not be used for screening in women younger than 30. Women who have negative test results for both cytology and HPV have a 1 in 1,000 chance of having CIN 2 or worse detected in the following 6 months. Prospective studies report less than 2 per 1,000 women will develop CIN 2 or greater in the following 3 years"-*Novak's Gyae 15th/5887*

191. Ans. e. Only one microscopically positive lymph node

[Ref: Shaw's Gynae 16th/480; Dutta Gynae 7th/277; Novak 15th/1142-43; Gynaecology by Robert Shaw 4th/41]

Post-op Radiation indicated for: *>1 LN+, LN with ECE, margin < 8-10 mm, lymphadenectomy not performed due to comorbid disease, LVSI*"-*en.wikibooks.org*

Post-op Indications for Radiotherapy

◈ *www.astro.org*

- ***Vulva (Heaps criteria): (+) margins, margin <8 mm pathologically or < 1 cm clinically, LVSI*** *(lymphovascular space involvement),* ***lesions > 5 mm deep***
- ***Inguinal/pelvic nodes*** *(Homesley GOG371986):* ***clinically + groin LN, >1 groin LN+, nodal ECE***

Postoperative Adjuvant Radiotherapy

◈ *Gynaecology by Robert Shaw 4th/41*

- Patient with risk factors for local recurrence such as a ***close surgical margin, lymphovascular space permeation,*** poorly differentiated tumor grade or diffuse infiltrative growth pattern, should be considered for **adjuvant external beam radiation therapy** to reduce the risk of recurrence
- With regard to the **nodal status,** ***no additional treatment is recommended if there is only one microscopically positive***

lymph node. However, if ***two or more metastatic nodes are present or there is capsular involvement in a single metastatic node***, **postoperative adjuvant radiotherapy** is usually recommended

Role of Radiation Therapy in Vulvar Carcinoma

◈ *Novak 15th/1142-43*

- It is important to remember that, with a rare exception, radiation therapy alone has little place in the primary management of vulvar cancer. It is indicated in conjunction with surgery.
- **Radiation seems to be indicated in the following situations:**
  - Preoperatively, in patients with advanced disease who would otherwise require pelvic exenteration or suffer loss of anal or urethral sphincteric function
  - Preoperatively, in patients with fixed, unresectable groin nodes
  - Postoperatively, to treat the pelvic lymph nodes and groins of patients with ***multiple microscopically positive groin nodes***, one or more ***macrometastasis (10 mm or larger***), or ***any evidence of extracapsular spread.***
- No additional treatment is recommended if ***one microscopically positive groin node (5 mm or less tumor deposit)*** is found in a fully dissected groin. The prognosis for this group of patients is excellent and only careful observation is required.
- If clinically evident **groin metastases** (any ***extracapsular spread or two or more microscopically positive groin nodes***) are found, the patient is at increased risk of groin and pelvic recurrence and should receive **postoperative groin and pelvic irradiation.**

192. Ans. a. Keep the IUCD, give antibiotic, follow up for antibiotic response and then take decision regarding IUCD removal

[Ref: Shaw's Gynae 16th/271; Novak's Gynae 15th/223-24]

"When PID is suspected in a woman wearing an IUD, *appropriate cultures should be obtained* and *antibiotic therapy should be administered. Removal of the IUD is not necessary unless symptoms do not improve after 72 hours of treatment.* Pelvic abscess, if suspected, should be ruled out by ultrasound examination. *Novak's Gynae 15th/223-24*

"Leaving an IUD in place is not thought to increase the chance of long-term complications from PID, although this cannot be guaranteed. In general the IUD can be left in place if the symptoms respond to antibiotic treatment within 48-72 hours"- www.fpnsw.org.au

193. Ans. a. KRAS; c. TP53; d. PTEN

[Ref: Shaw's Gynae 16th/436; Dutta Gynae 7th/304-05]

Two Important Carcinogenic Pathway

◈ *Dutta Gynae 7th/305*

- **Type I: Incorporation of Mullerian epithelial cells** on the ovary with formation of endometriosis or cortical inclusion cyst. **Type I ovarian tumors**, are borderline tumors, ***low grade serous ovarian cancers*** (LGSOC) or clear cell carcinoma. These patients ***harbor somatic gene mutations (KRAS, BRAF, or PTEN) but no association with p53 mutations.***
- **Type II: Incorporation of serous tubal intraepithelial carcinoma (STIC),** with exfoliation of cells, on to the surface of the ovary or both. This pathogenesis leads to development of ***high grade serous ovarian carcinoma*** (HGSOC). **HGSOC are aggressive from the outset as opposed to LGSOC that are indolent in nature.** Individuals with HGSOC harbor ***p53 mutations*** in about 100% of situation. *Currently the concept of distal fallopian tube origin of many pelvic serous carcinomas is considered indisputable.*
- Majority of epithelial ovarian cancers are not familial or hereditary. **Familial cancer account for 10-15% of all ovarian cancers**

"Low-grade serous carcinomas exhibit low-grade nuclei with infrequent mitotic figures. They evolve from adeno fibromas or borderline tumors, have frequent mutations of the **KRAS, BRAF, *or* ERBB2 *genes* and *lack* TP53 *mutations* (Type I pathway).** Low-grade tumors are indolent and have better outcome than high-grade tumors. In contrast**, high-grade serous carcinomas** have high-grade nuclei and numerous mitotic figures. More recently, studies have suggested that a proportion appear to originate from intraepithelial carcinoma in the fallopian tube. The development of these tumors is rapid (**Type II pathway**). The vast majority are characterized by ***TP53 mutations and lack mutations of KRAS, BRAF, or ERBB2"***- *www.ncbi.nlm.nih.gov*

"Mutations in the ARID1A gene have been found in many types of cancer, including ***cancers of the ovaries and lining of the uterus*** (endometrium) in women and cancers of the kidney, stomach, bladder, lung, breast and brain. These mutations are somatic, which means they are acquired during a person's lifetime and are present only in tumor cells"-ghr.nlm.nih.gov

"ARID1A is mutated in ~50% of ***ovarian clear cell carcinoma*** (OCCC)"-*www.ncbi.nlm.nih.gov*

"WT1: Wilms tumor, certain leukemias - *Robbins 9th/291*

Common Epithelial Tumour

◈ *Shaw's Gynae 16th/436*

- Serous
- Mucinous
- Endometrioid
- ***Clear cell***
- Brenner tumour
- Mixed epithelial tumor

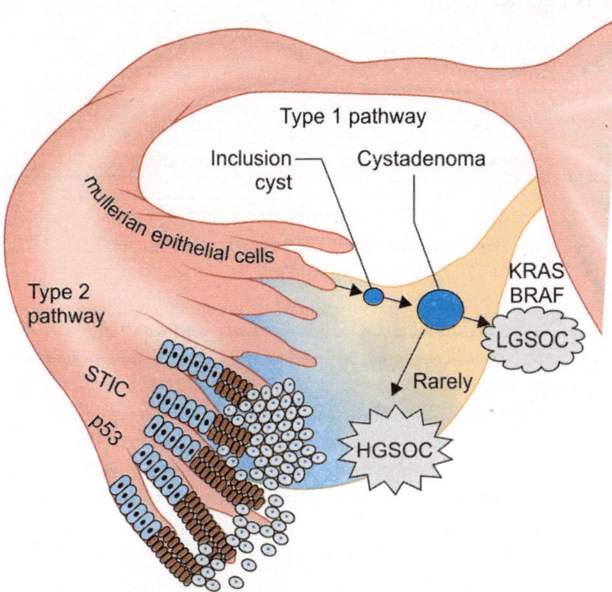

Fig: *(Dutta Gynae 7th/305)*: The schematic presentation of distal fallopian tube origin of ovarian carcinoma

PEDIATRICS

194. Ans. b. For making the diagnosis, the behavioral changes must begin before 5 year of age

[Ref: O.P.Ghai 8th/59-60; CPDT 17th/94-95; Nelson 20th (SAE)/200-205; Kaplan and Saddock 11th/1169-76]

"For making the diagnosis, the ***behavior must begin before 7 yr of age****, be present for at least 6 month"- O.P.Ghai 8th/59*

ADHD

◈ *Kaplan and Saddock 11th/1169-76*

- ADHD affects up to 5 to 8 percent of school-aged children, with 60 to 85 percent of those diagnosed as children continuing to meet criteria for the disorder in adolescence and up to ***60 percent continuing to be symptomatic into adulthood.***
- ADHD is frequently associated with comorbid disorders including learning disorders, anxiety disorders, ***mood disorders and disruptive behavior disorders***
- The Fifth Edition of the American Psychiatric Association's Diagnostic and Statistical Manual of Mental Disorders (DSM-5) has made several changes to the diagnostic criteria of ADHD in youth and in adults. Whereas in the past, ADHD symptoms had to be ***present by age 7 years, in DSM-5, "several inattentive or hyperactive impulsive symptoms" must be present by age 12 years.***
- Previously, there were two subtypes: Inattentive and Hyperactive/Impulsive type. In DSM-5, however, subtypes heen replaced by the following three specifiers, which essentially denote the same groups: (1) combined presentation, (2) predominantly inattentive presentation and (3) predominantly hyperactive/impulsive presentation
- ADHD is ***more prevalent in boys than in girls***, with the ratio ranging from 2: 1 to as high as 9: 1
- The course of ADHD is variable. Symptoms have been shown to ***persist into adolescence in 60 to 85 percent of cases and into adult life in approximately 60 percent of cases***. The remaining 40 percent of cases may remit at puberty, or in early adulthood.
- Most patients with the disorder, however, undergo partial remission and are vulnerable to antisocial behavior, substance use disorders and **mood disorders.**

"Busiprone is a relatively new anti-anxiety medication which ***shows some promise in treating ADHD*** when psychostimulant medications are not effective or their side effects cannot be tolerated. It can also "potentiate" benefits of the serotonergic antidepressants. The side-effects of Buspirone are often ***better tolerated than those of other medications used for ADHD."***- *www.healthyplace.com*

ADHD

◈ *Nelson 20th(SAE)/200-205*

- ***The prevalence rate in adolescent samples is 2–6%. Approximately 2% of adults have ADHD.***
- The most widely researched medications used in the treatment of ADHD are the psychostimulant medications, including methylphenidate, ***amphetamine and/or various dextroamphetamine preparations.***
- If satisfactory treatment results are not obtained with the 2nd stimulant, clinicians may choose to prescribe **atomoxetine**
- A childhood diagnosis of ADHD often leads to persistent ADHD throughout the life span. From 60–80% of children diagnosed with ADHD continue to experience symptoms in adolescence and up to ***40–60% of adolescents exhibit ADHD symptoms into adulthood.***

Attention-Deficit/Hyperactivity Disorder CPDT

◈ *17th/94-95*

- ADHD is a common neurodevelopmental disorder that ***may affect 2–10% of school-age children and may persist into adolescence and adulthood.***
- Although symptoms begin in early childhood, ***they can diminish between ages 10 and 25 years.***
- ***ADHD may be combined with other psychiatric conditions, such as mood disorder in approximately 20% of patients,*** conduct disorders in 20% and oppositionally defiant disorder in up to 40%.
- The use of medication, specifically stimulant medication such as ***methylphenidate (Ritalin) and dextroamphetamine,*** can be helpful. A new medication, **atomoxatine** a noncontrolled substance, has been found to be effective in some children with ADHD.

Table: *(O.P.Ghai 8th/59)*: **Examples of inattentive and hyperactive/ impulsive behavior includes within the criteria for diagnosis of ADHD**

Inattentive behavior
1. Early distraction by extraneous stimuli
2. Often makes careless mistakes in schoolwork or other activities
3. Often has difficulty sustaining attention in tasks or play
4. Often forgetful in daily activities
5. Does not seem to listen to what is being said to him
6. Often fails to finish schoolwork or other chores
7. Daydreams, becomes easily confused and move slowly
8. Difficulty in processing information as quickly and accurately as others
Hyperactive behavior
1. Runs about or climbs excessively in situations where it is inappropriate
2. Fidgets with hands and feet and squirms in seat
3. Talks nonstop
4. Has trouble sitting still during dinner, school and story time
5. Has difficulty doing quiet tasks or activities
Impulsive behavior
1. Has difficulty awaiting turn in games or group situations
2. Blurts out answers to questions
3. Often interrupts conversations or others' activities

195. Ans. a. HIV DNA PCR; e. HIV RNA PCR

[Ref: O.P.Ghai 8th/234; CPDT 17th/56; Nelson 20th (SAE)/1653-54]

Table: *(Nelson 20th (SAE)/1654; 18th)*: **Laboratory Diagnosis of HIV Infection**

Test	Comment
HIV DNA PCR	***Preferred test*** to diagnose HIV-1 subtype B infection in infants and children younger than 18 mo of age; highly sensitive and specific by 2 wk of age and available; performed on peripheral blood mononuclear cells. False negatives can occur in non-B subtype HIV-1 infections
HIV p24 Ag	Less sensitive, false-positive results during 1 mo of life, variable results; ***not recommended****(Nelson 18th, not given in Nelson 20th edition)*
ICD p24 Ag	Negative test result does not rule out infection; not recommended*(Nelson 18th, not given in Nelson 20th edition)*
HIV culture	Expensive, not easily available, requires up to 4 wk to do test; not recommended
HIV RNA PCR	***Preferred test*** to identify non-B subtype HIV-1 infections. Similar sensitivity and specificity to HIV DNA PCR in infants and children younger than 18 mo of age, DNA PCR is generally preferred because of greater clinical experience with that assay

Diagnosis of HIV

◈ *O.P.Ghai 8th/234*

- Although serological diagnostic tests were the most commonly used in the past, tests that allow for earlier definitive diagnosis in children have ***replaced antibody assays*** as the tests of choice for the diagnosis of HIV infection in infants.
- **Specific viral diagnostic assays**, such as ***HIV DNA or RNA PCR, HIV culture***, or ***HIV p24 antigen immune dissociated p24*** (ICD-p24), are essential for diagnosis of young infants born to HIV infected mothers.
- **By 6 months of age**, the ***HIV culture and/or PCR identifies all infected infants***, who are not having any continued exposure due to breast feeding. ***HIV DNA PCR*** is the preferred virologic assay in developed countries.
- Plasma **HIV RNA assays** may be more sensitive than DNA PCR for early diagnosis, but data are limited. ***HIV culture has similar sensitivity to HIV DNA PCR***; however, it is more technically complex and expensive and results are often not available for 2-4 week compared to 2-3 days with PCR.
- The ***p24 antigen assay is less sensitive than the other virologic tests.***
- The national program (Early Infant Diagnosis) now uses ***HIV DNA PCR*** test on dried blood spot samples; the positive tests need confirmation using a HIV DNA PCR on a whole blood sample.

"HIV Infection: Infants born to HIV-infected women should be tested by HIV DNA PCR at < 48 hours, at 1–2 months of age and at 2–4 months old. In an infant who is age 4 months with no positive PCR, infection can be reasonably excluded"- *CPDT 17th/56*

Diagnosis of HIV Infection

◈ *Nelson 20th (SAE)/1653-54*

- All infants born to HIV-infected mothers test antibody-positive at birth because of passive transfer of maternal HIV antibody across the placenta during gestation. ***Most uninfected infants lose maternal antibody between 6 and 12 mo of age and are known as seroreverters.***
- Because a small proportion of uninfected infants continues to test HIV antibody positive for up to 18 mo of age, positive IgG antibody tests, including the rapid tests, ***cannot be used to make a definitive diagnosis of HIV infection in infants younger than this age.***
- The presence of IgA or IgM anti-HIV in the infant's circulation can indicate HIV infection, because these immunoglobulin classes do not cross the placenta; however, IgA and IgM anti-HIV assays have been ***both insensitive and nonspecific and therefore are not valuable for clinical use.***
- In any child >18 mo of age, demonstration of IgG antibody to HIV by a repeatedly reactive enzyme immunoassay (**EIA**) and confirmatory test (immunoblot or immunofluorescence assay) establishes the diagnosis of HIV infection.
- Viral diagnostic assays, such as ***HIV DNA or RNA PCR or HIV culture, are considerably more useful in young infants***, allowing a definitive diagnosis in ***most infected infants by 1–6 mo of age.***

- By 3-4 month of age, the **HIV culture and/or PCR** identify all infected infants.
- **HIV DNA PCR** is the ***preferred virologic assay*** in developed countries. Almost 40% of infected newborns have positive test results in the 1st 2 days of life, with >90% testing positive by 2 wk of age.
- ***Plasma HIV RNA assays, which detect viral replication, may be more sensitive than DNA PCR for early diagnosis.***
- HIV culture has similar sensitivity to HIV DNA PCR; however, it is more technically complex and expensive and results are often not available for several weeks compared with 2–3 days for PCR.
- ***The p24 antigen assay is also highly specific and easy to perform, but it is less sensitive than the other virologic tests.*** It is not recommended for diagnosis of infection in infants <1 mo of age. ***In developing countries, the ICD-p24 test may be considered for older infants; however, if results are negative, it does not rule out infection(Nelson 18th, not given in Nelson 20th edition)***

196. Ans. c. Inhalational of aerosol

[Ref: O.P.Ghai 8th/250; Nelson 20th(SAE)/1446-47; CPDT 17th/56-57]

"**Mode of infection**: *The usual mode of infection is through* ***inhalation of droplets of infected secretions. Infection through ingestion of infected material*** *is rare. Rarely infection may be transmitted through skin, mucous membrane or transplacentally*"- *O.P.Ghai 8th/250*

Tuberculosis

◈ *CPDT 17th/56-57*

- Congenital tuberculosis (TB) is rare but may occur in the infant of a mother ***with hematogenously spread TB or by aspiration of infected amniotic fluid in cases of tuberculous endometritis***. Women with pulmonary TB are not likely to infect the fetus until after delivery.
- ***Postnatal acquisition is the most common mechanism of neonatal infection.***

Transmission of TB

◈ *Nelson 20th(SAE)/1446-47*

- Transmission of *M. tuberculosis* is person to person, usually by ***airborne mucus droplet nuclei***, particles 1–5 μm in diameter that contain *M. tuberculosis*.
- Transmission rarely occurs by ***direct contact with an infected discharge or a contaminated fomite***.
- The **chance of transmission** increases when the patient has an acid-fast smear of sputum, an extensive upper lobe infiltrate or cavity, copious production of thin sputum and severe and forceful cough. Environmental factors, especially poor air circulation, enhance transmission.
- Most adults no longer transmit the organism within several days to 2 weeks after beginning adequate chemotherapy, but some patients remain infectious for many weeks.
- Young children with tuberculosis rarely infect other children or adults.
- Tubercle bacilli are sparse in the endobronchial secretions of children with pulmonary tuberculosis and cough is often absent or lacks the tussive force required to suspend infectious particles of the correct size. However, children and adolescents with adult-type cavitary or endobronchial pulmonary tuberculosis can transmit the organism.

197. Ans. a. Most common cause of seizure in childhood; b. May persist beyond 5 years if associated with atypical feature; c. Family h/o is a risk factor

[Ref: O.P.Ghai 8th/556-57; Nelson 20th(SAE)/2829-30]

Febrile Convulsion

◈ *O.P.Ghai 8th/556-57*

- *It is* ***commonest provoked seizure*** *affecting 3-5% children*
- *It is defined as seizure during fever occurring b/w 6 months and 5 yr age in the absence of infection of the central nervous system in a* ***neurologically normal child***
- *Febrile seizures are frequently genetically determined*
- *Convulsions in a* ***developmentally challenged children*** *may be precipitated by fever, as the cerebral threshold for eizure is redued with the elevation of temperature. These are distinct from* ***febrile convulsions, which occur in neurodevelopmentally normal child***
- Prognosis: Recurrence risk of febrile convulsions varies from 30 to 50%.
- Risk factors that can predict the recurrence of simple and complex febrile seizures are early age of onset (<15 months), epilepsy or fevers in first-degree relatives, frequent fevers and low temperature at the onset of the febrile seizure.
- About 1-2% of children with simple febrile convulsions and up to 5% of those with recurrent complex seizures are ***likely to develop epilepsy***.
- Parents of the child should be reassured that the ***risk of epilepsy after simple febrile seizure is not significantly greater than the general population***.
- The risk of developing epilepsy is higher if the seizures are atypical, electroencephalogram is persistently abnormal, if the child has abnormal neurodevelopment or a family history of epilepsy.
- Complex partial seizures may manifest after several years of prolonged atypical febrile convulsions.

Febrile Seizures

◈ *Nelson 20th(SAE)/2829-30*

- Febrile convulsions, the ***most common seizure disorder during childhood***
- Febrile seizures are age dependent and are ***rare before 9 mo and after 5 yr of age.*** The peak age of onset is ≈14–18 mo of age and the incidence approaches 3–4% of young children.
- ***A strong family history of febrile convulsions*** in siblings and parents suggests a genetic predisposition.
- Approximately 30–50% of children have **recurrent seizures** with later episodes of fever and a small minority has numerous recurrent febrile seizures.
- Factors associated with increased recurrence risk include age <12 mo, lower temperature before seizure onset, a positive family history of febrile seizures and complex features.
- Febrile seizures are not associated with reduction in later intellectual performance and *most children with febrile*

seizures have only a slightly greater risk of later epilepsy than the general population.

- Factors that are associated with a substantially greater risk of later epilepsy include the presence of complex features during the seizure or postictal period, a ***positive family history of epilepsy***, an initial febrile seizure before 12 mo of age, delayed developmental milestones, or a pre-existing neurologic disorder.

Febrile Seizures

◈ *CPDT 17th/744-50*

- Febrile seizures occur in 2–3% of children. Rarely status epilepticus may occur during a febrile seizure.
- ***Febrile seizures rarely (1–2.4%) lead to epilepsy or recurrent nonfebrile seizures in later childhood and adult life.***

Table: *(CPDT 17th/746)*: **Seizures by age at onset, pattern and preferred treatment**

Seizure Type	Age at Onset	Clinical Manifestations	Causative Factors
Febrile convuls-ions	3m to 5y (maximum 6-18 m) Most common childhood seizure: incidence 2%	Usually generalized seizures, less than 15 mins; rarely focal in onset. May lead to status epilepticus. Latter usually benign. Recurrence risk of second febrile seizure 30%-50% if under 1 y of age; recurrence risk is same after status.	Non-neurologic febrile illness (temperature rises to 39°C or higher); positive family history, day care, slow development, prolonged neonatal hospitalization are other risk factors.

198. Ans. a. Galactosemia; d. Sostos syndrome; e. Morquio syndrome

[Ref: CPDT 17th/701; O.P.Ghai 8th/39-40]

"Morquio syndrome can cause *macrocephaly*"- *www.healthline.com*

"Rett Syndrome: *Microcephaly*"- *Kaplan and Saddock 11th/1166*

Table: *(O.P.Ghai 8th/40)*: **Causes of macrocephaly**

Megalencephaly
• Benign familial
• *Neurocutaneous syndromes:* Neurofibromatosis, tuberous sclerosis, Sturge-Weber, Klippel-Trenaunay-Weber, linear sebaceous nevus
• *Others:* ***Sotos,*** Fragile X syndrome
• *Leukodystrophies:* Alexander, Canavan, megalencephalic leukoencephalopathy
• *Lysosomal storage disease*: Tay-Sachs, mucopolysaccharidosis, gangliosidosis
Increased cerebrospinal fluid
• Hydrocephalus
• Benign enlargement of subarachnoid space
• Hydranencephaly, choroid plexus papilloma
Enlarged vascular compartment
• Arteriovenous malformation
• Subdural, epidural, subarachnoid or intraventricular hemorrhage
Increase in bony compartment
• *Bone disease*: Achondroplasia, osteogenesis imperfect, osteopetrosis, hyperphosphatasia, cleidocranial dysostosis
• *Bone marrow expansion*: Thalassemia major
Miscellaneous causes
• *Intracranial mass lesions*: Cyst, abscess or tumor
• *Raised intracranial pressure*: Idiopathic pseudotumor cerebri, lead poisoning, hypervitaminosis A, ***galactosemia***

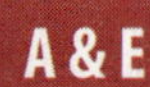

199. Ans. b. Loss of purposeful learned hand movements; c. Incoordinated gait; d. Expressive speech defect; e. Normal head circumference at birth

[Ref: CPDT 17th/191-92; Kaplan and Saddock 11th/1166; Nelson 20th(SAE)/2916-17]

Rett Syndrome: Diagnosis and Clinical Features

◈ *Kaplan and Saddock 11th/1166*

- ***During the first 5 months after birth, infants have age-appropriate motor skills, normal head circumference and normal growth.*** Social interactions show the expected reciprocal quality.
- At 6 months to 2 years of age, however, these children develop progressive encephalopathy with a number of characteristic features.
- The signs often include the ***loss of purposeful hand movements***, which are replaced by stereotypic motions, such as hand-wringing; the ***loss of previously acquired speech***; psychomotor retardation; and ataxia. Other stereotypical hand movements may occur, such as licking or biting the fingers and tapping or slapping. The head circumference growth decelerates and produces microcephaly.
- ***All language skills are lost*** and both receptive and ***expressive communicative*** and social skills seem to plateau at developmental levels between 6 months and 1 year.
- ***Poor muscle coordination and an apraxic gait*** with an unsteady and stiff quality develop.

Rett Syndrome

◈ *Kaplan and Saddock 11th/1166*

- ***It occurs almost exclusively in girls.***
- Most babies with Rett syndrome seem to develop normally at first, but after about **6 months** of age, ***they lose skills they previously had — such as the ability to crawl, walk, communicate or use their hands.***
- Over time, children with Rett syndrome have increasing problems with the use of muscles that control movement, coordination and communication. Rett syndrome can also cause seizures and intellectual disability.

- **Rett syndrome signs and symptoms include:**
  - **Slowed growth.** Brain growth slows after birth. Smaller than normal head size (***microcephaly***) is usually the first sign that a child has Rett syndrome.
  - Loss of normal movement and coordination
  - Loss of communication abilities
  - Abnormal hand movements.
  - Unusual eye movements
  - Breathing problems
  - Agitation and irritability
  - Cognitive disabilities
  - Seizures
  - Abnormal curvature of the spine (scoliosis)
  - Irregular heartbeat

Table: *(CPDT 17th/191)*: **Characteristics of nonautistic pervasive developmental disorders**

Disorder	Age at Onset	Clinical Features
Asperger's syndrome	Early childhood	"Odd" individuals (probably more common in males) with normal intelligence, motor clumsiness, eccentric interests and a limited ability to appreciate social nuances
Childhood disintegrative disorder	3-4 years	Profound deterioration to severe autistic disorder
Pervasive developmental disorder	Early childhood	Two to three times more common than autistic disorder, with similar but less severe symptoms
Rett syndrome	5 months to 4 years old	Females with reduced head circumference and loss of social relatedness who develop stereotyped hand movements and have impaired language and mental functioning

ORTHOPEDICS

200. Ans. b. Osteochondritis of lunate bone; c. Painful flexion and extension of wrist; d. Passive dorsiflexion of middle finger produces pain

[Ref: Maheshwari 5th/318; Apley's 9th/397-99; radiopaedia.org]

Kienbock Disease

◈ *Apley's 9th/397-99*

- R. Kienbock called it 'traumatic softening' of ***lunate bone***
- This is a form ischemic necrosis (probably d/t to stress or injury)
- Relative shortening of the ulna (***negative ulnar variance***) ***predisposes to stress overload of the lunate*** b/w the distal edge of the radius and the carpus, but this has not been proven convincingly

"There is a *significant association between* negative ulnar variance *and Kienbock disease*, although the majority of people with negative ulnar variance do not have the condition. A causal association is difficult to prove, however the effectiveness of decompressive procedures such as radial shortening or ulnar lengthening in relieving pain and preventing further collapse of the lunate is supportive. Overall, *negative ulnar variance is present as a predisposing factor in around 75% of cases of Kienbock disease*"-*radiopaedia.org*

- **"Positive ulnar variance** describes where the distal articular surface of the ulna is more distal when compared to the articular surface of the radius"-*radiopaedia.org*
- Patient complains of ache and stiffness
- ***Tenderness is localized over the lunate*** and grip strength is diminished
- In the ***later stages wrist movements are limited and painful***

Lunatomalacia: Characteristics *www.physio-pedia.com; www.wheelessonline.com*

- Typical symptoms of Kienböck's disease are activity-related ***dorsal wrist pain and weakness***, often accompanied by ***swelling dorsally around the lunate.***
- The complaints are in most cases longstanding and increase progressively. The pain can be described from just mild and occasional to severe and debilitating.
- The **range of motion of the joint** is nearly always decreased, with ***loss of flexion and extension***. Compared to the unaffected side there is ***loss of grip strength.***
- Symptoms are most commonly in the ***dominant wrist*** and a history of trauma may be present.

Kienböck's Disease: Clinical Manifestations

◈ *www.wheelessonline.com*

- Wrist pain that radiates up the forearm and stiffness, tenderness and swelling over lunate;
- ***Passive dorsiflexion of middle finger produces characteristic pain***
- ***Limitation of wrist motion, usually dorsiflexion***
- ***Weakness of grip***
- ***Pain and weakness increase as the lunate collapses*** and degenerative changes develop, making the disability both severe and chronic

Table: *(Maheshwari 5th/318)*: **Common osteochondritis**

Name	Site affected
Perthes' disease	Femoral head
Panner's disease	Capitulum
Kienbock's disease	Lunate bone
Osgood Shlatter's disease	Tibial tubercle
Sever's disease	Calcaneal tuberosity
Kohler's disease	Navicular bone
Freiberg's disease	Metatarsal head
Scheurmann's disease	Ring epiphysis of vertebrae
Calve's disease	Central bony nucleus of vertebral body
Iselin's disease	5th metatarsal

The Stahl classification of Kienbock disease, modified by Lichtman, is the most commonly used staging system and is useful in the treatment of Kienbock disease (avascular necrosis of the lunate). This system divides the disease into four stages: *radiopaedia.org*

- Stage I: Normal radiograph
- **Stage** II: Increased radiodensity of the lunate with possible decrease of lunate height on the radial side only
- **Stage** III
    - IIIa: Lunate collapse, no scaphoid rotation
    - IIIb: Lunate collapse, fixed scaphoid rotation
- **Stage** IV: Degenerative changes around lunate

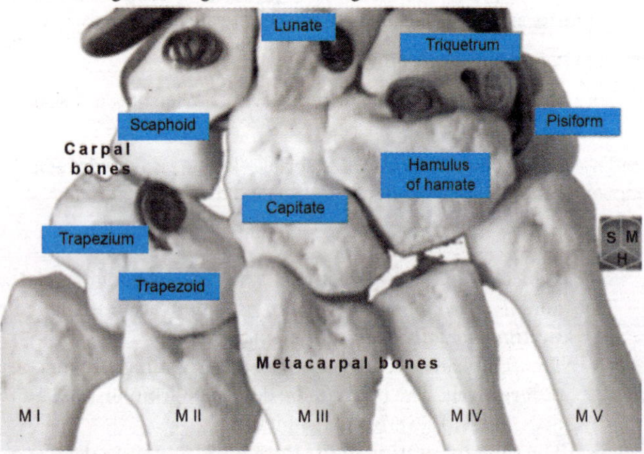

201. Ans. a. Fracture of C2 vertebrae; b. Neural arch disturbed; c. Traumatic spondylolisthesis of C2 on C3; d. C2-3 intervertebral disc may be torn

[Ref: L and B 26th/335; Apley's 9th/814; Sabiston 19th/444]

Hangman's Fracture

◈ *L and B 26th/335*

- The Hangman's fracture is a ***traumatic spondylolisthesis of*** C2 on C3.
- There are four types with varying degrees of instability
- Those with significant displacement or associated facet dislocation are treated operatively, usually with posterior stabilisation.
- C2 Hangman fracture: B***ilateral C2 pedicles with spondylol***isthesis"- *Sabiston 19th/444*
- *Spondylol*isthesis is a forward or backward slippage of one vertebra on an adjacent vertebra- www.med*icine*net.com

C2 Pars Interarticularis Fractures

◈ *Apley's 9th/814*

- *In* the true j**udicial 'hangman's f**racture' there are bilateral fractures of the pars interar***ticularis of C2 and the C2/3 disc i***s torn; the mechanism is extension with distraction.
- In **civilian in**juries (motor vehicle accidents), the mechanism is more complex, with varying degrees of extension, Compression and flexion.
- C2/3 fusion is sometimes required for persistent pain and instability ('**traumatic spondyloli**sthesis').
- Occasionally, the 'hangman's fracture' is associated with a C2/***3 facet dis***location. This is a severely unstable injury; open reduction and stabilization is required.

Traumatic Spondylolisthesis of the Axis (Hangman's Fractures)

◈ *Campbell's Operative Orthopedics, 11th ed./chap35*

- The term *hangman's* fracture originally referred to neck injuries incurred during the hanging of criminals. The most common cause of hangman's fracture now is a motor vehicle accident with hyperextension of the head on the neck.
- The occiput is forced down against the p***osterior arch of th***e atlas, which is forced against the ***pedicles*** of C2.
- Traumatic spondylolistheses of the axis is classified into four types. Type I fractures are minimally displaced and are believed to be caused by hyperextension and axial loading with ***failure of the neural arch in*** tension.
- **Type II** fractures:These injuries result from hyperextension and axial loading that cause the neural arch to fail with a predominantly vertical fracture line.The C***2-3 disc may be d***isrupted by the sudden flexion component involved in this injury.
- Type IIA fractures are a variant of type II fractures that show severe angulation between C2 and C3 with minimal translation.
- **Type III** injuries combine a bip***edicular fracture with posterior facet*** injuries. They usually hav***e severe angulation and translation of the neural arch*** fracture and an associated unilateral or bilateral facet dislocation at C2-3. These f***ractures frequently are associated with neurological*** def***icits.***

Hangman's fracture on X-ray: Spinal dislocation or slippage (also known as spondylolisthesis), kyphosis, scoliosis, as well as local and overall spine balance can be assessed with X-rays. Specific bony abnormalities such as ***bone spurs, disc space narrowing, vertebral body*** fracture, collapse or erosion can also be identified on plain film X-rays" -columbiaspine.org/condition

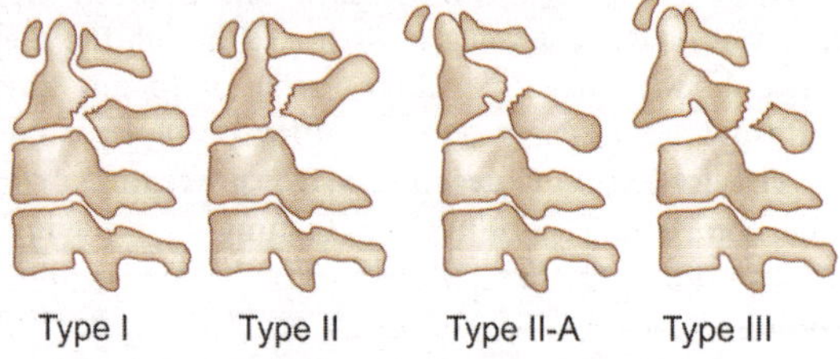

Fig: (Campbell's): Hangman's fracture

202. Ans. a. Osteomyelitis; b. Osteosarcoma

[Ref: Maheshwari 5th/168; Apley's 9th/207]

Metaphysis is Common Site for Osteomyelitis

◈ *Maheshwari 5th/168*

"Osteosarcoma: It may affect any bone but most commonly involves the long-bone metaphyses, especially around the knee and at the proximal end of humerus"- *Apley's 9th/207*

Table: Maheshwari 5th/237, 2.44

	Giant cell tumor	Ewing's sarcoma	Osteoclastoma
Location	Epiphysis	Diaphysis	Epiphysis

203. Ans. a. Knee is the most commonly affected joint in Indian population; c. Causes movement restriction and instability of the joint; d. Synovial thickening occur early; e. Heberden's nodes occur more commonly in female

[Ref: Maheshwari 5th/295-97; Apley's 9th/89-92; Robbins 9th(SAE)/1208-09]

*"Over a period of years osteophytes and soft tissue swelling produces a characteristic knobbly appearance of the distal interphalangeal joints (**Herberden nodes)** and less often, the proximal interphalangeal joints (Bouchard's nodes)"- Apley's 9th/94*

"***Heberden*** nodes, prominent osteophytes at the distal interphalangeal joints, are common in women (but not men). The wrists, elbows and shoulders are usually spared"-*Robbins 9th(SAE)/1209*

Heberden's nodes are 10 times more common* in** women. Also there is familial predisposition and can be found in many female members of some families"-**www.healthline.com; www. webmd.***boots.com**

"MRI can be used to evaluate the extent of synovitis, observed as ***synovial thi***ckening, in patients with early OA of the knee"- www.ncbi.nlm.nih.gov

"Instability *is common in late stages of articular* destruction, but it may be detected much earlier by special testing *Apley's* **9th/9***1*

"The ***hip joint is commonly affected in a population with western living*** habits, while the ***knee is involved more commonly in a population with Asian living*** habits i.e., the habit of squatting and sitting cross legged"- *Maheshwari* **5th/296**

"Other symptoms are: a feeling of ***instability of*** the joint and locking resulting from loose bodies and frayed menisci"- *Maheshwari 5th/296*

Osteoarthritis

◈ *Robbins 9th(SAE)/1208-09*

- *Osteoa***rthritis, also called degenerative joint disease, is characterized by degeneration of cartilage that results in structural and functional failure of synovial** joints. It is the most common type of joint disease.
- T***he knees and hands are more commonly affected in women and the hip***s ***in men.***
- ***The* lesions of osteoarthritis (OA) stem from degeneration of the articular cartilage and its disordered r**epair.
- The changes to chondrocytes can be divided into three phases: (1) chondrocyte injury, related to genetic and biochemical factors; (2) early OA, in which chondrocytes proliferate and secrete inflammatory mediators, collagens, proteoglycans and proteases, which act together to remodel the cartilaginous matrix and initiate secondary infl***ammatory changes in the*** synovium and subchondral bone; and (3) late OA, in which repetitive injury and chronic inflammation lead to chondrocyte drop out, marked loss of cartilage and extensive subchondral bone changes.
- Th***e joints commonly involved include the hips, knees, lower lumbar and cervical vertebrae, proximal and distal interphalangeal joints of the fingers, first carpometacarpal joints and first tarsometatars***al ***joints.***
- *"The joint **capsule usually shows thickening and** fibrosis. The synovial lining, as a rule, looks only mildly inflamed; sometimes, however, it is thick and red and covered by villi"- Apley's 9th/89*
- *"X-Ray: The cardinal signs are asymmetrical loss of cartilage(**narrowing of the joint space),** sclerosis of the subchondral bone under the area of cartilage loss, cysts close to the articular surface, osteophyte at the margins of the join and bone remodelling"- Apley's 9th/91*

*Osteoa***rthritis M***anual of Rheumatology and Outpatient Orthopedic Disorders by Stephen A. Paget 2000/Chap 44*

- *L***ocalized osteoar**thritis: Heberden's nodes without other joint involvement represent the most common form of primary OA. Family studies reveal that genetic factors are important in the development of Heberden's nodes. These nodes are ten times mor***e common*** in women than in men.

  Radiographic criteria for OA are as follows:

  a. Joint space narrowing secondary to degeneration and disappearance of articular cartilage.
  b. Osteophyte formation at joint margins or sites of ligamentous attachment.
  c. Subchondral bone sclerosis.
  d. Subchondral bone cysts.
  e. Altered shape of a bone end caused by bone remodeling.

204. Ans. a. Bone biopsy; d. Bone curettage, adjuvant treatment with phenol and bone cementing; e. PTH and serum calcium level measurement

[Ref: Maheshwari 5th/237-39; Apley's 9th/202-03; Robbins 9th/1203- 04]

It is a case of GCT. Nausea, vomiting and abdominal pain can be due to paraneoplastic syndrome

*Parane***oplastic** syndromes represent a group of nonmetastatic systemic disorders that accompany malignant disease and are usually the ***first or most prominent manifestation of an underlying malignancy- www.hindawi.com***

*"Gi***ant Cell Tumor***: It is prudent to obtain estimation of blood* ***calcium, phosphate and alkaline phosphatase concentration to*** *exclude an unusual 'brown tumor' associated with hyperparathyroidism"- Apley's* **9th***/203*

"Biopsy is essential. This can be done either as a frozen section before ***proceeding with operative*** treatment or (especially if a more extensive operation is contemplated) as a ***separate procedure-*** *Apley's* **9th/203**

Osteoclastoma (Giant Cell Tumor)

◈ *Maheshwari 5th/237-39*

- *Bones commonly affected are around the knee i.e., lower end of the femur and upper end of the tibia.* ***Lower end of radius*** *is another common site*
- ***X-ray: A*** *solitary, may be loculated, lyt**ic lesion; eccentric location; soap*** *bubble appearance;* ***cortex may be thinned***

out or perforated at places; No calcification within tumor; expansion of overlying cortex(expansile lesion)

Treatment of Osteoclastoma

◈ *Maheshwari 5th/238-39*

- ***Excision***
- ***Excision with reconstruction:*** *Arthrodesis by the turn-o-plasty procedure, arthrodesis by bridging the gap by double fibula and arthroplasty(Excision with graft-allograft, autograft or an artificial joint)*
- ***Curettage with or without supplementary procedures like cryotherapy or bone cement. Curettage performed alone has the disadvantage of a high recurrence rate*** *because some cells are always left along the walls of cavity. Supplementary procedures such as cryotherapy(Liquid nitrogen) and thermal burning(using cauterization) are used with curettage to reduce recurrence. Lately,* ***thermal effect of bone cement has been used.*** *The cavity is filled with bone cement, which by the heat it produces while setting, kills the residual cells*
- *Amputation: More aggressive lesion or following recurrence*
- *Radiotherapy:* ***Preferred treatment for GCT affecting*** *vertebrae*

Giant Cell Tumor: Treatment

◈ *Apley's 9th/203*

- *Well*-**confined, slow-growing** lesions with benign histology can safely be treated by ***thorough curettage and 'stripping' of the cavity with burrs and gouges, followed by swabbing with hydrogen peroxide or by the application of liquid*** nitrogen; the cavity is then packed with bone chips.
- More ag**gressive tumors and recurrent** lesions, should be treated by excision followed, if necessary, by bone grafting or prosthetic replacement.

◈ *Treatment Adams Outline of Orthopedics 14th/110-114*

- This depends upon the site of the tumor. C***urettage of the contents with a high-speed burr is the standard method of treatment for most giant cell turn ours, though this is associated with a high rate (20-25%) of*** recurrence. This rate can be reduced to less than 10% by the use of **adjuvant** treatment applied to the lining of the cavity after curettage. Methods used include the c***hemical phenol, freezing with liquid nitrogen, or the insertion of polymethylmethacrylate bo***ne cement.
- In addition to its exothermic reaction on any residual cells, the ce***ment has the added advantage of providing*** support to the subchondral bone and cartilage of the articular surface of the joint.

Giant Cell

◈ *Tumors Campbell's Operative Orthopedics 11th/883-85*

- *They* ***typically occur in patients 20 to 40 years old and there is a slight female predominance. The most common location for this tumor is the distal femur, followed closely by the proxim***al tibia.
- Most manifest as stage 2 or stage 3 lesions. Historically, t***reatment consisted of simple*** curettage; however, subsequent recurrence rates were greater than 50%. The use of a***djuvants, such as liquid nitrogen, phenol, bone cement, electrocautery, or an argon beam coagulator, theoretically help to kill any remaining tumor*** cells.
- To fill the defect after curettage, the surgeon has several options, i***ncluding autograft bone, allograft bone, an artificial bone graft substitute, or methylmethacrylate*** bo***ne cement.***
- Bone ***cement provides immediate stability***
- ***Curettage may not be effective in some stage 3 tumors and primary resection may be required after*** biopsy.
- For aggressive lesions of the distal **radius, *primary resection and reconstruction with a proximal fibular autograft (either as an arthroplasty or as an arthrodesis) may be in***dicated

---

205. Ans. a. Malunion;... b. Nonunion;... d. Ulnar nerve palsy; ... e. Recurrent dislocation

---

[Ref: Maheshwari 5th/103-04; Apley's 9th/761-62]

- C***hild, in this question is suffering from fracture of lateral condyle of*** humerus

Fracture of Lateral Condyle of the Humerus

◈ *Maheshwari 5th/103-04*

- A common fracture in children, it results from a varus injury to the elbow
- There is mild ***swelling and pain over the outer aspect of*** the elbow. This is associated with te***nderness over the lateral epicondyle***
- ***Complication: non-union, cubitus valgus deformity(result in tardy ulnar nerv***e palsy) and osteoarthritis

◈ *Apley's 9th/761-62*

- *The child fall on hand with the elbow extended and forced into varus*
- *The elbow is swollen and deformed. There is tenderness over lateral condyle. Passive flexion of the wrist(pulling on the extensors) may be painful*
- *Complication: N****on-union and malunion,(may later result in ulnar nerve palsy);*** *recurrent dislocation*
- *If the condyle is left capsized, non-union is inevitable*
- ***Recurrent dislocation- Occa****sionally condylar displacement results in posterolateral dislocation of the* elbow

Supracondylar Fracture of the Humerus

◈ *Maheshwari 5th/97-102*

- This is one of the most serious fracture in c**h**ildhood as it is often associated with complications
- Complications are- immediate (occurring at time of fracture), early (occurring within first 2-3 days) and late(occurring weeks to months after the fracture)
- **Immediate: *injury to brachial*** artery and injury to nerve (***median nerve-most*** common, radial nerve-sometime affected)
- Early: *Volkmann's ischemia*
- *Late* **compl*ication:*** *Malunion(cubitus varus deformity), myositis ossificans and Volkmann's ischemic contracture*
- *Displacement:* ***The*** *distal fragment may be displaced in the following direction*
    - Posterior or backward shift
    - Posterior or backward tilt
    - Proximal shift

- Medial or lateral shift
- Medial tilt
- Internal rotation

206. Ans. b. Complete excision is the best treatment; c. Present both above and below the flexor retinaculum

[Ref: Apley's 9th/408-09; Adams's Outline of Orthopedics 14th/330-31]

Compound Palmar Ganglion

◈ *Apley's 9th/408-09*

- This lesion is neither a ganglion nor compound.
- Chronic inflammation distends the common sheath of the flexor tendons bo***th above and below the flexor retina***culum.
- Rheumatoid arthritis and tuberculosis are the commonest causes.
- The synovial membrane becomes thick and villous. The amount of fluid is increased and it may contain fibrin particles moulded by repeated movement to the shape of melon seeds. The tendons may eventually fray and rupture
- ***Pain is*** unusual but paraesthesia due to median nerve compression may occur.
- The ***swelling is hourglass*** in ***shape, bulging above and below the flexor ret***inanculum; it is not warm or tender; f***luid can be pushed from one part to the other (cross-fluct***uation)
- "Compound palmar ganglion:The swellings in the palm and at the front of the wrist are continuous deep to the flexor retinaculum and flu***ctuation can be elicited betwee***n them"- Adams's Outline of Orthopedics 14th/331
- If the condition is tuberculous, general treatment is begun. The contents of the sac are evacuated, streptomycin is instilled and the wrist rested in a splint. *If these measures fail, the entire flexor sheath is dissected out.* ***Complete excision is also the best treatment when the cause is rheumatoid*** disease.

207. Ans. b. Excessive ligamental laxity; c. Vastus medialis agenesis; d. High oblique insertion of the vastus medialis; e. Flattening of the intercondylar groove

[Ref: Maheshwari 5th/153; Apley's 9th/562; boneandspine.com]

Recurrent Dislocation of the Patella

◈ *Maheshwari 5th/153*

- After the first episode of dislocation, generally during adolescence, the dislocation tends to recur with more and more ease.
- The reason for recurrence may be laxity of the medial capsule or some underlying defect in the anatomy of the knee. These could be: (i) ***excessive join***t laxity; (ii) ***a small*** patella; (iii) a patella alta (i.e., the ***patella is high lying in the shallower part of intercondyla***r groove); and (iv) genu valgum.
- Predisposing factor include- Gen***eralized ligamentous laxity, under development of the lateral femoral condyle and flattening of the intercondylar groove, a primary muscle defect***- *Apley's 9th/562*
- *T*reatment consists of operative reconstruction where the insertion of the patellar tendon on the tibial tuberosity is shifted medially and downwards so that the line of pull of the quadriceps shifts medially (Hauser's operation).
- Prof. Baksi from Calcutta has described a useful operation for this condition whereby pes anserinus is transferred to lower pole of the patella to provide a 'checkrein' effect.
- The *curren*t trend is to precisely find the cause of the recurrence, which may be bony (genu valgus, increased Q-angle etc.), or soft tissue (***ruptured medial patella-femoral*** ligament)
- The corrective surgery is aimed at correcting the underlying cause. The operations are done arthroscopic assisted

Causes of Recurrent Dislocation of Patella

◈ *boneandspine.com*

- *L*igaments Laxity: In children with diseases that cause lig***amentous*** laxity (e.g. osteogenesis imperfecta, arachnodactyly, or the Ehlers-Danlos syndrome), lateral dislocation of patella is more common.
- **Lateral Soft Tissue Contracture:** Taut lateral patellar retinaculum and patellofemoral ligament, contracted and hyper***trophied vastus l***ateralis and tight iliotibial tract may contribute to dislocation of patella.
- **Muscular Imbalance:** ***Atrophy, weakness, or a high oblique insertion of the vastus*** medialis is a factor in most patients. The vastus medialis is a dynamic medial stabilizer of the patella.
- **Mal-alignment of the Lower Limb:** Lateral tibiofibular torsion and genu valgum will displace the insertion of the patellar ligament laterally and cause valgus position of the quadriceps mechanism.
- **Patella Alta:** This is a high riding patella. In this the normal but***tressing effect of the lateral femoral*** condyle, which serves to check the tendency to lateralpatellar displacement, will be lost.
- **Injury:** A traumatic lateral dislocation inadequately treated will result in stretching and weakening of the medial capsule of the knee and insufficiency of the vastus medialis, predisposing to recurrent lateralsubluxation.

208. Ans. a. Most common causal organism is staphylococcus aureus; d. Cloacae are holes in involucrum

[Ref: Maheshwari 5th/168-172; Apley's 8th/30-32; L and B 26th/547]

Acute Osteomyelitis

◈ *Maheshwari 5th/168-171*

- It can be primary (haematogenous) or secondary (following an open fracture or bone operation).
- Haematogenous osteomyelitis is the commonest
- Acute osteomyelitis is almost invariably a disease of children. The causal organism is usually Staphy***lococcus*** aureus
- Patients with sickle-cell disease are prone to *infection by salmonella* (Apley's)
- In acute osteomyelitis, the child presents with sev*ere* pain, malaise and fever and in neglected cases toxaemia. Typically the limb is held still and there is acute 'fingertip' tenderness

near one of the larger joints. Even gentlest manipulation is painful and joint movement is restricted. (Apley)

- On X-ray, the earliest sign to appear is a periosteal new bone deposition (**Periosteal reaction**) **at the metaphysis.** It takes ***about 7-10 days to appear***
- *Bone scan with TC99 is earliest positive within 24 hours of onset of* symptoms.
- In acute osteomyelitis, metaphyseal infection is usual, the growth disc acts as a barrier to spread.
- Indium-111 labelled leucocyte scan is most specific for diagnosis of bone infection
- "**Metaphysis** is *common site for osteomyelitis. The lower* ***femoral metaphysis*** *is the commonest site*"

Chronic Osteomyelitis

◈ *Maheshwari 5th/171-72*

- ***Involucrum is dense sclerotic bone overlying a sequestrum.*** *There are many holes called cloacae*
- ***Sequestrum is a piece of dead bone,*** *surrounded by infected granulation* tissue

ANESTHESIA

209. Ans. a. Caffeine; c. Epidural blood patch; d. Synthetic ACTH in refractory cases; e. NSAIDS

[Ref: Ajay Yadav 5th/159-60; Morgan 5th/969,853;Lee 13th/517-18,666-667]

Postdural Puncture Headache

◈ *Morgan 5th/969*

- Any breach of the dura may result in a postdural puncture headache (PDPH).
- This may follow a diagnostic lumbar puncture, a myelogram, a spinal anesthetic, or an epidural "wet tap" in which the epidural needle passed through the epidural space and entered the subarachnoid space. Similarly, an epidural catheter might puncture the dura at any time and result in PDPH.
- The hallmark of PDPH is its association with body position.
- The onset of headache is usually 12–72 hr following the procedure; however, it may be seen almost immediately.
- Conservative treatment involves ***recumbent positioning, analgesics, intravenous or oral fluid administration and caffeine.***
- Keeping the patient supine will decrease the hydrostatic pressure driving fluid out of the dural hole and minimize the headache. Analgesic medication may range from ***acetaminophen to NSAIDs and opioids.*** Hydration and caffeine work to stimulate production of CSF. Caff eine further helps by vasoconstricting intracranial vessels.
- An **epidural blood patch** is an effective treatment for PDPH. It involves injecting 15–20 mL of ***autologous blood into the epidural space*** at, or one interspace below, the level of the dural puncture. It is believed to stop further leakage of CSF by either mass effect or coagulation.

Patients who are unable or unwilling to await spontaneous resolution of PDPH should be offered **epidural blood patch**"- *Barash 6th/Chap 37*

Cosyntropin, a synthetic form of adrenocorticotropic hormone, has been used in the treatment of refractory PDPH. Adrenocorticotropic hormone is believed to work by stimulating the adrenal gland to increase CSF production and β-endorphin output"- *www.ncbi.nlm.nih.gov*

The serotonin type 1-d receptor agonist **sumatriptan is** *effective in the treatment of PDPH,* with complete resolution of symptoms"- *www.ncbi.nlm.nih.gov*

Many therapeutic agents have been tried, but all suffer from a lack of large, randomized, controlled clinical trials. ***Desmopressin (DDAVP) has no effect on PDPH following lumbar puncture*** and the ***evidence for ACTH is inconclusive.*** Sumitriptan, the 5-HT1D receptor agonist and migraine treatment, has been used for PDPH but a controlled trial found no evidence of benefit"- *www.oaa-anaes.ac.uk/assets*

210. Ans. b. Thiopentone; c. Etomidate; d. Fentanyl; e. Propofol

[Ref: Ajay Yadav 5th/109; Morgan 5th/183]

Cardiovascular: In contrast to other anesthetic agents, ***ketamine increases arterial blood pressure, heart rate and cardiac output,*** particularly after rapid bolus injections"- *Morgan 5th/183* ***(Ketamine will improve shock. As intubation is planned, respiratory depression is not an issue)***

Fentanyl: ***Decreases (↓↓) mean arterial pressure***- *Ajay Yadav 5th/109*

Table: *(Morgan 5th/183)*: **Summary of nonvolatile anesthetic effects on organ systems**

	Cardiovascular		Respiratory			Cerebral	
Agent	**HR**	**MAP**	**Vent**	**B'dil**	**CBF**	**$CMRO_2$**	**ICP**
Barbiturates							
Thiopental	↑↑	↓↓	↓↓↓	↓	↓↓↓	↓↓↓	↓↓↓
Thiamylal	↑↑	↓↓	↓↓↓	↓	↓↓↓	↓↓↓	↓↓↓
Methohexital	↑↑	↓↓	↓↓↓	0	↓↓↓	↓↓↓	↓↓↓
Benzodiazepines							
Diazepam	0/↑	↓	↓↓	0	↓↓	↓↓	↓↓
Lorazepam	0/↑	↓	↓↓	0	↓↓	↓↓	↓↓
Midazolam	↑	↓↓	↓↓	0	↓↓	↓↓	↓↓

Contd...

	Cardiovascular		Respiratory			Cerebral	
Agent	**HR**	**MAP**	**Vent**	**B'dil**	**CBF**	**$CMRO_2$**	**ICP**
Ketamine	↑↑	↑↑	↓	↑↑↑	↑↑[2]	↑	↑↑[2]
Etomidate	0	↓	↓	0	↓↓↓	↓↓↓	↓↓↓
Propofol	0	↓↓	↓↓↓	0	↓↓↓	↓↓↓	↓↓↓

Abbreviation: Vent, ventilatory drive; B'dil, bronchodilation; CBF, cerebral blood flow; CMRO 2 , cerebral oxygen consumption; ICP, intracranial pressure; 0, no effect; 0/↑, no change or mild increase; ↓, decrease (mild, moderate, marked); ↑, increase (mild, moderate, marked).

Table: *Ajay Yadav 5th/109*

Agent	Analgesia
Thiopentone	Antanalgesic
Propofol	0
Etomidate	0
Droperidol+Fentanyl	++
Ketamine	+++

211. Ans. b. Selectively binds to rocuronium

[Ref: Morgan 5th/231; Barash 6th/Chap 20]

Sugammadex

◈ *Morgan 5th/231*

- Sugammadex is a novel selective relaxant-binding agent
- Its three-dimensional structure resembles a hollow truncated cone or doughnut with a hydrophobic cavity and a hydrophilic exterior.
- ***Hydrophobic interactions trap the drug (e.g., rocuronium)*** in the cyclodextrin cavity (doughnut hole), resulting in tight formation of a water-soluble guest–host complex in a 1:1 ratio. ***This terminates the neuromuscular blocking action*** and restrains the drug in extracellular fluid where ***it cannot interact with nicotinic acetylcholine receptors.***
- It is essentially eliminated unchanged via the kidneys.
- It produces rapid and effective r***eversal of both shallow and profound rocuronium-induced neuromuscular blockade*** in a consistent manner.

◈ *Barash 6th/Chap 20*

- Sugammadex, previously called ORG 25969, leads to restoration of normal neuromuscular function ***not by interfering with acetylcholine,*** the ***nicotinic receptor or acetylcholinesterase***, but by ***selectively binding to rocuronium*** and to ***a lesser extent to vecuronium and pancuronium.***
- Selective relaxant binding agent for reversal of neuromuscular blockade (NMB) induced ***by rocuronium or vecuronium*** in adults undergoing surgery"-*reference. medscape.com*
- The compound is a cyclodextrin, made up of eight sugars arranged in a ring to make a center to accommodate the rocuronium molecule. Once bound, rocuronium is held in place by polar side chains attached to the ring.
- Because sugammadex ***does not bind to any known receptor,*** it is devoid of major cardiovascular or other side effects.
- It does not bind neuromuscular blocking drugs that do not have a steroid nucleus.
- ***The benzylisoquinolines, such as atracurium, cisatracurium and mivacurium and succinylcholine are unaffected by sugammadex.***
- After injection of sugammadex, evidence suggests that binding of rocuronium to sugammadex in plasma leads to a marked decrease in free (unbound) rocuronium concentration,[153] leading to the establishment of a concentration gradient of rocuronium between the neuromuscular junction and plasma. This favors movement of rocuronium from neuromuscular junction to plasma, producing less neuromuscular block. ***Vecuronium*** has less affinity for sugammadex than ***rocuronium*** does and ***pancuronium*** has less still.
- Sugammadex could also be used in the case of a failed intubation. If rocuronium 0.6 mg/kg was given, sugammadex 8 mg/kg might be effective as early as 3 minutes after rocuronium injection and if the dose of rocuronium is doubled to 1.2 mg/kg, one might need 16 mg/kg of sugammadex. The availability of sugammadex might make succinylcholine obsolete for intubation.

212. Ans. a. Hofmann Elimination; b. Non-specific esterase; e. Ester hydrolysis

[Ref: Ajay Yadav 5th/116; Morgan 5th/216; Lee 13th/191; Miller 7th/ Chap 29]

Atracurium

◈ *Morgan 5th/216*

- Like all muscle relaxants, atracurium has a quaternary group; however, a benzylisoquinoline structure is responsible for its unique method of degradation. The drug is a mixture of 10 stereoisomers.
- Atracurium is so extensively metabolized that its pharmacokinetics are independent of renal and hepatic function and less than 10% is excreted unchanged by renal and biliary routes. Two separate processes are responsible for metabolism.
    - **Ester Hydrolysis:** This action is catalyzed by ***nonspecific esterases, not by acetylcholinesterase or pseudocholinesterase.***
    - Hofmann Elimination: A ***spontaneous nonenzymatic chemical breakdown*** occurs at physiological pH and temperature.

Atracurium: The presence (in duplicate) of two-carbon separations between quaternary nitrogen and ester carbonyl provides the basis for a Hofmann elimination reaction. Furthermore, it can undergo ***ester hydrolysis***. In a Hofmann elimination reaction, a quaternary ammonium group is converted to a tertiary amine by cleavage of a carbon-nitrogen bond. This is a pH- and temperature-dependent reaction in which higher pH and temperature favor elimination"-Miller 7th/Chap 29

*"Atracurium is also metabolized by **ester hydrolysis**, producing a quaternary alcohol and quaternary acid"-Lee 13th/191*

213. Ans. a. For confirmation of intubation; c. For assessing pulmonary embolism; d. To check adequate ventilation

[Ref: Ajay Yadav 5th/61; Morgan 5th/125-27]

Uses of Capnography

◈ *Ajay Yadav 5th/61*

I-$ETCO_2$ = 0 and flat line on wave form is seen in:

1. Esophageal intubation - ***Capnography is the surest confirmatory sign of correct intubation***
2. Accidental extubation
3. Complete obstruction
4. Disconnection
5. ***Ventilation failure***
6. Cardiac arrest (there is no blood to carry CO_2 from tissues to lungs)

II-Decrease in $ETCO_2$ is seen in

- ***Pulmonary embolism*** by air, fat or thrombus (It may become zero if embolus is large enough to block total pulmonary circulation)

III-No change in $ETCO_2$

- **Bronchospasm:** CO_2 has got very high diffusibility therefore $ETCO_2$ remains normal even in severe bronchospasm

IV-Increase in $ETCO_2$ is seen in:

1. Exhausted sodalime or defective valves of closed circuit which impairs the absorption of CO_2 by soda lime
2. Increase production in hyper metabolic states like fever, malignant hyperthermia ($ETCO_2$ may even rise to more than 100 mmHg), Thyrotoxicosis, Neuroleptic malignant syndrome

V-Other uses

- To control level of hypocapnia during hyperventilation in neurosurgery.

Capnography

◈ *Morgan 5th/125-27*

- Determination of end-tidal CO_2 (**$ETCO_2$**) concentration to ***confirm adequate ventilation*** is mandatory during all anesthetic procedures, but particularly so for general anesthesia.
- A rapid fall of $ETCO_2$ is a sensitive indicator of ***air embolism***, a major complication of sitting craniotomies. There are no contraindications.
- Capnography is a valuable monitor of the pulmonary, cardiovascular and anesthetic breathing systems. Capnographs in common use rely on the absorption of infrared light by CO_2. Nondiverting (mainstream) capnographs measure
- ***Capnographs rapidly and reliably indicate esophageal intubation***—a common cause of anesthetic catastrophe—but do not reliably detect bronchial intubation.
- Although there may be some CO_2 in the stomach from swallowing expired air, this should be washed out within a few breaths. Sudden cessation of CO_2 during the expiratory phase may indicate a circuit disconnection.
- The increased metabolic rate caused by ***malignant hyperthermia*** causes a marked rise in $ETCO_2$. The gradient between Paco 2 and $ETCO_2$ (normally 2–5 mm Hg) reflects alveolar dead space (alveoli that are ventilated but not perfused).
- ***Any significant reduction in lung perfusion (e.g., air embolism, decreased cardiac output, or decreased blood pressure) increases alveolar dead space, dilutes expired CO_2 and lessens*** $ETCO_2$.
- True capnographs (as opposed to capnometers) display a waveform of CO_2 concentration that allows recognition of a variety of conditions

214. Ans. b. Low capacity for carrying oxygen at physiological pO_2 levels; c. Transported oxygen is more completely offloaded than blood-transported oxygen; e. All oxygen carried by the perfluorocarbon is in the dissolved state

[Ref: Ajay Yadav 5th/20; www.ncbi.nlm.nih.gov/pmc]

Other than Human Red Blood Cells (Blood)

◈ *Miller*

- Other various substances that carry or facilitate the transport of oxygen have been made. Two concepts of synthetic blood have been attempted.
- The first approach uses ***linear binding kinetics***, unlike the nonlinear binding of hemoglobin. The most notable is the **perfluorochemical emulsion** called Fluosol-DA. However, it had little use because ***it carries oxygen (i.e., a small amount) only when the Pao_2 is more than 300 mm Hg.*** A newer perfluoro compound, **perfluorooctyl bromide,** carries three to four times more oxygen and has a longer half-life and presumably fewer problems than are associated with Fluosol-DA. Other related products are Oxygent (Alliance), Oxycyte (synthetic blood) and several other perfluorocarbon emulsions.
- The remaining synthetic blood or oxygen therapeutics are labeled as **hemoglobin-based oxygen carriers (HBOCs).**
- ***Perfluorocarbon do not react with oxygen****-www.slideshare.net*
- ***PFCs can dissolve oxygen about 50 times more oxygen than blood plasma****-www.slideshare.net*

Table *(Miller)*: **Comparison of Synthetic Blood in General with Allogeneic Blood**

Parameter	Synthetic	Allogeneic
Oxygen delivery	Rapid and consistent	Dependent on 2,3-DPG
Risk of disease transmission	None	Risk
Storage	Room temperature Stable efficacy	Refrigeration Loss of efficacy

Contd...

Parameter	Synthetic	Allogeneic
Shelf life	1–3 years	42 days
Preparation	Ready to use	Cross-match
Compatibility	Universal	Type specific
Duration of action	1–3 days	60-90 days

Oxygen Transport

◈ *www.ncbi.nlm.nih.gov/pmc*

- ***Blood exhibits a sigmoidal oxygen dissociation curve.***
- In contrast, perfluorocarbon emulsions are characterized by a ***linear relationship between oxygen partial pressure and oxygen content***. Elevated arterial oxygen partial pressures are thus beneficial to maximize the oxygen transport capacity of perfluorocarbon emulsions.
- Ventilation with 100% oxygen may raise concerns regarding oxygen toxicity.
- Note also that ***PFC emulsion-transported oxygen is more completely offloaded than blood-transported oxygen***, resulting in an approximate oxygen extraction (O_2-Ex.) ratio of 90% for the PFC emulsion, as compared with approximately 25% for blood
- Due to the small size (< 0.2 µm in diameter) perfluorocarbon emulsion particles ***mainly flow in the peripheral plasma layer in larger vessel***s. In the microcirculation, perfluorocarbon emulsion particles perfuse even the tiniest capillaries (4-5 µm in diameter), where no red blood cells may flow under certain conditions. It is precisely this area in which ***perfluorocarbon emulsions exert their greatest effects***, because they augment local oxygen delivery much more than would be expected from the increase in oxygen content in the arterial blood (large vessel with red blood cells).
- Another important aspect that determines the efficacy of perfluorocarbon emulsions is the fact that all ***oxygen carried by the perfluorocarbon is in the dissolved state,*** resulting in a higher oxygen partial pressures in the microcirculation and thereby augmenting the driving pressure for the diffusion of dissolved oxygen into the tissue.

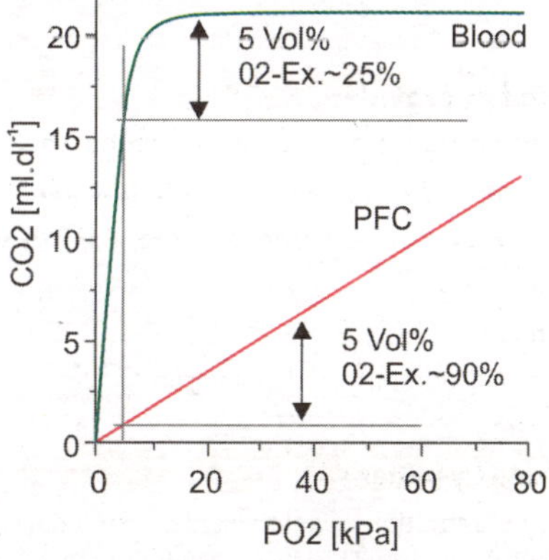

Fig: *Illumin.usc.edu*

"Fluosol DA serves as one of the original PFCs and it is comprised of 20 percent fluorocarbon [6]. A group of PFCs referred to as the **"new perflourochemicals"** has recently been developed. They include compounds such as ***perfluorooctyl bromide ($C_8F_{17}Br$) and perfluorodichorotane ($C_8F_{16}C_{12}$)***. Such molecular structures of the "new" perfluorocarbons allow the blood substitute to contain a higher concentration of PFCs, which ***subsequently increases the oxygen carrying capacity of the artificial blood***"- *illumin.usc.edu*

"**The advantages of PFCs** are their low cost, long shelf life (two years), lack of vasopressive effects, small size and synthetic nature (without the possibility of pathogen transfusion). The **disadvantages** are the flu-like symptoms, need for high oxygen concentration, rapid plasma clearance and ***low capacity for carrying oxygen at physiological pO_2 levels***"-*www.scielo.br*

Advantages of Perfluorocarbons (PFC) Emulsions

- PFCs do not react with oxygen.
- PFCs allow easy transportation of the oxygen to the body.
- They allow increased solubility of oxygen in plasma.
- PFCs minimize the effects of factors like pH and temperature in blood circulation.

Disadvantages of Perfluorocarbons (PFC) Emulsions

- Often causes flu-like symptoms.
- This is often caused by phagocytosis of the perfluorocarbons emulsion by the recipient organism's immune system
- Unable to remain mixed as aqueous solutions — thus, they must be prepared as emulsions for use in patients.
- A decrease in blood platelet count.
- PFC products cannot be used by the human body and must be discarded.
- This takes approximately 18-24 months.
- PFCs absorb oxygen passively, patients must breathe at a linear rate to ensure oxygenation of tissues.'

215. Ans. a. Reduction of secretion of saliva; b. Reduce anxiety and fear c. To produce amnesia; d. To prevent undesirable reflexes; e. Prevent vomiting

[Ref: KDT 8th/413; Ajay Yadav 6th/47]

Premedication: *Goals AjayYadav 6th/50*

- To relieve anxiety
- To produce hemodynamic stability
- To induce sedation(good sleep) & reduce metabolic rate
- To provide analgesia & amnesia
- To decrease the chance of aspiration
- To control oral & respiratory secretions
- To prevent postoperative nausea & vomiting
- To control infection

Preoperative Assessment: *Goals Ajay Yadav 6th/47*

- To reduce the anxiety & educate the patient about anesthesia
- To obtain information about patient's medical history
- To perform physical examination
- To determine which tests are required

- To plan anesthetic technique
- To obtain informed consent
- To give preoperative instructions

216. Ans. a. Spinal anaesthesia; b. Bier's block; e. Surface anaesthesia;

[Ref: Ajay Yadav 6th/xviii; Morgon 5th/263]

"In **regional anesthesia**, local anesthetics are typically injected or applied very close to their intended site of action; thus their pharmacokinetic profiles are much more important determinants of elimination and toxicity than of their desired clinical effect"-Morgon 5th/263

Methods of Regional Anesthesia

- *Spinal anesthesia*
- *Epidural anesthesia*
- *Conduction block(field block or nerve block)*
- *Intravenous regional anesthesia(Bier's Block)*
- *Infiltration anesthesia*
- *Topical anesthesia* ***(surface anesthesia)***

DERMATOLOGY

217. Ans. a. Demodex folliculorum; c. H.pylori

[Ref: Neena Khanna 5th/131; Roxburg 17th/166; Harrison 19th/352; Robbins 9th/1174]

Rosacea

◈ *Neena Khanna 5th/131*

- A pathogenic role for the follicular mite ***Demdex folliculorum*** and the microaerophilic gram-negative bacterium ***Heliobacter pylori*** is suspected
- It is chronic skin disorder characterized by- erythema and telangiectasia and punctuated by acute episodes of papules, pustules and swelling

Rosacea: Causes

◈ *www.medicalnewstoday.com*

Experts are not sure what causes rosacea. The following related factors are thought to contribute:

- **Abnormalities in facial blood vessels**
- **Light skin color**
- ***Demodex folliculorum*** **(microscopic mite):** *Demodex folliculorum* lives on human skin and usually causes no problems. However, patients with rosacea have much higher numbers of these mites than others do. It is unclear whether the mites cause the rosacea, or whether the rosacea causes the overpopulation of the mites.
- ***H. pylori*** **bacteria**: *H. pylori*, a bacteria found in the gut, stimulates the production of bradykinin, a small polypeptide known to cause blood vessels to dilate. ***Experts suggest that this bacterium may play a role in the development of rosacea.***
- **Family history (inheritance, genes)**

"A bug that causes infections in the intestines may play a role. This bug, *H pylori*, is common in people who have rosacea. Scientists cannot prove that *H pylori* can cause rosacea. Many people who do not have rosacea have an *H pylori* infection"- *www.aad.org*

"A mite that lives on everyone's skin, demodex, may play a role. This mite likes to live on the nose and cheeks and this is where rosacea often appears. Many studies found that people with rosacea have large numbers of this mite on their skin. The problem is some people who do not have rosacea also have large numbers of this mite on their skin"- *www.aad.org*

Acne Rosacea

◈ *Harrison 19th/352*

- Acne rosacea, commonly referred to simply as rosacea, is an inflammatory disorder predominantly affecting the central face.
- It is characterized by the presence of erythema, telangiectases and superficial pustules but is not associated with the presence of comedones.
- Rosacea of very long standing may lead to connective tissue overgrowth, particularly of the nose (*rhinophyma*) . Rosacea may also be complicated by various inflammatory disorders of the eye, including keratitis, blepharitis, iritis and recurrent chalazion. These ocular problems are potentially sight-threatening and warrant ophthalmologic evaluation.
- "**Acne vulgaris**: Microbial colonization (Organism implicated) includes- ***Propionibacterium spp. Especially P.acnes, malassezia furfur and staph. epidermidis***"- *Neena Khanna 5th/121*

218. Ans. b. 50–70% Tricholoroacetic acid; c. 10-25% Podophyllin resin; e. Imiquimod (5% cream)

[Ref: Neena Khanna 5th/339,291; Roxburg 17th/55; Harrison 19th/1201]

Anogenital warts: Treatment

◈ *Neena Khanna 5th/339*

- ***Topical podophyllin (25%)***
- ***Tricholoroacetic acid (50-100%)***
- *Cryotherapy with liquid nitrogen*
- *Topical podophyllotoxin (0.5%)*
- ***Imiquimod (5% cream)***

Table: *(Harrison 18th)*: **Treatment of External, Exophytic Anogenital Warts**

I. Administered by provider
A. Cryotherapy with liquid nitrogen or cryoprobe weekly
B. ***Podophyllin resin, 10–25% weekly for up to 4 weeks***
C. ***Trichloroacetic acid or bichloroacetic acid, 80–90% weekly***
D. Surgical excision
E. Other regimens
1. Intralesionally administered interferon
2. Laser surgery
II. Administered by patient
A. Podofilox, 0.5% solution or gel twice daily for 3 days, followed by 4 days without therapy. This cycle may be repeated four times.
B. ***Imiquimod, 5% cream 3 times per week for up to 16 weeks***

Therapeutic Options

◈ *Harrison 19th/1201*

- **Podophyllotoxin:** Podophyllotoxin (0.05% solution or gel and 0.15% cream) induces necrosis of genital wart tissue that heals within a few days.
- **Sinecatechins:** Sinecatechins (15% ointment) is used to treat genital warts but should not be used to treat vaginal, cervical, or anal lesions.
- **Imiquimod** (5% or 3.75% cream) is a patient-applied topical immunomodulatory agent thought to activate immune cells by binding to a Toll-like receptor—an event that leads to an inflammatory response.
- **Cryotherapy** (liquid nitrogen) for HPV-associated lesions causes cellular death. Genital warts usually disappear after two or three weekly sessions but often recur.

Table: *(Harrison 19th/1201)*: **Recommended Treatments That Must Be Administered by a Clinician for Genital Warts and Other Human Papilloma virus–Associated Lesions**

Variable	Cryo-therapy	Surgical Removal	Laser	Interferon
Effectiveness	Good	Excellent	Excellent	Good
Recurrence	Frequent	Frequent	Frequent	Frequent
Adverse effects	Mild, well tolerated	Mild, well tolerated	Mild to moderate, well tolerated	Frequent, moderately severe
Availability	Good	Good	Fair	Fair
Cost	Inexpen sive	Moderately expensive	Very expensive	Very expensive

219. Ans. a. Sporotrichosis; d. Fish tank granuloma; e. Lupus vulgaris

[Ref: Neena Khanna 5th/317,67; Roxburg 17th/; Harrison 19th/366]

"There are several infectious diseases that present as erythematous papules or nodules in a lymphocutaneous or sporotrichoid pattern, i.e., in a linear arrangement along the lymphatic channels. The two most common etiologies are Sporothrix schenckii (sporotrichosis) and the atypical mycobacterium Mycobacterium marinum. Additional causes include Nocardia, Leishmania and other atypical mycobacteria and dimorphic fungi; culture of lesional tissue will aid in the diagnosis"-*Harrison 19th/366*

Sporotrichoid lymphocutaneous infection is an uncommon syndrome that is often misdiagnosed and improperly treated. Of the several hundred cases seen each year in the United States, the majority are caused by Sporothrix schenckii, Nocardia brasiliensis, Mycobacterium marinum or Leishmania brasiliensis. The **"sporotrichoid" disease** begins at a site of distal inoculation and leads to the development of nodular lymphangitis"- *www.aafp.org*

Sporotrichosis: **Sporotrichoid pattern**- *Neena Khanna 5th/317*

DDx for Sporotrichoid spread *(www.coursehero.com):*

- *Cat Scratch*
- *Anthrax*
- *TB/Tularemia*
- *Nocardia*
- ***Sporotrichosis – mc***
- *Phaeohyphomycosis/Pyogenic bacteria*
- *Leishmania*
- ***Atypical mycobacteria – mc***
- *Tularemia*
- *Also, burkholderia mallei, cowpox, acanthomoeba spp, P. boydii)*

Differential Diagnosis of Sporotrichoid Spread

◈ *dermtuts.tripod.com*

- Atypical Mycobacteria: Mycobacterium avium complex (including Mycobacterium intracellulare and M avium), ***Mycobacterium marinum infection (fish tank granuloma)***, M kansasii
- lepromatous leprosy
- ***Lupus vulgaris***
- sarcoidosis
- Leishmania
- Blastomycosis
- histoplasmosis
- Pasteurella tularensis
- Nocardia brasiliensis
- Paecilomyces infection

220. Ans. a. Poison ivy; b. Nickel; d. Paraphenylene diamine; e. Rubber

[Ref: Neena Khanna 5th/113; Roxburg 17th/123; Harrison 19th/339; Nelson 20th/3152]

Agents causing allergic contract dermatitis: Nickel, poison ivy, rubber (mercaptobenzthiazole, thiouram), ethylene diamine, neomycin, lanolin etc"- *Roxburg 17th/123*

"Vesicle: A small, fluid-filled lesion, <0.5 cm in diameter, raised above the plane of surrounding skin. Fluid is often visible and the lesions are translucent (e.g., vesicles in allergic contact dermatitis caused by ***Toxicodendron* [poison ivy]**) "-*Harrison 19th/339*

Table: *Harrison 19th/341*

Allergic contact dermatitis	Anywhere	Localized erythema, vesicles, scale and pruritus (e.g., fingers, earlobes-nickel; dorsal aspect of foot- shoe; exposed surfaces – ***poison ivy***)

Table: *(Neena Khanna 5th/113)*: **Agents causing allergic contract dermatitis**

	Agent	Source
Plants	Parthenium	Airborne exposure (so called airborne contact dermatitis, ABCD)
Metals	Nickel	Costume jewelery and clips

Contd...

	Agent	Source
	Chromates	Chromium plating and cement Leather in footwear
Cosmetics	Paraphenylene diamine	Hair dyes
	Fragrances	Cosmetics, perfumes and shampoos
	Formaldehyde	Preservatives in cosmetics
	Parabens	Preservatives in cosmetics
Medicines	Neomycin	Topical antibiotics
	Benzocaine	Local anesthetics
Rubber	Mercapto mix (additives)	Shoe soles and uppers
	Thiuram mix (additives)	Rubber gloves

Contact Dermatitis

◈ *Harrison 19th/345*

- Contact dermatitis is an inflammatory skin process caused by an exogenous agent or agents that directly or indirectly injure the skin.
- In *irritant* contact dermatitis (ICD), this injury is caused by an inherent characteristic of a compound—for example, a concentrated acid or base.
- Agents that cause ACD induce an antigen-specific immune response (e.g., poison ivy dermatitis) . The clinical lesions of contact dermatitis may be acute (wet and edematous) or chronic (dry, thickened and scaly), depending on the persistence of the insult
- The most common irritants encountered are ***chronic wet work, soaps and detergents***. Treatment should be directed toward the avoidance of irritants and the use of protective gloves or clothing.
- The most common cause of ACD is exposure to plants, especially to members of the family Anacardiaceae, including the genus *Toxicodendron*. ***Poison ivy, poison oak and poison sumac*** are members of this genus and cause an allergic reaction marked by erythema, vesiculation and severe pruritus. The eruption is often linear or angular, corresponding to areas where plants have touched the skin. The sensitizing antigen common to these plants is urushiol, an oleoresin containing the active ingredient pentadecylcatechol. The **oleoresin** may adhere to skin, clothing, tools and pets and contaminated articles may cause dermatitis even after prolonged storage.

221. Ans. a. Campbell de Morgan spots; c. Angiokeratoma; e. Pyogenic granuloma

[Ref: Nelson 20th/3122-28; L and B 26th/599-600; Schwartz 10th/411-13; 1666-69; Roxburg 17th/194-97]

Campbell de Morgan spots: These are arteriovenous fistulas at the dermal capillary level in sun exposed skin of older patients"- *L and B 26th/599*

"Hutchinson freckle, also known as **lentigo maligna,** is a non-familial precursor to lentigo maligna melanoma, which accounts for 5-15% of cases of malignant melanoma. It is most frequent in the head and neck"- *radiopaedia.org/articles/hutchinson-freckle; Neena Khanna 5th/394*

"Pyogenic granuloma: These share many histological characteristics of haemangiomas and are probably a subtype thereof"- *L and B 26th/600*

"Pyogenic Granuloma (Lobular Capillary Hemangioma): A pyogenic granuloma is a small red, glistening, sessile, or pedunculated papule that often has a discernible epithelial collarette"- Nelson 20th/3127

Vascular Malformations (Angioma)/Capillary Naevi

◈ *Roxburg 17th/194-97*

- Stork mark
- Port-wine stains
- Capillary angioma
- Cavernous haemangioma
- Lymphangioma circumscriptum
- ***Angiokeratoma***
- Senile angioma (***Campbell de Morgan spots****, cherry angioma)*
- Capillary aneurysm
- Glomus cell tumour
- ***Pyogenic granuloma***

Keratoacanthoma: Skin coloured nodule which develops a central horny plug —*Neena Khanna 5th/386*

Other Capillary Vascular Malformations

◈ *www.dermnetnz.org*

- Angiokeratoma circumscriptum is a raised warty dark red-purple lesion that is most commonly found on the lower leg or foot. It is often covered with rough scaly patches of skin. In many cases, they are present at birth but may also develop in childhood or adulthood.
- Angiokeratomas are harmless lesions that usually require no treatment. For cosmetic reasons or concerns of possible melanoma, surgical removal or laser therapy may be performed.

Table: *(Nelson 20th/3122)*: **Vascular Malformations**

Type	Examples
Capillary	Port-wine stain
Venous	Venous malformation
	Angiokeratoma circumscriptum (hyperkeratotic venule)
	Cutis marmorata telangiectasia congenital (congenital phlebectasia)
Arterial	Arteriovenous malformation
Lymphatic	Small vessel lymphatic malformation (lymphangioma circumscriptum)
	Large vessel lymphatic malformation (cystic hygroma)

Keratoacanthoma (KA) is a relatively common low-grade tumor that originates in the pilosebaceous glands and closely ***resembles squamous cell carcinoma (SCC)***. In fact, strong arguments support classifying keratoacanthoma as a variant of invasive SCC. In most pathology/biopsy reports, dermatopathologists refer to the lesion as "squamous cell carcinoma, keratoacanthoma-type." emedicine.medscape.com

Dermatofibroma (Histiocytoma, sclerosing haemangioma): contain large number of small blood vessels- Roxburg 17th/197

Dermatofibroma: Benign tumor of fibrous tissue"- *Neena Khanna 5th/404*

222. Ans. a, Epidermis; c, Stratum spinosum; e. Prickle cell layer

[Ref: NeenaKhanna 5th/95;Behl 10th/265;Rook 7th/7.36;Harshmohan 8th/810]

- Spongiosis involves stratum spinosum (pricle cell layer of epidermis)

Layers of Epidermis

◈ *Harshmohan 8th/810(from top to down)*

- Stratum Corneum
- Stratum Lucidum
- Stratum Granulosum
- Stratum Spinosum(prickle cell layer)
- Stratum Basale(germinatum)

Stratum Basale

- ***Acantholytic cells of pemphigus vulgaris*** are derived from stratum basal.
- Basal cell degeneration occurs in ***Lichen planus.***

Stratum Spinosum

- Intercellular (in between the cells) edema → **Spongiosis**
- Thickening
  Acanthosis

Stratum Granulosum

- Thickening → **Hypergranulosis**

223. Ans. b. DLE; c. Lichen planus; e. Genital warts;

[Ref: Neena Khanna 6th/45;www.webmd.com]

Disorders showing Koebner's Phenomenon

Psoriasis
Lichen planus
Molluscum contagiosum
Warts
Vitiligo
Darrier disease (kertosisfollicularies)
Lichen nitidus
Pityriasisrubrapilaris

- **Rare causes are:** Erythema multiforme, Necrobiosislipoidica, **Hailey-hailey disease,** Xanthoma, **Leukemia & Carcinoma,** Vasculitis, **Lichen sclerosis**

PSYCHIATRY

224. Ans. a. Increased incidence of schizophrenia in genetically susceptible person with long term use of cannabis; d. Schizophrenic persons are more prone to cannabis use

[Ref: Ahuja 7th/46; Synopsis of Psychiatry by Kaplan and Sadock 11th/302; www.ncbi.nlm.nih.gov]

Substance Abuse: Substance abuse is common in schizophrenia. The lifetime prevalence of any drug abuse (other than **tobacco**) is often greater than 50 percent. For all drugs of abuse (other than tobacco), abuse is associated with poorer function. In one population based study, the *lifetime prevalence of alcohol within schizophrenia was 40 percent.* Alcohol abuse increases risk of hospitalization and, in some patients, may increase psychotic symptoms. People with schizophrenia have an increased prevalence of abuse of common street drugs. There has been ***particular interest in the association between cannabis and schizophrenia.*** Those reporting high levels of cannabis use (more than 50 occasions) were at ***six-fold increased risk of schizophrenia*** compared with nonusers. The use of amphetamines, cocaine and similar drugs should raise particular concern because of their marked ability to increase psychotic symptoms"- *Kaplan and Sadock 11th/302*

Complication of chronic cannabis use: ***worsenic or relapse*** *in schizophrenia"- Ahuja 7th/46*

Hemp insanity or **cannabis psychosis**: *Similar to an acute schizophreniform disorder with disorientation and confusion"- Ahuja 7th/46*

To date, the consensus is that ***cannabis use increases the risk of psychosis*** but, across the population, the effect is relatively small. However, the effect seems to be stronger in individuals who are already at risk, ***such as people with a family history of psychotic disorders or those who have experienced childhood abuse*** *www.medicalnewstoday.com*

Our research demonstrates that ***cannabis has a differential risk*** on susceptible versus non-susceptible individuals. In other words, young people with a **genetic susceptibility to schizophrenia** - those who have psychiatric disorders in their families - should bear in mind that ***they are playing with fire if they smoke pot during adolescence."*** *-www.medicalnewstoday.com*

"Recent research suggests that not only are people ***who are prone to schizophrenia more likely to try cannabis, but that cannabis may also increase the risk of developing symptoms.*** Its use has been linked to symptoms of psychosis, such as paranoia and delusional thinking, in up to 40 percent of users"- *www.medicalnewstoday.com*

225. Ans. b. Illness anxiety disorder; d. Somatic passivity disorders

[Ref: Ahuja 7th/104-09; Synopsis of Psychiatry by Kaplan and Sadock 11th/295,470-71; apps.who.int/classifications/icd10/browse/2016]

Illness anxiety disorder is a new diagnosis in the fifth edition of Diagnostic and Statistical Manual of Mental Disorders (DSM-5) that applies to those persons who are preoccupied with being sick or with developing a disease of some kind. ***It is a variant of somatic symptom disorder (hypochondriasis).*** As stated in DSM-5 : Most individuals with hypochondriasis are now classified as having somatic symptom disorder; however, in a minority of cases, the diagnosis of illness anxiety disorder applies instead. In describing the differential diagnosis between the two, according to DSM-5, somatic symptom disorder is diagnosed when somatic symptoms are present, whereas in illness anxiety disorder, there are few or no somatic symptoms and persons are "primarily concerned with the idea they are ill"- *Kaplan and Sadock 11th/471*

Illness Anxiety Disorder. Illness anxiety disorder is the fear of being sick with few or no somatic symptoms. It is a new diagnosis in DSM-5.

Somatic passivity: *Bodily sensations, especially sensory symptoms, are experienced as imposed on body by some external force. It is First Rank symptom of* ***schizophrenia****- Ahuja 7th/55*

Somatoform Disorder

◈ *Ahuja 7th/104-09*

- ***Somatisation disorder***
- ***Hypochondriasis***
- Somatoform autonomic dysfunction
- ***Persistent somatoform pain disorder***
- Other somatoform disorder- Globus hystericus, psychogenic torticollis, psychogenic pruritus, psychogenic dysmenorrhea, teeth-grinding

F45 Somatoform disorders

F45.0 ***Somatization disorder***

F45.1 Undifferentiated somatoform disorder

F45.2 ***Hypochondriacal disorders***

F45.3 Somatoform autonomic dysfunction

.30 Heart and cardiovascular system

.31 Upper gastrointestinal tract

.32 Lower gastrointestinal tract

.34 Genitourinary system

.38 Other organ or system

F45.4 ***Persistent somatoform pain disorder***

F45.8 Other somatoform disorders

F45.9 Somatoform disorder, unspecified

Somatoform Disorders

◈ *apps.who.int/classifications/icd10*

- The main feature is repeated presentation of physical symptoms together with persistent requests for medical investigations, in spite of repeated negative findings and reassurances by doctors that the symptoms have no physical basis.
- If any physical disorders are present, they do not explain the nature and extent of the symptoms or the distress and preoccupation of the patient

Somatic Symptom and Related Disorders

◈ *Kaplan and Sadock 11th/295*

This group of disorders (previously called somatoform disorders in DSM-IV) is characterized by marked preoccupation with the body and fears of disease or consequences of disease (e.g., death).

Somatic Symptom Disorder. Somatic symptom disorder is characterized by high levels of anxiety and persistent worry about somatic signs and symptoms that are misinterpreted as having a known medical disorder. It is also known as hypochondriasis.

A & E

226. Ans a. Duloxetine; b. Venlafaxine; c. Milnacipran

[Ref: Satoskar Pharmacology 25th/210-11; KDT 7th/454; Katzung 13th/515; Ahuja 7th/183; Kaplon 11th/1010]

Table: *(25th/210-11; KDT 7th/454; Katzung 13th/515)* **Classification of Antidepressants Satoskar**

I.	Reversible inhibitors of MAO-A (RIMAs) Moclobemide, Clorgyline
II.	Tricyclic antidepressants (TCAs) A. *NA* + 5-*HT* reuptake inhibitors Imipramine, Amitriptyline, Trimipramine, Doxepin, Dothiepin, Clomipramine B. *Predominantly NA reuptake inhibitors* Desipramine, Nortriptyline, Amoxapine, Reboxetine
III.	**Selective serotonin reuptake inhibitors (SSRIs)** Fluoxetine, Fluvoxamine, ***Paroxetine***, Sertraline, Citalopram, Escitalopram, **Dapoxetine**
IV.	**Serotonin and noradrenaline reuptake inhibitors (SNRIs)** ***Venlafaxine, Duloxetine, Milnacipran, Levomilnacipran,*** **desvenlafaxine**
V.	Atypical antidepressants Trazodone, Mianserin, Mirtazapine, Bupropion, Tianeptine, Amineptine, Atomoxetine

227. Ans. a. Seizures; b. Sedation; e. Constipation

[Ref: K. D. T 7th/441; Satoskar 25th/200; G and G 11th/481; Synopsis of Psychiatry by Kaplan and Sadock 11th/1030]

Side Effects of Clozapine

◈ *Kaplan and Sadock 11th/1030*

- The most common drug-related adverse effects are ***sedation***, dizziness, syncope, tachycardia, hypotension, electrocardiography (ECG) changes, nausea and vomiting.
- Other common adverse effects include fatigue, weight gain, various GI symptoms (most commonly ***constipation***), anticholinergic effects and subjective muscle weakness.
- **Sialorrhea, or hypersalivation**, is a side effect that begins early in treatment and is most evident at night. Patients report that their pillows are drenched with saliva. This side effect is most likely the result of impairment of swallowing. Although there are reports that clonidine or amitriptyline may help reduce hypersalivation, the most practical solution is to put a towel over the pillow.
- The risk of **seizures** is about 4 percent in patients talcing dosages greater than 600 mg a day. Leukopenia, granulocytopenia, agranulocytosis and **fever** occur in about 1 percent of patients

Clozapine

◈ *K. D. T 7th/441*

- It *produces* ***few or no extrapyramidal symptoms***; tardive dyskinesia is rare and prolactin level does not rise
- It is ***quite sedating***, moderately potent anticholinergic, but paradoxically induces hyperventilation

- Its major limitation is *higher incidence of agranulocytosis* (0. 8%) and other blood dyscrasias; weekly monitoring of leucocyte count is required
- Metabolic complication like weight gain, hyperlipidemia and precipitation of diabetes is *another major limitation*
- *High dose can* ***induce seizures even in non-epileptics***
- Other side-effects are **sedation**, unstable B. P, tachycardia and urinary incontinence
- Few cases of myocarditis have been reported which start like flu but may progress to death
- Cause **sialorrhoea**- *Satoskar 25th/200*
- *Clozapine is sufficiently anticholinergic to induce an atropine-like poisoning on overdose- G and G 11th/481*
- *Clozapine can decrease the efficiency of clearing saliva and severely impair intestinal motility.Clozapine can cause potentially severe ileus and* ***sialorrhea***- *G and G 11th/481*

228. Ans. a. ECT; b. Mood stabilizer; d. Antipsychotic drugs

[Ref: Ahuja 7th/77-80; Synopsis of Psychiatry by Kaplan and Sadock 11th/377]

"ECT can be used for **acute manic** *excitement, if it not adequately responding to* ***antipsychotics and mood stabilizers****"- Ahuja 7th/78*

Treatment of Acute Mania

Kaplan and Sadock's Textbook of Psychiatry 11th/378-79

- **Lithium Carbonate:** Lithium carbonate is considered the prototypical "mood stabilizer." Yet because the onset of antimanic action with lithium can be slow, it usually is supplemented in the early phases of treatment by atypical antipsychotics, mood-stabilizing anticonvulsants, or high-potency benzodiazepines. Therapeutic lithium levels are between 0.6 and 1.2 mEq/L.
- **Valproate** has surpassed lithium in use for acute mania. Unlike lithium, valproate is only indicated for acute mania, although most experts agree it also has prophylactic effects.
- Carbamazepine and Oxcarbazepine
- Clonazepam and Lorazepam: The high-potency benzodiazepine anticonvulsants used in acute mania include clonazepam (Klonopin) and lorazepam (Ativan).
- **Atypical and Typical Antipsychotics:** All of the atypical antipsychotics-olanzapine, risperidone, quetiapine, ziprasidone and aripiprazole have demonstrated ***antimanic efficacy*** and are approved by the Food and Drug Administration for this indication.

"ECT is at least equal to lithium in the treatment of acute manic episodes. The pharmacological treatment of manic episodes, however, is so effective in the short term and for prophylaxis that the use of ECT to treat manic episodes is generally limited to situations with specific contraindications to all available pharmacological approaches. The relative rapidity of the ECT response indicates its usefulness for patients whose manic behavior has produced dangerous levels of exhaustion. ECT should not be used for a patient who is receiving lithium, because lithium can lower the seizure threshold and cause a prolonged seizure"- *Kaplan and Sadock 11th/1068*

229. Ans. a. Delusion; b. Hallucination

[Ref: Parikh 7th/458-62; Reddy 34th/459-63; Ahuja 7th/229]

Delirium(with features of delusion and hallucination) is included in criminal responsibility of insane person

"Delirium: *A delirious person may commit criminal acts due to* ***delusions and hallucinations.*** *He is* ***not legally responsible for the acts committed during delirium****"- Reddy 34th/462*

Insanity Under Indian Penal Code

www.lawteacher.net

The ***defence of insanity*** is discussed in sec 84 of the Indian penal code which reads:

"Act of a person of unsound mind- Nothing is an offence which is done by a person who at the time of doing it, by reason of unsoundness of mind, is incapable of doing the act, or that he is doing what is either wrong or contrary in law."

Principles for the application of this section: The following principles are to be kept in mind in applying this section:

- ***Every type of insanity is not legal insanity;*** the cognitive faculty must be destroyed as to render one incapable of knowing the nature of his act or that what he is doing is wrong or contrary to law;
- The court shall presume the absence of such insanity;
- The burden of proof of legal insanity is on the accused, though it is not as heavy as the prosecution;
- The court must consider whether the accused suffered from legal insanity at the time when the offence was committed;
- In reaching such a conclusion, the circumstances which preceded, attended or followed the crime are relevant consideration; and
- The prosecution in discharging its burden of the plea of legal insanity has merely to prove the basic fact and rely upon the normal presumption of the law that everyone knows the law and the natural consequences of his act.

Delirium: This is a condition characterized by clouding of consciousness, impairment of mental processes, disorientation and abnormal experiences, such as ***delusions and hallucinations.*** The patient is therefore, impulsive and may commit suicide or some violent act. ***He is not legally responsible for such an act under section 84 of the Indian Penal Code*** which is done by a person who, at the time of doing it, is by reason of unsoundness of mind, incapable of knowing the nature of the act, or that he is doing what is either wrong or contrary to law"- Parikh 7th/460

MC Naughten Rule (Test For Determining Criminal Responsibility)

Reddy 34th/459-60

- **"An accused person is not legally responsible, if it is clearly proved, that at the time of committing the crime, he was suffering from such a defect of reason from abnormality of mind, that he did not know the nature and quality of the act he was doing, or that what he was doing was wrong".**
- This legal test has also been accepted in India as the law of criminal responsibility and is included in **Sec. 84, I.P.C** which is as follows: **"Nothing is an offence which is done**

A & E

by a person, who at the time of doing it, by reason of unsoundness of mind, is incapable of knowing the nature of the act, or that he is doing what is either wrong or contrary to law"

230. Ans. a. Waxy flexibility; b. Automatic obedience; c. Somatic passivity; d. Rigidity; e. Mutism

[Ref: Kaplan &Sadock11th/309, 781; NeerajAhuja 7th/59]

Catatonic Schizophrenia

◈ *NeerajAhuja 7th/59*

- It can be present in three clinical forms: excited catatonia, stuporous catatonia & catatonia alternating b/w excitement & stupor
- Excited catatonia: increase in psychomotor activity, increase in speech production
- Stuporous or retarded catatonia: Characterized by extreme retardation of psychomotor function; It includes- mutism, rigidity, negativitism, posturing, stupor, echolalia, echopraxia, waxy flexibility, ambitendency, automatic obedience, mannerism etc
- Somatic passivity: It is first rank symptom of schizophrenia- NeerajAhuja 7th/55 (so included in answer)

RADIOLOGY

231. Ans. b. Gray; d. Rad

[Ref: Sumer Sethi 6th/170-71; Grainger and Allison 6th/118; Radiology by S. Bhadury 2nd/197; Harrison 19th/263 e-1]

"The commonly used units of radiation are the rad and the gray (Gy). The *rad (radiation absorbed dose) is energy deposited within living matter* and is equal to 100 ergs/g of tissue. The traditional rad has been replaced by the Systeme Internationale (SI) unit of the gray; 100 rad = 1 Gy, while 1 Gy is equal to 1 joule/kg. The sievert (Sv) is the SI unit that refers to the equivalent radiation dose in biologic tissues. While 1 Sv is equal to 1 joule/kg, Sv and Gy are not interchangeable units: Sv refers to the biologic effect of the radiation, while Gy refers to the physical energy being transferred"- *Harrison 19th/263 e-1*

"Gray (Gy) is the SI unit of absorbed dose. One gray is equal to an absorbed dose of 1 Joule/kilogram (100 rads).

Rad is the special unit of absorbed dose. One rad is equal to an absorbed dose of 100 ergs/gram or 0.01 joule/kilogram (0.01 gray)"-*S. Bhadury 2nd/187-88*

Unit of Absorbed Radiation

◈ *Sumer Sethi 6th/170-71*

- Rad
- SI unit = Gray
- 1 gray (Gy) = 100 rads

Unit of Radioactivity

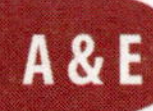

◈ *S. Bhadury 2nd/197*

- *It is measured by **Becquerel and Curie***
- *1Bq = 1 disintegration/second*
- *1 Curie (Ci) = 3.7 x 10^{10} disintegration/second*
- *1 Ci is equal to 37 gigabecquerel*

Unit of Biological Effectiveness or Equivalent Dose

◈ *Sumer Sethi 6th/170-71*

- Rem
- SI unit = Sievert
- 1 Sievert = 100 Rem

Unit of Radiation Exposure

◈ *Sumer Sethi 6th/170-71*

- Roentgen
- SI unit= coloumb/k

232. Ans. a. Cervical X-ray A-P view; b. Chest X-ray A–P view; c. Focused assessment with sonography for trauma (FAST); d. X-ray of visible injury site; e. X-ray pelvis AP view

[Ref: CSDT 14th/200, 211-12; L and B 26th/330;Schwartz 10th/162]

"A full **cervical spine** series includes ***anteroposterior and lateral views*** of the whole cervical spine and open mouth views. However, in many trauma centres ***computed tomography (CT) scanning,*** with sagittal reformats, is considered more accurate. This modality is particularly useful in visualising the cervicothoracic junction and in surveying the entire spine"-*L and B 26th/330*

"**Pelvic fracture radiological examination**: ***Pelvis with both hips-AP is the basic X-ray*** *required for screening purpose"- Maheshwari 5th/125*

"Chest X-ray: The AP shows magnification of the heart and widening of the mediastinum. Whenever possible the patient should be imaged in an upright PA position. **AP views** are less useful and should be reserved for very ill patients who cannot stand erect"- **www.med-ed.virginia.edu**

Imaging Studies

◈ *CSDT 14th/200*

- ***Radiographic plain films of the chest and pelvis are required in all major injuries.***
- **Lateral C-spine films** have been supplanted by formal CT scanning of the neck in patients with suspicion of or mechanism for cervical spine injury.
- Bedside focused assessment with ***sonography for trauma (FAST)*** is the preferred triage method for determining the presence of hemoperitoneum in blunt trauma patients or cardiac tamponade in blunt and penetrating trauma patients.
- Patients who have an **abnormal chest radiograph** with a mechanism for blunt aortic injury should undergo further screening with either helical chest CT done at the time of abdominal imaging or with aortography, if necessary.
- **Cervical spine CT scans** should be obtained for patients who are unconscious, have pain in the cervical region, have neurologic deficits, or have painful or distracting injuries.
- **CT scanning of the head** should be performed in all patients with loss of consciousness or more serious neurologic impairment.
- Radiographs of the long bones and noncervical spine can usually be deferred until the more critical injuries of the thorax and abdomen have been delineated and stabilized.

"A major advance in management of blunt trauma has been the FAST examination. *Ultrasound has proven to be an ideal modality in the immediate evaluation of the trauma patient* because it is rapid and accurate for the detection of intra-abdominal fluid or blood and is readily repeatable"- *CSDT 14th/211*

"Despite the many potential indications, *FAST followed by abdominal pelvic CT scanning* has replaced the need for most diagnostic peritoneal lavages. The only contraindication is a need for emergency laparotomy. A portion of the recovered fluid is sent for laboratory analysis of cell counts, the presence of particulate matter and amylase"- *CSDT 14th/212*

Table: *(CSDT 14th/213)*: **Comparison of diagnostic methods for abdominal trauma**

Methods	Time/Cost	Advantages/Disadvantages
Diagnostic peritoneal lavage (DRL)	Quick/ inexpensive	Rapid results in unstable patient but invasive and may be overly sensitive for blood and not specific for site of injury; requires experience and may be limited if previous surgery
Focused assessment with sonography for trauma (FAST)	Quick/ inexpensive	Rapid detection of intra abdominal fluid and pericardial tamponade; may be limited by operator experience, large body habitus, subcutaneous air; poor for detection of bowel injury. Fairly sensitive but bot highly specific
Helical computerized abdominal tomography (CT)	Slower/ expensive	Most specific for site of injury and can evaluate retro-peritoneum; very good sensitivity but may miss bowel injury; risk of reaction to contrast dye.

233. Ans. a. Gas under diaghragm- seen in perforated gastric ulcer; b. Rigler sign-seen in acute peritonistis with pneumoperitoneum; c. Differentiation of small and large bowel obstruction can be done by location of distended bowel loop; d. Large intestine- shows taenia coli and huastration

[Ref: Sumer Sethi 6th/122; Danhert Radiology Review Manual 7th/772; D/D by Chapman 4th/212]

Supine film signs of pneumoperitoneum: ***Rigler sign*** *(visualization of both aspects of bowel wall being outlined by air on either side)- Sumer Sethi 6th/122; Danhert 7th/772*

Gas under diaghragm: perforated gastric ulcer. Gas from perforation is usually bilateral, but may be asymmetrical. -WHO Radiology *Manual 2002/167*

Pneumoperitoneum: Erect position X-ray- free gas under diaphragm or liver. Can detect 10 ml air. Can take 10 min for all gas to rise"- D/D by Chapman 4th/212

Small Bowel Obstruction

◈ *Review of Radiology by Sumer Sethi 6th/123*

- ***Multiple centrally placed*** loops with ***valvulae connivates*** in jejunum and diameter 3-5 cm
- May show strings of beads appearance due to air trapped within valvulae and rest of loop being fluid filled

Large Bowel Obstruction

◈ *Review of Radiology by Sumer Sethi 6th/123*

- ***Few peripherally placed loops with haustra*** and diameter 5 cm+ and showing fecal matter within dilated loop
- A caecal diameter of > 9cm implies impending perforation
- Demonstration of the air in rectum implies a paralytic ileus rather than mechanical obstruction

The haustra (singular **haustrum**) of the colon are the small pouches caused by sacculation (sac formation), which give the colon its segmented appearance

The **taeniae coli** (also **teniae coli**) are three separate longitudinal ribbons of smooth muscle on the outside of the ascending, transverse, descending and sigmoid colons.

"The **circular folds (valves of Kerckring)** (also, **plicae circulares /valvulae conniventes**) are large valvular flaps projecting into the lumen of the small intestine.The space between circular folds are smaller than the haustra of the colon and, in contrast to haustra, *circular folds reach around the whole circumference of the intestine.* These differences can assist in distinguishing the small intestine from the colon on an abdominal x-ray"-wiki

Small bowel obstruction: Features of small bowel obstruction include the central position of gas-filled and distended loops of bowel. The ***white lines passing across the full width of the bowel are 'valvulae conniventes' - these are only found in the small bowel***-*www.radiologymasterclass.co.uk*

234. Ans. c. Strontium-89

[Ref: Sumer Sethi 6th/193; Harrison 19th/103e-4; news.cancerconnect.com/cancer]

Radiation therapy can slow down or stop sperm cell production if the testicle is in or near the target area for the radiation. A lead shield can help protect the testicles, but radiation "scatters" within the body, so it's impossible to shield the testicles completely. ***Total body irradiation used before some bone marrow transplants often causes permanent infertility***"-*www.livestrong.org*

"**Toxicity of Radiation Therapy:** Although radiation therapy is most often administered to a local region, systemic effects, including fatigue, anorexia, nausea and vomiting, may develop that are related in part to the volume of tissue irradiated, dose fractionation, radiation fields and individual susceptibility. Bone is among the most radioresistant organs, with radiation effects being manifested mainly in children through premature fusion of the epiphyseal growth plate. ***By contrast, the male testis, female ovary and bone marrow are the most sensitive organs***"-*Harrison 19th/103e-4*

Radiation therapy: Radiation therapy can damage the ovaries or testes. The risk is greatest when the radiation is focused in these areas: *www.cancer.net*

- ***The pelvis***
- The abdomen
- The spine
- The whole body

"Radiotherapy has by far the most damaging effect on reproductive ability by affecting both the part of the brain that contributes to testosterone levels as well as the testes. The harmful effect of irradiation depends on the ***total dose of radiation, the area irradiated, as well as the number and size of fractions (treatments) given***"

"**Alkylating agents:** The *alkylating agents* (nitrogen mustard, cyclophosphamide, chlorambucil, busulfan, procarbazine) are a ***major cause of late-testicular toxicity.*** Long-term infertility due to treatment with alkylating agents may be expected in more than 50% of the patients at a cumulative dose of cyclophosphamide greater that 6 g/m^2 and procarbazine greater than 4 g/m^2. Procarbazine-containing regimens (MOPP/ABVD) result in ***azoospermia*** in the vast majority of patients."

"**Radioactive iodine (I-131 therapy)** is a common therapy used in the treatment of thyroid cancer and hyperthyroidism. It is taken up and concentrated by the thyroid cells and the radiation, in turn, kills the cells. Much higher doses are used for the treatment of thyroid cancer than hyperthyroidism. Although generally well tolerated, a number of side effects may occur and there have been ***concerns about the effect of radioactive iodine on reproductive function and fertility***"-www.thyroid.org

"Although **radioactive iodine therapy** is associated with ***alterations in reproductive function in both men and women,*** these changes are usually short-lived. Pregnancies achieved after exposure to radioactive iodine treatment do not appear to be at increased risk for negative outcomes. Nevertheless, it is recommended that pregnancy be ***avoided for 1 year following radioactive iodine therapy to allow reproductive function to normalize***"-*www.thyroid.org*

"Men who receive large total doses because of many treatments with **RAI (also known as I-131)** may have ***lower sperm counts or, rarely, become infertile. Radioactive iodine may also affect a woman's ovaries*** and some women may have irregular periods for up to a year after treatment. Many doctors recommend that women avoid becoming pregnant for 6 months to a year after treatment. No ill effects have been noted in the children born to parents who received radioactive iodine in the past"-www.cancer.org

"Radioactive strontium-89 is given intravenously (by IV) for prostate cancer and advanced bone cancer"

A Clinician's Guide to Nuclear Oncology by Naomi P. Alazrak 2007/190

Side effects: Mild myelosuppression is commonly seen, necessitating weekly monitoring for at least 8 weeks. Flares in bone pain can occur hours to days after administration. This complication is seen in less than 10% of patients. Acute leukemia has been reported as a complication of therapy.

235. Ans. b. Decreased pulmonary vascularity; d. Coeur en sabot

[Ref: Sumer Sethi 6th/80; Radiology by S. Bhadury 2nd/47;Danhert Radiology Review Manual 7th/669;Harrison 19th/1527]

Tetralogy of Fallot

◈ *Sumer Sethi 6th/80*

- ***Boot shaped heart or cor-en sabot***
- ***Pulmonary oligaemia***
- Normal size heart
- 25% association with right sided aortic arch

"**TOF:** The ECG shows RV hypertrophy. Chest x-ray shows a normal-sized, ***boot-shaped heart (coeur en sabot)*** with a prominent RV and a concavity in the region of the pulmonary conus. ***Pulmonary vascular markings are typically diminished*** and the aortic arch and knob may be on the right side"-Harrison 19th/1527

Component of TOF

◈ *Sumer Sethi 6th/80*

- VSD
- Infundibular stenosis
- Aortic root over rides the VSD
- Right ventricular hypertrophy

236. Ans. b. Silicosis; d. Berylysosis; e. Coal worker pneumoconiosis

[Ref: Sumer Sethi 6th/64; Danhert Radiology Review Manual 7th/446; Harrison 19th/1690-91; Radiological differential Diagnosis by Chapman 4th/148]

"Patients with ***silicosis and coal miner's pneumoconiosis*** often develop small (<5 mm) diffuse lung parenchymal calcified nodules, often associated with ***egg-shell calcification of hilar or mediastinal lymph nodes***"-*www.ncbi.nlm.nih.gov*

"***Silicosis: Calcification of hilar nodes*** may occur in as many as 20% of cases and produces a characteristic "eggshell" pattern. Silicotic nodules may be identified more readily by HRCT"- *Harrison 19th/1690*

"**Chronic beryllium disease:** Chest imaging findings are similar to those of sarcoidosis (nodules along septal lines) except that ***hilar adenopathy is somewhat less common***"-Harrison 19th/1690

Bilateral hilar lymphadenopathy is a bilateral enlargement of the lymph nodes of pulmonary hila. It is a radiographic term that describes the enlargement of mediastinal lymph nodes and is most commonly identified by a chest x-ray.

Egg Shell Calcification

◈ *Radiological differential Diagnosis by Chapman 4th/148; Sumer Sethi 6th/64*

- ***Silicosis: Seen in approx. 5% of silicotics, predominantly hilar lymph nodes***
- ***Coal miner's pneumoconiosis***
- Sarcoidosis
- Lymphoma following radiotherapy

237. Ans. a. Images can be readily produced in axial, sagittal or coronal without changing position of the patient; c. Blood vessel can be seen without contrast

[Ref: Sumer Sethi 6th/14-19; Radiology and Imaging by Thayalan 1st/369]

Advantageof MRI

◈ *Sumer Sethi 6th/19*

- High soft tissue contrast
- No ionizing radiation(safe in pregnancy)
- Multiplanar imaging
- Doesn't use iodinated contrast so safe in iodine allergy

The Special Feature of MRI Includes

- *Thayalan 1st/369*
- ***Imaging of blood flow without contrast***
- ***High contrast sensitivity to soft tissues differences***
- ***Inherent safety t the patients(non-ionizing radiation)***
- ***To examine anatomic and physiological properties of the patients***

The limitations of MRI Includes

- *Thayalan 1st/369*
- High equipment cast
- Scan acquisition complexity
- Long imaging time
- Image artifacts
- Patient claustrophobia

Use and Advantage of MRI

- It is a non-invasive technique
- It is safe as it does not involve the use of ionizing radiation
- Images can be ***readily produced in any plane*** *(multi planner capabilities) e.g.,* axial, sagittal or coronal ***without changing position of the patient***
- It give high intrinsic contrast
- **Lack of artefact from adjacent bones:** This make MRI the modality of choice in areas such as the posterior fossa and pituitary fossa where the quality of CT image is degraded by artefact.
- MRI is imaging modality of *choice for most brain and spine disorders*

Limitations and Disadvantage of MRI

- Very high cost of imaging
- Inability to image bone and calcium
- It is unsuitable for patients with cardiac pacemakers and other ferromagnetic implants Imaging time is long, hence movement or motion artefacts are quite likely
- Highly operator dependent, hence require technical expertise

	CT	MRI
Scope of application:	CT can outline bone inside the body very accurately.	MRI is more versatile than the X-Ray and is used to examine a large variety of medical conditions.
Application	**Suited for** bone injuries, ***Lung*** and Chest imaging, cancer detection. Widely used in Emergency Room patient.	Suited for Soft tissue evaluation, *e.g.,* ligament and tendon injury, spinal cord injury, brain tumors etc.
Details of bony structures:	Provides good details about bony structures	Less detailed compared to X-ray
Details of soft tissues:	A major advantage of CT is that it is able to image bone, soft tissue and blood vessels all at the same time.	Much higher soft tissue detail as compare to CT scan.

238. Ans. a. Silicosis; b. Sarcoidosis; c. Lymphoma after treatment; e. T.B.

[Ref: Danhert Radiology Review manual 7th/454;Sumer Sethi 6th/64;Radiology by S.Bhadury 2nd/24]

Egg Shell Calcification

- *Danhert Radiology Review manual 7th/454*
- *Silicosis*
- *Coal worker pneumoconiosis*
- *Sarcoidosis*
- *Fungal+Bacterial infection: T.B, Histoplasmosis & Coccidioidomycosis*
- *Fibrosingmediastinitis*
- *Lymphoma following radiation therapy*
- *Not seen in: Asbestosis, berylliosis, talcosis&baritosis*

239. Ans. a. Radon-222 b. Radium-226 c. Iodine-125 d. Cobalt-60 e. Cesium-137

[Ref: Sumer Sethi 6th/177-78; Prez & Brandy's Radiation Oncology 5th/54; Grainger & Allison Radiology 6th/118;Dutta Gynaecology 5th/484, 4th/465; Merdith Radiation Physics & Nuclear Medicine/28]

Internal Radiotherapy or Brachytherapy

- *Prez & Brandy's Radiation Oncology 5th/54*
- In brachytherapy, the radiation source in close contact with tumor. The principle is to use an Intra or Juxtalesional radiation implant to irradiate the tumor in vicinity.
- **Sealed source in placed with in or near the tumor** i.e., **Short distance therapy.**
- Brachytherapy may be of following types: -
  - **Interstitial:** Artificial radioactive sources are inserted directly into tumor tissues. The radioactive sources (implant)may be either temporary/removable or permanent.
  - **Intracavitary**
  - **Mould**

Table: *(Dutta gynaecology 5th/484):* **Radioisotopes commonly used in gynaecological malignancies (as brachytherapy)**

Isotope	Energy (MeV)	Half life
Cesium 137 (Cs137)	0.662	30 years
Radium 226 (Ra226)	0.8	1620 years
Cobalt 60 (Co60)	1.173	5.3 years
Iridium 192 (Ir 192)	0.47	74 days
Gold 198 (Au 198)	0.411	2.96 days
Iodine 125 (I-125)	0.027	60 days
Phosphorus 32 (P32)	0.698	14.3 days

Table: *(Sumer Sethi 6th/177)*: **Brachytherapy Source**

Radionuclide	Radiation Emitted	Energy	Half-line
Radium-226	Gamma rays	1 MeV	1620 years
Caesium-137	Gamma rays	0.66 MeV	30 years

Contd...

Radionuclide	Radiation Emitted	Energy	Half-line
Cobalt-60	Gamma rays	1.25 MeV	5.26 years
Iridium-192	Gamma rays	0.4 MeV	74 days
Gold-198	Gamma rays	0.41 MeV	2.7 days
Strontium-90	Beta rays	2.27 MeV max	28.1 years
Yttrium-90	Beta rays	2.27 MeV max	64 hours

Intracavitary: Artificial radioactive sources are inserted into natural body cavities. **Most important use of intracavitary radiation is in patients with the cancer of the cervix after external radiation.** It is also used in cancer of ***uterus,esophageal cancer and lung cancer.***

Table: Intracavitary

Removable	Permanent
Radium	Colloidal radioactive gold
Cesium-137	Yttrium
Cobalt-60	Radioactive iodine (131_I)

240. Ans. b. Samarium-153; c. Phosphorus-32; e. Strontium-89;

[Ref: Sumer Sethi 6th/184;MD Anderson Manual of Medical Oncology/ Chap 41;Radiation Oncology 8th/141]

Metastatic Bone Pain

◈ *Radiation Oncology 8th/141*

- Bone metastases manifest through pain, which can arise even before the injury is radiologically detected. Relief of pain from bone metastasis can be achieved by treating the cancer itself; radiotherapy; conventional analgesics (NSAIDs opioids) and Bisphosphonates and calcitonin; and **bone-seeking radiopharmaceuticals.**
- Radiopharmaceuticals (radioactive isotopes) used for metastatic bone pain are **strontium** (Sr^{89}), **Samarium** (**Sm^{153}**), **rhenium** (**Re^{186}**), Phosphorus-32 and Tin-117 (Sn-177)
- "In refractory pain situations, drugs from other classes have been tried; some have been tried with a good response and others with only a minimal response. They include: psychotropic drugs, benzodiazepines, bisphosphonates, steroids (in spinal cord compression), lidocaine, intravenous and patch (39–41), ketamine (42,43), capsaicin (44) and radiopharmaceuticals (strontium 89, samarium)"-*MD Anderson Manual of Medical Oncology/Chap 41*

Table *(Sumer Sethi 6th/184)*: **Systemic radionuceotide for treatment of bone metastases**

Radionuclide	Half-Life	Emission	Energy (MeV)	Status
Phosphorus 32 (32P)	14.2 days	Beta	1.71	Approved
Strontium 89 (89Sr)	50.6 days	Beta	1.492	Approved
Samarium 153 (153Sm)	*46.3 hours*	Gamma	0.81	Approved 0.10
Rhenium 186 (186Re)	90.6 hours	Beta Gamma	1.071 0.131	Investigational
Rhenium 188 (188Re)	16.7 hours	Beta	2.116	Investigational

241. Ans. a. Amifostine; d. Pentoxiphylline;

[Ref: Sumer Sethi 6th/183; Devita 7th/275-76;Oxford Oncology 2nd/462; Harrison 20th/482]

Radioprotective *(Sumer Sethi 6th/183)*

- **Amifostine**
- *IL-1, GM –CSF*
- *keratinocyte growth factor*
- *Zinc oxide*
- *Pentoxiphylline*
- *Etramustine*
- *Potassium iodide*
- *Melatonin*
- *Chlorhexidine*
- *Antioxidants (Vitamin C, E & A)*

"Radiation causes breaks in DNA and generates free radicals from cell water that may damage cell membranes, proteins and organelles. *Radiation damage is augmented dependent on only oxygen; hypoxemic cells are more resistant.* Augmentation of oxygen is the basis for radiation sensitization. Sulfhydryl compounds interfere with free radical generation and may act as radiation protectors. Most radiation-induced cell damage is due to the formation of hydroxyl radicals"-Harrison 20th/482

Radiosensitizers *(Sumer Sethi 6th/183; Oxford Oncology 2nd/462)*

I. Hypoxic cell radiosensitizers

1. Hyperbaric oxygen (most potent)
2. Nitroimidazoles: **Metronidazole, Misonidazole**, Etanidazole, Nimorazole, Pimonidazole
3. Anticancers: **Actinomycin D (Dactinomycin)**, Bleomycin, Cisplatin, Doxorubicin, **5-FU,** Fludarabine, Gemcitabine, **Hydroxyurea**, Paclitaxel, itomycin-C, Topotecan, Vinorelbine.

Contd...

II Non hypoxic cell radiosensitizers

1. *Haloginatedpyrimidines:* **BUdR**, IUdR.

Note: *Cisplatin and 5-FU are two of the most commonly used* radiosensitizing agents.

Radioprotectors

◈ *Oxford Oncology 2nd/462*

- Radioprotectors are compounds that can protect oxygenated (not tumor) cells while having a limited effect on hypoxic (tumor)cells. This selective action serves to increase the therapeutic ratio by promoting the repair of irradiated normal tissues. Repairtakes place through the chemical ***process of reduction.***
- Free electrons are captured byradioprotectivesubstance, renderingthemunavailable to participate in further chen1ical reactions that might lead to cellular damage.
- The sulfhydryl (SH) groups contained in the non-protein fraction of most cells aid in the reduction process followingradiation damage. **Thiophosphate compounds (such as cysteine and cysteamine)** containing SH groups were among theearliest radioprotector synthesized.

ANSWER SHEET

1 – 50					
1	A	B	C	D	E
2	A	B	C	D	E
3	A	B	C	D	E
4	A	B	C	D	E
5	A	B	C	D	E
6	A	B	C	D	E
7	A	B	C	D	E
8	A	B	C	D	E
9	A	B	C	D	E
10	A	B	C	D	E
11	A	B	C	D	E
12	A	B	C	D	E
13	A	B	C	D	E
14	A	B	C	D	E
15	A	B	C	D	E
16	A	B	C	D	E
17	A	B	C	D	E
18	A	B	C	D	E
19	A	B	C	D	E
20	A	B	C	D	E
21	A	B	C	D	E
22	A	B	C	D	E
23	A	B	C	D	E
24	A	B	C	D	E
25	A	B	C	D	E
26	A	B	C	D	E
27	A	B	C	D	E
28	A	B	C	D	E
29	A	B	C	D	E
30	A	B	C	D	E
31	A	B	C	D	E
32	A	B	C	D	E
33	A	B	C	D	E
34	A	B	C	D	E
35	A	B	C	D	E
36	A	B	C	D	E
37	A	B	C	D	E
38	A	B	C	D	E
39	A	B	C	D	E
40	A	B	C	D	E
41	A	B	C	D	E
42	A	B	C	D	E
43	A	B	C	D	E
44	A	B	C	D	E
45	A	B	C	D	E
46	A	B	C	D	E
47	A	B	C	D	E
48	A	B	C	D	E
49	A	B	C	D	E
50	A	B	C	D	E

51 – 100					
51	A	B	C	D	E
52	A	B	C	D	E
53	A	B	C	D	E
54	A	B	C	D	E
55	A	B	C	D	E
56	A	B	C	D	E
57	A	B	C	D	E
58	A	B	C	D	E
59	A	B	C	D	E
60	A	B	C	D	E
61	A	B	C	D	E
62	A	B	C	D	E
63	A	B	C	D	E
64	A	B	C	D	E
65	A	B	C	D	E
66	A	B	C	D	E
67	A	B	C	D	E
68	A	B	C	D	E
69	A	B	C	D	E
70	A	B	C	D	E
71	A	B	C	D	E
72	A	B	C	D	E
73	A	B	C	D	E
74	A	B	C	D	E
75	A	B	C	D	E
76	A	B	C	D	E
77	A	B	C	D	E
78	A	B	C	D	E
79	A	B	C	D	E
80	A	B	C	D	E
81	A	B	C	D	E
82	A	B	C	D	E
83	A	B	C	D	E
84	A	B	C	D	E
85	A	B	C	D	E
86	A	B	C	D	E
87	A	B	C	D	E
88	A	B	C	D	E
89	A	B	C	D	E
90	A	B	C	D	E
91	A	B	C	D	E
92	A	B	C	D	E
93	A	B	C	D	E
94	A	B	C	D	E
95	A	B	C	D	E
96	A	B	C	D	E
97	A	B	C	D	E
98	A	B	C	D	E
99	A	B	C	D	E
100	A	B	C	D	E

101 – 150					
101	A	B	C	D	E
102	A	B	C	D	E
103	A	B	C	D	E
104	A	B	C	D	E
105	A	B	C	D	E
106	A	B	C	D	E
107	A	B	C	D	E
108	A	B	C	D	E
109	A	B	C	D	E
110	A	B	C	D	E
111	A	B	C	D	E
112	A	B	C	D	E
113	A	B	C	D	E
114	A	B	C	D	E
115	A	B	C	D	E
116	A	B	C	D	E
117	A	B	C	D	E
118	A	B	C	D	E
119	A	B	C	D	E
120	A	B	C	D	E
121	A	B	C	D	E
122	A	B	C	D	E
123	A	B	C	D	E
124	A	B	C	D	E
125	A	B	C	D	E
126	A	B	C	D	E
127	A	B	C	D	E
128	A	B	C	D	E
129	A	B	C	D	E
130	A	B	C	D	E
131	A	B	C	D	E
132	A	B	C	D	E
133	A	B	C	D	E
134	A	B	C	D	E
135	A	B	C	D	E
136	A	B	C	D	E
137	A	B	C	D	E
138	A	B	C	D	E
139	A	B	C	D	E
140	A	B	C	D	E
141	A	B	C	D	E
142	A	B	C	D	E
143	A	B	C	D	E
144	A	B	C	D	E
145	A	B	C	D	E
146	A	B	C	D	E
147	A	B	C	D	E
148	A	B	C	D	E
149	A	B	C	D	E
150	A	B	C	D	E

151 – 200					
151	A	B	C	D	E
152	A	B	C	D	E
153	A	B	C	D	E
154	A	B	C	D	E
155	A	B	C	D	E
156	A	B	C	D	E
157	A	B	C	D	E
158	A	B	C	D	E
159	A	B	C	D	E
160	A	B	C	D	E
161	A	B	C	D	E
162	A	B	C	D	E
163	A	B	C	D	E
164	A	B	C	D	E
165	A	B	C	D	E
166	A	B	C	D	E
167	A	B	C	D	E
168	A	B	C	D	E
169	A	B	C	D	E
170	A	B	C	D	E
171	A	B	C	D	E
172	A	B	C	D	E
173	A	B	C	D	E
174	A	B	C	D	E
175	A	B	C	D	E
176	A	B	C	D	E
177	A	B	C	D	E
178	A	B	C	D	E
179	A	B	C	D	E
180	A	B	C	D	E
181	A	B	C	D	E
182	A	B	C	D	E
183	A	B	C	D	E
184	A	B	C	D	E
185	A	B	C	D	E
186	A	B	C	D	E
187	A	B	C	D	E
188	A	B	C	D	E
189	A	B	C	D	E
190	A	B	C	D	E
191	A	B	C	D	E
192	A	B	C	D	E
193	A	B	C	D	E
194	A	B	C	D	E
195	A	B	C	D	E
196	A	B	C	D	E
197	A	B	C	D	E
198	A	B	C	D	E
199	A	B	C	D	E
200	A	B	C	D	E

201 – 250					
201	A	B	C	D	E
202	A	B	C	D	E
203	A	B	C	D	E
204	A	B	C	D	E
205	A	B	C	D	E
206	A	B	C	D	E
207	A	B	C	D	E
208	A	B	C	D	E
209	A	B	C	D	E
210	A	B	C	D	E
211	A	B	C	D	E
212	A	B	C	D	E
213	A	B	C	D	E
214	A	B	C	D	E
215	A	B	C	D	E
216	A	B	C	D	E
217	A	B	C	D	E
218	A	B	C	D	E
219	A	B	C	D	E
220	A	B	C	D	E
221	A	B	C	D	E
222	A	B	C	D	E
223	A	B	C	D	E
224	A	B	C	D	E
225	A	B	C	D	E
226	A	B	C	D	E
227	A	B	C	D	E
228	A	B	C	D	E
229	A	B	C	D	E
230	A	B	C	D	E
231	A	B	C	D	E
232	A	B	C	D	E
233	A	B	C	D	E
234	A	B	C	D	E
235	A	B	C	D	E
236	A	B	C	D	E
237	A	B	C	D	E
238	A	B	C	D	E
239	A	B	C	D	E
240	A	B	C	D	E
241	A	B	C	D	E
242	A	B	C	D	E
243	A	B	C	D	E
244	A	B	C	D	E
245	A	B	C	D	E
246	A	B	C	D	E
247	A	B	C	D	E
248	A	B	C	D	E
249	A	B	C	D	E
250	A	B	C	D	E

NAME OF THE CANDIDATE	ROLL NO.	CENTRE NO.	QUESTION BOOKLET NO.	BOOKLET CODE
CATEGORY SC ○ ST ○ OBC ○ GEN ○ CW ○ PH ○	0 0 0 0 0 1 1 1 1 1 2 2 2 2 2 3 3 3 3 3 4 4 4 4 4 5 5 5 5 5 6 6 6 6 6 7 7 7 7 7 8 8 8 8 8 9 9 9 9 9	0 0 1 1 2 2 3 3 4 4 5 5 6 6 7 7 8 8 9 9	0 0 0 0 0 1 1 1 1 1 2 2 2 2 2 3 3 3 3 3 4 4 4 4 4 5 5 5 5 5 6 6 6 6 6 7 7 7 7 7 8 8 8 8 8 9 9 9 9 9	A B C D

INSTRUCTIONS FOR FILLING THE SHEET

1. This sheet should not be folded or crushed.
2. Use only blue/black ball pen to fill the circles.
3. Use of pencil is strictly prohibited.
4. Circles should be darkened properly and completely.
5. Cutting & erasing on this sheet is not allowed.
6. Do not use any stray marks on the sheet.
7. Do not use marker, white fluid or any other device to hide the shading already done.

WRONG METHOD

CORRECT METHOD

CANDIDATE'S SIGNATURE
(in ball - point pen)

INVIGILATOR'S SIGNATURE
(in ball - point pen)

MAY

2017

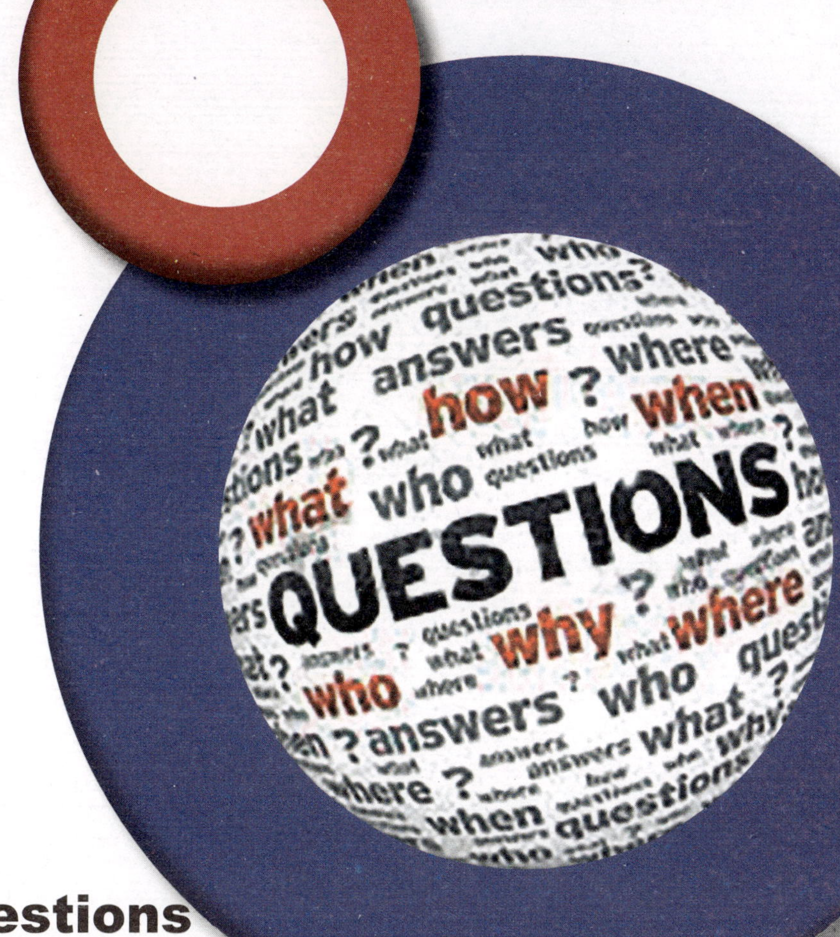

Multiple Choice Questions
Answers & Explanations

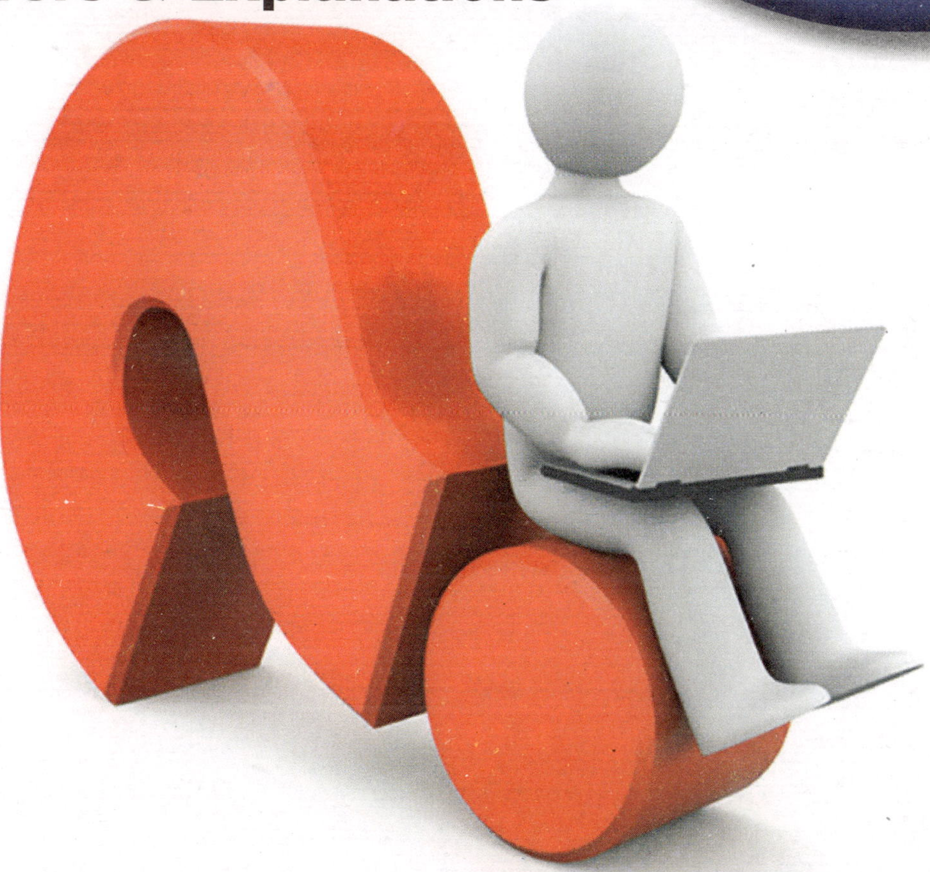

MAY 2017 MULTIPLE CHOICE QUESTIONS

ANATOMY

1. **Taste sensation from the tongue is/are carried by:**
   a. Facial nerve
   b. Glossopharyngeal nerve c. Hypoglossal nerve
   d. Vagus nerve e. Trigeminal nerve
2. **Which of the following statement(s) is/are true about phrenic nerve except:**
   a. It is primary motor supply to diaphragm
   b. Accessory phrenic nerve joins the phrenic nerve near the first rib
   c. Formed in front of scalenus medius muscle
   d. It descends posterior to sternocleidomastoid
   e. Gives sensory supply to central tendon of diaphragm
3. **True statement about shoulder joint:**
   a. Multipennate acromial fibres of deltoid are powerful abductor
   b. Axillary nerve injury has no effect on abduction
   c. Musculotendinous cuff stabilizes shoulder joint
   d. Supraspinatus initiates abduction
   e. Trapezius and serratus anterior act synergistically in abduction
4. **All are supplied by anterior interosseus nerve except:**
   a. Flexor carpi ulnaris b. Brachioradialis
   c. Abductor pollicis brevis d. Flexor pollicis longus
   e. Flexor digitorum superficialis
5. **All are true about parotid except:**
   a. 2nd largest salivary gland
   b. Stenson's duct opens into the vestibule of the mouth opposite 3rd upper molar
   c. Divided into superficial and deep lobes by facial nerve
   d. Majority of lymph nodes are embedded in deep lobe
   e. Deep lobe abscess can extend into parapharyngeal space
6. **True about epiglottis:**
   a. Contains serous gland
   b. Contains mucous secreting glands
   c. It is oval shaped
   d. Made up of elastic cartilage
   e. Has bilateral lymphatic supply
7. **True about Thyroid gland:**
   a. Thyroid lies in between 2 layers of deep cervical fascia
   b. Berry ligament derived from deep cervical fascia
   c. Left recurrent laryngeal nerve is larger than right recurrent laryngeal nerve
   d. Superior thyroid artery runs in close relation with superior laryngeal nerve
   e. The superior parathyroid glands are usually located ventral to the recurrent laryngeal nerve
8. **Which is attached most anteriorly on the intercondylar area of tibia (area b/w medial and lateral tibial plateau):**
   a. Anterior cruciate ligament
   b. Posterior cruciate ligament
   c. Anterior horn of the lateral meniscus
   d. Anterior horn of the medial meniscus
   e. Ligamentum patellae
9. **True about meiosis-I:**
   a. Homologous chromosomes separate
   b. Sister chromatids separate
   c. Haploid daughter cells
   d. Homologous chromosomes exchange material
   e. Sister chromatids replicate
10. **True about fibrous skeleton of heart:**
    a. Tendon of Todaro is between central fibrous parts to Eustachian valve
    b. Tendon of infundibulum is between pulmonary & aortic valve
    c. Trigonum fibrous dextrum is between mitral & tricuspid valve
    d. Trigonum fibrous sinistrum is between mitral and aortic valve
    e. Fibrous ring around mitral valve

PHYSIOLOGY

11. **Congenital adrenal hyperplasia is due to deficiency of enzyme:**
    a. 3β-Hydroxysteroid dehydrogenase deficiency
    b. 5α Reductase
    c. 17α-Hydroxylase deficiency
    d. 21-Hydroxylase deficiency
    e. Aromatase
12. **Which of the following is/are effect of increased 2,3-DPG on oxygen-hemoglobin dissociation curve:**
    a. ↑ed affinity of haemoglobin to oxygen
    b. ↓ed affinity of haemoglobin to oxygen
    c. Left shift of oxygen-hemoglobin dissociation curve
    d. Right shift of oxygen-hemoglobin dissociation curve
    e. No change in oxygen-hemoglobin dissociation curve
13. **Oxygen consumption by the heart is determined by:**
    a. Intramyocardial tension
    b. Contractile state of the myocardium
    c. Initial length of the myocardial muscle fiber
    d. Heart rate
    e. Basal oxygen consumption of myocardium

Answer

1.	a, b, d.	2.	c.	3.	a, c, d, e.	4.	a, b, c, e.	5.	a, b, d.	6.	b, d, e.	7.	a, b, c.
8.	d.	9.	a, c, d.	10.	a, b, d, e.	11.	a, c, d.	12.	b, d.	13.	All (a, b, c, d, e)		

14. True statement about male reproductive physiology:
a. Sertoli cells secrete Müllerian inhibiting substance (MIS)
b. Inhibin is released by sertoli cell
c. Primary spermatocyte is diploid
d. LH and FSH are steroidal in nature
e. Inhibin stimulates follicle-stimulating hormone (FSH)

15. Insulin causes intracellular shift of which of the following ion:
a. Na^+
b. K^+
c. Chloride
d. Calcium
e. Bicarbonate

16. Hypothalmic pituitary axis (HPA) controls all except:
a. Thyroid
b. Parathyroid
c. Pancreas
d. Testis
e. Adrenals

17. Stress hyperglycemia occurs due to all except:
a. Increased level of ACTH
b. Increased level of Cortisol
c. Decreased level of norepinephrine
d. Insulin resistance
e. Increased level of epinephrine

18. Erythropoietin is/are produced by:
a. Juxtaglomerular cells
b. Interstitial cells of the peritubular capillary bed of the kidneys
c. Pars recta of PCT
d. Macula densa
e. Mesangial cell

19. True about carotid sinus:
a. Chemoreceptor
b. Present in early part of internal carotid artery
c. Has glomus cells
d. Barorecptor
e. Supplied by glossopharyngeal nerve

BIOCHEMISTRY

20. Mechanisms for regulating enzyme activity is/are:
a. Covalent modification
b. Allosteric activation
c. Competitive inhibition
d. Induction of genes for enzyme synthesis
e. Repression of gene for inhibition of enzyme synthesis

21. All are true about glycosaminoglycans except:
a. Protein associated with glycosaminoglycans is called core proteins
b. May be associated with connective tissues
c. Highly positively charged
d. Negatively charged
e. Component of ECM

22. All are true about Hexose monophosphate pathway (HMP) except:
a. Produce NADPH in oxidative phase of pathway
b. Does not produce ATP
c. Occurs in testes, ovaries, placenta and adrenal cortex
d. Produces ribose 5-phosphate in oxidative phase of pathway
e. Glucose 6-phosphatase dehydrogenase enzyme is involved

23. Not useful in laboratory diagnosis of diabetic ketoacidosis (DKA):
a. Plasma ketones
b. Blood glucose
c. Urine ketones
d. Anion gap
e. Blood pH

24. Gluconeogenesis is favoured in fasting state by:
a. Activation of pyruvate carboxylase by acetyl CoA
b. Increased conversion of phosphoenol pyruvate to pyruvate by activation of pyruvate kinase
c. Increased fatty acid oxidation in liver
d. Hydrolysis of fructose 1, 6-bisphosphate by fructose 1, 6-bisphosphatase

25. Which is/are feature(s) of prostaglandins:
a. 20 carbon atom compound
b. 10 carbon atom compound
c. Cyclopentane ring
d. -OH group at 15th position
e. Trans double bond at 10th position

26. True statement(s) about lipid digestion and absorption:
a. Micelles play an important role in lipids absorption
b. Absorption of long-chain fatty acids is greatest in the upper parts of the small intestine
c. Bile acid has no role in fat absorption
d. Fatty acids after absorption are reesterified to triglycerides in the enterocytes

27. True statement are:
a. All lipid are fat
b. Linoleic acid is essential fatty acid
c. Hydrogenation converts unsaturated fatty acid to saturated fatty acid
d. Rancidity of food is due to lipid peroxidation
e. Hydrolysis of fat by acid is saponification

IMMUNOGENETICS & MOLECULAR BIOLOGY

28. Which of the following is/are pyrimidine(s):
a. Adenine
b. Cytosine
c. Uracil
d. Thymine
e. Guanine

MCQs

Answer

14. a, b, c.	15. b.	16. b, c.	17. c.	18. b.	19. b, d, e.	20. All.
21. c.	22. d.	23. None.	24. a, c, d.	25. a, c, d.	26. a, b, d.	27. b, c, d.
28. b, c, d						

29. True about telomerase:
a. It has reverse transcriptase activity
b. DNA-dependent RNA polymerase
c. Help in DNA replication at end of lagging strand
d. Also called terminal transferase

30. True about DNA Gyrase:
a. A type of topoisomerase I
b. A type of topoisomerase II
c. Act on circular DNA
d. Overcome the problem of supercoils

31. Ultraviolet radiation exposure can causes DNA damage by:
a. Pyrimidine dimers formation
b. DNA breakage
c. Thymine dimer formation
d. Acetylation of DNA
e. Methylation of DNA

32. Post-translation modification of protein includes all except:
a. Removal of peptide
b. 5' capping
c. Intein splicing
d. Protein folding
e. Covalent modification

33. Which of the following is not true about transcription:
a. Synthesis of precursors for the large and small ribosomal RNAs
b. Formation of tRNA transcript
c. RNA polymerase II is responsible for the synthesis of precursors for the large ribosomal RNAs
d. RNA polymerase I is responsible for the synthesis small ribosomal RNAs
e. Binding of RNA polymerase on DNA

34. True about DNA photolyase:
a. Repair damage caused by UV light
b. Found only in human
c. Use visible light
d. Breaks pyrimidine dimer

PATHOLOGY

35. PAX5 is/are marker for:
a. Acute myeloid leukemia
b. T-cell lymphomas
c. Anaplastic large cell lymphoma
d. Hodgkin's lymphoma
e. B-Lymphoblastic lymphoma

36. Which of the following is/are associated with synovial cell sarcoma:
a. Translocation (9;22) (q34;q11)
b. SS18-SSX4 fusion genes
c. Translocation t (X;18) (p11;q11)
d. SS18-SSX1 fusion genes

37. True about Dubin-Johnson syndrome:
a. ↑ed conjugated bilirubin
b. Usually associated with increased AST and ALT
c. Mutation in Uridine diphosphate-glucuronyltransferase peptide A1
d. Decreased biliary excretion of conjugated bilirubin
e. Autosomal dominant inheritance

38. Tumor marker for lung adenocarcinoma is/are:
a. Positive for cytokeratin 5
b. Positive for cytokeratin 7
c. Positive for cytokeratin 20
d. Transthyretin (TTR) mutation
e. EGFR mutation

39. Newer inclusion in 2015 WHO classification of Squamous cell carcinoma of lung include(s):
a. Clear cell variant
b. Papillary cell variant
c. Adenocarcinoma variant
d. Nonkeratinizing variant
e. Lymphoepithelioma-like carcinoma

40. True about RAS oncogene:
a. Tyrosine kinase has role in RAS activation
b. Most common form of oncogene in human tumors
c. It has an intrinsic GTPase activity
d. Mutation may result in carcinomatous growth
e. Belongs to growth factor category of oncogene

41. Which is/are not tumor suppressor gene(s):
a. TP53
b. RB
c. CD95
d. SKT11
e. RAS

42. Which of the following dyad of disease and inheritance pattern is/are true:
a. Sickle cell anaemia - autosomal recessive
b. Duchene muscle dystrophy- X-linked dominant
c. Vit D resistant rickets- X-linked dominant
d. Achondroplasia – autosomal dominant
e. Osteogenesis Imperfecta - autosomal recessive

43. True about Autosomal recessive polycystic kidney disease (ARPKD)
a. Can be diagnosed in utero by USG
b. Hypertension develops in late stages of the disease
c. May proceed to renal failure before preschool age
d. Enlargement of kidney
e. Hematuria is early feature

44. Multiple myeloma may be associated with:
a. Fanconi's syndrome
b. Amyloidosis
c. Mixed cryoglobinemia
d. Cast nephropathy
e. Interstitial nephritis

Answer

29. a, c, d.	30. b, c, d.	31. a, c.	32. b.	33. c, d.	34. a, c, d.	35. d, e.
36. b, c, d.	37. a, d.	38. b, e	39. d.	40. a, b, c, d.	41. c, e.	42. a, c, d.
43. a, b, c, d	44. All (a, b, c, d, e)					

45. True statement about primary myelofibrosis:
a. Hepatomegaly is the most common manifestation
b. Dry tap on bone marrow aspiration
c. Only potentially curative treatment is allogeneic stem cell transplantation
d. Splenomegaly is almost invariably present
e. Myeloblasts may be seen in peripheral blood

46. Which of the following can cause pulmonary embolism:
a. Pregnancy
b. OCP uses
c. Mitral regurgitation
d. Left ventricular failure
e. Excessive unaccustomed exercise

47. Most common translocation in acute promyelocytic leukemia (APML) is:
a. t (8:14)
b. t (9:22)
c. t (15:17)
d. t (8:21)
e. t (11:118)

48. Which of the following acute phase protein(s) decreases during acute inflammation:
a. Albumin
b. Transferrin
c. Ceruloplasmin
d. C-reactive protein
e. Haptoglobin

49. Which of the following is/are true about sideroblastic anaemia:
a. Basophils stippling in lead poisoning
b. Erythroid hypoplasia in bone marrow
c. Pappenheimer bodies is always present
d. Dimorphic RBC
e. Increased MCHC

50. Feature(s) of Type I membranoproliferative glomerulonephritis (MPGN):
a. Tram track appearance on light microscopy
b. Subendothelial electron-dense deposits on electron microscopy
c. Immunofluorescence microscopy show positive florescence of IgG and C3 on dense deposit
d. Intramembranous dense deposit on electron microscopy
e. Mesangial hypocellularity

51. True statement about asbestosis:
a. May involve hilar lymph node
b. Asbestosis begins in the lower lobes
c. Pleural plaques consists of calcified hyalinzed collagenous tissue
d. High resolution CT scanning is the best imaging method
e. No risk of lung carcinoma

52. True about silicosis:
a. Lower lobe is more commonly involved
b. Radiographically seen as eggshell calcification
c. Lobar pneumonia is common
d. Associated with an increased susceptibility to tuberculosis
e. Histologically silica nodules consists of hyalinised center surrounded by concentric laminations of collagen

53. Small vessel vasculitis is/are:
a. Kawasaki disease
b. IgA vasculitis
c. Carcinoma associated vasculitis
d. Anti–glomerular basement membrane (anti-GBM) disease
e. Takayasu arteritis

54. Feature(s) of antiphospholipid syndrome is/are except:
a. Recurrent thrombosis
b. SLE is associated with primary antiphospholipid syndrome
c. It includes two types of antibodies—lupus anticoagulant and anticardiolipin antibody
d. Foetus loss may occur
e. Occur d/t defect in prostacyclin metabolism

55. Prolongation of both— activated partial thromboplastin time (aPTT) and prothrombin time (PT) may be seen in factor deficiency of:
a. Factor 2
b. Factor 5
c. Factor 10
d. Factor 8
e. Factor 9

56. True about haematological disorder:
a. Cryoprecipitate is used in treatment in haemophilia B
b. Both PT and aPTT are increased in DIC
c. Intravenous gamma globulin is useful in immune thrombocytopenic purpura
d. Hemophilia C: X-linked disorder
e. Platelet count is decreased in DIC

57. Cancer(s) caused by viral infections:
a. Kaposi sarcoma
b. Nasopharyngeal carcinoma
c. Hepatocellular cancer
d. Hodgkin's lymphoma

58. Most common aneuploidy compatible with life is:
a. Down syndrome
b. Turner syndrome
c. Klinefelter's syndrome
d. Patau syndrome

59. Feature(s) of Turner syndrome is/are:
a. It is the aneuploidy compatible with life
b. Tall stature
c. High hairline
d. Causes miscarriage in early weeks of gestation
e. Wide chest

60. Inflammatory odontogenic cyst is/are:
a. Periapical cyst
b. Residual cyst
c. Paradental cyst
d. Eruption cyst
e. Dentigerous cyst

Answer

45. b, c, d, e.	46. a, b, d, e.	47. c.	48. a, b.	49. a, d.	50. a, b, c.	51. a, b, c, d.
52. b, d, e.	53. b, c, d.	54. b, e.	55. a, b, c.	56. b, c, e.	57. All.	58. a.
59. a, d, e.	60. a, b, c					

61. **True about prostaglandins:**
   a. Derived from lipooxygenase pathway
   b. First product is PGG2
   c. PG E2 causes vasoconstriction
   d. PG F2α causes bronchoconstriction
   e. PG I2 causes fall in BP

PHARMACOLOGY

62. **Drugs affecting purine synthesis:**
   a. Azathioprine
   b. Methotrexate
   c. Fludarabine
   d. 6-Mercaptopurine
   e. Capecitabine
63. **Methotrexate affects:**
   a. Purine synthesis
   b. Pyrimidine synthesis
   c. Conversion of DHFA to THFA
   d. Polymerization of mitotic tubule
64. **Drug of choice for Strongyloides stercoralis:**
   a. Mebendazole
   b. Albendazole
   c. Ivermectin
   d. Levamisole
   e. Diethylcarbamazine
65. **Which of the following drugs can be used in rifampicin-resistance Leprosy:**
   a. Rifapentine
   b. Moxifloxacin
   c. Clofazimine
   d. Minocycline
   e. Clarithromycin
66. **Long acting β agonist(s) which is/are used as once a day drug:**
   a. Salmeterol
   b. Formoterol
   c. Olodaterol
   d. Vilanterol
   e. Indacaterol
67. **Long acting Insulin is/are:**
   a. Lispro
   b. Detemir
   c. Glargine
   d. Isophane
   e. Glulisine
68. **DOC for mycoplasma is/are:**
   a. Doxycycline
   b. Ceftriaxone
   c. Azithromycin
   d. Penicillin
   e. Gentamycin
69. **Which of the following statement(s) is/are true about hepatotoxic drugs except:**
   a. Paracetamol toxicity is not dose dependent
   b. Tetracycline can cause liver toxicity in high dose
   c. Multiple exposure of halothane is important risk factor for halothane hepatitis
   d. Rifampicin cause hepatitis
   e. Chlorpropazine can cause cholestatic jaundice
70. **Which of the following is true about aminoglycoside associated acute kidney injury:**
   a. Seen in around 10-20% of patients treated with the drug
   b. May occur within 1 week of initiation of treatment
   c. Occur only after 3 weeks of treatment
   d. Interstitial nephritis occurs
   e. Usually develops within 72 hours of initiation of treatment
71. **Which of the following is true about antifungal drugs:**
   a. Echinocandins have very less side effects
   b. Flucanazole is first line drug for invasive aspergillosis
   c. Oral fluconazole has 100 % bioavailability
   d. Amphotericin B is fungistatic
   e. Nephrotoxicity is dose limiting side effect of amphotericin B
72. **Which of the following is/are not 5th generation Cephalosporin:**
   a. Cefoxitin
   b. Cefoperazone
   c. Ceftolozane
   d. Ceftaroline
   e. Ceftabiprole
73. **Which of the following drugs is excreted mainly by kidney:**
   a. Tetracycline
   b. Rifampicin
   c. Digoxin
   d. Penicillin
   e. Lithium
74. **Which of the following anti-tumor drug have high risk of gonadotoxicity:**
   a. Dactinomycin
   b. Cyclophosphamide
   c. Busulfan
   d. Vinblastine
   e. Ifosfamide
75. **Among ACE inhibitors, which of the following is/are prodrug(s):**
   a. Perindopril
   b. Captopril
   c. Lisinopril
   d. Ramipril
   e. Enalapril
76. **True statement(s) about albendazole:**
   a. Undergoes first-pass metabolism in the liver
   b. Active against both larva and adult of Nematodes
   c. Absorption increases with fatty meal
   d. Excreted in the urine
   e. Thiabendazole is less toxic than albendazole
77. **Which of the following dyad of anti-HIV drug and mechanism of action is/are correctly matched:**
   a. Maraviroc—Entry inhibitor
   b. Raltegravir—Intergase inhibitor
   c. Indinavir—Protease inhibitor
   d. Nevirapine - Nonnucleoside reverse transcriptase inhibitor
   e. Darunavir—Fusion inhibitor
78. **Drug(s) causing QT interval prolongation:**
   a. Amiodarone
   b. Cisapride
   c. Calcium gluconate
   d. Magnesium therapy
   e. Ketoconazole

Answer

61. b, d, e. 62. a, b, c, d. 63. a, c. 64. c. 65. all (a,b, c, d, e). 66. c, d, e. 67. b, c.
68. a, c. 69. a. 70. a, b. 71. a, e. 72. a, b 73. a, c, d, e. 74. b, c, e.
75. a, d, e 76. a, b, c, d 77. b, c, d 78. a, b

79. Anti-influenza drug which is/are given through inhalation route:
- a. Amantadine
- b. Oseltamivir
- c. Zanamivir
- d. Rimantadine

80. Adrenaline can be used in:
- a. Bronchial asthma
- b. Allergic disorder
- c. Cardio-pulmonary resuscitation
- d. Anaphylaxis
- e. As anti-analgesic medicine

81. Which of the following is true statement(s) about codeine:
- a. Used as anti-tussive agent
- b. Analgesic potency is equivalent to morphine
- c. Causes respiratory depression
- d. Partly metabolized to morphine
- e. Completely metabolized to morphine

82. Which of the following is/are true about First order kinetics:
- a. Applied to majority of drugs
- b. Rate of elimination is directly proportional to the drug concentration
- c. Very few drug follow it
- d. Clearance decreases with increase in concentration

MICROBIOLOGY

83. Which of the following is true about Malaria:
- a. Chloroquine resistance occurs in India
- b. Relapses is usual for vivax and ovale malaria
- c. Sexual cycle occurs in mosquito
- d. Not a public problem in India

84. Barrel shaped eggs is/are seen in:
- a. Hook worm
- b. Roundworm
- c. Pin worm
- d. Whipworm
- e. Strongyloides stercoralis

85. Which of the following dyad of disease and incubation period is/are correctly matched:
- a. Measles: 4-5 day
- b. Chicken pox: 3-20 day
- c. Bubonic plague: 2-5 day
- d. Leptospirosis: 4-20 days
- e. Hepatitis A: 45-180 day

86. True about Human papilloma virus:
- a. Belongs to family papovaviridae
- b. DNA virus
- c. RNA virus
- d. Enveloped
- e. Causes anal warts

87. All are true about Ebola virus infection except:
- a. Air droplet is most common mode of transmission
- b. Haemorrhagic manifestation may occur
- c. Thai forest type – most common species in epidemics
- d. Presents as sudden onset of fever and sore throat
- e. Case fatality rate may be high as 70%

88. Which of the following is/are Tick-borne disease:
- a. Murine typhus
- b. Epidemic typhus
- c. Lyme's disease
- d. Tularemia
- e. Trench fever

89. True about Actinomycosis:
- a. Caused by madurella mycetomatis
- b. Caused by anaerobic or microaerophilic bacteria
- c. Cervicofacial is the most common site affected
- d. Sulphur granules are present in lesion
- e. Actinomyces is non-acid fast

90. Not true about Donovanosis:
- a. Caused by Klebsiella granulomatis
- b. Associated with pseudobuboes
- c. Caused by Leishmania donovani
- d. Drug of choice is Miltefosine
- e. Drug of choice is sodium stibogluconate

91. Organism(s) commonly causing infection in cystic fibrosis patients:
- a. Burkholderia cepacia
- b. Pseudomonas aeruginosa
- c. Staphylococcus aureus
- d. Burkhodeleria pseduomallei
- e. Streptococus pyogenes

92. Antigen presenting cell(s) is/are:
- a. Skin langerhans cell
- b. T-lymphocytes
- c. Macrophages
- d. Kuffer cell
- e. Thymic epithelial cells

93. Dimorphic fungi is/are:
- a. Histoplasma capsulatum
- b. Sporothrix schenckii
- c. Malassezia furfur
- d. Cryptococcus neoformans
- e. Aspergillus

94. Which of the following is/are true about sand fly:
- a. Breed on overhead tanks
- b. Smaller than mosquito
- c. Female fly does not bites
- d. Don't fly by choice

Answer

79. c.	80. a, b, c, d.	81. a, c, d.	82. a, b.	83. a, b, c.	84. d.	85. c, d.
86. a, b, e.	87. a, c.	88. c, d.	89. b, c, d, e.	90. c, d, e.	91. a, b, c.	92. a, c, d, e.
93. a, b	94. b, d					

95. Deficiency of both T and B Lymphocyte involved in all except:
a. Chronic mucocutaneous candidiasis
b. Wiskott-Aldrich syndrome
c. DiGeorge Syndrome
d. Ataxia Telangiectasia
e. Common variable immunodeficiency

96. True about leptospirosis:
a. It is a zoonotic disease
b. Transmission may occurs through cuts and abraded skin
c. It is an arboviral disease
d. Rodents are the most important reservoir

97. Which of the following is/are true about Syphilis:
a. VDRL is the one of the most widely used nontreponemal antibody tests
b. Tabes dorsalis causes hypertonia
c. Jarisch Herxheimer reaction is due to IgE mediated action
d. Primary and secondary syphilis are treated by penicillin

98. Water loss of 500-1000 mL/hour in cholera is known as:
a. Cholera gravis
b. Cholera mitis
c. Cholera majoris

FORENSIC MEDICINE

99. Test used for blood stains detection is/are all except:
a. Barberio's test
b. Kastle-Meyer test
c. Benzidine test
d. Acid phosphatase test
e. Takayama test

100. Which of the following is/are dangerous injury in forensic science:
a. Injury causing endanger to life if not treated timely
b. Hearing loss
c. Loss of 2-3 teeth
d. Synonymous with grievous injury
e. Emasculation

101. Which of the following statement(s) is/are true about dying declaration:
a. Can be done in the presence of doctor if condition of the victim is serious and there is no time to call a Magistrate
b. Should be done by magistrate
c. If a declarant made more than one dying declarations and all are contradictory, then those all declarations lose their value or court can examine the statement of other witnesses toascertain the truth of the case
d. If incomplete, it is not valid
e. Even if the declarant survives, the declaration is of full value in the court

102. Saturated NaCl is not used in preservation of viscera in which of the following poisoning:
a. Sodium hydroxide
b. Aconite
c. Carbolic acid
d. Sulphuric acid

103. Which of the following Feature(s) is/are more common in strangulation rather than hanging:
a. Pale face
b. Fractures of trachea and larynx
c. Congested faces
d. Transverse ligature
e. Bruises at edges of the ligature mark

104. Which of the following is/are feature of Drowning:
a. Oedema aquosum in lung
b. Emphysema aquosum is presumptive evidence of death from drowning
c. Paltauf's haemorrhages is seen subpleurally
d. Gettler's test is used to test chloride content of blood from both sides of the heart
e. Lung is ballooned and light in sea water drowning

PREVENTIVE & SOCIAL MEDICINE

105. Period of communicability of measles is:
a. 3 days before and 10 days after appearance of rashes
b. 3 weeks after appearance of rashes
c. 1 week before appearance of rashes
d. 4 days before and 5 days after appearance of rashes
e. Up to 3 months after appearance of rashes

106. Vaccine contraindicated in AIDS patient:
a. MMR vaccine
b. Hepatitis A vaccine
c. Varicella vaccine
d. Hib vaccine
e. DPT vaccine

107. 9-valent HPV vaccine covers which type(s) HPV strain:
a. 6, 11
b. 16, 18
c. 31, 33
d. 41, 35
e. 42,58

108. True about Human development index (HDI):
a. Adult literacy rate range from 0 to 100
b. HDI score range is 0-10
c. Life expectancy at birth range from 25 years to 85 years
d. GDP per capita range from 25$ to 50000$
e. HDI score range is 0-1

109. Which of the following is/are true about Revised National Tuberculosis Control Programme (RNTCP):
a. TB is mandatory to notify
b. Suspicious TB patients are screened through 2 sputum smear examinations
c. MDR-TB is not included in RNTCP
d. Case finding is active
e. Covered the whole country since March 2006

Answer

95. a, c, e.	96. a, b, d.	97. a, d.	98. a.	99. a, d.	100. a.	101. a, b, c, d.
102. a, b, d.	103. b, c, d, e.	104. a, b, c, d.	105. d.	106. a, b, c.	107. a, b, c.	108. a, c, e.
109. a, b, e						

110. True statement about IPV vaccine:
a. Given through IM/SC route
b. Given through Intradermal route
c. Does not require stringent conditions
d. Dose is- 0.1 mL/dose
e. Dose is -0.5 mL/dose

111. True about Demographic cycle of India:
a. Entered into low stationary phase
b. Dependency ratio <40%
c. Year of Big divide-1921A.D
d. Population pyramid has a broad base and a tapering top
e. First regular census in India was carried in 1881

112. Which of the following is/are true about National Iron plus initiative:
a. Only school going adolescents are covered
b. Adolescents of age group 10-19 yr are covered
c. Preschool children are covered through aganwadi center
d. Biannual deworming through albendazole tablet
e. Screening of target groups for moderate/severe anaemia and referring these cases to an appropriate health facility

113. Which of the following is true about post exposure prophylaxis in rabies:
a. Category I- Both vaccine and immunoglobulin are given
b. Immunoglobulin not required if prior full vaccination is received
c. Local wound cleaning is done in all cases of dog wound
d. Category I- requires vaccination only
e. Vaccine is stopped if within 3 days of bite, dog dies

114. True about population coverage of primary health center:
a. 20000 in plain area
b. 30000 in plain area
c. 10000 in tribal area
d. 20000 in tribal area
e. 30000 in tribal area

OPHTHALMOLOGY

115. All are true about central retinal artery occlusion (CRAO) except:
a. Most commonly occurs due to thromboembolus
b. Anterior chamber paracentesis is used for treatment
c. Sudden painful loss of vision
d. Occurs due to obstruction of retinal artery at the level of lamina cribrosa
e. Macular area shows cherry-red spot

116. True about inferior opthalmic vein:
a. Smaller than superior ophthalmic vein
b. Connected to the pterygoid venous plexus
c. Formed at lateral wall and floor of orbit
d. Pass through superior orbital fissure
e. Empties into superior ophthalmic vein

117. All are true about congenital ptosis except:
a. Stimulus deprivation amblyopia may occur if treatment is delayed
b. Lid lag on downgaze
c. Prominence of lid crease
d. Loss of lid crease
e. Associated with weakness of the levator palpebrae superioris

118. Not true about Blue sclera:
a. Seen in Osteogenesis impertca
b. Does not seen in Ehlers-Danlos syndrome
c. Blue colour is produced by underlying uveal pigment
d. Seen in Marfan's syndrome
e. Sclera is thin

119. Which of the following statement(s) is/are true about Eyelid glands
a. Moll are modified sebaceous
b. Tarsal glands are meibomian glands
c. Gland of zeis are sweat gland
d. Meibomian glands are modified sebaceous glands
e. External hordeolum is an acute suppurative inflammation of gland of Zeis

120. Corneal ulcer is defined as:
a. Erosion of epithelium only
b. Erosion of endothelium only
c. Erosion of epithelium + underlying inflammation
d. Loss of endothelium with loss of corneal sensation

121. Which of the following can be ophthalmic complication of DM except:
a. Papillopathy
b. Snowflake cataract
c. Retinopathy
d. Rhegmatogenous retinal detachment
e. Cystoid macular oedema

122. Which of the following is/are true about medial longitudinal fasciculus (MLF) and its lesion except:
a. Unilateral lesion result in adduction palsy of opposite eye
b. MLF connects sixth cranial nerve nucleus of one side with the third cranial nerve nucleus of the other side
c. MLF is responsible for conjugate eye movements
d. It is an integral component of saccadic eye movements
e. Abducting nystagmus of the eye contralateral to the lesion

123. Postoperative endophthalmitis in cataract surgery can be prevented by use of:
a. Preoperative oral antibiotics
b. Intra-operative IV antibiotics
c. Use of povidone-iodine solution to paint the lids before surgery
d. Cleaning and sterilization of operation theatre
e. Postop topical antibiotics

Answer

110. a, c, e	111. c, d, e.	112. b, d, e.	113. b, c.	114. b, d.	115. c.	116. a, b, d, e.
117. c.	118. b.	119. b, d, e.	120. c.	121. d.	122. a.	123. c, d, e.

124. Which of the following is/are true about secondary cataract:
a. Treatment of thickened capsule can be done by discission with cystitome
b. Treatment by Nd-YAG laser posterior capsulotomy
c. More common after intracapsular cataract extraction than extracapsular cataract extraction
d. Posterior capsular opacification (PCO)
e. Anterior subcapsular cataract

ENT

125. Premalignant lesion of oral cavity include(s):
a. Lichen planus
b. Erythroplakia
c. Bowen's disease
d. Behchet's syndrome

126. True about foreign bodies of air passage in children except:
a. Vegetable foreign bodies are not common
b. Tracheal obstruction can causes sudden death
c. More common in right bronchus
d. More common in children of less than 4 yr of age
e. CT scan of chest is done in all cases

127. Deformities occurring in leprosy patients is/are:
a. Facies leonina
b. Low set ear
c. Saddle nose
d. Lagophthalmos
e. Micrognathia

128. Which of the following is/are true about Leforts fracture:
a. It is fracture of zygomatic bone
b. May cause CSF rhinorrhea
c. Type 1: complete separation of facial bones form the cranial bones
d. Classified as types 1 to 5

129. Which of the following is/are true about schwartz sign:
a. Sign of inactive disease
b. Indication for surgery
c. More common during pregnancy
d. Reddish hue over the promontory
e. Seen in the early stages of the otoscelerosis

130. Which of the following is/are true about the T-stage of maxillary sinus carcinoma:
a. Stage T4a- Frontal sinus involvement
b. Stage T3-Ethmoid sinus involvement
c. Stage T2-Sphenoid sinus involvement
d. Stage T2- bone of the posterior wall of maxillary sinus

131. Contraindication of cochlear implantation is/are:
a. Mondini deformity
b. Intracochlear ossification
c. Chronic suppurative otitis media
d. Agenesis of cochlear nerve

132. True about development of Cochlea:
a. Cochlea start developing from 3rd week of gestation
b. Semicircular canals develop after cochlea
c. Cochlea development completes by 20 week of gestation
d. Cochlea development completes at 2 year of age

MEDICINE

133. Components of APACHE-II score include(s):
a. Age
b. Glassgow comma scale
c. FiO_2
d. Alanine aminotransferase (*ALT*)
e. Serum lactate

134. Neurofibromatosis type 1 is/are associated with:
a. Café-au-lait spots
b. Cataracts
c. Axillary freckling
d. Facial nerve palsy
e. Optic nerve meningioma

135. Which of the following dyads are correct:
a. Pulsus paradoxus-Aortic regurgitation
b. Pulsus bisferiens- Mitral stenosis
c. Water-Hammer pulse- Aortic regurgitation
d. Pulsus parvus Et tardus -Aortic stenosis
e. Collapsing pulse- Aortic regurgitation

136. True about Ventilator associated pneumonia (VAP):
a. 2nd most common nosocomial infection in the intensive care unit
b. Colonization of the pharynx with bacteria is risk factor
c. Highest risk occur in the first 5 days
d. Gastric acid may play a role in protection against nosocomial pneumonias
e. Develops only after 1 week on mechanical ventilation

137. Which of the following is/are feature(s) of hypomagnesemia:
a. Tremors
b. Improvement seen with calcium supplementation
c. Athetoid movements
d. Seizure
e. Bradycardia

138. Which of the following is/are true about Jugular Venous Pressure (JVP) waveform:
a. a wave occur just after electrocardiographic P wave
b. Prominent x and y descents is seen in constrictive pericarditis
c. Canon a waves occur in atrioventricular (AV) dissociation
d. v wave occur in early systole of cardiac cycle
e. Prominent x descent but an absent y descent is seen in cardiac temponade

139. Feature(s) of Vitamin A toxicity include(s):
a. Hypercalcemia
b. Yellow skin
c. Anorexia
d. Poor wound healing
e. Papilledema and hepatomegaly

Answer

124. a, b, d. 125. a, b. 126. a, b, e. 127. a, c, d. 128. b. 129. b, c, d, e. 130. a, b.
131. c, d. 132. a, c. 133. a, b, c. 134. a, c. 135. c, d, e. 136. a, b, c, d. 137. a, b, c, d.
138. a, b, c, e 139. a, b, c, e

140. Which of the following statement(s) is/are true about Myasthenia Gravis with muscle-specific tyrosine kinase (MuSK) antibodies than anti-AChR Ab:

a. Disease onset is earlier with female predominance
b. Neck and facial muscle weakness are more common
c. More proximal muscle involvement
d. Associated with thymic hyperplasia
e. Poor response with acetylcholine esterase (AChE) inhibitors

141. Exudative pleural effusion is/are seen in all except:

a. Cirrhosis b. Carcinoma
c. Bacterial pneumonia d. Tuberculosis
e. Congestive heart failure

142. Clinical presentation of pituitary apoplexy include(s) all except:

a. Ophthalmoplegia b. Visual impairment
c. Fever d. Severe headache
e. Hypertension

143. Which of the following can occur in COPD:

a. Hypoxemia
b. Hypercarbia
c. Decreased gas exchange in terminal bronchioles
d. Acidosis

SURGERY

144. All are true about Succinate dehydrogenase deficient gastrointestinal stromal tumor (SDH-deficient GIST) except:

a. More common in children and young adult
b. Negative for DOG-1
c. Most common location is stomach
d. Associated with Carney-Stratakis syndrome
e. Absent c-kit mutation

145. Which of the following is/are true about Gastric lymphoma:

a. Associated with H.pylori infection
b. Majority belongs to B-cell Hodgkin lymphomas
c. Endoscopic ultrasound is performed to determine the depth of gastric wall invasion
d. Second most common tumor of stomach
e. Diagnosis is made on basis of endoscopic biopsy

146. All are true about bilateral breast cancer except:

a. Bilaterality is common when the tumor in the primary breast is lobular carcinoma
b. About 5% bilateral cancers are synchronous and 20% bilateral cancers are metachronous
c. More common in women of >50 year of age
d. BRCA mutation cancers are associated higher prevalence of bilateral breast cancer
e. Usually b/l if familial breast cancer present

147. Most accurate method for the diagnosis Gastroesophageal Reflux Disease (GERD) is:

a. Histological study
b. Manometry
c. 24-hour pH recording and electrical impedance measurement
d. Barium swallow studies
e. Upper GI endoscopy

148. Which of the following is/are true about appendicitis

a. Both diarrhea and constipation may present
b. Nausea and vomiting usually present
c. Pain on internal rotation of flexed hip
d. Pain on flexion and external rotation of hip
e. Initially pain is located in the periumbilical region

149. Risk Factors for thyroid carcinoma in patients with thyroid nodule include(s):

a. Female gender b. Exposure to radiation
c. Age b/w 20-60 year d. Nodule size >4 cm
e. Male gender

150. Only simple cholecystectomy is adequate in which stage of gallbladder cancer:

a. Stage IA b. Stage IB
c. Stage III d. Stage III
e. Stage IV

151. Not included in surgical safety checklist:

a. Sign in b. Sign out
c. Time in d. Time out
e. Pre-anesthetic checkup

152. All are true statement about hernias except:

a. Femoral hernia has the highest risk of strangulation of groin hernias
b. Direct inguinal hernia cause more symptoms than indirect
c. Direct inguinal hernia is most common in children
d. Indirect inguinal hernia occur due to patient processus vaginalis
e. Direct inguinal hernia occur due to defect in fascia transversalis

153. Which of the following is/are true about torsion of testis:

a. Most common type is extravaginal
b. Doppler USG may be used for diagnosis
c. Most common cause is trauma to testis
d. Differentiated from epididymitis by technetium-99m pertechnetate scan
e. Contralateral testis should also be explored on surgery

154. True about undescended testis:

a. U/L more common than B/L
b. Missing testis on palpation may be due to agenesis
c. 10% Bilateral
d. Undescended Testis may be associated with absent kidney
e. Stephen fowler technique involves renal artery ligation

Answer

140. a, b, c, e.	141. a, e.	142. e.	143. a, b, d.	144. b.	145. a, c, d, e.	146. c.
147. c.	148. a, b, c, e.	149. b, d, e.	150. a.	151. c, e.	152. b, c.	153. b, d, e.
154. a, b, c, d						

155. Mediastinal mass(s) which is/are more common in posterior mediastinum:
a. Lymphoma
b. Thymoma
c. Neurogenic tumor
d. Enterogenous cyst
e. Thyroid carcinoma

156. Condition(s) associated with esophageal carcinoma:
a. Achalsia
b. Post-cricoid web
c. Schatzki's ring
d. Paterson-Kelly syndrome
e. Lye ingestion

157. Hyperamylasemia is/are seen in all except:
a. Pancreatic pseudocyst
b. Cystic fibrosis
c. Macroamylasemia
d. Parotitis
e. Chronic pancreatitis

158. True about pseudocyst:
a. Pancreatic fluid collection
b. May be asymptomatic
c. Well-defined wall
d. Fluid collection is always infectious in nature
e. Rich in pancreatic enzymes

159. Indications of surgery in tuberculosis include(s):
a. Streaky hemoptysis
b. Tubercular empyema
c. Persistent bronchopleural fistula
d. Chronic cough
e. AFB +ve bacilli in sputum

160. True about tuberculosis:
a. Cavitatory lesion suggests inactive disease
b. Rasmussen aneurysm is a complication
c. High grade fever
d. Tubercular bronchiectasis occur in lower lobes

161. Raised intracranial pressure (ICP) in head injury is/are managed by:
a. Furosemide
b. Mannitol
c. Decompressive craniectomy is helpful in decreasing ICP but do not affect neurological outcome
d. Glucose free fluid
e. Hypotonic solution

162. True about Meckel's diverticulum:
a. Causes volvulus of intestine
b. Due to persistent remnant of the vitellointestinal duct
c. Commonly found on the mesenteric side of the ileum
d. Causes melena
e. Causes Haemoptysis

163. True about Endemic goiter:
a. Size may increase during pregnancy
b. Usually hypothyroid
c. Same as multinodular goiter
d. Can turn malignant

164. True about blunt abdominal trauma:
a. Liver is the most common organ affected
b. Abdominal pelvic CT scanning is helpful for evaluating intra-abdominal and retroperitoneal injuries
c. >100,000 red cells/μL in peritoneal lavage is considered positive and is indication for exploratory laparotomy
d. More than 2ml of free blood in the abdominal cavity is indication for exploratory laparotomy
e. FAST-USG is used for initial evaluation

165. All are true about basal cell carcinoma except:
a. Arises from basal cells of epidermis
b. On biopsy shows basaloid cells in a palisading arrangement
c. Noduloulcerative variant is k/a rodent ulcer
d. Xeroderma pigmentosum is a risk factor
e. More common in dark people

166. True about neurogenic claudication:
a. Low back pain is present
b. Fixed walking distance
c. Pain immediately relieved by rest
d. Shiny skin of foot
e. Pain relieved by leaning forward

167. Feature(s) of partial thickness burn (second degree) is/are:
a. Hairs easily pluckable
b. Severe pain
c. Thrombosed vessel
d. Leathery skin
e. Blistering of skin

168. Difference b/w Full thickness and partial thickness grafts:
a. Partial thickness graft have good cosmetic appearance
b. Full thickness graft are good for large area
c. Edema under graft may cause graft failure
d. Thin graft survive transplantation more reliably
e. Minimal contraction in full thickness graft

169. True about Hypertrophic scar:
a. Treated with Triamcinolone
b. Results from a prolonged inflammatory phase of wound healing
c. Most common in pigmented skin
d. Grow beyond margin
e. Improve spontaneously with time

170. True about surgical approach in thyroid surgery:
a. Incision is made 1 cm below cricoid cartilage
b. Usually vertical incision is used
c. Thoracic duct may be damaged
d. For lobectomy thyroid is dissected at the isthmus
e. Strap muscles are divided if greater exposure is needed

Answer

155. c, d.	156. a, b, d, e.	157. None.	158. a, b, c, e.	159. b, c.	160. b.	161. a, b, d.
162. a, b, d.	163. a, b, d.	164. b, c, e.	165. e.	166. a, c, e.	167. b, e.	168. c, d, e.
169. a, b, e	170. a, c, d, e					

OBSTETRICS & GYNECOLOGY

171. Which of the following statement(s) is/are true about cysts in ovary except:
- a. Follicular cyst is least common among functional cyst
- b. Corpus luteal cysts are often associated with pregnancy
- c. Dermoid cyst are germ cell tumor
- d. Fibroma of ovary is associated with Meig's syndrome
- e. Theca Leutin cyst is seen in association with hydatiform mole and GnRH analogue use

172. High-Grade Squamous Intraepithelial Lesions (HSIL) are found on pap smear. Next step(s) of management:
- a. Colposcopic study and biopsy of suspicious lesions
- b. Hysterectomy
- c. Radiotherapy
- d. Liquid based cytology
- e. HPV DNA testing

173. Screening test used to detect aneuploidy in 1st trimester includes:
- a. Estimation of PAAP-A and estradiol
- b. Estimation of PAAP-A and βhCG
- c. Estimation of PAAP-A and MSAFP
- d. Estimation of βhCG and Inhibin
- e. Estimation of MSAFP and βhCG

174. Vaginal prolapse following abdominal hysterectomy is/are caused by damage of:
- a. Level I support
- b. Level II support
- c. Level III support
- d. Urogenital diaphragm

175. True about $MgSO_4$ role in pre-eclampsia and eclampsia:
- a. Used for controlling hypertension in pre-eclampsia and eclampsia
- b. Therapeutic level for seizure control is 4–7 mEq/L
- c. Toxicity should be monitored
- d. Can be given as IV infusion
- e. Also can be given by intramuscular route

176. Contraindications for IUCD:
- a. Postabortal sepsis more than 1 year ago
- b. Present cervicitis and vaginitis
- c. Past history of ectopic pregnancy
- d. Unknown cause of vaginal bleeding
- e. Severe dysmenorrhea

177. Absolute Contraindications for medical abortion:
- a. Previous myomectomy
- b. Hypersensitivity to prostaglandin
- c. Previous LSCS
- d. Suspected ectopic pregnancy
- e. Undiagnosed adnexal mass

178. Finding(s) of atrophic vaginitis is/are:
- a. Low pH of vagina
- b. Occur due to estrogen deficiency
- c. Frequent intercourse is useful
- d. Intercourse causes painless bleeding
- e. Estradiol vaginal ring is helpful

179. True statement about vacuum extraction of baby:
- a. Pressure is maintained b/w 5 kg/cm^2 to 8 kg/cm^2
- b. Done when cervix is fully dilated
- c. Center of cup should be placed 1 cm in front of posterior fontanelle
- d. Cup rim should be placed 3 cm from the anterior fontanelle

180. Risk factors for abruptio placenta is/are:
- a. Traumatic separation of the placenta
- b. Mutigravida
- c. Diabetes
- d. Gestational hypertension
- e. Submucous fibroid

181. Pregnancy aggravates which of the following condition(s):
- a. Hypertension
- b. Anaemia
- c. Rheumatoid arthritis
- d. Acne

182. Feature(s) of HELP syndrome:
- a. Low platelets
- b. Increased AST and ALT
- c. Decreased lactate dehydrogenase
- d. Increased conjugated bilirubin
- e. Hemolysis

183. Contraindication of combined oral contraceptive (COC) include(s):
- a. Severe hypertension
- b. Ischemic heart disease
- c. Pre-menstrual tension
- d. Active liver disease

184. Chronic use of combine oral contraceptive (COC) helps in all except:
- a. Dysmenorrhea
- b. Breakthrough bleeding
- c. Menorrhagia
- d. Migraine
- e. Anaemia

185. Which of the following statement(s) is true about abdominal incision in women for various surgical procedures:
- a. Paramedian: best incision
- b. Transverse incision should be only used in exceptional cases
- c. Cherney incision is useful in uro-gynaecological procedures
- d. Maylard incision provide improved access to the pelvic side wall
- e. Rutherford-Morrison is particularly useful for approaching ovarian masses

Answer

171. a.	172. a.	173. b.	174. All (a,b, c, d).	175. b, c, d, e.	176. b, c, d, e.	177. b, d, e.
178. b, e.	179. b, d.	180. a, b, d, e.	181. a, b.	182. a, b, e.	183. a, b, d.	184. b, d.
185. c, d, e						

186. All is/are true about HIV in pregnancy except:
a. Vertical transmission to the neonate is about 15-30%
b. HAART therapy of pregnant woman reduces chance of transmission to neonates
c. Zidovudine therapy should be given to neonates
d. Elective caesarean section reduces the risk of vertical transmission
e. Zidovudine is given in place of stavudine in HAART therapy if mother is anaemic

187. True statement about primary dysmenorrhea:
a. Pain starts 2-3 day before menstruation and stops after 1 day of menstruation
b. Pain begins a few hours before or just after the onset of a menstrual period and may last 48 to 72 hours
c. May be associated with psychological factors
d. GnRH antagonists are always used in 1st line treatment

PEDIATRICS

188. A child is having Wilson disease. Which of the following statement(s) is/are not correct:
a. Kayser-Fleischer (KF) ring may be present in eye
b. Serum ceruloplasmin is <20 mg/dL
c. Hepatic copper is >250 μg/g dry weight of liver
d. In symptomatic patients, the 24 hr urinary copper excretion is less than 40 μg/day
e. Liver biopsy is of value for determining the extent and severity of liver disease

189. Which of the following is/are true about developmental milestones of 2 years old child:
a. Can walk up & down stairs with alternating feet
b. Walks up and down stairs, one step at a time
c. Rides tricycle
d. Knows age and sex
e. Weight quadruples of birth weight

190. Syndrome(s) related to paediatric brain tumors:
a. Tuberous sclerosis
b. Neurofibromatosis-2
c. Cokayne syndrome
d. Fanconi syndrome
e. Turcot syndrome

191. True about benign Idiopathic neonatal seizures:
a. Called as 5th day fits
b. Seizure often occur later in life
c. Status epilepticus may occur
d. Family history is usually present
e. More common in preterm

192. All are true about Wilms tumor except:
a. Painless abdominal mass
b. Mostly asymptomatic
c. Swelling is ballotable
d. Stage I- tumour confined to kidney
e. Completely excision is treatment of choice in stage I & II

193. A 5 month old infant has massive hepatomegaly. Which of the following condition(s) presents with massive heapatomegaly:
a. Type I Glycogen storage disorder
b. Biliary atresia
c. Gaucher's disease
d. Biliary cirrhosis

194. A Child is presented with mediastinal mass, swelling of face, dyspnea & stridor. Next line of management is/are:
a. Administration of oxygen with ventimask
b. Tracheostomy
c. Biopsy of mass and fine needle aspiration cytology
d. Mediastinal radiation
e. Rasburicase

195. Complication(s) of H type of tracheo-esophageal fistula is/are:
a. Dysphagia
b. Aspiration pneumonia
c. Hematemesis
d. Paroxysms of coughing or cyanosis with feeding
e. Death usually occur in infancy

196. Cause of lower GI Bleed in children of age >2 year of age:
a. TB
b. Meckel's diverticulum
c. Aspirin
d. Esophageal varices
e. It is bleeding from a site distal to ligament of treitz

ORTHOPEDICS

197. True about ankylosing spondylitis:
a. Pain relives on rest
b. Association with HLA B-27
c. Enthesitis may occur
d. 30% cases have acute posterior uveitis
e. Cardiac conduction defect may present

198. In ponseti technique last deformity to get corrected in CTEV:
a. Equinus
b. Talipus
c. Varus
d. Cavus
e. All deformity corrected simultaneously

199. Test for anterior cruciate ligament is/are:
a. Lachmann test
b. Apley's grinding test
c. Pivot shift test
d. Anterior drawer
e. KT-1000 knee arthrometer is an objective instrument for ACL reconstruction

200. A person has injury on dorsal surface of proximal interphalengeal joint of right middle finger. Which of the following can occur:
a. Rupture of lateral ligament
b. Buttonhole deformity
c. Mallet finger
d. Laceration of the central slip of the extensor

Answer

186. e.	187. b, c.	188. d.	189. b, e.	190. a, b, e.	191. a, c.	192. e.
193. a, d.	194. a, b, c.	195. b, d.	196. a, b, c, e.	197. b, c, e.	198. a.	199. a, c, d, e.
200. a, b, d.						

201. True about avascular necrosis of femur:
a. Affected side hip allows weight bearing
b. Asymptomatic cases may occur
c. Radionucleotide scan show increased uptake due to new bone formation in the area around the infarct
d. Trendelenburg sign is negative

202. True about Pectus excavatum:
a. More common in female
b. In severe cases, mitral valve prolapse may occur
c. May be present at birth
d. Seen in Marfan syndrome
e. Impairment of respiratory function

203. True about Osteomalacia:
a. More common in male
b. Low PTH
c. ↑alkaline phosphatase
d. ↓ed Calcium level
e. Looser's zone on X-ray

204. True about Ganglion cyst:
a. Most common in young male
b. Contain synovial fluid
c. Arise from extensor retinaculum
d. It usually arise from the lunotriquetral joint
e. Surgical treatment is excision of cyst

ANESTHESIA

205. Drugs known to trigger malignant hyperthermia:
a. Halothane
b. Succinylcholine
c. Pancuronium
d. Fentanyl
e. Propofol

206. When will you suspect malignant hyperthermia in post appendectomy patient shifted to ICU with high fever &:
a. Hypotonia
b. Seizure
c. Masseter spasm
d. Metabolic acidosis
e. Hypokalemia

207. Anaesthesia used for induction is/are:
a. Propofol
b. Thiopentone
c. Ketamine
d. Diazepam
e. Midazolam

208. Which of the following is/are used in Bupivacaine toxicity:
a. $CaCl_2$
b. Bretylium
c. Intralipids
d. Esmolol
e. Epinephrine

209. Which of the following criteria is/are used for setting mechanical ventilator for adult in ICU:
a. Age
b. Gender
c. Weight
d. Height
e. Underlying condition of patient

210. True about endotracheal tube:
a. Non cuffed tube is used in pediatric age group
b. Made of PVC & disposable
c. Can be put either oral or nasal according to different situations
d. Cuffed PVC tubes- low pressure, low volume
e. More tendency to go to right bronchus thereby decreasing left lung ventilation

211. True about endotracheal intubation:
a. Head trauma patient presenting with a GCS score 8 or less should be intubated
b. Done in patients with increased risk of aspiration
c. Can be used in patient with full stomach
d. In cervical injury, patient neck is stabilized before intubation
e. Done in patients who need anaesthesia

212. Which of the following is/are feature(s) of epidural anaesthesia than spinal anaesthesia:
a. Smaller size of needle is used
b. Drug used is less in concentration
c. Less chance of spinal headache
d. Onset of action is delayed
e. Density of anaesthetic agent is less in epidural than spinal

SKIN

213. Desmoglein is associated with:
a. Arrhythmogenic right ventricular cardiomyopathy
b. Hypertrichosis
c. Pemphigus vulgaris
d. Psoriasis
e. Keratoderma with wooly hair

214. Subepidermal blisters is/are seen in:
a. Pemphigus vulgaris
b. Pemphigus vegetans
c. Pemphigoid
d. Dermatitis hepetiformis
e. Pemphigus Violaceous

215. Dermatologic manifestation of Lithium is/are:
a. Rash
b. Psoriasis exacerbation
c. Acneiform eruptions
d. Pustular dermatoses
e. Pemphigus

Answer

201. a, b, c.
202. b, c, d, e.
203. c, d, e.
204. b, c, e.
205. a, b.
206. b, c, d.
207. a, b, c, e.
208. b, c, e.
209. b, c, d, e.
210. a, b, c, e.
211. All.
212. b, d, e.
213. a, b, c, e.
214. c, d.
215. b, c,d

PSYCHIATRY

216. Maximum score in Mini mental status examination is:

a. 10 b. 15
c. 20 d. 25
e. 30

217. Which of the following is/are feature(s) of nicotine withdrawal:

a. Weight loss
b. Irritability
c. Impaired concentration
d. Anxiety
e. Insomnia

218. Naltrexone is/are used for:

a. Alcohol dependence
b. Opioid dependence
c. Cocaine dependence
d. Cannabis toxicity

219. True match of EEG pattern in Sleep EEG:

a. K-complex is seen in stage I of NREM sleep
b. Waking state show alpha wave
c. Alpha- wave occur in onset of sleep
d. Theta wave is the predominant wave in stage I of NREM sleep
e. Stage III-NREM sleep shows high amplitude slow waves

220. Essential criteria for major depression are all except:

a. Delusion of grandeur b. Loss of pleasure
c. Insomnia d. Hypersomnia
e. Anorexia

221. True about generalized anxiety disorder:

a. Insomnia
b. Clear history of past traumatic event
c. Excessive anxiety and worry
d. Benzodiazepines is drugs of choice

RADIOLOGY

222. Features of strontium 89 in comparison to phosphorus-32:

a. Longer t-1/2
b. Deeper penetration
c. Emits Beta rays while P-32 emits alpha rays
d. Lesser toxicity

223. True about concomitant chemoradiotherapy:

a. Chemotherapy and radiotherapy both given simultaneously
b. Radiotherapy acts locoregionally and chemotherapy acts against distant micrometastases
c. Radiotherapy acts as sensitizing agent
d. Chemotherapy may act as sensitizing agent

224. Neoadjuvant chemotherapy stands for:

a. Chemotherapy along with surgery
b. Chemotherapy before surgery
c. Chemotherapy after surgery
d. Chemotherapy along with radiation therapy
e. Chemotherapy after radiation therapy

225. Which of the following is/are true about brachytherapy than teletherapy:

a. More effective in carcinoma cervix
b. Same Proportion of radiation is delivered to both-tumour & normal tissue
c. Better than teletherapy for large & bulky tumour
d. Deliver higher dose of radiation to tumour
e. Less damage to normal tissue

226. Feature(s) of Crohn's disease is/are:

a. Pipestem colon
b. Pseudosacculation
c. Loss of haustrasion
d. Cobblestone appearance
e. String sign of kantor

Answer

216. e. 217. b, c, d, e. 218. a, b, c. 219. b, d, e. 220. a. 221. a, c, d. 222. a, d.
223. a, b, d. 224. b. 225. a, d, e. 226. b, d, e

MAY 2017 ANSWERS & EXPLANATIONS

ANATOMY

1. **Ans. a. Facial nerve, b. Glossopharyngeal nerve d. Vagus nerve**

[Ref: BDC 7th/ Vol.III 278-79]

"**Hypoglossal nerve:** It is motor supply to all intrinsic and extrinsic muscle of tongue except palatoglossus (supplied by the cranial root of the accessory nerve through the pharyngeal plexus)- *BDC 7th/ Vol.III 278*

Chorda tympani is a branch of facial nerve *(BDC 7th/ Vol.IV 71)*

***Lingual nerve** is branch of mandibular division of **trigeminal nerve**-Snell 9th/625*

Table *(BDC 7th/ Vol.III 279)*: **Comparison of the parts of the tongue**

	Anterior two-thirds	Posterior one-third	Posteriormost part and vallecula
Situation	Lies in mouth cavity	Oropharynx	Oropharynx
Structure	Contains papillae	Contains lymphoid tissue	—
Function	Chewing	Deglutition	Deglutition
Sensory nerve	***Lingual*** (post-trematic branch of 1st arch)	Glossopharyngeal (nerve of 3rd arch)	Internal laryngeal branch of *vagus* (nerve of 4th arch)
Sensation of taste	***Chorda tympani*** except circumvallate papillae (pre-trematic branch of 1st arch)	***Glossopharyngeal*** including the vallate papillae	***Internal laryngeal branch of vagus***
Development of epithelium from endoderm	Lingual swellings of 1st arch. Tuberculum impar which soon disappears	Third arch which forms large ventral part of hypobranchial eminence	Fourth arch which forms small dorsal part of hypobranchial eminence

2. **Ans. c. Formed in front of scalenus medius muscle**

[Ref: BDC 7th/ Vol II 363-64; Moore 2nd/105-06; Gray's 40th/456-57, 1010; Snell's 9th/618]

Phrenic Nerve

Snell's 9th/618, 99

- The phrenic nerve arises from C3-5 nerves of the cervical plexus.
- It run vertically downward across the ***front of the scalenus anterior muscle*** and enter the thorax by passing in front of the subclavian artery.
- It passes in front of the root of the lung (left phrenic— of left lung; right phrenic- of right lung).
- The phrenic nerve is a mixed nerve that provides the ***sole motor supply to the diaphragm***.
- It also send sensory branches to the pericardium, the mediastinal parietal pleura and the pleura and peritoneum covering the upper and lower surfaces of the central part of the diaphragm.
- "Sensory fibres from the phrenic nerve supply the ***central part of the diaphragm***, including the surrounding **pleura** and **peritoneum**. The nerve also supplies sensation to the **mediastinal pleura** and the **pericardium"**-teachmeanatomy.info

"The phrenic nerves contain motor, sensory and sympathetic nerve fibers. These nerves provide the ***only motor supply to the diaphragm as well as sensation to the central tendon*** (except the most peripheral diaphragm, which is supplied by intercostal nerves). In the thorax, each phrenic nerve supplies the mediastinal pleura and pericardium"-wiki

Phrenic Nerve

Gray's 40th/456-57

- The phrenic nerve arises chiefly from the fourth cervical ventral ramus, but also has contributions from the third and fifth.
- It is **formed at** the upper part of the lateral border of **scalenus anterior** and descends almost vertically across its anterior surface behind the prevertebral fascia.
- It descends posterior to ***sternocleidomastoid, the interior belly of omohyoid*** (near its intermediate tendon), the internal jugular vein, transverse cervical and suprascapular arteries and, on the left, the thoracic duct.
- At the root of the neck, it runs anterior to the second part of the subclavian artery, from which it is separated by the ***scalenus anterior*** (some accounts state that on the left side the nerve passes anteriror to the first part of the subclavian artery), posterior to the subclavian vein.
- The phrenic nerve enters the thorax by crossing medially in front of the internal thoracic artery.

Accessory Phrenic Nerve

Gray's 40th/456

- The accessory phrenic nerve is composed of fibres from the fifth cervical ventral ramus which run in a branch of the nerve to subclavius.
- This lies lateral to the phrenic nerve and descends posterior (occasionally anterior) to the subclavian vein.
- The accessory phrenic nerve usually ***joins the phrenic nerve near the first rib,*** but may not do so until near the pulmonary hilum or beyond.
- The accessory phrenic nerve may be derived from the fourth or sixth cervical ventral rami or from the ansa cervicalis.

3. **Ans. a. Multipennate acromial...c. Musculotendinous cuff... d. Supraspinatus initiates... e. Trapezius and serratus anterior...**

[Ref: BDC 7th/Vol. I 70, 73, 77; Snell 9th/364-65; Essential Anatomy by Moore 2nd/484; Gray's 40th/812]

"The conventional view is that ***supraspinatus initiates abduction of shoulder*** *and assists deltoid in abduction thereafter. However, there is evidence that both supraspinatus and deltoid are involved throughout the range of abduction, including the initiation of the movement" (Gray's 40th/812)*

"The ***multipennate acromial fibres are powerful abductors*** *of arm at the shoulder joint from beginning to 900. A multipennate arrangement allows a large number of muscle fibres to be packed into a relatively small volume. As the strength of contraction of a muscle is proportional to the number of muscle fibres present in it (not on their length),* ***a multipennate muscle is much stronger than other muscles having the same volume*** *" (BDC 7th/ Vol. I 70-71)*

*"****Axillary nerve damage:*** *Deltoid is paralyzed, with loss of the power of abduction up to 90° at the shoulder, rounded contour of shoulder is lost and there is sensory loss over the lower half of the deltoid in a badge-like area called regimental badge" (BDC 7th/ Vol. I 72-73)*

*"****Musculotendinous cuff of the shoulder or rotator cuff*** *gives strength to the capsule of shoulder joint all around except inferiorly" (BDC 7th/ Vol. I 74)*

"Trapezius upper and lower fibres act with ***serratus anterior to*** *rotate the scapula forwards round the chest wall thus playing an* ***important role in abduction of the arm beyond 90°"*** *(BDC 7th/ Vol. I 64, 105)*

The deltoid originates in **three distinct sets of fibers**, often referred to as "heads"

- The **anterior or clavicular** fibers assist Pectoralis Major to flex the shoulder.
- The **lateral fibers or acromial fibers** perform basic shoulder abduction when the shoulder is internally rotated and perform ***shoulder transverse abduction*** when the shoulder is externally rotated.
- The **posterior fibers or spinal fibers** assist Latissimus Dorsi to extend the shoulder.

4. **Ans. a. Flexor carpi ulnaris..., b. Brachioradialis, c. Abductor pollicis brevis, e. Flexor digitorum superficialis**

[Ref: BDC 7th/ Vol. I 114]

Anterior Interosseous Nerve

◈ *BDC 7th/ Vol. I 114, 110*

- Branch of median nerve
- Supplies- ***flexor pollicis longus, flexor digitorum profundus (lateral half) and pronator quadratus***
- Also supplies- distal radioulnar and wrist joints

Muscles and Their Supply

"***Flexor carpi ulnaris-Ulnar nerve***"- *BDC 7th/ Vol. I 108*

"***Flexor digitorum superficialis- median nerve***"- *BDC 7th/ Vol. I 108*

"***Abductor pollicis brevis-median nerve***"- *BDC 7th/ Vol. I 124*

"***Brachioradialis-radial nerve***"- *BDC 7th/ Vol. I 101*

5. **Ans. a. 2nd largest salivary gland, b. Stenson's duct opens into the vestibule of the mouth..., d. Majority of lymph nodes are embedded in deep lobe**

[Ref: BDC 7th/ Vol. III 108-13; Snell 9th/630-32; Essential Anatomy by Moore 2nd/954-55; Gray's 40th/495-97]

"The facial nerve divides the gland into superficial and deep lobes"- *Snell 9th/630*

"Facial layer is very thick superficially but very thin on the deep side of the parotid gland where ***parotid abscess can burst to form a parapharyngeal abscess*** and thence spread to the mediastinum"-*P.L.Dingra 6th/263*

Parotid Gland

◈ *BDC 7th/ Vol. III 108-13*

- It is the largest of salivary glands.
- Stenson's duct opens into the vestibule of the mouth opposite the crown of the upper second molar teeth
- "Superficial surface of parotid is covered with a few deep parotid lymph nodes embedded in the glans"- *BDC 7th/ Vol. III 110*
- Facial nerve lies in relation to isthmus of the gland which separates large superficial part from small deep part of the gland. Facial nerve divides into two branches—temporofacial and cervicofacial nerve"- *BDC 7th/ Vol. III 111*

◈ *Gray's 40th/495-97*

- The paired parotid glands are ***the largest of the salivary glands.***
- The gland also projects forwards onto the surface of masseter.
- Lymph nodes occur in the skin overlying the parotid gland (preauricular nodes) and in the substance of the gland. There are usually 10 lymph nodes present in the gland, ***the majority lie in the superficial part of the gland*** above the plane related to the facial nerve. Lymph from the parotid gland drains to the upper deep cervical lymph nodes.

Parotid: The parotid lymph nodes are a small group of nodes located superficially to the parotid gland. They collect lymph from the nose, the nasal cavity, the external acoustic meatus, the tympanic cavity and the lateral borders of the orbit. There are also ***parotid lymph nodes deep to the parotid gland*** that drain the nasal cavities and the nasopharynx"-teachmeanatomy.info

6. **Ans. b. Contains mucous secreting glands, d. Made up of elastic cartilage, e. Has bilateral lymphatic supply**

[Ref: BDC 7th/ Vol. III 264; Snell's 8th/ 802; Moore 2nd/628; Gray's 40th/ 577-78, 588; Dhingra 6th/283-85; H and N Cancer by Louis B Harrison 3rd/368; H and N Surgery by Robert Satalof 1st /693]

Epiglottis/Epiglottic Cartilage

◈ *BDC 7th/ Vol. III 264*

- The epiglottis is a *leaf-shaped structure.*
- It is a flap that is made of elastic cartilage tissue covered with a mucous membrane, attached to the entrance of the larynx.
- The epiglottis is one of nine cartilaginous structures that make up the larynx (voice box). While one is breathing, it lies completely within the pharynx. When one is swallowing it serves as part of the anterior of the larynx.
- The epiglottis has two surfaces, a lingual and a laryngeal surface, related to the oral cavity and the larynx respectively
- The entire lingual surface and the apical portion of the laryngeal surface (since it is vulnerable to abrasion due to

its relation to the digestive tract) are covered by *a stratified squamous non-keratinized epithelium.*

- The rest of the laryngeal surface on the other hand, which is in relation to the respiratory system, has respiratory epithelium: pseudostratified, ciliated columnar cells and ***mucus secreting Goblet cells.***

Lymphatic Drainage

◈ *Gray's 40th/ 588; Moore 2nd/628*

- The vocal cords, with their firmly bound mucosa and paucity of lymphatics, provide a clear demarcation between the upper and lower areas of the larynx.
- **Above the vocal cords**, the lymph vessels draining the supraglottic part of the larynx accompany the superior laryngeal artery, pierce the thyrohyoid membrane and end in the upper deep cervical lymph nodes, ***often bilaterally.*** The supraglottic lymphatics also communicate with those at the base of the tongue. (Note: ***Epiglottis is supraglottic part of larynx***- *Dhingra 6th/283*)
- **Below the vocal cords**, some of the lymph vessels pass through the conus elasticus to reach the prelaryngeal (Delphian) and/or pretracheal and paratracheal lymph nodes, while others accompany the inferior laryngeal artery and join the ***lower deep cervical nodes.***
- "The supraglottis has **extensive bilateral network** of lymphatics that result in frequent regional metastases"-*H and N Cancer by Louis B Harrison 3rd/368*

"Unlike the other two anatomic sites (glottis and subglottis) of the larynx, the supraglottis is formed without midline union and consequently has ***bilateral lymphatic drainage****"-H and N Surgery by Robert Satalof 1st /693*

---

7. Ans. a. Thyroid lies in between 2 layers of deep cervical fascia, b. Berry ligament derived from deep cervical fascia, c. Left recurrent laryngeal nerve is larger than right recurrent laryngeal nerve

---

[Ref: L and B 26th/742; Schwartz 10th/1523]

Thyroid Gland

◈ *Schwartz 10th/1523-25*

- ***The thyroid gland is enveloped by a loosely connecting fascia that is formed from the partition of the deep cervical fascia into anterior and posterior divisions (false capsule)***
- The true capsule of the thyroid is a thin, densely adherent fibrous layer that sends out septa that invaginate into the gland, forming pseudolobules.
- The thyroid capsule is condensed into the ***posterior suspensory or Berry's ligament*** near the cricoid cartilage and upper tracheal rings.
- *"The* ***false capsule*** *is derived from the pretracheal layer of the deep cervical fascia. It is thin along the posterior border of the lobes, but thick on the inner surface of the gland where it forms a* ***suspensory ligament (of berry),*** *which connects the lobe to the cricoid cartilage"- BDC 7th/Vol III 145*

"The course of the recurrent laryngeal nerves on the right and left sides is different. ***The left RLN is longer than the right***, because it crosses under the arch of the aorta at the ligamentum arteriosum. The lower origin and consequently, a longer course of the left RLN makes it more vulnerable to injury than the right RLN."- emedicine.medscape.com; *BDC 7th/Vol IV 83*

"Superior thyroid artery: It runs downwards and forwards in intimate relation to external laryngeal nerve"- *BDC 7th/Vol III 147*

"About 85% of individuals have four parathyroid glands that can be found within 1 cm of the junction of the inferior thyroid artery and the RLN. ***The superior glands are usually located dorsal to the RLN, whereas the inferior glands are usually found ventral to the RLN****"-Schwartz 10th/1523*

---

8. Ans. d. Anterior horn of the medial meniscus

[Ref: BDC 7th/ Vol. II 26-27; Snell's 8th/470; Gray's 40th/1397]

Attachments on the intercondylar area (b/w medial and lateral tibial plateaus): Attachment from before backward *BDC 7th/ Vol. II 26-27*

1. Anterior horn of the medial meniscus
2. Anterior cruciate ligament
3. Anterior horn of the lateral meniscus
4. Posterior horn of the lateral meniscus
5. Posterior horn of the medial meniscus
6. Posterior cruciate ligament

Intercondylar Area

◈ *Gray's 40th/1397*

- The rough-surfaced area between the condylar articular surfaces is narrowest centrally where there is an intercondylar eminence, the edges of which project slightly proximally as the lateral and medial intercondylar tubercles.
- The anterior intercondylar area is widest anteriorly. Anteromedially, anterior to the medial articular surface, a depression marks the site of attachment of the ***anterior horn of the medial meniscus.*** Behind this a smooth area receives the anterior cruciate ligament.
- The **anterior horn of the lateral meniscus** is attached anterior to the intercondylar eminence, lateral to the ***anterior cruciate ligament***.
- The posterior horn of the lateral meniscus is attached to the posterior slope of the intercondylar area. The posterior intercondylar area inclines down and backwards behind the posterior horn of the lateral meniscus.
- A depression behind the base of the medial intercondylar tubercle is for the posterior horn of the ***medial meniscus.*** The rest of the area is smooth and provides attachment for the posterior cruciate ligament, spreading back to a ridge to which the capsule is attached

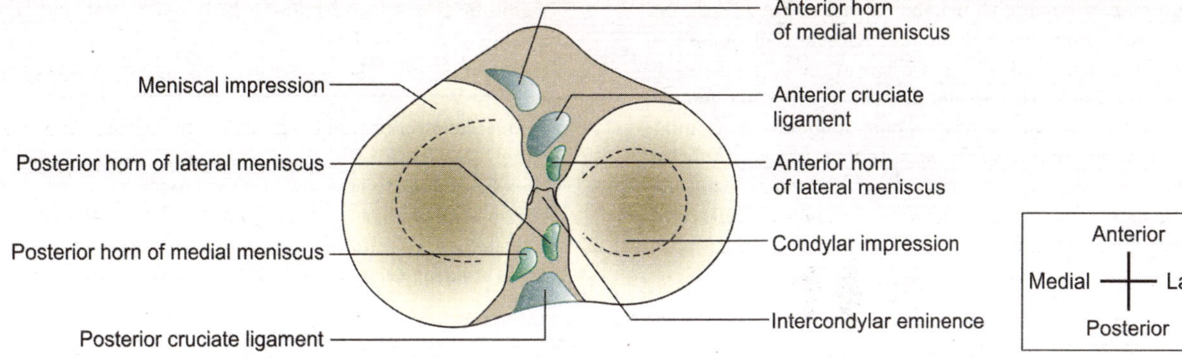

Fig: *(BDC 7th/ Vol. II 26-27):* Superior view of the upper end of the right tibia

9. Ans. a. Homologous chromosomes separate; c. Haploid daughter cells; d. Homologous chromosomes exchange material;

[Ref: Gray's 40th/22-23;I B Singh 10th/ 13-15;Langman's Medical Embryology 9th/6-7]

- *Meiosis consists of two consecutive divisions, meiosis I & meiosis, to yield four haploid gametes from a single diploid grand parent cell. Hence, the meiosis is called heterotypical or reduction division*
- *Characteristic of meiosis:* ***No DNA replication*** *b/w meiosis I & meiosis II*
- ***During diplotene stage of prophase I, pairs of homologous chromosome separates***
- ***In meiosis I: Homologous chromosome separate***
- ***In meiosis II: Sister chromatids of same chromosome separate***

Meiosis I

◈ *Gray's 40th/22-23; I B Singh 10th/ 13-15*

- Meiosis I consists of Prophase I (Leptotene, Zygotene, Pachytene, Diplotene & Diakinesis), metaphase I, Anaphase I and telophase I
- ***Prophase of Meiosis I-Contains 5 steps Gray's 40th/22-23;I B Singh 10th/ 13-15***
  - **During leptotene**, homologous chromosomes (maternal and paternal copies of the same chromosome), which were replicated in a preceding S phase and each ***consist of sister chromatids joined at the centromere***, locate one another within the nucleus and the process of ***genetic recombination is initiated.*** Cytologically, chromosomes begin to condense, appearing as individual threads that are attached via their telomeres to the nuclear membrane.
  - **Zygotene stage:** Duringzygotene, the homologous chromosomes initiate a process known as synapsis, during which they become intimately associated with one another. The pairs of synapsed homologues, also known as bivalents, are linked together by a highly structured fibrillar band, the synaptonemalcomplex.
  - **Pachytene stage:** When synapsis is complete for all chromosomes, the cell is said to be in pachytene. Each bivalent looks like a single structure, but is actually ***two pairs of sister chromatids held together by the synaptonemal complex. Genetic recombination is completed at this point***, with sites where it has occurred (usually one per chromosome arm) appearing as nodules in the center of the synaptonemalcomplex.
  - **Diplotene stage:** Duringdiplotene, the synaptonemal complex disassembles and ***pairs of homologous chromosomes, now much shortened,separate except where crossing over has occurred*** (chiasmata). At least one chiasma forms between each homologous pair, exchanging maternal and paternal sequences and up to five have been observed.
  - **Diakinesis:** Diakinesis is the prometaphase of the first meiotic division.
- Metaphase I resembles mitotic metaphase, except that the bodies attaching to the spindle microtubules are ***bivalents, not single chromosomes.***These become arranged so that the homologous pairs occupy theequatorial plane of the spindle.
- Anaphase I of meiosis begins with the ***release of cohesion between the arms of sister chromatids, much as it does during mitosis.*** In meiosis, this 'unties' the topological knots of the chiasmata and ***allows homologous chromosomes to separate and migrate to opposite spindle poles.*** As positioning of bivalent pairs is random, assortment of maternal and paternal chromosomes in each telophase nucleus is also random. ***Critically, sister centromeres and thus chromatids, do not separate during anaphase I.***
- In Telophase I, two daughter nuclei are formed. The division of nucleus is followed by division of the cytoplasm
- During meiosis I, cytoplasmic division occurs by specialized mechanisms. In females, the division is highly asymmetric, producing one egg and ***one tiny cell known as a polar body***. In males, the process does not go to full completion, resulting in ***production of spermatocytes*** that remain joined by small cytoplasmic bridges.

Meiosis II

◈ *Gray's 40th/22-23; I B Singh 10th/ 13-15*

- "Meiosis II is similar to mitosis. However, because of crossing over that has occurred during the meiosis I, the daughter cells are not identical in genetic content"- I B Singh 10th/ 15
- Meiosis II commences after only a short interval during which no DNA synthesis occurs. The centromeres of sister

chromatids remain paired, but rotate so that each one can face an opposite spindle pole. Onset of anaphase II is triggered by loss of cohesion between the centromeres, as it is in mitosis. This ***second division is more like mitosis, in that chromatids separate during anaphase***, but, unlike mitosis, ***the separating chromatids are genetically different*** (the result of genetic recombination). ***Cytoplasmic division also occurs and thus, in the male, four haploid cells result from meiosis I and II.***

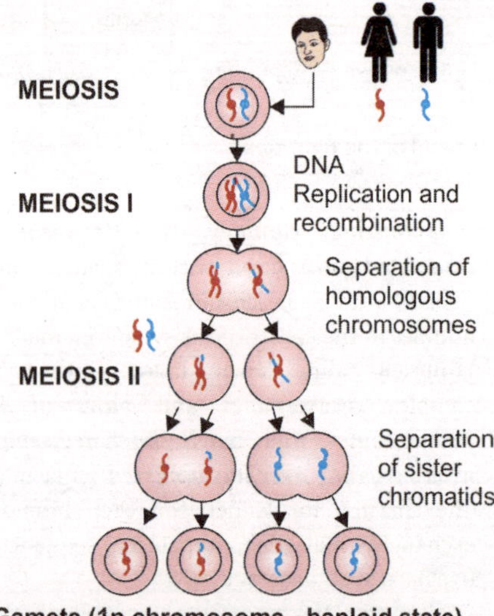

10. Ans. a. Tendon of Todaro is between central fibrous parts to Eustachian valve; b Tendon of infundibulum is between pulmonary & aortic valve; d Trigonum fibrous sinistrum is between mitral and aortic valve; e Fibrous ring around mitral valve

[Ref: BDC 7th/ Vol. I 274-76 ; Snell 9th/85 ;Gray's 40th/977]

Trigonum fibrous dextrum is fibrous tissue b/w atrioventricular rings(mitral & tricuspid) behind & the aortic ring in front- *BDC 7th/ Vol. I 276*

Trigonum fibrous sinistrum is between mitral and aortic valve- BDC 7th/ Vol. I 276

Tendon of infundibulum is between pulmonary & aortic valve- BDC 7th/ Vol. I 276

Fibrous skeleton of heart consists of fibrous ring surrounding orifices of AV orifices (**mitral** & tricuspid valve), pulmonary orifices & aortic orifices- BDC 7th/ Vol. I 275

Tendon of Todaro is a part of fibrous skeleton of heart which originates from central fibrous body & runs upto inferomedial part of inferior vena cava(Eustachian valve)-www.vhlab.umn.edu

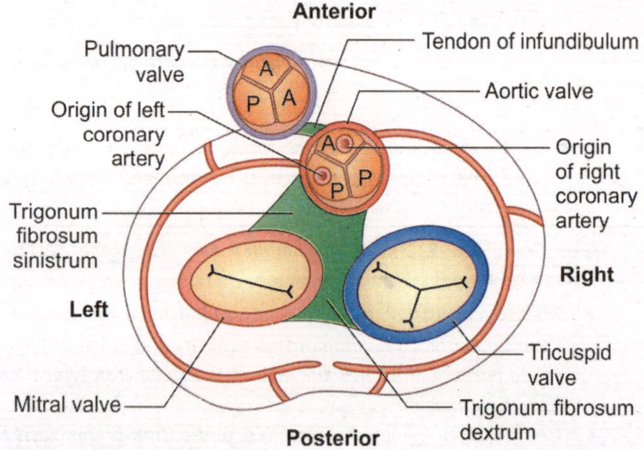

Fig: *(BDC 7th/ Vol. I 276)*: Valves & fibrous skeleton of heart

PHYSIOLOGY

11. Ans. a. 3β-Hydroxysteroid dehydrogenase deficiency, c. 17α-Hydroxylase deficiency, d. 21-Hydroxylase deficiency

[Ref: Davison 22nd/782; Harrison 19th/2327-28]

Table ***(Harrison 19th/2328)*: Variants of Congenital Adrenal Hyperplasia**

Variant	Gene	Impact on Steroid Synthesis
21-Hydroxylase deficiency (21OHD)	*CYP21A2*	Glucocorticoid deficiency, mineralocorticoid deficiency, adrenal androgen excess
11β-Hydroxylase deficiency (11OHD)	*CYP11B1*	Glucocorticoid deficiency, mineralocorticoid excess, adrenal androgen excess
17α-Hydroxylase deficiency (17OHD)	*CYP17A1*	(Glucocorticoid deficiency), mineralocorticoid excess androgen deficiency
3β-Hydroxysteroid dehydrogenase deficiency (3bHSDD)	*HSD3B2*	Glucocorticoid deficiency, (mineralocorticoid deficiency), adrenal androgen excess
P450 oxidoreductase deficiency (ORD)	*POR*	Glucocorticoid deficiency, (mineralocorticoid excess) androgen deficiency, skeletal malformations

"**Aromatase deficiency** and *17α-hydroxylase deficiency* are associated with ***decreased estrogen and elevated gonadotropins*** and with hyperandrogenism and hypertension, respectively"-*Harrison 19th/337*

Testosterone can be converted to the more potent DHT by **5α-reductase,** or it can be aromatized to estradiol by CYP19 (aromatase)"-*Harrison 19th/2358*

Congenital Adrenal Hyperplasia

◈ *Harrison 19th/2327-28*

- Congenital adrenal hyperplasia (CAH) is caused by mutations in genes encoding steroidogenic enzymes involved in glucocorticoid synthesis (*CYP21A2, CYP17A1, HSD3B2, CYP11B1*) or in the cofactor enzyme P450 oxidoreductase that serves as an electron donor to CYP21A2 and CYP17A1
- "The most common enzyme defect is 21-hydroxylase deficiency"-*Davison 22nd/782*
- Invariably, patients affected by CAH exhibit glucocorticoid deficiency. Depending on the exact step of enzymatic block, they may also have excess production of mineralocorticoids or deficient production of sex steroids
- The diagnosis of CAH is readily established by measurement of the steroids accumulating before the distinct enzymatic block, either in serum or in urine, preferably by the use of mass spectrometry–based assays
- Mutations in *CYP21A2* are the most prevalent cause of CAH, responsible for 90–95% of cases. 21-Hydroxylase deficiency disrupts glucocorticoid and mineralocorticoid synthesis

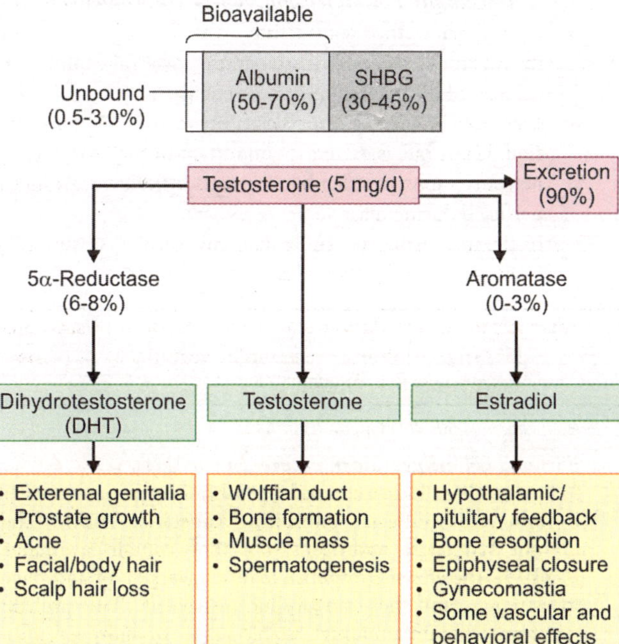

Fig. *(Harrison 19th/2359)*: Androgen metabolism and actions. SHBG, sex hormone–binding globulin.

12. Ans. b. ↑ed affinity of haemoglobin to oxygen, d. Right shift of oxygen-hemoglobin dissociation curve

[Ref: Ganong 25th/640-41; Guyton 12th/356-57; A K Jain 6th/430]

"*All the factors which shift the* **oxygen-hemoglobin dissociation curve to right, decreases the affinity of haemoglobin for oxygen, therefore, a higher pO_2 is required for Hb to bind a given amount of oxygen"**- *A K Jain 6th/430*

2,3-DPG and oxygen-hemoglobin dissociation curve *Ganong 25th/641*

- 2, 3-DPG is very plentiful in red cells. It is formed from 3-phosphoglyceraldehyde, which is a product of glycolysis via the Embden-Meyerhof pathway.
- It is a highly charged anion that binds to the β chains of deoxyhemoglobin. One mole of deoxyhemoglobin binds 1 mol of 2, 3-DPG.
- An increase in the concentration of ***2,3-DPG shifts the reaction to the right, causing more O2 to be liberated.***

Effect of BPG to Cause Rightward Shift of the Oxygen-Hemoglobin Dissociation Curve

◈ *Guyton 12th/357*

- The normal **BPG** in the blood keeps the oxygen-hemoglobin dissociation ***curve shifted slightly to the right all the time***.
- In hypoxic conditions that last longer than a few hours, the quantity of BPG in the blood increases considerably, thus shifting the oxygen-hemoglobin dissociation ***curve even farther to the right***.
- This causes ***oxygen to be released to the tissues at as much as 10 mm Hg higher tissue oxygen pressure than would be the case without this increased BPG***. Therefore, under some conditions, the BPG mechanism can be important for adaptation to hypoxia, especially to hypoxia caused by poor tissue blood flow.
- ***Red cell 2,3-DPG concentration is increased in anemia*** and in a variety of diseases in which there is chronic hypoxia. ***This facilitates the delivery of O2 to the tissues*** by raising the Po_2 at which O_2 is released in peripheral capillaries.
- In banked blood that is stored, the 2, 3-DPG level falls and the ability of this blood to release O_2 to the tissues is reduced.

Hb-O_2 Dissociation Curve	
Left shifting	**Right Shifting**
• ↓2, 3-BPG	• ↑2, 3-BPG
• Alkalosis	• **Acidosis**
• **Hypothermia**	• Hyperthermia
• **Foetal Hb**	• High altitude
• Hypocarbia	• Exercise
• Stored blood	• **Hypercarbia**
• Hb Chesapeake	• Anaemia
• Hb Ranier	• Sickle cell anaemia
	• HbM
	• Diabetic Ketoacidosis
	• Thyroid hormone
	• Growth hormone
	• Androgen
	• Diseases causing chronic hypoxia

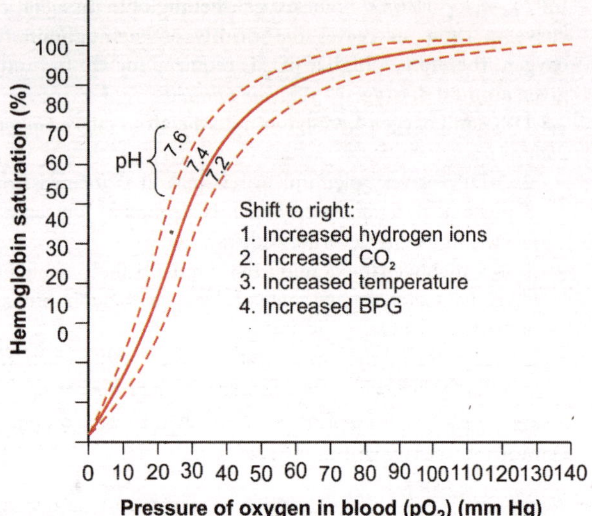

Fig: Shift of the oxygen-hemoglobin dissociation curve to the right caused by an increase in hydrogen ion concentration (decrease in pH). BPG, 2,3-biphosphoglycerate.

13. Ans. All (a, b, c, d, e)

[Ref: Ganong 25th/550; Guyton 12th/216-17]

"Frank-Starling law: The ***force of muscle contraction is directly proportional to the initial length of the muscle fiber,*** *within physiological limits. In the heart, the* ***initial length is at the end of diastole****"- Guyton 12th/216*

"**Increasing preload** (e.g., ***ventricular end-diastolic volume***) also increases ***myocardial oxygen consumption***; however, the increase is much less than what might be expected because of the LaPlace relationship"- *www.cvphysiology.com*

OXYGEN CONSUMPTION BY THE HEART

◈ *Ganong 25th/550*

- **Basal O_2 consumption** by the myocardium is ***about 2 mL/100 g/min***. O_2 consumption by the beating heart is about 9 mL/100 g/min at rest. Increases occur ***during exercise and in a number of different states.***
- O_2 consumption by the heart is determined primarily by the ***intramyocardial tension, the contractile state of the myocardium and the heart rate.***
- **Ventricular work** ***per beat correlates with O2 consumption.*** The *work is the product of stroke volume and mean arterial pressure* in the pulmonary artery or the aorta (for the right and left ventricle, respectively).
- Because aortic pressure is seven times greater than pulmonary artery pressure, the *stroke work of the left ventricle is approximately seven times the stroke work of the right.*
- In theory, a 25% increase in stroke volume without a change in arterial pressure should produce the same increase in O_2 consumption as a 25% increase in arterial pressure without a change in stroke volume. However, for reasons that are incompletely understood, pressure work produces a greater increase in O_2 consumption than volume work.
- In other words, ***an increase in afterload causes a greater increase in cardiac O_2 consumption than does an increase in preload.*** This is why angina pectoris due to deficient delivery of O_2 to the myocardium is more common in aortic stenosis than in aortic regurgitation. In aortic stenosis, intraventricular pressure must be increased to force blood through the stenotic valve, whereas in aortic regurgitation, an increase in stroke volume with little change in aortic impedance occurs.

Chemical Energy Required for Cardiac Contraction: Oxygen Utilization by the Heart

◈ *Guyton 12th/204-05*

- Oxygen consumption has also been shown to be nearly proportional to the ***tension*** that occurs in the heart muscle during contraction multiplied by the *duration of time* that the contraction persists, called the ***tension-time index.***
- Because tension is high when systolic pressure is high, correspondingly more oxygen is used.

Myocardial O_2 Consumption Determinants

◈ *www.openanesthesia.or*

- The amount of oxygen consumed is determined by the ***basal O_2 consumption, wall tension, contractility and heart rate.***
- The greater the contractility, the more oxygen the myocardium consumes. Faster, more powerful contractions (increased dP/dT) requires more energy.
- ***Increased HR leads to increased myocardial O_2 consumption.*** Heart rate is extremely important in that it influences not only supply, but demand as well, as the myocardium is perfused during diastole.
- In the unanesthetized individual, myocardial consumption is the main determinant of myocardial supply.

14. Ans. a. Sertoli cells secrete Mullerian inhibiting substance (MIS), b. Inhibin is released by sertoli cell, c. Primary spermatocyte is diploid

[Ref: Ganong 25th/409; Guyton 12th/537]

FSH and LH are ***peptide in nature****- Guyton 12th/537*

"The Sertoli cells secrete **androgen-binding protein (ABP), inhibin** and **Mullerian inhibiting substance (MIS).** They do not synthesize androgens, but they contain **aromatase (CYP19),** the enzyme responsible for conversion of androgens to estrogens and they can produce estrogens. ABP probably functions to maintain a high, stable supply of androgen in the tubular fluid. ***Inhibin inhibits follicle-stimulating hormone (FSH) secretion***"- *Ganong 25th/419*

Spermatogenesis

◈ *Ganong 25th/418*

- **Spermatogonia,** the primitive germ cells next to the basal lamina of the seminiferous tubules, mature into **primary spermatocytes.** This process begins during adolescence. The primary spermatocytes undergo meiotic division, reducing the number of chromosomes.

- In this two-stage process, they divide into **secondary spermatocytes** and then into **spermatids,** which contain the ***haploid number of 23 chromosomes***. The spermatids mature into **spermatozoa (sperm).**

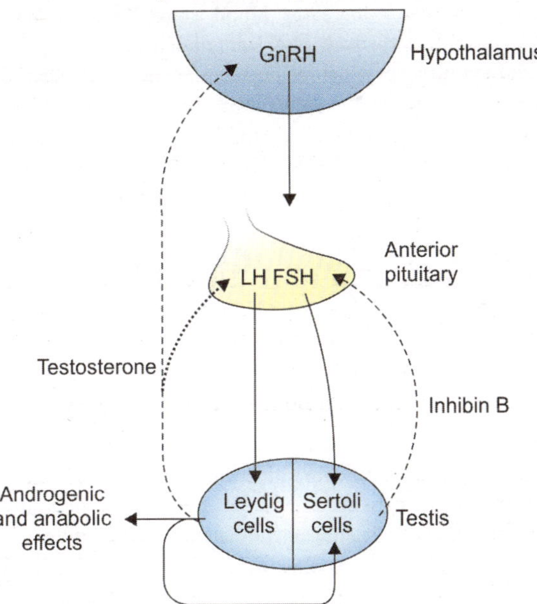

Fig: *(Ganong 25th/409)*: Postulated interrelationships between the hypothalamus, anterior pituitary and testes. Solid arrows indicate excitatory effects; dashed arrows indicate inhibitory effects

15. Ans. b. K^+

[Ref: Ganong 25th/433-34; Guyton 12th/613; A K Jain 6th/748]

Relation to Potassium

Ganong 25th/433-34; Guyton 12th/613

- ***Insulin causes K^+ to enter cells***, with a resultant lowering of the extracellular K^+ concentration.
- Infusions of insulin and glucose significantly lower the plasma K^+ level in normal individuals and are very effective for the temporary relief of hyperkalemia in patients with renal failure.
- **Hypokalemia** often develops when patients with diabetic acidosis are treated with insulin.
- The reason for the intracellular migration of K^+ is still uncertain. However, insulin increases the activity of Na, K ATPase in cell membranes, so that more K^+ is pumped into cells.

16. Ans. b. Parathyroid, c. Pancreas

[Ref: Ganong 25th/308-14; Harrison 19th/401e-2]

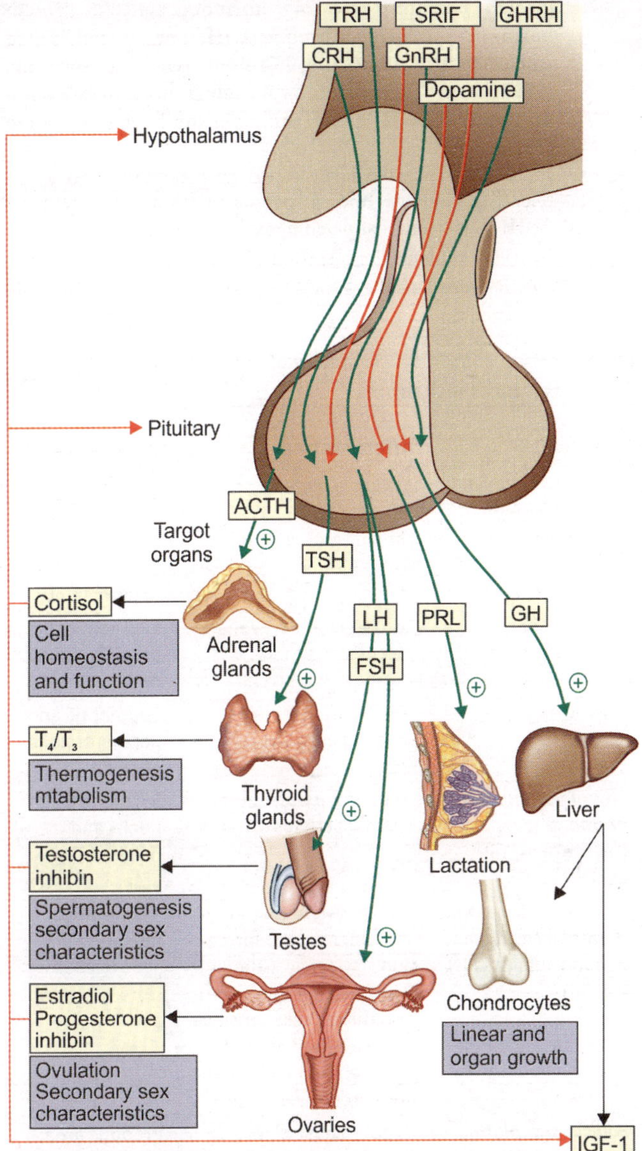

Fig: *(Harrison 19th/401e-2)*: Diagram of pituitary axes. Hypothalamic hormones regulate anterior pituitary trophic hormones that in turn determine target gland secretion. Peripheral hormones feedback to regulate hypothalamic and pituitary hormones.

Hypophysiotropic Hormones

Ganong 25th/314

- There are six established hypothalamic releasing and inhibiting hormones: **corticotropin-releasing hormone (CRH); thyrotropin-releasing hormone (TRH);**

growth hormone–releasing hormone (GRH); growth hormone–inhibiting hormone (GIH, now generally called **somatostatin); luteinizing hormone–releasing hormone (LHRH,** now generally known as **gonadotropin-releasing hormone [GnRH]);** and **prolactin-inhibiting hormone (PIH).**

- In addition, hypothalamic extracts contain prolactin-releasing activity and a **prolactin-releasing hormone (PRH)** has been postulated to exist.
- GnRH stimulates the secretion of FSH as well as that of LH and it seems unlikely that a separate FSH-releasing hormone exists.

Table *(Ganong 25th/309)*: **Summary of principal hypothalamic regulatory mechanisms**

Function	Afferents from	Integrating Areas
Neuroendocrine control of:		
Catecholamines	Limbic areas concerned with emotion	Dorsal and posterior hypothalamus
Vasopressin	Osmoreceptors, "volume receptors", others	Supraoptic and paraventricular nuclei
Oxytocin	Touch receptors in breast, uterus, genitalia	Supraoptic and paraventricular nuclei
Thyroid-stimulating hormone (thyrotropin, TSH) via TRH	Temperature receptors in infants, perhaps others	Paraventricular nuclei and neighboring areas
Adranocoriticotropic hormone (ACTH) and β -lipotropin (β-LPH) via CRH	Limbic system (emotional stimuli); reticular formation ("systemic" stimuli); Hypothalamic and anterior pituitary cells sensitive to circulating blood cortisol level; suprachiasmatic nuclei (diurnal rhythm)	Paraventricular nuclei
Follicle-stimulating hormone (FSH) and luteinizing hormone (LH) via GnRH	Hypothalamic cells sensitive to estrogens, eyes, touch receptors in skin and genitalia or reflex ovulating species	Preoptic area; other areas
Prolactin via PIH and PRH	Touch receptors in breasts, other unknown receptors	Arcuate nucleus; other areas (hypothalamus inhibits secretion)
Growth hormones via somatostatin and GRH	Unknown receptors	Periventricular nucleus, arcuate nucleus

17. Ans. c. Decreased level of norepinephrine

[Ref: Ganong 25th/364; Guyton 12th/598,556; Schwartz 9th/17-20; A K Jain 6th/606; L and B 26th/4-9; CSDT 11th/103-05]

Hormone which **increases blood sugar level***:* ***epinephrine, glucagon, GH, cortisol****"- A K Jain 6th/606*

"**Following injury**, neural impulses carried via spinothalamic pathways activate the brain stem and thalamic and cortical centers, which stimulate the hypothalamus. Hypothalamic stimulation triggers combined neural and endocrine discharges. ***Norepinephrine*** is released from sympathetic nerve endings, *epinephrine from the adrenal medulla*, aldosterone from the adrenal cortex, ADH from the posterior pituitary, glucagon from the pancreas and *ACTH*, TSH and growth hormone from the anterior pituitary. These hormones produce secondary *elevations of cortisol*, thyroid hormone and somatomedins"- *CSDT 11th/104*

Mediators of the Metabolic Response to Injury

◈ *L and B 26th/4-9*

- The classical neuroendocrine pathways of the **stress response** consist of afferent nociceptive neurones, the spinal cord, thalamus, hypothalamus and pituitary.
- Corticotrophinreleasing factor (CRF) released from the hypothalamus increases adrenocorticotrophic hormone **(ACTH)** release from the anterior pituitary.
- ***ACTH then acts on the adrenal to increase the secretion of cortisol.*** Hypothalamic activation of the sympathetic nervous system causes release of adrenalin and also stimulates release of glucagon.
- There are, however, many other players, including *alterations in insulin release and sensitivity, hypersecretion of prolactin and growth hormone (GH) in the presence of low circulatory insulin-like growth factor-1 (IGF-1)* and inactivation of peripheral thyroid hormones and gonadal function.
- Of note, GH has direct lipolytic, insulin-antagonising and proinflammatory properties

Insulin Resistance

◈ *L and B 26th/9*

- Following surgery or trauma, **postoperative hyperglycaemia** develops as a result of increased glucose production combined with decreased glucose uptake in peripheral tissues. Decreased glucose uptake is a ***result of insulin resistance*** which is transiently induced within the stressed patient.
- Suggested mechanisms for this phenomenon include the action of proinflammatory cytokines and the decreased responsiveness of insulin-regulated glucose transporter proteins. The degree of ***insulin resistance*** is proportional to the magnitude of the injurious process.

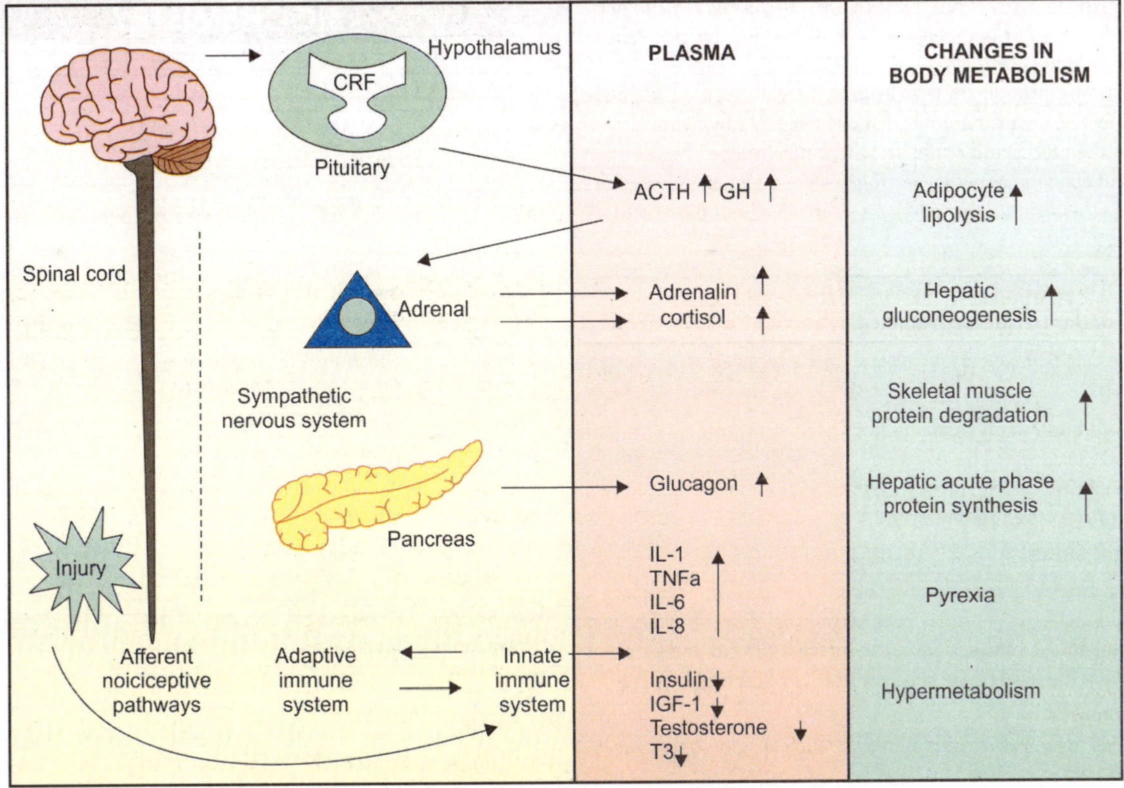

Fig: *(L and B 26th/5)*: The integrated response to surgical injury (first 24–48hr)

Insulin

◈ *Schwartz 9th/20*

- Hyperglycemia and insulin resistance are hallmarks of injury and critical illness due to the catabolic effects of circulating mediators, including ***catecholamines, cortisol, glucagon and GH.*** The increase in these circulating proglycemic factors, particularly ***epinephrine***, induces glycogenolysis, lipolysis and increased lactate production independent of available oxygen in a process that is termed "aerobic glycolysis."
- Although there is an increase in insulin production at the same time, severe stress is frequently associated with **insulin resistance,** leading to decreased glucose uptake in the liver and the periphery contributing to acute hyperglycemia.

Catecholamines

◈ *Schwartz 9th/20*

- The hypermetabolic state observed following severe injury is attributed to activation of the adrenergic system. ***Both norepinephrine (NE) and epinephrine (EPI) are increased*** three- to fourfold in plasma immediately following injury, with elevations lasting 24 to 48 hours before returning toward baseline levels.
- In the liver, **EPI promotes glycogenolysis, gluconeogenesis,** lipolysis and ketogenesis. It also causes decreased insulin release, but increases glucagon secretion. Peripherally, EPI increases lipolysis in adipose tissues and induces insulin resistance in skeletal muscle. These ***collectively manifest as stress-induced hyperglycemia***, not unlike the effects of cortisol on blood sugar.

18. Ans. b. Interstitial cells of the peritubular capillary bed of the kidneys

[Ref: Ganong 25th/706; Guyton 12th/461; A K Jain 6th/68]

The juxtaglomerular apparatus (JGA) consists of three types of cells: *A K Jain 6th/68*

- *the* **macula densa,** *a part of the distal convoluted tubule of the same nephron*
- **juxtaglomerular cells,** *(also known as granular cells) which* ***secrete renin***
- **mesangial cells** *or lacis cell: supporting cell*

Erythropoietin

◈ *Ganong 25th/706*

- In adults, about ***85% of the erythropoietin comes from the kidneys and 15% from the liver***. Both these organs contain the mRNA for erythropoietin.
- Erythropoietin can also be extracted from the ***spleen and salivary glands***, but these tissues do not contain its mRNA and consequently do not appear to manufacture the hormone. When renal mass is reduced in adults by kidney disease or nephrectomy, the liver cannot compensate and anemia develops.

- Erythropoietin is produced by ***interstitial cells in the peritubular capillary bed of the kidneys*** and by ***perivenous hepatocytes in the liver***.
- It is also produced in the **brain,** where it exerts a protective effect against excitotoxic damage triggered by hypoxia; and in the uterus and oviducts, where it is induced by estrogen and appears to mediate estrogen-dependent angiogenesis.

PCT *is divided into two parts: pars convolute and* ***pars recta****- A K Jain 6th/504*

19. Ans. b. Present in early part of internal carotid arterym, d. Barorecptor, e. Supplied by glossopharyngel nerve

[Ref: Ganong 25th/658; Guyton 12th/251-52; A K Jain 6th/327-29; Gray's 40th/447]

"Carotid bodies and aortic bodies are chemorecptor"- A K Jain 6th/331-32

"Each carotid and aortic body (glomus) contains islands of two types of cell, type I (glomus) and type II cells"- Ganong 25th/658

Carotid Sinus

◈ *A K Jain 6th/327-29*

It is dilated area at initial part of internal carotid artery just superior to the bifurcation of the internal carotid and external carotid at the level of the superior border of thyroid cartilage

Barorecptor

Supplied by carotid sinus nerve (branch of glossopharyngeal nerve)

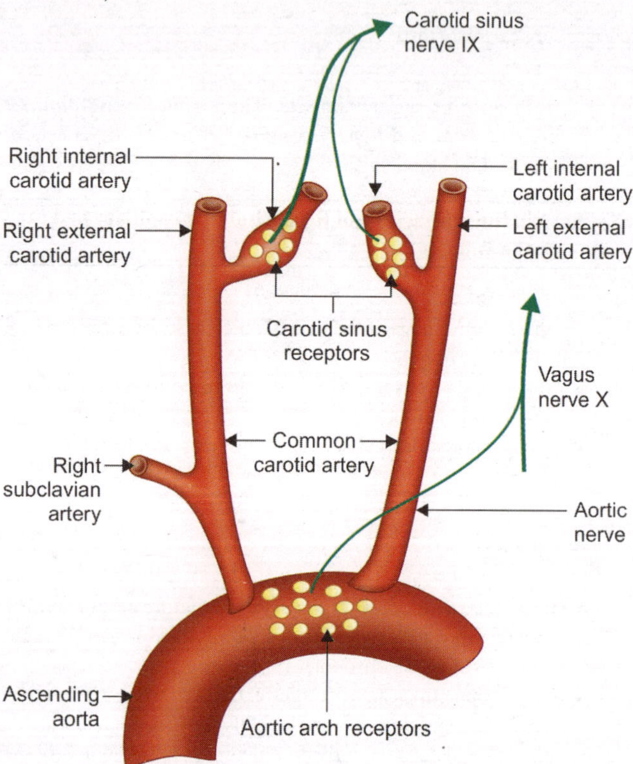

Fig: *(A K Jain 6th/329): Systemic arterial barorecptors (location and innervation)*

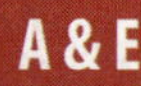

BIOCHEMISTRY

20. Ans. All (a, b, c, d, e)

[Ref: Harper 30th/ 89-94; Lippincott 6th/62-64; Vasudevan 5th/42-50; Shinde 7th/119-20; Satyanarayan 4th/100]

Table *(Lippincott 6th/64)*: **Mechanisms for regulating enzyme activity**

Regulator Event	Typical Effector	Results	Time required for change
Substrate inhibition	Substrate	Change in velocity (v_o)	Immediate
Product inhibition	Reaction product	Change in V_{max} and /or $K_{0.5}$	Immediate
Allosteric control	Pathway end product	Change in V_{max} and/or K_m	Immediate
Covalent modification	Another enzyme	Change in V_{max} and /or K_m	Immediate to minutes
Synthesis or degradation of enzyme	Hormone or metabolite	Change in the amount of enzyme	Hours to days

"**Allosteric regulation** may be either ***allosteric activation or allosteric inhibition***"- *Vasudevan 5th/48*

"In case of inhibition, the inhibitors acts on the enzyme activity directly. On the contrary, ***repression*** *acts at the* ***gene level and number of enzyme molecule is reduced in presence of repressor molecule****"- Vasudevan 5th/49-50*

"***Induction is turning 'on' the switch of the gene. Repression is turning 'off' the gene expression***"- *Vasudevan 5th/444*

Factor Influencing Enzyme Activity

◈ *Shinde 7th/119-20; Vasudevan 5th/42-50*

- *Enzyme concentration*
- *Product concentration*
- *Substrate concentration*
- *Activators and coenzymes*
- *Inhibitors (competitive, non-competitive and allosteric inhibition)*
- *Repressor or depressor*
- *Time*
- *pH*
- *Temperature*
- *Covalent modification*

Regulation of Enzyme Activity

◈ *Lippincott 6th/62-64*

- The regulation of the reaction velocity of enzymes is essential if an organism is to coordinate its numerous metabolic processes.
- The rates of most enzymes are responsive to changes in substrate concentration
- In addition, some enzymes with specialized regulatory functions respond to ***allosteric effectors or covalent modification***, or they ***show altered rates of enzyme synthesis (or degradation)*** when physiologic conditions are changed.

- **Regulation of allosteric enzymes**
- **Regulation of enzymes by covalent modification**
- **Induction and repression of enzyme synthesis:**The regulatory mechanisms described above modify the activity of existing enzyme molecules. However, cells can also regulate the amount of enzyme present by ***altering the rate of enzyme degradation*** or, more typically, the ***rate of enzyme synthesis. The increase (induction) or decrease (repression) of enzyme synthesis*** leads to an alteration in the total population of active sites.

21. Ans. c. Highly positively charged

[Ref: Harper 30th/634-36; Lippincott 6th/ 157-60; Shinde 7th/; Satyanarayan 4th/22,281]

"Hyaluronic acid is present in connective tissues, tendon, synovial fluid and vitreous fluid"-Vasudevan 5th/69

Glycosaminoglycans (GAGs)/Mucopolysaccharides

◈ *Lippincott 6th/ 157-60*

- They are large complexes of ***negatively charged*** hetero-polysaccharide chains. They are generally associated with a ***small amount of protein***, forming proteoglycans, which typically consist of over 95% carbohydrate. [Note: This is in comparison to the glyco proteins, which consist primarily of protein with a small amount of carbohydrate.]
- They have the special ability to bind large amounts of water, thereby producing the gel-like matrix that forms the basis of the body's ground substance, which, along with fibrous structural proteins such as ***collagen and elastin*** and adhesive proteins such as fibronectin, make up the ***extracellular matrix (ECM).***
- The viscous, ***lubricating properties of mucous secretions*** also result from the presence of glycosaminoglycans, which led to the original naming of these compounds as mucopolysaccharides.

Table *(Harper 30th/638)*: **Some Functions of Glycosaminoglycans and Proteoglycans**

- Act as ***structural components of the ECM***
- Have specific interactions with collagen, elastin, fibronectin, laminin and other proteins such as growth factors
- ***As polyanions, bind polycations and cations***
- Contribute to the characteristic turgor of various tissues
- Act as sieves in the ECM
- *Facilitate cell migration (HA)*
- Have role in compressibility of cartilage in weight-bearing (HA,CS)
- Play role in corneal transparency (KS I and DS)
- Have structural role in sclera (DS)
- Act as anticoagulant (heparin)
- Are components of plasma membranes, where they may act as receptors and participate in cell adhesion and cell-cell interactions (e.g., HS)
- Determine charge selectiveness of renal glomerulus (HS)
- Are components of synaptic and other vesicles (eg, HS)

The Glycosaminoglycans Found in Proteoglycans are Built up of Repeating Disaccharides

◈ *Harper 30th/634-35*

- **Proteoglycans** are proteins that contain covalently linked **glycosaminoglycans** (GAGs).
- At least 30 have been characterized and given names such as syndecan, betaglycan, serglycin, perlecan, aggrecan, versican, decorin, biglycan and fibromodulin.
- The proteins bound covalently to glycosaminoglycans are called **"core proteins."**
- Proteoglycans vary in tissue distribution, nature of the core protein, attached glycosaminoglycans and their function; they have proved difficult to isolate and characterize
- There are at least seven GAGs: **hyaluronic acid (hyaluronan), chondroitin sulfate, keratan sulfates I and II, heparin, heparan sulfate and dermatan sulfate.**

22. Ans. d. Produces ribose 5-phosphate in oxidative phase of pathway

[Ref: Harper 30th/ 196-200; Lippincott 6th/145-45; Satyanarayan 4th/270-71]

Hexose Monophosphate Pathway (HMP) or HMP Shunt

◈ *Satyanarayan 4th/270-71*

- *This is an alternative pathway to glycolysis and TCA cycle for the oxidation of glucose*
- *The sequence of reactions of HMP shunt is divided into 2 phases- oxidative and non-oxidative*
- *Oxidative phase:NADPH is produced*
- *Non-oxidative:* ***ribose 5-phosphate***
- *The first reaction (occur in oxidative phase) catalysed by G6PD is most regulatory in the HMP shunt*

Hexose Monophosphate Pathway (HMP)

◈ *Lippincott 6th/145*

- Also called as pentose phosphate pathway or 6-phosphoglu-conate pathway
- It occurs in the cytosol of the cell.
- It includes two, irreversible oxidative reactions, followed by a series of reversible sugar–phosphate interconversions
- ***No ATP is directly consumed or produced in the cycle.***
- Carbon 1 of glucose 6-phosphate is released as CO2 and ***two NADPH are produced*** for each glucose 6-phosphate molecule entering the oxidative part of the pathway.
- The ***pathway provides a major portion of the body's NADPH***, which functions as a biochemical reductant.
- It ***also produces ribose 5-phosphate***, required for the biosynthesis of nucleotides
- This portion of the pathway is particularly important in the **liver, lactating mammary glands and adipose**, which are active in the NADPH-dependent biosynthesis of fatty acids, in the **testes, ovaries, placenta and adrenal cortex**, which are active in the NADPH-dependent biosynthesis of steroid hormones and in **erythrocytes**, which require NADPH to keep glutathione reduced

23. Ans. None

[Ref: Harrison 19th/ 2417-18; Davidson 22nd /812-13; Lippincott 6th/339, 345]

All are useful in diagnosis of diabetic ketoacidosis (DKA)

Table *(Harrison 19th/2417)*: **Laboratory Values in Diabetic Ketoacidosis (DKA) and Hyperglycemic Hyperosmolar State (HHS) (Representative Ranges at Presentation)**

	DKA	HHS
Chloride	Normal	Normal
Phosphate	Normal	Normal
Creatinine	Slightly ↑	Moderately ↑
Osmolality (mOsm/ mL)	300–320	330–380
Plasma ketones	++++	+/–
Serum bicarbonate, mEq/L	<15 mEq/L	Normal to slightly ↓
Arterial pH	6.8–7.3	>7.3
Glucose, mmol/L	13.9–33.3	33.3–66.6
Sodium, mEq/L	125–135	135–145
Potassium	Normal to ↑	Normal
Magnesium	Normal	Normal
Arterial PCO_2, mmHg	20–30	Normal
Anion gap [Na– (Cl + HCO3)]	↑	Normal to slightly ↑
Glucose (mg/dl)	250–600	600–1200

Diabetic Ketoacidosis (DKA)– *Investigations*

◈ *Davidson 22nd /812–13*

The following are important but should not delay the institution of intravenous fluid and insulin replacement:

- *Venous blood*: for urea and electrolytes, ***glucose and bicarbonate*** (severe acidosis is indicated by a venous plasma bicarbonate < 12 mmol/L).
- ***Urine or blood analysis for ketones***
- *ECG.*
- *Infection screen*: full blood count, blood and urine culture, C-reactive protein, chest X-ray. Although leucocytosis invariably occurs in DKA, this represents a stress response and does not necessarily indicate infection.

Diabetic Ketoacidosis (DKA)

◈ *Harrison 19th/ 2417-18*

- DKA is characterized by hyperglycemia, ***ketosis and metabolic acidosis (increased anion gap)*** along with a number of secondary metabolic derangements
- Leukocytosis, ***hypertriglyceridemia*** and ***hyperlipoproteinemia*** are commonly found as well
- Ketosis results from a marked ***increase in free fatty acid release from adipocytes,*** with a resulting shift toward ketone body synthesis in the liver.
- Reduced insulin levels, in combination with elevations in catecholamines and growth hormone, ***increase lipolysis and the release of free fatty acids.***
- Increased lactic acid production also contributes to the acidosis. The ***increased free fatty acids increase triglyceride and VLDL production.***

24. Ans. a. Activation of pyruvate carboxylase by acetye CoA, c. Increased fatty acid oxidation in liver, d. Hydrolysis of fructose 1,6-bisphosphate by fructose 1,6-bisphosphatase

[Ref: Satyanarayan 4th/ 258-63; Harper 30th/188; Lippincott 6th/117-123; Shinde 7th/347]

*"**Acetyl CoA promotes gluconeogenesis**: During **starvation**-due to excessive lipolysis in adipose tissue, acetyl CoA accumulates in liver. **Acetyl CoA allosterically activates pyruvate carboxylase** resulting in enhanced glucose production"- Satyanarayan 4th/ 263*

Reactions Unique to Gluconeogenesis

◈ *Lippincott 6th/118-123*

- Seven glycolytic reactions are reversible and are used in the synthesis of glucose from lactate or pyruvate. However, three of the reactions are irreversible and must be circumvented by four alternate reactions that energetically favor the synthesis of glucose. ***These reactions, unique to gluconeogenesis, are described below.***
  A. **Carboxylation of pyruvate:** The first "roadblock" to overcome in the synthesis of glucose from pyruvate is the irreversible conversion in glycolysis of ***PEP to pyruvate by pyruvate kinase***. In gluconeogenesis, pyruvate is first carboxylated by pyruvate carboxylase to OAA, which is then converted to PEP by the action of PEP- carboxykinase
  B. **Transport of oxaloacetate to the cytosol:** OAA must be converted to PEP for gluconeogenesis to continue. The enzyme that catalyzes this conversion is found in both the mitochondria and the cytosol in humans. The PEP that is generated in the mitochondria is transported to the cytosol by a specific transporter, whereas that generated in the cytosol requires the transport of OAA from the mitochondria to the cytosol. However, OAA is unable to directly cross the inner mitochondrial membrane; it must first be reduced to malate by mitochondrial malate dehydro genase. ***Malate can be transported from the mitochondria to the cytosol, where it is reoxidized to oxaloacetate by cytosolic malate dehydrogenase as NAD+ is reduced***. The NADH produced is used in the reduction of 1,3-BPG to glyceraldehyde 3-phosphate, a step common to both glycolysis and gluconeogenesis.
  C. **Decarboxylation of cytosolic oxaloacetate:** Oxaloacetate is decarboxylated and phosphorylated to PEP in the cytosol by PEP-carboxykinase. The reaction is driven by hydrolysis of guanosine triphosphate. The combined actions of pyruvate carboxylase and PEPcarboxy kinase provide an energetically favorable pathway from pyruvate to PEP. Then, PEP is acted on by the reactions of glycolysis running in the reverse direction until it becomes fructose 1,6-bisphosphate
  D. **Dephosphorylation of fructose 1,6-bisphosphate: *Hydrolysis of fructose 1,6-bisphosphate by fructose 1,6-bisphosphatase*** bypasses the irreversible phosphofructokinase-1 reaction and provides an energetically favorable pathway for the formation of fructose 6-phosphate. ***This reaction is an important regulatory site of gluconeogenesis.***

Table *(Harper 30th/188)*: **Regulatory and Adaptive Enzymes Associated with Carbohydrate Metabolism**

	Activity in		Inducer	Repressor	Activator	Inhibitor
	Carbohydrate Feeding	**Fasting and Diabetes**				
Glycogenolysis, glycolysis and pyruvate oxidation						
Glycogen synthase	↑	↓			Insulin, glucose 6-phosphate	Glucagon
Hexokinase						Glucose 6-phosphate
Glucokinase	↑	↓	Insulin	Glucagon		
Phosphofructokinase-1	↑	↓	Insulin	Glucagon	5'AMP, fructose 6-phosphate, fructose 2,6-bisphosphate, P_i	Citrate, ATP, glucagon
Pyruvate kinase	↑	↓	Insulin, fructose	Glucagon	Fructose 1, 6-bisphosphate, insulin	ATP, alanine, glucagon, norepinephrine
Pyruvate dehydrogenase	↑	↓			CoA, NAD^+, insulin, ADP, pyruvate	Acetyl CoA, NADH, ATP (fatty acids, ketone bodies)
Gluconeogenesis						
Pyruvate carboxylase	↓	↑	Glucocorticoids, glucagon, epinephrine	Insulin	Acetyl CoA	ADP
Phosphoenolpyruvate carboxykinase	↓	↑	Glucocorticoids, glucagon, epinephrine	Insulin	Glucagon	
Glucose 6-phosphatase	↓	↑	Glucocorticoids, glucagon, epinephrine	Insulin		

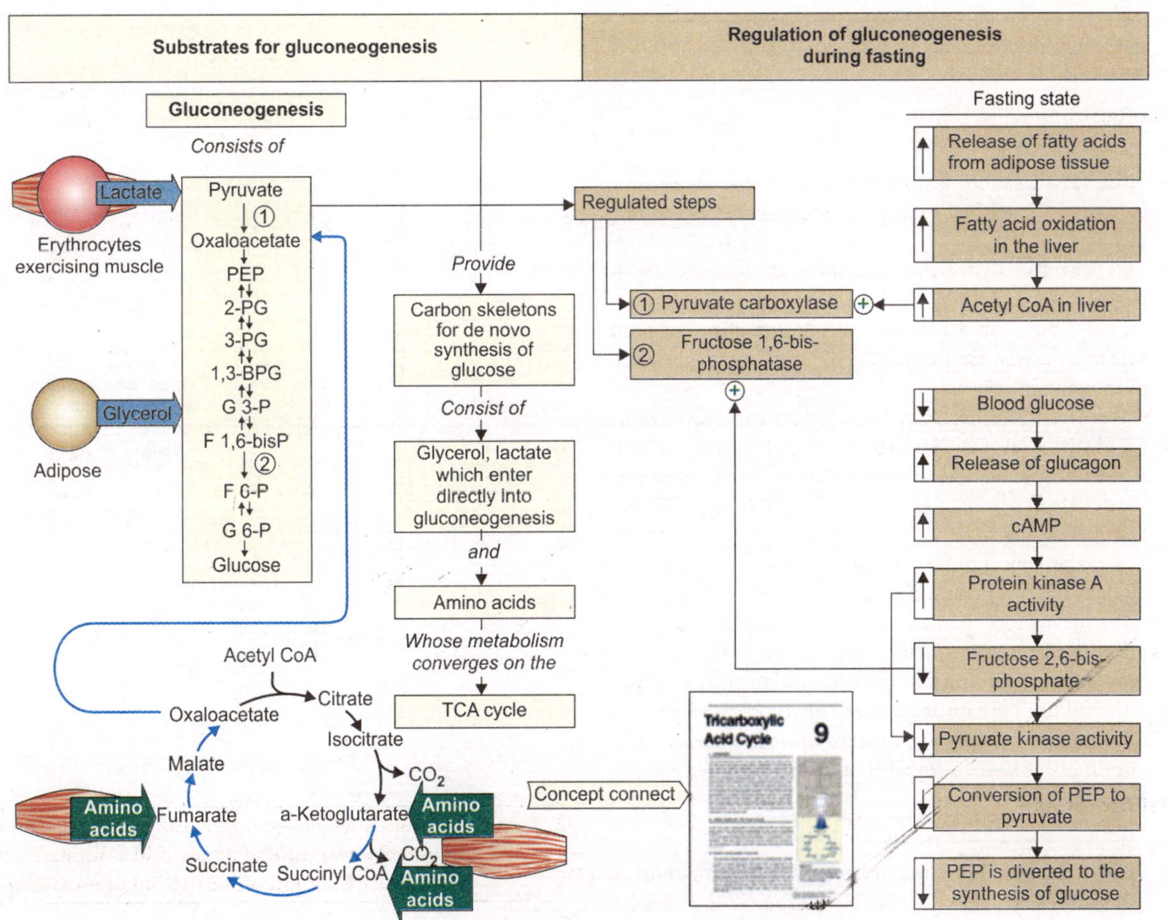

Fig: *(Lippincott 6th/123):* Key concept map for gluconeogenesis

25. Ans. a. 20 carbon atom compound, c. Cyclopentane ring, d. -OH group at 15th position

[Ref: Harper 30th/ 239-40; Lippincott 6th/ 213-15; Vasudevan 5th/167; Shinde 7th/64-65; Satyanarayan 4th/644]

Prostaglandins (PG)

◈ *Shinde 7th/64-65; Vasudevan 5th/167*

- *All naturally occurring PG are **20C fatty acids** containing a **cyclopentane ring** (formed by carbon atom 8 to 12)*
- *All PGs have following salient structural features: **-OH group at 15 position and trans double bond at 13 position***

Prostaglandins and Related Compounds

◈ *Lippincott 6th/ 213-15*

- Prostaglandins and the related compounds thromboxanes and leukotrienes, are collectively known as eicosanoids to reflect their origin from polyunsaturated fatty acids with ***20 carbons.***
- They are extremely potent compounds that elicit a wide range of responses, both physiologic (inflammatory response) and pathologic (hypersensitivity).

26. Ans. a. Micelles play an important role in lipids absorption, b. Absorption of long-chain fatty acids is greatest in the upper parts of the small intestine, d. Fatty acids after absorption are reesterified to triglycerides in the enterocytes

[Ref: Ganong 25th/481-83; Harper 30th/253-54; Guyton 12th/421-23; Lippincott 6th/176]

Fat Digestion

◈ *Ganong 25th/481-82*

- Most fat digestion therefore begins in the duodenum, **pancreatic lipase** being one of the most important enzymes involved.
- This **enzyme hydrolyzes** the 1- and 3-bonds of the ***triglycerides (triacylglycerols)*** with relative ease but acts on the 2-bonds at a very low rate, so the principal products of its action are free fatty acids and 2-monoglycerides (2-monoacylglycerols).
- Fats are relatively insoluble, which limits their ability to cross the unstirred layer and reach the surface of the mucosal cells. However, they are finely ***emulsified in the small intestine by the detergent action of bile acids, phosphatidylcholine and monoglycerides.***
- When the concentration of **bile acids** in the intestine is high, as it is after contraction of the gallbladder, lipids and bile acids interact spontaneously to form **micelles**.
- ***Micellar formation further solubilizes the lipids and provides a mechanism for their transport to the enterocytes.***
- The ***micelles play an important role in keeping lipids in solution and transporting them to the brush border of the intestinal epithelial cells, where they are absorbed.***

Fat Absorption

◈ *Ganong 25th/482-83*

- Fatty acids containing less than 10–12 carbon atoms are water-soluble enough that they pass through the enterocyte unmodified and are actively transported into the portal blood. They circulate as free (unesterified) fatty acids. The fatty acids containing more than 10–12 carbon atoms are too insoluble for this. ***They are reesterified to triglycerides in the enterocytes.***
- In addition, some of the absorbed cholesterol is esterified. The triglycerides and cholesterol esters are then coated with a layer of protein, cholesterol and phospholipid to form ***chylomicrons***. These leave the cell and enter the lymphatics, because they are too large to pass through the junctions between capillary endothelial cells
- ***Absorption of long-chain fatty acids is greatest in the upper parts of the small intestine***, but appreciable amounts are also absorbed in the ileum.

Absorption of Lipids by Intestinal Mucosal Cells (Enterocytes)

◈ *Lippincott 6th/176*

- Free fatty acids, free cholesterol and 2-monoacylglycerol are the primary products of lipid digestion in the jejunum. These, plus bile salts and fat-soluble vitamins (A, D, E and K), form ***mixed micelles***
- ***Mixed micelles are, therefore, soluble in the aqueous environment of the intestinal lumen.***
- ***Short- and medium chain length fatty acids do not require the assistance of mixed micelles for absorption by the intestinal mucosa.***

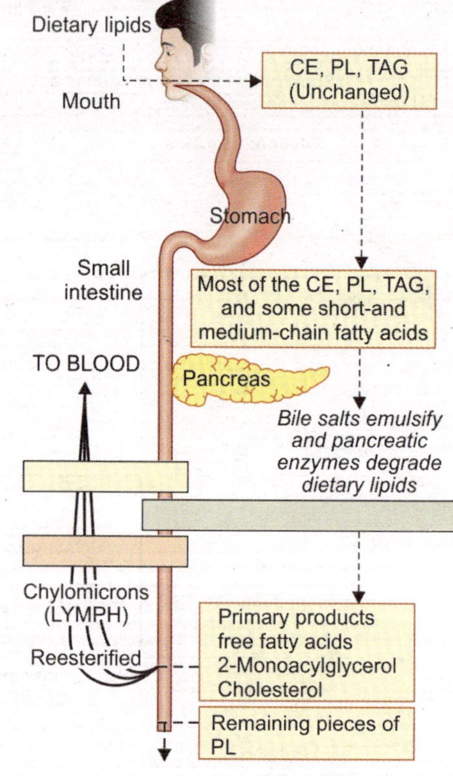

Fig: Lippincott 6th/ 174

27. Ans. b. Linoleic acid is essential fatty acid, c. Hydrogenation converts unsaturated fatty acid to saturated fatty acid, d. Rancidity of food is due to lipid peroxidation

[Ref: Harper 30th/ 211-15; Lippincott 6th/181-82; Satyanarayan 4th/28-29]

"During process of **hydrogenation**, ***unsaturated fatty acids are converted into saturated acids*** *and EFA content is drastically reduced"-Park 24th/650*

Classification of lipids: *(1) Simple lipids- Fats and oils (Triacylglycerols).* ***The difference b/w fat and oil is only physical****; (2) Complex (or compound) lipid; (3) Derived lipids; (4) Miscellaneous lipids"- Satyanarayan 4th/28-29*

Fatty Acids

◈ *Harper 30th/ 211-15*

- Fatty acids occur in the body mainly as esters in natural fats and oils, but are found in the unesterified form as **free fatty acids**, a transport form in the plasma. Fatty acids that occur in natural fats usually contain an even number of carbon atoms.
- The chain may be **saturated** (containing no double bonds) or **unsaturated** (containing one or more double bonds)

◈ *Lippincott 6th/181-82*

- **Fatty acid chains may contain no double bonds**—that is, be ***saturated— or contain one or more double bonds—that is, be mono- or polyunsaturated***. When double bonds are present, they are nearly always in the cis rather than in the trans configuration.
- **Essential fatty acids** Two fatty acids are dietary essentials in humans because of our inability to synthesize them: ***linoleic acid and α-linolenic acid***. Plants provide us with the essential fatty acids. [Note: Arachidonic acid becomes essential if linoleic acid is deficient in the diet.]

Hydrogenation, Saponification, Peroxidation of Fatty Acids

Hydrogenation

- Addition of hydrogen atoms to ***unsaturated*** fatty acid refers to hydrogenation. It reduces the number of double bonds in the unsaturated fats
- Hydrogenation of unsaturated fats in the presence of a catalyst (nickel) in known as ***"hardening"***, because it converts liquid vegetable oils into solid fats e.g. margarines, vegetable ghee, etc.
- As hydrogenation reduces number of double bonds, ***unsaturated fatty acids may get converted to saturated fatty*** acid, if all double bonds are reduced.

Saponification

- **Hydrolysis of a fat by alkali is known as saponification.** The products are glycerol and the alkali salts of the fatty acids which are called **soaps**

Peroxidation (Auto-oxidation)

- Peroxidation (auto-oxidation) of lipids exposed to oxygen is responsible not only for deterioration of foods (rancidity) but also for damage to tissues in vivo. Lipid peroxidation is a chain of reaction generating free radicals that initiate further peroxidation
- **Polyunsaturated fatty acids (PUFAs) can undergo peroxidation (auto-oxidation) and produce harmful free radicals.**

Rancidity

- The unpleasant odor and taste, developed by natural fats upon aging, is referred to as **"rancidity"**. Rancidity may be due to ***hydrolysis*** (by lipase) or ***oxidation*** of fat

IMMUNOGENETICS & MOLECULAR BIOLOGY

28. Ans. b. Cytosine, c. Uracil, d. Thymine

[Ref: Harper 30th /360; Lippincott 6th /291-92]

"Both DNA and RNA contain the same **purine bases**: ***adenine (A) and guanine (G)***. Both DNA and RNA contain the pyrimidine **cytosine (C),** but they differ in their second pyrimidine base: DNA contains ***thymine (T)***, whereas RNA contains ***uracil (U).*** T and U differ in that only T has a methyl group" *(Lippincott 6th /291)*

29. Ans. a. It has reverse trans..., c. Help in DNA replication at end..., d. Also called terminal transferase

[Ref: Harper 30th/745; Lippincott 6th /408; Satynarayan 4th/530-31; Vasudevan 5th/421-22]

Telomerase

◈ *www.khanacademy.org*

- Some cells have the ability to reverse telomere shortening by expressing **telomerase**, an enzyme that extends the telomeres of chromosomes.
- ***Telomerase is an RNA-dependent DNA polymerase***, meaning an enzyme that can make DNA using RNA as a template.
- ***It help in DNA replication at telomere (end of lagging strand)***

Telomerase

◈ *Satynarayan 4th/530-31*

- **Telomerase**, also called ***terminal transferase***, is a ***ribonucleoprotein*** that adds a species-dependent telomere repeat sequence to the 3' end of telomeres.
- A telomere is a region of repetitive sequences at each end of eukaryotic chromosomes in most eukaryotes

"Telomerase: This complex contains a protein that acts as a ***reverse transcriptase*** ***and a short piece of RNA that acts as a template***. The CA-rich RNA template base-pairs with the GT-rich, single-stranded 3'-end of telomeric DNA. The reverse transcriptase uses the RNA template to ***synthesize DNA in the usual 5'→3' direction,*** extending the already longer 3'-end. Telomerase then translocates to the newly synthesized end and the process is repeated. Once the GT-rich strand has been lengthened, primase can use it as a template to synthesize an RNA primer. The RNA primer is extended by DNA polymerase and the primer is removed"- *Lippincott 6th /408*

"Telomeres: Structures at the ends of chromosome that contain multiple repeats of specific hexanucleotide DNA sequences.

The telomeres of normal cells shorten on repeated cell division, which may result in cell death. The enzyme telomerase replicates telomeres and is often expressed in cancer cells, helping them to evade cell death. ***Telomerase is usually not detected in normal somatic cells***"-*Harper 30th/745*

30. Ans. b. A type of topoisomerase II, c. Act on circular DNA, d. Overcome the problem of supercoils

[Ref: Lippincott 6th /401; Satyanarayan 4th/528]

Gyrase

- *Satyanarayan 4th/528*
- *Bacteria contain a specific type II topoisomerase namely gyrase*
- *This **enzyme cuts and reseals the circular DNA** (of bacteria) and thus **overcome the problem of supercoils***

Type II DNA Topoisomerases

- *Lippincott 6th /401*
- These enzymes bind tightly to the DNA double helix and make transient breaks in both strands. The enzyme then causes a second stretch of the DNA double helix to pass through the break and, finally, reseals the break. As a result, both negative and positive supercoils can be relieved by this ATP-requiring process.
- **Type II DNA topoisomerases** are also required in both prokaryotes and eukaryotes for the separation of interlocked molecules of DNA following chromosomal replication.
- ***DNA gyrase, a Type II topoisomerase*** found in bacteria and plants, has the unusual property of being able to introduce negative supercoils into relaxed ***circular DNA*** using energy from the hydrolysis of ATP. This ***facilitates the future replication of DNA*** because the negative supercoils neutralize the positive supercoils introduced during opening of the double helix. It also aids in the transient strand separation required during transcription
- *Lippincott 6th /401*
- These enzymes reversibly cut one strand of the double helix. They have both nuclease (strand-cutting) and ligase (strand-resealing) activities. They do not require ATP, but rather appear to store the energy from the phosphodiester bond they cleave, reusing the energy to reseal the strand.
- Each time a transient "nick" is created in one DNA strand, the intact DNA strand is passed through the break before it is resealed, thus relieving ("relaxing") accumulated supercoils.
- **Type I topoisomerases** relax negative supercoils (that is, those that contain fewer turns of the helix than relaxed DNA) in E. coli and both negative and positive supercoils (that is, those that contain fewer or more turns of the helix than relaxed DNA) in eukaryotic cells.

31. Ans. a. Pyrimidine dimers formation, c. Thymine dimer formation

[Ref: Harper 30th /761; Lippincott 6th /412]

Ultraviolet Radiation can be Extremely Damaging

- *Harper 30th /761*
- Absorption of this short wavelength, high-energy light can cause the ***rupture of covalent bonds in proteins, DNA and RNA***; the ***formation of thymine dimers in DNA***

Repair of Damage caused by Ultraviolet (UV) Light

- *Lippincott 6th /412*
- Exposure of a cell to UV light can result in the covalent ***joining of two adjacent pyrimidines (usually thymines), producing a dimer***. These **thymine dimers** prevent DNA polymerase from replicating the DNA strand beyond the site of dimer formation. Thymine dimers are excised in bacteria by UvrABC proteins in a process known as nucleotide excision repair.
- A related pathway involving XP (xeroderma pigmentosum) proteins is present in humans.
  1. **Recognition and excision of dimers by UV-specific endonuclease:** First, a UV-specific endonuclease (called uvrABC excinuclease) recognizes the dimer and cleaves the damaged strand on both the 5'-side and 3'-side of the dimer. A short oligonucleotide containing the dimer is released, leaving a gap in the DNA strand that formerly contained the dimer. This gap is filled in using the same process described previously.
  2. **UV radiation and cancer:** ***Pyrimidine dimers can be formed in the skin cells of humans exposed to unfiltered sunlight***. In the rare genetic disease xeroderma pigmentosum (XP), the cells cannot repair the damaged DNA, resulting in ***extensive accumulation of mutations*** and, consequently, early and numerous skin cancers.

"Certain DNA sequences are particularly susceptible to mutagenesis. Successive pyrimidine residues (e.g., T-T or C-C) are subject to the formation of ultraviolet light–induced photoadducts. If these **pyrimidine dimers** are not repaired by the nucleotide excision repair pathway, mutations will be introduced after DNA synthesis."-*Harrison 19th/432-33*

32. Ans. b. 5' capping

[Ref: Satyanarayan 4th/561-62; Harper 30th /426; Lippincott 6th / 443-44]

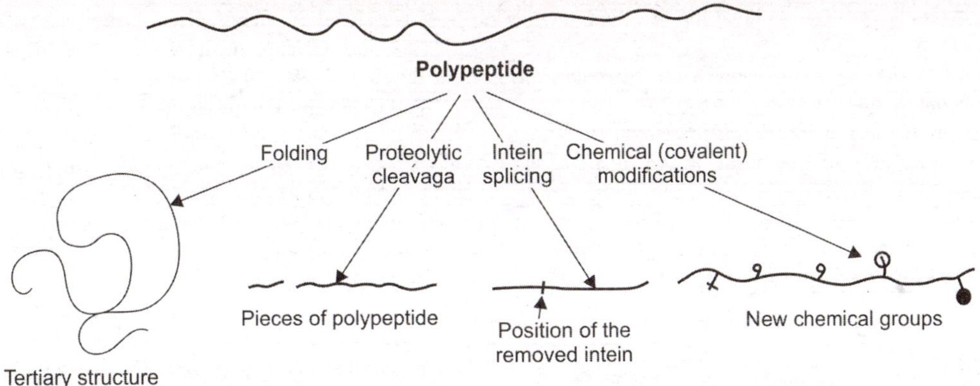

Fig: *(Satyanarayan 4th/561)*: An outline of Post-translation modification of proteins

Co- and Post-translational Modification of Polypeptide Chains

◈ *Lippincott 6th / 443-44*

- Many polypeptide chains are covalently modified, either while they are still attached to the ribosome (cotranslational) or after their synthesis has been completed (posttranslational). These modifications may include ***removal of part of the translated sequence***, or the ***covalent addition of one or more chemical groups*** required for protein activity.
- Some types of posttranslational modifications are:
  - A. **Trimming:** Many proteins destined for secretion from the cell are initially made as large, precursor molecules that are not functionally active. ***Portions of the protein chain must be removed*** by specialized endoproteases, resulting in the release of an active molecule.
  - B. **Covalent attachments:** Proteins may be activated or inactivated by the covalent attachment of a variety of ***chemical groups.***
  - C. **Protein folding:** Proteins must fold to assume their functional state. Folding can be spontaneous (as a result of the primary structure), or facilitated by proteins known as "chaperones"
  - D. **Protein degradation:** Proteins that are defective, for example, misfolded, or destined for rapid turnover are often marked for destruction by ubiquitination—the attachment of chains of a small, highly conserved protein, called ubiquitin

Post-transcriptional Modifications

◈ *Vasudevan 5th/426*

- *Poly-A tailing*
- *5' capping*
- *Methylation*
- *Removal of introns*
- *Spicing of exons (connect together)*
- *Endonuclease cleavage*

33. Ans. c. RNA polymerase II is responsible for the synthesis of precursors for the large ribosomal RNAs, d. RNA polymerase I is responsible for the synthesis small ribosomal RNAs

[Ref: Harrison 19th/427-28; Satyanarayan 4th/546, 566-68]

"The RNA copies of the active protein coding genes represent transcriptome. Thus transcriptome is initial product of gene expression which directs the protein synthesis"- *Satyanarayan 4th/543*

RNA Polymerase in Eukaryotes

◈ *Satyanarayan 4th/546*

- ***RNA polymerase I is responsible for the synthesis of precursors for the large ribosomal RNAs***
- ***RNA polymerase II synthesizes the precursors for mRNAs and small nuclear RNAs***
- ***RNA polymerase II participates in the formation of tRNAs and small ribosomal RNAs***

Transcription: The binding of the enzyme RNA polymerase to DNA is the prerequisite for the transcription to start. The specific region on DNA where the enzyme binds in known as promotor region"- *Satyanarayan 4th/544*

Genes

◈ *Harrison 19th/427-28*

- A *gene* is a functional unit that is regulated by transcription and ***encodes an RNA product,*** which is most commonly, ***but not always, translated into a protein*** that exerts activity within or outside the cell.
- Historically, genes were identified because they conferred specific traits that are transmitted from one generation to the next. Increasingly, they are characterized based on expression in various tissues (*transcriptome*).
- The number of genes greatly underestimates the complexity of genetic expression, because single genes can generate ***multiple spliced messenger RNA (mRNA) products*** (*isoforms*), which are translated into proteins that are

subject to complex posttranslational modification such as phosphorylation.

- *Exons refer to the portion of genes that are eventually spliced together to form mRNA*.
- *Introns* refer to the spacing regions between the exons that are spliced out of precursor RNAs during RNA processing.

34. Ans. a. Repair damage caused by UV light, c. Use visible light, d. Breaks pyrimidine dimer

[Ref: www.pnas.org; www.ncbi.nlm.nih.gov]

Photolyases

◈ *www.ncbi.nlm.nih.gov*

Photolyases are ***DNA repair enzymes*** that ***repair damage caused by exposure to ultraviolet light***.

This enzyme ***requires visible light***, preferentially from the violet/blue end of the spectrum and the mechanism known as **photoreactivation**.

Photolyase is a phylogenetically old enzyme which is present and functional in many species, from the bacteria to the fungi to plants and to the animals.

Photolyase is particularly important in repairing UV induced damage in plants. The ***photolyase mechanism is no longer working in humans and other placental mammals*** who instead rely on the less efficient nucleotide excision repair mechanism.

Photolyases bind complementary DNA strands and break certain types of pyrimidine dimers that arise when a pair of thymine or cytosine bases on the same strand of DNA become covalently linked.

Photolyases have a high affinity for these lesions and reversibly bind and ***convert them back to the original bases.***

◈ *www.pnas.org*

- **DNA photolyases are highly efficient light-driven DNA repair enzymes** which revert the genome-damaging effects caused by ***ultraviolet (UV) radiation***.
- These enzymes occur in almost all living organisms exposed to sunlight, the ***only exception being placental mammals like humans and mice.*** Their catalytic mechanism employs the ***light-driven injection of an electron onto the DNA lesion*** to trigger the cleavage of cyclobutane- pyrimidine dimers.

PATHOLOGY

35. Ans. d. Hodgkin's lymphoma, e. B-Lymphoblastic lymphoma

[Ref: Robbins 9th (SAE)/590; Harrison 19th/699]

"A high fraction of **B-ALLs** have loss-of-function mutations in genes that are required for B-cell development, such as ***PAX5***, *E2A* and *EBF*, or a balanced t (12; 21) involving the genes *ETV6* and *RUNX1*"- *Robbins 9th (SAE)/590*

"The Reed-Sternberg cells in nodular sclerosis and other "classical" **HL** subtypes have a characteristic immunophenotype; they are positive for ***PAX5*** (a B-cell transcription factor), CD15 and CD30 and negative for other B-cell markers, T-cell markers and CD45 (leukocyte common antigen)"-*Robbins 9th (SAE)/608*

"PAX5 has been reported as being frequently altered in both childhood and adult ***B-ALL***. PAX5 mutation was also reported in ***both Hodgkin lymphoma and non-Hodgkin lymphoma***"-*www.hindawi.com*

"**PAX-5,** a transcription factor expressed throughout B-cell maturation, is detected in most B-cell neoplasms including those that lack expression of mature B-cell markers, such as ***classical Hodgkin lymphoma (cHL), B-lymphoblastic leukemia and B-cell lymphomas*** following rituximab therapy. The **lack of PAX-5 expression** in most ***CD30-positive non-hematopoietic malignancies (embryonal carcinoma and seminoma) and T-cell lymphomas, such as anaplastic large cell lymphoma (ALCL)***, suggests that the absence of PAX-5 may be used to confirm non-B-cell lineage"-*www.ncbi.nlm.nih.gov*

"**Pax5, or B-cell-specific activator protein,** ***is mostly expressed in B lymphocytes and B-cell lymphomas***, although recent data have shown expression in the developing central nervous system, some neuroendocrine tumors and occasional myeloid leukemias. ***Pax5 staining is positive in most Hodgkin and B-cell non-Hodgkin lymphomas and also precursor B-cell lymphoblastic neoplasms***. **Plasma cell neoplasms, multiple myeloma and plasmablastic lymphomas typically are negative. T-cell lymphomas** are, to date, consistently negative. Recently, **Pax5** expression has been described in the majority of ***small cell carcinomas and Merkel cell carcinomas***"-*www.ncbi.nlm.nih.gov*

"***Lymphoplascytid lymphoma*** *is associated with* ***PAX 5 oncogene***"- *Harrison 19th/699 (Table)*

"t (9; 14) (p13; q32)	**PAX5** (BSAP)/ IgH:	*Lymphoplasmacytic lymphoma, plasma cell myeloma"*

◈ *Devita 8th /chap 51*

Table *(Harrison 19th/699)*: **Cytogenetic translocation and associated oncogenes often seen in lymphoid malignancies**

Disease	Cytogenetic Abnormality	Oncogene
CLL/small lymphocytic lymphoma	t (14; 15 ((q32; q13)	–
MALT lymphoma	t (11; 18) (q21; q21)	API2/MALT, BCL–10
Precursor B-cell acute lymphoid leukemia	t (9; 22) (q34; q11) or variant t (4; 11) (q21; q23) t (12; 21)	BCR/ABL AF4, MLLI TEL, AMLI
Precursor acute lymphoid leukemia	t (9; 22) t (1; 19) t (17; 19) t (5; 14)	BCR, ABL E2A, PBX HLF, E2A HOXI IL2, CTIP2

Contd...

Disease	Cytogenetic Abnormality	Oncogene
Mantle cell lymphoma	t (11; 14) (q13; q32)	BCL-I, IgH
Follicular lymphoma	t (14; 18) (q32; q21)	BCL-2, IgH
Diffuse large cell lymphoma	t (3; -) (q27; -)[a] t (17; -) (p13; -)[a]	BCL-6 P53
Burkitt's lymphoma, Burkitt's leukermia	t (8; -) (q24; -)[a]	C-MYC
CD30+ anaplastic large cell lymphoma	t (2; 5) (p23; q35)	ALK, NPM
Lymphoplasmacytoid lymphoma	t (9; 14) (p13; q32)	***PAX5***, *IgH*

36. Ans. b. SS18-SSX4 fusion genes, c. Translocation t (X; 18) (p11; q11), d. SS18-SSX1 fusion genes

[Ref: Robbins 9th (SAE)/1223-24; Harshmohan 7th/861; Harrison 19th/119e-1]

"**Chronic myelogenous leukemia (CML):** Translocation involving ***(9; 22) (q34; q11)"***- *Robbins 9th (SAE)/317*

"Ninety percent of synovial sarcomas contain a characteristic ***chromosomal translocation t (X; 18) (p11; q11)*** involving a nuclear transcription factor on chromosome 18 called *SYT* and two breakpoints on X.

Patients with translocations to the ***second X breakpoint (SSX2)*** may have longer survival than those with translocations involving ***SSX1***"-*Harrison 19th/119e-1*

"Most synovial sarcomas show a characteristic ***chromosomal translocation t (x; 18) (p11; q11)*** producing **SS18-SSX1, -SSX2 or -SSX-4 fusion genes** that encodes chimeric transcription factors"- *Robbins 9th (SAE)/1223-24*

Table *(MD Anderson Manual of Medical Oncology/Chap 33)*: ***Cytogenetic Translocation and Other Abnormalities in Sarcoma***

Tumor	Cytogenetic Abnormality	Gene Product
Synovial sarcoma	T(X; 18)(p11; q11)	SYT-SSX

37. Ans. a. ↑ed conjugated bilirubin, d. Decreased biliary excretion of conjugated bilirubin

[Ref: Robbins 9th (SAE)/854; Harrison 19th/2003-04]

Dubin-Johnson Syndrome (DJS)

◈ *Harrison 19th/2003-04*

- This benign, relatively rare disorder is characterized by low-grade, ***predominantly conjugated hyperbilirubinemia.***
- Total bilirubin concentrations are typically between 34 and 85 μmol/L (2 and 5 mg/dL) but on occasion can be in the normal range or as high as 340–430 μmol/L (20–25 mg/dL) and can fluctuate widely in any given patient.
- Because the hyperbilirubinemia is due to a ***predominant rise in conjugated bilirubin***, bilirubinuria is characteristically present. ***Aside from elevated serum bilirubin levels, other routine laboratory tests are normal.***
- Physical examination is usually normal except for jaundice, although an occasional patient may have hepatosplenomegaly.
- ***Routine liver function tests, including serum alkaline phosphatase and transaminase activities are usually normal.***
- Several different mutations in the ***MRP2* gene** produce the Dubin-Johnson phenotype, which has an ***autosomal recessive*** pattern of inheritance.
- MRP2 is play a ***important role in the biliary excretion of conjugated bilirubin***
- Patients with DJS also have a diagnostic abnormality in urinary coproporphyrin excretion. There are two naturally occurring coproporphyrin isomers, I and III. Normally, ~75% of the coproporphyrin in urine is isomer III. In urine from DJS patients, total coproporphyrin content is normal, but >80% is isomer I.

"Isolated ***bilirubin rise (other LFTs normal)***, normal ultrasound, urobilinogen present, conjugated bilirubin rise"- *Davidson 22nd/938 (Flow chart)*

Table *(Robbins 9th (SAE)/854)*: **Hereditary Hyperbilirubinemias**

Disorder	Inheritance	Defects in Bilirubin Metabolism	Liver Pathology	Clinical Course
Unconjugated Hyperbilirubinemia				
Crigler-Najjar syndrome type I	Autosomal recessive	Absent UGT1A1 activity	None	Fatal in neonatal period
Crigler-Najjar syndrome type II	Autosomal dominant with variable penetrance	Decreased UGT1A1 activity	None	Generally mild, occasional kernicterus
Gilbert syndrome	Autosomal recessive	Decreased UGT1A1 activity	None	Innocuous
Conjugated Hyperbilirubinemia				
Dubin-Johnson syndrome	Autosomal recessive	Impaired biliary excretion of bilirubin glucuronldes due to mutation in canallcular multidrug resistance protein 2 (MRP2)	Pigmented cytoplasmic globules	Innocuous
Rotor syndrome	Autosomal recessive	Decreased hepatic uptake and storage? Decreased biliary excretion?	None	Innocuous

UGT1A1, Uridine diphosphate –glucuronyttransferese family, peptide A1

38. Ans. **b. Positive for cytokeratin 7, e. EGFR mutation**

[Ref: Robbins 9th (SAE)/714; Harrison 19th/507-09]

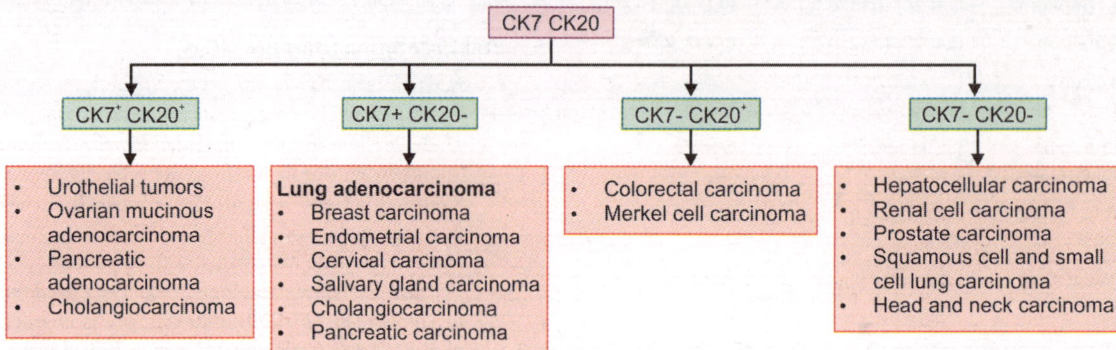

Fig: *(Harrison 19th/102e-2)*: Approach to cytokeratin (CK7 and CK20) markers used in adenocarcinoma of unknown primary

"**Transthyretin (TTR):** *Single amino acid substitution mutation in structure of TTR result in variant form of protein which is responsible for amyloidosis (Familial amyloid polyneuropathies, senile cardiac amyloidosis)"-Harshmohan 7th/68*

"The **epithelioid type of mesothelioma** consists of cuboidal, columnar, or flattened cells forming tubular or papillary structures resembling adenocarcinoma. Immunohistochemical stains are very helpful in differentiating it from pulmonary adenocarcinoma. Most **mesotheliomas show strong positivity** for ***keratin proteins, calretinin, Wilms tumor 1 (WT-1), cytokeratin 5/6 and D2-40***"*-Robbins 9th (SAE)/724*

Table *(Harrison 19th/507)*: **Driver Mutations in Non-Small-Cell Lung Cancer (NSCLC)**

Gene	Alteration	Frequency in NSCLC	Typical Histology
AKT1	Mutation	1%	Adenocarcinoma, squamous
ALK	Rearrangement	3–7%	Adenocarcinoma
BRAF	Mutation	1–3%	Adenocarcinoma
DDR2	Mutation	~4%	Squamous
EGFR	Mutation	10–35%	Adenocarcinoma
EGFR1	Amplification	~20%	Squamous
HER2	Mutation	2–4%	Adenocarcinoma
KRAS	Mutation	15–25%	Adenocarcinoma
MEK1	Mutation	1%	Adenocarcinoma
MET	Amplification	2–4%	Adenocarcinoma
NRAS	Mutation	1%	Adenocarcinoma
PIK3CA	Mutation	1–3%	Squamous
PTEN	Mutation	4–8%	Squamous

Lung Carcinoma

◈ *Harrison 19th/508-09*

- Lung cancer cells harbor multiple chromosomal abnormalities, including mutations, amplifications, insertions, deletions and translocations.
- One of the earliest sets of oncogenes found to be aberrant was the MYC family of transcription factors (*MYC, MYCN* and *MYCL*).*MYC* is most frequently activated via gene amplification or transcriptional dysregulation in both SCLC and NSCLC.
- Adenocarcinomas driver mutations involves ***EGFR***, which belongs to the ERBB (HER) family of protooncogenes, including ***EGFR*** **(ERBB1),** ***HER2/neu*** **(ERBB2),** ***HER3*** **(ERBB3) and** ***HER4*** **(ERBB4).**
- Additional examples of driver mutations in lung adenocarcinoma include the **GTPase** ***KRAS***, the serine-threonine kinase *BRAF* and the lipid kinase *PIK3CA*.
- More recently, more subsets of lung adenocarcinoma have been identifed as defined by the presence of specific chromsomal rearrangements resulting in the abberant activation of the ***TKs ALK, ROS1 and RET***.
- Although driver mutations have mostly been found in adenocarinomas, three potential molecular targets recently have been identified in **squamous cell lung carcinomas**: *FGFR1* amplification, *DDR2* mutations and *PIK3CA* mutations/*PTEN* loss. Together, these potentially "actionable" defects occur in up to 50% of squamous carcinomas.
- A large number of **tumor-suppressor genes** have also been identified that are inactivated during the pathogenesis of lung cancer. These include *TP53*, *RB1*, *RASSF1A*, *CDKN2A/B*, *LKB1* (*STK11*) and *FHIT*. Nearly 90% of SCLCs harbor mutations in *TP53* and *RB1*.

"**Adenocarcinoma of lung** is marked by oncogenic gain-of-function mutations involving components of growth factor receptor signaling pathways. These include gain-of-function mutations in multiple genes encoding receptor tyrosine kinases, including ***EGFR, ALK, ROS, MET*** **and** ***RET***, which are all also mutated in other forms of cancer"*-Robbins 9th (SAE)/714*

39. Ans. **d. Nonkeratinizing variant**

[Ref: Robbins 9th (SAE)/714; www.sciencedirect.com/scienc]

Clear and papillary cell variant** are **type of squamous cell carcinoma in old classification (not included in 2015 WHO classification)

Lymphoepithelioma-like carcinoma is classified as ***neuroendocrine tumors (Other and Unclassified carcinomas)*** in *2015 WHO classification of lung tumour"- www.sciencedirect.com/scienc*

2015 World Health Organization (WHO) Classification of Tumors of the Lung, Pleura, Thymus and Heart

- This classification is published in 2015
- This follows previous WHO Classifications of Lung Tumors in 1967 and 1981, of Lung and Pleural Tumors in 1999 and Tumors of the Lung, Pleura, Thymus and Heart in 2004.
- Compared with the 2004 WHO Classification, there are multiple major changes for the common lung cancers most of which follow the 2011 lung adenocarcinoma classification sponsored by the International Association for the Study of Lung Cancer (IASLC), American Thoracic Society (ATS) and European Respiratory Society (ERS), which has essentially been adopted with only minor changes.
- The **most significant changes in this edition compared with 2004 involve:**
  - Use of immunohistochemistry throughout the classification including for resected lung cancers
  - A new emphasis on genetic studies, in particular integration of molecular testing to help personalize treatment strategies for advanced lung cancer patients
  - A new classification for small biopsies and cytology as proposed by the 2011 IASLC/ATS/ERS Classification with a different approach to classification of resected lung cancers
  - A completely different approach to lung adenocarcinoma as proposed by the 2011 IASLC/ATS/ERS classification
  - Restricting the diagnosis of large cell carcinoma only to resected tumors that lack any clear morphologic or immunohistochemical differentiation with reclassification of the remaining former large cell carcinoma subtypes into different categories
  - Re-**classifying squamous cell carcinomas** into ***keratinizing, nonkeratinizing and basaloid subtypes*** with the nonkeratinizing tumors requiring immunohistochemistry proof of squamous differentiation
  - Grouping ofneuroendocrine tumors together in one category
  - Adding nuclear protein intestis (NUT) carcinoma to a category of other and unclassified tumors
  - Changing the term sclerosing hemangioma to sclerosing pneumocytoma and moving this tumor to the adenoma category
  - Changing the name hamartomato "pulmonary hamartoma,"
  - Creating a group of PEComatous tumors that include (a) lymphangioleiomyomatosis (LAM), (b) PEComa, benign (with clear cell tumor as a variant) and (c) PEComa, malignant
  - Introducing the entity pulmonary myxoid sarcoma with an *EWSR1–CREB1* translocation
  - Adding the entities myoepithelioma and myoepithelial carcinomas which can show*EWSR1* gene rearrangements
  - Recognition of usefulness of *WWTR1–CAMTA1* fusions in diagnosis of epithelioid hemangioendotheliomas
  - AddingErdheim–Chester disease to the lymphoproliferative tumors, and
  - A new group of tumors of ectopic origin was created to include germ cell tumors intrapulmonary thymoma, melanoma and meningioma.

Table: 2015 WHO Classification of Lung Tumors (Partial list-only squamous and adenocarcinoma)

Squamous cell carcinoma	***Keratinizing squamous cell carcinoma[e]; Nonkeratinizing squamous cell carcinoma[e]; Basaloid squamous cell carcinoma[e]; Preinvasive lesion- Squamous cell carcinoma in situ***
Adenocarcinoma	Lepidic adenocarcinoma[e]; Acinar adenocarcinoma; Papillary adenocarcinoma; Micropapillary adenocarcinoma[e]; Solid adenocarcinoma; Invasive mucinous adenocarcinoma[e]- Mixed invasive mucinous and nonmucinous adenocarcinoma; nonmucinous adenocarcinoma; Fetal adenocarcinoma; Enteric adenocarcinoma[e]; Minimally invasive adenocarcinoma[e]- Nonmucinous and Mucinous; Preinvasive lesions- Atypical adenomatous hyperplasia and Adenocarcinoma in situ[e] (mucinous and nonmucinous)

Note-e: New terms changed or entities added since 2004 WHO Classification

Table *(Robbins 9th (SAE)/714)*: **Histologic Classification of Malignant Epithelial Lung Tumors (Old classification-2004)**

Tumor Classification
Squamous cell carcinoma: Papillary, clear cell, small cell, basaloid
Small-cell carcinoma: Combined small-cell carcinoma
Adenocarcinoma: Minimally invasive adenocarcinoma (nonmucinous, mucinous) Lepidic, Acinar; papillary, solid (according to predominant pattern) Mucinous adenocarcinoma
Large-cell carcinoma: Large-cell neuroendocrine carcinoma
Adenosquamous carcinoma
Carcinomas with pleomorphic, sarcomatoid, or sarcomatous elements
Carcinoid tumor: Typical, atypical
Carcinomas of salivary gland type

40. Ans. a. Tyrosine kinase has role in RAS activation,
b. Most common form of oncogene in human tumors,
c. It has an intrinsic GTPase activity,
d. Mutation may result in carcinomatous growth

[Ref: Robbins 9th (SAE)/284; Harshmohan 7th/203-04]

RAS Oncogene

◈ *Harshmohan 7th/203-04*

- *This is the **most common form of oncogene in human tumors**, the abnormality being induced by point mutation in RAS gene*
- ***About a third of all human tumors carry mutated RAS gene**, seen in examples such as carcinoma colon, lung and pancreas*
- *Normally, the **inactive form of RAS protein is GDP-bound while the activated form is bound to GTP.***

RAS Mutations

◈ *Robbins 9th (SAE)/286*

- **Point mutations of *RAS* family genes constitute the most common type of abnormality involving proto-oncogenes in human tumors.**
- Approximately 15% to 20% of all human tumors express mutated RAS proteins, but in some types of cancers the frequency of *RAS* mutations is much higher.
- RAS proteins are members of a family of membrane-associated small G proteins that ***bind guanosine nucleotides (guanosine triphosphate [GTP] and guanosine diphosphate [GDP])***, similar to the larger trimolecular G proteins.
- They normally flip back and forth between an excited signal-transmitting state in which they are bound to GTP and a quiescent state in which they are bound to GDP.
- ***Stimulation of receptor tyrosine kinases by growth factors leads to exchange of GDP for GTP*** and subsequent conformational changes that generate ***active RAS***, which in turn stimulates both the MAPK and PI3K/AKT arms of the receptor ***tyrosine kinase signaling pathway***. These downstream kinases phosphorylate and activate a number of cytoplasmic effectors as well as several transcription factors that turn on genes that support rapid cell growth.
- Activation of RAS is transient because **RAS has an intrinsic GTPase activity** that is accelerated by *GTPase-activating proteins (GAPs)*, which bind to the active RAS and augment its GTPase activity by more than 1000-fold, thereby terminating signal transduction. Thus, GAPs prevent uncontrolled RAS activity.

Table *(Robbins 9th (SAE)/284)*: **Selected Oncogene, their mode of activation and associated Human tumors**

Category	Proto-Onco-gene	Mode of Activation in Tumor	Associated Human Tumor
Growth Factors			
PDGF-β chain	PDGFB	Overexpression	Astrocytoma
Fibroblast growth factors	HST1 FGF3	Overexpression Amplification	Osteosarcoma Stomach cancer Bladder cancer Breast cancer Melanoma
TGF-α	TGFA	Overexpression	Astrocytomas
HGF	HGF	Overexpression	Hepatocellular carcinomas Thyroid cancer
Growth Factor Receptors			
EGF-receptor family	ERBB1 (EGFR) ERBB2 (HER)	Mutation Amplification	Adenocarcinoma of lung Breast carcinoma
FMS-like tyrosine kinase 3	FLT3	Point mutation	Leukemia
Receptor for neurotrophic factors	RET	Point mutation	Multiple endocrine neoplasia 2A and B, familial medullary thyroid carcinomas
PDGF receptor	PDGFRB	Overexpression, translocation	Gliomas, leukemias
Receptor for KIT ligand	KIT	Point mutation	Gastrointestinal stromal tumors, seminomas, leukemias
ALK receptor	ALK	Translocation, fusion gene formation	Adenocarcinoma of lung, certain lymphomas Neuroblastoma
Proteins Involved in Signal Transduction			
GTP-binding (G) proteins	***KRAS*** ***HRAS*** ***NRAS*** *GNAO* *GNAS*	Point mutation Point mutation Point mutation Point mutation Point mutation	Colon, lung and pancreatic tumors Bladder and kidney tumors Melanomas, hematologic malignancies Uveal melanoma Pituitary adenoma, other endocrine tumors

Contd...

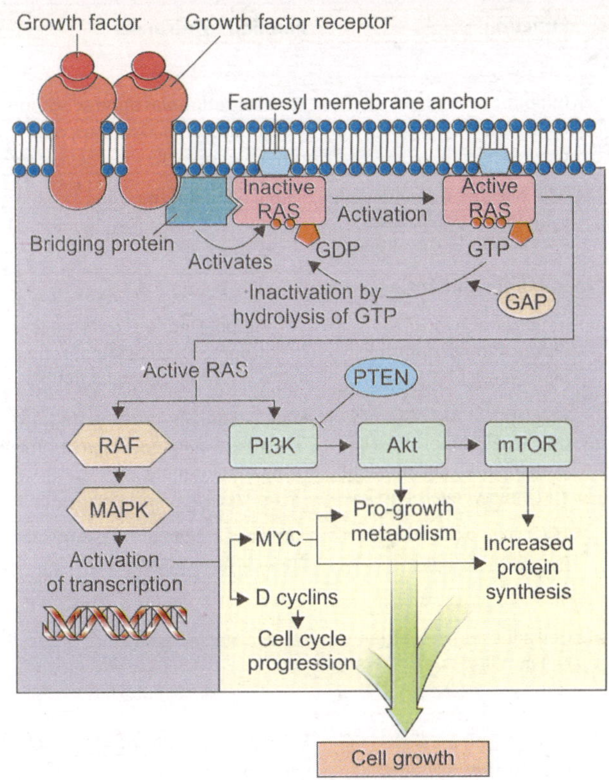

Fig. *(Robbins 9th (SAE)/285)*: Growth factor signaling pathways in cancer. Growth factor receptors, RAS, PI3K, MYC and D cyclins are oncoproteins that are activated by mutations in various cancers. GAPs apply brakes to RAS activation and PTEN serves the same function for PI3K.

41. Ans. c. CD95 e. RAS

[Ref: Robbins 9th (SAE)/291; Harshmohan 7th/205]

RAS is an proto-oncogene- Harshmohan 7th/203

CD95 (Fas) is a death receptor that has a role in apoptosis- Robbins 9th (SAE)/56

Table *(Robbins 9th (SAE)/291)*: **Selected Tumor Suppressor Genes and Associated Familial Syndromes and Cancers, Sorted by Cancer Hallmarks**

Gene	Protein	Function	Familial Syndromes	Sporadic Cancers
Inhibitors of Mitogenic Signaling Pathways				
APC	Adenomatous polyposis cdi protein	Inhibitor of WNT signaling	Familial colonic polyps and carcinomas	Carcinomas of stomach, colon, pancreas; melanoma
NF1	Neurofibromin-1	Inhibitor of RAS/MAPK signaling	Neurofibromatosis type 1 (neurofibromas and malignant peripheral nerve sheath tumors)	Neuroblastoma, juvenile myeloid leukemia
NF2	Merlin	Cytoskeletal stability, Hippo pathway signaling	Neurofibromatosis type 2 (acoustic schwannoma and meningioma)	Schwannoma, meningioma
PTCH	Patched	Inhibitor of Hedgehog signaling	Gorlin syndrome (basal cell carcinoma, medulloblastoma, several benign tumors)	Basal cell carcinoma medulloblastoma
PTEN	Phosphatase and tensin homologue	Inhibitor of PI3K/AKT signaling	Cowden syndrome (variety of benign skin, GI and CNS prowths; breast, endometrial and thyroid carcinoma)	Diverse cancers, particularly carcinomas and lymphoid tumors
SMAD2, SMAD4	SMAD2, SMAD4	Component of the TGFβ signaling pathway, repressors of MYC and CDK4 expression, inducers of CDK inhibitor expression	Juvenile polyposis	Frequently mutated (along with other components of the TGFβ signaling pathway) in colonic and pancreatic carcinoma

A & E

Contd...

Gene	Protein	Function	Familial Syndromes	Sporadic Cancers
Inhibitors of Cell Cycle Progression				
RB	Retinoblastoma (RB) protein	Inhibitor of G_1/S transition during cell cycle progression	Familial retinoblastoma syndrome (retinoblastoma, osteosarcoma, other sarcomas)	Retinoblastoma; osteosarcoma carcinomas of breast, colon, lung
CDKN2A	P16/INK4a and p14/ARF	P16: Negative regulator of cyclin-dependent kinases; p14, indirect activator of p53	Familial melanoma	Pancreatic, breast and esophageal carcinoma, melanoma, certain leukemias
Inhibitors of "Pro-growth" Programs of Metabolism and Anglogenesis				
VHL	Von Hip pel Lindau (VHL) protein	Inhibitor of hypoxia-induced transcription factors (e.g., HIF1α)	Von Hippel Lindau syndrome (cere bellar hemangioblastoma, retinal angioma, renal cell carcinoma)	Renal cell carcinoma
STK11	Liver kinase B1 (LKB1) or STK11	Activator of AMPK family of kinases; suppresses cell growth when cell nutrient and energy levels and low	Peutz-Jeghers syndrome (GI polyps, GI cancers, pancreatic carcinoma and other carcinomas)	Diverse carcinomas (5–20% of cases, depending on type)
SDHB, SDHD	Succinate dehydrogenase complex subunits B and D	TCA cycle, oxidative phosphorylation	Familial paraganglioma, familial pheochromocytoma	Paraganglioma
Inhibitors of Invasion and Metastasis				
CDH1	E-cadherin	Cell adhesion, inhibition of cell motility	Familial gastric cancer	Gastric carcinoma, lobular breast carcinoma
Enablers of Genomic Stability				
TP53	P53 protein	Cell cycle arrest and apoptosis in response to DNA damage	Li-Fraumeni syndrome (diverse cancers)	Most human cancers
DNA Repair Factors				
BRCA1, BRCA2	Breast cancer-1 and breast cancer-2 (BRCA1 and BRCA2)	Repair of double-stranded breaks in DNA	Familial breast and ovarian carcinoma; carcinomas of male breast; chronic lymphocytic leukemia (BRCA2)	Rare
MSH2, MLH1, MSH6	MSH1, MLH1, MSH6	DNA mismatch repair	Hereditary nonpolyposis colon carcinoma	Colonic and endometrial carcinoma
Unknown Mechanisms				
WT1	Wilms tumor-1 (WT1)	Transcription factor	Familial Wilms tumor	Wilms tumor, certain leukemias
MEN1	Menin	Transcription factor	Multiple endocrine neoplasia-1 (MEN 1; pituitary, parathyroid and pancreatic endocrine tumors)	Pituitary, parathyroid and pancreatic endocrine tumors

42. Ans. a. Sickle cell anaemia - autosomal recessive, c. Vit D resistant rickets- X-linked dominant, d. Achondroplasia – autosomal dominant

[Ref: Robbins 9th (SAE)/141-42]

Mendelian Disorders

◈ *Robbins 9th (SAE)/141-42*

- Sickle cell anaemia - autosomal recessive
- Duchene muscle dystrophy- X-linked recessive
- Vit D resistant rickets- X-linked dominant
- Achondroplasia – autosomal dominant
- Osteogenesis Imperfecta - autosomal dominant

43. Ans. a. Can be diagnosed in utero by USG, b. Hypertension develops in late stages of the disease, c. May proceed to renal failure before preschool age, d. Enlargement of kidney

[Ref: Robbins 9th (SAE)/945,947-48; Harshmohan 7th/645; Harrison 19th/1853; O.P.Ghai 8th/507; CMDT 2016/914]

"***ARPKD:*** *The age at presentation may be perinatal, neonatal, infantile or juvenile, but frequently serious manifestations are present at birth and result in death from renal failure in early childhood"- Harshmohan 7th/645*

A & E

Autosomal Recessive Polycystic Kidney Disease

◈ *O.P.Ghai 8th/507*

- *Affected children usually present in the neonatal period with oliguria, respiratory insufficiency and palpable kidney*
- *It is sometimes diagnosed in **young children** presenting with **hypertension, renal insufficiency** or **enlarged kidney**, or with portal hypertension due to associated congenital hepatic fibrosis*

Autosomal Recessive Polycystic Kidney Disease

◈ *Harrison 19th/1853*

- Classic ARPKD is ***generally diagnosed in utero or within the neonatal period*** and characterized by ***greatly enlarged echogenic kidneys*** in diseased fetuses.
- Some patients are diagnosed after the neonatal stage and form the older group. Morbidity and mortality in this group often involve ***systemic hypertension, progressive renal insufficiency and liver manifestations.***
- Some patients with the diagnosis of ARPKD at 1 year of age with nephromegaly exhibit ***slowly declining renal function over 20 years with only minimally enlarged kidneys at ESRD*** and markedly atrophic kidneys following renal transplantation. The slow progression of renal disease is likely due to increasing fibrosis rather than the development of cysts.
- ***Systemic hypertension is common in all ARPKD patients***, even those with normal renal function.
- Diagnosis:***Ultrasonography, CT and MRI all can be used for diagnosis.*** Ultrasonography reveals large, echogenic kidneys with poor corticomedullary differentiation. ***The diagnosis can be made in utero after 24 weeks of gestation in severe cases.***

Table *(Robbins 9th (SAE)/945)*: **Summary of Renal Cystic Diseases (Partial list)**

Disease	Inheritance	Pathologic Features	Clinical Features of Complications	Typical outcome
Adult polycystic kidney disease	Autosomal dominant	Large multicystic kidneys, liver cysts, berry aneurysms	***Hematuria***, flank pain, urinary tract infection, renal stones, ***hypertension***	Chronic renal failure beginning at age 40–60 years
Childhood polycystic kidney disease	Autosomal recessive	Enlarged, cystic kidneys at birth	Hepatic fibrosis	Variable, death in infancy or childhood

44. Ans. All (a, b, c, d, e)

[Ref: Robbins 9th (SAE)/937; Harrison 19th/714; Harshmohan 7th/363]

Type I cryoglobulinemia is composed of a single mono-clonal Ig, usually IgM. Type I cryoglobulinemia accounts for 10% to 15% of people with cryoglobulinemia. It is mainly found in patients with lymphoproliferative disorders (immunocytoma/ Waldenström macroglobulinemia, ***multiple myeloma***)"- *asheducationbook.hematologylibrary.org*

Light-Chain Cast Nephropathy ("Myeloma Kidney")

◈ *Robbins 9th (SAE)/937*

Overt renal insufficiency occurs in half of those with multiple myeloma and related lymphoplasmacytic disorders. Several factors contribute to renal damage:

- **Bence-Jones proteinuria and cast nephropathy:** The main cause of renal dysfunction is related to Bence-Jones (light-chain) proteinuria and correlates with the degree of proteinuria. Bence-Jones proteins combine with the urinary glycoprotein (Tamm-Horsfall protein) under acidic conditions to form large, histologically distinct tubular casts that obstruct the tubular lumens and induce a characteristic inflammatory reaction (***lightchain cast nephropathy***).
- **Amyloidosis of AL type,** formed from free light chains (usually of λ type), which occurs in 6% to 24% of individuals with myeloma.
- **Light-chain deposition disease**: In some patients, light chains (usually of κ type) deposit in GBMs and mesangium in nonfibrillar forms, causing a glomerulopathy and in tubular basement membranes, which may cause ***tubulointerstitial nephritis.***
- *Hypercalcemia* and *hyperuricemia* are often present in these patients.

"**Multiple myeloma**: With the increase in the amount of light chains presented to the tubule, the tubular cells become overloaded with these proteins and tubular damage results either directly from light chain toxic effects or indirectly from the release of intracellular lysosomal enzymes. The ***earliest manifestation of this tubular damage is the adult Fanconi's syndrome*** (a type 2 proximal renal tubular acidosis), with loss of glucose and amino acids, as well as defects in the ability of the kidney to acidify and concentrate the urine"-*Harrison 19th/714; Nelson 20th/2530*

45. Ans. b. Dry tap on bone marrow aspiration, c. Only potentially curative treatment is allogeneic stem cell transplantation, d. Splenomegaly is almost invariably present, e. Myeloblasts may be seen in peripheral blood

[Ref: Robbins 9th (SAE)/620-21; Harshmohan 7th/339-40; Harrison 19th/674-76; Davidson 22nd/]

"**Primary myelofibrosis**: On examination, splenomegaly is almost invariably present and is commonly massive. The

liver is enlarged in more than 50% of cases. Nucleated red blood cells are present and the myeloid series is shifted, with immature forms including a small percentage of ***promyelocytes or myeloblasts.*** Splenectomy is not routinely performed but is indicated for medication-refractory splenic enlargement causing recurrent painful episodes, severe thrombocytopenia, or an unacceptable transfusion requirement The ***only potentially curative option for this disease is allogeneic stem cell transplantation*** in selected patients, especially those with a matched sibling donor"- *CMDT 2016/518-19*

"**Primary myelofibrosis:*Massive splenomegaly*** *produce abdominal discomfort, pain and discomfort.* ***Hepatomegaly is present in half the cases.*** *Bone marrow aspiration is generally unsuccessful and yields* ***'dry tap'.*** **Peripheral blood smear** *shows bizarre red cell shapes, tear drop poikilocytes, basophilic stippling, nucleated red cells,* ***immature leucocytes*** *(i.e. leucoerythroblastic reaction), basophilia and giant platelet forms"- Harshmohan 7th/340*

Primary myelofibrosis or Chronic PMF or idiopathic myelofibrosis or agnogenic myeloid metaplasia, or myelofibrosis with myeloid metaplasia) *Harrison 19th/674-76*

- No signs or symptoms are specific for PMF. Many patients are asymptomatic at presentation and the disease is usually detected by the discovery of ***splenic enlargement and/or abnormal blood counts*** during a routine examination.
- A blood smear will show the characteristic features of extramedullary hematopoiesis: teardrop-shaped red cells, ***nucleated red cells, myelocytes and promyelocytes; myeloblasts*** may also be present.
- ***Mild hepatomegaly may accompany the splenomegaly but is unusual in the absence of splenic enlargement***
- ***Marrow is usually inaspirable due to the myelofibrosis***
- For unexplained reasons, ***splenectomy increases the risk of blastic transformation.*** Splenic irradiation is best
- ***Allogeneic bone marrow transplantation is the only curative treatment for PMF***

46. Ans. a. Pregnancy, b. OCP uses, d. Left ventricular failure, e. Excessive unaccustomed exercise

[Ref: Robbins 9th (SAE)/127; Harshmohan 7th/106; L and B 26th/914; Schwartz 10th/918; Davidson 22nd/721]

"**Pulmonary embolism** *is* ***7-10 times more common in OCP user*** *than in nonusers in first year of use"-Shaw's Gynae 16th/274*

"**Stress or fatigue fracture**: *occur mainly in lower limb after excessive or unaccustomed exercise. Fat embolism is a complication of Stress fracture"- Applied Basic Science for Basic Surgical Training by Andrew T. Raftery 2008/394*

Venous thromboembolism (VTE) *is a disease that includes both deep vein thrombosis (DVT) and* ***pulmonary embolism*** *(PE)"- www.clevelandclinicmeded.com*

Table *(L and B 26th/914)*: **Risk factors for venous thromboembolism**

Patient factors	Disease or surgical procedure
• Age • Obesity • Varicose veins • Immobility • Pregnancy • Puerperium • High-dose oestrogen therapy • Previous deep vein thrombosis or pulmonary embolism • Thrombophilia	• Trauma or surgery, especially of pelvis, hip and lower limb • Malignancy, especially pelvic and abdominal metastatic • Heart failure • Recent myocardial infarction • Paralysis of lower limb (s) infection • Inflammatory bowel disease • Nephrotic syndrome • Polycythaemia • Paraproteinaemia • Paroxysmal nocturnal haemoglobinuria antibody or lupus anticoagulant • Behçet's disease • Homocystinaemia

Recurrent pulmonary emboli, sometimes with infarction, are an important cause of morbidity and mortality late in the course of **mitral stenosis**"- *Harrison 19th/1540,Davidson 22nd/616*

Risk Factors for Venous Thromboembolism

(Schwartz 10th/918)

Acquired

- Advanced age
- Hospitalization/immobilization
- Hormone replacement therapy and ***oral contraceptive use***
- ***Pregnancy and puerperium***
- Prior venous thromboembolism
- Malignancy
- Major surgery
- Obesity
- Nephrotic syndrome
- Trauma or spinal cord injury
- Long-haul travel (>6 hours)
- Varicose veins
- Antiphospholipid antibody syndrome
- Myeloproliferative disease
- Polycythemia

Inherited

- Factor V Leiden
- Prothrombin 20210A
- Antithrombin deficiency
- Protein C deficiency
- Protein S deficiency
- Factor XI elevation
- Dysfibrinogenemia

Mixed Etiology

- Homocysteinemia
- Factor VII, VIII, IX, XI elevation

- Hyperfibrinogenemia
- Activated protein C resistance without factor V Leiden

47. Ans. c. t(15:17)

[Ref: Robbins 9th (SAE)/317; Harrison 19th/679, 102e-5-7]

"The **promyelocytic leukemia**–retinoic acid receptor (PML-RAR) fusion protein, generated by the ***t (15; 17)*** observed in most cases of ***acute promyelocytic leukemia (APML)***"-*Harrison 19th/102e-7*

"**Acute promyelocytic leukemia (APML)** is virtually always associated with a reciprocal translocation between chromosomes 15 and 17 that produces a *PML-RARA* fusion gene"-*Robbins 9th (SAE)/317*

Table *(Robbins 9th (SAE)/317)*: **Selected examples of oncogenes caused by translocations**

Malignancy	Translocation	Affected Genes
Chronic myelogenous leukemia (CML)	(9; 22) (q34; q11)	ABL 9q34 BCR 22q11
Acute myeloid leukemia (AML)	(8; 21) (q22; q22) (15; 17) (q22; q21)	AML 8q22 ETO 21q22 PML 15q22 RARA 17 q21

AML with recurrent genetic abnormalities *(Harrison 19th/679)*
AML with t (8; 21) (q22; q22); *RUNX1-RUNX1T1*
AML with inv (16) (pl3.1q22) or t (16; 16) (p13.1; q22); *CBFB-MYH11*
Acute promyelocytic leukemia with t (15; 17) (q22; q12); PML-RARA
AML with t (9; 11) (p22; q23); *MLLT3-MLL*
AML with t (6; 9) (p23; q34); *DEK-NUP214*
AML with inv (3) (q21q26.2) or t (3; 3) (q21; q26.2); *RPN1-EVI1*
AML (megakaryoblastic) with t (1; 22) (p13; q13); *RBM15-MKL1*

48. Ans. a. Albumin, b. Transferrin

[Ref: www.ncbi.nlm.nih.go; wiki; Robbins 9th (SAE)/99]

Acute-phase Proteins: Positive and Negative www.ncbi.nlm.nih.go; wiki

"**Negative acute-phase proteins** ***decrease in inflammation***. The physiological role of decreased synthesis of such proteins is generally to save amino acids for producing "positive" acute-phase proteins more efficiently.

Positive acute-phase proteins ***increase in plasma concentration in response to inflammation*** (usually within 1-2 days).

Table: *www.eclinpath.com/chemistry*

Positive APPs	Negative APPs
C-reactive protein (CRP)	***Albumin***
Serum Amyloid A (SAA)	*Transferrin*
Haptoglobin (Hp)	Transthyretin
Ceruloplasmin	Retinol-binding protein
α2-Macroglobulin	
α1-Acid glycoprotein (AGP)	
Fibrinogen	
Complement (C3, C4)	

"Positive" acute-phase Proteins *(Wiki)*
C-reactive protein
Serum amyloid P component
Serum amyloid A
Complement factors
Mannan-binding lectin
Fibrinogen, prothrombin, factor VIII, von Willebrand factor
Plasminogen activator inhibitor-1 (PAI-1)
Alpha 2-macroglobulin
Ferritin
Hepcidin
Ceruloplasmin
Haptoglobin
Orosomucoid (Alpha-1-acid glycoprotein, AGP)
Alpha 1-antitrypsin
Alpha 1-antichymotrypsin

49. Ans. a. Basophils stippling in lead poisoning, d. Dimorphic RBC

[Ref: Harshmohan 7th/277-78; Wintrobe's Clinical Hematology 12th/845-46]

Sideroblastic Anaemia

◈ *Harshmohan 7th/277-78*

- *Bone marrow examination show **erythroid hyperplasia** with usually macronormoblastic erythropoiesis*
- *MCV, MCH and MCHC are very low (except MCV raised in acquired type)*
- *The blood picture shows hypochromic anaemia which may be microcytic or there may be some normocytic red cells as well (dimorphic)*
- *Lead may cause sideroblastic anaemia*

Sideroblastic Anaemia: Laboratory Findings

◈ *Wintrobe's Clinical Hematology 12th/845-46*

- The anemia is usually moderate and may be normocytic but more often is macrocytic
- The **mean corpuscular hemoglobin concentration** is ***normal or slightly reduced*** and a variable population of hypochromic cells is found on blood smear.
- A particularly characteristic finding is the presence of **occasional basophilic stippling** in hypochromic cells that stains positive for iron.
- Typical **Pappenheimer bodies** are uncommon unless there is associated hyposplenism or the spleen is absent.
- **Erythroid hyperplasia** is found on bone marrow examination.

"**Siderocyte:** *These are red cells containing granules of non-haem iron. These granules stain positively with Prussian blue reaction as well as stain with Romanowsky dyes when they are referred to as* ***Pappenheimer bodies****. Siderocytes are normally not present in the human peripheral blood but a small number may appear following splenectomy"- Harshmohan 7th/277*

"**Punctate basophilia or basophilic stippling** *(presence of many dark blue-coloured pinhead-sized spots in cytoplasm of RBC) is present in* ***lead poisoning****"-Reddy Forensic 33rd/544*

Diagnosis of Microcytic Anemia

◈ *(Harrison 19th/628)*

Tests	Iron Deficiency	Inflammation	Thalassemia	Sideroblastic Anemia
Smear	Micro/hypo	Normal micro/hypo	Micro/hypo with targeting	Variable
Serum iron (μg/dL)	<30	<50	Normal to high	Normal to high
TIBC (μg/dL)	>360	<300	Normal	Normal
Percent saturation	<10	10–20	30–80	30–80
Ferritin (μg/L)	<15	30–200	50–300	50–300
Hemoglobin pattern on electrophoresis	Normal	Normal	Abnormal with αβ thalassemia; can be normal with a thalassemia	Normal

50. Ans. a. Tram track appearance on light microscopy, b. Subendothelial electron-dense deposits on electron microscopy, c. Immunofluorescence microscopy show positive florescence of IgG and C3 on dense deposit

[Ref: Robbins 9th (SAE)/910,920; Harshmohan 7th/658-59]

"**Type I MPGN** is characterized by the presence of discrete **subendothelial electron-dense deposits.** Mesangial and occasional subepithelial deposits may also be present. By immunofluorescence, ***IgG and C3*** are ***deposited in a granular pattern*** and early complement components (C1q and C4) are often also present, indicative of an immune complex pathogenesis"- *Robbins 9th (SAE)/920*

"**In type II MPGN,** ***C3 is present on GBM but not in the dense deposist****"- Robbins 9th (SAE)/920*

"***Grossly and by light microscopy, all the three type of MPGN are similar****. By electron microscopy and immunofluorescence microscopy, the changes are different in three types of MPGN"- Harshmohan 7th/658-59*

MPGN: Light Microscopy Feature (Feature Common to all 3 types)

◈ *Robbins 9th (SAE)/920*

- The **glomeruli are large and hypercellular**. The ***hypercellularity*** is produced both by ***proliferation of cells in the mesangium*** and so-called endocapillary proliferation involving capillary endothelium and infiltrating leukocytes.
- The glomeruli have an accentuated "lobular" appearance due to the **proliferating mesangial cells and increased mesangial matrix**.
- The GBM is thickened and often shows a **"doublecontour" or "tram-track" appearance**, especially evident in silver or PAS stains. This is caused by **"duplication" of the basement membrane** (also commonly referred to as splitting), usually as the result of new basement membrane synthesis in response to subendothelial deposits of immune complexes.
- Between the duplicated basement membranes there is inclusion or interposition of cellular elements, which can be of mesangial, endothelial, or leukocytic origin. Such interposition also gives rise to the appearance of ***"split" basement membranes.***
- Crescents are present in many cases.

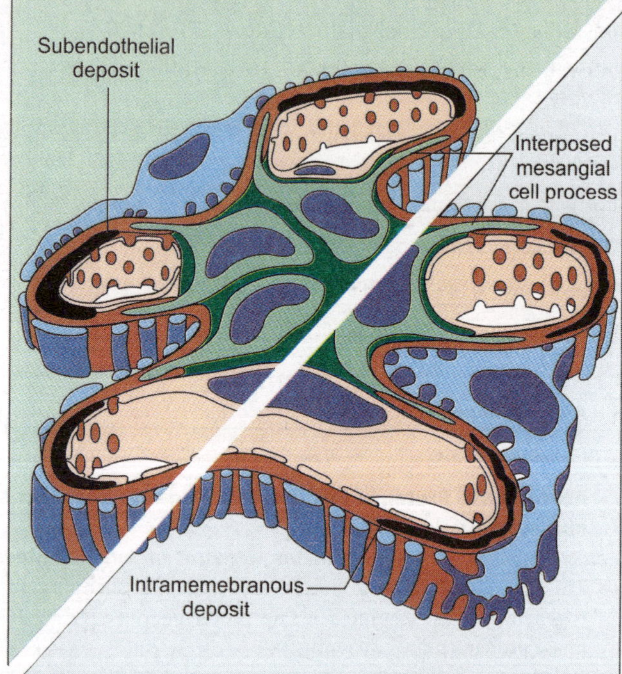

Fig. *(Robbins 9th (SAE)/921)*: Schematic representation of patterns in the two types of membranoproliferative glomerulonephritis. In type I there are ***subendothelial deposits***; type II is characterized by ***intramembranous dense deposits (dense-deposit disease)***. In both, the basement membranes appear split when viewed in the light microscope

Table (*Robbins 9th (SAE)/910*): **Summary of MPGN**

Disease	Most Frequent Clinical Presentation	Pathogenesis	Glomerular Pathology		
			Light Microscopy	Fluorescence Microscopy	Electron Microscopy
Membranoproliferative glomerulonephritis (MPGN) Type I	Nephritic/ Nephrotic syndrome	Immune complex	Mesangial proliferative or membranoproliferative pattern of proliferation; GBM thickening; splitting	IgG + +C3; C1q + C4	***Subendothelial deposits***
Dense deposit disease (MPGN Type II)	Hematuria Chronic renal failure	Autoantibody: alternative complement pathway	Mesangial proliferative or membranoproliferative pattern of proliferation; GBM thickening; splitting	C3; no C1q or C4	Dense deposits

51. Ans. a. May involve hilar lymph node, b. Asbestosis begins in the lower lobes, c. Pleural plaques consists of calcified hyalinzed collagenous tissue, d. High resolution CT scanning is the best imaging method

[Ref: Robbins 9th (SAE)/723-24; Park 24th/844; Harshmohan 7th/472-74; Danhert Radiology Manual 7th/472-73]

"***High resolution CT scanning is the best imaging method*** for asbestosis because of its ability to detect parenchymal fibrosis and define the presence of coexisting pleural plaques"-*CMDT 2016/306*

Asbestosis

◈ *Harshmohan 7th/472-74*

- *The* ***involvement of hilar lymph nodes*** *is not as significant as in silicosis*
- ***Fibrocalcific pleural plaques*** *are the most common lesion associated with asbestos exposure. Microscopically, they consists of* ***hyalinzed collagenous*** *tissue which may be calcified so that they are visible on chest x-ray*

Asbestosis and Asbestos-Related Diseases

◈ *Robbins 9th (SAE)/723-24*

- Occupational exposure to asbestos is linked to (1) parenchymal interstitial fibrosis (*asbestosis*); (2) ***localized fibrous plaques*** or, rarely, diffuse fibrosis in the pleura; (3) pleural effusions; (4) ***lung carcinomas;*** (5) malignant pleural and peritoneal mesotheliomas; and (6) laryngeal carcinoma.
- In addition to cellular and fibrotic lung reactions, asbestos probably also functions as both a tumor initiator and a promoter.
- In contrast with coal worker's pneumoconiasis and silicosis, ***asbestosis begins in the lower lobes and subpleurally***, but the middle and upper lobes of the lungs become affected as fibrosis progresses.
- **Pleural plaques** are the most common manifestation of asbestos exposure and are well-circumscribed plaques of dense collagen, often containing calcium. They develop most frequently on the anterior and posterolateral aspects of the **parietal pleura** and over the domes of the diaphragm.
- The presenting complaints are chest pain, dyspnea and, as noted, recurrent pleural effusions. Concurrent pulmonary asbestosis (fibrosis) is present in only 20% of individuals with pleural mesothelioma.
- The lung is invaded directly and there ***is often metastatic spread to the hilar lymph nodes*** and, eventually, to the liver and other distant organs.

52. Ans. b. Radiographically seen as eggshell calcification, d. Associated with an increased susceptibility to tuberculosis, e. Histologically silica nodules consists of hyalinised center surrounded by concentric laminations of collagen

[Ref: Robbins 9th (SAE)/690; Park 24th/843; Harshmohan 7th/471; Harrison 19th/1688; Davidson 22nd/717]

"Histologically ***silicotic nodules*** *consists of* ***hyalinised center surrounded by concentric laminations of collagen****"-Harshmohan 7th/471*

Silicosis

◈ *Robbins 9th (SAE)/690*

- Silicosis is characterized grossly in its early stages by tiny, barely palpable, discrete pale to blackened (if coal dust is also present) nodules in the hilar lymph nodes and ***upper zones of the lungs.***
- As the disease progresses, these nodules coalesce into **hard, collagenous scars.**
- Some nodules may undergo central softening and cavitation due to superimposed tuberculosis or to ischemia. Fibrotic lesions may also occur in the hilar lymph nodes and pleura.
- Sometimes, thin ***sheets of calcification occur in the lymph nodes and are seen radiographically as eggshell calcification*** (i.e., calcium surrounding a zone lacking calcification).
- If the disease continues to progress, expansion and coalescence of lesions may produce progressive ***massive fibrosis.***
- Histologic examination reveals the hallmark lesion characterized by a central area of ***whorled collagen fibers*** with a more peripheral zone of dust-laden macrophages.
- Examination of the nodules by polarized microscopy reveals the birefringent silicate particles (silica is weakly birefringent).

- Chest radiographs typically show a fine nodularity in the ***upper zones of the lung***.
- It is associated with an increased susceptibility to *tuberculosis*.
- Patients with silicosis have double the risk for developing lung cancer.

Silicosis

◈ *Park 24th/843*

- *The longer the duration of exposure, the greater the risk of developing silicosis*
- *It is found that the incubation period may vary from a few month up to 6 years of exposure, depending upon the above factors*
- *Pathologically, silicosis is characterized by a dense nodular fibrosis, the nodule ranging from 3 to 4 mm in diameter*
- *Some of the early manifestations are irritant cough, dyspnea on exertion and pain in chest*
- *With more advanced disease, impairment of total lung capacity (TLC) is commonly present*
- *A X-ray of chest shows "snow storm" appearance in the lung fields*
- *Silicosis is progressive and what is more important is that silicotics are prone to pulmonary tuberculosis, a conditional called **"silico-tuberculosis"***
- *There is no effective treatment for silicosis. Fibrotic change that have already taken place cannot be reversed*

*"Characteristic lung tissue pathology in nodular silicosis consists of fibrotic nodules with concentric "onion-skinned" arrangement of collagen fibers, central hyalinization and a cellular peripheral zone, with **lightly birefringent particles** seen under polarized light" (www. askdrwiki. com/mediawik)*

Table *(Harrison 19th/1688)*: **Categories of Occupational Exposure and Associated Respiratory Conditions**

Asbestos: mining, processing, construction, ship repair	Fibrosis (asbestosis), pleural disease, cancer, mesothelioma
Silica: mining, stone cutting, sandblasting, quarrying	Fibrosis (silicosis), PMF, cancer, silicotuberculosis, COPD

53. Ans. b. IgA vasculitis, c. Carcinoma associated vasculitis, d. Anti-glomerular basement membrane (anti-GBM) disease

[Ref: Robbins 9th (SAE)/506-12; Harshmohan 7th/382-84]

"Goodpasture's disease or **Anti-glomerular basement membrane (anti-GBM)** disease is a ***rare small vessel vasculitis*** that affects the capillary beds of the kidneys and lungs"- *cjasn. asnjournals.org*

Microscopic Polyangiitis (Microscopic Polyarteritis, Hypersensitivity, or Leukocytoclastic Vasculitis)

◈ *Robbins 9th (SAE)/510; Harshmohan 7th/383*

- *This type of necrotizing vasculitis generally affects arterioles, capillaries and venules—smallest vessel*
- **Tumor antigens** may be the precipitating cause- *Robbins 9th (SAE)/510*
- ***Vasculitis associated with malignancy***- *Harshmohan 7th/383*

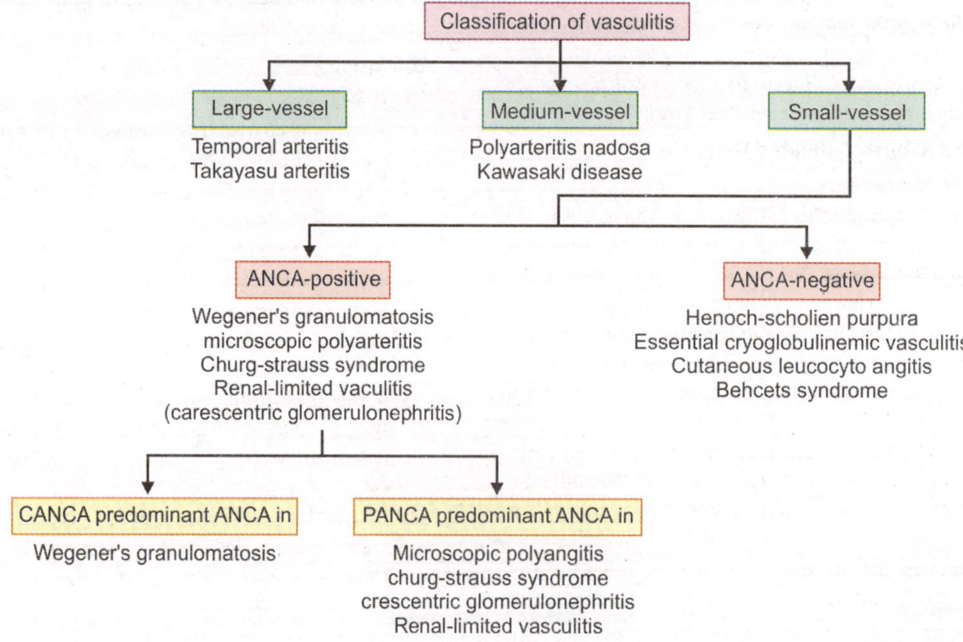

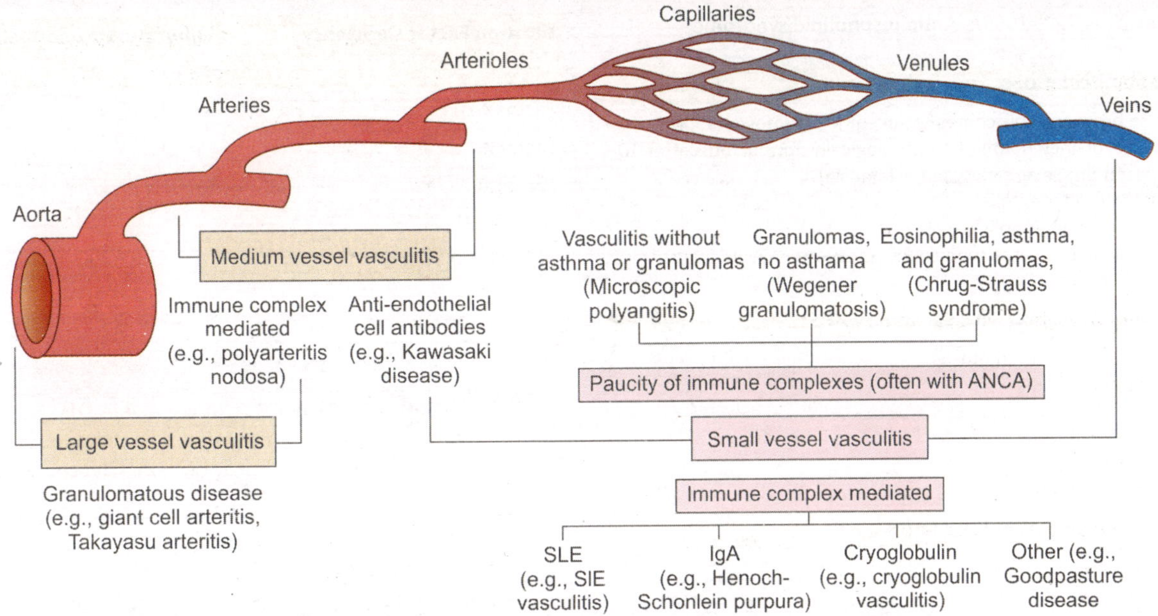

54. Ans. b. SLE is associated with primary antiphospholipid syndrome, e. Occur d/t defect in prostacyclin metabolism

[Ref: Robbins 9th (SAE)/124-25; William's Obs 23rd/1151-53; Davidson 22nd/1009,1055]

Antiphospholipid Antibody Syndrome

◈ *Robbins 9th (SAE)/124-25*

- This syndrome (previously called the ***lupus anticoagulant syndrome***) has protean clinical manifestations, including ***recurrent thromboses, repeated miscarriages***, cardiac valve vegetations and thrombocytopenia.
- Depending on the vascular bed involved, the clinical presentations can include pulmonary embolism (PE) (following lower extremity venous thrombosis), pulmonary hypertension (from recurrent subclinical pulmonary emboli), stroke, bowel infarction, or renovascular hypertension.
- Suspected antibody targets include *β2-glycoprotein I, a plasma protein that associates with the surfaces of endothelial cells and trophoblasts and thrombin.*
- Antiphospholipid antibody syndrome has **primary and secondary forms**. Individuals with a well-defined autoimmune disease, such as **systemic lupus erythematosus**, are designated as ***having secondary antiphospholipid syndrome*** (hence the earlier term *lupus anticoagulant syndrome*).
- In *primary antiphospholipid syndrome*, patients exhibit only the manifestations of a hypercoagulable state and lack evidence of ***other autoimmune disorders***; occasionally, it appears following exposure to certain drugs or infections.

Antiphospholipid Syndrome

◈ *William's Obs 23rd/1151-53*

- These antiphospholipid antibodies include ***lupus anticoagulant (LAC)*** **and** ***anticardiolipin antibodies (ACAs)***. They may be of IgG, IgM and IgA classes, alone or in combination. Although they may be found in normal persons, they also are associated with the *antiphospholipid antibody syndrome (APS)*.
- This is characterized by recurrent arterial or ***venous thromboses, thrombocytopenia and fetal losses***—especially stillbirths—during the second half of pregnancy

◈ *Davidson 22nd/1055*

- The antiphospholipid antibodies are heterogeneous and typically are directed against proteins which bind to phospholipids. Although causal roles for these antibodies have been proposed, the mechanisms underlying the clinical features of APS are not clear.
- In clinical practice, **two types of test are used**, which detect:
  - Antibodies which bind to negatively charged phospholipid on an ELISA plate (called an ***anticardiolipin antibody test***)
  - Those which interfere with phospholipid-dependent coagulation tests like the APTT or the dilute Russell viper venom time (DRVVT; called a ***lupus anticoagulant test***).
- The term antiphospholipid antibody encompasses both a lupus anticoagulant and an anticardiolipin antibody; individuals may be positive for one or both of these activities.
- **Lupus anticoagulant** (more strongly associated with thrombosis than anticardiolipin antibodies)

Table *(Davidson 22nd/1055)*: **Antiphospholipid syndrome**

Clinical Manifestations
• Adverse pregnancy outcome [Recurrent first trimester abortion (≥ 3); Unexplained death of morphologically normal fetus after 10 wks' gestation; Severe early pre-eclampsia] • Venous thromboembolism • Arterial thromboembolism • Livedo reticularis, catastrophic APS, transverse myelitis, skin necrosis, chorea
Conditions Associated with Secondary APS
• Systemic lupus erythematosus • Rheumatoid arthritis • Systemic sclerosis • Behçet's syndrome • Temporal arteritis • Sjögren's syndrome
Targets for Antiphospholipid Antibodies
• β2-glycoprotein 1 • Protein C • Annexin V • Prothrombin (may result in haemorrhagic presentation)

55. Ans. a. Factor 2, b. Factor 5, c. Factor 10

[Ref: Robbins 9th (SAE)/663; Harrison 19th/733]

"Factor 8 (Hemophilia A) and Factor 9 (Hemophilia B) deficiency: ***PT is normal and aPTT is prolonged***" *Robbins 9th (SAE)/663*

Prothrombin Time (PT)

◈ *Robbins 9th/656*
- This assay tests the extrinsic and common coagulation pathways
- A prolonged PT can results from deficiency or dysfunction of factor V, factor VII, factor X, prothrombin or fibrinogen

Partial Tromboplastin Time (PTT)

◈ *Robbins 9th/656*
- This assay tests intrinsic and common clotting pathways
- Prolongation of the PTT can be due to deficiency or dysfunction of factor ***V, VIII, IX, X, XI or XII, prothrombin or fibrinogen.***

Table *(Harrison 19th/733)*: **Laboratory Characteristics of Inherited Coagulation Disorders**

Clotting Factor Deficiency	Laboratory Abnormality[a]		
	aPTT	PT	TT
Fibrinogen(Factor I)	+	+	+
Prothrombin(Factor II)	+	+	–
Factor V	+/–	+/–	–
Factor VII	–	+	–
Factor VIII	+	–	–
Factor IX	+	–	–
Factor X	+/–	+/–	–
Factor XI	+	–	–
Factor XII	+	–	–
HK	+	–	–
Prekallikrein	+	–	–
Factor XIII	–	–	+/–

[a]Values within normal range (–) or prolonged (+)

56. Ans. b. Both PT and aPTT are increased in DIC, c. Intravenous gamma globulin is useful in Immune Thrombocytopenic Purpura, e. Platelet count is decreased in DIC

[Ref: CMDT 2016/549; Harrison 19th/ 737,728; Davidson 22nd/1051-52; Robbins 9th (SAE)/663]

"**Cryoprecipitat**e is enriched with ***FVIII protein*** (each bag contains ~80 IU of FVIII) and was commonly used for the treatment of hemophilia A decades ago; it is still in use in some developing countries, but because of the risk of bloodborne diseases, this product should be avoided in hemophilia patients when factor concentrates are available"- *Harrison 19th/ 734*

"**Immune Thrombocytopenic Purpura**: ***Intravenous gamma globulin (IVIgG),*** which is pooled, primarily IgG antibodies, has more efficacy than anti-Rh0 (D) in post-splenectomized patients. IVIgG is dosed at 1–2 g/kg total, given over 1–5 days"- *Harrison 19th/ 728*

"**DIC**: Common findings include the ***prolongation of PT and/or aPTT; platelet counts μ100,000/μL, or a rapid decline in platelet numbers***; the presence of schistocytes (fragmented red cells) in the blood smear; and elevated levels of FDP. The most sensitive test for DIC is the FDP level. DIC is an unlikely diagnosis in the presence of normal levels of FDP"-*Harrison 19th/ 737*

"**Disseminated intravascular coagulation (DIC):** There is progressive thrombocytopenia (rarely severe), ***prolongation of the activated partial thromboplastin time (aPTT) and prothrombin time (PT) a***nd low levels of fibrinogen."- *CMDT 2016/549*

"**Factor XI (FXI) deficiency, also called hemophilia** C, plasma thromboplastin antecedent deficiency and Rosenthal syndrome. ***FXI deficiency is inherited in an autosomal recessive pattern, meaning both parents must carry the gene to pass it on to their children; men and women are affected equally***"- *www.hemophilia.org/Bleeding-Disorders*

"Mutations in the **factor XI gene** cause the congenital deficiency of factor XI clotting activity. The inheritance pattern of factor XI is ***autosomal but not completely recessive***, because heterozygotes may have bleeding"

"In severe **haemophilia A**, bleeding episodes should be treated by raising the factor VIII level, usually by ***intravenous infusion of factor VIII concentrate***"- *Davidson 22nd/1051-52*

"**Haemophilia B:** The disease is treated with infusions of recombinant factor IX"- *Robbins 9th (SAE)/663*

57. Ans. All (a, b, c, d)

[Ref: Robbins 9th (SAE)/326-27; Harrison 19th/697]

Epstein-Barr virus *is closely associated with* ***nasopharyngeal cancer*** *" (P.L.Dhingra 6th/250)*

Oncogenic Viruses

◈ *Robbins 9th (SAE)/326-27*

- Four DNA viruses—HPV, Epstein-Barr virus (EBV), Kaposi sarcoma herpesvirus (KSHV, also called human herpesvirus-8 [HHV-8]) and hepatitis B virus (HBV)—are of special interest because they are strongly associated with human cancer.
- **Epstein-Barr Virus associated cancer:** Burkitt lymphoma; B cell lymphomas; a subset of Hodgkin lymphoma; ***nasopharyngeal carcinoma***; a subset of T cell lymphomas; gastric carcinomas; NK cell lymphomas; and even, in rare instances, sarcomas, mainly in the immunosuppressed.
- The epidemiologic evidence linking chronic HBV and hepatitis C virus (HCV) infection with hepatocellular carcinoma is strong. It is estimated that 70% to 85% of hepatocellular carcinomas worldwide are due to infection with HBV or HCV.

Table *(Harrison 19th/697)*: **Infectious Agents Associated with the Development of Lymphoid Malignancies**

Infectious Agent	Lymphoid Malignancy
Epstein-Barr virus	Burkitt's lymphoma Post-organ transplant lymphoma Primary CNS diffuse large B-cell lymphoma Hodgkin's lymphoma Extranodal NK/T-cell lymphoma, nasal type
HTLV-1	Adult T-cell leukemia/lymphoma
HIV	Diffuse large B-cell leukemia/lymphoma Burkitt's lymphoma
Hepatitis C virus	Lymphoplasmacytic lymphoma
Helicobacter pylori	Gastric MALT lymphoma
Human herpesvirus 8	Primary effusion lymphoma Multicentric Castleman's disease

58. Ans. a. Down syndrome

[Ref: Robbins 9th (SAE)/161-66; Harshmohan 7th/253]

Most embryos cannot survive with a missing or extra autosome (numbered chromosome) and are spontaneously aborted. The ***most frequent aneuploidy in humans is trisomy 16, although fetuses affected with the full version of this chromosome abnormality do not survive to term*** (it is possible for surviving individuals to have the mosaic form, where trisomy 16 exists in some cells but not all). ***The most common aneuploidy that infants can survive with is trisomy 21***, which is found in **Down syndrome**, affecting 1 in 800 births. Trisomy 18 (Edwards syndrome) affects 1 in 6,000 births and trisomy 13 (Patau syndrome) affects 1 in 10,000 births. 10% of infants with trisomy 18 or 13 reach 1 year of age"- *en.wikipedia.org*

Trisomy of Sex Chromosomes can also Occur and Include

◈ *en.wikipedia.org*

XXX (Triple X syndrome)
XXY (Klinefelter syndrome)
XYY

Trisomy 21 (Down Syndrome)

◈ *Robbins 9th (SAE)/161*

- ***Down syndrome is the most common of the chromosomal disorders and is a major cause of mental retardation***.
- In the United States the incidence in newborns is **about 1 in 700**. Approximately 95% of affected individuals have trisomy 21, so their chromosome count is 47. FISH with chromosome 21–specific probes reveals the extra copy of chromosome 21 in such cases
- "***Down syndrome is the most common chromosomal disorder***"- *Harshmohan 7th/253*

Klinefelter Syndrome

◈ *Robbins 9th (SAE)/165*

- *Klinefelter syndrome is best defined as male hypogonadism that occurs when there are two or more X chromosomes and one or more Y chromosomes.*
- It is one of the most frequent forms of genetic disease involving the sex chromosomes as well as one of the most common causes of hypogonadism in the male. The incidence of this condition is approximately ***1 in 660 live male births.***

Turner Syndrome

◈ *Robbins 9th (SAE)/166*

- *Turner syndrome results from complete or partial monosomy of the X chromosome and is characterized primarily by hypogonadism in phenotypic females.*
- It is the most common sex chromosome abnormality in females, affecting ***about 1 in 2500 live-born females.***

Structural Abnormalities of Chromosomes

◈ *Robbins 9th (SAE)/159*

- If an error occurs in meiosis or mitosis and a cell acquires a chromosome complement that is not an exact multiple of 23, it is referred to as *aneuploidy.*
- The usual causes for aneuploidy are *nondisjunction* and *anaphase lag.* When nondisjunction occurs during gametogenesis, the gametes formed have either an extra chromosome (n + 1) or one less chromosome (n – 1).
- Fertilization of such gametes by normal gametes results in two types of zygotes—trisomic (2n + 1) or monosomic (2n – 1). In anaphase lag, one homologous chromosome in meiosis or one chromatid in mitosis lags behind and is left out of the cell nucleus. The result is one normal cell and one cell with monosomy. As seen subsequently, monosomy or trisomy involving the sex chromosomes, or even more bizarre aberrations, are compatible with life and are usually associated with variable degrees of phenotypic abnormalities.
- **Monosomy involving an autosome generally causes loss of too much genetic information to permit live birth or even embryogenesis, but several autosomal trisomies do permit survival.**

- ***With the exception of trisomy 21, all yield severely handicapped infants who almost invariably die at an early age***

59. Ans. a. It is the aneuploidy compatible with life, d. Causes miscarriage in early weeks of gestation, e. Wide chest

[Ref: Robbins 9th (SAE)/166-67; Harshmohan 7th/253]

"**Monosomy X (45,X)** *is the single* ***most common chromosomal abnormality in miscarriage***"*-Dutta Obs 8th/186*

"**Turner syndrome**: *About* ***70-90% of pregnancies abort in early weeks of gestation***"*-Shaw's Gynae 16th/146*

Turner Syndrome

◈ *Robbins 9th (SAE)/166*

- With routine cytogenetic methods, three types of karyotypic abnormalities are seen in individuals with Turner syndrome. *Approximately 57% are missing an entire X chromosome, resulting in a 45,X karyotype* of the remaining 43%, approximately one third (approximately 14%) have structural abnormalities of the X chromosomes and two thirds (approximately 29%) are mosaics.
- Left-sided cardiovascular abnormalities, particularly preductal coarctation of the aorta and bicuspid aortic valve, are seen most frequently.
- At puberty there is *failure to develop normal secondary sex characteristics.* The genitalia remain infantile, breast development is inadequate and there is little pubic hair. The mental status of these patients is usually normal, but subtle defects in nonverbal, visual-spatial information processing have been noted.

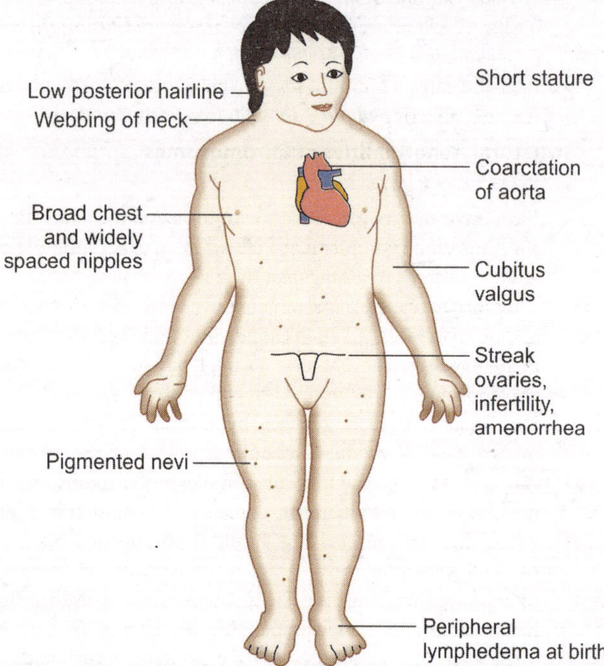

Fig: *(Robbins 9th (SAE)/167)*: Clinical features and karyotypes of Turner syndrome

- Of particular importance in establishing the diagnosis in the adult is the ***shortness of stature*** (rarely exceeding 150 cm in height) and amenorrhea.
- *Turner syndrome is the single most important cause of primary amenorrhea*, accounting for approximately one third of the cases.

60. Ans. a. Periapical cyst, b. Residual cyst, c. Paradental cyst

[Ref: Robbins 9th/ 734; Manipal Surgery 4th/292-93; Harshmohan 7th/511-12]

Table *(Robbins 9th/ 734)*: **Histologic Classification of Odontogenic cyst**

Inflammatory	Developmental
• Periapical cyst • Residual cyst • Paradental cyst	• Dentigerous cyst • Odontogenic keratocyst • Gingival cyst of newborn • Gingival cyst of adult • Eruption cyst • Lateral periodontal cyst • Glandular odontogenic cyst • Calcifying epithelial odontogenic cyst (Gorlin cyst)

61. Ans. b. First product is PGG_2; d. PG $F_{2\alpha}$ causes bronchoconstriction; e. PG I_2 causes fall in BP;

[Ref: Robbins 9th/83-84]

Prostaglandins (PGs)

◈ *Robbins 9th/83-84*

- PGs are produced by mast cells, macrophages, endothelial cells and many other cell types and are involved in the vascular and systemic reactions of inflammation.
- They are generated by the actions of two *cyclooxgenases,* called COX1 and COX2.
- Prostaglandins are divided into series based on structural features as coded by a letter (PGD, PGE, PGF, PGG and PGH) and a subscript numeral (e.g., 1, 2), which indicates the number of double bonds in the compound.
- TxA2, a potent platelet aggregating agent and vasoconstrictor
- Prostacyclin (PGI_2) is a vasodilator and a potent inhibitor of platelet aggregation and also markedly potentiates the permeability increasing and chemotactic effects of other mediators.
- PGD2 is the major prostaglandin made by mast cells; along with **PGE_2** (which is more widely distributed), it causes ***vasodilation*** and increases the permeability of postcapillary venules, thus potentiating edema formation.
- **$PGF_{2\alpha}$** stimulates the ***contraction of uterine and bronchial smooth muscle*** and small arterioles and PGD_2 is a chemoattractant for neutrophils.

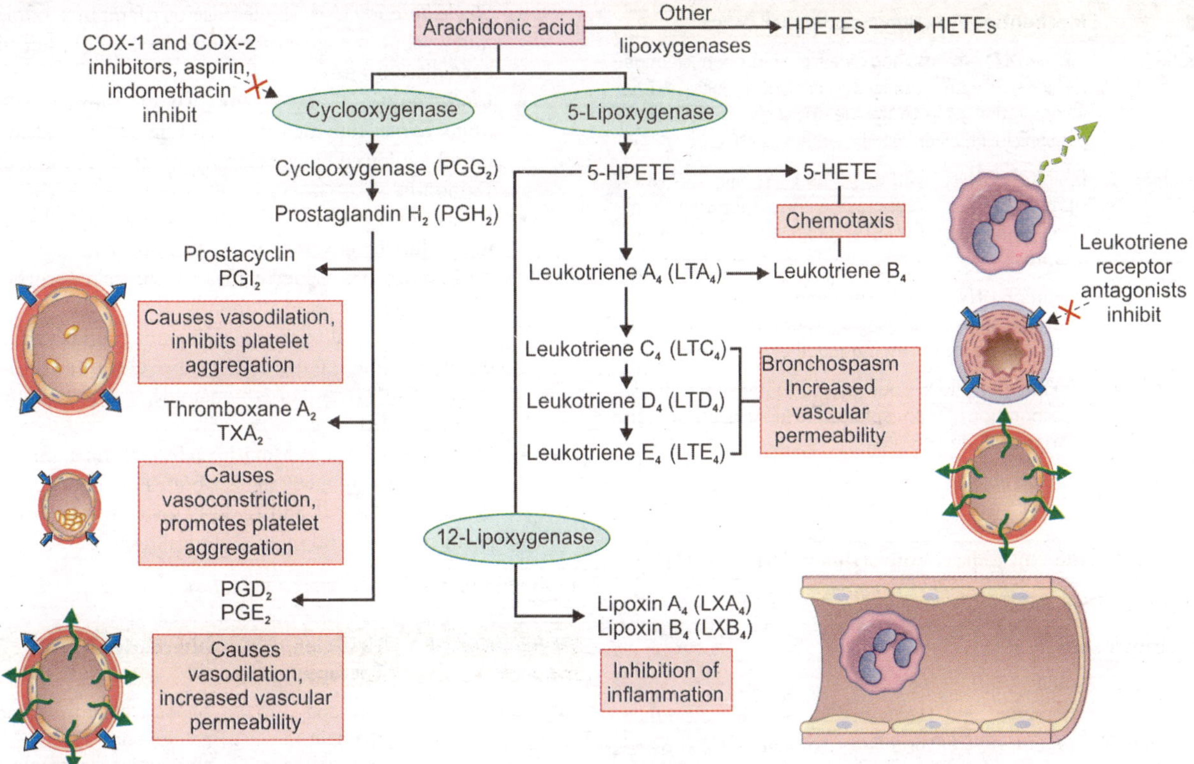

Fig: (Robbins 9th/84): Production of arachidonic acid metabolites & their role in inflammation

PHARMACOLOGY

62. Ans. a. Azathioprine, b. Methotrexate, c. Fludarabine, d. 6-Mercaptopurine

[Ref: K.D.T 7th/858; Katzung 13th/928, 931; Goodman and Gilman's 11th/1336, 1346-48; Satoskar Pharma 24th/829; Rang and Dale 8th/681]

Methotrexate is not purine antagonist but affect purine synthesis

***Capecitabine is pyrimidine antagonist**- K. D. T 7th/864*

*"Methotrexate blocks conversion of DHFA to THFA. **THFA is an essential coenzyme required for one carbon transfer reaction in de novo purine synthesis**"- K. D. T 7th/858*

Purine Antagonists

- *Satoskar Pharma 24th/829; K. D. T 7th/858*
- ***6-Mercaptopurine***
- ***Azathioprine***
- *6-Thioguanine*
- ***Fludarabine***
- *Cladribine*

Anticancer drug affecting Purine pathway: *Cladribine, clofarabrine, fludarabine, mercaptopurine, nelarabine, pentostatin, tioguanine"- Rang and Dale 8th/681 (Table)*

Antimetabolite Drug

- *Rang and Dale 8th/681 (Table)*

Folate antagonists	Methotrexate, pemetrexed, raltitrexed
Pyrimdine pathway	Azacitidine, capecitabine, cytarabine, decitabine, fluorouracil gemcitabine, tegafur
Purine pathway	Cladribine, clofarabrine, fludarabine, mercaptopurine, nelarabine, pentostatin, tioguanine

Drug	Mechanism of Action *(Katzung 13th /928)*
Capecitabine	Inhibits Thymidylate synthease (TS); resulting in alteration in RNA processing; incorporation of FdUPT into DNA resulting in inhibition of DNA synthesis and function
5-Fluorouracil	Inhibits TS, incorporation of FUTP into RNA resulting in alteration in RNA pro-cessing; incorporation of FdUTP into DNA resulting in inhibition of DNA syn-thesis and function
Methotrexate	Inhibits DHFR; inhibit TS; inhibit de novo purine nucleotide synthesis
Pemetrexed	Inhibits TS, inhibits de novo purine nucleotide synthesis
Cytarabine	Inhibits DNA synthesis and repair, inhibit ribonucleotide reductase with reduced formation of dNTPs, incorporation of cytarabine triphosphate into DNA

Contd...

Drug	Mechanism of Action *(Katzung 13th /928)*
Gemcitabine	Inhibits DNA synthesis and repair; inhibits ribonucleotide reductase with reduced formation of dNTPs; incorporation of gemcitabine triphosphate into DNA resulting in inhibition of DNA synthesis and function
Fludarabine	Inhibits DNA synthesis and repair, inhibits ribonucleotide reductase; incorporation of fludarabine triphosphaste into DNA, induction of apoptosis
Cladribine	Inhibits DNA synthesis and repair, inhibits ribonucleotide reductase; incorporation of cladribine triphosphate into DNA; induction of apoptosis
6-MERCAPTOPURINE	Inhibits de novo purine nucleotide synthesis; incorporation of triphosphate into RNA; incorporation of triphosphate into DNA
6- THIOGUANINE	Same as above

63. Ans. a. Purine synthesis, c. Conversion of DHFA to THFA

[Ref: K. D. T 7th/ 862; Katzung 13th/928]

Methotrexate

- *K. D. T 7th/ 862*
- *Folate antagonist*
- *Acts by inhibiting dihydrofolate reductase (DHFRase)- **blocking the conversion of DHFA to THFA***
- ***THFA is an essential coenzyme required for one carbon transfer reaction in de novo purine synthesis***

64. Ans. c. Ivermectin

[Ref: K. D. T 7th/850; Katzung 13th/909; Satoskar Pharma 24th/816; Rang and Dale 8th/673]

Strongyloides stercoralis (thread worm): ***First choice of drugs is ivermectin.*** *Alternative drug is albendazole and thiabendazole"- Satoskar Pharma 24th/816 K. D. T 7th/850*

Table: *Katzung 13th/909*

Infecting Organism	Drug of Choice	Alternative Drugs
Strongyloides stercoralis (threadworm)	Ivermectin	Albendazole or thiabendazole

65. Ans. All (a, b, c, d, e)

[Ref: K. D. T 7th/786; Park 24th/340-41; Goodman and Gilman's 11th/1204; Satoskar Pharma 24th/771-72; Rang and Dale 8th/640]

Alternative Regimens

- *K. D. T 7th/786*

Many alternative regimens incorporating newer antileprotic drugs have been investigated. However, these are used only in case of ***rifampin-resistance*** or when it is impossible/inadvisable to employ the standard MDT regimen. Some of these are:

- *Intermittent ROM:* Rifampin 600 mg + ofloxacin 400 mg + ***minocycline*** 100 mg are given once a month for 3–6 month for PBL and for 12 or 24 month for MBL cases, without any drug in between
- *Single dose ROM:* A single dose of rifampin + ofloxacin + minocycline was given for single lesion PBL, but this has been discontinued.
- ***Cloflazimine*** 50 mg + any two of ofloxacin 400 mg/ ***minocycline*** 100 mg/clarithromycin 500 mg daily for 6 month, followed by clofazimine 50 mg daily for additional 18 months.
- Four durg regimen of rifampin 600 mg + sparfloxacin 200 mg + **clarithromycin** 500 mg + minocycline 100 mg daily for 12 weeks has yielded equivalent clinical improvement in MBL cases to standard 12 month MDT.
- In case of refusal to accept clofazimine: ofloxacin 400 mg or minocycline 100 mg daily can be substituted for it in the standard MDT. Use of ethionamide as a substitute is not recommended.
- Intermittent RMMx: **Moxifloxacin** 400 mg + minocycline 200 mg + rifampin 600 mg is administered once a month: 6 doses given for PBL and 12 doses given for MBL cases have produced rapid and marked clinical response.

Table: *(Goodman and Gilman's 11th/1204)*

Mycobacterial Species	First-Line Therapy	Alternative Agents
M. leprae	Dapsone + rifampin +/- clofazimine	Minocycline; moxifloxacin or gatifloxacin; clofazimine clarithromycin; ethionamide

"Other antimicrobial agents active against *M. leprae* in animal models and at the usual daily doses used in clinical trials include ***ethionamide/prothionamide;*** the aminoglycosides streptomycin, kanamycin and amikacin (but not gentamicin or tobramycin); ***minocycline; clarithromycin***; and several fluoroquinolones, particularly ofloxacin. Next to rifampin, ***minocycline, clarithromycin and ofloxacin*** appear to be most bactericidal for *M. leprae*, but these drugs have not been used extensively in leprosy control programs. Most recently, ***rifapentine and moxifloxacin*** have been found to be especially potent against *M. leprae* in mice. In a clinical trial in lepromatous leprosy, moxifloxacin was profoundly bactericidal, matched in potency only by rifampin"- *Harrison 19th/1126*

In case the reference laboratory reports that the patient is harbouring rifampicin resistant M. leprae the following treatment should be given *www.leprosy-ila.org/sit*

- Administration of 50 mg of clofazimine, together with 400 mg of ofloxacin and 100 mg of minocycline, daily for six months;
- Administration of 50 mg of clofazimine, together with 100 mg of minocycline or 400 mg of ofloxacin daily for at least an additional 18 months.
- The above-mentioned treatment regimen is also to be used for patients reported to be harbouring both rifampicin and dapsone resistant M. leprae.

66. Ans. c. Olodaterol, d. Vilanterol, e. Indacaterol

[Ref: K. D. T 7th/ 222-24; Katzung 13th/340; Rang and Dale 8th/348]

β Agonists

- *Katzung 13th/340*
- "Ultra-long acting β agonists, ***indacaterol, olodaterol and vilanterol***, need to be taken only once a day"
- Long acting β agonists ***salmeterol and formoterol*** (duration of action, 8-12 hr) are given twice daily- *Rang and Dale 8th/348*
- Short acting β agonists are salbutamol and terbutaline (duration of action 3-5 hr)

67. Ans. b. Detemir, c. Glargine

[Ref: K. D. T 7th/263; Satoskar Pharma 24th/893]

Isophane insulin (Neutral protamine hagedorn) is intermediate acting insulin- K. D. T 7th/263

Table *(Satoskar Pharma 24th/893)*: **Currently available human insulins**

1. **Standard Recombinant (SR) insulins:**
   a. Rapid acting regular (Actrapid)
   b. Intermediate acting (NPH, Insulatard)
   c. Premade mixture of (a) and (b) (Mixtard)
2. **Human Insulin analogues, recombinant:**
   a. Very Rapid Acting (VRA): Lispro; (Humalog); Aspart (Novolog), Glulisine (Apidra)
   b. Intermediate acting premade mixtures; Lispro-protamine + Lispro (Humalog Mix); Aspart-protamine + Aspart (Novolog Mix)
   c. Long acting insulins: ***Glargine (Lantus); Detemir (Levemir)***
   d. Ultra-long acting insulin: Insulin Degludec

68. Ans. a. Doxycycline, c. Azithromycin

[Ref: K. D. T 7th/737; Jawetz 27th/337; Satoskar Pharma 24th/718, 676; Rang and Dale 8th/633]

Tetracyclines (e.g doxycycline) are the first choice drug *for atypical pneumonia due to mycoplasma pneumonia- K. D. T 7th/737*

*Macrolide (**Erythromycin,Azithromycin**): It is **drug of choice in treatment of mycoplasma pneumonia**- Satoskar Pharma 24th/676*

"Many strains of mycoplasmas are inhibited by a variety of antimicrobial drugs, but most strains are resistant to penicillins, cephalosporins and vancomycin. ***Tetracyclines and erythromycins are*** effective both in vitro and in vivo and are, at present, the ***drugs of choice*** in mycoplasmal pneumonia. Some ureaplasmas are resistant to tetracycline"- *Jawetz 27th/337*

Treatment options for acute *M. pneumoniae* infection include ***macrolides*** (e.g., oral **azithromycin**), **tetracyclines** (e.g.,oral **doxycycline**) and respiratory fluoroquinolones. However, ciprofloxacin and ofloxacin are *not* recommended because of their high minimal inhibitory concentrations against *M. pneumoniae* isolates and their poor performance in experimental studies"- *Harrison 19th/1164*

"In the treatment of mycoplasmal pneumonia, antimicrobials against *M pneumoniae*are bacteriostatic, not bactericidal. Tetracycline and erythromycin compounds are very effective. The ***second-generation tetracyclines (doxycycline) and macrolides are the drugs of choice.*** Macrolide resistance has been reported in several areas of the world, but most experts agree that macrolides are the antibiotics of choice for treating *M pneumoniae* infections in adults and children.If a patient does not respond appropriately to a macrolide, a fluoroquinolone should be added to the treatment regimen. ***Penicillins and cephalosporins are ineffective, because the organism lacks a cell wall"***-*emedicine.medscape.com*

Organism *Satoskar Pharma 24th/718*	First choice drug	Other effective drug
Mycoplasma pneumoniae	***Azithromycin/ Clarithromycin*** Fluoroquinolones	3rd Generation cephalosporin Doxycycline

Table *(Harrison 19th/1164)*: **Antimicrobial agents of choice for mycoplasma infection**

Organism	Drug (s)
M. pneumonie	Azithromycin, clarithromycin, erythromycin, doxycycline, levofloxacin, moxifloxacin, gemifloxacin (not ciprofloxacin or ofloxacin)
U. urealyticum, U. parvum	Axithromycin, clarithromycin, erythromycin, doxycycline
M. hominis	Doxycycline, clindamycin
M. genitalium	Azithromycin

69. Ans. a. Paracetamol toxicity is not dose dependent

[Ref: K. D. T 7th/768, 207,379; Katzung 13th/791; Goodman and Gilman's 11th/357, 430, 1178; Satoskar Pharma 24th/177]

"***Acute PCM poisoning***: *Early manifestation includes liver tenderness. After 12-18 hours centrilobular hepatic necrosis occurs. Jaundice starts after 2 days. **Further course depends on dose taken.** Fulminant hepatic failure and death are likely if plasma levels are the line joining 200 µg/ml at 4 hr and 30 µg/ml at 15 hr. If the levels are lower-recovery with supportive treatment is the rule"- K. D. T 7th/207*

"**PCM:** ***Large dose*** **(>6 g)** as in acute poisoning produce extensive heaptocelluar damage"- *Satoskar Pharma 24th/177*

"**Halothane** reduces splanchnic and hepatic blood flow. ***Halothane can produce fulminant hepatic necrosis*** in a small number of patients.There is a rapid progression to hepatic failure, with a fatality rate of ~50%.This syndrome occurs in about 1 in 10,000 patients receiving halothane and is referred to as halothane hepatitis."- *Goodman and Gilman's 11th/357*

"Multiple exposure of halothane is single most important risk factor for halothane hepatitis"-*Ajay Yadav 5th/80*

"Reversible intrahepatic ***obstructive (choestatic)*** jaundice occurs in about 0.5 to 2% of the patients receiving ***chlorpromazine***. It is probably allergic in origin"- *Satoskar Pharma 24th/199*

"**Tetracyclines** can probably impair hepatic function, especially during pregnancy, in patients with preexisting hepatic insufficiency and when ***high doses*** are given intravenously.

Hepatic necrosis has been reported with daily doses of 4 g or more intravenously"- *Katzung 13th/791; Goodman and Gilman's 11th/1178*

"Rifampin: Hepatitis, a major adverse effect, generally occurs in patients with pre-existing liver disease and ***is dose-related****; infrequent with ≤ 600 mg/day dose"-K. D. T 7th/768*

70. Ans. a. Seen in around 10-20% of patients treated with the drug, b. May occur within 1 week of initiation of treatment

[Ref: K. D. T 7th/ 745; Katzung 13th/802; Goodman and Gilman's 11th/1163; Satoskar Pharma 24th/684; Rang and Dale 8th/635; Harrison 19th/1806]

"Several antimicrobial agents are commonly associated with **Acute kidney injury (AKI).** *Aminoglycosides and amphotericin B* both cause tubular necrosis. Nonoliguric AKI (i.e., without a significant reduction in urine volume) accompanies ***10–30%*** of courses of aminoglycoside antibiotics, even when plasma levels are in the therapeutic range. Aminoglycosides are freely filtered across the glomerulus and then accumulate within the renal cortex, where concentrations can greatly exceed those of the plasma. ***AKI typically manifests after 5–7 days of therapy*** and can present even after the drug has been discontinued"- *Harrison 19th/1803*

"With many of the epithelial cell toxins such as aminoglycoside antibiotics and cisplatin, the rise in S.Cr is characteristically delayed for ***3–5 days to 2 weeks*** after initial exposure"-*Harrison 19th/1807*

"**Aminoglycosides** cause some degree of acute tubular necrosis in up to ***25% of hospitalized patients*** receiving therapeutic levels of the drugs. Nonoliguric kidney injury typically starts to occur ***after 5–10 days of exposure***.

Predisposing factors include underlying kidney damage, volume depletion and advanced age"-*CMDT 2016/904*

Adverse Effects of Aminoglycosides

◈ *Katzung 13th/802*

- Ototoxicity and nephrotoxicity are more likely to be encountered when therapy is continued ***for more than 5 days,*** at higher doses, in the elderly and in the setting of renal insufficiency. Concurrent use with loop diuretics (e.g., furosemide, ethacrynic acid) or other nephrotoxic antimicrobial agents (e.g., vancomycin or amphotericin) can potentiate nephrotoxicity and should be avoided if possible.
- Nephrotoxicity results in rising serum creatinine levels or reduced creatinine clearance, although the earliest indication often is an increase in trough serum aminoglycoside concentrations.
- Neomycin, tobramycin and gentamicin are the most nephrotoxic.

Nephrotoxicity

◈ *Goodman and Gilman's 11th/1163*

- ***Approximately 8–26%*** of patients who receive an aminoglycoside for more than several days will develop mild renal impairment that almost always is reversible.
- The toxicity results from accumulation and retention of aminoglycoside in the ***proximal tubular cells.*** The initial manifestation is excretion of enzymes of the renal tubular brush border, followed by a defect in renal concentrating ability, ***mild proteinuria and the appearance of hyaline and granular casts***.
- The ***glomerular filtration rate is reduced*** after several additional days.
- While severe ***acute tubular necrosis*** may occur rarely, the most common finding is a mild rise in plasma creatinine.
- Toxicity correlates with the total amount of drug administered and is more likely to be encountered with ***longer courses of therapy***.

Drug-induced Renal Disease/Dysfunction

◈ *Davidson 22nd/522*

- **Acute tubular necrosis** Aminoglycosides, amphotericin
  - Paracetamol overdose
  - Radiographic contrast media
- **Loss of tubular/collecting duct function**
  - Lithium; Cisplatin
  - Aminoglycosides, amphotericin
- **Glomerulonephritis (immune-mediated)**
  - Penicillamine, gold Membranous nephropathy
  - Penicillamine Crescentic or focal necrotising glomerulonephritis in association with ANCA and systemic small-vessel vasculitis
  - NSAIDs Minimal change nephropathy
- **Interstitial nephritis (immune-mediated)**
  - NSAIDs, penicillins, proton pump inhibitors, many others
- **Interstitial nephritis (toxicity)**
  - Lithium Ciclosporin, tacrolimus
- **Interstitial nephritis (with papillary necrosis)**
  - Various NSAIDs

71. Ans. a. Echinocandins have very less side effects, e. Nephrotoxicity is dose limiting side effect of amphotericin B

[Ref: K. D. T 7th/ 787-95; Katzung 13th/825-31]

Antifungal Drugs

◈ *Katzung 13th/825-31*

- Amphotericin B is selective in its ***fungicidal*** effect because it exploits the difference in lipid composition of fungal and mammalian cell membranes.
- **Ergosterol,** a cell membrane sterol, is found in the cell membrane of fungi, whereas the predominant sterol of bacteria and human cells is **cholesterol.** Amphotericin B binds to ergosterol and alters the permeability of the cell by forming amphotericin B-associated pores in the cell membrane
- Therapy with amphotericin B is ***often limited by toxicity, especially drug-induced renal impairment***.
- ***Fluconazole displays no activity against aspergillus*** or other filamentous fungi.
- *Itraconazole is the azole of choice for treatment of disease due to the dimorphic fungi* histoplasma, Blastomyces and sporothrix.

A & E

- ***Itraconazole has activity against Aspergillus sp***, but it has been replaced by voriconazole as the azole of choice for aspergillosis. Itraconazole is used extensively in the treatment of dermatophytoses and onychomycosis.
- "***Fluconazole is 94% absorbed***; *oral bioavailability is not affected by food or gastric pH*" - *K. D. T 7th/ 793*
- ***Echinocandin agents are extremely well tolerated, with minor gastrointestinal side effects and flushing reported infrequently.***

72. Ans. a. Cefoxitin, b. Cefoperazone

[Ref: K. D. T 7th/726; Katzung 13th/779; Goodman and Gilman's 11th/781; Satoskar Pharma 24th/693]

Table *(KDT 7th/ 726; medimoon.com; Wiki)*: **Cephalosprorins**

Generation	Parenteral	Oral
1st generation	Cefazolin	Cephalexin, Cefadroxil
2nd generation	Cefuroxime, **Cefoxitin**	Cefaclor, Cefuroxime axetil, Cefprozil
3rd generation	*Cefotaxime*, Ceftizoxime, *Ceftazidine*, Cefoperazone	*Cefixime*, Cefpodoxime Proxetil, Cefdinir Pivoxil
4th generation	Cefepime, ***Cefpirome***	
5th generation	**Ceftaroline, Ceftolozane**	
	Ceftabiprole	

73. Ans. a. Tetracycline, c. Digoxin, d. Penicillin, e. Lithium

[Ref: K. D. T 7th/695; Katzung 13th/790; Satoskar Pharma 24th/225]

"***Lithium is handled by kidney in much the same way as Na+.*** *Renal clearance of lithium is 1/5 of creatinine clearnace -K. D. T 7th/449*

"*The pharmacokinetics of* **penicillin G** *is dominated by* ***very rapid renal excretion****; about 10% by glomerular filtration and rest by tubular secretion*"- *K. D. T 7th/718*

"**Digoxin** *is primarily* ***excreted unchanged by the kidney****: mainly by glomerular filtration; rate of excretion is altered parallel to creatinine clearance. Its t1/2 is prolonged in elderely patients and in those with renal insufficiency: dose has to be reduced*"- *K. D. T 7th/615-16*

"***Most tetracyclines are primarily excreted in urine*** *by glomerular filtration; dose has to be reduced in renal failure; doxycyline is an exception*" *(K. D. T 7th/735)*

"**Rifampicin**: *It is metabolized in liver to an active deacetylated metabolite which is excreted mainly in bile, some in urine. Urine and secretions may become orange-red*" *(KDT 7th/768)*

"Rifampin is well absorbed after oral administration and *excreted mainly through the liver into bile.* It then undergoes enterohepatic recirculation, with the bulk excreted as a deacylated metabolite in feces and a ***small amount in the urine.*** Dosage adjustment for renal or hepatic insufficiency is not necessary" - *(Katzung 12th/841)*

74. Ans. b. Cyclophosphamide, c. Busulfan, e. Ifosfamide

[Ref: K. D. T 7th/859,; Katzung 13th/924; Goodman and Gilman's 11th/1326; Satoskar Pharma 24th/830]

Ifosamide, busulfan and cyclophosphamide are alkylating agent

"**All alkylating agents** *have toxic effects on the male and female reproductive systems, causing* ***premature ovarian failure*** *in women and irreversible* ***azoospermia in men***"*-Goodman and Gilman's 11th/1326*

"The adverse effects usually associated with **alkylating agents** are generally dose-related and occur primarily in rapidly growing tissues such as bone marrow, the gastrointestinal tract and the ***reproductive system***"*- Katzung 13th/924*

"**Alkylating agents** *impair* ***spermatogenesis irreversibly in males and can cause amenorrhoea***"*- Satoskar Pharma 24th/830*

"**Alkylating agents**, the ***most gonadotoxic chemotherapeutic medications***, cause dose-dependent, direct destruction of oocytes and follicular depletion and may bring about cortical fibrosis and ovarian blood-vessel damage"*-www.ncbi.nlm.nih.gov*

"Busulfan (Alkylating Agent)-*Causes Sterility*"

◈ *K. D. T 7th/861*

"**Busulfan**:*Cause amenorrhoea and gynaecomastia*"- *Satoskar Pharma 24th/831*

"**Busulfan:** *Long term use leads to* ***impotence, sterility, amenorrhea*** *and fetal malformation*"*-Goodman and Gilman's 11th/1331*

Caution is advised when ***cyclophosphamide*** *is used because of its potential for* ***inducing sterility****, teratogenic effects and leukemia.* ***Ifosfamide*** *has virtually the same toxicity profile as cyclophosphamide, although it causes greater platelet suppression, neurotoxicity, nephrotoxicity and in the absence of mesna, urothelial damage. Goodman and Gilman's 11th/1328*

- **The gonadotoxic risk of common anticancer chemotherapeutic agents** *(Tableonlinelibrary.wiley.com)*

Chemotherapy	Type of agent	Risk category
Cyclophosphamide	Alkylating agents	High risk
Ifosfamide	Alkylating agents	High risk
Prosfamide	Alkylating agents	High risk
Procarbazine	Alkylating agents	High risk
Busulfan	Alkylating agents	High risk
Melphalan	Alkylating agents	High risk
Chlorambucil	Alkylating agents	High risk
Carboplatin	Platinum analogue	Medium risk
Doxorubicin	Antibiotics	Medium risk
Vincristine	Vinca alkaloids	Low risk
Vinblastine	Vinca alkaloids	Low risk
Methotrexate	Antimetabolites	Low risk
Mercaptopurine	Antimetabolites	Low risk
Dactinomycin	Antibiotics	Low risk
Bleomycin	Antibiotics	Low risk

*"**Dactinomycin:** Toxic manifestations include anorexia, nausea and vomiting, usually beginning a few hours after administration. Hematopoietic suppression with pancytopenia may occur in the first week after completion of therapy. Proctitis, diarrhea, glossitis, cheilitis and ulcerations of the oral mucosa are common; dermatological manifestations include alopecia, as well as erythema, desquamation and increased inflammation and pigmentation in areas previously or concomitantly subjected to x-ray radiation. Severe injury may occur as a result of local toxic extravasation"-Goodman and Gilman's 11th/1357*

75. Ans. a. Perindopril, d. Ramipril, e. Enalapril

[Ref: K. D. T 7th/23,501]

Table: *K. D. T 7th/501*

Drug	Captopril	Enalapril	Lisinopril	Fosinopril	Perindopril	Ramipril
Activity status	Active	Prodrug	Active	Prodrug	Prodrug	Prodrug

76. Ans. a. Undergoes first-pass metabolism in the liver, b. Active against both larva and adult of Nematodes, c. Absorption increases with fatty meal, d. Excreted in the urine

[Ref: K. D. T 7th/ 850-51; Katzung 13th/908-09; Goodman and Gilman's 11th/1079; Satoskar Pharma 24th/818]

Albendazole

◈ *K. D. T 7th/ 850-51*

- Absorption after oral administration is significant, but inconsistent. It is ***enhanced when the drug is taken with fatty meal***
- "Given orally, it is rapidly absorbed and has better availability than mebendazole"- *Satoskar Pharma 24th/818*
- ***"Thiabendazole has gone out of use, due to the availability of better tolerated mebendazole and albendazole"**-K. D. T 7th/ 852*
- *Helminth includes nematodes, cestodes, trematodes, flukes etc.*
- *Thiabendazole is active against a wide range of nematodes that infect the GI tract, but its clinical use has declined markedly because of its toxicity relative to other equally effective drugs. Goodman and Gilman's 11th/1079*
- "*Albendazole is active against both larval and adult stages of nematodes and is ovicidal for* Ascaris *and* Trichuris*"-Goodman and Gilman's 11th/1079*

◈ *Katzung 13th/908-09*

- Albendazole, a broad-spectrum oral antihelminthic, is the drug of choice and is approved in the USA for treatment of hydatid disease and cysticercosis. It is also used in the treatment of pinworm and hookworm infections, ascariasis, trichuriasis and strongyloidiasis.
- ***After oral administration, it is erratically absorbed*** (increased with a fatty meal) and then rapidly ***undergoes first-pass metabolism in the liver*** to the active metabolite albendazole sulfoxide.
- Albendazole metabolites are ***excreted in the urine***.
- Albendazole also has ***larvicidal effects in hydatid disease, cysticercosis, ascariasis and hookworm infection and ovicidal effects in ascariasis, ancylostomiasis and trichuriasis.***

77. Ans. b. Raltegravir - Intergase inhibitor, c. Indinavir - Protease inhibitor, d. Nevirapine - Nonnucleoside reverse transcriptase inhibitor

[Ref: K. D. T 7th/798; Park 24th/369; Katzung 13th/842-55]

Anti-Retrovirus Drug

◈ *K. D. T 7th/798; Katzung 13th/842-55*

(a) Nucleoside reverse transcriptase inhibitors (NRTIs): Zidovudine, Didanosine, Stavudine Lamivudine, Abacavir, Emtriitabine, Tenofovir (Nt RTI)
(b) Nonnucleoside reverse transcriptase inhibitors (NNRTIs): ***Nevirapine***, Efavirenz, Delavirdine,Etravirine,Rilpivirine
(c) Protease inhibitor: Ritonavir**,** Atazanair, ***Indinavir***, Nelfinavir, Saquinavir, Amprenavir, Lopinavir ***Darunavir***, Fosamprenavir,Tipranavir
(d) **Entry (fusion) inhibitor**: Enfuvirtide
(e) **CCR5 receptor inhibitor**: ***Maraviroc***
(f) **Integrase inhibitor**: ***Raltegravir,*** Elvitegravir, Dolutegravir

78. Ans. a. Amiodarone, b. Cisapride

[Ref: K. D. T 7th/528; Davidson 22nd/571]

Table *(Davidson 22nd/571)*: **Causes of long QT interval and torsades de pointes**

Bradycardia

- Bradycardia compounds other factors that cause torsades de pointes

Electrolyte disturbance

- Hyypokalaemia
- Hypomagnesaemia
- Hypocalcaemia

Drugs

- Disopyramide, flecainide (and other class Ia, Ic antiarrhythmic drugs)
- Amitriptyline (and other tricyclic antidepressants)
- Chlorpromazine (and other phenothiazines)
- Erythromycin (and other phenothiazines)

Table *(KDT 7th/528)*: **Drug that can potentiate torsades de pointes**

Antiarrhythmics	Quinidine, procainamids, disopyramide, propafenone, ***amiodarone***
Antimalarials	Quinine, mefloquine, artemisinin, halofantrine
Antibacterials	Sparfloxacin, mosifloxacin
Antihistaminics	Terfenadine, astemizole, ebastine
Antidepressants	Amitryptyline and other tricyclics
Anitpsychotics	Thioridazine, pimozide, aripiprazole
Prokinetic	Cisapride

Table (*ECG by Hampton 8th/157*): **Drug that can potentiate Torsades de pointes**

Congenital	Other drugs
Jervell-Lange-Nielson syndrome Romano-ward syndrome	Tricyclic antidepressants Erythromycin
Antiarrhythmic drugs	Plasma electrolyte
Procainamide Disopyramide Amiodarone Sotalol	Low potassium Low magnesium Low calcium

79. Ans. c. Zanamivir

[Ref: K. D. T 7th/801-03; Park 24th/169; Katzung 13th/862-63]

Anti-influenza Drugs

◈ *K. D. T 7th/801*

- Zanamavir
- Oseltamivir
- Rimantadine
- Amantadine

Zanamavir is administered by inhalation as a powder due to very low oral bioavailability- *K. D. T 7th/802; Park 24th/169*

- Oseltamivir is given through oral and i.v route- *Katzung 13th/862-63*
- Rimantadine and Amantadine are given through oral route- *Katzung 13th/862*

80. Ans. a. Bronchial asthma, b. Allergic disorder, c. Cardio-pulmonary resuscitation, d. Anaphylaxis

[Ref: Ajay Yadav 5th/266-67; K. D. T 7th/138; Satoskar Pharma 24th/270]

Adrenaline

◈ *Ajay Yadav 5th/267; Satoskar Pharma 24th/270*

- CPR (**cardio-pulmonary resuscitation)**
- ***Anaphylaxis*** and angioneurotic edema
- For producing vasoconstriction with local anaesthetics
- For producing local ischemia/to decrease blood loss
- ***Allergies disorders***: It afford quick relief in urticarial, angioedema; is life saving in laryngeal edema and anaphylaxis- *K. D. T 7th/138*
- *Insulin hypoglycaemia: Adr may be used as an expedient measure, but glucose should be given as soon as possible- K. D. T 7th/139*
- ***Bronchial asthma****-Adrenaline, given s.c is a potent bronchodilator- Satoskar Pharma 24th/270*

81. Ans a. Used as anti-tussive agent, c. Causes respiratory depression, d. Partly metabolized to morphine

[Ref: K. D. T 7th/474; Katzung 13th/545-49; Goodman and Gilman's 11th/566; Satoskar Pharma 24th/159; Rang and Dale 8th/525]

Codeine

◈ *K. D. T 7th/474*

- It is ***partly converted in the body to morphine***
- "About 10% codeine is converted to morphine in the liver"- *Satoskar Pharma 24th/159*
- It is ***less potent than morphine (1/10th as analgesic)***, also less efficacious
- It is a partial agonist at opioid receptor with a low ceiling effect
- It is ***more selective cough (antitussive)*** suppressant (1/3rd as potent as morphine)
- Constipation is a prominent side effect
- In relation to its analgesic effect, codeine produces the same degree of depression as morphine, but the limited response even at high doses means that is seldom a problem in practice"- *Rang and Dale 8th/525*

82. Ans. a. Applied to majority of drugs, b. Rate of elimination is directly proportional to the drug concentration

[Ref: K. D. T 7th/30-31; Satoskar Pharma 24th/22-23]

First Order Kinetic

◈ *K. D. T 7th/30-31*

- The rate of elimination is ***directly proportional to the drug concentration, CL (clearance) remain constant;*** or a constant fraction of the drug present in the body is eliminated in unit time
- This ***applied to majority of drugs*** which do not saturate the elimination processes (transporters,enzymes,blood flow etc.) over the therapeutic concentration range
- However, if the dose is high enough, elimination pathways of all drugs will get saturated

Zero Order Kinetic

◈ *K. D. T 7th/31*

- ***Few drugs*** normally saturate eliminating mechanisms and handled by zero order kinetics
- The ***rate of elimination remain constant irrespective of the drug concentration***, CL decreases with increase in concentration; or a constant amount is eliminated in unit time

MICROBIOLOGY

83. Ans. a. Chloroquine resistance occurs in India, b. Relapses is usual for vivax and ovale malaria, c. Sexual cycle occurs in mosquito

[Ref: KDT 7th/822; Park 24th/272-75]

*"**Chloroquine-resistant among P.falciparum is now widespread in India** and no entirely sensitive areas can be identified. The largest number of CQ failures are reported from the northeastern part of India where 24-83% P.falciparum cases are resistant to CQ and some of these (particularly in areas bordering Myanmar) are multidrug resistant"-KDT 7th/822*

Malaria

◈ *Park 24th/272-75*

- *"**Malaria continues to pose a major public health threat in India**, particularly due to plasmodium falciparum which is prone to complication"- Park 24th/272*

- *"The malaria parasite undergoes 2 cycles of development- the human cycle (asexual cycle) and the* ***mosquito cycle (sexual cycle)****"- Park 24th/273*
- ***"Relapses: It is usual for vivax and ovale malaria to relapse*** *more than 3 years after the first attack. Recurrence of falciparum malaria usually disappear within 1-2 years. P.malariae has a tendency to cause prolonged low-level, asymptomatic parasitaemia"- Park 24th/275*

84. Ans. d. Whipworm

[Ref: Paniker's Parasitology 7th/117; Chatterjee Parasitology 13th/205, 209, 213]

Egg of whipworm: ***Barrel-shaped*** *with a mucous plug at each pole"-Chatterjee Parasitology 13th/205*

Helminth egg	Shape
*Trichuris trichurra (human **whipworm**)*	***Barrel shaped**, triple shell and bile-stained- Paniker's 7th/173*
Pinworm	Planoconvex- *Paniker's 7th/191*
Roundworm (Ascaris lumbricoides)	Elliptical (Unfertilized); Round or oval (fertilized)- *Paniker's 7th/196*
Strongyloides stercoralis	Oval -*Paniker's Parasitology 7th/117*
Hookworm (A.duodenaleand N.americanus)	Oval or elliptical- *Paniker's 7th/183*

85. Ans. c. Bubonic plague: 2-5 day, d. Leptospirosis: 4-20 days

[Ref: Park 24th/157, 154; Ananthanarayan 9th/322, 512, 381; Harrison 19th/1183]

"Incubation period of Hepatitis A: ***10 to 50 days (usually 14-28 days)****"- Park 24th/226*

"Leptospira: *Incubation period is usually about* ***10 days (range 2-26 days)****- Ananthanarayan 9th/381 (Range 4-20 days:Park 24th/309)*

"Leptospira: The incubation period is ***usually 1–2 weeks but ranges from 1 to 30 days***"-- *Harrison 19th/1144*

Measles: *Incubation period is commonly* ***10 days from exposure to onset of fever and 14 days to appearance of rash****"-Park 24th/157; Harrison 19th/1296*

"Measles: *It takes about* ***9-11 days*** *from the time of exposure to infection for the first signs of clinical disease to appear"- Ananthanarayan 9th/512*

"Chicken pox: *Incubation period is usually* ***14 to 16 days*** *(14-17 days:Harrison 19th/1183), although extremes as wide as 10 to 21 days have been reported"-Park 24th/154; Harrison 19th/1183*

Plague (Yersinia Pestis)

- *Incubation period Park 24th/312*
- ***Bubonic: 2–7 days (2–5 days:*** *Ananthanarayan 9th/322)*
- Septicemic: 2–7 days
- Pneumonic: 1–3 days

86. Ans. a. Belongs to family papovaviridae, b. DNA virus, e. Causes anal warts

[Ref: Ananthanarayan 9th/ 553; Harrison 19th/1197-99; Robbins (SEA) 9th/ 326]

Human Papillomavirus

- *Ananthanarayan 9th/ 553*
- ***Belong to family papovaviridae***
- ***They are small, non-enveloped, icosahedral DNA tumour viruses***
- *Harrison 19th/1197-99*
- HPV is an icosahedral, ***nonenveloped,*** 8000-base-pair, ***double-stranded DNA virus*** with a diameter of 55 nm. Like those of other papillomaviruses, HPV's genome consists of an early (E) gene region, a late (L) gene region and a noncoding region that contains regulatory elements
- A cell-mediated immune response plays an important role in controlling the progression of natural HPV infection.
- *Robbins (SEA) 9th/ 326*
- At least 70 genetically distinct types of HPV have been identified. Some types (e.g., 1, 2, 4 and 7) cause **benign squamous papillomas (warts) in humans**.
- In contrast, high-risk HPVs (e.g., types 16 and 18) have been implicated in the genesis of **squamous cell carcinomas of the cervix, anogenital region and head and neck (particularly tumors arising in the tonsillar mucosa).**
- "HPV: Invasive cervical cancer and other squamous cell carcinoma and dysplasia such as anus, perianal region, vagina, vulva, penis and oral cavity" *(Harshmohan 7th/218)*

Disease	HPV type
Common warts	2, 7
Plantar warts	1, 2, 4, 63
Flat warts	3, 10, 8
Anal lesions	6, 16, 18, 31, 53, 58

87. Ans. a. Air droplet is most common mode of transmission, c. Thai forest type – most common species in epidemics

[Ref: Ananthanarayan 9th/559; Park 24th/374; Harrison 19th/1323-29; www.cdc.gov]

"The virus **family Filoviridae** includes three genera: Cuevavirus, Marburgvirus and Ebolavirus. Within the genus Ebolavirus, five species have been identified: Zaire, Bundibugyo, Sudan, Reston and ***Taï Forest.*** The first three, ***Bundibugyo ebolavirus, Zaire ebolavirus and Sudan ebolavirus*** have been associated with large outbreaks in Africa. The virus causing the 2014–2016 West African outbreak belongs to the Zaire ebolavirus species"-*www.who.int/mediacentre (so* ***Taï Forest species is not most common in epidemics)***

Symptoms of Ebola Virus Disease

- *www.who.int/mediacentre*
- The incubation period, that is, the time interval from infection with the virus to onset of symptoms is 2 to 21 days. Humans are not infectious until they develop symptoms.
- First symptoms are the ***sudden onset of fever fatigue, muscle pain, headache and sore throat***. This is followed by vomiting, diarrhoea, rash, symptoms of impaired kidney and liver function and in some cases, ***both internal and external bleeding*** (e.g. oozing from the gums, blood in the stools).

- Laboratory findings include low white blood cell and platelet counts and elevated liver enzymes.

"**Haemorrhagic manifestations** arise during the peak of the illness and include petechiae, ecchymoses, uncontrolled oozing from venepuncture sites, mucosal haemorrhages and post-mortem evidence of visceral haemorrhagic effusions. A macropapular rash associated with varying severity of erythema and desquamate can often be noted by day 5–7 of the illness; this symptom is a valuable differential diagnostic feature and is usually followed by desquamation in survivors"- *www.ncbi.nlm.nih.gov*

Ebola Virus

◈ *Park 24th/374*

- Incubation period is 2-21 days and is not infective during this period
- It is member of family filoviridae and comprises of 5 distinct species- Zaire ebolavirus, Reston ebolavirus, Sudan ebolavirus, ***Tai ebolavirus*** and Bundibugyo ebolavirus
- ***Case fatality rate may be as high as 70%***
- The virus is transmitted through ***direct contact with blood,*** organs, body secretions or other body fluids of infected animals like chimpanzees, gorillas, monkeys, fruit bats etc.
- Human to human transmission is through blood or body fluids of an infected symptomatic person or through exposure to objects (such as needle) that have been contaminated with infected secretions
- *It is **not transmitted through air, water, or food***
- The illness is characterized by ***sudden onset of fever, intense weakness, muscle pain, headache, sorethroat, vomiting, diarrhea, rash, impaired kidney and liver function*** and in ***some both internal and external bleeding***
- Currently there is ***no specific treatment for this disease***
- There is ***no vaccine against ebola***

"Human infections typically occur through ***direct exposure of skin lesions or mucosal surfaces to contaminated bodily fluids or material or by parenteral inoculation (e.g., via accidental needle sticks or reuse of needles in poorly equipped hospitals)"*** *(Harrison 19th/1326-27)*

88. Ans. c. Lyme's disease, d. Tularemia

[Ref: Park 24th/817,805; Ananthanarayan 9th/407; Greenwood 16th/350]

Trench Fever Transmitted by Louse

◈ *Park 24th/807*

Epidemic typhus transmitted by louse- *Park 24th/805*

"Endemic typhus (murine) is transmitted by rat flea"- *Ananthanarayan 9th/407*

"Lyme's disease is transmitted by the bite of Ixodid ticks"- *Ananthanarayan 9th/380; Greenwood 16th/350*

Disease Transmitted by Tick

◈ *(Park 24th/817, 805)*

Tick	Disease Transmitted
Hard tick	*Tick typhus, viral encephalitis, viral fevers, viral haemorrhagic fever, (e.g., Kyasanur forest disease),* ***tularemia****, tick paralysis, human babesiosis*
Soft tick	Q fever, relapsing fever, KFD

89. Ans. b. Caused by anaerobic or microaerophilic bacteria, c. Cervicofacial is the most common site affected, d. Sulphur granules are present in lesion, e. Actinomyces is non-acid fast

[Ref: Ananthanarayan 9th/391-93,600-01; Greenwood 16th/221-22; Harrison 19th/1088]

"**Mycetoma is of 3 types**- *eumycetoma (maduramycosis=Madura foot), actinomycetoma and botryomycosis. Eumycetoma is caused by madurella mycetomatis and other fungi*"- *Ananthanarayan 9th/600-01*

Actinomyces

◈ *Greenwood 16th/221-22*

- *They are **facultative anaerobes,** but often fail to grow aerobically on primary culture. They grow best under anaerobic or micro-aerophilic conditions with the addition of 5-10% carbon dioxide*
- They are responsible for the disease known as ***actinomycosis***
- Around 98% of cases of actinomycosis occur in cervicofacial region; the jaw is often involved

◈ *Harrison 19th/1088*

- Actinomycosis is an indolent, slowly progressive infection caused by ***anaerobic or microaerophilic bacteria***, primarily of the genus *Actinomyces*, that colonize the mouth, colon and vagina. Mucosal disruption may lead to infection at virtually any site in the body.
- In vivo growth of actinomycetes usually results in the formation of characteristic clumps called ***grains* or *sulfur granules.***
- Three "classic" clinical presentations that should prompt consideration of this unique infection are (1) the combination of chronicity, progression across tissue boundaries and mass-like features (mimicking malignancy, with which it is often confused); (2) the development of a sinus tract, which may spontaneously resolve and recur; and (3) a refractory or relapsing infection after a short course of therapy, since cure of established actinomycosis requires prolonged treatment.
- **Oral-Cervicofacial Disease**: Actinomycosis occurs most frequently at an oral, cervical, or facial site, usually as a soft tissue swelling, abscess, or mass lesion that is often mistaken for a neoplasm. The angle of the jaw is generally involved, but a diagnosis of actinomycosis should be considered with any mass lesion or relapsing infection in the head and neck

Table *(Greenwood 16th/222)*: **Differences b/w the genera Actinomyces and Nocardia**

Actinomyces spp.	Noardia spp.
• Facultative anaerobes	• Strict aerobes
• Grow at 35–37°C	• Wide temperature range of growth
• Oral commensals	• Environmental saprophytes
• Non-acid fast mycelia	• Usually weakly acid-fast
• Endogenous cause of disease	• Exogenous cause of disease

A & E

Summarized form of Text

Ananthanarayan 9th/391-93

Actinomyces	Nocardia
• Anaerobic/microaerophilic	• Aerobic
• Non-acid fast	• May be acid fast
• Endogenous in origin	• Exogenous

90. Ans. c. Caused by Leishmania donovani, d. Drug of choice is Miltefosine, e. Drug of choice is sodium stibogluconate

[Ref: Ananthanarayan 9th/397; Harrison 19th/298e1-2; Greenwood 16th/310; Park 24th/350]

*"**Leishmania donovani is cause of Kala-azar**. Miltefosine, sodium stibogluconate, amphotericin B, paromomycin etc are used for treatment of kala-azar"-KDT 7th/844-45*

Donovanosis or Granuloma inguinale or Klebsiella granulomatis (Formerly known as Donovania granulomatis and Calymmatobacterium granulomatis)- *Ananthanarayan 9th/397*

- Tetracycline given for at least thrice week is usually curative.
- Cotrimoxazole, chloramphenicol, gentamycin, quinolones and the newer macrolides are also effective

Donovanosis: The four main types of cutaneous lesions are as follows: *emedicine.medscape.com*

- **Nodular**: The initial granuloma inguinale lesion is a papule or nodule that arises at the site of inoculation. The nodule is soft, often pruritic and erythematous and eventually ulcerates. ***A nodule may be mistaken for a lymph node*** [i.e., ***pseudobubo***].
- **Ulcerovegetative (most common):** These granuloma inguinale lesions develop from nodular lesions and consist of large, usually painless, expanding, suppurative ulcers.
- **Cicatricial:** Dry ulcers evolve into cicatricial plaques and may be associated with lymphedema.

Hypertrophic or Verrucous (Relatively Rare)

Table *(Harrison 19th/800)*: **Clinical Features of Genital Ulcers**

Feature	Donovanosis
Incubation period	1–4 Weeks (up to 6 months)
Early primary	Papule
Early primary lesions	Papule
No. of lesions	Variable
Diameter	Variable
Edges	Elevated, irregular
Depth	Elevated
Base	Red and velvety, bleeds readily
Induration	Firm
Pain	Uncommon
Lymphadenopathy	None; Pseudobuboes

91. Ans. a. Burkholderia cepacia, b. Pseudomonas aeruginosa, c. Staphylococcus aureus

[Ref: Ananthanarayan 9th/315-16; Greenwood 16th/286-88; Robbins 9th/470]

*"**Burkholderia cepacia** is increasingly being recognized as an opportunist environmental pathogen, particularly in those with **cystic fibrosis** or chronic granulomatous disease, in whom it causes fatal necrotizing pneumonia" (Ananthanarayan 9th/316; Greenwood 16th/286-88)*

*"**Pseudomonas aeruginosa**: It is a common cause of respiratory act infection in **cystic fibrosa** patients"*- Ananthanarayan 9th/315

"**Cystic fibrosis**: The lungs are macroscopically normal at birth, but bronchiolar inflammation and infections usually lead to bronchiectasis in childhood. At this stage, the lungs are most commonly infected with ***Staphylococcus aureus***; however, in adulthood, many patients become colonised with ***Pseudomonas aeruginosa***"-Davidson 22nd/680

"**Burkhodeleria pseduomallei** is causative agent of melioidosis. Diabetes mellitus increases risk"- *Ananthanarayan 9th/317*

Table *(Robbins 9th/470)*: **Clinical features of cystic fibrosis**

- ***Chronic sinopulmonary disease*** manifested by Persistent colonization/infection with typical cystic fibrosis *pathogens, including Staphylococcus aureus, nontypeable Hemophilus influenzae*, mucoid and nonmucoid *Pseudomonas aeruginosa, Burkholderia cepacia*
- "**Cystic fibrosis**: Poor prognostic indicators such as sputum culture containing ***B. cepacia, mucoid P. aeruginosa, or atypical mycobacteria*** are rigorously monitored in the CF patient population. An increasing incidence of **methicillin-resistant *S. aureus*** has also been observed, although the clinical significance of this finding has not been fully elucidated"- *Harrison 19th/1699*

92. Ans. a. Skin langerhans cell, c. Macrophages, d. Kuffer cell, e. Thymic epithelial cells

[Ref: Ananthanarayan 9th/137-38; Greenwood 16th/133-34]

*Antigen presenting cells are **specialized dendritic cells, macrophagesand B lymphocyte**"- Ananthanarayan 9th/138*

*Macrophages named according to different location are- **alveolar macrophages, histiocytes, kuffer cells, osteoclasts and mesangial cells**"- Ananthanarayan 9th/137*

"Although **monocytes-macrophages** were originally thought to be the major antigen-presenting cells (APCs) of the immune system, it is now clear that cell types called *dendritic cells* are the most potent and effective APCs in the body"-*Harrison 19th/372e-4*

"The first site of TCR-MHC-peptide interaction in the life of a T cell occurs in the thymus, where self-peptides are presented to developing **thymocytes** by MHC molecules expressed on thymic epithelium and hematopoietically derived **antigen-presenting cells**, which are primarily responsible for positive and negative selection, respectively"- *Harrison 19th/373e-3*

"Human skin exposure to modest doses of UV-B can deplete the epidermal ***antigen-presenting cells*** known as **Langerhans cells**, thereby reducing the degree of allergic sensitization to application of the potent contact allergen dinitrochlorobenzene at the irradiated skin site"- *Harrison 19th/388*

Table *(Greenwood 16th/134)*: **Antigen-presenting cells in the lymph nodes**

Area	Antigen-presenting cell	Antigen
Sub-capsular marginal sinus	Marginal zone macrophage	T-independent antigens
Follicles and B cell areas	Follicular dendritic cells	Antigen-antibody complexes
Medulla	Classical macrophages	Most antigens
T cell areas	Interdigitating dendritic cells	Most antigens

Antigen-Presenting Cells

◈ *www. sciencedirect.com*

- Antigen-presenting cells (APC) are cells that can process a protein antigen, break it into peptides and present it in conjunction with class II MHC molecules on the cell surface where it may interact with appropriate T cell receptors.
- Professional APCs include dendritic cells, macrophages and B cells, whereas nonprofessional APCs that function in antigen presentation for only brief periods include ***thymic epithelial cells and vascular endothelial cells.***

93. Ans. a. Histoplasma capsulatum, b. Sporothrix schenckii

[Ref: Harrison 19th/1329; Ananthanarayan 9th/589-90; Jawetz 27th/853]

Cryptococcus is a Yeast

◈ *(Ananthanarayan 9th/589)*

Dimorphic Fungi

◈ *(Jawetz 27th/853)*

- *Blastomycosis dermatitidis*
- Paracoccidioides brasiliensis
- Coccidioides posadasii and *Coccidioides immitis*
- ***Histoplasma capsulatum***
- ***Sporothrix schenckii***
- Penicillium marneffei

Fungus Classification

◈ *(Harrison 19th/ 1329)*

- Three terms frequently used in clinical discussions of fungal infections are ***yeast, mold and dimorphic fungus.***
- ***Yeasts*** are seen as rounded single cells or as budding organisms. *Candida* and *Cryptococcus* are traditionally classified as yeasts.
- **Molds** grow as filamentous forms called *hyphae* both at room temperature and in invaded tissue. *Aspergillus, Rhizopus* (the genus that causes mucormycosis, also known as zygomycosis) and fungi commonly infecting the skin to cause ringworm and related cutaneous conditions are classified as molds.
- Variations occur within this classification of yeasts and molds. For instance, when *Candida* infects tissue, both yeasts and filamentous forms may be present (except with *C. glabrata*, which forms only yeasts in tissue); in contrast, *Cryptococcus* exists only in yeast form.
- **Dimorphic** is the term used to describe fungi that grow as yeasts or large spherical structures in tissue but as filamentous forms at room temperature in the environment. Classified in this group are the organisms causing ***blastomycosis, paracoccidioidomycosis, coccidioidomycosis, histoplasmosis and sporotrichosis.***

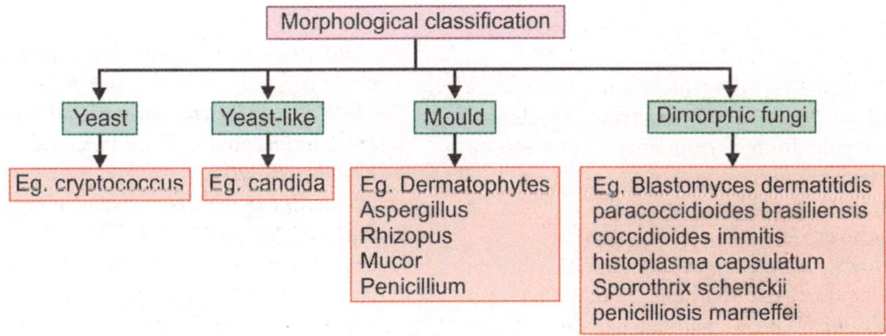

Fig: *(Ananthanarayan 9th/589)*: Morphological Classification of fungus

94. Ans. b. Smaller than mosquito, d. Don't fly by choice

[Ref: Park 24th/812-13]

Sandflies

◈ *Park 24th/812-13*

- ***Only the females bite***, the males live on vegetable juice
- Sandflies may be distinguished from mosquitoes by the following characteristics:
    - *Size*: ***Sandflies are smaller than mosquitoes.***
    - *Wings*: The wings of the sand fly are up-right and lanceolate in shape; the second longitudinal vein branches twice, the first branching taking place in the middle of the wing.
    - *Legs*: The legs of the sand fly are longer compared with the size of the body.
    - *Hairs*: Sand fly is a hairy insect
    - *Hopping*: Sandflies hop about and ***do not fly by choice***.

"Three important factors are required for the gravid female sand fly to lay eggs. These are presence of moisture, organic matter and eration of the soil. In that way, the backyard of the houses and the ground near cattle sheds and the like constitute the peridomestic breeding place. The dust accumulatins with moisture and organic matter in the ***cracks and crevices of the walls of the house constitute intradomestic breeding place***"- Community Medicine by *Suryakant 4th/132*

95. Ans. a. Chronic mucocutaneous candidiasis c. DiGeorge Syndrome e. Common variable immunodeficiency

[Ref: Ananthanarayan 9th/174-75; Robbins 9th/239-40]

Table *(Ananthanarayan 9th/174; 8th/156)*: **Disorder of specific immunity**

Humoral immunodeficiency (B cell defect)	Cellular immunodeficiency (T cell defect)	Combined immune deficiency (B and T cell defect)
X-linked Agammaglobulinemia ***Common variable Immunodeficiency*** Selective Ig deficiency	DiGeorge Syndrome Chronic mucocutaneous candidiasis	Nezel of Syndrome ***Ataxia Telangiectasia*** ***Wiskott-Aldrich syndrome*** Severe Combined Immunodeficiency (SCID)

96. Ans. a. It is a zoonotic disease, b. Transmission may occurs through cuts and abraded skin, d. Rodents are the most important reservoir

[Ref: Harrison 19th/1140-45; Ananthanarayan 9th/380-82]

Leptospira is a Spirochetes (not Arbovirus)

Leptospirosis

◈ *Harrison 19th/1140-45*

- Leptospirosis is a globally important ***zoonotic disease*** whose apparent reemergence is illustrated by recent outbreaks on virtually all continents.
- The disease is caused by pathogenic *Leptospira* species and is characterized by a broad spectrum of clinical manifestations, varying from asymptomatic infection to fulminant, fatal disease.
- In its **mild form**, leptospirosis may present as nonspecific symptoms such as fever, headache and myalgia.
- **Severe leptospirosis**, characterized by jaundice, renal dysfunction and hemorrhagic diathesis, is often referred to as ***Weil's syndrome.*** With or without jaundice, severe pulmonary hemorrhage is increasingly recognized as an important presentation of severe disease.
- **As a zoonosis**, leptospirosis affects almost all mammalian species and represents a significant veterinary burden. ***Rodents, especially rats, are the most important reservoir,*** although other wild mammals as well as domestic and farm animals may also harbor these microorganisms
- Leptospirosis presents as both an *endemic and an epidemic disease.*
- **Transmission of leptospires** may follow ***direct contact with urine, blood, or tissue from an infected animal*** or, more commonly, exposure to environmental contamination. The dogma that human-to-human transmission is very rare is challenged by recent findings on household clustering, asymptomatic renal colonization and prolonged excretion of leptospires.
- ***Transmission occurs through cuts, abraded skin***, or mucous membranes, especially the conjunctival and oral mucosa. After entry, the organisms proliferate, cross tissue barriers and disseminate hematogenously to all organs (*leptospiremic phase*).

97. Ans. a. VDRL is the one of the most widely used nontreponemal antibody tests, d. Primary and secondary syphilis are treated by penicillin

[Ref: Ananthanarayan 9th/372-77; Neena Khanna 6th/320-27]

"**Tabes Dorsalis:** *Hypotonia*"-*PJM 20th/372*

"**Lipoproteins** released from treatment of *Treponema pallidum* infections are believed to induce the Jarisch-Herxheimer reaction. The **Herxheimer reaction** has shown an increase in inflammatory cytokines during the period of exacerbation, including ***tumor necrosis factor alpha, interleukin-6 and interleukin-8***"-wikipedia

"**Jarisch-herxheimer reaction**: A dramatic although usually mild reaction consisting of fever, chills, myalgias, headache, tachycardia, increased respiratory rate, increased circulating neutrophil count and vasodilation with mild hypotension may follow the initiation of treatment for syphilis. This reaction is thought to be a response to ***lipoproteins released by dying T. pallidum organisms***. The Jarisch-Herxheimer reaction occurs in 50% of patients with primary syphilis, 90% of those with secondary syphilis and a lower proportion of persons with later stage disease."- *Harrison 19th/1140*

Jarisch-herxheimer reaction occurs due to release of exotoxin from dead organism"- *books.google.co.in/books.isbn=1451148631*

"***Anaphylactic reaction of penicillin is IgE mediation action***"- *books.google.co.in/books.isbn=1451148631*

"***TPHA is most frequently used treponemal test. Commonly used nontreponemal test include VDRL and RPR***"- *Neena Khanna 6th/320*

"***Penicillin is the drug of choice for treatment of all stages of syphilis***"-*Jawetz 27th/326*

"**Tabes dorsalis** is a late manifestation of syphilis that presents as symptoms and signs of demyelination of the posterior columns, dorsal roots *and* dorsal root ganglia. Symptoms include ataxic wide-based gait and foot drop; ***paresthesia***; bladder disturbances; impotence; areflexia; and loss of positional, deep-pain and temperature sensations"-*Harrison 19th/1136*

"The ***most widely used nontreponemal antibody tests for syphilis are the RPR and VDRL tests***, which measure IgG and IgM directed against a cardiolipin-lecithin-cholesterol antigen complex. The RPR test is easier to perform and uses unheated serum or plasma; it is the test of choice for rapid serologic diagnosis in a clinical setting. The VDRL test remains the standard for examining CSF and is superior to the RPR for this purpose"- *Harrison 19th/1137*

Table *(Harrison 19th/1139)*: **Recommendation of treatment of syphilis**

Stage of Syphilis	Patients without Penicillin Allergy
Primary, secondary, or early latent	Penicillin G benzathine
Late latent (or latent of uncertain duration), cardiovascular, or benign tertiary	Penicillin G benzathine
Neurosyphilis (asymptomatic or symptomatic)	Aqueous crystalline penicillin G or Aqueous procaine penicillin G plus oral probenecid

98. Ans. a. Cholera gravis

[Ref: Harrison 19th/1063; www.ncbi.nlm.nih.gov]

Despite exhaustive search I could not find terms like cholera mitis and majoris

Clinical Spectrum of V. Cholerae Infection

◈ *www.ncbi.nlm.nih.gov*

- Infection with *V. cholerae* produces a clinical spectrum that ranges from asymptomatic colonization to **cholera gravis**, the most severe form of the disease
- Following host ingestion of contaminated food or water, *V. cholerae* colonizes the small intestine for 12 to 72 hours before symptoms appear. Cholera often begins with stomach cramps and vomiting followed by diarrhoea, which may progress to ***fluid losses of up to 1 litre per hour***

"Individuals infected with *V. cholerae* O1 or O139 exhibit a range of clinical manifestations. Some individuals are asymptomatic or have only mild diarrhea; others present with the sudden onset of explosive and life-threatening diarrhea (***cholera gravis***). ***In severe cases, volume loss can exceed 250 mL/ kg in the first 24 h.*** If fluids and electrolytes are not replaced, hypovolemic shock and death may ensue"-*Harrison 19th/1063*

"Few diseases have a clinical presentation as striking as that of cholera. Massive watery diarrhoea, ***up to 1 L per hour, can lead to hypotensive shock and death within hours of the first symptom (so-called cholera gravis)***"- thelancet.com/journals

Clinical spectrum of Vibrio Cholerae Infection

◈ *www.ncbi.nlm.nih.gov*

	Asymptomatic infection	Mild infection	Severe infection
Symptoms	None	Diarrhoea	Vomiting and profuse diarrhoea
Dehydration	None	None to mild	Moderate to severe (hypovolaemic shock)
Stool characteristics	Normal	Loose or watery	Rice water
Vibrios per gram of stool	Up to 10^5	Up to 10^8	10^7 to 10^9 in stool (and vomitus)
Treatment	None	Oral rehydration solution (ORS)	ORS, intravenous fluids and antibiotics
Mortality	None	None	Untreated: up to 50% Treated: less than 1%

FORENSIC MEDICINE

99. Ans. a. Barberio's test, d. Acid phosphatase test

[Ref: Reddy 33rd/450-51,435-36; Parikh 7th/492-93,484-86]

Examination of Blood

◈ *Reddy 33rd/450-51; Parikh 7th/484-86*

- Chemical examination: ***Benzidine test, Phenolphthalein test (Kastle-Meyer test)***
- Microchemical test: ***Haemin crystal test (Teihmann's test), Haemochromogen crystal test (Takayama test)***

Chemical Examination of Seminal Fluid

◈ *Reddy 33rd/435-36; Parikh 7th/492-93*

- ***Florence test***
- ***Barberio's test***
- ***Acid phosphatase test***
- ***Creatine phosphokinase***

100. Ans. a. Injury causing endanger to life if not treated timely

[Ref: Reddy 33rd/ 293; Parikh 7th/ 263]

Dangerous Injuries

◈ *Reddy 33rd/ 293*

- **Dangerous injuries** are those which cause ***imminent danger to life***, either by involvement of important organs or structures, or extensive area of the body. ***If no surgical aid is available, such injuries may prove fatal.***
- The concept of **injury dangerous to life** is not very precise. As such, it is not enough if the medical witness makes simple statement that the injury in a particular part is dangerous to human life. He should place all relevant data, namely the nature and extent of injury, the kind of weapon used, the part of the body struck, whether the injury caused haemorrhage or shock, affected important structures or organs, or was very extensive, or otherwise caused imminent danger and should also state the various grounds on which he considers the injury to be a dangerous one.
- **Some examples of injuries which endanger life** are: *stab on the abdomen or head or vital part, hurt causing rupture of spleen, squeezing testicles, incised wound on the neck, compound fracture of the skull, rupture of an internal organ, injury of a large blood vessel.*

◈ *Parikh 7th/ 263*

- **A dangerous injury** ***is a variety of grievous injury.***
- It is ***an injury which endangers***, i.e. poses an immediate danger to life. It is either extensive or serious in relation to the organ or part wounded. The injury is fatal in the absence of surgical aid.
- **Common examples** of such injuries are: *gun shot wounds, compound fractures of the skull, trauma to a large or important blood vessel and rupture of some internal organ, e.g. spleen.*
- This is generally caused by a shooting, stabbing or cutting implement.

The following kinds of hurt only are designated as "grievous" (S.320,I.P.C):

- **First:** ***Emasculation;***
- **Secondly:** Permanent privation of the sight of either eye;
- **Thirdly:** ***Permanent privation of the hearing of either ear;***
- **Fourthly:** Privation of any member or joint;
- **Fifthly:** Destruction or permanent impairing of the powers of any member or joint;
- **Sixthly:** Permanent disfiguration of the head or face;
- **Seventhly:** ***Fracture or dislocation of a bone or tooth;***
- **Eighthly:** *Any hurt which endangers life or which causes the sufferer to be during the space of twenty days in severe bodily pain or unable to follow his ordinary pursuits*

101. Ans. a. Can be done in the presence..., b. Should be done by magistrate, c. If a declarant made more than one..., d. If incomplete,...

[Ref: Reddy 33rd/10-11]

Dying Declaration

◈ *Reddy 33rd/10-11*

- It is a written or oral statement of a person, who is dying as a result of some unlawful act, relating to the material facts of cause of his death or bearing on the circumstances (S.32, I.E.A.). **If there is time, Executive magistrate should be called to record the declaration.**
- Before recording the statement, the doctor should certify that the person is conscious and his mental faculties are normal (*compos mentis*).
- If the condition of the victim is serious and there is no time to call a Magistrate, ***the doctor should take the declaration in the presence of two witnesses.***
- The statement can also be recorded by the village headman, police or any other person, but its evidential value will be less.
- While recording the dying declaration, **oath is not administered, because of the belief that the dying person tells the truth.**
- **Statement:** The statement should be recorded in the man's own words, without any alteration of terms or phrases. Leading questions should not be put. The declarant should be permitted to give his statement without any undue influence, outside prompting or assistance. If a point is not clear, question may be asked to make it clear, but the actual question and the answer received should be recorded
- **If the declarant survives, the declaration is not admitted, but has corroborative value and the person is called to give oral evidence**

Incomplete Statement

◈ *www.legalservicesindia.com*

- The Apex Court had held that ***if a deceased fails to complete the main sentence*** (as for instance, the genesis or motive for the crime) ***a dying declaration would be unreliable.*** However, if the deceased has narrated the full story, but fails to answer the last formal question as to what more he wanted to say, the declaration can be relied upon.
- "***Incomplete declaration: dying declaration must be complete***"-www.ourlaw.in

Multiple Dying Declarations

◈ *blog.ipleaders.in*

- Supreme Court Of India held that multiple dying declarations can be relied upon without corroboration if there is consistency in all the dying declaration. ***If all the dying declarations are similar to each other than it can be admissible.***
- But if the ***dying declaration is different from each other*** than the court will examine the ***facts of the case or can examine the statement of other witnesses to ascertain the truth of the case.***
- In Kushal Rao v state of Bombay, this case set the importance of dying declaration and what is the right process to record it. In this case, if the dying declaration is recorded in question-answer form, if the medical certificate is given by the doctor, if it is recorded by the authorized person, then it is admissible and reliable. If there are multiple dying declarations, then court looks into all these points to see ***which dying declaration holds more evidentiary value.***
- The Supreme Court has held that multiple dying declarations can be relied upon without corroboration if consistency is maintained throughout. ***Otherwise, the courts would have to examine the statement of other witnesses to ascertain the truth in a criminal trial.***
- "Contradictory statements: ***if a declarant made more than one dying declarations and all are contradictory, then those all declarations lose their value***"- *www.legalservicesindia.com*

102. Ans. a. Sodium hydroxide, b.Aconite, d. Sulphuric acid

[Ref: Reddy 33rd/124; Parikh 7th/108-09]

"In all cases of poisoning, ***inclusive of carbolic acid*** *but exclusive of other acids, saturated solution of common salt should be used"- Parikh 7th/108*

Sulphuric acid is a corrosive acid*- Reddy 33rd/530*

"Sodium hydroxide is an alkali"*- Reddy 33rd/536*

Preservatives

◈ *Reddy 33rd/124*

- Saturated **sodium chloride** solution, ***except in poisoning from corrosive acids, alkalis, corrosive sublimate*** **(mercuric chloride)** ***and aconite.***

- **Rectified spirit**, except in cases of suspected poisoning by (a) alcohol, kerosene, (b) chloroform, ether, (c) chloral hydrate, (d) formic acid, (e) formaldehyde, acetic acid, (f) phenol, (g) phosphorus and h) paraldehyde, because the organic acids and paraldehyde are soluble in alcohol and the phosphorescence of phosphorus is diminished by alcohol.
- Ten. mg./ml of sodium or **potassium fluoride**. (Prevents glycolysis, inhibits enzyme enolase and inhibits bacterial growth) and 3 mg. potassium oxalate (anti-coagulant) should be used for preserving blood.
  - Fluoride should also be added to urine, CSF and vitreous humour if alcohol estimation is required and also to samples for analysis for cocaine, cyanide and CO.
  - In poisoning by oxalic acid, ethylene glycol, fluoride and CO, 30 mg. sodium citrate should be added for 10 ml. of blood as preservative.
  - One ml of concentrated hydrochloric acid or 100 mg. of thymol or 100 mg. of sodium fluoride can be used for 10 ml urine as a preservative. Toluene is better.
  - Preservative is not necessary if (1) viscera can be analysed within 24 hours, (2) if sample can be kept in a refrigerator or ice box, (3) bone, hair, nails, (4) lung for detecting inhaled poisons.
  - N.B. The viscera **should not be preserved in formaldehyde** because extraction of poison, especially non-volatile organic compounds becomes difficult

103. Ans. b. Fractures of trachea and larynx, c. Congested faces, d. Transverse ligature, e. Bruises at edges of the ligature mark

[Ref: Reddy 33rd/351]

Table *(Reddy 33rd/351)*: **Difference between handing and strangulation**

Trait	Hanging	Strangulation by ligature
Ligature mark:	It is oblique, does not completely encircle the neck; usually seen high up in the neck between the chin and larynx. The base is pale, hard and parchment-like	It is **transverse,** completely encircling the neck below the thyroid cartilage. The base is soft and reddish.
Abrasions and ecchymoses:	About the edges of ligature mark not common	About the edges of the ligature mark are common.
Bruising:	Of the neck muscles less common	Of the neck muscles more common
Neck:	Stretched and elongated	Not stretched or elongated
Subcutaneous tissues:	White, hard and glistening under the mark.	Ecchymosed under the mark.
Hyoid bone:	Fracture may occur.	Fracture is uncommon
Thyroid cartilage:	Fracture is less common.	Fracture is more common.
Larynx and trachea:	Fracture rare	Fracture may be found
Emphysematous bullae:	Not present on the surface of the lungs	Very common on the surface of the lungs
Carotid arteries:	Damage may be seen	Damage is very rare
Face:	***Usually pale and petechiae are not common***	*Congested, **livid and marked with petechiae***
Signs of asphyxia:	External signs less marked	External signs well-marked
Tongue:	Swelling and protrusion is less marked	Swelling and protrusion is more marked.
Saliva:	Often runs out of mouth	Absent
Bleeding:	From the nose, mouth and ears not common	From the nose, mouth and ears common
Involuntary discharge:	Of faeces and urine less common	Of faeces and urine more common
Seminal fluid:	At glans is more common	At glans is less common

Contd...

104. Ans. a. Oedema aquosum in lung, b. Emphysema aquosum is presumptive evidence of death from drowning, c. Paltauf's haemorrhages is seen subpleurally, d. Gettler's test is used to test chloride content of blood from both sides of the heart

[Ref: Reddy 33rd/369-70; Parikh 7th/ 192-93]

Drowning

◈ *Reddy 33rd/364-75*

- On section, an oedematous condition due to the presence of watery, frothy, sometimes blood-stained fluid is seen. Drowning fluid actually penetrates alveolar walls to enter the tissues and the blood vessels. This has been described as **emphysema aquosum**. It is present in about 80% of cases and is ***presumptive evidence of death from drowning.***
- ***"Sea water drowning: Lung is ballooned and heavy"***- *Reddy 33rd/370*
- If the victim is unconscious at the time of drowning, mere flooding of the lungs with water, but without formation of columns of froth occurs, which is known as **oedema aquosum**. The foam acts as a "check valve".
- The more powerful inspiratory efforts allow air entry to the lungs, but expiratory efforts are insufficient to expel air, water and foam. The lungs feel doughy and readily pit on pressure. The alveolar Walls may rupture due to increased pressure during Forced expirations and produce haemorrhages, which when ***present subpleurally*** are called **"Paltauf's haemorrhages"**.
- **Paltaufs haemorrhages** are shining, pale pink or bluish-red and may be minute or 3 to 5 cm in diameter. They are usually present in about 50 percent of cases in the lower lobes of the lungs, but may be seen on the anterior surfaces of lungs and the interlobar surfaces.

Positive Sign of Drowning

◈ *Parikh 7th/ 197*

- Froth-fine, foamy, copious, lathery
- Positive diatoms test
- Weeds or grass in cadaveric spasm of hands, if present
- Emphysema aqosum or hydremia of lung
- Rib marking on the lungs
- ***Gettler's test** is used to test chloride content of blood from both sides of the heart"- Parikh 7th/193*

PREVENTIVE & SOCIAL MEDICINE

105. Ans. d. 4 days before and 5 days after appearance of rashes

[Ref: Park 24th/157; Community Medicine with Recent Advances by Suryakantha 4th/328]

"**Communicability of measles**: The period of communicability is approx. ***4 days before and 4 days after the appearance of the rash***"- *Park 24th/157*

"**Period of communicability**: ***4 days before and 5 days after the appearance of rashes***. Measles is highly infectious during this period"- *Suryakantha 4th/328*

106. Ans. a. MMR vaccine, b. Hepatitis A vaccine, c. Varicella vaccine

[Ref: Park 24th/108; Community Medicine by Piyush Gupta 1st/428; Community Medicine with Recent Advances by Suryakantha 4th/287; O.P.Ghai 8th/189-90]

*Live **attenuated vaccines are contraindicated in AIDS patients***

*Two type of **Hepatitis A vaccine** is available-**inactivated (killed) and live attenuated vaccine**- Piyush Gupta 1st/428; Park 24th/227*

***DPT- Toxoid** -Park 24th/108*

***MMR, Varicella:Live vaccine**- Park 24th/108*

***Hib: Glycoconjugate**- Park 24th/108*

"Haemophilus influenza b vaccine (Hib): capsular polysaccharide is used as agent. C/I- hypersensitivity to previous dose"- O.P.Ghai 8th/189-90

C/I for Vaccines

◈ *Park 24th/108; Suryakantha 4th/287*

- ***Live vaccines should not be administered to persons with immunodeficiency disease*** or to persons whose immune response may be suppressed because of leukemia,***HIV***, lymphoma or malignancy or because of therapy with cortiocosteriods, alkylating agents, antimetabolic agents or radiation
- Pregnancy is another C/I, for live vaccines unless the risk of infection exceeds the risk of harm to the foetus of some live vaccines
- The only absolute C/I for killed vaccine is severe local or general reaction to a previous dose.

107. Ans. a. 6, 11, b. 16, 18, c. 31, 33

[Ref: www.ncbi.nlm.nih.gov; www.merckvaccines.com]

◈ *9-valent HPV vaccine www.ncbi.nlm.nih.gov*

- The 9-valent HPV vaccine, which protects against HPV ***types 6, 11, 16, 18, 31, 33, 45, 52 and 58***, is safe and effective and will further reduce the incidence of HPV infection, as well as HPV-related cancers.
- It can also indirectly protect unvaccinated individuals through herd immunity. With an effective vaccination program, most cervical cancers can be prevented.
- Analyses show that the cost-effectiveness of the 9-valent HPV vaccine in female patients is comparable to the original quadrivalent HPV vaccine (which protects against HPV types 6, 11, 16 and 18) currently in use.
- However, the usefulness of vaccinating male patients with the 9-valent HPV vaccine needs further investigation.

Indication for GARDASIL 9

◈ *www.merckvaccines.com*

- **GARDASIL 9** is a vaccine indicated in females 9 through 26 years of age for the prevention of cervical, vulvar, vaginal and anal cancers caused by human papillomavirus (HPV) Types 16, 18, 31, 33, 45, 52 and 58; precancerous or dysplastic lesions caused by HPV Types 6, 11, 16, 18, 31, 33, 45, 52 and 58; and genital warts caused by HPV Types 6 and 11.
- **GARDASIL 9** is indicated in males 9 through 26 years of age for the prevention of anal cancer caused by HPV Types 16, 18, 31, 33, 45, 52 and 58; precancerous or dysplastic lesions caused by HPV Types 6, 11, 16, 18, 31, 33, 45, 52 and 58; and genital warts caused by HPV Types 6 and 11.
- **GARDASIL 9** (Human Papillomavirus 9-valent Vaccine, Recombinant) does not eliminate the necessity for girls to continue to undergo recommended cervical cancer screening later in life. Recipients of GARDASIL 9 should not discontinue anal cancer screening if it has been recommended by a health care professional.
- Not all vulvar, vaginal and anal cancers are caused by HPV and GARDASIL 9 protects only against those vulvar, vaginal and anal cancers caused by HPV Types 16, 18, 31, 33, 45, 52 and 58.
- Vaccination with GARDASIL 9 may not result in protection in all vaccine recipients.

108. Ans. a. Adult literacy rate range from 0 to 100, c. Life expectancy at birth range from 25 years to 85 years, e. HDI score range is 0-1

[Ref: Park 24th/17-18; Community Medicine with Recent Advances by Suryakantha 4th/7]

Human Development Index

◈ *Park 24th/17*

- The ***HDI value range b/w 0 to 1***
- Minimum and maximum values (goalposts) are set in order to transform the indicators into indices b/w 0 and 1
- The maximums are the observed values in the time series (1980-2011)

- The **minimum values** are set at ***20 years for expectancy, at 0 years for both education variables and at $ 100 for per capita gross national income (GNI)***

Human Development Index

◈ *Suryakantha 4th/7*

- **Minimum and maximum value:** ***Life expectancy at birth (25 years and 85 years); Adult literacy rate (0 percent and 100 percent); Combined gross enrolment ratio-school (0 percent and 100 percent); Real GDP per capita (100 and 40000 $)***

109. Ans. a. TB is mandatory to notify, b. Suspicious TB patients are screened through 2 sputum smear examinations, e. Covered the whole country since March 2006

[Ref: Park 24th/427-30; Community Medicine by Piyush Gupta 1st/826-30; Suryakantha 4th/921-23; National Health Programs of India by Jugal Kishore 7th/91]

"Under RNTCP case finding is passive. Patients presenting themselves with symptoms suspicious of TB are screened ***through 2 sputum smear examinations****" (Park 24th/429)*

"After diagnosis, the treatment of MDR-TB is initiated at designated DOTS-Plus sites, which are established in tertiary care centers at least one in each state" (Park 24th/190)

TB Notification

◈ *Piyush Gupta 1st/826*

*"**GOI declared TB a notifiable disease on 7th may 2012** with following objective*

- *To have establish TB surveillance system in the country*
- *To extent mechanism of TB treatment adherence and contact tracing of patients treated in private sector*
- *To ensure proper TB diagnosis and case management and further accelerate reduction of TB transmission*
- *To mitigate the impending drug resistant TB epidemic in the country*

Revised National Tuberculosis Control Programme (RNTCP)

◈ *Park 24th/427*

The government of India, WHO and World Bank together reviewed the NTP (Operated since 1962) in the year 1992

The salient features are:

- Achievement of ***at least 85% cure rate*** of infectious cases through the supervised short course chemotherapy involving peripheral health functionaries.
- Augmentation of ***case finding activities*** through high quality sputum microcopy to detect at ***least 70%*** estimated cases.
- Involvement of ***NGOs***, information, education and communication and improved operational research.
- Direct observed therapy short-term (DOTS)- a community based TB treatment and care strategy

Note:

- ***The RNTCP covers the whole country since March 2006***
- ***DOTS-Plus is a strategy under development for the management of multi-drug resistant TB (MDR-TB)***
- *The first phase of the World Bank assisted RNTCP ended on 30th Sept. 2006. The second phase of the project has started on 1st Oct. 2006 for a further period of 5 years*

National Tuberculosis Programme (NTP)

◈ *Park 22rd/390*

Long term objectives: to reduce TB in the community to that level when it ceases to be a public health problem i, e

- *One case infects less than one new person annually*
- *The prevalence of infection in the age group below 14 years is brought down to less than 1%*

110. Ans. a. Given through IM/SC route, c. Does not require stringent conditions e. Dose is -0.5 ml/dose

[Ref: Park 24th/221-22; O.P.Ghai 8th/192]

"IPV dose: 0.5 ml; IM/SC" *O.P.Ghai 8th/192*

Differences between IPV and OPV

◈ *Park 24th/222*

IPV (Salk type)	OPV (Sabin type)
Killed formalised virus	Live attenuated virus
Given ***subcutaneously (SC) or intramuscular (IM)***	Given orally
Induces circulating antibody, but no local (intestinal) immunity	Immunity is both humoral and intestinal. Induces antibody quickly
Prevents paralysis, but does not prevent reinfection by wild polio viruses	Prevents not only paralysis, but also intestinal reinfection
Not useful in controlling epidemics	Can be effectively used in controlling epidemics. Even a single dose elicits substantial immunity (except in tropical countries)
More difficult to manufacture	Easy to manufacture
The virus content is 10,000 times more than OPV,hence costlier	Cheaper
Does not require stringent conditions during storage and transportation. I las a longer shelf—life	Requires to be stored and transported at sub-zero temperatures, unless stabilized

111. Ans. c. Year of Big divide-1921A.D, d. Population pyramid has a broad base and a tapering top, e. First regular census in India was carried in 1881

[Ref: Park 24th/513-518; Community Medicine by Piyush Gupta 1st/610-12; Community Medicine with Recent Advances by Suryakantha 4th/651-57]

Demographic Cycle of India

◈ *Park 24th/513-518*

- India's population has been steadily increasing since 1921. ***The year 1921 is called the "big divide"*** because the absolute number of people added to the population during each decade has been on the increase since 1921

- For India, the **dependency ratio** (0–14 yrs and >65 yr) for the year mid 2016 is- ***52.4%*** *-Park 24th/518*
- *The age pyramid of India is typical of developing countries, with **a broad base and a tapering top***
- *Demographic cycle phases- First phase (High stationary), Second phase (Early expanding), Third phase (Late expanding), Fourth stage (Low stationary) and Fifth stage (Declining)*
- ***India has entered into third stage (late expanding)****- Park 24th/513*
- The ***first regular census in India was taken in 1881****- Park 24th/877*

Developing country *Suryakantha 4th/656*	**Developed country**
Broad base (High birth rate)	Narrow base (low birth rate)
Concave border (Concave facing outwards)	Convex border (facing outward)
Acute apex (indicating less number of elderly people)	Obtuse apex (more of elderly people)

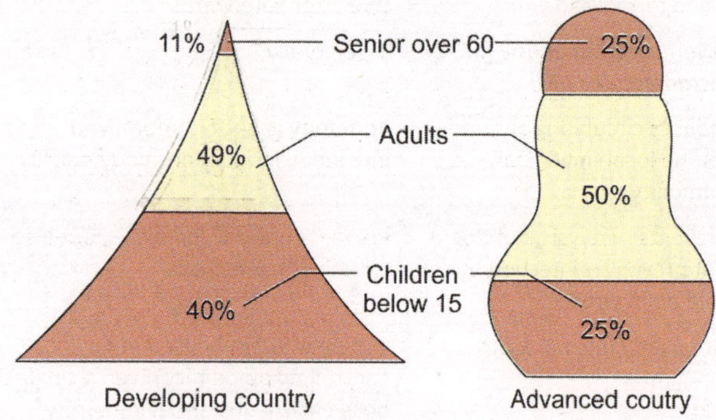

Fig *(Suryakantha 4th/ 656)*: Population pyramid of developing and advanced country

112. Ans. b. Adolescents of age group 10-19 yr are covered, d. Biannual deworming through albendazole tablet, e. Screening of target groups for moderate/severe anaemia and referring these cases to an appropriate health facility

[Ref: Park 24th/471; http://nhm.gov.in/nrhmcomponnetsCommunity Medicine by Piyush Gupta 1st/814-15; Community Medicine with Recent Advances by Suryakantha 4th/196-97]

Weekly Iron and Folic Acid Supplementation (WIFS) Programme covers only adolescent girls and boys

National Iron Plus Initiative

Piyush Gupta 1st/814

- National Iron plus initiative include, ***adolescent (10-19 yr), both in and out of school***
- Those in ***school is covered by Weekly Iron and Folic Acid Supplementation Scheme (WIFS), while out of school adolescent is reached through Anganwadi centers***
- Weekly Iron and Folic Acid Supplementation Scheme (WIFS) component
  - ***Supervised administration of weekly iron and folic supplements of 100 mg elemental iron and 500 mcg folic acid***
  - ***Bi-annual de-worming (albendazole 400 mg)***
  - ***Screening of target group for moderate and severe anaemia***

Weekly Iron and Folic Acid Supplementation (WIFS) Programme

nhm.gov.in/nrhmcomponnets

- The Ministry of Health and Family Welfare has launched the WIFS Programme to meet the challenge of high prevalence and incidence of anaemia amongst adolescent girls and boys.
- WIFS is evidence based programmatic response to the prevailing anaemia situation amongst adolescent girls and boys through supervised weekly ingestion of IFA supplementation and biannual helminthic control.
- The long term goal is to break the intergenerational cycle of anaemia, the short term benefits is of a nutritionally improved human capital. The programme, implemented across the country both in rural and urban areas.

Salient Features of WIFS

- **Objective** of Weekly Iron Folic acid Supplementation (WIFS) To reduce the prevalence and severity of anaemia in adolescent population (10-19 years).
- **Target groups**
  - School going adolescent girls and boys in 6th to 12th class enrolled in government/government aided/ municipal schools.
  - Out of school adolescent girls.
- **Intervention**
  - Administration of supervised **Weekly Iron-folic Acid Supplements** of 100mg elemental iron and 500ug Folic acid using a fixed day approach.
  - Screening of target groups for moderate/severe anaemia and referring these cases to an appropriate health facility.
  - ***Biannual de-worming (Albendazole 400mg), six months apart, for control of helminthic infestation.***
  - Information and counselling for improving dietary intake and for taking actions for prevention of intestinal worm infestation.
- **Convergence** with key stakeholder ministries like the Ministry of Women and Child Development and Ministry of Human Resource Development is an essential part of implantation plan of the WIFS programme. Key convergent areas include: joint programme planning, capacity building of nodal service providers including Medical Officers, Anganwadi Worker (AWW) Staff Nurses, School teachers, monitoring and a comprehensive communication component.

113. Ans. b. Immunoglobulin not required if prior full vaccination is received, c. Local wound cleaning is done in all cases of dog wound

[Ref: Park 24th/296-97; Community Medicine by Piyush Gupta 1st/323]

Post Exposure Prophylaxis

◈ *Park 24th/296-97*

- First aid: Immediately, the wound should be flushed thoroughly and washed with soap and water, detergent or water alone. This procedure is recommended for all bite wounds"- *Piyush Gupta 1st/323*
- In case where the vaccine is started with the bitting animal kept under observation, an alternative recommendation is ***to stop treatment after five days.*** The ***animal is observed for a further five days, the vaccine being started again if the animal becomes ill or dies during the period***"- Ananthanarayan 9th/536
- Rabies immunoglobulin is not required if complete pre-exposure vaccination is done
- If complete pre-exposure vaccination is done, give only two booster dosage (1.0 ml) on day 0 and 3- *Piyush Gupta 1st/324*

Table *(Park 24th/296)*: **Categories of contact and recommended post-exposure prophylaxis**

Categories of contact with suspect rabid animal	Post–exposure prophylaxis measures
Category I– touching or feeding animals, licks on intact skin	None
Category II– nibbling of uncovered skin, minor scratches or abrasion without bleeding	Immediate vaccination and local treatment of the wound
Category III–single or multiple transdermal bites or scratches, licks on broken skin; contamination of mucous membrane with saliva from licks, contacts with bats	Immediate vaccination and administration or rabies immunoglobulin; local treatment of the wound

114. Ans. b. 30000 in plain area, d. 20000 tribal area

[Ref: Park 24th/941; Community Medicine by Piyush Gupta 1st/806]

"The **National Health Plan (1983)** proposed reorganisation of PHC on the basis of ***one PHC for every 30,000 rural population in plains and one PHC for every 20,000 population in hilly, tribal and backward areas*** for more effective coverage"- *Park 24th/941; Piyush Gupta 1st/806*

OPHTHALMOLOGY

115. Ans. c. Sudden painful loss of vision

[Ref: A K Khurana 6th/269; Parson 22nd/320-21; Ophthalmic Diagnosis and Treatment by Yanoff 3rd/65-67]

"The ***most common cause of CRAO is thromboembolus***, which occurs at the narrowest part of the central retinal artery, where it pierces the dural sheath of the optic nerve. It could also occur as a result of an occlusive thrombus at the level immediately posterior to the ***lamina cribrosa***"- *www.merckmanuals.com*

"Standard non-invasive therapies include: Intravenous acetazolamide and mannitol, plus ***anterior chamber paracentesis***, followed by withdrawal of a small amount of aqueous fluid from the eye to increase retinal artery perfusion pressure by reducing intraocular pressure"- www.nature.com/eye

Central Retinal Artery Occlusion (CRAO)

◈ *A K Khurana 6th/269*

- It ***occurs due to obstruction at the level of lamina cribrosa***
- *Symptoms.* Patient complains of ***sudden painless loss of vision***
- Direct pupillary light reflex is absent.
- On ophthalmoscopic examination retinal arteries are markedly narrowed but retinal veins look almost normal. Retina becomes milky white due to oedema.
- ***Central part of the macular area shows cherry-red spot*** due to vascular choroid shining through the thin retina of this region.
- In eyes with a cilioretinal artery, part of the macular will remain normal. Blood column within the retinal veins is segmented (***cattletrucking***).
- **Central Retinal Artery Occlusion** *Ophthalmic Diagnosis and Treatment* by Yanoff 3rd/65-67
- ***Thrombosis or embolic blockage to the central retinal artery***; the most common source of emboli comes from the carotid arteries.
- Sign
  - Retinal whitening
  - **Cherry-red spot** in the fovea (xanthophyllic pigment of fovea stands out in an otherwise white macula)
  - Narrowing or segmentation of retinal arterioles
  - Optic nerve pallor: can be seen in the late stages.
- **Investigation**
  - *Fluorescein angiography*: demonstrates delayed or even complete lack of retinal arterial filling
  - *Echoretinography (ERG)*: shows a reduction in the B-wave amplitude
  - *Systemic workup*: carotid artery noninvasive testing, echocardiography, erythrocyte sedimentation rate if temporal arteritis suspected

Central Retinal Artery Occlusion (CRAO)

◈ *Parson 22nd/320-21*

- It is ***nearly always at the lamina cribrosa***, where the vessels normally become slightly narrowed.
- Such an accident causes sudden and complete retinal ischaemia and this tissue rapidly dies.
- The ***eye becomes suddenly blind***, although when the causative factor is minute emboli, premonitory obscurations of vision may occur.
- There is ***no direct pupillary reaction and light perception is lost.***

116. Ans. a. Smaller than superior ophthalmic vein, b. Connected to the pterygoid venous plexus, d. Pass through superior orbital fissure, e. Empties into superior ophthalmic vein

[Ref: A K Khurana 6th/6; www.mananatomy.com; www.sciencedirect.com]

Inferior Ophthalmic Vein

◈ *www.sciencedirect.com/topic*

- The **inferior ophthalmic vein** begins as a ***plexus near the anterior floor of the orbit***.
- It drains blood from the lower and lateral muscles, the inferior conjunctiva, the lacrimal sac and the inferior vortex veins
- It may form **two branches**: ***one that empties into either the superior ophthalmic vein*** or the cavernous sinus and ***one that empties into the pterygoid venous plexus***.
- The latter branch exits the orbit through the inferior orbital fissure and the other branch passes through the ***superior orbital fissure*** either to join the superior ophthalmic vein or to empty directly into the cavernous sinus.

Inferior Ophthalmic Vein

◈ *www.mananatomy.com*

- It is one of the two veins that drain the orbital cavity and structures within it.
- The inferior ophthalmic vein begins in a venous network in the ***anterior part of the floor of the orbit.***
- The **Inferior Ophthalmic Vein** (*v. ophthalmica inferior*) begins in a venous net-work at the forepart of the ***floor and medial wall of the orbit***- www.imaios.com
- The inferior ophthalmic vein then runs backward in the inferior part of the orbit and divides into two branches
- One of these branches passes through the inferior orbital fissure and ***joins the pterygoid venous plexus.***
- The other branch passes through the superior orbital fissure and ends in the cavernous sinus with the superior ophthalmic vein.

"The ***superior ophthalmic vein, the larger of the two ophthalmic veins***, runs with the ophthalmic artery and, as it passes posteriorly, receives blood from veins that drain the superior orbital structures"-www.sciencedirect.com

"**Superior Ophthalmic Vein**: Provides the ***main venous drainage of the orbit***. Originates in the superonasal quadrant of the orbit and extends posteriorly through the medial part of the superior orbital fissure into the cavernous sinus"-eyewiki.aao.org

117. Ans. c. Prominence of lid crease

[Ref: A K Khurana 6th/379-81; Parson 22nd/461-64]

"Congenital ptosis:It almost always needs surgical correction. In severe ptosis, surgery should be performed at the earliest to prevent stimulus deprivation amblyopia"- *A K Khurana 6th/381*

Congenital Ptosis

◈ *A K Khurana 6th/379*

- It is associated with ***congenital weakness (maldevelopment) of the levator palpebrae superioris (LPS)***.
- Characteristic feature
  - Drooping of one or more upper lids
  - ***Lid crease is either diminished or absent***
  - ***Lid lag on downgaze***
  - LPS function may be poor, fair or good
- It may occur in the following forms:
  - *Simple congenital ptosis* (not associated with any other anomaly)
  - Congenital ptosis with associated weakness of superior rectus muscle.
  - As a part of *blepharophimosis syndrome*, which comprises congenital ptosis, blepharophimosis, telecanthus and epicanthus inversus
  - *Congenital synkinetic ptosis* (Marcus Gunn jawwinking ptosis). In this condition there occurs retraction of the ptotic lid with jaw movements i.e., with stimulation of ipsilateral pterygoid muscle.

◈ *Parson 22nd/461-64*

- ***It is usually, but not invariably, bilateral*** and is due in most cases to defective development of the muscles.
- Abnormal synkineses such as the jaw winking phenomenon or Marcus Gunn ptosis may be seen, in which **lid retraction** is observed on opening the mouth or moving the jaw to the opposite side.
- Dystrophy of the levator may also be recognized by ***looking at the palpebral aperture in down gaze,*** where the ptotic eye will have a wider aperture as compared to the opposite normal one.
- Surgery is the *treatment of choice*
- *The Fasanella-Servat operation* is indicated for cases of minimal ptosis of 1.5-2 mm with good function of the levator and a good lid fold.

118. Ans. b. Does not seen in Ehlers-Danlos syndrome

[Ref: A K Khurana 6th/144; Parson 22nd/230-31]

Blue Sclera

◈ *A K Khurana 6th/144*

- It is an asymptomatic condition characterised by marked, generalised blue discolouration of sclera ***due to thinning.***
- It is a typical association of ***osteogenesis imperfecta.*** Its other causes are ***Marfan's syndrome, Ehlers-Danlos syndrome***, pseudoxanthoma elasticum, buphthalmos, high myopia and healed scleritis.

Blue Sclera

◈ *Parson 22nd/230-31*

- The sclera is bluish in babies, but the effect reduces with age. A much more pronounced blue coloration is sometimes seen in several members of the same family as a hereditary condition that persists throughout life. This disease is known as osteogenesis imperfecta and is characterized by frequent bone fractures (*fragilitas ossium*), blue sclera and deafness.
- Both sexes are equally involved; only those affected can transmit the disease. Histologically, ***the sclera and cornea are thin.***

- The *uveal pigment shines through the thin sclera and produces the blue colour*. Other systemic diseases that may be associated with blue sclera are ***Ehlers-Danlos syndrome, Marfan syndrome and pseudoxanthoma elasticum.***
- Local ocular diseases such as keratoconus and keratoglobus can also have blue sclera as an additional feature.

119. Ans. b. Tarsal glands are meibomian glands, d. Meibomian glands are modified sebaceous glands, e. External hordeolum is an acute suppurative inflammation of gland of Zeis

[Ref: A K Khurana 6th/363; Parson 22nd/449]

Glands of Eyelids

◈ *A K Khurana 6th/363*

- *Meibomian glands.* These are **also known as *tarsal glands*** and are present in the stroma of tarsal plate arranged vertically. They are about 30-40 in the upper lid and about 20-30 in the lower lid. They are ***modified sebaceous glands***. Their ducts open at the lid margin. Their secretion constitutes the oily layer of tear film.
- *Glands of Zeis.* These are also ***sebaceous glands*** which open into the follicles of eyelashes
- *Glands of Moll.* These are ***modified sweat glands*** situated near the hair follicle. They open into the hair follicles or into the ducts of Zeis glands. They do not open directly onto the skin surface as elsewhere.
- *Accessory lacrimal glands of Wolfring.* These are ***present near the upper border of the tarsal plate.***

"EXTERNAL HORDEOLUM (STYE): It is an acute suppurative inflammation of gland of the Zeis or Moll"-*A K Khurana 6th/367*

120. Ans. c. Erosion of epithelium + underlying inflammation

[Ref: A K Khurana 6th/98; Parson 22nd/ 194]

Pathology of Cornea

◈ *Parson 22nd/ 194*

- **Keratitis** is the descriptive term used for any type of corneal inflammation. Inflammation anterior to Bowman's membrane (involving the epithelium and Bowman's membrane) is called ***superficial keratitis.***
- The major pathological changes that occur are broadly categorized as ***keratitis and corneal 'ulceration', 'scarring' and 'opacification'.***
- A loss of epithelium is termed an **epithelial defect** and can be demonstrated clearly by staining with1% sodium fluorescein dye and viewed with cobalt blue filtered light.
- If superficial, without any inflammation, an epithelial defect is also called ***abrasion* or *erosion*** and usually heals within 12-24 hours by regeneration of the epithelial cells from the periphery, which slide over to cover the defect.
- ***A loss of epithelium with inflammation in the surrounding cornea is called a corneal ulcer.*** Inflammation in the cornea is visible as a greyish haze or loss of clarity. If accompanied by an outpouring of leucocytes the appearance is more off-white or yellowish and this hazy area is termed as an infiltration. Corneal ulcers can be infective or sterile.
- A ***corneal scar*** is the final outcome of any inflammation.

"ULCERATIVE KERATITIS: *Corneal ulcer* may be defined as ***discontinuation in normal epithelial surface of cornea*** associated with necrosis of the surrounding corneal tissue. Pathologically it is characterised by oedema and cellular infiltration"- *A K Khurana 6th/98*

121. Ans. d. Rhegmatogenous retinal detachment

[Ref: A K Khurana 6th/276-80,193; Parson 22nd/312-17,369]

DM causes tractional retinal detachment

Predisposing factors for Rhegmatogenous retinal detachment are: myopia, aphakia, pseudophakia, trauma senile posterior vitreous detachment- *A K Khurana 6th/299*

"Diabetic papillopathy: This is an uncommon condition seen in young patients in their teens or twenties who are suffering from juvenile insulin-dependent diabetes. They present with unilateral or bilateral blurred vision of insidious onset, or may be asymptomatic and the condition detected incidentally in these patients"-*Parson 22nd/369*

"True diabetic cataract. It is also called *'snow flake cataract'* or *'snow-storm cataract'.* It is a rare condition, usually occurring in young adults due to osmotic over-hydration of the lens. Initially a large number of fluid vacuoles appear underneath the anterior and posterior capsules, which is soon followed by appearance of bilateral snowflake-like white opacities in the cortex"-*A K Khurana 6th/193; Parson 22nd/268*

Feature of Diabetic Eye

- **Cystoid macular edema** (*A K Khurana 6th/280)*
- ***Tractional retinal detachment*** (*A K Khurana 6th/280; Parson 22nd/315)*
- Diabetic retinopathy (Proliferative and Non-proliferative)

122. Ans. a. Unilateral lesion result in adduction palsy of opposite eye

[Ref: A K Khurana 6th/355; Parson 22nd/409; Ophthalmic Diagnosis and Treatment by Yanoff 3rd/242]

"One of the most important among such connections is the group of fibres which link up the ***sixth nucleus of one side with the third nucleus of the other (i.e. the medial longitudinal fasciculus or the MLF)"***-*Parson 22nd/409*

"The **medial longitudinal fasciculus** carries information about the direction that the eyes should move. It connects the cranial nerve nuclei III (Oculomotor nerve), IV (Trochlear nerve) and VI (Abducens nerve) together and integrates movements directed by the gaze centers (frontal eye field) and information about head movement (from cranial nerve VIII, Vestibulocochlear nerve). ***It is an integral component of saccadic eye movements*** as well as vestibulo-ocular and optokinetic reflexes"-wiki

Internuclear ophthalmoplegia. In this condition there is lesion of the ***medial longitudinal bundle***. It is the pathway by which various ocular motor nuclei are linked. Internuclear ophthalmoplegia is characterised by: ***defective action of medial rectus on the side of lesion, horizontal nystagmus of the opposite eye and defective convergence"***-*A K Khurana 6th/355*

Internuclear Ophthalmoplegia *Ophthalmic Diagnosis and*

Treatment by Yanoff 3rd/242

- A lesion of the medial longitudinal fasciculus (MLF) resulting in paresis of adduction and dissociated nystagmus.
- **Symptoms**-Blurred vision, Double vision (vertical and horizontal) and Oscillopsia.
- **Signs**
  - *Adduction deficit that varies from the absence of adduction to a mild decrease in the velocity of adduction without any limitation in the extent of movement*
  - *Abducting nystagmus with an inward drift with an outward corrective saccade that may be hypermetric, hypometric or orthometric*
  - *Hypertropic eye*
  - *Convergence failure*: suggests that the lesion involves the MLF in the midbrain; this is labeled an "anterior" INO
  - *Intact convergence*: implies that the lesion has involved the MLF more caudally in the pons, sparing the medial rectus subnucleus; this is termed a "posterior" INO.

Medial Longitudinal Fasciculus Pathway

◈ *medicscenter.com*

- It links the cranial nerve nuclei composing of the oculomotor nerve, trochlear nerve and abducens nerve respectively and consolidates movements targeted by the eye (frontal eye field) and give details about the head movement (from the cranial nerve, vestibulocochlear nerve).
- ***It is an essential part of saccadic eye actions along with vestibular-ocular and optokinetic reflexes.***

Medial Longitudinal Fasciculus Syndrome: Signs of this Syndrome

- ***Medial rectus muscle weakness ipsilateral to the side of the lesion with paresis of adduction or adduction lag.***

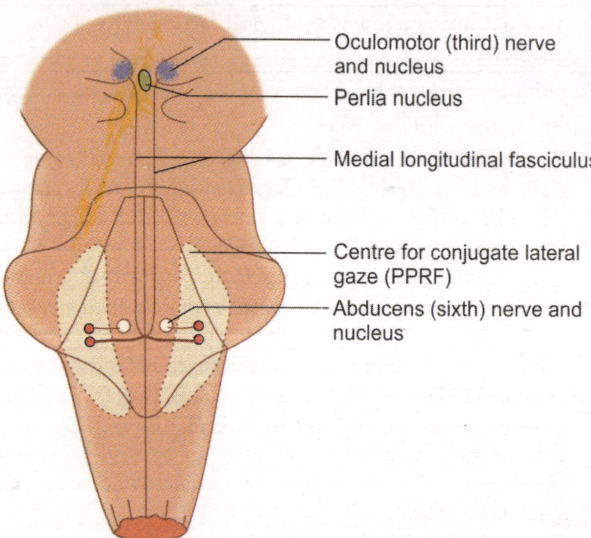

Fig: *(Parson 22nd/409):* Diagrammatic representation of the dorsal surface of the brainstem showing the connection of the pontine centres for conjugate lateral gaze (pontine paramedian reticular formation or PPRF) with the abducens nuclei and the oculomotor nuclei by way of the ***medial longitudinal fasciculus.***

- ***Abducting nystagmus of the eye contralateral to the lesion*** *– Dissociated nystagmus.*
- Dissociated vertical nystagmus – downbeat occuring with greater torsional component rate in the contralateral eye.
- Skew deviation – rapid production o fhypertropia on the lower side of the lesion.
- Normal convergence.
- Gaze evoked upright nystagmus Exacerbated top to bottom pursuit.
- Lessened vertically vestibular capability.
- Reducing in the amplitude saccadic intrusions that involve to the brainstem right next to the MLF.

123. Ans. c. Use of povidone-iodine solution to paint the lids before surgery, d. Cleaning and sterilization of operation theatre, e. Postop topical antibiotics

[Ref: Khurana 6th/197; Yanoff's Ophthalmology 3rd/435-37; Parson 21st/282,20th/265]

Bacterial Endophthalmitis

◈ *Khurana 6th/214*

- This is one of the most dreaded post-operative complications with an incidence of 0.2 to 0.5 percent.
- The principal sources of infection are contaminated solutions, instruments, surgeon's hands, patient's own flora from conjunctiva, eyelids and ***air-borne bacteria.***

Preoperative medications and preparations for cataract surgery *Khurana 6th/ 197*

- **Topical antibiotics** such as fourth generation fluoroquinolone (moxifloaxacin or gatifloxacin) may be used QID for 3 days before surgery to eradicate conjunctival bacterial flora
- **Povidone-iodine** (10%) solution should be ***used to paint the lids and facial skin preferably 2-3 hours before surgery***
- **Povidone-iodine** (5%) solution as a single drop 10-30 minutes before surgery is one of the most effective measure to decrease bacterial flora
- Preparation of the eye to be operated. Eyelashes of upper lid should be trimmed at night and the eye to be operated should be marked.
- **Scrub bath and care of hair.** Each patient should be instructed to have a scrub bath including face and hair wash with soap and water. Male patients must get their beard cleaned and hair trimmed. Female patients should comb their hair properly.

YANOFF'S Ophthalmology 3rd/435-37: *Writes*

- "***Before cataract surgery, topical anti-infective regimens*** have included gramicidin-neomycin-polymyxin B sulfate, aminoglycosides such as gentamicin or tobramycin (which provide gram-negative and Pseudomonas coverage) and the fluoroquinolones- ciprofloxacin, norfloxacin, ofloxacin or levofloxacin. Dosage is 1 drop 4 times over 1 h preceding surgery"
- "The **intraoperative use of antibiotics** *in irrigating solutions is **a controversial issue in cataract surgery***"
- *"Antibiotics in dose of 0.1 ml intracapsularly via sideport at end of procedure is given in cataract surgery"*

- "**Postoperative regimens of topical antibiotics** vary but generally consist of one drop to the operated eye 4-6 times daily for 1-2 weeks. The duration of treatment varies from 5 days in uncomplicated surgery to weeks if prolonged inflammation occurs"

"**Systemic administration**: Role of systemic antibiotics has been *severely questioned by* the endophthalmitis vitrectomy study at least for the cases of post cataract surgery endophthalmitis"- Clinical Practice in Ophthalmology *by Sandeep Saxena 1st/414*

"**Postop cataract management**: ***Antibiotic-steroid eyedrops*** are used for four times, three times, two times and then once a day for 2 weeks each"- *Khurana 6th/2104th/ 197*

124. Ans. a. Treatment of thickened capsule can be done by discission with cystitome, b. Treatment by Nd-YAG laser posterior capsulotomy, d. Posterior capsular opacification (PCO)

[Ref: A K Khurana 6th/214-15; Parson 22nd/268; Review of ophthalmology by Trattler 2nd/281]

Posterior Capsular Opacification (PCO; Secondary Cataract)

◈ *Review of ophthalmology by Trattler 2nd/281*

- Proliferation of residual lens epithelial cells (Elschnig's pearls) and fibrosis
- Incidence: up to 50% of patients within 2 years of ***extracapsular cataract surgery***; influenced by optic material (acrylic < silicone < PMMA) and edge design (square edge < round edge); with newer IOLs, the incidence has decreased to ~10%. Incidence approaches 100% in children and patients with uveitis
- Treatment: ***Nd-YAG laser posterior capsulotomy*** when visually significant. In young children, primary posterior capsulotomy and anterior vitrectomy are performed at the time of cataract surgery

Secondary Cataract; Posterior Capsular Opacification (PCO)

◈ *Ophthalmic Diagnosis and Treatment by Yanoff 3rd/65-67*

- A late complication of ***extracapsular cataract extraction*** (ECCE) in which the capsular epithelium proliferates and opacifies the posterior lens capsule.

Symptoms

- Symptoms follow ECCE, either nuclear expression or phacoemulsification
- *Obscuration of vision*: may occur as early as a few weeks after ECCE, but usually occurs months to years later
- Blurred vision
- *Dim vision*: patients often complain of a combination of dim vision (vision used to be brighter) and blurred vision
- Hazy vision
- Halos at night.

Signs

- *Opacification of posterior lens capsule:*
- *Cellular reaction on anterior surface of intraocular lens implant*
- *Fibrinous reaction on anterior surface of intraocular lens implant*
- *Elschnig's pearls*
- *Soemmerring's ring*

Pharmacologic Treatment

- No medical treatment is available to prevent, stabilize, or reverse posterior capsular lens opacities
- An early fibrinous inflammatory reaction on the anterior surface of the lens implant usually responds well to 1% corticosteroid solutions given topically, one drop every 2–4 hours daily.

Nonpharmacologic Treatment

Neodymium:Yttrium-Aluminum-Garnet (Nd:YAG) Laser

Other Treatments

- *Surgical incision of posterior capsule*: rarely performed since the advent of Nd:YAG laser treatment.

After Cataract

◈ *A K Khurana 6th/214-15*

- It is ***also known as 'secondary cataract'***. It is the opacity which persists or develops ***after extracapsular lens extraction.***
- *Clinical types.* After cataract may present as thickened posterior capsule, or dense membranous after cataract or *Soemmering's ring* which refers to a thick ring of after cataract formed behind the iris, enclosed between the two layers of capsule or *Elschnig's pearls* in which the vacuolated subcapsular epithelial cells are clustered like soap bubbles along the posterior capsule
- ***Treatment* is as follows:**
  - Thin membranous after cataract and thickened posterior capsule are ***best treated by YAG-laser capsulotomy or discission with cystitome or Zeigler's knife.***
  - Dense membranous after cataract needs surgical membranectomy.
  - Soemmering's ring after cataract with clean central posterior capsule needs no treatment.
  - Elschnig's pearls involving the central part of the posterior capsule can be treated by YAGlaser capsulotomy or discission with cystitome.

Complicated Cataract

◈ *Parson 22nd/268*

- In inflammations or degenerations affecting the posterior segment a *characteristic opacification usually commences in the posterior part of the cortex in the axial region* (***posterior cortical cataract*** **or** ***posterior subcapsular cataract***).
- Ophthalmoscopically, it appears as a vaguely defined, dark area and with the slit-lamp the opacity is seen to have irregular borders extending diffusely towards the equator and often axially forwards towards the nucleus.

ENT

125. Ans. a. Lichen planus, b. Erythroplekia

[Ref: Dhingra 6th/224-25; L and B 26th/707; Logan and Turner 10th /126; ENT by Hazarika 3rd/502; Neena Khanna 5th/387]

Premalignant Lesion for Oral Cavity Cancer

◈ *Dhingra 6th/224-25; Hazarika 3rd/502*

- ***Leukoplakia*** ("white patch") is induced by the same factors (tobacco, alcohol) that cause carcinomas. The ***malignant potential of leukoplakia corresponds to the degree of cellular dysplasia seen on biopsy.***
- ***Erythroplakia*** ("red patch") usually shows severe cellular dysplasia and carries a ***50% risk of malignant degeneration***
- ***Melanosis and mucosal hyperpigmentation:*** *may transform into malignant melanoma*
- ***Submucous fibrosis***
- Lichen planus

"**Bowen disease (squamous cell carcinoma in situ)** is a form of intraepidermal carcinoma, a malignant tumor of keratinocytes. Bowen disease may ultimately ***progress to an invasive squamous cell carcinoma***"- *Neena Khanna 5th/387; emedicine.medscape.com*

"**Behchets *syndrome (Oculo-oro-genital syndrome)*:** *It is characterized by a triad of aphthous-like ulcer in oral cavity, genital ulceration and uveitis*"- *Dhingra 6th/218*

126. Ans. a. Vegetable foreign bodies are not common, b. Tracheal obstruction can causes sudden death, e. CT scan of chest is done in all cases.

[Ref: Dhingra 6th/321-23; ENT by Maqbool 11th/344-48; ENT by Hazarika 3rd/651]

Foreign Bodies of Air Passages

◈ *Dhingra 6th/321-23*

- *Children are more often affected;* ***more than half of them are below 4 yr of age***
- *"Most foreign bodies enter the* ***right bronchus*** *because it is wider and more in line with the tracheal lumen"- Dhingra 6th/321; ENT by Maqbool 11th/344*

Foreign Body Aspiration

◈ *O.P.Ghai 8th/391*

- *"Foreign bodies most commonly* ***aspirated are food and coins****"-O.P.Ghai 8th/369*
- ***Young children b/w 1 and 4 yr*** *of age are especially prone to aspirate small object*

Investigation for Foreign Bodies

◈ *ENT by Maqbool 11th/345*

- ***X-rays of the chest are of great help***
- ***Bronchoscopy may be done as diagnostic investigation*** *and as a therapeutic procedure in cases where X-rays are not helpful but the history is suggestive*
- *Fluoroscopy/videofluoroscopy*
- ***CT chest***

Table *(Dhingra 6th/321)*: **Symptoms and signs of foreign bodies at different levels**

Site of foreign bodies	Symptoms and signs
Larynx	• ***Complete obstruction leading to death*** • Partial obstruction: stridor, hoarseness, cough, respiratory difficulty
Trachea	• ***Choking, stridor, wheeze, cough, palpatory thud, audible slap***
Bronchi	• Cough, wheeze and diminished air entry to lung forms a "triad" • Respiratory distress with swelling of foreign body • Lung collapse, emphysema, pneumonitis, bronchiectasis or lung abscess are late features

127. Ans. a. Facies leonina, c. Saddle nose, d. Lagophthalmos

[Ref: Park 24th/345; Dhingra 6th/157; Neena Khanna 5th/280]

Saddle nose: *Sometime occur due to* **leprosy**,*tuberculosisor syphilis"-P.L.Dhingra 6th/143*

Table *(Park 24th/345)*: **Deformities occurring in leprosy**

Face	Mask face, ***facies leonina***, sagging face, ***lagophthalmos***, loss of eyebrows (superciliary madarosis) and eyelashes (ciliary madarosis), corneal ulcer and opacities, perforated nose, depressed nose, ear deformities, e.g. nodules on the ear and elongated lobules.
Hands	Claw hand, wrist-drop, ulcers, absorption of digits thumb-web contracture, hollowing of the interosseous spaces and swollen hand.
Feet	Plantar ulcers, foot–drop, inversion of the foot, clawing of the toes, absorption of the toes, collapsed foot, swollen foot and callosities.
Other deformities	Gynaecomastia and perforation of the palate

"**Micrognathia** is a condition in which the jaw is undersized. It is a symptom of a variety of craniofacial conditions. Micrognathia can present as a birth defect in numerous syndromes, including *cleft lip, cleft palate, Pierre Robin sequence or syndrome, Stickler's syndrome, Beckwith-Wiedemann syndrome, hemifacial microsomia, Treacher-Collins syndrome and others*"- *www.chop.edu/conditions-disease*

"**Low-set ears** are ears with depressed positioning of the pinna two or more standard deviations below the population average. It can be associated with conditions such as:*Down's syndrome, Turner Syndrome, Noonan syndrome, Patau syndrome, DiGeorge syndrome, Cri du chat syndrome, Edwards syndrome, Fragile X syndrome etc*"-*wikipedia.org*

128. Ans. b. May cause CSF rhinorrhea

[Ref: Dhingra 6th/185; Logan and Turner 10th /27-28; Schwartz 10th/577]

Fracture of Zygoma is Called Tripod Fracture: *Dhingra 6th/183*
FRACTURES OF MAXILLA They are ***classified into three types***: *Dhingra 6th/185*

- **Le Fort I (transverse)** fracture runs above and parallel to the palate. It crosses lower part of nasal septum, maxillary antra and the pterygoid plates
- **Le Fort II (pyramidal)** fracture passes through the root of nose, lacrimal bone, floor of orbit, upper part of maxillary sinus and pterygoid plates. This fracture has some features common with the zygomatic fractures.
- **Le Fort III** (craniofacial dysjunction). There is ***complete separation of facial bones form the cranial bones***. The fracture line passes through root of nose, ethmofrontal junction, superior orbital fissure, lateral wall of orbit, frontozygomatic and temporozygomatic sutures and the upper part of pterygoid plates.

Clinical Features

◈ *Dhingra 6th/185*

- Malocclusion of teeth with anterior open bite
- Elongation of midface
- Mobility in the maxilla
- ***CSF rhinorrhea***. Cribriform plate is injured in Le Fort II and Le For III fractures.

Diagnosis

◈ *Dhingra 6th/185*

X-rays, helpful in diagnosis of maxillary fractures are Water's view, posteroanterior view, lateral view and the CT scans. They help to delineate fracture lines and the displacement of fragments.

Midface Fractures

◈ *Schwartz 10th/577*

- Midface fractures are classically described in three patterns: Le Fort I, II and III.
- **Le Fort I fractures** occur transversely across the alveolus, above the level of the teeth apices. In a pure Le Fort I fracture, the palatal vault is mobile while the nasal pyramid and orbital rims are stable.
- **The Le Fort II fracture** extends through the nasofrontal buttress, medial wall of the orbit, across the infraorbital rim and through the zygomaticomaxillary articulation. The nasal dorsum, palate and medial part of the infraorbital rim are mobile.
- **The Le Fort III fracture** is also known as ***craniofacial disjunction***. The frontozygomaticomaxillary, frontomaxillary and frontonasal suture lines are disrupted. The entire face is mobile from the cranium. It is convenient to conceptualize complex midface fractures according to these patterns; however, in reality, fractures reflect a combination of these three types.

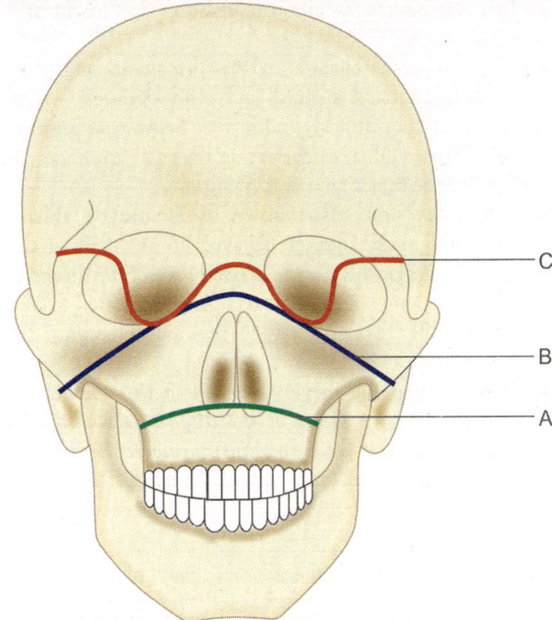

Fig *(Dhingra 6th/185)*: Fracture of maxilla (A) Le Fort I, (B) Le Fort II and (C) Le Fort III

129. Ans. b. Indication for surgery, c. More common during pregnancy, d. Reddish hue over the promontory, e. Seen in the early stages of the otosclerosis

[Ref: Dhingra 6th/450; ENT by Hazarika 3rd/179; Ballenger's Otorhinolaryngology 16th/318]

"**Schwartze's sign**, a ***reddish hue over the promontory*** caused by increased vascularity of the bone immediately under the periosteum, may be ***seen in the early stages of the disease*** but is not present in all patients"- *Ballenger's Otorhinolaryngology 16th/318*

"**Schwartz sign** is a pink reflex, seen through intact tympanic membrane, in the area of oval window. It indicates ***active otosclerosis*** usually during pregnancy"- *Dhingra 6th/450*

Schwartz Sign

◈ *wiki*

It also known as Flemingo's pink sign, is a ***diagnostic indicator for otosclerosis***, a disease of the bones of the middle or inner ear. In clinical examination of the ear drum, ***increased vascularity of the promontory*** may be seen through the ear drum. This sign is ***known as Flemingo's flush sign or Schwartz's sign***. This ***indicates otospongiosis (active otosclerosis)***.

In about 10% of cases of otosclerosis, there is a redness of the promontory of the cochlea seen through the tympanic membrane due to prominent vascularity associated with an otospongiotic focus

◈ *www.ncbi.nlm.nih.gov*

- Otosclerosis is an ***otic capsule disorder*** that leads to progressive conductive and/or sensorineural hearing loss due to stapes footplate fixation and cochlear bone involvement.

- The disorder is bilateral in 70% of patients and it usually starts between the third and fifth decade. One of its characteristic clinical findings is **Schwartze sign** which refers to a reddish discoloration over the promontory seen beyond the intact tympanic membrane.
- **Schwartze sign, also known as Flemingo's flush sign or Rising sun sign** is believed to be associated with otospongiosis which is the ***active phase of the disease***.
- The prevalence of **Schwartze sign** is estimated to be 10%. The prevalence of bilateral sign has not been reported, but it is presumed to be too low.
- It seems that the ***surgery remains a therapeutic option, when the active phase of the disease is stabilized even following a short course of pharmacologic therapy***.

130. Ans. a. Stage T_{4a}- Frontal sinus involvement, b. Stage T_3- Ethmoid sinus involvement

[Ref: Dhingra 6th/208; Logan and Turner 10th /210; ENT by Hazarika 3rd/375]

Table *(Dhingra 6th/208)*: **TNM classification and staging system of cancer of maxillary sinus**

Maxillary Sinus	
T_1	Tumour limited to maxillary sinus mucosa with no erosion or destruction of bone.
T_2	Tumour causing bone erosion or destruction including extension into the hard palate and/or middle nasal meatus, except extension to posterior wall of maxillary sinus and pterygoid plates
T_3	Tumour invades any of the following: ***bone of the posterior wall of maxillary sinus***, subcutaneous tissues, floor or medial wall of orbit, pterygoid fossa and ***ethmoid sinuses.***
T_{4a}	Tumour invades anterior orbital contents, skin of cheek, pterygoid plates, infratemporal fossa, cribriform plate, ***sphenoid or frontal sinuses.***
T_{4b}	Tumour invades any of the following: orbital apex, dura, brain, middle cranial fossa, cranial nerves other than maxillary division of trigeminal nerve (V_2), nasopharynx or clivus.

Maxillary sinus primary tumor (T) American joint committee on cancer Atlas 2006/55-56

- **TX** Primary tumor cannot be assessed
- T_0 No evidence of primary tumor
- **Tis** Carcinoma *in situ*
- T_1 Tumor limited to the maxillary sinus mucosa with no erosion or destruction of bone
- T_2 Tumor causing bone erosion or destruction including extension into the hard palate and/or middle nasal meatus, except extension to posterior wall of maxillary sinus and pterygoid plates
- T_3 Tumor invades any of the following: bone of the posterior wall of maxillary sinus, subcutaneous tissues, floor or medial wall of orbit, pterygoid fossa, ethmoid sinuses
- T_{4a} Tumor invades anterior orbital contents, skin of cheek, pterygoid plates, infratemporal fossa, cribriform plate, sphenoid or frontal sinuses
- T_{4b} Tumor invades any of the following: orbital apex, dura, brain, middle cranial fossa, cranial nerves other than maxillary division of trigeminal nerve V2, nasopharynx, or clivus

131. Ans. c. Chronic suppurative otitis media, d. Agenesis of cochlear nerve

[Ref: Ballenger's Otorhinolaryngology 16th/476-83; Dhingra 6th/124-26; Logan and Turner 10th /327; ENT by Hazarika 3rd/89]

"Mondini deformity refers to the absence of the apical modiolus and interscalar septum, resulting in an incomplete partitioning of the cochlea together with an enlarged vestibular aqueduct (EVA) and dilated vestibule.It was first described in 1791 by Carlo Mondini after dissecting the inner ear of an 8-year-old deaf boy.***Cochlear implantation has been described as an effective tool*** for treating sensorineural hearing loss due to incomplete partitioning"-*emedicine.medscape.com*

"The use of ***cochlear implantation to treat patients with inner ear malformations such as Mondini dysplasia*** has been increasingly successful"- *www.ncbi.nlm.nih.go*

Table *(www.researchgate.net)*: ***Contraindications for the cochlear implantation***

Absolute	Relative
Agenesia of Cochlea	Inappropiate medical conditions (e.g. pulmonary, cardiac, hematologic)
Agenesia of Cochlear Nerve	Uncontrolled epilepsy
Severe mental disease	Not being available for postoperative rehabilition
Acute/chronic otitis media and mastoiditis without eradication of the disease	
Mental retardation to cooperate with speech training	

Cochlear Implantation

◈ *Ballenger's Otorhinolaryngology 16th/476-83*

- ***Intracochlear ossification is not a contraindication to cochlear implantation*** but can limit the type and insertion depth of the electrode array that can be introduced into the cochlea.
- ***Congenital malformations of the cochlea are likewise not contraindications to cochlear implantation.***
- When an effusion occurs in an ear with a cochlear implant, no treatment is required as long as the effusion remains uninfected. ***Chronic otitis media, with or without cholesteatoma, must be resolved before implantation***; this is accomplished with conventional otologic treatments.
- **Prior ear surgery** that has resulted in a mastoid cavity ***does not contraindicate cochlear implantation***, but this situation may require mastoid obliteration with closure of the external auditory canal or reconstruction of the posterior bony ear canal

Table *(Ballenger 16th/479)*: **Pediatric Candidacy Criteria for Cochlear Implantation**

Children Aged 12 to 23 Mo	Children Aged 24 Mo to 17 Yr, 11 Mo
Bilateral profound hearing loss	Bilateral severe-to-profound hearing loss
Lack of auditory skills development and minimal hearing aid benefit (documented by parent questionnaire)	Lack of auditory skills development and minimal hearing aid benefit (eg. Word recognition scores < 30% correct)
No medical contraindications	No medical contraindications
Enrolment in a therapy of education program emphasizing auditory development	Enrolment in a therapy of education program emphasizing auditory development

Contraindications

◈ *emedicine.medscape.com*

- Contraindications to cochlear implantation may include ***deafness due to lesions of the eighth cranial nerve or brain stem***. In addition, ***chronic infections of the middle ear and mastoid cavity or tympanic membrane perforation can be contraindications***. The ***absence of cochlear development as demonstrated on CT scans remains an absolute contraindication***.

Certain medical conditions that preclude cochlear implant surgery (e.g., specific hematologic, pulmonary and cardiac conditions) also may be contraindications.

The lack of realistic expectations regarding the benefits of cochlear implantation and/or a lack of strong desire to develop enhanced oral communication skills poses a strong contraindication for implant surgery.

132. Ans. a. Cochlea start developing from 3rd week of gestation, c. Cochlea development completes by 20…

[Ref: Dhingra 6th/12; Logan and Turner 10th /410; Gray's 40th/651,633-34]

*"Development of phylogenetically older part of labyrinth-pars superior (**semicircular canals** and utricles) takes place earlier than pars inferior (saccule and **cochlear**)"- Dhingra 6th/12*

*Cochlea: **Development begins at 3rd week and complete by 20th week**- Dhingra 6th/12*

"6 week:The cochlea and semicircular canals start forming"- I.B.Singh Embryology 10th/374

***"Cochlea fully formed by the eleventh week"**- Logan and Turner 10th /410*

Table *(Dhingra 6th/12)*: **Timing of development of the ear in the week of gestation**

Development	Middle ear	Vestibular labyrinth	Cochlea
Begins	3rd	3rd	3rd
Complete	30th	20th	20th

MEDICINE

133. Ans. a. Age, b. Glasgow comma scale, c. FiO_2

[Ref: Harrison 19th/1729-30; Davidson 22nd/204]

Assessment of Illness Severity

◈ *Harrison 19th/1729-30*

- The most commonly utilized scoring systems are the APACHE (Acute Physiology and Chronic Health Evaluation) and the SAPS (Simplified Acute Physiology Score) systems.
- The **APACHE II system** is the most commonly used severity-of-illness (SOI) scoring system in North America.
- The **APACHE II score** is the ***sum of the acute physiology score (vital signs, oxygenation, laboratory values), the Glasgow coma score, age and chronic health points.*** The worst values during the first 24 h in the ICU should be used

Table *(Harrison 19th/1730)*: **Calculation of Acute Physiology and Chronic Health Evaluation II (APACHE II) Score**

Acute Physiology Score									
Score	4	3	2	1	0	1	2	3	4
Rectal temperature (°C)	≥41	39.0–40.9		38.5–38.9	36.0–38.4	34.0–35.9	32.0–33.9	30.0–31.9	≤29.9
Mean blood pressure (mmHg)	≥ 160	130–159	110–129		70–109		50–69		≤ 49
Heart rate (beats/min)	≥ 180	140–179	110–139		70–109		55–69	40–54	≤ 39
Respiratory rate (breaths/min)	≥ 50	35–49		25–34	12–24	10–11	6–9		
Arterial pH	≥ 7.70	7.60–7.69		7.50–7.59	7.33–7.49		7.25–7.32	7.15–7.24	≤ 7.15
Oxygenation If FiO_2 > 0.5, use $(A - 2) DO_2$ If $FiO_2 \leq 0.5$, use paO_2	≥ 500	350–499	200–349		<200 >70	61–70		55–60	<55

Contd...

Acute Physiology Score									
Score	**4**	**3**	**2**	**1**	**0**	**1**	**2**	**3**	**4**
Serum sodium (mEq/L)	≥ 180	160–179	155–159	150–154	130–149		120–129	111–119	≤ 110
Serum potassium (mEq/L)	≥ 7.0	6.0–6.9		5.5–5.9	3.5–5.4	3.0–3.4	2.5–2.9		<2.5
Serum creatinine (mg/dL)	≥ 3.5	2.0–3.4	1.5–1.9		0.6–1.4		<0.6		
Hematocrit (%)	≥ 60		50–59.9	46–49.9	30–45.9		20–29.9		<20
WBC count (10^3/mL)	≥ 40		20–39.9	15–199	3–14.9		1–2.9		<1
Glasgow Coma Score[a,b]									
Eye Opening		Verbal (Nonintubated)			Verbal intubated		Motor Activity		
4–Spontaneous		5–Oriented and talks			5–Seems able to talk		6–Verbal command		
3–Verbal Stimull		4–Disoriented and talks			3–Questionable ability to talk		5–Localizes to pain		
2–Painful stimull		3–Inappropriate words			1–Generally unresponsive		4–Withdraws from pain		
1–No response		2–Incomprehensible sounds					3–Decorticate		
		1–No response					2–Decerebrate		
							1–No response		
Points Assigned to Age and Chronic Disease									
Age, Years		Score							
<45		0							
45–54		2							
55–64		3							
65–74		5							
≥ 75		6							
Chronic Health (History of Chronic Conditions)[c]					**Score**				
None					0				
If patient is admitted after elective surgery					2				
If patient is admitted after emergency surgery or for reason other than after elective surgery					5				

*a*Glasgow coma score (GCS) = eye-opening score + verbal (intubated or nonintubated) score + motor score.

*b*For GCS component of acute physiology score, subtract GCS from 15 to obtain points assigned.

*c*Hepatic: cirrhosis with portal hypertension or encephalopathy; cardiovascular: class IV angina (at rest or with minimal self-care activities); pulmonary: chronic hypoxemia or hypercapnia, polycythemia, ventilator dependence; renal: chronic peritoneal or hemodialysis; immune: immunocompromised host.

Abbreviations: (A – a) DO_2, alveolar-arterial oxygen difference; FiO_2, *fraction of inspired oxygen*

A & E

134. Ans. a. Café-au-lait spots, c. Axillary freckling

[Ref: Harrison 19th/603; Davidson 22nd/1216]

Neurofibromatosis Type 1 (NF1) (von Recklinghausen's Disease)

◈ *Harrison 19th/603*

- NF1 is an autosomal dominant disorder
- Mutations of *NF1* result in a large number of nervous system tumors including neurofibromas, plexiform neurofibromas, *optic nerve gliomas*, astrocytomas and meningiomas.
- In addition to neurofibromas, which appear as multiple, soft, rubbery cutaneous tumors, other cutaneous manifestations of NF1 include ***cafe-au-lait spots and axillary freckling***.
- NF1 is also associated with hamartomas of the iris termed Lisch nodules, pheochromocytomas, pseudoarthrosis of the tibia, scoliosis, epilepsy and mental retardation.

Neurofibromatosis 1 and Neurofibromatosis 2: Clinical Feature

◈ *Davidson 22nd/1216*

Neurofibromatosis 1	Neurofibromatosis 2
Skin Cutaneous/subcutaneous neurofibromas Angiomas ***Café au lait patches (> 6)*** ***Axillary/groin freckling*** Hypopigmented patches	Much less commonly affected then NF1 Cafè au lait patches (usually <6) Cutaneous schwannomas: plaque lesions Subcutaneous schwannomas
Eyes Lisch nodules (iris fibromas) Glaucoma Congenital ptosis	***Cataracts*** Retinal hamartoma ***Optic nerve meningioma***
Nervous system Plexiform neurofibromas Malignant peripheral nerve sheath tumours Aqueduct stenosis Slight tonsillar descent Cognitive impairment Epilepsy	Vestibular schwannomas Cranial nerve schwannomas (not 1 and 2) Spinal schwannomas Peripheral nerve schwannomas Cranial meningiomas Spinal meningiomas Spinal/brainstem ependymomas Spinal/cranial astrocytoma
Bone Scoliosis Osteoporosis Pseudoarthrosis	
Cardiorespiratory systems Pulmonary stenosis Hypertension Renal artery stenosis Compression from neurofibroma causing restrictive lung defect	
Gastrointestinal system Gastrointestinal stromal tumour Dysplasia Duodenal carcinoid tumour	

135. Ans. c. Water-Hammer pulse- Aortic regurgitation, d. Pulsus parvus Et tardus -Aortic stenosis, e. Collapsing pulse- Aortic regurgitation

[Ref: Harrison 19th/1445-46; Kundu 4th/295-97; P.J.M 20th/40-42]

Different Types of Pulses

◈ *P.J.M 20th/40-42; Kundu 4th/295-97*

Pulse type	Condition
Anacrotic pulse	Aortic stenosis
Pulsus bisferiens	*Idiopathic hypertrophic subaortic stenosis;* ***Severe AR with mild AS***
Dicrotic pulse	Fever like typhoid fever, congestive cardiac failure, cardiac temponade, following open heart surgery
Pulsus parvus Et Tardus	Severe AS
Pulsus alternans	LVF, Toxic myocarditis, Paroxymal tachycardias
Pulsus paradoxus	SVC obstruction; Lung conditions- asthma,emphysema, airway obstruction; Cardiac- pericardial effusion, constrictive pericarditis, severe CCF
Pulsus bigeminus	A.V block, sinoatrial block with ventricular escape
Thready pulse	Shock especially cardiogenic
Waterhammer pulse (High volume collapsing pulse)	High output states like anaemia, beri-beri, thyrotoxicosis; Cardiac lesions- AR, PDA, Rupture of sinus of valsalva into the heart chambers, aortopulmonary window

Contd...

136. Ans. a. 2nd most common nosocomial infection in the intensive care unit, b. Colonization of the pharynx with bacteria is risk factor, c. Highest risk occur in the first 5 days, d. Gastric acid may play a role in protection against nosocomial pneumonias

[Ref: Harrison 19th/809-11; Davidson 22nd/685-86; CMDT 2016/272-75]

HAP (not VAP) is the second most common cause of infection among hospital inpatients

Ventilator-associated and hospital-acquired pneumonia *emedicine.medscape.com; ccforum.biomedcentral.com*

- "***VAP is the second most common nosocomial infection in the intensive care unit (ICU) and the most common in mechanically ventilated patients***"- *ccforum.biomedcentral.com*
- **Ventilator-associated pneumonia (VAP)** is pneumonia that ***develops 48 hours or longer after mechanical ventilation*** is given by means of an endotracheal tube or tracheostomy.
- **VAP** results from the ***invasion of the lower respiratory tract and lung parenchyma by microorganisms. Intubation compromises the integrity of the oropharynx and trachea and allows oral and gastric secretions to enter the lower airways***"- *emedicine.medscape.com*
- ***Risk for VAP is greatest during the first 5 days of mechanical ventilation***
- **Early onset VAP** is defined as pneumonia that ***occurs within 4 days*** and this is usually attributed to antibiotic sensitive pathogens whereas **late onset VAP** is more likely caused by multidrug resistant (MDR) bacteria and ***emerges after 4 days of intubation***
- Infectious bacteria obtain direct access to the lower respiratory tract via: (1) ***micro aspiration***, which can occur during intubation itself; (2) development of a biofilm laden with bacteria (typically Gram-negative bacteria and fungal species) within the endotracheal tube; (3) pooling and trickling of secretions around the cuff; and (4) impairment of mucociliary clearance of secretions with gravity dependence of mucus flow within the airways

VAP

◈ *www.ncbi.nlm.nih.gov*

- ***Pneumonia is the second most common nosocomial infection in critically ill patients, affecting 27% of all critically ill patients***
- ***Eighty-six percent of nosocomial pneumonias are associated with mechanical ventilation and are termed ventilator-associated pneumonia (VAP)***
- **Ventilator-associated pneumonia** is defined as pneumonia ***occurring more than 48 h after patients*** have been intubated and received mechanical ventilation.
- Reasonable clinical criteria for the suspicion of VAP include a new and persistent (>48-h) or progressive radiographic infiltrate plus two of the following: temperature of >38°C or <36°C, blood leukocyte count of >10,000 cells/ml or <5,000 cells/ml, purulent tracheal secretions and gas exchange degradation

Nosocomial Pneumonia (Hospital-Acquired, Ventilator-Associated and Health Care–Associated)

◈ *CMDT 2016/272-75*

- **Hospital-acquired pneumonia (HAP)** occurs > 48 hours after admission to the hospital or other health care facility and excludes any infection present at the time of admission.
- **Health care–associated pneumonia (HCAP)** occurs in community members whose extensive contact with healthcare has changed their risk for virulent and drug resistant organisms.
- ***HAP is the second most common cause of infection among hospital inpatients*** and is the leading cause of death due to infection with mortality rates ranging from 20% to 50%-*CMDT 2016/273*
- HAP develops more than 48 hours after admission to the hospital and ***VAP develops in a mechanically ventilated patient more than 48 hours after endotracheal intubation.***
- Colonization of the pharynx and possibly the stomach with bacteria is the most important step in the pathogenesis of nosocomial pneumonia.
- ***Gastric acid may play a role in protection against nosocomial pneumonias***. Observational studies have suggested that ***elevation of gastric pH due to antacids, H2-receptor antagonists, proton pump inhibitors (PPIs), or enteral feeding is associated with gastric microbial overgrowth, tracheobronchial colonization and HAP/VAP.***

Ventilator-Associated Pneumonia

◈ *Harrison 19th/809-11*

- The frequency of diagnosis is not static but changes with the duration of mechanical ventilation, with the ***highest hazard ratio in the first 5 days*** and a plateau in additional cases (1% per day) after ~2 weeks.

Hospital-Acquired Pneumonia

◈ *Davidson 22nd/685-86*

- Hospital-acquired or nosocomial pneumonia is a new episode of pneumonia occurring ***at least 2 days after admission to hospital.***
- It is the ***second most common hospital-acquired infection (HAI)*** and the leading cause of HAI-associated death.

137. Ans. a. Tremors, b. Improvement seen with calcium supplementation, c. Athetoid movements, d. Seizure

[Ref: Harrison 19th/2461-62; Davidson 22nd/448]

"**Hypermagnesaemia**: Clinical features include ***bradycardia***, hypotension, *reduced consciousness* and respiratory depression"-*Davidson 22nd/448*

Hypomagnesemia

◈ *Harrison 19th/2461-62*

- Hypomagnesemia may cause generalized alterations in neuromuscular function, including tetany, ***tremor, seizures***, muscle weakness, ataxia, nystagmus, vertigo, apathy, depression, irritability, delirium and psychosis.
- Cardiac arrhythmias may occur, including ***sinus tachycardia***, other supraventricular tachycardias and ventricular arrhythmias.
- Other electrolyte abnormalities often seen with ***hypomagnesemia, including hypocalcemia (with hypocalciuria) and hypokalemia***, may not be easily corrected unless magnesium is administered as well. The hypocalcemia may be a result of concurrent vitamin D deficiency
- Mild, asymptomatic hypomagnesemia may be treated with oral magnesium salts ($MgCl_2$, MgO, $Mg[OH]_2$) in divided doses
- It is important to consider the need for ***calcium, potassium and phosphate supplementation in patients with hypomagnesemia.***
- Vitamin D deficiency frequently coexists and should be treated with ***oral or parenteral vitamin D or 25 (OH)D*** (but not with 1,25[OH]2D

Hypomagnesemia: Common symptoms are those of hypokalemia and hypocalcemia, with weakness and muscle cramps. Marked neuromuscular and central nervous system hyperirritability may produce *tremors*, ***athetoid movements***, *jerking, nystagmus, Babinski response, confusion, disorientation,tetany,*, seizures, muscle weakness, ataxia, vertigo, apathy,depression, irritability, delirium and psychosis"-*CMDT 2016/887*

138. Ans. a. a wave occur just after electrocardiographic P wave, b. Prominent x and y descents is seen in constrictive pericarditis, c. Canon a waves occur in atrioventricular (AV) dissociation, e. Prominent x descent but an absent y descent is seen in cardiac temponade

[Ref: Harrison 19th/1444,1573; Davidson 22nd/527]

"The three principal features of **cardiac tamponade** (*Beck's triad*) are hypotension, soft or absent heart sounds and jugular venous distention with a ***prominent x descent but an absent y descent***"-*Harrison 19th/1476*

"In **constrictive pericarditis**, the right and left atrial pressure pulses display an M-shaped contour, with **prominent *x* and *y* descents**. The *y* descent, which is absent or diminished in cardiac tamponade, is the most prominent deflection in constrictive pericarditis; it reflects rapid early filling of the ventricles"- *Harrison 19th/1476*

"The first peak is the **a-wave**, which immediately ***follows the p wave of the ECG waveform***. The a-wave is a pressure increase that is due to atrial contraction at end-diastole. Shortly after the a-wave there is a second peak, the **c-wave**. The c-wave immediately follows the r wave of the ECG waveform. This is a pressure increase due to tricuspid bulging into the atrium as a result of ***isovolumic ventricular contraction*** (IVC). Note that a and c-waves are split by the r wave of the ECG waveform. This is because the a-wave always represents end-diastole and the c-wave represents early ventricular systole"- www.openanesthesia.org

Jugular Venous Pressure and Waveform

◈ *Harrison 19th/1444*

- The ***a wave reflects right atrial presystolic contraction and occurs just after the electrocardiographic P wave***, preceding the first heart sound (S1).
- A **prominent *a* wave** is seen in patients with reduced right ventricular compliance; **a cannon *a* wave** occurs with ***atrioventricular (AV) dissociation and right atrial contraction against a closed tricuspid valve.***
- In a patient with a wide complex tachycardia, the appreciation of cannon *a* waves in the jugular venous waveform identifies the rhythm as ventricular in origin.
- The *a* wave is not present with atrial fibrillation.
- The ***x* descent** defines the fall in right atrial pressure after inscription of the *a* wave. The *c* wave interrupts this *x* descent and is followed by a further descent.
- The ***v* wave** represents ***atrial filling (atrial diastole)*** and ***occurs during ventricular systole***. In patients with TR, the *v* wave is accentuated and the subsequent fall in pressure (*y* descent) is rapid. With progressive degrees of TR, the *v* wave merges with the *c* wave and the right atrial and jugular vein waveforms become "ventricularized."
- The ***y* descent,** which follows the peak of the *v* wave, can become prolonged or blunted with obstruction to right ventricular inflow, as may occur with tricuspid stenosis or ***pericardial tamponade***.

Jugular Venous Pressure and Waveform

◈ *Davidson 22nd/527*

- In normal sinus rhythm, the two venous peaks, the *a* and *v* waves, approximate to atrial and ventricular systole respectively.
- The *x* descent reflects atrial relaxation and apical displacement of the tricuspid valve ring. The *y* descent reflects atrial emptying early in diastole. These signs are subtle.
- Tricuspid regurgitation produces giant *v* waves that coincide with ventricular systole.

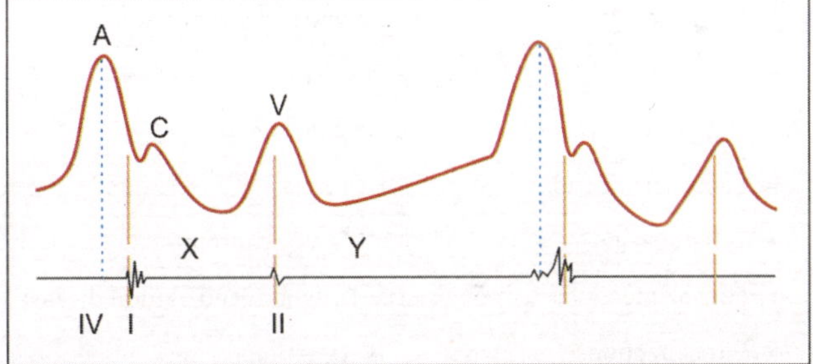

Fig: *(Harrison 19th/1444):* Jugular venous pulse wave tracing (*top*) with heart sounds (*bottom*)

Table: Central venous pressure Waveform components

Waveform Component	Phase of Cardiac Cycle	Mechanical Event
a wave	End diastole	Atrial contraction
c wave	Early systole	Tricuspid bulging (IVC)
v wave	Late systole	Systolic filling of the atrium
x descent	Mid systole	Atrial relaxation
y descent	Early diastole	Early ventricular filling

139. Ans. a. Hypercalcemia, b. Yellow skin, c. Anorexia, e. Papilledema and hepatomegaly

[Ref: Harrison 19th/96e-7; Davidson 22nd/127; Robbins 9th/438; CMDT 2016/1258]

Vitamin A Toxicity

◈ *Harrison 19th/96e-7*

- Acute toxicity is manifested by ***increased intracranial pressure, vertigo, diplopia, bulging fontanels (in children), seizures and exfoliative dermatitis***; it may result in death.
- Among children being treated for vitamin A deficiency according to the protocols outlined above, ***transient bulging of fontanels*** occurs in 2% of infants and ***transient nausea, vomiting and headache*** occur in 5% of preschoolers.
- **Chronic vitamin A intoxication**:Manifestations include ***dry skin, cheilosis, glossitis, vomiting, alopecia, bone demineralization and pain, hypercalcemia, lymph node enlargement, hyperlipidemia, amenorrhea and features of pseudotumor cerebri with increased intracranial pressure and papilledema. Liver fibrosis with portal hypertension and bone demineralization*** may result from chronic vitamin A intoxication.
- ***Carotenemia, which is characterized by a yellowing of the skin (in creases of the palms and soles) but not the sclerae, may follow ingestion of >30 mg of β-carotene daily.***

Vitamin A Toxicity

◈ *Robbins 9th/438*

- The symptoms of acute vitamin A toxicity include ***headache, dizziness, vomiting, stupor and blurred vision***, symptoms that may be confused with those of a brain tumor (*pseudotumor cerebri*).
- **Chronic toxicity** is associated with ***weight loss, anorexia, nausea, vomiting and bone and joint pain.***

Hypervitaminosis A

◈ *CMDT 2016/1258*

- Early manifestations include dry, scaly skin, hair loss, mouth sores, painful hyperostoses, anorexia and vomiting.
- More serious findings include ***hypercalcemia***; increased intracranial pressure, with papilledema, headaches and decreased cognition; and ***hepatomegaly***, occasionally progressing to cirrhosis. Excessive vitamin A has also recently been related to increased risk of hip fracture.
- Acute toxicity can result from ingestion of massive doses of vitamin A, such as in drug overdoses or consumption of polar bear liver. Manifestations include nausea, vomiting, abdominal pain, headache, ***papilledema*** and lethargy.

140. Ans. a. Disease onset is earlier with female predominance, b. Neck and facial muscle weakness are more common, c. More proximal muscle involvement, e. Poor response with acetylcholine esterase (AChE) inhibitors

[Ref: Harrison 19th/2701-03; Davidson 22nd/1226; CMDT 2016/1028; onlinelibrary.wiley.com]

Anti-MuSK Antibody

◈ *onlinelibrary.wiley.com*

- MG patients with anti-MuSK have atypical clinical features, such as ***selective facial, bulbar, neck or respiratory muscle weaknesses with occasional marked muscle atrophy, with relative sparing of the ocular muscles.***
- Respiratory crises are more common with involvement of muscle groups like paraspinal and upper esophageal muscles.
- Enhanced sensitivity, non-responsiveness or even clinically adverse reactions to anticholinesterase medications have also been reported.
- ***Disease onset is earlier with female predominance and thymus histology is usually normal.***
- The immune response in MuSK MG patients is dominated by immunoglobulin G (IgG)4 autoantibodies, instead of IgG1 or IgG3, as observed in AChR MG patients
- ***Anti-MuSK antibody occurs in about 40% of patients without AChR antibody***"- *Harrison 19th/2701*

"Certain patients without antibodies to acetylcholine receptors have serum antibodies to muscle-specific tyrosine kinase (MuSK), which should therefore be determined; these patients ***are more likely to have facial, respiratory and proximal muscle weakness*** than those with antibodies to acetylcholine receptors"-*CMDT 2016/1028*

Anti-MuSK Antibody

◈ *emedicine.medscape.com*

- About half of the patients with negative results for anti-AChR Ab (seronegative MG) may have positive test results for antibody to muscle-specific kinase (MuSK), a receptor tyrosine kinase that is essential for neuromuscular junction development. These patients may represent a distinct group of autoimmune MG, in that they show some collective characteristics that are different from those of anti-AChR–positive patients.
- Anti-MuSK–positive individuals tend to have ***more pronounced bulbar weakness and may have tongue and facial atrophy.*** They may have ***neck, shoulder and respiratory involvement without ocular weakness.***
- ***They are also less likely to respond to acetylcholine esterase (AChE) inhibitors and their symptoms may actually worsen with these medications***

Diagnosis of Myasthenia Gravis (MG)

◈ *Harrison 19th/2702*

History

- Diplopia, ptosis, dysarthria, dysphagia, dyspnea
- Weakness in characteristic distribution: ***proximal limbs***, neck extensors, generalized
- Fluctuation and fatigue: worse with repeated activity, improved by rest
- Effects of previous treatments

Physical Examination

- Ptosis, diplopia
- Motor power survey: quantitative testing of muscle strength
- Forward arm abduction time (5 min)
- Vital capacity measurement
- Absence of other neurologic signs

Laboratory Testing

- **Anti-AChR radioimmunoassay:** ~85% positive in generalized MG; 50% in ocular MG; definite diagnosis if positive; negative result does not exclude MG; ~40% of AChR antibody–negative patients with generalized MG have anti-MuSK antibodies
- **Repetitive nerve stimulation:** decrement of >15% at 3 Hz: highly probable
- **Single-fiber electromyography:** blocking and jitter, with normal fiber density; confirmatory, but not specific
- Edrophonium chloride (EnlonR) 2 mg + 8 mg IV; highly probable diagnosis if unequivocally positive
- **For ocular or cranial MG:** Exclude intracranial lesions by CT or MRI

141. Ans. a. Cirrhosis, e. Congestive heart failure

[Ref: Harrison 19th/1718; Robbins 9th/722; CMDT 2016/310]

"**Parapneumonic effusions** are associated with ***bacterial pneumonia***, lung abscess, or bronchiectasis and are probably the most common cause of ***exudative pleural effusion*** in the United States"-*Harrison 19th/1717*

Table *(Harrison 19th/1718)*: **Differential diagnoses of pleural effusions**

Transudative Pleural Effusions	
Congestive heart failure	Peritoneal dialysis
Cirrhosis	Superior vena cava obstruction (!! It is removed in 19th edition)
Pulmonary embolization	*Myxedema*
Nephrotic syndrome	*Urinothorax*
Exudative Pleural Effusion	
1. Neoplastic diseases	6. Post-coronary artery bypass surgery
▪ Metastatic Disease	7. Yellow nail syndrome
▪ Mesothelioma	8. Asbestos exposure
2. Infectious diseases	9. Sarcoidosis
▪ Bacterial infections	10. Uremia
▪ Tuberculosis	11. Meigs' syndrome
▪ Fungal infections	***12. Drug-induced pleural disease***
▪ Viral infections	▪ Dasatinib

Contd...

▪ Parasitic infections	▪ Nitrofurantoin
3. Pulmonary embolization	▪ Dantrolene
4. Gastrointestinal disease	▪ Methysergide
▪ Esophageal perforation	▪ Bromocriptine
▪ Pancreatic disease	▪ Procarbazine
▪ Intraabdominal abscesses	▪ Amiodarone
▪ Diaphragmatic hernia	13. Hemothorax
▪ After abdominal surgery	14. Trapped lung
▪ Endoscopic variceal Sclerotherapy	15. Radiation therapy
▪ After liver transplant	16. Post-cardiac injury syndrome
5. Collagen vascular diseases	17. Chylothorax
▪ Sjogren's syndrome	18. Iatrogenic injury
▪ Rheumatoid pleuritis	19. Ovarian hyperstimulation syndrome
▪ Systemic lupus Erythematosus	20. Pericardial disease
▪ Churg-Strauss syndrome	
▪ Drug-induced lupus	
▪ Immunoblastic Lymphadenopathy	
▪ Granulomatosis with polyangiitis (Wegener's)	

142. Ans. e. Hypertension

[Ref: Harrison 19th/2257; Oxford Textbook of Medicine 4th edition]

Pituitary Apoplexy

◈ *Harrison 19th/2257*

- Acute intrapituitary hemorrhagic vascular events can cause substantial damage to the pituitary and surrounding sellar structures.
- Pituitary apoplexy may occur spontaneously in a preexisting adenoma; postpartum (Sheehan's syndrome); or in association with diabetes, hypertension, sickle cell anemia, or acute shock. The hyperplastic enlargement of the pituitary, which occurs normally during pregnancy, increases the risk for hemorrhage and infarction.
- Apoplexy is an endocrine emergency that may result in ***severe hypoglycemia, hypotension and shock, central nervous system (CNS) hemorrhage and death.***
- Acute symptoms may include ***severe headache*** with signs of meningeal irritation, ***bilateral visual changes, ophthalmoplegia*** and, in severe cases, cardiovascular collapse and loss of consciousness.
- Pituitary computed tomography (CT) or MRI may reveal signs of intratumoral or sellar hemorrhage, with pituitary stalk deviation and compression of pituitary tissue.
- Visual recovery after sellar surgery is inversely correlated with the length of time after the acute event. Therefore, severe ophthalmoplegia or visual deficits are indications for early surgery. Hypopituitarism is common after apoplexy.

"Pituitary apoplexy is a rare but life-threatening disorder. Clinical presentation of this condition includes ***severe headaches, impaired consciousness, fever, visual disturbance and variable ocular paresis.*** The clinical presentation of meningeal irritation is very rare. Nonetheless, if present and associated with fever, pituitary apoplexy may be misdiagnosed as a meningitis"-www.ncbi.nlm.nih.go

Most common clinical presentation *Oxford Textbook of Medicine 4th edition*

- Sudden onset retro-orbital headache
- Visual field defect

Sometimes

- Nausea and vomiting
- Meningism
- Altered conscious level
- Diplopia

Also

- Compatible with hypopituitarism or hyperprolactinaemia: lethargy, reduced libido, oligomenorrhoea/ amenorrhoea, impotence, galactorrhoea

143. Ans. a. Hypoxemia, b. Hypercarbia, d. Acidosis

[Ref: Harrison 19th/1704-05; Robbins 9th/675; CMDT2016/258-60]

"**Hypercarbia** can accompany severe airway obstruction (e.g., COPD) or progressive restrictive physiology, as in patients with neuromuscular weakness"- *Harrison 19th/1663*

"**Emphysema (a component of COPD) is characterized by irreversible enlargement of the airspaces distal to the terminal bronchiole,** *accompanied by destruction of their walls without obvious fibrosis"- Robbins 9th/675*

COPD

◈ *Harrison 19th/1704-05*

- Accompanying worsening airflow obstruction is an increased frequency of exacerbations. Patients may also develop resting ***hypoxemia*** and require institution of supplemental oxygen
- Arterial blood gases and oximetry may demonstrate ***resting or exertional hypoxemia.***

COPD

◈ *CMDT2016/258-60*

- Arterial blood gas measurements characteristically show no abnormalities early in COPD other than an increased a–a–Do2. Indeed, they are unnecessary unless (1) ***hypoxemia or hypercapnia*** is suspected, (2) the FEV1 is < 40% of predicted, or (3) there are clinical signs of right heart failure.
- ***Hypoxemia occurs in advanced disease,*** particularly when chronic bronchitis predominates. ***Compensated respiratory acidosis*** occurs in patients with chronic respiratory failure, particularly in chronic bronchitis, with worsening of academia during acute exacerbations
- Most patients with COPD have features of both emphysema and chronic bronchitis.

- **Chronic bronchitis** is a clinical diagnosis defined by excessive secretion of bronchial mucus and is manifested by daily productive cough for 3 months or more in at least 2 consecutive years.
- **Emphysema** is a pathologic diagnosis that denotes abnormal permanent enlargement of air spaces distal to the terminal bronchiole, with destruction of their walls and without obvious fibrosis.

Table *(CMDT2016/258)*: **Patterns of disease in advanced COPD**

	Type A: Pink Puffer (Emphysema Predominant)	Type B: Blue Bloater (Bronchitis Predominant)
Laboratory studies	Hemoglobin usually normal (12–15 g/dL). PaO_2 normal to slightly reduced (65–75 mm Hg) but SaO_2 normal at rest. $PaCO_2$ normal to slightly reduced (35–40 mm Hg). Chest radiograph shows hyperinflation with flattened diaphragms. Vascular markings are diminished, particularly at the apices.	Hemoglobin usually elevated (15–18 g/dL). PaO_2 reduced (45–60 mm Hg) and $Paco_2$ slightly to markedly elevated (50–60 mm Hg). Chest radiograph shows increased interstitial markings ("dirty lungs"), especially at bases. Diaphragms are not flattened.
Pulmonary function tests	Airflow obstruction ubiquitous. Total lung capacity increased, sometimes markedly so. DICO reduced. Static lung compliance increased.	Airflow obstruction ubiquitous. Total lung capacity generally normal but may be slightly increased. DICO normal. Static lung compliance normal
(V/Q) matching	Increased ventilation to high (V/Q) areas, i.e, high dead space ventilation.	Increased perfusion to low (V/Q) areas

DICO, single-breath diffusing capacity for carbon monoxide; (V)

SURGERY

144. Ans. b. Negative for DOG-1

[Ref: L and B 26th/1054; Sabiston 19th/1220; Schwartz 9th/1297; Nelson 20th/1903]

"Succinate dehydrogenase-deficient gastrointestinal stromal tumors (GISTs) demonstrate unique pathological and clinical features, including the absence of activating mutations of *KIT* and *PDGFRA* and primary resistance to imatinib. The great majority of pediatric GISTs and all the GISTs that occur in Carney Triad (the non-familial association of gastric GIST, pulmonary chondroma and extra-adrenal paraganglioma) and Carney–Stratakis Syndrome (the familial association of GIST and paraganglioma) represent specific examples of SDH-deficient GISTs"-www.nature.com/modpathol

"Histologically, SDH-deficient GISTs are typically composed of multiple tumor islands of epithelioid tumor cells spaced by muscularis propria elements. Lymphovascular invasion and lymph node metastases occur almost exclusively in these GISTs. Immunohistochemically diagnostic is loss of SDHB in tumor cells in all cases, whereas loss of SDHA is specific to examples with loss of SDHA. Similar to KIT-mutant GISTs, SDH-deficient GISTs also ***strongly express KIT and DOG1/Ano-1*** and usually also CD34, ***but these GISTs do not have KIT or PDGFRA mutations***. Their genetic basis includes loss of function in SDH subunit genes (most commonly SDHA) and possibly epigenetic silencing and genomic methylation is a typical feature of SDH-deficient GISTs. Succinate dehydrogenase–deficient GISTs should be specifically recognized, as these tumors may not respond to the standard KIT tyrosine kinase inhibitors, such as imatinib mesylate, in contrast to KIT-mutant GISTs- journals.lww.com

Clinical and Morphological Features of Sdh-Deficient Gists

◈ *www.ncbi.nlm.nih.gov*

- SDH-deficient GISTs account for 5% to 7.5% of all unselected GISTs.
- These tumors have a tendency to appear in ***children and young adults.*** Nearly all gastric GISTs patients < 18 years old and a substantial percentage of patients < 30 years old belonged to this group. However, the older adult patients rarely displayed an SDH-deficient pattern.
- ***SDH-deficient GISTs occur exclusively in the stomach*** and although any part of the stomach can be involved, there is some predilection to the distal stomach and antrum.
- **Carney's triad,** which is commonly found in girls and young women, is a rare non-heritable syndrome consisting of gastric GIST, paraganglioma and pulmonary chondroma. ***KIT or PDGFRA mutations were undetectable in GISTs associated with Carney's triad,*** although the loss of expression of *SDHB* can be observed within the tumors.
- **Carney-Stratakis syndrome** is characterized by the development of gastric GISTs and paragangliomas. Unlike Carney's triad, it is inherited in an autosomal dominant manner and affects both men and women. These tumors also lack *KIT* and *PDGFRA* mutations and have been proven to be ***SDH-deficient***, according to immunohistochemical staining results, which indicates defects in SDHB.
- Pediatric GISTs, which account for 1% to 2% of GISTs, often occur in young girls. The majority of pediatric GISTs, despite showing strong KIT immunoreactivity, ***lack KIT and PDGFRA mutations*** and display a characteristic similar to GISTs associated with Carney triad and Carney-Stratakis syndrome patients

SDH-Deficient GISTs

◈ *www.nature.com/modpathol*

- Approximately half of all wild-type GISTs show loss of respiratory chain complex II enzymatic activity. This complex comprises four subunits ***(SDHA, SDHB, SDHC and SDHD)*** and serves to oxidize succinate to fumarate as part of the mitochondrial Krebs cycle.

- Germline mutations in *SDHA*, *SDHB*, or *SDHC* increase the risk not only for the development of one or more SDH-deficient GISTs but also for ***paragangliomas (Carney-Stratakis syndrome).***
- ***GISTs that arise in pediatric patients*** (~1–2% of all GISTs) are predominantly SDHB immunonegative, but rarely harbor an *SDH* gene mutation. These tumors, which often metastasize but tend to grow slowly, have a different gene expression signature from ***KIT/PDGFRA-mutant GISTs.***

145. Ans. a. Associated with H.pylori infection, c. Endoscopic ultrasound is performed to determine the depth of gastric wall invasion, d. Second most common tumor of stomach, e. Diagnosis is made on basis of endoscopic biopsy

[Ref: L and B 26th/1054; Sabiston 19th/1218-20; Schwartz 10th/1084]

Gastric Lymphoma

◈ *CSDT 14th/537*

- Lymphoma is the ***second-most common primary cancer of the stomach*** but constitutes only 2% of the total number, 95% being adenocarcinomas.
- ***Almost all are non-Hodgkin lymphomas*** and are generally classified as B cell mucosaassociated lymphoid tissue (MALT) lymphomas. About 20% of patients manifest a second primary cancer in another organ.

"*About 85% of stomach cancers are adenocarcinomas, with 15% due to lymphomas, gastrointestinal stromal tumors (GISTs) and leiomyosarcomas.*Primary lymphoma of the stomach is relatively uncommon, accounting for <15% of gastric malignancies and ~2% of all lymphomas. The ***stomach is, however, the most frequent extranodal site for lymphoma***"-*Harrison 19th/534-35*

"***Like gastric adenocarcinoma, infection with H. pylori increases the risk for gastric lymphoma in general and MALT lymphomas in particular***"-*Harrison 19th/536*

◈ *Schwartz 10th/1084*

- Gastric lymphomas generally account for about 4% of gastric malignancies. ***Over half of patients with non-Hodgkin's lymphoma have involvement of the GI tract.***
- The stomach is the most common site of primary GI lymphoma a***nd over 95% are non- Hodgkin's type.*** Most are B-cell type, thought to arise in mucosa associated lymphoid tissue (MALT), although most high-grade gastric lymphomas are without any characteristics of the low grade MALT neoplasm.
- In populations with a high incidence of gastric lymphoma, there is a ***high incidence of H. pylori infection***; patients with gastric lymphoma also usually have *H. pylori* infection

Primary Gastric Lymphoma

◈ *L and B 26th/1054*

- At an early stage, the disease takes the form of a diffuse mucosal thickening, which may ulcerate. ***Diagnosis is made as a result of the endoscopic biopsy*** and seldom on the basis of the endoscopic features alone, which are not specific.
- Some of the more controversial aspects of gastric lymphoma concern the role of ***H. pylori.*** It has also been shown that ***early gastric lymphomas may regress and disappear when the Helicobacter infection is treated.***

Gastric Lymphoma

◈ *Sabiston 19th/1218-20*

- The stomach is the ***most common site of lymphomas in the GI system.*** However, primary gastric lymphoma is still relatively uncommon, ***accounting for less than 15% of gastric*** malignancies and 2% of lymphomas.
- Patients often present with vague symptoms, namely epigastric pain, early satiety and fatigue. Constitutional B symptoms are very rare.
- ***The most common gastric lymphoma is diffuse large B-cell lymphoma*** (55%), followed by extranodal marginal cell lymphoma (MALT) (40%), Burkitt's lymphoma (3%) and mantle cell and follicular lymphomas (each <1%).
- Immunodeficiencies and ***H. pylori* infection** are risk factors for the development of primary diffuse large B-cell lymphoma.
- ***Endoscopic ultrasound is useful to determine the depth of gastric wall invasion***, specifically to identify patients at risk for perforation secondary to full-thickness involvement of the gastric wall.

146. Ans. c. More common in women of >50 year of age

[Ref: Schwartz 10th/515-25; CSDT 14th/314; academic.oup.com]

"Bilateral breast cancer has an overall incidence of 4–20% in patients with primary operable breast cancer. The risk factors associated with bilateral occurrence are: ***familial or hereditary breast cancer, young age at primary breast cancer diagnosis, lobular invasive carcinoma, multicentricity and radiation exposure.***

Contralateral breast cancer is either a metastatic lesion or the second primary cancer and occurs either ***synchronously or metachronously***"- *academic.oup.com*

Bilateral Breast Cancer

◈ *CSDT 14th/314*

- ***Bilateral breast cancer occurs in less than 5% of cases***, but there is as ***high as a 20%-25% incidence of later occurrence of cancer in the second breast.***
- Bilaterality occurs more often in ***familial breast cancer, in women under age 50 years and when the tumor in the primary breast is lobular.***
- The incidence of second breast cancers increases directly with the length of time the patient is alive after her first cancer—about 1%-2% per year.

"Bilateral breast cancer was defined as **synchronous** when ***contralateral cancer was identified within 6 months after the first breast cancer.*** Contralateral breast cancer, diagnosed with the interval of ***more than 6 months***, was defined as **metachronous** bilateral breast cancer"

"It is estimated that 5 to 10% of all breast cancers are hereditary, half of which are related to a germ-line mutation in BRCA1 or BRCA2. ***Women with BRCA mutations are at risk for bilateral breast cancer*** and bilateral disease increases the likelihood of identifying a mutation"-medind.nic.in/ici

"***LCIS occurs bilaterally in 50% to 70% of cases, whereas DCIS occurs bilaterally in 10% to 20% of cases.*** Invasive lobular carcinoma accounts for 10% of breast cancers. It is frequently multifocal, multicentric and bilateral"- *Schwartz 10th/519,522*

Breast Cancer

◈ *Schwartz 10th/515*

- *BRCA1*-associated breast cancers have a number of distinguishing clinical features, such as an early age of onset compared with sporadic cases and a ***higher prevalence of bilateral breast cancer***
- ***BRCA2*-associated breast** cancer has a number of distinguishing clinical features, such as an early age of onset compared with sporadic cases and a higher prevalence of ***bilateral breast cancer***

Table *(Schwartz 10th/520)*: **Salient characteristics on in situ ductal (DCIS) and lobular (LCIS) carcinoma of the breast**

	LCIS	DCIS
Incidence of synchronous invasive carcinoma	5%	2%–46%
Multicentricity	60%–90%	40%–80%
Bilaterality	50%–70%	10%–20%
Axillary metastasis	1%	1%–2%
Subsequent carcinomas:		
Incidence	25% –35%	25%–70%
Laterality	Bilateral	Ipsilateral

147. Ans. c. 24-hour pH recording and electrical impedance measurement

[Ref: L and B 26th/989-90,996; Manipal 4th/433; CSDT 14th/458]

"Prolonged measurement of pH is now accepted as the most accurate method for the diagnosis of gastro-oesophageal reflux. In the last few years, the introduction of catheter assemblies that incorporate multiple electrodes along the length of the catheter as well as a pH probe has resulted in ***combined measurement of pH and electrical impedance.*** Impedance measurement differentiates antegrade from retrograde bolus transit, gas from liquid and provides a reliable measure of non-acid or weakly acidic events that cause symptoms. This may be important in the ***identification of patients with non-erosive reflux disease on endoscopy***"-*L and B 26th/989*

Diagnostic Measurement in GORD

◈ *L and B 26th/996*

- ***24-hour pH recording is the 'gold standard' for diagnosis of GORD***
- TLOSRs (transient lower oesophageal sphincter relaxations) are the most important manometric findings in GORD
- The length and pressure of the LOS are also important

Gastroesophageal Reflux Disease (GERD)

◈ *Harrison 19th/1894*

- **Endoscopy** is a sensitive test for diagnosis of esophagitis, but will miss nonerosive reflux disease (NERD) because some patients have symptomatic reflux without esophagitis.
- The ***most sensitive test for diagnosis of GERD is 24-h ambulatory pH monitoring.***

GERD

◈ *Investigation Manipal 4th/433*

- *Barium swallow can demonstrate the reverse flow of barium into the lower end of the oesophagus (from the stomach)*
- *Oesophagoscopy*
- *Oesophageal manometry to detect motility disorder*
- ***24-hour pH monitoring is gold standard***

Ambulatory 24-Hour pH Monitoring

◈ *CSDT 14th/458*

- This test measures reflux of acid from the stomach into the esophagus and it ***is considered the gold standard for the diagnosis of GERD.***
- **Esophageal impedance** is a technique that measures flow of liquids and gas across the gastroesophageal junction, independently of the pH of the gastric refluxate. In ***association with pH monitoring, impedance*** is indicated in patients with proton pump inhibitors (PPIs)—resistant typical reflux symptoms and chronic unexplained cough.

Upper Gastrointestinal Series

◈ *CSDT 14th/458*

- The upper gastrointestinal series test is performed by giving the patient barium to swallow.
- This test ***characterizes a hiatal hernia, an esophageal stricture, an esophageal diverticulum, or an intraluminal mass.***

Upper Endoscopy

◈ *CSDT 14th/458*

- This test allows visualization of the mucosal surface of the esophagus, the stomach and the duodenum.
- The presence and degree of ***esophagitis and the presence of an intraluminal mass*** can be determined and biopsies taken.

Esophageal Manometry

◈ *CSDT 14th/458*

- Esophageal manometry allows determination of: (1) ***LES location, length, pressure and relaxation in response to swallowing***; (2) pressure, duration and velocity of propagation of the peristaltic waves; and (3) location, pressure, relaxation of the UES and coordination with the pharyngeal contraction.

148. Ans. a. Both diarrhea and constipation may present, b. Nausea and vomiting usually present, c. Pain on internal rotation of flexed hip, e. Initially pain is located in the periumbilical region

[Ref: L and B 26th/1202-05; Sabiston 19th/1280; Harrison 19th/1987]

Acute appendicitis: Physical Examination

◈ *Sabiston 19th/1280*

- The exact location of the tenderness is directly over the appendix, which is most commonly at **McBurney's point** (located one third of the distance along a line drawn from the anterior superior iliac spine to the umbilicus).
- Any movement, including coughing (*Dunphy's sign*), may cause increased pain. Other findings may include pain in

the right lower quadrant during palpation of the left lower quadrant (*Rovsing's sign*), ***pain on internal rotation of the hip (obturator sign, suggesting a pelvic appendix) and pain on extension of the right hip (iliopsoas sign, typical of a retrocecal appendix).***

Table *(Harrison 19th/1987)*: **Relative Frequency of Common Presenting Symptoms**

Symptoms	Frequency
Abdominal pain	>95%
Anorexia	>70%
Constipation	4–16%
Diarrhea	4–16%
Fever	10–20%
Migration of pain to right lower quadrant	50–60%
Nausea	>65%
Vomiting	50–75%

Table *(Harrison 19th/1987)*: **Classic Signs of Appendicitis in Patients with Abdominal pain**

Maneuver	Findings
Rovsing's sign	Palpating in the left lower quadrant causes pain in the right lower quadrant
Obturator sign	***Internal rotation of the hip*** causes pain, suggesting the possibility of an inflamed appendix located in the pelvis
Iliopsoas sign	***Extending the right hip*** causes pain along posterolateral back and hip, suggesting retrocecal appendicitis

"Typically, the illness begins with vague midabdominal or periumbilical discomfort followed by ***nausea, anorexia*** and indigestion. The pain is continuous but not severe, with occasional mild cramping. The patient may ***feel constipated or may vomit***. Importantly, within several hours of the onset of symptoms the pain shifts to the right-lower quadrant, becoming localized and causing discomfort on moving, walking, or coughing"- CSDT 14th/651

Acute Appendicitis

◈ *History L and B 26th/1202-03*

- The ***pain is frequently first noticed in the periumbilical region*** and is similar to, but less intense than, the colic of small bowel obstruction.
- Central abdominal pain is associated with ***anorexia, nausea and usually one or two episodes of vomiting that follow the onset of pain (Murphy).***
- Anorexia is a useful and constant clinical feature, particularly in children. The patient often gives a history of similar discomfort that settled spontaneously.

*"Pain is initially felt in umbilical region. **After a few hours, the pain localizes to the right iliac fossa**. This is called shifting pain of acute appendicitis" (Manipal 4th/828)*

149. Ans. b. Exposure to radiation, d. Nodule size >4 cm, e. Male gender

[Ref: L and B 26th/ 763-66; CSDT14th/282; Harrison 19th/2303]

Risk Factors for Thyroid Carcinoma in Patients with Thyroid Nodule

◈ *Harrison 19th/2303*

- History of head and neck irradiation, including total-body irradiation for bone marrow transplant and brain radiation for childhood leukemia
- Exposure to ionizing radiation from fallout in childhood or adolescence
- ***Age <20 or >65 years***
- ***Increased nodule size (>4 cm)***
- New or enlarging neck mass
- ***Male gender***
- Family history of thyroid cancer, MEN 2, or other genetic syndromes associated with thyroid malignancy (e.g.,Cowden's syndrome, familial polyposis, Carney complex)
- Vocal cord paralysis, hoarse voice
- Nodule fixed to adjacent structures
- Extrathyroidal extension
- Lateral cervical lymphadenopathy

Thyroid Cancer

◈ *Harrison 19th/2303*

- Prognosis is worse in older persons (>65 years). Thyroid cancer is twice as common in women as men, but male gender is associated with a worse prognosis.
- Additional important risk factors include a ***history of childhood head or neck irradiation, large nodule size (≥4 cm), evidence for local tumor fixation or invasion into lymph nodes and the presence of metastases***

"Clinical groups with the highest risk for malignancy in a thyroid nodule are ***children, males, adults younger than 30 or older than 60 years and those exposed to radiation therapy, especially during childhood***"- *Sabiston 19th/899*

150. Ans. a. Stage IA

[Ref: L and B 26th/ 1117; Sabiston 19th/1509; Schwartz 10th/ 1335]

Gallbladder Carcinoma

◈ *Schwartz 10th/ 1335*

- Tumors limited to the muscular layer of the gallbladder (T1) are usually identified incidentally, after cholecystectomy for gallstone disease. ***There is near universal agreement that simple cholecystectomy is an adequate treatment for T1 lesions and results in a near 100% overall 5-year survival rate.***
- When the tumor invades the perimuscular connective tissue without extension beyond the serosa or into the liver (**T2 tumors**), ***an extended cholecystectomy*** should be performed. That includes resection of liver segments IVB and V and lymphadenectomy of the cystic duct and pericholedochal, portal, right celiac and posterior pancreatoduodenal lymph nodes.

- One half of patients with T2 tumors are found to have nodal disease on pathologic examination. Therefore, regional lymphadenectomy is an important part of surgery for T2 cancers.
- For tumors that grow beyond the serosa or invade the liver or other organs (**T3 and T4 tumors**), there is a high likelihood of intraperitoneal and distant spread. If no peritoneal or nodal involvement is found, ***complete tumor excision with an extended right hepatectomy*** (segments IV, V, VI, VII and VIII) must be performed for adequate tumor clearance.

Management

◈ *Sabiston 19th/1508*

- The appropriate operative procedure for the patient with localized gallbladder cancer is determined by the pathologic stage.
- Patients with tumors confined to the ***gallbladder mucosa or submucosa (T1a) or confined to the gallbladder muscularis (T1b)*** are usually identified after cholecystectomy for gallstone disease and have an overall 5-year survival rate approaching 100% and 85%, respectively. Therefore, ***cholecystectomy is adequate therapy for patients with T1 tumors.***
- Cancer of the gallbladder with invasion beyond (**stages II and III**) the gallbladder muscularis is associated with an increased ***incidence of regional lymph node metastases and should be managed with an "extended cholecystectomy."***

Table *(Sabiston 19th/1509)*: **TNM Staging for Gallbladder Cancer**

Stage	Stage Grouping
IA	T1 N0 M0
IB	T2 N0 M0
IIA	T3 N0 M0
IIB	T1 N1 M0 T2 N1 M0 T3 N1 M0
III	T4 Any N M0
IV	Any T Any N M1

151. Ans. c. Time in, e. Pre-anesthetic checkup

[Ref: L and B 26th/166-67; en.wikipedia.org/wiki]

Checklists

◈ *L and B 26th/166-67*

- Checklists in the operating theatre environment are now accepted as standard safety protocols since the 'Safe Surgery Saves Lives' Study Group at the World Health Organization published their results.
- The use of a perioperative surgical safety checklist in eight hospitals around the world was associated with a reduction in major complications from 11.0 per cent before, to 7.0 per cent after, the introduction of the checklist.
- The surgical safety checklist identifies specific checks to be carried out at ***three obligatory time points.*** The items are not intended to be comprehensive and additions and modifications are encouraged.

Table *(L and B 26th/167)*: **WHO Surgical Safety Checklist**

Before induction of anaesthesia: SIGN IN

- Patient has confirmed
  - Identify
  - Site
  - Procedure
  - Consent
- Site marked/not applicable
- Anaesthesia safety check completed
- Pulse oximeter on patient and functioning

Does patient have a:

Know allergy
- No
- Yes

Difficult airway/aspiration risk
- No
- Yes and equipment/assistance available

Risk of > 500 ml blood loss (7 ml/kg in children)
- No
- Yes and adequate intravenous access and fluids planned

Before skin incision: Time out

- Confirm all team members have introduced themselves by name and role
- Surgeon, anaesthesia professional and nurse verbally confirm
  - Patient
  - Site
  - Procedure

Anticipated critical events
- **Surgeon reviews:** what are the critical or unexpected steps, operative duration, anticipated blood loss
- **Nursing team reviews:** has sterility (including indicator results) been confirmed Ş are there equipment issue or any concerns

Has antibiotic prophylaxis been given within the last 60 minutes
- Yes
- Not applicable

Is essential imaging displayed
- Yes
- Not applicable

Before patient leaves operating room: SIGN OUT

Nurse verbally confirms with the team:
- The name of the procedure recorded
- That instrument, sponge and needle counts are correct (or not applicable)
- How the specimen in labelled (including patient name)
- Whether there are any equipment problems to be addressed

- Surgeon, anaesthesia professional and nurse review they key concerns for recovery and management of this patient

WHO Surgical Safety Checklist

◈ *en.wikipedia.org/wiki*

The World Health Organization (WHO) published the *WHO Surgical Safety Checklist and Implementation Manual* in 2008 in order to increase the safety of patients undergoing surgery.

The checklist essentially **identifies three distinct phases of an operation**, each corresponding to a specific period in the normal flow of work: ***Before the induction of anaesthesia, before the incision of the skin and before the patient leaves the operating facility***.

In each phase, a 'checklist coordinator' must confirm that the surgical team has completed the listed tasks before it proceeds with the procedure.

Before induction of anaesthesia Before the patient undergoes anaesthesia, the patient must confirm his/her identity, the site of operation, what procedure is to be carried out and that he/she has consented for the procedure.

Time Out: Before the surgical procedure begins (i.e. before the first incision), the entire team must take a ***'time out' (stop and pause).***

Sign Out: Before the patient leaves the operating room there is a further check, usually conducted by the nursing staff.

152. Ans. b. Direct inguinal hernia cause more symptoms than indirect, c. Direct inguinal hernia is most common in children

[Ref: L and B 26th/954-60; CSDT 14th/768-70]

"In general, ***direct hernias produce fewer symptoms than indirect inguinal*** hernias and are less likely to become incarcerated or strangulated"-*CSDT 14th/770*

"In the groin, an **indirect inguinal hernia** results ***when obliteration of the processus vaginalis***, the peritoneal extension accompanying the testis in its descent into the scrotum, fails to occur. The resultant hernia sac passes through the internal inguinal ring, a ***defect in the transversalis fascia*** halfway between the anterior iliac spine and the pubic tubercle"-*CSDT 14th/768*

"The **Hesselbach triangle** is bounded by the inguinal ligament, the inferior epigastric vessels and the lateral border of the rectus muscle. ***A weakness or defect in the transversalis fascia, which forms the floor of this triangle, results in a direct inguinal hernia***. In most **direct hernias**, the ***transversalis fascia*** is diffusely attenuated, though a discrete defect in the fascia may occasionally occur. This funicular type of direct inguinal hernia is more likely to become incarcerated,since it has distinct borders"-*CSDT 14th/769*

"A femoral hernia passes beneath the iliopubic tract and inguinal ligament into the upper thigh. The predisposing anatomic feature for femoral hernias is a small empty space between the lacunar ligament medially and the femoral vein laterally—the femoral canal. Because its borders are distinct and unyielding, a ***femoral hernia has the highest risk of incarceration and strangulation of groin hernias***"-*CSDT 14th/769*

"***Nearly all inguinal hernias in infants, children and young adults are indirect inguinal hernias***. Although these "congenital" hernias most often present during the first year of life, the first clinical evidence of hernia may not appear until middle or old age, when increased intra-abdominal pressure and dilation of the internal inguinal ring allow abdominal contents to enter the previously empty peritoneal diverticulum"-*CSDT 14th/769*

153. Ans. b. Doppler USG may be used for diagnosis, d. Differentiated from epididymitis by technetium-99m pertechnetate scan, e. Contralateral testis should also be explored on surgery

[Ref: L and B 26th/1379-80; CSDT 14th/982]

Torsion of Testis

◈ *CSDT 14th/982*

- In children and adolescents, testicular torsion is either idiopathic or occurs after activity or trauma.
- **Epididymitis** must be differentiated from torsion of the testis, testicular tumor and tuberculous epididymitis. A **technetium-99m pertechnetate scan** reveals ***increased uptake with epididymitis but decreased uptake with torsion.***
- **Scrotal ultrasound** distinguishes between the ***solid mass of a testicular tumor and an enlarged, inflamed epididymis*** and can also identify epididymal or testicular abscess, which requires operative treatment.
- ***Increased blood flow on Doppler ultrasound*** also helps ***distinguish epididymitis from torsion***, though it is not completely reliable.
- If the diagnosis is strongly suspected, the best "test" is **operative scrotal exploration.** The testicular salvage rate if detorsion is performed within 6 hours after onset of symptoms is up to 97%, versus less than 10% if delayed more than 24 hours. At operation, the torsion is corrected and the gonad, if viable, is fixed to the hemiscrotum in three places.
- Because the paired testicle is at risk for torsion since the testicular anatomy tends to mirror itself, ***contralateral orchiopexy (suture fixation) should be performed in all cases.***

"The blood supply to the testicle is compromised due to twisting of the spermatic cord within the ***tunica vaginalis***, resulting in ischemia to the epididymis and the testis. ***In newborns, an extravaginal torsion also*** can occur with twisting of the tunica vaginalis and spermatic cord together. Risk factors for torsion include undescended testis, testicular tumor and a "bell-clapper" deformity—poor gubernacular fixation of the testicles to the scrotal wall"-*Schwartz 10th/1662*

"***Contralateral testes also must be explored and fixed*** to the dartos fascia due to the possibility that the same anatomic defect allowing torsion exists on the contralateral side"- *Schwartz 10th/1663*

"The **diagnosis of testicular torsion** is based mainly on clinical examination. Although one may utilize ***Doppler ultrasonography*** *and radionuclide scanning* to aid in the diagnosis, these tests are time consuming and, in the case of ultrasound, operator specific"-CSDT 14th/982

"**Testicular torsion** is most frequent in late childhood and early adolescence, though the range can include the fetus and the adult. Anatomically, there are two forms of testicular torsion depending on where the spermatic cord is twisted with respect to the tunica vaginalis: ***intravaginal torsion (bell-clapper deformity), the most common form and extravaginal torsion that occurs principally in neonates and in children with an undescended testis***. Rarely, the testis may twist on a long epididymal mesentery. In children and adolescents, testicular torsion is ***either idiopathic or occurs after activity or trauma***"- *CSDT 14th/982*

Torsion of the Testis

◈ *L and B 26th/1379-80*

For torsion to occur, one of several abnormalities must be present:

- ***Inversion of the testis is the most common predisposing cause***. The testis is rotated so that it lies transversely or upside down.
- ***High investment of the tunica vaginalis causes the testis to hang within the tunica like a clapper in a bell***

Management

- If there is any doubt as to the diagnosis, then urgent scrotal exploration is indicated. ***While Doppler ultrasound scanning can confirm the absence of the blood supply to the affected testis, false positive results can be seen, so it is not routinely recommended.***
- If the testis is viable when the cord is untwisted it should be prevented from twisting again by fixation with nonabsorbable sutures between the tunica vaginalis and the tunica albuginea. ***The other testis should also be fixed because the anatomical predisposition is likely to be bilateral***

154. Ans. a. U/L more common than B/L, b. Missing testis on palpation may be due to agenesis, c. 10% Bilateral, d. Undescended Testis may be associated with absent kidney

[Ref: CSDT14th/1257; L and B 26th/1377-79; 25th/1377-79; Nelson 20th/2592-93]

Fowler-Stephens Orchidopexy

◈ *Opearive Urology at Clevland 2006/516-17*

- High intraabdominal testes offer a particular challenge. There is often inadequate vascular length to bring these testicles into the scrotum. To facilitate mobilization, the vessels may be divided high in the abdomen and the testis brought down on the pedicle of ***vasal vessels*** and collaterals in the peritoneum ***between the vas and distal spermatic vessels***.
- For high intraabdominal testicles, an autotransplantation may be considered as an adjunct to the Fowler-Stephens orchidopexy.
- Following division of the vessels and mobilization of the testicle, a microvascular anastomosis is performed between the ***testicular vessels and the inferior epigastric vessels***

Unescended Testis

◈ *Nelson 20th/2592-93*

- Failure to find the testis in the scrotum indicates that the testis is undescended, absent, or retractile
- Cryptorchidism is ***bilateral in 10% of cases***
- Approximately ***10% of cryptorchid boys have a nonpalpable testis; in these boys the testis is present in abdominal or inguinal region in 50% and it is absent or atrophic, almost always in scrotum, secondary to spermatic cord torsion in utero (vanishing testis) in remaining 50%.***
- In a newborn phenotypic male with bilateral nonpalpable testes, ***one should consider the possibility that the child could be a virilized female with congenital adrenal hyperplasia***.
- The incidence of undescended or partially descended testis is 1%-2% in full-term infants and up to 30% in premature babies. The ***right testis is affected in 45% of cases, the left testis in 30% and both testes in 25%.***
- A patent processus vaginalis is present in 95% of patients with cryptorchidism and approximately 25% develop a clinical hernia.
- Anomalies associated with cryptorchidism occur in about 15% of cases and include a wide variety of syndromes such as Klinefelter syndrome, hypogonadotropic hypogonadism, the prune belly syndrome, ***horseshoe kidneys, renal agenesis or hypoplasia, exstrophy of the bladder, ureteral reflux, gastroschisis and cloacal exstrophy.***

◈ *Schwartz 10th/1636*

- If an abdominal testis is identified that is too far to reach the scrotum, a two-stage ***Fowler-Stephens approach*** is used.
- In the first stage, the ***testicular vessels*** can be clipped via laparotomy or laparoscopically. This promotes neovasculogenesis along the vas deferens.
- Several months later, the second stage is performed during which the testis is mobilized intra-abdominally along with a swath of peritoneum with ***collateralized blood supply along the vas.*** Preservation of the gubernacular attachments with its collaterals to the testicle may confer improved testicular survival following orchidopexy in over 90% of cases.

Incompletely Descended Testis

◈ *L and B 26th/1377-79*

- About 4 per cent of boys are born with one or both testes incompletely descended. About two thirds of these reach the scrotum during the first three months of life, but full descent after that is uncommon. The ***incidence of testicular maldescent at the age of one year is around 1 per cent.***
- The condition is more common on the right and is ***bilateral in 20 per cent of cases.***

155. Ans. c. Neurogenic tumor, d. Enterogenous cyst

[Ref: L and B 26th/ 868-69; Harrison 19th/1720; Schwartz 10th/673]

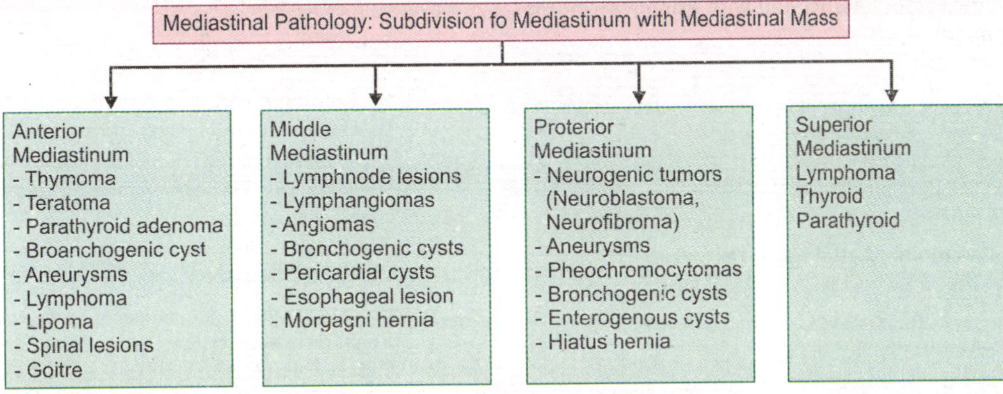

Table *(Schwartz 10th/673)*: **Mediastinal Tumors in Adults**

Tumor Type	Incidence (%)	Location
Neurogenic tumors	21	Posterior
Cysts	20	All
Thymomas	19	Anterior
Lymphoma	13	Anterior/middle
Germ cell tumors	11	Anterior
Mesenchymal tumors	7	All
Endocrine tumors	6	Anterior/middle

Table *(Harrison 19th/1720)*: **The Three compartment of the mediastinum**

	Anterior Compartment	Middle Compartment	Posterior Compartment
Contents	Thymus gland, anterior mediastinal lymph nodes, internal mammary arteries and veins	Pericardium, heart, ascending and transverse arch of aorta, superior and inferior vena Cavae, brachiocephalic arteries and veins, phrenic nerves, trachea and main bronchi and their contiguous lymph nodes, pulmonary arteries and veins	Descending thoracic aorta, esophagus, thoracic duct, azygos and hemiazygos veins, sympathetic chains and the posterior group of mediastinal lymph nodes
Common abnormalities	Thymoma, lymphomas, teratomatous neoplasms, thyroid masses, parathyroid masses, mesenchymal tumors, glant lymph node hyperplasia, hernia through foramen of Morgagni	Metastatic lymph node enlargement, granulomatous lymph node enlargement, pleuropericardial cysts, bronchogenic cysts, masses of vascular origin	***Neurogenic tumors***, meningocele, meningomyelocele, ***gastroenteric cysts***, esophgeal diverticula, hernia through foramen of Bochdalek, extramedullary hematopolesis

156. Ans. a. Achalsia, b. Post-cricoid web, d. Paterson-Kelly syndrome, e. Lye ingestion

[Ref: L and B 26th/1019; Sabiston 19th/1050-51; Harrison 19th/532; CSDT 14th/474]

"**Schatzki's ring** is a thin submucosal circumferential ring in the lower esophagus at the squamocolumnar junction, often associated with a ***hiatal hernia***. Its significance and pathogenesis are unclear"-*Schwartz 10th/984*

"**Schatzki's ring** is a ***non-neoplastic condition***"-*L and B 26th/1019*

Some etiologic factors associated with squamous cell cancer of the esophagus *Harrison 19th/532*

Excess alcohol consumption
Cigarette smoking
Other ingested carcinogens: Nitrates (converted to nitrites), Smoked opiates, Fungal toxins in pickled vegetables
Mucosal damage from physical agents: Hot tea, ***Lye ingestion***, Radiation-induced strictures, ***Chronic achalasia***
Host susceptibility
Esophageal web with glossitis and iron deficiency (i.e., ***Plummer-Vinson or Paterson-Kelly syndrome***)
Congenital hyperkeratosis and pitting of the palms and soles (i.e., tylosis palmaris et plantaris)
? Dietary deficiencies of selenium, molybdenum, zinc and vitamin A

Some Etiologic Factors Associated with Adenocarcinoma of the Esophagus

- *Harrison 19th/533*
- Chronic gastroesophageal reflux
- Obesity
- Barrett's esophagus
- Male sex
- Cigarette smoking

Squamous Carcinoma: Aetiological Factors

- *Davidson 22nd/870*
- Smoking
- Alcohol excess
- Chewing betel nuts or tobacco
- ***Achalasia of the oesophagus***
- Coeliac disease
- ***Post-cricoid web***
- Post-caustic stricture
- Tylosis (familial hyperkeratosis of palms and soles)

Table *(Maingot's Abdominal Operations -Chapter 9)*: **Factors Associated with Pathogenesis of Esophageal Cancer**

Factor	Squamous Cell Cancer	Adenocarcinoma
Smoking	+++	+
Alcohol consumption	+++	–
Hot beverages	+	–
N-nitroso compounds (e.g., pickled vegetables)	+	–
Betel nut chewing	+	–
Maté drinking	+	–
Deficiencies of green vegetables and vitamins	+	–
Low socioeconomic class	+	–
Fungal toxin or virus	+	–
History of radiation to the mediastinum	+	+
Lye corrosive stricture	+	–
History of aerodigestive malignancy	+++	–
Plummer-Vinson syndrome	+	–
Obesity	–	++
Achalasia	+	–
Gastroesophageal reflux	–	+++
Barrett's esophagus	–	++++

157. Ans. None

[Ref: L and B 26th/1133; Davidson 22nd/891; Harrison 231e-3]

Hyperamylasemia is seen in all above Conditions

Causes of Hyperamylasemia and Hyperamylasuria

- *Harrison 19th/2089*

Pancreatic Disease

I. Pancreatitis
   A. Acute
   B. Chronic: ductal obstruction
   C. Complications of pancreatitis
      1. ***Pancreatic pseudocyst***
      2. Ascites caused by pancreatic duct disruption
      3. Pancreatic necrosis

II. Pancreatic trauma

III. Pancreatic carcinoma

Nonpancreatic Disorders

I. Renal insufficiency

II. Salivary gland lesions
   A. ***Mumps***
   B. Calculus
   C. Irradiation sialadenitis
   D. Maxillofacial surgery

III. "Tumor" hyperamylasemia
   A. Carcinoma of the lung, esophagus, breast, or ovary

IV. *Macroamylasemia*

V. Burns

VI. Diabetic ketoacidosis

VII. Pregnancy

VIII. Renal transplantation

IX. Cerebral trauma

X. Drugs: opiates

Other Abdominal Disorders

I. Biliary tract disease: cholecystitis, choledocholithiasis

II. Intraabdominal disease
   A. Perforated or penetrating peptic ulcer
   B. Intestinal obstruction or inflammation
   C. Ruptured ectopic pregnancy
   D. Peritonitis
   E. Aortic aneurysm
   F. Postoperative hyperamylasemia

Cystic fibrosis involvement of Pancrease: ***pancreatic insufficiency, recurrent acute pancreatitis, chronic pancreatitis***"-Robbins 9th/470

"***Pseudocyst fluid usually has a high amylase level***, but that is not diagnostic, as a tumour that communicates with the duct system may yield similar findings"- *L and B 26th/ 1133*

"**Mumps pancreatitis**, which may present as abdominal pain, occurs in ~4% of infections but is difficult to diagnose because an ***elevated serum amylase level*** can be associated with ***either parotitis or pancreatitis***"-*Harrison 231e-3*

"A **persistently elevated** serum amylase concentration suggests ***pseudocyst formation.*** Peritoneal amylase concentrations are massively elevated in ***pancreatic ascites***. Serum amylase concentrations are also elevated (but less so) in ***intestinal ischaemia, perforated peptic ulcer and ruptured ovarian cyst, whilst the salivary isoenzyme of amylase is elevated in parotitis***. If available, serum lipase measurements are preferable to amylase, as they have greater diagnostic accuracy for acute pancreatitis"- *Davidson 22nd/891*

158. Ans. a. Pancreatic fluid collection, b. May be asymptomatic, c. Well-defined wall e. Rich in pancreatic enzymes

[Ref: L and B 26th/1127,1133; Robbins 9th/889-90]

Pseudocyst

◈ *L and B 26th/ 1133*

- A pseudocyst is a ***collection of amylase-rich fluid*** enclosed in a ***wall of fibrous or granulation tissue***.
- ***Pseudocysts typically arise following an attack of acute pancreatitis***, but ***can develop in chronic pancreatitis or after pancreatic trauma***.
- ***Formation of a pseudocyst requires 4 weeks or more from the onset of acute pancreatitis.***
- "The **two major causes of acute pancreatitis** are *biliary calculi, which occur in 50–70 per cent of patients and alcohol abuse, which accounts for 25 per cent of cases"-L and B 26th/ 1127*
- They are often single but, occasionally, patients will develop multiple pseudocysts.
- If carefully investigated, more than half will be found to have a communication with the main pancreatic duct
- ***Pseudocysts will resolve spontaneously in most instances, but complications can develop***. *Pseudocysts that are thick-walled or large (over 6 cm in diameter), have lasted for a long time (over 12 weeks) or have arisen in the context of chronic pancreatitis are less likely to resolve spontaneously*, but these factors are not specific indications for intervention.
- Therapeutic interventions are advised only if the pseudocyst causes symptoms, if complications develop or a distinction has to be made between a pseudocyst and a tumour- *L and B 26th/ 1133*

Pancreatic Pseudocyst

◈ *Harrison 19th/2093*

- An encapsulated collection of fluid with a well-defined ***inflammatory wall*** usually outside the pancreas with minimal or no necrosis. This entity usually occurs >4 weeks after onset of interstitial edematous pancreatitis.
- **Computed tomography criteria**: Well circumscribed, usually round or oval; Homogeneous fluid density; No nonliquid component; **Well-defined wall** that is, completely encapsulated; Maturation usually requires >4 weeks after onset of acute pancreatitis; occurs after interstitial edematous pancreatitis

Pseudocysts

◈ *Robbins 9th/889-90*

- Pseudocysts are localized collections of necrotic and hemorrhagic material that are ***rich in pancreatic enzymes and lack an epithelial lining*** (hence the prefix "pseudo").
- ***Pseudocysts account for approximately 75% of cysts in the pancreas***. They usually arise following a bout of acute pancreatitis, particularly one superimposed on chronic alcoholic pancreatitis. Traumatic injury to the pancreas can also give rise to pseudocysts.
- ***While many pseudocysts spontaneously resolve***, they may ***become secondarily infected and larger pseudocysts may compress or even perforate into adjacent structures***.
- ***Pseudocysts are usually solitary*** and may be situated within the pancreas, or, more commonly, in the lesser omental sac or in the retroperitoneum between the stomach and transverse colon or between the stomach and liver. They can even be subdiaphragmatic.
- Pseudocysts are formed when areas of intrapancreatic or peripancreatic hemorrhagic fat necrosis are walled off by fibrous tissue and granulation tissue

159. Ans. b. Tubercular empyemam, c. Persistent bronchopleural fistula

[Ref: L and B 26th/ 870; CSDT 14th/372]

Coughing up blood from the respiratory tract is called hemoptysis. The amount of blood produced can vary from a ***few streaks of blood mixed*** with normal sputum to large amounts of pure blood. ***Blood-streaked sputum is common in many minor respiratory illnesses***, such as upper respiratory infections and viral bronchitis. Massive hemoptysis is the production of more than a pint (about 600 milliliters) of blood within 24 hours. The most common causes include- Lung cancer, Bronchiectasis and Some pneumonias, including tuberculosis"- *www.msdmanuals.com*

Surgical Treatment of Tuberculosis

◈ *L and B 26th/ 870*

Surgery is rarely indicated for tuberculosis in developed countries but, when it is, it must be combined with adequate antitubercular chemotherapy or the benefit of surgery will be lost

Tuberculosis: indications for surgery

◈ *L and B 26th/ 870*

- Suspicious lesion on chest radiograph in which neoplasia cannot be excluded
- Chronic tuberculous abscess, resistant to chemotherapy
- Aspergilloma within a tuberculous cavity
- ***Life-threatening haemoptysis***

Surgical Treatment of Tuberculosis

◈ *CSDT 14th/372*

- The role of surgery in treatment of tuberculosis has diminished dramatically since chemotherapy became available.
- It is now confined to the following indications: ***(1) failure of chemotherapy; (2) performance of diagnostic procedures; (3) destroyed lung; (4) postsurgical complications; (5) persistent bronchopleural fistula; and (6) intractable hemorrhage.***
- The most common parenchymal resections include **lobectomy**, followed by ***pneumonectomy***. Pulmonary resection is adjunctive to chemotherapy.
- The ***rationale for lung resection of parenchyma affected by MDR-TB*** is to remove a large focal burden of organisms present in destroyed nonviable lung tissue.
- ***Surgery is recommended in MDR-TB patients with extensive drug resistance***—those with localized disease amenable to resection and those with high drug activity.

- **Diagnostic lung resection** may be necessary to rule out other diseases, such as cancer, or to obtain material for cultures.

"**Tuberculous empyema** is a chronic, active infection of the pleural space characterized by thick rind of pleura with thick and irregular calcification of both parietal and visceral pleura usually surrounding a loculated pleural fluid which contains a large number of tubercle bacilli.**Treatment** consists of pleural space drainage, decortication to allow re-expansion of the trapped lung and ***decortication plus pneumonectomy*** to remove a lung"- *radiopaedia.org*

160. Ans. b. Rasmussen aneurysm is a complication

[Ref: Harrison 19th/1108; Robbins 9th/373]

"**Acute tuberculous cavitation: *Thin walled cavity*.** When the ***cavity become chronic, the wall thicken*** and the cavity usually shrinks, followed by fibrosis"-*WHO Basic Radiological Manual 1st/58*

"***Cavitation and fibrosis do not always mean active tuberculosis***"- *WHO Basic Radiological Manual 1st/58*

"**Cavitary tuberculosis: *Hallmark of reactivation tuberculosis***"-*Dahnert Radiology Manual 7th/549*

"**Cavitation,** the radiological hallmark of PTB, is radiographically evident in 20–45% of patients, while air-fluid levels in the cavity occur in 10% of cases. Cavitation may progress to endobronchial spread and results in a typical 'tree-in-bud' distribution of nodules in addition to cavitation; ***this is considered a reliable marker of active TB***"- *www.sciencedirect.com*

"Early in the course of disease, symptoms and signs are often nonspecific and insidious, consisting mainly of **diurnal fever** and night sweats due to defervescence, weight loss, anorexia, general malaise and weakness.

Hemoptysis develops in 20–30% of cases and massive hemoptysis may ensue as a consequence of the erosion of a blood vessel in the wall of a cavity. Hemoptysis, however, may also result from rupture of a dilated vessel in a cavity (***Rasmussen's aneurysm***) or from aspergilloma formation in an old cavity"- *Harrison 19th/1108*

"Systemic features include ***fever (often low-grade and intermittent) in up to 80% of cases*** and wasting"-*Harrison 19th/1108*

"Commonly, the ***fever is low grade and remittent*** (appearing late each afternoon and then subsiding) and night sweats occur. Some degree of hemoptysis is present in about half of all cases of pulmonary tuberculosis"-*Robbins 9th/373*

"**Rasmussen's aneurysm** is an inflammatory pseudo-aneurysmal dilatation of a branch of pulmonary artery adjacent to a tuberculous cavity. Life threatening massive hemoptysis from the rupture of a Rasmussen's aneurysm is an uncommon yet life threatening complication of cavitary tuberculosis (TB)"-*www.ncbi.nlm. nih.gov*

"Distribution of bronchiectasis can help in narrowing the differential diagnosis. **Upper lobe bronchiectasis** is typically seen in: cystic fibrosis and ***tuberculosis***"- *radiopaedia.org*

161. Ans. a. Furosemide, b. Mannitol, d. Glucose free fluid

[Ref: L and B 26th/318-19; ; Ajay Yadav 5th/15; Harrison 19th/1780]

"***As hyperglycemia can increase cerebral edema***, therefore ***glucose containing solution must not be used for head injuries***"-*Ajay Yadav 5th/15*

"**Hypotonic solution** *can aggravate edema therefore should* ***not be used for cerebral and pulmonary edema***"- *Ajay Yadav 5th/15*

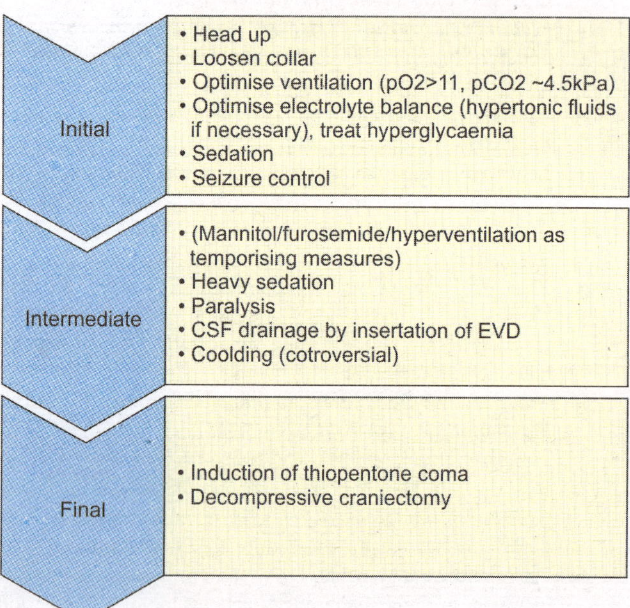

Fig: *(L and B 26th/319):* A hierarchy of intracranial pressure management strategies in ventilated head injury patients. CSF, cerebrospinal fluid; EVD, external ventricular drainage

"**Decompressive craniectomy**—Decompressive craniectomy is the surgical removal a large portion of the cranial vault to allow for the edematous intracranial contents to expand and subsequently reduce ICP. At the time of the procedure any mass lesion (neoplasm or hematoma) is also removed. ***Decompressive craniectomy has been considered a last resort; some evidence suggests that it does improve outcomes***"-CSDT 14th/855-856.

Stepwise Approach to Treatment of Elevated Intracranial Pressure (ICP)

◈ *Harrison 19th/1780*

Insert ICP monitor—ventriculostomy versus parenchymal device

General goals: maintain ICP <20 mmHg and CPP ≥60 mmHg.

For ICP >20–25 mmHg for >5 min:

- Elevate head of the bed; midline head position
- Drain CSF via ventriculostomy (if in place)
- **Osmotherapy**—***mannitol*** 25–100 g q4h
- Glucocorticoids—dexamethasone 4 mg q6h for vasogenic edema from tumor, abscess (avoid glucocorticoids in head trauma, ischemic and hemorrhagic stroke)

- Sedation (e.g., morphine, propofol, or midazolam); add neuromuscular paralysis if necessary
- Hyperventilation—to $PaCO_2$ 30–35 mmHg (short-term use or skip this step)
- Pressor therapy—phenylephrine, dopamine, or norepinephrine to maintain adequate MAP to ensure CPP ≥60 mmHg (maintain euvolemia to minimize deleterious systemic effects of pressors).
- Consider second-tier therapies for refractory elevated ICP
    - **Decompressive craniectomy**
    - High-dose barbiturate therapy ("pentobarb coma")
    - Hypothermia to 33°C

162. Ans. a. Causes volvulus of intestine, b. Due to persistent remnant of the vitellointestinal duct, d. Causes melena

[Ref: L and B 26th/1169-70; CSDT 14th/1249-50; Schwartz 10th/1164]

Intestinal obstruction associated with Meckel's diverticulum can result from several mechanisms: *Schwartz 10th/1164*

- ***Volvulus of the intestine*** around the fibrous band attaching the diverticulum to the umbilicus
- Entrapment of intestine by a mesodiverticular band
- Intussusception with the diverticulum acting as a lead point
- Stricture secondary to chronic diverticulitis

Meckel's Diverticulum

◈ *L and B 26th/1169-70*

- A Meckel's diverticulum is a ***persistent remnant of the vitellointestinal duct*** and is present in about 2 per cent of the population.
- It is found on the antimesenteric side of the ileum, commonly at 60 cm from the ileocaecal valve and is classically 5 cm long.
- In around 20 per cent of cases, the mucosa of a Meckel's diverticulum contains heterotopic epithelium of gastric, colonic or pancreatic type.
- A Meckel's diverticulum can present clinically in the following ways:
    - **Haemorrhage**: If gastric mucosa is present, peptic ulceration can occur and present as ***painless maroon rectal bleeding or melaena.*** If the stomach, duodenum and colon are cleared by endoscopy, radioisotope scanning with technetium-99m may demonstrate a Meckel's. (A Meckel's is notoriously difficult to see with contrast radiology.)
    - **Diverticulitis**. Meckel's diverticulitis presents like appendicitis, although if perforation occurs the presentation may resemble a perforated duodenal ulcer.
    - **Intussusception**. A ***Meckel's can be the lead point for ileoileal or ileocolic intussusception.***
    - **Chronic ulceration**. Pain is felt around the umbilicus, as the site of the diverticulum is midgut in origin.
    - **Intestinal obstruction**. A band between the apex of the diverticulum and the umbilicus (also part of the vitellointestinal duct) may cause obstruction directly or by a volvulus around it.
    - **Perforation**.
- The vast majority of Meckel's are asymptomatic. When found in the course of abdominal surgery, a Meckel's can safely be left alone provided it has a wide mouth and is not thickened. When there is doubt, it can be resected. The finding of a Meckel's diverticulum in an inguinal or femoral hernia has been described as ***Littre's hernia***.

163. Ans. a. Size may increase during pregnancy, b. Usually hypothyroid, d. Can turn malignant

[Ref: L and B 26th/747-50; Manipal 4th/326-28; Sabiston 19th/898; CSDT 14th/283; Harrison 19th/2301]

Simple Goitre

◈ *L and B 26th/747*

- Simple goitre may develop as a result of stimulation of the thyroid gland by TSH, either as a result of inappropriate secretion from a microadenoma in the anterior pituitary (which is rare), or in response to a chronically low level of circulating thyroid hormones.
- The ***most important factor in endemic goitre is dietary deficiency of iodine*** but defective hormone synthesis probably accounts for many sporadic goiters

"**An increased incidence of cancer** (usually follicular) has been reported from ***endemic areas***. Dominant or rapidly growing nodules in ***long-standing goitres*** should always be subjected to aspiration cytology"-*L and B 26th/749*

"**Complication of multinodular goiter**: ***Follicular carcinoma in a long-standing goiter***"- *Manipal 4th/326 Sabiston 19th/898*

Simple or Nontoxic Goiter (Diffuse and Multinodular Goiter)

◈ *CSDT 14th/283*

- Simple goiter may be physiologic, occurring during puberty or pregnancy, or it may occur in patients from endemic (iodine-poor) regions or as a result of prolonged exposure to goitrogenic foods or drugs. As the goiter persists, there is a tendency to form nodules.
- Goiter may also occur early in life as a consequence of a congenital defect in thyroid hormone production or in patients with Hashimoto thyroiditis.

Diffuse Nontoxic (Simple) Goiter

◈ *Harrison 19th/2301*

- When diffuse enlargement of the thyroid occurs in the ***absence of nodules and hyperthyroidism***, it is referred to as a *diffuse nontoxic goiter*. This is sometimes called *simple goiter*, because of the absence of nodules, or *colloid goiter*, because of the presence of uniform follicles that are filled with colloid.
- Worldwide, ***diffuse goiter is most commonly caused by iodine deficiency and is termed endemic goiter*** when it affects >5% of the population.
- In nonendemic regions, *sporadic goiter* occurs and the cause is usually unknown.
- Thyroid enlargement in teenagers is sometimes referred to as *juvenile goiter*.
- In general, goiter is more common in women than men, probably because of the greater prevalence of underlying autoimmune disease and the ***increased iodine demands associated with pregnancy.***

Nontoxic Multinodular Goiter

◈ *Harrison 19th/2301*

- Depending on the population studied, MNG or nodular enlargement of the thyroid occurs in up to 12% of adults.
- MNG is more common in women than men and increases in prevalence with age. It is more common in ***iodine-deficient regions but also occurs in regions of iodine sufficiency***, reflecting multiple genetic, autoimmune and environmental influences on the pathogenesis.
- ***Most patients with nontoxic MNG are asymptomatic and euthyroid.***
- Sudden pain in an MNG is usually caused by hemorrhage into a nodule but should raise the possibility of invasive ***malignancy. Hoarseness, reflecting laryngeal nerve involvement, also suggests malignancy.***

164. Ans. b. Abdominal pelvic CT scanning is helpful for evaluating intra-abdominal and retroperitoneal injuries, c. >100,000 red cells/μL in peritoneal lavage is considered positive and is indication for exploratory laparotomy, e. FAST-USG is used for initial evaluation

[Ref: L and B 26th/358-59; Manipal 4th/885-89; Sabiston 19th/; CSDT 14th/209-10; Schwartz 10th/181-82]

"The ***spleen is the most commonly injured organ in cases of blunt abdominal trauma***"- *CSDT 14th/213*

Table *(CSDT 14th/212)*: **Criteria for evaluation of peritoneal lavage fluid**

I. Positive
- 100,000 red cells/μL; = 500 white cells/μL; = 175 units amylase/dL;
- Bacteria on Gram-stained smear
- Bile; Food particles

II. Intermediate
- Pink fluid on free aspiration
- 50,000–100,000 red cells/μL in blunt trauma
- 100–500 white cells/μL
- 75–175 units amylase/dL

III. Negative
- Clear aspirate
- <100 white cells/μL
- <75 units amylase/dL

Diagnostic Peritoneal Lavage

◈ *L and B 26th/358*

- Diagnostic peritoneal lavage (DPL) is a test used to assess the presence of blood in the abdomen.
- The presence of >100 000 red cells/μL or >500 white cells/μL is deemed positive (***this is equivalent to 20 mL of free blood in the abdominal cavity***).
- DPL is especially useful in the hypotensive, unstable patient with multiple injuries as a means of excluding intraabdominal bleeding.

"**After the initial FAST examination**, patients who are stable or who respond to initial fluid resuscitation should have a **CT scan** of the abdomen and pelvis to evaluate for intra-abdominal and retroperitoneal injuries. Patients with persistent hypotension requiring fluid and blood resuscitation in the face of a **positive FAST** or **diagnostic peritoneal lavage** should be ***transported to the operating room emergently for exploratory laparotomy***"- *CSDT 14th/210*

"A major advance in management of blunt trauma has been the **FAST examination**. ***Ultrasound has proven to be an ideal modality in the immediate evaluation of the trauma patient*** because it is rapid and accurate for the detection of intra-abdominal fluid or blood and is readily repeatable"-*CSDT 14th/211*

"Despite the many potential indications, ***FAST followed by abdominal pelvic CT scanning*** has replaced the need for most diagnostic peritoneal lavages. The only contraindication is a need for emergency laparotomy. A portion of the recovered fluid is sent for laboratory analysis of cell counts, the presence of particulate matter and amylase"- *CSDT 14th/212*

Table *(CSDT 14th/213)*: **Comparison of diagnostic methods for abdominal trauma**

Methods	Time/Cost	Advantages/ Disadvantages
Physical examination	Quick/no cost	Useful for serial examinations, very limited by other injuries, coma, drug intoxication, poor sensitivity and specificity
Diagnostic peritoneal lavage (DRL)	Quick/inexpensive	Rapid results in unstable patient but invasive and may be overly sensitive for blood and not specific for site of injury; requires experience and may be limited if previous surgery
Focused assessment with sonography for trauma (FAST)	Quick/inexpensive	Rapid detection of intra abdominal fluid and pericardial tamponade; may be limited by operator experience, large body habitus, subcutaneous air; poor for detection of bowel injury. Fairly sensitive but bot highly specific
Helical computerized abdominal tomography (CT)	Slower/expensive	Most specific for site of injury and can evaluate retro-peritoneum; very good sensitivity but may miss bowel injury; risk of reaction to contrast dye.

165. Ans. e. More common in dark people

[Ref: L and B 26th/591-93; Harrison 19th/500; CSDT 14th/1159; Neena Khanna 5th/388-92]

Basal Cell Carcinomas (BCCs)

◈ *Robbins 9th/1156-58*

- Basal cell carcinomas usually present as **pearly papules** containing prominent dilated subepidermal blood vessels (**telangiectasias**)
- ***Some tumors contain melanin*** and ***superficially resemble melanocytic nevi or melanomas.***
- Advanced lesions may **ulcerate** and extensive local invasion of bone or facial sinuses may occur after many years of neglect or in unusually aggressive tumors, explaining the archaic designation ***rodent ulcers.***
- ***Histologically, the tumor cells resemble those in the normal basal cell layer of the epidermis.***
- As with squamous cell carcinoma, the incidence of basal cell carcinoma is increased in the setting of immunosuppression and in disorders of DNA repair, such as ***xeroderma pigmentosum***

◈ *Neena Khanna 5th/388-92*

- ***Noduloulcerative variant of BCC is k/a rodent ulcer***
- ***In whites, it is commonest malignant tumour; infrequent in blacks***
- ***Xeroderma pigmentosum-risk factor***
- Biopsy diagnostic. ***Shows islands and lobules of basaloid cells in a palisading arrangement***

"**Squamous cell carcinoma:** Primary *cutaneous SCC* is a malignant neoplasm of ***keratinizing epidermal cells***"*-Harrison 19th/500*

"**Nonmelanoma skin cancer (NMSC):** *Basal cell carcinomas (BCCs) account for 70–80% of NMSCs.*

Squamous cell carcinomas (SCCs), which comprise ~20% of NMSCs"-Harrison 19th/500

"Types of cells in epidermis- ***squamous cell, basal cell and melanocyte***"- www.cancer.org

◈ *L and B 26th/591-93*

- Usually a slow growing, locally invasive malignant tumour of ***pluripotential epithelial cells*** arising from ***basal epidermis*** and hair follicles, hence affecting the pilosebaceous skin
- ***White-skinned people are almost exclusively affected.***
- BCCs rarely metastasise, are hard to culture and resist transplantation.
- Microscopic: Twenty-six histological types have been described. The characteristic finding is of ovoid cells in nests with a single 'palisading' layer. It is only the outer layer of cells that actively divide.

166. Ans. a. Low back pain is present, c. Pain immediately relieved by rest, e. Pain relieved by leaning forward

[Ref: CSDT 14th/1139; Schwartz 10th/1742]

Fixed walking distance and shiny skin are feature of intermittent claudication (vascular)

Neurogenic Claudication

◈ *Schwartz 10th/1742*

- Neurogenic claudication is characterized by **low back and leg pain** that ***occurs while walking and is relieved by stopping, leaning forward, or sitting.***
- It is normally caused by degenerative lumbar stenosis causing compression of the cauda equina.
- Neurogenic claudication must be **distinguished from vascular claudication**, ***which tends to resolve quickly with cessation of walking.*** There is typically no need to change position and the ***pain follows a stocking distribution rather than a dermatomal distribution. Pallor and coldness of the feet*** and normal neurologic examination are also typical, though diabetic patients may present a challenge with microvascular neuropathy.
- **Patients with neurogenic claudication** have a *slowly progressive course* and may be surgical candidates when their pain interferes with their lifestyle.
- The usual surgery is an L3 to L5 lumbar laminectomy to decompress the nerve roots

"**Neurogenic claudication** (***back pain with radiating leg pain*** that is ***worse with activity*** and ***immediately relieved by rest***) is a common complaint. This can be ***differentiated from vascular claudication by the immediacy of relief with rest*** (for vascular claudication, pain relief occurs only after minutes of rest)"- *CSDT 14th/1139*

◈ *SDT 14th/799-801*

Most commonly, intermittent (or vascular or arterial) claudication is due to ***peripheral arterial disease*** which implies significant atherosclerotic blockages resulting in arterial insufficiency.

It is distinct from neurogenic claudication, which is associated with lumbar spinal stenosis.

It is strongly associated with smoking, hypertension and diabetes

Typically, symptoms are completely relieved after 2–5 minutes of inactivity.

It generally occurs after a relatively consistent distance traveled (fixed distance) and it is relieved by cessation of walking. Relief of symptoms is not dependent upon sitting or other positional change. The severity of claudication is traditionally expressed in terms of city blocks

Integumentary changes: With more advanced ischemia, there is ***atrophy of the skin and subcutaneous tissue so that the foot becomes shiny, scaly and skeletonized***

167. Ans. b. Severe pain, e. Blistering of skin

[Ref: L and B 26th/389-90; Harrison 19th/; CSDT 14th/227-28; Schwartz 10th/229-30]

Burn Classification

◈ *CSDT 14th/227-28*

- Traditionally, burns have been classified as ***first-, second- and third-degree***, but the current emphasis on burn healing has led to classification as **partial-thickness burns**, which can heal spontaneously and **full-thickness burns**, which require skin grafting, although deep partial-thickness burns are usually excised and grafted as well.

- A **first-degree burn** involves only the epidermis and is characterized by ***erythema and minor microscopic changes; tissue damage is minimal, protective functions of the skin are intact, skin edema is minimal and systemic effects are rare.*** Pain, the chief symptom, usually resolves in 48-72 hours and healing takes place uneventfully. In 5-10 days, the damaged epithelium peels off in small scales, leaving no residual scarring. The most common causes of first-degree burns are overexposure to sunlight and brief scalding.
- **Second-degree or partial-thickness (Superficial and deep)** burns are deeper, involving ***all of the epidermis*** and some of the corium or dermis. The systemic severity of the burn and the quality of subsequent healing are directly related to the amount of undamaged dermis.
- **Superficial burns** ***are often characterized by blister formation***, while ***deeper partial-thickness burns have a reddish appearance or a layer of whitish, nonviable dermis firmly adherent to the remaining viable tissue.*** Blisters, when present, continue to increase in size in the postburn period as the osmotically active particles in the blister fluid attract water. ***Complications from superficial second-degree burns are mainly severe pain related.*** These burns usually heal with minimal scarring in 10-14 days unless they become infected.
- **Deep dermal burns** heal over a period of 4-8 weeks with only a fragile epithelial covering developing that arises from the residual uninjured epithelium of the deep dermal sweat glands and ***hair follicles.*** Severe hypertrophic scarring occurs when such an injury heals; the resulting epithelial covering is prone to blistering and breakdown. Evaporative losses after healing remain high compared with losses in normal skin.
- **Full-thickness (third-degree) burns** have a characteristic white, dry, waxy appearance and may appear to the untrained eye as unburned skin. Burns caused by prolonged exposure to heat, with involvement of fat and underlying tissue, may be brown, dark red, or black. ***The diagnostic findings of full-thickness burns are lack of sensation in the burned skin, lack of capillary refill and a leathery texture that is unlike normal skin. All dermal epithelial elements are destroyed, leaving no potential for reepithelialization.***

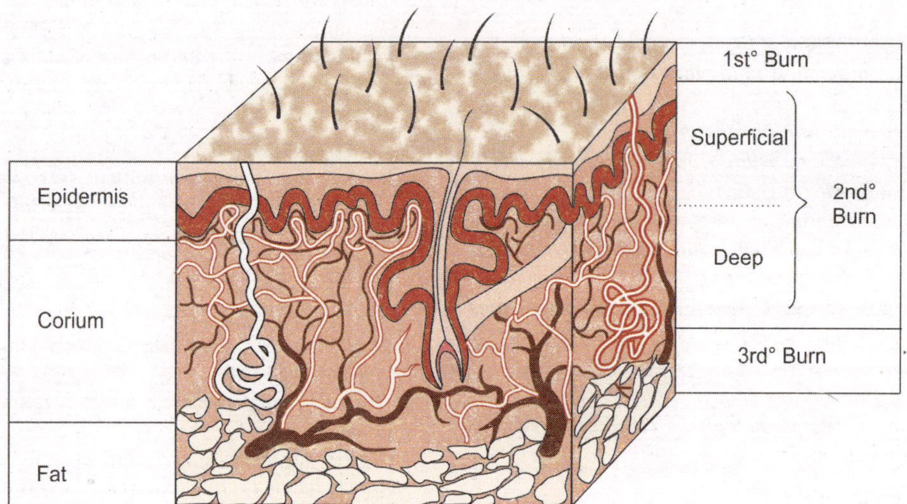

Fig: *(CSDT 14th/228):* Layers of the skin showing depth of first-degree, second-degree and third-degree burns

Burn Depth

◈ *Schwartz 10th/229-30*

- Based on the original burn depth classification by Dupuytren, burn wounds are commonly classified as superficial (first-degree), partial-thickness (second-degree), fullthickness (third-degree) and fourth-degree burns, which affect underlying soft tissue.
- **Partial-thickness burns** are classified as either ***superficial or deep partial-thickness*** burns by depth of involved dermis.
- Clinically, **first-degree burns** are ***painful but do not blister,*** **second-degree** burns have ***dermal involvement and are extremely painful with weeping and blisters*** and **third degree burns** are ***leathery, painless and nonblanching.***

Superficial Partial-thickness Burns

◈ *L and B 26th/389*

- The damage in these burns goes no deeper than the papillary dermis.
- The clinical features are ***blistering and/or loss of the epidermis.***

Deep Partial-thickness Burn

◈ *L and B 26th/389*

- These burns involve damage to the deeper parts of the reticular dermis. Clinically, the epidermis is usually lost.
- Sensation is reduced and the patient is unable to distinguish sharp from blunt pressure when examined with a needle.

Full-Thickness Burns

◈ *L and B 26th/389*

- The whole of the dermis is destroyed in these burns
- Clinically, they have a ***hard, leathery feel.*** The appearance can vary from that similar to the patient's normal skin to charred black, depending upon the intensity of the heat. There is no capillary return. ***Often, thrombosed vessels can be seen under the skin.*** These ***burns are completely anaesthetised: a needle can be stuck deep into the dermis without any pain or bleeding.***

168. Ans. c. Edema under graft may cause graft failure, d. Thin graft survive transplantation more reliably, e. Minimal contraction in full thickness graft

[Ref: Schwartz 10th/266; L and B 26th/ 402-03; CSDT 14th/1149-50]

Types of Skin Grafts

◈ *CSDT 14th/1149-50*

- Skin grafts can be either split-thickness (Partial thickness) or full-thickness grafts. Each type has advantages and disadvantages and is indicated or contraindicated for different kinds of wounds

Split-Thickness Grafts

- **Thinner split-thickness grafts** (0.01-0.015 inch) ***become vascularized more rapidly and survive transplantation more reliably.*** A ***second advantage is that donor sites heal more rapidly and can be reused within a relatively short time (7-10 days) in critical cases such as major burns.***
- Thin grafts ***exhibit the highest degree of postgraft contraction***, offer the least amount of resistance to surface trauma and are ***least like normal skin in texture***, suppleness, pore pattern, hair growth and other characteristics. Hence, they are ***usually aesthetically unacceptable***.
- **Thicker split-thickness skin grafts** (> 0.015 inch) contract less, are more resistant to surface trauma and are more similar to normal skin than are thin split-thickness grafts. They are also aesthetically more acceptable but not as acceptable as full-thickness grafts.
- The disadvantages of thick split-thickness grafts are relatively few but can be significant. They are less easily vascularized than thin grafts and thus result in fewer successful takes when used on less than ideal surfaces.Their donor sites are slower to heal (requiring 10-18 days) and heal with more scarring than donor sites for thin split-thickness grafts—a factor that may prevent reuse of the area.

Full-Thickness Grafts

- Full-thickness skin grafts include the epidermis and all the dermis.
- They are the ***most aesthetically desirable of the free grafts*** because they include the highest number of skin appendage elements, undergo the least amount of contracture and have a greater ability to withstand trauma.
- There are several limiting factors in the use of full-thickness grafts. Since no epidermal elements remain to produce epithelialization in the donor site, it must be closed primarily and a scar will result. The ***size and number of available donor sites is therefore limited.*** Furthermore, conditions at the recipient site must be optimal in order for transplantation to be successful.

"***The dermal component of full-thickness grafts lends mechanical strength and resists wound contraction better, resulting in improved cosmesis***. The use of skin grafts or bioengineered skin substitutes and other innovative treatments (e.g., topically applied growth factors, systemic agents and gene therapy) ***cannot be effective unless the wound bed is adequately prepared. This may include débridement to remove necrotic or fibrinous tissue, control of edema,*** revascularization of the wound bed, decreasing the bacterial burden and minimizing or eliminating exudate"- *Schwartz 10th/266*

Table *(CSDT 14th/1150)*: **Advantages and disadvantages of various types of skin grafts**

Type of Graft	Advantages	Disadvantages
Thin split-thickness	Survive transplantation most easily. Door sites heal most rapidly.	Fewest qualities of normal skin. Maximum contraction. Least resistance to trauma. Sensation poor. ***Aesthetically poor.***
Thick split-thickness	More qualities of normal skin. Less contraction. More resistant to trauma. Sensation fair. Aesthetically more acceptable	Survive transplantation less well. Donor site heals slowly
Full thickness	***Nearly all qualities of normal skin. Minimal contraction***. Very resistant to trauma. Sensation good. Aesthetically good.	***Survive transplantation least well***. Donor site must be closed surgically. Donor sites are limited.

169. Ans. a. Treated with Triamcinolone, b. Results from a prolonged inflammatory phase of wound healing, e. Improve spontaneously with time

[Ref: Schwartz 10th/261-62; L and B 26th/30; CSDT 14th/67]

Table *(Schwartz 10th/262)*: **Characteristics of keloids and hypertrophic scars**

	Keloid	Hypertrophic Scar
Incidence	Rare	Frequent
Ethnic groups	African American, Asian, Hispanic	No predilection
Prior injury	Yes	Yes
Site predilection	Neck, chest, ear lobes, shoulders, upper back	Anywhere

Contd...

	Keloid	Hypertrophic Scar
Genetics	Autosomal dominant with incomplete penetration	No
Timing	Symptom-free interval; may appear year after injury	4–6 weeks post injury
Symptoms	Pain, pruritus, hyperesthesia, ***growth beyond wound margins***	Raised, some pruritus, ***respects wound confines***
Regression	No	Frequent spontaneous
Contracture	Rare	Frequent
Histology	Hypocellular, thick, wavy collagen fibers in random orientation	Parallel orientation of collagen fibers

Treatment of Hypertrophic and Keloid Scars

◈ *L and B 26th/30*

- Pressure – local moulds or elasticated garments
- Silicone gel sheeting (mechanism unknown)
- Intralesional steroid injection (***triamcinolone)***
- Excision and steroid injectionsa
- Excision and postoperative radiation (external beam or brachytherapy)
- Intralesional excision (keloids only)
- Laser – to reduce redness (which may resolve in any event)
- Vitamin E or palm oil massage (unproven)

"A hypertrophic scar is defined as ***excessive scar tissue that does not extend beyond the boundary of the original incision or wound***. It ***results from a prolonged inflammatory phase of wound healing*** and from ***unfavourable scar siting*** (i.e. across the lines of skin tension). In the face, these are known as the lines of facial expression. ***Hypertrophic scars improve spontaneously with time, whereas keloid scars do not***"-*L and B 26th/30*

Scar Formation Versus Regeneration

◈ *CSDT 14th/67*

- ***Hypertrophic scars are generally self-limited,*** are related to residual inflammation and may regress after a year or so. ***Keloids by definition extend beyond the borders of the wound and are most common in pigmented skin.***
- ***Excessive or hypertrophic scarring is rare in burn injuries that heal within 21 days.***

Hypertrophic Scars (HTSs) and Keloids

◈ *Schwartz 10th/261-62*

- ***HTSs rise above the skin level but stay within the confines of the original wound*** and often regress over time.
- ***Keloids rise above the skin level as well, but extend beyond the border of the original wound and rarely regress spontaneously.***
- ***Both HTSs and keloids occur after trauma to the skin and may be tender, pruritic and cause a burning sensation. Keloids are 15 times more common in darker-pigmented ethnicities,*** with individuals of African, Spanish and Asian ethnicities being especially susceptible.

170. Ans. a. Incision is made 1 cm below cricoid cartilage, c. Thoracic duct may be damaged, d. For lobectomy thyroid is dissected at the isthmus, e. Strap muscles are divided if greater exposure is needed

[Ref: L and B 26th/760-61; Schwartz 10th/1251-54]

Technique of Thyroid Surgery

◈ *L and B 26th/760-61*

- The patient is supine on the operating table with the table tilted up 15° at the head end to reduce venous engorgement (reverse Trendelenburg).
- A gently curved skin crease ***incision is made midway between the notch of the thyroid cartilage*** and the suprasternal notch: a lower incision is easier to hide but is more likely to result in a hypertrophic scar.
- ***The strap muscles are not divided as a routine but may be if greater exposure is required.***
- The strap muscles (sternohyoid, sternothyroid and superior belly of the omohyoid) are located anteriorly and are innervated by the ansa cervicalis (ansa hypoglossi)-*Schwartz 10th/1523*
- ***In subtotal thyroidectomy the isthmus is transected*** and the lobe resected obliquely from the medial and lateral aspects to produce a V-shaped surface

Thyroid Surgery

◈ *Schwartz 10th/1251-54*

- A ***Kocher transverse collar incision***, typically ***4 to 5 cm in length***, is placed in or parallel to a natural skin crease ***1 cm below the cricoid cartilage***, although longer incisions may be needed.
- The subcutaneous tissues and ***platysma are incised sharply*** and subplatysmal flaps are raised superiorly to the level of the thyroid cartilage and inferiorly to the suprasternal notch.
- The ***strap muscles are divided in the midline along the entire length of the mobilized flaps*** and the thyroid gland is exposed.
- On the side to be approached first, the sternohyoid muscles are separated from the underlying sternothyroid muscle by blunt dissection until the ***internal jugular vein and ansa cervicalis nerve are identified.***
- ***The strap muscles rarely need to be divided to gain exposure to the thyroid gland.*** If this maneuver is necessary, the muscles should be divided high to preserve their innervation by branches of the ansa cervicalis.
- The RLNs should then be identified. ***The course of the right RLN is more oblique than the left RLN***. The nerves can be most consistently identified at the level of the cricoid cartilage. ***The RLN is most vulnerable to injury in the vicinity of the ligament of Berry.***
- ***If a lobectomy is to be performed, the isthmus is divided flush with the trachea on the contralateral side and suture ligated***. The procedure is repeated on the opposite side for a total thyroidectomy.

"***Thoracic duct injury is a rare complication of thyroid surgery*** whose incidence tends to increase with the extent of the procedure performed. Thoracic duct injury could be identified and managed intraoperatively, or may be diagnosed postoperatively"- *www.ncbi.nlm.nih.go*

OBSTETRICS & GYNECOLOGY

171. Ans. a. Follicular cyst is least common among functional cyst

[Ref: Shaw's 16th/444; Dutta Gynae 6th/289-90 Robert Shaw Gynae 4th/673]

The combination of an **ovarian fibroma** *with ascites and hydrothorax, usually right side is known as* **Meig's syndrome**-*Shaw's 16th/444*

"**Theca Lutein cysts** *are often found in association with* ***hydatiform moles, choriocarcinoma, gonadotropin (hCG) or clomiphene therapy***"-*Shaw's Gynae 16th/430*

Corpus luteal cyst- *It may be* ***often associated with pregnancy*** *and persists for about 12 weeks- Dutta Gynae 6th/290*

Dermoid cyst ***arises from the germ cells*** *arrested after the first meiotic division- Dutta Gynae 6th/290*

Nonneoplastic Ovarian Masses

◈ *Novak's Gyae 15th/411-12*

- **Functional ovarian cysts include follicular cysts, corpus luteum cysts and thecalutein cysts. All are benign and usually do not cause symptoms or requiresurgical management.**
- Cigarette and marijuana smoking are associated with anincreased risk of functional cysts, although the increased risk may be attenuated inoverweight or obese women.
- **Oral contraceptive** use is associated with adecreased risk of developing ovarian cysts, although low-dose pills may have a smaller benefit and oral contraceptives do not hasten the resolution of ovarian cysts
- **The most common functional cyst is the follicular cyst, which rarely is larger than 8 cm.**
- **Corpus luteum cysts are less common than follicular cysts.** Corpus luteum cystsmay rupture, leading to a hemoperitoneum and requiring surgical management.
- **Theca lutein cysts are the least common of functional ovarian cysts. They areusually bilateral and occur with pregnancy, including molar pregnancies.** Theymay be associated with multiple gestations, molar pregnancies, choriocarcinoma,diabetes, Rh sensitization, clomiphene citrate use, human menopausal gonadotropin–human chorionic gonadotropin ovulation induction and the use of ***GnRH analogues***.
- Most benign cystic teratomas (**dermoid cysts**) occur during the reproductive years, although dermoid cysts have a wider age distribution than other ovarian ***germ cell tumors***; in some case series, up to 25% of dermoids occur inpostmenopausal women and they can occur in newborns"- *Novak's Gyae 15th/413*
- "**Follicular cyst**:It is ***most common type of benign ovarian tumor*** and is most often found incidently in women of reproductive age, particularly during early ear of menarche"- *Robert Shaw Gynae 4th/673*

172. Ans. a. Colposcopic study and biopsy of suspicious lesions

[Ref: Shaw's 16th/88-90; Dutta Gynae 6th/111-15, 323-28; Novak's Gyae 15th/588]

HSIL *includes* ***CINII, CINIII and CIS****- Shaw's 16th/88*

High-Grade Squamous Intraepithelial Lesions *Novak's Gyae 15th/588*

- ***Any woman with a cytologic specimen suggesting the presence of HSIL should undergo colposcopy and directed biopsy.*** This is because two-thirds of patients with this cytologic finding will have CIN 2 or greater.
- After colposcopically directed biopsy and determination of the distribution of the lesion, excisional or ablative therapy that addresses the entire transformation zone should be performed

"Since cytology alone does not give a clue to which abnormal cells progress to invasive cancer and aneuploidy which suggest the risk of progression is not routinely performed, it is necessary to submit all women with HSIL ***cytology for colposcopic study and biopsy of suspicious lesions****"- Shaw's 16th/489*

"A ***combined HPV testing*** *and* ***pap smear yields 96% sensitivity*** *as compared to only 60-70% with* ***pap smear*** *alone. PCR, southern blot or hybrid capture detects HPV DNA"-Shaw's 16th/491*

"A single pap smear has a diagnostic sensitivity of about 60%. False negative results may be upto 25%. False negative rate of Pap smear after 3 consecutive negative tests is less than 1%. ***Error in cytology could be reduced further by liquid-based thin layer slide preparation*** *and automated (computer) screening methods.* ***Abnormal cytology is an indication of colposcopic evaluation and directed biopsy****"-Dutta Gynae 6th/113*

173. Ans. b. Estimation of PAAP-A and βhCG

[Ref: Dutta Obs 8th/128,132; J B Sharma 1st/155]

First Trimester Screening

◈ *J B Sharma 1st/155; Dutta Obs 8th/128*

- It uses ***PAPP-A (lower in Down syndrome) and free β-hCG (higher in Down's syndrome)*** b/w 11 and 14 weeks
- It can detects 62% Down's syndrome pregnancies with a 5% false-positive rate

Second Trimester Screening

◈ *J B Sharma 1st/155*

- Double test (MSAFP is lower while total hCG or free β-hCG is raised in Down's syndrome
- Triple test- MSAFP, hCG and uE3 (unconjugated estriol)
- Quadruple test- MSAFP, hCG, uE3 and inhibin-A
- Penta screen- AFP, hCG, uE3, diameric inhibin-A and hyperglycosylated hCG

174. Ans. All (a, b, c, d)

[Ref: Shaw's 16th/349-51; Dutta Gynae 6th/599; Novak's Gyae 15th/102-03]

Vaginal prolapse may occur as a complication of ***abdominal hysterectomy***-*Dutta Gynae 6th/599*

"**Hysterectomy:** The uterus is an important part of the support structure at the top of the vagina. ***Without the uterus, the top of the vagina may gradually fall toward the vaginal opening. This condition is called a vaginal vault prolapse.*** As the top of the vagina falls, added stress is placed on other ligaments. ***Hysterectomy is also commonly associated with an enterocele,*** in which the small intestine herniates downward near the top of the vagina"- www.emedicinehealth.com

Supports of Vagina

◈ *Snell's Anatomy 8th/373*

- The upper part of the vagina is supported by lavatories ai muscles and the transvers cervical, pubocervical and sacrocervical ligaments
- The middle part of vagina is supported by the ***urogenital diaphragm***
- The lower part of vagina, especially the posterior wall, is supported by perineal body

Prolapse of the Vagina

◈ *Snell's Anatomy 9th/406*

- The vaginal vault is supported by the same structures that support the uterine cervix.
- ***Prolapse of the uterus is necessarily associated with some degree of sagging of the vaginal walls.*** However, if the supports of the bladder, urethra, or anterior rectal wall are damaged in childbirth, prolapse of the vaginal walls occurs, with the uterus remaining in its correct position.

Supports of the Genital Tract

◈ *Shaw's 16th/349*

DeLancey introduced **three level system of support**

- **Level I:** Uterosacral and cardinal ligaments support the uterus and vaginal vault. The cervix remains at or just above the ischial spines and the vagina lies horizontally.
- **Level II:** Pelvic fascias and paracolpos which connects the vagina to the white line on the lateral pelvic wall through the arcus tendineus. This includes the pubocervical fascia anteriorly and the rectovaginal fascia and septum posteriorly.
- **Level III:** Levator ani muscle supports the ***lower one-third of the vagina.*** The levator muscle forms a platform against which the pelvic organs (uterus and upper vagina) gets compressed during straining.
- **Level I:** damage causes uterine descent, **enterocele**, vault descent.
- ***Level II damage causes cystocele, rectocele***
- ***Level III damage causes urethrocele, gaping introitus and deficient perineum***

Vaginal Prolapse

◈ *Shaw's 16th/350-51*

- **Anterior vaginal wall** (Cystourethrocele): ***Upper two-third (Cystocele) and Lower one-third (Urethrocele)***
- **Posterior vaginal wall**: ***Upper one-third (enterocele) and lower two-third (rectocele)***

Clinical Relevance

◈ *Novak's Gyae 15th/102-03*

- **Disruption of level I support** may lead to prolapse of the uterus or ***vaginal vault***, while damage to ***level II and III supports predispose to anterior and posterior vaginal prolapse***. All levels of defective support should be repaired during reconstructive surgery.
- There are three levels of vaginal support as described by DeLancey.
- **Level I support** consists of paracolpium that suspends the ***apical portion of the vagina*** and is comprised of the cardinal-uterosacral ligament complex.
- **Level II** support comprises the paracolpium that is attached to the ***vagina laterally*** via the arcus tendineus fasciae pelvis and superior fascia of the levator ani.
- **Level III** support consists of the ***distal vaginal attachments***: anteriorly, via fusion of the urethra to the vagina, laterally, to the levators and posteriorly, with the perineal body.

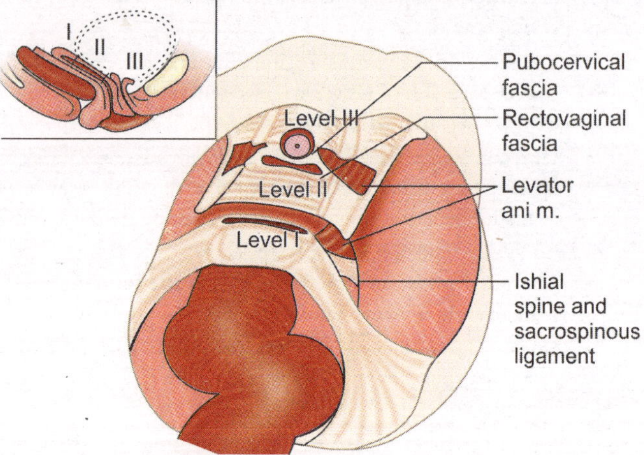

Fig: DeLancey levels of support

175. Ans. b. Therapeutic level for seizure control is 4-7 mEq/L, c. Toxicity should be monitored, d. Can be given as IV infusion, e. Also can be given by intramuscular route

[Ref: Dutta Obs 8th/273,583; J B Sharma 1st/437-39]

Magnesium Sulphate

◈ *Dutta Obs 8th/273; J B Sharma 1st/437-39*

- Magnesium sulphate is drug of choice as ***anticonvulsant in eclampsia***

- It ***does not control hypertension***
- The ***therapeutic level of serum magnesium is 4-7 mEq/L***
- ***Various regimens: Pritchard (IV+IM), Sibai (IV), Zuspan (IV) and Dhaka regimen (IV+IM).***
- ***In India, most hospital use Pritchard regimen (magnesium sulphate4 g is given IV slowly over 3-4 min immediately followed by 5 g in each buttock IM) as it is safer***
- Serum magnesium level may be monitored in selected cases (renal insufficiency, absent deep tendon reflex)
- Magnesium toxicity and serum magnesium level is seen in (a) loss of deep tendon reflex > 7 mEq/L (b) respiratory depression more than 10 mEq and (c) cardiac arrest more than 25 mEq/L

176. Ans. b. Present cervicitis and vaginitis, d. Unknown cause of vaginal bleeding, e. Severe dysmenorrhea

[Ref: Dutta Obs 8th/616; J B Sharma 1st/682; William's Obs 23rd/; Novak's Gyae 15th/224]

"**Relative contraindication:** ***purulent cervical discharge***"-Park 24th/531

WHO Category 4: Do not use (Absolute contraindications of IUDs in Gynecologic/Obstetric conditions) J B Sharma 1st/682

- PID, current or within past 3 months
- Current STD or STD within past 3 months
- Known pelvic tuberculosis
- ***Unexplained or suspicious vaginal bleeding***
- Malignant gestational trophoblastic disease
- Cervical and endometrial cancer
- Uterine/cervical abnormality incompatible with IUD insertion
- Uterine fibroids with distortion of uterine cavity.
- ***Puerperal or postabortal sepsis***
- =Suspected pregnancy

Contraindications for Insertion of IUCD

◈ *Dutta Obs 8th/616*

- ***Presence of pelvic infection, current or within 3 months***
- ***Undiagnosed genital tract bleeding***
- Suspected pregnancy
- Distortion of the shape of the uterine cavity as in fibroid or congenital uterine malformation;
- ***Severe dysmenorrhea***
- Past history of ectopic pregnancy
- Within 6 weeks following cesarean section
- ***STIs—Current or recurrent***;
- Trophoblastic disease;
- Significant immunosuppression.

Additionally for CuT are:

- Wilson disease and
- Copper allergy.

For LNG-IUS are:

- Hepatic tumor or hepatocellular disease (active);
- Current breast cancer and (15) Severe arterial disease.

177. Ans. b. Hypersensitivity to prostaglandin, d. Suspected ectopic pregnancy, e. Undiagnosed adnexal mass

[Ref: Dutta Obs 8th/204,206; J B Sharma 1st/126; William's Obs 23rd/232; Novak's Gyae 15th/256-57; Robert Shaw Gynae 4th/435]

Absolute C/I of medical abortion: ***Suspected ectopic pregnancy*** or ***undiagnosed adnexal mass***; ***Allergy to any drug***"-*J B Sharma 1st/126*

Contraindications to Medical Abortion

◈ *Novak's Gyae 15th/256-57*

- Contraindications to medical abortion with mifepristone/misoprostol include **ectopic pregnancy; an IUD in place (remove IUD first); chronic adrenal failure; concurrent long-term corticosteroid therapy; history of allergy to mifepristone, misoprostol, or other prostaglandin; and the inherited porphyrias**.
- The mifepristone–misoprostol combination was studied for gestations at 9 to 13 weeks; although it is almost as effective as earlier in pregnancy, a larger proportion of patients will experience heavy bleeding and require vacuum curettage

Table: *Robert Shaw Gynae 4th/435*

Absolute contraindications
- Adrenal insufficiency
- *Ectopic pregnancy*
- Asthma
- Cardiac disease
- Heavy smoker
- Older than 35 years
- On anticoagulants or bleeding disorder

Relative contraindications
- Heavy smoker
- >35 years
- Obesity
- Hypertension (diastolic > 100 mmHg)

Contraindications to Medical Abortion

◈ *William's Obs 23rd/232*

- In addition to specific allergies to the medicines, they have included an in situ intrauterine device, ***severe anemia, coagulopathy or anticoagulant use and significant medical conditions, such as active liver disease, cardiovascular disease and uncontrolled seizure disorders***.
- Additionally, because misoprostol can lower glucocorticoid activity, women with adrenal disease or with disorders requiring glucocorticoid therapy should be excluded.

178. Ans. b. Occur due to estrogen deficiency, e. Estradiol vaginal ring is helpful

[Ref: Shaw's 16th/ 386-87; Dutta Gynae 6th/165-66; Novak Gynae 15th/563]

Atrophic Vaginitis or Senile Vaginitis

◈ *Shaw's 16th/ 386-87; Dutta Gynae 6th/165-66*

- *The **acidity of vagina is lowered (i.e pH is increased)***
- *Dry vagina, **dyspareunia (difficult or painful sexual intercourse) and** a purulent, often **slightly blood tinged, discharge are evident***
- *There is atrophy of the vulvovaginal structure due to **estrogen deficiency***
- *Vaginal examination is often painful and the walls are found inflamed*

- ***Estrogen in form of oral, pessary** or cream raises the glycogen content and lower the vaginal pH*

Atrophic Vaginitis

◈ *Novak Gynae 15th/563*

- Estrogen plays an important role in the maintenance of normal vaginal ecology.
- **Women undergoing menopause, either naturally or secondary to surgical removal of the ovaries, may develop inflammatory vaginitis, which may be accompanied by an increased, purulent vaginal discharge.**
- **In addition, they *may have dyspareunia and postcoital bleeding resulting* from atrophy of the vaginal andvulvar epithelium.**
- Examination reveals atrophy of the external genitalia, along with aloss of the vaginal rugae. The vaginal mucosa may be somewhat friable in areas.
- Microscopy of the vaginal secretions shows a predominance of parabasal epithelial cellsand an increased number of leukocytes.
- **Atrophic vaginitis is treated with topical estrogen vaginal cream. Use of 1 g of conjugated estrogen cream intravaginally each day for 1 to 2 weeks generally provides relief.** Maintenance estrogen therapy, either topical or systemic, should be considered to prevent recurrence of this disorder.

Atrophic Vaginitis

◈ *COGDT 2006/Chap 37*

- Prepubertal, lactating and postmenopausal women lack the vaginal effects of estrogen production. The ***pH of the vagina is abnormally high*** and the normally acidogenic flora of the vagina may be replaced by mixed flora.
- Although most patients are asymptomatic, many postmenopausal women report vaginal dryness, spotting, presence of a ***serosanguineous or watery discharge and/or dyspareunia.***
- On examination, the vaginal mucosa is thin, with few or absent vaginal folds. ***The pH is 5.0–7.0.***
- **Treatment** includes intravaginal application of estrogen cream, ***estradiol vaginal ring*** and Systemic estrogen therapy

179. Ans. b. Done when cervix is fully dilated, d. Cup rim should be placed 3 cm from the anterior fontanelle

[Ref: Dutta Obs 8th/660-63,654; J B Sharma 1st/634-37; William's Obs 23rd/522-23]

Vacuum Extractor or Ventouse

◈ *J B Sharma 1st/634-37*

- Pre-requisites includes- **cervix fully dilated** or almost so
- The center of cup should be over the saggital suture and ***2 to 3 cm in front of posterior fontanelle*** (flexion point) with nob of the cup pointing in the direction of the occiput
- ***Pressure is maintained b/w 0.2 kg/cm² to 0.8 kg/cm²***

Vacuum Extraction

◈ *William's Obs 23rd/522-23*

- An important step in vacuum extraction is proper cup placement over the *flexion point*. This pivot point maximizes traction, minimizes cup detachment, flexes but averts twisting of the fetal head and delivers the smallest head diameter through the pelvic outlet. This improves success rates, lowers fetal scalp injury rates and lessens perineal trauma because the smallest fetal head diameter distends the vulva
- The flexion point is found along the sagittal suture, ***approximately 3 cm in front of the posterior fontanel and approximately 6 cm from the anterior fontanel.*** Because cup diameters range from 5 to 6cm, when properly placed, the ***cup rim lies 3 cm from the anterior fontanel.***
- Gradual vacuum creation is advocated by some and is generated by increasing the suction in**increments of 0.2 kg/cm2 every 2 minutes** until a ***total negative pressure of 0.8 kg/cm2 is reached.*** That said, other studies have shown that negative pressure can be ***increased to 0.8***kg/cm2 in < 2 minutes without a significant difference in efficacy or in maternal and fetal outcomes

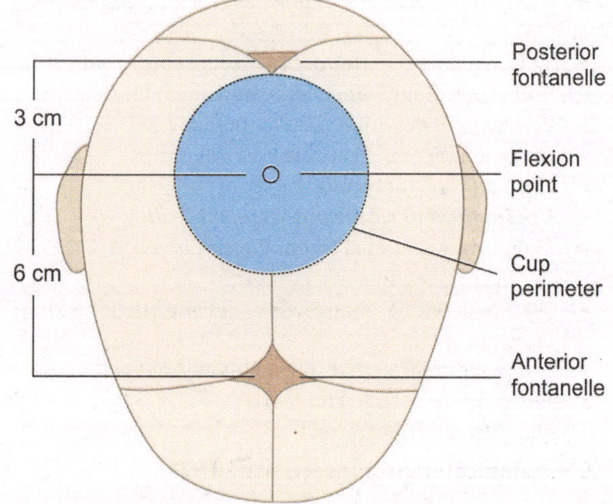

Fig: *(William)*: Drawing demonstrates correct cup placement at the flexion point. Along the sagittal suture, this spot lies 3 cm from the posterior fontanel and 6 cm from the anterior fontanel.

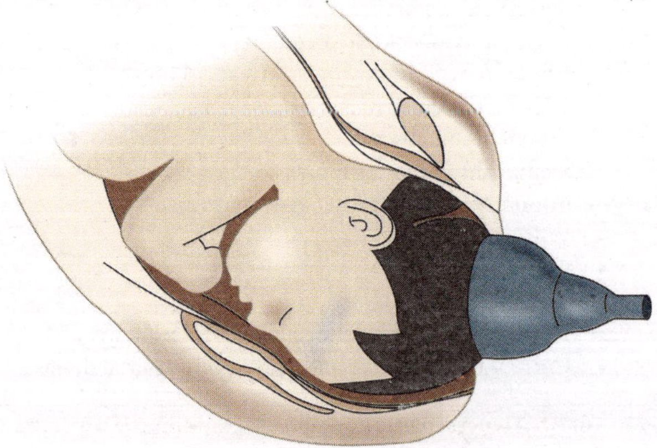

Fig: *(William)*: Cup placed before application of traction.

180. Ans. a. Traumatic separation of the placenta, b. Mutigravida, d. Gestational hypertension, e. Submucous fibroid

[Ref: Dutta Obs 8th/295; J B Sharma 1st/ 414; William's Obs 23rd/764]

Table *(William's Obs 23rd/764)*: **Risk Factors for Placental Abruption**

Risk factor	Relative Risk
Prior abruption	10–50
Increased age and parity	1.3 –2.3
Preeclampsia	2.1–4.0
Chorioamnionitis	3.0
Preterm ruptured membranes	2.4–4.9
Multifetal gestation	2.1
Low birthweight	14.0
Hydramnios	2.0
Cigarette smoking	1.4–1.9
Thrombophilias	3–7
Cocaine use	NA
Uterine leiomyoma	NA

Placental Abruption: Etiology

◈ *Dutta Obs 8th/295*

- The exact cause of separation of a normally situated placenta remains obscure in majority of cases.
- **Risk factors are:** (a) **high birth order** ***pregnancies with gravida 5 and above***—three times more common than in first birth (b) **Advancing age** of the mother (c) poor socio-economic condition (d) malnutrition (e) smoking (vasospasm).
- *Hypertension in pregnancy* is the important predisposing factor. ***Preeclampsia, gestational hypertension and essential hypertension***, all are associated with placental abruption.
- **Trauma:** ***Traumatic separation of the placenta*** usually leads to its marginal separation with escape of blood outside. The trauma may be due to: (i) Attempted external cephalic version specially under anesthesia using great force (ii) Road traffic accidents or blow on the abdomen (iii) Needle puncture at amniocentesis.
- **Sudden uterine decompression:** Sudden decompression of the uterus leads to diminished surface area of the uterus adjacent to the placental attachment and results in separation of the placenta. This may occur following— (a) delivery of the first baby of twins (b) sudden escape of liquor amnii in hydramnios and (c) premature rupture of membranes.
- **Short cord,** either relativeor absolute, can bring about placental separation during labour by mechanical pull.
- **Supine hypotension syndrome:** In this condition which occurs in pregnancy there is passive engorgement of the uterine and placental vessels resulting in rupture and extravasation of the blood.
- ***Placental anomaly:*** Circumvallate placenta
- ***Sick placenta:*** Poor placentation, evidenced by abnormal uterine artery Doppler waveforms is associated with placental abruption.
- **Folic acid deficiency:** Even without evidence of overt megaloblastic erythropoiesis--this has been observed to be associated.
- ***Uterine factor:*** Placenta implanted over a septum (septate Uterus) or a ***submucous fibroid.***
- Torsion of the uterus: leads to increased venous pressure and rupture of the veins with separation of the placenta.
- Cocaine abuse: is associated with increased risk of transient hypertension, vasospasm and placental abruption.
- Thrombophilias inherited or acquired have been associated with increased risk of placental infarts or abruption
- **Prior abruption:** Risk of recurrence for a woman with previous abruption varies between 5% and 17%

181. Ans. a. Hypertension, b. Anaemia

[Ref: Dutta Obs 8th/255,303; J B Sharma 1st/541; William Obs 23rd/1156]

"***Acne usually improves in pregnancy***"*-J B Sharma 1st/543*

"There are ***no obvious adverse effects of rheumatoid arthritis on pregnancy outcome***. The ***disease improves in majority (90%) of women during pregnancy***"*-J B Sharma 1st/541*

Most women with **rheumatoid arthritis,** perhaps as many as ***80% to 90%, experience improvement in their disease during pregnancy***. Improvement in joint stiffness and pain generally begins in the first trimester and persists until several weeks postpartum"- Obstetrics by G.Gabbe 6th/1006-07

"Up to 90 percent of women with **rheumatoid arthritis** will experience improvement during pregnancy"- *William Obs 23rd/1156*

Hypertension is one of the common medical complications of pregnancy"-Dutta Obs 8th/255

"**Anemia** is the commonest haematological disorder that ***may occur in pregnancy***, the others being rhesus isoimmunisation and blood coagulation disorders"- *Dutta Obs 8th/303*

182. Ans. a. Low platelets, b. Increased AST and ALT, e. Hemolysis

[Ref: Dutta Obs 8th/258; J B Sharma 1st/427; William's Obs 23rd/732]

HELLP Syndrome

◈ *Dutta Obs 8th/258*

- This is an acronym for ***Hemolysis (H), Elevated Liver enzymes (EL) and Low platelet count (LP) (<100, 000/ mm³).***
- This is a rare complication of preeclampsia (10–15%).
- HELLP syndrome may develop even without maternal hypertension. This syndrome is manifested by nausea, vomiting, epigastric or right upper quadrant pain, along with biochemical and hematological changes.
- Parenchymal necrosis of liver causes elevation in hepatic enzymes (**AST and ALT**> 70 IU/L, **LDH**> 600 IU/L) and **bilirubin** (> 1.2 mg/dL).

- There may be subcapsular hematoma formation (which is diagnosed by CT scan) and abnormal peripheral blood smear.
- Eventually liver may rupture to cause sudden hypotension, due to hemoperitoneum.

HELLP: ***Elevated serum biliubin (indirect form),*** low serum haptoglobin, elevated lactate dehydrogenase (LDH)"- Obstetrics by G.Gabbe 6th/790

183. Ans. a. Severe hypertension, b. Ischemic heart disease, d. Active liver disease

[Ref: Dutta Obs 8th/623; Shaw's Gynae16th/273-75; Harrison19th/2391; Katzung10th/668- 670]

"**OCP:** *As it cause regular andscanty menstruation, it is* ***useful inmenorrhgia*** *and polymenorrhoea. By virtu of non-ovulation, it can* ***relieve dysmenorrhoea*** *and* ***pre menstrual tension"*** *(Shaw's 16th/274)*

Table *(Harrison19th/2391)*: **Oral Contraceptives–C/I and Disease Risk**

Contraindications
Absolute
Previous thromboembolic event or stroke
History of an estrogen-dependent tumor
Active liver disease
Pregnancy
Undiagnosed abnormal uterine bleeding
Hypertriglyceridemia
Women over age 35 who smoke heavily (>15cigarettes per day)
Relative
Hypertension; Women following bariatric surgery
Women receiving anticonvulsant drug therapy

Table *(Dutta Obstetrics 8th/623)*: **Contraindication of Combined Oral Pills**

Absolute			Relative
• **Circulatory disease (past or present)**	• **Disease of the liver**	• **Others**	
▪ Arterial or venous thrombosis ▪ ***Severe hypertension***, stroke ▪ Valvular heart disease, ***Ischaemic heart disease***, Angina ▪ Diabetics with vascular complications ▪ Severe hypercholesterolemia ▪ Smoker over age 35 ▪ Focal migraine	▪ ***Active liver disease*** ▪ **Liver adenoma,** ▪ Carcinoma	▪ Pregnancy ▪ Undiagnosed genital tract bleeding ▪ Oestrogen dependent neoplasm *e.g.,*breast cancer ▪ Breastfeeding (within6 weeks postpartum) ▪ Major surgery or pro-longed immobilization	▪ Age >40 years ▪ Smoker or <35 years ▪ History of jaundice ▪ Diabetes ▪ Gall bladder disease ▪ Hyperlipidemia ▪ Post breast cancer ▪ Breastfeeding (Post partum 6wk to 6month) ▪ Sickle cell disease ▪ CIN

184. Ans. b. Breakthrough bleeding, d. Migraine

[Ref: Dutta Obs 8th/625; Dutta Gynae 6th/489; J B Sharma 1st/687-88; Novak's Gynae 15th/236]

"**OCP:***As it cause regular andscanty menstruation, it is* ***useful in menorrhgia*** *and polymenorrhoea. By virtu of non-ovulation, it can* ***relieve dysmenorrhoea*** *and* ***pre menstrual tension"*** *(Shaw's 16th/274)*

Noncontraceptive Benefit of COC

◈ *Dutta Gynae 6th/489*
- ***Reduction of dysmenorrhea (40%)***
- ***Reduction of menorrhagia (50%)***
- ***Protection against iron-deficiency anaemia***

Adverse Effect of COC

◈ *Dutta Gynae 6th/489; Dutta Obs 8th/625-26*
- Breakthrough bleeding: It is commonly due to subthreshold blood level of hormones
- Menorrhagia
- Headache

"**Indication of withdrawal of COC**: ***Severe migraine***"-Dutta Gynae 6th/487

Table *(Novak's Gynae 15th/236)*: **Established and Emerging Non-contraceptive Benefits of Oral Contraceptives**

Established Benefits
Menses-related
Increased menstrual cycle regularity
Reduced blood loss
Reduced iron-deficiency anemia
Reduced dysmenorrhea
Reduced symptoms of premenstrual dysphoric disorder
Inhibition of ovulation
Fewer ovarian cysts
Fewer ectopic pregnancies
Other
Reduced fibroadenomas/fibrocystic breast changes
Reduced acute pelvic inflammatory disease
Reduced endometrial cancer
Reduced ovarian cancer

Contd...

Emerging Benefits

Increased bone mass
Reduced acne
Reduced colorectal cancer
Reduced uterine leiomyomata
Reduced rheumatoid arthritis
Treatment of bleeding disorders
Treatment of hyperandrogenic anovulation
Treatment of endometriosis
Treatment of perimenopausal changes

185. Ans. c. Cherney incision is useful in uro-gynaecological procedures, d. Maylard incision provide improved access to the pelvic side wall, e. Rutherford-Morrison is particularly useful for approaching ovarian masses

[Ref: J B Sharma 1st/651; William's Obs 23rd/ 549-52; Robert W. Shaw Gynae 4th/105-06]

Abdominal Incision Robert

◈ *W. Shaw Gynae 4th/105-06*

- "The **vertical midline incision** avoids all major nerves, vessels and muscles by dividing rectus sheath. It gives good access to the whole abdomen except the subdiaphragmatic areas and is a very fast incision to make. It should always be closed using 'mass technique"
- The **Paramedian incision** is ***only included for historical intrest. It is inferior to the 'mass closure technique' of vertical median incision*** and does not provide improved access to either side of the abdomen"
- "The ***majority of gynaecological surgery is performed through a transverse incision***, usually a Pfannenstiel incision. If correctly placed, access to pelvis is good,although access to the pelvic brim is limited
- "The **Maylard incision** provide improved access to the ***pelvic side wall*** when compared with Pfannenstiel incision and is useful for oncological surgery"

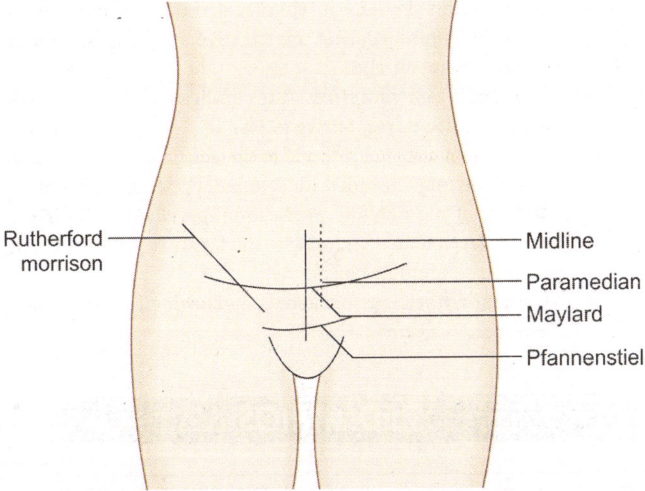

Fig: *(Robert W. Shaw Gynae 4th/105-06)*: Abdominal incision

- "The **Cherney incision** is similar to Pfannenstiel incision but the rectus muscles are divided 1 cm from their insertion into the symphysis pubis. This incision can also be useful in oncological surgey or if placed lower, is useful for complex urogynaecological procedures"
- "The **Rutherford-Morrison** is particularly useful for approaching ovarian masses in the second half of the pregnancy"

"**Two basic skin incisions** are used: ***suprapubic transverse and midline vertical***. *Paraumbilical (right or left) incision is not usually used for caesarean delivery*"*-J B Sharma 1st/651*

Technique for Cesarean Delivery

◈ *William's Obs 23rd/ 549-52*

With minor variations, surgical performance of cesarean delivery is comparable worldwide.

Abdominal Incisions

- Usually either a **midline vertical or a suprapubic transverse incision** is used. Only in especial circumstances would a **paramedian or midtransverse incision** be employed.
- An infraumbilical midline vertical incision is quickest to make. The incision should be of sufficient length to allow delivery of the infant without difficulty. Therefore, its length should correspond with the estimated fetal size.
- **Transverse Incisions:**With the modified *Pfannenstiel incision*, the skin and subcutaneous tissue are incised using a lower transverse, slightly curvilinear incision. The incision is made at the level of the pubic hairline and is extended somewhat beyond the lateral borders of the rectus muscles. The cosmetic advantage of the transverse skin incision is apparent.
- When a transverse incision is desired and more room is needed, the ***Maylard incision*** provides a safe option.

186. Ans. e. Zidovudine is given in place of stavudine in HAART therapy if mother is anaemic

[Ref: Dutta Obs 8th/350-52; J B Sharma 1st/551-53; William's Obs 23rd/1246-53]

"In the absence of prophylactic antiretroviral therapy to the mother during pregnancy, labor and delivery and to the fetus following birth, the probability of transmission of HIV from mother to infant/ fetus ranges from ***15% to 25% in industrialized countries and from 25% to 35% in developing countries***"-Harrison 19th/1223

HIV and AIDS in Pregnancy

◈ *Dutta Obs 8th/350-52; J B Sharma 1st/551-53*

- ***Vertical transmission to the neonate is about 14-25%.*** Transmission of HIV2 is less frequent (1-4%) than for HIV 1 (15–40%)"- Dutta Obs 8th/351
- "***Vertical transmission to the neonate is about 30%*** (13-25% in developed countries; 35% is developing countries)"- J B Sharma 1st/551
- Women with CD4+ count (≤ 350 cells/mm^3) or HIV RNA level ≥50,000 copies/mm^3 should be initiated with HAART
- **Highly active antiretroviral therapy (HAART):** Triple therapy is preferred as a first line defence and to be started any time b/w 14 weeks and 28 weeks and then continued throughout pregnancy, labour and postpartum period

- "**Zidovudine:** anaemia and neutropenia are most important and dose-related side effect. ***Stavudine is substituted for zidovudine if patient is anaemic***"-KDT 7th/807
- ***Elective caesarean section reduces the risk of vertical transmission by about 50%.*** Avoidance of breastfeeding, HAART therapy and appropriate mode of delivery has reduced MTCT rates from 25-30% to <1%. Baby should be bathed immediately
- **Neonatal care**: Antiretroviral therapy should be given to all neonates within 4 hours of birth. Usually ***zidovudine montherapy (Zidovudine syrup)*** is started. It is continued for first 6 week of life. High risk neonate should be treated with HAART
- HIV diagnosis is made by detecting HIV viral RNA in blood by PCR testing or by detecting antibodies to HIV (enzyme immunoassay). Western blot is specific test

187. Ans. b. Pain begins a few hours before or just after the onset of a menstrual period and may last 48 to 72 hours
c. May be associated with psychological factors

[Ref: Shaw's 16th/471-73; Dutta Gynae 6th/178-80; Novak's Gyae 15th/481-83]

Primary Dysmenorrhea

◈ *Dutta Gynae 6th/178-80; Shaw's 16th/471-73*

- *The **pain begin few hour before or just with onset of menstruation***
- *The severity of pain usually lasts for few hours, may extend to 24 hours but seldom persists beyond 48 hours*

***GnRH antagonists** (Leuprolide, buserelin, nafarelin) are used for pelvic endometriosis (**cause of secondary dysmenorrhea**)-Shaw's 16th/4713*

*"**Premenstrual syndrome** is associated with **psychological symptoms** (like emotional liability, irritability,mood swing, depression)"-Shaw's 16th/471*

Table *(Shaw's 16th/472)*: **Differentiating features of primary and secondary dysmenorrhea**

Differentiating features	Primary	Secondary
Onset	Within 2 years of menarche	20–30 years, may be pre-and postmenstrual
Description	Cramping–hypogastrium, back, inner thighs	Variable dull ahce
Symptomatology	Nausea, vomiting, diarrhea, headache, fatigue	Dyspareunia, infertility, menstrual disorders
Pelvic findings	Normal	Variable, depending on cause
Aetiology	Excessive myometrial contraction, ischaemia, excessive prostaglandin production	***Endometriosis***, PID, adenomyosis, fibroids, pelvic vein congestion
Management	Reassurance, analgesics, NSAIDs, antispasmodics, OC pills, in rare cases, surgery–Cotte's operation or laparoscopic uterisacral nerve ablation (LUNA)	Treatment directed to the cause

Contd...

Cyclic Pain: Primary and Secondary Dysmenorrhea

◈ *Novak's Gyae15th/481*

- Dysmenorrhea is a common gynecologic disorder affecting as many as 60% of menstruating women.
- **Primary dysmenorrhea** refers to menstrual pain without pelvic pathology, whereas secondary dysmenorrhea is defined as painful menses associated with underlying pathology.
- The pain of primary dysmenorrhea ***usually begins a few hours before or just after the onset of a menstrual period and may last 48 to 72 hours.***
- The pain is similar to labor, with suprapubic cramping and may be accompanied by lumbosacral backache, pain radiating down the anterior thigh, nausea, vomiting, diarrhea and rarely syncopal episodes.
- Primary dysmenorrhea usually appears within 1 to 2 years of menarche, when ovulatory cycles are established. The disorder affects younger women but may persist into their 40s.
- Secondary dysmenorrhea usually develops years after menarche and can occur with anovulatory cycles.
- The etiology of primary dysmenorrhea includes excessive or imbalanced amount of prostanoids secreted from the endometrium during menstruation. The prostanoids result in increased uterine contractions with a dysrhythmic pattern, increased basal tone and increased active pressure. Uterine hypercontractility, decreased uterine blood flow and increased peripheral nerve hypersensitivity contribute to pain
- Prostaglandin synthase inhibitors, also called ***nonsteroidal anti-inflammatoryagents***, are effective for the treatment of primary dysmenorrhea
- ***Hormonal contraceptives*** are indicated for primary dysmenorrhea unresponsive to NSAIDs
- If the patient does not respond to this regimen, hydrocodone or codeine may be added for 2 to 3 days per month; before addition of the narcotic medication, ***psychological factors*** should be evaluated and diagnostic laparoscopy to rule out pathology should be considered.
- **Dysmenorrhoea** is associated with ***neurological symptoms***-Robert Shaw's Gynae 4th/455

PEDIATRICS

188. Ans. d. In symptomatic patients, the 24 hr urinary copper excretion is less than 40 μg/day

[Ref: Robbins 9th (SAE)/849-50; O.P.Ghai 8th/320-21; Nelson 20th/1940-41]

Wilson Disease

◈ *O.P. Ghai 8th/320-21*

- *Serum* **ceruloplasmin is decreased (<20mg/dL) in most patients**
- *In symptomatic patients, the 24 hr* ***urinary copper excretion is more than 100 µg/day***
- **Kayser-Fleischer (KF) ring** *indicates long standing disease and severe copper load*
- **Hepatic copper** *is the single best predictive marker and is considered to be the gold standard, with values usually* ***above 250 µg/g dry weight of liver***
- *Liver biopsy is required for hepatic copper estimation*

"Most patients with Wilson disease have decreased ceruloplasmin levels **(<20 mg/dL)**.The serum free copper level may be elevated in early Wilson disease (>1.6 µmol/L and ***urinary copper excretion (usually <40 µg/day) is increased to >100 µg/day and often up to 1,000 µg or more per day. Liver biopsy is of value for determining the extent and severity of liver disease*** and for measurement of the hepatic copper content (normally <10 µg/g dry weight). In Wilson disease, **hepatic copper content exceeds 250 µg/g dry weight**"- *Nelson 20th/1940-41*

Wilson Disease

◈ *Robbins 9th (SAE)/849-50*

- Wilson disease is an autosomal recessive disorder caused by mutation of the *ATP7B* gene, resulting in impaired copper excretion into bile and a failure to incorporate copper into ceruloplasmin.
- The liver often bears the brunt of injury, but the disease may also present as a neurologic disorder. The hepatic changes are variable, ranging from relatively minor to massive damage and mimic many other disease processes.
- **Fatty change (steatosis)** may be mild to moderate with focal hepatocyte necrosis. An acute, fulminant hepatitis can mimic acute viral hepatitis. Chronic hepatitis in Wilson disease exhibits moderate to severe inflammation and ***hepatocyte necrosis***, admixed with fatty change and features of ***steatohepatitis*** (hepatocyte ballooning with prominent Mallory-Denk bodies). Eventually cirrhosis supervenes.
- Demonstration of ***Kayser-Fleischer rings*** further favors the diagnosis.

189. Ans. b. Walks up and down stairs, one step at a time, e. Weight quadruples of birth weight

[Ref: O.P.Ghai 8th/49; Nelson 20th/ 75]

"**Weight** at 6 month-doubles (6 kg), at 1 yr -triples (9 kg) and at ***2 yr- quadruples (12 kg) of birth weight (3 kg)***"- *O.P.Ghai 8th/13*

Developmental Milestones

◈ *O.P.Ghai 8th/49*

- ***2 yr: Walks up and downstairs (2 feet/step); Jumps***
- **3 yr:** Rides tricycle; alternate feet going upstairs
- 4 yr: Hopes on one foot; alternate feet going downstairs

24 Month *Nelson 20th/75*	
Motor	Runs well, ***walks up and down stairs, one step at a time***; opens doors; climbs on furniture; jumps
Adaptive	Makes tower of 7 cubes (6 at 21 mo); scribbles in circular pattern; imitates horizontal stroke; folds paper once imitatively
Language	Puts 3 words together (subject, verb, object)
Social	Handles spoon well; often tells about immediate experiences; helps to undress; listens to stories when shown pictures

30 Month *Nelson 20th/75*	
Motor:	Goes up stairs alternating feet
Adaptive:	Makes tower of 9 cubes; makes vertical and horizontal strokes, but generally will not join them to make cross; imitates circular stroke, forming closed Fig.
Language:	Refers to self by pronoun "I"; knows full name
Social:	Helps put things away; pretends in play

36 Month *Nelson 20th/75*	
Motor	***Rides tricycle***; stands momentarily on one foot
Adaptive	Makes tower of 10 cubes; imitates construction of "bridge" of 3 cubes; copies circle; imitates cross
Language	***Knows age and sex***; counts 3 objects correctly; repeats 3 numbers or a sentence of 6 syllables
Social	Plays simple games (in "parallel" with other children); helps in dressing (unbuttons clothing and puts on shoes); washes hands

15 Month *Nelson 20th/75*	
Motor:	Walks alone; crawls up stairs
Adaptive:	Makes tower of 3 cubes; makes a line with crayon; inserts raisin in bottle
Language:	Jargon; follows simple commands; may name a familiar object (e.g., ball)
Social:	Indicates some desires or needs by pointing; hugs parents

18 Month *Nelson 20th/75*	
Motor:	Runs stiffly; sits on small chair; walks up stairs with one hand held; explores drawers and wastebaskets
Adaptive:	Makes tower of 4 cubes; imitates scribbling; imitates vertical stroke; dumps raisin from bottle
Language:	10 words (average); names pictures; identifies one or more parts of body
Social:	Feeds self; seeks help when in trouble; may complain when wet or soiled; kisses parent with pucker

48 Month *Nelson 20th/75*	
Motor:	Hops on one foot; throws ball overhand; uses scissors to cut out pictures; climbs well
Adaptive:	Copies bridge from model; imitates construction of "gate" of 5 cubes; copies cross and square; draws man with 2 to 4 parts besides head; identifies longer of 2 lines
Language:	Counts 4 pennies accurately; tells story
Social:	Plays with several children, with beginning of social interaction and role-playing; goes to toilet alone

60 Month *Nelson 20th/ 75*	
Motor:	Skips
Adaptive:	Draws triangle from copy; names heavier of 2 weights
Language:	Names 4 colors; repeats sentence of 10 syllables; counts 10 pennies correctly
Social:	Dresses and undresses; asks questions about meaning of words; engages in domestic role-playing

190. Ans. a. Tuberous sclerosis, b. Neurofibromatosis-2, e. Turcot syndrome

[Ref: O.P.Ghai 8th/613; Nelson 20th/2454]

Cockayne syndrome – ***predispose to skin cancer***- *Nelson 20th/3159*

Fanconi syndrome: *Proximal RTA, phosphaturia, glycosuria, proteinuria, aminoaciduria*"- *Nelson 20th/2529*

Table *(O.P.Ghai 8th/613; Nelson 20th/2454)*: **Familial Syndromes Associated with Pediatric Brain Tumors**

Syndrome	CNS Manifestations
Neurofibromatosis type 1 (autosomal dominant)	Optic pathway gliomas, astrocytoma, malignant peripheral nerve sheath tumors, neurofibromas
Neurofibromatosis type 2 (autosomal dominant)	Vestibular schwannomas, meningiomas, spinal cord ependymoma, spinal cord astrocytoma, hamartomas
von Hippel-Lindau (autosomal dominant)	Hemangioblastoma
Tuberous sclerosis (autosomal dominant)	Subependymal giant cell astrocytoma, cortical tubers
Bilateral retinoblastoma	Pineal tumor
Li-Fraumeni (autosomal dominant)	Astrocytoma, primitive neuroectodermal tumor
Cowden (autosomal dominant)	Dysplastic gangliocytoma of the cerebellum (Lhermitte-Duclos disease)
Turcot (autosomal dominant)	Medulloblastoma, Glioblastoma
Gorlin syndrome	Medulloblastoma
Nevoid basal cell carcinoma (autosomal dominant)	Medulloblastoma

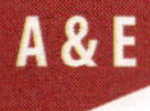

191. Ans. a. Called as 5th day fits, c. Status epilepticus may occur

[Ref: Nelson 20th/2851-52]

Benign Idiopathic Neonatal Seizures (Fifth Day Fits)

◈ *Nelson 20th/2851*

- Apneic and focal motor seizures that start around the ***fifth day of life***
- Interictal EEG shows a distinctive pattern called theta pointu alternant (runs of sharp 4-7 Hz activity) and ictal EEG shows multifocal electrographic seizures
- Patients have a ***good response to medications and a good prognosis***
- **Fifth-day fits** occur on day 5 of life (4–6 days) in normal-appearing neonates. ***The seizures are multifocal and are present for less than 24 hr.*** The diagnosis requires exclusion of other causes of seizures"- *Nelson 20th/2852*

"The diagnosis of BINS is made in **full-term babies** who are neurologically normal and have ***no familial history of neonatal convulsions***"- *link.springer.com*

"**Benign nonfamilial neonatal seizures** usually begin when the baby is four to six days old. There is ***no family history of seizures***. The baby will usually have partial, clonic seizures, often limited to one side of the body. The ***seizures may lead to status epilepticus***, lasting from two hours to three days. There is not much information available on outcomes for children with benign nonfamilial neonatal seizures, ***but the seizures do not often continue in later life***"-*www.aboutkidshealth.ca*

Benign Neonatal Seizures

◈ *journals.lww.com/clinicalneurophy*

- It is a rare but increasingly recognized syndrome characterized by seizures in the neonatal or infantile period.
- **Two forms** are recognized: **familial and nonfamilial**
- **In both instances,** the seizures may be quite severe and ***status epilepticus is common.***
- The **nonfamilial form** is characterized by ***idiopathic, self-limited seizures occurring in previously normal neonates.*** The seizures most commonly ***occur at day 5 and have been called "fifth-day fits" by some authors.***
- **Familial seizures** most frequently have their onset during the first week of life, but onset may occur as late as early infancy. These seizures may recur for several months before resolving. No cause is found for the seizures and the patient appears healthy during the interictal period. The family history reveals benign neonatal seizures in other family members.
- ***Although the prognosis is favorable in both syndromes, seizures may occasionally occur later in life in the familial form.*** The familial form of benign neonatal seizures is autosomal dominant and the gene has been localized to chromosome 20

Benign Familial Neonatal Seizures

◈ *Nelson 20th/2851*

- An autosomal dominant condition have onset at ***2-4 days of age and usually remit at 2-15 wk of age***
- The seizure consists of ocular deviation, tone posturing, clonic jerks and at times, motor automatisms

- Interictal EEG is usually normal
- ***Approximately 16% of patients develop later epilepsy***

"The occurrence of ***status epilepticus is common in benign idiopathic neonatal convulsions (BINC)*** but is uncommon in benign familial neonatal convulsions (BFNC). Because the condition benign idiopathic neonatal convulsions is a diagnosis of exclusion, it is nearly always made in retrospect, ***when the seizures spontaneously resolve and the infant is found to have neurologically normal development***"-*emedicine.medscape.com*

"Interestingly, unaffected family members of ***patients with benign familial neonatal convulsions have a higher-than-expected risk of developing epilepsy in later life***"-emedicine. medscape.com

Benign neonatal seizures is a rare but increasingly recognized syndrome characterized by seizures in the neonatal or infantile period. Two forms are recognized: familial and nonfamilial. ***In both instances, the seizures may be quite severe and status epilepticus is common. The nonfamilial form is characterized by idiopathic, self-limited seizures occurring in previously normal neonates.*** Although the prognosis is favorable in both syndromes, seizures may occasionally occur later in life in the familial form."- *www.researchgate.ne*

192. Ans. b. Mostly asymptomatic, c. Swelling is ballotable, d. Stage I- tumour confined to kidney, e. Completely excision is treatment of choice in stage I and II

[Ref: O.P.Ghai 8th/617-18; Nelson 20th/2464-68]

Wilms Tumor

◈ *O.P.Ghai 8th/617-18*

- *At diagnosis* ***30% presents with abdominal pain***
- ***Most patients presents with a asymptomatic abdominal mass***
- ***Renal lump is ballottable****-Kundu 4th/255*
- ***Stages: I-IV.***
- ***Stage I- tumour confined to kidney and completely excised***

Clinical Manifestations

◈ *Nelson 20th/2464-68*

- Wilms tumor usually presents as an abdominal mass. Some patients ***may present with abdominal pain*** and vomiting and hematuria is seen in 12–25% of patients.
- Wilms tumor, also known as **nephroblastoma,** is a complex mixed embryonal neoplasm of the kidney composed of three elements: blastema, epithelia and stroma.
- Familial predisposition to Wilms tumor is inherited in an **autosomal dominant manner.**

Table *(Nelson 20th/2467)*: **Staging System Developed by the Third National Wilms Tumor Study**

Stage	Description
Stage I	Tumor is limited to kidney and is completely excised. Capsular surface intact; no tumor rupture; no residual tumor apparent beyond margins of excision
Stage II	Tumor extends beyond kidney but is completely excised. Regional extension of tumor; vessel infiltration; tumor biopsied or local spillage of tumor confined to the flank. No residual tumor apparent at or beyond margins of excision
Stage III	Residual non-hematogenous tumor confined to the abdomen. Lymph node involvement of hilus, periaortic chains, or beyond; diffuse peritoneal contamination by tumor spillage; peritoneal implants of tumor, tumor extends beyond surgical margins microscopically or macroscopically; tumor not completely removable because of local infiltration into vital structures
Stage IV	Deposits beyond stage III (e.g., lung, liver, bone, brain)
Stage V	Bilateral renal involvement at diagnosis

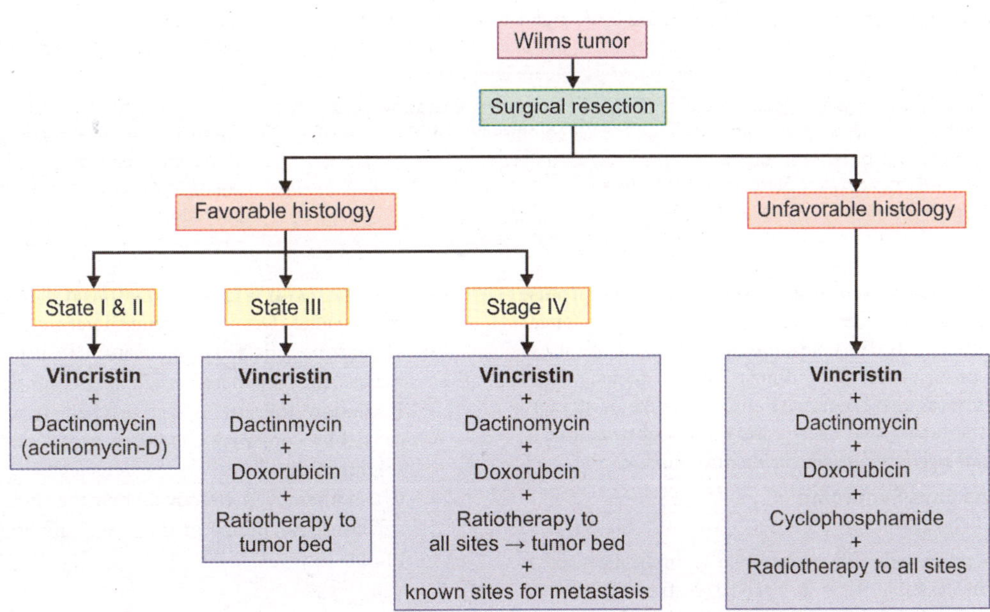

193. Ans. a. Type I Glycogen storage disorder, d. Biliary cirrhosis

[Ref: O.P.Ghai 8th/310; Nelson 20th/ 1922]

"**Gaucher disease**: The spleen is markedly enlarged. The ***liver is enlarged***"- O.P.Ghai 8th/661

"**Gaucher disease**: Painless hepatomegaly and splenomegaly: the ***size of the spleen can be 1500-3000 mL, as opposed to the normal size of 50-200 mL***"-wiki

"Patients with **type I glycogen storage disease** may present in the neonatal period with hypoglycemia and lactic acidosis; however, they more commonly present at 3–4 mo of age with hepatomegaly or hypoglycemic seizures, or both. These children often have doll-like faces with fat cheeks, relatively thin extremities, short stature and a protuberant abdomen that is due to ***massive hepatomegaly***"-*Nelson 20th/718*

Biliary cirrhosis becomes symptomatic in only 2–3% of patients. Manifestations may include icterus, ascites, hematemesis from esophageal varices and evidence of hypersplenism. A neonatal hepatitis-like picture and **massive hepatomegaly** owing to steatosis have been reported. Biliary colic secondary to cholelithiasis may occur in the 2nd decade of life. Liver disease occurs independent of genotype"- *Nelson 20th*

"Biliary atresia: Hepatosplenomegaly and ascites – late sign, suggestive of cirrhosis and portal hypertension"- *pedclerk.bsd.uchicago.edu*

Cause of Massive Hepatomegaly

- Chronic extrahepatic cholestasis cholestasise.g., congenital biliary atresia
- Malaria, kala-azar for long duration
- ***Glycogen storage disease***
- Congenital hepatic fibrosis
- Amoebic liver abscess
- Hepatoma or secondary malignant deposits
- Cysts of liver
- ***Biliary cirrhosis***
- Chronic congestive hepatomegaly: VSD with heart failure, Cardiomyopathy with congestive heart failure, Constrictive pericarditis

194. Ans. a. Administration of oxygen with ventimaskm, b. Tracheostomy, c. Biopsy of mass and fine needle aspiration cytology

[Ref: O.P.Ghai 8th/ 622; Nelson 20th/2433]

This is case of superior vena cave syndrome

Next line of management should include-oxygen administration with ventimask, tracheostomy (if respiratory distress is not relieved by ventimask) and biopsy and aspiration cytology (for confirmation of diagnosis)

Mediastinal radiation therapy should be included later after confirmation of diagnosis. Rasburicase (for tumor lysis syndrome) should be considered only after confirmation of diagnosis, if risk of tumour lysis syndrome is present

"The treatment of SVCS depends on the severity of the symptoms and the cause of the obstruction, as well as on the histological type and stage of the tumor produced. ***Measures such as reclining the patient and elevating the head, as well as controlling the volume of oxygen administered and the oxygen supplementation***, are valid alternatives for use prior to diagnosis and initiation of the definitive treatment"- *www.scielo.br; emedicine.medscape.com*

Table *(O.P.Ghai 8th/ 622)*: **Presentation and treatment of common oncologic emergencies**

Oncologic emergency	Manifestation	Underlying disease	Treatment
Tumor lysis syndrome	Hyperkalemia leading to arrhythmias; hyperphosphatemia; hyperuricemia; acute kidney injury; hypocalcemia with tetany; metastatic calcifications	Acute lymphoblastic leukemia, non-Hodgkin lymphoma (most commonly Burkitt lymphoma), acute lymphoblastic leukemia	Hydration, alkalinization, allopurinol, ***rasburicase*** (if uric acid >10mg/dl), dialysis for renal failure
Superior vena cava or mediastinal syndrome	***Swelling of face*** and neck, dyspnea; orthopnea; dysphagia; hoarse voice; proptosis; Horner syndrome; chest pain; wheezing; pleural or pericardial effusion; type II respiratory failure	**Superior mediastinal mass,** most commonly NHL, ALL or germ cell tumor	Establish histological diagnosis by tissue sampling; administer corticosteroids. Avoid intravenous access in upper limbs; ***monitor for tumor lysis;*** chemotherapy; radiation

"**Superior Vena Cava Syndrome**: **Respiratory symptoms**: initially started as orthopnea, later on progressed to dyspnea. Dyspnea together with dry nonproductive cough is the most common symptom observed in almost 75 % of patients with SVCS. Sometimes is also hoarseness and dysphonia or ***stridor***, shortness of the breath and chest pain.**Venous obstruction** is present as ***facial swelling***"- *telemedicina.med.muni.cz*

Superior Vena Cava Syndrome

◈ *Harrison 19th/1788*

- The one potentially life-threatening complication of a superior mediastinal mass is tracheal obstruction. Upper airway obstruction demands emergent therapy.
- Diuretics with a low-salt diet, head elevation and **oxygen** may produce temporary symptomatic relief.
- Glucocorticoids may be useful at shrinking lymphoma masses; they are of no benefit in patients with lung cancer.
- **Radiation therapy** is the primary treatment for SVCS caused by non-small-cell lung cancer and other metastatic solid tumors.
- Chemotherapy is effective when the underlying cancer is small-cell carcinoma of the lung, lymphoma, or germ cell tumor.

Superior Mediastinal Compression (SMC) Syndrome Initial Management

◈ *www.starship.org.nz/*

- **Prevention of tumour lysis syndrome**: Start hyperhydration and recombinant urate oxidase (or allopurinol if this is not available) with 6 hourly monitoring of electrolyte and urate levels (refer to tumour lysis syndrome).
- **Avoid accessing veins draining into the SVC.** Do not insert central venous catheter until SMC syndrome resolved. Do not insert IV cannula into a vein draining into SVC, i.e., put into foot vein or greater saphenous.
- **Try to establish the diagnosis** without resorting to sedation or a general anaesthetic:
  - Full Blood Count - immunophenotyping on peripheral blood.
  - ***Fine needle aspirate or core biopsy of palpable, pathological lymph node*** under local anaesthetic. In addition to cytology/histology, specimens must be sent for immunophenotyping.
  - ***Aspirate of pleural effusion***. Procedures such as diagnostic pleural aspiration should not be performed on the ward without the presence of an anesthetist or intensivist and resuscitation equipment ready. Guidelines need to be followed, including avoidance of drainage of large volumes of pleural fluid, due to the risks of re-expansion pulmonary oedema and precipitating airway collapse, risks which are higher in children.
  - Lumbar Puncture by an experienced clinician for CSF cytospin.
  - ***Bone marrow aspiration*** should be performed as soon as possible. Older children may tolerate a bone marrow aspirate with local anaesthetic only.
  - If there is no detectable extrathoracic disease, discuss alternative means of diagnosis with a surgeon e.g., ***mediastinal thoracoscopy and biopsy.***
  - A general anaesthetic is often high risk and should be avoided if possible.
  - Systemic steroids may be necessary to shrink the mass and reduce medistinal compression prior to biopsy. Systemic steroids can rapidly reduce the size of a mass but significantly alters tissue quality, due to its oncolytic effects. This can delay accurate diagnosis on biopsy and staging. **This decision should involve a paediatric oncologist, with multi-disciplinary consultation.**

195. Ans. b. Aspiration pneumonia, d. Paroxysms of coughing or cyanosis with feeding

[Ref: Nelson 20th/1783; O.P. Ghai 8th/176; CSDT 14th/1233-34; Neonatology by Tricia Lacy Gomella 5th/572]

Dysphagia is not present because of patency of esophagus

H-type TEF accounts for 4-5% of all congenital tracheoesophageal malformations. The clinical features are variable; common being the ***recurrent respiratory symptoms, aspiration during feeding with cyanosis and abdominal distension***. The ***early diagnosis of this disorder is difficult and some cases may remain undiagnosed until late in infancy or childhood***. H-type TEF is associated with other malformations in about 30% of cases, including VACTERL/VATER, CHARGE syndrome, Goldenhar's syndrome, esophageal stenosis and syndactyly"- *www.ncbi.nlm.nih.gov*

"The **neonate with EA** typically has frothing and bubbling at the mouth and nose after birth as well as episodes of coughing, cyanosis and respiratory distress. ***Feeding exacerbates these symptoms, causes regurgitation and may precipitate aspiration.*** Aspiration of gastric contents via a distal fistula causes more damaging pneumonitis than aspiration of pharyngeal secretions from the blind upper pouch. The infant with an isolated TEF in the absence of EA ("H-type" fistula) may come to medical attention later in life with ***chronic respiratory problems, including refractory bronchospasm and recurrent pneumonias***"-*Nelson 20th/1783*

"The clinical diagnosis of an H-type TEF has been associated with the ***triad of paroxysms of coughing or cyanosis with feeding, gaseous distension of the gastrointestinal tract and recurrent pneumonia or bronchitis***"- *www.nature.com/jp/journa*

"Overall survival in patients with H-type TEF without esophageal atresia (ie, congenital isolated TEF) appears ***to be good, with a multicenter retrospective reporting a 97% overall survival and a 16% in-hospital complication rate*** (excluded vocal cord issues; the main complication was postoperative leak [8%]) in 102 patients"-emedicine.medscape.com

H-Type Tracheoesophageal Fistula

◈ *Neonatology by Tricia Lacy Gomella 5th/572*

- This anomaly is the third most common type of TEF, making up 5% of cases. Esophageal continuity is intact, but there is a fistulous communication between the posterior trachea and the anterior esophagus.
- **Pathophysiology.** If the fistula is small, as is usually the case, **"silent" aspiration** occurs during feedings with resulting ***pneumonitis***. If the fistula is unusually large, coughing and choking may accompany each feeding
- **Diagnosis.** Barium swallow is the initial diagnostic study and may identify the fistula. The most accurate procedure, however, is bronchoscopy (perhaps combined with esophagoscopy); this should allow discovery and perhaps cannulation of the fistula.

TEF Without Esophageal Atresia:There is an "H"-type tracheoesophageal fistula that is usually present in the low cervical region (type E, 4%-5% of cases). ***Diagnosis may be delayed (several months) in cases*** of ***H-type tracheoesophageal fistula who are able to feed but may present with recurrent***

upper respiratory infections due to aspiration"-*CSDT 14th/1233-34*

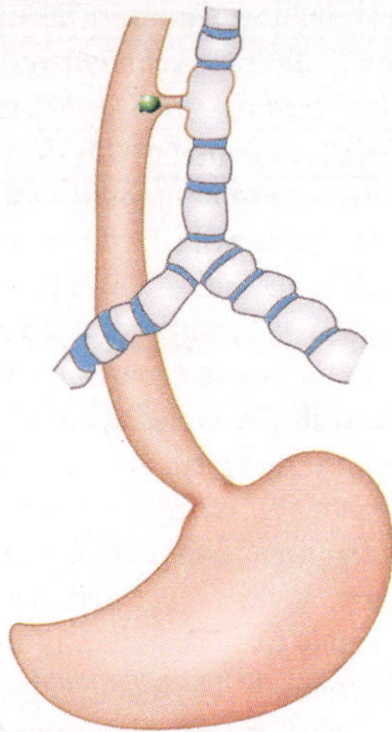

Fig: *(emedicine.medscape.com)*: Tracheoesophageal fistula. H-type of tracheoesophageal fistula

196. Ans. a. TB, b. Meckel's diverticulum, c. Aspirin, e. It is bleeding from a site distal to ligament of treitz

[Ref: O.P.Ghai 8th/306-08; Nelson 20th/1767, 1925; CSDT 14th/1251]

Paracetamol is Safer Drug

Gastrointestinal Bleeding

- *O.P.Ghai 8th/306*
- *Upper GI bleeding is defined as bleeding from a site proximal to the ligament of treitz (at the level of duodenojejunal flexure).*
- *Lower GI bleeding is defined as bleeding from a site distal to ligament of treitz*

Table *(O.P.Ghai 8th/306-08)*: **Causes of lower gastrointestinal bleeding**

Neonate or infant	Children >2 years
Noncolitic	
Infectious colitis	Infectious colitis
Cow milk protein allergy	Inflammatory bowel disease
Necrotising enterocolitis	***Tuberculosis***
Hirschsprung	Pseudomembranous colitis
Enterocolitis	Cow milk protein allergy
Systemic vasculitis	Uncommon: Amebiasis, cytomegalovirus, neutropenic colitis
Noncolitic	
Anal fissure	Fissure; Arteriovenous malformation
Intussusception	Polyp or polyposis syndrome
Duplication cyst	Solitary rectal ulcer syndrome

Contd...

Neonate or infant	Children >2 years
Noncolitic	
Arteriovenous malformation	*Meckel's diverticulum*
Coagulopathy	Rectal varices or colopathy
Rectal prolapse	***NSAID induced ulcer***
Meckel's diverticulum	Hemorrhoids; Coagulopathy
Hemorrhagic disease of newborn	Henoch-Schonlein purpura

Table *(CPDT 17th/653)*: **Differential diagnosis of gastrointestinal bleeding in children by symptoms and age at presentation**

	Infant	Child (2–12 years)
Hematemesis	Swallowed maternal blood peptic esophagitis Mallory–Weiss tear Gastritis Gastric ulcer Duodenal ulcer Gastric, duodenal ulcer	Epistaxis Peptic esophagitis Caustic ingestion Mallory–Weiss tear Esophageal varices Gastritis Gastric ulcer Duodenal ulcer Heraditary hemorrhagic telangiectasia Hemobilia Henoch–Schonlein purpura
Painless melena	Duodenal ulcer Duodenal duplication Ileal duplication Meckel diverticulum Gastric heterotopia	Duodenal ulcer Duodenal duplication Ileal duplication Meckel diverticulum Gastric heterotopia
Melena with pain, obstruction, peritonitis, perforation	Necrotizing enterocolitis Intussusception Volvulus	Duodental ulcer Hemobilia Intussusception Volvulus Ileal ulcer (isolated)
Hematochezia with diarrhea, crampy abdominal pain	Infectious colitis Pseudomembranous colitis Eosinophilic colitis Hirschsprung enterocolitis	Infectious colitis Pseudomembranous colitis Granulomatous (Crohn) colitis Hemolytic-uremic syndrome Henoch-Schonlein purpura Lymphonodular hyperplasia

ORTHOPEDICS

197. Ans. b. Association with HLA B-27, c. Enthesitis may occur, e. Cardiac conduction defect may present

[Ref: Apley 9th/66-70; Harrison 19th/ 2169-72; Davidson 22nd/1105-06]

"Eye involvement is the most common, with ***anterior uveitis (or iritis) seen in 25% to 40%*** of patients who have ankylosing spondylitis"- *www.clevelandclinicmeded.com*

Aortic valve regurgitation is ***present in 3% to 5% of patients.*** When present, it should be followed closely, as it often progresses to heart failure. ***Complete heart block*** may develop when fibrosis extends from the aortic root to the electrical conduction system"- *Manual of Rheumatology and Outpatient Orthopedic Disorders by Stephen A. Paget 2000 /Chap 33*

Ankylosing Spondylitis (AS)

- *Apley 9th/66-70*
- *HLA-B27 is present in 95% of cases*
- ***Rest and immobilisation are contraindicated*** *because they tend to increase the general feeling of stiffness*
- ***Acute anterior uveitis occurs in about 25% of patients***

"The onset is insidious, with early symptoms including pain in the buttocks, heels and lower back. ***Patients complain typically of morning stiffness, the improvement of symptoms with activity during the day*** and the return of symptoms in the evening. **Enthesitis** occurs at the insertion of the annulus fibrosus on the vertebral body with eventual calcification that results in the characteristic "bamboo spine." ***Approximately 30% of patients develop uveitis and 30% have chest tightness***. Limited chest expansion indicates thoracic involvement. ***Fewer than 5% of patients have involvement of the aorta, characterized by dilation and possible conduction defects***. In addition, patients may suffer from renal amyloidosis and pulmonary fibrosis"- *Current Diagnosis and Treatment in Orthopedics 4th/Chap 5*

Ankylosing Spondylitis (AS)

- *Davidson 22nd/1105-06*
- The onset is typically between the ages of 20 and 30, with a male preponderance of about 3: 1.
- ***The cardinal feature is low back pain*** and early morning stiffness with radiation to the buttocks or posterior thighs.

- *Harrison 19th/ 2169-72*
- ***In most ethnic groups, HLAB27 is present in 80–90% of patients.***
- The initial symptom is usually dull pain, insidious in onset, felt deep in the lower lumbar or gluteal region, accompanied by ***low-back morning stiffness of up to a few hours' duration*** that improves with activity and returns following inactivity. Within a few months, the pain has usually become persistent and bilateral.
- The most common extraarticular manifestation is ***acute anterior uveitis, which occurs in up to 40% of patients***
- ***Aortic insufficiency***, sometimes leading to congestive heart failure, occurs in a small percentage of patients, occasionally early. ***Third-degree heart block may occur alone or together with aortic insufficiency.*** Subclinical pulmonary lesions and cardiac dysfunction may be relatively common.
- To **qualify as the criterion for inflammatory back pain of axial SpA**, *the chronic (≥3 months) back pain should have four or more of the following characteristic features: (1) age of onset <40 years old; (2) insidious onset; (3) improvement with exercise; (4) no improvement with rest; and (5) pain at night with improvement upon getting up.*

Extra-articular Features of Ankylosing Spondylitis

- *(Davidson 22nd/1105)*
- ***Anterior uveitis (25%)*** and conjunctivitis (20%)
- Prostatitis (80% men): usually asymptomatic
- Cardiovascular disease: Aortic incompetence, Mitral incompetence, ***Cardiac conduction defects***, Pericarditis
- Amyloidosis
- Atypical upper lobe pulmonary fibrosis

198. Ans. a. Equinus

[Ref: surgicaltechniques.jbjs.org/content/6/3/e28]

The three main components of the deformity are always corrected in the following order *Apley 9th/593*

- First the forefoot must be brought into rotational alignment with the hind foot
- Next both hind foot and forefoot are together gradually brought out of ***varus and supination***; correction is assisted by keeping the fulcrum on the lateral side of the head of the talus.
- ***Finally, equinus is corrected by bringing the heel down and dorsiflexing the foot.***

Application of Ponseti Casts

- *Campbell's Operative Orthopaedics, 11th/Chap26*
- The Ponseti method consists of two phases: treatment and maintenance.
- Generally **five to six casts** are required to correct the alignment of the foot and ankle fully.
- The ***first cast application corrects the cavus deformity*** by aligning the forefoot with the hindfoot, supinating the forefoot to bring it in line with the heel and elevating (dorsiflexing) the first metatarsal
- A crucial point in the Ponseti technique is that the heel is never directly manipulated. With reduction of the talar head beneath the navicular, ***correction of the talus, navicular and cuboid causes the calcaneus to abduct and evert.***

Ponseti Method

- *surgicaltechniques.jbjs.org*
- The Ponseti method consists of a specific technique of ***manipulation of the clubfoot deformity, followed by the application of a plaster cast*** with the foot in the corrected position.
- A percutaneous tenotomy of the Achilles tendon is done prior to the final cast to gain complete correction in most patients. Bracing with a foot abduction orthosis is necessary to minimize relapse of the deformity.
- The method begins with the Ponseti manipulation and consists of the **following steps**:
  - Identify the head of the talus by palpation.
  - ***Supinate the forefoot to eliminate the cavus deformity*** and create a normal-appearing arch.
  - ***Abduct the forefoot*** with the vector of force parallel to the sole of the foot while using the lateral head of the talus as the fulcrum and maintaining the reduction of the cavus deformity.
  - This manipulation is followed by the application of an above-the-knee cast with the foot in the corrected position.

- The manipulation and casting steps are repeated every 5 to 7 days until the foot is abducted approximately 50° from the frontal plane of the tibia.
- In most patients (60% to >90%), a percutaneous tenotomy of the Achilles tendon is necessary to correct the residual ankle ***equinus after gaining full abduction of the foot with the manipulations.***
- The final cast is applied and worn for three weeks.

199. Ans. a. Lachmann test, c. Pivot shift test, d. Anterior drawer, e. KT-1000 knee arthrometer is an objective instrument for ACL reconstruction

[Ref: Maheswari 5th/367; Apley 9th/877]

- **Apley's grinding test**: *for meniscal injury- Maheswari 5th/367*
- **Pivot shift test**: *for* ***ACL injury****- Maheswari 5th/368*
- **Reverse pivot shift manoeuvre**-*Probable structures damaged: PCL,poplitues tendon and arcuate ligament- Apley 9th/877*
- **Pivot shift manoeuvre**-*Probable structures damaged: ACL,LCL and lateral aspect of knee capsule - Apley 9th/877*

"The **anterior cruciate ligament (ACL)** is the primary restraint to anterior tibial motion in relation to the femur. ACL deficiency can be evaluated using clinical tests (namely the ***anterior drawer test, Lachman test and pivot shift test***), magnetic resonance imaging, arthroscopy and arthrometric testing. Comparing surgical outcomes using imaging modalities or arthroscopy is not objective. Although clinical tests are useful for diagnosis and treatment, their interpretation can vary among clinicians. The **KT-1000 knee arthrometer (KT-1000)** is an ***objective instrument for ACL reconstruction,*** which measures anterior tibial motion relative to the femur. The test involves strapping the KT-1000 to the leg, pulling the tibia anteriorly and quantifying the amount of movement in millimeters (mm)"- *pdfs.semanticscholar.org*

Table *(Maheshwari 5th/149)*: **Essential features of knee ligament injury**

Name of the ligament	Mechanism of injury	Tests
Medial collateral	Valgus force	Valgue stress + at 30° knee flexion
Lateral collateral	Varus force	Varus stress + at 30° knee flexion
Anterior cruciate	Twisting extension	Anterior drawer test + Lachmann test +
Posterior cruciate	Backward force on tibia	Posterior drawer test +

200. Ans. a. Rupture of lateral ligament, b. Buttonhole deformity, d. Laceration of the central slip of the extensor

[Ref: Apley 9th/ 418-19; orthoinfo.aaos.org/topic.cfm]

"Mallet finger (baseball finger) is ***an injury of the extensor digitorum tendon of the fingers at the distal interphalangeal joint (Zone I)****" (orthoinfo.aaos.org/topic.cfm)*

Zone III *Campbell's Operative Orthopaedics, 11th ed. Chap/63*

Zone III is the area of the proximal interphalangeal joint

Rupture or Acute Transection of the Central Slip of the Extensor Expansion (Buttonhole Deformity)

- **Rupture or laceration of the *central slip of the*** extensor expansion at or near its insertion results in loss of active extension of the proximal interphalangeal joint and consequently persistent flexion of the joint.
- ***Buttonholing*** also can be caused by traumatic rotation of a digit at the proximal interphalangeal joint while partially flexed. Rotation can cause a condyle of the proximal phalanx to protrude through the capsule and disrupt the triangular ligament area between the lateral band and the central tendon. After such an injury, the proximal interphalangeal joint cannot be fully extended because of hemorrhage and swelling. The joint remains in its flexed position and the subluxated lateral band contracts, allowing the transverse retinacular ligament also to contract, securely holding the subluxated lateral band.
- Spinner and Choi have shown experimentally that with ***anterior dislocation of the proximal interphalangeal joint, complete rupture of the central slip and lateral ligament may*** occur

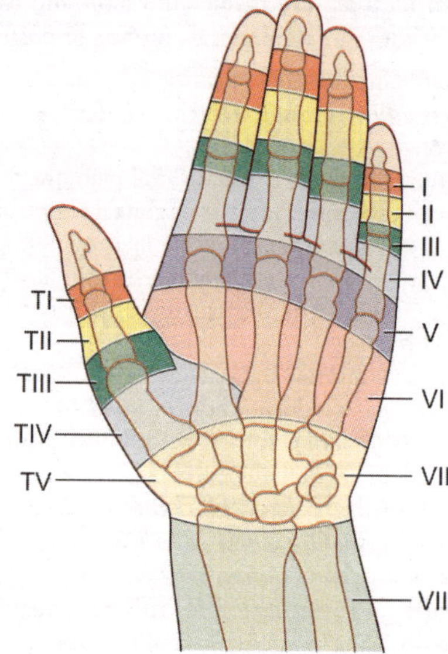

Fig: *(Campbell's)*: Indications for surgery of extensor tendon lacerations vary according to level of pathological condition

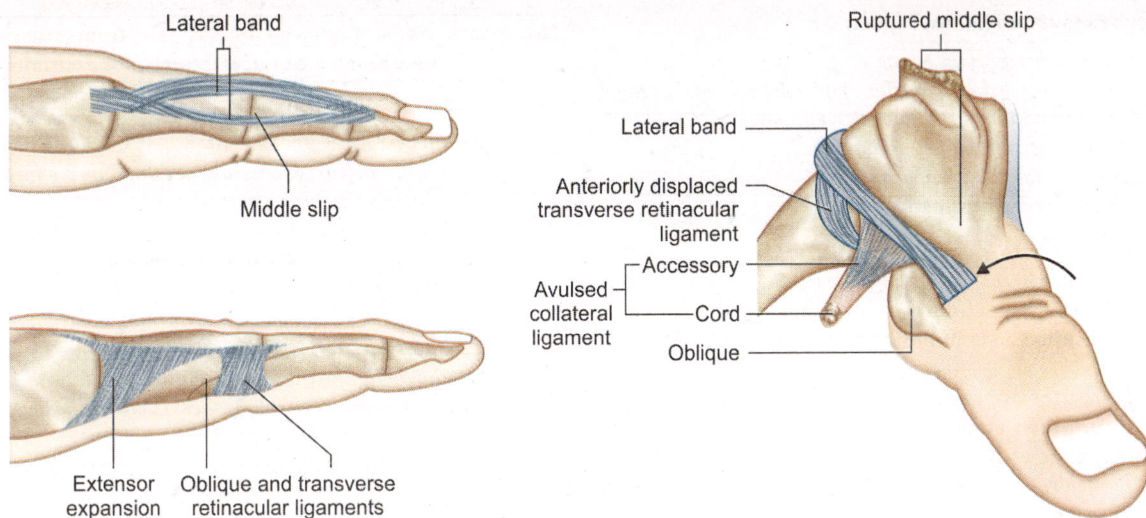

Fig: *(Campbell's):* A and B, Dorsolateral and lateral views of extensor mechanism. C, ***Anterior dislocation of proximal interphalangeal joint*** with *rupture of middle slip, avulsed collateral ligament and partial tear of distal fibers of transverse retinacular ligament. Lateral band is displaced anteriorly.*

Hand injury

◈ *Campbell's Operative Orthopaedics, 11th ed. Chap/63*

An extensor tendon is presumed to be divided between the proximal and distal interphalangeal joints when active extension of the ***distal interphalangeal joint*** is lost. Initially, a gross **mallet finger deformity** may be absent because the surrounding capsule and other soft tissues have not yet been stretched by the strong flexor digitorum profundus.

Zone I

- Zone I is at the level of the distal interphalangeal joint. ***Mallet finger deformities*** usually result from closed avulsion of the insertion of the tendon, sometimes with a small bone fragment and can be treated by splinting alone. An open transection of the central slip insertion at the distal phalanx usually is repaired with a roll stitch, or a dermotenodermal suture and protected with a small transarticular Kirschner wire.

201. Ans. a. Affected side of hip allow wt. bearing, b. Asymptomatic cases may occur, c. Radionucleotide scan show increased uptake due to new bone formation in the area around the infarct

[Ref: Maheswari 5th/318-19, Apley 9th/528-30; 103-08]

"The earliest stage of bone death is asymptomatic*; by the time the patient presents, the lesion is usually well advanced"-Apley 9th/105*

"**Radioscintography: *99mTc-HDP scan*** (in bone phase) may show a cold area, particularly if a large segment of bone is avascular (e.g., after fracture of the femoral neck). More often, however, the picture is dominated by increased activity, reflecting hyperaemia and ***new bone formation in the area around the infarct****"- Apley 9th/107*

Osteonecrosis or Avascular Necrosis

◈ *Apley 9th/528-30*

- The presenting complaint is ***usually pain in the hip*** (or, in over 50% of cases, both hips), which ***progress over a period of 2-3 years to become quite severe***
- However, ***in over 10% of cases the condition is asymptomatic***
- Adult patients come from both sexes and all ages
- The thigh is wasted and the limb may be 1-2 cm short
- On examination, the patient walks with a limp and may have a ***positive Trendelenburg sign***

AVN of femoral head *occurs in fracture of the femoral neck- Maheshwari 5th/318*

Table *(Maheshwari 5th/318-19)*: **Cause of avascular necrosis of femoral head**

- Idiopathic-commonest
- Alcoholism
- Steroid therapy
- Sickle cell disease
- Patient of renal dialysis
- Patient on anticancer drug
- Post-partum necrosis
- Gaucher's disease
- Caisson's disease

202. Ans. b. In severe cases, mitral valve prolapse may occur, c. May be present at birth, d. Seen in Marfan syndrome, e. Impairment of respiratory function

[Ref: Dahnert Radiolog Review Manual 7th/17; Davidson 22nd/731]

Pectus Excavatum (Funnel Chest)

◈ *Dahnert Radiolog Review Manual 7th/17*

- *May be associated with **Marfan syndrome**,Poland syndrome, Noonan syndrome, fetal alcohol syndrome, homocystinuria, prematurity, congenital heart disease*
- ***Decreased total lung capacity***
- ***Decreased cardiac stroke volume***

Pectus Excavatum

◈ *Davidson 22nd/731*

- Pectus excavatum (funnel chest) is an idiopathic condition in which the body of the sternum, usually only the lower end, is curved inwards.
- The heart is displaced to the left and may be compressed between the sternum and the vertebral column but only rarely is there associated disturbance of cardiac function.
- The ***deformity may restrict chest expansion and reduce vital capacity***.
- Operative correction is rarely performed and then only for cosmetic reasons.

Pectus Excavatum

◈ *emedicine.medscape.com*

Pectus excavatum is the most common type of congenital chest wall abnormality (90%), followed by pectus carinatum (5-7%), cleft sternum, pentalogy of Cantrell, asphyxiating thoracic dystrophy and spondylothoracic dysplasia.

Pectus excavatum occurs in an estimated 1 in 300-400 births, with **male predominance** (male-to-female ratio of 3:1).

The condition is typically noticed at birth and more than 90% of cases are diagnosed within the first year of life.

"It can either be present at birth or not develop until puberty"*-wiki*

Pectus excavatum is sometimes considered to be cosmetic, but depending on the severity, it can impair cardiac and respiratory function and cause pain in the chest and back.

In mild cases, cardiorespiratory function is normal, although the heart can be displaced and/or rotated.

In ***severe cases, mitral valve prolapse*** may be present and physical capability may be limited due to base lung capacity being decreased

203. Ans. c. ↑alkaline phosphatase, d. ↓ed Calcium level, e. Looser's zone on X-ray

[Ref: Maheswari 5th/312, Apley 9th/138; Davidson 22nd/768]

"Osteomalacia: PTH is raised"*- Davidson 22nd/768*

*"Changes common to almost all types of vitamin D related rickets and osteomalacia are **diminished levels of serum calcium and phosphate, increased alkaline phosphatase** and diminished urinary excretion of calcium. **In vitamin D deficiency 25-OH D levels also are low**"- Apley 9th/138*

Osteomalacia *Maheswari 5th/312*

- It is common in women who live in purdah and lack exposure to sunlight
- *The serum **calcium level is low**, the **phosphates are low** and the **alkaline phosphatase high**"*
- ***Radiological examination: Looser's zone (pseudo-fractures)***

204. Ans. b. Contain synovial fluid, c. Arise from extensor retinaculum, e. Surgical treatment is excision of cyst

[Ref: Maheswari 5th/ 303, Apley 9th/ 407-08]

Ganglion cyst *Apley 9th/ 407-08*

- *It arises from leakage of **synovial fluid** from a joint or tendon sheath and contains a glariy, viscous fluid*
- *Although it can appear anywhere around the carpus, it usually develops on the **dorsal surface of the scapho-lunate ligament***
- *Palmar wrist ganglia usually arise from the **scapho-lunate or scapho-trapezio-trapezoid joint***
- *The patient, often a **young adult**, presents with a painless lump, although occasionally there is slight ache and weakness*
- *It does not move with the tendons*
- *Treatment is usually unnessary. The lump can be safely be left alone; it often disappears spontaneously. It can be aspirated or excised*
- "Ganglion cysts, are ***more common in women and 70% occur in people between the ages of 20-40***. Rarely, ganglion cysts can occur in children younger than 10 years"- *www.webmd.com/a-to-z*
- "They are most common in younger people between the ***ages of 15 and 40 years and women are more likely to be affected than men***"-orthoinfo.aaos.org
- Ganglion cysts, also known as Bible cysts, Bible bumps, Gideon's disease and synovial cyst

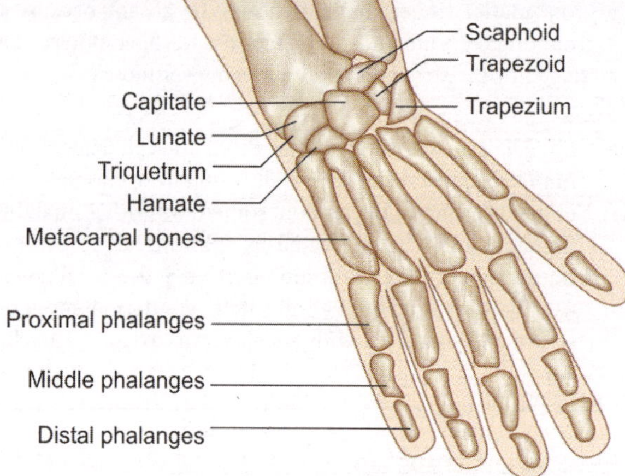

Fig: Bones and joints of hand

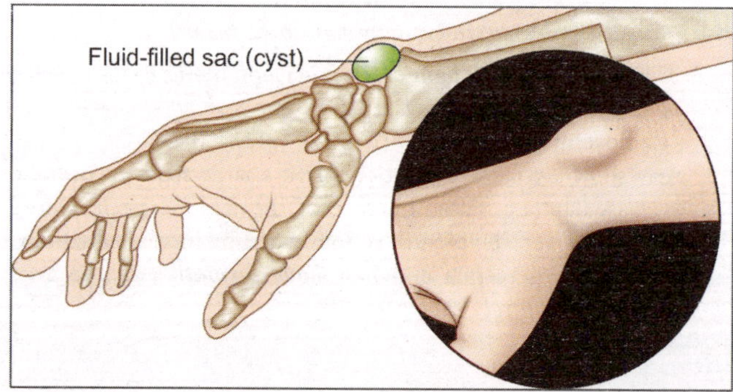

ANESTHESIA

205. Ans. a. Halothane, b. Succinylcholine

[Ref: Morgan Anaesthesia 5th/1187-90; Ajay Yadav 5th/133-35; Miller 7th/ 1187-89; Lee 13th/ 353; Wylie's Anaesthesia 7th/365, 367]

Drug known to Trigger MH

- Ether
- Cyclopropane
- *Halothane*
- Methoxyflurane
- Enflurane
- Isoflurane
- Desflurane
- Sevoflurane
- ***Succinylcholine***

Safe Anaesthetic Drug in Patient who are Susceptible to MH

- **Thiopentone sodium**
  - Pancuronium
  - *Nitrons oxide*
  - Propofol
  - Etomidate
  - *Benzodiazepines*
  - *Ketamine*
  - Opiates
  - Droperidol

206. Ans. b. Seizure, c. Masseter spasm, d. Metabolic acidosis

[Ref: Morgan Anaesthesia 5th/1187-90; Ajay Yadav 5th/133-35; Miller 7th/ 1187-89; Lee 13th/ 353; Wylie's Anaesthesia 7th/365, 367]

"Other complications of MH include **cerebral edema with seizures** and hepatic failure"- *Morgan Anaesthesia 5th/1187*

Malignant Hyperthermia: Clinical Feature

◈ *Ajay Yadav 5th/134*

- ***Hyperthermia***
- Increased End tidal CO_2
- Hypoxia, cyanosis and decrease in mixed venous oxygen saturation
- ***Severe metabolic acidosis***
- ***Masseter spasm***
- ***Hyperkalemia, muscle rigidity***, increased creatinine phosphokinase, increased myoglobin, myoglobinuria
- Renal failure, DIC, pulmonary and cerebral edema
- Death-ventricular fibrillation is most common cause of death
- Due to sympathetic stimulation- Tachycardia, hypertension and cardiac arrhythmias

Table *(Morgan Anaesthesia 5th/1187)*: **Signs of malignant hyperthermia**

Markedly Increased Metabolism
- Increased CO_2 production
- Increased oxygen consumption
- Reduced mixed venous oxygen tension
- Metabolic acidosis
- Cyanosis
- Mottling

Increased sympathetic activity
- Tachycardia
- Hypertension
- Arrhythmias

Muscle damage
- *Masseter spasm*
- *Generalized rigidity*
- Increased serum creatine kinase
- Hyperkalemia
- Hypernatremia
- Hyperphosphatemia
- Myoglobinemia
- Myoglobinuria

Hyperthermia
- Fever
- Sweating

207. Ans. a. Propofol, b. Thiopentone, c. Ketamine, e. Midazolam

[Ref: Morgan Anaesthesia 5th/175-82; Ajay Yadav 5th/92; Lee 13th/155]

"Diazepam: ***Parenteral diazepam has now been almost obsolete****"- Ajay Yadav 5th/99*

Table *(Lee 13th/155)*: **Pharmacokinetic parameters for induction agents**

Agent	Protein bound %	T½ (h)	Active metabolites
Thiopental	85	10	Pentobarbital
Thiamylal	85	14	Quinalbarbital
Methohexital	85	4	Hydroxymethohexital
Etomidate	76	3	None
Midazolam	98	2	1-and 4-Hydroxymidazolam
Propofol	98	6	None
Ketamine	60	3	Norketamine, dehydronorketamine

208. Ans. b. Bretylium, c. Intralipids, e. Epinephrine

[Ref: Morgan Anaesthesia 5th/273-74; Ajay Yadav 5th/144; Miller 6th/933; Lee 13th/384; Barash Anesthesia 6th/545]

Treatment of Bupivacaine Induced Cardiotoxicity: *Bretylium, phenytoin, amiodarone, lignocaine,20% of lipid emulsion, adrenaline, vasopressin*- *Ajay Yadav 5th/144*

Treatment of Bupivacaine Induced Cardiotoxicity

◈ *Miller 6th/933*

- Beyond the established uses of **epinephrine, vasopressin, atropine and Intralipid**, there is no established role for antiarrhythmic drugs or other traditional resuscitation drugs in the setting of bupivacaine-induced cardiac arrest.

- It is *not recommended that bupivacaine-induced ventricular arrhythmias be treated with* ***lidocaine or amiodarone***

Treatment of Bupivacaine Induced Cardiotoxicity

◈ *Barash Anesthesia 6th/545*

- Ventricular dysrhythmias may be difficult to treat and may need large and multiple doses of electrical **cardioversion, epinephrine, vasopressin and amiodarone.**
- The use of ***calcium channel blockers*** *in this setting is not recommended, as its cardio depressant effect is exaggerated*

209. Ans. b. Gender, c. Weight, d. Height, e. Underlying condition of patient

[Ref: Morgan Anaesthesia 5th/1288; emedicine.medscape.com]

In ICU, weighing of patient is difficult, so predicted body weight (PBW) is used for calculation of tidal volume

Protective Lung Ventilation

◈ *lifeinthefastlane.com; emcrit.org*

- Protective lung ventilation is the current standard of care for mechanical ventilation
- It is synonymous with low tidal volume ventilation (4–8 mL/kg) and often includes permissive hypercapnia
- 6 mL/kg predicted body weight (not actual body weight) is most commonly quoted as this was the intervention arm of the practice defining ARDSNet ARMA trial and is physiologically normal for a healthy person
- NB. **PBW** in **men** is calculated as 50 (45 in **women**) + 0.91 (**Height in** cm −152.4)
- Protective lung ventilation should be used for mechanically ventilated patients with ARDS and those with risk factors for developing ARDS
- There is also a reasonable default ventilation strategy in all mechanically ventilated patients
- Set a tidal volume of 6mL/kg based on ***predicted body weight (PBW) and target plateau pressures <30 cmH20***
- It can be combined with an open lung approach in moderate-severe ARDS (i.e. higher PEEP and recruitment manoeuvres)
- The ventilation strategy should be modified in patients with obstructive lung disease to prevent dynamic hyperinflation (COPD and asthma)

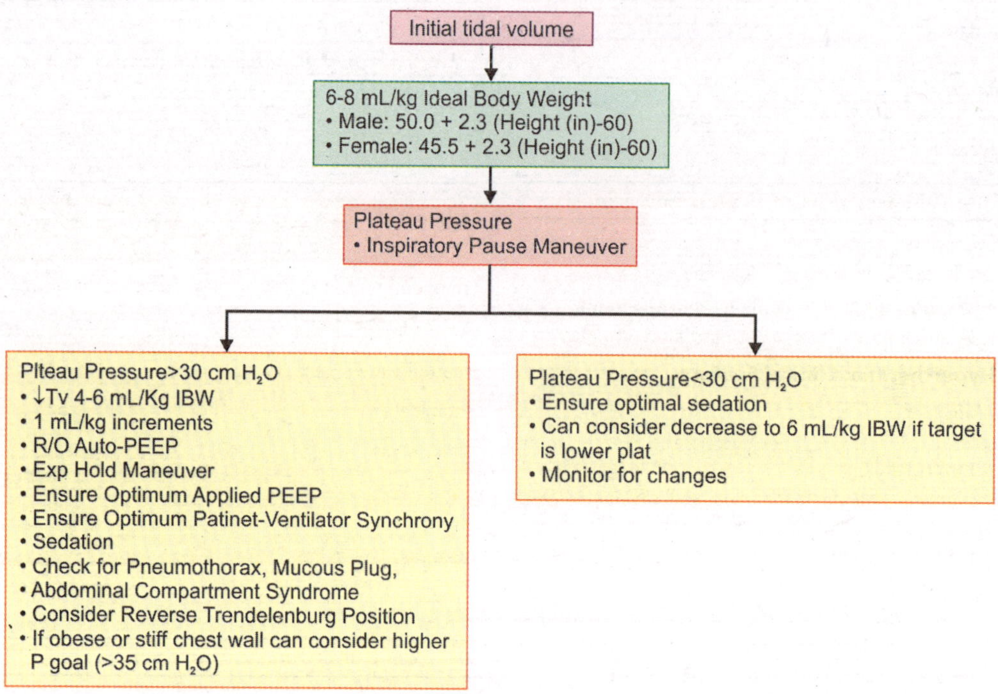

Fig: *(emcrit.org)*: Algorithm for initiating initial mechanical ventilation settings in the Emergency department

Table: Initial ventilator setting in different conditions

	Tidal volume	RR	I/E ratio	PEEP	FIO_2
Normal lungs	8 mL/kg	10–12	1:2	4	1.0
Asthma/COPD	6 mL/kg	5–8	1:4	4	1.0
ARDS	6 mL/kg	10–12	1:2	4–15	1.0
Hypovolemia	8 mL/kg	10–12	1:2	0-4	1.0

Table *(Harrison 19th/1742)*: **Characteristics of the Most Commonly Used Forms of Mechanical Ventilation**

Ventilatory Mode	Variables Set by User (Independent)	Variables Monitored by User (Dependent)	Trigger Cycle Limit	Advantages
ACMV (assist-control ventilation)	Tidal volume Ventillator rate FIO_2 PEEP level Pressure limit	Peak, mean and plateau airway pressures VE ABG I/E ratio	Patient effort Timer Pressure limit	Patient control Guaranteed ventilation
IMV (Intermittent mandatory ventilation)	Tidal volume Mandatory ventilator rate FIO_2 PEEP level Pressure limit Spontaneous breaths between assisted breaths	Peak, mean and plateau airway pressure VE ABG I/E ratio	Patient effort Timer Pressure limit	Patient control Comfort from spontaneous breaths Guaranteed ventilation
PSV (pressure-support ventilation)	Inspiratory pressure level Flo_2 PEEP Pressure limit	Tidal volume Respiratory rate VE ABG	Pressure limit Inspiratory flow	Patient control Comfort Assures synchrony
NIV (noninvasive ventilation)	Inspiratory and expiratory pressure level FIO_2	Tidal volume Respiratory rate VE ABG	Pressure limit Inspiratory flow	Patient control

210. Ans. a. Non cuffed tube is used in pediatric age group, b. Made of PVC and disposable, c. Can be put either oral or nasal according to different situations, e. More tendency to go to right bronchus thereby decreasing left lung ventilation

[Ref: Morgan Anaesthesia 5th/320-25; Ajay Yadav 5th/43-46; Lee 13th/208-09]

Endotracheal Tube and Intubation

◈ *Ajay Yadav 5th/43-46; Morgan Anaesthesia 5th/320-25*

- *There are* **two major type of cuffs**: *high pressure (low volume) and low pressure (high volume)*
- **PVC tube:** ***Transparent, Cuff (low pressure and high volume)***
- **Red rubber tube:** *Non-transparent,* ***Cuff (high pressure and low volume)***
- ***Used both for oral and nasal intubation***

Overly "deep" insertion usually results in intubation of the right (rather than left) main-stem bronchus because of the **right bronchus'** less acute angle with the trachea. Clues to the diagnosis of bronchial intubation include unilateral breath sounds, ***unexpected hypoxia with pulse oximetry*** (unreliable with high inspired oxygen concentrations), inability to palpate the TT cuff in the sternal notch during cuff inflation and decreased breathing-bag compliance (high peak inspiratory pressures)"-*Morgan Anaesthesia 5th/335*

"**Nasotracheal intubation (NTI)** is necessary when the ***oral route is not possible (e.g., limited mouth opening) or would impede surgical access***. NTI was formerly considered the technique of choice for resuscitation, but orotracheal intubation using the rapid-sequence technique is now usually the first choice"-*Miller 7th/1586*

211. Ans. a. Head trauma patient presenting with a GCS score 8 or less should be intubated, b. Done in patients with increased risk of aspiration, c. Can be used in patient with full stomach, d. In cervical injury, patient neck is stabilized before intubation, e. Done in patients who need anaesthesia

[Ref: Lee 13th/208; Miller 7th/1586; CSDT 14th/814]

"A ***patient presenting with a GCS score 8 or less should be intubated***. Mechanical ventilation should be used if necessary to provide adequate oxygenation and ventilation"-*CSDT 14th/814*

"**Indication of tracheal intubation**: ***To protect the airway against aspiration aspiration of stomach contents*** or blood and debris from operations on the head and upper airways"- *Lee 13th/208*

"**Rapid sequence induction-indication**: A*ny* ***"full stomach" patient has an indication for a rapid sequence intubation***"-*www.sarasotaanesthesia.com*

"The safety of orotracheal intubation for patients with potential C-spine injury has been documented in recent years. For patients requiring immediate and/or urgent airway control, ***rapid sequence induction followed by orotracheal intubation with cricoid pressure and manual in-line immobilization of the head and neck is recommended***"- *www.openanesthesia.org*

Indication for Tracheal intubation

◈ (*Miller 7th/1586*)

Surgical and Anesthetic Indications

Surgical requirement for neuromuscular blocking drugs, e.g., abdominal surgery

Airway access shared with the surgeon, including ear, nose and throat surgery

Patient position in which access to the airway is restricted or precludes rapid tracheal intubation, e.g., lateral, prone

Predicted difficult airway

Risk of aspiration of gastric contents or blood, e.g., upper gastrointestinal obstruction or sepsis, facial trauma, bleeding into the respiratory tract from any cause

Surgery that impairs gas exchange

Prolonged surgery

Other airway techniques ineffective

Critical Illness

Inability to protect the airway, e.g., coma from any cause

Impaired respiratory function (hypoxemia or hypercapnia) unresponsive to noninvasive management

Prevention of hypercapnia, e.g., raised intracranial pressure

212. Ans. b. Drug used is less in concentration, d. Onset of action is delayed, e. Density of anaesthetic agent is less in epidural than spinal

[Ref: Morgan Anaesthesia 5th/959,969; Ajay Yadav 5th/162; Miller 7th/1626]

"**Epidural:** *Onset of effect takes place in 15-20 min*"- *Ajay Yadav 5th/162*

Lidocaine concentration: *epidural (1-2%); spinal (5%).* **Bupivacine**: *epidural (0.125-0.5%), spinal (0.5%)-Ajay Yadav 5th/162,156*

Regional Anesthesia

◈ *Barash Anaesthesia 6th/932,947*

- The outside diameter of both epidural and spinal needles is used to determine their gauge. **Larger gauge (i.e., smaller diameter) spinal needles** are ***less likely to cause postdural puncture headaches (PDPH),*** but are more readily deflected than smaller gauge needles.
- ***Epidural needles are typically sized 16 to 19 gauge and spinal needles 22 to 29 gauge.***
- PDPH is a common complication of spinal anesthesia with a reported incidence as high as 25% in some studies. The ***risk of PDPH is less with epidural anesthesia, but it occurs in up to 50% of young patients following accidental meningeal puncture with large-diameter epidural needles.***

Epidural Needles

◈ *Morgan Anaesthesia 5th/959, 969*

- The standard epidural needle is typically 17–18 gauge, 3 or 3.5 inches long and has a blunt bevel with a gentle curve of 15–30° at the tip. The Tuohy needle is most commonly used
- ***Epidural anesthesia is slower in onset*** (10–20 min) and may ***not be as dense as spinal anesthesia.*** This can be manifested as a ***more pronounced differential block or a segmental block,*** a feature that can be useful clinically.
- PDPH is believed to result from leakage of CSF from a dural defect and intracranial hypotension.
- The incidence of PDPH is strongly related to ***needle size, needle type and patient population. Th e larger the needle, the greater the likelihood of PDPH.*** Cutting-point needles are associated with a higher incidence of PDPH than pencil-point needles of the same gauge. Factors that increase the risk of PDPH include young age, female sex and pregnancy. The ***greatest risk,*** then, would be expected following an accidental wet tap with a ***large epidural needle*** in a young woman (perhaps as high as 20% to 50%). The ***lowest incidence would be expected in an elderly male using a 27-gauge pencil-point needle*** (<1%). Studies of obstetric patients undergoing spinal anesthesia for cesarean section with small-gauge pencil-point needles have shown rates as low as 3% or 4%.

SKIN

213. Ans. a. Arrhythmogenic right ventricular cardiomyopathy, b. Hypertrichosis, c. Pemphigus vulgaris, e. Keratoderma with wooly hair

[Ref: Neena Khanna 5th/79; www.ncbi.nlm.nih.gov/pmc; Harrison 19th/370-71]

Desmogleins (Dsg): Dsgs are present in desmosomes which are involved in keratinocyte-keratinocyte adhesion in the epidermis. Dsg1and 3 are important in ***pemphigus. Antibodies to Dsg 3 and 1 are pathogenic in pemphigus vulgaris while antibodies to Dsg1 are pathogenic in pemphigus foliaceus***"- *Neena Khanna 5th/79;* Harrison 19th/370-71 (Table)

"**Desmoglein-2** is a protein that in humans is encoded by the *DSG2*gene. Desmoglein-2 is highly expressed in epithelial cells and cardiomyocytes. Desmoglein-2 is localized to desmosome structures at regions of cell-cell contact and functions to structurally adhere adjacent cells together. In cardiac muscle, these regions are specialized regions known as intercalated discs. Mutations in desmoglein-2 have been associated with ***arrhythmogenic right ventricular cardiomyopathy*** and familial dilated cardiomyopathy.

Mutations in *DSG2* have been identified in patients with arrhythmogenic right ventricular cardiomyopathy, along with other desmosomal proteins PKP2 and DSP"-wiki

"**Keratoderma with woolly hair** comprises several related conditions with overlapping signs and symptoms. Researchers have recently proposed classifying keratoderma with ***woolly hair*** into **four types**, based on the underlying genetic cause. **Type I**, also known as Naxos disease, is characterized by palmoplantar keratoderma, woolly hair and a form of cardiomyopathy called arrhythmogenic right ventricular cardiomyopathy (ARVC). **Type II**, also known as Carvajal syndrome, has hair and skin abnormalities similar to type I but features a different form of cardiomyopathy, called dilated left ventricular cardiomyopathy.

Type III also has signs and symptoms similar to those of type I, including ARVC, although the hair and skin abnormalities are often milder. **Type IV** is characterized by **palmoplantar keratoderma** and woolly and sparse hair, as well as abnormal fingernails and toenails. Type IV does not appear to cause cardiomyopathy"- *ghr.nlm.nih.gov*

Desmogleins Targeted in Human Diseases

◈ *www.ncbi.nlm.nih.gov/pmc*

Isoform	Type	Diseases
Desmoglein 1	Autoimmune	pemphgius foliaceus pemphigus vulgaris (mucocutaneous type) paraneoplastic pemphigus
	Infection	Staphylococcal scalded skin syndrome bullous impetigo
	Genetic	Striate ***palmoplantar keratoderma***

Contd...

Isoform	Type	Diseases
Desmoglein 2	Infection	Respiratory and urinary tract infection (receptors for adenovirus serotypes 3, 7, 11 and 14)
	Genetic	Arrythmogenic right ventricular cardiomyopathy dilated cardiomyopathy
Desmoglein 3	Autoimmune	Pemphigus vulgaris (mucosal dominant type, mucocutaneous type) paraneoplastic pemphigus
Desmoglein 4	Genetic	Hypotrichosis

214. Ans. c. Pemphigoid, d. Dermatitis hepetiformis

[Ref: Neena Khanna 5th/76]

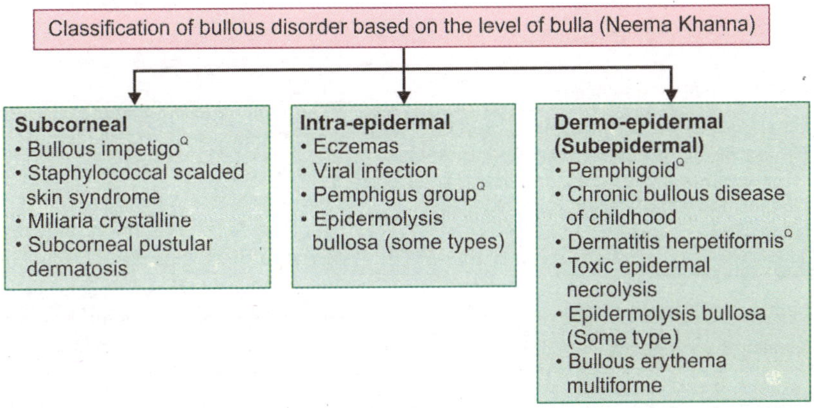

Classification of bullous disorder based on the level of bulla (Neema Khanna)

Subcorneal
- Bullous impetigo[Q]
- Staphylococcal scalded skin syndrome
- Miliaria crystalline
- Subcorneal pustular dermatosis

Intra-epidermal
- Eczemas
- Viral infection
- Pemphigus group[Q]
- Epidermolysis bullosa (some types)

Dermo-epidermal (Subepidermal)
- Pemphigoid[Q]
- Chronic bullous disease of childhood
- Dermatitis herpetiformis[Q]
- Toxic epidermal necrolysis
- Epidermolysis bullosa (Some type)
- Bullous erythema multiforme

215. Ans. b. Psoriasis exacerbation, c. Acneiform eruptions, d. Pustular dermatoses

[Ref: Neena Khanna 5th/45; K. D. T 7th/449]

Dermatological side effect of Lithium: ***Acneiform eruptions, popular eruptions and exacerbation of psoriaisis***"-*Neeraj Ahuja 7th/190*

*"Lithium can cause **dermatitis and worsen acne**"- K. D. T 7th/449*

Lithium Side Effect

- "DRUG-INDUCED LUPUS: Lithium"- *H19th/2134*
- "**May exacerbate psoriasis**"-*Harrison 19th/347*
- May produce ***acneiform eruptions*** or aggravate preexisting acne"- *Harrison 19th/352*
- "Alopecia is a side effect"-*Harrison 19th/354*
- **PUSTULAR LESIONS**: *Acneiform eruptions* and *folliculitis* represent the most common ***pustular dermatoses***. Noninfectious forms of folliculitis is associated with ***lithium***"- *Harrison 19th/356*

Drug Implicated in Aetiology of Psoriasis

◈ *Neena Khanna 5th/45*

- ***Lithium***
- Antimalarial
- β-adrenergic blockers
- NSAIDs
- Corticosteroid withdrawal

PSYCHIATRY

216. Ans. e. 30

[Ref: Kaplon and Sadock 11th/2537]

Cognitive Function

◈ *Davidson 22nd/234*

The Mini-Mental State Examination (MMSE) is a useful screening questionnaire to detect cognitive impairment. A **score of less than 24 out of 30** typically suggests cognitive impairment.

How you are Scored and what it Means

◈ *www.unforgettable.org*

- The mini mental health state examination is scored out of 30.
- A score of
  - 27-30 usually means your memory is normal

- 10-26 could indicate mild to moderate dementia Less than 10 suggests you may have quite severe symptoms of dementia

"The **Folstein mini-mental status examination (MMSE)** is a standardized screening examination of cognitive function that is extremely easy to administer and takes <10 min to complete. Using age-adjusted values for defining normal performance, the test is ~85% sensitive and 85% specific for making the diagnosis of dementia that is moderate or severe, especially in educated patients."-*Kaplon and Sadock 11th/2537*

Table: Mini-mental status examination (MMSE)

Category	Possible points	Description
Orientation to time	5	From broadest to most narrow. Orientation to time has been correlated with future decline.
Orientation to place	5	From broadest to most narrow. This is sometimes narrowed down to streets and sometimes to floor.
Registration	3	Repeating named prompts
Attention and calculation	5	Serial sevens, or spelling "world" backwards. It has been suggested that serial sevens may be more appropriate in a population where English is not the first language.
Recall	3	Registration recall
Language	2	Naming a pencil and a watch
Repetition	1	Speaking back a phrase
Complex commands	6	Varies. Can involve drawing

217. Ans. b. Irritability, c. Impaired concentration, d. Anxiety, e. Insomnia

[Ref: Reddy 33th/615; Niraj Ahuja 7th/52; Kaplon and Sadock 11th /682]

"**Nicotine withdrawal symptoms:** Intense urge to smoke, ***anxiety***, ***impaired concentration and memory***, depression or hostility, headache, muscle cramps, ***sleep disturbances (decreased sleep***- *Niraj Ahuja 7th/52)*, increased appetite and ***weight gain***, diaphoresis and rapid respirations. A short period (6 to 12 weeks) of maintenance often followed by a gradual reduction in 6 to 12 weeks is adopted"- *Reddy 33th/615*

Tobacco Withdrawal: The DSM-5 does not have a diagnostic category for tobacco intoxication, but it does have a diagnostic category for nicotine withdrawal. Withdrawal symptoms can develop within 2 hours of smoking the last cigarette; they generally peak in the first 24 to 48 hours and can last for weeks or months. The common symptoms include an intense craving for tobacco, tension, ***irritability***, ***difficulty concentrating***, drowsiness and ***paradoxical trouble sleeping***, decreased heart rate and blood pressure, increased appetite and ***weight gain***, decreased motor performance and increased muscle tension. A mild syndrome of tobacco withdrawal can appear when a smoker switches from regular to low-nicotine cigarettes"- *Kaplon and Sadock 11th /682*

218. Ans. a. Alcohol dependence, b. Opioid dependence, c. Cocaine dependence

[Ref: Katzung 13th/ 564; Niraj Ahuja 7th/42,44,132; Pharmacology by Satoskar 24th/165]

"The μ opioid receptor antagonist and partial agonist **naltrexone** is FDA-approved for indication in ***opioid and alcohol addiction***. Its effect is modest and may involve a modulation of endogenous opioid systems"- *Katzung 13th/ 564*

"Since its introduction, **naltrexone** has been tried for the treatment of a wide range of psychiatric disorders, including, among others, ***eating disorders, autism, self-injurious behavior, cocaine dependence, gambling and alcoholism.*** Naltrexone was approved for the treatment of ***alcohol dependence*** in 1994"-*Kaplon and Sadock 11th/1004*

"**Alcohol Dependence**: Opioid receptor antagonists are also used as adjuncts to cognitive-behavioral programs for treatment of alcohol dependence. Opioid receptor antagonists ***reduce alcohol craving and alcohol consumption*** and they ***ameliorate the severity of relapses***"- *Kaplon and Sadock 11th/1006*

219. Ans. b. Waking state show alpha wave, d. Theta wave is the predominant wave in stage I of NREM sleep, e. Stage III-NREM sleep shows high amplitude slow waves

[Ref: Niraj Ahuja 7th/132-34; Kaplon and Sadock 11th/534]

Stages of Sleep-Electrophysiological Criteria

(Kaplon and Sadock 11th/ 534)

Electroencephalogram	
Wakefulness	Low-voltage, mixed frequency activity; Alpha (8–13 cps) activity with eyes closed
Nonrapid eye movement sleep (NREM)	
Stage I	Low-voltage, mixed frequency activity; Theta (3–7 cps) activity, vertex sharp waves
Stage II	Low-voltage, mixed frequency background with sleep spindles (12–14 cps bursts) and K complexes (negative sharp wave followed by positive slow wave)
Stage III	High-amplitude (≥75 μV) slow waves (≤2 cps) occupying 20 to 50% of epoch
Stage IV	High-amplitude slow waves occupy >50% of epoch
REM sleep	Low-voltage, mixed frequency activity; Saw-tooth waves, theta activity and slow alpha activity

220. Ans. a. Delusion of grandeur

[Ref: Niraj Ahuja 7th/71-72; Kaplon and Sadock 11th/357]

Table *(Kaplon and Sadock 11th/357)*: **DSM-IV-TR Criteria for Major Depressive Episode**

- Five (or more) of the following symptoms have been present during the same 2-week period and represent a change from previous functioning; at least one of the symptoms is either ***(1) depressed mood or (2) loss of interest or pleasure.***
  - Depressed mood most of the day, nearly every day, as indicated by either subjective report (e.g., feels sad or empty) or observation made by others (e.g., appears tearful). **Note:** In children and adolescents, can be irritable mood
  - ***Markedly diminished interest or pleasure in all***, or almost all, activities most of the day, nearly every day (as indicated by either subjective account or observation made by others)
  - Significant weight loss when not dieting or weight gain (e.g., a change of more than 5% of body weight in a month), or ***decrease or increase in appetite*** nearly every day. **Note:** In children, consider failure to make expected weight gains.
  - ***Insomnia or hypersomnia nearly*** every day
  - ***Psychomotor agitation or retardation*** nearly every day (observable by others, not merely subjective feelings of restlessness or being slowed down)
  - Fatigue or loss of energy nearly every day
  - Feelings of worthlessness or excessive or inappropriate guilt (which may be delusional) nearly every day (not merely self-reproach or guilt about being sick)
  - Diminished ability to think or concentrate, or indecisiveness, nearly every day (either by subjective account or as observed by others)
  - Recurrent thoughts of death (not just fear of dying), recurrent suicidal ideation without a specific plan, or a suicide attempt or a specific plan for committing suicide
- The symptoms do not meet criteria for a mixed episode.
- The symptoms cause clinically significant distress or impairment in social, occupational, or other important areas of functioning.
- The symptoms are not due to the direct physiological effects of a substance (e.g., a drug of abuse, a medication) or a general medical condition (e.g., hypothyroidism).
- The symptoms are not better accounted for by bereavement, i.e., after the loss of a loved one, the symptoms persist for longer than 2 months or are characterized by marked functional impairment, morbid preoccupation with worthlessness, suicidal ideation, psychotic symptoms, or psychomotor retardation.

221. Ans. a. Insomnia, c. Excessive anxiety and worry, d. Benzodiazepines is drugs of choice

[Ref: Niraj Ahuja 7th/90-91; Kaplon and Sadock 11th/409]

"Benzodiazepines have been the drugs of choice for generalized anxiety disorder"- *Kaplon and Sadock 11th/411*

Table *(Kaplon and Sadock 11th/409)*: **DSM-5 Diagnostic Criteria for Generalized Anxiety Disorder**

- ***Excessive anxiety and worry*** (apprehensive expectation), occurring more days than not for at least 6 months, about a number of events or activities (such as work or school performance).
- The individual finds it difficult to control the worry.
- **The anxiety and worry are associated with three (or more) of the following six symptoms** (with at least some symptoms having been present for more days than not for the past 6 months): Note: Only one item is required in children.
  - *Restlessness or feeling keyed up or on edge.*
  - *Being easily fatigued.*
  - ***Difficulty concentrating or mind going blank.***
  - ***Irritability***
  - *Muscle tension*
  - ***Sleep disturbance (difficulty falling or staying asleep, or restless, unsatisfying sleep).***
- The anxiety, worry, or physical symptoms cause clinically significant distress or impairment in social, occupational, or other areas of functioning.
- The disturbance is not attributable to the physiological effects of a substance (e.g., a drug of abuse, a medication) or another medical condition (e.g., hyperthyroidism).
- The **disturbance is not better explained by another medical disorder** (e.g., anxiety or worry about having panic attacks in panic disorder, negative evaluation in social anxiety disorder [social phobia], contamination or obsessions in obsessive-compulsive disorder, separation from attachment Fig. s in separation anxiety disorder, ***reminders of traumatic events in posttraumatic stress disorder***, gaining weight in anorexia nervosa, physical complaints in somatic symptom disorder, perceived appearance flaws in body dysmorphic disorder, having a serious illness in ill ness anxiety disorder, or the content of delusional beliefs in schizophrenia or delusional disorder).

RADIOLOGY

222. Ans. a. Longer t-1/2, d. Lesser toxicity

[Ref: Review of Radiology by Sumer Sethi 6th/184; Harrison 19th/363e-3; Bonica's Management of Pain by Scott Fishman/655]

Table *(www.scielo.br/scielo.php)*: **Physical and nuclear characteristics of bone-seeking therapeutic radionuclides**

Isotope	Emission	Mean Half- Life	Mean b Energy	Soft Tissue Penetration
Phosphorus (^{32}P)	β	14.4 days	695 KeV	8 mm
Strontium (^{89}Sr)	β	50.5 days	583 KeV	2.4 mm

Table *(Scott Fishman/655)*: **Bonica's Management of Pain by**

Physical Characteristics and Clinical Data for Radionuclides

Radionuclide	Half-life (days)	Beta energy (MeV)	Gamma energy (keV	Response rage (%)	Duration of response (mo	Toxicity
^{32}P	14.26	1.7	0	77	5.1	Moderate
^{89}Sr	50.53	1.5	0	80	3-6	Low

"The tumor-to-marrow absorbed dose ratio for **Sr-89** is greater than 10:1, suggesting that patients would experience ***minimal myelosuppression***. This is indeed what is observed clinically. In addition, ***Sr-89 is a pure beta-emitter*** with a maximum beta energy of 1.46 MeV and a ***longer half-life (50.5 days) than P-32*** (14.3 days), characteristics that result in minimal irradiation of healthy tissues and a duration of at least 100 days in osteoblastic target sites. These properties provide the rationale for Sr-89 as a therapeutic isotope."- *www.cancernetwork.com*

"^{32}P as sodium phosphate is no longer approved in many countries because of ***documented myelotoxocity associated with therapeutic administration***. More recently, a clinical trial comparing ^{89}Sr and ^{32}P in patients suffering from bone metastases reported slightly ***higher toxicity in the ^{32}P group but comparable efficacy in terms of pain palliation***"- *www.ncbi.nlm.nih.gov*

223. Ans. a. Chemotherapy and radiotherapy both given simultaneously, b. Radiotherapy acts locoregionally and chemotherapy acts against distant micrometastases, d. Chemotherapy may act as sensitizing agent

[Ref: www.wisegeek.com; www.medscape.com]

"**Concurrent chemotherapy** is ***chemotherapy provided alongside radiation therapy*** for cancer patients"- *www.wisegeek.com*

Concomitant Chemoradiotherapy

◈ *link.springer.com*

- The use of chemotherapy delivered concurrently with radiation. ***Either chemotherapy can act as a radiosensitizer***, improving the probability of local control and potentially the survival, by aiding the destruction of radio-resistant clones, or it can be used with organ-preserving intent, resulting in improved function and/or cosmetic results compared with surgical resection with/without adjuvant treatment.
- In addition, chemotherapy given as part of concurrent chemoradiation may act ***systemically and potentially prevent distant metastases***.

Concomitant Chemoradiotherapy

◈ *www.medscape.com*

- Three clinical rationales support the use of chemotherapy delivered concurrently with radiation.
- First, concomitant chemoradiotherapy can be used with organ-preserving intent, resulting in improved cosmesis and function compared with surgical resection with or without adjuvant treatment.
- Second, **chemotherapy can act as a radiosensitizer**, improving the probability of local control and, in some cases, survival, by aiding the destruction of radioresistant clones.
- Third, chemotherapy given as part of concurrent chemoradiation may act systemically and potentially ***eradicate distant micrometastases***
- Currently, concomitant chemoradiotherapy is widely used in the treatment of solid tumors. In almost all malignancies in which locoregional control is necessary, concurrent chemoradiotherapy is either an established treatment modality or is actively being investigated.
- The term spatial cooperation is used to describe the scenario whereby radiotherapy **acts locoregionally** and chemotherapy acts against distant micrometastases, without interaction between the agents
- This cooperative effect requires the ***agents to have non-overlapping toxicity profiles*** in order that both modalities can be ***used at effective doses without increasing normal tissue*** effects.
- When combined concurrently with radiotherapy, however, ***few chemotherapeutic agents meet this criterion***, because limited single-agent activity or toxicity-driven dose reductions preclude the delivery of systemic dosing schedules.
- Many trials of concomitant chemoradiotherapy, however, have ***demonstrated decreased incidence of distant metastases compared with radiation alone***. This evidence could indicate that chemotherapy delivered at radiosensitizing doses has some systemic spatial cooperative effect, or that the improved local control of chemoradiotherapy decreases subsequent metastases.

224. Ans. b. Chemotherapy before surgery

[Ref: Katzung 13th/919-20; chemoth.com/neoadjuvant-chemotherapy]

"Chemotherapy uses drugs to destroy cancer cells, stop their growth, or ameliorate symptoms. In **neoadjuvant** (also called **preoperative** or **primary**) chemotherapy, ***drug treatment takes place before surgical extraction of a tumor***. This is in contrast with **adjuvant chemotherapy**, which is drug treatment *after* surgery"- *chemoth.com/neoadjuvant-chemotherapy*

225. Ans. a. More effective in carcinoma cervix, d. Deliver higher dose of radiation to tumour, e. Less damage to normal tissue

[Ref: Review of Radiology by Sumer Sethi 6th/176-78; Dutta Gynae 6th/506-07]

Brachytherapy

◈ *Sumer Sethi 6th/176-78*

- This technique is particularly useful in treating ***cancers of cervix, uterus, vagina*** and certain H and N cancers. It can also be used to treat breast, brain, skin, esophageal, soft tissue, lung, bladder and prostate cancer
- Sometimes brachytherapy is done in conjunction with external beam therapy.
- The **external beam radiation** destroys cancerous cell in a ***large area surrounding the tumour.***
- **Brachytherapy** delivers a boost, or ***higher dose of radiation, to help destroy the main mass of tumour cells***

◈ *Dutta Gynae 6th/506-07*

- ***Damage to normal tissue is less*** as there is rapid fall-off of radiation around the source (inverse square law)
- Application may be- intracavity, interstitial or surface (skin)
- It gives a very high dose of radiation where the source of radiation is placed within, or close to the tumor
- ***Advantage: Localised high radiation dose to a small tumour volume with high local control***
- **Disadvantage**: *Large tumours are usually unsuitable unless used following EBRT and/or chemotherapy*; Risks of exposure to medical and nursing personnel due to gamma rays

"**External Beam radiotherapy (EBRT) or Teletherapy**: It is designed to ***deliver uniform radiation dose to the tumor volume without hot (excess dose) or cold (under dose) spots***"- *Dutta Gynae 6th/507*

"**Carcinoma cervix:** ***High dose brachytherapy is safe and effective***"- *Dutta Gynae 6th/350*

226. Ans. b. Pseudosacculation, d. Cobblestone appearance, e. String sign of kantor

[Ref: Review of Radiology by Sumer Sethi 6th/120-21; Danhert Radiology Review Manual 7th/; Harrison 19th/1956]

Crohn's Disease

◈ *Sumer Sethi 6th/120-21*

- HALO SIGN on CT
- ***String sign of kantor***
- Skip lesions
- Transmural involvement
- ***Cobblestone appearance***
- Raspberry/rose thorn appearance
- Strictures and fistula more common
- ***Pseudosacculation***
- Earliest change is apthoid ulceration

Ulcerative Colitis

◈ *Sumer Sethi 6th/120*

- ***Pipestem colon (ahaustral)***
- Continuous, mucosal involvement
- Pseudopolyp
- Toxic megacolon (>5.5 cm)
- Collar button ulcer
- Reflex ileitis

Table *(Harrison 19th/1956)*: **Different Clinical, Endoscopic and Radiographic Features**

	Ulcerative Colitis	Crohn's Disease
Endoscopic		
Rectal sparing	Rarely	Frequently
Continuous disease	Yes	Occasionally
"Cobblestoning"	No	Yes
Granuloma on biopsy	No	Occasionally
Radiographic		
Small bowel significantly abnormal	No	Yes
Abnormal terminal ileum	No	Yes
Segmental colitis	No	Yes
Asymmetric colitis	No	Yes
Stricture	Occasionally	Frequently

ANSWER SHEET

1 – 50						51 – 100						101 – 150						151 – 200						201 – 250					
1	A	B	C	D	E	51	A	B	C	D	E	101	A	B	C	D	E	151	A	B	C	D	E	201	A	B	C	D	E
2	A	B	C	D	E	52	A	B	C	D	E	102	A	B	C	D	E	152	A	B	C	D	E	202	A	B	C	D	E
3	A	B	C	D	E	53	A	B	C	D	E	103	A	B	C	D	E	153	A	B	C	D	E	203	A	B	C	D	E
4	A	B	C	D	E	54	A	B	C	D	E	104	A	B	C	D	E	154	A	B	C	D	E	204	A	B	C	D	E
5	A	B	C	D	E	55	A	B	C	D	E	105	A	B	C	D	E	155	A	B	C	D	E	205	A	B	C	D	E
6	A	B	C	D	E	56	A	B	C	D	E	106	A	B	C	D	E	156	A	B	C	D	E	206	A	B	C	D	E
7	A	B	C	D	E	57	A	B	C	D	E	107	A	B	C	D	E	157	A	B	C	D	E	207	A	B	C	D	E
8	A	B	C	D	E	58	A	B	C	D	E	108	A	B	C	D	E	158	A	B	C	D	E	208	A	B	C	D	E
9	A	B	C	D	E	59	A	B	C	D	E	109	A	B	C	D	E	159	A	B	C	D	E	209	A	B	C	D	E
10	A	B	C	D	E	60	A	B	C	D	E	110	A	B	C	D	E	160	A	B	C	D	E	210	A	B	C	D	E
11	A	B	C	D	E	61	A	B	C	D	E	111	A	B	C	D	E	161	A	B	C	D	E	211	A	B	C	D	E
12	A	B	C	D	E	62	A	B	C	D	E	112	A	B	C	D	E	162	A	B	C	D	E	212	A	B	C	D	E
13	A	B	C	D	E	63	A	B	C	D	E	113	A	B	C	D	E	163	A	B	C	D	E	213	A	B	C	D	E
14	A	B	C	D	E	64	A	B	C	D	E	114	A	B	C	D	E	164	A	B	C	D	E	214	A	B	C	D	E
15	A	B	C	D	E	65	A	B	C	D	E	115	A	B	C	D	E	165	A	B	C	D	E	215	A	B	C	D	E
16	A	B	C	D	E	66	A	B	C	D	E	116	A	B	C	D	E	166	A	B	C	D	E	216	A	B	C	D	E
17	A	B	C	D	E	67	A	B	C	D	E	117	A	B	C	D	E	167	A	B	C	D	E	217	A	B	C	D	E
18	A	B	C	D	E	68	A	B	C	D	E	118	A	B	C	D	E	168	A	B	C	D	E	218	A	B	C	D	E
19	A	B	C	D	E	69	A	B	C	D	E	119	A	B	C	D	E	169	A	B	C	D	E	219	A	B	C	D	E
20	A	B	C	D	E	70	A	B	C	D	E	120	A	B	C	D	E	170	A	B	C	D	E	220	A	B	C	D	E
21	A	B	C	D	E	71	A	B	C	D	E	121	A	B	C	D	E	171	A	B	C	D	E	221	A	B	C	D	E
22	A	B	C	D	E	72	A	B	C	D	E	122	A	B	C	D	E	172	A	B	C	D	E	222	A	B	C	D	E
23	A	B	C	D	E	73	A	B	C	D	E	123	A	B	C	D	E	173	A	B	C	D	E	223	A	B	C	D	E
24	A	B	C	D	E	74	A	B	C	D	E	124	A	B	C	D	E	174	A	B	C	D	E	224	A	B	C	D	E
25	A	B	C	D	E	75	A	B	C	D	E	125	A	B	C	D	E	175	A	B	C	D	E	225	A	B	C	D	E
26	A	B	C	D	E	76	A	B	C	D	E	126	A	B	C	D	E	176	A	B	C	D	E	226	A	B	C	D	E
27	A	B	C	D	E	77	A	B	C	D	E	127	A	B	C	D	E	177	A	B	C	D	E	227	A	B	C	D	E
28	A	B	C	D	E	78	A	B	C	D	E	128	A	B	C	D	E	178	A	B	C	D	E	228	A	B	C	D	E
29	A	B	C	D	E	79	A	B	C	D	E	129	A	B	C	D	E	179	A	B	C	D	E	229	A	B	C	D	E
30	A	B	C	D	E	80	A	B	C	D	E	130	A	B	C	D	E	180	A	B	C	D	E	230	A	B	C	D	E
31	A	B	C	D	E	81	A	B	C	D	E	131	A	B	C	D	E	181	A	B	C	D	E	231	A	B	C	D	E
32	A	B	C	D	E	82	A	B	C	D	E	132	A	B	C	D	E	182	A	B	C	D	E	232	A	B	C	D	E
33	A	B	C	D	E	83	A	B	C	D	E	133	A	B	C	D	E	183	A	B	C	D	E	233	A	B	C	D	E
34	A	B	C	D	E	84	A	B	C	D	E	134	A	B	C	D	E	184	A	B	C	D	E	234	A	B	C	D	E
35	A	B	C	D	E	85	A	B	C	D	E	135	A	B	C	D	E	185	A	B	C	D	E	235	A	B	C	D	E
36	A	B	C	D	E	86	A	B	C	D	E	136	A	B	C	D	E	186	A	B	C	D	E	236	A	B	C	D	E
37	A	B	C	D	E	87	A	B	C	D	E	137	A	B	C	D	E	187	A	B	C	D	E	237	A	B	C	D	E
38	A	B	C	D	E	88	A	B	C	D	E	138	A	B	C	D	E	188	A	B	C	D	E	238	A	B	C	D	E
39	A	B	C	D	E	89	A	B	C	D	E	139	A	B	C	D	E	189	A	B	C	D	E	239	A	B	C	D	E
40	A	B	C	D	E	90	A	B	C	D	E	140	A	B	C	D	E	190	A	B	C	D	E	240	A	B	C	D	E
41	A	B	C	D	E	91	A	B	C	D	E	141	A	B	C	D	E	191	A	B	C	D	E	241	A	B	C	D	E
42	A	B	C	D	E	92	A	B	C	D	E	142	A	B	C	D	E	192	A	B	C	D	E	242	A	B	C	D	E
43	A	B	C	D	E	93	A	B	C	D	E	143	A	B	C	D	E	193	A	B	C	D	E	243	A	B	C	D	E
44	A	B	C	D	E	94	A	B	C	D	E	144	A	B	C	D	E	194	A	B	C	D	E	244	A	B	C	D	E
45	A	B	C	D	E	95	A	B	C	D	E	145	A	B	C	D	E	195	A	B	C	D	E	245	A	B	C	D	E
46	A	B	C	D	E	96	A	B	C	D	E	146	A	B	C	D	E	196	A	B	C	D	E	246	A	B	C	D	E
47	A	B	C	D	E	97	A	B	C	D	E	147	A	B	C	D	E	197	A	B	C	D	E	247	A	B	C	D	E
48	A	B	C	D	E	98	A	B	C	D	E	148	A	B	C	D	E	198	A	B	C	D	E	248	A	B	C	D	E
49	A	B	C	D	E	99	A	B	C	D	E	149	A	B	C	D	E	199	A	B	C	D	E	249	A	B	C	D	E
50	A	B	C	D	E	100	A	B	C	D	E	150	A	B	C	D	E	200	A	B	C	D	E	250	A	B	C	D	E

NAME OF THE CANDIDATE	ROLL NO.					CENTRE NO.		QUESTION BOOKLET NO.					BOOKLET CODE
CATEGORY	0	0	0	0	0	0	0	0	0	0	0	0	A
	1	1	1	1	1	1	1	1	1	1	1	1	B
	2	2	2	2	2	2	2	2	2	2	2	2	C
SC ○	3	3	3	3	3	3	3	3	3	3	3	3	D
ST ○	4	4	4	4	4	4	4	4	4	4	4	4	
OBC ○	5	5	5	5	5	5	5	5	5	5	5	5	
GEN ○	6	6	6	6	6	6	6	6	6	6	6	6	
CW ○	7	7	7	7	7	7	7	7	7	7	7	7	
PH ○	8	8	8	8	8	8	8	8	8	8	8	8	
	9	9	9	9	9	9	9	9	9	9	9	9	

INSTRUCTIONS FOR FILLING THE SHEET

1. This sheet should not be folded or crushed.
2. Use only blue/black ball pen to fill the circles.
3. Use of pencil is strictly prohibited.
4. Circles should be darkened properly and completely.
5. Cutting & erasing on this sheet is not allowed.
6. Do not use any stray marks on the sheet.
7. Do not use marker, white fluid or any other device to hide the shading already done.

WRONG METHOD

× ● ✓ ◌ ○

CORRECT METHOD

○ ○ ○ ● ○

CANDIDATE'S SIGNATURE
(in ball - point pen)

INVIGILATOR'S SIGNATURE
(in ball - point pen)

NOVEMBER
2016

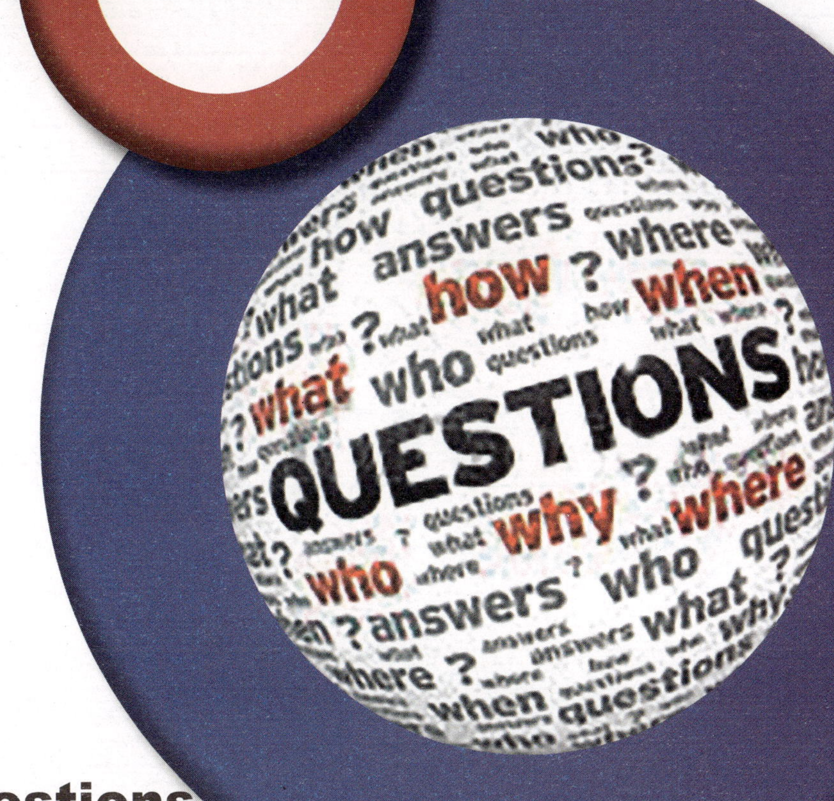

Multiple Choice Questions
Answers & Explanations

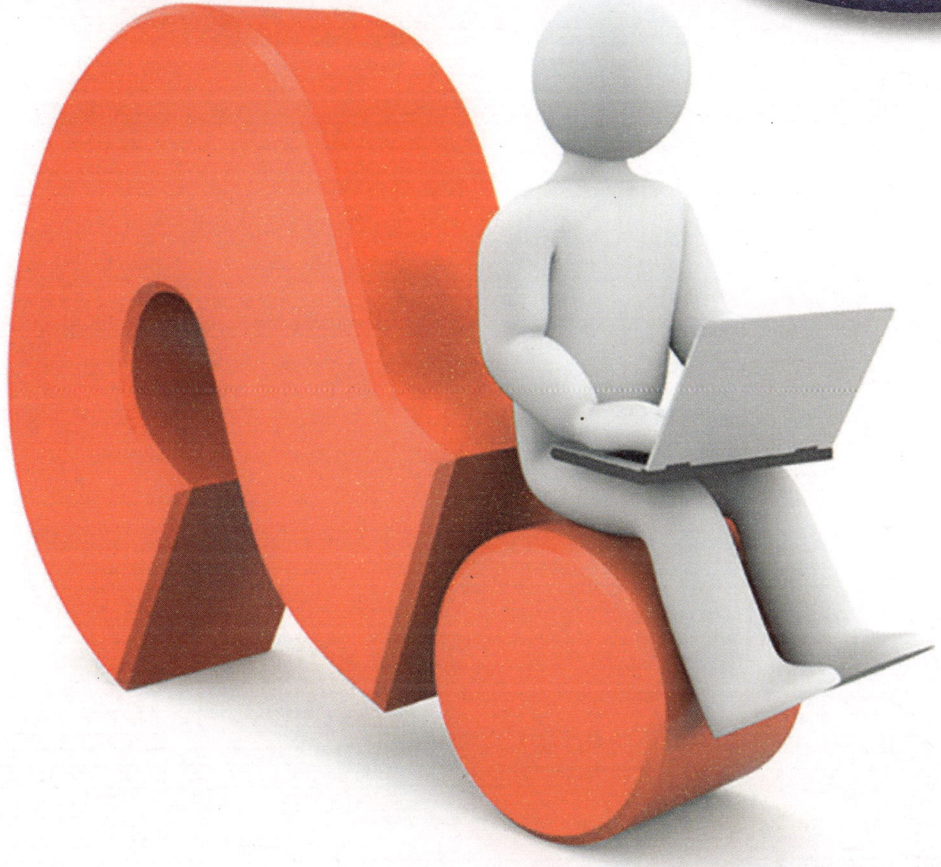

NOVEMBER 2016 MULTIPLE CHOICE QUESTIONS

ANATOMY

1. **Posterior interosseous nerve supplies all except:**
   a. Extensor carpi radialis longus
   b. Extensor carpi ulnaris
   c. Extensor digitorum
   d. Extensor indices
   e. Flexor carpi ulnaris
2. **Muscle(s) of anterior compartment of leg is/are:**
   a. Peroneus tertius
   b. Peroneus brevis
   c. Peroneus longus
   d. Flexor digitorum longus
   e. Flexor hallucis longus
3. **Branch(es) of Internal carotid artery directly arising from it:**
   a. Posterior communicating artery
   b. Superior hypophyseal artery
   c. Inferior hypophyseal artery
   d. Posterior cerebral Artery
   e. Recurrent artery of Heubner
4. **All are true about vestibular nerve except:**
   a. It has two division- superior and inferior vestibular
   b. Vestibular nuclei situated at junction of pons and medulla
   c. Nerve fibres relay at scarpa's ganglion
   d. Nucleus lies in midbrain near aqueduct
5. **True about Trochlear Nerve**
   a. Arise from ventral aspect of brainstem
   b. Enters orbit through annulus of Zinn
   c. Lesion causes diplopia
   d. Nucleus of the trochlear nerve is located in the caudal mesencephalon beneath the cerebral aqueduct
   e. Damage causes ipsilateral palsy of superior oblique muscle
6. **Content(s) of aortic hiatus:**
   a. Thoracic duct
   b. Aorta
   c. Vagus nerve
   d. Inferior vena cava
   e. Azygos vein
7. **Which flexor tendon zone in hand is known as "No man's land":**
   a. Zone I
   b. Zone II
   c. Zone III
   d. Zone IV
   e. Zone V
8. **Correct statement(s) about meiosis:**
   a. Somatic cells not divide by meiosis because number of chromosomes reduces to half
   b. Occur in germ cell which result in haploid cells
   c. One spermatocyte produces one sperm and one oocyte produces one ovum
   d. Germ cell undergoes division to form diploid cell and increase their number
   e. Body needs meiosis to produce large no. of eggs and sperms
9. **Cross section through medulla at the level of mid-olivary section through floor of fourth ventricle contains which of the following structures:**
   a. Trapezoid body
   b. Dorsal nucleus of vagus
   c. Nucleus of tractus solitarius
   d. Nucleus ambiguus
   e. Superior vestibular nucleus

PHYSIOLOGY

10. **True statement(s) about Olfactory system:**
    a. Olfactory mucosa cover upper 1/3 of nasal cavity
    b. Olfactory pathway passes via thalamus to orbitofrontal cortex
    c. Adaptation to odour develop only after 1–2 minutes
    d. Olfactory receptors act via cAMP
    e. Rate of olfactory nerve impulses change approximately in proportion to the logarithm of stimulus strength
11. **True about special anatomy and physiology of lung:**
    a. Surfactant prevent collapse of small alveoli into larger one
    b. Larger alveoli has more tendency to collapse than smaller alveoli in absence of surfactant
    c. Surfactant decrease chance of collapse
    d. Surfactant increases surface tension
    e. With surfactant, large alveoli tend to become smaller and smaller ones tend to become larger
12. **All are true about acromegaly except:**
    a. Increased IGF-1 levels
    b. Excessive growth occurs before fusion of the epiphyses of the long bones
    c. Somatostatin analogues can be used
    d. Growth hormone levels increased
    e. Trans sphenoidal surgical resection is the preferred primary treatment for pituitary adenoma
13. **True statement(s) is/are:**
    a. Vasopressin increase only water reabsorption, not solute reabsorption
    b. Aldosterone increase Na^+ reabsorption from tubules
    c. Glomerular filtrate of PCT has similar osmolarity as of plasma
    d. Urine is hyperosmolar in early DCT
    e. Generally urine osmolarity equals to plasma osmolarity

Answer 

1.	a, e.	2.	a.	3.	a, b, c.	4.	d.	5.	c, d.	6.	a, b, e.	7.	b.
8.	a, b, e.	9.	b, c, d.	10.	a, b, d. e.	11.	a, c, e.	12.	b.	13.	a, b, c.		

14. Rapidly adapting receptor(s) is/are:

a. Pain receptor
b. Pacinian corpuscles
c. Muscle spindle
d. Golgi tendon organs
e. Meissner corpuscles

15. Which of the following is/are true about normal blood level:

a. Total Calcium: 8.5–10.5 mg/dL
b. Sodium:135–145 mmol/L
c. Potassium: 3.5–5.1 mmol/L
d. Creatinine: 0.6–2.6 mg/dL
e. TSH level: 0.1–3.1 mIU/L

16. True about Action potential in skeletal muscle fibers and nerve fibres:

a. Skeletal muscle fibres conduction velocity is ¼ of thick myelinated nerve fiber
b. Action potential of both qualitatively similar
c. Resting membrane potential almost same
d. Duration of action potential same in both
e. Action potential of both quantitatively similar

17. Tissue elevation of which of the following cause vasoconstriction:

a. Na^+
b. K^+
c. Mg
d. Ca^{2+}
e. H^+

18. Which of the following statement(s) is/are true about changes at time of ovulation:

a. GnRH level decreases
b. Gonadotropin hormone surge
c. hCG surge
d. ↑ Prostaglandins
e. Activation of proteolytic enzymes

19. Comprehension preserved in which of the following aphasia:

a. Broca's aphasia
b. Conduction aphasia
c. Wernicke's aphasia
d. Gobal aphasia
e. Anomic aphasia

20. Vomiting centre(s) involved in post-operative vomiting:

a. Area postrema
b. Chemoreceptor trigger zone (CTZ)
c. Reticular formation located in medulla
d. Nucleus tractus solitarius
e. Basal ganglia

BIOCHEMISTRY

21. Hyperuricemia is/are associated with:

a. HGPRT deficiency
b. HGPRT overactivity
c. PRPP synthetase deficiency
d. Glucose 6- phosphatase deficiency
e. Glucose phosphate dehydrogenase deficiency

22. Hyperphenylalaninemia occurs due to:

a. Phenylalanine hydroxylase deficiency
b. Phenylalanine hydroxylase overactivity
c. Dihydrobiopterin reductase deficiency
d. Tyrosine hydroxylase deficiency
e. Defect in dihydrobiopterin biosynthesis

23. Oxidative phosphorylation not inhibited by:

a. Fluoride
b. 2, 4-dinitrophenol (DNP)
c. Oligomycin
d. Carboxin
e. Ouabin

24. True about Apolipoproteins:

a. Constitute peripheral region of plasma lipoproteins
b. Divided into A, B, C only
c. Apo A-I is the major protein component of high density lipoprotein (HDL)
d. Apo A,B and C are further divided
e. Role in enzyme activation

25. Amino acids containing hydroxyl group:

a. Threonine
b. Tyrosine
c. Serine
d. Tryptophan
e. Valine

26. Cytochrome P450 is/are involved in:

a. Hydroxylation of xenobiotics
b. Methylation of xenobiotics
c. Deamination reaction
d. Involved in hydroxylation of steroids
e. Drug interaction

27. True about role of phospholipids:

a. Cell to cell recognition
b. Cell signaling
c. Precursor of Second Messengers
d. Mediators of inflammation
e. Regulate membrane permeability

28. Correct statement about membrane:

a. Phospholipids undergo rapid lateral diffusion
b. Transverse movement of lipids across the membrane is faster than protein
c. Hydrophobic core of the phospholipid bilayer remains constantly in motion because of rotations around the bonds of lipid tails
d. Phospholipids that have one fatty acyl group, cannot form the bilayer
e. Phospholipids span whole bilayer

IMMUNOGENETICS & MOLECULAR BIOLOGY

29. During DNA replication which bond breaks:

a. Phosphodiester bonds
b. Phosphate bond
c. Hydrogen bond
d. Glycosidic bonds

Answer

14. b, d, e.	15. a, b, c.	16. b, c.	17. d.	18. b, d, e.	19. a, b, e.	20. a, b, d.
21. a, d.	22. a, c, e.	23. a, d, e.	24. a, c, d, e.	25. a, b, c.	26. a, c, d, e.	27. b, c, d, e.
28. a, c, d.	29. c.					

30. Which RNA contains abnormal purine and pyrimidine:
a. tRNA b. 23SrRNA
c. 16SrRNA d. 5SrRNA
e. mRNA

31. Component of 50S ribosomal subunit:
a. 16S RNA b. 18S RNA
c. 5.8 RNA d. 5S RNA
e. 23S RNA

32. True about chromatin remodeling:
a. Energy is required to displace the histone octamers from DNA or translocate them onto neighboring DNA segments
b. Histone modifications by specific enzyme
c. Do not involve enzymes
d. Aberrations in chromatin remodeling proteins may be associated with cancer

33. Best assessment of protein binding regions on a DNA molecule can be done by:
a. DNA footprinting b. RT PCR
c. Microarray d. Western blotting
e. Northern blotting

PATHOLOGY

34. Feature(s) of Chronic myelogenous leukemia (CML):
a. Bone narrow biopsy is necessary for diagnosis
b. Presence of BCR-ABL gene which directs the synthesis of BCR-ABL tyrosine kinase
c. Dasatinib is used in imatinib resistant cases
d. Generalized painful lymphadenopathy is presenting feature in most cases
e. Myeloblasts usually constitute more than 10% of all white cells in chronic phase

35. True about Cystic fibrosis:
a. Occurs due CFTR gene mutation on chromosome 7
b. Meconium ileus is present in >90% cases
c. CFTR gene can be detected antenately
d. Poor body growth

36. True about caspases:
a. Caspases initiate apoptosis by extrinsic and intrinsic pathway
b. Caspases are protease enzyme
c. Caspases are receptor
d. Caspases inhibit apoptosis
e. Causes non enzymatic degradation of critical cellular components

37. True about minimal change disease:
a. Hypertension is commonly present
b. Most common cause of nephrotic syndrome in adults
c. High dose steroids results in remission in most cases
d. Commonly progress to chronic renal failure
e. Reversible loss of podocyte function

38. Feature(s) of Adult polycystic kidney disease is/are:
a. Renal enlargement
b. Small kidney
c. Spider leg deformity on intravenous urography
d. Ultrasound shows multiple cysts

39. Which is/are caused by protein misfolding:
a. Creutzfeldt–Jakob disease
b. Bovine spongiform encephalopathy
c. Huntington disease
d. Alzheimer disease e. Parkinson disease

40. True about Creutzfeldt-Jakob disease:
a. Gliosis in thalamus
b. Spongiform swelling in cerebral cortex
c. Brain atrophy in late stage
d. Slow and irregular background rhythm on EEG

41. Hereditary non-polyposis colorectal cancer (HNPCC) is/are commonly associated with:
a. Endometrial cancer b. Cervical cancer
c. Ovarian cancer d. Breast cancer
e. Thyroid cancer

42. Feature of nonbacterial thrombotic endocarditis (NBTE):
a. Common in SLE
b. Present on undersurface of valve
c. Vegetative growth is large and loosely attached to valve
d. May occur after post-cardiac catheterization
e. Source of systemic emboli

43. True about Alzheimer disease:
a. Most common cause of dementia in elderly
b Unusual before 45 years of age
c. Plaques consists of tau protein
d. May have family history
e. Short term memory is affected less than long-term memory

44. Negri bodies in animal can be best seen in:
a. Hippocampus b. Basal ganglia
c. Cerebral cortex d. Cerebellum
e. Thalamus

45. True about p53:
a. Has tyrosine kinase activity
b. Has pro-apoptotic activity
c. Tumour suppressor gene
d. Has anti-apoptotic activity

46. True about Takayasu syndrome:
a. Involves small and Medium sized vessels
b. Shares many clinical features of giant cell arteritis if involves aorta
c. More common in male than female
d. Granulomatous vasculitis
e. Also called pulseless disease

47. Which are inheritable malignancies:
a. Breast cancer b. Thyroid cancer
c. Wilm's tumour d. Retinoblastoma
e. Prostate cancer

Answer

30. a.	31. d, e.	32. a, b, d.	33. a.	34. a, b, c.	35. a, c, d.	36. a, b.
37. c, e.	38. a, c, d.	39. All (a, b, c, d, e)	40. b, c, d.	41. a, c.	42. b, d, e.	43. a, b, d.
44. a, d.	45. a, b, c.	46. b, d, e.	47. All (a, b, c, d, e)			

48. **Cause(s) of Non-megaloblastic macrocytic anemia:**
   a. Folate deficiency
   b. Lead toxicity
   c. Hypothyroidism
   d. Liver disease
   e. Vit B_{12} deficiency
49. **True statement(s) about Wilm's tumor:**
   a. Most commonly presents as asymptomatic abdominal mass
   b. Hereditary predisposition is present in 50% cases
   c. Bilateral in 25% cases
   d. Classic triphasic combination of blastemal, stromal, and epithelial cell types is observed
   e. Most common in children
50. **Which of following is not classified as Primitive neuroectodermal tumour (PNET):**
   a. Retinoblastoma
   b. Medulloblastoma
   c. Rhabdomyosarcoma
   d. Ewing sarcoma
   e. Carcinoid tumour
51. **Glucose level in CSF is/are reduced in:**
   a. Bacterial meningitis
   b. Fungal meningitis
   c. Viral meningitis
   d. Tubercular meningitis
   e. Spirochetal meningitis
52. **True about proliferative phase of wound healing**
   a. Neutrophils increases gradually
   b. Macrophage increases gradually
   c. Collagen type I present predominantly
   d. Collagen type III present predominantly
   e. Angiogenesis occurs
53. **Correct match of stain with tissue is/are:**
   a. Perls' Prussian blue-iron in tissue
   b. Von Kossa-collagen
   c. Masson's trichrome –elastin fiber
   d. PAS- glycogen
   e. PAS- Acidic and neutral mucin

PHARMACOLOGY

54. **Which of the following is/are action of estrogen except:**
   a. Development of the alveolar system
   b. Proliferation of stroma of breast
   c. Ductal growth of the breast
   d. ↓ Bone resorption
   e. Development of lobules of breast
55. **All are true about bisphosphonates except:**
   a. Prevent reabsorption of bone by osteoclast
   b. Structurally similar to pyrophosphate
   c. Absorption increases with food
   d. Can be safely given in liver disease
56. **Which of the following is/are newer drugs for TB:**
   a. Bedaquiline
   b. Clofazimine
   c. Coftaroline
   d. Rifapentine
   e. Etanercept
57. **All are true about oral iron therapy in anemia except:**
   a. May worsen inflammatory bowel disease
   b. It takes minimum 2 weeks for reticulocyte count to increase
   c. Generally 3-6 month therapy is required to replenish iron stores
   d. Gastrointestinal side-effects limits its dose
   e. Hb level is generally attained in 1-3 month
58. **Drug which can be given by inhalation route:**
   a. Zileuton
   b. Steroid
   c. Salbutamol
   d. Tobramycin
59. **Liver function test (LFT) monitoring is/are required in use of which of the following Disease Modifying Antirheumatic Drugs (DMARDs):**
   a. Methotrexate
   b. Hydroxychloroquine
   c. Sulfasalazine
   d. Leflunomide
   e. Gold
60. **Drugs which can be used in gestational hypertension:**
   a. Metoprolol
   b. Labetalol
   c. Methyldopa
   d. Sustained release nifedipine
   e. Losartan
61. **Adverse effects of mirtazapine is/are:**
   a. Insomnia
   b. Sedation
   c. Sexual dysfunction
   d. Vomiting
   e. Weight gain
62. **Carbonic anhydrase inhibitor(s) is/are:**
   a. Acetazolamide
   b. Amiloride
   c. Nitrofurantoin
   d. Topiramate
63. **Which of the following is/are true about Tacrolimus:**
   a. A macrolides antibiotic
   b. Structure similar to cyclosporine
   c. Derived from a fungus
   d. T cell inhibitor
   e. Hirsutism less evident than cyclosporine
64. **True about Low molecular weight heparin (LMWH):**
   a. Anti-factor Xa assay monitoring required in every patient
   b. It increases aPTT more than UFH
   c. Can be safely given in renal failure
   d. Toxicity is totally reversed by protamine sulphate
   e. Inactivate factor Xa selectively

Answer

48. c, d. 49. a, d, e. 50. a, c, d, e. 51. a, b, d. 52. d, e. 53. a, d, e. 54. a, e.
55. c. 56. a, b, d. 57. b. 58. b, c. 59. a, d, e. 60. a, b, c, d. 61. b, e.
62. a, d. 63. a, d, e. 64. e.

65. True about Mafenide:
a. Can penetrate eschars
b. Doesn't cause burning sensation when applied to raw surface
c. Can be used orally
d. May cause metabolic acidosis

66. Which of the following is/are true about pharmacodynamics of drugs:
a. Affinity means how strongly drug binds to receptor
b. Efficacy means maximal effect by a drug
c. Irreversible antagonist mainly forms ionic bonds with receptor
d. Agonist potency depends on two parameters: affinity and efficacy
e. For antagonists, efficacy is zero

67. All are true about plasma protein binding except:
a. Acidic drugs generally bind to plasma albumin and basic drugs to α_1 acid glycoprotein
b. Plasma binding determines volume of distribution
c. More plasma protein binding means more storage in liver
d. More plasma protein binding means less penetration in vascular membrane
e. High degree of protein binding generally makes the drug long acting

68. First pass metabolism is significant problem in drug given through:
a. Sublingual route
b. Rectal route
c. Intramuscular route
d. Directly into stomach
e. Directly into large intestine

69. Which of the following dyads show clinically significant drug interactions:
a. Vancomycin—Amphotericin B
b. Rantidine–Atorvastatin
c. Warfarin—Aspirin
d. Allopurinol—Azathioprine
e. Aminoglycoside—Vancomycin

70. True about osmotic diuretics:
a. Osmotic diuretics have their major effect in the distal convoluted tubule
b. Contraindicated in congestive heart failure
c. Causes Hyperkalemia
d. Increases renal blood flow

71. True about effect of steroid intake in inflammatory conditions:
a. Proanabolic effect on muscles
b. ↑ glucose in plasma
c. –ve feedback on corticotropin-releasing hormone (CRH) production
d. May cause osteoporosis

72. Drug that can potentiate Torsades de pointes:
a. Amiodarone
b. Sotalol
c. Chlorpromazine
d. Cisapride
e. Aspirin

MICROBIOLOGY

73. All is/are true about Rotavirus infection except:
a. Most commonly seen in adult of > 30 year age group
b. Person to person transmission may occur
c. Severity of disease decreases with each repeat infection
d. Commonest cause of diarrhea in infants and children
e. Single infection provide lifelong immunity against reinfection

74. True about pseudomonas aeruginosa:
a. Not lysine decarboxylase positive
b. Oxidase positive
c. Produce pyocyanin pigment
d. Gram-negative bacilli
e. Has 6–12 flagella

75. Which of the following is/are DNA viruses:
a. Herpes virus
b. Hepadnaviridae
c. Parvovirus
d. Orthomyxoviridae
e. Enteroviruses

76. True about ZIKA virus:
a. Belong to flavivirus
b. First case detected in 1953 in Nigeria
c. RT PCR is useful in diagnosis
d. Causes macrocephaly
e. May presents with conjunctivitis

77. Parasite which infects through ingestion of aquatic vegetation:
a. Fasciola hepatica
b. Fasciolopsis buski
c. Paragonimus westermani
d. Watsonius watsoni
e. Gastrodiscoides hominis

78. Which of the following dyads of vector with disease is/are correctly matched:
a. Rat flea– Endemic typhus
b. Sand flea—Oriental sore
c. Black fly—Kala azar
d. Cyclops—Dracunculosis
e. Louse—Chagas disease

79. All are feature of Scrub typhus except:
a. Black eschar
b. Maculo-papular rash
c. More common in rural areas
d. Ciprofloxacin is drug of choice
e. Tick borne disease

Answer

65. d. 66. a, b, d, e. 67. c. 68. d, e. 69. a, c, d, e. 70. b, c, d. 71. b, c, d.
72. a, b, c, d. 73. a, e. 74. a, b, c, d. 75. a, b, c. 76. a, c, e. 77. a, b, d, e. 78. a, b, d.
79. d, e.

80. Unlike nocardia, Actinomyoses is:
a. Facultative anaerobes
b. Not acid fast
c. Endogenous cause of disease
d. Environmental saprophyte
e. Grow at wide range of temperature range

81. Which of the following is/are caused by dermatophytes:
a. Madura foot
b. Athlete's foot
c. Kerion
d. Favus

82. Which of the following has least minimum infective dose (MID) required for causing infection:
a. *Salmonella typhi*
b. *Campylobacter jejuni*
c. *Shigella dysentery*
d. *Vibrio cholera*

83. Which type of bacteria can not survive in absence of oxygen:
a. Obligate aerobe
b. Facultative anaerobes
c. Microaerophilic
d. Obligate Anaerobes
e. Facultative aerobes

84. All are true about H1N1 influenza except:
a. Zanamivir commonly given through IV route
b. Fatality more in some high risk group
c. RT-PCR is used for investigation
d. WHO latest trivalent influenza vaccine contains two influenza A subtypes (H3N2 and H1N1) and one influenza B component
e. CDC latest quadrivalent influenza vaccine contains two influenza A subtypes (H3N2 and H1N1) and two influenza B component

85. True about serum marker of inactive carrier phase of chronic Hepatitis B:
a. Hbs Ag +ve
b. Hbe Ag +ve
c. Anti-HBe antibody positive
d. Low level DNA
e. Increased ALT

86. Which of the following mechanism is/are used by bacteria to escape host defence mechanism:
a. *Mycobaterium tuberculsosis* prevent intracellular killing by inhibiting phagolysosome formation
b. *Streptococcus pyogenes* by M protein
c. *Neisseria meningitides* by capsular polysaccharide
d. *Staphlococcus aureus* by iron-regulated outer membrane proteins
e. Polysaccharide capsules of *H. influenzae*

87. True about gas gangrene:
a. Onset is usually acute
b. Painless condition
c. Wound is swollen
d. At first wound is dusky or red, later becomes pale
e. Caused by gram +ve organism

88. All are true about Dengu virus except:
a. Belong to flaviviridae
b. Type DEN 4 is most common in India
c. Main vectors are aedes aegypti and aedes albopictus
d. Virus has positive sense RNA
e. Vector is sensitive to DDT

89. Which of the following is/are true about Dengu fever:
a. Positive Tourniquet test means more than 10 petechiae per square inch
b. Caused by flavivirus
c. Aedes aegypticus and albopictus are most important vector in India
d. IgM/IgG ratios may be used to distinguish primary from secondary infection
e. No vaccine available at present

90. Autoclave is/are used for sterilization of:
a. Wooden material
b. Metallic instrument
c. Plastic
d. Glasswares
e. Fibro-optic bronchoscope

FORENSIC MEDICINE

91. Valid ground of divorce for female:
a. Impotence of male partner
b. Extramarital affair of male partner
c. Infertility of female
d. Unemployment of male partner
e. If she was married before the age of fifteen and she want to renounces the marriage before she attains eighteen years of age

92. Bite mark may aid in:
a. Assessment of age
b. Identification of accused
c. Assessment of height
d. Assessment of type of teeth
e. Collection of DNA sample

93. Feature of gunshot injury is/are:
a. Gutter injury
b. Grease collar
c. Radiating wound
d. Tissue opening on opposite end

94. Which of the following is/are true regarding Per jury:
a. Willfully giving false statement under oath which he/she either knows or believes to be false or does not believe to be true
b. S. 190 IPC deals with perjury
c. Voluntarily giving false evidence under oath which he/she either knows or believes to be false or does not believe to be true
d. The witness is liable to be prosecuted for perjury

Answer 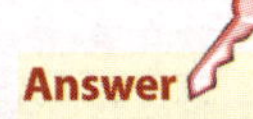

80. a, b, c.	81. b, c, d.	82. c.	83. a.	84. a.	85. a, c, d.	86. a, b, c, e.
87. a, c, e.	88. b.	89. All (a, b, c, d, e)	90. b.	91. a, b, e.	92. b, d, e.	93. All (a, b, c, d)
94. a, c, d.						

95. True about corpus delicti:
a. Medical negligence
b. Body of offence
c. It includes body of the victim and other facts which are conclusive of death by foul play
d. The essence of crime

96. Which is not a method of crime scene examination:
a. Grid
b. Strip
c. Wheel
d. Composite
e. Point to point

PREVENTIVE & SOCIAL MEDICINE

97. Which of the following is/are true about tuberculosis in India:
a. India has approximately 1/4th of Global load of TB
b. MDR-TB among notified new pulmonary TB patients is about 5%
c. 5% of TB patients estimated to be HIV positive
d. MDR-TB among retreatment cases is about 15%
e. Incidence is around 2 million new TB cases annually

98. Importance of lepromin test are all except:
a. Only has epidemiological significance
b. Prognostic value
c. Tells about immunity status of leprosy patients
d. Differentiate between different types of leprosy
e. Predictive value

99. A leprosy person is presented with involvements of sural and radial nerve. Which type of regimen you will give:
a. Multibacillary treatment × 9 month
b. Multibacillary treatment × 12 month
c. Multibacillary treatment × 15 month
d. Paucibacillary treatment × 6 month
e. Single dose treatment of Rifampicin, Ofloxacin and Minocycline (ROM)

100. Which of the following is true about data representation:
a. Histogram is used for presentation of discrete data
b. Random dots in scatter diagram— no correlation
c. Pictogram is represented by small pictures or symbols
d. Pie chart is represented by quadrangular figures
e. Regression graph is said linear when the increase or decrease in the variables remains proportional in different subjects

101. True about program evaluation and review technique (PERT):
a. Better than critical path method for small project
b. Recurrent activities is better monitored than CPM
c. Activities are divided into small goals
d. Main objective to monitor cost
e. It is a management technique better for non-research activities than CPM

102. Which of the following content is/are more in Human milk than cow's milk:
a. Protein
b. Iron
c. Carbohydrate
d. Fat
e. Energy

103. Which of the following is/are true:
a. Serial interval = gap in time b/w invasion by an infectious agent and appearance of clinical feature
b. Latent period = the period from disease initiation to disease detection in non-infectious disease
c. Incubation period = time b/w the onset of the primary case and the secondary case
d. Generation time = time period between the onset of the infection and the maximum infectivity of the host
e. Communicable period = It is a period during which the reservoir is infectious to others

104. Tests to check pasteurization of milk:
a. Phosphatase test
b. Standard plate count
c. Methylene blue test
d. Nitric acid test
e. Coliform count

OPHTHALMOLOGY

105. True about component of vision 2020:
a. Cataract surgery should be performed at primary level
b. Retinal surgery should be performed at tertiary level
c. Need to develop 10 centre of excellence at tertiary level and 100 training centre at advanced tertiary level
d. Ophthalmia neonatorum is included in childhood blindness
e. Primary vision center covers a population of 50000

106. True about Nodular episcleritis:
a. Can be associated with SLE
b. Take longer time to resolve than diffuse variety
c. More symptomatic than diffuse type
d. Painless
e. Elevated hard nodule

107. Which type of cataract is/are associated with Myotonic dystrophy:
a. Posterior subcapsular
b. Anterior subcapsular
c. Nuclear cataract
d. Cortical cataract

108. What is the WHO criteria for defining blindness:
a. <3/60 vision with available correction
b. <6/60 vision with available correction
c. <3/60 vision with best correction
d. <6/60 vision with best correction
e. <3/60 vision without correction

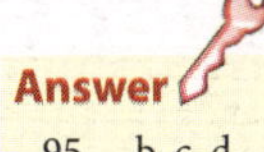
Answer

95. b, c, d. 96. d, e. 97. a, c, d, e. 98. a. 99. b. 100. b, c, e. 101. c.
102. b, c. 103. b, d, e. 104. a, b, c, e. 105. b, d, e. 106. a, b, c, e. 107. a. 108. c.

109. True about Acanthamoebic keratitis:
- a. More in those wearing rigid gas permeable than soft contact lenses user
- b. Can occur as opportunistic infection in patients with herpetic keratitis
- c. Can be cultured on non-nutrient agar enriched with E. coli
- d. Painful condition
- e. Radial kerato-neuritis may occur

110. True about ferritin line in eye:
- a. Ferry's Line-corneal epithelial iron line at the edge of filtering blebs
- b. Stockers Line-Corneal epithelial iron line at the edge of pterygium
- c. Hudson-Stahli line- visible all around the base of cone in Keratoconus
- d. Fleischer's ring: Horizontal corneal epithelial iron line at the inferior one third of cornea due to aging
- e. Coat's white ring- A form of iron deposit at the level of Bowman's layer of cornea

111. Which of the following is the feature of sodium fluorescein angiography compared to indocyanine green angiography:
- a. In choroidal circulation it passes freely across the endothelium
- b. Diffuse freely through retinal *capillaries*
- c. Albumin binding is less than indocyanine green
- d. Bind < 50% to albumin
- e. Stimulated by a longer wavelength of light

112. True about phthisis bulbi:
- a. Size of eye decreases
- b. Removed by enucleation operation especially if painful
- c. IOP increases in late stage
- d. Calcification may occur in Bowman's layer of cornea

113. Advantage of continuous curvilinear capsulorhexis over can opener technique:
- a. Preferred method of anterior capsulotomy in phacoemulsification
- b. More chances of posterior capsular opacification
- c. Keeps the nucleus in place
- d. Resists radial tears
- e. Helps in stabilizing and centering the lens implant

ENT

114. All is true about foreign body impaction in ear except:
- a. Objects located medial to isthmus of canal is difficult to remove
- b. Syringing is used for removal of vegetative foreign body
- c. Syringing uses room temperature water
- d. Blunt hook is used to remove rounded foreign body
- e. GA is preferred in children to remove foreign bodies

115. All are true about epistaxis except:
- a. Keisselbach's plexus is source in 90% cases
- b. If anterior packing is left in nose for more than 48 hrs antibiotic coverage is given
- c. Anterior nasal pack is easy to insert and less traumatic than balloon temponade
- d. Trotter method is first aid method
- e. Cauteristaion is done in refractory cases under general anaesthesia

116. True about Secretory otitis media:
- a. Type C tympanogram may be seen in early stage of otitis media with effusion
- b. Flat tympanogram is present
- c. Leads to conductive deafness
- d. Presence of cleft palate reduces its chance
- e. Most common cause is Eustachian tube dysfunction

117. Which cause reddish lesion on tongue:
- a. Median rhomboid glossitis
- b. Hairy leukoplakia
- c. Lichen planus
- d. Geographic tongue
- e. Fordyce's spots

118. True statement regarding wax in ear:
- a. Syringing and instrumental manipulation are generally done to remove impacted wax
- b. If wax is hard and impacted, ceruminolytic substances is used to soften wax
- c. In syringing fluid is injected along the lower wall of the meatus
- d. Wax has antibacterial property

119. True about spasmodic dysphonia:
- a. A neurological problem
- b. Mostly psychogenic in origin
- c. Hyperadduction of vocal cord may be seen
- d. Botulinum toxin relives spasm
- e. Speech therapy is beneficial

120. Feature(s) of peritonsillar abscess:
- a. Foul breath
- b. Hot potato voice
- c. Shifting of uvula in opposite side
- d. Difficulty in swallowing even own saliva
- e. Always presents as b/l severe pain in throat

121. True about antrochoanal polyp:
- a. Starts as edema of maxillary sinus mucosa
- b. Suppressed by steroids
- c. Comes out via accessory ostium and grows in the choana and nasal cavity
- d. More common in adults than children
- e. Commonly presents as unilateral nasal obstruction

Answer

109. b, c, d, e.	110. a, b, e.	111. a, c.	112. a, b, d.	113. a, c, d, e.	114. b.	115. c.
116. a, b, c, e.	117. a, d.	118. a, b, d.	119. a, c, d, e.	120. a, b, c, d.	121. a, c, e.	

MEDICINE

122. Which of the following is/are feature of aortic stenosis:
a. Duration between onset of symptom and death is generally 10–15 year
b. Angina occurs mainly because of fixed coronary blood flows
c. No increase in cardiac output despite exercise
d. Ejection systolic murmur radiating to neck may present
e. Left ventricular hypertrophy

123. True about organophosphate-induced delayed polyneuropathy:
a. Usually occurs after 2–3 month of acute exposure
b. Involves both sensory and motor nerve
c. Steroid is used for treatment
d. Incomplete recovery

124. Unlike Child Pugh scoring, MELD score have:
a. Bedside assessment easy
b. Prothrombin time expressed as international normalized ratio (INR)
c. Serum creatinine estimation
d. Four component is used in scoring
e. Albumin level estimation

125. Risk factors associated with health care associated pneumonia (HCAP):
a. Acute care hospitalization for at least 2 days in the preceding 90 days
b. Home infusion therapy
c. Immunosuppressive disease or immunosuppressive therapy
d. Antibiotic therapy in the preceding 90 days
e. Hospitalization for ≥ 48 h

126. All are feature(s) of sarcoidosis except:
a. High CD4: CD8 ratio
b. Hypercalciuria and hypercalcimia may be present
c. ↑ Serum levels of angiotensin-converting enzyme (ACE)
d. Schauman and asteroid bodies are pathognomic

127. Transudative pleural effusion occurs in:
a. Urinothorax
b. Dressler syndrome
c. Nephrotic syndrome
d. Myxedema
e. Congestive heart failure

128. True about primary sclerosing cholangitis:
a. Involves only intrahepatic bile duct, not extrahepatic bile duct
b. Associated with Inflammatory bowel disease
c. Causes macronodular cirrhosis
d. Periductal fibrosis of smaller bile ducts

129. True about insulinoma:
a. Encapsulated
b. Mostly multiple
c. Associated with MEN-I
d. Enucleation is the treatment of choice for benign tumour
e. Histology similar to normal β-cells

130. True about Hypersensitivity pneumonitis:
a. Occurs due to inorganic antigen
b. Increased CD8+ T cells in bronchoalveolar lavage
c. Manifests mainly as an occupational and environment disease
d. For severe acute cases, oral steroids is given for 3–4 weeks
e. Interstitial inflammatory infiltrate is seen in lung

131. All are true about Sjögren's syndrome except:
a. Bilateral parotid gland enlargement
b. Parotid gland enlargement may be painful
c. Xerostomia may present
d. Progression to lymphoma
e. Males are affected more than females

132. Feature(s) of Felty's syndrome is/are:
a. Seropositive for rheumatoid factor
b. Splenomegaly
c. Long standing rheumatoid arthritis
d. Neutrophilia
e. Keratoconjunctivitis sicca

133. Malignancies associated with AIDS:
a. Primary CNS lymphoma
b. Cervical cancer
c. Kaposi sarcoma
d. Ovarian cancer
e. Endometrial cancer

134. Malignancy associated with hypercalcemia:
a. Breast cancer
b. Small cell lung cancer
c. Non-small lung cancer
d. Prostate cancer
e. Multiple myeloma

135. True about Severe Combined Immunodeficiency (SCID):
a. Adenosine deaminase enzyme may be given for treatment
b. Haematopoietic stem cell transplant (HSCT) is curative
c. Most common inheritance is X linked recessive and autosomal recessive
d. Lymphocytosis is present in most cases
e. Increased risk of infection by *pneumocystis jiroveci*

136. Proximal renal tubular acidosis(RTA) is/are associated with:
a. Fanconi anemia
b. Multiple myeloma
c. Lead poisoning
d. Sjogren's syndrome
e. SLE

137. High anion gap acidosis is/are associated with:
a. Lactic acidosis
b. Ethylene glycol poisoning
c. Aspirin overdose
d. Diarrhea
e. Renal tubular acidosis

138. Tubular proteinuria is/are seen in:
a. Multiple myeloma
b. Wilson disease
c. Lead poisoning
d. Fanconi syndrome

Answer

122. c, d, e. 123. a, b, d. 124. b, c. 125. All (a, b, c, d, e) 126. d. 127. a, c, d, e. 128. b, d.
129. a, c, d, e. 130. b, c, d, e. 131. e. 132. a, b, c, e. 133. a, b, c, d. 134. a, c, d, e. 135. a, b, c, e.
136. a, b, c. 137. a, b, c. 138. b, c, d.

139. All are true about Celiac disease except:
a. Antiendomysial antibody is present
b. Oat, rye and barley can be safely given
c. Associated with dermatitis herpetiformis
d. Associated with gliadin
e. No risk for development of cancer

140. Respiratory failure type II is/are seen in:
a. Myasthenia gravis
b. Acute exacerbation in COPD
c. Acute severe asthma
d. Pulmonary edema
e. Pulmonary embolism

141. Photosensitivity is/are not seen in:
a. Acute intermittent porphyria
b. Variegate porphyria
c. Porphyria cutanea tarda
d. Congenital erythropoietic porphyria
e. Erythropoietic protoporphyria

142. True about 4th heart sound:
a. Low pitch
b. Present during early diastole
c. Absent in atrial fibrillation
d. Produced in the ventricle during ventricular filling phase
e. Present in severe left ventricular hypertrophy

143. True about atrial flutter:
a. Narrow-complex tachycardia of up to 150/min
b. P wave absent
c. Associated with 2: 1, 3: 1 or 4: 1 AV block
d. Best therapy is catheter ablation
e. Occur due to macro re-entry circuit within the right atrium

144. Positive ECG sign(s) of ischemia in Tread mill test is/are:
a. Upsloping depression of the ST segment >0.1 mV below baseline
b. Downsloping depression of the ST segment >0.1 mV below baseline
c. Junctional ST-segment
d. Tachycardia
e. Ventricular premature beats

145. Which of the following is/are included in management of acute ischemic stroke:
a. Unfractioned Heparin
b. LMWH
c. Streptokinase
d. Aspirin
e. Recombinant tissue plasminogen activator (rt-PA)

146. Finding(s) in hemolytic anemia is/are:
a. Increase in conjugated bilirubin
b. Increase in unconjugated bilirubin
c. Increase in urine urobilinogen
d. Increase in faecal stercobilinogen
e. Increased bilirubin in urine

147. True about idiopathic thrombocytopenic purpura:
a. In children, it is usually a chronic disease
b. Self-limited course in acute form
c. In adults, it is a more acute disease
d. Immune-mediated destruction of platelets

148. True about coagulation disorders:
a. In DIC both PT and aPTT increase
b. Hemophilia C is a X linked recessive condition
c. Factor VIII can be given in hemophilia B
d. Hemophilia A is inherited as X-linked recessive

149. Plexiform lesion is prominent in which group of pulmonary hypertension:
a. Recurrent thromboemboli
b. Interstitial lung diseases
c. Familial pulmonary HTN
d. Congenital heart disease with left-to-right shunts
e. Pulmonary hypertension associated with human immunodeficiency

150. In which of the following condition, non-hepatic surgery is associated with most adverse outcome:
a. Child-Pugh score B
b. Child-Pugh score C
c. Acute viral hepatitis
d. Acute alcoholic hepatitis
e. Chronic viral hepatitis

151. True about multiple sclerosis:
a. Periventricular involvement can't be seen by imaging studies
b. May produce mass lesion
c. Autoimmune inflammatory condition
d. Oligoclonal bands may be present in CSF
e. Spinal cord involvement may occur

152. Safest transplantation approach in liver disease:
a. Directly transplanting embryonic stem cell in the liver
b. Transplanting donor hepatocytes into liver
c. Transplanting mesenchymal stem cell from adipose tissue to liver
d. Injecting erythropoietin into body

SURGERY

153. True about postoperative ileus:
a. Colon recovers earlier than small intestine
b. Small intestine most commonly affected
c. Adhesion is most common cause
d. Usually resolves within 48–72 hour
e. Radiographs show diffusely dilated bowel with air in the colon and rectum

MCQs

Answer 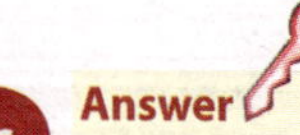

139. b, e. 140. a, b, c. 141. b. 142. a, c, d, e. 143. a, c, d, e. 144. b. 145. d, e,
146. b, c, d. 147. b, d. 148. a, d. 149. c, d, e. 150. b. 151. b, c, d, e. 152. c,
153. d, e.

154. True about secondary bacterial peritonitis:
a. Marked leukocytosis with left shift of the WBCs to band forms
b. Usually caused by polymicrobial infection
c. May be associated with appendicular perforation
d. Associated with cirrhosis of the liver

155. Correct statement about intestinal ischemia:
a. Watershed zones are usually affected
b. Arterial ischemic lesion has better demarcation than ischemia caused by impaired venous drainage
c. Crypts may be hyperproliferative
d. Microscopic examination may show coagulative necrosis of the muscularis propria
e. Surface epithelium is normal

156. True about Colorectal cancer:
a. Right side cancer usually presents with obstructive symptoms
b. May be associated with HNPCC
c. Left-sided cancer presents with alteration in bowel habit
d. Left side colon is more commonly involved

157. True about thyroid cancer:
a. Follicular cancer is more common in radiation exposed patient
b. Hürthle cell carcinoma has better prognosis than follicular cancer
c. Follicular cancer have better prognosis than pupillary cancer
d. Insular variant of papillary carcinoma has better prognosis than papillary cancer
e. Medullary carcinoma is associated with MEN-2b

158. True about Schatzki ring:
a. Contain true esophageal muscle
b. Concentric symmetric narrowing of lower esophagus
c. Consists of esophageal mucosa above and gastric mucosa below
d. Dysphagia is usually to solid foods
e. Association with reflux disease

159. True about intestinal type of gastric cancer:
a. Incidence decreased nowadays
b. Associated with *H. pylori* infection
c. More common in male than female
d. Better prognosis than diffuse
e. More common than diffuse type

160. Correct statement about Intussusception in children is/are all except:
a. Appendix is the most common leading point
b. Ileocolic is the most common site
c. Usually presents with pain without vomiting
d. Can be corrected by air and barium enema
e. Diagnosis is confirmed on abdominal ultrasound

161. Non-absorbable suture(s) is/are:
a. Silk
b. Catgut
c. Polypropylene
d. Polyester
e. Nylon

162. Correct statement(s) about surgical site infection:
a. Can occurs due to environmental flora in OT
b. Superficial infection require re-surgical exploration of wound
c. Does not occur later than 14 days post-operative
d. Shaving is beneficial for prevention
e. Can occur even after 1 yr in case of implant left in situ

163. Regarding pre-operative antibiotic prophylaxis, which of the following statement(s) is/are correct:
a. Should be started 2 days before surgery
b. Should be given half an hour prior to surgery
c. Not needed in clean surgery
d. Should be given more than 1 hour before surgery

164. Grade III (contaminated) wound is/are
a. Appendicular perforation
b. Wound contaminated with gross fecal material spillage
c. Wound in urinary tract without unusual contamination
d. Surgery over a clean site
e. Incision through abscess

165. True about testicular cancer:
a. Seminoma is more common than non-seminoma
b. Cryptorchidism is associated with seminoma
c. Retroperitoneal LN dissection is done for grade II testicular tumour
d. Usually presents as painless testicular lump
e. Seminomas metastasise mainly via haematogenous route

166. True about obstructive jaundice:
a. Cholangiocarcinoma cause intermittent jaundice
b. Courvoisier law related to pancreatic head cancer
c. Cholangitis presents with fever and jaundice
d. Increase in urine urobilinogen
e. Increase in fecal urobilinogen

167. True statement regarding surviving sepsis guideline:
a. Activated protein C is useful
b. qSOFA should be assessed in case of prolong stay of patient in ICU
c. Suggest against the use of IV immunoglobulins in patients with sepsis
d. Recommend the use of erythropoietin for treatment of anemia associated with sepsis
e. Recommend empiric broad-spectrum therapy

Answer 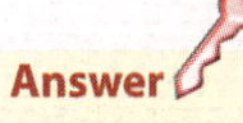

154. a, b, c.	155. a, b, c, d.	156. b, c, d.	157. e.	158. b, c, d, e.	159. a, b, c, d.	160. a, c.
161. a, c, d, e.	162. a, b.	163. b.	164. b.	165. a, b, c, d.	166. b, c.	167. b, c, e.

168. True about management of Peptic ulcer:
a. Vagotomy- decreases acid secretion
b. Early dumping syndrome occurs due to hypoglycaemia
c. Late dumping consists of abdominal and vasomotor symptoms
d. Billroth I gastrectomy has high rate of morbidity and mortality
e. Highly selective vagotomy has low incidence of side effects

169. True about surgical occlusive dressing:
a. Maintain moisture in wound
b. Provides mechanical support
c. Prevents microbial entry
d. Wide Mesh is helpful
e. Used for highly exudative wounds

170. Which of the following nipple discharge is most probably physiological:
a. B/L spontaneous discharge
b. B/L milky discharge with squeezing from multiple ducts
c. U/L bloody discharge
d. U/L bloody discharge with squeezing from a single duct
e. U/L spontaneous serous discharge

171. True about Fat necrosis in women:
a. History of trauma can be elicited in >90% cases
b. More common in lactating women
c. Can be easily differentiated from malignancy on mammography
d. No malignant potential
e. Biopsy is required for diagnosis

172. True about omphalocele:
a. Viscera covered by peritoneum
b. Viscera covered by amniotic membrane
c. Most commonly associated with cardiovascular congenital anomalies
d. Commonly associated with Beckwith-Wiedemann syndrome
e. Viscera is not covered

173. Feature(s) of oesophageal atresia with trachea-oesophageal fistula:
a. Drooling of saliva
b. Associated with oligohydramnios
c. Nasogastric tube cannot passes into stomach
d. May be associated with VACTERL anomalies
e. Abdominal distension

174. Correct statement(s) about hypospadias is/are:
a. Urethral opening on ventral aspect
b. Chordae on dorsal aspect
c. May be associated with penile torsion
d. Proximal varieties are more common
e. Coupons spongiosum is deficient

175. True about Bronchogenic cyst:
a. More common in anterior mediastinum than middle mediastinum
b. May have malignant potential
c. Produce symptoms which are usually compressive in nature
d. Air-fluid may be seen on chest X-ray
e. Mostly asymptomatic

176. A patient has Glasgow coma scale score -$E_1 V_T M_2$. What is not required for his/her management:
a. Head end elevation
b. Total parenteral nutrition
c. Stress ulcer prophylaxis
d. Central line placement
e. DVT prophylaxis

177. True about pyomyositis:
a. *Staphylococcus aureus* is the most common causative organism
b. *Streptococcus pyogens* is the most common causative organism
c. Quadriceps is one of the most commonly affected muscle
d. Treatment involves drainage of abscess without antibiotic coverage
e. Best detected by MRI

178. True about Prostate-Specific Antigen:
a. Serum level >4nmol/ml occur in >90% of those with prostate malignancy
b. Only produces by prostate
c. >10 mg/mL suggestive of prostate cancer
d. Useful in prognosis and follow-up
e. Cannot be used to monitoring for recurrence

179. Feature(s) of Patterson Kelly syndrome:
a. Dysphagia
b. More common in male than female
c. Achlorhydria
d. Treatment consists of dilation of oesophagus by oesophageal bougies

180. All are feature(s) of Beckwidth-Wide man syndrome except:
a. Omphalocele
b. Macrosomia
c. Hyperglycemia
d. Visceromegaly

181. Correct statement about electrocautery:
a. In monopolar mode one electrode used at surgical field and second electrode is attached to patient plate
b. Patient plate should have conductive jelly to ensure proper contact with body
c. Burn may be seen at site of patient plate
d. Cutting has more voltage than coagulation

182. Most common post-operatives complaints of patients is/are:
a. Pain
b. Nausea
c. Vomiting
d. Shivering
e. Sedation

Answer

168. a, d, e. 169. a, b, c. 170. b. 171. d, e. 172. a, b, d. 173. a, c, d, e. 174. a, c,
175. b, c, d, e. 176. None 177. a, c, e. 178. b, c, d. 179. a, c, d. 180. c. 181. All (a, b, c, d)
182. a, b, c.

183. True about abdominal aortic aneurysm:
a. Most common below renal artery
b. May presents as pulsatile abdominal mass
c. Atherosclerosis is most common cause
d. For asymptomatic aneurysms repair is indicated if the diameter is >4 cm.

OBSTETRICS & GYNAECOLOGY

184. During external radiation therapy for cervical cancer which lymph node is/are excluded:
a. External iliac lymph node
b. Common iliac lymph node
c. Internal iliac lymph node
d. Sacral lymph node
e. Obturator lymph node

185. Which of the following is true about vulvodynia:
a. Surgery is usually done for localized vulval lesion
b. Pain without any significant lesion
c. May be associated with irritable bowel syndrome
d. Tricyclic antidepressant is useful
e. Psychological factor is associated

186. Indications for in-vitro fertilization(IVF):
a. Bilateral tube blockage
b. Normal male factor
c. Hostile cervical factor
d. Proximal tubal block
e. Premature ovarian insufficiency

187. Which of the following is/are true about management of pregnancy with NYHA class 3 or 4 heart disease:
a. Delivery should be done in specialised hospitals
b. Often tolerate major surgical procedures poorly
c. Caesarean delivery is limited to obstetrical indications
d. Mortality is 5-20%
e. Epidural is preferred for delivery and labour pain management

188. Which of the following is changes during pregnancy:
a. In last trimester blood volume increase by 50%
b. Cardiac output increase by 20% in last trimester
c. Hemodynamic changes in pregnancy can cause CHF following during labour and following delivery in pre-existing cardiac lesions
d. Hypercoagulability occurs

189. True statement about Breech delivery:
a. Vasa previa is a complication
b. Fetal congenital malformation increases breech risk
c. Increases fetal and maternal morbidity
d. Oligohydramnios increases breech risk
e. Increases risk of hip joint dislocation of baby

190. Complications of shoulder dystocia is/are:
a. Humerus fracture
b. Brachial plexus injury
c. Birth asphyxia
d. Sacroiliac joint dislocation of mother

191. Which of the following is/are true about monozygotic twin formation:
a. If division occurs after embryonic disc formation, it results in conjoint twin
b. If division occur before 72 hrs, it results in formation of diamniotic- dichorionic twins
c. If division occurs b/w 4–8 days, it results in formation of monochorionic monoamniotic twin
d. If division occurs after 8 days—it results in formation of monochorionic monoamniotic twin

192. Which of the following is/are true about combined oral contraceptive pills:
a. Reduces risk of venous thromboembolism
b. Reduces risk of benign breast disease
c. Protects against endometrial cancer
d. ↓ Bone density

193. True about amniocentesis and Chorionic villus sampling:
a. In 1st trimester, amniocentesis is better than Chorionic villus sampling
b. 2nd trimester amniocentesis has less foetal loss than Chorionic villus sampling
c. Amniocentesis may result in oligohydraminos
d. Amniocentesis in 1st trimester has lower risk of foetal loss than 2nd trimester amniocentesis
e. Amniocentesis in 1st trimester has more risk of talipes

194. True about anatomy of vagina:
a. Covered by columnar epithelium
b. Covered by non keratinized stratified squamous epithelium
c. Vaginal secretion is from transudation of vaginal epithelium
d. Supplied by cervicovaginal branch of the uterine artery
e. Anterior wall is longer than posterior wall

195. Which of following is/are not fertility awareness based methods:
a. Withdrawal method
b. Rhythm method
c. Cervical mucus method
d. MTP pill
e. Sympto-thermal method

196. Predisposing factor(s) for obstetrical haemorrhage is/are:
a. Obesity
b. Placental abruption
c. Oligohydramnios
d. Smoking
e. Instrumental delivery

197. All are true about puerperal sepsis except:
a. Temperature >38°C (100.4°F)
b. Caesarean section has no increased risk for sepsis
c. Group A beta-hemolytic streptococcus is one of the common causative organism
d. Instrument delivery increases risk
e. Retained placenta is a cause

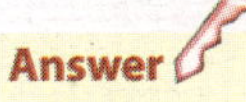

183. a, b, c. 184. c. 185. b, c, d, e. 186. a, d, e. 187. All a b c d e. 188. a, c, d. 189. b, c, d, e.
190. All (a b c d) 191. a, b, d. 192. b, c. 193. b, c, e. 194. b, c, d. 195. a, d. 196. a, b, d, e.
197. b.

198. True statement(s) regarding investigation in endometrial cancer:
a. MRI is superior to CT in detecting myometrial involvement
b. CT is superior to MRI in detecting omental metastasis
c. USG is initial investigation to be performed
d. USG is the best investigation

199. True about Delivery of HIV +ve woman
a. Vaginal delivery has lower risk for transmission of HIV to child than CS
b. Vaginal delivery has higher risk for transmission of HIV to child than CS
c. Instrumentation has no risk of increased infection
d. Vertical transmission is less in cases with preterm birth

PAEDIATRICS

200. True about Constitutional growth delay:
a. Baseline growth hormone decreased
b. IGF-1 levels is low for chronological age
c. Growth delay only occurs after 2–3 years of age
d. Puberty spurt is delayed
e. Final height is within normal limits

201. Feature of pallid breath holding spell in comparison to cyanotic breath holding spell:
a. More common than cyanotic breath holding spell
b. Elicited by painful stimulus
c. Bradycardia is prominent
d. Atropine is given in refractory cases

202. Which of the following finding is normal in infants:
a. Papilledema is rare in raised intracranial pressure
b. Floppy infant
c. Stroking patellar tendon of one side leads to contraction on opposite side
d. Elbow cross midline if passively done by examiner
e. Parachute reflex

203. Which vaccines recommended at 2 year of age according to latest IAP guideline:
a. MMR
b. Pneumococcal conjugate
c. Varicella Rubella
d. Booster of Typhoid Conjugate Vaccine
e. IPV booster

204. A child is presenting features of rickets including rachitic changes on bones and has hypophosphatemia. Which of the following is true:
a. It is commonly caused by X linked recessive disorder
b. Normal zone of provisional calcification adjacent to the metaphysis is present
c. There is defect of mineralization of matrix
d. CRF may be the cause
e. Renal tubule dysfuction leads to hypophosphatemia

205. Which of the following is/are true about atrial septal defect(ASD):
a. Ostium primum is most common type
b. Surgery usually done before 3 year
c. Second heart sound-Wide and fixed
d. Soft delayed diastolic rumble at the lower left sternal border

206. Risk factor for Neural tube defect is/are:
a. Diabetic mother
b. MTHFR mutation
c. Antiepileptic drug intake
d. Methotrexate intake

207. True about breast milk jaundice:
a. Appears after 1 week
b. Typically bilirubin level is around 10–20 mg/dl
c. Phototherapy is useful
d. Managed conservatively
e. Diaper staining is presenting feature

208. High risk infants are:
a. Birth order >3
b. Twinning
c. Birth weight <3 kg
d. Failure to gain weight for 3 consecutive months
e. Artificial feeding

209. True about Cephalohematoma:
a. Maximum at birth then regress
b. Occurs due to forcep injury to periosteum
c. Edematous swelling of soft tissue
d. Localized collection of blood below periosteum
e. May extend across the midline and across suture lines

210. True about newborns:
a. Apgar score provide an immediate estimate of the physical condition of the baby
b. Apgar scoring is done at 1min
c. Apgar scoring at 5 min has no prognostic value
d. Normal respiratory rate is RR is 30-60 breaths/min
e. Normal heart rate >100 beats/min

211. Maximum risk to foetus occur when maternal infection with rubella occurs during which of the following time:
a. 6–12 weeks
b. 12–18 weeks
c. 14–20 weeks
d. 20–24 weeks
e. 32–36 weeks

212. True about paracetamol toxicity in children:
a. Hypernatremia is common side effect of N-acetylcysteine
b. Liver failure may occur after 3-4 days
c. N-acetylcysteine is very less effective if given after 24 hours of paracetamol ingestion
d. N-acetylcysteine can be given orally or IV
e. Renal damage also may occur

MCQs

Answer

198. a, b, c. 199. b. 200. b, d, e. 201. b, c, d. 202. a, c, e. 203. d. 204. c, e.
205. b, c, d. 206. All (a, b, c, d) 207. a, b, c, d. 208. b, d, e. 209. b, d. 210. a, b, d, e. 211. a.
212. b, c, d, e.

ORTHOPAEDICS

213. All are true about Anterior Cruciate ligament except:
- a. Commonly occurs as a result of twisting force
- b. May be associated with Segond fracture
- c. Rarely associated with meniscal injury
- d. Lachman test is highly sensitive test for tear

214. Pirani scoring for CTEV includes all except:
- a. Curvature of the medial border of the foot
- b. Severity of the medial crease
- c. Position of the lateral part of the head of the talus
- d. Emptiness of the heel
- e. Severity of the posterior crease

215. True about tuberculosis of Spine:
- a. Middle path regimen is used in management
- b. Posterior elements of the spine is most commonly affected
- c. Commonly spread by hematogenous route from lung
- d. Acute onset paraplegia has worse prognosis
- e. Lower thoracic and upper lumbar is most common site

216. Which of the following is/are indication of surgical management of fracture shaft humerus:
- a. Fracture in elderly
- b. Radial nerve involvement after manipulation
- c. Pathological fractures
- d. Vascular injury
- e. Multiple fractures

217. Which of the following is/are true about Ewing sarcoma:
- a. Vascular origin
- b. Ewing's sarcoma is second most common primary malignant bone tumour in children and adolescent after Osteosarcoma
- c. Metaphysis of long bone is most common site
- d. Fever and weight loss may be present
- e. Surgery is very useful in management

218. True about giant cell tumour:
- a. Most common age group affected is 20–40 year
- b. Proximal femur is most common site affected
- c. Pulmonary metastasis occur in <3% of cases
- d. A locally aggressive tumour
- e. May involve sacrum

219. Spur sign is/are seen in:
- a. Supracondylar fracture of humerus
- b. Radial head fracture
- c. Acetabulum fracture of pelvis
- d. Talus fracture

220. Cause(s) of avascular necrosis of femoral Head:
- a. Fracture of femoral neck b. Steroid use
- c. Alcohol use d. Sickle cell disease
- e. Caisson disease

221. Which of the followings are not included in Gurd's criteria for fat embolism:
- a. Central nervous system depression disproportionate to hypoxaemia
- b. Tachycardia <110 bpm
- c. Deep vein thrombosis
- d. Axillary or subconjunctival petechiae
- e. Hypoxaemia Pa_{O2} <60 mm Hg, $Fi_{O2} = 0.4$

222. Correct statement about hand infection:
- a. Opening of Felon by fish month incision is preferred incision technique
- b. Felon is middle volar pulp infection
- c. Apical subungual infection- V-shaped piece is removed from the center of the free edge of the nail along with a little wedge of the full thickness of the skin overlying the abscess
- d. When the pus extends beneath the nail, it is necessary to remove the some part of nail for adequate drainage of pus

ANAESTHESIA

223. Component of Advanced cardiovascular life support (ACLS) in accordance to AHA 2015 guideline:
- a. Chest compression 100–150 per minute
- b. Chest compression at least 5 cm/2 inch
- c. Vasopressors is used to maintain MAP > 70 mmHg in non-responsive to fluids
- d. 1 Breath every 8 seconds
- e. Vasopressin is used as vasopressor

224. Anaesthetic agents(s) having epileptogenic potential:
- a. Atracurium b. Etomidate
- c. Enflurane d. Pethidine
- e. Propofol

225. True about xenon is are:
- a. Environment friendly b. Cheap
- c. Low blood solubility d. Inert
- e. Stable

226. In gas tubing, flow rate of turbulent flow depends upon:
- a. Viscosity of gas
- b. Pressure gradient
- c. Length of tube
- d. Radius of tube
- e. Density of gas

227. Gas stored in liquid state in cylinders:
- a. Nitrogen
- b. Helium
- c. CO_2
- d. Cyclopropane
- e. Nitrous oxide

Answer

213. c. 214. a. 215. a, c, e. 216. b, c, d, e. 217. b, d. 218. a, c, d, e. 219. c.
220. All (a, b, c, d, e) 221. c. 222. c, d. 223. b. 224. a, c, d. 225. a, c, d, e. 226. b, e.
227. c, d, e.

228. True about caudal anesthesia in children:
a. Average distance from the skin to the anterior wall of the sacral canal is 21 mm
b. 0.5 mL/kg dose of bupivacaine is sufficient for lumber and sacral dermatomes block
c. Beyond 6–7 years of age, it is difficult to give and is less successful in comparison to younger children
d. 2–3 cm of epidural catheter is advances through epidural space in continuos infusion
e. Distance from the upper border of the sacral hiatus to the dural sac is 30±10.4mm

SKIN

229. Acantholysis is/are not seen in :
a. Lichen planus
b. Bullous pemphigoid
c. Dermatitis herpetiformis
d. Hailey-Hailey disease
e. Pemphigus vulgaris

230. Cutaneous marker(s) of internal malignancy is/are all except:
a. Tripe palms
b. Sign of Leser-Trelat
c. Dermatomyositis
d. Migratory thrombophlebitis
e. Seborrheic patch at back

231. Nikolsky's sign is/are seen in all except:
a. Pemphigus
b. Hailey-Hailey disease
c. Staphylococcal scalded skin syndrome
d. Toxic epidermal necrolysis
e. Grover disease

232. True about acute paronychia:
a. Pus under nail bed
b. Pus may extend to base of nail
c. Swelling of nail fold
d. Candida is most common causative organism

PSYCHIATRY

233. Defence mechanism in obsessive-compulsive disorder (OCD) is/are:
a. Undoing
b. Reaction formation
c. Suppression
d. Isolation of affect
e. Projection

234. Beck's cognitive triad of depression includes:
a. Self
b. Future
c. Past experience
d. World and environment
e. Others

235. Which is not a brain stimulation technique:
a. Electroconvulsive therapy
b. Magnetic seizure therapy
c. Deep brain stimulation
d. Rapid transcranial magnetic stimulation
e. Cognitive therapy

236. Feature(s) of delirium tremens is/are:
a. Most common complication in alcohol withdrawal
b. Auditory hallucination may occur
c. Visual hallucination may be present
d. Predominantly low-voltage fast activity on EEG
e. Most severe alcohol withdrawal syndrome

237. Personality type associated with coronary artery disease:
a. A
b. B
c. C
d. D
e. E

RADIOLOGY

238. Chest roentgenogram feature(s) of stage-2 Sarcoidosis in Scadding scoring system:
a. Bilateral hilar lymphadenopathy
b. Mediastinal lymphadenopathy
c. Upper lobe parenchymal infiltrates
d. Enlarged paratracheal nodes
e. Pulmonary fibrosis

239. Standard treatment of whole-brain radiotherapy (WBRT) for brain Metastasis:
a. 20 grays (Gy) in 10 fractions
b. 30 grays (Gy) in 10 fractions
c. 30 grays (Gy) in 5 fractions
d. 15 grays (Gy) in 10 fractions

Answer

228. a, c, d, e. 229. a, b, c. 230. e. 231. b, e. 232. a, b, c. 233. a, b, d. 234. a, b, d.
235. e. 236. b, c, d, e. 237. a. 238. a, c. 239. b.

NOVEMBER 2016 ANSWERS & EXPLANATIONS

ANATOMY

1. Ans. (a) Extensor carpi radialis longus, (e) Flexor carpi ulnaris

[Ref: BDC 7th/ Vol. I 140; Moore 2nd/458-59 and Gray's 40th/784]

Extensor carpi radialis longus is supplied by radial nerve and Flexor carpi ulnaris is supplied by ulnar nerve. All other 3 muscles given in question are supplied by Posterior interosseous nerve

Posterior interosseous nerve: *Branches* *BDC 7th/ Vol. I 140 and Moore* 2nd*/458-59*

Branch	Supply
Muscular	• Extensor carpi radialis brevis • Supinator • Extensor digitorum • Extensor digiti minimi • Extensor carpi ulnaris • Abductor pollicis longus • Extensor pollicis brevis • Extensor pollicis longus • Extensor indicis
Articular	Wrist, distal radioulnar joint, Intercarpal and intermetacarpal joint
Sensory	Interossous membrane, radius and ulna

Table *(Gray's 40th/784):* **Movements, muscles and segmental innervation in the upper limb**

Joint	Movement	Muscle	Innervation
Elbow	Flexion	Biceps brachii	Musculocutaneous n.
		Brachialis	Musculocutaneous and radial n.
		Brachioradialis	Radial n.
	Extension	Triceps	Radial n.
	Supination	Biceps brachii	Musculocutaneous n.
		Supinator	Posterior interosseous n.
	Pronation	Pronator quadratus	Anterior interosseous n.
		Pronator teres	Median n.
Wrist	Flexion	Flexor carpi radialis	Median n.
		Palmaris longus	Median n.
		Flexor carpi ulnaris	Ulnar n.
	Extension	Extensor carpi radialis longus	Radial n.
		Extensor carpi radialis brevis	Posterior interosseous n.
		Extension carpi ulnaris	Posterior interosseous n.
	Abduction	Extensor carpi radials longus	Radial n.
		Extensor carpi radials brevis	Posterior interosseous n.
		Flexor carpi radialis	Median n.
	Adduction	Extensor carpi ulnaris	Posterior interosseous n.
		Flexor carpi ulnaris	Ulnar n.
Fingers	Flexion (Mp/pp joints)	Flexor digitorum superficialis	Median n.
		Dorsal interossei	Unlar n.
		Palmar interossei	Ulnar n.
	Flexion (DIP Joints)	Flexor digitorum profundus (lateral)	Anterior interosseous n.
		Flexor digitorum profundus (medial)	Ulnar n.
	Flexion (MP joint)	Flexor digiti minimi brevis	Ulnar n.
	Extension (MP/PIP/DIP joints)	Extensor digitorum	Posterior interosseous n.
		Extensor indicis	Posterior interosseous n.

Contd...

Joint	Movement	Muscle	Innervation
	Extension (MP/PIP/DIP	Flexor digiti minimi	Posterior interosseous n.
	Extension (PIP/DIP Joints)	Lumbricals I and II	Usually Median n.
		Lumbricals II and IV	Usually Ulnar n.
	Abduction	Dorsal interossei	Ulnar n.
	Abduction (thumb fixed)	Abductor pollicis brevis	Median n.
	Abduction	Abductor digiti minimi	Ulnar n.
	Adduction	Palmar interossei	Ulnar n.
	Opposition	Opponens digiti minimi	Ulnar n.
Thumb	Flexion (IP Joint)	Flexor pollicis longus	Anterior interosseous n.
	Flexion/Rotation (MP joint)	Flexor pollicls brevis	Median n. and/or ulnar n.
	Extension (MP joint)	Extensor pollicls brevis	Posterior interosseous n.
	Extension (IP Joint)	Extensor pollicis longus	Posterior internosseous n.
	Abduction	Abductor pollicis longus	Posterior interosseous n.
	Abduction/Rotation	Abductor pollicis brevis	Median n.
	Adduction/Rotation	Adductor pollicis	Ulnar n.
	Adduction/Flexion (MP Joint)	Palmar interosseous I	Ulnar n.
	Apposition	Opponens pollicis	Medlan n. and ulnar n.

2. Ans. (a) Peroneus tertius

[Ref: BDC 7th/ Vol. II 101-02; Essential Anatomy by Moore 2nd/360-63]

"The four muscles in the anterior compartment of the leg are—the ***tibialis anterior, extensor digitorum longus, extensor hallucis longus, and fibularis (Peroneus) tertius***"- *Moore 2nd/360*

Table *(Essential Anatomy by Moore 2nd/360-63)*: **Muscles of anterior and lateral compartment of leg**

Muscle	Proximal Attachment	Distal Attachment	Innervation	Main Action(s)
Anterior compartment				
Tibialis anterior	Lateral condyle and superior half of lateral surface of tibia and interosseous membrane	Medial and inferior surfaces of medial cuneiform and base of 1st metatarsal	Deep fibular (peroneal) nerve (L4 and L5)	Dorsiflexes ankle and inverts foot
Extensor hallucis longus	Middle part of anterior surface of fibula and interosseous membrane	Dorsal aspect of base of distal phalanx of great toe (hallux)	Deep fibular (peroneal) nerve (L5 and S1)	Extends great toe and dorsiflexes ankle
Extensor digitorum longus	Lateral condyle of tibia and superior three fourths of anterior surface of interosseous membrane	Middle and distal phalanges of lateral four digits	Deep fibular (peroneal) nerve (L5 and S1)	Extends lateral four digits and dorsiflexes ankle
Fibularis(Peroneus) Tertius	Inferior third of anterior surface of fibula and interosseous membrane	Dorsum of base of 5th metatarsal	Deep fibular (peroneal) nerve (L5 and S1)	Dorsiflexes ankle and aids in eversion of foot
Lateral compartment				
Fibularis (peroneus) longus	Head and superior two thirds of lateral surface of fibula	Base of 1st metatarsal and medial cuneiform	Superficial fibular (peroneal) nerve (L5, S1, and S2)	Evert foot and weakly plantarflex ankle
Fibularis (peroneus) brevis	Inferior two thirds of lateral surface of fibula	Dorsal surface of tuberosity on lateral side of base of 5th metatarsal	Superficial fibular (peroneal) nerve (L5, S1, and S2)	Evert foot and weakly plantarflex ankle

3. Ans. (a) Posterior communicating artery, (b), Superior hypophyseal artery, (c) Inferior hypophyseal artery

[Ref: BDC 7th/ Vol. IV 170-71; Snell 9th/598-99; Gray's 40th/323,248; Essential Anatomy by Moore 2nd/528]

Posterior cerebral artery *is branch of* ***basilar artery and*** Recurrent artery of Heubner is branch from the anterior cerebral artery (ACA)

"**Posterior cerebral artery** *is branch of* **basilar artery**"*- Snell 9th/699*

"**Recurrent artery of Heubner,** also known as the **medial striate artery** or **long central artery**, is the largest perforating branch from the proximal **anterior cerebral artery** (ACA)" *- radiopaedia.org*

Blood supply of pituitary gland: Arteries are derived from the ***superior and inferior hypophyseal arteries, branches of the internal carotid artery***"*- Snell 9th/654*

"The arteries of the ***pituitary arise from the internal carotid arteries*** via a single ***inferior and several superior hypophysial arteries*** on each side. The former come from the cavernous part of the internal carotid artery, the latter from its supraclinoid part and from the anterior and posterior cerebral arteries"*-Gray's 40th/323*

"The **inferior hypophyseal artery** is an artery supplying the neurohypophysis of the pituitary gland. It is a branch of the cavernous carotid artery (***internal carotid artery***). The **superior hypophyseal artery** is a branch of the cerebral part of the **internal carotid artery**"*-Wikipedia*

Internal Carotid Artery

Branches BDC 7th/ Vol. IV 170-71; Moore 2nd/528

- Ophthalmic artery
- ***Posterior communication artery***
- *Anterior choroidal artery*
- ***Anterior cerebral artery:*** *Orbital; Frontal and Parietal branches*
- **Middle cerebral artery:** Deep or perforating branch; temporal branch; Frontal branch and Parietal branches

Branches of the External Carotid Artery

◈ *Snell 9th/598*

- *Superior thyroid artery*
- *Ascending pharyngeal artery*
- *Lingual artery*
- *Facial artery*
- *Occipital artery*
- *Posterior auricular artery*
- *Superficial temporal artery*
- *Maxillary artery*

4. Ans. (d) Nucleus lies in midbrain near aqueduct

[Ref: BDC 7th/ Vol. IV 74-75; Snell 9th/569; Gray's 40th/642-43; P.L.Dhingra 6th/16-17;Essential Anatomy by Moore 2nd/661]

"Axons of the vestibular nerve synapse in the vestibular nucleus that are found on the ***lateral floor and wall of the fourth ventricle in the pons and medulla.*** It arises from ***bipolar cells in the vestibular ganglion (ganglion of Scarpa)***, which is situated in the upper part of the outer end of the internal auditory meatus"*-en.wikipedia.org*

Vestibulocochlear Nerve

◈ *radiopaedia.org*

- It ***emerges between the pons and the medulla***, lateral to the facial nerve and nervus intermedius, passing laterally through the cerebellopontine angle to the internal acoustic meatus (IAM) with two other nerves.
- In the IAM the nerve splits into 4 bundles: *cochlear nerve, superior and inferior division of the vestibular nerve and nerve from the posterior semicircular canal*
- The ***vestibular nerve relays in the vestibular ganglion*** (also k/a **ganglion of Scarpa**), from there three bundles emerge:
    - The superior division of the vestibular nerve carries sensory fibres from the hair cells of the anterior and lateral semicircular canals and utricle.
    - The **inferior division** carries sensory fibres from the saccule.

Vestibulocochlear Nerve

◈ *teachmeanatomy.info*

The vestibular and cochlear portions of the vestibulocochlear nerve are functionally discrete, and so originate from different nuclei in the brain:

- **Vestibular component:** Arises from the vestibular nuclei complex in the ***pons and medulla.***
- **Cochlear component:** Arises from the ventral and dorsal cochlear nuclei, situated in the inferior cerebellar peduncle.

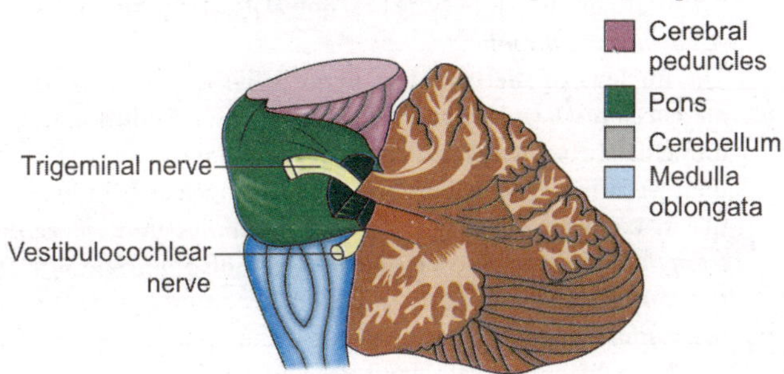

Fig: *(Teachmeanatomy.info):* The origin of the vestibulocochlear nerve from the cerebellopontine angle

Vestibular Nerve

◈ *Gray's 40th/642-43*

- The main nerve **divides at and within the vestibular (Scarpa's) ganglion** into ***superior and inferior divisions***, which are connected by an isthmus
- The **superior division**, the larger of the two, passes through the small holes in the superior vestibular area at the fundus of the internal acoustic meatus and supplies the lateral and anterior ampullary nerves, respectively.
- The **inferior division of the vestibular nerve** passes through small holes in the inferior vestibular area to supply the remainder of the saccule and the posterior ampullary crest via saccular and singular branches, respectively
- *Occasionally, a very small supplementary or accessory branch innervates the posterior crest*; it is probably a vestigial remnant of the crista neglecta, an additional area of sensory epithelium found in some other mammals but seldom in man.

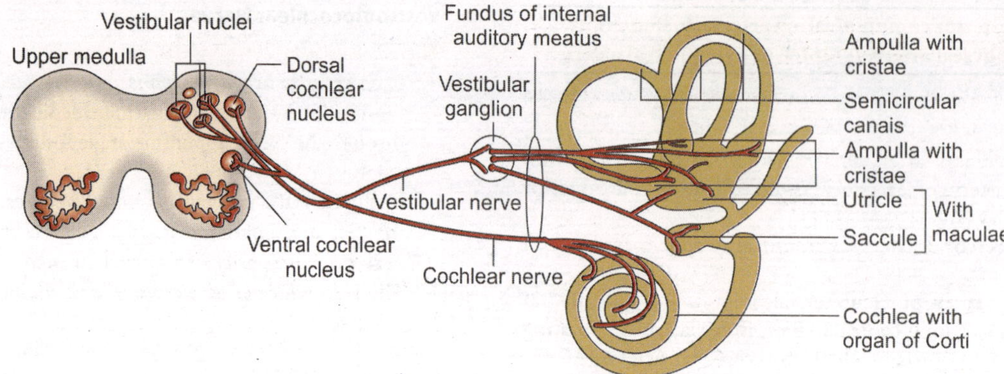

Fig: *(BDC 7th/ Vol. IV 75):* Course of cochlear and vestibular nerves

5. Ans. (c) Lesion causes diplopia, (d) Nucleus of the trochlear nerve is located in the caudal mesencephalon ....

[Ref: BDC 7th/ Vol. II 101-02; Essential Anatomy by Moore 2nd/360-63]

"The trochlear nerve arises from the trochlear nucleus of the brain, emerging from the posterior aspect of the midbrain (it is the ***only cranial nerve to exit from the posterior midbrain***). The trochlear nerve innervates a single muscle – the superior oblique, which is a muscle of oculomotion. As the fibres from the trochlear nucleus cross in the midbrain before they exit, the trochlear neurones innervate the contralateral superior oblique" *-teachmeanatomy.info*

The **nucleus of the trochlear nerve** is located in the ***caudal mesencephalon (midbrain) beneath the cerebral aqueduct***. It is immediately below the nucleus of the oculomotor nerve (III) in the rostral mesencephalon. The trochlear nucleus is unique in that its axons run ***dorsally and cross the midline before emerging from the brainstem***—so a ***lesion of the trochlear nucleus affects the contralateral eye. Lesions of all other cranial nuclei affect the ipsilateral side*** (except of course the optic nerve, cranial nerve II, which innervates both eyes)"- *www.boundless.com*

Trochlear Nerve

◈ *BDC 7th/ Vol. IV 63-65*

- *It supply only the superior oblique muscle of the eyeball*
- *It is the **only cranial nerve which emerges on the dorsal aspect of the brain stem***
- *Paralysis of trochlear nerve results in: defective depression of the adducted eye and diplopia*

Trochlear Nerve

◈ *Gray's 40th/666*

- The trochlear nerve is the fourth cranial nerve and ***innervates superior oblique exclusively***.
- It is the ***only cranial nerve to emerge from the dorsal surface of the brain stem***, passing from ***the midbrain onto the lateral surface of the crus of the cerebral peduncle.***
- It runs through the lateral dural wall of the cavernous sinus and then crosses the oculomotor nerve to enter the orbit through the superior orbital fissure, ***above the common tendinous ring*** and levator palpebrae superioris, and medial to the frontal and lacrimal nerves.
- The trochlear nerve travels but a short distance to ***enter the superior (orbital) surface of superior oblique.***

The **tendinous ring**, also known as the **annulus of Zinn (also k/a annular tendon** or **common tendinous ring)**, situated at its entrance at the apex of the orbit, is the common origin of the four rectus muscles (extraocular muscles). It can be used to divide the regions of the superior orbital fissure -radiopaedia.org

The tendinous ring straddles the superior orbital fissure and through it (from superior to inferior) pass:

- *Superior division of the oculomotor nerve (CN III)*
- *Nasociliary nerve (a branch of the ophthalmic nerve)*
- *Inferior division of the oculomotor nerve (CN III)*
- *Abducens nerve (CN VI)*

6. Ans. (a) Thoracic duct, (b) Aorta, (e) Azygos vein

[Ref: BDC 7th/ Vol.I 201-02; Snell 9th/46; Gray's 40th/1007-08]

Table *(BDC 7th/ Vol.I 202):* **Large openings in thoraco-abdominal diaphragm**

Opening	Situation	Shape	Structures passing	Effect on contraction
Vena cava	T8, junction of right and median leaflet of central tendon	Quadrilateral	IVC Right phrenic nerve Lymphatic of liver	Dilation
Oesophageal	T10, splitting of right crus	Elliptical	Oesophagus, Both vagal trunks, Left gastric vessel	Constriction
Aortic	T12, behind median arcuate ligament	Rounded	Aorta , Thoracic duct, Azygos vein	No change

7. Ans. (b) Zone II

[Ref: medical-dictionary.thefreedictionary; boneandspine.com/flexor-tendon-zones-of-hand]

Zone II *boneandspine.com/flexor-tendon-zones-of-hand*

- Zone II extends from the middle of the middle phalanx to distal palmar crease. It contains both flexor tendon superficialis and flexor tendon profundus.
- ***It has been called "No Man's Land" or "No Man's Zone" because repair in this zone is very difficult.***
- Both the tendons are interwoven and surrounded by a number of pulleys in this zone

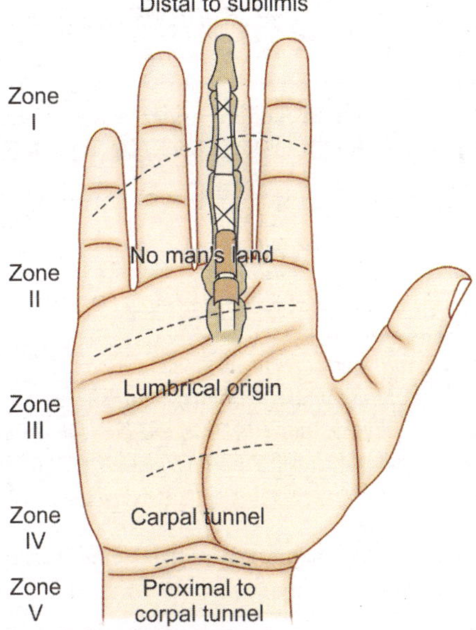

Fig: *(boneandspine.com):* Flexor tendon zones

No Man's Land

◈ *medical-dictionary.thefreedictionary*

- A fanciful term for the fibrous sheath of the flexor tendons of the hand, specifically in the zone from the distal palmar creaseto the proximal interphalangeal joint.
- Any tendon injury to the distal forearm, wrist or hand could be a 'No Man's land' if
  - The facilities and/or equipment are inadequate
  - The operator is inexperienced or exhausted or
  - The tendon is potentially damaged beyond salvage

8. Ans. (a) Somatic cells not divide..., (b) Occur in germ cell which result, (e) Body needs meiosis to produce

[Ref: Embryology by I.B.Singh 10th/ 11,13-15; Gray's 40th/20-23]

Meiosis

◈ *www.nature.com*

- Meiosis is a type of cell division that ***reduces the number of chromosomes in the parent cell by half and produces four gamete cells.***
- This process is required to produce ***egg and sperm cells for sexual reproduction.*** During reproduction, when the sperm and egg unite to form a single cell, the number of chromosomes is restored in the offspring.
- Meiosis begins with a **parent cell that is diploid**, meaning it has two copies of each chromosome. The parent cell undergoes one round of DNA replication followed by two separate cycles of nuclear division. The process results in ***four daughter cells that are haploid,*** which means they ***contain half the number of chromosomes of the diploid parent cell.***
- Meiosis has both similarities to and differences from **mitosis,** which is a cell division process in which a ***parent cell produces two identical daughter cells.***
- Meiosis begins following one round of DNA replication in cells in the ***male or female sex organs.*** The process is split into meiosis I and meiosis II, and both meiotic divisions have multiple phases. ***Meiosis I is a type of cell division unique to germ cells, while meiosis II is similar to mitosis.***

Cell Division

◈ *I.B.Singh 10th/ 11*

- When a cell divides, it is essential that the entire genetic information within it be passed on to both the daughter cells resulting from the division. In other words, the daughter cells must have chromosomes identical in number (and in genetic content) to those in the mother cell. This type of cell division is called ***mitosis.***
- A different kind of cell division called ***meiosis*** occurs ***during the formation of the gametes.*** This consists of two successive divisions called the ***first and second meiotic divisions.*** The cells resulting from these division (i.e., gametes) differ from other cells of the body in that–The ***number of chromosomes is reduced to half the normal number*** and the *genetic information in the various gametes produced is not identical*

Significance of Meiosis

◈ *I.B.Singh 10th/15*

- In this kind of cell division, there is reduction of the number of chromosomes from ***diploid to haploid.*** At the time of fertilization, the diploid number (46) is restored. This provides consistency of chromosome number from generation to generation.
- The forty-six chromosomes of a cell consist of twenty-three pairs, one chromosome of each pair being derived from the mother and one from the father. During the first meiotic division, the chromosomes derived from the father and those derived from the mother are distributed between the daughter cells entirely at random.
- This, along with the phenomenon of crossing over, results in thorough shuffling of the genetic material so that the cells produced as a result of various meiotic divisions (i.e., ***ova or spermatozoa***) all have a distinctive genetic content.
- A third step in this process of genetic shuffling takes place at fertilization when there is a combination of randomly selected spermatozoa and ova. It is, therefore, not surprising that no two persons (except identical twins) are alike.

Mitosis and Meiosis

◈ *Gray's 40th/21*

- **Mitosis** is the process that results in the distribution of ***identical copies of the parent cell genome to the two daughter somatic cells.***
- In **meiosis**, the divisions immediately before the final production of gametes ***halve the number of chromosomes to the haploid number,*** so that at fertilization the diploid number is restored. Moreover, meiosis includes a phase

in which exchange of genetic material occurs between homologous chromosomes. This allows a reassortment of genes to take place, which means that the *daughter cells differ from the parental cell in both their precise genetic sequence and their haploid state.*

MEIOSIS

MEIOSIS I

DNA Replication and recombination

Separation of homologous chromosomes

MEIOSIS II

Separation of sister chromatids

Gamete (1n chromosome - haploid state)

Fig: *(www.google.co.in/search):* Meiosis

- Mitosis and meiosis are alike in many respects, and ***differ principally in chromosomal behaviour*** during the early stages of cell division. In **meiosis,** two divisions occur in succession, without an intervening S phase. *Meiosis I is distinct from mitosis, whereas meiosis II is more like mitosis.*

9. Ans. (b) Dorsal nucleus of vagus, (c) Nucleus of tractus solitarius, (d) Nucleus ambiguous

[Ref: BDC 7th/ Vol. IV 95-96; Snell 9th/547; Gray's 40th/278-79]

Trapezoid body is present in white matter of lower part pons *when cut at level of tegmentus- BDC 7th/ Vol. IV 98*

Superior Vestibular nucleus is located in pons*-en.wikipedia; BDC 7th/ Vol. IV 97-98*

Transverse section through the upper part of medulla passing through the floor of fourth ventricle/Open part: Grey Matter *BDC 7th/ Vol. IV 95-96*

- *Hypoglossal nuclei*
- ***Dorsal nucleus of vagus***
- ***Nucleus of tractus solitaries***
- ***Inferior and medial vestibular nuclei***
- ***Nucleus ambigus***
- *Dorsal and ventral cochlear nucleus*
- *Nucleus of the spinal tract of trigeminal nerve*
- *Inferior olivary nucleus (responsible for producing the elevation of olive). Close to inferior olivary nucleus there are medial and dorsal accessory olivary nucleus*
- *Arcuate nucleus*
- *Visceral centers: respiratory center, cardiac center and vaso-motor center*

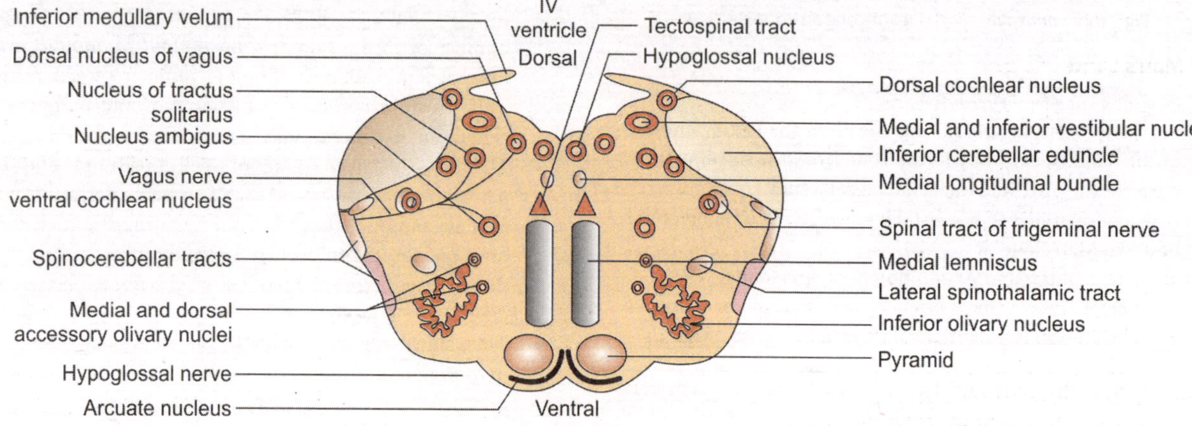

Fig: *(BDC 7th/ Vol. IV 95): T.S of medulla oblongata at the level of olivary nucleus passing through floor of fourth ventricle*

Transverse section of the medulla at the caudal end of the fourth ventricle *Gray's 40th/278-79*

- The total area of grey matter is increased by the presence of the ***large olivary nuclear complex and nuclei of the vestibulocochlear, glossopharyngeal, vagus and accessory nerves.***
- A smooth, oval elevation, **the olive,** lies between the ventrolateral and dorsolateral sulci of the medulla. It is formed by the underlying inferior olivary complex of nuclei, and lies lateral to the pyramid, separated from it by the ventrolateral sulcus and emerging hypoglossal nerve fibres.
- The **central grey matter** at this level constitutes the ventricular floor. It contains (sequentially from medial to lateral): ***the hypoglossal nucleus, dorsal motor nucleus of the vagus, nucleus solitarius, and the caudal ends of the inferior and medial vestibular nuclei.***
- The ***tractus solitarius and the associated nucleus solitarius*** extend throughout the length of the medulla.
- The spinocerebellar, spinotectal, vestibulospinal, rubrospinal and lateral spinothalamic (spinal lemniscal) tracts all lie in the ventrolateral area of the medulla at this level.

PHYSIOLOGY

10. Ans. (a) Olfactory mucosa cover ..., (b) Olfactory pathway passes..., (d) Olfactory receptors... (e) Rate of olfactory nerve ...

[Ref: BDC 7th/Vol. IV 248;A.K.Jain 6th/1055-59;Guyton 12th/716-20;Ganong 25th/217-21;Dhingra 6th/142; L and T 10 th/10-11]

"Over a wide range, the ***rate of olfactory nerve impulses change approximately in proportion to the logarithm of stimulus strength***, which states that the olfactory receptors obey principles of transduction similar to those of other sensory receptors"- *Guyton 12th/718*

"The olfactory receptors ***adapt about 50% in the first second or so after stimulation****. Thereafter, they adapt very little and very slowly"- Guyton 12th/718*

"**Adaptation**: *It develops within* ***seconds or minutes****, depending on the nature of the substance"- A.K.Jain 6th/1058*

"**Webner-Fechner Law** states that the subjective sensation (of odor, sound or light intensity) is ***proportional to the logarithm of the stimulus intensity***"- books.google.co.in/books

"There are **3 olfactory pathway**: the Very Old, the Less Old, and the Newer Olfactory Pathways into the Central Nervous System. The *very old* olfactory system subserves the basic olfactory reflexes, a *less old* system provides automatic but partially learned control of food intake and aversion to toxic and unhealthy foods, and a *newer* system is comparable to most of the other cortical sensory systems and is used for conscious perception and analysis of olfaction. The ***newer olfactory pathway passes through the thalamus***, passing to the ***dorsomedial thalamic nucleus*** and then to the lateroposterior quadrant of the orbitofrontale cortex. Based on studies in monkeys, this newer system probably helps in the conscious analysis of odor"- *Guyton 12th/718*

"The receptor for smell are placed in ***upper one-third of the nasal cavity*** *including the roof formed by cribriform plate and the medial and lateral walls up to the level of the superior concha. This part is lined by olfactory mucosa. The rest of the nasal cavity is lined by respiratory mucosa"- BDC 7th/Vol. IV 248*

"The ***receptor in the olfactory mucous membrane are coupled to G-proteins****. Some act via adenyl cyclase and cAMP and others act via phospholipase C. All of them are cation channels causing Na+ and Ca2+ influx"-A.K.Jain 6th/1058*

"Adaptation: The first step may be mediated by a calcium-binding protein (calcium/calmodulin) that binds to the receptor channel protein to lower its affinity for cyclic nucleotides. The next step is called **short-term adaptation, *which occurs in response to cAMP*** and implicates a feedback pathway involving calcium/calmodulin-dependent protein kinase II acting on adenylyl cyclase. The next step is called **long-term adaptation,** which includes activation of ***guanylyl cyclase and cGMP production***. A Na^+/Ca^{2+} exchanger to restore ion balance also contributes to long-term adaptation"- *Ganong 25th/221*

Olfactory region: *Upper 1/3 of lateral wall* *(upto superior concha), corresponding part of the nasal septum and the roof of nasal cavity from the olfactory region. Here, mucous membrane is paler in color"-Dhingra 6th/138*

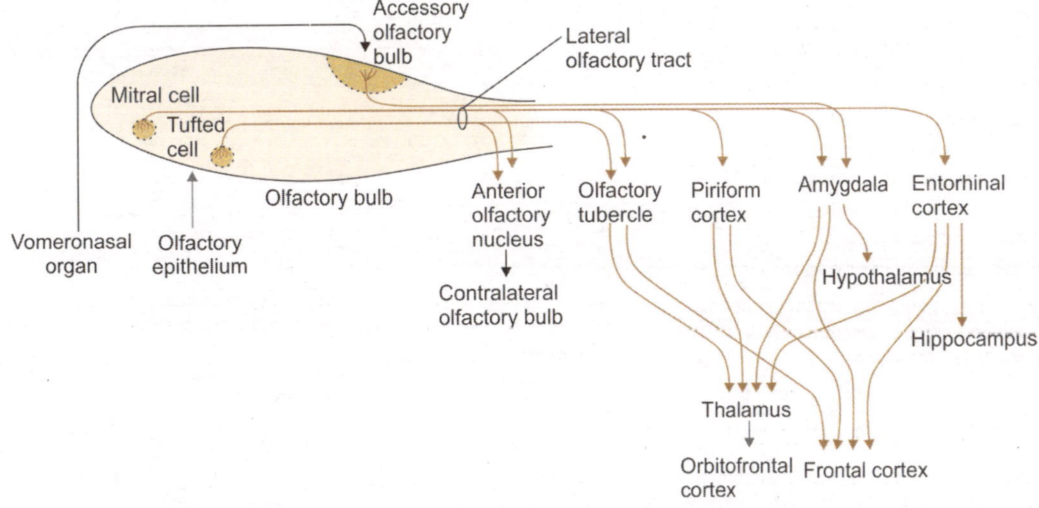

Fig: *(Ganong 25th/219):* Diagram of the olfactory pathway

11. Ans. (a) Surfactant prevent collapse of..., (c) Surfactant decrease chance..., (e) With surfactant, large alveoli tend to...

[Ref: Ganong 25th/630-32; Guyton 12th (SAE)/320-21; https://www.google.co.in]

Regional Variation of Compliance and Effect of Gravity

- *Guyton 12th(SAE)/320*
- ***Upper region alveoli have larger volumes*** as compared to those in the basal and more dependent regions. The alveoli in the ***upper regions are already filled with air and are less***

compliant compared to those in the dependent regions, which are more compliant and are able to increase their volume with each breath.

Alveolar Surface Tension

- *Ganong 25th/630-32*
- The ***low surface tension when the alveoli are small*** is due to the presence in the fluid lining the alveoli of **surfactant,** a lipid surface-tension-lowering agent. ***If the surface tension is not kept low when the alveoli become smaller during expiration, they collapse in accordance with the law of Laplace.***
- Surfactant deficiency is an important cause of **infant respiratory distress syndrome** (IRDS, also known as **hyaline membrane disease**), the serious pulmonary disease that develops in infants born before their surfactant system is functional.
- ***Surface tension in the lungs of these infants is high, and the alveoli are collapsed in many areas*** **(atelectasis).**
- "Surfactant is a *surface active agent in water,* which means that it greatly reduces the surface tension of water. It is secreted by special surfactant-secreting epithelial cells called *type II alveolar epithelial cells,* which constitute about 10 percent of the surface area of the alveoli"- *Guyton 12th(SAE)/320-21*

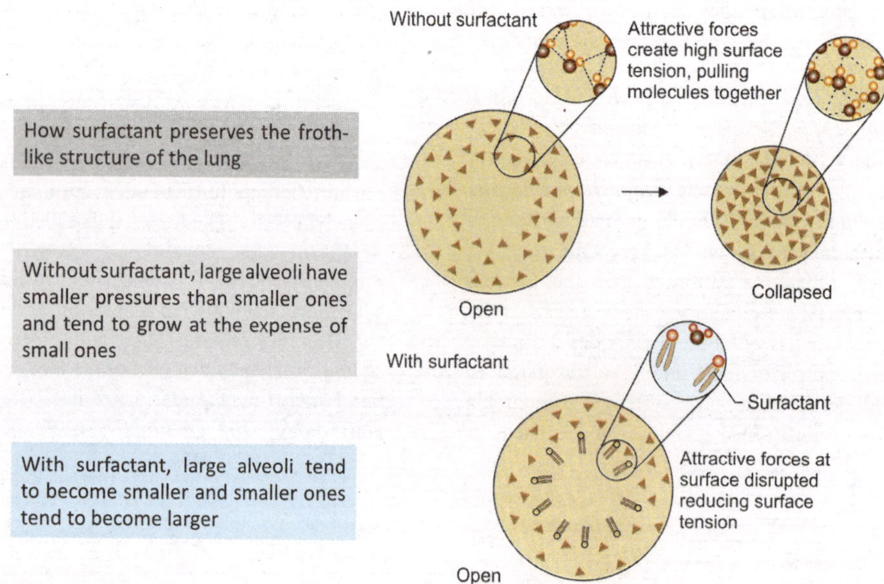

Roles of Surfactant

- Reduces "stiffness" of the lungs
- Protects patency of small airways
- Prevents total collapse of the alveoli (i.e. stabilises alveoli)
- Reduces work of breathing
- Prevents small alveoli emptying into larger ones

    - According to the law of Laplace: the smaller alveoli (with smaller radius - r) have a higher tendency to collapse
    - Pulmonary surfactant is a complex mixture of lipids and proteins secreted by type II alveoli
    - It lowers alveolar surface tension by interspersing between the water molecules lining the alveoli
    - Surfactant lowers the surface tension of smaller alveoli more than that of large alveoli
    - This prevent the smaller alveoli form collapsing and emptying their air contents into the larger alveoli

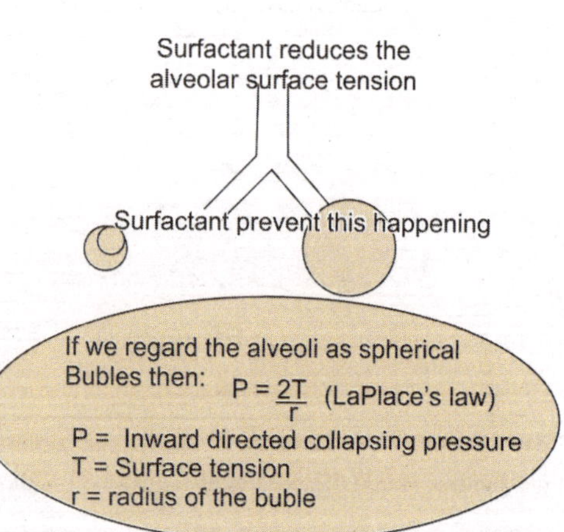

12. **Ans. (b) Excessive growth occurs before fusion of the epiphyses of the long bones**

[Ref: Harrison 19th/2269-70;Ganong 25th/326; Guyton 12th(SAE)/557-58]

"In acromegaly, ***IGF-I levels are invariably high*** and reflect a ***log-linear relationship with circulating GH concentrations***"-*Harrison 19th/401e-3*

"For acromegaly, ***somatostatin analogues*** and GH receptor antagonists are indicated"-*Harrison 19th/2264*

Acromegaly

◈ *Harrison 19th/2269-70*

- ***Age-matched serum IGF-I levels are elevated in acromegaly***. Consequently, an IGF-I level provides a useful laboratory screening measure when clinical features raise the possibility of acromegaly.
- The goal of treatment is to control GH and IGF-I hypersecretion, ablate or arrest tumor growth, ameliorate comorbidities, restore mortality rates to normal, and preserve pituitary function.
- Surgical resection of GH-secreting adenomas is the initial treatment for most patients.***Somatostatin analogues are used as adjuvant treatment for preoperative shrinkage*** of large invasive macroadenomas.
- Irradiation or repeat surgery may be required for patients who cannot tolerate or do not respond to adjunctive medical therapy.
- ***Transsphenoidal surgical resection by an experienced surgeon is the preferred primary treatment*** for both microadenomas (remission rate ~70%) and macroadenomas (<50% in remission).

Gigantism and Acromegaly

◈ *Ganong 25th/326*

- Tumors of the somatotropes of the anterior pituitary (pituitary adenomas) ***secrete large amounts of growth hormone,*** leading to ***gigantism in children and to acromegaly in adults.***
- ***Hypersecretion of growth hormone*** is accompanied by hypersecretion of prolactin in 20–40% of patients with acromegaly. About 25% of patients have abnormal glucose tolerance tests, and 4% develop lactation in the absence of pregnancy.
- Acromegaly can be caused by extrapituitary as well as intrapituitary growth hormone–secreting tumors and by hypothalamic tumors that secrete GHRH, but the latter are rare.

Acromegaly

◈ *Guyton 12th(SAE)/557-58*

- If an acidophilic tumor occurs after adolescence-that is, ***after the epiphyses of the long bones have fused with the shafts***-the person cannot grow taller, but the bones can become thicker and the soft tissues can continue to grow. This condition, is known as *acromegaly.*

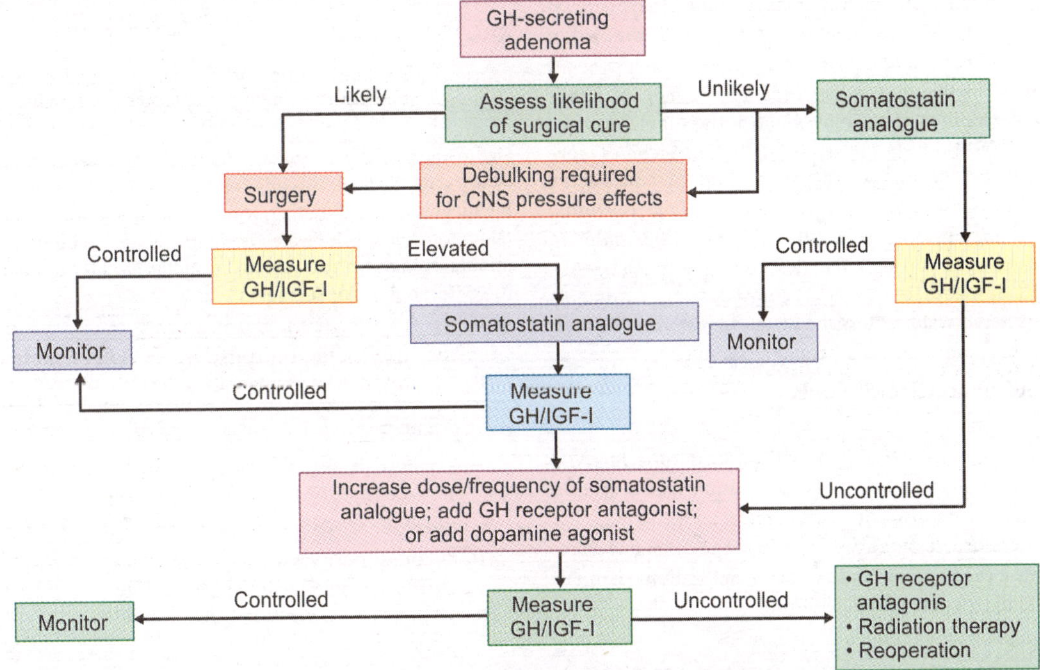

Fig: *(Harrison 19th/2270):* Management of acromegaly

13. Ans. (a) Vasopressin increase only water reabsorption..., (b) Aldosterone increase Na⁺..., (c) Glomerular filtrate of PCT has

[Ref: Ganong 25th/701; Guyton 12th(SAE)/ 480-88; AK Jain 6th/527,558]

"**Antidiuretic hormone (ADH, also k/a Vasopressin)** *increases permeability of distal tubules(mild action) and collecting ducts(mainly) to water→**increases water reabsorption**"- AK Jain 6th/673*

"**Aldosterone** *causes **retention of sodium from the kidney and increased urinary excretion of potassium**; it has **little effect on water excretion**"- AK Jain 6th/724*

Water Reabsorption

◈ *AK Jain 6th/527*

- ***"PCT: The osmolality of the fluid in tubule is unchanged at approx. 300mosm i.e, isotonicity is maintained"***
- ***"The tubular fluid entering the DCT is always hypotonic to plasma**, regardless of the hydration state"*
- *Early part of DCT is relatively impermeable to water and continued removal of solute in excess of solvent further dilutes the tubular fluid. However, Na+ absorption in this segment is variable and being regulated by aldosterone. Approx. 5-8% of the filtered water is removed passively in this segment*
- *In Terminal DCT and CT, the osmolarity in the tubular fluid changes according to water permeability of the tubule to ADH. Under the influence of ADH, another 10-12% of filtered water is reabsorbed*

"Active transport of many substances occurs from the fluid in the proximal tubule, but micropuncture studies have shown that the fluid remains essentially ***iso-osmotic until the end of the proximal tubule***"*- Ganong 25th/683*

"The fluid in the ***descending limb of the loop of Henle becomes hypertonic*** as water moves out of the tubule into the hypertonic interstitium. ***In the ascending limb it becomes more dilute*** because of the movement of Na+ and Cl− out of the tubular lumen, and ***when fluid reaches the top of the ascending limb (called the diluting segment) it is now hypotonic to plasma***. In passing through the descending loop of Henle, another 15% of the filtered water is removed, so approximately 20% of the filtered water enters the distal tubule, and the TF/P of inulin at this point is about 5"*-Ganong 25th/684*

Effects of Adrenocortical Steroids

◈ *Ganong 25th/701*

- Adrenal mineralocorticoids such as ***aldosterone increase tubular reabsorption of Na⁺ in association with secretion of K⁺ and H⁺ and also Na⁺ reabsorption with Cl⁻***.
- The mineralocorticoids act primarily in the collecting ducts to increase the number of active epithelial sodium channels (ENaCs) in this part of the nephron.

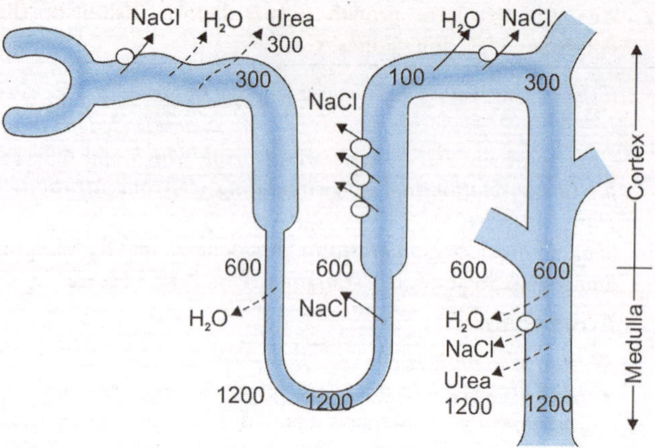

Fig: *(Guyton 12th(SAE)/ 484):* Formation of a concentrated urine when antidiuretic hormone (ADH) levels are high.

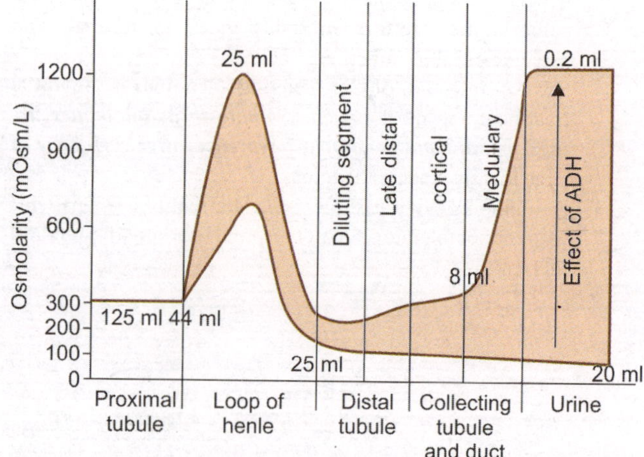

Fig: *(Guyton 12th(SAE)/486)*: Changes in osmolarity of the tubular fluid as it passes through the different tubular segments in the presence of high levels of antidiuretic hormone (ADH) and in the absence of ADH. (Numerical values indicate the approximate volumes in milliliters per minute or in osmolarities in milliosmoles per liter of fluid flowing along the different tubular segments.)

14. Ans. (b) Pacinian corpuscles, (d) Golgi tendon organs (e) Meissner corpuscles

[Ref: Ganong 25th/160; Guyton 12th(SAE)/688; AK Jain 6th/864]

"**Merkel's discs and Meissner's corpuscles** *are tactile receptors. They are **rapidly adapting receptors**. This is why we do not feel our clothes once they are put on"-AK Jain 6th/864*

"**Pacinian corpuscles**: *They respond to deformation caused by firm pressure and are **quickly adapting**. This is why we do not feel seat pressure when sitting"- AK Jain 6th/864*

"**Joint receptors** *are mainly the pacinian corpuscles,* **Golgi tendon organs** *and Ruffini's end organs which are situated in the ligaments of the joint. They are* **quickly adapting receptors**"*- AK Jain 6th/865*

"The ***pacinian corpuscle adapts very rapidly***, hair receptors adapt within a second or so, and ***some joint capsule and muscle spindle receptors adapt slowly***. Furthermore, some sensory receptors adapt to a far greater extent than others. *Guyton 12th(SAE)/688*

Adaptation of Receptors

◈ *Two types AK Jain 6th/870*

- **Tonic receptors***: They are poor,* ***slow and incompletely adapting receptors****, therefore, they can continue to transmit the information for many hours even if the intensity of stimulus remains absolutely constant over many days. E.g* ***Muscle spindle; Sensation of pain and cold; Baroreceptors and chemoreceptors***
- **Phasic (or rate) receptors***: These are* ***rapidly adapting receptors*** *and transmits signals only when the stimulus strength is changed e.g* ***touch, olfactory and pressure***

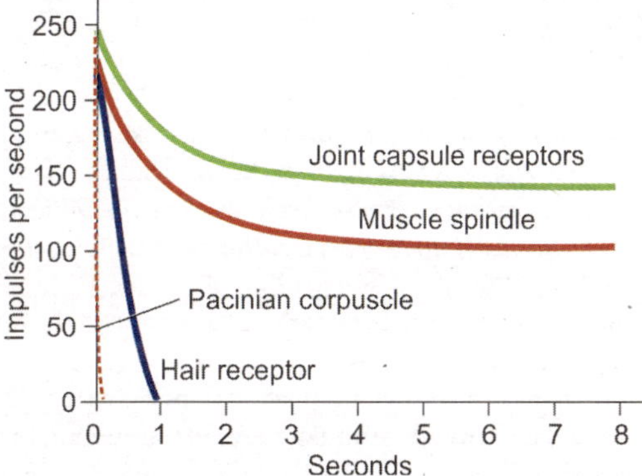

Fig: *(Guyton 12th(SAE)/688):* Adaptation of different types of receptors, showing rapid adaptation of some receptors and slow adaptation of others.

Classification of Receptor by Rate of Adaptation

◈ *wikipedia*

- **Slowly adapting**: Slowly adapting mechanoreceptors include Merkel and Ruffini corpuscle end-organs, and some free nerve endings.
    - Slowly adapting type I mechanoreceptors have multiple Merkel corpuscle end-organs.
    - Slowly adapting type II mechanoreceptors have single Ruffini corpuscle end-organs.
- **Intermediate adapting**: Some free nerve endings are intermediate adapting.
- **Rapidly adapting**: Rapidly adapting mechanoreceptors include ***Meissner corpuscle end-organs, Pacinian corpuscle end-organs, hair follicle receptors and some free nerve endings.***
    - Rapidly adapting type I mechanoreceptors have multiple Meissner corpuscle end-organs.
    - Rapidly adapting type II mechanoreceptors (usually called Pacinian) have single Pacinian corpuscle end-organs

15. Ans. (a) Total Calcium: 8.5–10.5 mg/dL, (b) Sodium:135–145 mmol/L (c) Potassium: 3.5–5.1 mmol/L

[Ref: Harrison 19th/ 2762-63,2758;Davidson 22nd/1308-09]

*"**TSH 0.2-4.5mU/L**"-Davidson 22nd/1308*
*"**Calcium (total): 8.5 -10.5 mg/dL**"-Davidson 22nd/1310*

Parameter	Normal value
Serum creatinine	0.6–1.6 mg/dl (Harrison 19th/464)
Thyroid stimulating Hormone (TSH)	***0.34–4.25 mIU/L*** (Harrison 19th/2763)
Calcium Ionized calcium	**8.7–10.2 mg/dL** (Harrison 19th/2758) 4.5–5.3 mg/dL
Potassium	3.5–5.0 meq/L (Harrison 19th/2762)
Sodium	136–146 meq/L (Harrison 19th/2763)

Table (Davidson 22nd/1308): **Urea and electrolytes in venous blood**

Analysis	Reference range	
	SI units	Non-SI units
Sodium	135–145 mmol/L	135–145 meq/L
Potassium	3.6–5.0 mmol/L	3.6–5.0 meq/L
Chloride	95–107 mmol/L	95–107 meq/L
Urea	2.5–6.6 mmol/L	15–40 mg/dL
Creatinine	60–120 mmol/L	0.68–1.36 mg/dL

*serum values are, on average, 0.3 mmol/L higher than plasma

16. Ans. (b) Action potential of both qualitatively similar, (c) Resting membrane potential almost same

[Ref: Guyton 12th(SAE)/81; Guyton 11th/89]

Muscle Action Potential-Comparison with Nerve Action Potential

◈ *Guyton 11th/89*

Almost everything regarding initiation and conduction of action potentials in nerve fibers applies equally to skeletal muscle fibers, ***except for quantitative differences***. Some of the quantitative aspects of muscle potentials are the following:

- Resting membrane potential: ***about -80 to -90 millivolts in skeletal fibers-the same as in large myelinated nerve fibers.***
- Duration of action potential: ***1 to 5 milliseconds in skeletal muscle-about five times as long as in large myelinated nerves.***
- Velocity of conduction: ***3 to 5 m/sec-about 1/13 the velocity of conduction in the large myelinated nerve fibers that excite skeletal muscle.***

Table *(Guyton 12th(SAE)/81)*: **Comparison of the nerve and muscle action potential**

	Nerve Action Potential	Muscle Action Potential
Resting membrane potential	–70 mV	–80 to –90 mV
Duration of action potential	0.2–0.3 msec	1–5 msec
Velocity of conduction	70–120 m/sec	3–5 m/sec

All values for the nerve in Table refer to large myelinated nerves

17. Ans. (d) Ca^{2+}

[Ref: Ganong 25th/586; Guyton 12th(SAE)/269;A.K.Jain 6th/322]

Vascular Control by Ions and Other Chemical Factors

◈ *Guyton 12th(SAE)/269*

Many different ions and other chemical factors can either dilate or constrict local blood vessels. Most of them have little function in *overall regulation* of the circulation, but some specific effects are:

- An increase in ***calcium ion*** concentration causes ***vasoconstriction***. This results from the general effect of calcium to stimulate smooth muscle contraction
- An increase in ***potassium ion*** concentration, within the physiological range, causes *vasodilation*. This results from the ability of potassium ions to inhibit smooth muscle contraction.
- An increase in ***magnesium ion*** concentration causes *powerful vasodilation* because magnesium ions inhibit smooth muscle contraction.
- An ***increase in hydrogen ion*** concentration (decrease in pH) causes dilation of the arterioles. Conversely, *slight decrease in hydrogen ion* concentration causes arteriolar constriction.
- *Anions* that have significant effects on blood vessels are ***acetate*** **and** ***citrate***, both of which cause mild degrees of vasodilation.
- An ***increase in carbon dioxide concentratio***n causes moderate vasodilation in most tissues but marked vasodilation in the brain.

Table *(Ganong 25th/586)*: **Summary of factors affecting the caliber of the arterioles**

Vasoconstriction	Vasodilation
Local factors	
Decreased local temperature Autoregulation	Increased CO_2 and decreased O_2 Increased K^+, adenosine, lactate Decreased local pH Increased local temperature
Endothelial products	
Endothelin-1 Locally released platelet Serotonin Thromboxane A_2	Nitric oxide Kinins Prostacyclin
Circulating neurohumoral agents	
Epinephrine (except in skeletal muscle and liver) Norepinephrine Arginine vasopressin Angiotensin II Endogenous digitalis-like substance Neuropeptide Y	Epinephrine in skeletal muscle and liver Calcitonin G-related protein Substance P Histamine Atrial natriuretic peptide Vasoactive intestinal polypeptide
Neural factors	
Increased discharge of sympathetic nerves	Decreased discharge of sympathetic nerves Activation of sympathetic cholinergic vasodilator nerves to vasculature of skeletal muscles of the limbs

Contd...

18. Ans. (b) Gonadotropin hormone surge, (d) ↑ Prostaglandins, (e) Activation of proteolytic enzymes

[Ref: Ganong 25th/ 408–09; Guyton 12th(SAE)/ 639–41; AK Jain 6th/803–05]

Ovulation

◈ *Novak's Gynae 15th/155*

- **The midcycle LH surge is responsible for a dramatic increase in local concentrations of prostaglandins and proteolytic enzymes in the follicular wall**
- These ***substances progressively weaken the follicular wall and ultimately allow a perforation to form***. Ovulation most likely represents a slow extrusion of the oocyte through this opening in the follicle rather than a rupture of the follicular structure.

"If pregnancy does occur, placental hCG will mimic LH action and continually stimulate the corpus luteum to secrete progesterone. Successful implantation results in hormonal support to allow continued maintenance of the corpus luteum and the endometrium"- *Novak's Gynae 15th/155*

Ovulation

◈ *Ganong 25th/ 409*

- Once luteolysis begins, the estrogen and progesterone levels fall and the ***secretion of FSH and LH increases***. A new crop of follicles develops, and then a single dominant follicle matures as a result of the action of FSH and LH.
- ***Near midcycle, estrogen secretion from the follicle rises.*** This rise augments the responsiveness of the pituitary to ***GnRH and triggers a burst of LH secretion.***

Feedback Effects

◈ *Ganong 25th/ 408*

- At 36–48 h before ovulation, the estrogen feedback effect becomes positive, and this ***initiates the burst of LH secretion (LH surge) that produces ovulation.***
- ***Ovulation occurs about 9 h after the LH peak. FSH secretion also peaks***, despite a small rise in inhibin, probably because of the ***strong stimulation of gonadotropes by GnRH***. During the luteal phase, the secretion of LH and FSH is low because of the elevated levels of estrogen, progesterone, and inhibin.

Initiation of Ovulation

◈ *Guyton 12th(SAE)/ 639-40*

- Within a few hours, two events occur, both of which are necessary for ovulation: (1) The *theca externa* (the capsule of the follicle) begins to ***release proteolytic enzymes*** from lysosomes, and these cause dissolution of the follicular capsular wall and consequent weakening of the wall, resulting in further swelling of the entire follicle and degeneration of the stigma. (2) Simultaneously there is rapid growth of new blood vessels into the follicle wall, and at the same time, ***prostaglandins (local hormones that cause vasodilation)*** are secreted into the follicular tissues. These two effects cause plasma transudation into the follicle, which contributes to follicle swelling.
- ***Finally, the combination of follicle swelling and simultaneous degeneration of the stigma causes follicle rupture, with discharge of the ovum.***

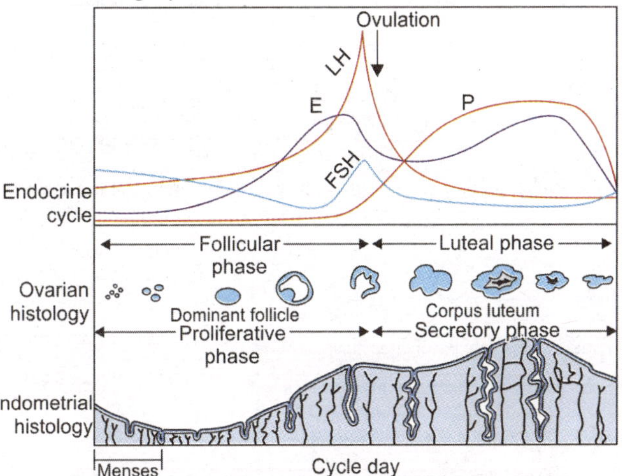

Fig: *(Novak's Gynae 15th/148):* Menstrual cycle

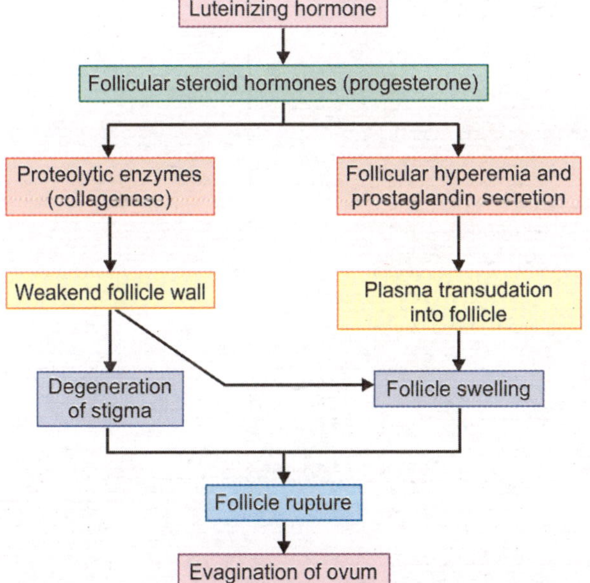

Fig: *(Guyton 12th(SAE)/ 640):* Postulated mechanism of ovulation

19. Ans. (a) Broca's aphasia, (b) Conduction aphasia, (e) Anomic aphasia

[Ref: Harrison 19th/177; AK Jain 6th/1034-35]

Table *(Harrison 19th/177):* **Clinical Features of Aphasias and Related Conditions commonly seen in cerebrovascular accidents**

	Comprehension	Repetition of Spoken Language	Naming	Fluency
Wernicke's	Impaired	Impaired	Impaired	Preserved or increased
Broca's	Preserved (except grammar)	Impaired	Impaired	Decreased
Global	Impaired	Impaired	Impaired	Decreased
Conduction	Preserved	Impaired	Impaired	Preserved
Nonfluent (motor) transcortical	Preserved	Preserved	Impaired	Impaired
Fluent (sensory) transcortical	Impaired	Preserved	Impaired	Preserved
Isolation	Impaired	Echolalia	Impaired	No purposeful speech
Anomic	Preserved	Preserved	Impaired	Preserved except for word-finding pauses
Pure word deafness	Impaired only for spoken language	Impaired	Preserved	Preserved
Pure alexia	Impaired only for reading	Preserved	Preserved	Preserved

20. Ans. (a) Area postrema, (b) CTZ, (d) Nucleus tractus solitarius

[Ref: Ganong 25th/501; Guyton 12th(SAE)/456-57; AK Jain 6th/226; Ajay yadav 5th/132;KDT 7th/662]

Postoperative Nausea and Vomiting (PONV)

◈ *www.academic.oup.com*

- **PONV** is defined as any nausea, retching, or vomiting occurring during the ***first 24–48 h after surgery in inpatients***.
- PONV is one of the most common causes of patient dissatisfaction after anaesthesia, with reported incidences of 30% in all post-surgical patients and up to 80% in high-risk patients.
- The physiology of PONV is complex and not perfectly understood. According to our current model, the brain

structures involved in the pathophysiology of vomiting are distributed throughout the ***medulla oblongata of the brainstem, not centralized in an anatomically defined 'vomiting centre'***. Such structures include the ***chemoreceptor trigger zone (CRTZ), located at the caudal end of the fourth ventricle in the area postrema***, and the ***nucleus tractus solitarius (NTS), located in the area postrema and lower pons***.

- The CRTZ receives input from vagal afferents in the gastrointestinal tract, and it can also detect emetogenic toxins, metabolites, and drugs circulating in the blood and cerebrospinal fluid due to its lack of the blood–brain barrier. The ***CRTZ projects neurons to the NTS***, which receives input from vagal afferents and from the vestibular and limbic systems. The NTS triggers vomiting by stimulating the r***ostral nucleus, the nucleus ambiguous, the ventral respiratory group, and the dorsal motor nucleus of the vagus***

PONV

◈ *www.medscape.com*

- **PONV** can be triggered by several ***perioperative stimuli, including opioids, volatile anaesthetics, anxiety, adverse drug reactions, and motion***. Multiple neurotransmitter pathways are implicated in the physiology of nausea and vomiting. Enterochromaffin cells in the gastrointestinal tract release serotonin, and the vagus nerve communicates with the **CRTZ** via 5-HT_3 receptors.
- The CRTZ communicates with the **NTS** primarily via dopamine-2 (D2) receptors.

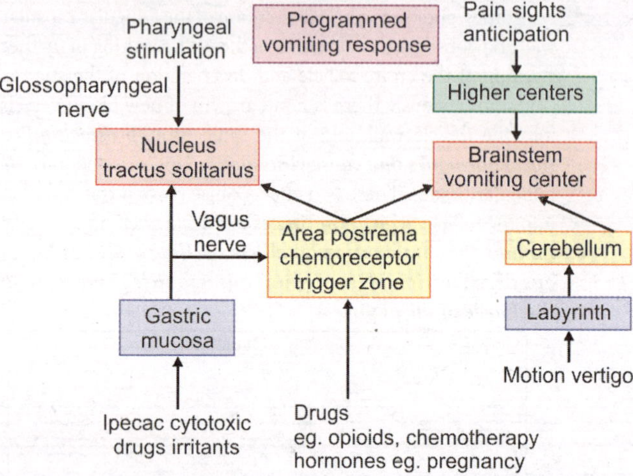

Fig: *(Ganong 25th/501):* Neural pathways leading to the initiation of vomiting in response to various stimuli

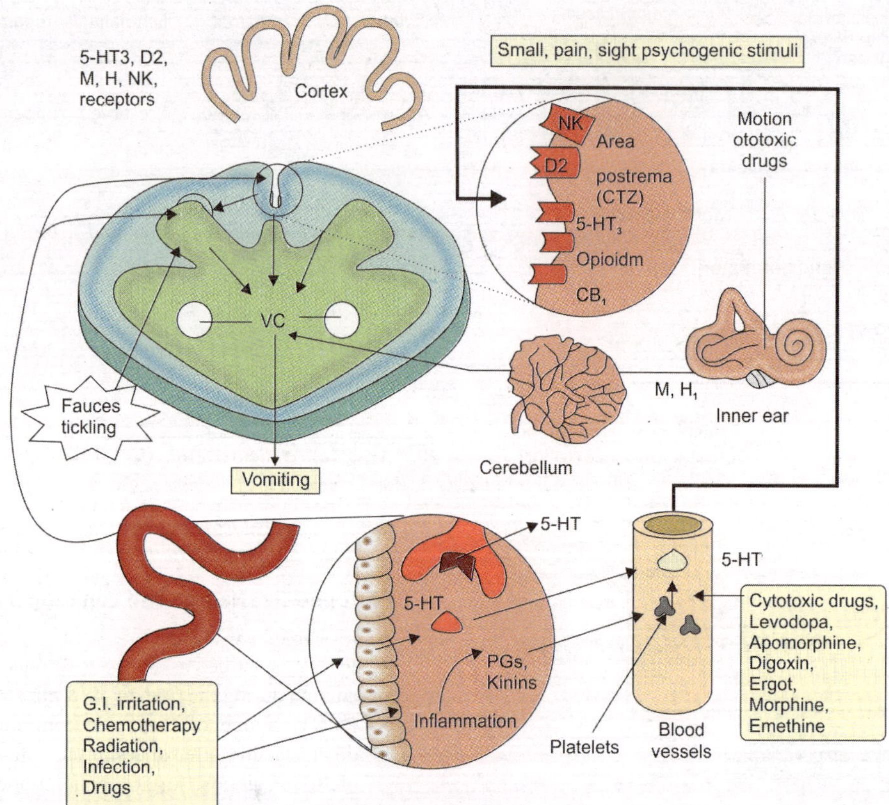

Fig: *(KDT 7th/662):* Major central and visceral structures involved in emesis and the neurohumoral receptors mediating the emetic response; NTS-Nucleus tractus solitarius; VC-Vomiting center; CTZ –Chemoreceptor zone

BIOCHEMISTRY

21. Ans. (a) HGPRT deficiency, (d) Glucose 6- phosphatase deficiency

[Ref: Harper 30th/354-56; Satyanarayan 4th/269-70, 394-95]

"Von Gierke's disease (Type 1 glycogen storage disease): ***Hyperuricemia occurs due to Glucose 6-phosphatase enzyme defect"*** *- Satyanarayan 4th/269-70*

Primary gout (overproduction of uric acid): Important metabolic defects(enzymes) *Satyanarayan 4th/394-95*

- ↑ **PRPP synthetase**: *Increased production of purines*
- ↑*PRPP glutamylamidotransferase: Increased production of purines*
- ***HGPRT deficiency****(as seen in Lesch-Nyhan syndrome): Increased production of purines*
- ***Glucose 6-phosphatase deficiency****:Purine overproduction*
- *Elevation of glutathione reductase*

Gout is a Metabolic Disorder of Purine Catabolism

◈ *Harper 30th/354*

- Various genetic defects in ***PRPP synthase*** present clinically as gout. Each defect—for example, an elevated *V*max, increased affinity for ribose 5-phosphate, or resistance to feedback inhibition—results in ***overproduction and overexcretion of purine catabolites.***
- When serum urate levels exceed the solubility limit, sodium urate crystalizes in soft tissues and joints and causes an inflammatory reaction, **gouty arthritis.**

Gout

◈ *Harper 30th/354-56; Satyanarayan 4th/394*

- Gout is usually preceded and accompanied by **hyperuricemia** (plasma uric acid level >0.41 mmol/L).
- Hyperuricemia is caused by ***decreased renal excretion, increased production, or increased intake of uric acid.***
- Increased production can occur due to certain ***enzyme abnormalities (eg, deficiency of hypoxanthine-guanine phosphoribosyl transferase [HGPRT] and over-activity of PRPP synthetase)***, although these are uncommon
- In Lesch-Nyhan syndrome, mutations of the gene encoding HGPRT are involve, and gout can be a feature.

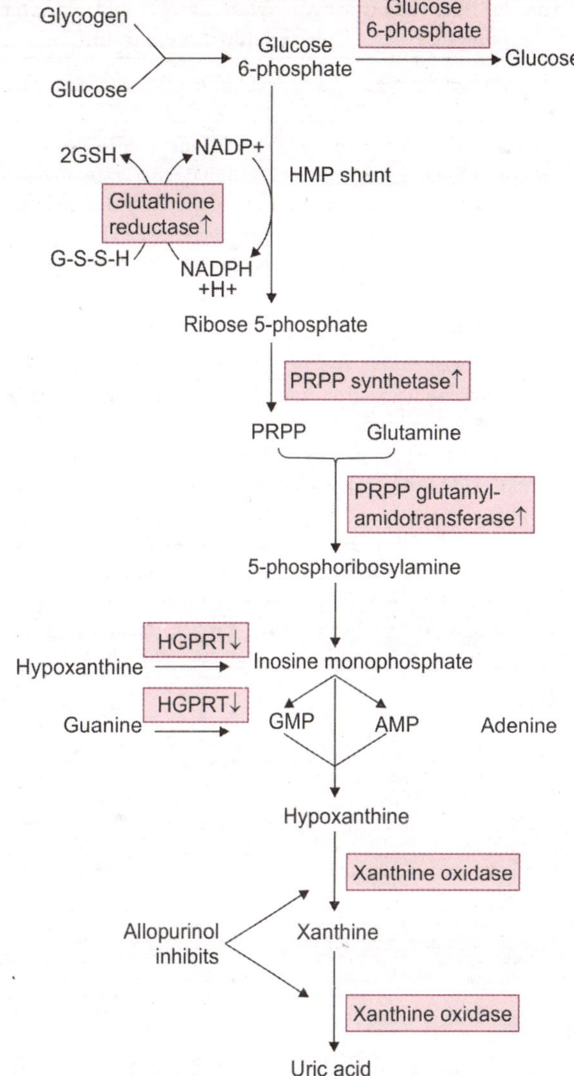

Fig: *(Satyanarayan 4th/395)*: Summary of possible enzymes alternation causing gout; GSSG-oxidized glutathione; GSH-reduced glutathione

Table *(Harper 30th/356)*: **Metabolic Disorders of Purine and Pyrimidine Metabolism**

Defective Enzyme	Major Signs and Symptoms
Purine Metabolism	
Hypoxanthine-guanine phosphoribosyl transferase	Lesch-Nyhan syndrome Uricemia, self-mutalation
PRPP synthase	Gout; gouty arthritis
Adenosine deaminase	Severely compromised immune system
Purine nucleoside phosphorylase	Autoimmune disorders; benign and opportunistic infections
Pyrimidine Metabolism	
Dihydropyrimidine dehydrogenase	Can develop toxicity to 5-fluorouracil, also a substrate for this dehydrogenase
Orotate phosphoribosyl transferase and orotidylic acid decarboxylase	Orotic acid aciduria type 1; megaloblastic anemia
Orotidylic acid decarboxylase	Orotic acid aciduria type 2

22. Ans. (a) Phenylalanine hydroxylase..., (c) Dihydrobiopterin reductase..., (e) Defect in dihydrobiopterin...

[Ref: Harper 30th/304-06; Lippincott 6th/270-71; Satyanarayan 4th/345-47]

"**Tyrosine Hydroxylase (TH) deficiency** (also known as Recessive Dopa- Responsive Dystonia) is a rare metabolic disorder characterized by the lack of the enzyme involved in converting the amino acid tyrosine to L-dopa. TH is a critical enzyme in normal dopamine production"- *www.pndassoc.org/diseases*

Phenylalanine

◈ *Harper 30th/304-06*

- Phenylalanine is first converted to tyrosine. Subsequent reactions are those of tyrosine
- Hyperphenylalaninemias arise from ***defects in phenylalanine hydroxylase*** itself (type I, classic phenylketonuria or PKU), in ***dihydrobiopterin reductase*** (types II and III), or in ***dihydrobiopterin biosynthesis*** (types IV and V). Alternative catabolites are excreted.
- A diet low in phenylalanine can prevent the mental retardation of PKU. DNA probes facilitate prenatal diagnosis of defects in ***phenylalanine hydroxylase or dihydrobiopterin reductase***. Elevated blood phenylalanine may not be detectable until 3–4 days postpartum. False-positives in premature infants may reflect delayed maturation of enzymes of phenylalanine catabolism.

Phenylketonuria (PKU)

◈ *Lippincott 6th/ 270-71*

- PKU is caused by a ***deficiency of phenylalanine hydroxylase***, is the most common clinically encountered inborn error of amino acid metabolism
- Biochemically, it is characterized by ***accumulation of phenylalanine*** (and a deficiency of tyrosine). Hyper phenyl alaninemia may also be caused by deficiencies in any of the ***several enzymes required to synthesize BH4***, or in ***dihydropteridine reductase***, which regenerates BH4 from BH2.
- Such deficiencies ***indirectly raise phenylalanine concentrations***, because phenyl alanine hydroxylase requires BH4 as a coenzyme. BH4 is also required for tyrosine hydroxylase and tryptophan hydroxylase, which catalyze reactions leading to the synthesis of neurotransmitters, such as serotonin and reverse the central nervous system (CNS) effects due to deficiencies in neurotransmitters.

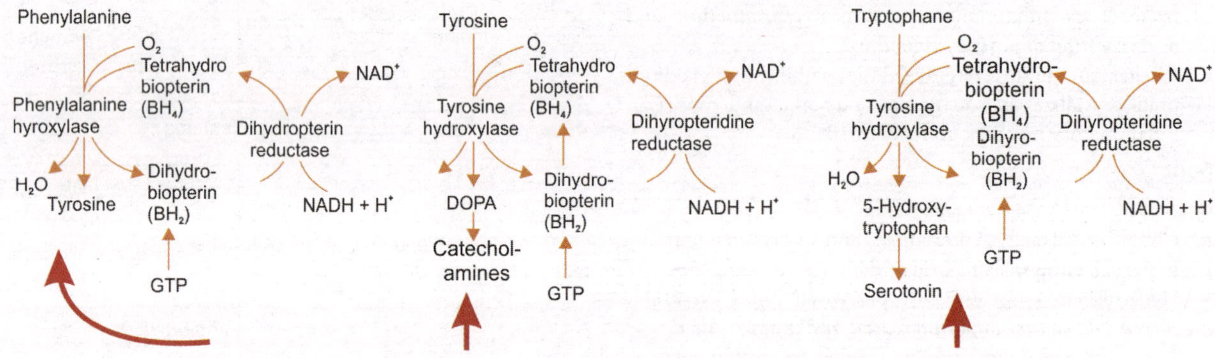

A deficiency in dihydropteridine reductase or any of the enzymes of BH_4 synthesis leads to Hyperphenylalaninemia, and decreased synthesis of catecholamines and serotonin.

Fig: *(Lippincott 6th/270):* Biosynthetic reactions involving amino acids and tetrahydrobiopterin

O_2 Phynlalanine hydroxylase H_2O
Phenylalanine ($CH_2-CH(NH_3^+)-COO^-$) → Tyrosine ($HO-C_6H_4-CH_2-CH(NH_3^+)-COO^-$)
Tetrahydro-biopterin
Dihydro-biopterin
Dihydrobiopterin reductase
NADP$^+$
NADH + H$^+$

Fig: *(Satyanarayan 4th/346):* Synthesis of tyrosine from phenylalanine (■: Block in phenylketonuria)

23. Ans. (a) Fluoride, (d) Carboxin, (e) Ouabin

[Ref: Harper 30th/132-33; Lippincott 6th/79; Satyanarayan 4th/233-34; Chatterjea 7th/132-34]

"Carboxin inhibit complex II, which is not involved in oxidative phosphorylation (so not included in answer)"- *Chatterjea 7th/134*

"**Ouabain** is a cardiac glycoside that acts by inhibiting the ***Na^+/K^+-ATPase*** sodium-potassium ion pump"-Harper 30th/491

"**Fluoride**: *It inhibits the activities of certain enzymes. Sodium fluoride* ***inhibits enolase*** *(of glycolysis) while fluoroacetate inhibits* ***aconitase*** *(of citric acid cycle)"- Satyanarayan 4th/420*

Inhibitors of Oxidative Phosphorylation

◈ *Satyanarayan 4th/233-34*

- *Uncouplers: The uncouplers allow oxidation of substrates without ATP formation*
  - **2,4-dinitrophenol (DNP)**
  - *Dinitrocresol*
  - *Trifluorocarbonylcyanide phenylhydrazone*
  - *Pentachlorophenol*
  - *Aspirin (in high dose)*
  - *Physiological uncouplers: High concentration of thermogenin, thyroxine and long chain free fatty acids*
  - *Antibiotics- valinomycin, gramicidin A and nigercin*
- *Other inhibitors of oxidative phosphorylation*
  - ***Oligomycin***
  - *Atractyloside*

Oxidative Phosphorylation

- In this ATP is produced by combining ADP and Pi with the energy generated by the flow of electrons of NADH to molecular oxygen in the electron transport chain
- There are three sites in respiratory chain where ATP is formed by oxidative phosphorylation
- Three sites are- Site I (Complex-I), Site II (Complex III) and Site III (Complex IV). Complex II (Succinate dehydrogenase FAD) is not involved in oxidative phosphorylation

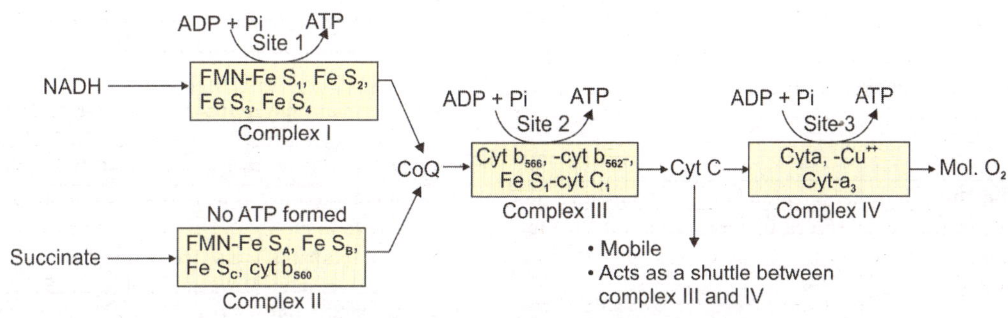

Fig: *(Chatterjea 7th/132):* Showing four complex of Electron transport chain

Table *(Chatterjea 7th/134): Inhibitors of ETC*

Inhibitors of ETC	
Site–I (Complex-I):	
• **Rotenone:** A fish poison and also insecticide. Inhibits transfer of electrons through complex-I- NADH-Q-reductase. • **Amobarbital (Amytal) and Secobarbital:** Inhibits electron transfer through NADH-Q reductase • **Piericidin A:** An antibiotic. Blocks electron transfer by competing with CoQ. • **Drugs:** Chlorpromazine and hypotensive drug like guanethidine	
Site-II (Complex III): • Antimycin A • BAL (Dimer-Coprol) • Hypoglycaemic drugs: like phenformin	Blocks electron transfer from cyt b to C_1
Site-III (Complex IV): • **Cyanide** • **H_2S to** • **Azide**	Inhibits terminal transfer of electrons molecular O_2
• **CO (Carbon monoxide):** Inhibits cyt. Oxidase by combining with O_2 binding site. It can be reversed by illumination with light	
Complex II: Succinate dehydrogenase FAD: • **Carboxin** • **TTFA**	Specifically inhibit transfer of reducing equivalent from succinate dehydrogen ase
• **Malonate:** A competitive inhibitor of succinate dahydrogenase	

Many Poisons Inhibit the Respiratory Chain

◈ *Harper 30th/132*

- They may be classified as inhibitors of the ***respiratory chain, inhibitors of oxidative phosphorylation, and uncouplers of oxidative phosphorylation.***
- **Barbiturates such as amobarbital** inhibit electron transport via Complex I by blocking the transfer from Fe-S to Q. At sufficient dosage, they are fatal in vivo. ***Antimycin A and dimercaprol*** inhibit the respiratory chain at Complex III. The classic poisons ***H 2 S, carbon monoxide and cyanide*** inhibit Complex IV and can therefore totally arrest respiration.
- **Malonate** is a competitive inhibitor of Complex II.
- **Atractyloside** inhibits ***oxidative phosphorylation***
- The antibiotic **oligomycin** completely blocks oxidation and phosphorylation
- The uncoupler that has been used most frequently is **2, 4-dinitrophenol**, but other compounds act in a similar manner. **Thermogenin** (or the uncoupling protein) is a physiological uncoupler found in brown adipose tissue that functions to generate body heat

24. Ans. (a) Constitute peripheral region of..., (c) Apo A-I is the major protein..., (d) Apo A, B and C are..., (e) Role in enzyme ...

[Ref: Harper 30th/254-55; Satyanarayan 4th/318; http://nopr.niscair.res.in/bitstream; onlinelibrary.wiley.com]

Apolipoproteins (apo)

◈ *onlinelibrary.wiley.com*

- Apolipoproteins (apo) play very important roles in the synthesis and catabolism of plasma lipoproteins, in lipid transport, and as activators of certain enzymes associated with lipid and lipoprotein metabolism. They are also involved in various metabolic states or diseases.
- Apolipoproteins are the protein components of **plasma lipoproteins** which consist of a ***core of triglyceride and cholesterol esters*** and a ***peripheral region of phospholipid, sphingolipid and protein.***
- They are designated: ***apo A-I, apo A-II, apo A-IV; apo B-48, apo B-100; apo C-I, apo C-II, apo C-III; apo D; apo E-l, apo E-II, apo E-Ill, apo E-IV; apo F, apo G and apo H.***
- They also play very important roles in the synthesis and catabolism of lipoproteins, and as cofactors, inhibitors or ***activators of certain enzymes*** (eg lecithin cholesterol acyltransferase, hepatic lipase, lipoprotein lipase) associated with lipid and lipoprotein metabolism conditions in which there is excess or deficiency of one or other of the apolipoprotein lead to or are associated with specific diseases or syndromes.
- ***Apo A-I is the major protein component of high density lipoprotein (HDL)*** and a minor component of chylomicrons and very low density lipoprotein (VLDL).
- Apo A-II is the second most abundant protein in HDL, comprising approximately 20% of its protein while apo A-I constitutes 70% of it. ***Thus, high levels of apo A-I or A-II, or both, are predictive of a decreased risk of coronary artery disease (CAD).***

Apolipoproteins

◈ *Lippincott 6th/227*

- ***Apolipo proteins are divided by structure and function into five major classes, A through E, with most classes having subclasses, for example, apolipoprotein (or apo) A-I and apo C-II. [Note: Functions of all of the apolipoproteins are not yet known.]***

The Distribution of Apolipoproteins Characterizes the Lipoprotein

◈ *Harper 30th/255*

- ***Some apolipoproteins are integral and cannot be removed (e.g., apo B)***, whereas ***others are bound to the surface and are free to transfer to other lipoproteins, eg, apos C and E).***
- The ***major apolipoproteins of HDL (α-lipoprotein) are apoAs***
- The main **apolipoprotein of LDL** (β-lipoprotein) is apo B (B-100), which is found also in VLDL. Chylomicrons contain a truncated form of apo B (B-48) that is synthesized in the intestine, while B-100 is synthesized in the liver.
- Apo E, found in VLDL, HDL, chylomicrons, and chylomicron remnants, is also freely transferable; it accounts for 5% to 10% of total VLDL apolipoproteins in normal subjects.
- Apolipoproteins carry out several roles: (1) they ***can form part of the structure of the lipoprotein***, for ***example, apo B***;(2) they are ***enzyme cofactors***, for example, C-II for ***lipoprotein lipase***, A-I for ***lecithin:cholesterol acyltransferase***, or **enzyme inhibitors**, for example, apo A-II and apo C-III for lipoprotein lipase, apo C-I for cholesteryl ester transfer protein; and (3) they act as ligands for interaction with lipoprotein receptors in tissues, for example, apo B-100 and apo E for the LDL receptor, apo E for the LDL-receptor-related protein-1 (LRP-1), which has been identified as the remnant receptor, and apo A-I for the HDL receptor.

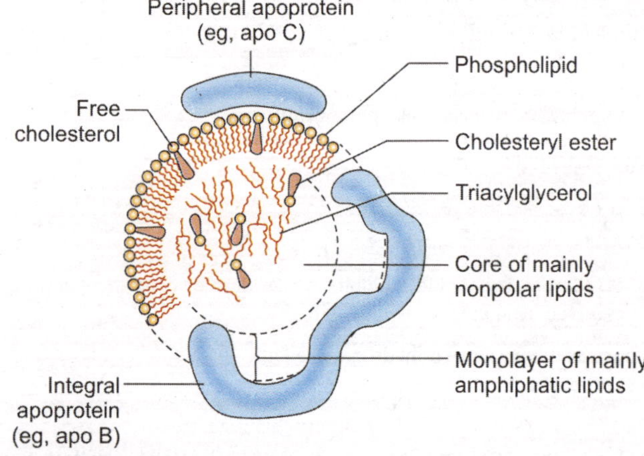

Fig: *(Harper 30th/255):* Generalized structure of a plasma lipoprotein

Table: **Major apolipoproteins** *(nopr.niscair.res.in/bitstream)*

Apolipo-protein	Chromo-somal	Functional activity	Lipoprotein carrier(s)
Apo A-I	11	Cofactor LCAT	Chylomicrom, HDL
Apo A-II	1	Not known	HDL
Apo A-IV	11	Activation of LCAT	Chylomicrom, HDL
	2	Secretion of triglyceride from liver binding protein to LDL receptor	
Apo B-48	2	Secretion of triglyyceride from intestine	Chylomicron
Apo B-100	2	Cholesterol transport from liver	LDL
Ppo C-I	19	Activation of LCAT (?)	Chylomiron, VLDL, HDL
Ppo C-II	19	Cofactor of LPL	Chylomiron, VLDL, HDL
Ppo C-III	11	Inhibition of apo CIII, activation of LPL	Chylomiron, VLDL, HDL
Apo D	3	Unknown	HDL
Apo E	19	Facilitation of uptake of chylomicrom remnant and LDL	Chylomiron, VLDL, HDL
Apo (a)	6	Unknown	Lp (a)

25. Ans. (a) Threonine, (b) Tyrosine, (c) Serine

[Ref: Harper 30th/16-17; Lippincott 6th/4; Satyanarayan 4th/45]

"***Serine, threonine, and tyrosine*** each contain a polar hydroxyl group that can participate in hydrogen bond formation. The side chains of asparagine and glutamine each contain a carbonyl group and an amide group, both of which can also participate in hydrogen bonds"-*Lippincott 6th/4*

Table *(Harper 30th/16-17):* **L-α-Amino Acids Present in Proteins**

Name
With Aliphatic Side Chains
Glycine
Alanine
Valine
Leucine
Isoleucine
With Side Chains Containing Hydroxylic (OH) Groups
Serine
Threonine
Tyrosine
With Side Chains Containing Sulfur Atoms
Cysteine
Methionine
With Side Chains Containing Acidic Groups or Their Amides
Aspartic acid
Asparagine
Glutamic acid
Glutamine
With Side Chains Containing Basic Groups
Arginine
Lysine
Histidine
Containing Aromatic Rings
Histidine
Phenylalanine
Tyrosine
Tryptophan
Imino Acid
Proline

26. Ans. (a) Hydroxylation of xenobiotics, (c) Deamination reaction, (d) Involved in hydroxylation of steroids, (e) Drug interaction

[Ref: Harper 30th/584-85; KDT 7th/23-26; Satyanarayan 4th/639-40]

Cytochrome P450s are involved in phase I (hydroxylation) of the metabolism of xenobiotics, not in phase II. Methylation of xenobiotics occur in phase II by methyltransferase

Table *(Harper 30th/585):* **Some properties of human cytochrome P450s.**

Involved in phase I of the metabolism of innumerable xenobiotics, including perhaps 50% of the drugs administered to humans
Involved in the metabolism of many endogenous compounds (e.g., **steroids**)
All are hemoproteins
Often exhibit broad substrate specificity, thus acting on many compounds; consequently, different P450s may catalyze formation of the same product
Extremely versatile catalysts, perhaps catalyzing about 60 types of reactions
However, basically they catalyze reactions involving introduction of one atom of oxygen into the substrate and one into water
Their hydroxylated products are more water-soluble than their generally lipophilic substrates, facilitating excretion
Liver contains highest amounts, but found in most if not all tissues, including small intestine, brain, and lung
Located in the smooth endoplasmic reticulum or in mitochondria (***steroidogenic hormones***)
In some cases, their products are mutagenic or carcinogenic
Many have a molecular mass of about 55 kDa
Many are inducible, resulting in one cause of ***drug interactions***
Many are inhibited by various drugs or their metabolic products, providing another ***cause of drug interactions***

Contd...

Some exhibit genetic polymorphisms, which can result in atypical drug metabolism

Their activities may be altered in diseased tissues (e.g, cirrhosis), ***affecting drug metabolism***

Genotyping the P450 profile of patients (e.g., to detect polymorphisms) may in the future permit ***individualization of drug therapy***

Table *(Harper 30th/584)*: **The Families of cytochrome P450 in human tissues**

Family	Function
CYP1	Drug and steroid (especially estrogen) metabolism
CYP2	Drug and steroid metabolism
CYP3	Drug and steroid (including testosterone) metabolism
CYP4	Arachidonic acid and fatty acid metabolism
CYP5	Thromboxane A_2 synthase
CYP7	Bile acid biosynthesis and steroid 7α hydroxylase
CYP8	Various, including prostacyclin synthase and bile acid synthesis
CYP11	Steroid biosynthesis
CYP17	Steroid biosynthesis, 17α hydroxylase
CYP19	Steroid biosynthesis, aromatase
CYP20	Unknown function
CYP21	Steroid biosynthesis
CYP24	Vitamin D catabolism
CYP26	Retinoic acid hydroxylase
CYP27	Various, including bile acid synthesis and calcidiol 1 α hydroxylase
CYP39	7-Alphahydroxylation of 24-hydroxycholesterol
CYP46	Cholesterol 24-hydroxylase
CYP17	Cholesterol biosynthesis

Reactions Catalyzed by P450

◈ *www.angelfire.com*

Aliphatic hydroxylation
Aromatic hydroxylation
N-dealkylation
O-dealkylation
S-demethylation
Epoxidation
Deamination
Sulkfoxide formation
N-oxidation
dealogenation

Cytochromes P450

◈ *Harper 30th/583-86*

- Cytochromes P450 Are Monooxygenases: Important for the ***Detoxification of Many Drugs and for the Hydroxylation of Steroids.***
- The metabolism of xenobiotics is generally considered in two phases. In **phase 1,** the major reaction involved is **hydroxylation,** catalyzed mainly by members of a class of enzymes referred to as **monooxygenases** or **cytochromes P450**.
- Hydroxylation may terminate the action of a drug, though this is not always the case. In addition to hydroxylation, these enzymes catalyze a **wide range of reactions**, including those involving ***deamination, dehalogenation, desulfuration, epoxidation, peroxygenation, and reduction***. Reactions involving hydrolysis (eg, catalyzed by esterases) and certain other non- P450-catalyzed reactions also occur in phase 1.
- ***Phase 1 metabolism renders compounds more reactive, introducing groups that can be conjugated with glucuronic acid, sulfate, acetate, glutathione, or amino acids in phase 2 metabolism***. This produces **polar compounds** that are water soluble and can therefore readily be excreted in urine or bile. Very hydrophobic xenobiotics would persist in adipose tissue almost indefinitely if they were not converted to more polar forms.
- **Methylation**—A ***few xenobiotics are subject to methylation by methyltransferases***, employing S-adenosylmethionine as the methyl donor.
- Induction of cytochrome P450 underlies **drug interactions,** when the effects of one drug are altered by prior, concurrent, or later administration of another

Role of Cytochrome P_{450}

◈ *Satyanarayan 4th/639-40*

- Most of oxidation reations of detoxication are catalyzed by monooxygenase or cytochrome P450. This enzyme, also called **Mixed function oxidase**, is associated with the microsomes. The usage P_{450} refers to the absorption peak (at 450 nm), exhibited by the enzyme when exposed to carbon monoxide.
- Most of the reactions of cytochrome P_{450} involve the ***addition of a hydroxyl group to aliphatic or aromatic compounds*** which may be represented as
  $RH + O_2 + NADPH \rightarrow ROH + H_2O + NADP^+$

Salient Features of Cytochrome P_{450}

◈ *Satyanarayan 4th/639-40*

- Multiple forms of cytochrome P_{450} are believed to exist, ranging from 20 to 200.
- They are all ***hemoproteins***, containing heme as the prosthetic group.
- Cytochrome P_{450} species are found in the highest concentration in the microsomes of liver. In the adrenal gland, they occur in mitochondria.
- The mechanism of action of cytochrome P_{450} is complex and is dependent on NADPH.
- The phospholipid-phosphatidylcholine is a constituent of cytochrome P_{450} system which is necessary for the action of this enzyme.
- Cytochrome P_{450} is an ***inducible enzyme.*** Its synthesis is increased by the administration of drugs such as phenobarbitol.
- A distinct species namely cytochrome P_{448} (with absorption peak at 448 nm) has been studied. It is specific for the metabolism of ***polycyclic aromatic hydrocarbons***, hence it is also known as aromatic hydrocarbon hydroxylase.

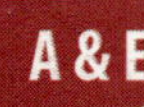

27. Ans. (b) Cell signaling, (c) Precursor of Second Messengers, (d) Mediators of inflammation, (e) Regulate membrane permeability

[Ref: Harper 30th/212,216,253-54; Robbins 9th/83-84; Satyanarayan 4th/36-37]

*"Glycoprotein (fibronectin, laminin) is involve in **cell-cell recognition** and adhesion"- Satyanarayan 4th/25; www.78stepshealth.us*

Phospholipids are the Main Constituents of Membranes

◈ *Harper 30th/215-16*

- "Sphingomyelins are found in the outer leaflet of the cell membrane lipid bilayer and are particularly abundant in specialized areas of the plasma membrane known as **lipid rafts**. They are also found in large quantities in the **myelin sheath** that surrounds nerve fibers. They are believed to play a role in ***cell signaling*** and in **apoptosis"**- *Harper 30th/216*
- **"Phosphatidylinositol Is a Precursor of Second Messengers:** The inositol is present in **phosphatidylinositol** as the stereoisomer, myoinositol. Phosphorylated phosphatidylinositols (**phosphoinositides**) are minor components of cell membranes, but play an important part *in **cell signaling and membrane trafficking**"-Harper 30th/216*

Functions of Phospholipids

◈ *Satyanarayan 4th/36-37*

Phospholipids constitute an important group of compound lipids that perform a wide variety of functions

- In association with proteins, phospholipids form the structural ***components of membranes*** and ***regulate membrane permeability.***
- Phospholipids participate in the ***absorption of fat*** from the intestine.
- Phospholipids are essential for the synthesis of different lipoproteins, and thus participate in the ***transport of lipids.***
- Accumulation of fat in liver (fatty liver) can be prevented by phospholipids, hence they are regarded as ***lipotropic factors.***
- Arachidonic acid, an unsaturated fatty acid les of liberated from phospholipids, serves as a precursor for the synthesis of ***eicosanoids (prostaglandins, prostacyclins, thromboxanes*** etc.).
- Phospholipids participate in the reverse cholesterol transport and thus help in the cholesterol from the body.
- Phospholipids act as surfactants (agents lowering surface tension). For instance, dipalmitoyl phosphatidylcholine is an important lung surfactant. ***Respiratory distress syndrome*** in infants is associated with insufficient production of this surfactant.
- Cephalins, an important group of phospholipids participate in ***blood clothing.***
- Phosphatidylinositol is the source of ***second messengers***— inositol triphosphate and diacylglyceol, that are involved the action of some hormones.

"The immediate precursor of the ***eicosianoids is arachidonic acid***, present in the ***beta position of phospholipids*** in cell membranes and membranes of subcellular particles. Eicosanoids are synthesized via two major pathways:((1)The cyclooxygenase pathway, from which ***thromboxane A2, prostacyclin (PGI2), and PGD2, PGE2 and PGF2 are synthesized and (2)The 5-lipoxygenase pathway, from which the leukotrienes*** (LTB4, LTC4, LTD4 and LTE4) are synthesized. Arachidonic acid is hydrolyzed from phospholipids by Phospholipase A2, also a membrane component. Aspirin and other NSAIDs inhibit cyclooxygenase but not lipoxygenase. *Anti-inflammatory steroids stabilize membranes and prevent phospholipid hydrolysis thereby inhibiting both pathways"- pro2services.com* and *Robbins 9th/83-84*

28. Ans. (a) Phospholipids undergo..., (c) Hydrophobic core of the phospholipid..., (d) Phospholipids that have one fatty acyl...

[Ref: Harper 30th/215-17,478-90; Satyanarayan 4th/650-51; en.wikibooks.org]

"Membranes are mainly made up of lipids, proteins and small amount of carbohydrate. Phospholipids are the most common lipids present and they are amphipathic in nature"- Vasudevan 5th/12

*"Some of the **intergral membrane proteins span the whole bilayer** and they are called **transmembrane protein.** The transmembrane proteins can serve as receptor, tissue specific antigens, ion channels, membrane-based enzymes, etc"-Vasudevan 5th/12*

*"Not all lipid can form bilayer. The **lysophospholipids have only one fatty acyl group, it cannot form the bilayer** as the polarheads are too large, similarly cholesterol also cannot form bilayers as the rigid fused ring systems and additional nonpolar tails are too large"- Chatterjea 7th/12*

*"It is not only the integral protein, the phospholipids also undergo rapid redistribution in the plane of membrane. This diffusion within the plane of the membrane is termed **transitional diffusion**. It can be quite rapid for a phospholipid molecule. Within the plane of membrane, one molecule of phospholipid can move several micrometers per second. The phase changes and thus the fluidity of the membrane are highly dependent upon the lipid composition of the membrane"-Chatterjea 7th/12-13*

"The ***hydrophobic core of the phospholipid bilayer is constantly in motion*** because of rotations around the bonds of lipid tails. Hydrophobic tails of a bilayer bend and lock together. However, because of ***hydrogen bonding with water, the hydrophilic head groups exhibit less movement as their rotation and mobility are constrained***. This results in increasing viscosity of the lipid bilayer closer to the hydrophilic heads"-wikipedia

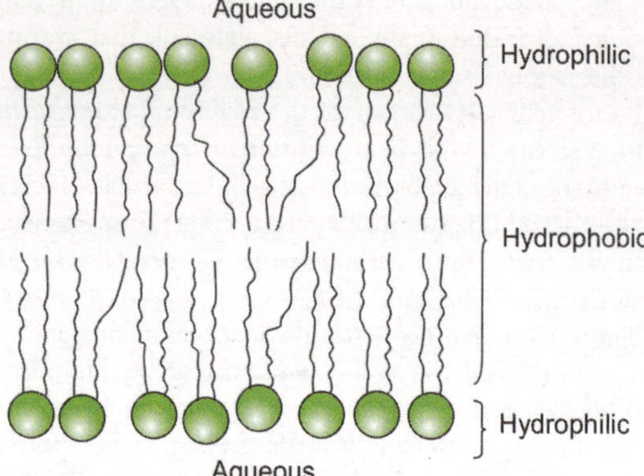

Fig: *(30th/480, 29th/):* **Diagram of a section of a bilayer membrane formed from phospholipid molecules.** The unsaturated fatty acid tails are kinked and lead to more spacing between the polar head groups, ***hence to more room for movement.*** This in turn results in increased membrane fluidity.

The Fluid Mosaic Model of Membrane Structure is Widely Accepted

◈ *Harper 30th/483*

- The model is often likened to *integral membrane protein "icebergs" floating in a sea of (predominantly) fluid phospholipid molecules.*
- **Phospholipids** undergo even more ***rapid lateral diffusion*** with subsequent redistribution within the plane of the membrane. Measurements indicate that within the plane of the membrane, one molecule of phospholipid can move several micrometers per second.
- The **phase changes**—and thus the **fluidity** of membranes—are ***largely dependent upon the lipid composition of the membrane.***
- The **fluidity of a membrane significantly affects its functions.** As membrane fluidity increases, so does its permeability to water and other small hydrophilic molecules. ***The lateral mobility of integral proteins increases as the fluidity of the membrane increases.***

Membranes are Dynamic Structures

◈ *Harper 30th/481-82*

- **Membranes and their components are dynamic structures.** Membrane lipids and proteins undergo turnover
- Another indicator of the dynamic nature of membranes is that a variety of studies have shown that **lipids and certain proteins** exhibit ***lateral diffusion in the plane of their membranes.***
- Many nonmobile proteins do not exhibit lateral diffusion because they are anchored to the underlying actin cytoskeleton. By contrast, the ***transverse movement of lipids across the membrane*** **(flip-flop)** ***is extremely slow and does not appear to occur at an appreciable rate in the case of membrane proteins.***

"**Lateral diffusion** refers to the ***lateral movement of lipids and proteins found in the membrane.*** Membrane lipids and proteins are generally free to move laterally if they are not restricted by certain interactions. Lateral diffusion is a fairly quick and spontaneous process"

"**Transverse diffusion** or **flip-flop** involves the ***movement of a lipid or protein from one membrane surface to the other.*** Unlike lateral diffusion, transverse diffusion is a fairly slow process due to the fact that a relatively significant amount of energy is required for flip-flopping to occur. Most large proteins do not flip-flop due to their extensive polar regions, which are unfavorable in the hydrophobic core of a membrane bilayer. This allows the asymmetry of membranes to be retained for long periods, which is an important aspect of cell regulation"

IMMUNOGENETICS & MOLECULAR BIOLOGY

29. Ans. (c) Hydrogen bond

[Ref: Lippincott 6th/397-400; Harper 30th/381-86; Satyanarayana 4th/524-29]

"When DNA replicates, a ***helicase enzyme "unzips" the double helix, breaking the hydrogen bonds*** that hold it together in the center"- www.boundless.com/physics

"**Separation of the two DNA strands in the double helix:** ***The two strands of the double helix separate when hydrogen bonds between the paired bases are disrupted.*** Disruption can occur in the laboratory if the pH of the DNA solution is altered so that the nucleotide bases ionize, or if the solution is heated. [Note: ***Phosphodiester bonds are not broken by such treatment.***] ***Separation of the two strands over short regions occurs during both DNA and RNA synthesis***"- *Lippincott 6th/397-98*

DNA Structure

◈ *Lippincott 6th/396-98*

- **Phosphodiester bonds** join the 3'-hydroxyl group of the deoxy pentose of one nucleotide to the 5'-hydroxyl group of the deoxy pentose of an adjacent nucleotide through a phosphate group.
- Phosphodiester linkages between nucleotides (in DNA or RNA) can be cleaved hydrolytically by chemicals, or hydrolyzed enzymatically by a family of nucleases: deoxyribonucleases for DNA and ribonucleases for RNA. [Note: Only RNA is cleaved by alkali.]
- In the DNA helix, the **hydrophilic deoxyribose-phosphate backbone** of each chain is on the outside of the molecule, whereas the hydrophobic bases are stacked inside. The overall structure resembles a twisted ladder
- The ***base pairs*** are held together by **hydrogen bonds:** two between A and T and three between G and C. These hydrogen bonds, plus the hydrophobic interactions between the stacked bases, stabilize the structure of the double helix.

DNA Replication

◈ *serc.carleton.edu/microbelife*

- In general, DNA is replicated by uncoiling of the helix, ***strand separation by breaking of the hydrogen bonds between the complementary strands,*** and synthesis of two new strands by complementary base pairing.

- As the strands continue to unwind and separate in both directions around the entire DNA molecule, ***the hydrogen bonding of free DNA nucleotides with those on each parent strand produce new complementary strands.***
- As the new nucleotides line up opposite each parent strand by hydrogen bonding, enzymes called **DNA polymerases** ***join the nucleotides by way of phosphodiester bonds.***

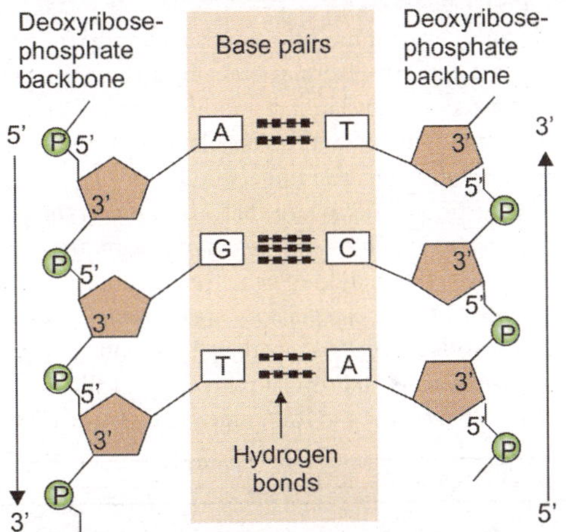

Fig: *(Lippincott 6th/397):* Two complementary DNA

Table *(Harper 30th/382):* **Classes of proteins involved in replication**

Protein	Function
DNA polymerases	Deoxynucleotide polymerization
Helicases	Processive unwinding of DNA
Topoisomerases	Relieve torsional strain that results from helicase-induced unwinding
DNA primase	Initiates synthesis of RNA primers
Single-strand binding proteins	Prevent premature reannealing of dsDNA
DNA ligase	Seals the single strand nick between the nascent chain and Okazaki fragments on lagging strand

Table *(Harper 30th/382):* **Steps Involved in DNA Replication in Eukaryotes**

- Identification of the origins of replication
- Unwinding (denaturation) of dsDNA to provide an ssDNA template
- Formation of the replication fork
- Initiation of DNA synthesis and elongation
- Formation of replication bubbles with ligation of the newly synthesized DNA segments
- Reconstitution of chromatin structure

30. Ans. (a) tRNA

[Ref: Harper 30th/394,411; Lippincott 6th/ 418]

*"tRNA molecule contain a high percentage of **unusual bases**, for example, **dihydrouracil** and have extensive intra-chain base pairing that leads to characteristic secondary and tertiary structure"- Lippincott 6th/ 418*

Transfer RNA

◈ *Lippincott 6th/ 418*

- tRNAs are the smallest (4S) of the three major types of RNA molecules. There is at least one specific type of tRNA molecule for each of the 20 amino acids commonly found in proteins. Together, tRNAs make up about 15% of the total RNA in the cell.
- ***The tRNA molecules contain a high percentage of unusual bases (for example, dihydro uracil)*** and have extensive intrachain base-pairing that leads to characteristic secondary and tertiary structure.

"**Transfer RNA** is unique among nucleic acids in its content of ***"unusual" bases***. An ***unusual base is any purine or pyrimidine ring except the usual A, G, C, and U*** from which all RNAs are synthesized. All other bases are produced by modification of one of the four bases after it has been incorporated into the polyribonucleotide chain.

"There are three distinct size species of ***rRNA (23S, 16S and 5S)***"*- Lippincott 6th/418*

31. Ans. (d) 5S RNA, (e) 23S RNA

[Ref: Lippincott 6th/436]

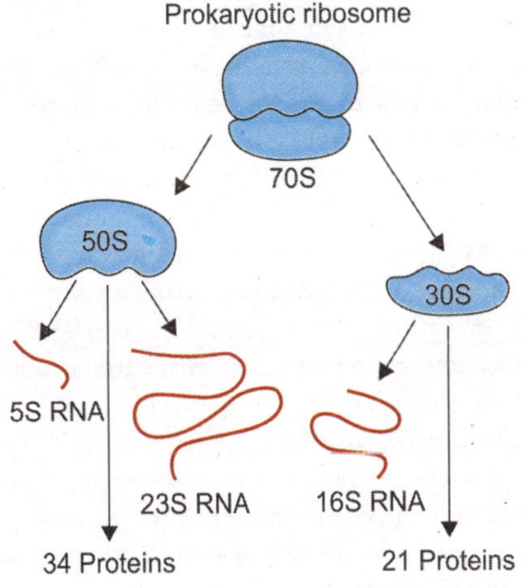

Fig: *(Lippincott 6th/436):* Ribosomal composition of prokaryotic ribosome

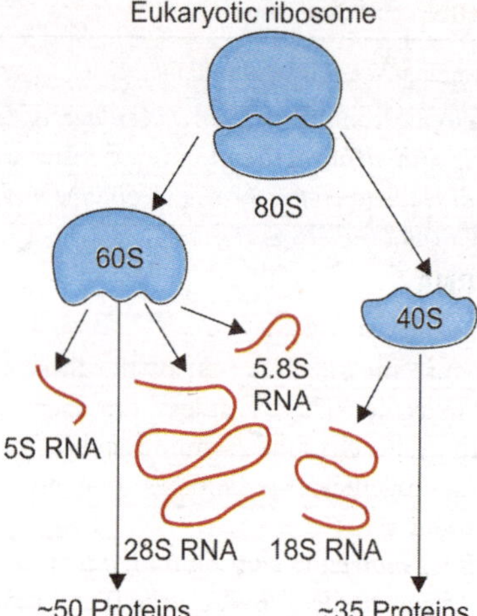

Fig: *(Lippincott 6th/436):* Ribosomal composition of eukaryotic ribosomal subunits varies somewhat from species to species.)

32. Ans. (a) Energy is required to displace the histone..., (b) Histone modifications by..., (d) Aberrations in ...

[Ref: Harper 30th/735, 438-39; Lippincott 6th/422, 460; Harrison 19th/102e-7]

Chromatin Remodeling

◈ *wikipedia*

- **Chromatin remodeling** is the dynamic modification of chromatin architecture to allow access of condensed genomic DNA to the regulatory transcription machinery proteins, and thereby control gene expression.
- Such remodeling is principally carried out by 1) ***covalent histone modifications by specific enzymes***, e.g., histone acetyltransferases (HATs), deacetylases, methyltransferases, and kinases, and 2) ***ATP-dependent chromatin remodeling complexes*** which either move, eject or restructure nucleosomes.
- Besides actively regulating gene expression, dynamic remodeling of chromatin imparts an epigenetic regulatory role in several key biological processes, egg cells DNA replication and repair; apoptosis; chromosome segregation as well as development and pluripotency.
- ***Aberrations in chromatin remodeling proteins*** are found to be associated with human diseases, including ***cancer.***
- Targeting chromatin remodeling pathways is currently evolving as a ***major therapeutic strategy in the treatment of several cancers***

Chromatin Remodelers

◈ *www.ncbi.nlm.nih.gov*

- In general, **two major mechanisms** exist which regulate chromatin accessibility: **First,** histones can be post-translationally modified enabling the recruitment of specific effector proteins to chromatin, thereby changing the activity state of chromatin domains.
- **Second,** specific chromatin remodeling complexes ***displace the histone octamers from DNA or translocate them onto neighboring DNA segments***, thereby exposing underlying DNA sequences to sequence specific regulatory factors. The ***ATP-dependent chromatin remodeling enzymes*** are highly abundant in the cell, with about one remodeling complex per 10 nucleosomes and also and remarkably diverse

Chromatin Remodeling is an Important Aspect of Eukaryotic Gene Expression

◈ *Harper 30th/437-38*

- Histone covalent modification is an important determinant of gene activity. Histones are subjected to a wide range of specific post-translational modifications. These modifications are dynamic and reversible. Histone ***acetylation and deacetylation*** are best understood.
- The surprising discovery that ***histone acetylase*** and other enzymatic activities are associated with the coregulators involved in regulation of gene transcription.
- Together then coregulators (***chromatin modifiers and chromatin remodellers***), working in conjunction, can open up gene promoters and regulatory regions, facilitating binding of other trans factors and RNA polymerase II and GTFs.

33. Ans. (a) DNA footprinting

[Ref: www.biotecharticles.com; www.biologyexams4u.com Lippincott 6th/473]

"**DNA footprinting**- An in-vitro technique ***to find out protein binding regions on a DNA molecule.*** The technique is also called as **DNAse I footprinting**. Thousands of proteins (enzymes) are interacting with DNA in the nucleus for regulating activities like replication, transcription, translation etc. The technique to find out this ***protein binding regions in DNA molecule is called DNA footprinting***"- *www.biologyexams4u.com*

DNA Footprinting

◈ *www.biotecharticles.com*

- It is a molecular technique used to identify the specific ***DNA sequence (binding site) that binds to a protein.***
- This technique mainly used to identify the transcription factors which bind to promoter, enhancer or silencer region of gene to regulate its expression. Therefore the regulation of transcript ion of a gene can be studied using this method.

Application of DNA Footprinting

◈ *www.biotecharticles.com*

- DNA footprinting can be used to ***determine the sequence specific DNA-binding protein site.***
- Interaction between protein and DNA can be studied using this technique both in-vivo and ex-vivo of a cell.
- Transcriptional regulations can be studied using DNA footprinting technique.
- Promoter, enhancer and silencer sequence of a gene can be identified
- Scientists and researchers can use this technique to identify the functional genes present in the large genome of human.

DNA Footprinting Procedure

◈ *www.biotecharticles.com*

- DNA fragment thought to contain protein binding sequence is extracted, amplified and labelled at one end of the double helix using polymerase chain reaction technique.

- Labelled DNA fragments with DNA binding protein and cleavage agent are mixed in a test tube.

Table *(Lippincott's 6th/473)*: **Techniques used to analyse DNA, RNA and proteins**

Technique	Sample Analysed	Gel Used	Purpose
Southern blot	*DNA*	Yes	Detect DNA changes
Northern blot	*RNA*	Yes	Measures mRNA amounts and size
Western blot	*Protein*	Yes	Measures protein amounts
ASO	*DN*	No	Detects *DNA mutations*
Microarray	*RNA or cDNA*	No	Measures many mRNA levels at once

PATHOLOGY

34. Ans. (a) Bone narrow biopsy necessary..., (b) Presence of BCR-ABL gene which directs..., (c) Dasatinib is used in imatinib resistant...

[Ref: Robbins 9th/616-18; Harrison 19th/687-92; Davidson 22nd/1039-40]

Chronic Myelogenous Leukemia

◈ *Davidson 22nd/1039-40*

- Splenomegaly is present in 90%; in about 10%, the enlargement is massive, extending to over 15 cm below the costal margin. Hepatomegaly occurs in about 50%. ***Lymphadenopathy is unusual.***
- ***Myeloblasts usually constitute less than 10% of all white cells.***
- ***Bone marrow should be obtained to confirm the diagnosis*** and phase of disease by morphology, chromosome analysis to demonstrate the presence of the Ph chromosome.
- ***Imatinib, dasatinib and nilotinib*** specifically inhibit BCR ABL tyrosine kinase activity and reduce the uncontrolled proliferation of white cells. They are recommended as first-line therapy in chronic-phase CML, producing complete cytogenetic response (disappearance of the Ph chromosome) in 76% at 18 months of therapy
- ***For those failing to respond or progress on imatinib***, options include second-generation tyrosine kinase inhibitors, such as ***dasatinib*** or nilotinib, allogeneic Transplantation of haematopoietic stem cells (HSCT), or classical cytotoxic drugs such as hydroxycarbamide (hydroxyurea) or interferon

Chronic Myelogenous Leukemia

◈ *Robbins 9th/616-18*

- CML is distinguished from other myeloproliferative disorders by the presence of a chimeric ***BCR-ABL gene*** derived from portions of the *BCR* gene on chromosome 22 and the *ABL* gene on chromosome 9.
- *BCR-ABL* directs the synthesis of a constitutively active ***BCR-ABL tyrosine kinase***
- ***Blasts usually make up less than 10% of the circulating cells.***

Chronic Myeloid Leukemia (CML)

◈ *Harrison 19th/687-89*

- The disease is ***driven by the BCR-ABL1 chimeric gene product, a constitutively active tyrosine kinase,***
- CML accounts for 15% of all cases of leukemia.
- There is a slight male preponderance (**male:** female ratio 1.6:1).
- The median age at diagnosis is 55–65 years.
- Untreated, the course of CML may be biphasic or triphasic, with an early indolent or chronic phase, followed often by an accelerated phase and a terminal blastic phase.
- In geographic locations where access to health care is more limited, patients often present with high CML burden including ***splenomegaly, anemia, and related symptoms (abdominal pain, weight loss, fatigue)***, as well as a higher frequency of high-risk CML.
- Most patients with CML (90%) present in the indolent or chronic phase.
- ***Common symptoms, when present, are manifestations of anemia and splenomegaly.***
- ***Splenomegaly is the most common physical finding, occurring in 20–70% of patients*** depending on health care screening frequency. Other less common findings include hepatomegaly (10–20%), ***lymphadenopathy (5–10%),*** and extramedullary disease (skin or subcutaneous lesions).
- The peripheral blood differential shows left-shifted hematopoiesis with predominance of neutrophils and the presence of bands, myelocytes, metamyelocytes, promyelocytes, and ***blasts (usually ≤5%).***
- Biochemical abnormalities include a low leukocyte alkaline phosphatase score and high levels of vitamin B12, uric acid, lactic dehydrogenase, and lysozyme.
- ***The bone marrow is hypercellular with marked myeloid hyperplasia and a high myeloid-to-erythroid ratio of 15–20:1. Marrow blasts are 5% or less; when higher***, they carry a worse prognosis or represent acceleration (if they are ≥15%).

Table *(Harrison 19th/689)*: **Presenting signs and symptoms of newly diagnosed Philadelphia chromosome– Positive chronic myeloid Leukemia in chronic phase**

Parameter	Percentage
Age≥ 60 years (median)	18 (46)
Female gender	35–45
Splenomegaly	30
Hepatomegaly	5
Lymphadenopathy	5
Other extramedullary disease	2

Contd...

Parameter	Percentage
Hemoglobin <10 g/dL	10-15
Platelets >450 × 10^9 cells/L <100 × 10^9 cells/L	 30–35 3–5
White blood cells ≥50 × 10^9 cells/L	35–40
Marrow ≥5% blasts ≥5% basophils	 5 10×15
Peripheral blood ≥3% blasts ≥7% basophils	 8–10 10
Cytogenetic clonal evolution other than the Philadelphia chromosome	4–5
Sokal risk Low Intermediate High	 60–65 25–30 10

35. Ans. (a) Occurs due CFTR gene mutation on chromosome 7, (c) CFTR gene can be detected antenataly, (d) Poor body growth

[Ref: Robbins 9th/466-71;Harrison 19th/ 1697-1700; Davidson 22nd/680-85]

*"Patients with cystic fibrosis are often malnourished with **low body mass index**"-CMDT 2016/266*

Cystic Fibrosis

◈ *Robbins 9th/466-71*

- **The primary defect in cystic fibrosis results from abnormal function of an epithelial chloride channel protein encoded by the cystic fibrosis transmembrane conductance regulator (CFTR) gene on chromosome 7q31.2.**
- Approximately 5% to 10% of the cases come to clinical attention at birth or soon after because of *meconium ileus.*
- Sequencing the *CFTR* gene is the gold standard for diagnosis of cystic fibrosis. Therefore, in patients with suggestive clinical findings or family history (or both), ***genetic analysis may be warranted.***

Cystic Fibrosis

◈ *Harrison 19th/ 1697-1700*

- The diagnosis of CF is based in part on clinical symptoms, family history, or positive newborn screening. *CFTR* mutation analysis together with sweat electrolyte measurements represent cardinal diagnostic tests.
- "The most common mutation in the CFTR gene (~70% of CF chromosomes) is a 3-bp deletion (a class II mutation) that results in an absence of phenylalanine at amino acid position 508 (ΔF508) of the CF gene protein product, known as cystic fibrosis transmembrane conductance regulator (CFTR)"-*Harrison 19th/1697*
- Contents of the intestinal lumen are often difficult to excrete, leading to ***meconium ileus (a presentation in approximately 10–20% of newborns with CF)*** or distal intestinal obstructive syndrome in older individuals.

Cystic Fibrosis

◈ *Davidson 22nd/680-85*

- CF is the result of mutations affecting a gene on the long arm of chromosome 7
- ***Neonatal screening*** for CF using immunoreactive trypsin and genetic testing of newborn blood samples is now routine in the UK, and should reduce delayed diagnosis and improve outcomes
- Prenatal screening by amniocentesis may be offered to those known to be at high risk.

Table *(Robbins 9th/470):* **Clinical features of cystic fibrosis**

- ***Chronic sinopulmonary disease*** manifested by
  - Persistent colonization/infection with typical cystic fibrosis *pathogens, including Staphylococcus aureus, nontypeable Hemophilus influenzae*, mucoid and nonmucoid *Pseudomonas aeruginosa, Burkholderia cepacia*
  - Chronic cough and sputum production
  - Persistent chest radiograph abnormalities (e.g., bronchiectasis, atelectasis, infiltrates, hyperinflation)
  - Airway obstruction manifested by wheezing and air trapping
  - Nasal polyps; radiographic or computed tomographic abnormalities of paranasal sinuses
  - Digital clubbing
- ***Gastrointestinal and nutritional abnormalities***, including
  - **Intestinal:** meconium ileus, distal intestinal obstruction syndrome, rectal prolapsed
  - **Pancreatic:** pancreatic insufficiency, recurrent pancreatitis
  - **Hepatic:** chronic hepatic disease manifested by clinical or histologic evidence of focal biliary cirrhosis, or multilobular cirrhosis
  - **Nutritional:** ***failure to thrive*** (protein-calorie malnutrition), hypoproteinemia, edema, complications secondary to fat-soluble vitamin deficiency
- **Salt-loss syndromes:** *acute salt depletion, chronic metabolic acidosis*
- ***Male urogenital abnormalities*** *resulting in obstructive azoospermia (congenital bilateral absence of vas deferens)*

36. Ans. (a) Caspases initiate apoptosis by extrinsic and intrinsic pathway (b) Caspases are protease enzyme

[Ref: Robbins 9th/52-57;Harrison 19th/3726-26]

Mechanisms of Apoptosis

◈ *Robbins 9th/53*

- **Apoptosis results from the activation of enzymes called *caspases* (so named because they are cysteine proteases that cleave proteins after aspartic residues).** Like many proteases, caspases exist as inactive proenzymes, or zymogens, and must undergo ***enzymatic cleavage to become active.*** The presence of cleaved, active caspases is a marker for cells undergoing apoptosis.
- The process of apoptosis may be divided into an *initiation phase,* during which some caspases become catalytically active, and an *execution phase,* during which other caspases trigger the degradation of critical cellular components.

- The activation of caspases depends on a finely tuned balance between production of pro-apoptotic and anti-apoptotic proteins.
- **Two distinct pathways converge on caspase activation: the mitochondrial pathway and the death receptor pathway**.
- "Apoptosis: ***Characterized by enzymatic degradation of proteins*** and DNA, initiated by caspases; and by recognition and removal of dead cells by phagocytes"- *Robbins 9th/58*
- *"The* **fundamental event in apoptosis** *is the activation of enzymes called Caspases which are cystein proteases involved in apoptosis by initiating apoptotic signals (via intrinsic or extrinsic pathway) and executing apoptotic program (via execution phase)"*

"Caspases are a family of ***endoproteases*** that provide critical links in cell regulatory networks controlling inflammation and cell death. The ***activation of these enzymes*** is tightly controlled by their production as inactive zymogens that gain catalytic activity following signaling events promoting their aggregation into dimers or macromolecular complexes"-*www.cshperspectives.cshlp.org*

37. Ans. (c) High dose steroids results in remission in most cases, (e) Reversible loss of podocyte function

[Ref: Robbins 9th/917-18; Harrison 19th/1842-43; CMDT 2016/928; O.P. Ghai 8th/477-78; Nelson (SAE) 20th/2521-26]

Minimal-Change Disease

◈ *Robbins 9th/917-18*

- This relatively benign disorder is characterized by ***diffuse effacement of foot processes of visceral epithelial cells (podocytes)***, detectable only by electron microscopy, in glomeruli that appear virtually normal by light microscopy.
- It is the ***most frequent cause of nephrotic syndrome in children, but it is less common in adults***
- **The principal lesion is in the visceral epithelial cells, which show a uniform and diffuse effacement of foot processes,** these being reduced to a rim of cytoplasm with loss of recognizable intervening slit diaphragms. This change, often incorrectly termed "fusion" of foot processes, actually represents simplification of the epithelial cell architecture with flattening, retraction, and swelling of foot processes. The ***visceral epithelial changes are completely reversible after corticosteroid therapy***, concomitant with remission of the proteinuria.
- Despite massive proteinuria, ***renal function remains good,*** and there is ***commonly no hypertension*** or hematuria. The proteinuria usually is highly selective, most of the protein consisting of albumin.
- ***Most children (more than 90%) with minimal change disease respond rapidly to corticosteroid therapy***. However, the nephrotic phase may recur, and some patients may become steroid dependent or resistant. Nevertheless, the ***long-term prognosis for patients is excellent, and even steroid-dependent disease resolves when children reach puberty. Although adults are slower to respond, the long-term prognosis is also excellent.***

Minimal Change Disease

◈ *Harrison 19th/1842-43*

- Minimal change disease (MCD), sometimes known as *nil lesion,* causes ***70–90% of nephrotic syndrome in childhood but only 10–15% of nephrotic syndrome in adults.***
- Focal segmental glomerulosclerosis (FSGS) represents up to ***one-third of cases of nephrotic syndrome in adults***
- Membranous glomerulonephritis (MGN) accounts for ***approximately 30% of cases of nephrotic syndrome in adults***. It is rare in childhood and the most common cause of nephrotic syndrome in the elderly.
- "Minimal change disease ***can rarely cause acute renal failure*** due to tubular changes and interstitial edema" - *CMDT 2016/928*
- Less common clinical features include ***hypertension (30% in children, 50% in adults),*** microscopic hematuria (20% in children, 33% in adults), atopy or allergic symptoms (40% in children, 30% in adults), and decreased renal function (<5% in children, 30% in adults).
- The appearance of ***acute renal failure*** in adults is often seen more commonly in patients with low serum albumin and intrarenal edema (nephrosarca) that is responsive to intravenous albumin and diuretics. This presentation must be distinguished from acute renal failure secondary to hypovolemia
- ***Ninety to 95% of children will develop a complete remission after 8 weeks of steroid therapy***, and ***80–85% of adults will achieve complete remission***, but only after a longer course of 20–24 weeks.

Minimal Change NS

◈ *Nelson (SAE) 20th/2523–24*

- More than 95% of children with minimal change disease respond to corticosteroid therapy
- "Important features are absence of hypertension and gross hematuria (the so called nephritic feature)

Table *(Nelson 20th/2523)*: **Minimal change nephrotic syndrome**

Clinical Manifestations	
Age (Yr)	2–6, some adults
Sex	2:1 male
Nephrotic syndrome	100%
Asymptomatic proteinuria	0
Hematuria	10–20%
Hypertension	10%
Rate of progression to renal failure	Does not progress
Renal Pathology	
Light microscopy	Normal
Immunofluorescence	Negative
Electron microscopy	Foot process fusion
Response to steroids	90%

A & E

38. Ans. (a) Renal enlargement (c) Spider leg deformity on intravenous..., (d) Ultrasound shows multiple cysts

[Ref: Robbins 9th/945-47; L & B 26th/1284-85; Manipal Surgery 4th/934; Harrison 19th/1851-52]

"**Intravenous urography** *of polycystic kidney disease: The* ***spider leg deformity of the calyces***"*-Manipal Surgery* 4th*/934*

Clinical Manifestations

◈ *Harrison 19th/1851-52*

- ADPKD is characterized by the progressive ***bilateral formation of renal cysts.***
- ***Enlarged kidneys*** can each reach a fourfold increase in length and weigh up to 20 times the normal weight
- Although many patients are asymptomatic until the fourth to fifth decade of life and are diagnosed by incidental discoveries of hypertension or abdominal masses, back or flank pain is a frequent symptom in ~60% of patients with ADPKD.
- The pain may result from renal cyst infection, hemorrhage, or nephrolithiasis.
- Gross hematuria resulting from cyst rupture occurs in ~40% of patients during the course of their disease, and many of them will have recurrent episodes.
- Liver cysts derived from the biliary epithelia are the most common extrarenal complication

Autosomal-Dominant (Adult) Polycystic Kidney Disease (ADPKD)

◈ *Robbins 9th/945-47*

- It is a hereditary disorder characterized by ***multiple expanding cysts of both kidneys*** that ultimately destroy the renal parenchyma and cause renal failure.
- The disease is ***universally bilateral***; reported unilateral cases probably ***represent multicystic dysplasia.*** The cysts initially involve only portions of the nephrons, so renal function is retained until about the fourth or fifth decade of life.
- In gross appearance, the ***kidneys are bilaterally enlarged and may achieve enormous sizes***; weights as much as 4 kg for each kidney have been reported. The external surface appears to be composed solely of a mass of cysts, up to 3 to 4 cm in diameter, with no intervening parenchyma

Table *(Robbins 9th/945):* ***Summary of renal cystic diseases***

	Inheritance	Pathologic Features	Clinical Features or Complications	Typical Outcome
Adult polycystic kidney disease	Autosomal dominant	Large multicystic kidneys, liver cysts, berry aneurysms	Hematuria, flank pain, urinary tract infection, renal stones, hypertension	Chronic renal failure beginning at age 40–60 yr
Childhood polycystic kidney disease	Autosomal recessive	Enlarged, cystic kidneys at birth	Hepatic fibrosis	Variable, death in infancy or childhood

39. Ans. a. Creutzfeldt–Jakob..., b. Bovine spongiform..., c. Huntington disease, d. Alzheimer disease, e. Parkinson disease

[Ref: Robbins 9th/1281,1286-1300; www.nature.com]

"In medicine, **proteopathy** refers to a class of diseases in which ***certain proteins become structurally abnormal, and thereby disrupt the function of cells***, tissues and organsof the body. Often the proteins fail to fold into their normal configuration; in this misfolded state, the proteins can become toxic in some way (a gain of toxic function) or they can lose their normal function. The proteopathies (also known as **proteinopathies, protein conformational disorders**, or **protein misfolding diseases**) include such diseases as ***Creutzfeldt–Jakob disease, Alzheimer's disease, Parkinson's disease, prion disease, amyloidosis, and a wide range of other disorders***"-wikipedia

"**Misfolded Proteins and Neurodegenerative Diseases:** Accumulation of misfolded proteins can cause disease, and unfortunately some of these diseases, known as amyloid diseases, are very common. The most prevalent one is Alzheimer's disease, Parkinson's disease and Huntington's disease have similar amyloid origins"- *www.nature.com*

Neurodegenerative diseases: The pathological process that is common across most of the neurodegenerative diseases is the ***accumulation of protein aggregates***, which can be used as a morphological hallmark of the disease (hence the occasional use of term '***proteinopathy***')"- *Robbins 9th/1285*

Table *(Robbins 9th/1287):* **Features of the Major Neurodegenerative Diseases**

Disease	Clinical pattern	Inclusions
Alzheimer disease (AD)	Dementia	Aβ (plaques) Tau (tangles)
Frontotemporal lobar degeneration (FTLD)	Behavioral changes, language disturbance	Tau, TDP-43, FUS
Parkinson disease (PD)	Hypokinetic movement disorder	α-synuclein Tau
Progressive supranuclear palsy (PSP	Parkinsonism with abnormal eye movements	Tau

Contd...

Disease	Clinical pattern	Inclusions
Corticobasal degeneration (CBD)	Parkinsonism with asymmetric movement disorder	Tau
Multiple system atrophy (MSA)	Parkinsonism, cerebellar ataxia, autonomic failure	α- synuclein
Huntington disease (HD)	Hyperkinetic movement disorder	Huntington (polyglutamine)
Spinocerebellar ataxias (SCA1, 2, 3, 7, 17 and DRPLA)	Cerebellar ataxia	Various proteins (prolyglutamine containing)
Amyotrophic lateral sclerosis (ALS)	Weakness with upper and lower motor neurons signs	SOD1 TDP-43 FUS
Spinal bulbar muscular atrophy (SBMA)	Lower motor neuron weakness, diminished androgen	Androgen receptor (polyglutamine containing)

Prion Diseases

◈ *Robbins 9th/1281*

- **Prions are abnormal forms of a cellular protein that cause rapidly progressive neurodegenerative disorders that may be sporadic, familial or transmitted.** This group of diseases includes ***Creutzfeldt-Jakob disease, Gerstmann-Sträussler-Scheinker syndrome, fatal familial insomnia, and kuru in humans; scrapie in sheep and goats; mink-transmissible encephalopathy; chronic wasting disease of deer and elk; and bovine spongiform encephalopathy.***
- *Pathogenesis and Molecular Genetics.* Prion diseases are conceptually important because they exemplify degenerative disorders that are caused by "spreading" of ***misfolded proteins***, a remarkable phenomenon that allows a pathogenic protein to acquire many of the characteristics of an infectious organism

40. Ans. (b) Spongiform swelling in cerebral cortex, (c) Brain atrophy in late.., (d) Slow and irregular background...

[Ref: Robbins 9th/1282; Kaplon and Saddock's synopsis of Psychiatry 11th/730; Harshmohan 7th/870]

Spongiform Encephalopathy (Creutzfeldt-Jakob Disease

◈ *Harshmohan 7th/870*

- Grossly, the changes are too rapid to become noticeable but ***brain atrophy may be seen in long-standing cases***
- ***Microscopically, the hallmark is spongiform change.*** These changes are predominantly seen in the cortex and other grey matter areas.

Creutzfeldt-Jakob Disease (CJD)

◈ *Kaplon and Saddock's 11th/730*

- Diagnosis requires pathological examination of the cortex, which reveals the classic triad of ***spongiform vacuolation, loss of neurons, and astrocyte cell proliferation***. The ***cortex and basal ganglia are most affected.***
- Although not specific for CJD, **EEG abnormalities** are present in nearly all patients, ***consisting of a slow and irregular background rhythm with periodic complex discharges***.
- Computed tomography (CT) and MRI studies may reveal ***cortical atrophy*** later in the course of disease.

Creutzfeldt-Jakob Disease (CJD)

◈ *Robbins 9th/1282*

- Although the most common prion disease, CJD is a rare disorder that manifests clinically as a rapidly progressive dementia.
- The disease has a peak incidence in the seventh decade.
- The clinical picture is usually typical, with the initial subtle changes in memory and behavior followed by a rapidly progressive dementia, often with pronounced involuntary jerking muscle contractions on sudden stimulation (startle myoclonus).
- Signs of cerebellar dysfunction, usually manifested as ataxia, are present in a minority of patients. The disease is uniformly fatal, with an average duration of only 7 months, although a few patients have survived for several years. These cases exhibit extensive atrophy of involved gray matter.
- The progression of the dementia in CJD is usually so rapid that there is ***little if any grossly evident brain atrophy***.
- The pathognomonic finding is a **spongiform** transformation of the ***cerebral cortex*** and, often, deep gray matter structures (caudate, putamen); this multifocal process results in the uneven formation of small, apparently empty, microscopic vacuoles of varying sizes within the neuropile and sometimes in the perikaryon of neurons.
- In advanced cases there is severe neuronal loss, ***reactive gliosis***, and sometimes expansion of the vacuolated areas into cystlike spaces ("***status spongiosus***").
- Inflammation is notably absent.

41. Ans. (a) Endometrial cancer, (c) Ovarian cancer

[Ref: Robbins 9th/810; Davidson 22nd/267; Harriosn 19th/538]

Table *(Davidson 22nd)/267*

Syndrome	Malignancies	Inheritance	Gene
Hereditary non-polyposis colon cancer (HNPCC)	Colonic, endometrial, ovarian, pancreatic, gastric	*AD*	AD *MSH2, MLH1, MSH6, PMS1, PMS2*

Hereditary Non-Polyposis Colorectal Cancer

◈ *Robbins 9th/810*

- Hereditary non-polyposis colorectal cancer (HNPCC), also known as Lynch syndrome, was originally described based on familial clustering of cancers at several sites including the ***colorectum, endometrium, stomach, ovary, ureters, brain, small bowel, hepatobiliary tract, pancreas, and skin***
- HNPCC is thought to account for 2% to 4% of all colorectal cancers, making it the most common syndromic form of colon cancer.
- **HNPCC is caused by inherited mutations in genes that encode proteins responsible for the detection, excision, and repair of errors that occur during DNA replication.**

Table *(Harrison 19th/538)*: **Hereditable (Autosomal Dominant) Gastrointestinal Polyposis Syndromes**

Syndrome	Distribution of Polyps	Histologic Type	Malignant Potential	Associated Lesions
Nonpolyposis syndrome (Lynch syndrome)	Large intestine (often proximal)	Adenoma	Common	Endometrial and ovarian tumors (most frequently); gastric, genitourinary, pancreatic, biliary cancers (less frequently)
Peutz-Jeghers syndrome	Small and large intestines, stomach	Hamartoma	Rare	Mucocutaneous pigmentation; tumors of the ovary, breast, pancreas, endometrium

42. Ans. (b) Present on undersurface of valve, (d) May occur after post-cardiac..., (e) Source of systemic emboli

[Ref: Robbins 9th/561-62; Harshmohan 7th/425]

Vegetation of NBTE is small and loosely attached to the underlying valve

Nonbacterial Thrombotic Endocarditis (NBTE)

◈ *Robbins 9th/561-62*

- **NBTE is characterized by the deposition of small sterile thrombi on the leaflets of the cardiac valves.**
- The lesions are 1 to 5 mm in size, and ***occur as single or multiple vegetations along the line of closure of the leaflets or cusps.***
- Histologically, they ***comprise bland thrombi*** that are ***loosely attached to the underlying valve***; the vegetations are not invasive and do not elicit any inflammatory reaction. Thus, although the local effect of the vegetations is usually trivial, they can be the ***source of systemic emboli that produce significant infarcts in the brain, heart, or elsewhere.***
- NBTE is often encountered in debilitated patients, such as those with cancer or sepsis—hence the previous term *marantic endocarditis* (root word *marasmus*, relating to malnutrition).
- It frequently occurs concomitantly with ***deep venous thromboses,*** pulmonary emboli, or other findings suggesting an underlying systemic hypercoagulable state.
- ***Endocardial trauma, as from an indwelling catheter, is another well-recognized predisposing condition***, and right-sided valvular and endocardial thrombotic lesions frequently track along the course of pulmonary artery catheters.

Nonbacterial Thrombotic Endocarditis (NBTE)

◈ *Harshmohan 7th/425*

- **These verrucae are typically small (1 to 5 mm in diameter), single or multiple, brownish and occur along the line of closure of the leaflet but more friable than the vegetations of RHD**
- **Embolic phenomenon is seen in many cases of NBTE and result in infarcts in the brain, lungs, spleen and kidneys**

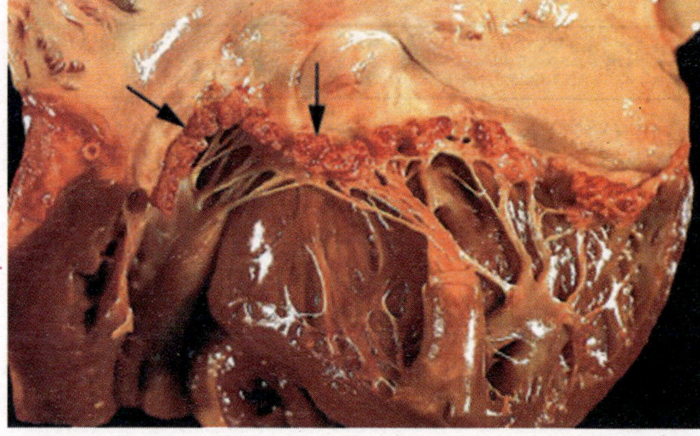

Fig: *(Robbins 9th/561)* Nonbacterial thrombotic endocarditis (NBTE). Nearly complete row of thrombotic vegetations along the line of closure of the mitral valve leaflets *(arrows)*.

43. Ans. (a) Most common cause of dementia in..., (b) Unusual before 45 years of age, (d) May have family history

[Ref: Robbins 9th/1287-92; Harrison 19th/2598-2602; Harshmohan 7th/876-77; CMDT 2016/1003; Niraj Ahuja 6th/26; Kaplan and Saddok's Synopsis of Psychiatry 11th/ 705-06]

Alzheimer Disease

◈ *Kaplan and Saddok's 11th/ 705-06*

- Some studies have indicated that as many as ***40 percent of patients have a family history of dementia of the Alzheimer's type***; thus, genetic factors are presumed to play a part in the development of the disorder, at least in some cases.
- Additional support for a **genetic influence** is the concordance rate for ***monozygotic twins***, which is higher than the rate for dizygotic twins (43 percent vs. 8 percent, respectively). In several well-documented cases, the disorder has been transmitted in families through an ***autosomal dominant gene***, although such transmission is rare. Alzheimer's type dementia has shown linkage to chromosomes 1, 14, and 21.
- Of all patients with dementia, ***50 to 60 percent have the most common type of dementia, dementia of the Alzheimer's type (Alzheimer's disease).***
- ***Dementia of the Alzheimer's type increases in prevalence with increasing age.***

"**Alzheimer disease:** The key clinical feature is ***impairment of the ability to remember new information.*** Hence, patients present with gradual impairment of memory, usually in association with disorders of other cortical functions. ***Short-term and long-term memory are both affected, but the defects in former are usually more obvious*** *(Davidson 22nd/252)*

"Alzheimer disease (AD):***Short-term memory impairment is early and prominent in most cases***." *(CMDT 2016/1003)*

"Alzheimer disease (AD) is the ***most common cause of dementia in the elderly***" *(Robbins 9th/1287)*

"Macroscopic examination of the brain shows a variable degree of **cortical atrophy** with widening of the cerebral sulci that is most pronounced in the ***frontal, temporal, and parietal lobes.*** With significant atrophy, there is compensatory ventricular enlargement (hydrocephalus ex vacuo) secondary to loss of parenchyma. The major microscopic abnormalities of Alzheimer disease are **neuritic (senile) plaques, neurofibrillary tangles, and amyloid angiopathy"** *(Robbins 9th/1288)*

"Approximately 10% of all persons over the age of 70 years have significant memory loss, and in more than half, the cause is Alzheimer's disease (AD). ***AD can manifest as young as the third decade, but it is the most common cause of dementia in the elderly"*** *- Harrison 19th/2598-2602*

Table *(CMDT 2016/1003)*: **Common Causes of Age-related Dementia**

Disorder	Pathology	Clinical Features
Alzheimer disease	***Plaques containing beta-amyloid peptide, and neurofibrillary tangles containing tau*** protein, occur throughout the neocortex	Most common age-related neurodegenerative disease; incidence doubles every 5 years after age 60 Short-term memory impairment is early and prominent in most cases Uriable deficits of executive function, visuospatial function, and language

44. Ans. (a) Hippocampus, (d) Cerebellum

[Ref: Robbins 9th/1277; Ananthanarayan 9th/531;Harshmohan 7th/178]

*"Rabies: Intracytoplasmic inclusion bodies (**Negri bodies**) can be demonstrated in the brain of animals dying of street virus infection. Negri bodies are composed of a finely fibrillar matrix and rabies virus particles and are most abundant in the **cerebellum and hippocampus**"-Ananthanarayan 9th/531*

"External examination of the brain shows intense edema and vascular congestion. On microscopic examination, there is widespread neuronal degeneration and an inflammatory reaction that is most severe in the rhombencephalon (midbrain, and floor of the fourth ventricle, particularly in the medulla). The basal ganglia, spinal cord, and dorsal root ganglia may also be involved. **Negri bodies**, the pathognomonic microscopic finding, are cytoplasmic, round to oval, eosinophilic inclusions that can be found in pyramidal neurons of the ***hippocampus and Purkinje cells of the cerebellum,*** sites usually devoid of inflammation. The presence of rabies virus can be detected within Negri bodies by ultrastructural and immunohistochemical examination"*- Robbins 9th/1277*

45. Ans. (a) Has tyrosine..., (b) Has pro-apoptotic..., (c) Tumour suppressor...

[Ref: Robbins 9th/293-95; Harshmohan 7th/206-07]

"P53 gene(TP53): Two major function of p53 in normal cell cycle are: (1) In blocking mitotic activity and (2) In promoting apoptosis"*- Harshmohan 7th/206*

Tp53 (Guardian of the Genome)

◈ *Robbins 9th/293-95*

- ***TP53*, a tumor suppressor gene that regulates cell cycle progression, DNA repair, cellular senescence, and apoptosis, is the most frequently mutated gene in human cancers.**
- Loss-of-function mutations in *TP53*, located on chromosome 17p13.1, are found in more than 50% of cancers.
- Moreover, *TP53* mutations occur with some frequency in virtually every type of cancer, including carcinomas of the lung, colon, and breast—the three leading causes of cancer death.
- **Once activated, p53 thwarts neoplastic transformation by inducing either transient cell cycle arrest, senescence (permanent cell cycle arrest), or programmed cell death (apoptosis).**
- The key target genes that execute the functions of p53 are not completely defined, but appear to fall into three major categories: (1) ***those that cause cell cycle arrest***; (2) ***those that cause apoptosis***; and (3) *those that enhance catabolic metabolism or inhibit anabolic metabolism.*

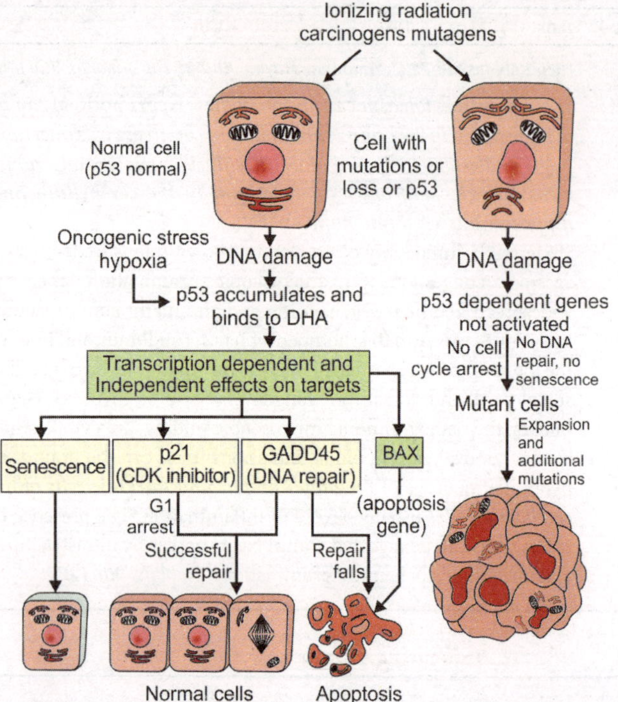

Fig: *(Robbins 9th/295):* The role of p53 in maintaining the integrity of the genome.

- **p53-induced apoptosis.** Apoptosis of cells with irreversible DNA damage is the ultimate protective mechanism against neoplastic transformation. p53 directs the transcription of several pro-apoptotic genes such as *BAX* and *PUMA* , which are believed to tip the balance in favor of cell death via the intrinsic (mitochondrial) pathway.

46. Ans. (b) Shares many clinical features of giant cell arteritis if involves aorta, (d) Granulomatous vasculitis, (e) Also called pulseless disease

[Ref: Robbins 9th/508-09; Harshmohan 7th/384; Harrison 19th/2189-90; Davidson 22nd/1116]

"**Giant cell arteritis (GCA)** is a ***granulomatous arteritis*** that predominantly affects medium-sized arteries in the head and neck"- *Davidson 22nd/1117*

"Takayasu arteritis (**Pulseless disease**): The disease affects ***chiefly young women***"-*Harshmohan 7th/384*

Takayasu's Disease

◈ *Davidson 22nd/1116*

- It ***predominantly affects the aorta***, its major branches and occasionally the pulmonary arteries.
- The typical age at onset is between 25 and 30 years, with an ***8: 1 female preponderance***.
- Clinical examination may reveal ***loss of pulses***, bruits, hypertension and aortic incompetence

Takayasu Arteritis

◈ *Robbins 9th/508-09*

- Takayasu arteritis is a ***granulomatous vasculitis*** of ***medium sized and larger arteries*** *characterized principally by ocular disturbances and marked weakening of the pulses in the upper extremities* (hence the alternate name, *pulseless disease*).
- This disorder manifests with *transmural scarring and thickening of the aorta—particularly the aortic arch and great vessels—with severe luminal narrowing of the major branch vessels.*
- ***Aortic lesions share many of the clinical and histologic features of giant cell aortitis***. Indeed, the distinction between the two entities is made largely on the basis of a patient's age; those older than 50 years are designated giant cell aortitis, and those younger than 50 years, Takayasu aortitis.
- Pulmonary arteries are involved in 50% of patients, and renal and coronary arteries also can be affected.
- The histologic picture encompasses a spectrum ranging from adventitial mononuclear infiltrates and perivascular cuffing of the vasa vasorum, to intense transmural mononuclear inflammation, to ***granulomatous inflammation***, replete with giant cells and patchy medial necrosis.
- **Clinical Features of Takayasu Aortitis**: Initial signs and symptoms usually are nonspecific, including fatigue, weight loss, and fever. With progression, vascular signs and symptoms appear and dominate the clinical picture. These include reduced upper extremity blood pressure and pulse strength; neurologic deficits; and ocular disturbances, including visual field defects, retinal hemorrhages, and total blindness.

47. Ans. a. Breast cancer, b. Thyroid cancer, c. Wilm's tumour, d. Retinoblastoma & e. Prostate cancer

[Ref: Davidson 22nd/267; Harrison 19th/ 101e-2; Robbins 9th/279; Harshmohan 7th/198]

Genetic Factors

◈ *Davidson 22nd/267*

- A number of ***inherited cancer syndromes*** are recognized that account for 5–10% of all cancers.
- In general they result from inherited mutations in genes that regulate cell growth, cell death and apoptosis. Examples include the *BRCA1*, *BRCA2* and *AT* (ataxia telangiectasia) genes that cause breast and some other cancers, the *FAP* gene that causes bowel cancer, and the ***Rb gene that causes retinoblastoma.***
- Although carriers of these gene mutations have a greatly elevated risk of cancer, none has 100% penetrance and additional modulating factors, both genetic and environmental, are likely to be operative. Exploration of a possible genetic contribution is a key part of cancer management, especially with regard to ascertaining the risk for an affected patient's offspring.

Table *(Davidson 22nd/267)*: **Inherited cancer predisposition syndromes**

Syndrome	Malignancies	Inheritance	Gene
Ataxia telangiectasia	Leukaemia, lymphoma, ovarian, gastric, brain, colon	AR	AT
Breast/ovarian	***Breast,*** ovarian, colonic, prostatic, pancreatic	AD	BRCA1, BRCA2
Bloom's syndrome	Leukaemia, tongue, oesophageal, coloni, wilms' tumour	AR	BLM
Cowden's syndrome	Breast, ***thyroid,*** gastrointestinal tract, pancreatic	AD	PTEN
Familial adenomatous polyposis	Colonic, upper gastronintestinal tract	AD	APC, MUTYH
Fanconi anaemia	Leukamie, oesophageal, skin, hepatoma	AR	FACA, FACC, FACD
Gorlin's syndrome	Basal cell skin, brain	AD	PTCH
Hereditary non-polyposis colon cancer (HNPCC)	Colonic, endometrial, ovarian, pancreatic, gastric	AD	MSH2, MLH1, MSH6, PMS1, PMS2
Li-Fraumeni syndrome	Sarcoma, ***breast,*** osteosarcoma, leukaemia, glioma, adrenocortical	AD	TP53
Melanoma	Melanoma	AD	CDK2 (TP16)
Multiple endocrine neoplasia (MEN)-1	Pancreatic, islet cell, pituitary adenoma, parathyroid adenoma and hyperplasia	AD	MEN1
MEN-2	Medullary thyroid, phaeochromocytoma, parathyroid hyperplasia	AD	RET
Neurofibromatosis 1	Neurofibrosarcoma, phaeocytoma, optic glioma	AD	NF1
Neurofibromatosis 2	Vestibular schwannoma	AD	NF2
Papillary renal cell cancer syndrome	Renal cell cancer	AD	MET
Peutz-Jeghers syndrome	Colonic, ileal, breast, ovarian	AD	STK11
Prostate cancer	Prostate	AD	HPC1
Retinoblastoma	Retinoblastoma, osteosarcoma	AD	RB1
Von Hippel–Lindau syndrome	Haemangioblastoma of retina and CNS, renal cell, phaeochromocytoma	AD	VHL
Wilms' tumour	Nephroblastoma, neuroblastoma, hepatoblastoma, rhabdomyosarcoma	AD	WT1
Xeroderma pigmentosum	Skin leukaemia, melanoma	AR	XPA, XPC, XPD (ERCC2) XPF

Table *(Harrison 19th/ 101e-2)*: **Common oncogenes altered in human cancers**

Oncogene	Function	Alteration in cancer	Neoplasm
AKT1	Serine/threonine kinase	Amplification	Stomach
AKT2	Serine/threonine kinase	Amplification	Ovarian, breast, pancreatic
BRAF	Serine/threonine kinase	Point mutation	Melanoma, lung, colorectal
CDK4	Cyclin-dependent kinase	Point mutation, amplification	Breast, melanoma, myeloma, others
CTNNB1	Signal transduction	Point mutation	Colon, prostate, melanoma, skin, others
FOS	Transcription factor	Overexpression	Osteosarcomas
FRBB2	Receptor tyrosine kinase	Point mutation, amplification	Breast, ovary, stomach, neuroblastoma
JUN	Transcription factor	Overexpression	Lung
MET	Receptor tyrosine kinase	Point mutation, rearrangement	Osteocarcinoma, kidney, glioma
MYB	Transcription factor	Amplification	ANL, CML, colorectal, melanoma
C-MYC	Transcription factor	Amplification	Breast, colon, gastric, lung
L-MYC	Transcription factor	Amplification	Lung, bladder

Contd...

Oncogene	Function	Alteration in cancer	Neoplasm
N-MYC	Transcription factor	Amplification	Neuroblastoma, lung
PIK3A	Phosphoinosital-3-kinase	Point Mutation	Multiple cancers
HRAS	GTPase	Point mutation	Colon, lung, pancreas
KRAS	GTPase	Point mutation	Melanoma, colorectal, AML
NRAS	GTPase	Point mutation	Various carcinomas, melanoma
REL	Transcription factor	Rearrangement, amplification	Lymphomas
WNTI	Growth factor	Amplification	Retinoblastoma

48. Ans. (c) Hypothyroidism (d) Liver disease

[Ref: www.newhealthadvisor.com/macrocytic-anemia-causes; Harrison 19th/640-49; Davidson 22nd/1002-03,1022-24]

"The anemia of lead intoxication is hypochromic, and **normo- or microcytic** with associated reticulocytosis"- www.atsdr.cdc.gov

Macrocytic Anemia Causes

◈ *www.newhealthadvisor.com/macrocytic-anemia-causes*

Macrocytic anemias can be classified further into two main groups. First, you have the megaloblastic macrocytic anemia, which is the more common type. Then you have the ***non-megaloblastic macrocytic anemia,*** which is usually associated with various serious medical problems, such as liver or bone marrow disease. In some cases, no causes can be identified with the non-megaloblastic type of anemia.

Megaloblastic Macrocytic Anemia Causes

◈ *newhealthadvisor.com*

- DNA production disrupted
- **Medications:** One of the common macrocytic anemia causes is medication, especially those that interfere with ***folate metabolism and absorption.*** These include ***methotrexate,*** a drug used to treat cancer and rheumatoid arthritis, ***anticonvulsants, anti-cancer drugs, HIV medications, antidiabetic drugs (metformin) and antimicrobials.***
- Vitamin B12 deficiency
- **Folate deficiency:** Drugs causing folate deficiency include anticonvulsants, alcohol, methotrexate, trimethoprim and sulfasalazine.

Non-Megaloblastic Macrocytic Anemia Causes

◈ *newhealthadvisor.com*

Causes of non-megaloblastic macrocytic anemia are not related to defective DNA synthesis. Non-megaloblastic macrocytic anemia is less common and is characterized by the absence of megaloblasts, and instead, the presence of mature but large red blood cells. This type of red blood cells is normally seen in newborns only. Causes include:

- ***Chronic alcoholism***
- ***Liver disease***
- ***Hypothyroidism***
- ***Reticulocytosis***
- ***Blood disorders like red-cell aplasia, aplastic anemia, myelodysplastic syndromes, and myeloid leukemia***
- ***Drugs such as azathioprine***
- ***Pregnancy***

49. Ans. (a) Most commonly presents as..., (d) Classic triphasic combination of..., (e) Most common in children

[Ref: Nelson(SAE) 20th/2464-68; O.P.Ghai 8th/617-18;Robbins 9th/479-81; Harshmohan 7th/683-84; L and B 26th/124]

Wilms Tumor

◈ *O.P.Ghai 8th/617-18*

- Most common malignant tumour of kidney, accounting for 6–7% of all childhood malignancy
- 80% of patients with Wilm's tumour present under age of 5 yr
- The peak age at diagnosis is 2–4 yr
- 6% patient have bilateral disease
- While a vast majority of tumour is sporadic, 1–2% may be familial
- Most patients present with an asymptomatic abdominal mass detected by parents or physician during routine examination
- Features of congenital syndrome may be present in 13–28% of patients

Wilms Tumor

◈ *Nelson(SAE) 20th/2464-68*

- Wilms tumor, also known as **nephroblastoma,** is a complex mixed embryonal neoplasm of the kidney composed of ***three elements: blastema, epithelia, and stroma.***
- Most cases of Wilms tumor are sporadic, ***although 1–2% of patients have a family history.***
- It ***usually occurs in children between 2–5 yr of age,*** although it has also been encountered in neonates, adolescents, and adults.
- It accounts for approximately ***6% of pediatric cancers and is the second most common malignant abdominal tumor in childhood.***
- It may arise in one or both kidneys; the incidence of ***bilateral Wilms tumor is 7%.***
- Wilms tumor ***usually presents as an abdominal mass.*** It generally is discovered fortuitously, and it is not uncommon for the parent to notice it while bathing the infant

Wilms Tumor

◈ *Robbins 9th/479-81*

- The peak incidence for Wilms tumor is between 2 and 5 years of age, and 95% of tumors occur before the age of 10 years.
- ***Approximately 5% to 10% of Wilms tumors involve both kidneys,*** either simultaneously *(synchronous)* or one after the other *(metachronous).*

- Most children with Wilms tumors present with a ***large abdominal mass that may be unilateral or, when very large, may extend across the midline and down into the pelvis***.
- Grossly, Wilms tumor tends to present as a large, solitary, well circumscribed mass, ***although 10% are either bilateral or multicentric at the time of diagnosis.***
- Microscopically, Wilms tumors are characterized by recognizable attempts to recapitulate different stages of nephrogenesis. **The classic triphasic combination of blastemal, stromal, and epithelial cell types is observed in the vast majority of lesions,** although the percentage of each component is variable.

50. Ans. (a) Retinoblastoma, (c) Rhabdomyosarcoma, (d) Ewing sarcoma, (e) Carcinoid tumour

[Ref: radiopaedia.org;Nelson (SAE) 20th/ 2458; Danhert Radiology 7th/327;Harshmohan 7th/483-84,839-40;emedicine.medscape.com]

Ewing's sarcoma is closely related to PNET, but not PNET *(Robbins and Schwartz)*

"Embryonal tumors or **primitive neuroectodermal tumors (PNET)** are the most common group of malignant CNS tumors of childhood, accounting for 20–25% of pediatric CNS tumors. These tumors have the potential to metastasize to the neuraxis. This group includes ***medulloblastoma, supratentorial PNET, ependymoblastoma, medulloepithelioblastoma, and atypical teratoid/rhabdoid tumor (ATRT),*** all of which are histologically classified as WHO grade IV tumors"- *Nelson (SAE) 20th/ 2458*

Ewing Sarcoma Family Tumors: **Ewing sarcoma** is a malignant bone tumor characterized by primitive round cells without obvious differentiation. Recently, Ewing sarcoma and **primitive neuroectodermal tumor** (PNET) have been unified into a single category: the **Ewing sarcoma family tumors** (ESFT) based on shared clinical, morphologic, biochemical and molecular features. Although PNET demonstrates more neuroectodermal differentiation than Ewing sarcoma, the distinction is not clinically significant"- *Robbins 9th/1203*

"PNETs (***neuroblastomas, ganglioneuroblastomas, and ganglioneuromas***) derive from primordial neural crest cells that migrate from the mantle layer of the developing spinal cord. ***Ewing's sarcoma and Askin's tumour are closely related to PNET***. Histologically, PNETs and Ewing's sarcomas are small, round cell tumors."-Schwartz 9th/565

"Medulloblastoma (an infratentorial PNET)"- L and B 26th/616

Primitive Neuroectodermal Tumours (or CNS PNET)

◈ *radiopaedia.org*

- These are aggressive neoplasms of the brain, most frequently encountered in the paediatric population. The term no longer appears in the current WHO classification of CNS tumours.
- The term has fallen out of favour and has been removed from the 2016 update to the WHO classification of CNS tumours, now incorporated into the term embryonal tumors with multilayered rosettes (ETMR).
- Traditionally a number of tumours variably **fell under the umbrella term CNS PNET**:
  - **Medulloblastoma:** by far the most common (discussed separately)
  - **Supratentorial PNET:** 15% of all CNS PNET
    - **Pineoblastoma:** most common supratentorial PNET
    - **Ependymoblastoma:** also removed from the WHO in 2016
    - Medulloepithelioma
  - **Spinal PNET:** rare

Primitive Neuroectodermal Tumors (PNETs)

◈ *emedicine.medscape.com*

- PNET are a group of highly malignant tumors composed of small round cells of neuroectodermal origin that affect soft tissue and bone.
- Primitive neuroectodermal tumors (PNETs) exhibit great diversity in their clinical manifestations and pathologic similarities with other small, round cell tumors.
- This has made classifying this family of tumors challenging and controversial. Batsakis et al divided the primitive neuroectodermal tumor (PNET) family of tumors into the following 3 groups based on the tissue of origin:
  - CNS primitive neuroectodermal tumors (PNETs) - Tumors derived from the central nervous system
  - Neuroblastoma - Tumors derived from the autonomic nervous system
  - **Peripheral primitive neuroectodermal tumors** (pPNETs) - Tumors derived from tissues outside the central and autonomic nervous system. These includes -***Ewing sarcoma*** (osseus and extraosseous), Malignant peripheral primitive neuroectodermal tumors (pPNETs) or peripheral neuroepithelioma of bone and soft tissues, ***Askin tumor*** (peripheral neuroepithelioma of the thoracopulmonary region) and Other less common tumors (e.g., *neuroectodermal tumor, ectomesenchymoma, peripheral medulloepithelioma*)

51. Ans. (a) Bacterial meningitis, (b) Fungal meningitis, (d) Tubercular meningitis

[Ref: Robbins 9th/1272-74; CMDT 2016/1277; Harshmohan 7th/867-68; Ananthanarayan 9th/669]

Table *(CMDT 2016/1277)*: **Typical cerebrospinal fluid findings in various CNS diseases**

Diagnosis	Cells/mcL	Glucose (mg/dL)	Protein (mg/dL)	Opening Pressure
Normal	0–5 lymphocytes	45–85	15–45	70–180 mm H_2O
Purulent meningitis (bacterial) community-acquired	200–20,000 polymorphonuclear neutrophils	Low (< 45)	High (> 50)	Markedly elevated

Contd...

Diagnosis	Cells/mcL	Glucose (mg/dL)	Protein (mg/dL)	Opening Pressure
Granulomatous meningitis (mycobacterial, fungal)	100–1000, mostly lymphocytes	Low (< 45)	High (> 50)	Moderately elevated
Spirochetal meningitis	100–1000, mostly lymphocytes	Normal	Moderately high (> 50)	Normal to slightly elevated
Aseptic meningitis, viral or meningoencephalitis	25–2000, mostly lymphocytes	Normal or low	High (> 50)	Slightly elevated
"Neighborhood reaction"	Variably increased	Normal	Normal or high	Variable

Table *(Harshmohan 7th/868)*: **CSF findings in health and various types of meningitis**

Feature	Normal	Acute pyogenic (bacterial) meningitis	Acute lymphocytic (viral) meningitis	Chronic (tuberculous) meningitis
• *Naked eye appearance*	Clean and colourless	Cloudy or frankly purulent	Clear or slightly turbid	Clear or slightly turbid, forms fibrin coagulum on standing
• *CSF pressure*	60–150 mm water	Elevated (above 180 mm water)	Elevated (above 250 mm water)	Elevated (above 300 mm water)
• *Cells*	4–0 lymphocytes/mL	10–10,000 neurtrophils/ mL	10–100 lymphocytes/mL	100–1000 lymphocytes/mL
• *Proteins*	15–45 mg/dL	Markedly raised	Mildly raised	Raised
• ***Glucose***	50–80 mg/dL	Markedly reduced	Normal	Reduced
• *Bacteriology*	Sterile	Causative organisms present	Sterile	Tubercle bacilli present

52. Ans. (d) Collagen type III present predominantly, (e) Angiogenesis occurs

[Ref: Robbins 9th/106-08; Harshmohan 7th/157-59]

The Phases of Wound Healing

- *www.clinimed.co.uk*
- Inflammatory phase
- Proliferation phase
- Maturation phase
- The **inflammatory phase** is the body's natural response to injury. After initial wounding, the blood vessels in the wound bed contract and a clot is formed. The predominant cells at work here are the phagocytic cells; '***neutrophils and macrophages***'; mounting a host response and autolysing any devitalised 'necrotic / sloughy' tissue.
- During **proliferation**, the wound is 'rebuilt' with new granulation tissue which is comprised of collagen and extracellular matrix and into which a ***new network of blood vessels develop***, a process known as '**angiogenesis**'. Healthy granulation tissue is dependent upon the fibroblast receiving sufficient levels of oxygen and nutrients supplied by the blood vessels. Healthy granulation tissue is granular and uneven in texture; it does not bleed easily and is pink / red in colour.Epithelial cells finally resurface the wound, a process known as '**epithelialisation**'.
- **Maturation** is the final phase and occurs once the wound has closed. This phase involves remodelling of ***collagen from type III to type I***. Cellular activity reduces and the number of blood vessels in the wounded area regress and decrease.

"**Proliferative phase**: Approximately 80% of the collagen in normal skin is type I collagen; the remaining is mostly type III. In contrast, ***type III collagen is the primary component of early granulation tissue*** and is abundant in embryonic tissue. Collagen fibers are deposited in a framework of fibronectin"emedicine.medscape.com

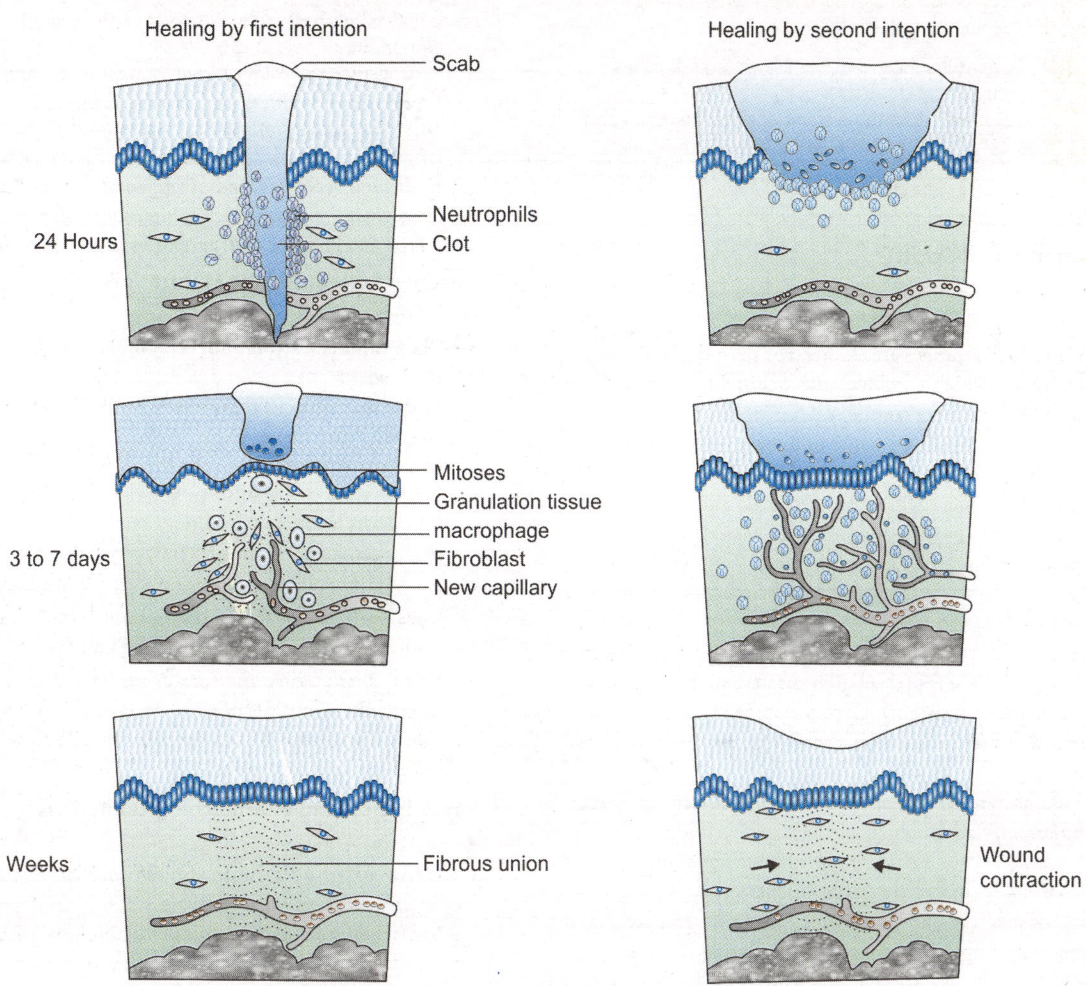

Fig: *(Robbins 9th/107):* Steps in wound healing by first intention (left) and second intention (right). In the latter, note the large amount of granulation tissue and wound contraction

53. Ans. (a) Perls' Prussian blue-iron..., (d) PAS- glycogen, (e) PAS- Acidic and neutral...

[Ref: bitesizebio.com; www.ivyroses.com]

"**Perls' Prussian blue** is used to detect the presence of iron in tissues. It is an extremely sensitive test, and can even detect single granules of iron in cells"- bitesizebio.com

Masson's Trichrome Staining:This method is used for the detection of collagen fibers in tissues"- *www.ihcworld.com*

"There are many elastin special stain techniques such as Weigert-Type, Orcein, Aldehyde-Fuchsin and Verhoeff's. The most common is Verhoeff's technique of staining elastin due to its quick method and strong elastin colour result"- skinpathonline.wordpress.com

Table *(www.ivyroses.com):* **Histology stain**

Masson trichrome	• Trichrome histology stains are formed from a mixture of three dyes • Can be used to distinguish between cellular items and extracellular items • Can be used on connective tissue
Von kossa stain	• Used to indicate calcium and calcium deposits
Periodic Acid Schiff (PAS)	• A Mucin stain (listed above) • Used for staining glycogen and other carbohydrates • Used to show glomeruli, basement membranes, and glycogen in the liver

Contd...

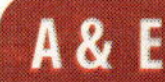

Perl's Iron stain	• Can be used to reveal the presence of iron in biological tissues.
Gomori trichrome	• Trichrome histology stains are formed from a mixture of three dyes • Gomori's trichrome stains connective tissue and collagen (green or blue), muscle, keratin and cytoplasm (red) and nuclei (grey/blue/black)
Orcein stain	• Can be used to stain for elastin fibres

PAS (Periodic Acid-Schiff)

◈ *www.pathologyoutlines.com*

- Substances with nearby glycol groups or their amino or alkylamino derivatives are oxidized by periodic acid to form dialdehydes, which combine with Schiff's reagent to form an insoluble magenta compound
- Used for formalin fixed tissue and enzyme cytochemistry; can be used for frozen sections with modifications
- Stains basement membrane (normal and in tumors), ***glycogen,*** some mucins and mucopolysaccharides
- A routine stain in brain (with Luxol fast blue), cornea, kidney, liver and skeletal muscle specimens for nontumor pathology
- Some mucins are PASD (PAS with predigestion with diastase) positive (i.e. stain is present after diastase predigestion; also called diastase resistant); glycogen is PASD negative (also called diastase sensitive because diastase removes PAS staining)
- PAS stains ***neutral and acid-simple non-sulfated and acid-complex sulfated mucins***
- PAS does **NOT** stain ***acid-simple mesenchymal mucins and acid-complex connective tissue mucins***
- Also stains various inclusions, bodies, granules and secretions composed of mucopolysaccharides or mucins

"The PAS technique is particularly sensitive for the detection of ***neutral mucins as well as acid mucins*** that contain significant quantities of sialic acid. In addition to mucins, the PAS technique is also widely used for the detection of **glycogen** and various glycoproteins"- www.leicabiosystems.com

PHARMACOLOGY

54. Ans. (a) Development of the alveolar system,
(e) Development of lobules of breast

[Ref: KDT 7th/ 306-12; Katzung 13th/699-702; G and G 11th/1543-53; Pharmacology by Satoskar 24th/947-49]

"Oestrogen causes only duct development. Progesterone is responsible for glandular development, i.e it promotes the growth of the lobules and alveolar tissue in breast"*-A.K.Jain 6th/838*

"Progesterone promotes the development of the ***alveolar (acinar) system of the breast****"- Satoskar 24th/955; KDT 7th/ 317*

Estrogen

◈ *KDT 7th/ 306-12*

- *"It is important in maintaining* ***bone mass primarily by retarding bone resorption****. Osteoclast pit formation is inhibited and there is increased expression of bone matrix proteins such as osteonectin, osteocalcin, collagen and alkaline phosphatase*
- *"Estrogens produced at puberty cause growth of breasts-* ***proliferation of ducts and stroma, accumulation of fat"***
- *"It brings about pubertal changes in the female including growth of uterus, fallopian tube and vagina. Vaginal epithelium gets thickened, stratified and cornified"*
- *"It augment rhythmic contractions of the fallopian tubes and uterus and induce a watery alkaline secretion from the cervix"*

Estrogen Action: Female Maturation

◈ *Katzung 13th/700*

- They stimulate ***stromal development and ductal growth in the breast***
- They contribute to the growth of ***axillary and pubic hair*** and alter the distribution of body fat to produce typical female body contours.
- Larger quantities also stimulate development of ***pigmentation in the skin, most prominent in the region of the nipples and areolae*** and in the genital region.
- Continuous exposure to estrogens for prolonged periods leads to ***hyperplasia of the endometrium*** that is usually associated with abnormal bleeding patterns.
- Estrogens ***decrease the rate of resorption of bone*** by promoting the apoptosis of osteoclasts and by antagonizing the osteoclastogenic and pro-osteoclastic effects of parathyroid hormone and interleukin-6.

Physiological and Pharmacological Actions

◈ *G and G 11th/1543, 1547,1553*

- Estrogens in girls cause ***growth and development of the vagina, uterus, and fallopian tubes, and contribute to breast enlargement, molding the body contours, shaping the skeleton, and causing the pubertal growth spurt of the long bones and epiphyseal closure.***
- ***Estrogens increase bone mass****, largely by* ***decreasing the number and activity of osteoclasts****, thereby* ***decreasing bone resorption.***
- *Estrogen therapy is clearly efficacious in decreasing the incidence of fractures, although bone loss resumes when treatment is discontinued.*
- ***Estrogens are more effective in preventing than restoring bone loss*** *and are most effective if initiated before significant bone loss occurs.*

55. Ans. (c) Absorption increases with food

[Ref: KDT 7th/ 343-46; Katzung 13th/ 754-55; Pharmacology by Satoskar 24th/1006-07]

Liver related adverse effects are not mentioned in the given references. So can be given in liver diseases

Biphosphonates (BPNs)

◈ *KDT 7th/ 343-46*

- BPNs are ***analogues of pyrophosphate***; carbon atom replacing oxygen in the P-O-P skeleton
- *"****All oral BNPs are poorly absorbed*** and produce ***gastric irritation, esophagitis as the major side effect.*** They are

contraindicated in gastroesophageal reflux, peptic ulcer and renal impairment"

- They ***inhibit bone resorption*** and have recently attracted considerable attention because of their ability to prevent osteoporosis in addition to their usefulness in metabolic bone diseases and hypercalcemia

Bisphosphonates

◈ *Katzung 13th/ 754-55*

- The bisphosphonates are ***analogs of pyrophosphate*** in which the P-O-P bond has been replaced with a nonhydrolyzable PC- P bond
- **Etidronate, pamidronate,** and **alendronate** have now been joined by **risedronate, tiludronate, ibandronate,** and **zoledronate** for clinical use.
- They ***localize to regions of bone resorption and so exert their greatest effects on osteoclasts***. However, the exact mechanism by which they ***selectively inhibit bone resorption*** is not clear.
- The results from animal and clinical studies indicate that less than 10% of an oral dose of these drugs is absorbed. ***Food reduces absorption*** even further, ***necessitating their administration on an empty stomach.***
- Nearly half of the absorbed drug accumulates in bone; the remainder is excreted unchanged in the urine. ***Decreased renal function, esophageal motility disorders, and peptic ulcer disease are the main contraindications to the use of these drugs***
- ***Esophageal irritation*** can be minimized by taking the drug with a full glass of water and remaining upright for 30 minutes.
- Of the other complications, **osteonecrosis of the jaw (ONJ)** has received considerable attention, but is rare in patients receiving the usual doses of bisphosphonates.

56. Ans. (a) Bedaquiline, (b) Clofazimine, (d) Rifapentine

[Ref: Community Medicine with Recent Advances by Suryakantha 4th/371; KDT 7th/765-76; Katzung 13th/816-21; Pharmacology by Satoskar 24th/748-49; Rang and Dale 8th/638;Park 23rd/191-92]

Coftaroline is a cephalosporin active against MRSA- *Katzung 13th/779*

Etanercept: It is a ***TNF-α inhibitor.*** It is used in rheumatoid arthritis, ankylosing spondylitis, plaque psoriasis etc"- *KDT 7th/884*

Newer Anti-TB Drugs

◈ *Community Medicine with Recent Advances by Suryakantha 4th/371*

- *Rifabutin*
- ***Rifapentine***
- *Macrolides:Roxithromycin,Clarithromycin, Azithromycin*
- *Amikacin*
- *Fluoroquinolones:Ciprofloxacin, ofloxacin and sparfloxacin*
- *B-lactum antibiotics: trials are going on with amoxicillin-clavulanic acid*
- ***Clofazimine***
- *Paramomycin*
- *Cytokine immunotherapy:IL-2, cytokine gamma interferon and cytokine IL-12*

Bedaquiline

◈ *Katzung 13th/21 www.who.int/tb/challenges/mdr/bedaquiline*

- The last time a drug was introduced specifically for the treatment of TB was in the late 1960s. That drug was rifampicin. Since then, resistance to rifampicin has been increasingly reported in the world. This is a major concern given that it remains among the most effective anti-TB drugs available today.
- Bedaquiline has been released specifically to treat TB patients with bacteria that are resistant to rifampicin as well as to isoniazid, another core anti-TB drug, and thus suffer from ***multidrug-resistant tuberculosis (MDR-TB).***
- Bedaquiline is a bactericidal drug which belongs to a new class of antibiotics (diarylquinolines). Although the drug is active against many different bacteria, it has been registered ***specifically for the treatment of MDR-TB.***
- The drug is unique among the anti-tuberculosis drugs currently used in that it interferes with the function of an enzyme required by the tuberculosis bacterium to produce energy and to replicate.

Table *(Katzung 13th/816)*: **Antimicrobials used in the treatment of tuberculosis**

First-line agents
Isoniazid 300 mg/d
Rifampin 600 mg/d
Pyrazinamide 25 mg/kg/d
Ethambutol 15–25 mg/kg/d
Streptomycin 15 mg/kg/d
Second-line agents
Amikacin 15 mg/kg/d
Aminosalicylic acid 8–12 g/d
Bedaquiline 400mg/d
Capreomycin 15 mg/kg/d
Ciprofloxacin 1500 mg/d, divided
Clofazimine 200 mg/d
Cycloserine 500–1000 mg/d, divided
Ethionamide 500–750 mg/d
Levofloxacin 500 mg/d
Moxifloxacin 400 mg/d
Rifabutin 300 mg/d
Rifapentine 600 mg once or twice weekly

Table *(Park 23rd/192):* **Drugs for XDR-TB**

Drugs
Inj. Capreomycin (Cm)
PAS
Moxifloxacin (Mfx)
High dose INH (High dose-H)
Clofazimine (Cfz)
Linezolid (Lzd)
Amoxyclav (Amx/Clv)
Pyridoxine
Reserve/Substitute drugs
Clarithromycin (Clr)
Thiacetazone (Thz)[#]

57. Ans. (b) It takes minimum 2 weeks for reticulocyte count to increase

[Ref: KDT 7th/ 603; Katzung 13th/571; Pharmacology by Satoskar 24th/504-07; G and G 11th/1447-49]

"Following oral iron, ***normal Hb level is usually attained within 1 to 3 months****, depending mainly on the initial Hb level. It is important, however, to continue with the therapy for* ***12-20 weeks after the Hb level has returned to normal, in order to replenish the depleted iron stores****"-Satoskar 24th/504-05*

"The response to iron therapy is quite predictable. The ***reticulocyte count in the peripheral blood begins to rise within a week, reaches a peak at 10 to 14 days*** *and* ***returns to normal after 3 weeks****"- Satoskar 24th/505*

"A rise in Hb level by 0.5–1 g/dl per week is an optimum response to iron therapy. It is faster in the beginning and when anaemia is severe. Later, the rate of increase in Hb% declines. However, therapy should be continued till normal Hb level is attained (***generally takes 1–3 months depending on the severity***) and ***2–3 months or more thereafter to replenish the stores***"-*KDT 7th/ 605*

Oral Iron Therapy: *Adverse Effects of Oral Iron*

◈ *KDT 7th/ 603*

- These are common at therapeutic doses and are related to elemental iron content. Individuals differ in susceptibility. Side effects are: ***Epigastric pain, heartburn, nausea, vomiting, bloating, staining of teeth, metallic taste, colic***, etc.
- Tolerance to oral iron can be improved by initiating therapy at low dose and gradually escalating to the optimum dose.
- Constipation is more common (believed to the due to astringent action of iron) than diarrhoea (thought to reflect irritant action). However, these may be caused by ***alteration of intestinal flora as well.***
- "***Gastric irritation and constipation*** (the most important side effects of oral iron) are related to the total quantity of elemental iron administered. If viewed in terms of iron content, nearly all preparations have the same degree of gastric tolerance, the limits of which are fairly well defined in individual patients."

Oral Iron Therapy

◈ *Katzung 13th/571*

- Patients unable to tolerate large doses of iron can be given lower daily doses of iron, which results in slower but still complete correction of iron deficiency.
- ***Treatment with oral iron should be continued for 3–6 months after correction of the cause of the iron loss***. This corrects the anemia and replenishes iron stores.
- Common adverse effects of oral iron therapy include ***nausea, epigastric discomfort, abdominal cramps, constipation, and diarrhea***. These effects are usually dose-related and can often be overcome by lowering the daily dose of iron or by taking the tablets immediately after or with meals.

Treatment of Iron Deficiency

◈ *G and G 11th/1447,1149*

- The response of iron-deficiency anemia to iron therapy is influenced by several factors, including the severity of anemia, ***the ability of the patient to tolerate and absorb medicinal iron***, and the presence of other complicating illnesses.
- ***The patient's ability to tolerate and absorb medicinal iron is a key factor in determining the rate of response to therapy.***
- *Clinically, the effectiveness of iron therapy is best evaluated by tracking the reticulocyte response and the rise in the Hb or the hematocrit.* ***An increase in the reticulocyte count is not observed for at least 4–7 days after beginning therapy.***
- ***Intolerance to oral preparations of iron primarily is a function of the amount of soluble iron in the upper GI tract and of psychological factors.*** Side effects include heartburn, nausea, upper gastric discomfort, and diarrhea or constipation.

"Patients with IBD are commonly found to have iron deficiency anemia (IDA) secondary to chronic blood loss, and impaired iron absorption due to tissue inflammation. IDA is often associated with inflammation in patients with IBD. Oral iron preparations are available and are used in patients with mild disease activity. These preparations are inexpensive and convenient, but can produce ***gastrointestinal side effects, such as abdominal pain and diarrhea, that limit their use and patient compliance***. These preparations are partly absorbed due to inflammation. ***Non-absorbed iron can be toxic and worsen IBD disease activity*** as a result of oxidative stress, neutrophilic infiltration, increased cytokines, and activation of NF-kappa"- *www.ncbi.nlm.nih.gov/pmc*

58. Ans. (b) Steroid, (c) Salbutamol

[Ref: KDT 7th/ 229,222,747; Katzung 13th/327; G and G 11th/724; Pharmacology by Satoskar 24th/368; Rang and Dale 8th/218,723]

"**Inhalational steroids**: *Beclomethasone, dipropionate, budesonide, fluticasone propionate, flunisolide and ciclesonide*"- *KDT 7th/ 222*

"**Salbutamol**: *used in form of – oral, i.m/s.c and* ***inhalation***"- *KDT 7th/ 223*

"**Tobramycin**: Used in form of- ***i.m/i.v, eye drop***"- *Katzung 13th/804 and KDT 7th/749*

"**Zileuton**: *It is* ***available only as extended release (oral) formulation***"- *Satoskar 24th/368; reference.medscape.com*

59. Ans. (a) Methotrexate, (d) Leflunomide, (e) Gold

[Ref: Harrison 19th/2146-47;KDT 7th/210-16; Katzung 13th/626-28; Pharmacology by Satoskar 24th/1077]

For sulfasalazine, initial evaluation includes LFT but LFT is not required for monitoring for drug use(according to Harrison)

Table *(Harrison 19th/2146-47)*: **DMARDs Used for the treatment of rheumatoid arthritis**

Drug	Serious toxicities	Other common side effects	Initial evaluation	Monitoring
Hydroxychloroquine	Irreversible retinal damage Cardiotoxicity Blood dyscrasia	Nausea Diarrhea Headache Rash	Eye examination if > 40 years old or prior ocular disease	Funduscopic and visual field testing every 12 months
Sulfasalazine	Granulocytopenia Hemolytic anemia (with G6PD deficiency)	Nausea Diarrhea Headache	CBC, ***LFTs*** G6PD level	CBC every 2–4 weeks for first 3 months, then every 3 months
Methotrexate	Hepatotoxicity Myelosuppression Infection Interstitial pneumonitis Pregnancy category X	Nausea Diarrhea Stomatitis/mouth ulcers Alopecia Fatigue	CBC, ***LFTs*** Viral hepatitis panel* Chest x-ray	CBC, creatinine, ***LFTs every 2–3 months***
Leflunomide	Hepatotoxicity Myelosuppression Infection Pregnancy category X	Alopecia Diarrhea	CBC, ***LFTs*** Viral hepatitis panel	CBC, creatinine, ***LFTs every 2–3 months***
Tocilizumab	Risk of infection Infusion reaction LFT elevation Dyslipidemia Cytopenias		PPD skin test	CBC and ***LFTs at regular intervals***

Abbreviations: CBC, complete blood count; PPD, purified peptide derivative; SQ, subcutaneous

"**Gold salt**: It can cause dermatitis, nephropathy, oral ulceration, bone marrow depression, peripheral neuropathy and ***liver damage***"- *Satoskar 24th/1077*

"***Hepatotoxicity is a rare but potentially serious complication of gold sodium thiomalate therapy***. Jaundice, cholestatic hepatitis, hepatic necrosis, and granulomatous hepatitis have been associated with gold therapy. Cholestasis is the most common form of gold-induced hepatotoxicity and typically presents early in the course of gold therapy. While usually reversible upon discontinuation of the drug, fatal cases of intrahepatic cholestasis have been reported. The presence of rash and eosinophilia in many cases suggests that this form of hepatotoxicity is due to a hypersensitivity reaction. Several cases of massive hepatic necrosis have also been reported in the literature."-www.drugs.com

"***Sulfasalazine:*** *Neutropenia/thrombocytopenia occurs in about 10% patients and* ***hepatitis is possible***"*- KDT 7th/211*

"Approximately 30% of patients using **sulfasalazine** discontinue the drug because of toxicity. Common adverse effects include nausea, vomiting, headache, and rash. Hemolytic anemia and methemoglobinemia also occur, but rarely. Neutropenia occurs in 1–5% of patients, while thrombocytopenia is very rare. Pulmonary toxicity and positive double-stranded DNA are occasionally seen, but drug-induced lupus is rare. Reversible infertility occurs in men, but sulfasalazine does not affect fertility in women. The drug does not appear to be teratogenic"- *Katzung 13th/628*

"With prolonged therapy, dose dependent progressive liver damage leading to cirrhosis occurs in some patients (this is not seen with short courses used in cancer). ***Mtx is contraindicated*** in pregnancy, breast-feeding, ***liver disease***, active infection, leucopenia and peptic ulcer"- *KDT 7th/211*

"**Mtx**- ***Progressive dose-related hepatotoxicity in the form of enzyme elevation*** occurs frequently, but cirrhosis is rare (< 1%). Liver toxicity is not related to serum methotrexate concentrations, and liver biopsy follow-up is only recommended every 5 years.

"Adverse effects of **leflunomide** are diarrhoes, headache, nausea, rashes, loss of hair, thrombocytopenia, leucopenia, increased chances of chest infection and ***raised hepatic transaminases***. It is not to be used in children and pregnant/lactating women. ***Leflunomide is an alternative to Mtx or can be added to it, but the combination is more hepatotoxic***. Combination with sulfasalazine improves benefit"- *KDT 7th/212*

"Diarrhea occurs in approximately 25% of patients given **leflunomide,** although only about 3–5% discontinue the drug because of this effect. ***Elevation in liver enzymes also occurs***"- *Katzung 13th/627*

"Although ocular toxicity may occur at dosages greater than 250 mg/d for chloroquine and greater than 6.4 mg/ kg/d for **hydroxychloroquine**, it rarely occurs at lower doses. Nevertheless, ophthalmologic monitoring every 6–12 months is advised. Other toxicities include dyspepsia, nausea, vomiting, abdominal pain, rashes, and nightmares. These drugs appear to be relatively safe in pregnancy"- *Katzung 13th/626*

60. Ans. (a) Metoprolol, (b) Labetalol, (c) Methyldopa, (d) Sustained release nifedipine

[Ref: KDT 7th/573; Pharmacology by Satoskar 24th/440; Obs by JB Sharma 1st/430,433]

Anti-hypertensive agents used in pregnancy: ***Methyldopa, hydralazine, labetalol, Nifedipine, atenolol****"-Obs by JB Sharma 1st/430,433*

Antihypertensives to be Avoided During Pregnancy

◈ *KDT 7th/573*

ACE inhibitors, ARBs (e.g., **losartan**): Risk of foetal damage, growth retardation.

Diuretics: Tend to reduce blood volume–accentuate uteroplacental perfusion deficit (of toxaemia)– increase risk of foetal wastage, placental infarcts, miscarriage, stillbirth.

Nonselective β blockers: Propranolol has been implicated to cause low birth weight, decreased placental size, neonatal bradycardia and hypoglycaemia.

Sod. Nitroprusside: Contraindicated in eclampsia

Antihypertensives Found Safer During Pregnancy

◈ *KDT 7th/573*

Hydralazine

Methyldopa (a positive Coombs' test occurs, but has no adverse implication)

Dihydropyridine CCBs (e.g **Nifedipine**): if used, they should be discontinued before labour as they weaken uterine contractions

Cardioselective β blockers and those with ISA, e.g., atenolol, ***metoprolol,*** pindolol, acebutolol: may be used if no other choice.

Prazosin and clonidine: Provided that postural hypotension can be avoided

"Drug used in severe hypertension in pregnancy: **Nifedipine**: 5-10 mg capsule to be bitten and swallowed, or just swallowed, every 30 min. There are three types of nifedipine preparations-capsules, intermediate-release tablets (PA), and slow-release tablets"- www.ncbi.nlm.nih.gov

61. Ans. (b) Sedation, (e) Weight gain

[Ref: Kaplan and Sadock's Psychiatry 11th/993; KDT 7th/ 458; Katzung 13th/525, 528; Pharmacology by Satoskar 24th/216, 221; G and G 11th/436, 447-48]

"**Mirtazepine**: *Important adverse drug reactions are-* ***marked sedation, increased appetite and weight gain****"- Satoskar 24th/221*

"***Mirtazapine has significant sedative effect and*** weight gain"- *Katzung 13th/525*

Table *(Kaplan and Sadock's 11th/993):* **Adverse Reactions Reported with Mirtazapine**

Event	Patients (%)
Somnolence	54
Dry mouth	25
Increased appetite	17
Constipation	13
Weight gain	12
Dizziness	7
Myalgias	5
Distrubing dreams	4

Precautions and Adverse Reactions

◈ *Kaplan and Sadock's Psychiatry 11th/993*

- ***Somnolence, the most common adverse effect of mirtazapine***, occurs in more than 50 percent of persons. This adverse effect is why mirtazapine is almost always given before sleep.
- Mirtazapine also causes dizziness in 7 percent of persons. It ***does not appear to increase the risk for seizures.*** Mania or hypomania occurred in clinical trials at a rate similar to that of other antidepressant drugs.
- Mirtazapine ***increases appetite*** in about one-third of patients.
- Mirtazapine may also ***increase serum cholesterol concentration*** to 20 percent or more above the upper limit of normal in 1 5 percent of persons
- A small number of persons experience ***orthostatic hypotension*** while taking mirtazapine.
- Although no data exist regarding the effects on fetal development, mirtazapine should be used with caution during pregnancy.
- Because of the risk of ***agranulocytosis*** associated with mirtazapine use, persons should be attuned to signs of infection. Because of the sedating effects of mirtazapine, persons should determine the degree to which they are affected before engaging in driving or other potentially dangerous activities.

Table *(G and G 11th/436):* **Mirtazapine**

	Side-effect								
	Agitation	Seizures	Sedation	Hypotension	Anti-cholinergic effect	Gastrointestinal effect	Weight gain	Sexual effects	Cardiac effect
Mirtazapine	0	0	4+	0/+	0	0/+	0/+	0	0

0, negligible; 0/+, minimal; +, mild; 2+, moderate; 3+, moderately severe; 4+, severe.

62. Ans. (a) Acetazolamide (d) Topiramate

[Ref: KDT 7th/587,420,155; Katzung 13th/255-56]

"***Amiloride***(*Potassium sparing diuretics)-Inhibitor of renal epithelial Na+ channel*"- *KDT* 7th*/579*
"***Nitrofurantoin***: *Urinary antiseptic*"- *KDT* 7th*/760*
Carbonic anhydrase inhibitor: ***Topiramate, Acetazolamide, methazolamide, dichlorphenamide, dorzolamide, brinzolamide***"- *KDT* 7th*/ 587,420,155*
"**Topically active carbonic anhydrase inhibitors** (***dorzolamide, brinzolamide***) are available and reduce intraocular pressure without producing detectable plasma levels. Thus, diuretic and systemic metabolic effects are eliminated for the topical agents"- *Katzung* 13th*/255*
"**Carbonic anhydrase inhibitors** used orally in the treatment of glaucoma- ***Acetazolamide, dichlorphenamide and methazolamide***"- *Katzung* 13th*/255*

63. Ans. (a) A macrolides antibiotic, (d) T cell inhibitor, (e) Hirsutism less evident than cyclosporine

[Ref: KDT 7th/881; Katzung 13th/955]

Tacrolimus (FK506)

◈ *KDT 7th/881*

- This immunosuppressant is ***chemically different from cyclosporine***, but has ***the same mechanism of action, and is ~ 100 times more potent.***
- It binds to a different cytoplasmic immunophilin protein labelled 'FK 506 binding protein (FKBP)' but the subsequent steps are the same, i.e. ***inhibition of helper T cells via calcineurin.***
- Tacrolimus is administered orally as well as by i.v. infusion. Oral absorption is variable and decreased by food.
- It is metabolized by CYP3A4 and excreted in bile with a T½ of 12 hours.
- ***Therapeutic application, clinical efficacy as well as toxicity profile are similar to cyclosporine.***
- Tacrolimus also requires blood level monitoring for dose adjustment. However, due to higher potency and easier monitoring of blood levels, it is generally preferred now for organ transplantations. Tacrolimus may be useful in patients whose rejection reaction is not suppressed by cyclosporine.
- It is particularly valuable in liver transplantation because its absorption is not dependent on bile. Being more potent, it is also suitable for suppressing acute rejection that has set in.
- ***Hypertension, hirsutism, gum hyperplasia and hyperuricaemia are less marked*** than with cyclosporine, but tacrolimus is ***more likely to precipitate diabetes, cause neurotoxicity alopecia and diarrhoea***. Dose limiting toxicity is renal.

Tacrolimus

◈ *Katzung 13th/955*

- Tacrolimus (FK 506) is an immunosuppressant ***macrolide antibiotic*** produced by Streptomyces tsukubaensis(a bacteria)
- It is ***not chemically related to cyclosporine***, but their mechanisms of action are similar. Both drugs bind to cytoplasmic peptidylprolyl isomerases that are abundant in all tissues. ***While cyclosporine binds to cyclophilin, tacrolimus binds to the immunophilin*** FK-binding protein (FKBP). Both complexes inhibit calcineurin, which is necessary for the activation of the T-cellspecific transcription factor NF-AT.
- On a weight basis, tacrolimus is 10–100 times more potent than cyclosporine in inhibiting immune responses.
- Tacrolimus is utilized for the same indications as cyclosporine, particularly in organ and stem cell transplantation.
- Like cyclosporine, tacrolimus is metabolized primarily by P450 enzymes in the liver, and there is potential for drug interactions.
- The dosage is determined by trough blood level at steady state. Its toxic effects are similar to those of cyclosporine and include nephrotoxicity, neurotoxicity, hyperglycemia, hypertension, hyperkalemia, and gastrointestinal complaints.
- Because of the effectiveness of systemic tacrolimus in some dermatologic diseases, a topical preparation is now available.
- Tacrolimus ointment is currently used in the therapy of atopic dermatitis and psoriasis.

"*Cyclosporine:* It is a ***cyclic polypeptide with 11 amino acids, obtained from a fungus***"- *KDT* 7th*/878*

64. Ans. (e) Inactivate factor Xa selectively

[Ref: KDT 7th/619; Katzung 13th/588-89; Pharmacology by Satoskar 24th/481-83]

"**LMWH**: *Since they have a minimal effect on tests of clotting in vitro,* ***monitoring is not done routinely. Patients with end-stage renal failure may require monitoring with an anti-factor Xa assay because this condition may prolong the half life of LMW heparin***"*-G and G* 11th*/1473*

Low Molecular Weight (LMW) Heparins and UFH

- "*Protamine does not neutralize fondaparinux and it* ***only partially reverses the anticoagulant effect of LMW heparins***"- *KDT* 7th*/620*
- "*Heparin can be promptly arrest by administration of protamine sulfate*"- *Satoskar* 24th*/484*
- ***Inactivate factor Xa selectively****; their action against thrombin is minimal(ratio of anti-Xa to anti-IIa activity is 2:1 to 4:1; c.f Heparin 1:1)- Satoskar* 24th*/481,483*
- "*Low concentration of heparin prolong aPTT without significantly prolonging PT. High concentration significantly prolong both*"- *KDT* 7th*/617*

Low Molecular Weight (LMW) Heparins

◈ *KDT 7th/619*

- Heparin has been fractionated into LMW forms (MW 3000–7000) by different techniques.
- LMW heparins have a different anticoagulant profile; i.e. ***selectively inhibit factor Xa with little effect on IIa.***

- They act only by inducing ***conformational change in AT III*** and not by providing a scaffolding for interaction of AT III with thrombin. As a result, ***LMW heparins have smaller effect on aPTT and whole blood clotting time than unfractionated heparin (UFH)*** relative to antifactor Xa activity. Also, they have lesser antiplatelet action–less interference with haemostasis.
- ***Thrombocytopenia is less frequent***. A lower incidence of haemorrhagic complications compared to UFH has been reported in some studies, but not in others. However, major bleeding may be less frequent.
- They are ***eliminated primarily by renal excretion; are not to be used in patients with renal failure.***
- The more important advantages of LMW heparins are pharmacokinetic:
  - Better subcutaneous bioavailability (70–90%) compared to UFH (20–30%): Variability in response in minimized.
  - Longer and more consistent monoexponential t½: (4–6 hours), making possible once daily s.c. administration
  - ***Since aPTT/clotting times are not prolonged, laboratory monitoring is not needed***; dose is calculated on body weight basis.
  - Risk of osteoporosis after long term use is much less with LMW heparin compared with UFH.
- Most studies have found LMW heparins to be equally efficacious to UFH except during cardiopulmonary bypass surgery, in which high dose UFH is still the preferred anticoagulant, because LMW heparin and fondaparinux are less effective in preventing catheter thrombosis and their effects are not fully reversed by protamine.
- Indications of LMW heparins are:
  - Prophylaxis of deep vein thrombosis and pulmonary embolism in high-risk patients undergoing surgery; stroke or other immobilized patients
  - Treatment of established deep vein thrombosis.
  - Unstable angina and MI: they have largely replaced continuous infusion of UFH
  - To maintain patency of cannula and shunts in dialysis patients

Monitoring of Heparin Effect *Katzung 13th/588*

- Close monitoring of the **activated partial thromboplastin time (aPTT or PTT)** is necessary in patients receiving UFH. Levels of UFH may also be determined by protamine titration (therapeutic levels 0.2–0.4 unit/mL) or ***anti-Xa units*** (therapeutic levels 0.3–0.7 unit/mL).
- Weight-based dosing of the LMW heparins results in predictable pharmacokinetics and plasma levels in patients with normal renal function. Therefore, ***LMW heparin levels are not generally measured except in the setting of renal insufficiency, obesity, and pregnancy.***
- LMW heparin levels can be determined by anti-Xa units.

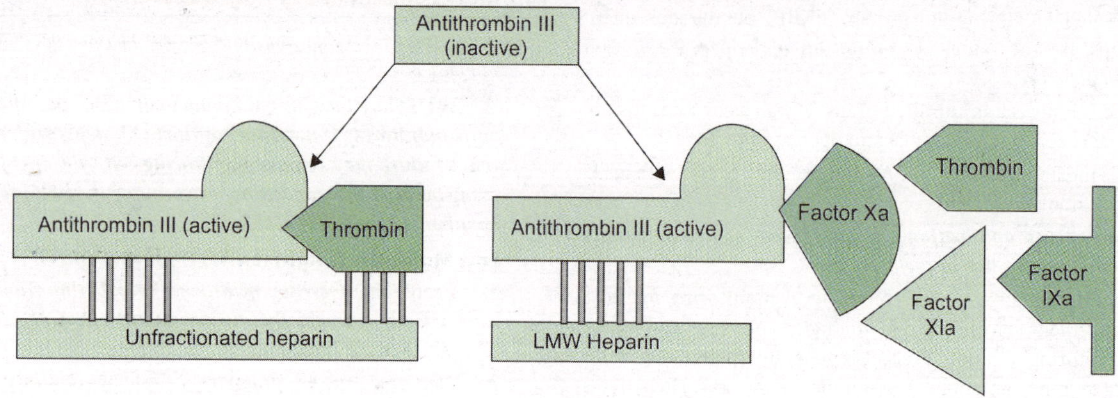

Fig: *(Katzung 13th/588):* Cartoon illustrating differences between fondaparinux, low-molecular-weight heparins (LMWH), and high-molecular-weight heparin (HMWH, unfractionated heparin). Activated antithrombin III (AT III) degrades thrombin, factor X, and several other factors. Binding of these drugs to AT III can increase the catalytic action of AT III 1000-fold. The combination of AT III with unfractionated heparin increases degradation of both factor Xa and thrombin. Combination with fondaparinux or LMWH more selectively increases degradation of Xa.

65. Ans. (d) May cause metabolic acidosis

[Ref: KDT 7th/704-05;G and G 11th/1115; Pharmacology by Satoskar 24th/650]

Mafenide

◈ *KDT 7th/704-05*

- It is not a typical sulfonamide, because a $-CH_2-$bridge separates the benzene ring and the amino group.
- It is ***used only topically***–inhibits a variety of gram-positive and gram-negative bacteria.
- In contrast to typical sulfonamides, it is active in the presence of pus and against *Pseudomonas*, clostridia which are not inhibited by typical sulfonamides.
- It has been mainly employed for ***burn dressing*** to prevent infection, but not to treat already infected cases.
- The **biggest limitation** is that mafenide produces ***burning sensation and severe pain when applied to raw surface.***

- It is rapidly absorbed from the raw surface, metabolized and excreted in urine.
- Mafenide and its metabolite are carbonic anhydrase inhibitors. Accordingly, they alkalinize urine, can cause acidosis and hyperventilation.
- Mafenide must not be applied over large areas. Allergic reactions, particularly rashes also occur.

Mafenide

◈ *G and G 11th/1115*

- *It is used topically to prevent colonization of burns by a large variety of gram-negative and gram-positive bacteria.*
- *Cleansing of wound and removal of debris should be carried out before each application of the drug*
- *It is associated with significant adverse effects, including **intense pain at sites of application**, allergic reactions, loss of fluid by evaporation from the burn surface, and **metabolic acidosis** secondary to inhibition of carbonic anhydrase.*

66. Ans. (a) Affinity means how strongly..., (b) Efficacy means maximal..., (d) Agonist potency depends..., (e) For antagonists,...

[Ref: KDT 7th/ 40-42; Katzung 13th/5-6,23-24; Pharmacology by Satoskar 24th/32-34,41; Rang and Dale 8th/12]

*"**Irreversible competitive (non-equilibrium) antagonism** occurs with drugs that possess reactive groups **that form covalent bonds with receptor**.* Irreversible, or non-equilibrium, competitive antagonism occurs when the antagonist dissociates very slowly, or not at all, from the receptors, with the result that no change in the antagonist occupancy takes place when the agonist is applied"- *Rang and Dale 8th/12*

Receptor Block Antagonism Involves two Important Mechanisms

◈ *Rang and Dale 8th/11*

- *Reversible competitive antagonism*
- *Irreversible, or non-equilibrium, competitive antagonism.*

Agonists, Antagonists and Efficacy

◈ *Rang and Dale 8th/15*

- Drugs acting on receptors may be ***agonists*** or ***antagonists***.
- Agonists initiate changes in cell function, producing effects of various types; antagonists bind to receptors without initiating such changes.
- **Agonist potency** depends on two parameters: ***affinity*** (i.e. tendency to bind to receptors) and ***efficacy*** (i.e. ability, once bound, to initiate changes that lead to effects).
- ***For antagonists, efficacy is zero.***
- **Full agonists** (which can produce maximal effects) have high efficacy; partial agonists (which can produce only submaximal effects) have intermediate efficacy.
- According to the two-state model, efficacy reflects the relative affinity of the compound for the resting and activated states of the receptor. Agonists show selectivity for the activated state; antagonists show no selectivity. This model, although helpful, fails to account for the complexity of agonist action.
- **Inverse agonists** show selectivity for the resting state of the receptor, this being of significance only in unusual situations where the receptors show constitutive activity.

Receptor Pharmacology

◈ *KDT 7th/ 40-42*

- **Agonist:** An agent which activates a receptor to produce an effect similar to that of the physiological signal molecule.
- **Inverse agonist** An agent which activates a receptor to produce an effect in the opposite direction to that of the agonist
- **Antagonist** An agent which prevents the action of an agonist on a receptor or the subsequent response, but does not have any effect of its own
- **Competitive antagonists** have affinity but no intrinsic activity (IA=0), e.g., propranolol, atropine, chlorpheniramine, naloxone.
- ***Partial agonists*** have affinity and submaximal intrinsic activity (IA between 0 and I), e.g. dichloroisoproterenol (on β adrenergic receptor) pentazocine (on μ opioid receptor)
- ***Inverse agonists*** have affinity but intrinsic activity with a minus sign (IA between 0 and –1)
- The ability to bind with the receptor designated as *affinity*, and the capacity to induce a functional change in the receptor designated as *intrinsic activity* (IA) or *efficacy* are independent properties.
- Competitive antagonists occupy the receptor but do not activate it. Moreover, certain drugs are partial agonists which occupy and submaximally active the receptor. An all or none action is not a must at the receptor.
- The upper limit of DRC is the index of *drug efficacy* and refers to the maximal response that can be elicited by the drug. Efficacy is a more decisive factor in the choice of a drug.
- Often the terms 'drug potency' and 'drug efficacy' are used interchangeably, but these are not synonymous and refer to different characteristics of the drug.

67. Ans. (c) More plasma protein binding means more storage in liver

[Ref: KDT 7th/19-22; Katzung 13th/53; G and G 11th/7-8; Pharmacology by Satoskar 24th/16; Rang and Dale 8th/ 108]

"**Drugs which are highly protein bound** *or ionized remain largely within the vascular compartment and have very* ***low volume of distribution****. Nonionized, lipid soluble drugs(the vast majority) readily cross membranes and are distributed throughout the body, they have large volume of distribution"-Pharmacology by Satoskar 24th/16*

Plasma Protein Binding

◈ *KDT 7th/19-20*

- Most drugs possess physiochemical affinity for plasma proteins and get reversibly bound to these.
- ***Acidic drugs generally bind to plasma albumin and basic drugs to a_1 acid glycoprotein.***

- Binding to albumin is quantitatively more important. Extent of binding depends on the individual compound; no generalization for a pharmacological or chemical class can be made (even small chemical change can markedly alter protein binding)
- Increasing concentrations of the drug can ***progressively saturate the binding sites***: fractional binding may be lower when large amounts of the drug are given. The generally expressed percentage binding refers to the usual therapeutic plasma concentrations of a drug.
- The **clinically significant implications** of plasma protein binding are:
  - Highly plasma protein bound drugs are largely restricted to the vascular compartment because ***protein bound drug does not cross membranes*** (except through large paracellular spaces, such as in capillaries). ***They tend to have smaller volumes of distribution.***
  - The ***bound fraction in not available for action***. However, it is in equilibrium with the free drug in plasma and dissociated when the concentration of the latter is reduced due to elimination. ***Plasma protein binding thus tantamounts to temporary storage of the drug.***
  - ***High degree of protein binding generally makes the drug long acting***, because bound fraction is not available for metabolism or excretion, unless it is actively extracted by liver or by kidney tubules. ***Highly protein bound drugs are not removed by haemodialysis and need special techniques for treatment of poisoning.***
  - The generally expressed plasma concentrations of the drug refer to bound as well as free drug.
  - In hypoalbuminemia, binding may be reduced and high concentration of free drug may be attained

Plasma Proteins

◈ G and G 11th/7-8

- Many drugs circulate in the bloodstream reversibly bound to plasma proteins. ***Albumin is a major carrier for acidic drugs; a1-acid glycoprotein binds basic drugs.***
- The fraction of total drug in plasma that is bound is *determined by the drug concentration, the affinity of binding sites for the drug, and the number of binding sites.*
- *Importantly, binding of a drug to plasma proteins limits its concentration in tissues and at its site of action because only unbound drug is in equilibrium across membranes. Accordingly, after* ***distribution equilibrium*** *is achieved, the concentration of active, unbound drug in intracellular water is the same as that in plasma except when carrier-mediated transport is involved.*
- ***Binding of a drug to plasma protein also limits the drug's glomerular filtration*** *because this process does not immediately change the concentration of free drug in the plasma (water is also filtered).* ***Drug transport and metabolism also are limited by binding to plasma proteins,*** *except when these are especially efficient, and drug clearance, calculated on the basis of unbound drug, exceeds organ plasma flow.*

68. Ans. (d) Directly into stomach, (e) Directly into large intestine

[Ref: KDT 7th/27; Katzung 13th/47-48; Pharmacology by Satoskar 24th/10; G and G 11th/5-6]

Drug given directly into stomach and intestine still have to pass through first pass metabolism in the intestinal wall and in the liver

"Trans-Rectal Route Advantage: *Avoids First Pass Metabolism*"

◈ Satoskar 24th/10

"The ***rectal route****, though less predictable, can be used when oral ingestion is precluded because the patient is unconscious or when vomiting is present.* ***Approximately 50% of the drug that is absorbed from the rectum will bypass the liver****, thus reducing* ***the hepatic first-pass effect****"- G and G 11th/5-6*

First Pass (Presystemic) Metabolism

◈ KDT 7th/27

- This refers to metabolism of a drug during its passage from the site of absorption into the systemic circulation. ***All orally administered drugs*** are exposed to ***drug metabolizing enzymes in the intestinal wall and liver (where they first reach through the portal vein).***
- ***Presystemic metabolism in the gut and liver can be avoided by administering the drug through sublingual, transdermal or parenteral (i.v/i.m/intradermal/s.c) routes.*** However, limited presystemic metabolism can occur in the skin (transdermally administered drug) and in lungs (for drug reaching venous blood through and route).
- ***The extent of first pass metabolism differs for different drugs and is an important determinant of oral bioavailability.***

Attributes of Drugs with High First Pass Metabolism

◈ KDT 7th/27

- *Oral dose is considerably higher than sublingual or parenteral dose*
- *There is marked individual variation in the oral dose due to differences in the extent of first pass metabolism*
- *Oral bioavailability is apparently increased in patients with severe liver disease*

Alternative Routes of Administration and the First-Pass Effect

◈ Katzung 13th/48

- **"First-Pass Elimination***:* Following absorption across the gut wall, the portal blood delivers the drug to the liver prior to entry into the systemic circulation"- *Katzung 13th/47*
- ***The hepatic first-pass effect can be avoided to a great extent by use of sublingual tablets and transdermal preparations and to a lesser extent by use of rectal suppositories.***
- ***Sublingual absorption provides direct access to systemic—not portal—veins. The transdermal route offers the same advantage. Drugs absorbed from suppositories in the lower rectum enter vessels that drain into the inferior vena cava, thus bypassing the liver.***
- Although drugs administered by inhalation bypass the hepatic first-pass effect, the lung may also serve as a site of first-pass loss by excretion and possibly metabolism for drugs administered by nongastrointestinal ("parenteral") routes.

Table *(Katzung 13th/47)*: **Routes of administration, bioavailability, and general characteristics**

Route	Bioavailability(%)	Characteristics
Intravenous (IV)	100 (by definition)	Most rapid onset
Intramuscular (IM)	75 to ≤ 100	Large volumes often feasible; may be painful
Subcutaneous (SC)	75 to ≤ 100	Smaller volumes than IM; may be painful
Oral (PO)	5 to <100	Most convenient; first-pass effect may be significant
Rectal (PR)	30 to <100	Less first-pass effect than oral
Inhalation	5 to <100	Often very rapid onset
Transdermal	80 to ≤ 100	Usually very slow absorption; used for lack of first-pass effect; prolonged duration of action

69. Ans. (a) Vancomycin—Amphotericin B, (c) Warfarin— Aspirin, (d) Allopurinol— Azathioprine, (e) Aminoglycoside—Vancomycin

[Ref: KDT 7th/25-26, 789, 216; Katzung 13th/1119-30; G and G 11th/121-24, 951-52, 972]

"**Drug interaction:** One of the factors that can alter the response to drugs is the concurrent administration of other drugs. There are several mechanisms by which **drugs may interact**, but most can be categorized as ***pharmacokinetic (absorption, distribution, metabolism, excretion), pharmacodynamic (additive or antagonistic effects), or combined interactions***"- *Katzung 13th/1118*

Table *(Katzung 13th/1119-30)*: **Important drug interactions**

Drug or drug group	Properties promoting drug interaction	Clinically documented interactions
Allopurinol	Inhibits hepatic drug-metabolizing enzymes.	**Azathioprine:** [P] Decreased azathioprine detoxification resulting in increased azathioprine toxicity.
Anticoagulants, Oral (Warfarin).	Metabolism inducible. Susceptible to inhibition of metabolism by CYP2C9. Highly bound to plasma proteins. Anticoagulation response altered by drugs that affect clotting factor synthesis or catabolism	**Salicylates:** [HP] Platelet inhibition with aspirin but not with other salicylates; [P] large doses have hypoprothrombinemic effect.
HMG-CoA reductase inhibitors	Lovastatin, simvastatin, and, to a lesser extent, atorvastatin are susceptible to CYP3A4 inhibitors; lovastatin, simvastatin, and, to a lesser extent, atorvastatin are susceptible to CYP3A4 inducers; increased risk of additive myopathy risk with other drugs that can cause myopathy.	(Not mentioned Ranitidine in drug list)

Note: HP, Highly predictable. Interaction occurs in almost all patients receiving the interacting combination; P, Predictable. Interaction occurs in most patients receiving the combination; NP, Not predictable. Interaction occurs only in some patients receiving the combination; NE, Not established. Insufficient data available on which to base estimate of predictability.

"**Allopurinol** *inhibits the degradation of 6-mercaptopurine and* **azathioprine**; *their doses should be reduced to 1/3rd"-KDT 7th/216*

"Aminoglycosides, ***vancomycin,*** *cyclosporine and other nephrotoxic drug enhance the renal impairment caused by* ***amphotericin B****"- KDT 7th/789*

"Enhanced anticoagulant action of ***warfarin:*** *Aspirin-inhibit platelet aggregation and causes g.i.bledding- this may be hazardous in anticoagulated patients.* ***High doses of salicylates have synergistic hypoprothrombinemic action and also displace warfarin from protein binding site****"- KDT 7th/623*

It is cimetidine which has significant drug interaction with others drug, not ranitidine

- "Cimetidine inhibit several cytochromes P-450 isoenzymes- *KDT 7th/650*
- ***"Cimetidine inhibits CYPs and thereby can increase the levels of a variety of drugs that are substrates for these enzymes. Ranitidine also interacts with hepatic CYPs, but with an affinity of only 10% of that of cimetidine; thus ranitidine interferes only minimally with hepatic metabolism of other drugs"****- G and G 11th/972*

All statins (including atorvastatin), except rosuvastatin metabolized primarily by CYP3A4. Inhibitors and inducers of this isoenzyme respectively increase and decrease statin blood level"- *KDT 7th/637*

Table: Drugs that inhibit drug metabolizing enzymes *(KDT 7th/26)*

Allopurinol	Amiodarone
Omeparazole	Propaxyphene
Erythromycin	Isoniazid
Clarithromycin	Cimetidine
Chloramphenicol	Quinidine
Ketoconazole	Disulfiram
Itraconazole	Diltiazem
Metronixazole	Verapamil
Ciprofloxacin	MAO inhibitors
Sulfonamides	Ritonavir (and other HIV protease inhibitors
Fluoxetine (and other SSRIs)	

70. Ans. (b) Contraindicated in congestive heart failure, (c) Causes Hyperkalemia, (d) Increases renal blood flow

[Ref: KDT 7th/590-91; Katzung 13th/262; Pharmacology by Satoskar 24th/557]

Mannitol

◈ *KDT 7th/590-91*

- Mannitol is a nonelectrolyte of low molecular weight that is pharmacologically inert can be given in large quantities sufficient to raise osmolarity of plasma and tubular fluid.
- Though the primary action of mannitol is to increase urinary volume, *excretion of the cations (Na^+, K^+, Ca^{2+}, Mg^{2+}, Mg^{2+}) and anions (Cl^-, HCO^-_3, PO_4^{3-}) is also enhanced*
- *Most common side effect is headache. Nausea and vomiting may occur*
- ***Contraindiacted in CHF***
- It is minimally metabolized in the body; freely filtered at the glomerulus and undergoes limited reabsorption: therefore excellently suited to be used as osmotic diuretic. Mannitol appears to limit tubular water and electrolyte reabsorption in a variety of ways:
  - Retains water isoosmotically in PT–dilutes luminal fluid which opposes NaCl reabsorption
  - ***Inhibits transport processes in the thick AscLH*** by an unknown mechanism. Quantitatively this appears to be the largest contributor to the diuresis
  - ***Expands extracellular fluid volume*** (because it does not enter cells, mannitol draws water from the intracellular compartment)–increases g.f.r and inhibits renin release
  - ***Increases renal blood flow***, especially to the medulla–medullary hypertonicity is reduced (due to washing off)–corticomedullary osmotic gradient is dissipated–passive salt reabsorption is reduced.

Osmotic Diuretics

◈ *Katzung 13th/ 262*

- ***Osmotic diuretics have their major effect in the proximal tubule and the descending limb of Henle's loop.*** Through osmotic effects, they also oppose the action of ADH in the collecting tubule.

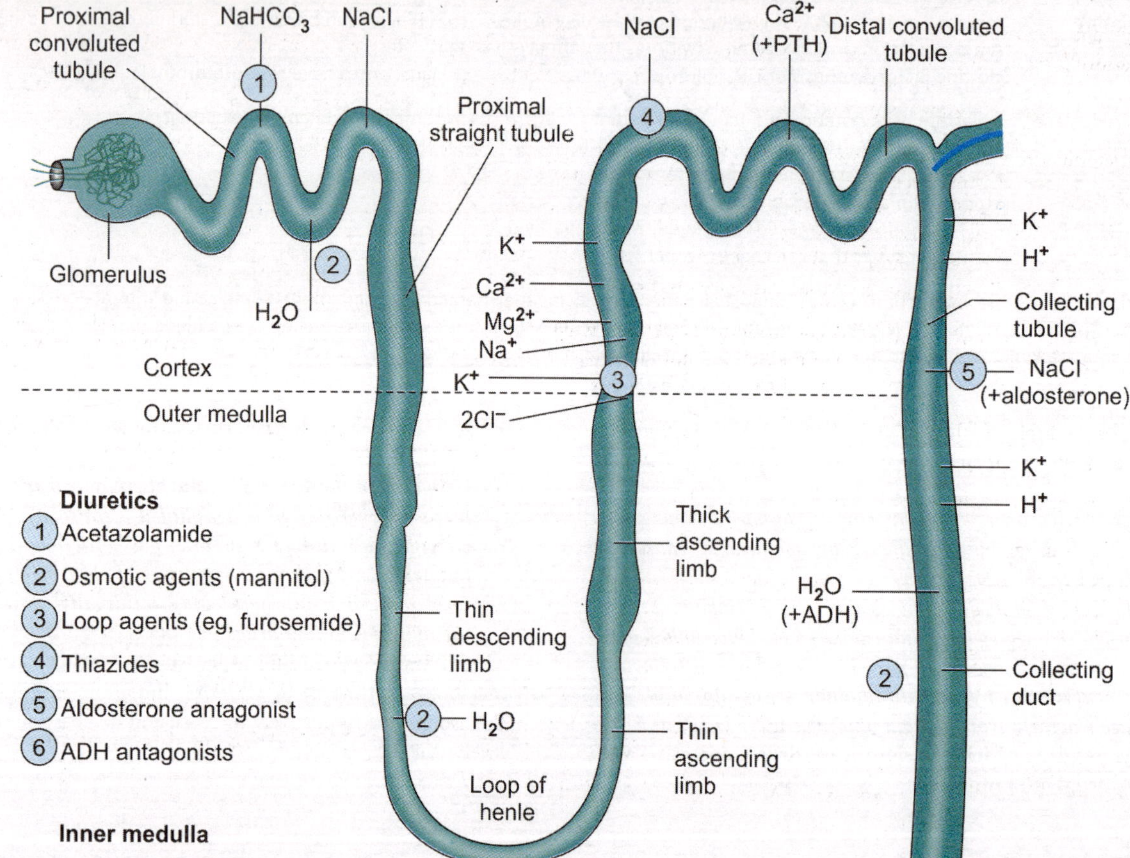

Fig: *(Katzung 13th/250):* Tubule transport systems and sites of action of diuretics. ADH, antidiuretic hormone.

- The presence of a nonrecoverable solute such as mannitol prevents the normal absorption of water by interposing a countervailing osmotic force. As a result, urine volume increases. The increase in urine flow rate decreases the contact time between fluid and the tubular epithelium, thus reducing Na+ as well as water reabsorption. The resulting natriuresis is of lesser magnitude than the water diuresis, leading ***eventually to excessive water loss and hypernatremia.***
- Osmotic diuretics are used to ***increase water excretion in preference to sodium excretion***. This effect can be useful when avid Na^+ retention limits the response to conventional agents.
- **Extracellular Volume Expansion** Mannitol is rapidly distributed in the extracellular compartment and extracts water from cells. Prior to the diuresis, this leads to expansion of the extracellular volume and hyponatremia. This effect can ***complicate heart failure*** and may produce ***florid pulmonary edema***. ***Headache, nausea, and vomiting*** are commonly observed in patients treated with osmotic diuretics.
- **Dehydration, Hyperkalemia, and Hypernatremia:** Excessive use of mannitol without adequate water replacement can ultimately lead to severe dehydration, free water losses, and ***hypernatremia***. As water is extracted from cells, intracellular K^+ concentration rises, leading to cellular losses and ***hyperkalemia.***
- **Hyponatremia:** When used in patients with diminished renal function, parenterally administered mannitol is retained intravenously and causes osmotic extraction of water from cells, leading to hyponatremia.

71. Ans (b) ↑ glucose in plasma, (c) –ve feedback on corticotropin-releasing..., (d) May cause osteoporosis

[Ref: KDT 7th/282-87; Katzung 13th/682-85; A.K.Jain 6th/723]

Cortisol has a negative feedback on ACTH and CRH production. Thus when GC production is impaired as in Addison disease, ACTH is elevated. Similarly, excess GC (either endogenous or exogenous) suppresses ACTH"- medind.nic.in

Glucocorticoids

◈ *Katzung 13th/682-85*

- ***Glucocorticoids given chronically suppress the pituitary release of ACTH***, growth hormone, thyroid-stimulating hormone, and luteinizing hormone.
- ***Glucocorticoids increase serum glucose levels*** and thus stimulate insulin release and inhibit the uptake of glucose by muscle cells, while they stimulate hormone sensitive lipase and thus lipolysis.
- Although glucocorticoids stimulate RNA and protein synthesis in the liver, they ***have catabolic and antianabolic effects in lymphoid and connective tissue, muscle, peripheral fat, and skin***.
- Supraphysiologic amounts of glucocorticoids lead to decreased muscle mass and weakness and thinning of the skin.
- Catabolic and antianabolic effects on bone are the cause of osteoporosis in Cushing's syndrome and impose a major limitation in the long-term therapeutic use of glucocorticoids. In children, glucocorticoids reduce growth.

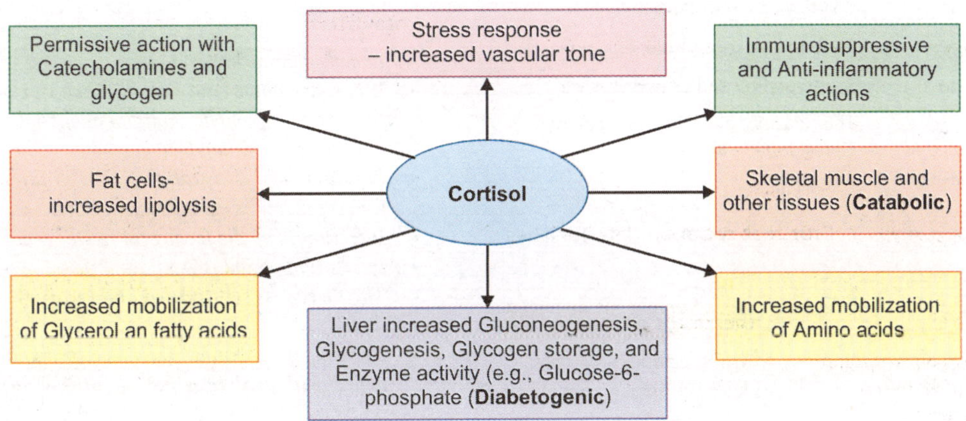

Fig: *A.K.Jain 6th/723*

72. Ans. (a) Amiodarone, (b) Sotalol, (c) Chlorpromazine, (d) Cisapride

[Ref: Davidson 22nd/570-71;KDT 7th/528; ECG by Hampton 8th/157]

Torsades de Pointes (Ventricular Tachycardia)

◈ *Davidson 22nd/570-71*

- This form of polymorphic VT is a complication of prolonged ventricular repolarisation (prolonged QT interval).
- The ECG shows rapid irregular complexes that oscillate from an upright to an inverted position and seem to twist around the baseline as the mean QRS axis changes. The arrhythmia is usually nonsustained and repetitive, but may degenerate into ventricular fibrillation.
- During periods of sinus rhythm, the ECG will usually show a prolonged QT interval (> 0.43 s in men, > 0.45 s in women when corrected to a heart rate of 60/min).

Table *(Davidson 22nd/571)*: **Causes of long QT interval and torsades de pointes**

Bradycardia
• Bradycardia compounds other factors that cause torsades de pointes
Electrolyte disturbance
• Hyypokalaemia • Hypomagnesaemia • Hypocalcaemia
Drugs
• Disopyramide, flecainide (and other class Ia, Ic anti-arrhythmic drugs, p. 574) • Amitriptyline (and other tricyclic antidepressants) • Chlorpromazine (and other phenothiazines) • Erythromycin (and other phenothiazines)
Congenital syndromes
• Long QT1: gene affected KCHQl: K^+ channel, 30–35% • Long QT2: gene affected HERG: K^+ channel, 25–30% • Long QT3: gene affected SCNSA: Na^+ channel, 5–10% • Long QT4–12: rare

Table *(KDT 7th/528)*: **Drug that can potentiate torsades de pointes**

1.	*Antiarrhythmics*	Quinidine, procainamide, disopyramide, propafenone, amiodarone
2.	*Antimalarials*	Quinine, mefloquine, artemisinin, halofantrine
3.	*Antibacterials*	Sparfloxacin, mosifloxacin
4.	*Antihistaminics*	Terfenadine, astemizole, ebastine
5.	*Antidepressants*	Amitryptyline and other tricyclics
6	*Anitpsychotics*	Thioridazine, pimozide, aripiprazole, ziprasidone
7.	*Prokinetic*	Cisapride

Table *(ECG by Hampton 8th/157)*: **Drug that can potentiate Torsades de pointes**

Congenital	**Other drugs**
• Jervell-Lange-Nielson syndrome • Romano-ward syndrome • Several other genetic abnormalities also identified	• Tricyclic antidepressants • Erythromycin
Antiarrhythmic drugs	**Plasma electrolyte abnormalities**
• Procainamide • Disopyramide • Amiodarone • Sotalol	• Low potassium • Low magnesium • Low calcium

MICROBIOLOGY

73. Ans. (a) Most commonly seen in... (e) Single infection provide...

[Ref: Ananthanarayan 9th/560-61; Park 23rd/223; Harrison 19th/1287-88; Jawetz 27th/534-35; Greenwood 16th/525-26]

Rotavirus

◈ *Ananthanarayan 9th/560-61*

- *It is* ***commonest cause of diarrhea in infants and children*** *the world over and accounts for about half the cases of children hospitalized for diarrhea*
- *Rota diarrhea is* ***usually seen in children below the age of five years****, but is most frequent b/w 6 and 24 months of age*
- ***Infection is by the fecal-oral route***
- *Incubation period is 2-3 days*
- *The* ***disease is self-limited and recovery occurs within 5-10 days***
- *"In temperate climate there is a pronounced seasonal incidence,* ***with peak in winter months*** *occurring with clockwise precision"- Greenwood 16th/525; Park 23rd/223*
- *"Transmission occur primarily by the feco-oral route,* ***directly from person to person*** *or indirectly by contaminated fomites"- Park 23rd/223*

Rotavirus

◈ *Harrison 19th/1287-88*

- Worldwide, nearly all children are infected with ***rotavirus by 3–5 years of age.***

- ***Reinfections are common, but the severity of disease decreases with each repeat infection***. Therefore, severe rotavirus infections are less common among older children and adults than among younger individuals.
- The clinical spectrum of rotavirus infection ranges from subclinical infection to severe gastroenteritis leading to life-threatening dehydration.
- After an ***incubation period of 1–3 days***, the illness has an abrupt onset, with vomiting frequently preceding the onset of diarrhea.
- Up to one-third of patients may have a temperature of >39°C. The stools are characteristically loose and watery and only infrequently contain red or white cells. Gastrointestinal symptoms generally resolve in 3–7 days.
- Respiratory and neurologic features in children with rotavirus infection have been reported, but causal associations have not been proven. Moreover, rotavirus infection has been associated with a variety of other clinical conditions (e.g., sudden infant death syndrome, necrotizing enterocolitis, intussusception, Kawasaki's disease, and type 1 diabetes), but no causal relationship has been confirmed with any of these syndromes.

74. Ans. (a) Not lysine... (b) Oxidase positive (c) Produce pyocyanin... (d) Gram-negative

[Ref: Ananthanarayan 9th/314-16; Harrison 19th/1042-43; Jawetz 27th/137-39; Greenwood 16th/282,16]

"**P. aeruginosa** is a ***Gram-negative bacillus*** that is typically 1–3 μm in length. It grows on many solid media and can grow at both 37 and 42°. Most strains have a characteristic grapelike odor. It does not ferment carbohydrates. It is positive in the indophenol oxidase test, and is Simmon's citrate positive, l-arginine dehydrolase positive, ***l-lysine decarboxylase negative***, and l-ornithine decarboxylase negative"- *link.springer.com*

"Lysine Decarboxylase Test (LDC): To assist in the identification of Salmonellae (+ve) and Shigellae (-ve)"

Bacteria that are Lysine Decarboxylase (LDC) Positive *microbeonline.com*

- *Escherichia coli*
- *Salmonella typhi* and Most other salmonellae species (except Salmonella paratyphi A).
- *Klebsiella pneumoniae*
- *Serratia marcescens*
- *Vibrio cholerae*
- *Vibrio Parahemolyticus*

*"P. aeruginosa: Motile by virtue of **one or two polar flagella**"- Greenwood 16th/282*

P. aeruginosa

◈ *Ananthanarayan 9th/314-16*

- *It is a **Gram-negative bacillus** actively motile by a polar flagellum*
- *It is an obligate aerobes*
- *Produces a number of pigments, the best known being **pyocyanin (bluish-green)** and fluorescein (greenish-yellow). Other pigments produced are pyorubin (red) andpyomelanin (brown)*
- *The metabolism is oxidative and non-fermentative. It is catalase positive, **oxidase positive** and motile. Glucose is utilized oxidatively, forming only acid*

Biochemical Test and Identification of Pseudomonas aeruginosa*www.microbiologyinfo.com*

Enzymatic Reactions	
Amidase	–
Arginine dehydrolase	Positive (+ve)
Lecithinase	–
Lipase	Positive (+ve)
Lysine	Negative (–ve)

Pseudomonads

◈ *Harrison 19th/1042-43*

- The pseudomonads are a heterogeneous group of ***gram-negative bacteria*** that have in common an inability to ferment lactose.
- *P. aeruginosa* is a nonfastidious, ***motile, gram-negative rod*** that grows on most common laboratory media, including blood and MacConkey agars.
- It is easily identified in the laboratory on primary-isolation agar plates by ***pigment production*** that confers a ***yellow to dark green or even bluish appearance.*** Colonies have a shiny "gun-metal" appearance and a characteristic fruity odor. Two of the identifying biochemical characteristics of *P. aeruginosa* are an inability to ferment lactose on MacConkey agar and a ***positive reaction in the oxidase test.***

75. Ans. (a) Herpes virus, (b) Hepadnaviridae, (c) Parvovirus

[Ref: Ananthanarayan 9th/428,439-40; Harrison 19th/214e-1; Jawetz 27th/852]

Table *(Harrision 19th 214e-1)*: **Virus Families pathogenic for Humans**

Family	Representative Viruses	Type of RNA/DNA	Lipid Envelope
RNA Viruses			
Picornaviridae	Poliovirus Coxsackievirus Echovirus ***Enterovirus*** Rhinovirus Hepatitis A virus	(+) RNA	No
Caliciviridae	Norwalk agent Hepatitis E virus	(+) RNA	No

Contd...

Family	Representative Viruses	Type of RNA/DNA	Lipid Envelope
Togaviridae	Rubella virus Eastern equine encephalitis virus Western equine encephalitis virus	(+) RNA	Yes
Flaviviridae	Yellow fever virus Dengue virus St. Louis encephalitis virus West Nile virus Hepatitis C virus Hepatitis G virus	(+) RNA	Yes
Coronaviridae	Coronaviruses[a]	(+) RNA	Yes
Rhabdoviridae	Rabies virus Vesicular stomatitis virus	(–) RNA	Yes
Filoviridae	Marburg virus Ebola virus	(–) RNA	Yes
Paramyxoviridae	Parainfluenza virus Respiratory syncytial virus Newcastle disease virus Mumps virus Rubeola (measles) virus	(–) RNA	Yes
Orthomyxoviridae	Influenza A, B, and C viruses	(–) RNA, 8 segments	Yes
Bunyaviridae	Hantavirus California encephalitis virus Sandfly fever virus	(–) RNA, 3 circular segments	Yes
Arenaviridae	Lymphocytic choriomeningitis virus Lassa fever virus South American hemorrhagic fever virus	(–) RNA, 2 circular segments	Yes
Reoviridae	Rotavirus Reovirus Colorado tick fever virus	ds RNA, 10–12 segments	No
Retroviridae	Human T lymphotropicvirus types I and II Human immunodeficiency virus types 1 and 2	(+) RNA, 2 identical segments	Yes
DNA Viruses			
Hepadnaviridae	Hepatitis B virus	ds DNA with ss portions	Yes
Parvoviridae	Parvovirus B19	ss DNA	No
Papovaviridae	Human papillomaviruses JC virus BK virus	ds DNA	No
Adenoviridae	Human adenoviruses	ds DNA	No
Herpesviridae	Herpes simplex virus types 1 and 2 Varicella-zoster virus Epstein-Barr virus Cytomegaloviruse Human herpesvirus 6 Human herpesvirus 7 Kaposi's sarcoma—associated herpesvirus	ds DNA	Yes
Poxviridae	Variola (smallpox) virus Orf virus Molluscumcontagiosum virus	ds DNA	Yes

76. Ans. (a) Belong to flavivirus, (c) RT PCR is useful in diagnosis, (e) May presents with conjunctivitis

[Ref: Harrison 19th/1314; www. cdc. gov;www. nytimes. com]

Zika Virus Infection

◈ *www. cdc. govand other sites*

- It is spread mostly by the bite of an infected *Aedes* species mosquito (*A. aegypti* and *A. albopictus*). These mosquitoes are aggressive daytime biters. They can also bite at night.
- It can be ***passed from a pregnant woman to her fetus.*** Infection during pregnancy can cause certain birth defects.
- It can be ***passed through sex*** from a person who has Zika to his or her partners. It can be passed through sex, even if the infected person does not have symptoms at the time.
- ***The majority of people infected with Zika virus do not display any symptoms***
- According to the Pan American Health Organization (PAHO), **only 1 in 4 people infected with Zika virus develop symptoms.** In contrast, the CDC state the figure is **1 in 5.** According to the Pan American Health Organization (PAHO), **only 1 in 4 people infected with Zika virus develop symptoms. 5** In contrast, the CDC state the figure is **1 in 5.**
- The infections in adults may result rarely in Guillain–Barré syndrome
- A blood or urine test can confirm Zika infection diagnosis.
- ***Real-time reverse transcription-polymerase chain reaction (rRT-PCR)*** testing should be performed on serum collected during the first two weeks after symptom onset.
- A negative rRT-PCR result does not exclude Zika virus infection and serum should be analyzed by IgM antibody (serological) testing.
- Zika virus-specific IgM and neutralizing antibodies typically develop toward the end of the first week of illness.
- ***There's no vaccine or specific treatment for the disease.*** Treatment instead focuses on relieving symptoms and includes rest, rehydration and medications for fever and pain.

Zika Virus

◈ *www.who.int/mediacentre*

- There is scientific consensus that Zika virus is a cause of ***microcephaly*** and Guillain-Barré syndrome.
- Zika virus is a ***mosquito-borne flavivirus*** that was ***first identified in Uganda in 1947 in monkeys through a network that monitored yellow fever. It was later identified in humans in 1952 in Uganda and the United Republic of Tanzania.***
- Outbreaks of Zika virus disease have been recorded in Africa, the Americas, Asia and the Pacific. From the 1960s to 1980s, human infections were found across Africa and Asia, typically accompanied by mild illness.
- The first large outbreak of disease caused by Zika infection was reported from the Island of Yap (Federated States of Micronesia) in 2007. In July 2015 Brazil reported an association between Zika virus infection and Guillain-Barré syndrome. In October 2015 Brazil reported an association between Zika virus infection and ***microcephaly.***

Zika Virus Infection

◈ *Harrison 19th/1314*

- Zika virus is an emerging pathogen that is transmitted among nonhuman primates and humans by ***Aedes mosquitoes.***
- A maculopapular rash, ***conjunctivitis***, myalgia, and arthralgia usually accompany or follow those manifestations.
- Zika virus infection was first documented in Africa in 1947 and was later recognized in southeastern and southern Asia.
- In recent years, the number of Zika virus infections reported from Micronesia and Polynesia has increased steadily

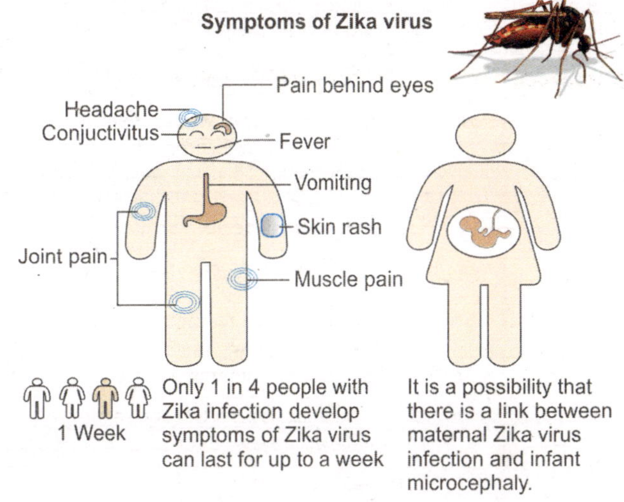

77. Ans. (a) Fasciola hepatica, (b) Fasciolopsis buski, (d) Watsonius watsoni, (e) Gastrodiscoides hominis

[Ref: Paniker's Parasitology 7th/151; Chatterjee Parasitology 13th/174; Harrison 19th/245e-1]

Mode of infection: *Tramatode infection may occur in the following ways (Paniker's Parasitology 7th/140; Chatterjee Parasitology 13th/174)*

- By ingestion of encysted cercariae in
  - Vegetables, as in F.hepatica, F.buski, W.watsoni
  - Fish, as in C.sinensis, H.heterophyses, M.yokogawi
  - *Flesh of crab or crayfish, as in **P.westermani***
- Free cercariae penetrating directly through the skin, as in S.heamatobium, S.mansoni, S.japonicum

"**Mode of infection of Fasciola hepatica**: *The definitive host, sheep and man, get infection by ingestion of metacerceriae encysted on **aquatic vegetation**"-Paniker's Parasitology 7th/151*

"Intermediate host of **Fasciola hepatica:** *Snails of genus lymnaea and succinea. Encystment occurs on **aquatic plants**, which act as second intermediate host"-Paniker's Parasitology 7th/151*

"Infective form of **Fasciolopsis Buski**: *Encysted metacercariate on **aquatic vegetation**"-Paniker's Parasitology 7th/154*

"Second intermediate host of **Fasciolopsis Buski:** *Encystment occurs on **aquatic plants**, roots of the lotus, bulb of water chestnut which act as second intermediate host"-Paniker's Parasitology 7th/154*

*"Mode of infection of **Paragonimus Westermani**: Man acquires infection by eating undercooked crab or cray fish containing metacercariae"-Paniker's Parasitology 7th/156*

"Second intermediate host of Gastrodiscoides hominis: *aquatic plant.* *The cercariae encyst on water plants. Man and* *animals become infected by feeding upon vegetations harbouring the metacercaria"- Paniker's Parasitology 7th/157*

78. Ans. (a) Rat flea– Endemic typhus, (b) Sand flea—Oriental sore, (d) Cyclops—Dracunculosis

[Ref: Park 23rd/768; Paniker's Parasitology 7th/223]

Table *(Park 23rd/768):* **Arthropad-borne diseases**

Arthropod		Disease transmitted
1.	Mosquito	Malaria, filaria, viral encephalitis (e.g., Japanese encephalitis), viral fevers (e.g., dengue, West Nile, viral haemorrhagic fevers (e.g., yellow fever, dengue haemorrhagic fever)
2.	*Housefly*	Typhoid and paratyphoid fever, diarrhoea, dysentery, cholera, gastroenteritis, amoebiasis, helminthic infestations, poliomyelitis, conjunctivitis, trachoma, anthrax, yaws, etc.
3.	Sandfly	***Kala-azar***, ***oriental sore***, sandfly fever, orayafever
4.	Tsetse fly	Sleeping sickness
5.	Louse	Epidemic typhus, relapsing fever, trench fever, pediculosis
6.	Rat flea	Bubonic plague, ***endemic typhus,*** chiggerosis, hymenolepisdiminuata
7.	Blackfly	Onchocerciasis.
8.	Reduviid bug	Chagas disease.
9.	Hard tick	Tick typhus, viral encephalitis, viral fevers, viral haemorrhagic fever, (e.g., Kyasanur forest disease), tularemia, tick paralysis, human babesiosis.
10.	Soft tick	Q fever, relapsing fever.
11.	Trombiculid mite	Scrub typhus, Rickettsial-pox.
12.	Itch-mite	Scabies
13.	Cyclops	Guinea-worm disease, fish tapeworm (D. latus).
14.	Cockroaches	Enteric pathogens.

Table *(Paniker's Parasitology 7th/223):* **Parasites requiring one intermediate host to complete their life cycle**

Intermediate host	Parasite
• Man	Plasmodium species Echinococcus granulosus Echinococcus multilocularis Taeniamulticeps
• Pig	Taenia solium Taeniasaginata asiatica Sarcocystis suihominis Trichinella spiralis
• Cow	Taeniasaginata Sarcocystishominis
• Snail	Schistosoma species
• Cyclops	Dracunculus medinensis (Dracunculosis)
• Sandfly	Leishmania species
• Tsetse fly	Trypanosoma species
• Chrysops	Loa loa
• Mosquito	Wuchereria bancrofti Brugia spp. Mansonella spp.
• Tick	Babesia species
• Triatomine bug	Trypanosoma cruzi
• Flea	Hymenolepis nana Hymenolepis diminuta Dipylidium caninum

79. Ans. (d) Ciprofloxacin is drug of choice, (e) Tick borne disease

[Ref: Ananthanarayan 9th/408; Harrison 19th/1159; Park 23rd/300; Medical microbiology by Greenwood 16th /372]

*"**Scrub typhus:** One typical feature is the punched-out ulcer covered with a **blackened scab (eschar)** which indicates the location of mite bite"- Park 23rd/300*

*"**Scrub typhus**: Most travel-acquired cases occur during visits to **rural areas** in endemic countries for activities such as **camping, hiking or rafting**, but urban cases have also been described. **Tetracycline is drug of choice**"- Park 23rd/300*

*"**Scrub typhus,** originally found in scrub jungles, has also been identified in a variety of other habitats, such as sandy beaches, **mountain deserts** and equatorial rain-forests"- Ananthanarayan 9th/408*

Scrub Typhus

- *Ananthanarayan 9th/408*
- *The vectors are **trombiculid mites** of genus Leptotrombidium*
- ***Incubation period is 1-3 week***
- *Originally found in scrub jungles, has also been identified in a variety of other habitats, such as **sandy beaches, mountain deserts and equatorial rain-forests***
- "Human beings are infected *when they are beaten by the mite larva (chigger). Adult mites feed only on plant"*
- "Zoonotic terad of Scrub typhus: *It consists of Orien tatsutsugamushi, chiggers, rats, secondary or transitional forms of vegetation"*
- "Three major antigenic types have been recognized- Gilliam, Karp and Kato"- *Ananthanarayan 8th/ 409*

Contd...

Scrub Typhus

◈ *(Chigger-borne Typhus) Harrison 19th/1159*

- *O. tsutsugamushi* is maintained by transovarial transmission ***intrombiculid mites.***
- After hatching, infected larval mites (chiggers, the only stage that feeds on a host) inoculate organisms into the skin. Infected chiggers are particularly likely to be found in areas of heavy scrub vegetation during the wet season, when mites lay eggs.
- Scrub typhus is endemic and reemerging in eastern and southern Asia, northern Australia, and islands of the western Pacific and Indian Oceans. Infections are prevalent in these regions; in some areas, >3% of the population is infected or reinfected each month.
- *Illness varies from mild and self-limiting to fatal. After an incubation period of 6–21 days, onset is characterized by fever, headache, myalgia, cough, and gastrointestinal symptoms.*
- Some patients recover spontaneously after a few days. The classic case description includes an **eschar** where the chigger has fed, regional lymphadenopathy, and a ***maculopapular rash***—signs that are seldom seen in indigenous patients. Fewer than 50% of Westerners develop an eschar, and fewer than 40% develop a rash (on day 4–6 of illness).
- Patients are treated with doxycycline, azithromycin, or chloramphenicol

Table (*Jawetz 27th/342*): **Scrub typhus**

Organism	Disease	Geographic Distribution	Vector	Mammalian Resevoir	Clinical Features
Orientia tsutsugamushi	Scrub typhus	Asia, South Pacific, northern Australia	Mite	Rodents, birds	Fever, headache, rash (50% have eschar), lymphadenopathy, atypical lymphocytes

80. Ans. (a) Facultative anaerobes, (b) Not acid fast, (c) Endogenous cause of disease

[Ref: Ananthanarayan 9th/391-93;Jawetz 27th/295,198-99; Greenwood 16th/221-22; Harrison 19th/1088]

Actinomyces

◈ *Greenwood 16th/221-22*

- *They are* ***facultative anaerobes,*** *but often fail to grow aerobically on primary culture. They grow best under anaerobic or micro-aerophilic conditions with the addition of 5-10% carbon dioxide*
- They are responsible for the disease known as actinomycosis

Table (*Greenwood 16th/222*): **Differences b/w the genera Actinomyces and Nocardia**

Actinomyces spp.	Nocardia app
• Facultative anaerobes • Grow at 35–37°C • Oral commensals • Non-acid fast mycelia • Endogenous cause of disease	• Strict aerobes • Wide temperature range of growth • Environmental saprophytes • Usually weakly acid-fast • Exogenous cause of disease

Summarized form of Test

◈ *Ananthanarayan 9th/391-93*

Actinomyces	Nocardia
• Anaerobic/microaerophilic • Non-acid fast • Endogenous in origin (Greenwood 16th/222)	• Aerobic • May be acid fast • Exogenous

Actinomycosis

◈ *Harrison 19th/1088*

- Actinomycosis is an indolent, slowly progressive infection caused by ***anaerobic or microaerophilic bacteria***, primarily of the genus *Actinomyces*, that colonize the mouth, colon, and vagina. Mucosal disruption may lead to infection at virtually any site in the body.
- In vivo growth of actinomycetes usually results in the formation of characteristic clumps called *grains* or *sulfur granules*.
- Three "classic" clinical presentations that should prompt consideration of this unique infection are (1) the combination of chronicity, progression across tissue boundaries, and mass-like features (mimicking malignancy, with which it is often confused); (2) the development of a sinus tract, which may spontaneously resolve and recur; and (3) a refractory or relapsing infection after a short course of therapy, since cure of established actinomycosis requires prolonged treatment.

Nocardia

◈ *Harrison 19th/1084*

- *Nocardia*, a genus of ***saprophytic aerobic actinomycetes*** that are common worldwide, resides in soil, contributing to the decay of organic matter.
- Nearly 100 species have been identified, mostly on the basis of 16S rRNA gene sequences.

81. Ans. (b) Athlete's foot, (c) Kerion, (d) Favus

[Ref: Ananthanarayan 9th/596-97; Harrison 19th/1358]

"Madura foot (eumycetoma or maduramycosis) is caused by fungi- *scedosporium, madurella mycetomatis and M.grisea,* *acremonium spp., exophiala spp., aspergillus spp. and fusarium spp."- Ananthanarayan 9th/600-601*

Clinical Aspect of Dermatophytosis

◈ *Ananthanarayan 9th/596*

Dermnatophytosis is twice as common in males as in females. Clinical classification is according to the anatomic site involved:

- *Tinea barbae* (barber's itch) involves the bearded areas of the face and neck
- *Tinea corporis* (Tinea glabrosa) is ringworm of the smooth or non-hairy skin of the body
- *Tinea imbricate* is a special type of *Tinea corporis* found in the tropics, which presents with characteristic extensive concentric rings of papulosquamous scaly patches
- *Tinea capitis* is ringworm of the scalp; ***favus and kerion*** are variants
- *Tinea cruris* (jock itch) involves the groin and perineum
- *Tinea pedis* (***athlete's foot***) is ringworm of the foot
- *Tinea manuum* involves the hand
- *Tinea unguinum* involves the nails

"Favus: A chronic type of ringworm in which dense crusts (scutula) develop in the hair follicles, leading to alopecia and scarring"- *Ananthanarayan 9th/596*

"Kerion: Severe boggy lesions with marked inflammatory reaction that sometimes develops in scalp infection due to dermatophytes"-*Ananthanarayan 9th/596*

Dermatophyte (Mold) Infections

◈ *Harrison 19th/1358*

- The molds that cause skin infections in humans include the genera *Trichophyton*, *Microsporum*, and *Epidermophyton*.
- These organisms, which are not components of the normal skin flora, can live within the keratinized structures of the skin—hence the term *dermatophytes*.

Table *(Annanthanaryan 9th/596):* **Clinical types of dermatophytoses and their common causative agents**

Disease	Common causative agents
Tinea capitis	Microsporum any species Trichophyton most species
Favus	T. Schoenleinii, T. violaceum M. gypseum
Tinea barbae	T. rubrum, T. mentagrophytes, T. verrucosum
Tinea imbricate	T. Concentricum
Tinea corporis	T. rubrum and any other dermatophyte
T cruris	E. floccosum, T.rubrum
T pedis	T. rubrum, E. floccosum
Ectothrix hair	Microsporum species,
Infection	T. rubrum, T. mentagrophytes
Endothrix hair	T. schoenleinii, T. tonsurans,
Infection	T. violaceum

82. Ans. (c) Shigella dysentery

[Ref: Ananthanarayan 9th/287, 295; Greenwood 16th/261, 252, 289]

*"**Shigella cause bacillary dysentery**. Infection occur by ingestion. The minimum infective dose is low: as few as **10-100 bacilli** are capable of initiating the disease, probably because they survive gastric acidity better than other enterobacterium"-Ananthanarayan 9th/287*

"Bacillary dysentery may follow the ingestion of as few as 10 viable bacteria"- Greenwood 16th/261

"**Campylobacter jejuni**: *In volunteer studies, infection has been established with as few as **500-800 organisms**"-Greenwood 16th/289*

Cholera (Vibrio cholera): *It has been shown that **10^6 pathogenic vibrios** administered to fasting normochlorohydric volunteers, without food or buffer, did not produce infection, while the same dose given along with food or sodium bicarbonate caused clinical cholera in 80-100 percent of them"- Ananthanarayan 9th/307*

"**Enteric fever (S.typhi, S.paratyphi -A, B, C)**: *The infection is acquired by ingestion. In human volunteer experiments, ID50 was found to be about **10^3 to 10^6 bacilli**"- Ananthanarayan 9th/295*

83. Ans. (a) Obligate aerobe

[Ref: Ananthanarayan 9th/ 24-25;Greenwood 16th/41]

Oxygen Requirement and Metabolism

◈ *Ananthanarayan 9th/ 24*

- Depending on the influence of oxygen on growth and viability, bacteria are divided into aerobes and anaerobes.
- **Aerobic bacteria** require oxygen for growth. They may be ***obligate aerobes*** like the cholera vibrio, which will ***grow only in the presence of oxygen***, or ***facultative anaerobes*** which are ordinarily aerobic but can also grow in the absence of oxygen, though less abundantly.
- Most bacteria of medical importance are facultative anaerobes. Anaerobic bacteria, such as clostridia, grow in the absence of oxygen and the **obligate anaerobes** may even die on exposure to oxygen. **Microaerophilic** bacteria are those that grow best in the presence of **low oxygen tension**.
- The reason for the apparent toxicity of oxygen for anaerobic bacteria is not well understood. It has been suggested that in the presence of oxygen, hydrogen peroxide and other toxic peroxides accumulate. The enzyme catalase which splits hydrogen peroxide is present in most aerobic bacteria but is absent in anaerobes. Another reason is that obligate anaerobes possess essential enzymes that are active only in the reduced state.
- The influence of free oxygen is related to the metabolic character of the bacterium. Aerobic bacteria obtain their energy and intermediates only through oxidation, involving oxygen as the ultimate hydrogen acceptor, while the anaerobes use hydrogen acceptors other than oxygen. Facultative anaerobes may act in both ways. In the case of aerobes, where the ultimate electron acceptor is atmospheric oxygen (aerobic respiration)

- The carbon and energy source may be completely oxidized to carbon dioxide and water. Energy is provided by the production of energy-rich phosphate bonds and the conversion of adenosine diphosphate (ADP) to adenosine triphosphate (ATP). This process is known as **oxidative phosphorylation**. Anaerobic bacteria use as electron acceptors compounds such as nitrates or sulphates instead of oxygen (anaerobic respiration)

84. Ans. (a) Zanamivir commonly given...

[Ref: Park 23rd/156-59; Ananthanarayan 9th/499-504; Harrison 19th/1209-14; KDT 7th/802-03]

WHO: It is recommended that trivalent vaccines for use in the 2016-2017 influenza season (northern hemisphere winter) contain the following: *www.who.int/influenza/vaccine*

- An A/California/7/2009 (H1N1) pdm09-like virus;
- An A/Hong Kong/4801/2014 (H3N2)-like virus;
- A B/Brisbane/60/2008-like virus.

It is recommended that quadrivalent vaccines containing two influenza B viruses contain the above three viruses and a B/Phuket/3073/2013-like virus.

WHO: It is recommended that *trivalent vaccines* for use in the 2017 southern hemisphere influenza season contain the following: *www.who.int/influenza/vaccine*

- An A/Michigan/45/2015 (H1N1) pdm09-like virus;
- An A/Hong Kong/4801/2014 (H3N2)-like virus; and
- A B/Brisbane/60/2008-like virus.

It is recommended that ***quadrivalent vaccines*** containing ***two influenza B viruses contain the above three viruses and a B/Phuket/3073/2013-like virus.***

"CDC guideline: Vaccine virus strains included in the 2016–17 U.S. **trivalent influenza** *vaccines will be an* ***A/California/7/2009 (H1N1)–like virus, an A/Hong Kong/4801/2014 (H3N2)–like virus, and a B/Brisbane/60/2008–like virus (Victoria lineage).*** **Quadrivalent vaccines** *will include an* ***additional influenza B virus strain, a B/Phuket/3073/2013***–*like virus (Yamagata lineage)"- www.cdc.gov/mmwr*

Pandemic Influenza A (H_1n_1) 2009

◈ *Park 23rd/156-59*

- Currently susceptible to *oseltamivir and zanamivir* but resistant to amantadine or rimantadine
- Treatment: oseltamivir adult oral dose is 75 mg twice daily for 5 days. ***Zanamivir dose is two inhalation*** (2 × 5 mg) twice daily for 5 days
- In patient who have persistent severe illness despite oseltamivir, there are few licensed alternative antiviral treatments. In these situations, clinician have ***considered intravenous administration*** of alternative antiviral drugs such as zanamivir, peramivir and ribavirin"- *Park 23rd/159*
- Chemoprophylaxis: Oseltamivir is drug of choice for chromoprophylaxis. It should be given till 10 days after last exposure
- "**Zanamivir:** ***10 mg through breath actuated inhaler,*** *BDX5 days for treatment and OD for prophylaxis"-KDT 7th/803*
- ***Influenza vaccine only become effective about 14 days after vaccination.*** Those infected shortly before (1-3 days) or shortly after immunization can still get the disease.
- Vaccinated individuals can also get influenza caused by a *different strain of influenza virus*, for which the vaccine does not provide protection

Pandemic Influenza A (H_1n_1) 2009

◈ *Park 23rd/156-59*

- ***Case fatality rate*** *is similar to seasonal influenza i.e about 0.5%; however this could change*
- ***RT-PCR provides the most timely and sensitive detection of the infection***
- *Age and sex for seasonal influenza (also similar to H1N1 pandemic):* ***Influenza affects all ages and both sexes. In general attack rate is lower among adults.*** *Children constitute an important link in the transmission chain. The* ***highest mortality rate during an epidemic occur among certain high-risk groups*** *in population such as old people (generally over 65 years of age), children under 18 months, and person with diabetes or chronic health disease, kidney and respiratory ailments. - Park 23rd/154*

Etiologic Agent

◈ *Harrison 19th/1209-11*

- Influenza outbreaks occur virtually every year, although their extent and severity vary widely. The most recent ***pandemic emerged in March of 2009*** and was caused by an **influenza A/H_1N_1** virus that rapidly spread worldwide over the next several months.
- A 5-day course of oseltamivir or zanamivir reduces the duration of signs and symptoms of uncomplicated influenza by 1–1.5 days if treatment is started within 2 days of the onset of illness and may be effective if started up to 5 days after onset of symptoms.
- ***Zanamivir is administered via an oral inhalation device*** and may exacerbate bronchospasm in asthmatic patients. Oseltamivir has been associated with nausea and vomiting, whose frequency can be reduced by administration of the drug with food. Oseltamivir has also been associated with neuropsychiatric side effects in children. ***Peramivir, an investigational neuraminidase inhibitor that can be administered intravenously, is being evaluated in clinical trials, as is an intravenous form of zanamivir.***

85. Ans. (a) Hbs Ag +ve, (c) Anti-HBe antibody positive, (d) Low level DNA

[Ref: Ananthanarayan 9th/543-48; Harrison 19th/2032-33,2007; Davidson 22nd/950-52; Park 23rd/215]

"**Chronic HBV infection**: **Inactive carriers** are patients with circulating ***hepatitis B surface antigen (HBsAg), normal serum aminotransferase levels, undetectable HBeAg, and levels of HBV DNA that are either undetectable or present at a threshold of ≤103 IU/mL.*** This serologic profile can occur not only in inactive carriers but also in patients with HBeAg-negative chronic hepatitis B during periods of relative inactivity; distinguishing between the two requires sequential biochemical and virologic monitoring over many months"- Harrison 19th/33

Table *(Davidson 22nd/951)*: **The five phases of chronic hepatitis B virus infection**

Phase	HBsAg	HBeAg	Anti-HBe Ab	Viral load	ALT	Histology	Notes
'Immune tolerant' Phase	+	+	–	+++	Normal/Low	Normal/minimal necroinflammation	Prolonged in perinatally infected individuals; may be short or absent if infected as an adult. High viral load and so very infectious
'Immune reactive' HBeAg-positive chronic hepatitis phase	+	+	–	++	Raised	Moderate/severe necroinflammation	May last weeks or years. High risk of cirrhosis or HCC if prolonged. Increased chance of spontaneous loss of HBeAg with seroconversion to anti-HBe Ab-positive state
'Inactive carrier' phase	+	–	+	–/+	Normal	Normal/minimal necroinflammation	Low risk of cirrhosis or HCC in majority
HBeAg-negative chronic hepatitis phase	+	–	+	Fluctuating +/++	Raised/ Fluctuating	Moderate/severe necroinflammation	May represent late immune reactivation or presence of 'pre-core mutant' HBV. High risk of cirrhosis or HCC
HBsAg-negative phase	–	–	+	–/±	Normal	Normal	Ultrasensitive techniques may detect low-level HBV even after HBsAg loss

Table *(Harrison 19th/2017)*: **Commonly Encountered serologic patterns of Hepatitis B Infection**

HBsAg	Anti-HBs	Anti-HBc	HBeAg	Anti-HBe	Interpretation
+	–	IgM	+	–	Acute hepatitis B, high infectivity
+	–	IgG	+	–	Chronic hepatitis B, high infectivity
+	–	IgG	–	+	• Late acute or chronic hepatitis B, low infectivity • HBeAg-negative ("precore- mutant") hepatitis B (chronic or, rarely, acute)
+	+	+	+/–	+/–	• HBsAg of one subtype and heterotypic anti-HBs (common) • Process of seroconversion from HBsAg to anti-HBs (rare)
–	–	IgM	+/–	+/–	• Acute hepatitis B • Anti-HBc "window"
–	–	IgG	–	+/–	• Low-level hepatitis B carrier • Hepatitis B in remote past
–	+	IgG	–	+/–	Recovery from hepatitis B
–	+	–	–	–	• Immunization with HBsAg (after vaccination) • Hepatitis B in the remote past (?) • False-positive

Chronic HBV Infection

◈ *Harrison 19th/2032-33*

- Chronic HBV infection can occur in the presence or absence of serum hepatitis B e antigen (HBeAg), and generally, for both HBeAg-reactive and HBeAg-negative chronic hepatitis B, the level of HBV DNA correlates with the level of liver injury and risk of progression. In *HBeAg-reactive chronic hepatitis B*, two phases have been recognized based on the relative level of HBV replication
- The relatively ***replicative phase*** is characterized by the presence in the serum of HBeAg and HBV DNA levels well in excess of 103–104 IU/mL, sometimes exceeding 109 IU/mL; by the presence in the liver of detectable intrahepatocyte nucleocapsid antigens (primarily hepatitis B core antigen [HBcAg]); by high infectivity; and by accompanying liver injury.
- In contrast, the relatively ***nonreplicative phase*** is characterized by the absence of the conventional serum marker of HBV replication (HBeAg), the appearance of anti-HBe, levels of HBV DNA below a threshold of ~103 IU/mL, the absence of intrahepatocytic HBcAg, limited infectivity, and minimal liver injury. Patients in the replicative phase

tend to have more severe chronic hepatitis, whereas those in the nonreplicative phase tend to have minimal or mild chronic hepatitis or to be inactive hepatitis B carriers.

- The likelihood in a patient with HBeAg-reactive chronic hepatitis B of converting spontaneously from relatively replicative to nonreplicative infection is approximately 10% per year.
- ***HBeAg-negative chronic hepatitis B*** (i.e., chronic HBV infection with active virus replication, readily detectable HBV DNA but without HBeAg [anti-HBe-reactive]), is more common than HBeAg-reactive chronic hepatitis B in Mediterranean and European countries and in Asia (and, correspondingly, in HBV genotypes other than A). Compared to patients with HBeAg-reactive chronic hepatitis B, patients with HBeAg-negative chronic hepatitis B have levels of HBV DNA that are several orders of magnitude lower (no more than 105–106 IU/mL) than those observed in the HBeAg-reactive subset.

86. Ans. (a) Mycobaterium tuber.. (b) Streptococcus pyogenes... (c) Neisseia meningtitides... (e) Polysaccharide...

[Ref: Ananthanarayan 9th/350,212; textbookofbacteriology.net/antiphago;Jawetz 27th/158-65; Greenwood 16th/244]

*"The virulence determinants of **invasive meningococci** seem to be the **LPS capsule**(all pathogenic meningococci are capsulated), IgA proteases and **iron utilization from transferrin**"- Greenwood 16th/244*

The Requirement for Iron

◈ *Jawetz 27th/165*

- Some bacteria have evolved high-affinity iron assimilation systems. Part of these high-affinity systems involves **siderophores**
- Some bacteria do not have demonstrable siderophores. *Y pestis* can utilize iron from hemin and may be able to initiate infection using iron from hemin in the gut of the biting flea. *N gonorrhoeae* makes a series of ***iron-regulated outer membrane proteins***, but the mechanism by which these proteins function to capture and internalize iron is not well understood. Other bacteria (e.g., *Legionella pneumophila*, *Listeria* species, *Salmonella* species, and other bacteria) can obtain iron from the host's intracellular iron pools.
- The ***availability of iron affects the virulence of pathogens***. For example, the **virulence of *N meningitidis*** for mice is increased 1000-fold or more when the bacteria are ***grown under iron-limited conditions***.

*"**S.pyogenes typing by M protein**: This is the **most important protein used for typing as well as for virulence**. It acts as a **virulence factor by inhibiting phagocytosis**. It is antigenic. The antibody to the M protein promotes phagocytosis of the coccus and is therefore protective"- Ananthanarayan 9th/212*

*"There are three main surface antigens. The major antigenic determinant of capsulated strains is the **capsular polysaccharide** based on which H.influenzae strains have been classified into capsular types- a to f. Other two surface antigens are- outer membrane protein(OMP) andlipooligosaccharides (LOS). OMP and LOS subtyping may be epidemiological value"-Ananthanarayan 9th/328-29*

Inhibition of Phagocytic Engulfment

◈ ***Textbook of Bacteriology.net/Antiphago***

- Many important pathogenic bacteria bear on their ***surfaces substances that inhibit phagocytic adsorption or engulfment***. Resistance to phagocytic ingestion is usually due to a component of the bacterial cell surface (***cell wall, or fimbriae, or a capsule***).
- Classical examples of antiphagocytic substances on bacterial surfaces include:
    - **Polysaccharide capsules** of *S. pneumoniae*, ***Haemophilus influenzae***, *Treponema pallidum* and *Klebsiella pneumoniae*
    - **M protein** and **fimbriae** of Group A streptococci
    - **Surface slime** (polysaccharide) produced as a **biofilm** by *Pseudomonas aeruginosa*
    - **O polysaccharide** associated with LPS of *E. coli*
    - **K antigen** (acidic polysaccharides) of *E. coli* or the analogous **Vi antigen** of *Salmonella typhi*
    - Cell-bound or soluble **Protein A** produced by *Staphylococcus aureus*.

Survival Inside of Cells

- **Inhibition of fusion of the phagocytic lysosomes (granules) with the phagosome**. The bacteria survive inside of phagosomes because they prevent the discharge of lysosomal contents into the phagosome environment. Specifically, ***phagolysosome formation is inhibited in the phagocyte***. This is the strategy employed by *Salmonella*, ***M. tuberculosis***, *Legionella* and the chlamydiae.
- **Survival inside the phagolysosome**-Mycobacteria (including *M. tuberculosis* and *Mycobacterium leprae*).

Table: Bacterial interference with phagocytes textbook of bacteriology, (net)

Bacterium	Type Of Interference	Mechanism
Streptococcus pyogenes	Kill phagocyte	Streptolysin induces lysosomal discharge into cell cytoplasm
	Inhibit neutrophil chemotaxis	Streptolysin is chemotactic repellent
	Resist engulfment (unless Ab is present)	M Protein on fimbriae
	Avoid detection by phagocytes	Hyaluronic acid capsule
Staphylococcus aureus	Kill phagocyte	Leukocidin lyses phagocytes and induces lysosomal discharge into cytoplasm

Contd...

Bacterium	Type Of Interference	Mechanism
	Inhibit opsonized phagocytosis	Protein A blocks Fc portion of Ab; polysaccharide capsule in some strains
	Resist killing	Carotenoids, catalase, superoxide dismutase detoxify toxic oxygen radicals produced in phagocytes
	Inhibit engulfment	Cell-bound coagulase hides ligands for phagocytic contact
Bacillus anthracis	Kill phagocytes or undermine phagocytic activity	Anthrax toxin EF
	Resist engulfment and killing	Capsular poly-D-glutamate
Streptococcus pneumoniae	Resist engulfment (unless Ab is present)	Capsular polysaccharide
Klebsiella pneumoniae	Resist engulfment	Polysaccharide capsule
Haemophilus influenzae	Resist engulfment	***Polysaccharide capsule***
Pseudomonas aeruginosa	Kill phagocyte	Exotoxin A kills macrophages; Cell-bound leukocidin
	Resist engulfment	Alginate slime and biofilm polymers
Salmonella typhi	Resist engulfment and killing	Vi (K) antigen (microcapsule)
Salmonella enterica (typhimurium)	Survival inside phagocytes	Bacteria develop resistance to low pH, reactive forms of oxygen, and host "defensins" (cationic proteins)
Listeria monocytogenes	Escape from phagosome	Listeriolysin, phospholipase C lyse phagosome membrane
Clostridium perfringens	Inhibit phagocyte chemotaxis	ø toxin
	Inhibit engulfment	Capsule
Yersinia pestis	Resist engulfment and/or killing	Protein capsule on cell surface
Yersinia enterocolitica	Kill phagocytes	Yop proteins injected directly into neutrophils
Mycobacteria	Resist killing and digestion	Cell wall components prevent permeation of cells; soluble substances detoxify of toxic oxygen radicals and prevent acidification of phagolysosome
Mycobacterium tuberculosis	***Inhibit lysosomal fusion***	***Mycobacterial sulfatides modify lysosomes***
Legionella pneumophila	Inhibit phagosome-lysosomal fusion	Unknown
Neisseria gonorrhoeae	Inhibit phagolysosome formation; possibly reduce respiratory burst	***Involves outer membrane protein (porin) P.I***
Rickettsia	Escape from phagosome	Phospholipase A
Chlamydia	Inhibit lysosomal fusion	Bacterial substance modifies phagosome
Brucella abortus	Resist killing	Cell wall substance (LPS?)
Treponema pallidum	Resist engulfment	Polysaccharide capsule material
Escherichia coli	Resist engulfment	O antigen (smooth strains); K antigen (acid polysaccharide)
	Resist engulfment and possibly killing	K antigen

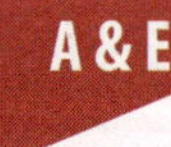

Bacterial Virulence Factors

◈ *Jawetz 27th/158-65*

- Biofilms are important in human infections that are persistent and difficult to treat.e.g. *Staphylococcus epidermidis*, ***Staphylococcus aureus***, *Pseudomonas aeruginosa* etc
- Antigenic Heterogeneity: **N meningitidis capsular polysaccharide types A and C are associated with epidemic meningitis**
- Intracellular Pathogenicity:Some bacteria (e.g., ***M tuberculosis***, *Brucella* species, and *Legionella* species) live and grow in the hostile environment within polymorphonuclear

cells, macrophages, or monocytes. The bacteria accomplish this feat by several mechanisms: They may ***avoid entry into phagolysosomes*** and live within the cytosol of the phagocyte; they may prevent phagosome-lysosome fusion and live within the phagosome; or they may be resistant to lysosomal enzymes and survive within the phagolysosome.

- **Antiphagocytic Factors**: **S aureus has surface protein A**, which binds to the Fc portion of IgG. Other pathogens have surface factors that impede phagocytosis—eg, *S pneumoniae, N meningitidis;* many other bacteria have polysaccharide capsules. **S pyogenes (group A streptococci) has M protein.**
- **Enzymes**: The best-characterized are enzymes from *C perfringens* , ***S aureus* , *group A streptococc*us**, and, to a lesser extent, anaerobic bacteria In addition to **lecithinase,** *C perfringens* produces the proteolytic enzyme **collagenase. Hyaluronidases** are produced by many bacteria (eg, staphylococci, streptococci, and anaerobes) and aid in their spread through tissues.
- **IgA1 Proteases**: ***IgA1 protease*** is an important virulence factor of the pathogens *N gonorrhoeae, N meningitidis, H influenzae,* and *S pneumoniae*

87. Ans. (a) Onset is usually acute, (c) Wound is swollen, (e) Caused by gram +ve organism

[Ref: Davidson 22nd/305;L and B 26th/57; Harrison 19th/990-95; Ananthanarayan 9th/257-59; Jawetz 27th/186-87; Greenwood 16th /231-35]

Gas Gangrene (Clostridial Myonecrosis)

◈ *Davidson 22nd/305*

- It is defined as acute invasion of healthy living muscle undamaged by previous trauma, and is most commonly caused by *C. perfringens*.
- In at least 70% of cases, it follows deep penetrating injury sufficient to create an anaerobic (ischaemic) environment and allow clostridial introduction and proliferation. ***Severe pain at the site of the injury progresses rapidly over 18–24 hours.***
- Skin colour changes from ***pallor to bronze/purple discoloration and the skin is tense, swollen, oedematous and exquisitely tender.***

Gas Gangrene

◈ *L and B 26th/57*

- This is caused by *C. perfringens*. These **Gram-positive**, anaerobic, spore-bearing bacilli are widely found in nature, particularly in soil and faeces.
- Gas gangrene wound infections are associated with ***severe local wound pain and crepitus*** (gas in the tissues, which may also be noted on plain radiographs). The wound produces ***a thin, brown, sweet-smelling exudate, in which Gram staining will reveal bacteria. Oedema and spreading gangrene*** follow the release of collagenase, hyaluronidase, other proteases and alpha toxin. **5**

Clostridial Myonecrosis (Gas Gangrene)

◈ *Harrison 19th/990-95*

- ***Severe pain, crepitus, brawny induration with rapid progression to skin sloughing, violaceous bullae***, and marked tachycardia are characteristics found in the majority of patients.
- *Traumatic gas gangrene C. perfringens* myonecrosis (gas gangrene) is one of the most fulminant ***gram-positive bacterial*** infections of humans.
- The incubation period for traumatic gas gangrene can be as short as 6 h and is usually <4 days. The infection is characterized by ***the sudden onset of excruciating pain at the affected site*** and the rapid development of a foul-smelling wound containing a thin serosanguineous discharge and gas bubbles. ***Brawny edema and induration develop and give way to cutaneous blisters containing bluish to maroon-colored fluid. Such tissue later may become liquefied and slough.***
- The first symptom of spontaneous gas gangrene may be confusion followed by the abrupt onset of excruciating pain in the absence of trauma. These findings, along with ***fever, should heighten suspicion of spontaneous gas gangrene.***
- ***Swelling increases, and bullae filled with clear, cloudy, hemorrhagic, or purplish fluid appear.*** The surrounding skin has a **purple hue**, which may reflect vascular compromise resulting from the diffusion of bacterial toxins into surrounding tissues.

88. Ans. (b) Type DEN 4 is most common...

[Ref: Park 23rd /246-56; Ananthanarayan 9th/523; Harrison 19th/1318-19; Jawetz 27th/552-54]

Dengu Virus

◈ *Park 23rd /246-56*

- Belong to ***genus flavivirus*** with positive sense RNA (Harrison 19th 214e-1 table)
- All the 4 serotypes i.e dengu 1, 2, 3 and 4 have been isolated in India but at ***present DENV-1 and DENV-2 serotypes are widespread***
- Vector- ***Aedes aegypti and Aedes albopictus*** are the ***two most important vectors of dengu***
- "Adult mosquito are most commonly controlled by spraying house with residual insecticide. ***DDT is insecticide of choice***"- Park 23rd /773

Dengue

◈ *Harrison 19th/1318-19*

- The most clinically important ***flaviviruses*** that cause the fever and myalgia syndrome are dengue viruses 1–4.
- ***All four viruses have A. aegyptias their principal vector.***
- The range of a lesser dengue virus vector, ***A. albopictus,*** now extends from Asia to the United States, the Indian Ocean, parts of Europe, and Hawaii. *A. aegypti* typically breeds near human habitation, using relatively fresh water from sources such as water jars, vases, discarded containers, coconut husks, and old tires. The mosquito usually inhabits dwellings and bites during the day.

Table *(Harrison 19th 214e-1):* **Virus Families Pathogenic for Humans**

Family	Representative Viruses	Type of RNA/DNA	Lipid Envelope
Flaviviridae	Yellow fever virus Dengue virus St. Louis encephalitis virus West Nile virus Hepatitis C virus Hepatitis G virus	(+) RNA	Yes

89. Ans. a. Positive tourniquet..., b. Caused by..., c. Aedes aegypticus..., d. IgM/IgG ratios... & e. No vaccine...

[Ref: Park 23rd /246-56; Davidson 22nd/323; Ananthanarayan 9th/523; Harrison 19th/1318-19; Jawetz 27th/552-54]

Dengue

Park 23rd

- **Positive torniquet test** (i,e. ***10 or more petechiae per square inch***) is most common hemorrhagic phenomenon. In DHF the test usually gives a definite positive with 20 petechiae or more- Park 23rd /249
- *Vaccine- **So far there is no satisfactory vaccine** and no immediate prospect of preventing the disease by immunization-* Park 23rd /254
- "The diagnosis is made by IgM ELISA or paired serology during recovery or by antigen-detection ELISA or RT-PCR during the acute phase"- *Harrison 19th/1318-19*

"The diagnosis can be confirmed by seroconversion of IgM or a fourfold rise in IgG antibody titres. Serological tests may detect cross-reacting antibodies against other flaviviruses, including yellow fever vaccine. ***IgM/IgG ratios may be used to distinguish primary from secondary infection***. Isolation of dengue virus from blood or detection of dengue virus RNA by PCR"- Davidson 22nd/323

90. Ans. (b) Metallic instrument

[Ref: Ananthanarayan 9th/37,30-32; Greenwood 16th/77-78;Chakraborty 2nd/45-46; en.wikipedia.org]

*"Autoclaves in operation theaters is used to sterilize **surgical instrument, OT garments, linen, gloves, masks, gown** etc. However, it is **not suitable for plastics**"-Community Medicine with Recent Advances by Suryakantha 4th/310*

*"Glutaraldehyde: Used for **Cystoscope and bronchoscopes**"- Ananthanarayan 9th/34*

Materials	Methods of sterilization and disinfection
• Glasswares- syringes, petridishes, test tubes, flasks, surgical instrument, oily fluids and powders	Hot air oven
• Serum, body fluids, bacterial vaccines	Waterbath, vaccine bath
• Milk	Pasteurisation, 63°C × 30 min. or 72°C × 20 sec.

Contd...

Materials	Methods of sterilization and disinfection
• Materials	Methods of sterilization and disinfection
• Cystoscope and endoscope	Glutaraldehyde (Cridex-2%) or ethylene oxide
• Most of the culture media	Autoclaving
• Culture media containing egg, serum or sugar	Tyndallisation
• Rubber, plastic and polythene tubes, disposable syringes	Glutaradehyde, Ethylene oxide gas
• Dressings, aprons, gloves, catheters, surgical instruments except sharp instruments.	Autoclaving
• Sharp instruments	5% cresol
• Suture meterials except catgut	Autoclaving
• Catgut	Ionising radiation
• Rubber or plastic disposable goods, disposable syringes, bone and tissue graft, adhesive dressings	Ionising radiation
• Materials	Methods of sterilization and disinfection
• Faeces and urine, vomitus Sputum	Bleaching powder cresols, formalin, Burning, autoclaving
• Sterilisation of operation theatre	Formaldehyde gas
• Wards and laboratory or Operation theatre floor space	Formaldehyde gas and cresols (Lysol)
• Skin	Tincture iodine, spirit (70% ethanol), savlon (phenol derivative)

Table *(Ananthanarayan 9th/37):* **Commonly used methods of sterilization and disinfection**

Name of the article	Method
Surgical linen	Autoclaving
Syringes, needles, catheters, gloves	Gamma radiations or ethylene oxide gas sterilization
Culture media in microbiology	Autoclaving
Glassware, paraffin, glove powder, jellies	Hot-air oven
Serum sugars	Filtration
Stethoscope, probes, thermometer	Alcohol

FORENSIC MEDICINE

91. Ans. (a) Impotence of male partner, (b) Extramarital affair of male partner, (e) If she was married before the age of fifteen…

[Ref: http://www.indidivorce.com/grounds-for-divorce-in-india.html: Parikh 7th/367, 386. 6th/5.1.5.24]

"Adultery is the act of indulging in any type of consensual physical relationship with a person other than the spouse. An adulterous relationship is established between two individuals who are not married to each other. Since this correlation is voluntary, ***it can also be termed as an extra marital affair*** or infidelity towards one's partner. ***Adultery is considered as an offence against marriage by both the Penal law and the Matrimonial law in India and anyone committing an adulterous act can be punished under law***"- http://www.advocatekhoj.com/

"***Impotency and infertility are completely distinct terms. Unlike impotency, infertility cannot be grounds for divorce***, the Bombay high court (HC) ruled on Monday. http://www.hindustantimes.com/ Jul 24, 2012

Following are the grounds for divorce in India mentioned under the Hindu Marriage Act, 1955 *http://www. indidivorce.com/grounds-for-divorce-in-india.html*

- Adultery
- **Cruelty**
- **Desertion**
- **Conversion:** Incase either of the two converts himself/herself into another religion
- **Mental Disorder:** Mental disorder can become a ground for filing a divorce if the spouse of the petitioner suffers from ***incurable mental disorder and insanity*** and therefore cannot be expected from the couple to stay together.
- **Leprosy:** In case of a 'virulent and incurable' form of leprosy, a petition can be filed by the other spouse based on this ground
- **Venereal Disease:** If one of the spouses is suffering from a serious disease that is easily communicable, a divorce can be filed by the other spouse. The sexually transmitted diseases like AIDS are accounted to be **venereal Disease**
- **Renunciation**
- Not Heard Alive
- No Resumption of Co-habitation

The following are the grounds for divorce in India on which a petition can be filed only by the wife

- The husband has indulged in ***rape, bestiality and sodomy.***
- If the marriage is solemnized before the Hindu Marriage Act and the husband has again married another woman in spite of the first wife being alive, the first wife can seek for a divorce.
- A girl is entitled to file for a divorce ***if she was married before the age of fifteen*** *and renounces the marriage before she attains eighteen years of age.*
- If there is no co-habitation for one year and the husband neglects the judgment of maintenance awarded to the wife by the court, the wife can contest for a divorce.

Note (***Sterile female*** *is not a ground for divorce* (***Premature ejaculation***, *if leads to impotency then ground for divorce, otherwise not ground for divorce*)

Impotent Man: a ground for divorce *refhttp://indiankanoon. org/doc*

"Impotency is a ground for annulling marriage. In *Parmaswami pillai v. Sornathammal AIR1969* it was held that the marriage of a woman with an impotent man is voidable"

"*Siraj mohmedkhan Janmohamadkhan v. Hafizunnisa Yasinkhan and Anr on 14 Sept 1981* HELD: Proved **impotence** of the husband and his inability to discharge his marital obligations amount to both legal and mental cruelty make it a just ground for the wife to refuse to live with the husband……… **impotence** under the civil law is a good ground for granting divorce or for refusing restitution of conjugal rights"

Divorce

◈ *Parikh 7th/367, 386; 6th/ 5.1,5.24*

- *This means dissolution of a previously valid marriage. If the intrauterine age of the child is proved to be greater than the period of access b/w the parents, the dissolution of marriage is allowed by the court on* ***ground of adultery.***
- *The other grounds for divorce includes- (a) desertion (b) cruelty (c) criminal sex practices(e.g, rape, sodomy, or bestiality) and (d)* ***incurable insanity,*** *HIV infection, leprosy or venereal disease in a communicable form*

92. Ans. (b) Identification of…, (d) Assessment of…, (e) Collection of…

[Ref: Ready 33rd/98-100: Parikh 7th/83-84]

"The first step in analyzing the bite is to identify it as human. Animal teeth are very different from humans' teeth, so they leave very different bite-mark patterns. Next, ***the bite is swabbed for DNA***, which may ***have been left in the saliva of the biter***. The dentist must also determine whether the bite was self-inflicted"- science.howstuffworks.com

"**Bite mark analysis for** Size, shape and arrangement of teeth: ***Human incisor teeth produce rectangular marks whereas canine teeth produce triangular marks in the cross-section***. Animal bites (dogs, cats) usually puncture the skin and the cross sectional size of the tooth is small and circular. Number of incisor teeth and the distance between individual teeth may be greater with animal bites"-www.medind.nic.in

Bite Marks

◈ *Parikh 7th/83-84*

- **Bite marks** ***can permit precise identification*** because the alignment of teeth is ***peculiar to each individual.***
- The mark may be on the articles of food found at the scene of crime or on human beings involved in sexual crimes, and may be found on the skin of neck, breast, shoulder or buttock. It is important to realise that a bite on human flesh can leave a mark not necessarily due to a break in the continuity of the skin but due to a small subdermal or thin deep haemorrhage.
- Bite marks are ***always contaminated by saliva*** and, therefore, contain *amylase, ptyalin and blood groups which can be determined, if the biter is a secretor.*

- The ***identity of the biter can also be determined***, if the cast of the suspect's mouth is made and a transparency of his bite compared with that of the unknown bite.
- It should be remembered that bite marks on skin are apt to be modified by its elasticity when the teeth are withdrawn.
- Generally, it is ***easier to exclude a certain person than to identify one conclusively from the bite mark***. However, the pattern of teeth marks with the arrangement of teeth within a dental arch provides a *valid and simple method of demonstrating points of similarity and dissimilarity to a court.*
- On a number of occasions, abnormalities of tooth position or arrangement within a dental arch of a suspect confirm or completely eliminate the accused as a perpetrator of a bite mark.

Bite Marks

◈ *Reddy 33rd/98-100*

- Swabs of the bite mark should be taken immediately, using a swab moistened with sterile water
- Recording and reproducing method of bite marks-***photographic method, casts and digital imaging***
- They are ***useful in identification*** because the alignment of teeth is peculiar to the individual.
- **ML importance:** Bite marks may be found in materials left at the place of crime, e.g., foodstuffs, such as cheese, bread, butter, sandwiches, fruit, or in humans involved in assaults, when either the victim or the accused may show the marks, usually on the hands, fingers, forearms, nose and ears.
- **Charting of teeth:** There are more than 150 different methods of identifying, numbering, and charting of teeth. The one of the widely used systems for permanent teeth is **Universal system:** Teeth are numbered l to 16 from upper right to upper left, and 17 to 32 from lower left to lower right. This follows the plan advocated by the American and International Society of Forensic Odontology.

93. Ans. All (a, b, c, d)

[Ref: Reddy 33rd/ 224,32nd/205,235; Parikh 7th/ 249-53, 6th/ 4.43-44; Forensic Anthropology by Steven Byers 4th/256]

"The ***impact of bullets*** on bone may cause **fracture lines** to form. The **two type** of fracture lines are distinguishable on cranial vault: ***radiating and concentric***. **Radiating fracture** lines originate from the site of impact where they move outward in any direction(this is ***especially seen in entrance wound***). Concentric fracturing: Concentric lines appear as part of a circle whose center is at the point of bullet impact"- *Forensic Anthropology by Steven Byers 4th/256*

Bullet wound: In exit wound, size is bigger than bullet- Reddy 33rd/ 226

Smudge Ring/Lead Ring/Grease Collar/Dirt Collar

◈ *Parikh 7th/ 249-50; Reddy 33rd/ 224*

- *This is **due to the wipe of the soft metal of the bullet**, or dirt present on it, or grease carried from the barrel and is deposited round the entrance wound internal to the abraded collar*
- *The smudge ring may therefore be absent when the jacketed bullet has passed through clothing*
- The smudging in case of lead shot or unjacketed bullets can be detected microchemically on the target (skin/cloth)
- The forensic value of bullet wipe is to establish a hole as a bullet hole, to determine the entry site, and on occasion the sequence of shots or bullet's passage through multiple objects
- "**Abrasion collar (Marginal abrasion):** *Abrasion collar surrounds the dirt collar. The abraded collar is reddish at first, but becomes reddish brown as it dries. Some contusion is present in abraded collar and as such, it is also called "contusion collar". These two features are proof of an entrance firearm wound"- Reddy 33rd/ 224*

Gutter fracture: *They are formed when part of the thickness of the bone is removed so as to form a gutter, e.g., in **oblique bullet wound**"- Reddy 33rd/246,32nd/235*

Firearm Wound

◈ *Reddy 33rd/ 224-231*

- **Glancing wounds** (striking someone or something at an angle rather than directly and with full force) ***may simulate incised or lacerated wounds.***
- A bullet that pass through glass or some other object and then strikes the body may produce a ***wound resembling a laceration***
- Firearm wounds cause crushing of the tissues and produce an actual hole

Firearm Injuries

◈ *Parikh 7th/ 249-53*

- Firearm injuries are wounds caused to the body tissue due to impact, entry and passage of a missile discharged from a firearm. They generally ***simulate contused wounds***
- When a missile pass tangentially, the wound ***may simulate an abrasion or a gutter***
- Slit like exit wounds are occasionally encountered. They are due to the bullet exiting on its board side or due to exit of a fragmented bone. Such injuries ***may simulate incised wounds or stab wounds***

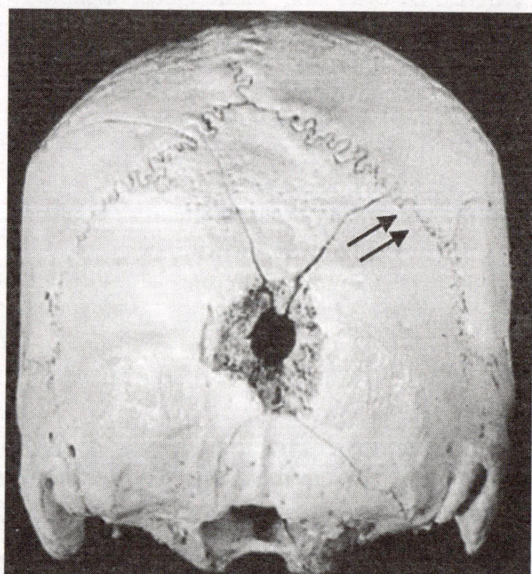

Fig: *(Forensic Anthropology by Steven Byers 4th/256):* Classifical radiating fracture lines from exit wound

94. Ans. (a) Wilfully giving false statement..., (c) Voluntarily giving false evidence under..., (d) The witness is liable to be ...

[Ref: Reddy 33rd/13; Parikh 7th/10]

Perjury

◈ *Reddy 33rd/13*

- *It means **giving wilful false/fabricated evidence***
- *Whoever, being legally bound by an oath, or by an express provision of law to state the truth, or being bound by law to make a declaration upon any subject, makes **any statement which is false** and which he either knows or believes to be false or does not believe to be true, is said to give false evidence(S. 191 and 192- I.P.C., 344-CrPC)*
- *It occurs if the person's earlier statement regarding the facts on oath and subsequent statement on oath are opposed to each other and they cannot be reconciled. The witness is liable to be prosecuted for perjury and imprisonment may extend to seven years (S.193 I.P.C)*

"**Perjury**: A witness who after taking oath or making a solemn affirmation, wilfully makes a statement which he knows or believes to be false is ***guilty of the crime of perjury under section 193 IPC***"- *Parikh 7th/10*

Section 191 in the Indian Penal Code

◈ *indiankanoon.org*

"**191. Giving false evidence.**—Whoever, being legally bound by an oath or by an express provision of law to state the truth, or being bound by law to make a declaration upon any subject, makes any statement which is false, and which he either knows or believes to be false or does not believe to be true, is said to give false evidence. Explanation 1.—A statement is within the meaning of this section, whether it is made verbally or otherwise. Explanation 2.—A false statement as to the belief of the person attesting is within the meaning of this section, and a person may be guilty of giving false evidence by stating that he believes a thing which he does not believe, as well as by stating that he knows a thing which he does not know"

Section 192 in the Indian Penal Code

◈ *indiankanoon.org*

"192. **Fabricating false evidence.**—Whoever causes any circumstance to exist or makes any false entry in any book or record, or electronic record or makes any document or electronic record containing a false statement, intending that such circumstance, false entry or false statement may appear in evidence in a judicial proceeding, or in a proceeding taken by law before a public servant as such, or before an arbitrator, and that such circumstance, false entry or false statement, so appearing in evidence, may cause any person who in such proceeding is to form an opinion upon the evidence, to entertain an erroneous opinion touching any point material to the result of such proceeding, is said "to fabricate false evidence"

Section 193 in the Indian Penal Code

◈ *indiankanoon.org*

"**193. Punishment for false evidence.**—Whoever intentionally gives ***false evidence*** in any stage of a judicial proceeding, or fabricates false evidence for the purpose of being used in any stage of a judicial proceeding, shall be punished with imprisonment of either description for a term which may extend to seven years, and shall also be liable to fine, and whoever intentionally gives or fabricates false evidence in any other case, shall be punished with imprisonment of either description for a term which may extend to three years, and shall also be liable to fine"

95. Ans. (b) Body of offence, (c) It includes body of the victim and..., (d) The essence of crime

[Ref: Ready 33rd/57; Parikh 7th/55]

The Corpus Delicti

◈ *Reddy 33rd/57*

- **The corpus delicti (delicti=fault; offence) (the body of offence; the essence of crime) means, the facts of any criminal offence, e.g., murder.**
- **The corpus delicti of murder is the fact that a person died from unlawful violence.**
- It includes the ***body of the victim and other facts*** which are conclusive of death by foul play, such as a ***bullet or a broken knife-blade found in the body*** and responsible for death.
- ***Clothings*** showing marks of the weapon, and ***drawings and photographs*** of the deceased showing fatal injuries are also included in this term.
- The ***main part of corpus delicti is the establishment of identity of the dead body*** and infliction of violence in a particular way, at a particular time and place, by the person or persons charged with the crime and none other. The ***case against the accused cannot be established unless there is convincing proof of these points.***
- If the victim's identity is not known, it becomes difficult for the police to solve the crime.
- The identification of a dead body and proof of corpus delicti is important before a sentence is passed in murder trials, as unclaimed, decomposed bodies, or portions of a dead body or bones are sometimes produced to support false charge. However, a conviction for an offence does not necessarily depend upon the corpus delicti, if there are eye-witnesses or strong corroborative evidence.

96. Ans. (d) Composite, (e) Point to point

[Ref:www.universalclass.com/articles/law/processing-a-crime-scene.htm; www.policeone.com/investigation; wps.prenhall.com]

Processing a Crime Scene

◈ *www.universalclass.com*

- To properly analyze and interpret any crime scene, ***certain basic steps*** must be followed in order to create a sense of beginning and a sensible conclusion to the examination.
- There are several methods used by law enforcement agencies throughout the world that follow **six basic crime scene search patterns**- ***Strip method, Wheel method,*** Spiral method, ***Zone method,Grid method and Line method***
- The use of any or a number of these search methods will be determined by the location and size of the particular

crime scene; the one that is chosen is less important than the fact that the search is carried out with due diligence and attention to detail.

- The **strip method** requires that crime scene personnel walk a path from one end of the crime scene, over to the other side of the room or area, and then return in the direction from which he or she first started.
- The **wheel method** employs the use of several crime scene personnel or searchers. Starting in the middle of an imaginary circle, each investigator moves in a direction straight out from the center, or "hub" of the wheel, much like the spokes of a bicycle wheel.
- The **spiral method** has the investigator(s) examining the area for evidence in an ever-widening circle, from the position of the core crime scene or on the perimeter and then moves in an outward direction.
- The **zone method** breaks the crime scene area into squares.
- The **grid method** is best used in large crime scenes such as fields or woods. Several searchers, or a line of them, move alongside each other from one end of the area to be searched to the other.
- The **line method** is best used outdoors as well, and is similar to the grid search with the exception that searchers generally only move in one direction, from one side of the search area to the other.

PREVENTIVE & SOCIAL MEDICINE

97. Ans. (a) India has approximately... (c) 5% of TB patients ..., (d) MDR-TB among retreatment ..., (e) Incidence is around ...

[Ref: Park 23rd/176-77; Community Medicine by Piyush Gupta 1st/192-97; Community Medicine with Recent Advances by Suryakantha 4th/364-70]

Tuberculosis in India

◈ *Park 23rd/176-77*

- *"India is the highest TB burden country in the world in term of absolute number of incident cases that occur each year. It accounts for **one-fourth of the estimated global incident TB cases in 2013**"*
- *"MDR-TB among notified new pulmonary TB patients was **about 2.2%** and among **retreatment cases was about 15%***

*"India has the highest TB burden in the world accounting for **about a fourth** of the estimated incident cases globally, in 2013"-Piyush Gupta 1st/193*

"Of the 9 million new cases in 2013, 56% were reported from south east asia and western pacific regions. India alone contributed about ***24% of the total new cases***"- *Piyush Gupta 1st/192*

*"It is estimated that an **average 2% of new patients have MDR**, representing nearly 20,000 cases in the country every year"- Suryakantha 4th/364*

"Currently, **multidrug-resistant TB** is a global concern and is encountered in ***3% of all new cases and 12% of retreatment cases***. Multidrug-resistant tuberculosis is defined as a resistant organism to rifampicin and isoniazid while 'other drug resistance' is defined as any resistance to another drug. Lack of clinical or radiological improvement, development of a new lesion or a cold abscess, or an increase in bone destruction in spite of medical treatment for 3 to 5 months may indicate multidrug-resistant TB"- www.ncbi.nlm.nih.gov/pmc

Box *(Piyush Gupta 1st/194)*: **Problem of Tuberculosis in India (2014)**

- *Incidence:* 2.2 million new TB cases annually-176 cases per 100,000 population
- Prevalence: 2.8 million cases-230 cases per 100,000 population
- Deaths: About 270,000 deaths each year-22 deaths per 100,000 population
- Approximately ***5% of TB patients estimated to be HIV positive*** – *Piyush Gupta 1st/194;*Park 23rd/177
- *DR-TB (Drug resistant-TB)*: 2.2% in new cases and 15% in previously treated cases

T.B: Indian Scenario

◈ *Suryakantha 4th/364*

- India accounts for ***nearly one-fifth of the global problem***
- About 40 percent of the population are infected with TB bacilli (40 crores).
- About 14 million people are suffering from the disease (1.4 crore).
- Annual incidence in India during 2009 was ***1.98 million cases*** (***1/5 of global problem***).
- About 4 million cases are infectious (sputum positive for AFB) (40 lakhs).
- About 1.5 million new cases are added every year (15 lakhs).
- About 0.37 million cases are dying every year (3.7 lakhs).
- About 12,000 crores is economic loss to Government of India every year.

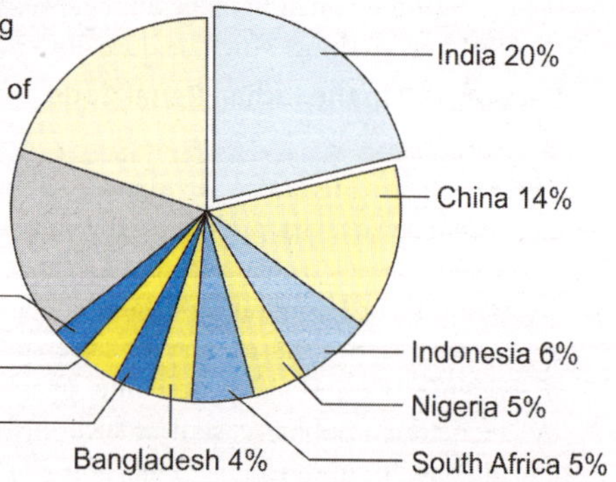

Fig: *(Suryakantha 4th/364)*: India is the largest TB burden country accounting for one-fifth of the global incidence

98. Ans. (a) Only has epidemiological significance

[Ref: Park 23rd/320-21; Community Medicine with Recent Advances by Suryakantha 4th/539-40]

Value of Lepromin Test

- Park 23rd/320-21
- *It is not a diagnostic test. The two drawbacks that stand in the way of this test bring used for diagnosis are:(i) positive results in non-cases, and (ii) negative results in lepromatous and near-lepromatous cases*
- *The test has been generally accepted as a useful tool in* ***evaluating the immune status (CMI) of leprosy patients.***
- *It is of considerable value in confirming the results of classification of cases of leprosy on clinical and bacteriological grounds. In other words, the test is widely used as an* ***aid to classify the types of disease***
- *The test is also of great value in* ***estimating the prognosis in case of leprosy of all types.*** *The test is usually strongly positive in the typical tuberculoid cases, and the positivity getting weaker as one passes through the spectrum to the lepromatous end, the typical lepromatous cases being lepromin negative indicating a failure of CMI*

Lepromin Test

- *Suryakantha 4th/539*
- It is an intradermal test ***employed for detecting the cell mediated immunity against leprosy.***
- It is ***not a diagnostic test*** as it may give positive result in non-cases and negative results in lepromatous patient. However, ***it helps in classifying leprosy patients and also in assessing prognosis with treatment and vaccine.***

Applications of Lepromin Test

- *Suryakantha 4th/539-40*
- In lepromin test, Midsuda reaction is preferred over Fernandez reaction. The test has a limited diagnostic value because it gives positive reaction among non-cases (false-positive). However, ***it helps in classification of leprosy.***
- The test is strongly positive in tuberculoid leprosy (showing good CMI) and negative in lepromatous leprosy (showing failure of CMI). It is variable in borderline and indeterminate leprosy.
- The ***test has a prognostic value***, because it shows an immunological shift in the behavior of a case. For example, the reaction which is negative in lepromatous leprosy, when becomes positive after treatment, it indicates that the patient has developed immunity and has improved.
- The ***test has predictive value as well.*** It gives an indication of the risk of the disease among contacts of open cases.
- The ***test has an epidemiological value as well.*** It indicates the incidence and prevalence of infection among children. In the first 6 months of life, most children are lepromin negative. They become positive progressively as their age advances.

99. Ans. (b) Multibacillary treatment × 12 month

[Ref: Park 23rd/323-24; Community Medicine by Piyush Gupta 1st/282-83; Community Medicine with Recent Advances by Suryakantha 4th/535-45; Neena Khanna 5th/ 272-84]

It is a pure neuritic type of leprosy.It is a case of Multibacillary leprosy for therapeutic purpose (according to WHO classification, more than one nerve trunk involvement is termed as multibacillary for treatment purpose)

Is pure neuritic leprosy-paucibacillary or multibacillary for therapeutic purposes? *www.ijdvl.com/article.asp*

- The only classification which the WHO advocates for leprosy from the year 1982 is paucibacillary/multibacillary for therapeutic purposes, based on skin smear status and number of skin lesions.
- There are no guidelines from the WHO about the classification of pure neuritic leprosy depending on number of nerves involved and, therefore, its treatment. However, ***many consider that pure neuritic leprosy belongs to the paucibacillary group*** since all of them are acid-fast bacilli negative on skin smears by definition and are mostly lepromin positive. This was also the recommendation made by the National Leprosy Eradication Programme (NLEP) of India in 1987, which grouped pure neuritic leprosy within paucibacillary leprosy for therapeutic purposes.
- Although skin smears are always negative, nerve biopsy in several cases of pure neuritic leprosy has revealed features of borderline or even lepromatous leprosy along with acid-fast bacilli. However, it would be impractical to perform nerve biopsy routinely in patients of pure neuritic leprosy to classify the disease for treatment purpose as most common nerves affected are mixed nerves.
- Hence, the ***number of nerve trunks*** involved is taken as a ***clinical criterion for determining the multidrug therapy regimen (paucibacillary/multibacillary).***
- According to present NLEP guidelines in India, when ***one nerve trunk is involved in leprosy it is considered as paucibacillary***, and ***when more than one nerve trunk is involved, it is considered as multibacillary for therapeutic purposes***. This definition for therapy is being applied at present, both to pure neuritic as well as paucibacillary leprosy in India

Table *(Neena Khanna 5th/284)*: **WHO recommendation for treatment of leprosy in adults**

	PB	MB
Definition	≤5 lesions	>5 lesions
Duration of therapy	6 months (can be completed in 9 months)	12 months (can be completed in 18 months)

Contd...

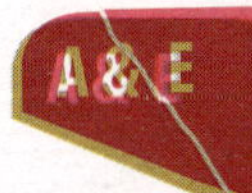

	PB	MB
Drugs		
Supervised (monthly)	Rifampicin, 600 mg	Rifampicin, 600 mg + Clofazimine, 300 mg
Not supervised (daily)	Dapsone, 100 mg	Dapsone, 100 mg + Clofazimine, 50 mg

Table *(Suryakantha 4th/545):* **The WHO-recommended MDT Regimen of Leprosy (Adults)**

Type of leprosy	Drugs used	Dosage (adults)	Frequency of administration	Duration of treatment	Follow-up
Multibacillary (MB)	Dapsone Rifampicin Clofazimine	100 mg 600 mg 300 mg 50 mg	Daily Once monthly Once monthly Daily	12 months	Once a year for 5 years
Paucibacillary (PB)	Dapsone Rifampicin	100 mg 600 mg	Daily Once monthly	6 months	Once a year for 2 years
Single skin lesion paucibacillary (SSLPB)	Rifampicin Ofloxacin Minocycline	600 mg 400 mg 100 mg	Single dose Single dose Single dose	Single dose treatment of ROM	–

"**Paucibacillary leprosy:** *A person having 1-5 skin lesions and/or only one nerve involvement" (Park 23rd/322)*

*"**Multibacillary leprosy:** A person having 6 or more skin lesions and/or more than one nerve involvement"- (Park 23rd/322)*

Table *(KDT 7th/784):* **National leprosy eradication programme (2009) classification of leprosy**

Paucibacillary (PB)	Multibacillary (MB)
1-5 skin lesions No nerve/only one nerve involvement ± 1-5 skin lesions Skin smear negative at all sites	6 or more skin lesions > 1 nerve involved irrespective of number of skin lesions Skin smear positive at any one site

The WHO Classification

◈ *Suryakantha 4th/535-36*

This is based on the number of skin lesions and bacteriological status.

- Single skin lesion, paucibacillary leprosy
  - Single skin lesion
  - No nerve involvement
  - Skin smear for AFB negative
- Paucibacillary leprosy (PBL)
  - 2-5 lesions (skin and nerves)
  - Only one nerve trunk
  - Skin smear for AFB negative
- Multibacillary leprosy (MBL)
  - More than 5 lesions (i.e. 6 and above)
  - More than one nerve trunk involvement.
  - Skin smear positive.

100. Ans. (b) Random dots in scatter diagram..., (c) Pictogram is represented..., (e) Regression graph is said linear...

[Ref: Park 23rd/845-47; Community Medicine by Piyush Gupta 1st/652; Community Medicine with Recent Advances by Suryakantha 4th/694-99, 729-30]

Histogram

◈ *Park 23rd/845-45*

- *It is a **pictorial diagram of frequency distribution**. It consists of series of blocks*
- *The class intervals are given along the horizontal axis and the frequencies along the vertical axis*
- *Area of each blocks or rectangle is proportional to the frequency*

Histogram

◈ *Suryakantha 4th/695-96*

- It is a graphic representation of a ***frequency distribution*** table in which the vertical axis represents the frequency and the horizontal axis the class interval.
- It consists of series of bars adjoining to each other, the length of each bar is being ***proportional to the frequency and the width to the class interval***
- Histograms are ideally suited to represent the ***distribution of anthropometric values like height, weight, mid-arm circumference, etc.*** They can also represent ***other types continuous data*** series such as blood pressure, pulse rate and hemoglobin level.

- Histograms provide a ***better understanding of quantitative data of continuous type than frequency distribution tables.***

Table *(Piyush Gupta 1st/652)*: **Conditions under which various types of diagrams are appropriate**

Categories on x-axis	Quantity to be represented on y-axis	Appropriate diagram
Continuous	Additive (frequency or percentage)	Pie if proportional contribution of the categories is to be represented, otherwise histogram
	Non-additive (number, rate or ratio)	Line for depiction of trend, otherwise bar
Discrete or categorial	Additive (frequency or percentage)	Pie if proportional contribution of the categories is to be represented, otherwise bar
	Non-additive (number, rate or ratio)	Bar

Pie Charts

◈ *Park 23rd/846*

- *Instead of comparing the length of a bar, **the areas of segments of a circle are compared**. The area of each segments depends upon the angle*
- It is often necessary to indicate the percentage in the segments as it may not be sometimes very easy, virtually, to compare the areas of segments

Pie Diagram

◈ *Suryakantha 4th/698*

- It is a ***circular diagram*** in which the frequencies of observations are shown as sectors or wedges in a circle, the size of each sector being proportional to the frequency.
- Degrees of angle denote the frequency and the area of the sector gives comparative difference at a glance.

Scatter Diagram or Dot Diagram

◈ *Suryakantha 4th/698*

- One variable is represented on X-axis and another variable on Y-axis. Perpendiculars drawn from these readings meet, to give one scatter point.
- There will be as many points as there are individuals in the observation. When all the point are plotted, the diagram gives the picture of a scatter. Hence the name 'Scatter diagram' (Dot diagram).
- The direction of scatter helps to determine presence or absence of the association. ***If the scatter takes the direction midway between the two axes, it signifies positive association (correlation).***
- If it takes a direction at right angles to midway scatter it indicates negative association.
- A haphazard scatter represents neither positive nor negative association.

Pictogram

◈ *Park 23rd/846*

- This is a popular method of presenting data to the "man in the street" and to those who cannot understand orthodox charts
- ***Small pictures or symbols*** are used to present the data. Fractions of the picture can be used to represent numbers smaller than the value of a whole symbol

Pictogram

◈ *Suryakantha 4th/699*

- It is also called as ***picture diagram or pictorial diagram***. It consists of a series of small pictures or symbols or silhouettes, each representing a group of data.
- This method is used to impress a lay person, who cannot understand the orthodox charts

Regression

◈ *Suryakantha 4th/729-30*

- This change of dependent variable with respect to change in independent variable is known as 'Regression'.
- **Regression Equation:**The relationship between the two variables can be represented by a mathematical equation, known as 'Regression equation'.
- ***Regression can be linear (depicted by line) or curvilinear (depicted by curve). Linear means the increase or decrease in the variables remains proportional in different subjects*** *- Piyush Gupta 1st/652*

101. Ans. (c) Activities are divided into small goals

[Ref: Park 23rd/872; Community Medicine by Piyush Gupta 1st/783; Community Medicine with Recent Advances by Suryakantha 4th/860]

"There are two methods of network analysis namely Program Evaluation and Review Technique (PERT) and Critical Path Method (CPM)"- *Suryakantha 4th/860; Park 23rd/872*

"Limitation of PERT: It is not suitable for relatively simple and repetitive precesses"–*www.yourarticlelibrary.com*

PERT(Programme Evaluation and Review Technique)

◈ *Park 23rd/872*

- It is a ***management technique*** which makes ***possible more detailed planning*** and ***more comprehensive supervision***
- The essence of PERT is to construct an ***Arrow Diagram***. The diagram represents the logical sequence in which events must take place.
- It is possible with such a diagram to ***calculate the time*** by which each activity must be completed and to ***identify those activities that are critical***
- It is a useful management technique which can be ***applied to a great variety of projects***
- It ***aids in planning, scheduling and monitoring the project***; it allows better communication b/w the various levels of management; it identifies potential problems; it furnishes continuous, timely progress reports; it forms a solid foundation upon which to build an evaluation and checking system

CPM (Critical Path Method)

- *Park 23rd/872*
- The longest path of the network is called critical path. If any activity along the critical path is delayed, the entire project will be delayed

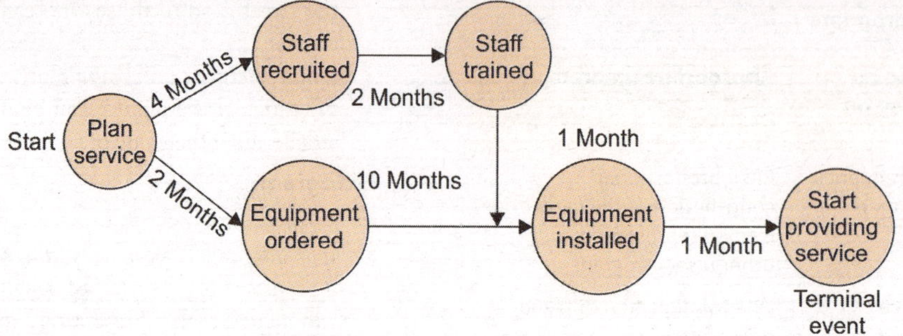

Fig: *(Park 23rd/872):* Network analysis

Table *(Suryakantha 4th/860):* **Differences between PERT and CPM**

	Program evaluation and review technique (PERT)	Critical path method (CPM)
1.	Design is based on event	Design is based on activity
2.	Time requirement is estimated	Time requirement is taken from previous experience
3.	Main objective is to ***take shortest time***	There is ***mixture of time and cost***
4.	Activity time is ***not subjective***	Activity time is ***subjective***
5.	Slack time* cannot be identified	Slack time can be identified

*Slack time is the difference between the minimum time required and the maximum time taken up for the activity.

Program Evaluation and Review Technique

- *Suryakantha 4th/860*
- This method is adopted when a project work consists of a ***large number of processes*** which should be brought together into an integrated plan.
- This involves the numbering of series of process (events) in a serial order and the time required for completion of each event.
- This helps to prepare a schedule to identify the crucial problems and also to know the total duration required for the completion of the work

PERT(Programme Evaluation and Review Technique)

- *Community Medicine by Piyush Gupta 1st/783*
- It specifies techniques and procedures to assist the manager in *planning schedules and costs, determining timing and cost status, forecasting manpower skill requirements, predicting schedule slippages and cost overruns, developing alternate time cost plans and allocating resources among tasks*
- PERT uses probability and linear programming for planning and controlling activities

Table *(www.keydifferences.com):* **Comparision b/w PERT and CPM**

Basis for comparison	PERT	CPM
Meaning	PERT is a project management technique, used to manage uncertain activities of a project.	CPM is a statistical technique of project management that manages well defined activities of a project
What is it?	A techniques of planning and control of time	A method to control cost and time
Focus on	Event	Activity
Model	Probabilistic model	Deterministic model
Estimates	Three time estimates	One time estimate
Appropriate for	High precision time estimate	Reasonable time estimate
Management of	Unpredictable activities	Predictable activities
Nature of jobs	Non-repetitive nature	Repetitive nature
Critical and non-critical activities	No differentiation	Differentiated
Suitable for	Research and development project	Non-research projects like civil construction, ship building etc.
Crashing concept	Not applicable	Applicable

Key Differences Between PERT and CPM

- *www.keydifferences.com*
- PERT is a project management technique, whereby planning, scheduling, organising, coordinating and controlling of uncertain activities is done. CPM is a statistical technique of project management in which planning, scheduling, organising, coordination and control of well-defined activities takes place.

- PERT is a technique of ***planning and control of time.*** Unlike ***CPM, which is a method to control costs and time.***
- PERT is set according to events while CPM is aligned towards activities.
- A ***deterministic model is used in CPM***. Conversely, ***PERT uses probabilistic model.***
- There are three times estimates in PERT i.e. optimistic time (to), most likely time ™, pessimistic time (tp). On the other hand, there is only one estimate in CPM.
- PERT technique is best suited for a high precision time estimate, whereas CPM is appropriate for a reasonable time estimate.
- PERT ***deals with unpredictable activities***, but ***CPM deals with predictable activities.***
- ***PERT is used where the nature of the job is non-repetitive***. In contrast to, CPM involves the job of repetitive nature.
- There is a demarcation between critical and non-critical activities in CPM, which is not in the case of PERT.
- PERT is best for research and development projects, but CPM is for non-research projects like construction projects.
- Crashing is a compression technique applied to CPM, to shorten the project duration, along with least additional cost. The crashing concept is not applicable to PERT.

102. Ans. (b) Iron, (c) Carbohydate

[Ref: Park 23rd/630; Community Medicine with Recent Advances by Suryakantha 4th/620]

Table *(Park 23rd/630):* **Nutritive value of milks compared (Value per 1000 grams)**

		Buffalo	Cow	Goat	Human
Fat	(g)	6.5	4.1	4.5	3.4
Protein	(g)	4.3	3.2	3.3	1.1
Lactose	(g)	5.1	4.4	4.6	7.4
Calcium	(mg)	210	120	170	28
Iron	(mg)	0.2	0.2	0.3	
Vitamin C	(mg)	1	2	1	3
Minerals	(g)	0.8	0.8	0.8	0.1
Water	(g)	81.0	87	86.8	88
Energy	(kcal)	117	67	72	65

Table *(Suryakantha 4th/620):* **Composition of the milk (per 100mL)**

	Proteins (g)	Fats (g)	Carbohydrate (g)	Vitamin C	Vitamin D	Calcium	Iron	Energy
Human milk	1.1	3.1	7.1	6 mg	5 IU	0.03 mg	0.1 mg	65 kcals
Cow's milk	3.3	3.5	5.0	2 mg	2.5 IU	0.1 mg	0.04 mg	67 kcals

103. Ans. (b) Latent period = the period from..., (d) Generation time = time..., (e) Communicable period = It...

[Ref: Park 23rd/99-100; Community Medicine with Recent Advances by Suryakantha 4th/281-82]

Serial Interval

◈ *Park 23rd/100*

- The gap in time ***b/w the onset of the primary case and the secondary case is called serial interval***
- Primary case is followed by 2 or 3 secondary cases within a short time

Incubation Period

◈ *Park 23rd/99*

- The time interval ***b/w invasion by an infectious agent and appearance of first sign or symptom of disease in question***
- The length of the incubation period is characteristic of each disease

Latent Period

◈ *Park 23rd/99*

- The term latent period is used in non-infectious as the ***equivalent of incubation period*** in infectious disease
- Latent period has been defined as "***the period from disease initiation to disease detection***"
- In chronic disease, the agent-host interactions leading to a sequence of cellular changes are not well understood

Generation time

◈ *Park 23rd/100*

- It is defined as "the interval of time b/w ***receipt of infection by a host and maximal infectivity of that host***"
- In general, generation time is roughly equal to the incubation period. However, these two terms are not the same
- With person-to-person transmission of infection, the interval b/w cases is determined by generation time

Communicable Period

◈ *Park 23rd/100*

- It is defined as "the time during which an infectious agent may be transferred directly or indirectly from an infected person to another person, from an infected animal to man, or from an infected person to an animal, including arthropods

Secondary Attack Rate

◈ *(SAR) Park 23rd/100*

- SAR is defined as "the number of exposed persons developing the disease within the range of the incubation period, following exposure to the primary case"

Incubation Period and Related Terms

◈ *Suryakantha 4th/281-82*

- **Extrinsic incubation period:** It is the period between the entrance of the pathogen inside the body of the arthropod till the arthropod (vector) becomes infective. For example, 10 to 14 days in malaria, filariasis and yellow fever.

- **Window period:** It is the period between the entry of the pathogen and the production of the antibodies. It is 2 to 8 weeks in HIV/AIDS. ELISA test is negative during this period. But infected person is infectious to others during this period.
- **Prepatent period:** It is the interval between the entrance of the parasite (infective larvae of the *Wuchereria bancrofti*) and the first appearance of the microfilariae in the blood as in filariasis. It varies from 12 to18 months.
- **Minimum and maximum incubation period:** Since the incubation period always varies, every infectious disease has a minimum and a maximum incubation period. But it is almost constant in diseases like smallpox (14 days) and measles (10 days).
- **Median incubation period:** It is the time required for 50 percent of the cases to occur following exposure

104. Ans. **(a) Phosphatase test, (b) Standard plate count, (c) Methylene blue test, (e) Coliform count**

[Ref: Park 23rd/655; Community Medicine with Recent Advances by Suryakantha 4th/186]

"Nitric acid test is done epidemic dropsy (argemone oil detection)"- *Park 23rd/658*

Test of Pasteurized Milk

◈ *Park 23rd/ 655; Suryakantha 4th/186*

- ***Phosphatase test***: This test is widely used to check the efficiency of pasteurization. This test is based on the fact that raw milk contains an enzyme called phosphatase which is destroyed on heating at a temperature which corresponds closely with the standard time and temperature required for pasteurization
- **Standard plate count**: The bacteriolocial quality of pasteurized milk is determined by the standard plate count. Most countries in the west enforce a ***limit of 30,000 bacterial count per ml*** of pasteurized milk
- **Coliform count:** Coliform organism is usually completely destroyed by pasteurization
- **Methylene blue test**

Pasteurization of Milk

◈ *Park 23rd/655*

- It kills nearly 90% of the bacteria in milk including the more heat-resistant tubercle bacillus and the Q fever organisms. But it will not kill thermoduric bacteria nor the bacterial spores
- **Three methods are commonly used for pasteurization**
  1. Holder (Vat method)
  2. High temperature and short time method (HTST)
  3. Ultra high temperature: Milk is heated in usually 2 stages (the second stage usually being under pressure) to 125 °C for a few seconds. It is then rapidly cooled and bottled as quickly as possible

OPHTHALMOLOGY

105. Ans. **(b) Retinal surgery should be..., (d) Ophthalmia neonatorum..., (e) Primary vision center covers a...**

[Ref: Khurana 6th/480-82; Parson 22nd/566-71]

Interventions For prevention and Treatment

◈ *Parson 22nd/566*

- No effective preventive measures in the form of drugs or otherwise have been conclusively established. At the **primary level**, the health worker ***screens for cataract*** and reports those with vision less than a locally determined guideline (usually <3/60 or <6/60) for surgery. He or she plays a role in counselling and motivating those affected to undergo surgery.
- At the **secondary level,** ***cataract surgery should be performed*** with equal emphasis on the quality and quantity of surgery. At the **tertiary level** lies the provision of facilities for ***surgical treatment of complicated cases such as congenital cataract, subluxated lens, complicated cataracts and cataract associated with systemic diseases*** such as uncontrolled or inadequately controlled diabetes.
- In addition, tertiary care centres have the responsibility of ***training staff at other centres,*** providing outreach facilities and services, and providing organizational leadership and technical expertise in programmes to eliminate cataract-related blindness.

Tertiary Eye Care

◈ *Parson 22nd/566*

- Tertiary care units are large institutes in urban centres usually linked to major hospitals and medical colleges, which have all the state-of-the-art diagnostic and therapeutic facilities. These provide the following services:
  - Management of less common blinding conditions which require highly specialized staff and expensive, sophisticated equipment;
  - A focus on the care of diseases that need specialized treatment such as ***corneal grafting, paediatric cataract surgery, retinal detachment surgery, management of ocular and orbital malignancies*** and any other disorders that could not be treated or did not respond to treatment at the secondary level;
  - Provision of expert technical leadership, training of personnel involved at the secondary level, promotion of ophthalmology in relation to public health and conducting research to improve the delivery of eye health services.

Strategic Plan for Vision 2020: the Right to Sight in India

◈ *Khurana 6th/482*

- The Government of India has adopted 'Vision 2020: Right to Sight' under 'National Programme for Control of Blindness' at a meeting held in Goa on October 10- 13, 2001 and constituted a working group.

- The draft plan of action submitted by the 'Working Group' to the Ministry of Health and Family Welfare Govt. of India in August, 2002 includes following strategies: Strengthening advocacy, Reduction of disease burden Human resource development, and Eye care infrastructure development
- **Reduction of disease burden (disease-specific approach):** Target diseases identified for intervention under 'Vision 2020' initiative in India include:
  - Cataract
  - Childhood blindness
  - Refractive errors and low vision
  - Corneal blindness
  - Diabetic retinopathy
  - Glaucoma, and
  - Trachoma (focal)

Childhood Blindness

◈ *Khurana 6th/483-84*

- *Common causes* of childhood blindness are vitamin A deficiency, measles, conjunctivitis, ***ophthalmia neonatorum,*** injuries, congenital cataract, retinopathy of prematurity (ROP), and childhood glaucoma. Refractive errors are the commonest cause of visual impairment in children.
- ***Aim*** is to eliminate avoidable causes of childhood blindness by the year 2020.

Eye Care Infrastructure Development

◈ *Khurana 6th/485-86*

Based on the recommendations of WHO, there is need to develop the infrastructure pyramid which includes:

- **Primary level Vision Centres:** There is a need to develop ***20000 vision centres***, each with one Ophthalmic Assistant or equivalent (Community based MLOP) covering a ***population of 50000.***

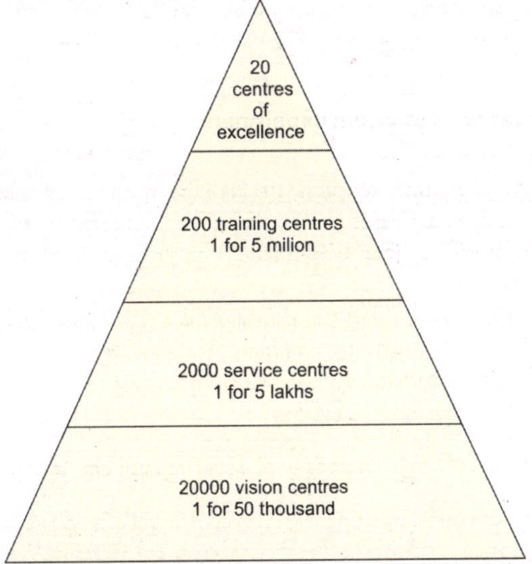

Fig: *(Khurana 6th/486)*: The infrastructure pyramid, based on the recommendations of WHO

- **Service centres**: There is need to develop ***2000 service centres*** at ***secondary level*** — each with two ophthalmologists and 8 paramedics (Hospital based MLOP), covering a ***population of 500000***. One eye care manager will be required at each service centre.
- **Training Centres:** There is a need to ***develop 200 'Training Centres'*** for the training of Ophthalmologists. Each ***tertiary level training centre*** will cater to a population of 5 million.
- **Centre of Excellence (COE):** There is need to develop ***20 COE*** with well developed all sub specialities of Ophthalmology. Each ***advanced tertiary level*** center of excellence will cater to a population of 50 millions

106. Ans. (a) Can be associated with... (b) Take longer time to..., (c) More symptomatic..., (e) Elevated hard nodule

[Ref: Khurana 6th/141-42 Parson 22nd/225-26]

"Both **episcleritis and scleritis** are mainly seen in adults. They can initially look similar but they do not feel similar and they do not behave similarly. Both are slightly more common in women than in men. Both can be associated with other conditions such as rheumatoid arthritis and ***systemic lupus erythematosus (SLE)***, although ***this is more likely in the case of scleritis.*** Episcleritis does not cause scleritis, although scleritis can lead to associated episcleritis"- *patient.info/in/health/episcleritis*

Episcleritis

◈ *Parson 22nd/225-26*

- This is a benign inflammatory affectation of the deep subconjunctival connective tissues, including the superficial scleral lamellae, and frequently affects both eyes, though their involvement may not be simultaneous.
- Anatomically, dense lymphocytic infiltration of the subconjunctival and episcleral tissues is found. It is often regarded as an allergic reaction to an endogenous toxin. The condition falls within the vague category of collagenous diseases. ***A history of rheumatoid arthritis*** is commonly obtained.
- Patients-usually young adults and commonly females.
- Present with an acute onset of redness, ***mild or no pain in one or both eyes,*** with no discharge. A history of recurrent episodes is common. Clinically, two types of presentations may occur: (i) simple or diffuse episcleritis; and (ii) nodular episcleritis.
- On examination, patients with **simple or diffuse episcleritis** have a sectoral or diffuse redness of one or both eyes mostly due to the engorgement of the large episcleral vessels which run in a radial direction beneath the conjunctiva. There is mild-to-moderate tenderness over the area of episcleral injection.
- In **nodular episcleritis** ***a circumscribed nodule of dense leucocytic infiltration, which may be as large as a lentil, appears usually 2 or 3 mm from the limbus. It is hard, tender and immovable (or at most can be moved slightly over the underlying sclera, with the conjunctiva moving freely over it). It is traversed by the deeper episcleral vessels so that it looks purple, not bright red.***
- There may be little or no pain, but usually there is a feeling of discomfort and tenderness on pressure, and sometimes severe neuralgia.

- ***Nodular episcleritis tends to be more symptomatic and takes longer to resolve.***
- In the worst cases the disease extends into the deeper parts of the sclera and thus passes almost imperceptibly into scleritis. The ***involvement of the eye is nearly always temporal in location.***
- It is usually transient lasting several days or some weeks but has a strong tendency to recur; thus the disease may drag on for months. Occasionally the attacks are fleeting but frequently repeated *(episcleritis periodica fugax).*
- **Treatment:** This is difficult and often unrewarding.

Episcleritis

◈ *Khurana 6th/141-42*

- It is found in association with gout, rosacea and Psoriasis and connective tissue disease
- Simple episcleritis is characterized by sectoral(occasionally diffuse) inflammation of episclera.
- ***Nodular episcleritis*** *is characterized by* a **pink or purple flat nodule** surrounded by injection is seen, usually situated 2-3 mm away from the limbus.The nodule is ***firm, tender,*** can be ***moved separated from the sclera*** and the overlying conjunctiva also moves freely

107. Ans. (a) Posterior subcapsulcar

[Ref: Khurana 6th/183; Parson 22nd/269]

"**Myotonic dystrophy** is associated with ***posterior subcapsular type of presenile cataract. Christmas tree cataract*** is typically seen in this condition"- *Khurana 6th/183*

Myotonic Dystrophy

◈ *Parson 22nd/269*

- Characteristic cataracts may develop with myotonic dystrophy and may be an early and prominent feature in 90% of patients. In a sharply limited zone of the cortex underneath the capsule both anteriorly and posteriorly, fine dust-like opacities appear interspersed with tiny iridescent spots. The polychromatic dots and flakes in the superficial cortex resemble a ***'Christmas tree' in appearance.***
- The cataract may remain stationary or progress. As the opacities mature a characteristic stellate opacity appears at the ***posterior pole***. The operative prognosis is good.

Type of cataract	Cause
Snow flake/Snow storm cataract	*Diabetes mellitus*
Sunflower/Petals of flower cataract	*Wilson disease* *Chalcosis* *Penetrating trauma*
Vossius ring on anterior surface of lens *Rossette shaped cataract*	*Blunt trauma*
Christmas tree cataract	***Myotonic dystrophica***
Oil drop cataract *Dust like lenticular opacity*	*Galactosemia*
Posterior cortical Bread's crumb appearance *Polychromatic lusture /Rainbow cataract*	*Complicated cataract*
Morgagnian cataract	*Hypermature senile cataract*

108. Ans. (c) <3/60 vision with best correction

[Ref: Khurana 6th/475-78; Parson 22nd/562-63]

"Applying the WHO criteria for definition of blindness, i.e. a ***visual acuity of less than 3/60 in the better eye with best possible refractive correction***, approximately 45 million people in the world are estimated to be blind. Another 135 million people are deemed to be visually disabled, i.e. are either visually impaired or severely visually impaired"- *Parson 22nd/562*

WHO Definition of Blindness

◈ *Khurana 6th/475*

- In order to have comparable national and international statistics, the WHO in 1972 proposed a uniform criterion and defined blindness as, "***Visual acuity of less than 3/60 (Snellen) or its equivalent***". In order to facilitate the screening of visual acuity by non-specialised persons, in the absence of appropriate vision charts, the WHO in 1979 added the "*Inability to count fingers in day-light at a distance of 3 metres*" to indicate vision less than 3/60 or its equivalent.
- Visual filed less than 10°, irrespective of the level of visual acuity in also labelled as blindness (WHO, 19774).

Other Definitions of Blindness in Vogue are

◈ *Khurana 6th/476*

- *Economic blindness:* vision in better eye <6/60 to 3/60
- *Social blindness:* Vision in better eye <3/60 to 1/ 60
- *Legal blindness:* Vision in better eye <1/60 to perception light
- *Total blindness:* No light perception (PL -ve).

Categories of Visual Impairment

◈ *Khurana 6th/475*

- In the Ninth Revision (1977) of the International Classification of Diseases (ICD), the visual impairment (maximum vision less than 6/18 Snellen) has been divided into 5 categories.
- Categories 1 and 2 constitute "*low vision*" and categories 3, 4 and 5 constitute "*blindness*". Patients with the visual fields between 5° and 10° are placed in category 3 and those with less than 5° in category 4.

Table *(Khurana 6th/476)*: **Categories of visual impairment (WHO, 1977)**

Category of visual impairment	Level of visual acuity (Snellen)
Normal vision	0-6/6 to 6/18
Low vision	• Less than 6/18 to 6/60 • Less than 6/60 to 3/60

Contd...

Blindness	• Less than 3/60 (FC at 3 m) to 1/60 (FC at 1m) or visual field between 5° and 10° • Less than 1/60 (FC at 1 m) to light perception or visual field less than 5° • No light perception

Note: FC- Finger count

Table *(Parson 22nd/563):* **Classification of visual impairment and blindness**

Category of visual impairment*	Best corrected visual acuity (BCVA) in the better eye
0 'Normal'	6/6 to 6/18, i.e. can see 6/18 or better
1 'Visual impairment'	<6/18 to 6/60, i.e. cannot see 6/18, can see 6/60
2 'Severe visual impairment'	<6/60 to 3/60, i.e. cannot see 6/60, can see 3/60
3 'Blind'	<3/60 to 1/60, i.e. cannot see 3/60, can see 1/60
4 'Blind'	<1/60 to only light perception, i.e. cannot see 3/60, can see light
5 'Blind'	No light perception, i.e. cannot see light
9 'Undetermined or unspecified'	

** Adapted from International Statistical Classification of Disease and Related Health Problems, tenth revision. Geneva, World Health Organization, 1992.*

109. Ans. (b) Can occur as opportunistic..., (c) Can be cultured on non-nutrient..., (d) Painful condition (e) Radial kerato-neuritis...

[Ref: Khurana 6th/112-14; Parson 22nd/208; Harrison 19th/1367-68]

Acanthamoebic Keratitis

◈ *Khurana 6th/112-14*

- Corneal infection with acanthamoeba results from direct corneal contact with any material or water contaminated with the organism.
- ***Contact lens wearers*** using home-made saline (from contaminated tap water and saline tablets) is the commonest situation recognised for acanthamoeba infection in western countries.
- *Opportunistic infection.* Acanthamoeba keratitis can also occur as opportunistic infection in patients with herpetic keratitis, bacterial keratitis, bullous keratopathy and neuroparalytic keratitis
- ***Symptoms:*** These include ***very severe pain*** (out of proportion to the degree of inflammation), watering, photophobia, blepharospasm and blurred vision.
- ***Signs:*** Acanthamoeba keratitis evolves over several months as a gradual worsening keratitis with periods of temporary remission. Presentation is markedly variable, making diagnosis difficult.
- *Initial lesions* of acanthamoeba keratitis are in the form of limbitis, coarse, opaque streaks, fine epithelial and subepithelial opacities, and ***radial kerato-neuritis***, in the form of infiltrates along corneal nerves.
- *Advanced cases* show a central or paracentral ring-shaped lesion with stromal infiltrates and an overlying epithelial defect, ultimately presenting as ring abscess. Hypopyon may also be present.
- ***Laboratory diagnosis: Culture on non-nutrient agar*** **(*E. coli* enriched)** may show trophozoites within 48 hours, *which gradually turn into cysts.*

Acanthamoebic Keratitis

◈ *Parson 22nd/208*

- Acanthamoebic keratitis can be a devastating infection if not recognized early. Its occurrence is frequently associated with the wearing of ***soft contact lenses.***
- ***Ocular pain is severe***, perhaps due to deep linear stromal infiltrates localized along the ***corneal nerves***..

Acanthamoeba Infections

◈ *Harrison 19th/1367-68*

- Demonstration of the trophozoites and cysts of *Acanthamoeba* on wet mounts or in biopsy specimens establishes the diagnosis. ***Culture on nonnutrient agar plates seeded with Escherichia coli*** also may be helpful.
- Risk factors include the use of homemade saline, the wearing of lenses while swimming, and inadequate disinfection. Since contact lenses presumably cause microscopic trauma, the early corneal findings may be nonspecific. The first symptoms usually include tearing and the ***painful sensation*** of a foreign body.

110. Ans. (a) Ferry's Line-corneal epithelial iron line..., (b) Stockers Line-Corneal epithelial... (e) Coat's white ring- A form of iron ...

[Ref: www.eophtha.com; Khurana 6th/434; Parson 22nd/395-96]

"There are **four types of known iron lines: *Hudson-Stahli Line, Fleischer's Ring, Stocker's Line, and Ferry's Line.*** Additionally, in the last two decades there have been reports of iron lines following radial keratotomy, refractive keratoplasty, intrastromal corneal ring insertion, as well as another iron line, Coat's Ring, that develops in Bowman's layer after metallic foreign body in the cornea"- www.ncbi.nlm.nih.gov

"Coat's white ring- A form of iron deposit at the level of Bowman's layer of cornea"-*dro.hs.columbia.edu*

Lines in Ophthalmology

◈ *www.eophtha.com*

Arlt's Line = conjunctival scar in sulcus subtarsalis.
Ehrlich-Turck Line = linear deposition of KPs in ueitis
Ferry's Line = corneal epithelial iron line at the edge of filtering blebs.
Hudson-Stahil Line= Horizonatl corneal epithelial iron line at the inferior one third of cornea due to aging.
Khodadoust Line = corneal graft endothelial rejection line composed of inflammatory cells.
Paton's Line = Circumferential retinal folds due to optic nerve edema.

Sampaoelesi line = Increased pigmentation anterior to Schwalbe›s line in pseudoexfoliation syndrome.
Scheie's Line = pigment on lens equator and posterior capsule in pigment dispersion syndrome.
Schwalbe's Line = Angle structure representing peripheral edge of Descemets membrane.
Stockers Line = Corneal epithelial iron line at the edge of pterygium
White lines of Vogt = Sheathed or sclerosed vessels seen in Lattice degeneration

Lines and Rings in Ophthalmology

dhavalpatel.wordpress.com

- Arlt's Line = conjunctival scar in sulcus subtarsalis in Trachoma.
- Ehrlich-Turck Line = linear deposition of KPs in uveitis
- **Ferry's Line** = corneal epithelial iron line at the edge of filtering blebs.
- **Hudson-Stahil Line** = Horizonatl corneal epithelial iron line at the inferior one third of cornea due to aging.
- Khodadoust Line = corneal graft endothelial rejection line composed of inflammatory cells.
- Paton's Line = Circumferential retinal folds due to optic nerve edema.
- Sampaoelesi line = Increased pigmentation anterior to Schwalbe's line in pseudoexfoliation syndrome.
- Zentmeyer line (Scheie's Line): on the equatorial surface of the lens pigment dispersion syndrome
- Schwalbe's Line = Angle structure representing peripheral edge of Descemets membrane.
- Stockers Line = Corneal epithelial iron line at the edge of pterygium
- White lines of Vogt = Sheathed or sclerosed vessels seen in Lattice degeneration
- Fingerprint lines: The map-dot fingerprint dystrophy
- LASIK Iron Line
- Vogt's striae
- The Descemet's breaks or Haab's striae
- Ring Keratitis: The hallmark of Acanthamoeba keratitis
- Kayser-Fleischer's ring: Wilson's disease
- **Coats' ring:** remnants of a foreign body. The remnants are fine ***iron deposits in the cornea.***
- **Fleischer's ring:** Visible all around the base of cone in Keratoconus
- Pseudo-Fleischer's ring: iron deposition can be seen in Hyperopia
- Soemmering's ring: early opacification of lens capsule in cataract
- Vossius' ring: on lens in concussion injury to eye
- Weiss ring: epipapillary glial tissue torn from the optic disc in Posterior vitreous detachment (PVD)
- Double ring sign

Spots in Ophthalmology

www.eophtha.com

Bitot's spot = White, foamy area of keratinising squamous metaplasia of bulbar conjunctiva,seen in vitamin A deficiency.
Brushfield spot = Whitish grey spot in peripheral iris,seen in Down's syndrome.
Fuch's spot = pigmented (RPE hyperplasia) macular leisons in pathological myopia.
Roth spots = haemorrhages with white centres, seen in SABE, severe anaemia,collagen vascular disorders.

Dots in ophthalmology

www.eophtha.com

Gunn's dot = light reflectios from internal limiting membrane around disc and macula

Horner-Trantras Dot = Collections of eosinophils at limbus in vernal conjunctivitis.

Kayes' dot = subepithelial infiltrates seen in corneal graft rejection

Mittendorf's dot = whitish spot at posterior lens surface, remnant of hyaloid artery.

---

111. Ans. (a) In choroidal circulation it passes..., (c) Albumin binding is less ...

[Ref: Khurana 6th/517-18; Parson 22nd/142-43]

"**Sodium fluorescein:** Upon entering the circulation, ***approximately 80% of the dye molecules bind to plasma proteins***, which significantly reduces fluorescence because the free electrons that form this chemical bond are subsequently unavailable for excitation. The remaining unbound or free fluorescein molecules fluoresce when excited with light of the appropriate wavelength. With a molecular weight of 376, fluorescein ***diffuses freely out of all capillaries except those of the central nervous system, including the retina***"-"- http://www.opsweb.org/
"The percentage of total **fluorescein** bound by human ***serum proteins ranged from 83% to 53%***"-jamanetwork.com
Indocyanine green: ***binds primarily (95%) to albumin***, with lesser binding to α_2-globulins"- clinchem.aaccjnls.org
ICG binds tightly to plasma proteins and becomes confined to the vascular system"-*wikipedia*

Fluorescein Angiography

Parson 22nd/142-43

- Fluorescein angiography of the fundus is based on the detection of fluorescent light emitted by a dye in circulation.
- This fluorescence is produced by irradiation of the dye with light of a wavelength within the absorption band of the fluorescein and blood mixture (***420-490 nm***). The ***emitted fluorescence (510-530 nm)*** is passed through a barrier filter to the film, with complete exclusion of the irradiating light.
- ***Fluorescein is readily bound to the albumin in the blood stream.*** The **blood-retinal barrier**, by ***preventing dye leakage*** in the physiological state, facilitates the delineation of retinal vessels of all calibres. In the **choroidal circulation**, fluorescein ***passes freely across the endothelium*** of the capillaries to the extravascular spaces. ***A physiological barrier to the dye prevents the passage across Bruch's membrane and the intact retinal pigment epithelium.***
- When the dye enters the eye initially ***there is a choroidal blush*** and then the dye can be followed through the retinal

arterioles, the capillary bed and into the veins, which are at first laminated due to a differential flow of blood. A late phase is usually recorded 5-30 minutes after injection

- Fluorescein angiography is particularly ***helpful in exposing the depth of pathological involvement in diabetic retinopathy and reveals neovascularization occurring in any area of the fundus***
- Fluorescein angiography is ***also helpful in the interpretation of neovascularization of the iris when leakage from the vessels of the iris may be the first sign of rubeosis.***

Indocyanine Green (ICG) Angiography

◈ *Parson 22nd/142-43*

- ***Indocyanine green stays within the choroidal circulation*** and is ***stimulated by a longer wavelength of light than fluorescein dye. This provides a better resolution of the choroidal vasculature***, especially choroidal neovascular membranes (CNVM).
- "***ICG absorbs mainly between 600 nm and 900 nm and emits fluorescence between 750 nm and 950 nm***. The large overlapping of the absorption and fluorescence spectra leads to a marked reabsorption of the fluorescence by ICG itself. The fluorescence spectrum is very wide. Its maximum values are approx. 810 nm in water and approx. 830 nm in blood"- en.wikipedia.org

Fundus Fluorescein Angiography (FFA)

◈ *Khurana 6th/517-18*

- Basically, FFA gives information by allowing the examiner to study the changes, produced by various fundus disorders, in the ***flow of fluorescein dye along the vasculature of the retina and choroid.***
- ***Indications***: It is indicated in many disorders of ocular fundus, viz., (1) Diabetic retinopathy (2) Vascular occlusions; (3) Eales' disease. (4) Central serous retinopathy, (5) Cystoid macular oedema.
- ***Technique***: The technique of FFA comprises rapidly injecting 5 ml of 10 per cent solution of sterile ***sodium fluorescein dye*** in the antecubital vein and taking serial photographs (with fundus camera) of the fundus of the patient who is seated with pupils fully dilated. The fundus camera has a mechanism to use ***blue light (420-490 nm wavelength)*** for exciting the fluorescein present in blood vessels and to use ***yellow-green filter for receiving the fluorescent light (510-530 nm wavelength)*** back for photography. The first photograph is taken after 5 seconds, then every second for next 20 seconds and every 3-5 seconds for next one minute. The last pictures are taken after 10 minutes.
- *Abnormalities detected by FFA*:In the ***blood, fluorescein is readily bound to the albumin. Normally the dye remains confined to the intravascular space due to the barriers formed by the tight junctions between the endothelial cells of retinal capillaries (inner blood-retinal barrier)*** and that between the pigment epithelial cells (outer blood-retinal barrier). In diseased states abnormalities in the form of hyperfluorescence and hypofluorescence may be detected on FFA.

112. Ans. (a) Size of eye decrease, (b) Removed by enucleation..., (d) Calcification may occur ...

[Ref: Khurana 6th/157-58]

Phthisis Bulbi

◈ *Khurana 6th/157-58*

- It is the ***final stage end result of any form of chronic uveitis.***
- In this condition, ciliary body is disorganised and so ***aqueous production is hampered***. As a result of it the eye becomes soft, shrinks and eventually becomes a small atrophic globe (phthisis bulbi).
- Development of phthisis bulbi can be divided into three overlapping stages
    - Stage of phthisis bulbi without shrinkage is the initial stage:
    - *Stage of atrophic bulbi with shrinkage* continued ciliary body dysfunction. In this stage:
    - *Atrophic bulbi with disorganization* is the final stage known as phthisis bulbi. In this stage due to Continued disorganization of ciliary body:***IOP is markedly lowered, Size of eyeball is markedly decreased, and Cornea becomes sclera like.***
- *Histopathological examination* at this stages reveals: Disorganization of all the intraocular tissues,***Calcification may occur in Bowman's layer of cornea***, lens and retina.
- ***Phthisis bulbi*** especially when painful, requires removal by ***enucleation operation.***

◈ *radiopaedia.org/articles/phthisis-bulbi*

- **Phthisis bulbi**, also known as **end-stage eye**, is an atrophic scarred and disorganised globe that may result from a variety of severe ocular insults.
- The ***globe is reduced in size (usually < 20 mm)*** with a thickened/folded posterior sclera. ***Dystrophic calcification is common***, and osseous metaplasia sometimes occurs, forming what is called «intraocular bone».
- The globe is non-functioning thus the patient is blind in that eye. ***Enucleation +/- prosthesis insertion*** is performed if there is associated chronic pain or for cosmetic reasons.

113. Ans. (a) Preferred method of..., (c) Keeps the nucleus..., (d) Resists radial tears, (e) Helps in stabilizing...

[Ref: Khurana 6th/201, 203; Parson 22nd/278-79]

Anterior Capsulotomy in ECCE

It can be performed by any of the following methods: *Khurana 6th/201*

- **Can-opener's technique**. In it, an irrigating cystitome (or simply a 26 gauge needle, bent at its tip) is introduced into the anterior chamber and multiple small radial cuts are made in the anterior capsule for 360o
- **Linear capsulotomy**
- **Continuous circular capsulorrhexis (CCC)**. Recently this is the most commonly performed procedure. In this the anterior capsule is torn in a circular fashion either with the help of an irrigating bent-needle cystitome or with a capsulorrhexis forceps

Continuous Curvilinear Capsulorrhexis (CCC)

◈ *www.aao.org*

- Although a ***can-opener capsulotomy can be used with phacoemulsification, continuous-tear curvilinear capsulorrhexis (CCC) is the capsular opening that allows a wider range of safer phaco techniques.***
- ***CCC resists radial tears*** that could extend around and open the posterior capsule, setting the stage for the development of complications.
- In addition, ***CCC stabilizes the nucleus***, allowing maneuvers to disassemble the nucleus within the capsular bag. Disassembling the nucleus in the capsular bag decreases endothelial trauma.
- ***CCC also helps stabilize and center the lens implant.*** Further, CCC transfers the haptic forces circumferentially and prevents lens implant decentration if YAG posterior capsulotomy is performed.
- A CCC sized just smaller than the IOL optic may allow a tighter contact between the posterior surface of the posterior chamber IOL and the posterior capsule, possibly ***reducing posterior capsule opacification***. Lastly, certain lens implants designed to provide multifocality require a CCC of a certain size.
- ***If a CCC cannot be completed, conversion to a can-opener anterior capsulotomy is an acceptable strategy.*** However, this type of ***anterior capsulotomy makes hydrodissection, hydrodelineation, and endocapsular phacoemulsification more challenging.***

Table *(Clinical Atlas of Procedures in Ophthalmic and Oculofacial Surgery by Daniel 2nd):* **Indications for Anterior Capsulotomy Techniques**

Continuous Curvilinear Capsulorhexis	Can-Opener Capsulotomy
Phacoemulsification Utilize capsular staining techniques with mature, white cataracts	Planned extracapsular cataract extraction Useful for mature, white cataracts ***if capsular stain not available***

Capsulorhexis

◈ *en.wikipedia.org*

- Prior to the advent of the CCC, a "**can opener" approach** was used, with a ***small bent needle making small incisions around the anterior surface of the lens, forming a somewhat continuous hole that the lens could be removed through.*** However, any of these ragged edges could promote a tear that could proceed outwards.
- A ***CCC when done correctly, does not have any edges, and any forces applied to the capsule during surgery are distributed and do not result in a tear.***

ENT

114. Ans. (b) Syringing is used for removal of vegetative foreign body

[Ref: Dhingra 6th/54; L and T 10th/267, 345-46; ENT by Maqbool 11th/54-55]

*"**Syringing is contraindicated for living vegetable** foreign body"- ENT by Hazarika 3rd/125*

Foreign bodies of ear *For young children, it is best to use general anesthesia*. Inanimate objects located lateral to the isthmus of the canal are removed with an alligator forceps or by placing a hook or ring curette behind it and pulling it out. Suctioning with Frazier suction catheters is useful in removing an object with a smooth surface that is hard to grasp. Irrigation can be used in certain instances. Objects ***located medial to the isthmus of the canal are more difficult to remove*** and may require local or general anesthesia."- *Ballenger's Otorhinolaryngology 16th/233-34*

Foreign Bodies of Ear

◈ *Dhingra 6th/54*

- *Methods of removing a foreign body include: forceps removal, syringing, suction, microscopic removal with special instruments andpostaural approach*
- *Soft and irregular foreign bodies like a piece of paper, swab or a piece of sponge can be removed with fine crocodile foreceps*
- *In all impacted foreign bodies or in those where earlier attempts at extraction have been made, it is preferable to use **general anaesthesia** and an operating microscope*
- *"Syringing of ear may be necessary to remove the wax or a foreign body.The water for irrigation(usually tap water) is **brought to the body temperature.** If the water used is not at body temperature, it produces caloric stimulation with symptoms of giddiness and vomiting. The jet of water from the nozzle is directed **along the posterosuperior canal wall.** If the wax or foreign body is directly hit by the stream of water it moves deeper and may get impacted. **Excessive force used while syringing may damage the canal wall or the tympanic membrane***

Foreign Bodies in External Auditory Canal

◈ *ENT by Maqbool 11th/54-55*

- ***Metallic foreign bodies, glass beads and small sized foodgrains may be removed by syringing***
- *A **living foreign body** may be killed by installing some oily drops into the ear. This suffocates and kills the insect which can be then removed by foreceps or syringe*
- ***The foreign bodies lying deep in the meatus in children and in patients who are apprehensive are removed under general anaesthesia.** Impacted foreign bodies may need a postaural approach for removal*

Foreign Bodies in the Ear

◈ *L and T 10 th/345-46*

- Gentle inspection will reveal the object in most cases. If it is not seen, the ear may be gently syringed, as a very small foreign body may lie out of sight in the ***anterior recess of the meatus.***
- In removing foreign bodies three facts should be remembered. First, the ***narrowest part of the external auditory meatus, the isthmus***, is situated near its mid-point in the bony part.
- Secondly, ***foreign bodies of vegetable origin, such as nuts, peas and beans, are hygroscopic and should not be syringed***, as if the first attempt fails, they will swell up and impact against the meatal walls.

- Thirdly, ***no attempts should be made to remove smooth spherical objects such as beads by forceps***: As the forceps close the object will inevitably be pushed deeper down the meatus.
- As a general rule, most foreign material can be removed by gentle syringing. This is particularly so if it consists of several particles. ***Larger objects lying superficial to the isthmus should not be syringed, as there is a risk of wedging them in that area***. They, and all material of vegetable origin, should be removed with a fine hook.
- ***Beads which have a diameter less than that of the isthmus can be syringed; larger ones are better removed with a hook***. Attempts at removal of foreign bodies in children should not be prolonged because of the pain produced and the fright engendered. ***In such cases it is wiser to remove it under general anaesthetic with the help of the operating microscope***. In rare instances repeated attempts at removal may drive the object into the middle ear, and an external operation may be required for its extraction.
- It is useless to attempt to syringe animal foreign bodies out as they are firmly attached the meatal walls. Chloroform water or vapour must be applied to the meatus in order to anaesthetize or kill the maggots and so release their grip on the skin. Thereafter they may be removed by syringing.

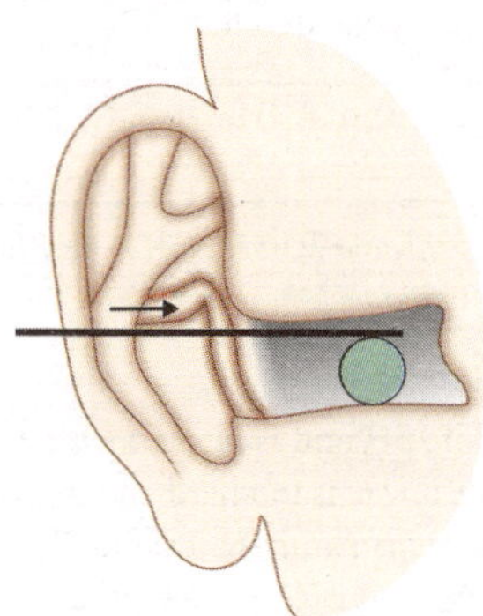

Fig: *(Smooth or rounded objects are best removed with use of right-angled blunt hook such as a Day hook"):* Essential Guide to primary care procedures by E.J. Mayeaux 2007/346

115. Ans. (c) Anterior nasal pack is easy to insert and less traumatic than balloon temponade

[Ref: Dhingra 6th/176-80; L and T 10th/30-33; ENT by P.Hazarika 3rd/272-78; www.entsho.com/epistaxis]

Epistaxis

◈ *P.Hazarika 3rd/272-78*

- **"Kiesselbach's plexus:** This plexus is the ***commonest site of bleeding(90% of cases)"***
- Patient may put in the sitting position with the head bending forwards with mouth open(**Trotter's method**)
- **Anterior nasal packing:** ***Prophylactic antibodies should be used if pack is in a place for more than 24 hours***
- A **balloon tamponade** may be used as an alternative to anterior nasal packing. ***This is less traumatic*** and is best suited in epistaxis due to bleeding or clotting disorders
- ***Nasal endoscopy assisted bipolar cauterization under general anaesthesia may be done to coagulate the bleeder in case of epistaxis is refractory to conservative measures***

Epistaxis

◈ *Dhingra 6th/176-80*

- ***In 90% cases of epistaxis, bleeding occurs from Little's area***. It is situated in the anterior inferior part of nasal septum, just above the vestibule. Four arteries anastomose here to form a vascular plexus called "***Kiesselbach's plexus***"
- Woodruff's plexus: It is a plexus of veins situated inferior to posterior end of inferior turbinate. It is a site of posterior epistaxis in adults
- Anterior nasal pack can be removed after 24 hr, if bleeding has stopped. Sometimes, ***it has to be kept for 2-3 days; in that case, systemic antibiotics should be given*** to prevent sinus infection and toxic shock syndrome

First Aid

- Little's area-pinching the nose with thumb and index finger for about 5 minutes compression of vessels.
- Trotter's method-patientis made to sit, leaning a little forward over a basin to spit any blood, and breathe quietly from mouth- cold compresses should be applied to nose to cause reflex vasoconstriction.

116. Ans. (a) Type C tympanogram may..., (b) Flat tympanogram..., (c) Leads to conductive..., (e) Most common cause is Eustachian...

[Ref: Dhingra 6th/64-65; L and T 10th/432-40; ENT by P.Hazarika 3rd/145-48]

*"Impedance audiometry show a **flat curve** with a shift in compliance to the negative side"- P.Hazarika 3rd/147-48*

"Eustachian tube (ET) dysfunction is considered the ***major etiologic factor*** in the development of middle ear disease. Politzer first proposed the ex vacuo theory of OM in 1867. The theory postulates that chronic negative pressure, secondary to ET malfunction, results in the development of a transudate into the middle ear space. Numerous experiments have been carried out by many authors to substantiate this theory. It is traditionally maintained that the effusion is sterile; therefore, ***therapy should be aimed chiefly at relieving ET dysfunction***"-*Ballenger's Otorhinolaryngology 16th/250*

Otitis media with effusion (Syn. Serous Otitis Media, Secretory Otitis Media, Mucoid Otitis Media, "Glue Ear") *(Dhingra 6th/64-65)*

- This is an insidious condition characterized by accumulation of non-purulent effusion in the middle ear cleft. Often the effusion is thick and viscid but sometimes it may be thin and serous. The fluid is nearly sterile. The condition is commonly seen in school-going children.
- **"Type B tympanogram**: A ***flat or dome-shaped graph***. Seen in ***middle ear fluid*** or thick tympanic membrane"-*Dhingra 6th/24*
- **"Type C tympanogram**: Seen in Eustachian tube obstruction or ***early stage of otitis media with effusion***"-*Dhingra 6th/25*
- Two main mechanism are thought to be responsible: ***Malfunctioning of Eustachian tube*** (causes include palatal

defects e.g. ***cleft palate***, palatal paralysis) and increased secretory activity of middle ear mucosa

- Hearing loss: This is presenting and sometimes only symptom. Hearing loss is of ***conductive type*** of 20-40 dB. Sometimes, there is associated sensorineural hearing loss due to fluid pressing on the round window membrane. This disappear with evacuation of fluid
- Because of hearing loss, development of speech is delayed or defective

Serous Otitis Media

◈ *L and T 10th/434*

- "Middle ear fluid and conductive hearing loss are frequent in children with a cleft palate and it has been quoted in upto 90% of cases"
- Deafness-conductive. It is usually bilateral in children and unilateral in adults"- *ENT by P.Hazarika 3rd/145-48*

Tymanogram

◈ *Dhingra 6th/24*

A — Normal

As — Reduced compliance at ambient pressure (otosclerosis). 's' stands for shallow tympanogram but remember for stiffness.

AD — Increased compliance at ambient pressure (ossicular discontinuity). 'd' stands for deep tympanogram. Remember disruption of ossicular chain.

B — Flat or dome-shaped (***fluid in middle ear***).

C — Maximum compliance at pressures more than –200 mm H_2O (negative pressure in middle ear), e.g. ***eustachian tube obstruction or early stage of otitis media with effusion.***

117. Ans. (a) Median rhomboid glossitis, (d) Geographic tongue

[Ref: Dhingra 6th/220; L and T 10 th/126-27; Robbins 9th/730]

"Hairy leukoplakia is usually seen in immunocompromised patients and is caused by Epstein-Barr virus (EBV). *Hairy leukoplakia takes the form of* *white, confluent patches of fluffy ("hairy"), hyperkeratotic thickenings, almost always situated on the lateral border of the tongue"-Robbins 9th/730*

White Lesions of Oral Cavity

◈ *L and T 10th/126*

- ***Fordyces's granules***
- ***Lichen planus***
- *Moniliasis*
- *Leukoplakia*

Red Lesions of Oral Cavity

◈ *L and T 10th/126*

- Papillomas
- Pemphigoid
- Erythroplakia
- Granular-cell tumour
- Epulides
- Hemangioma

Specific Tongue Lesions

◈ *L and T 10th/126*

- ***Median rhomboid glossitis: reddish*** *rhomboid-shaped area*
- ***Geographic tongue: smooth red*** *mucosal surface in which the fungiform papillae become visible as* ***red elevations***
- ***Hairy tongue: Hairy black-brown or yellow*** *aspect of the dorsal surface of the tongue*

Median Rhomboid Glossitis

◈ *Dhingra 6th/220*

- It is red rhomboid area, devoid of papilla, seen on dorsum of tongue in front of foramen caecum
- It is a developmental anomaly that occurs due to persistence of tuberculum impair, which fails to invaginate
- Recent studies reveal this condition to be due to chronic candida infection

Geographical Tongue

◈ *Dhingra 6th/220*

- It is characterized by ***erythematous areas,*** devoid of papillae, surrounded by an irregular keratotic white outline
- The lesions keep changing their shape and hence the condition is also called "migratory glossitis." The condition is asymptomatic and may not require any treatment.

Fordyce Spots

◈ *Dhingra 6th/220*

- They are aberrant sebaceous glands present under the buccal or labial mucosa and shine through it as ***yellowish or yellow-brown spots.***
- They are seen with equal frequency in both males and females and are considered normal.

118. Ans. (a) Syringing and instrumental..., (b) If wax is hard and impacted, cerom..., (d) Wax has antibacterial property

[Ref: Dhingra 6th/53; L and T 10th/265-67; ENT by P.Hazarika 3rd/123]

Impacted Wax or Cerumen

◈ *Dhingra 6th/53*

- Wax has acidic pH and is ***bacteriostatic and fungistatic***
- Occasionally, if wax is too hard and impacted, to be removed by ***syringing or instruments***, it should be softened by drops of 5% sodium bicarbonate in equal parts of glycerine and water. Hydrogen peroxide, liquid paraffin or olive oil may also achieve the same result. Commercial drops containing ceruminolytic agents paradichlorobenxene 2% can also be used
- Patient usually presents with impairment of hearing or sense of blocked ear
- Long standing impacted wax may result in wax granuloma
- It is necessary before syringing to ask for any past history of ear discharge or an existing perforation. A quiescent otitis media may be reactivated by syringing

Wax/Cerumen

◈ *ENT by P.Hazarika 3rd/123*

- Function of wax: antibacterial action; traps dust and foreign body
- ***Waxolytic agents for impacted wax to soften the wax. It can then be removed by syringing/suctioning***

Impacted Wax

◈ *L and T 10th/265-67*

- ***Tinnitus and disturbance of balance may occur from pressure of the wax on the drumhead***, and a cough reflex due to stimulation of the auricular branch of the vagus has been described.

- ***Wax is removed either by instrumental manipulation or by syringing***. The former method should be reserved for special situations and performed only by an otologist.
- Sterile saline solution, or boracic lotion (1: 40), or a solution of sodium bicarbonate, warmed to blood heat, should be employed for syringing.
- The patient's head is inclined slightly downwards and towards the same side to prevent the fluid from running down the neck. It is a natural reaction or patient to tilt his head away from the stream of fluid. The *auricle is pulled up wards and backwards to straighten out the meatus, and the* ***fluid is injected along the upper wall of the meatus***

119. Ans. (a) A neurological..., (c) Hyperadduction of vocal..., (d) Botulinum toxin..., (e) Speech therapy is...

[Ref: Dhingra 6th/314-15; www.nidcd.nih.gov;L and T 10th/158; ENT by P.Hazarika 3rd/635; Ballenger's Otorhinolaryngology 16th/1124-25]

"Spasmodic dysphonia is a ***neurological disorder*** affecting the voice muscles in the larynx, or voice box"- www.nidcd.nih.gov

"The cause of spasmodic dysphonia is unknown. Because the voice can sound normal or near normal at times, ***spasmodic dysphonia was once thought to be psychogenic***, or originating in a person's mind, rather than from a physical cause. In rare cases, psychogenic forms of spasmodic dysphonia do exist; however, ***in most instances, the muscle spasms are caused by abnormalities in the central nervous system*** (the brain)"- www.nidcd.nih.gov

"The **three types of spasmodic dysphonia** (SD) are adductor spasmodic dysphonia, abductor spasmodic dysphonia and mixed spasmodic dysphonia"- *www.nidcd.nih.gov, Wikipedia; Ballenger's Otorhinolaryngology 16th/1124-25; Dhingra 6th/314-15*

Spastic Dysphonia

◈ *L and T 10th/158*

- This is a relatively recently described condition which gives the voice a peculiar grating quality. It is ***usually stress-related*** but this is probably the only point of general agreement.
- The usual treatment is ***speech therapy*** but decompression of the recurrent laryngeal nerve has been described.

Spastic Dysphonia

◈ *ENT by P.Hazarika 3rd/635*

- It is a condition associated with a harsh and soft voice alternatively, as a result of severe vocal disability, with ***excessive adduction of vocal cords during phonation***.
- Exact etiology is not known. The patient may have ***strained, cricking or choked vocal attacks***.
- *Indirect laryngoscopy:* ***Excessive adduction of vocal cords may be seen on phonation***.
- They ***respond poorly to psychotherapy and speech therapy***.
- ***Botulinum toxin injection*** into the laryngeal muscles has been tried in the treatment of spastic dysphonia

Adductor Dysphonia

◈ *Dhingra 6th/314*

- The adductor muscle go into spasm causing vocal cords to go into adduction
- Aetiology of this condition is uncertain but one should exclude neurological conditions
- Treatment consists of ***botulinum toxin injection*** in the thyroarytenoid muscle
- ***Voice therapy is useful*** to improve voice only when combined with injection
- ***Earlier disease was considered to be psychological in origin but psychotherapy was not found useful***

Abductor Dysphonia

◈ *Dhingra 6th/314-15*

- It is due to spasm of abductor muscle(posterior cricoarytenoid muscle)
- Symptom get aggravated during periods of stress
- Like adductor spasm dysphonia, cause of this is not known
- Treatment consists of ***botulinum toxin*** injection in the posterior cricoarytenoid muscle
- ***Voice therapy is useful to improve voice only when combined with injection***

Spasmodic Dysphonia

◈ *Ballenger's Otorhinolaryngology 16th/1124-25*

- It is probably an ***organic movement disorder with an unknown cause***.
- The closure form of the disorder is often referred to as ***adductor spasmodic dysphonia and the open form as abductor spasmodic dysphonia***.
- ***The adductor form is more common than the abductor***, but both may be heard in a single patient.
- ***Inconsistency of symptoms undoubtedly contributes to the traditional assumption that spasmodic dysphonia is psychogenic.Indeed, it may be, but research evidence indicates the possibility of a neural etiologic component***
- ***Differing concepts are mentioned simply because the neurogenic theory has led to surgical therapeutic procedures that have been more successful in treating the adductor type than other approaches***.
- The tenacious persistence of spasmodic dysphonia has caused patients to seek help from ***psychiatry, clinical psychology, speech therapy, hypnosis, drugs of many varieties, and bizarre remedies of every type, all unsuccessfully.***
- The underlying rationalization for the temporary paralysis procedures is that ***if spasmodic dysphonia is psychogenic***, the fluent speech practiced during the period of paralysis should persist after recovery from the paralysis. *Unfortunately, the speech symptoms tend to recur with return of function.* When unilateral paralysis is permanent after section of one recurrent nerve, the voice is almost always normally fluent for at least the first year, but as time passes, more and more patients report recurrence of their symptoms.
- These varying results lead to the speculation that spasmodic dysphonia symptoms are probably the result of ***multiple causes.***
- The **abductor type of spasmodic dysphonia** is not helped by intentional unilateral vocal fold paralysis. This procedure simply exaggerates the undesired glottal

opening. Patients with this problem report considerable variation in symptoms, ***with the disorder worsening with anxiety and worry***. Psychiatry, clinical psychology, speech-language pathology, medicine, and many exotic approaches have been as unsuccessful with this form of spasmodic dysphonia as with the adductor form. Unfortunately, there is no known temporary alleviation of the abductor symptoms that parallels the anesthetic blocking of one recurrent laryngeal nerve used with the adductor form of the disorder. ***There is substantial evidence of neurogenic disorder with the abductor as well as the adductor form of the dysphonia. Support for neural involvement*** has been found in electromyography, electroencephalography, magnetic resonance imaging, auditory brainstem response, and various clinical neurologic tests.

120. Ans. (a) Foul breath, (b) Hot potato voice, (c) Shifting of uvula in opposite side, (d) Difficulty in swallowing even own saliva

[Ref: Dhingra 6th/264-65; L and T 10th/85-86; ENT by P.Hazarika 3rd/485-86]

"**Peritonsillar abscess:**Acute severe ***unilateral odynophagia is present***"- *ENT by P.Hazarika 3rd/486*

Peritonsillar Abscess (Quinsy)

◈ *Dhingra 6th/264-65*

- It is a collection of pus in the peritonsillar space which lies between the capsule of tonsil and the superior constrictor muscle.
- Peritonsillar abscess usually follows acute tonsillitis though it may arise de novo without previous history of sore throats. First, one of the tonsillar crypts, usually the crypta magna, gets infected and sealed off. It forms an intratonsillar abscess which then bursts through the tonsillar capsule to set up peritonsillitis and then an abscess.
- Culture of pus form the abscess may reveal pure growth of *streptococcs pyyogenes, S. aureus* or anaerobic organisms. More often the growth is mixed, with both aerobic and anaerobic organisms.
- Peritonsillar abscess mostly affects adults and rarely the children though acute tonsillitis is more common in children.
- ***Usually, it is unilateral though occasionally bilateral abscesses are recorded.***
- Clinical features are divided into:
    - **General** They are due to septicaemia and resemble any acute infection. They included fever (up to 104°F), chills and rigors, general malaise, body aches, headache, nausea and constipation.
    - **Local**
        - ***Severe pain in throat***. Usually unilateral
        - ***Odynophagia.*** It is so marked that the ***patient cannot even swallow his own saliva*** which dribbles from the angle of his mouth. Patient is usually dehydrated
        - Muffled and thick speech, often called "***hot potato voice***"
        - ***Foul breath due to sepsis*** in the oral cavity and poor hygiene
- Examination: ***Uvula is swollen and oedematous and pushed to the opposite side***

121. Ans. (a) Starts as edema of maxillary..., (c) Comes out via accessory..., (e) Commonly presents as unilateral...

[Ref: Dhingra 6th/173-75; L and T 10th/55; ENT by P.Hazarika 3rd/346-48]

Antrochoanal Polyp (Syn, Killian's Polyp) *Dhingra 6th/173-74*

- This polyp ***arises from the mucosa of maxillary antrum near its accessory ostium***, comes out of it and ***grows in the choana and nasal cavity.*** Thus it has three parts
    - Antral, which is a thin stalk
    - Choanal, which is round and globular
    - Nasal, which is flat from side to side
- **Aetiology:** Exact cause is unknown. Nasal allergy coupled with sinus infection is incriminated. Antrochoanal polypi are ***seen in children and young adults. Usually they are single and unilateral.***
- **Symptoms:** ***Unilateral nasal obstruction is the presenting symptoms.*** Obstruction may become bilateral when polyp grown into the nasopharynx and starts obstructing the opposite choana. Voice may become thick and dull due to hyponasality. ***Nasal discharge, mostly mucoid, may be seen on one or both sides.***
- **Signs:** As the antrochoanal polyp grows posteriorly it may be missed on anterior rhinoscopy. When large, a smooth greyish mas covered with nasal discharge may be seen. It is soft and can be moved up and down with a probe. A large polyp may protrude from the nostril and show a pink congested look on its exposed part

Antrochoanal Polyp

◈ *P. Hazarika 3rd/346-48*

- "***Commonly seen in children***"- *P.Hazarika 3rd/346*
- "***Common in adolescence***"- *L and T 10th/55*
- "Nasal polyp: It is defined as a prolapsed, edematous, pediculated nasal mucosa, which may arise from the sinuses or the nasal cavity"- *P.Hazarika 3rd/342*
- Unilateral nasal obstruction is the most common presentation
- **Treatment:** Complete surgical removal of polyp is commonly employed treatment and incomplete resection is associated with a relatively high recurrence rate- *Dhingra 6th/175, P.Hazarika 3rd/348*

Ethmoidal polypi: *Medical treatment following surgery with steroid nasal spray helps in preventing recurrence. Antifungal treatment should be given if allergic/invasive fungal sinusitis is suspected or proved"- P.Hazarika 3rd/346*

Table *(Dhingra 6th/175)*: **Differences b/w antrochoanal polyp and ethmoidal polyp**

	Antrochoanal polypi	Ethmoidal polypi
Age	Common in children	Common in adults
Aetiology	Infection	Allergy or multifactorial
Number	Solitary	Multiple
Laterality	Unilateral	Bilateral
Origin	Maxillary sinus near the ostium	Ethmoidal sinuses, uncinate process, middle turbinate and middle meatus

Contd...

	Antrochoanal polypi	Ethmoidal polypi
Growth	Grows backwards to the choana; may hang down behind the soft palate	Mostly grow anteriorly and may present at the nares
Size and shape	Trilobed with antral, nasal and choanal parts. Choanal part may protrude through the choana and fill the nasopharynx obstructiong both sides	Usually small and grape–like masses
Recurrence	Uncommon, if removed completely	Common
Treatment	Polypectomy; endoscopic removal or Caldwell–Luc operation if recurrent	Polypectomy. Endoscopic surgery or ethmoidectomy (which may be intranasal, extranasal or transantral)

MEDICINE

122. Ans. (c) No increase in cardiac output despite exercise, (d) Ejection systolic murmur radiating to neck may present, (e) Left ventricular hypertrophy

[Ref: Harrison 19th/1529-33; Davidson 22nd/620-22, 616-17]

"The **average time to death** after the onset of various symptoms is as follows: ***angina pectoris, 3 years; syncope, 3 years; dyspnea, 2 years; congestive heart failure, 1.5–2 years***. Moreover, in >80% of patients who died with AS, symptoms had existed for <4 years"- *Harrison 19th/1532*

"The **murmur of AS** is characteristically an ***ejection (mid) systolic murmur*** that commences shortly after the S1, increases in intensity to reach a peak toward the middle of ejection, and ends just before aortic valve closure. It is characteristically low-pitched, rough and rasping in character, and loudest at the base of the heart, most commonly in the second right intercostal space. It is ***transmitted upward along the carotid arteries***"- *Harrison 19th/1531*

"*Angina pectoris* usually develops somewhat later and reflects an imbalance between the augmented myocardial oxygen requirements and reduced oxygen availability. ***CAD may or may not be present***, although its coexistence is common among AS patients older than age 65"- *Harrison 19th/1530-31*

Aortic Stenosis

◈ *Davidson 22nd/620-22*

- Cardiac output is initially maintained at the cost of a steadily increasing pressure gradient across the aortic valve. ***The LV becomes increasingly hypertrophied and coronary blood flow may then be inadequate; patientsmay therefore develop angina, even in the absence of concomitant coronary disease.***
- ***The fixed outflow obstruction limits the increase in cardiac output required on exercise.*** Eventually, the LV can no longer overcome the outflow tract obstruction and pulmonary oedema supervenes.
- In **contrast to patients with mitral stenosis**, which tends to progress very slowly, those with aortic stenosis typically ***remain asymptomatic for many years but deteriorate rapidly when symptoms develop, and death usually ensues within 3–5 years of these.***
- Aortic stenosis is commonly picked up in asymptomatic patients at routine clinical examination but the three cardinal symptoms are angina, breathlessness and syncope.
- ***Angina arises because of the increased demands of the hypertrophied LV*** working against the high-pressure outflow tract obstruction, leading to a ***mismatch between oxygen demand and supply,*** but may also be due to coexisting coronary artery disease, especially in old age, when it affects over 50% of patients.
- Exertional breathlessness suggests cardiac decompensation as a consequence of the excessive pressure overload placed on the LV.
- ***Syncope usually occurs on exertion when cardiac output fails to rise to meet demand, leading to a fall in BP.***
- ***A harsh ejection systolic murmur radiates to the neck***, with a soft second heart sound, particularly in those with calcific valves.

Clinical Features of Aortic Stenosis

◈ *Davidson 22nd/620*

Symptoms

- Mild or moderate stenosis:usually asymptomatic
- Exertional dyspnoea
- Angina
- Exertional syncope
- Sudden death
- Episodes of acute pulmonary oedema

Signs

- Ejection systolic murmur
- Slow-rising carotid pulse
- Thrusting apex beat (LVpressure overload)
- Narrow pulse pressure
- Signs of pulmonary venous congestion (e.g. crepitations)

123. Ans. (a) Usually occurs after 2–3 month of acute exposure, (b) Involves both sensory and motor nerve, (d) Incomplete recovery

[Ref: Harrison 19th/2688; Davidson 22nd/222]

Organophosphate-induced Delayed Polyneuropathy

◈ *Davidson 22nd/222*

- Organophosphate-induced delayed polyneuropathy (OPIDN) is a rare complication that usually occurs ***2–3 weeks after acute exposure.*** It is a ***mixed sensory/motor polyneuropathy***, especially affecting long myelinated neurons, and appears to result from inhibition of enzymes other than AChE.
- It is a feature of poisoning with some OPs such as trichlorocresylphosphate, but is less common with nerve agents.

- Early clinical features are muscle cramps followed by numbness and paraesthesiae, proceeding to ***flaccid paralysis of the lower and subsequently the upper limbs***. Paralysis of the lower limbs is associated with foot drop and a high-stepping gait, progressing to paraplegia.Paralysis of the arms leads to wrist drop.
- **Sensory loss** may also be present but is variable. Initially, tendon reflexes are reduced or lost but mild spasticity may develop later.
- There is ***no specific therapy for OPIDN***. Regular physiotherapy may limit deformity caused by muscle wasting.
- ***Recovery is often incomplete*** and may be limited to the hands and feet, although substantial functional recovery after 1–2 years may occur, especially in younger patients.

"**Organophosphate induced delayed polyneuropathy (OPIDP)** is a rare, delayed neurotoxic effect, which occurs ***1-5 weeks*** after *severe* toxicity from some cholinesterase inhibitors. ***No specific treatment has been identified***. The early administration of pralidoxime and atropine does not seem to prevent the condition. ***Patients with mild cases recover over several months; those with more serious polyneuropathies have persistent effects***. Recovery affects only sensory nerves, while motor neurons may permanently lose function"-*www.atsdr.cdc.gov*

Table *(Harrison 19th/2688)*: **Toxic neuropathies (partial list)**

Drug	Mechanism of Neurotoxicity	Clinical Features	Nerve Histopathology	EMG/NCS
Organophosphates	Bind and inhibit neuropathy target esterase	Early features are those of neuromuscular blockade with generalized weakness; later axonal sensorimotor PN ensues	Axonal degeneration along with degeneration of gracile fasciculus and corticospinal tracts	**Early**: repetitive firing of CMAPs and decrement with repetitive nerve stimulation; **late**: ***axonal sensorimotor PN***

124. Ans. (b) Prothrombin time expressed as international normalized.., (c) Serum creatinine estimation

[Ref: Harrison 19th/1995-96,2069; CMDT 2016/693-94;Davidson 22nd/944]

Model for End-Stage Liver Disease (MELD) System

◈ *Harrison 19th/1995*

- Recently, the Child-Pugh system has been replaced by MELD system for the liver transplantation. The MELD score is a prospectively derived system designed to predict the prognosis of patients with liver disease and portal hypertension.
- This score is ***calculated from* three *noninvasive variables***: the ***prothrombin time expressed as the international normalized ratio (INR), the serum bilirubin level, and the serum creatinine concentration***.
- The MELD system provides a ***more objective means of assessing disease severity and has less center-to-center variation*** than the Child- Pugh score as well as a ***wider range of values***.
- MELD is currently used to establish priority listing for liver transplantation. A similar system, PELD (pediatric end-stage liver disease), is based on bilirubin, INR, serum albumin, age, and nutritional status and is used for children <12 years of age.

"The Child–Pugh score and, more recently, the MELD (Model for End-stage Liver Disease) score can be used to assess prognosis. ***The MELD is more difficult to calculate at the bedside*** *but, unlike the Child–Pugh score, includes renal function; if this is impaired, it is known to be a poor prognostic feature in end-stage disease.* Although these scores give a guide to prognosis, the course of cirrhosis can be unpredictable, as complications such as variceal bleeding may occur"- *Davidson 22nd/944*

Prognosis of Cirrhosis

◈ *CMDT 2016/693-94*

- The consistency of the MELD score among different hospitals may be improved when the INR is calibrated based on ***prothrombin time control*** samples that ***include patients with liver disease*** rather than those taking oral anticoagulants.
- A MELD score of >14 is required for liver transplant listing. In patients with a relatively low MELD score (<21) and a low priority for liver transplantation, a low serum sodium concentration (<130 mEq/L [130 mmol/L]), an elevated hepatic venous pressure gradient, persistent ascites, and a low health-related quality of life appear to be additional independent predictors of mortality, and ***modifications of the MELD score, including one that incorporates the serum sodium (MELDNa), are under consideration***.

Table *(Davidson 22nd/944)*: **One-year survival rate depending on MELD score**

MELD score	One-year survival (%)	
	No complications	Complications
<9	97	90
10–19	90	85
20–29	70	65
30–39	70	50

MELD From SI units

10× (0.378 [In serum bilirubin (μMol/L) + 1.12 [In INR] + 0.957 [In serum creatinine (mmol/L)] + 0.643)

Table *(CMDT 2016/693):* **Child-turcotte-pugh scoring system and MELD for staging cirrhosis**

	Child-Turcotte-Pugh scoring system		
	Numerical Score		
Parameter	**1**	**2**	**3**
Ascites	None	Slight	Moderate to severe
Encephalopathy	None	Slight to moderate	Moderate to severe
Bilirubin (mg/dL)	< 2.0	2–3	> 3.0
Albumin (g/dL)	> 3.5	2.8–3.5	< 2.8
Prothrombin time (seconds increased)	1–3	4–6	> 6.0
	Total numerical score and corresponding Child-Turcotte-Pugh class		
	Score		**Class**
	5–6		A
	7–9		B
	10–15		C

125. Ans. a. Acute care..., b. Home infusion ..., c. Immunosuppressive..., d. Antibiotic ... & e. Hospitalization...

[Ref: Harrison 19th/803; CMDT 2016/273; Davidson 22nd/146]

Health care–associated pneumonia (HCAP) occurs in ***community members*** whose extensive contact with healthcare has changed their risk for virulent and drug-resistant organisms"- *CMDT 2016/272*

Hospital-acquired pneumonia (HAP) occurs more than 48 hours after admission ***to the hospital or other health care facility*** and excludes any infection present at the time of admission"- *CMDT 2016/272*

Table *(CMDT 2016/273):* **Risk factors for health care–associated pneumonia**

- Antibiotic therapy in the preceding 90 days.
- Acute care hospitalization for at least 2 days in the preceding 90 days
- Residence in a nursing home or extended care facility
- Home infusion therapy, including chemotherapy, within the past 30 days
- Long-term dialysis within the past 30 days
- Home wound care
- Family member with an infection involving a multiple drug-resistant pathogen
- Immunosuppressive disease or immunosuppressive therapy

Table *(Harrison 19th/803):* **Clinical conditions associated with and likely pathogens in health care–associated pneumonia**

	Pathogen			
Condition	**MRSA**	***Pseudomonas aeruginosa***	***Acinetobacter* spp.**	**MDR Enterobacteriaceae**
Hospitalization for ≥48 h	✓	✓	✓	✓
Hospitalization for ≥2 days in prior 3 months	✓	✓	✓	✓
Nursing home or extended-care-facility residence	✓	✓	✓	✓
Antibiotic therapy in preceding 3 months		✓		✓
Chronic dialysis	✓			
Home infusion therapy	✓			
Home wound care	✓			
Family member with MDR infection	✓			✓

Abbreviations: MDR, multidrug-resistant; MRSA, methicillin-resistant *Staphylococcus aureus.*

"Healthcare-associated pneumonia (HCAP) is a category of nosocomial pneumonia defined by the 2005 American Thoracic Society/Infectious Diseases Society of America (ATS/IDSA) guidelines to include any patient who has been hospitalized in an acute care hospital for 2 or more days within the past 90 days; residents of a nursing home or long-term care facility; ***recipients of recent intravenous antibiotic therapy, chemotherapy, or wound care within the past 30 days***; or patients who have attended a hospital or hemodialysis clinic. In creating this relatively new category the ATS/IDSA acknowledged that these patients are at *increased risk for infection with antibiotic-resistant organisms and that initial inadequate antibiotic coverage leads to increased mortality*" *www.ncbi.nlm.nih.gov*

126. Ans. (d) Schauman and asteroid bodies are pathognomic

[Ref: Davidson 22nd/709-11;Harrison 19th/ 2205-12; Robbins(SAE) 9th/693-94;CMDT 2016/292-93]

Sarcoidosis

"***Hypercalcemia and/or hypercalciuria*** occurs in about 10% of sarcoidosis patients.The mechanism of abnormal calcium metabolism is increased production of 1,25-dihydroxyvitamin D by the granuloma itself."- *Harrison 19th/ 2208*

- ***"Bronchoalveolar lavage fluid in sarcoidosis is usually characterized by an increase in lymphocyte and a high CD4/ CD8 ratio"*** *(CMDT 2016/293)*

- "The use of the lymphocyte markers CD4 and CD8 can be used to determine the CD4/CD8 ratio of these increased lymphocytes in the **BAL fluid**. A ***ratio of > 3.5 is strongly supportive of sarcoidosis*** but is less sensitive than an increase in lymphocytes alone" *(Harrison 19th/2210)*
- "**Sarcoidosis**: *Intra-alveolar and interstitial accumulation of CD4+ T cells, resulting in* CD4: CD8 *ratios ranging from* ***5:1 to 15:1**" (Robbins 9th/693)*
- "Serum levels of **angiotensin-converting enzyme (ACE)** can be ***helpful in the diagnosis of sarcoidosis.*** However, the test has somewhat low sensitivity and specificity. Elevated levels of ACE are reported in 60% of patients with acute disease and only 20% of patients with chronic disease. Although there are several causes for mild elevation of ACE, including diabetes, elevations of >50% of the upper limit of normal are seen in only a few conditions including sarcoidosis, leprosy, Gaucher's disease, hyperthyroidism, and disseminated granulomatous infections such as miliary tuberculosis."- *Harrison 19th/ 2209*
- **"Schauman and asteroid bodies:*Although characteristic, these cells are not pathognomic of sarcoidosis*** because they may be ***encountered in other granulomatous diseases (e.g., tuberculosis)"*** *(Robbins 9th/693)*
- The ***granuloma is the pathologic hallmark of sarcoidosis***
- A positive gallium scan can support the diagnosis if increased activity is noted in the parotids and lacrimal glands (***Panda sign***) or in the right paratracheal and left hilar area (*lambda sign*)
- The ***Kviem-Siltzbach procedure*** is a specific diagnostic test for sarcoidosis

127. Ans. (a) Urinothorax, (c) Nephrotic syndrome, (d) Myxedema, (e) Congestive heart failure

[Ref: Harrison 19th/1718; CMDT 2016/310; Davidson 22nd/661-62]

Post-cardiac injury (Dressler's) syndrome (PCIS) causes exudative pleural effusion

Table *(Harrison 19th/1718):* **Differential diagnoses of pleural effusions**

Transudative Pleural Effusions	
• ***Congestive heart failure*** • Cirrhosis • Pulmonary embolization • ***Nephrotic synd***rome	• Peritoneal dialysis • Superior vena cava obstruction(!! It is removed in 19th edition) • ***Myxedema*** • ***Urinoth***orax
Exudative Pleural Effusions	
• Neoplastic diseases ▪ Metastatic disease ▪ Mesothelioma • Infectious diseases ▪ Bacterial infections ▪ Tuberculosis ▪ Fungal infections ▪ Viral infections ▪ Parasitic infections • Pulmonary embolization • Gastrointestinal disease ▪ Esophageal perforation ▪ Pancreatic disease ▪ Intraabdominal abscesses ▪ Diaphragmatic hernia ▪ After abdominal surgery ▪ Endoscopic variceal sclerotherapy ▪ After liver transplant	• Post-coronary artery bypass surgery • Asbestos exposure • Sarcoidosis • Uremia • Meigs' syndrome • Yellow nail syndrome • Drug-induced pleural disease ▪ Nitrofurantoin ▪ Dantrolene ▪ Methysergide ▪ Bromocriptine ▪ Procarbazine ▪ Amiodarone ▪ Dasatinib
Exudative Pleural Effusions	
• Collagen vascular diseases ▪ Rheumatoid pleuritis ▪ Systemic lupus erythematosus ▪ Drug-induced lupus ▪ Immunoblastic lymphadenopathy ▪ Sjögren's syndrome ▪ Granulomatosis with polyangiitis (Wegener's) ▪ Churg-Strauss syndrome	• Trapped lung • Radiation therapy • ***Post-cardiac*** injury syndrome • Hemothorax • Iatrogenic injury • Ovarian hyperstimulation syndrome • Pericardial disease • Chylothorax

Contd...

"The **post-cardiac injury (Dressler's) syndrome (PCIS)** can occur after any type of cardiac injury and is thought to be due to anti-myocardial antibodies. Pleural effusions are common with PCIS. Following CABG surgery, most patients will have a small unilateral left-sided pleural effusion, and approximately 10% of patients will have a larger effusion. These large effusions can be separated into early effusions occurring within the first 30 days of surgery that are ***bloody exudates*** with a high percentage of eosinophils, and late effusions occurring more than 30 days after surgery that are ***clear yellow lymphocytic exudates***"- *www.ncbi.nlm.nih.gov*

128. Ans. (b) Associated with inflammatory bowel disease, (d) Periductal fibrosis of smaller bile ducts

[Ref: Davidson 22nd/965-66;Robbins 9th/858-60]

Cirrhosis due to primary sclerosing cholangitis: Following changes are seen-fibrosing cholangitis, ***periductal fibrosis***, dilation of intervening bile ducts and cholestatis with full blown picture of biliary cirrhosis"-*Harshmohan 7th/611*

Primary sclerosing cholangitis causes ***micronodular cirrhosis***-*Harshmohan 7th/611; www.cirrhosisoftheliver.co*

Primary Sclerosing Cholangitis

◈ *Robbins 9th/859-60*

- **PSC is characterized by inflammation and obliterative fibrosis of intrahepatic and extrahepatic bile ducts with dilation of preserved segments.**
- Characteristic "beading" on radiographs of the intrahepatic and extrahepatic biliary tree is attributable to these irregular, biliary strictures and dilations.
- *Inflammatory bowel disease , particularly ulcerative colitis, coexists in approximately 70% of individuals with PSC*
- Morphologic changes differ between the large ducts (***intrahepatic and extrahepatic***) and the smaller ***intrahepatic ducts.***
- The **smaller ducts,** often have little inflammation and show a striking **circumferential "onion skin" fibrosis** around

an increasingly atrophic duct lumen , eventually leading to obliteration by a "tombstone" scar.

- As the disease progresses the liver becomes markedly cholestatic, culminating in ***biliary cirrhosis*** much like that seen with chronic obstruction and primary biliary cirrhosis.
- Biliary intraepithelial neoplasia may develop and cholangiocarcinoma appears usually with a fatal outcomes.

Primary Sclerosing Cholangitis (PSC)

◈ *Davidson 22nd/965-66*

- Primary sclerosing cholangitis (PSC) is a cholestatic liver disease caused by diffuse inflammation and fibrosis; it can involve the entire biliary tree and leads to the gradual obliteration of ***intrahepatic and extrahepatic bile ducts***, and ultimately biliary cirrhosis, portal hypertension and hepatic failure.
- The cause of PSC is unknown but there is a close association with ***inflammatory bowel disease***, particularly ulcerative colitis. About two-thirds of patients have coexisting ulcerative colitis, and ***PSC is the most common form of chronic liver disease in ulcerative colitis.***
- PSC is twice as common in young men. Most patients present at age 25–40 years, although the condition may be diagnosed at any age and is an important cause of chronic liver disease in children.

Diseases Associated with Primary Sclerosing Cholangitis

◈ *Davidson 22nd/965*

- ***Ulcerative colitis***
- ***Crohn's colitis***
- Chronic pancreatitis
- Retroperitoneal fibrosis
- Riedel's thyroiditis
- Retro-orbital tumours
- Immune deficiency states
- Sjögren's syndrome
- Angio-immunoplastic lymphadenopathy
- Histiocytosis X
- Autoimmune haemolytic anaemia
- Autoimmune pancreatitis/ IgG4-associated cholangitis

129. Ans. (a) Encapsulated, (c) Associated with MEN-I, (d) Enucleation is the treatment..., (e) Histology similar to normal β-cells

[Ref: Harrison 19th/569;Robbins 9th/1121; L and B 26th/787-89]

"**Benign insulinoma**: ***Tumour enucleation is the technique of choice***"*-L and B 26th/789*

*"Grossly insulinoma is **usually solitary** and **well-encapsulated tumour** which may vary in size from 0.5 to 10 cm. **Rarely, they are multiple**. Microscopically, the tumour is composed of cords and **sheet of well-differentiated** β**-cells which do not differ from normal cells**"-Harshmohan 7th/818*

"Insulinoma: *About 90% are solitary and about* ***10% are multiple*** *and are* ***associated with MEN1. About 10% are malignant"****-L and B 26th/788*

*"**Majority of the insulinomas occur in the tail and body of pancreas** and **majority of them are benign**, one third are malignant and one-third are multiple"-Manipal manual of Surgery 3rd/501*

Insulinomas

◈ *Robbins 9th/1121*

- "**β-cell tumors (insulinomas)** are the ***most common of pancreatic endocrine neoplasms*** and may be responsible for the elaboration of sufficient insulin to induce clinically significant hypoglycemia.
- There is a characteristic **clinical triad** resulting from these pancreatic lesions: (1) Attacks of hypoglycemia occur with blood glucose levels below 50 mg/dL of serum; (2) the attacks consist principally of such ***central nervous system manifestations*** as confusion, stupor, and loss of consciousness; and (3) the attacks are precipitated by fasting or exercise and are promptly relieved by feeding or parenteral administration of glucose"
- Insulinomas are most often found within the pancreas and are ***generally benign***.
- ***Most are solitary, although multiple tumors may be encountered***.
- **Solitary tumors** are usually small (often < 2 cm in diameter), ***encapsulated,*** pale to red-brown nodules located anywhere in the pancreas.
- Histologically, these benign tumors look ***remarkably like giant islets***, with preservation of the regular cords of monotonous cells and their orientation to the vasculature. Not even the malignant lesions present much evidence of anaplasia, and they may be ***deceptively encapsulated***. **Deposition of amyloid** is a characteristic feature of many insulinomas

Insulinomas

◈ *Harrison 19th/569*

- Insulinomas are generally small (>90% are <2 cm) and ***usually not multiple (90%)***; only 5–15% are malignant, and they almost invariably occur only in the pancreas, distributed equally in the pancreatic head, body, and tail.
- Insulinomas should be suspected in all patients with hypoglycemia, especially when there is a history suggesting that attacks are provoked by fasting, or ***with a family history of MEN 1.***
- Only 5–15% of insulinomas are malignant; therefore, after appropriate imaging , surgery should be performed. In different studies, 75–100% of patients are cured by surgery.

130. Ans. (b) Increased CD8+ T cells in..., (c) Manifests mainly as an..., (d) For severe acute cases..., (e) Interstitial inflammatory...

[Ref: Robbins 9th/694-95;Davidson 22nd/719-20; Harrison 19th/ 1681-83;CMDT 2016/306-07]

Hypersensitivity Pneumonitis

◈ *Robbins 9th/694-95*

- Most commonly, hypersensitivity results from the ***inhalation of organic dust*** containing antigens made up of the spores of thermophilic bacteria, fungi, animal proteins, or bacterial products.
- ***Bronchoalveolar lavage*** specimens also consistently demonstrate ***increased numbers of both CD4+ and CD8+ T lymphocytes***.

- The clinical manifestations are varied. Acute attacks, which follow inhalation of antigenic dust in sensitized patients, consist of ***recurring episodes of fever, dyspnea, cough, and leukocytosis***.

Hypersensitivity Pneumonitis

❖ *CMDT 2016/306-07*

- It is ***manifested mainly as an occupational disease***, in which exposure to ***inhaled organic agents*** leads to acute and eventually chronic pulmonary disease
- Treatment of hypersensitivity pneumonitis consists of identification of the offending agent, avoidance of further exposure and in severe acute or protracted cases, ***oral corticosteroids*** (prednisone, 0.5 mg/kg daily as a single morning dose ***for 2 weeks***, tapered to nil over ***4–6 weeks***) may be given

Hypersensitivity Pneumonitis (HP)

❖ *Davidson 22nd/719-20*

- BAL fluid usually shows an ***increase in the number of CD8+ T lymphocytes***
- HRCT showing typical patchy ground glass opacification.
- Histology shows evidence of an ***interstitial inflammatory infiltrate in the lung***, expanding alveolar walls, with a peribronchial distribution.
- In acute cases, ***prednisolone should be given for 3–4 weeks***, starting with an oral dose of 40 mg per day.

Hypersensitivity Pneumonitis (HP)

❖ *Harrison 19th/ 1681-83*

- The incidence and prevalence of HP are variable, depending on geography, occupation, avocation, and environment
- The various ***antigens and environmental conditions*** associated with HP give rise to an expansive list of monikers given to specific forms of HP.
- Most cases of HP have a ***CD4+/CD8+ lymphocyte ratio of less than 1***, but again, this is not a specific finding and has limited utility in the diagnosis of HP(Note: ***Normal CD4+/CD8+ ratio is 2***)
- Within the alveolar spaces and ***in the interstitium, a mixed cellular infiltrate*** with a lymphocytic predominance is observed that is frequently patchy in distribution.
- Although glucocorticoids do not change the long-term outcome in these patients, they can accelerate the resolution of symptoms. While there is significant variability in the approach to glucocorticoid therapy by individual clinicians, prednisone therapy can be initiated at 0.5–1 mg/kg of ideal body weight per day (not to exceed 60 mg/d or alternative glucocorticoid equivalent) over a ***duration of 1–2 weeks***, followed by a ***taper over the next 2–6 weeks***.

131. Ans. (e) Males are affected more than females

[Ref: Harrison 19th/2166-68; CMDT 2016/836-37; Davidson 22nd/1114; Robbins 9th/226-27; L and B 26th/737]

Sjögren's Syndrome

❖ *Harrison 19th/2166-67*

- "***Females are affected more than males*** in the ratio 10:1"- *L and B 26th/737*
- "***Middle-aged women*** (female-to-male ratio, 9:1) are primarily affected, although Sjögren's syndrome may occur at any age, including childhood"-*Harrison*
- The ***principal oral symptom of Sjögren's syndrome is dryness (xerostomia)***. Patients report difficulty in swallowing dry food, an inability to speak continuously, a burning sensation, an increase in dental caries, and problems in wearing complete dentures
- ***Enlargement of the parotid or other major salivary glands*** occurs in two-thirds of patients with primary Sjögren's syndrome but is uncommon in those with the secondary syndrome.
- Sjögren's syndrome causes ***bilateral parotid enlargement***-*Harrison 19th/2167(table)*
- "Occasionally, there is enlargement of the salivary glands, more commonly the parotid rather than the submandibular glands. The ***glands are occasionally painful,*** and the patient sometimes develops a bacterial sialadenitis due to ascending infection from the associated ***xerostomia***"-*L and B 26th/737*
- ***Lymphoma is a well-known manifestation of Sjögren's syndrome*** that usually presents later in the illness. Persistent parotid gland enlargement, purpura, leukopenia, cryoglobulinemia, low C4 complement levels, and ectopic germinal centers in minor salivary gland biopsy samples are manifestations suggesting the development of lymphoma

Table *(Davidson 22nd /1114)*: **Features of sjogren's syndrome**

Risk Factors	
• Age of onset 40-60 • Female > male	• HLA-B8/DR3
Common Clinical Features	
• Keratoconjunctivitis sicca • Xerostomia • Salivary gland enlargement	• Non-erosive arthritis • Raynaud's phenomenon • Fatigue
Less Common Features	
• Low-Grade Fever • Interstitial Lung Disease • Anaemia, Leucopenia • Thrombocytopenia • Cryoglobulinaemia • Vasculitis	• Peripheral neuropathy • Lymphadenopathy • Lymphoreticular lymphoma • Glomerulonephritis • Renal tubular acidosis
Autoantibodies Frequently Detected	
• RF • ANA • SS-A (anti-Ro)	• SS-B (anti-La) • Gastric parietal cell • Thyroid
Associated Autoimmune Disorders	
• SLE • Progressive systemic sclerosis	• Primary biliary cirrhosis • Chronic active hepatitis • Myasthenia gravis

132. Ans. (a) Seropositive for..., (b) Splenomegaly, (c) Long standing... (e) Keratoconjunctivitis sicca

❖ *[Ref: Robbins 9th/606; CMT 2016/821; Harrison 19th/418,2138; Davidson 22nd/1100]*

Felty's Syndrome

◈ *Harrison 19th/418*

- *"Felty's syndrome* is defined by the **clinical triad** of ***neutropenia, splenomegaly, and nodular RA*** and is seen in less than 1% of patients, although its incidence appears to be declining in the face of more aggressive treatment of the joint disease. It typically occurs in the ***late stages of severe RA***"*-Harrison 19th/2138*
- Spleen-produced antibodies can shorten neutrophil life span, while large granular lymphocytes can attack marrow neutrophil precursors.
- Splenectomy may increase the neutrophil count in Felty's syndrome and lower serum neutrophil binding IgG.
- Some Felty's syndrome patients also have neutropenia associated with an increased number of LGLs.

Table *(davidson 22nd/1100):* **Felty's syndrome**

Risk factors	
• Age of onset 50-70 yrs • Female > male • Caucasians> blacks • Long-standing RA	• Deforming but inactive disease • Seropositive for RF
Common clinical features	
• Splenomegaly • Lymphadenopathy • Weight loss • Skin pigmentation	• Keratoconjunctivitis sicca • Vasculitis, leg ulcers • Recurrent infections • Nodules
Laboratory findings	
• Normochromic, normocytic anaemia • Neutropenia • Abnormal liver function	• Thrombocytopenia • Impaired T-and B-cell immunity

133. Ans. (a) Primary CNS lymphoma, (b) Cervical cancer, (c) Kaposi sarcoma, (d) Ovarian cancer

[Ref: Davidson 22nd/405; CMDT 2016/1322; Harrison 19th/1268; Davidson 22nd/405; Ananthanarayan 9th/576-77; Lippincott Microbiology 3rd/ 302]

Neoplastic Diseases

◈ *Harrison 19th/1268*

- The neoplastic diseases considered to be AIDS defining conditions are ***Kaposi's sarcoma, non-Hodgkin's lymphoma, and invasive cervical carcinoma.***
- In addition, there is also an increase in the incidence of a variety of **non-AIDS-defining malignancies** including ***Hodgkin's disease; multiple myeloma; leukemia; melanoma;and cervical, brain, testicular, oral, lung, gastric, liver, renal, and anal cancers.***

HIV-Related Malignancies

◈ *CMDT 2016/1322*

- Four cancers are currently included in the CDC classification of AIDS: ***Kaposi sarcoma, non-Hodgkin lymphoma, primary lymphoma of the brain, and invasive cervical carcinoma.***
- ***Non-Hodgkin's lymphoma: The best studied example is Burkitt's lymphoma"***

"The AIDS-defining cancers are ***Kaposi's sarcoma, cervical cancer and non-Hodgkin lymphoma (NHL).*** NHL may occur at any CD4 count but is more commonly seen below 200 cells/mm3. Almost all NHL are B-cell tumours and most are stage 4 when the patient presents. The incidence of a number of other cancers induced by viruses is also increased in HIV-infected people"- *Davidson 22nd/405*

Table *(Davidson 22nd/405):* **Approximate incidence ratio of virus-related cancers in HIV patients compared to the general population**

Viral cancers	Incidence ratio
Human herpesvirus 8-related	
Kaposi's sarcoma	3600
Epstein–Barr virus-related	
Non-Hodgkin lymphoma	80
Hodgkin lymphoma	10
Human papillomavirus-related	
Cervical cancer	6
Vulval cancer	6
Anal cancer	30
Penile cancer	4
Hepatitis B/C virus-related	
Hepatoma	5

134. Ans. (a) Breast cancer, (c) Non-small lung cancer, (d) Prostate cancer, (e) Multiple myeloma

[Ref: Davidson 22nd/271; Williams Textbook of Endocrinology, 11th ed; Harrison 19th/608-09; CMDT 2016/ 1586-88; Robbins 9th/330- 31]

"**Hypercalcemia** is probably the most common paraneoplastic syndrome; overtly symptomatic hypercalcemia is most often related to some form of cancer rather than to hyperparathyroidism. Two general processes are involved in cancer-associated hypercalcemia: osteolysis induced by cancer, whether primary in bone, such as ***multiple myeloma***, or metastatic to bone from any primary lesion, and, the production of calcemic humoral substances by extraosseous neoplasms. *Hypercalcemia owing to skeletal metastases is not a paraneoplastic syndrome" (Robbins 9th/330)*

Table *(Harrison 19th/609):* **Paraneoplastic syndromes caused by ectopic hormone production**

Paraneoplastic Syndrome	Ectopic hormone	Typical tumor types
Hypercalcemia of malignancy	Parathyroid hormone-related protein (PTHrP)	Squamous cell (head and neck, lung, skin), breast, genitourinary, gastrointestinal

Contd...

Paraneoplastic Syndrome	Ectopic hormone	Typical tumor types
	1, 25 dihydroxyvitamin D	Lymphomas
	Parathyroid hormone (rare)	Lung, ovary
	Prostaglandin E2 (PGE2) (rare)	Renal, lung

"***Lung carcinoma, breast carcinoma, and multiple myeloma*** account for more than 50% of all cases of malignancy-associated hypercalcemia. **Lung carcinomas** that produce hypercalcemia have ***squamous or large cell histology, whereas small cell carcinoma almost never causes hypercalcemia.*** Among other solid tumors, the most common are *squamous and renal carcinomas.* ***Gastrointestinal tumors*** and ***prostate carcinoma*** are less common causes of hypercalcemia"- *Williams Textbook of Endocrinology, 11thed*

Table: *(Williams Textbook of Endocrinology11th ed.):* **Malignancy-associated hypercalcemia**

Primary Site	No. (%) of Cases
Lung	111 (25.0)
Breast	87 (19.6)
Multiple myeloma	43 (9.7)
Head and neck	36 (8.1)
Renal and urinary tract	35 (7.9)
Esophagus	25 (5.6)
Female genitalia	24 (5.2)
Unknown primary	23 (5.2)
Lymphoma	14 (3.2)
Colon	8 (1.8)
Liver, biliary	7 (1.6)
Skin	6 (1.4)
Other	25 (5.6)

Table *(Robbins 9th/331):* **Paraneoplastic syndromes**

Clinical Syndromes	Major Forms of Underlying Cancer	Causal Mechanism
Hypercalcemia	Squamous cell carcinoma of lung Breast carcinoma; Renal carcinoma Adult T-cell leukemia/ lymphoma	Parathyroid hormone-related protein (PTHRP), TGF-α, TNF, IL-1

135. Ans. (a) Adenosine deaminase..., (b) Haematopoietic stem..., (c) Most common inheritance...., (e) Increased risk of infection...

[Ref: Robbins 9th/239- 40; Harrison 19th/2107-08; Ananthanarayan 9th/ 174-75]

Severe Combined Immunodeficiency (SCID)

❖ *Harrison 19th/2107-08*

- SCID is characterized by a profound block in T cell development and thus the complete absence of these cells.
- The most frequent clinical manifestations are recurrent oral candidiasis, failure to thrive, and protracted diarrhea and/ or acute interstitial pneumonitis caused by *Pneumocystis jiroveci*
- Diagnosis of SCID can be suspected based on the patient's clinical history and, possibly, a family history of deaths in very young children (suggestive of ***either X-linked or recessive inheritance***).
- Lymphocytopenia is strongly suggestive of SCID in more than 90% of cases.
- The absence of a thymic shadow on a chest x-ray can also be suggestive of SCID. An accurate diagnosis relies on precise determination of the number of circulatingT, B, and NK lymphocytes and their subsets.
- Although counts are usually low (<500/μL of blood), higher maternal T cell counts may, under some circumstances, initially mask the presence of SCID.
- **Severe combined immunodeficiency caused by a cytokine-signaling deficiency**: The most frequent SCID phenotype (accounting for 40–50% of all cases) is the absence of both T and NK cells
- **Purine metabolism deficiency:** Ten to 20% of SCID patients exhibit a ***deficiency in adenosine deaminase*** (ADA), an enzyme of purine metabolism that deaminates adenosine (ado) and deoxyadenosine (dAdo).
- Patients with SCID require appropriate care with aggressive antiinfective therapies, immunoglobulin replacement, and (when necessary) parenteral nutrition support. In most cases, ***curative treatment relies on HSCT.*** Today, HSCT provides a very high curative potential for SCID patients who are otherwise in reasonably good condition.
- Gene therapy has been found to be successful for cases of X-linked SCID (γc deficiency) and SCID caused by an ADA deficiency,although toxicity has become an issue in the treatment of the former disease that may now be overcome by use of newly generated vectors.
- Lastly, a third option for the treatment of ***ADA deficiency consists of enzyme substitution with a pegylated enzyme.***

Severe Combined Immunodeficiency

❖ *Ananthanarayan 9th/ 174-75*

- They are inherited in the ***autosomal recessive*** mode
- **Adenosine deaminase deficiency**: *This the first immunodeficiency disease associated with an enzyme deficiency*
- *Deficiency of both humoral and CMI response*

Severe Combined Immunodeficiency

❖ *Robbins 9th/239- 40*

- Persons with SCID are extremely susceptible to recurrent, severe infections by a wide range of pathogens, including *Candida albicans*, ***Pneumocystis jiroveci***, *Pseudomonas*, cytomegalovirus, varicella, and a whole host of bacteria.

- Without HSC transplantation, *death occurs within the first year of life.*
- The ***most common form, accounting for 50% to 60% of cases, is X-linked***, and hence SCID is more common in boys than in girls. The genetic defect in the X-linked form is a **mutation in the common γ-chain (γc) subunit of cytokine receptors**
- Autosomal recessive SCID: The remaining forms of SCID are autosomal recessive disorders. The most common cause of autosomal recessive SCID is a deficiency of the enzyme ***adenosine deaminase (ADA).***
- *Currently, HSC transplantation is the mainstay of treatment*, but X-linked SCID is the first human disease in which gene therapy has been successful.

136. Ans. **(a) Fanconi anemia, (b) Multiple myeloma, (c) Lead poisoning**

[Ref: Harrison 19th/320; Davidson 22nd/446]

Renal Tubular Acidosis

◈ *Davidson 22nd/446*

- Renal tubular acidosis (RTA) should be suspected when there is a hyperchloraemic acidosis with a normal anion gap and no evidence of gastrointestinal disturbance.
- The urine pH is inappropriately high (> 5.5) in the presence of systemic acidosis.
- **RTA can be caused by a defect in one of three processes**: impaired bicarbonate reabsorption in the proximal tubule (proximal RTA); impaired acid secretion in the late distal tubule or cortical collecting duct intercalated cells (classical distal RTA); or impaired sodium reabsorption in the late distal tubule or cortical collecting duct, which is associated with reduced secretion of both potassium and H+ ions (hyperkalaemic distal RTA).

Table *(Davidson 22nd/446)*: **Causes of renal tubular acidosis**

Proximal renal tubular acidosis	
• Inherited Fanconi's syndrome Cystinosis Wilson's disease • Paraproteinaemia Myeloma • Amyloidosis • Hyperparathyroidism	• Heavy metal toxicity Lead, cadmium and mercury poisoning • Drugs Carbonic anhydrase Inhibitors Ifosfamide
Classical distal renal tubular acidosis	
• Inherited • Autoimmune diseases Systemic lupus Erythematosus Sjogren's syndrome	• Hyperglobulinaemia • Toxins and drugs Toluene Lithium Amphotericin
Hyperkalaemic distal renal tubular acidosis	
• Hypoaldosteronism (primary or secondary) • Obstructive nephropathy • Renal transplant rejection	• Drugs Amiloride Spironolactone

137. Ans. **(a) Lactic acidosis, (b) Ethylene glycol... (c) Aspirin overdose**

[Ref: Harrison 19th/318; CMDT 2016/890; Davidson 22nd/445]

Table *(Harrison 19th/318)*: **Causes of high anion–gap metabolic acidosis**

- Lactic acidosis
- Ketoacidosis (diabetic, alcoholic, starvation)
- Toxins (ethylene glycol, methanol, starvation, propylene glycol, pyroglutamic acid)
- Renal failure (acute and chronic)

Table *(Davidson 22nd/445)*: **Causes of metabolic acidosis**

Disorder	Mechanism
A. Normal anion gap	
Ingestion or infusion of inorganic acid	Therapeutic infusion of or poisoning with NH4Cl, HCl
Gastrointestinal HCO_3 loss	Loss of HCO3 in ***diarrhoea***, small bowel fistula, urinary diversion procedure
Renal tubular acidosis (RTA)	Urinary loss of HCO3 in proximal RTA; impaired tubular acid secretion in distal RTA
B. Increased anion gap	
Endogenous acid load	
Diabetic ketoacidosis	Accumulation of ketones with hyperglycaemia
Starvation ketosis	Accumulation of ketones without hyperglycaemia
Lactic acidosis	Shock, liver disease, drugs
Renal failure	Accumulation of organic acids
Exogenous acid load	
Aspirin poisoning	Accumulation of salicylate
Methanol poisoning	Accumulation of formate
Ethylene glycol poisoning	Accumulation of glycolate, oxalate

Table *(CMDT2016/890)*: **Anion gap in metabolic acidosis**

Increased (> 12 mEq)
A. Metabolic anion
Diabetic ketoacidosis
Alcoholic ketoacidosis
Lactic acidosis
Chronic kidney disease (advanced stages)
Starvation
Metabolic alkalosis (increased number of negative charges on protein)
5–oxoproline acidosis from acetaminophen toxicity

Increased (> 12 mEq)
B. Drug or chemical anion
Salicylate intoxication
Sodium carbenicillin therapy
Methanol (formic acid)
Ethylene glycol (oxalic acid)
Normal (6–12 mEq)
A. Loss of HCO3
Diarrhea
B. Chloride retention
Renal tubular acidosis

138. Ans. (b) Wilson disease, (c) Lead poisoning, (d) Fanconi syndrome

[Ref: Harrison 19th/293; CMDT 2016/898-99]

Proteinuria

◈ *CMDT 2016/898-99*

- Proteinuria is defined as excessive protein excretion in the urine, generally greater than 150–160 mg/24 h in adults.
- Significant proteinuria is a sign of an underlying renal abnormality, usually glomerular in origin when greater than 1 g/d.
- There are four primary reasons for development of proteinuria:
  - **Functional proteinuria** is a benign process stemming from stressors such as acute illness, exercise, and "orthostatic proteinuria."
  - **Overload proteinuria** can result from overproduction of circulating, filterable plasma proteins (monoclonal gammopathies), such as Bence Jones proteins associated with ***multiple myeloma***. Urinary protein electrophoresis will exhibit a discrete protein peak. Other examples of overload proteinuria include myoglobinuria in rhabdomyolysis and hemoglobinuria in hemolysis.
  - **Glomerular proteinuria** results from effacement of epithelial cell foot processes and altered glomerular permeability with an increased filtration fraction of normal plasma proteins. Glomerular diseases exhibit some degree of proteinuria. The urinary electrophoresis will have a pattern exhibiting a large albumin spike indicative of increased permeability of albumin across a damaged glomerular basement membrane (GBM).
  - **Tubular proteinuria** occurs as a result of faulty reabsorption of normally filtered proteins in the proximal tubule, such as β_2-microglobulin and immunoglobulin light chains. Causes include ***acute tubular necrosis, toxic injury (lead, aminoglycosides), drug-induced interstitial nephritis, and hereditary metabolic disorders (Wilson disease and Fanconi syndrome).***

Table: Causes of Proteinuria (Excluding glomerular cause) *patient.info/in/doctor*

Transient proteinuria
• Emotional stress. • Exercise. • Fever. • Urinary tract infection. • Orthostatic (postural) proteinuria. • Seizures. • Persistent proteinuria.
Tubular causes
• Aminoaciduria. • Drugs (eg, NSAIDs, antibiotics). • Fanconi's syndrome. • Heavy metal ingestion.
Overflow causes
• Haemoglobinuria. • Multiple myeloma. • Myoglobinuria.
Other important causes (likely to have multiple pathologies)
• Pre-eclampsia/eclampsia.

139. Ans. (b) Oat, rye and barley can be safely given, (e) No risk for development of cancer

[Ref: Harrison 19th/1940-42;Davidson 22nd/880-82]

Celiac Disease

◈ *Harrison 19th/1940-42*

- "It is an inflammatory disorder of the small bowel occurring in genetically susceptible individuals, which results from intolerance to wheat gluten and similar proteins found in ***rye, barley and, to a lesser extent, oats***"- *Davidson 22nd/880*
- The symptoms range from significant malabsorption of multiple nutrients, with diarrhea, steatorrhea, weight loss, and the consequences of nutrient depletion (i.e., anemia and metabolic bone disease), to the absence of gastrointestinal symptoms despite evidence of the depletion of a single nutrient (e.g., iron or folate deficiency, osteomalacia, edema from protein loss).
- One *environmental* factor is the clear association of the disease with ***gliadin***, a component of gluten that is present in ***wheat, barley, and rye***.
- An *immunologic* component in the pathogenesis of celiac disease is critical and involves both adaptive and innate immune responses. ***Serum antibodies—IgA antigliadin, antiendomysial, and anti-tTG antibodies— are present***, but it is not known whether such antibodies are primary or secondary to the tissue damage. The presence of ***antiendomysial antibody is 90–95% sensitive and 90–95% specific***
- A **small-intestinal biopsy** is required to establish a diagnosis of celiac disease. A biopsy should be performed when patients have symptoms and laboratory findings suggestive of nutrient malabsorption and/or deficiency as well as a positive tTG antibody test.
- **Gluten** is ubiquitous, and a significant effort must be made to exclude all gluten from the diet. ***Use of rice flour*** in place of wheat flour is very helpful, and several support groups

A & E

provide important aid to patients with celiac disease and to their families. More than 90% of patients who have the characteristic findings of celiac disease respond to complete dietary gluten restriction.

- Celiac disease is ***associated with dermatitis herpetiformis (DH),*** but this association has not been explained
- The most important complication of ***celiac disease is the development of cancer***. The incidences of both gastrointestinal and nongastrointestinal neoplasms as well as intestinal lymphoma are elevated among patients with celiac disease.

140. Ans. (a) Myasthenia gravis, (b) Acute exacerbation in COPD, (c) Acute severe asthma

[Ref: Harrison 19th/1731-32; Davidson 22nd/663-65]

Type II Respiratory Failure

◈ *Harrison 19th/1732*

- This type of respiratory failure is a consequence of **alveolar hypoventilation** and results from the inability to eliminate carbon dioxide effectively.
- Mechanisms are categorized by impaired central nervous system (CNS) drive to breathe, impaired strength with failure of neuromuscular function in the respiratory system, and increased load(s) on the respiratory system.
- Reasons for diminished CNS drive to breathe include ***drug overdose, brainstem injury, sleep-disordered breathing, and severe hypothyroidism.***
- Reduced strength can be due to impaired neuromuscular transmission (e.g., ***myasthenia gravis, Guillain-Barre syndrome, amyotrophic lateral sclerosis) or respiratory muscle weakness (e.g., myopathy, electrolyte derangements, fatigue).***

Table *(Davidson 22nd/664)*: **How to interpret blood gas abnormalities in respiratory failure**

	Type I		**Type II**	
	Hypoxia (PaO_2 <8.0kPa (60 mmHg) Normal or low $PaCO_2$ (<6.6 kPa (50 mmHg)		Hypoxia (PaO_2 <8.0 kPa (60 mmHg) Raised $PaCO_2$ (> 6.6 kPa (50 mmHg)	
	Acute	**Chronic**	**Acute**	**Chronic**
H^+	→	→	↑	→ or ↑
Bicarbonate	→	→	→	↑
Causes	Acute asthma Pulmonary oedema Pneumonia Lobar collapse Pneumothorax Pulmonary embolus ARDS	COPD Lung fibrosis Lymphangitis Carcinomatosa Right-to-left shunts	***Acute severe asthma*** ***Acute exacerbation of COPD*** Upper airway obstruction Acute ***neuropathies/ paralysis*** Narcotic drugs Primary alveolar hypoventilation Flail chest injury	COPD Sleep apnoea Kyphoscoliosis ***Myopathies/ muscular dystrophy*** Ankylosing spondylitis

141. Ans. (b) Acute intermittent porphyria

[Ref: Davidson 22nd/459, 1260; Harrison 19th/ 2521-30; CMDT 2016/1655-56]

"In contrast to other forms of porphyria, ***cutaneous photosensitivity is absent in AIP***" - *CMDT 2016/1655*

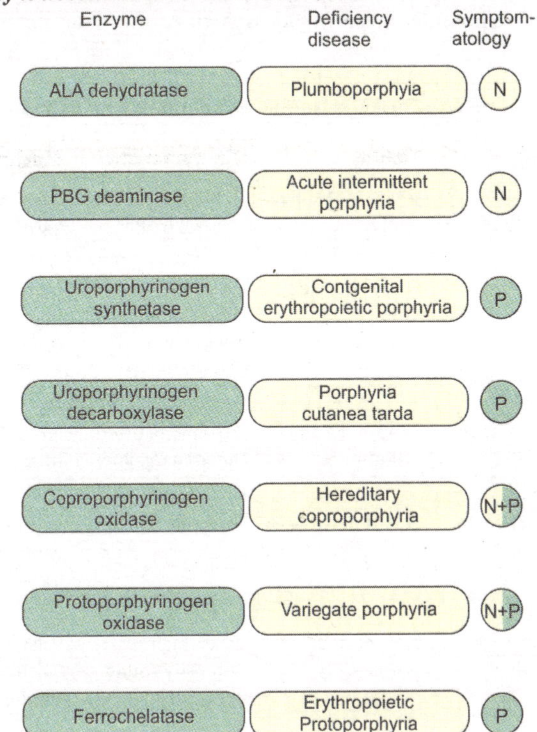

Fig: *(Davidson 22nd/459):* Enzyme defects responsible for the porphyrias. (N = neurovisceral; P = photosensitive)

142. Ans. (a) Low pitch, (c) Absent in atrial..., (d) Produced in the ventricle..., (e) Present in severe left ventricular...

[Ref: Harrison 19th/1448;Davidson 22nd/560; Braunward 8th/136]

Fourth Heart Sound (S4)

◈ *Harrison 19th/1448*

- The fourth heart sound (S4) occurs during the ***atrial filling phase of ventricular diastole and indicates LV presystolic expansion.***
- S4 is more common among patients who derive significant benefit from the atrial contribution to ventricular filling, such as those with chronic LV hypertrophy or active myocardial ischemia.
- ***S4 is not present with atrial fibrillation.***

Fourth Heart Sound (S4)

◈ *Braunward 8th/136*

- It is a ***low-pitched, presystolic sound produced in the ventricle during ventricular filling***; it is associated with an effective atrial contraction and is best heard with the *bell piece of the stethoscope.*
- The sound is ***absent in patients with atrial fibrillation.***

- The S4 occurs when diminished ventricular compliance increases the resistance to ventricular filling; it is frequently present in patients with *systemic hypertension, aortic stenosis, hypertrophic cardiomyopathy, ischemic heart disease, and acute mitral regurgitation.*
- The right-sided S4 is present in patients with ***right ventricular hypertrophy secondary*** to either pulmonic stenosis or pulmonary hypertension and frequently accompanies a prominent presystolic a wave in the JVP.
- The incidence of an audible S4 increases with increasing age. Whether an audible S4 in adults without other evidence of cardiac disease is abnormal remains controversial.

Table *(Davidson 22nd/560):* **Normal and abnormal heart sounds**

Sound	Timing	Characteristics	Mechanisms	Variable features
First heart sound (S1)	Onset of systole	Usually single of narrowly split	Closure of mitral and tricuspid valves	Loud: hyperdynamic circulation (anaemia, pregnancy, thyrotoxicosis); mitral stenosis Soft: heart failure; mitral regurgitation
Second heart sound (S2)	End of systole	Split on inspiration Single of expiration (p. 532)	Closure of aortic and pulmonary valve A_2 first P_2 second	Fixed wide splitting with atrial septal defect Wide but variable splitting with delayed right heart emptying (e.g. right bundle branch block) Reversed splitting due to delayed left heart emptying (e.g. left bundle branch block)
Third heart sound (S3)	Early in diastole, just after S2	Low pitch, often heard as 'gallop'	From ventricular wall due to abrupt cessation of rapid filling	**Physiological:** yound people, pregnancy **Pathological:** heart failure, mitral regurgitation
Fourth heart sound (S4)	**End of diastole,** just before S1	Low pitch	Ventricular origin (stiff ventricle and augmented atrial contraction) related to atrial filling	*Absent in atrial fibrillation* A feature of ***severe left ventricular hypertrophy*** (e.g. hypertrophic cardiomyopathy)
Systolic clicks	Early or mid-systole	Brief, high-intensity sound	Valvular aortic stenosis Valvular pulmonary stenosis Floppy mitral valve Prosthetic heart sounds from opening and closing of normally functioning mechanical valves	Click may be lost when stenotic valve becomes thickened or calcified Prosthetic clicks lost when valve obstructed by thrombus or vegetations
Opening snap (OS)	Early in diastole	High pitch, brief duration	Opening of stenosed leaflets of mitral valve Prosthetic heart sounds	Moves closer to S2 as mitral stenosis becomes more severs. May be absent in calcific mitral stenosis

143. Ans. (a) Narrow-complex..., (c) Associated with 2: 1, 3: 1 or 4:..., (d) Best therapy is catheter..., (e) Occur due to macro...

[Ref: Harrison 19th/1484-85; CMDT 2016/393; Davidson 22nd/564]

P wave is absent in atrial fibrillation-*The ECG by Hampton 8th/78*

Atrial Flutter

◈ *Davidson 22nd/564*

- Atrial flutter is ***characterised by a large (macro) re-entry circuit***, usually within the right atrium encircling the tricuspid annulus.
- The ***atrial rate is approximately 300/min***, and is usually associated with ***2: 1, 3: 1 or 4: 1 AV block*** (with corresponding ***heart rates of 150, 100 or 75/min***).
- Rarely, in young patients, every beat is conducted, producing a rate of 300/min and, potentially, haemodynamic compromise. The ECG shows sawtoothed flutter waves. When there is regular 2: 1 AV block, it may be difficult to identify flutter waves that are buried in QRS complexes and T waves.
- Atrial flutter should always be suspected when there is a ***narrow-complex tachycardia of 150/min***. Carotid sinus pressure or intravenous adenosine may help to establish the diagnosis by temporarily increasing the degree of AV block and revealing flutter waves
- Digoxin, β-blockers or verapamil can control the ventricular rate. However, in many cases, it may be preferable to try to restore sinus rhythm by direct current (DC) cardioversion or by using intravenous amiodarone.
- ***Catheter ablation offers a 90% chance of complete cure and is the treatment of choice for patients with persistent symptoms.***

"The atrial rate is typically 240–300 beats/min but may be slower in the presence of atrial disease or antiarrhythmic drugs. It ***often conducts to the ventricles with 2:1 AV block, creating a regular tachycardia at 150 beats/min***, with p waves that may be difficult to discern. For recurrent episodes of common atrial flutter, ***catheter ablation of the cavotricuspid isthmus abolishes the arrhythmia in over 90% of patients***"- *Harrison 19th/1484-85*

Essentials of Diagnosis

◈ *CMDT 2016/393*

- Usually regular heart rhythm.
- ***Often tachycardic (100–150 beats/min)***.
- Often associated with palpitations (acute onset) or fatigue (chronic).
- ECG shows "sawtooth" pattern of atrial activity in leads II, III, and AVF.
- Often seen in conjunction with structural heart disease or chronic obstructive pulmonary disease (COPD).

144. Ans. (b) Downsloping depression of the ST segment >0.1 mV below baseline

[Ref: Harrison 19th/1582; Davidson 22nd/534]

"If the ST segments are depressed but upward sloping, there is probably no ischemia"-*ECG by Hampton 8th/144*

Stress Testing

◈ *Harrison 19th/1582*

- Exercise duration is usually symptom-limited, and the test is **discontinued** upon evidence of chest discomfort, severe shortness of breath, dizziness, severe fatigue, ST-segment depression >0.2 mV (2 mm), a fall in systolic blood pressure >10 mmHg, or the development of a ***ventricular tachyarrhythmia***.
- This test is used to discover any limitation in exercise performance, detect typical ECG signs of myocardial ischemia, and establish their relationship to chest discomfort.
- ***The ischemic ST-segment response generally is defined as flat or downsloping depression of the ST segment >0.1 mV below baseline (i.e., the PR segment) and lasting longer than 0.08 s.***
- ***Upsloping or junctional ST-segment changes are not considered characteristic of ischemia and do not constitute a positive test.***
- Although T-wave abnormalities, conduction disturbances, and ***ventricular arrhythmias that*** develop during exercise should be noted, they are ***also not diagnostic***.
- ***Negative exercise tests in which the target heart rate (85% of maximal predicted heart rate for age and sex) is not achieved are considered nondiagnostic.***
- The **normal response** to graded exercise includes progressive ***increases in heart rate and blood pressure***. Failure of the blood pressure to increase or an actual decrease with signs of ischemia during the test is an important adverse prognostic sign, since it may reflect ischemia-induced global left ventricular dysfunction.
- ***The development of angina and/or severe (>0.2 mV) ST-segment depression at a low workload, i.e., before completion of stage II of the Bruce protocol, and/or ST-segment depression that persists >5 min after the termination of exercise increases the specificity of the test and suggests severe IHD and a high risk of future adverse events.***

Exercise (Stress) ECG

◈ *Davidson 22nd/534*

- Exercise electrocardiography is used to detect myocardial ischaemia during physical stress and is helpful in the diagnosis of coronary artery disease.
- A 12-lead ECG is recorded during exercise on a treadmill or bicycle ergometer.
- The Bruce Protocol is the most commonly used for testing. BP is recorded and symptoms assessed throughout the test.
- ***A test is 'positive' if anginal pain occurs, BP falls or fails to increase, or if there are ST segment shifts of more than 1 mm.***
- False-negative results can occur in patients with coronary artery disease, and some patients with a positive test will not have coronary disease (false-positive).

Table *(Exercise testing): Davidson 22nd/534*

Indications
• To confirm the diagnosis of angina • To evaluate stable angina • To assesses prognosis following myocardial infarction • To assess outcome after coronary revascularization, e.g. coronary angioplasty • To diagnose and evaluate the treatment of exercise-induced arrhythmias
High-risk findings
• Low threshold for ischaemia (i.e within stage 1 or 2 of the Bruce protocol) • Fall in BP on exercise • Widespread, marked or prolonged ischaemic ECG changes • Exercise-induced arrhythmia

145. Ans. (d) Aspirin, (e) Recombinant tissue plasminogen...

[Ref: Harrison 19th/2561-63; CMDT 2016/981; Davidson 22nd/ 1244]

"**Acute Ischemic Stroke**: In patients not eligible for thrombolytic therapy, and in whom hemorrhage has been excluded by CT, the immediate administration of ***aspirin*** 325 mg orally daily is indicated. ***Anticoagulant drugs are started without delay in the setting of atrial fibrillation or other source of cardioembolism when hemorrhage*** has been excluded by CT. Treatment is with ***warfarin (target INR 2.0–3.0) or dabigatran (150 mg twice daily); bridging warfarin with heparin is not necessary,*** but some experts advocate treatment with aspirin until the INR becomes therapeutic. Aspirin therapy should not continue after achieving therapeutic anticoagulation because of an increased risk of hemorrhage"-*CMDT 2016/981*

"**Thrombolytic agents** are- ***Streptokinase, urokinase and recombinant tissue plasminogen activator***(rt-PA e.g alteplase, reteplase, tenecteplase)"-*KDT 7th/627*

"**Streptokinas**: It is not employed now except for consideration of cost. Compared to newer more fibrin-specifc tissue plasminogen activators (e.g alteplase) it is ***less effective in opening occluded coronary arteries*** and cause less reduction in MI related mortality. There are several other disadvantages as well with streptokinase"- *KDT 7th/627*

Acute Ischemic Stroke

◈ *Harrison 19th/2561-63*

- Treatments designed to reverse or lessen the amount of tissue infarction and improve clinical outcome fall within six categories: (1) medical support, (2) ***IV thrombolysis,*** (3) endovascular revascularization, (4) antithrombotic treatment, (5) neuroprotection, and (6) stroke centers and rehabilitation.
- **Intravenous thrombolysis:** Treatment with IV rtPA ***within 3 h of the onset of ischemic stroke improved clinical outcome.***
- **Platelet Inhibition: *Aspirin*** is the only antiplatelet agent that has been proven effective for the acute treatment of ischemic stroke. The use ***of aspirin within 48 h of stroke onset reduced both stroke recurrence risk and mortality minimally***
- Anticoagulation: Numerous clinical trials have ***failed to demonstrate any benefit of anticoagulation in the primary treatment of atherothrombotic cerebral ischemia.*** Several trials have investigated antiplatelet versus anticoagulant medications given within 12–24 h of the initial event. The U.S. Trial of Organon 10172 in Acute Stroke Treatment (TOAST), an investigational ***low-molecular-weight heparin (LMWH), failed to show any benefit over aspirin.*** Use of SC unfractionated heparin versus aspirin was tested in IST. Heparin given SC afforded no additional benefit over aspirin and increased bleeding rates. Several trials of ***LMWHs have also shown no consistent benefit in AIS.*** Furthermore, trials generally have shown an excess risk of brain and systemic hemorrhage with acute anticoagulation. A recent meta-analysis of all forms of heparin found no benefit for acute stroke patients at high or low risk of thrombotic events. Therefore, ***trials do not support the use of heparin or other anticoagulants for patients with atherothrombotic stroke.***

"**Thrombolysis**: If with recombinant tissue plasminogen activator ***(rt-PA) is given within 4.5 hours*** of symptom onset to carefully selected patients, the haemorrhagic risk is offset by an improvement in overall outcome. The earlier treatment is given, the greater the benefit"- *Davidson 22nd/ 1244*

"**Aspirin**: In the absence of contraindications, ***aspirin (300 mg daily) should be started immediately after an ischaemic stroke unless rt-PA has been given, in which case it should be withheld for at least 24 hours.*** Aspirin reduces the risk of early recurrence and has a small but clinically worthwhile effect on long-term outcome"- *Davidson 22nd/ 1244*

"**Heparin**: Anticoagulation with heparin has been widely used to treat acute ischaemic stroke in the past. Whilst it reduces the risk of early ischaemic recurrence and venous thromboembolism, it ***increases the risk of both intracranial and extracranial haemorrhage.*** Furthermore, routine use of heparin does not result in better long-term outcomes, and ***therefore it should not be used in the routine management of acute stroke.*** It is unclear whether heparin might provide benefit in selected patients, such as those with recent myocardial infarction, arterial dissection or progressing strokes. Intracranial haemorrhage must be excluded on brain imaging before considering anticoagulation"- *Davidson 22nd/ 1244*

Table *(Davidson 22nd/ 1244):* **Role of Treatments in Acute Stroke**

Treatment	Target group	Approx. proportion of patients eligible for treatment	NNT to prevent 1 death or disability in those treated
Aspirin	Acute ischaemic stroke	90%	80
Thrombolysis with rt-PA	Acute ischaemic stroke Treatment within 3 hrs of onset Treatment within 3–4.5 hrs of onset	10% 10%	9 20
Decompressive hemi-craniectomy	Large cerebral infarction	< 1%	2
Stroke unit care	Acute stroke	80%	20

NNT-number needed to treat

146. Ans. (b) Increase in unconjugated bilirubin, (c) Increase in urine... (d) Increase in faecal stercobilinogen

[Ref: Harrison 19th/649-50; Davidson 22nd/1026-31]

Investigation Results Indicating Active Haemolysis

◈ *Davidson 22nd/1026*

Hallmarks of Haemolysis

- ↓Haemoglobin
- ↑***Unconjugated bilirubin***
- ↑Lactate dehydrogenase
- ↑Reticulocytes
- ↑***Urinary urobilinogen***

Additional Features of Intravascular Haemolysis

- ↓Haptoglobin
- ↑Methaemalbumin
- Positive urinary haemosiderin
- Haemoglobinuria

Haemolytic Anaemia

◈ *Davidson 22nd/1026-31*

- Haemolysis indicates that there is shortening of the normal red cell lifespan of 120 days.
- Red cell destruction overloads pathways for haemoglobin breakdown in the liver, causing a ***modest rise in unconjugated bilirubin*** in the blood and mild jaundice.
- ***Increased reabsorption of urobilinogen from the gut results in an increase in urinary urobilinogen.***
- Red cell destruction releases LDH into the serum.
- The bone marrow compensation results in a reticulocytosis, and sometimes nucleated red cell precursors appear in the blood.

Intravascular Hemolysis

- Whatever the mechanism, *intravascular hemolysis is manifested by (1) hemoglobinemia, (2) hemoglobinuria, (3) jaundice,* and *(4)* ***hemosiderinuria.***

- Free hemoglobin in plasma is promptly bound by an α2-globulin (haptoglobin), producing a complex that is rapidly cleared by the mononuclear phagocyte system, thus preventing excretion into the urine. ***Decreased serum haptoglobin is characteristic of intravascular hemolysis.***
- When the liver is normal, jaundice is rarely severe. Excessive bilirubin excreted by the liver into the gastrointestinal tract leads to ***increased formation and fecal excretion of urobilin***

Table *(PJM 20th/20)*: **Differential diagnosis of jaundice**

	Hepatocellular	Obstructive	Hemolytic
I. History			
1. Abdominal pain	Absent	Present	Present in crisis
2. Pruritus	Transient	Marked	Absent
3. Past history	(a) Contact with jaundice patient (b) Drugs	(a) Pain (**Stones**)	(a) Of crisis (b) Drugs, blood transfusion, etc.
II. Examination			
1. Tender liver	May be present	Absent	Absent
2. Spleen	May be present	Absent	Present
3. Gallbladder	Not palpable	Palpable if due to neoplasm	Not palpable
4. Pallor	Absent	Present	Present
III. Investigations			
1. Urine: Bilirubin Urobilinogen	Present Present	Present Absent	Absent Present
2. Stools: Stercobilinogen	Present	Absent	Present
3. Peripheral smear	Leucopenia in infective hepatitis	Normal	Reticulocytosis, Spherocytosis
4. LFT			
(a) Bilirubin	++	++	+
(b) Alkaline phosphate	Raised	Markedly raised	Normal
(c) SGOT	Markedly raised	Raised	Normal
5. Barium meal and cholangiography	Normal	May reveal pancreatic growth	Normal
6. RBC Survival	Normal	Normal	Decreased

147. Ans. (b) Self-limited course in acute form, (d) Immune-mediated destruction of platelets

[Ref: Robbins 9th/Vol.I 658-59; Harrison 19th/72-29]

Immune Thrombocytopenic Purpura (ITP; a/k Idiopathic Thrombocytopenic purpura)

◈ *Harrison 19th/72-29*

- It is an acquired disorder in which there is immune-mediated destruction of platelets and possibly inhibition of platelet release from the megakaryocyte.
- In ***children, it is usually an acute disease***, most commonly following an infection, and with a ***self-limited course.***
- In ***adults, it is a more chronic disease***, although in some adults, spontaneous remission occurs, usually within months of diagnosis.
- ITP is termed *secondary* if it is associated with an underlying disorder; autoimmune disorders, particularly systemic lupus erythematosus (SLE), and infections, such as HIV and hepatitis C, are common causes. The association of ITP with *Helicobacter pylori* infection is unclear.
- ITP is characterized by mucocutaneous bleeding and a low, often very low, platelet count, with an otherwise normal peripheral blood cells and smear.
- Patients usually ***present either with ecchymoses and petechiae***, or with thrombocytopenia incidentally found on a routine CBC.
- Mucocutaneous bleeding, such as oral mucosa, gastrointestinal, or heavy menstrual bleeding, may be present. Rarely, life-threatening, including central nervous system, bleeding can occur.
- Wet purpura (blood blisters in the mouth) and retinal hemorrhages may herald lifethreatening bleeding.
- Bone marrow examination can be reserved for those who have other signs or laboratory abnormalities not explained by ITP or in patients who do not respond to initial therapy. The peripheral blood smear may show large platelets, with otherwise normal morphology. Depending on the bleeding history, iron-deficiency anemia may be present.
- **Laboratory testing** is performed to evaluate for secondary causes of ITP and should include testing for HIV infection and hepatitis C (and other infections if indicated).

148. Ans. (a) In DIC both PT and aPTT increase, (d) Hemophilia A is inherited as X-linked recessive

[Ref: CMDT 2016/549,553; Robbins 9th/661-64; Harrison 19th/ 732-38; Davidson 22nd/1050-56]

"Hemophilia A: ***Inheritance is X-linked recessive***,leading to affected males and carrier females"- *CMDT 2016/553*

"In early **Disseminated intravascular coagulation(DIC)**, the platelet count and fibrinogen levels may remain within the normal range, albeit reduced from baseline levels. There is progressive thrombocytopenia (rarely severe), ***prolongation of the activated partial thromboplastin time (aPTT) and prothrombin time (PT),*** and low levels of fibrinogen. D-dimer levels typically are elevated due to the activation of coagulation and diffuse cross-linking of fibrin. Schistocytes on the blood smear, due to shearing of red cells through the microvasculature, are present in 10–20% of patients"- *CMDT 2016/549*

"Factor XI (FXI) deficiency, also called hemophilia C, plasma thromboplastin antecedent deficiency and Rosenthal syndrome. ***FXI deficiency is inherited in an autosomal recessive pattern, meaning both parents must carry the gene to pass it on to their children; men and women are affected equally***"-*www.hemophilia.org/Bleeding-Disorders*

"Mutations in the **factor XI gene** cause the congenital deficiency of factor XI clotting activity. The inheritance pattern of factor XI is ***autosomal but not completely recessive***, because heterozygotes may have bleeding.

"**DIC**: Common findings include the ***prolongation of PT and/or aPTT***; platelet counts µ100,000/µL, or a rapid decline in platelet numbers; the presence of schistocytes (fragmented red cells) in the blood smear; and elevated levels of FDP. The most sensitive test for DIC is the FDP level"-*Harrison 19th/ 737*

Hemophilia B (Christmas Disease, Factor IX Deficiency): As with hemophilia A, the PTT is prolonged and the PT is normal. Diagnosis of Christmas disease is possible only by assay of the factor levels. ***The disease is treated with infusions of recombinant factor IX***"- *Robbins 9th/663*

"In severe **haemophilia A**, bleeding episodes should be treated by raising the factor VIII level, usually by ***intravenous infusion of factor VIII concentrate***"- *Davidson 22nd/1051-52*

Table *(Davidson 22nd/1051):* **Congenital Causes of coagulopathy**

X-linked	
• Haemophilia A and B	
Autosomal	
• Von willebrand disease • Factor II, V, VII, X, XI and XIII deficiencies • Combined II, VII, IX and X deficiency	• Combined V and VIII deficiency • Hypofibrinogenaemia • Dysfibrinogenaemia

149. Ans. (c) Familial pulmonary HTN, (d) Congenital heart disease with left-to... (e) Pulmonary hypertension...

[Ref: Robbins 9th/700; Harshmohan 7th/447-48; Harrison 19th/1658; Davidson 22nd/724]

"**Morphology of pulmonary hypertension**: One extreme in the spectrum of pathologic changes is the ***plexiform lesion***, so called because a tuft of capillary formations is present, producing a network, or web, that spans the lumens of dilated thin-walled, small arteries and may extend outside the vessel. **Plexiform lesions are most prominent** in ***idiopathic and familial pulmonary hypertension (group 1), unrepaired congenital heart disease with left-to-right shunts (group 2), and pulmonary hypertension associated with human immunodeficiency***"- *Robbins 9th/700*

Pulmonary Hypertension

◈ *Robbins 9th/700*

- Based on underlying mechanisms, the World Health Organization has classified pulmonary hypertension into five groups. These groups are: ***(1) pulmonary arterial hypertension, a diverse collection of disorders that all primarily impact small pulmonary muscular arteries; (2) pulmonary hypertension secondary to left-heart failure; (3) pulmonary hypertension stemming from lung parenchymal disease or hypoxemia; (4) chronic thromboembolic pulmonary hypertension;***
- As can be gathered from the classification above, pulmonary hypertension has diverse causes. It is most frequently associated with structural cardiopulmonary conditions that increase pulmonary blood flow, pulmonary vascular resistance, or left heart resistance to blood flow. Some of the more common causes are:***Chronic obstructive or interstitial lung diseases (Group 3),Antecedent congenital or acquired heart disease Group 2), Recurrent thromboemboli (Group 4), Autoimmune diseases (Group 1) and Obstructive sleep apnea (also group 3)***

150. Ans. (b) Child-Pugh score C

[Ref: Harrison 19th/1995; Davidson 22nd/978; www.ncbi.nlm.nih.gov]

Surgery in the Patient with Liver Disease

◈ *www.ncbi.nlm.nih.gov*

- In a patient with liver disease, *surgical risk* depends on the severity of liver disease, nature of the surgical procedure and presence of comorbid conditions. There are a number of liver-related contraindications to elective surgery
- Once liver disease is identified in a patient in need of surgery, an assessment of the severity of liver disease should be undertaken, as should an evaluation for other known risk factors for perioperative mortality. Data from studies of patients with cirrhosis suggest that the severity of liver disease can best be assessed by the ***Child-Turcotte-Pugh (CTP) score (Child, or Child-Pugh, class) and MELD score***
- In general, patients with compensated cirrhosis who have normal synthetic function have a low overall risk, and the ***risk increases for patients with decompensated cirrhosis.***
- Two of the most important studies, separated by 13 years, reported nearly identical results: mortality rates for patients undergoing surgery were 10% for those with Child class A, ***30% for those with Child class B, and 76–82% for those with Child class C cirrhosis.***

- In addition to predicting perioperative mortality, the Child class correlates with the frequency of postoperative complications, which include liver failure, worsening encephalopathy, bleeding, infection, renal failure, hypoxia and intractable ascites.
- A general consensus is that ***elective surgery is well tolerated in patients with Child class A cirrhosis, permissible with preoperative preparation in patients with Child class B cirrhosis (except those undergoing extensive hepatic resection or cardiac surgery), and contraindicated in patients with Child class C cirrhosis***

*"The **Child-Pugh score** is calculated by adding the scores of the five factors and can range from 5–15. Child-Pugh class is either A (a score of 5–6), B (7–9), or C (10 or above). **Decompensation indicates cirrhosis with a Child-Pugh score of 7 or more (class B). This level has been the accepted criterion for listing for liver transplantation**"- Harrison 19th/1995*

Table *(www.ncbi.nlm.nih.gov)*: **Factors predictive of perioperative complications and of postoperative mortality**

Predictor of complications	Predictor of mortality
Child-pugh class B and C	Male gender
Ascites	***Child-Pugh class B and C***
Etiology of cirrhosis other than primary biliary cirrhosis	Etiology of cirrhosis other than primary biliary cirrhosis
Elevated creatinine	Ascites
Preoperative infection	Preoperative infection
Chronic obstructive pulmonary disease	Respiratory surgery
Preoperative upper gastrointestinal bleed	American Society of Anaesthesiologists physical status IV and V
Invasiveness of surgical procedure	
Intraoperative hypotension (20% decrease of base line blood pressure line blood pressure for 10 min or more)	
American society of Anaesthesiologists physical status IV and V	

151. Ans. (b) May produce..., (c) Autoimmune inflammatory condition, (d) Oligoclonal bands may..., (e) Spinal cord involvement ...

[Ref: Harrison 19th/2661-67; CMDT 2016/1007-09; Davidson 22nd/1188-92; Robbins 9th/1284-85]

"Elevated IgG in cerebrospinal fluid and ***discrete bands of IgG (oligoclonal bands)*** are present in many patients. The presence of such bands is not specific, however, since they have been found in a variety of inflammatory neurologic disorders and occasionally in patients with vascular or neoplastic disorders of the nervous system"-*CMDT 2016/1008*

Multiple Sclerosis-lesion Size of 1-25 (Majority b/w 5 and 10) mm

◈ *Danhert Radiology Manual 7th/314*

- ***Large lesions may masquerade as brain tumours***
- ***Mass effect/edema in active lesion*** *(infrequent)*

Diagnosis of Multiple Sclerosis

◈ *CMDT 2016/1008*

- Multiple sclerosis should not be diagnosed unless there is evidence that two or more different regions of the central white matter (dissemination in space) have been affected at different times (dissemination in time). The diagnosis may be made in a patient with two or more typical attacks and ***two or more MRI lesions***.
- To fulfill the criterion of dissemination in space in a patient with only one lesion, repeat imaging in a few months should demonstrate at least one lesion in at least two of four typical sites (***periventricular, juxtacortical, infratentorial, or spinal***); alternatively, an additional attack localized to a different site suffices.
- Primary progressive disease requires at least a year of progressive disease, plus two of three of the following: at least one typical brain lesion, at least two spinal lesions, or ***oligoclonal banding in the cerebrospinal fluid***

Multiple Sclerosis (MS)

◈ *Harrison 19th/2661-67*

- It is an ***autoimmune disease*** of the CNS characterized by ***chronic inflammation***, demyelination, gliosis (scarring), and neuronal loss; the course can be relapsing-remitting or progressive.
- There is no definitive diagnostic test for MS. Diagnostic criteria for clinically definite MS require documentation ***of two or more episodes of symptoms and two or more signs that reflect pathology in anatomically noncontiguous white matter tracts of the CNS***
- Symptoms must last for >24 h and occur as distinct episodes that are separated by a month or more.
- MRI or the simultaneous presence of both an enhancing lesion and a nonenhancing lesion in an asymptomatic location. In patients whose course is progressive from onset for ≥6 months without superimposed relapses, documentation of intrathecal IgG synthesis may be used to support a diagnosis of PPMS.

Partial Table *(Harrison 19th/2665)*: **Diagnostic criteria for multiple sclerosis (MS)**

Clinical Presentation	Additional Data Needed for MS Diagnosis
2 or more attacks, objective Clinical evidence of 2 or more lesions or objective clinical evidence of 1 lesion with reasonable historical evidence of a prior attack	None
2 or more attacks; objective clinical evidence of 1 lesion	Dissemination in space, demonstrated by • ≥ 1 T2 lesion on MRI in at least 2 out of 4 MS-typical regions of the CNS (***periventricular, juxtacortical, infratentorial, or spinal cord***) OR • Await a further clinical attack implicating a different CNS site

A & E

Table *(Harrison 19th/2663)*: **Initial symptoms of MS**

Symptom	Percentage of cases	Symptom	Percentage of cases
Sensory loss	37	Lhermitte	3
Optic neuritis	36	Pain	3
Weakness	35	Dementia	2
Paresthesias	24	Visual loss	2
Diplopia	15	Facial palsy	1
Ataxia	11	Impotence	1
Vertigo	6	Myokymia	1
Paroxysmal attacks	4	Epilepsy	1
Bladder	4	Falling	1

152. Ans. (c) Transplanting mesenchymal stem cell from adipose tissue to liver

[Ref: www.hindawi.com/journals/ijh/2012/307165/; Harrison 19th/90e1-3; L and B 26th/1427-29; Schwartz 9th/1124-28]

√ ***Safer approach means. Lesser chance of rejection, lesser transmission of disease and lesser risk of cancerous growth***

Among all options c, is best

Option a	*More regenerative capacity, so more chance of abnormal growth (including tumour formation)* *Allograft risk*
Option b	*Hepatocyte carries allograft risk, risk of transmission of donor disease*
Option c	*Autograft so less immune risk* *No transmission of disease from donor*
Option d	*Eryhropoietin is used in haematopietic tissue generation*

Liver Transplantation

◈ *Harrison 19th/90e-3*

- Clinical trials of **hepatocyte transplantation** demonstrate its potential as a substitute for organ transplantation, but ***this approach is limited by the paucity of available cells.***
- Potential sources of stem cells for regenerative strategies include endogenous ***liver stem cells (such as oval cells), ES cells, MSCs, and USCs.***
- Although a series of studies in humans as well as animals suggested that transplanted ***MSCs and HSCs can generate hepatocytes***, fusion of the transplanted cells with endogenous liver cells, giving the erroneous appearance of new hepatocytes, appears to be the underlying event in most circumstances.
- The available evidence suggests that ***transplanted HSCs and MSCs can generate hepatocyte-like cells in the liver only at a very low frequency, but there are beneficial consequences presumably related to indirect paracrine effects.***
- ES cells can be differentiated into hepatocytes and transplanted in animal models of liver failure without the ***formation of teratomas.*** Clinical trials are in progress in cirrhosis with numerous cell types, including ***MSCs, USCs, HSCs, and ASCs.***

How Stem Cells can help in Liver Disease Treatment?

◈ *www.startstemcells.com*

- As far back as 2000, researchers showed that hepatocytes could grow in the body on non-liver cell sources. This phenomenon is called ***transdifferentiation.***
- Today, autologous (from the patient) ***adipose tissue stem cells are the only stem cells that have been used clinically for treating liver disease.*** The major advantage with using these cells is that because they come from the patient, there is ***no risk of rejection when they are transplanted back.***
- The stem cells are transdifferentiating into hepatocytes as well as producing soluble factors that promote regeneration and repair. There is also the possibility that the stem cells may be fusing with resident hepatocytes to direct their regeneration.
- Mesenchymal stem cells are found throughout the adult body in tissues such as bone, muscle, cartilage and fat.
- Mesenchymal stem cells are among the most ***'multipotent' stem cells*** that remain in our bodies after birth. This means that they are still able to make a variety of different cell types.
- Many trials have shown that patients with liver cirrhosis have benefitted from ***autologous adipose tissue derived mesenchymal stem cells.*** We have proven results reversing the effects of hepatitis, cirrhosis and liver damage due to chemo and other drug therapies.

Advantages of Stem Cell therapy in Swiss Medica Clinics for Liver Disease

◈ *www.startstemcells.com/*

- Side effects and rejection free (use the patient's very own stem cells from their abdomen)
- Avoidance of any allergic and immune reactions (own cells suit chromosomal and genetic structure)
- No risk of contamination by transmissible diseases
- ***No oncological complication as adult stem cells in the comparison with embryonic cells are rather mature***
- Small quantity of fat tissue is needed (that is why after activation process the stem cells can be at once injected to patient without necessity of growing them on substances. Embryonic stem cells are grown during several months)
- The period of time between getting lipoaspirate and injection of the activated stem cells is only a few hours
- Adipose tissue stem cells are easily accessible and yielding up to ten times more stem cells than patients bone marrow

General Strategies for Stem cell Replacement

◈ *Harrison 19th/90e1*

- At least **three different** therapeutic concepts for cell replacement can be envisaged
- One therapeutic approach involves direct **administration of stem cells**. The cells may be injected directly into the damaged organ or ***injected systemically***
- A second approach involves ***transplantation of differentiated cells derived from stem cells.***
- A third approach involves ***stimulation of endogenous stem cells*** to facilitate repair. Therapeutic stimulation of precursor cells is already a clinical reality in the hematopoietic system, where factors such as ***erythropoietin***, *granulocyte colony-stimulating factor, and granulocyte-macrophage colony-*

stimulating factor are used to increase production of specific blood elements.

- In addition to these strategies for cell replacement, a number of other approaches could involve stem cells for ex vivo or in situ generation of tissues, a process termed ***tissue engineering***
- Stem cell transplantation is not a new concept but rather is already part of established medical practice.

Embryonic Stem Cells

◈ *Harrison 19th/90e1*

- Embryonic stem cells have the ***potential to generate all the cell types in the body***; thus, in theory, there are no restrictions on the organs that could be regenerated.
- Cells tend to develop ***abnormal karyotypes and other abnormalities with increased time in culture***, and ES cells have the ***potential to form teratomas*** if all cells are not committed to the desired cell types before transplantation.

Organ-Specific Multipotent Stem Cells

◈ *Harrison 19th/90e2*

- Cells potentially could be obtained from the patient and amplified in cell culture, circumventing the problems associated with immune rejection.
- Moreover, these populations of cells are ***more limited in potentiality than are pluripotent ES or iPS cells***, and they may be difficult to obtain in large quantities from many organs.
- A number of early studies of ***MSCs transplanted into heart, liver, and other organs suggested that the cells had differentiated into organ-specific cell types with beneficial effects in animal models of disease.***
- Regardless of the source of the stem cells used in regenerative strategies, a number of generic problems must be overcome for the development of successful clinical applications. These **problems** include the devising of methods to ***reliably generate large numbers of specific cell types, to minimize the risk of tumor formation or proliferation of inappropriate cell types, to ensure the viability and function of the engrafted cells, to overcome immune rejection when autografts are not used, and to facilitate revascularization of regenerated tissue.***

Sources of Stem Cells for Tissue Repair

◈ *Harrison 19th/90e1*

- A variety of different types of stem cells could be used in regenerative strategies, including embryonic stem (ES) cells, induced pluripotent stem (iPS) cells, umbilical-cord blood stem cells (USCs), organ-specific somatic stem cells (e.g., neural stem cells for treatment of the brain), and somatic stem cells that generate cell types specific for the target organ rather than the donor organ (e.g., ***bone marrow mesenchymal stem cells or CD34+ hematopoietic stem cells for cardiac repair***).
- Although each cell type has potential advantages and disadvantages, there are a number of generic problems in developing any of these cell types into a useful and reliable clinical tool

Hepatocyte Transplantation and Stem Cell Transplantation

◈ *www.hindawi.com/journals/ijh/2012/307165/*

- The widespread application of hepatocyte transplantation, however, is also limited by organ availability, by problems with viability of isolated hepatocytes after cryopreservation, and by the ***potential formation of hepatocyte aggregates*** during injection subsequently obstructing ***liver sinusoids and resulting in portal hypertension or fatal emboli.***
- The **BM compartment** is largely made up of ***HSCs, committed progenitor cells***, and ***noncirculating stromal cells called mesenchymal stem cells (MSC)*** which have the ability to develop into mesenchymal lineages.
- ***Unlike hepatocytes, the use of BMSCs for liver regeneration does not depend on the procurement of cadaveric livers whose donors are often immunologically disparate and also in short supply***. The use of ***adult stem cells*** is attractive as it overcomes the moral and ethical barriers of ES cell manipulation.
- Further advantages of the use of **BMSCs** are that they are ***multipotent,*** there is already considerable experience in their use, they are ***easily accessible, and there is unlimited supply***. Conversely, concerns have been raised about the adverse long-term effects of stem cell therapy.
- There is evidence to suggest that treatment with ***BMSCs may provide liver fibrogenic cells*** (hepatic stellate cells and myofibroblasts) which contribute to fibrosis and could have a deleterious effect on already decompensated cirrhotic livers. ***Similarly, there are concerns that hepatocellular carcinoma (HCC) originates from hepatic oval cells and BMSCs***. Much of the data concerning the malignant potential of BMSCs, however, originates from genetically modified rodent models and may not be present in humans

Table: Autologous Stem cell therapies and clinical studies in Liver disease (Contributing to the hepatocyte population direct cell administration)

	Cell Source	Intended Mechanism	Evidence	Comments
Undifferentiated cell	ESCs Adult stem/ progenitor cells	Hepatic engraftment and hepatocyte differentiation and function	Engraftment and differentiation demonstrated but limited hepatocyte function	Risk of malignancy with ESCs Clinical trials unrealistic currently Concerns regarding phenotypic stability

Contd...

	Cell Source	Intended Mechanism	Evidence	Comments
Ex vivo differentiated hepatocytes	ESCS Adult stem/ progenitor cells IPSCs	Hepatic engraftment and hepatocyte function	Low level of engraftment with limited cell function	Risk of malignancy with ESCs Limited function of ex vivo differentiated hepatocytes are present Clinical trials Unrealistic currently
Bioartificial liver support (BALS) systems	Ex vivo differentiated hepatocytes	Extracorporeal hepatocytes contact-infuse blood via a semipermeable membrane	Improved survival in fulminant/subfulminant hepatic failure with procine-derived hepatocytes	Further advances required in efficient hepatocyte generation from human cells Most potential in this field
Promoting endogenous processes **Bone marrow derived stem cells**	HSCs	Matrix remodeling, vascular remodeling, immunomodulation, and facilitation of resident hepatocyte differentiation	Improved physiological parameters in phase 1 clinical trials	Therapeutic potential demonstrated Further cautious clinical investigation required
	Bone marrow MSCs	Matrix remodeling, immunomodulation, and facilitation and facilitation of resident hepatocyte differentiation	Improved physical parameters in a phase 1 clilnical trial	Limited clinical evidence MSC isolation problematic Potential for increased hepatic fibrosis

SURGERY

153. Ans. (d) Usually resolves within 48–72 hour, (e) Radiographs show diffusely dilated bowel with air in the...

[Ref: Manipal Surgery 4th/765; L and B 26th/276; Schwartz 9th/992-93; Sabiston 19th/307-08]

Illeus and Early Postoperative Bowel Obstruction

◈ *Sabiston 19th/307-08*

- Early postoperative bowel obstruction denotes obstruction occurring ***within 30 days after surgery***. The obstruction may be ***functional (i.e., ileus)***, due to inhibition of propulsive bowel activity, or mechanical as a result of a barrier.
- Ileus that occurs immediately after surgery in the absence of precipitating factors and resolves ***within 2 to 4 days*** is referred to as *primary* or *postoperative ileus*.
- On the other hand, ileus that occurs as a result of a precipitating factor and is associated with a delay in return of bowel function is referred to as *secondary* or *adynamic* or *paralytic ileus*.
- **Mechanical bowel** obstruction may be caused by a ***luminal, mural, or extraintestinal barrier***.
- In the *immediate postoperative period, restricted oral intake and postoperative narcotic analgesia also contribute to altered small bowel motility*.
- **Mechanical** early postoperative small bowel obstruction is ***commonly caused by adhesions (92%)***, a phlegmon or abscess, internal hernia, intestinal ischemia, or intussusception.
- Postoperative ileus affects the stomach and colon primarily.
- After laparotomy, ***small bowel motility returns within several hours, gastric motility within 24 to 48 hours, and colonic motility in 48 to 72 hours***.
- Secretions and swallowed air are not emptied from the stomach, and gastric dilation and vomiting may occur. Return of bowel activity is heralded by the presence of bowel sounds, flatus, and bowel movements.
- In ***adynamic ileus, the stomach, small bowel, and colon are affected***.
- The **diagnosis of bowel obstruction** is usually based on clinical findings and plain radiographs of the abdomen.
- A CT scan, abdominal radiographs, and small bowel follow-through are variably used to establish the diagnosis and assist in treatment decision making.
- In **adynamic ileus**, ***abdominal radiographs reveal diffusely dilated bowel throughout the intestinal tract with air in the colon and rectum***.
- A ***CT scan is more accurate*** in differentiating functional from mechanical obstruction by identifying the so-called transition point or cutoff at the obstruction site in cases of mechanical obstruction.

Paralytic ileus

◈ *L and B 26th/276*

- Paralytic ileus may present with ***nausea, vomiting, loss of appetite, bowel distension and absence of flatus or bowel movements.***
- Following laparotomy, gastrointestinal motility temporarily decreases.
- Treatment is usually supportive with maintenance of adequate hydration and electrolyte levels. However, intestinal complications may present as prolonged ileus and so should be actively sought and treated.
- **Return of function of the intestine** occurs in the following order: ***small bowel, large bowel and then stomach***. This pattern allows the passage of faeces despite continuing lack

of stomach emptying and, therefore, vomiting may continue even when the lower bowel has already started functioning normally.

154. Ans. (a) Marked leukocytosis with left shift..., (b) Usually caused by..., (c) May be associated with...

[Ref: Manipal Surgery 4th/634-44; Harrison 19th/846-48; L and B 26th/971-75; Schwartz 9th/124-25; Sabiston 19th/1100-02]

Secondary Peritonitis

◈ *Harrison 19th/846-48*

- Secondary peritonitis develops when bacteria contaminate the peritoneum as a result of spillage from an ***intraabdominal viscus (e.g. appendicular perforation).***
- ***The organisms found almost always constitute a mixed flora*** in which facultative gram-negative bacilli and anaerobes predominate, especially when the contaminating source is colonic.
- Patients with secondary peritonitis generally have abnormal findings on abdominal examination, with marked voluntary and involuntary guarding of the anterior abdominal musculature. ***Later findings include tenderness, especially rebound tenderness.*** In addition, there may be localized findings in the area of the inciting event.
- In general, ***patients are febrile***, with marked leukocytosis and a ***left shift of the WBCs to band forms.***

Primary and Secondary Microbial Peritonitis

◈ *Schwartz 9th/124-25*

- *Primary microbial peritonitis* occurs when microbes invade the normally sterile confines of the peritoneal cavity via hematogenous dissemination from a distant source of infection or direct inoculation. This process is more common among patients who retain large amounts of peritoneal fluid due to ascites, and among those individuals who are being treated for ***renal failure via peritoneal dialysis. These infections invariably are monomicrobial*** and rarely require surgical intervention.
- *Secondary microbial peritonitis* occurs subsequent to contamination of the peritoneal cavity due to perforation or severe inflammation and infection of an intra-abdominal organ. Examples include a***ppendicitis, perforation of any portion of the gastrointestinal tract,*** or diverticulitis.

Peritonitis

◈ *L and B 26th/971-75*

- ***Peritoneal infection is usually caused by two or more bacterial strains.***
- There are also less common forms in which the aetiology is a **primary 'spontaneous' peritonitis**, in which a ***pure infection*** with streptococcal, pneumococcal or haemophilus bacteria occurs.

Primary (Spontaneous) Bacterial Peritonitis

◈ *Harrison 19th/846*

- Peritonitis is either primary (***without an apparent source of contamination***) or secondary.
- The types of organisms found and the clinical presentations of these two processes are different. In adults, **primary bacterial peritonitis (PBP)** occurs most commonly in conjunction with ***cirrhosis of the liver*** (frequently the result of alcoholism).
- However, the disease has been reported in adults with metastatic malignant disease, ***postnecrotic cirrhosis***, chronic active hepatitis, acute viral hepatitis, congestive heart failure, systemic lupus erythematosus, and lymphedema as well as in patients with no underlying disease.
- Although PBP virtually always develops in patients with preexisting ascites, it is, in general, an uncommon event, occurring in ≤10% of ***cirrhotic patients***

Table *(L and B 25th/973):* **Clinical features in Peritonitis**

Clinical features in Peritonitis
Abdominal pain, worse on movement
Guarding/rigidity of abdominal wall
Pain/tenderness on rectal/vaginal examination (pelvic peritonitis)
Pyrexia (may be absent)
Raised pulse rate
Absent or reduced bowel sounds
Septic shock' [systemic inflammatory response syndrome (SIRS)] in later stages

155. Ans. (a) Watershed zones..., (b) Arterial ischemic lesion..., (c) Crypts may be..., (d) Microscopic examination ...

[Ref: Robbins 9th/779-80; L and B 26th/1173;Sabiston 19th/1177]

Ischemic Bowel Disease

◈ *Robbins 9th/779-80*

- Intestinal responses to ischemia occur in **two phases**. The initial ***hypoxic injury*** occurs at the onset of vascular compromise. The second phase, *reperfusion injury*, is initiated by restoration of the blood supply and it is at this time that the greatest damage occurs.
- ***Intestinal segments at the end of their respective arterial supplies are particularly susceptible to ischemia. These watershed zones include the splenic flexure***, where the superior and inferior mesenteric arterial circulations terminate, and, to a lesser extent, the sigmoid colon and rectum where inferior mesenteric, pudendal, and iliac arterial circulations end.
- Although the ***colon is the most common site of gastrointestinal ischemia***, mucosal and mural infarction may involve any level of the gut from stomach to anus.
- Substantial portions of the bowel are generally involved in **transmural infarction** due to **acute arterial obstruction.** The ***demarcation between normal and ischemic bowel is sharply defined*** and the infarcted bowel is initially intensely congested and dusky to purple-red. ***There is coagulative necrosis of the muscularis propria*** within 1 to 4 days, and perforation may occur.

- In **mesenteric venous thrombosis**, arterial blood continues to flow for a time, resulting in a ***less abrupt transition*** from affected to normal bowel. However, propagation of the thrombus may lead to secondary involvement of the splanchnic bed. The ultimate result is similar to that produced by acute arterial obstruction because ***impaired venous drainage*** eventually prevents oxygenated arterial blood from entering the capillaries.
- **Microscopic examination** of ischemic intestine demonstrates the ***characteristic atrophy or sloughing of surface epithelium***. In contrast, ***crypts may be hyperproliferative***. Inflammatory infiltrates are initially absent in acute ischemia, but ***neutrophils are recruited within hours of reperfusion.***

Mesenteric Ischemia

◈ *Sabiston 19th/1177*

- Mesenteric ischemia can be secondary to either ***acute or chronic arterial or venous insufficiency***
- ***Acute colonic ischemia*** is the ***most common form of mesenteric ischemia.***
- It tends to occur in the ***watershed areas of the splenic flexure and the rectosigmoid colon***, but can be right-sided in up to 40% of patients.
- The diagnosis is generally confirmed with flexible endoscopy, which reveals edema, hemorrhage, and a demarcation between the normal and abnormal mucosa.
- In 85% of cases, ***the ischemia is self-limited*** and resolves without incident.

156. Ans. (b) May be associated with HNPCC, (c) Left-sided cancer presents..., (d) Left side colon is more commonly involved

[Ref: L and B 26th/ 1163-65; Schwartz 9th/1041-50; CSDT11th/ 719]

"Tumours of the left side of the colon which are far more common. It usually present with a change in bowel habit or rectal bleeding, while more proximal lesions typically present later with iron deficiency anaemia or a mass"- *L and B 26th/1164*

Table *(L and B 25th/ 1180)*: **Symptoms and signs of colorectal cancer**

- **Right-sided tumours:** Iron deficiency anaemia, abdominal mass
- **Left-sided tumours:** Rectal bleeding, alteration in bowel habit, tenesmus, obstruction
- **Metastatic disease:** Jaundice, ascites, hepatomegaly; other symptoms and signs from rarer sites of metastasis
- There may be considerable overlap between these symptoms

Carcinoma Right Colon

◈ *CSDT11th/ 719*

- The right colon has a large caliber and a thin and distensible wall, and the fecal content is fluid.
- Patients often see a physician for complaints of fatigue and weakness due to severe anemia. ***Unexplained microcytic hypochromic anemia should always raise the question of carcinoma of the colon.***
- *Alterations in bowel habits are not characteristic of carcinoma of the right colon,* and ***obstruction is uncommon.***

Carcinoma Left Colon

◈ *CSDT11th/ 719*

- The left colon has a smaller lumen than the right, and the feces are semisolid.
- Tumors of the left colon can gradually occlude the lumen, causing ***changes in bowel habits with alternating constipation and increased frequency of defecation*** (not true watery diarrhea).
- ***Partial or complete obstruction may be the initial picture.***

Colon and Rectal Cancers: HNPCC Association

◈ *Schwartz 9th/1046*

- **Hereditary Nonpolyposis Colon Cancer (Lynch's Syndrome)**: It is characterized by the ***development of colorectal carcinoma at an early age (average age, 40–45 years).***
- Approximately 70% of affected individuals will develop colorectal cancer. The risk of synchronous or metachronous colorectal carcinoma is 40%.

157. Ans. (e) Medullary carcinoma is associated with MEN-2b

[Ref: Harrison 19th/2305-08; Manipal Surgery 4th/339-45; L and B 26th/763-70; Sabiston 19th/904-11]

"Histologically, **papillary carcinomas** may exhibit papillary projections, a mixed pattern of papillary and follicular structures, or a pure follicular pattern ***(follicular variant).*** Other variants of papillary carcinoma include tall cell, ***insular***, columnar, diffuse sclerosing, clear cell, trabecular, and poorly differentiated types. These variants account for about 1% of all papillary carcinomas and are generally associated with a ***worse prognosis***"-*Schwartz 9th/1362*

*"**Irradiation to the neck during** childhood increases the risk of **papillary carcinoma**"- Manipal Surgery 4th/339*

*"**Follicular carcinoma** usually arise in a multinodular goiter especially in case of endemic goiter(**Iodine deficient areas**)"- Manipal Surgery 4th/343*

"**Follicular carcinomas** account for 10% of thyroid cancers and occur more commonly in ***iodine-deficient areas***"- *Schwartz 9th/1363*

Hürthle Cell Carcinoma

◈ *Sabiston 19th/ 912*

- Hürthle cell carcinoma is a subtype of follicular carcinoma that closely resembles FTC both grossly and on microscopic examination.
- Some studies have suggested that ***Hürthle cell carcinoma may have a worse clinical prognosis*** than standard FTC; however, there is no uniform agreement on these findings.
- ***Unlike papillary and follicular cancer, spread to local lymph nodes is a poor prognostic event associated with nearly 70% mortality***
- ***Higher chance of spread to lymph node compared to follicular carcinoma***-*Manipal 4th/347*

Follicular Carcinoma

◈ *L and B 26th/765*

- These appear to be macroscopically encapsulated but, ***microscopically, there is invasion of the capsule and of the vascular spaces in the capsular region***
- Blood-borne metastases are more common and the eventual ***mortality rate is twice that of papillary cancer.***
- Hurthle cell tumours are a variant of follicular neoplasm in which oxyphil (Hurthle, Askanazy) cells predominate histologically. ***Hurthle cell cancers are associated with a poorer prognosis*** and some hold that all Hurthle cell neoplasms are malignant

Medullary Carcinoma

◈ *Sabiston 19th/1005-06*

- MCT accounts for 3% to 9% of thyroid cancers and arises from ***parafollicular cell, or C cell***, derived from the neural crest.
- MCT is associated with the ***secretion of a biologic marker, calcitonin***.
- Medullary carcinoma can occur in a sporadic form or as part of ***MEN 2A or 2B***. MEN 2A usually has a more favorable long-term outcome than MEN 2B or sporadic MCT does

Table *(L and B)*: **Major differences between papillary and follicular carcinoma**

	Papillary(%)	Follicular (%)
Male incidence	22	35
Lymph node metastases	35	13
Blood vessel invasion	40	60
Recurrence rate	19	29
Overall mortality rate	11	24
Location of recurrent carcinoma		
Distant metastases	45	75
Nodal metastases	34	12
Local recurrence	20	12

158. Ans. (b) Concentric symmetric..., (c) Consists of esophageal mucosa..., (d) Dysphagia is usually..., (e) Association with...

[Ref: Manipal Surgery 4th/451; L and B 26th/1019-20; Schwartz 9th/845-46;Sabiston 19th/1037]

Schatzki Ring

◈ *Sabiston 19th/1037*

- Lying precisely at the squamocolumnar mucosal GEJ, this ring consists of a ***concentric symmetric narrowing*** representing an area of restricted distensibility of the lower esophagus.
- It consists of ***esophageal mucosa above and gastric mucosa below***, with variable amounts of muscularis mucosae, connective tissue, and submucosal fibrosis in between.
- It ***does not have a component of true esophageal muscle***, nor is it associated with esophagitis.
- It is often accompanied by a ***small hiatal hernia***, and some have advocated that it is a result of ***reflux esophagitis***
- Most patients with Schatzki's rings present with dysphagia. The ***dysphagia is usually to solid foods only*** and comes on abruptly with nearly complete obstruction.
- Diagnosis of a Schatzki's ring is made with a barium esophagram.

Most commonly it presents as ***intermittent dysphagia, especially to solid food***. A history of food impaction is also very common. Dysphagia is more common in patients with an associated motility disorder"-radiopaedia.org

"**Pathology: The pathogenesis of the Schatzki ring is unclear with conflicting hypotheses that include redundant pleats of mucosa, congenital abnormalities and modified peptic strictures. Interestingly, there is a reduced incidence of Barrett oesophagus in patients with a Schatzki ring.** Schatzki rings are located at the gastro-oesophageal junction, illustrated by the fact that there is ***squamous epithelium above and columnar epithelial below the ring***"- *radiopaedia.org*

Schatzki's Ring

◈ *L and B 26th/1019*

- Schatzki's ring is a circular ring in the distal oesophagus, usually at the squamocolumnar junction. The cause is obscure, but there is a ***strong association with reflux disease***.
- The core of the ring consists of variable amounts of ***fibrous tissue and cellular infiltrate***.

Schatzki's Ring

◈ *Schwartz 9th/845-46*

- Schatzki's ring is a ***thin submucosal circumferential ring*** in the lower esophagus at the squamocolumnar junction, often associated with a hiatal hernia.
- Barium esophagogram showing Schatzki's ring (i.e., ***a thin circumferential ring in the distal esophagus at the squamocolumnar junction***).
- Symptoms associated with Schatzki's ring are brief ***episodes of dysphagia during hurried ingestion of solid foods***.
- Its treatment has varied from dilation alone to dilation with antireflux measures, antireflux procedure alone.

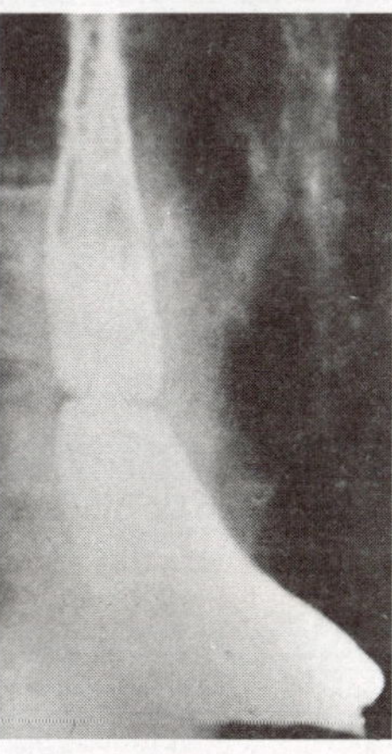

Fig: *(L and B 26th/ 1020)*: Schatzki's ring, a thin submucosal web ***completely encircling the whole of the lumen***, usually situated at the squamocolumnar junction

159. Ans. (a) Incidence decreased..., (b) Associated with H..., (c) More common in male..., (d) Better prognosis...

[Ref: Manipal Surgery 4th/487-90; L and B 26th/1045-48; Schwartz 9th/926-33; Sabiston 19th/1204-09]

The Diffuse form of Gastric Adenocarcinoma-linitis Plastica

◈ *Manipal Surgery 4th/491*

- ***Poorly differentiated***
- *Metastasis early*
- *More common in women*
- *Intraperitoneal metastases are frequent*
- *The* ***prognosis is less favourable*** *for patients with diffuse-subtype histology*

Gastric Carcinoma

◈ *Schwartz 9th/926-28*

- Over the past several decades, there has been a ***dramatic decrease in the gastric cancer*** incidence and death rate in most Western industrialized countries. This ***decrease has been largely in the so-called intestinal form rather than in the diffuse form*** of gastric cancer
- In younger patients, tumors are more often of the **diffuse variety** and tend to be ***large, aggressive, and more poorly differentiated, sometimes infiltrating*** the entire stomach (linitis plastic).

Pathology of Gastric Cancer

◈ *Sabiston 19th/1206-07*

- The Lauren system separates gastric adenocarcinoma into ***intestinal or diffuse types*** based on histology.
- The **intestinal variant** typically arises in the setting of a recognizable precancerous condition such as gastric atrophy or intestinal metaplasia. ***Men are more commonly affected than women***, and the incidence of the intestinal-type gastric adenocarcinoma ***increases with age***. The intestinal variety is ***well differentiated*** with a tendency to form glands. Metastatic spread is generally hematogenous to distant organs.
- The intestinal type is also the dominant histology in areas in which ***gastric cancer is epidemic, suggesting an environmental etiology.***
- An intermediate step in Correa's model of gastric cancer (intestinal type) development is intestinal metaplasia.
- **Intestinal metaplasia** occurs due to persistent irritation of the gastric mucosa, most commonly from ***H. pylori infection***.
- The risk for progression from ***intestinal metaplasia to gastric cancer*** is higher in the type III metaplasia than in type I

Table *(Sabiston 19th/1207)*: **Lauren classification system**

Intestinal	Diffuse
Environmental	Familial
Gastric atrophy, intestinal metaplasia	Blood type A
Men >women	Women >men
Increasing incidence with age	Younger age group
Gland formation	Poorly differentiated, signet ring cells
Hematogenous spread	Transmural/lymphatic spread
Microsatellite instability *APC* gene mutations	Decreased E-cadherin
p53, p16 inactivation	*p53, p16* inactivation

Table *(Schwartz 9th/928)*: **Factors increasing or decreasing the risk of gastric cancer**

Increase risk
Family history
Diet (high in nitrates, salt, fat)
Familial polyposis
Gastric adenomas
Hereditary nonpolyposis colorectal cancer
Helicobacter pylori infection: Atrophic gastritis, ***intestinal metaplasia***, dysplasia
Previous gastrectomy or gastrojejunostomy (>10 yr ago)
Tobacco use
Ménétrier's disease
Decrease risk
Aspirin
Diet (high fresh fruit and vegetable intake)
Vitamin C

160. Ans. (a) Appendix is the most common leading point, (c) Usually presents with pain without vomiting

[Ref: Manipal Surgery 4th/749-53; L and B 26th/114-15]

Intussusception in Children

◈ *L and B 26th/114-15*

- Most intussusceptions in children are seen from two months to two years of age. They are life-threatening.
- Intussusception typically causes a strangulating bowel obstruction, which can progress to gangrene and perforation.
- Intussusception is classified according to the site of the intussusceptum and intussuscipiens. In ***children, more than 80 per cent are ileocolic***, beginning several centimetres proximal to the ileocaecal valve with their apex found in the ascending or transverse colon.
- In the majority, the cause is hyperplasia of Peyer's patches (lymphoid tissue), which may be secondary to a viral infection. In 10 per cent of children, intussusception is secondary to a ***pathological lead point, such as a Meckel's diverticulum, enteric duplication cyst or even a small bowel lymphoma.*** Such cases are more likely in children over the age of two years and in those with recurrent intussusception.
- Classically, a previously healthy infant presents with ***colicky pain and vomiting*** (milk, then bile). Between episodes,

the child initially appears well. Later, they may pass a '*redcurrant jelly' stool.*

- Clinical signs include dehydration, abdominal distension and a palpable sausage-shaped mass in the right upper quadrant.
- A plain radiograph is rarely requested but if done it commonly shows signs of small bowel obstruction and a soft-tissue opacity. ***Diagnosis is confirmed on an abdominal ultrasound.***
- After resuscitation with intravenous fluids, broad-spectrum antibiotics and nasogastric drainage, non-operative reduction is attempted using an ***air enema***.
- ***More than 70 per cent of intussusceptions can be reduced nonoperatively***.
- If an operative reduction is needed, this is ***usually performed open***. The intussusception is milked distally by gentle compression from its apex. Both the intussusceptum and the intussuscipiens are inspected for areas of non-viability.
- *An irreducible intussusception or one complicated by infarction or a pathological lead point requires resection and primary anastomosis.*

Intussusception

- *Manipal Surgery 4th/749-53*
- Most common cause is idiopathic
- Most common type of non-operative ***reduction is by using air and barium enema***
- ***Most commonly used noninvasive test for diagnosis is ultrasound***-pseudokidney sign, target sign, duplex-assesses vascularity also

161. Ans. (a) Silk, (c) Polypropylene, (d) Polyester, (e) Nylon

[Ref: L and B 26th/37-38; Sabiston 19th/233]

Table *(L and B 26th/ 38)*: **Absorbable (Suture--Tensile strength retention in vivo)**

Catgut (Plain): Lost within 7–10 days

Catgut (Chromic): Lost within 21–28 days

Polyglactin: Approximately 60% remains at 2 weeks

Polyglyconate: Approximately 70% remains at 2 weeks

Polyglycolic: Approximately 40% remains at 1 week 2 weeks

Polydioxanone: Approximately 70% remains at 2 weeks

Polyglycaprone: 21 days maximum

Table *(L and B 26th/ 37)*: **Non-absorbable (Suture- Tensile strength)**

Nylon ***(Polyamide polymer):*** Loses 15–20% per year

Polyester: Infinite (>1 year)

Polybutester: Infinite (>1 year)

Polypropylene: Infinite (>1 year)

Table *(Sabiston 19th/233)*: **Comparison of absorbable sutures**

Suture	Types	Raw material	Tensile strength retention in vivo	Tissue reaction
Surgical Gut Suture	Chromic	Collagen derived from healthy beef and sheep	Individual patient characteristics can affect rate of tensile strength loss.	Moderate reaction
Monocryl Suture (poliglecaprone 25)	Monofilament	Copolymer of glycolide and epsilon-caprolactone	~50%-60% (violet: 60%-70%) remains at 1 week.	Minimal acute inflammatory reaction
Coated Vicryl Suture (polyglactin 910)	Braided Monofilament	Copolymer of lactide and glycolide coated with 370 and calcium stearate	~75% remains at 2 weeks. ~50% remains at 3 weeks.	Minimal acute inflammatory reaction
PDS II Suture (polydioxanone)	Monofilament	Polyester polymer	~70% remains at 2 weeks ~50% remains at 4 weeks ~25% remains at 6 weeks	Slight reaction

Table *(Sabiston 19th/233)*: **Comparison of Nonabsorbable Sutures**

Suture	Types	Raw Material	Tensile Strength Retention In Vivo	Tissue Reaction
Silk Suture	Braided	Organic protein called *fibroin*	Progressive degradation of fiber may result in gradual loss of tensile strength over time.	Acute inflammatory reaction
Nylon Suture	Monofilament	Long-chain aliphatic polymers Nylon 6 or Nylon 6,6	Progressive hydrolysis may result in gradual loss of tensile strength over time.	Minimal acute inflammatory reaction
Polyester Fiber Suture	Braided Monofilament	Poly (ethylene terephthalate)	No significant change known to occur in vivo.	Minimal acute inflammatory reaction
Polypropylene Suture	Monofilament	Isotactic crystalline stereoisomer of polypropylene	Not subject to degradation or weakening by action of tissue enzymes.	Minimal acute inflammatory reaction

A & E

162. Ans. (a) Can occurs due to environmental flora in OT, (b) Superficial infection require re-surgical...

[Ref: Manipal Surgery 4th/27-28; CSDT 14th/84-90; L and B 26th/50-66; Schwartz 9th/335-36,123-24; Sabiston 19th/244-46]

SSI: within 1 year if an implant is left in place (so option e is not correct as it mentioned after 1year)

Definition of SSI

◈ *CSDT 14th/84-90*

- The Centers for Disease Control and Prevention (CDC) define SSI as an infection that occurs at or near the surgical incision ***within 30 postoperative days of the surgical procedure***, or ***within 1 year if an implant is left in place*** (e.g., mesh, heart valve)
- The CDC further classifies SSI as: 1. Superficial incisional 2. Deep incisional 3. Organ/space SSI

Surgical Site Infection (SSI)

◈ *Manipal Surgery 4th/27-28*

- *Staph. aureus remains the most common pathogen in SSIs*
- *Main source of SSIs: Environment(this is from **operating room** and patient related)*
- ***Preoperative hair removal (clipping) should be done immediately before an operation***

Surgical Site Infection (SSI)

◈ *Sabiston 19th/244-46*

- By definition, they ***can occur anytime from 0 to 30 days after the operation or up to 1 year after a procedure that has involved the implantation of a foreign material (mesh, vascular graft, prosthetic joint, and so on).***
- Study has shown that *Staphylococcus aureus* remains the most common pathogen in SSIs, followed by coagulase-negative staphylococci, enterococci, and *Escherichia coli.*
- **Microorganisms** causing SSI can be either exogenous or endogenous. ***Exogenous microorganisms come from the operating team or from the environment around the surgical site*** (OR, equipment, air, water, and so on).
- ***Preoperative shaving has been shown to increase the incidence of SSI after clean procedures as well.***
- In general, the mainstay of treatment is source control or draining of the infected area. For a **superficial SSI** this involves ***opening the wound at the skin and subcutaneous levels and cleansing the wound***, along with dressing changes twice or three times a day.
- For organ/procedure-related SSI, source control can generally be achieved with percutaneous drainage.

"**Preoperative hair removal** has been correlated in several studies with a ***higher rate of SSI***, even when the procedure involves the scalp or the patient has abundant hair at the surgical site. A 2006 Cochrane database systematic review and meta-analysis concluded that ***preoperative shaving increases the rate of SSI by at least twofold***; it is noteworthy that there was no difference in the rates of SSI when hair clipping was compared to no hair removal. Therefore, ***if hair removal is deemed necessary, preoperative hair clipping is preferred to shaving***"-*CSDT 14th/87*

Table *(CSDT 14th/85):* **Criteria and definitions of surgical site infection**

Superficial incisional SSI	Deep incisional SSI	Organ/space SSI
Infection occurs *within 30 d* after the operative procedure *and* Involves only skin and subcutaneous tissue of the incision *and* Patient has at least one of the following: • Purulent drainage from the superficial incision. • Organisms isolated from an aseptically obtained culture of fluid or tissue from the superficial incision. • At least one of the following signs or symptoms of infection: pain or tenderness, localized swelling, redness, or heat, and superficial incision are deliberately opened by surgeon, and are culture-positive or not cultured. A culture-negative finding does not meet this criterion. • Diagnosis of superficial incisional SSI by the surgeon or attending physician.	Infection occurs *within 30 d* after the operative procedure if no implant is left in place or *within 1 y if implant* is in place and the infection appears to be related to the operative procedure *and* Involves deep soft tissues (eg, fascial and muscle layers) of the incision *and* Patient has at least one of the following: • Purulent drainage from the deep incision but not from the organ/space component of the surgical site. • A deep incision spontaneously dehisces or is deliberately opened by a surgeon and is culture-positive or not cultured and the patient has at least one of the following signs or symptoms: fever (> 38°C), or localized pain or tenderness. A culture-negative finding does not meet this criterion. • An abscess or other evidence of infection involving the deep incision is found on direct examination, during reoperation, or by histopathologic or radiologic examination. • Diagnosis of a deep incisional SSI by a surgeon or attending physician.	Infection occurs *within 30 d* after the operative procedure if no implant is left in place or *within 1 y if implant* is in place and the infection appears to be related to the operative procedure *and* Infection involves any part of the body, excluding the skin incision, fascia, or muscle layers, that is *opened or manipulated* during the operative procedure *and* Patient has at least one of the following: • Purulent drainage from a drain that is placed through a stab wound into the organ/space. • Organisms isolated from an aseptically obtained culture of fluid or tissue in the organ/space. • An abscess or other evidence of infection involving the organ/space that is found on direct examination, during reoperation, or by histopathologic or radiologic examination. • Diagnosis of an organ/space SSI by a surgeon or attending physician.

163. Ans. **(b) Should be given half an hour prior to surgery**

[Ref: CSDT 14th/88; L and B 26th/59-61; Manipal Surgery 4th/27-28; Sabiston 19th/250-55]

Table *(CSDT 14th/88)*: **Surgical Care Improvement Project (SCIP) measures aimed at prevention of surgical site infections.**

SCIP Infection Measure 1: Prophylactic antibiotic received within 1 h prior to surgical incision
SCIP Infection Measure 2: Appropriate prophylactic antibiotic selection for the surgical patient
SCIP Infection Measure 3: Prophylactic antibiotic discontinued within 24 h after surgery end time (within 48 h after cardiac surgery end time)
SCIP Infection Measure 4: Blood glucose level at 6 am < 200 mg/dL on postoperative days 1 and 2 in cardiac surgery
SCIP Infection Measure 6: ***No or appropriate hair removal (clippers not shaving)***
SCIP Infection Measure 7: Immediate postoperative normothermia (temperature > 96.8°F within 15 min postoperatively) in colorectal surgery

Prophylactic Antibiotic Therapy

◈ *Sabiston 19th/250-55; Sabiston 18th*

- "Antibiotic prophylaxis is ***indicated for most clean-contaminated and contaminated***(or potentially contaminated) operations.
- Antibiotic prophylaxis for **clean surgery is controversial.** ***When bone is incised (e.g. craniotomy, sternotomy) or a prosthesis is inserted, antibiotic prophylaxis is generally indicated***. Some controversy persists with clean surgery of soft tissue(e.g breast, hernia)"- *Sabiston 19th/251*
- Prophylactic antibiotic therapy is clearly ***more effective when begun preoperatively*** and ***continued through the intraoperative period***
- ***Antibiotics started as late as 1 to 2 hours after bacterial contamination are markedly less*** effective, and it is completely without value to start prophylactic antibiotics after the wound is closed.
- ***The optimal time to give parenteral antibiotic prophylaxis is within 1 hour prior to incision. Antibiotic given sooner are ineffective, as are agents given after incision is closed"- Sabiston 9th/252***
- ***It is unnecessary and may be detrimental to start them more than 1 hour preoperatively***, and it is ***unnecessary to give them after the patient leaves the operating room.***
- Prophylactic antibiotic coverage for ***more than 12 hours for a planned operation is never*** indicated.

Prophylactic Antibiotics

◈ *L and B 26th/59-61*

- If antibiotics are given to prevent infection after surgery or instrumentation, they should be used when local wound defenses are not established (the decisive period). ***Ideally, maximal blood and tissue levels should be present at the time at which the first incision is made and before contamination occurs. Intravenous administration at induction of anaesthesia is optimal.***
- In long operations or when there is excessive blood loss or when unexpected contamination occurs, ***antibiotics may be repeated at 4-hourly intervals during the surgery***, as tissue antibiotic levels often fall faster than serum levels.
- The ***use of the newer, broad-spectrum antibiotics for prophylaxis should be avoided***

Choice of Antibiotics for Prophylaxis

◈ *L and B 26th/61*

- Empirical cover against expected pathogens with local hospital guidelines
- Single-shot intravenous ***administration at induction of anaesthesia***
- Repeat only during long operations or if there is excessive blood loss

164. Ans. **(b) Wound contaminated with gross fecal material spillage**

[Ref: Schwartz 9th/123; L and B 26th/63; CSDT 14th/86]

Appendicular perforation- Type IV
Incision through abscess- Type IV
Surgery over a clean site-Type I
Wound in urinary tract without unusual contamination-type II

Wound Class

◈ *Schwartz 9th/123*

- *Clean wounds* (class I) include those in which no infection is present; only skin microflora potentially contaminate the wound, and ***no hollow viscus that contains microbes is entered***. Class I D wounds are similar except that a prosthetic device (e.g., mesh or valve) is inserted.
- *Clean/contaminated wounds* (class II) include those in which a ***hollow viscus such as the respiratory, alimentary, or genitourinary tracts with indigenous bacterial flora is opened under controlled circumstances without significant spillage of contents.***
- *Contaminated wounds* (class III) include open accidental wounds encountered early after injury, those with extensive introduction of bacteria into a normally sterile area of the body due to major breaks in sterile technique (e.g., open cardiac massage), ***gross spillage of viscus contents such as from the intestine, or incision through inflamed, albeit nonpurulent tissue.***
- *Dirty wounds* (class IV) include traumatic wounds in which a significant delay in treatment has occurred and in which necrotic tissue is present, those created in the presence of overt infection as evidenced by the presence of purulent material, and those created to ***access a perforated viscus*** accompanied by a high degree of contamination.

Table *(Schwartz 9th/123)*: **Wound class examples of cases expected infection rates**

Wound class	Example of class	Expected infection rate
Clean (class I)	Hernia repair, breast biopsy specimen	1-2%
Clean/contaminated (class II)	Cholecystectomy, elective GI surgery (not colon)	2.1%-9.5%
Clean/contaminated (class II)	Colorectal surgery	4-14%
Contaminated (class III)	Penetrating abdominal trauma, large tissue injury, enterotomy during bowel obstruction	3.4-13.2%
Dirty (class IV)	Perforated diverticulitis, necrotizing soft tissue infections	3.1-12.8%

Table *(L and B 26th/63)*: **Surgical site infection (SSI) rates relating to wound contamination**

Type of surgery	Infection rate (%)	Rate before prophylaxis
Clean (no viscus opened)	1–2	The same
Clean-contaminated (***viscus opened, minimal spillage***)	<10	Gastric surgery up to 30% Biliary surgery up to 200%
Contaminated (***open viscus with spillage or inflammatory disease)***	15–20	Variable but up to 60%
Dirty (pus or perforation, or incision through an abscess)	<40	Up to 60% or more

Table *(CSDT 14th/86)*: **Wound classification**

Clean	These are uninfected operative wounds in which no inflammation is encountered and the respiratory, alimentary, genital, or uninfected urinary tracts are not entered.
Clean/Contaminated	These are operative wounds in which the respiratory, alimentary, genital, or urinary tract is entered under controlled conditions and without unusual contamination.
Contaminated	These include open, fresh, accidental wounds, operations with major breaks in sterile technique or gross spillage from the gastrointestinal tract, and incisions in which acute, nonpurulent inflammation is encountered.
Dirty	These include old traumatic wounds with retained deviatlized tissue and those that involve existing clinical infection or perforated viscera.

165. Ans. (a) Seminoma is more..., (b) Cryptorchidism is associated..., (c) Retroperitoneal LN dissection..., (d) Usually presents as...

[Ref: Manipal Surgery 4th/994-99; L and B 26th/1385-87; Robbins 9th/975-79;Schwartz 9th/1462; Sabiston 19th/1858]

"Seminomas are the most common type of germ cell tumor, making up about 50% of these tumors. The peak incidence is the third decade and they almost never occur in infants"- *Robbins 9th/976*

Testicular Tumors

◈ *CSDT 14th/1008-09*

- Metastases first develop in the retroperitoneal nodes; right-sided tumors metastasize primarily to the interaortocaval region just below the renal vessels and left-sided tumors primarily to the left para-aortic area at the same level.
- Testicular tumors present as a ***painless firm mass*** within the testicular substance. They often have been present for several months before the patient seeks consultation. Occasionally (10%), a hydrocele is present
- ***Following orchiectomy, three management options*** are available: (i) active surveillance, (ii) ***retroperitoneal lymph node dissection (RPLND),*** and (iii) systemic chemotherapy
- ***RPLND is recommended for clinical stage I patients*** (no evidence of metastatic disease on imaging) or for those with ***retroperitoneal lymphadenopathy that is not bulky (stage IIA-IIB***).

Table *(CSDT 14th/1009)*: **Treatment and prognosis of testicular cancer related to tumor stage**

Conventional stage	TNM stage	Clinical findings	Treatment	Five-Year Survival (%)
I	T1	Confined to testicle	Nonseminoma: RPLND vs. Surveillance; Seminoma: irradiation	>95
IIA	N1	Regional nodes <2cm	Adjuvant chemotherapy Nonseminoma: RPLND or chemotherapy; Seminoma: XRT or chemotherapy	>90
IIB	N2	Nodes 2-5 cm	Adjuvant chemotherapy Nonseminoma; RPLND or adjuvant chemotherapy; Seminoma: XRT or chemotherapy	>85
IIC III	N3 M+	Nodes > 5 cm Distant metastases	Chemotherapy followed by resection of residual disease	~70

Contd...

Testicular Cancer

◈ *Schwartz 9th/1462*

- Most men are diagnosed with an ***asymptomatic enlarging mass.***
- A ***major risk for the development of testicular cancer is cryptorchidism***

Testicular Tumour

◈ *Manipal Surgery 4th/994-99*

- *Seminoma is the most common type of germ cell tumour*
- ***Undescended testis, undoubtedly predisposes to seminoma***

"***Nonseminomatous germ cell tumours are usually associated with dedescended testes***"*-Sabiston 19th/1858*

Tumours of the Teste

◈ *L and B 26th/1385-87*

- The peak incidence of seminomas is in the fourth decade of life with the non-seminomatous germ cell tumours being more common in the third decade of life. They are the most common form of tumour in young men.
- Risk factors include a history of ***testicular maldescent***, a history of a contralateral testicular tumour and Klinefelter's syndrome.
- ***Seminomas metastasise mainly via the lymphatics*** and haematogenous spread is uncommon.
- Usually the patient presents with a ***painless testicular lump***.
- A sensation of heaviness can occur if the testis is two or three times its normal size, but ***only a minority of patients experience pain***. Some cases may simulate epididymo-orchitis and rarely some patients present with severe pain and acute enlargement of the testis because of haemorrhage into the tumour. Such cases can occasionally mimic testicular torsion.
- In ***1–2 per cent of cases, the tumour is bilateral at the time of diagnosis***.
- *"**Radical inguinal orchidectomy** is the treatment of choice in all testicular tumour irrespective of the histological type and stage" (Manipal Surgery 4th/997)*

Classification and pathology-Tumours of the testis are classified according to their predominant cellular type:

- Germ cell tumours (90–95% per cent) (these include seminoma, embryonal cell carcinoma, yolk sac tumor, teratoma, and choriocarcinoma);
- Interstitial tumours (1–2 per cent) (these include Leydig cell tumours);
- Lymphoma (3–7 per cent);
- Other tumours (1–2 per cent).

166. Ans. (b) Courvoisier law related to pancreatic head cancer, (c) Cholangitis presents with fever and jaundice

[Ref: Manipal Surgery 4th/566; PJM 20th/20; Schwartz 9th/1149; Davidson 22nd/ 937-38; Land B 26th/1115]

Cholangiocarcinoma

◈ *L and B 26th/1115*

- Early symptoms of cholangiocarcinoma are often non-specific with abdominal pain, early satiety, anorexia and weight loss commonly seen. Symptoms associated with ***biliary obstruction*** (prurit's and jaundice) may be present in a minority of patients.
- In these patients, examination often demonstrates clinical signs of jaundice, cachexia is often noticeable and a palpable gall bladder is present if the obstruction is in the ***distal common bile duct (Courvoisier's sign)***.

"***Stone in CBD: Intermittent pain, intermittent fever and intermittent jaundice are classical of stone in CBD***"*-Manipal Surgery 4th/566*

"**Cholangitis**: The most common presentation is fever, epigastric or right upper quadrant pain, and jaundice. These classic symptoms, well known as *Charcot's triad*, are present in about two thirds of patients. The illness may progress rapidly with septicemia and disorientation, known as *Reynolds' pentad* (e.g., fever, jaundice, right upper quadrant pain, septic shock, and mental status changes)"- *Schwartz 9th/1149*

Obstructive (Cholestatic) Jaundice

◈ *Davidson 22nd/ 937-38*

- Obstruction of the bile duct drainage due to blockage of the extrahepatic biliary tree is characteristically associated with pale stools and dark urine.
- Pruritus may be a dominant feature and can be accompanied by skin excoriations. Peripheral stigmata of chronic liver disease are absent.
- ***If the gallbladder is palpable, the jaundice is unlikely to be caused by biliary obstruction due to gallstones, probably because a chronically inflamed stone-containing gallbladder cannot readily dilate. This is Courvoisier's Law, and suggests that jaundice is due to a malignant biliary obstruction (e.g. pancreatic cancer).***
- Cholestatic jaundice is characterised by a relatively greater elevation of ALP and GGT than the aminotransferases.

Table *(Davidson 22nd/ 937)*: **Clinical features suggesting an underlying cause of cholestatic jaundice**

Feature	Cause
Static or increasing jaundice:	Carcinoma, Primary biliary cirrhosis, Primary sclerosing cholangitis
Fluctuating jaundice:	Choledocholithiasis, Stricture, Pancreatitis, Choledochal cyst, Primary sclerosing cholangitis
Abdominal pain:	Choledocholithiasis, Pancreatitis, Choledochal cyst
Cholangitis:	Stone, Stricture, Choledochal cyst
Abdominal scar:	Stone, Stricture
Irregular hepatomegaly:	Hepatic carcinoma
Palpable gallbladder:	Carcinoma below cystic duct (usually pancreas)
Abdominal mass:	Carcinoma, Pancreatitis (cyst), Choledochal cyst
Occult blood in stools:	Ampullary tumour

Table *(PJM 20th/20)*: **Differential diagnosis of obstructive jaundice (partial list)**

- Urine Bilirubin: Present
- Urine Urobilinogen: Absent
- Stools Sterocobilinogen: Absent

167. Ans. (b) qSOFA should be assessed in..., (c) Suggest against the use of IV..., (e) Recommend empiric broad-...

[Ref: Harrison 19th/1758; www.foamcast.org/2017/01/19; jamanetwork.com/journal;Schwartz 9th/128-29]

As this Q is asked in November, 2016; we try to find answer of this Q according to 2012 Surviving Sepsis guidelines (Because latest, 2016 guideline issued in Jan, 2017)

"The **2016 Surviving Sepsis guidelines** produced by the Society of Critical Care Medicine and the European Society of Intensive Care Medicine have been released. Many of the guideline recommendations remain unchanged from previous versions but include in depth rationales from studies published since the 2012 guidelines were released. The 2016 guidelines cover the treatment of sepsis and septic shock in depth and include recommendations including ***fluid resuscitation, vasopressor selection, antimicrobial therapy, mechanical ventilation, blood and blood products, insulin adminstration, DVT and stress ulcer prophylaxis, and nutrition therapy***"

Surviving Sepsis Guidelines *2012*

❖ *jamanetwork.com/journal*

- "Notably, ***recombinant human activated protein C was completely omitted from the 2012 guidelines(in 2008 guideline it recommended for use in some selected situations)***, prompted by the voluntary removal of the drug by the manufacturer after failing to show benefit"-"- *www.the-hospitalist.org*
- "A ***higher SOFA score is associated with an increased probability of mortality***. The score grades abnormality by organ system and accounts for clinical interventions. However, laboratory variables, namely, ***Pao_2, platelet count, creatinine level, and bilirubin level, are needed for full computation***. Furthermore, selection of variables and cutoff values were developed by consensus, and *SOFA is not well known outside the critical care community*"- *jamanetwork.com/journal*
- Organ dysfunction can be identified as an acute change in total **SOFA score** ≥2 points consequent to the infection.
- A SOFA score ≥2 reflects an overall mortality risk of approximately 10% in a general hospital population with suspected infection.
- Patients with suspected infection who are likely to have a **prolonged ICU stay** or to die in the hospital can be promptly identified at the bedside with qSOFA, ie, alteration in mental status, systolic blood pressure ≤100 mm Hg, or respiratory rate ≥22/min.
- We recommend that administration of **IV antimicrobials** be initiated as soon as possible after recognition and ***within 1 h*** for both sepsis and septic shock (strong recommendation, moderate quality of evidence; grade applies to both conditions).
- We recommend **empiric broad-spectrum therapy** with one or more antimicrobials for patients presenting with sepsis or septic shock to cover all likely pathogens
- We suggest **against using IV hydrocortisone** to treat septic shock patients if adequate fluid resuscitation and vasopressor therapy are able to restore hemodynamic stability.
- We recommend **against the use of erythropoietin for treatment of anemia** associated with sepsis (strong recommendation, moderate quality of evidence).
- We suggest **against the use of IV immunoglobulins** in patients with sepsis or septic shock (weak recommendation, low quality of evidence).

Surviving Sepsis Campaign Recommendation Highlights

	2012	2016
Sepsis Definition	Systemic manifestation of infection + suspected infection Severe sepsis: sepsis + organ dysfunction	Life threatening organ dysfunction caused by dysregulated response to infection, No severe sepsis category
Initial Resuscitation	At least 30 cc/kg in first 3 hours Crystalloid fluid (no recommendations on 0.9% NaCl vs balanced solution) Albumin if patients require "substantial" fluids (weak)	
	Protocolized care including CVP $ScVO_2$ Normalize lactate	Use dynamic resuscitation markers (passive leg raise) Target MAP of 65 mmHg Reassess hemodynamic status to guide resuscitation Normalize lactate
Vasopressors	Target MAP of 65 mmHg • Norepinephrine • Epinephrine if not at target MAP OR vasopressin to reduce norepinephrine requirement • Avoid dopamine in most patients	
Steroids	Only indicated for patients with septic shock refractory to adequate fluids and vasopressors	
Antibiotics	One or more antibiotics active against presumed pathogen Combination therapy (double coverage) for neutropenic patients and pseudomonas	Initial broad spectrum antibiotics (ex: vancomycin+ piperacillin-tazobactam) Against combined therapy (i.e. do not double cover pseudomonas) May use procalcitonin to guide de-escalation

Contd...

Surviving Sepsis Campaign Recommendation Highlights		
	2012	**2016**
Source Control	Achieve within 12 hours, if feasible	Achieve as soon as medically and logically feasible
Ventilator	6 cc/kg tidal volume prone patients with severe ARDS (PF <150 in 2017 guidelines)	
	No recommendation	Against high frequency oscillatory ventilation (HFOV)
	Weak recommendation for noninvasive ventilation in select patients with sepsis induced ARDS	Unable to make recommendation on noninvasive ventilation

The New Surviving Sepsis Guideline 2016 (Earlier Guidelines Issued in 2012, 2008, 2004) is Being Rolled out in Nsw in January 2017: Summary of New Recommendations *emergencypedia.com*

- **Time to antibiotics** within 60 minutes for patients with Sepsis (SOFA>=2), septic shock patients which essentially implies anyone with qSOFA and/or organ dysfunction
- **Lactate** measurement and targeting lactate reduction in those who have an elevated as a serial marker
- **Blood cultures** before antibiotics (unless there is going to be significant delay)
- Early Empiric broad spectrum **Antibiotic** therapy for all sepsis patients (refer to local guidelines)
- There is no mention of C-reactive protein anywhere in document
- **Fluid Challenge** for fluid resuscitation (rather than '*drip*' method)
- What fluid? The usual crystalloids first, albumin next (NO 'GEL' and NO SPECIAL COLLOIDS)
- **Fluid Volume** – up to 30ml/kg
- What about **Inotropes**? – Norepinephrine – Vasopressin – Dobutamine OR Adrenaline in that order...
- No routine use **Steroids** unless specific other indication(s)

168. Ans. (a) Vagotomy- decreases acid..., (d) Billroth I gastrectomy has high rate..., (e) Highly selective vagotomy has low...

[Ref: Manipal Surgery 4th/471-75; L and B 26th/1036-40; Schwartz 9th/942]

"Typically, 15 to 30 minutes after a meal, the patient becomes diaphoretic, weak, light-headed, and tachycardic. These symptoms may be ameliorated by recumbence or saline infusion. Crampy abdominal pain is not uncommon and diarrhea often follows. This is referred to as ***early dumping,*** and should be distinguished from **postprandial (reactive) hypoglycemia,** *also called* ***late dumping,*** which usually occurs later (2–3 hours following a meal), and is relieved by the administration of sugar"- *Schwartz 9th/942*

Billroth I Gastrectomy

◈ *L and B 26th/1038*

- The distal stomach is mobilised and resected in the same way as in the Billroth II gastrectomy. This resection should include the ulcer that is usually situated on the lesser curve.
- The incidence of recurrent ulceration after this operation is low, ***but it carries with it the morbidity and mortality associated with any gastric resection.***

Truncal Vagotomy and Drainage

◈ *L and B 26th/1037*

- The principle of the operation is that section of the vagus nerves, ***which are critically involved in the secretion of gastric acid, reduces the maximal acid output by approximately 50 per cent.***

Highly Selective Vagotomy

◈ *L and B 26th/1037–38*

- In this only the parietal cell mass of the stomach was denervated
- ***This proved to be the most satisfactory operation for duodenal ulceration,*** with a low incidence of side effects and acceptable recurrence rates when performed to a high technical standard.

Early Dumping

◈ *L and B 26th/1039*

- Early dumping consists of ***abdominal and vasomotor symptoms***
- The principal treatment is dietary manipulation. Small, dry meals are best, and avoiding fluids with a high carbohydrate content also helps.

Late Dumping

◈ *L and B 26th/1039*

- This is ***reactive hypoglycaemia.*** The carbohydrate load in the small bowel causes a rise in the plasma glucose, which, in turn, causes insulin levels to rise, causing a ***secondary hypoglycaemia.***
- This can be easily demonstrated by serial measurements of blood glucose in a patient following a test meal. The treatment is essentially the same as for early dumping. Octreotide is very effective in dealing with this problem.

Table *(Land B 26th/1039)*: **Operative mortality, side effects and incidence of recurrence following duodenal ulcer operations.**

Operation	Operative mortality (%)	Significant side effects (%)	Recurrent ulceration (%)
Gastrectomy	1–2	20–40	1–4
Gastroenterostomy alone	< 1	10–20	50
Truncal vagotomy and drainage	< 1	10–20	2–7
Selective vagotomy and drainage	< 1	10–20	5–10

Contd...

A & E

Operation	Operative mortality (%)	Significant side effects (%)	Recurrent ulceration (%)
Highly selective vagotomy	<0.2	<5	2–10
Truncal vagotomy and antrectomy	1	10–20	1

Table *(L and B 26th/1039):* **Features of early and late dumping**

	Early	Late
Incidence	5–10%	5%
Relation to meals	Almost immediate	Second hour after meal
Duration of attack	30–40 minutes	30–40 minutes
Relief	Lying down	Food
Aggravated by	More food	Exercise
Precipitating factor	Food, especially carbohydrate-rich and wet	As early dumping
Major symptoms	Epigastric fullness, sweating, light-headedness, tachycardia, colic, sometimes diarrhoea	Tremor, faintness, prostration

169. Ans. (a) Maintain moisture in wound, (b) Provides mechanical support, (c) Prevents microbial entry

[Ref: L and B 26th/60; Schwartz 9th/229-30; Sabiston 19th/170-71]

"Occlusive dressing class provides moisture retention, mechanical protection and a barrier to bacteria"*- Sabiston 19th/170*

Wide mesh gauze is composition of absorptive dressing- *Sabiston 19th/171*

Wound Dressings

◈ *Sabiston 19th/170-71*

- Wound dressings can be categorized into **four classes:** ***nonadherent fabrics; absorptive dressings; occlusive dressings; and creams, ointments, and solutions.***
- The rate of epithelialization under an occlusive dressing was twice that of a wound that was left uncovered and allowed to dry.
- Placement of an occlusive dressing over the wound provides a ***mildly acidic pH and low oxygen tension on the wound*** surface. The steep oxygen gradient is a ***good environment for proliferation of fibroblasts and formation of granulation tissue.***
- A relatively occlusive dressing is a good choice for many wounds; however, ***other options would be beneficial in wounds that have a significant amount of exudate or wounds with high bacterial counts.***
- ***If the wound has a heavy amount of exudate, it is crucial to have a dressing that has a degree of absorption.*** The skin surrounding the wound can become macerated with large amounts of uncontrolled exudate. These wounds require a dressing that reduces the bacterial load within the wound while removing the exudate produced. ***Placement of a pure occlusive dressing without bactericidal properties will allow bacterial overgrowth and worsen the infection.***
- ***Occlusive dressing class can be divided into- biological and non-biological dressing***

Dressing

◈ *Schwartz 9th/229-30*

- **Absorbent Dressings:** Accumulation of wound fluid can lead to maceration and bacterial overgrowth. Ideally, the dressing should absorb without getting soaked through, as this would permit bacteria from the outside to enter the wound. The dressing must be designed ***to match the exudative properties of the wound*** and may include cotton, wool, and sponge.
- **Nonadherent Dressings:** Nonadherent dressings are impregnated with paraffin, petroleum jelly, or water-soluble jelly for use as nonadherent coverage.
- **Occlusive and Semiocclusive Dressings.** Occlusive and semiocclusive dressings provide a good environment for clean, minimally exudative wounds. ***These film dressings are waterproof and impervious to microbes but permeable to water vapor and oxygen.***
- **Hydrophilic and Hydrophobic Dressings:** These dressings are components of a composite dressing. Hydrophilic dressing aids in absorption, whereas a hydrophobic dressing is waterproof and prevents absorption.
- **Hydrocolloid and Hydrogel Dressings.** Hydrocolloid and hydrogel dressings attempt to ***combine the benefits of occlusion and absorbency.***

Table *(Sabiston 19th/171):* **Types of occlusive dressing (Non-biologic and biologic)**

Category	Composition and characteristic	Function	Comments
1. Nonbiologic		Insulation, moisture retention, protective barrier acts against bacteria	
Films	Clear polyurethane membranes with acrylic adhesive on one side	See above	Waterproof; permeable to oxygen, carbon dioxide, and water vapor; do not interfere with patient function; allow visualization of wound; nonabsorptive, can leak; require intact skin around wound area: wound contraction may be slowed, removal may disrupt new epithelium

Contd...

Category	Composition and characteristic	Function	Comments
Hydrocolloids	Hydrocolloid matrix (gelatin, pectin, carboxymethyl cellulose)	As above; absorbs water from wound exudates, swells, liquefies to form moist gel	Available as adhesive wafers, paste, powders; similar features as films, but bulkier; more protection but may interfere more with function
Algintes	Cellulose-like polysaccharide fibers derived from calcium salt of alginate (seaweed)	As above; calcium alginate conversion to soluble sodium salt following contact with wound exudates results in hydrophilic gel	Occlusive environment; various forms–ropes, ribbons, pads
Hydrogels	Polyethylene oxide or carboxymethyl cellulose polymer and water (80%)	As above; rehydrating agents for dry wounds; little water absorption (high water content	Available as gels, sheets, impregnated gauze; occlusive environment
2. Biologic		Similar to nonbiologics	
Homograft	Derived from genetically unique humans		Temporary dressing; is rejected if left on wound for extended period
Xenograft	Interspecies graft (e.g., pig)		Same as above
Amnion	Human placenta		Good biologic dressing
Skin substitutes	Different compositions		Integra–bilayered membrane skin substitute; AlloDerm–acelluler cadaveric dermis; apligraf–living, bilayered, biologic dressing composed of neonatal dermal fibroblasts on collagen matrix

170. Ans. (b) B/L milky discharge with squeezing from multiple ducts

[Ref: L and B 26th/802; Schwartz 9th/467; Sabiston 19th/828]

Pathologic Discharge

www.aafp.org/afp

- Nipple discharge is classified as pathologic if it is ***spontaneous, unilateral, bloody, serous, clear, or associated with a mass.***
- Mammography and subareolar ultrasonography should be performed in patients with nipple discharge that is unilateral, spontaneous, clear, serous, bloody, or associated with a mass.

Physiologic Discharge

www.aafp.org/afp

- ***Physiologic discharge is usually bilateral, involves multiple ducts, and is associated with nipple stimulation or breast compression.***
- ***Bilateral milky nipple discharge*** is appropriate during pregnancy and lactation, and may persist for up to one year postpartum or after cessation of breastfeeding.
- **Bilateral milky white discharge** in persons who are not pregnant or lactating is called ***galactorrhea***;
- A human chorionic gonadotropin pregnancy test should be performed in patients with galactorrhea to rule out pregnancy. If negative, prolactin and thyroid-stimulating hormone levels should be obtained to determine the presence of an endocrinopathy.
- Medications that inhibit dopamine and are associated with physiologic nipple discharge.

Unilateral Nipple Discharge

Schwartz 9th/467

- ***It may be suggestive of cancer if it is spontaneous, unilateral, localized to a single duct, present in women ≥40 years of age, bloody, or associated with a mass.***
- ***Nipple discharge associated with a cancer may be clear, bloody, or serous.***

Bilateral Nipple Discharge

Schwartz 9th/467

- ***Nipple discharge is suggestive of a benign condition if it is bilateral and multiductal in origin, occurs in women ≤39 years of age, or is milky or blue-green.***
- ***Prolactin-secreting pituitary adenomas are responsible for bilateral nipple discharge in <2% of cases.***

Discharges from the Nipple

L and B 26th/802

- ***A clear, serous discharge may be 'physiological' in a parous woman*** or may be associated with a duct papilloma or mammary dysplasia.

- ***Multiduct, multicoloured discharge is physiological and the patient may be reassured.***

Nipple Discharge

◈ *Sabiston 19th/828*

- A milky discharge from both breasts is termed ***galactorrhea.*** In the absence of lactation or a history of recent lactation, ***galactorrhea may be associated with increased production of prolactin***.
- However, true galactorrhea is rare and is diagnosed only when the discharge is milky (contains lactose, fat, and milk-specific proteins).
- ***Unilateral, nonmilky discharge coming from one duct orifice is surgically significant and warrants special attention. However, the underlying cause is rarely a breast malignancy.***
- The ***most common cause of spontaneous nipple discharge from a single duct is a solitary intraductal papilloma*** in one of the large subareolar ducts under the nipple.
- In summary, ***nipple discharge that is bilateral and comes from multiple ducts is not usually a surgical problem. Bloody discharge from a single duct, does require surgical biopsy to establish a diagnosis***. Intraductal papilloma is found in most of these cases.

Discharges from the Nipple

◈ *L and B 26th/802*

Discharge from a Single Duct

Blood-stained: Intraduct papilloma, Intraduct carcinoma, Duct ectasia

Serous (any colour): Fibrocystic disease, Duct ectasia, Carcinoma

Discharge from More than One Duct

Blood-stained: Carcinoma, Ectasia, Fibrocystic disease

Black or green: Duct ecstasia

Purulent: Infection

Serous: Fibrocystic disease, Duct ectasia, Carcinoma

Milk: Lactation, Rare causes (hypothyroidism, pituitary tumour)

Table *(CSDT 14th/300):* **Characteristics of nipple discharge in the nonpregnant, nonlactating woman**

Finding	Significance
Serous	Most likely benign FCC(fibrocystic condition), ie, duct ectasia
Bloody	More likely neoplastic–papilloma, carcinoma
Associated mass	More likely neoplastic
Unilateral	Either neoplastic or non-neoplastic
Bilateral	Most likely non-neoplastic
Single duct	More likely FCC
Milky	Endocrine disorders, medications
Spontaneous	Either neoplastic or non-neoplastic
Produced by pressure at single site	Either neoplastic or non-neoplastic

171. Ans. (d) No malignant potential, (e) Biopsy is required for diagnosis

[Ref: CSDT 14th/301; Robbins 9th/1047L and B 26th/803; Sabiston 19th/840]

Traumatic Fat Necrosis

◈ *L and B 26th/803*

- Traumatic fat necrosis may be acute or chronic and usually occurs in stout, middle-aged women.
- ***Following a blow, or even indirect violence*** (e.g. contraction of the pectoralis major), a lump, often painless, appears.
- This may mimic a carcinoma, even displaying skin tethering and nipple retraction, and ***biopsy is required for diagnosis. A history of trauma is not diagnostic*** as this may merely have drawn the patient's attention to a preexisting lump.

Fat Necrosis

◈ *CSDT 14th/301*

- Fat necrosis is a rare lesion of the breast but is of clinical importance because it produces a mass (often accompanied by skin or nipple retraction) that is ***usually indistinguishable from carcinoma even with imaging studies.***
- ***Trauma is presumed to be the cause, though only about 50% of patients give a history of injury. The safest course is to obtain a biopsy. Needle biopsy is often adequate,*** but frequently the entire mass must be excised, primarily to exclude carcinoma.

Fat Necrosis

◈ *Sabiston 19th/840*

- Fat necrosis can mimic cancer by producing a palpable mass or a ***density on mammography that may contain calcifications.***
- Fat necrosis may ***follow an episode of trauma to the breast, but frequently there is no history of trauma.***
- This lesion has ***no malignant potential.***

Fat Necrosis

◈ *Robbins 9th/1047*

- Fat necrosis can present as a painless palpable mass, skin thickening or retraction, a mammographic density, or ***mammographic calcifications.***
- The majority of women will give a history of trauma or prior surgery.
- The major clinical significance of the condition is ***its possible confusion with breast carcinoma as a palpable mass or mammographic calcifications.***

172. Ans. (a) Viscera covered by peritoneum, (b) Viscera covered by amniotic..., (d) Commonly associated with...

[Ref: CSDT 14th/1258-59; Schwartz 9th/1442-43;Nelson 19th(SAE)/891]

"Defects in abdominal wall closure may lead to omphalocele or gastroschisis. In **omphalocele**, viscera protrude through an open umbilical ring and are ***covered by a sac derived from the amnion***. In **gastroschisis**, the viscera protrude through a defect lateral to the umbilicus and ***no sac is present***"-*Schwartz 9th/1271*

*"The majority (~75%) of infants with omphalocele have associated congenital anomalies/syndrome, including **Beckwith-Wiedemann syndrome and other chromosomal (29%, including trisomies 13 and 18) and nonchromosomal (45%) multiple and isolated congenital anomalies (musculoskeletal-24%; urogenital-20%; cardiovascular-15% and central nervous system-9%)**"-Nelson 19th (SAE)/891*

Omphalocele

◈ *CSDT 14th/1258-59*

- This is a midline abdominal wall defect noted in 1:5000 live births. The abdominal viscera (commonly liver and bowel) are contained within a ***sac composed of peritoneum and amnion from which the umbilical cord arises at the apex and center***.
- When the defect is less than 4 cm, it is termed as hernia of the umbilical cord; when greater than 10 cm, it is termed a giant omphalocele.
- Associated abnormalities occur in 30%-70% of infants and include, in descending order of frequency, ***chromosomal abnormalities (trisomy 13, 18, 21)***, congenital heart disease (tetralogy of Fallot, atrial septal defect), ***Beckwith-Wiedemann syndrome*** (large-for-gestational-age baby; hyperinsulinism; visceromegaly of kidneys, adrenal glands, and pancreas; macroglossia, hepatorenal tumors, cloacal extrophy), pentalogy of Cantrell, and prune belly syndrome (absent abdominal wall muscles, genitourinary abnormalities, cryptorchidism).

Omphalocele

◈ *Schwartz 9th/1442-43*

- Omphalocele refers to a congenital defect of the abdominal wall in which the bowel and solid viscera are ***covered by peritoneum and amniotic membrane***
- Omphalocele occurs in association with special syndromes such as exstrophy of the cloaca (vesicointestinal fissure), the ***Beckwith-Wiedemann*** constellation of anomalies etc.

173. Ans. (a) Drooling of saliva, (c) Nasogastric tube cannot..., (d) May be associated with..., (e) Abdominal distension

[Ref: CSDT 14th/1233; L and B 26th/118; Schwartz 9th/1420-22]

Oesophageal Atresia

◈ *L and B 26th/118*

- Affected infants ***present soon after birth with drooling and cyanotic episodes on attempting to feed***.
- There may have been ***polyhydramnios*** due to failure to swallow amniotic fluid.
- The diagnosis is ***confirmed when a nasogastric tube goes no further than the upper oesophageal pouch on the chest x-ray and abdominal gas signifies the tracheo-oesophageal fistula***
- Associated anomalies are common and include ***cardiac, renal and skeletal defects.***
- "There is a **50% incidence of associated anomalies**: cardiac (patent ductus arteriosus, septal defects), GI (imperforate anus, duodenal atresia), genitourinary, and skeletal.
- The **VACTERL association (vertebral, anorectal, cardiac, tracheoesophageal, renal, and limb anomalies)** is present in 25% of cases. Isolated esophageal atresia has been associated with various genetic abnormalities, including trisomy 18 and trisomy 21"-*CSDT 14th/1233*
- Repair is usually via a right-sided extrapleural thoracotomy within a day or two of birth. The fistula is divided and the tracheal side closed. The oesophageal ends are then anastomosed.

Esophageal Atresia and Tracheoesophageal Fistula

◈ *Schwartz 9th/1420-22*

- Esophageal atresia (EA) with tracheoesophageal fistula (TEF) is one of the most gratifying pediatric surgical conditions to treat.
- There are five major varieties of EA and TEF. The most commonly seen variety is EA with distal TEF (type C), which occurs in approximately 85% of the cases in most series.
- When the esophagus ends either as a blind pouch or as a fistula into the trachea (as in types A, B, C, or D), infants present with ***excessive drooling, followed by chocking or coughing immediately after feeding is initiated as a result of aspiration through the fistula tract.***
- As the neonate coughs and cries, air is transmitted through the fistula into the stomach, resulting in ***abdominal distention***. As the abdomen distends, it becomes ***increasingly more difficult for the infant to breathe.***
- The **diagnosis of EA** is confirmed by the ***inability to pass an orogastric tube into the stomach***.
- If a soft feeding tube is used, the tube will coil in the upper pouch, which provides further diagnostic certainty.
- The presence of a TEF can be demonstrated clinically by finding ***air in the gastrointestinal tract***.
- ***There may be polyhydramnios****. These findings reflect the absence of efficient swallowing by the fetus.*

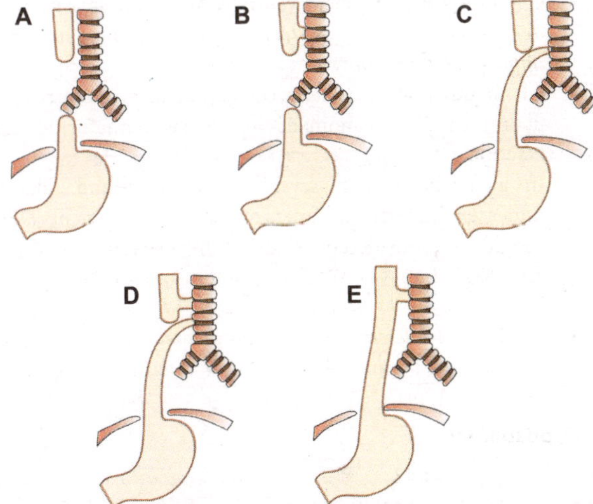

Fig: *(CSDT 14th/1233):* **A.** Pure (long gap) esophageal atresia. **B.** Esophageal atresia with proximal tracheoesophageal fistula. **C.** Esophageal atresia with distal tracheoesophageal fistula. **D.** Esophageal atresia with proximal and distal fistulas. **E.** Tracheoesophageal fistula without esophageal atresia

174. Ans. (a) Urethral opening on ventral aspect, (c) May be associated with penile torsion

[Ref: Manipal Surgery 4th/967; Nelson 20th/2586;CSDT 14th/968-69; L and B 26th/112]

"**Penile torsion** is a fairly common congenital (present from birth) condition that can affect any male infant. It can range from mild to severe. It is most likely to be seen in an uncircumcised penis. The penis is almost always rotated to the left (counter-clockwise). Penile torsion can be a stand-alone medical issue, or associated with other congenital conditions of the penis. These conditions include: ***Hypospadias***, Congenital chordee (penile curvature)and Hooded prepuce (a misshapen or incomplete foreskin)"- *my.clevelandclinic.org*

"**Hypospadia:** There is incomplete development of the prepuce, called a **dorsal hood,** in which the foreskin is on the ***sides and dorsal aspect of the penile shaft and absent ventrally***. Some boys with hypospadias, particularly those with proximal hypospadias, have **chordee,** in which there is ***ventral penile curvature*** during erection. ***Approximately 65% of cases are distal***, 25% are subcoronal or midpenile, and 10% are proximal. Complications of untreated hypospadias include (1) deformity of the urinary stream, either ventral deflection or severe splaying; (2) sexual dysfunction secondary to penile curvature; (3) infertility if the urethral meatus is proximal; and (4) meatal stenosis (congenital), which is rare"- *Nelson 20th/2586*

Hypospadias

◈ *L and B 26th/112*

- In hypospadias, seen in 1:300 boys, the ***urethra opens proximally and ventrally***. Most commonly, the opening is just proximal to the glans, but it can open on the penile shaft or onto the perineum.
- It is attributed to failure of complete urethral tubularisation in the fetus.
- The foreskin is deficient ventrally and there is a ***variable degree of chordee (a ventral curvature of the penis most apparent on erection)***.
- Glanular hypospadias needs correction for cosmetic reasons but more proximal anomalies interfere with micturition and erection.
- In a newborn with severe hypospadias and bilateral undescended testes, disorders of sexual development (DSD) should be considered. A distal hypospadias is usually repaired before two years of age in one or two stages.
- *Proximal varieties require complex staged procedures.*
- ***Ritual circumcision is contraindicated*** in infants with hypospadias because the foreskin is often required for the reconstruction.

Hypospadias

◈ *CSDT 14th/968-69*

- Hypospadias results from failure of fusion of the urethral folds on the undersurface of the genital tubercle. ***The urethral meatus is ventrally displaced*** on the glans on the shaft of the penis or more proximal at the level of the scrotum or perineum.
- With more proximal displacement, ***chordee (ventral curvature of the penile shaft)*** frequently occurs and requires treatment, or it precludes straight erections and normal intercourse.
- In hypospadias with the meatus positioned proximal to the corona, the ***prepuce is abnormal***—not forming a complete cylinder due to a ventral defect.
- The ***degree of hypospadias dictates the need for repair. If the opening is glandular or coronal (85% of patients)***, the penis is usually functional both for micturition and procreation, and repair is done primarily for cosmetic reasons.
- Surgical plastic repair of hypospadias is currently accomplished by a variety of highly successful one-stage operations and is routinely ***performed between 6 and 18 months of age***.
- ***"Denis-Browne's operation*** is still the *simple and most accepted operation"- Textbook of Surgery by S.Das 5th/ 1323*

175. Ans. (b) May have malignant..., (c) Produce symptoms which..., (d) Air-fluid may be seen on..., (e) Mostly asymptomatic

[Ref: Schwartz 9th/1419-20; Sabiston 19th/1602-03; CSDT 14th/1231]

"Anterior mediastinal masses make up one-third and are most commonly teratomas and lymphomas. ***Middle mediastinal masses are rare but when present are most likely to be bronchogenic cysts***"-*CSDT 14th/1231*

Bronchogenic Cyst

◈ *Schwartz 9th/1419-20*

- Bronchogenic cysts are duplication cysts originating from the airway, regardless of the identity of the epithelial lining.
- Histologically, they are hamartomatous and usually consist of a single cyst lined with an epithelium; ***the mesenchyme contains cartilage and smooth muscle.***
- ***Although they may be completely asymptomatic***, bronchogenic cysts ***may produce symptoms, usually compressive in nature,*** depending on the anatomic location and size
- In the paratracheal region of the neck, they can produce ***airway compression and respiratory distress***.
- In the lung parenchyma, they may become infected and ***present with fever and cough.*** In addition they may cause obstruction of the bronchial lumen with ***distal atelectasis and infection***, or they may cause mediastinal compression.
- **Chest x-ray** usually shows a dense mass, and CT scan or magnetic resonance imaging (MRI) delineates the precise anatomic location of the lesion.

Bronchogenic Cysts

◈ *CSDT 14th/363*

- When large, cysts can compress surrounding vital structures, including the aerodigestive tract causing *dysphagia, pneumothorax, cough, or hemoptysis or become infected.*
- The diagnosis is ***confirmed by CT as a spherical fluid- or mucus-filled nonenhancing mass.*** An ***air-fluid*** level may be present thus suggesting communication with the airway.

- In general, mediastinal bronchogenic cysts present with airway compression and parenchymal cysts are manifested by pulmonary infection.
- ***Rare cases of malignant transformation have been reported***. All bronchogenic cysts—regardless of location—are best treated with either ***simple or segmental resection by VATS or thoracotomy.*** Rarely, lobectomy is required.

Bronchogenic Cysts

◈ *Sabiston 19th/1602-03*

- Bronchogenic cysts are the ***most common primary cysts of the mediastinum***, representing 50% to 60% of these cysts.
- The ***cyst wall is composed of cartilage, mucous glands, smooth muscle, and fibrous tissue*** with a pathognomonic inner layer of ciliated respiratory epithelium.
- **Rarely,** a true communication between the cyst and the ***tracheobronchial tree exists***, and an ***air-fluid level may be observed on chest radiograph***.
- ***Two thirds of bronchogenic cysts are asymptomatic.*** In infants, ***these cysts may cause severe respiratory compromise by compressing the trachea or the bronchus; compression of the bronchus may cause bronchial stenosis and recurrent pneumonitis***.
- ***Malignant degeneration has been reported***, as has the presence of a bronchial adenoma within the cysts.

176. Ans. None

[Ref: Morgan 5th/100; SN Chugh 4th/232-33; Manipal Surgery 4th/1038-39; L and B 26th/303-20; Harrison 19th/1779-80;CSDT 11th/902]

*Patient given in question is in comatose stage (bcoz GCS ≤8). He/she should need care in ICU. Immediate/short-term management of this this patient consists of-**head end elvation** (to **decrease ICP**, **to prevent aspiration pneumonia**) and **CVP line placement** (**for fluid management, administering drugs, CVP measurement**) and long term management consists of **stress ulcer prophylaxis, DVT prophylaxis and adequate nutrition**(either through **enteric nutrition or through TPN**)*

"**Central venous catheterization** is indicated for monitoring ***central venous pressure (CVP) in critically ill patient, administration of fluid to treat hypovolemia and shock, infusion of caustic drugs and total parenteral nutrition, aspiration of air emboli, insertion of transcutaneous pacing leads, and gaining venous access in patients with poor peripheral veins.*** With specialized catheters, central venous catheterization can be used for ***continuous monitoring of central venous oxygen saturation***"*- Morgan 5th/100; www.nursingtimes.ne*

"Estimates of the incidence of overt gastrointestinal **(GI) bleeding range from 1.5 to 8.5 percent among all intensive care unit (ICU) patients**, but may be as ***high as 15 percent among patients who do not receive stress ulcer prophylaxis.*** Most episodes of overt GI bleeding in critically ill patients are due to gastric or esophageal ulceration. Stress ulceration can also cause perforation. However, this complication is rare, occurring in fewer than 1 percent of surgical ICU patients"- *www.uptodate.com*

"Stress-related mucosal disease (SRMD) is an acute, erosive gastritis representing conditions ranging from stress-related injury to stress ulcers. Mucosal damage has been reported to occur during the first 24 hours of hospital admission in 75% to 100% of intensive care unit (ICU) patients. ***Initiation of acid suppression therapy (AST) for stress ulcer prophylaxis (SUP) in the ICU setting is well established***"*- www.ncbi.nlm.nih.gov*

"**Venous thromboembolism (VTE)**, including pulmonary embolism (PE) and deep venous thrombosis (DVT), is a common and ***severe complication of critical illness.*** **Critically ill patients are at high risk of VTE** because they combine both *general risk factors together with specific ICU risk factors of VTE, like sedation, immobilization, vasopressors or central venous catheter.* ***Thromboprophylaxis is needed in all ICU patients***, mainly with low molecular weight heparin. Mechanical thromboprophylaxis has to be used if anticoagulation is not possible"*-www.ncbi.nlm.nih.gov*

"**Elevation of the head-of-bed (HOB)** of intubated patients is an ***effective method for reducing rates of aspiration pneumonia.*** It was demonstrated that the semirecumbent position decreased rates of aspiration of gastric contents four-fold. Kollef used multivariate analysis for risk factors of developing aspiration pneumonia and found that head position <30 degrees in the first 24 hrs of intubation was an independent risk factor for developing VAP"*- www.medscape.com*

"***Enteral nutrition is preferred to intravenous parenteral nutrition*** on grounds of cost and associated complications, and should be commenced within 72 hours of head injury. Prokinetics (e.g., metaclopramide, erythromycin) can be administered to promote absorption"*- L and B 26th/320*

Further Management of the Comatose

◈ *research.ncl.ac.uk/nsa/coma*

This care will often be delivered in a specialist unit, usually an intensive care/therapy unit. Long term management involves consideration of the problems suffered by a patient lying still for very prolonged periods with no protective reflexes. These include

- Pressure area care
- Care of the mouth, eyes and skin
- Physiotherapy to protect muscles and joints
- ***Risks of deep vein thrombosis***
- ***Risks of stress ulceration of the stomach***
- ***Nutrition and fluid balance***
- Urinary catheterization
- Monitoring of the CVS
- Infection control
- Maintenance of adequate oxygenation, with the assistance of artificial ventilation

Maintaining Patent Airway

◈ *nursingassignments.blogspot.in*

- Elevating the head end of the bed to 30 degree prevents aspiration.
- Positioning the patient in lateral or semi prone position.
- Suctioning.

"**Monitoring of ICP**: In general, patients who should be considered for ICP monitoring are those with primary neurologic disorders, such as stroke or traumatic brain injury, who are at significant risk for secondary brain injury due to elevated ICP and decreased CPP. Included are patients with the following: severe traumatic brain injury ***(Glasgow Coma Scale [GCS] score ≤8)***; large tissue shifts from supratentorial ischemic or hemorrhagic stroke; or hydrocephalus from subarachnoid hemorrhage (SAH), intraventricular hemorrhage, or posterior fossa stroke"- *Harrison 19th/1779*

Table *(Harrison 19th/1780)*: **Stepwise approach to treatment of elevated intracranial pressure(partial table)**

Elevate head of the bed; midline head position

The Glasgow Coma Score Can be Used as follows

- *ICU Book by Paul Marino 3rd*
- To define coma (GCS = 8).
- To stratify the severity of head injury (mild 13–15, moderate 9–12, severe = 8)
- To identify candidates for intubation (i.e., patients with GCS = 8 are usually unable to protect their airway and require endotracheal intubation).

Table *(L and B 26th/303)*: **Head injury severity-clinical classification**

Eyes open	Spontaneously	4
	To verbal command	3
	To painful stimulus	2
	Do not open	1
Verbal	Normal oriented conversation	5
	Confused	4
	Inappropriate/words only	3
	Sound only	2
	No sounds	1
	Intubated patient	T
Motor	Obeys commands	6
	Localises to pain	5
	Withdrawal/flexion	4
	Abnormal flexion	3
	Extension	2
	Non motor response	1

177. Ans. (a) Staphylococcus aureus is the most common..., (c) Quadriceps is one of..., (e) Best detected by MRI

[Ref: Harrison 19th/831;Manipal Surgery 4th/25-26; www.ncbi.nlm.nih.gov; jbjs.org/content/84 jbjs.org/content]

Acute Pyomyositis

- *Manipal Surgery 4th/25-26*
- *Localized area of suppuration within striated muscle is pyomyositis*
- ***Staphylococcus aureus (90%),*** *streptococcus pyogenes and E.coli*
- ***Classically quadriceps,*** *gluteus, shoulder and upper arm muscle are affected*
- Most pyomyositis cases involve only a single muscle group, but more diffuse involvement is described in 10 to 20% of cases. The large muscles of the lower extremities are ***most commonly affected (such as the quadriceps and gluteus muscle group)***, perhaps as a result of strenuous exercise or trauma leading to muscle injury. Any skeletal muscle group may be involved"- *www.ncbi.nlm.nih.gov*
- *Tenderness, induration and spasm of muscles are characteristic*
- *Renal failure follow soon*
- ***CT and MRI are ideal investigation*** *to know the spread of the infection*

"**Pyomyositis** is usually due to ***S. aureus,*** is common in tropical areas, and generally has no known portal of entry. Cases of pyomyositis caused by MRSA producing the PVL toxin have been described among children. Muscle infection begins at the exact site of *blunt trauma or muscle strain*. ***Infection remains localized.*** In contrast, ***S. pyogenes*** **may induce primary myositis** (referred to as *streptococcal necrotizing myositis*) in association with severe systemic toxicity"- *Harrison 19th/831*

Primary pyomyositis (also called tropical myositis, infective myositis, pyogenic myositis, suppurative myositis, myositis purulenta tropica, epidemic abscess, or bacterial myositis) *jbjs.org/content/84*

- Primary pyomyositis is a rare, subacute, primary muscle infection that is probably the result of a transient bacteremia in most patients.
- The ***quadriceps, gluteal, and iliopsoas muscles are the most commonly*** affected anatomic sites.
- ***Staphylococcus aureus*** is the culpable bacteria in >75% of cases.
- There are three consecutive stages of the disease: diffuse muscle infection, abscess formation, and sepsis.
- ***Magnetic resonance imaging is the preferred diagnostic imaging modality.***
- Treatment includes ***complete drainage of any abscess cavity combined with appropriate antibiotic therapy.***

Primary Pyomyositis

- *journals.lww.com*
- A bacterial infection of previously healthy skeletal muscle, it is usually caused by ***Staphylococcus aureus*** (methicillin sensitive).
- The pathology begins as a bacteremia that seeds ***deep muscles.***
- ***An MRI is usually required to diagnose and clarify the extent of the process.***
- ***Surgical drainage and prolonged antibiotic therapy are the norm.***

178. Ans. (b) Only produces by prostate, (c) >10 mg/mL suggestive of prostate cancer, (d) Useful in prognosis and follow-up

[Ref: Robbins 9th/988-89; Manipal Surgery 4th/977; L and B 26th/1341, 1345; Schwartz 9th/255-56]

Table: *Schwartz 9th/255*

Marker	Cancer	Sensitivity(%)	Specificity
PSA (4 g/L)	Prostate	57-93	55-68

"20% to 40% of patients with organ-confined prostate cancer have a PSA value of 4.0 ng/mL or less- *Robbins 9th/988*

PSA

Manipal Surgery 4th/977

- >4 nmol/mL: carcinoma to be suspected
- 10 nmol/mL: suggestive of prostatic cancer
- 35 nmol/mL: disseminated carcinoma

Prostate-Specific Antigen

CSDT 14th/1004-05

- PSA is elevated in the serum of most men with prostate cancer, but high-grade (Gleason 8-10) cancers and ductal variant adenocarcinomas can present with normal PSA levels.
- ***Values above 4 ng/mL are considered abnormal*** but rise normally with age and significant benign prostatic hypertrophy.
- **Methods for enhancing PSA specificity** include the following: (1) **age-specific PSA** (younger men [< age 50 years], normal < 2.5 ng/mL; older men [> age 70 years], normal > 6.5 ng/mL); (2) **PSA density** (PSA divided by prostate volume), where less than 0.15 ng/mL suggests cancer; (3) **percent-free PSA** (total PSA minus complexed PSA), where lower values signify an increased risk of cancer (useful for total PSA levels between 4 and 10).
- ***While total PSA is useful for staging, it is not absolute.*** PSA appears to be ***most helpful in following up on patients after treatment, as levels fall to undetectable after surgery and decrease dramatically after radiation*** therapy when there is a complete response.

Prostate-Specific Antigen

Schwartz 9th/256

- Prostate-specific antigen (PSA) is an androgen-regulated serine protease ***produced by the prostate epithelium.***
- PSA levels have been shown to be ***useful in evaluating the effectiveness of prostate cancer treatment*** and ***monitoring for recurrence after therapy.*** In ***monitoring for recurrence, a trend of increasing levels is considered more significant than a single absolute elevated value.***

PSA

Robbins 9th/988-89

- ***PSA is organ specific but not cancer specific.***
- A significant rise in serum PSA levels, despite the latest serum PSA test being below the normal cutoff (<4 ng/mL), is abnormal and should prompt a work-up.
- Furthermore, it appears that per cent free PSA is most valuable in discriminating between benign and malignant disease when the total PSA level is in the "gray zone" of 4 to 10 ng/mL. *When per cent free PSA is higher than 25%, it indicates a lower risk of cancer, whereas per cent free PSA values of less than 10% are worrisome for cancer*

Elaboration and Secretion of Prostate-specific Antigen

L and B 26th/1341

- It is a ***marker for prostatic disease.***
- There is no real normal upper limit.
- ***The levels increase with age, with prostate cancer and with BPH.***
- There are age-related values but, in general, ***in men aged 50–69 years, a level of about 3–4 ng/mL*** would prompt a discussion about the need for prostate biopsy. ***Its level in men with metastatic prostate cancer is usually increased to >30 ng/mL*** and falls to low levels after successful androgen ablation.
- ***Men with locally confined prostate cancer usually have serum PSA levels <10–15 ng/mL.***
- ***Although PSA is a reliable marker for the progression of advanced disease, it is neither specific nor sensitive in the differential diagnosis of early prostate cancer and BPH, as both diseases are compatible with PSA in the range of 3–15 ng/mL.***
- PSA measurement has superseded measurement of serum acid phosphatase. In summary, about 25 per cent of men with a PSA of 4–10 ng/mL have prostate cancer (i.e. it is not very specific), and about ***15–20 per cent of men with a PSA of 1–4 ng/mL have prostate cancer.***
- In general, one would advise men aged 50–69 years to undergo prostate biopsy if the PSA was more than ~3 ng/mL. The threshold would be lower in younger men with a strong family history.

179. Ans. (a) Dysphagia, (c) Achlorhydria, (d) Treatment consists...

[Ref: P.L.Dhingra 6th/343-44; Robbins 9th/652; Harrison 19th/532]

Plummer-Vinson (Patterson-Brown-Kelly) Syndrome

P.L.Dhingra 6th/343-44

- Classical features of this syndrome include dysphagia, iron-deficiency anaemia, glossitis, angular stomatitis, koilonychia (spooning of nails) and achlorhydria. There is atrophy of the mucous membrane of the alimentary tract.
- Predominantly, it ***affects females past 40 years.*** Barium swallow shows a web in the postcricoid region and the same can be seen on oesophagoscopy. It is due to subepithelial fibrosis in this region.
- About 10% of the cases with this syndrome will develop postcricoid carcinoma. It also predisposes to the development of carcinoma in the tongue, buccal mucosa, pharynx, oesophagus and the stomach.
- **Treatment**
  - To correct anaemia by oral/parenteral iron. Serum levels of iron are more important than haemoglobin level. Associated B_{12} and B_6 deficiency should also be corrected.
  - ***Dilatation of the webbed area by oesophageal bougies***

180. Ans. (c) Hyperglycemia

[Ref: Schwartz 9th/1448; Robbins 9th/480]

"In addition, there is an increased incidence of ***Wilms' tumor*** in certain overgrowth conditions, particularly Beckwith-Wiedemann syndrome and hemihypertrophy. Beckwith-Wiedemann syndrome is an overgrowth syndrome that is characterized by ***visceromegaly, macroglossia, macrosomia, omphalocele and hyperinsulinemic hypoglycemia***"- *Schwartz 9th/1448,1442*

"Hepatoblastoma may be associated **Beckwith-Wiedemann syndrome** as well. The treatment is surgical resection and chemotherapy. Untreated, the tumor is usually fatal within a few years, but therapy has raised the 5-year survival to 80%"-*Robbins 9th/480*

181. Ans. a. In monopolar mode..., b. Patient plate..., c. Burn may be... & d. Cutting has more...

[Ref: Manipal Surgery 4th/1180; L and B 26th/47-48; Schwartz 9th/77; S.Das textbook 5th/; Sabiston 19th/235]

Electrosurgery and Electrocautery

◈ *Sabiston 19th235*

- Since 1928, electrocautery and electrosurgery have become the most important and basic surgical tools in the operating room.
- ***High-frequency alternating current*** can be delivered in either unipolar or bipolar fashion.
- The **unipolar (or monopolar) device** is composed of a generator, an electrode for application, and an electrode for the returning current to complete the circuit. The patient's body becomes part of the circuit when the system is activated.
- Unipolar devices can be used to incise tissue when activated with a constant waveform and to coagulate when activated with an intermittent waveform.
- In the **cutting mode, *much heat is generated relatively quickly over the target with minimal lateral thermal spread***. As a result, the device cuts through tissue without coagulating any underlying vessels.
- In contrast, in the **coagulation mode**, electrocautery generates ***less heat on a slower frequency***, *with the potential for large lateral thermal spread*. Such spread results in tissue dehydration and vessel thrombosis. A *blended waveform can be chosen that will be able to take advantage of both the cutting and coagulation modes.*
- *A large **grounding pad** must be placed securely on the **patient for the unipolar electrosurgical/ electrocautery device** to function properly and to **prevent thermal burn injury** at the current reentry electrode site.*
- **Bipolar electrocautery** establishes a short circuit between the tips of the instrument, whether a tissue grasper or forceps, without the requirement for a grounding pad. The tissue grasped between the tips of the instrument completes the circuit. In generating heat that affects only the tissue within the short circuit, it provides precise thermal coagulation.
- *Bipolar electrocautery is more effective than the monopolar instrument in coagulating vessels* because it adds the mechanical advantage of compression of tissue between the tips of the instrument to the thermal coagulation.
- ***Bipolar electrocautery is particularly useful when conducting a procedure in which lateral thermal injury or an arcing phenomenon needs to be avoided.***

Electrocautery

◈ *Manipal Surgery 4th/1180*

- **Bipolar electrocautery:** Effective in wet fields, uses coagulation current only
- Monopolar electrocautery: Not effective in wet fields, use both cutting and coagulation current. There dissection is possible
- Bipolar cautery is safe with pacemakers

"In **cutting mode** electrode touches the tissue, and sufficiently ***high power density*** is applied to vaporize its water content. **Coagulation** is performed using waveforms with ***lower average power***, generating heat insufficient for explosive vaporization, but producing a thermal coagulum instead"-wikipedia

Electrosurgery and Electrocautery

◈ *www.ncbi.nlm.nih.gov*

- For the high power surgical uses during anesthesia the *monopolar modality* relies on a ***good electrical contact between a large area of the body*** (Typically at ***least the entire back of the patient***) and the ***return electrode or pad (Also known as dispersive pad or patient plate)***.
- **Severe burns** (3rd degree) can occur if the contact with the ***return electrode is insufficient***, or when a patient comes into contact with metal objects serving as an unintended (capacitative) leakage path to Earth/Ground.
- To prevent unintended burns, the skin is cleaned and a ***conductive gel is used to enhance the contact with the return electrode.***
- Proper electrical grounding practices must be followed in the electrical wiring of the building.
- The ***grounding plate should be applied on dry, hairless skin, using a conductive jelly***.

The Principles of Diathermy: Electrosurgery

◈ *L and B 26th/47-48*

- ***There are two basic types of diathermy system in use, monopolar diathermy and bipolar diathermy***
- In **monopolar diathermy**, which is the most commonly used form, an ***alternating current*** is produced by a suitable generator and passed to the patient via an active electrode which has a very small surface area.
- The current then passes through the tissues and returns via a very large surface plate (the indifferent electrode) back to the earth pole of the generator.
- *As the surface area of contact of the active electrode is small in comparison to the indifferent electrode, the concentrated powerful current produces heat at the operative site.* However, ***the large surface area electrode of the patient plate spreads the returning current over a wide surface area, so it is less concentrated and produces little heat.***
- In **bipolar diathermy**, the two active electrodes are usually represented by the limbs of a pair of diathermy forceps.
- In **coagulation**, a heating effect leads to cell death by dehydration and protein denaturation.
- **Cutting** occurs when sufficient heat is applied to the tissue to cause cell water to explode into steam. The ***cut current is a continuous wave form and the monopolar diathermy*** is

most effective when the active electrode is held a very short distance from the tissues.

- In **fulguration**, the diathermy matching is set to coagulation and a ***higher effective voltage is used*** to make larger sparks jump an air gap thus fulgurating the tissues. This is known as blended current and provides both forms of diathermy activity.
- **Complications of diathermy:** *Electrocution*, *Explosion* **and** *Burns*
- These are the most common type of diathermy accidents in both open and endoscopic surgery. They occur when the current flows in some way other than that in which the surgeon intended and are far ***more common in monopolar than bipolar*** diathermy.
- *Pacemakers:* Diathermy currents can interfere with the working of a pacemaker with its obvious potential danger to the patient's health.

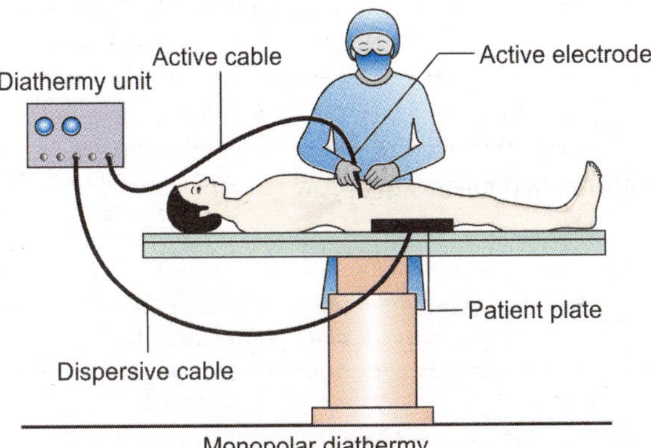

Fig: (Land B):The principles of monopolar diathermy

182. Ans. (a) Pain, (b) Nausea, (c) Vomiting

[Ref: L and B 26th/272-80; Schwartz 9th/1749-50;Sabiston 19th/410-11]

Nausea, vomiting and pain are most common post-op complications (Most probable answer)

Post-operative Complication

◈ *patient.info/in/doctor*

Immediate

- Primary haemorrhage (starting during surgery) or reactionary haemorrhage (following postoperative increase in blood pressure) - replace blood loss and may require return to theatre to re-explore the wound.
- Basal atelectasis: minor lung collapse.
- Shock: blood loss, acute myocardial infarction, pulmonary embolism or septicaemia.
- Low urine output: inadequate fluid replacement intra-operatively and postoperatively.

Early

- ***Pain.***
- Acute confusion: exclude dehydration and sepsis. May also be due to other various causes, including pain, sleep disturbance, medication or metabolic disturbances.
- ***Nausea and vomiting***: analgesia or anaesthetic-related; paralytic ileus.
- Fever
- Secondary haemorrhage: often as a result of infection.
- Pneumonia.
- Wound or anastomosis dehiscence.
- DVT.
- Acute urinary retention.
- Urinary tract infection (UTI).
- Postoperative wound infection.
- Pressure sores.
- Bowel obstruction due to fibrinous adhesions.
- Paralytic Ileus.

Late

- Bowel obstruction due to fibrous adhesions.
- Incisional hernia.
- Persistent sinus.
- Recurrence of reason for surgery - e.g., malignancy.
- Keloid formation.
- Cosmetic appearance - depends on many factors (best discussed with surgeon).

Postoperative Nausea and Vomiting

◈ *Sabiston 19th/410*

- ***Perhaps one of the most annoying problems for both patients and personnel in the PACU(Post anaesthesia care unit) is postoperative nausea and vomiting.***

Nausea and Vomiting

◈ *L and B 26th/277*

- ***Adequate treatment of pain, anxiety, hypotension and dehydration will minimise the risk of the patient developing PONV.***

Postoperative Nausea and Vomiting

◈ *Schwartz 9th/1749-50*

- PONV typically ***occurs in 20% to 30% of surgical cases***, with considerable variation in frequency reported between studies (range, 8%–92%).
- Troublesome PONV can prolong recovery room stay and hospitalization and is ***one of the most common causes of hospital admission following ambulatory surgery.***

Nearly everyone has some pain after surgery"-www.webmd.com

Pain: The Fifth Vital Sign

- ***Acute postoperative pain*** and its treatment (or prophylaxis) are significant challenges for the healthcare professional.
- Despite the recent development of new nonnarcotic analgesics and a better understanding of the side effects associated with pain medication of all types, ***acute postoperative pain remains a significant concern for patients and represents an extremely negative experience for patients undergoing surgery.***
- ***Many patients experience pain in the postoperative period*** despite the use of potent techniques such as patient-controlled analgesia, epidural analgesia, and regional anesthesia.

Acute Pain Management

◈ *Sabiston 19th/411*

- ***Pain, one of the most common symptoms experienced by surgical patients***, has historically been poorly evaluated and frequently undertreated.
- Surveys demonstrate that continued improvement is necessary to further reduce the high incidence of ***moderate to severe acute postoperative pain.***
- Acute pain occurs frequently in the setting of surgery and trauma.

Postoperative Period

◈ *L and B 26th/272*

- All vital parameters should be monitored and documented.
- ***Treat pain and nausea/vomiting.***

The patient can be discharged from the recovery room when they fulfill the following criteria: *L and B 26th/272*

- Patient is fully conscious.
- ***Patient is normothermic, not in pain nor nauseous.***

183. Ans. (a) Most common..., (b) May presents as pulsatile..., (c) Atherosclerosis is most...

[Ref: Harrison 19th/ 1639-40;CMDT 2016/476-78; L and B 26th/894- 99; Sabiston 19th/1697-99;CSDT 11th/ 829-35; Manipal 4th/1031-32]

Abdominal Aortic Aneurysm (AAA)

◈ *Harrison 19th/ 1639-40*

- 90% of abdominal aortic aneurysm (AAA) of ***size > 4cm*** in diameter is due to ***atherosclerosis.***
- ***Male*** are more frequently affected than female.
- An abdominal aortic aneurysm *commonly produces no symptoms*. It is usually detected on routine examination as a palpable, pulsatile, expansile, and nontender mass, or it is an incidental finding during an abdominal X-ray or ultrasound study performed for other reasons.
- As abdominal aortic aneurysms expand, however, they may become painful. Some patients complain of strong pulsations in the abdomen; others experience pain in the chest, lower back, or scrotum. Aneurysmal pain is usually a harbinger of rupture and represents a medical emergency
- The aneurysm **most commonly** arises ***below the level of renal artery.***
- Prognosis of abdominal aortic aneurysm is depends on size of the aneurysm and the severity of co-existing coronary artery and cerebrovascular disease. Most of the time they are asymptomatic
- Beta blocker decreases the perioperative cardiovascular morality.
- "Operative repair of the aneurysm with insertion of a ***prosthetic graft or endovascular placement of an aortic stent*** graft is indicated for abdominal aortic aneurysms of any size that are expanding rapidly or are associated with symptoms. For **asymptomatic aneurysms,** abdominal aortic aneurysm ***repair is indicated if the diameter is >5.5 cm***" *(Harrison 19th/1640)*

Abdominal Aortic Aneurysm

◈ *L and B 26th/894-99*

- Abdominal aortic aneurysm is by far the most common type of large vessel aneurysm and is found in 2 per cent of the population at autopsy; ***95 per cent have associated atheromatous degeneration and 95 per cent occur below the renal arteries.***
- An asymptomatic abdominal aortic aneurysm in an otherwise fit patient should be ***considered for repair if >55 mm in diameter*** (measured by ultrasonography).
- **Endovascular aneurysm repair** (EVAR) is now established in clinical practice and has been shown to have reduced mortality compared to ***open repair*** over the first six years. Currently, about 50 per cent of infrarenal aneurysms are suitable for EVAR which is dependent on the morphology of the aneurysm when assessed by CT scan.
- Less than 50 per cent of patients with rupture survive to reach hospital. Ruptured abdominal aortic aneurysm is a surgical emergency; it should be suspected in a patient with the ***triad of severe abdominal and/or back pain, hypotension and a pulsatile abdominal mass.***

Abdominal Aortic Aneurysm

◈ *Sabiston 18th/1906-20*

- The classic presentation of a ruptured AAA is the **triad** of ***sudden-onset midabdominal or flank pain, shock, and the presence of a pulsatile abdominal mass.*** However, ***only one third of patients with ruptured AAA present with this triad.***
- The pain may radiate into the groin or thigh and is usually severe, constant, and unaffected by position. It is more commonly located on the left side.

OBSTETRICS & GYNAECOLOGY

184. Ans. (c) Internal iliac lymph node

[Ref: Shaw's Gynae 16th/ 502-03; Dutta Gynae 6th/, 5th/488; Novak's gynae 15th/1325-27; Robert Shaw's Gynae 4th/592; CDTOG 10th; Novak's 14th/1427; Devita 7th/1297; The MD Anderson Manual of Medical Oncology]

I could not get explicit reference of inclusion of internal iliac lymph node in external irradiation therapy given in cervical cancer

Treatment Field for Carcinoma Cervix

◈ *Dutta's Gynae 5th/ 488*

- *Superior border: b/w L4 and L5 to include the* ***common iliac nodes***
- *Inferior border: At the inferior margin of obturator foramen to include the* ***obturator nodes***
- *Lateral border: 1 cm lateral to the margins of the bony pelvis*

"The extent of the irradiated fields encompasses the level of the midpubis or 3 to 4 cm below the cervical or vaginal lesions inferiorly, L5 to S1 level to cover the area of ***common iliac nodes*** *superiorly (or up to L4 to L5 if paraaortic nodes* are at high risk), and at least 1 cm lateral to bony pelvic margins" *(The MD Anderson Manual of Medical Oncology)*

"The goal of external irradiation in cervical cancer is to sterilize metastatic disease to *pelvic lymph nodes* and the parametria and/or to decrease the size of the cervix to allow optimal placement of intracavitary radioactive sources. Patients with known or suspected metastatic disease to ***periaortic lymph nodes*** may be considered for extended field irradiation. *(CDTOG 10th)*

"**Lymphatic Spread in cervical cancer**: The cervix is drained by preureteral, postureteral, and uterosacral lymphatic channels. The following are considered first station nodes: ***obturator, external iliac, hypogastric, parametrial, presacral, and common iliac***. *Para-aortic nodes* are second station, are rarely involved in the absence of primary nodal disease, and are considered metastases. The percentage of involved lymph nodes increases directly with primary tumor volume" *(Johns Hopkins Manual of Gynecology and Obstetrics, The, 3rd Edition)*

*"Ca cervix: When the lymphatics are involved, tumor cells are carried to the regional pelvic lymph nodes (**parametrial, hypogastric, obturator, external iliac, and sacral**)"-COGDT chap. 50*

Planning Treatment fields

◈ *Devita 7th/1297; The MD Anderson Manual of Medical Oncology*

- The anterior field margins should include, where indicated, possible extensions of the tumor into the body of the uterus. The posterior field margins should include tumor extension into the ***uterosacral ligament and presacral lymph nodes.*** Lateral field margins need to adequately include the pelvic lymph nodes.
- For lesions in the lower one third of the vagina, the *inguinal lymph nodes* need to be treated. The use of extended-field radiation to treat occult or macroscopic *para-aortic lymph node* disease needs to be carefully planned to ensure adequate dose (45 Gy for microscopic disease) without exceeding bowel, spinal cord, or renal tolerances.

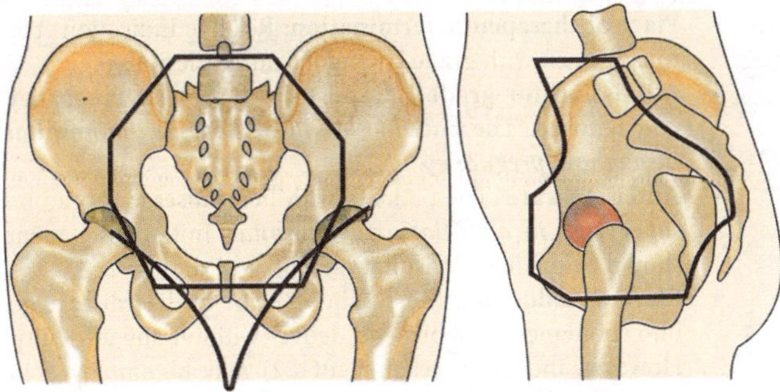

Fig: Typical fields used to treat the pelvis with a four-field technique. When lateral fields are used to treat cervical cancers, particular care must be taken to adequately encompass the primary tumor and potential sites of regional spread in the radiation fields

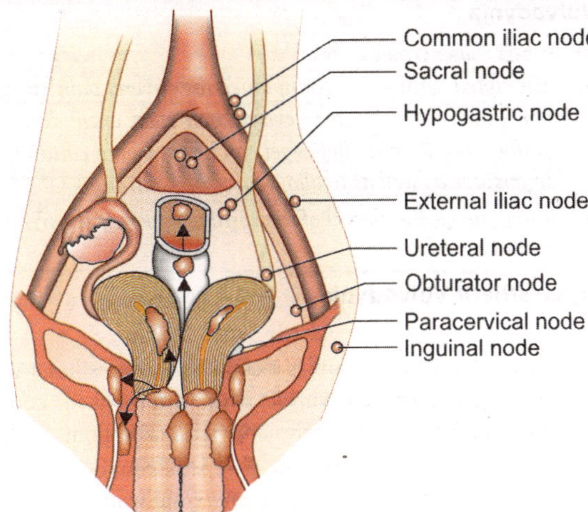

Fig: Possible sites of direct extension of cervical cancer to adjoining organs or metastases to regional lymph nodes. The uterus, cervix, and vagina are depicted bisected and opened to reveal the possible sites of tumor implantation

185. Ans. (b) Pain without any..., (c) May be associated with..., (d) Tricyclic antidepre..., (e) Psychological factor is...

[Ref: Shaw's Gynae 16th/374; Dutta Gynae 6th/265; Novak's Gynae 15th/425; Robert Shaw's Gynae 4th/605-06; www.mayoclinic.org]

"Vulvodynia is chronic pain of the vulva (external female genitalia) in the absence of localized infection. It is often associated with ***irritable bowel syndrome (IBS)"*** *- www.ncbi.nlm.nih.gov*

"Vulvodynia: Associated stress-related and chronic pain conditions such as headaches, face, tongue and mouth pain, fibromyalgia, ***irritable bowel syndrome***, painful bladder syndrome, bloating, fatigue, sleep problems and eating disorders"- www.dermnetnz.org

Vulvodynia

◈ *Dutta Gynae 6th/265*

- It is a severely painful socially debilitating disease where infection, invasive disease or inflammation have been excluded.
- It is **characterized by burning sensation over the vulva (burning vulva syndrome).** It is often seen in perimenopausal or postmenopausal women.
- Exact etiology is not known. Clinical examination does not reveal any abnormality in many cases.
- **Treatment is unsatisfactory.** Tricyclic antidepressant (amitriptyline) is found helpful.
- **Gabapentin is also beneficial**
- **Pyschosexual counselling and behaviour therapy are needed for some cases**
- **Surgery is contraindicated**

Vulvodynia

◈ *Robert Shaw's Gynae 4th/606*

- *Attempted coitus is accompanied by severe pain at entry. The pain may last for several hours or even days after contact. Local anaesthetics gel can be used on a cotton ball to desensitize as well as to allow coitus to continue*
- *Rarely surgical removal of the vestibular skin is the treatment of choice*

Dysaesthetic Vulvodynia

◈ *Shaw's Gynae 16th/374*

- Dysaesthetic vulvodynia is a cutaneous dysaesthesia which causes nonlocalized vulval pain, unprovoked constant ***neurologic pain*** in the vulva and perianal region.
- A burning ache similar to postherpetic pain occurs usually in perimenopausal and postmenopausal woman; therefore, history of dyspareunia is rarely reported.
- A woman is often ***psychologically disturbed and anxious***. This affects normal activity, walking, social life and sexual function.
- **Management:** **(a)** Remove and treat the cause, (b)Thirty percent have spontaneous remission in a year's time and (c) Medical—Topical lignocaine 1-2% may help, so also steroid creams.
- Amitriptyline for neuralgic pain
- Biofeedback therapy with electromyelography for pelvic floor muscles and Kegel exercise cures 80% cases.
- In a severe case, a woman may need vestibulectomy. It consists of excision of the horseshoe-shaped vestibule and inner labial fold and covering the raw area with vaginal mucosa dissected from the posterior vaginal wall.

186. Ans. (a) Bilateral tube blockage, (d) Proximal tubal block, (e) Premature ovarian insufficiency

[Ref: Shaw's Gynae 16th/247-47; Dutta Gynae 6th/250-53; Novak's Gynae 15th/1158; Robert Shaw's Gynae 4th/359]

For hostile cervical mucus artificial insemination is done

Premature ovarian insufficiency: IVF is indicated. Donor oocyte is used for IVF

*"**Proximal tubal occlusion**: If occulusion persists or recurs, IVF is usually recommended"- Novak's Gynae 15th/1158*

Indications of in-vitro Fertilization (IVF)

◈ *Shaw's Gynae 16th/247*

- *Mild endometriosis*
- *Blocked fallopian tubes or failed tubal surgery*
- *Failed intrauterine or fallopian insemimation*
- ***Immunological factor in male and female***
- ***Abnormal semen finding***
- *Idiopathic or unexplained male or female infertility*
- *Donor semen or sperm*

Table *(Dutta Gynae 6th/252)*: **Indications of in-vitro Fertilization (IVF)**

- Tubal disease
- Unexplained infertility

Contd...

- Endometriosis
- Male factor infertility
- Multiple factors (female and male)
- Failed ovulation induction
- Ovarian failure (Donor oocyte IVF)
- Women with normal ovaries but no functional uterus (Mullerian agenesis)
- Women with genetic risk (IVF and Preimplantation genetic diagnosis)

Indication of Artificial Insemination (IUI and Fallopian Tube Sperm Transfer)

◈ *Dutta Gynae 6th/250; Shaw's Gynae 16th/246-47*

- ***Hostile cervical mucus***
- *Cervical stenosis*
- *Oligospermia or asthenospermia*
- *Immune factor (male and female)*
- ***Male factor**- impotency or anatomical defect (hypospadias) but normal ejaculate can be obtained*
- *Unexplained infertility*
- *Chronic medical disorder*
- *HIV-positive male or female*

187. Ans. a. Delivery should be..., b. Often tolerate major ..., c. Caesarean..., d. Mortality is..., e. Epidural is preferred...

[Ref: Dutta Obs 8th/320-23; William's Obs 23rd/962-63; Obs by JB Sharma 1st/498-500; Normal and Problem Pregnancy by Gabbe 6th/830-38]

Management of Heart Disease in Pregnancy

◈ *Dutta Obs 8th/320-23*

- **General management: *Multidisplinary team approach*** (obstetrician, cardiologist and neonatologist) and mandatory hospital delivery
- **Place of therapeutic termination:** Relative indication- parous women with grade III and IV cardiac lesions
- **Admission for grade III and IV:** As soon as pregnancy is diagnosed. The ***patient should be kept in the hospital throughout pregnancy***
- **Antenatal care:** The patients with heart disease should be ***supervised in a tertiary care hospital***. Initial assessment should be made in consultation with a cardiologist
- **Place of induction:** Most patients with cardiac disease go into spontaneous labour and deliver without any difficulty. However, induction (vaginal PGE2) may be employed in very selected cases for obstetric indications
- **Place of caesarean section:** In general, there is ***no indication of CS for heart disease***
- **Cardiac indications of CS:** coarctation of aorta, aortic dissection or aneurysm, aortopathy with aortic root >4 cm and warfarin treatment within 2 weeks
- In coarctation of aorta, elective ES is indicated to prevent rupture of the aorta or myotic cerebral aneurysm. Anaestheisa should be given by expert anaesthetist using either ***epidural (preferred)*** or general anaestheisa

Management of Class III and IV Disease

◈ *Obs by JB Sharma 1st/498-500*

- Women with class III and IV disease ***should be admitted whenever diagnosed*** and should stay in hospital until delivery or until their functional cardiac status improves to lower grade

◈ *William's Obs 23rd/963*

- If women choose to become pregnant, they must understand the risks and cooperate fully with planned care. If seen early enough, women with some types of severe cardiac disease should consider pregnancy interruption. If the pregnancy is continued, prolonged hospitalization or bed rest is often necessary.
- ***Epidural analgesia for labor and delivery is usually recommended. Vaginal delivery is preferred in most cases, and labor induction can usually be done safely*** (Oron and associates, 2004).
- ***Cesarean delivery is limited to obstetrical indications.*** The decision for cesarean delivery must take into account the specific cardiac lesion, overall maternal condition, availability and experience of anesthetic support, as well as physical facilities.
- ***These women often tolerate major surgical procedures poorly*** and should be delivered in a facility with experience with complicated cardiac disease

Labor and Delivery

◈ *William's Obs 23rd/962-63*

- In general, delivery should be accomplished vaginally ***unless there are obstetrical indications for cesarean delivery.***
- ***Induction is generally safe.***
- Relief from pain and apprehension is especially important. Although intravenous analgesics provide satisfactory pain relief for some women, ***continuous epidural analgesia is recommended in most cases.***
- For vaginal delivery in women with only mild cardiovascular compromise, ***epidural analgesia given along with intravenous sedation*** often suffices. This has been shown to minimize intrapartum cardiac output fluctuations and allows forceps or vacuum-assisted delivery.
- ***Subarachnoid blockade is not generally recommended in women with significant heart disease.*** For cesarean delivery, ***epidural analgesia is preferred by most clinicians*** with caveats for its use with pulmonary hypertension.

Table *(Obs by JB Sharma 1st/498;Dutta Obs 8th/321)*: **Risk wise categorization of cardiac disease during pregnancy**

Cardiac Disorder	Mortality
Group 1 – Minimal Risk NYHA class I and II	0–1%
Group 2 – Moderate Risk	5–15%
Mitral stenosis, NYHA class III and IV	
Group 3 – Major Risk	25–50%

188. Ans. (a) In last trimester blood volume..., (c) Hemodynamic changes in pregnancy..., (d) Hypercoagulability occurs

[Ref: Dutta Obs 8th/58-63; William's Obs 23rd/120; Obs by JB Sharma 1st/49-51; Normal and Problem Pregnancy by Gabbe 6th/]

"Marked hemodynamic changes in pregnancy and cardiac output in particular, have profound effect on heart disease. The **cardiac failure** *occurs during pregnancy around 30 weeks,* ***during labour and mostly soon following delivery****"- Dutta Obs 8th/319*

"Cardiac output reach its peak 40-50% at about 30-34 weeks. CO increases futher during labour (+50%) and immediately following delivery (+70%) over the pre-labour values"- *Dutta Obs 8th/60*

*"***Blood volume***: It increases in pregnancy to maximun* ***40-50% above nonpregnant level at 30-34 weeks****"- Dutta Obs 8th/58*

*"***Blood volume***: It increases in pregnancy by* ***about 40-45%"****- JB Sharma 1st/47*

"Blood coagulation factors: Pregnancy is a state with most clotting factors increasing and the anticoagulants and fibrinolytic activity decreasing in pregnancy*"- JB Sharma 1st/48*

"Changes in pregnancy: Cardiac output increases by 40%, ***Stroke volume increase by 27%, heart rate increases by 17%,systemic vascular resistance decreases by 21% and pulmonary vascular resistance decreases by 34%"*** *(Dutta's Obstetrics 8th/60)*

Table *(Dutta's Obstetrics 8th/58)*: **Principal blood changes during pregnancy**

Parameters	Change
Blood Volume (ml)	+30–40%
Plasma volume (ml)	+40–50%
Red cell volume (ml)	+20–30%
Total Hb (g)	+18–20%
Hematocrit (whole body)	Diminished

Table *(William's Obstetrics 23rd/ 120)*: **Hemodyamics Changes during pregnancy**

Pregnant		Postpar-tum	Change
Cardiac output (L /min)	6.2 ± 1.0	4.3 ± 0.9	+ 43%

189. Ans. (b) Fetal congenital malformation..., (c) Increases fetal and..., (d) Oligohydramnios increases..., (e) Increases risk of hip ...

[Ref: Dutta Obs 8th/435-38; William's Obs 23rd/527; Obs by JB Sharma 1st/304]

*"***Breech:** *Labour is not prolonged. But because of increased frequency of operative delivery including caesarean section, the* ***maternal morbidity is increased****"- Dutta Obs 8th/438*

*"***Breech***: Fetal risk in term of* ***perinatal mortality*** *is considerable in vaginal breech delivery"- Dutta Obs 8th/438*

"Vasa previa occur in vilamentous placenta*"- Dutta Obs 8th/301*

"**Vasa previa** occurs when fetal blood vessel (s) from the placenta or umbilical cord cross the entrance to the birth canal, beneath the baby. ***Vasa previa can result in rapid fetal hemorrhage*** (occurs from the vessels tearing when the cervix dilates or membranes rupture) or lack of oxygen (if the vessels become pinched off as they are compressed between the baby and the walls of the birth canal). The aberrant vessels result from velamentous insertion of the cord, bilobed or succenturiate lobed placenta"-*vasaprevia.com*

Etiology of Breech Presentation

◈ *Dutta's Obstetrics 8th/435; Normal and Problem Pregnancy by Stevens G. Gabes 6th/396*

- *Prematurity: MC cause*
- *Factor preventing spontaneous version: Breech with extended legs; Twins;* ***Oligohydramnios****; Congenital malformation of uterus such as septate or bicornuate uterus; Short cord and IUD of fetus*
- *Favourable adaptation: Hydrocephalous; Placenta previa; Contracted pelvis and Cornu-fundal attachment of the placenta*
- *Undue mobility of fetus: Hydramnios and Multiparae with lax abdomen*
- ***Fetal abnormalities****: Trisomies 13,18,21; Anencephaly and myotonic dystrophy due to alternation of fetal muscular tone and mobility*

Causes of Breech Presentation

◈ *COGDT*

- It includes oligohydramnios, hydramnios, ***uterine anomalies such as bicornuate or septate uterus***, pelvic tumors obstructing the birth canal, abnormal placentation, ***advanced multiparity***, and a ***contracted maternal pelvis.***
- Additionally, 6% of breech presentations are found to have **congenital malformations**, which include *congenital hip dislocation, hydrocephalus, anencephalus, familial dysautonomia, spina bifida, meningomyelocele, and chromosomal trisomies 13, 18, and 21.* Thus, those conditions that alter fetal muscular tone and mobility increase the likelihood of breech presentation.

190. Ans. a. Humerus..., b. Brachial plexus..., c. Birth asphyxia, & d. Sacroiliac joint...

[Ref: Dutta Obs 8th/469; William's Obs 23rd/482; Obs by JB Sharma 1st/317; Normal and Problem Pregnancy by Gabbe 6th/411,493]

Complications *of shoulder dystocia* *Obs by JB Sharma 1st/317; Dutta Obs 8th/469*

Maternal Complication

- Postpartum hemorrhage (both atonic and traumatic)
- Lacerations of vagina, cervix and perineum
- Rupture uterus and bladder
- Sacroiliac joint dislocation

Fetal Complication

Shoulder dystocia may be associated with significant fetal morbidity and even mortality in up to 25% cases.

- Risk of fetal death ***due to asphyxia and injuries.***
- Meconium aspiration syndrome can occur.
- Erb's palsy is due to injury to the spinal nerves C_5, C_6 and C_7 from downward traction on the brachial plexus during delivery of the anterior shoulder
- Klumpke's paralysis is due to injury to C_8 and T_1, spinal nerves and results in claw hand deformity.
- ***Fracture of the clavicle*** is relatively common but is not of much clinical significance.
- There can also be ***fracture of humerus.***

Complications of Shoulder Dystocia

◈ *www.aafp.org*

- Maternal
- Postpartum hemorrhage
- Rectovaginal fistula
- Symphyseal separation or diathesis, with or without transient femoral neuropathy
- Third- or fourth-degree episiotomy or tear
- Uterine rupture
- Fetal
- Brachial plexus palsy
- Clavicle fracture
- Fetal death
- Fetal hypoxia, with or without permanent neurologic damage
- Fracture of the humerus

191. Ans. (a) If division occurs after embryonic disc..., (b) If division occur before 72 hrs, it ..., (d) If division occurs after 8 days, it ...

[Ref: Dutta Obs 8th/233-37; William's Obs 23rd/859-61; Obs by JB Sharma 1st/446-47]

Dizygotic twins (80%): It is most common and result from fertilisation of 2 ova. Monozygotic twins (20%) is formed from fertilization of single ovum- *Dutta Obs 8th/233*

Monozygotic or Uniovular Twins or Identical Twins

◈ *Obs by JB Sharma 1st/446*

- It results from fertilization of a single ovum by a single sperm and occurs in 1/3rd (33%) of all twin pregnancies.
- It is of many types depending upon the 'time' when splitting occurs in the embryo as described below:
    - If cleavage takes place at about the 8 cells stage, i.e. **within 3 days (72 hours)** after fertilization, the resulting embryo will have two separate or a single fused placenta, two chorions and two amnions **(dichorionic diamniotic).** It accounts for nearly one-third of monozygotic twin pregnancies
    - If the division occurs when the inner cell mass is forming **(4-7 days, Dutta obs- 4 to 8 days),** the two embryos will develop enclosed by a single chorion, have a single placenta but two separate amniotic sacs **(monochorionic-diamniotic). It is the most common variety accounting for about two-thirds of monozygotic twins**
    - If the splitting occurs between **8-12 days(Dutta obs – after 8 days)** after fertilization, i.e. after differentiation of amnion there is a single amniotic cavity, single chorion and a single placenta **(monochorionic-monoamniotic).** These account for only 1-5% of monozygotic twins (Fig. 33.1 D).

- On very rare occasions, when splitting occurs after the **appearance of the primitive streak**, i.e. after the 13th day (Dutta obs- after 2 week of development of embryonic disc) of fertilization, it results in the formation of conjoint twins within a single amnion and chorion

Dizygotic Twins or Binovular or Fraternal Twins

◈ *Obs by JB Sharma 1st/446*

- It results from fertilization of two ova which have most probably ruptured from two distinct graafian follicles, usually of the same ovary or one from each ovary, by two sperms.
- The babies bear only fraternal resemblance to each other. It is the most common variety and nearly two-thirds (67%) of all twins are dizygotic.
- All dizygotic twins have two placentae which are dichorionic and diamnioitic. Rarely they may he fused.

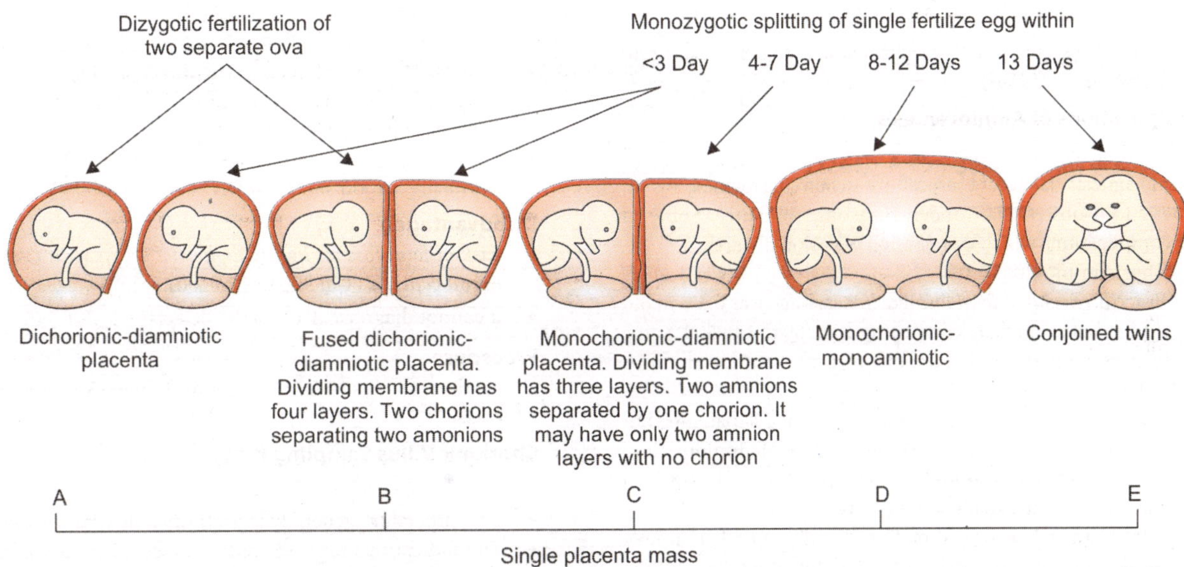

Fig: *(JB Sharma 1st/446):* Type and genesis of twinning

192. Ans. (b) Reduces risk of benign breast disease, (c) Protects against endometrial cancer

[Ref: Shaw's Gynae 16th/273-75; Obs by JB Sharma 1st/688; Dutta Gynae 6th/488-89;Dutta Obsterics 8th/622-27]

"**Non contraceptive benefits of OCP**- ***increased bone density and prevention of osteoporosis***"-*Obs by JB Sharma 1st/688*

"**Thromboembolic disorders**: Pulmonary embolism and cerebral thrombosis, both venous and arterial, are ***7 to 10 times more frequent in the pill(OCP) users*** than in the non-users in the first year of use"- *Shaws Gynaecology 16th/274*

"**OCP**: It has proved to lower the incidence of ***benign breast neoplasia such as fibrocystic disease***"- *Shaws Gynaecology 16th/274*

*"OCP: It **reduces the incidence of ovarian and uterine malignancy**. The incidence of ovarian cancer is reduced by 40% and uterine malignancy by 50% if taken for 1 year"- Shaws Gynaecology 16th/274*

*"**OCP protects from osteopenia and postmenopausal osteoporotic fracture**"- Dutta Gynaecology 6th/489*

"**Combined oral pills** *are highly effective,* ***protect against ovarian and endometrial cancer.*** *Although there remains controversy, most data suggest that* ***no link exists between COC use and breast cancer risk*** *yet* ***COC should not be given to female suffering from breast carcinoma***"- *Novak's Gynaecology 14th /274*

Table *(Harrison 19th/2391):* **Oral contraceptives disease risk**

Cervical cancer—relative risk 2–4 times
Ovarian cancer—50% reduction in risk
Endometrial cancer—40% reduction in risk

Table *(Harrison 19th/2391)*

Oral contraceptives - contraindications and disease
Increased
Coronary heart disease—increased only in smokers >35; no relation to progestin type
Hypertension—relative risk 1.8 (current users) and 1.2 (previous users)
Venous thrombosis—***relative risk ~4***; markedly increased with factor V Leiden or prothrombin-gene mutations
Stroke—increased only in combination with hypertension; unclear relation to migraine headache

Contd...

Cerebral vein thrombosis—relative risk ~13–15; synergistic with prothrombin-gene mutation

Cervical cancer—relative risk 2–4

Decreased

Ovarian cancer—50% reduction in risk

Endometrial cancer—40% reduction in risk

193. Ans. (b) 2nd trimester amniocentesis has less foetal…, (c) Amniocentesis may result in…, (e) Amniocentesis in 1st trimester…

[Ref: William's Obs 23rd/299-300; Obs by JB Sharma 1st/157-61]

"Amniocentesis: It is usually ***performed b/w 15-18 weeks***"- *Obs by JB Sharma 1st/157-61*

Complications of Amniocentesis

◈ *Obs by JB Sharma 1st/160*

Amniocentesis is a safe procedure when performed by an experienced obstetrician under ultrasonic guidance. Some of the complications which can develop occasionally are:

- Chorioamnionitis (0.1%)
- ***Procedure related fetal loss*** like miscarriage was 0.5% in old studies but is much less now being 1 in 300 to 1 in 500. Some losses are unrelated and are due to pre-existing conditions or fetal anomalies.
- Leakage of amniotic fluid occurs in about 2% patients, but is usually self resolving. Persistent leakage of amniotic fluid ***causing oligohydramnios*** leading to pulmonary, hypoplasia and fetal pressure deformities is rare.
- Fetal trauma like skin dimpling, fistula, cord hematoma, corneal perforation and postural deformities like ***talipes equinovarus.***
- Vaginal bleeding (2–3%)
- Rh isoimmunization
- Preterm labor
- Respiratory distress
- Intrauterine death (IUD)

Early Amniocentesis

◈ *Obs by JB Sharma 1st/160*

- Early amniocentesis is performed <15 weeks of gestation, but the technique has been largely abandoned due to the ***increased fetal loss rates, fetal talipes and reduced amniocyte culture rate*** **(level IA evidence).**

Second-Trimester Amniocentesis

◈ *William's Obs 23rd/299*

- Amniocentesis for genetic diagnosis usually is performed ***between 15 and 20 weeks.***
- Complications are infrequent and include transient vaginal spotting or amnionic fluid leakage in 1 to 2 percent and chorioamnionitis in less than 0.1 percent.
- ***Fetal loss of 0.5 percent or less*** has been reported by many investigators, and it does not appear possible to reduce this further

Early Amniocentesis

◈ *William's Obs 23rd/299-300*

- This procedure is performed between 11 and 14 weeks
- Early amniocentesis has higher rates of postprocedural pregnancy loss. One fetal complication that stand out is ***talipes equinovarus-clubfoot***
- Amniotic fluid leak, fetal loss and talipes equinovarus are significantly higher following early compared with traditional amniocentesis

Chorionic (Chorion) Villus Sampling

◈ *Obs by JB Sharma 1st/160*

Advantages

- Its results are ***available prior to 14 weeks*** of gestation and hence early termination can be performed causing lesser morbidity and substantial psychological benefit
- Results can be obtained from direct analysis as well as culture in contrast to amniocentesis where diagnosis requires cultured cells.
- Preferred procedure for diagnosis requiring DNA analysis as villi are a good source of DNA.

Disadvantages

- ***Risk of fetal loss is slightly higher*** (0.5-1%) ***with CVS than amniocentesis*** (1 in 300 to 1 in 500).
- It cannot diagnose neural tube defects.

Procedure

CVS is done for ***first trimester prenatal diagnosis between 10-14 weeks.***

Chorionic Villus Sampling (CVS)

◈ *William's Obs 23rd/300*

- This procedure generally is ***performed at 10 to 13 weeks.***
- The indications for CVS and amniocentesis are essentially the same, except for a few analyses that specifically require either amnionic fluid or placental tissue.
- The **primary advantage of CVS** is that ***results are available earlier in pregnancy,*** which lessens parental anxiety when results are normal. It also ***allows earlier and safer methods of pregnancy termination*** when they are abnormal.
- Complications of CVS are similar to those of amniocentesis. Several randomized and case-control trials have compared the safety of CVS with that of early and midtrimester amniocentesis as well as the safety of ***transabdominal versus transcervical CVS.***
- ***Transcervical CVS has a procedure-related fetal death rate 3.7 percent greater than that of either transabdominal CVS or traditional amniocentesis. This rate is similar to that for early amniocentesis.***
- The fetal loss rate associated with ***transabdominal CVS before 20 weeks was 1.5 percent, compared with that of 0.9 percent for early amniocentesis.***
- ***Midtrimester amniocentesis was safer than either transcervical CVS or early amniocentesis.*** They ***recommend transabdominal CVS if early diagnosis is required.***
- Early reports of an association between CVS and limb-reduction defects, oromandibular defects, and cavernous hemangiomas have been disproved. When CVS is performed after 9 weeks, the incidence of limb-reduction defects to be 6 per 10,000—the same as the background incidence. The frequency of oromandibular-limb hypogenesis, however,

was increased after CVS when the procedure was performed before 9 weeks

194. Ans. (b) Covered by non keratinized…, (c) Vaginal secretion is from…, (d) Supplied by cervicovaginal branch…

[Ref: Obs by JB Sharma 1st/5; Shaw's Gynae 16th/3-5; Dutta Gynae 6th/4-6; Novak's Gynae 15th/90; Robert Shaw's Gynae 4th/]

*"**Vaginal lubrication occurs primarily by transudation**, with contributions from cervical and bartholin gland secretion"- Novak's Gynae 15th/90*

Vagina

◈ *Obs by JB Sharma 1st/5*

- *Vaginal wall: It has four walls- **an anterior wall (6-8 cm long), a posterior wall(7-10 cm long)** and two lateral walls*
- *Mucous membrane is **non-cornified stratified squamous epithelium** with rugae but is devoid of secreting glands*
- *Arterial supply: **Upper 1/3-cervicovaginal branch of the uterine artery**, Middle 1/3- vaginal artery and Lower 1/3- middle rectal artery and internal pudendal artery*

Vagina

◈ *Dutta Gynae 6th/4-6*

- *Length of the anterior wall is about 7 cm and that of the posterior wall is about 9 cm*
- ***Epithelium- stratified squamous***
- *Secretion: Mainly derived from the glands of cervix and uterus and **transudation of vaginal epithelium and Bartholin's gland** (during sexual excitation)*
- *Arterial supply:**cervicovaginal branch of the uterine artery**, vaginal artery, middle rectal artery and internal pudendal artery*

Vagina

◈ *Shaw's Gynae 16th/3-5*

- *Posterior wall 4.5 inch(11.5 cm) and anterior wall 3.5 inch (9cm)*
- *Secretion: **Derived from mucous discharge of cervix and transudation of vaginal epithelium***

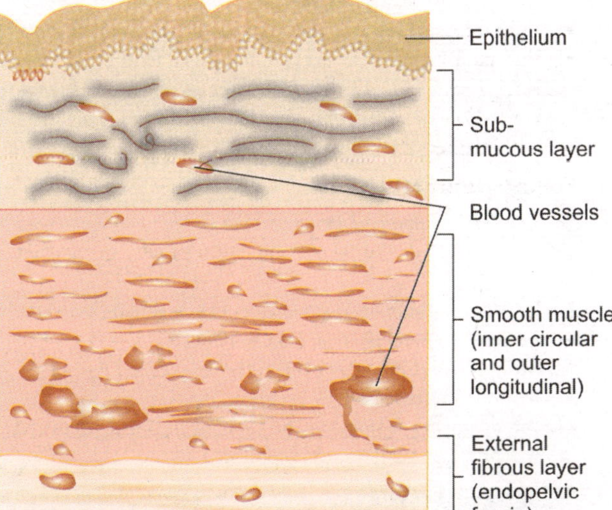

Fig: *(Dutta Gynae 6th/6):* Structure of vaginal wall

195. Ans. (a) Withdrawal method, (d) MTP pill

[Ref: Shaw's Gynae 16th/264-65; Obs by JB Sharma 1st/673; Dutta Obstetrics 8th/ 611-12; Dutta Gynae 6th/476]

Fertility Awareness Based Methods (FAB)

◈ *Obs by JB Sharma 1st/673*

- All family planning methods that attempt to identify fertile time in each cycle and then modify sexual behaviour are called ***Fertility Awareness Based Methods (FAB).***
- When fertility awareness methods involve sexual abstinence during fertile period, they are called Natural Family Planning Methods (NFP). They are as follows:
  - ***Rhythm method /calendar method***
  - ***Basal body temperature method***
  - ***Cervical mucus method/Billing method***
  - ***Sympto-Thermal method***
  - Standard days method using cycle beads
  - Two day method
  - Ovulation detection
  - Coitus interruptus
  - Lactation amenorrhoea method (LAM)
  - Abstinence

Table *(Dutta Obstetrics 8th/ 611; Dutta Gynae 6th/476):* **Failure rate of contraceptive methods in first 12 months of use**

Methods	Pregnancy rate per 100 women years (approx.)
No method	85
Natural (Calender, temperature, mucus)	25
Withdrawl	27
Lactational amenorrhoea	2
Condom (male)	15
Condom (female)	21
Diaphragm	16
CuT 380A	0.8
LNG 20 (IUCD)	0.1
Combined oral pills	0.1
Progestin only pills	1
DMPA and NET injectables	0.3
Norplant	0.05
Implanon	0.01
Vasectomy	0.15
Tubectomy	0.15

196. Ans. (a) Obesity, (b) Placental abruption, (d) Smoking, (e) Instrumental delivery

[Ref: Dutta Obs 8th/283; William's Obs 23rd/757-60; Obs by JB Sharma 1st/335; Normal and Problem Pregnancy by Gabbe 6th/426]

*"**Smoking is risk factor for placenta praevia**"- Dutta Obs 8th/283*

"Smoking is a risk factor for abruption placentae"- Dutta Obs 8th/285
So smoking is risk for obstetrical haemorrhage

Table *(William's Obs 23rd/759)*: **Conditions that predispose to or worsen obstetrical hemorrhage**

Abnormal Placentation

- Placenta previa
- *Placental abruption*
- Placenta accreta/increta/percreta
- Ectopic pregnancy
- Hydatidiform mole

Trauma During Labor and Delivery

- Episiotomy
- Complicated vaginal delivery
- Low- or midforceps delivery
- Cesarean delivery or hysterectomy
- Uterine rupture—risk increased by:
- Previously scarred uterus
- High parity
- Hyperstimulation
- Obstructed labor
- Intrauterine manipulation
- Midforceps rotation

Small Maternal Blood Volume

- Small women
- Pregnancy hypervolemia not yet maximal
- Pregnancy hypervolemia constricted
- Severe preeclampsia
- Eclampsia

Other Factors

- Obesity
- Native American ethnicity
- Previous postpartum hemorrhage

Uterine Atony

- Overdistended uterus
- Large fetus
- Multiple fetuses
- Hydramnios
- Distention with clots
- Anesthesia or analgesia
- Halogenated agents
- Conduction analgesia with hypotension
- Exhausted myometrium
- Rapid labor

Contd...

- Prolonged labor
- Oxytocin or prostaglandin stimulation
- Chorioamnionitis
- Previous uterine atony

Coagulation Defects—Intensify Other Causes

- Placental abruption
- Prolonged retention of dead fetus
- Amnionic fluid embolism
- Saline-induced abortion
- Sepsis syndrome
- Severe intravascular hemolysis
- Massive transfusions
- Severe preeclampsia and eclampsia
- Congenital coagulopathies
- Anticoagulant treatment

197. Ans. (b) Caesarean section has no increased risk for sepsis

[Ref: Dutta Obs 8th/500-504; William's Obs 23rd/661-65; Obs by JB Sharma 1st/392-96]

Microorganisms Responsible for Puerperal Sepsis

◈ *Dutta Obs 8th/501*

- *Most of the infection in the genital tract are polymicrobial with a mixture of aerobic and anaerobic organisms*
- *Aerobic:* ***Group A beta-hemolytic streptococcus, Group B beta-hemolytic streptococcus****and Methicillin-resistant S.aureus(MRSA). Others- Staphlococcus pyogenes, s.aureus, E.coli, Klebsiella, Pseudomonas, proteus, chlamydia*
- *Anaerobic- Streptococcus, peptococcus, bacteroides, fusobacterium, mobiluncus and clostridia*

Puerperal Sepsis

◈ *Obs by JB Sharma 1st/392-96*

- Puerperal sepsis is one of the cause of Puerperal pyrexia
- Puerperal pyrexia (fever) is defined as a temperature elevation of 38°C (100.4°F) or more after 24 hours of delivery recorded on two different occasions, 24 hours apart, usually within 10 days following childbirth

Predisposing Factors

◈ *Obs by JB Sharma 1st/393*

Certain factors may influence the pathogenicity of the vaginal flora.

- Introduction of organisms from outside during delivery.
- Lowered general or local host resistance.
- Multiplication of organisms in the devitalized tissues.
- Relative increase in drug resistant organisms.

The predisposing factors can be divided into antepartum and intrapartum factors. They are as follows:

Antepartum Factors

◈ *Obs by JB Sharma 1st/393*

- Poor general condition and malnutrition
- Anemia

- Lower socio-economic status
- Extremes of age
- Premature labor
- Preterm rupture of membranes
- Antepartum hemorrhage
- Immuno-suppressive states, like HIV, AIDS patients with renal transplant
- Medical conditions like diabetes, obesity and other chronic illnesses
- "*Retained bits of placental tissue or membrane*"- *Dutta Obs 8th/501*

Intrapartum and Postpartum Factors

◈ *Obs by JB Sharma 1st/393*

- **Cesarean delivery** It is the single most important risk factor for the development of puerperal sepsis. The incidence is 1-3% with vaginal delivery, 5-15% with elective caesarean delivery and 30-35% with emergency cesarean deliveries. In high-risk patients (diabetic, anemic and obese women etc.), the incidence is even higher.
- Serial vaginal examinations especially if not performed aseptically.
- Prolonged rupture of membranes
- Postpartum hemorrhage
- ***Operative and instrumental delivery***
- Handling by traditional birth attendants (TBAs, Dais)
- Intrauterine manipulations like manual removal of placenta
- Twin delivery
- Prolonged or obstructed labour

198. Ans. (a) MRI is superior to CT in detecting..., (b) CT is superior to MRI in detecting..., (c) USG is initial investigation...

[Ref: Shaw's Gynae 16th/510; Dutta Gynae 6th/356-57, 118-19; Novak'sgynae 15th/1257-58; Robert Shaw's Gynae 4th/637-38]

"**USG in endometrial carcinoma**: *Patients with suspicious symptoms* ***should initially be investigated*** *with a transvaginal USG to investigate the endometrial cavity*"- *Robert Shaw's Gynae 4th/637*

Diagnosis of Endometrial Carcinoma

◈ *Dutta Gynae 6th/356-57*

- "CT scan of pelvis and abdomen may be used to detect lymph node metastases"
- "***MRI can detect myocardial invasion***"
- "Sensitivity of PET in detecting pelvic node metastases is 80% compared to MRI(70%0 and CT(48%)"- *Dutta Gynae 6th/119*
- "*CT is useful in the diagnosis of lymph node metastasis and depth of myometrial invasion in endometrial cancer*"- *Dutta Gynae 6th/119*
- "***MRI is superior to CT or ultrasound in diagnosing adenomyosis, myomas and endometrial caner(including myometrial invasion)***"- *Dutta Gynae 6th/118*

Diagnosis of Endometrial Carcinoma

◈ *Shaw's Gynae 16th/510*

- "Ultrasound is useful in studying the endometrial thickness, irregular line, detecting polypi and associated ovarian tumour or ovarian metastasis"
- "**MRI is superior to CT in detecting myometrial involvement** and nodal enlargement with 90% detection rate and without radiation hazard. Normally, between the endometrial and ometrial junction, a low-intensity zone exists and if this zone is intact, myometrial invasion can be ruled out, and the amour is staged as Stage I. MRI is more expensive and time-consuming but accurate staging is possible in 80-90% (sensitivity 72% and specificity 96%)"
- *CT* has a predictable rate of 85% in studying the extent of spread of the lesion. Hypodensity in the myometrium suggests myometrial infiltration. The pelvic and aortic nodes are defined if enlarged to more than 1 cm. ***CT is superior to MRI in detecting ascites, bowel and omental metastasis***, but radiation exposure is the disadvantage.

166) Delivery of HIV +ve woman – vaginal delivery has higher risk than CS for transmission of HIV to child

199. Ans. (b) Vaginal delivery has higher risk for transmission of HIV to child than CS

[Ref: Dutta Obs 8th/350-53; William's Obs 23rd/; Obs by JB Sharma 1st/553-54

"**Elective CS** ***reduces the risk of vertical transmission*** *by about 50%. Avoidance of breastfeeding, HAART therapy and appropriate mode of delivery has reduced MTCT rate from 25-30% to <1%.* Baby should be bathed immediately"- *Dutta Obs 8th/352*

"**Risk factors for increased perinatal transmission** are: ***vaginal delivery, preterm delivery*** etc"- *Dutta Obs 8th/353*

"***Elective cesarean delivery decreases transmission by 87%*** if used in conjunction with zidovudine therapy in the mother and infant" *(Nelson 18th 1429)*

"**Invasive** ***procedures*** *that might result in break in the skin or mucous membrane of the infants(procedures like attachment of scalp electrode and determination of scalp blood pH) are* ***contraindicated. Instrumentation(ventouse) is avoided***"- *Dutta Obs 8th/352*

"Vertical transmission to the neonates is about *14-25%*. Transmission of HIV-2 is less frequent (1–4%) than for HIV- 1 (15–40%). Transplacental transmission occurs: 20% before 36 weeks, over 80% of transmission occur around the time of labour and delivery"- *Dutta Obs 8th/351*

"Vertical transmission is more in cases with preterm birth and with prolonged membrane rupture. Risk of vertical transmission is directly related to maternal viral load (measured by HIV RNA) and inversely to maternal immune status (CD4 count)"- *Dutta Obs 8th/351*

PAEDIATRICS

200. Ans. (b) IGF-1 levels is low for chronological age, (d) Puberty spurt is..., (e) Final height is within...

[Ref: O.P.Ghai 8th/37; Nelson (SAE) 20th/2643]

"Children with constitutional delay of growth and puberty ***do not have growth hormone deficiency*** and treating them with growth hormone is not as effective at increasing their growth rate as administering sex steroids.

Constitutional Growth Delay

◈ O.P.Ghai 8th/37

- These children are born with a normal length and weight and ***grow normally for the first 6-12 months*** of life. Their growth then ***shows a deceleration so that the height and weight fall below the 3rd centile.***
- **By 3 yr of age, *normal height velocity is resumed*** and ***they continue to grow just below and parallel to the 3rd centile with a normal height velocity.***
- The ***onset of puberty and adolescent growth spurt is also delayed*** in these children but ***final height is within normal limits.***
- Bone age is lower than chronological age and corresponds to the height age. History of delayed puberty and delayed height spurt is usually present in one or both parents.

Constitutional Growth Delay

◈ Nelson (SAE) 20th/2643

- Constitutional growth delay is a common variant of normal growth. Length and weight measurements of affected children are normal at birth, and growth is ***normal for the first 4–12 months of life***. Height is sustained at a lower percentile during childhood. The ***pubertal growth spurt is delayed***, so their growth rates continue to decline after their classmates have begun to accelerate.
- Detailed questioning often reveals other family members (frequently 1 or both parents) with histories of short stature in childhood, delayed puberty, and eventual normal stature.
- ***IGF-I levels tend to be low for chronological age but within the normal range for bone age.***
- ***Growth hormone responses to provocative testing tend to be lower than in children*** with a more typical timing of puberty. The prognosis for normal adult height in these children is guarded.
- Predictions based on height and bone age tend to overestimate eventual height to a greater extent in boys than in girls.
- Boys with more than 2 yr of pubertal delay may benefit from a short course of ***testosterone therapy*** to hasten puberty after 14 yr of age.
- The cause of this variant of normal growth is thought to be persistence of the relatively hypogonadotropic state of childhood

Table *(O.P.Ghai 8th/37)*: **Distinction between constitutional delay in growth and familial short stature**

Feature	Constitutional growth delay	Familial short stature
Height	Short	Short
Height velocity	Normal	Normal
Family history	Delayed puberty	Short stature
Bone age	Less than chronological age	Normal
Puberty	Delayed	Normal
Final height	Normal	Low but normal for target height

201. Ans. (b) Elicited by painful stimulus, (c) Bradycardia is prominent, (d) Atropine is given in refractory cases

[Ref: O.P.Ghai 8th/411,58-59; Nelson (SAE) 20th/2858,175; www.childneurologyfoundation.org/disorders/breath-holding-spells]

"**Subtypes of breath holding spells** *include* ***cyanotic, pallid or mixed episode. Cyanotic are the dominant type***"- Nelson (SAE) 20th/175

Although, bradycardia may present in cyanotic spells, but it is not prominent and also there is no need of atropine treatment in cyanotic spells

Pallid Spells

◈ Nelson (SAE) 20th/2858 10th/2477

- These spells are ***much less common than cyanotic breath-holding spells***, but they share several characteristics.
- Pallid spells are ***typically initiated by a painful experience***, such as falling and striking the head or a sudden startle. The child stops breathing, rapidly loses consciousness, becomes pale and hypotonic, and may have a tonic seizure.
- ***Bradycardia with periods of asystole of >2 sec may be recorded.***
- The interictal EEG is normal.
- Most children respond to conservative measures as outlined for cyanotic spells, ***but a trial of an anticholinergic, oral atropine sulfate*** 0.01 mg/kg/24 hr in divided doses with a maximum daily dose of 0.4 mg, which increases the heart rate by blocking the vagus nerve, may be considered in refractory cases.
- Atropine should not be prescribed during very hot weather because an episode of hyperpyrexia may be initiated.

Cyanotic Spells

◈ Nelson (SAE) 20th/2858, 18th/2476-77

- A cyanotic breath-holding spell is usually predictable and is ***always provoked by upsetting or scolding an infant.***
- The episode is heralded by ***a brief, shrill cry*** followed by forced expiration and apnea. There is rapid onset of generalized cyanosis and a loss of consciousness that may be associated with repeated generalized clonic jerks, opisthotonos, and bradycardia.
- Results of an interictal electroencephalogram (EEG) are normal. A breath-holding spell can occur repeatedly within a few hours or it can recur sporadically, but it is always stereotyped.
- Breath-holding spells are rare before 6 mo of age, peak at about 2 yr of age, and abate by 5 yr of age.
- The **management** of breath-holding spells concentrates on the support and reassurance of the parents. Some parents feel that whatever the physician recommends, they must splash cold water on the face, turn the child upside down, or initiate mouth-to-mouth resuscitation and even cardiopulmonary resuscitation.

Pallid Breath-holding Spells

◈ www.childneurologyfoundation.org

- The ***most common stimulus is a painful event.*** The child turns pale (as opposed to blue) and loses consciousness with little if any crying. The EEG is also normal, and again there is no post ictal phase, nor incontinence.

- The child is usually alert within a minute or so. There may be some relationship with adulthood syncope in children with this type of spell.

Two Types of Breath-holding Spells

Pallid: child turns a pale color	**Cyanotic:** child turns a blue color, especially around the lips
Characteristics include: • Triggered by ***sudden fright or pain*** or falling with a minor injury to the head • Child may gasp and give a brief cry • Child becomes pale, loses consciousness and becomes limp • Child may become sweaty and may stiffen and have a few body jerks or lose bladder control	Characteristics include: • Triggered by becoming ***frustrated or angry*** • The child may cry vigorously, usually less than 15 seconds • After crying, the child becomes silent, stops breathing, and rapidly turns blue • The child usually loses consciousness, goes limp, or stiffens and arches his back • Recovery happens in less than one minute • May gasp and return to regular breathing • Regain consciousness and returns to normal • May seem tired • It is rare for the child to be upset and cry again triggering another episode

202. Ans. (a) Papilledema is rare in raised, (c) Stroking patellar tendon of one side leads to… (e) Parachute reflex

[Ref: O.P.Ghai 8th/142, 570; Nelson (SAE) 20th/2796, 2798]

Option c: Stroking patellar tendon of one side leads to contraction on opposite side: Normal until 6–7 months. So included in answer

*"The MacEwen or crackpot sign indicates **raised intracranial pressure** after sutures have closed. **Papilledema is unusal in infancy** unless intracranial pressure is very high"- O.P.Ghai 8th/570*

"The "**floppy infant**" represents a diagnostic challenge to general pediatricians. Infants can present with hypotonia that is due to ***central or peripheral nervous system abnormalities, myopathies, genetic disorders, endocrinopathies, metabolic diseases, and acute or chronic illness***. A systematic approach to a child who has hypotonia, paying attention to the history and clinical examination, is paramount in localizing the problem to a specific region of the nervous system"- pedsinreview.aappublications.org

"The knee jerk in an infant may produce a **crossed adductor response** (tapping the patellar tendon in one leg causes contraction in the opposite extremity), which, if present, ***does not become abnormal until 6–7 months of age***. The deep tendon reflexes are absent or decreased in primary disorders of the muscle (myopathy), nerve (neuropathy), and myoneural junction and in abnormalities of the cerebellum. They are characteristically increased in upper motor neuron lesions. Asymmetry of deep tendon reflexes suggests a lateralizing lesion"- *Nelson (SAE) 20th/2798*

"When the upper extremity of a normal term infant is pulled gently across the chest, the elbow normally does not quite reach the midsternum (scarf sign). ***The elbow of a hypotonic infant extends beyond the midline with ease***"- *Nelson (SAE) 20th/2796*

"The **parachute reflex** is demonstrated by suspending the child by the trunk and by suddenly producing forward flexion as if the child were to fall. The child spontaneously extends the upper extremities as a protective mechanism. The parachute reflex appears before the onset of walking"- *Nelson (SAE) 20th/2798*

Table *(Nelson (SAE) 20th/2798)*: **Timing of selected primitive reflexes**

Reflex	Onset	Fully developed	Duration
Palmar grasp	28 wk	32 wk	2–3 mo
Rooting	32 wk	36 wk	Less prominent after 1 mo
Moro	28–32 wk	37 wk	5–6 mo
Tonic neck	35 wk	1 mo	6–7 mo
Parachute	7–8 mo	10–11 mo	Remains throughout life

203. Ans. (d) Booster of Typhoid Conjugate Vaccine

[Ref: O.P. Ghai 8th/206; Park 23rd/122-24]

AP Immunization Schedule 2016 (Tabular form)

◈ *http://acvip.org*

Age (completed)	Vaccines	Comments
Birth	BCG; OPV 0; Hep-B 1	Administer these vaccines to all newborns before hospital discharge
6 weeks	DTwP 1; IPV 1; Hep-B 2; Hib 1; Rotavirus 1; PCV 1	**DTP:** • DTaP vaccine/combinations should preferably be avoided for the primary series • DTaP vaccine/combinations should be preferred in certain specific circumstances/ conditions only **Polio:** • All doses of IPV may be replaced with OPV if administration of the former is unfeasible **Rotavirus:** • 2 doses of RV1 and 3 doses of RV5 and RV 116E

Contd...

Age (completed)	Vaccines	Comments
10 weeks	DTwP 2; IPV 2; Hib 2; Rotavirus 2; PCV 2	**Rotavirus:** • If RV1 is chosen, the first dose should be given at 10 weeks
14 weeks	DTwP 3; IPV 3; Hib 3; Rotavirus 3; PCV 3	**Rotavirus:** • Only 2 doses of RV1 are recommended. • If RV1 is chosen, the 2nd dose should be given at 14 weeks
6 months	OPV 1 Hep-B 3	**Hepatitis-B:** • The final (3rd or 4th) dose in theHepB vaccine series should be administered no earlier than age 24 weeks and at least 16 weeks after the first dose.
9 Months	OPV 2; MMR-1	
9-12 months	Typhoid Conjugate Vaccine	• Currently, two typhoid conjugate vaccines, Typbar-TCV® and PedaTyph® available in Indian market;either can be used • An interval of at least 4 weeks with the MMR vaccine should be maintained while administering this vaccine
12 months	Hep-A 1	
15 months	MMR 2 Varicella 1 PCV booster	**MMR:** • The 2nd dose must follow in 2nd year of life • However, it can be given at anytime 4-8 weeks after the 1st dose **Varicella:** The risk of breakthrough varicella is lower if given 15 months onwards
16 to 18 Months	DTwP B1/DTaP B1; IPV B1: Hib B1	
18 months	Hep-A 2	Hepatitis A: 2nd dose for inactivated vaccines only
2 years	Booster of Typhoid Conjugate Vaccine	• A booster dose of Typhoid conjugate vaccine (TCV), if primary dose is given at 9-12 months • A dose of Typhoid Vi-polysaccharide(Vi-PS) vaccine can be given if conjugate vaccine is not available or feasible; • Revaccination every 3 years with Vi-polysaccharide vaccine • Typhoid conjugate vaccine should be preferred over Vi-PS vaccine
4 to 6 years	DTwP B2/DTaP B2 OPV 3 Varicella 2 MMR 3	**Varicella:** The 2nd dose can be given at anytime 3 months after the 1st dose. MMR: The 3rd dose is recommended at 4-6 years of age.
10 to 12 years	Tdap/Td HPV	**Tdap:** Is preferred Td followed by Td devery 10 years

Typhoid Vaccines Routine Vaccination

- *acvip.org/professional*
- Both Vi-PS conjugate and Vi-PS (polysaccharide) vaccines are available
- Minimum ages:
  - Vi-PS conjugate (Typbar-TCV®): 6 months; oVi-PS conjugate (Pedatyph®): 6 months;
  - Vi-PS (polysaccharide) vaccines: 2 years
- Vaccination schedule:
  - Typhoid conjugate vaccines (Vi-PS):
    - Typbar-TCV®: Single dose at 9-12 through 23 months followed by a booster at 2 years of age
    - Pedatyph®: Single dose at 9-12 through 23 months followed by a booster at 2 years of age
  - Vi-PS (polysaccharide) vaccines: Single dose at 2 years; revaccination every 3 years;

Table *(Ghai 8th/206)*: **Comparison of the vaccinations scheduled in the National immunization Program and the 2012 recommendations of the Indian Academy of Paediatrics (IAP)**

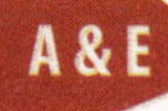

Age	National Immunization Program	IAP Recommendations
0 (at birth)	BCG, OPV0, Hep B0*	BCG, OPV0, Hep B1
6 weeks	DTwP1, OPV1, HepB1*, Hib1*	DTwP1/ DTaP1,IPV1$, Hep B2, Hib1, Rotavirus 1, PCV1

Contd...

Age	National Immunization Program	IAP Recommendations
10 weeks	DTwP2, OPV2, HepB2*, Hib2*	DTwP2/ DTaP2,IPV2[$], Hib2, Rotavirus 2, PCV2
14 weeks	DTwP3, OPV3, HepB3*, Hib3*	DTwP3/ DTaP3,IPV3[$], Hib3, Rotavirus 2, PCV3
6 mo	-	OPV1/Hep B3
9 mo	Measles, vitamin A1	OPV2, Measles
12 mo	-	Hep A1
15 mo	MMR*	MMR1, Varicella, PCV B1
16-24 mo	DTwP B1, OPV B1, vitamin A2, Japanese encephalitis**	(16-18 mo) DTwB1/ DTaP B1, IPV B1[$], Hib B1
2 yr	-	Typhoid 1 **
5 yr	DTwP B2	DTwP B2/DTaP B2, OPV3, MMR2, Varicella 2, Typhoid 2
10 yr	TT	Tda/Td[$$], HPV
16 yr TT		

B1 first booster dose; B2 second booster dose; BCG Bacillus Calmette Guerin vaccine; DT diphtheria toxoid with tetanus toxoid; DTwP diphtheria toxoid, tetanus toxoid, whole cell killed pertussis vaccine; DTaP diphtheria toxoid, acellular pertussis vaccine; Td tetanus toxoid with reduced dose diphtheria; Tdap tetanus toxoid dose diphtheria and pertussis vaccine; Hep B hepatitis B vaccine; Hib Haemophilia influenza b vaccine; HPV human papilloma virus vaccine; MMR measles; mumps and rubella and rubella vaccine; PCV pneumococcal conjugate vaccine, TT tetanus toxoid.*Implemented in selected states, districts and cities; **SA 14-14-2 vaccine, in select endemic districts; [$]OPV if an inactivated polio vaccine (IPV) is not affordable. [$$]dT preferred over TT

204. Ans. (c) There is defect of mineralization of matrix, (e) Renal tubule dysfuction leads to hypophosphatemia

[Ref: O.P.Ghai 8th/ 113-15; Nelson (SAE) 20th/333-36]

X-linked hypophosphatemic rickets (XLH) inherited in dominant manner(not recessive)

"Among the genetic disorders causing rickets due to hypophosphatemia, X-***linked hypophosphatemic rickets (XLH) is the most common***. The defective gene is on the X chromosome, but female carriers are affected, so it is an ***X-linked dominant disorder***"- *Nelson (SAE) 20th/333*

*"Radiological changes are characteristically seen at metaphysis. The first change is **loss of normal zone of provisional calcification adjacent to the metaphysis**"- O.P.Ghai 8th/ 113*

"In **chronic renal failure**, unlike the other causes of vitamin D deficiency, patients have ***hyperphosphatemia*** as a result of decreased renal excretion"- *Nelson (SAE) 20th/337*

"**Rickets,** a disease of growing bone, occurs in children only before fusion of the epiphyses, and is due to ***unmineralized matrix at the growth plates***. - *Nelson (SAE) 20th/331*

"**Fanconi syndrome** is secondary to generalized dysfunction of the renal proximal tubule. There are renal losses of phosphate, amino acids, bicarbonate, glucose, urate, and other molecules that are normally reabsorbed in the proximal tubule. The most clinically relevant consequences are hypophosphatemia due to phosphate losses and proximal renal tubular acidosis due to bicarbonate losses"- *Nelson (SAE) 20th/339*

"**Proximal or distal renal tubular acidosis(RTA**) *is important cause of* ***refractory ricket in children****.Patient with* ***proximal RTA show low level of phosphate****"- O.P.Ghai 8th/ 113*

Clinical Manifestations of Rickets

Nelson (SAE) 20th/333

- Most manifestations of rickets are due to skeletal changes. **Craniotabes,** a softening of the cranial bones, can be detected by applying pressure at the occiput or over the parietal bones.
- Widening of the costochondral junctions results in a **rachitic rosary;** this feels like the beads of a rosary as the examiner's fingers move along the costochondral junctions from rib to rib
- Decreased calcification leads to ***thickening of the growth plate***. The edge of the metaphysis loses its sharp border, which is described as fraying. In addition, the edge of the metaphysis changes from a convex or flat surface to a more concave surface. This is termed *cupping*, and is most easily seen at the distal ends of the radius, ulna, and fibula.
- Other radiologic features include ***coarse trabeculation of the diaphysis and generalized rarefaction.***

Table *(Nelson)*: **Laboratory findings in disorders causing rickets**

Disorder	Ca	Pi	PTH	25-OHD	1, 25-(OH) 2D	ALK PHOS	URINE Ca	URINE Pi
Vitamin D deficiency	N, ↓	↓	↑	↓	↓, N, ↑	↑	↓	↑
VDDR, type 1	N, ↓	↓	↑	N	↓	↑	↓	↑
VDDR, type 2	N, ↓	↓	↑	N	↑↑	↑	↓	↑

Contd...

Disorder	Ca	Pi	PTH	25-OHD	1, 25- (OH) 2D	ALK PHOS	URINE Ca	URINE Pi
Chronic renal failure	N, ↓	↑	↑	N	↓	↑	N, ↓	↓
Dietary Pi deficiency	N	↓	N, ↓	N	↑	↑	↑	↓
XLH	N	↓	N	N	RD	↑	↓	↑
ADHR	N	↓	N	N	RD	↑	↓	↑
HHRH	N	↓	N, ↓	N	RD	↑	↑	↑
Tumor-induced rickets	N	↓	N	N	RD	↑	↓	↑
Fanconi syndrome	N	↓	N	N	RD or ↑	↑	↓ or ↑	↑
Dietary Ca deficiency	N, ↓	↓	↑	N	↑	↑	↓	↑

ADHR, autosomal dominant hypophosphatemic rickets; AlkPhos, alkaline phosphatase; Ca, calcium; HHRH, hereditary hypophosphatemic rickets with hypercalicuria; N, normal; Pi, phosphorus; PTH, parathyroid hormone; RD, relatively decreased (because it should be increased given the concurrent hypophosphatemia); VDDR, vitamin D–dependent rickets; XLH, X-linked hypophosphatemic rickets; 1, 25- (OH) 2D, 1, 25-dihydroxy vitamin D; 25-OHD, 25-hydroxy vitamin D; ↓, decreased; ↑, increased; ↑↑, extremely increased.

205. Ans. (b) Surgery usually done before 3 year, (c) Second heart sound-Wide and..., (d) Soft delayed diastolic rumble ...

[Ref: O.P.Ghai 8th/413-14; Nelson (SAE) 20th/2189-91,2246-47; Harison 19th/1520-21; Robbins 9th/534]

Atrial Septal Defect (ASD)

◈ *O.P.Ghai 8th/413-14*

- "An increased flow through the tricuspid valve may result in a ***soft delayed diastolic rumble at the lower left sternal border***"
- *"S2: Wide fixed split, P2++"*

Atrial Septal Defect

◈ *Robbins 9th/534*

- ***Secundum ASD (90% of all ASD)***
- ***Primum anomalies (5% of all ASD) occur adjacent to the AV valve*** and ***are often associated with AV valve abnormalities*** and/***or a VSD***

Atrial Septal Defect

◈ *Nelson (SAE) 20th/2189-91*

- An ***ostium secundum defect in the region of the fossa ovalis is the most common form of ASD*** and is associated with structurally normal atrioventricular (AV) valves
- Examination of the chest may reveal a ***mild left precordial bulge. A right ventricular systolic lift is generally palpable at the left sternal border.***
- A loud 1st heart sound and sometimes a pulmonic ejection click can be heard. In most patients, the **2nd heart sound** is characteristically ***widely split and fixed in its splitting*** in all phases of respiration.
- A ***systolic ejection murmur is heard.***
- A ***short, rumbling mid-diastolic murmur***
- ***The timing for elective closure is usually after the 1st yr and before entry into school.*** Closure carried out at open heart surgery is associated with a mortality rate of <1%. Repair is preferred during early childhood because surgical mortality and morbidity are significantly greater in adulthood; the long-term risk of arrhythmia is also greater after ASD repair in adults.

206. Ans. All (a, b, c, d)

[Ref: William's Obs 23rd/288; O.P.Ghai 8th/575-76; Nelson (SAE) 20th/2802-03]

TABLE *(William's Obs 23rd/288):* **Risk factors for neural-tube defects**

Genetic cause
• Family history—multifactorial inheritance
• MTHFR (MTHFR = methylene tetrahydrofolate reductase) mutation—677C →T
• Syndromes with autosomal recessive inheritance—Meckel Gruber, Roberts, Joubert, Jarcho-
• Levin, HARDE (hydrocephalus-agyria-retinal dysplasia-encephalocele)
• Aneuploidy—trisomy 13 and 18, triploidy
Environmental exposures
• Diabetes—hyperglycemia
• Hyperthermia—hot tub or sauna, fever (controversial)
• Medications—valproic acid, carbamazepine, coumadin, thalidomide, efavirenz
Geographical—Ethnicity, Diet, and other factors
• United Kingdom, India, China, Egypt, Mexico, Southern Appalachian United States

"***Anticonvulsants***, most notably *valproic acid* and *carbamazepine*, significantly ***increase malformation risk***. *Aminopterin* and *isotretinoin* have been associated with a constellation of abnormalities that can include anencephaly or encephalocele"- *William's Obs 23rd/288*

"Well-established evidence shows that women who are obese, have poorly controlled diabetes, or take certain antiseizure medications, such as phenytoin (Dilantin), carbamazepine (Tegretol), and valproic acid (Depakote), or anti-folate (such as

aminopterin, methotrexate) are at greater risk than are other women of having an infant with spina bifida or anencephaly"- www.rightdiagnosis.com

Neural Tube Defect

◈ *O.P.Ghai 8th/575–76*

- Maternal risk factors include zinc and ***folate deficiency***, alcohol, radiation exposure, ***insulin dependent diabetes mellitus(IDDM),*** and use of valproate and carbamazepine during pregnancy
- Patients with trisomy 13 and 15 shows these defects

Neural Tube Defects (Dysraphism)

◈ *Nelson (SAE) 20th/2802–03*

- Although the precise cause of neural tube defects remains unknown, evidence suggests that many factors, including ***hyperthermia, drugs, malnutrition, chemicals, maternal obesity or diabetes, and genetic determinants (mutations in folate-responsive or folate-dependent pathways)*** may adversely affect normal development of the CNS from the time of conception.
- In some cases, an abnormal maternal nutritional state or exposure to radiation before conception may increase the likelihood of a CNS congenital malformation. The **major neural tube defects *include spina bifida occulta, meningocele, myelomeningocele, encephalocele, anencephaly, dermal sinus, tethered cord, syringomyelia, diastematomyelia, and lipoma*** involving the conus medullaris and/or filum terminale.

207. Ans. (a) Appears after 1 week, (b) Typically bilirubin…, (c) Phototherapy is useful, (d) Managed conservatively

[Ref: O.P.Ghai 8th/172; Nelson (SAE) 20th/288,871-75]

Breast Silk Jaundice

◈ *O.P.Ghai 8th/172*

- Approximately 2–4% of exclusively breastfed term babies have jaundice in ***excess of 10 mg/dl*** beyond ***third-fourth weeks*** of life. These babies should be investigated for prolonged jaundice.
- A diagnosis of breast milk jaundice should be considered if this is ***unconjugated (not staining nappies)***; and other causes for prolongation such as inadequate feeding, continuing hemolysis, extravasated blood, G-6PD deficiency and hypothyroidism have been ruled out.
- Mothers should be advised to continue at frequent intervals and TSB levels usually decline over a period of time. ***Some babies may require phototherapy.***
- Breastfeeding should not be stopped either for diagnosis or treatment of breast milk jaundice.

Breast-milk Jaundice

◈ *Nelson (SAE) 20th/874*

- Significant elevation in unconjugated bilirubin (breast-milk jaundice) develops in an estimated 2% of breast-fed term infants after the 7th day of life, with maximal concentrations as high as ***10–30 mg/dL reached during the 2nd–3rd week.***
- If breast-feeding is continued, the bilirubin gradually decreases but may persist for 3–10 week at lower levels. If nursing is discontinued, the serum bilirubin level falls rapidly, reaching normal levels within a few days.
- With resumption of breast-feeding, bilirubin levels seldom return to previously high levels.
- Phototherapy may be of benefit. Although uncommon, kernicterus can occur in patients with breast-milk jaundice.
- The etiology of breast-milk jaundice is not entirely clear, but may be attributed to the presence of glucuronidase in some breast milk.

Breast-feeding Jaundice

◈ *Nelson (SAE) 20th/874–75*

- Breast-milk jaundice should be distinguished from an early-onset, accentuated unconjugated hyperbilirubinemia known as breast-feeding jaundice which occurs in the ***1st week of life***, in breast-fed infants who normally have higher bilirubin levels than formula-fed infants.
- ***Hyperbilirubinemia (>12 mg/dL)*** develops in 13% of breast-fed infants in the 1st wk of life and may be due to decreased milk intake with dehydration and/or reduced caloric intake.
- Frequent breast-feeding (>10/24 hr), rooming-in with night feeding, discouraging 5% dextrose or water supplementation, and ongoing lactation support may reduce the incidence of early breast-feeding jaundice

208. Ans. (b) Twinning, (d) Failure to gain weight for 3 consecutive months, (e) Artificial feeding

[Ref: Park 23rd/535;O.P.Ghai 8th/178-79;Nelson (SAE) 20th/818-19]

Identification of at Risk Infants

◈ *Park 23rd/535*

- Birth weight less than 2.5 kg
- Twins
- Birth order 5 or more
- Artificial feeding
- ***Weight below 70% of expected weight(i.e II*** and ***III degree of malnutrition)***
- ***Failure to gain weight during three successive months***
- ***Children with PEM, diarrhea***
- ***Working mother/one parent***

Table *(O.P.Ghai 8th/178):* **Common newborn conditions requiring high risk follow up care**

Birth weight < 1500 g and/or gestation < 32 weeks Perinatal asphyxia: Apgar score < 3 at 5 min and/or hypoxic ischemic encephalopathy
Mechanical ventilation for >24 hr
Metabolic problems: Symptomatic hypoglycemia and hypocalcemia
Infections: Meningitis and/or culture positive sepsis
Hyperbilirubinemia >20 mg/dl or requirement of exchange transfusion

Table *(Nelson (SAE) 20th/819)*: **High-risk Infants(Partial list)**

Demographic Social Factors
Maternal age <16 or >40 yr, Illicit drug, alcohol, cigarette use
Emotional or physical stress, Unmarried, Poverty
Present Pregnancy
Vaginal bleeding (abruptio placentae, placenta previa)
Sexually transmitted infections (colonization: herpes simplex, group B streptococcus), chlamydia, syphilis, hepatitis B, HIV
Multiple gestation
Preeclampsia
Premature rupture of membranes
Short interpregnancy time
Poly/oligohydramnios
Labor and Delivery
Premature labor (<37 week)
Postdates (>42 week)
Fetal distress
Immature L: S ratio; absent phosphatidylglycerol
Breech presentation
Meconium-stained fluid
Nuchal cord
Cesarean section
Forceps delivery
Apgar score <4 at 1 min
Neonate
Birthweight <2, 500 or >4,000 g
Birth before 37 or after 42 week of gestation
SGA, LGA growth status
Tachypnea, cyanosis
Congenital malformation
Pallor, plethora, petechiae

209. Ans. (b) Occurs due to forcep injury to periosteum, (d) Localized collection of blood below periosteum

[Ref: Dutta Obs. 8th/558-59; O.P.Ghai 8th/138,141; Nelson (SAE) 20th/834]

Cephalohematoma

◈ *Dutta Obs. 8th/558-59*

- *It is a* ***collection of blood in b/w the pericranium*** and ***the flat bone(subperiosteal)*** *of the skull, usually unilateral* and *over a parietal bone*
- *It is due to rupture of a small emissary vein from the skull* and *may be associated with fracture of the skull bone*
- *This may be caused by forcep delivery but may also be met with following a normal labour*
- *It is never present at birth but gradullay develop after 12-24 hours*
- *The swelling is limited by the suture lines of the skull as the pericranium is fixed to the margins of the bone*
- *Blood is absorbed in course of time(6-8 weeks) leaving an entirely normal skull*
- *No active treatment is necessary*

Caput Succedaneum

◈ *Nelson (SAE) 20th/ 834*

- **Caput succedaneum** is a diffuse, sometimes ecchymotic, ***edematous swelling of the soft tissues of the scalp*** involving the area presenting during vertex delivery. ***It may extend across the midline and across suture lines.***
- The ***edema disappears within the 1st few days of life.*** Molding of the head and overriding of the parietal bones are frequently associated with caput succedaneum and become more evident after the caput has receded; they disappear during the 1st weeks of life. Rarely, a hemorrhagic caput may result in shock and require blood transfusion. Analogous swelling, discoloration, and distortion of the face are seen in face presentations.
- No specific treatment is needed, but if extensive ecchymoses are present, hyperbilirubinemia may develop

Table *(O.P.Ghai 8th/14)*: **Difference b/w caput succedaneum and cephalohematoma**

Characteristic	Caput succedaneum	Cephalohematoma
Incidence	Common	Less common
Location	Subcutaneous plane	Over parietal bones, b/w skull and periosteum
Time of presentation	**Maximum size** and **firmness at birth**	Increasing size for 12-24 hr and then stable
Time course	**Softens progressively from birth** and **resolves within 2–3 days**	Takes 3–6 weeks to resolve
Characteristic findings	Diffuse; cross suture line	Does not cross suture line; has distinct margins
Association	None	Linear skull fracture (5-25%); hyperbilirubinemia

210. Ans. (a) Apgar score provide an immediate..., (b) Apgar scoring is..., (d) Normal respiratory..., (e) Normal heart rate >100...

[Ref: Park 23rd/532; O.P.Ghai 8th/126; Nelson (SAE) 20th/798]

"Newnates have a ***normal respiratory rate of 40-60 breaths/min. Normal rate of heart rate is 110-160 beats/min.*** *Bradycardia is heart rate <100 beats/min"- O.P.Ghai 8th/137*

Apgar Scores

◈ *Park 23rd/532*

- *Today it is considered as negligence to omit apgar scoring of a newborn infant, especially LBW babies*
- ***It provide an immediate estimate of the physical condition of the baby***
- *A score* ***below 5 needs prompt action***

- ***Infants with low apgar scores at 5 minutes of age are subject to a high-risk of complications*** and ***death during the neonatal period***

Role of Apgar Scores in Resuscitation

◈ *O.P.Ghai 8th/126*

- The Apgar score is an objective method of evaluating the newborn's condition. It is generally performed 1 minute and again at 5 minutes after birth. However, resuscitation must be initiated before the 1-minute score is assigned. Therefore, the ***Apgar score is not used to guide the resuscitation.***
- While the Apgar score is not useful for decision making at the beginning of resuscitation, the change of score at sequential time points following birth can ***reflect how well the baby is responding to resuscitative efforts***. Hence, Apgar scores should be obtained every 5 minutes for up to 20 minutes, if the 5-minute Apgar score is less than 7.

Apgar Score

◈ *Nelson (SAE) 20th/798*

- The **Apgar score** is a practical method of systematically assessing newborn infants immediately after birth to help identify those requiring resuscitation and to predict survival in the neonatal period.
- The 1-min Apgar score may signal the need for immediate resuscitation, and the 5-, 10-, 15-, and 20-min scores may indicate the probability of successfully resuscitating an infant. A low score may be due to a number of factors, including drugs given to the mother during labor and immaturity
- The ***Apgar score was not designed to predict neurologic outcome***. Indeed, the score is normal in most patients in whom cerebral palsy subsequently develops, and the incidence of cerebral palsy is low in infants with Apgar scores of 0–3 at 5 min (but higher than in infants with Apgar scores of 7–10).
- The Apgar score and umbilical artery blood pH both predict neonatal death. An Apgar score of 0–3 at 5 min is uncommon but is a better predictor of neonatal death (in both term and preterm infants) than an umbilical artery pH of 7.0 or less; the presence of both variables increases the relative risk of neonatal mortality in term and preterm infants

Table *(Nelson (SAE) 20th/798):* **Apgar evaluation of newborn infants**

SIGN	0	1	2
Heart rate	Absent	Below 100	Over 100
Respiratory effort	Absent	Slow, irregular	Good, crying
Muscle tone	Limp	Some flexion of extremities	Active motion
Response to catheter in nostril (tested after oropharynx is clear)	No response	Grimace	Cough or sneeze
Color	Blue, pale	Body pink, extremities blue	Completely pink

Sixty sec after complete birth of the infant (disregarding the cord and placenta), the five objective signs above are evaluated, and each is given a score of 0, 1, or 2. A total score of 10 indicates an infant in the best possible condition. An infant with a score of 0-3 requires immediate resuscitation.

211. Ans. (a) 6–12 weeks

[Ref: William's Obs 23rd/1214; Park 23rd/151; O.P.Ghai 8th/272; Nelson (SAE) 20th/1550-51]

"**80 percent** of pregnant women with rubella infection and a rash during the ***first 12 weeks*** have a fetus with congenital infection. At **13 to 14 weeks**, this incidence was ***54 percent***, and by the ***end of the second trimester, it was 25 percent***. As the duration of pregnancy increases, fetal infections are less likely to cause congenital malformations"- *William's Obs 23rd/1214*

"The **first trimester of pregnancy** is the ***most disastrous time*** for the foetus as the organs are developing. Infection during this period results in abnormalities in the ***infant in about 85 per cent of cases***, whereas detectable defects are found in about 16 per cent of infants, who acquired infection during the second trimester. Birth defects are uncommon if maternal infection occurs after 20 weeks of gestation. Inapparent maternal infections can produce these anomalies as well. It can result in foetal death and spontaneous abortion"- *Park 23rd/151*

"Classical triad of **congenital rubella syndrome consists of deafness, cataract** and **congenital heart disease"** *(O.P. Ghai 8th/ 272)*

Congenital Rubella Syndrome

◈ *Nelson (SAE) 20th/1549-51*

- "Transmissibility is highest in the first trimester and so the rate of fetal disease (90% at <11 weeks). The fetus completely spared if infection occurs beyond 16 weeks"
- Nerve deafness is the single most common finding among infants with CRS. Most infants have some degree of intrauterine growth restriction. Retinal findings described as **salt-and-pepper retinopathy** are the most common ocular abnormality, but it has little early effect on vision.
- ***Unilateral or bilateral cataracts*** are the most serious eye finding, occurring in about ⅓ of infants.
- **Cardiac abnormalities** occur in half of the children infected during the 1st 8 wk of gestation. ***Patent ductus arteriosus*** is the most frequently reported cardiac defect, followed by lesions of the pulmonary arteries and valvular disease. Interstitial pneumonitis leading to death in some cases has been reported.
- **Neurologic abnormalities** are common and may progress following birth. ***Meningoencephalitis*** is present in 10– 20% of infants with CRS and may persist for up to 12 mo.

Table *(Nelson (SAE) 20th/1549):* **Pathologic findings of congenital rubella syndrome(partial list)**

System	Pathologic Findings
Cardiovascular	Patent ductus arteriosus Pulmonary artery stenosis Ventriculo septal defect Myocarditis

Contd...

System	Pathologic Findings
Central nervous system	Chronic meningitis Parenchymal necrosis Vasculitis with calcification
Eye	Microphthalmia Cataract Iridocyclitis Ciliary body necrosis Glaucoma Retinopathy
Bone	Malformed osteoid Poor mineralization of osteoid Thinning cartilage

212. Ans. (b) Liver failure may occur..., (c) N-acetylcysteine is..., (d) N-acetylcysteine can..., (e) Renal damage may...

[Ref: Nelson (SAE) 20th/456-57, 453; KDT 7th/ 206-07; Katzung 13th/1006-07]

TABLE *(Nelson (SAE) 20th/456)*: **Classic stages in the clinical course of acetaminophen toxicity**

State	Time after ingestion	Characteristics
I	0.5–24 hr	Anorexia, vomiting, malaise, Labs typically normal except for acetaminophen level
II	24–48 hr	Resolution of earlier symptoms; right upper quadrant abdominal pain and tenderness; elevated hepatic transaminases (aspartate aminotransferase > alanine aminotransferase), Elevated INR
III	3–5 days.	Peak transaminase elevations; ***development of liver failure,*** multi organ-system failure, death or recovery begins
IV	4 days-2 wk	Resolution of liver function abnormalities, Clinical recovery precedes histologic recovery

Acetaminophen

◈ *Nelson(SAE) 20th/456-57*

- ***Acetaminophen intoxication is a common cause of acute liver failure in adolescents and adults.***
- Acetaminophen toxicity results from the formation of a highly reactive intermediate metabolite, ***N-acetyl-p-benzoquinoneimine (NAPQI).***
- When therapeutic doses are administered, only a small amount (≈4%) of a dose is metabolized by the hepatic cytochrome P450 enzyme CYP2E1 to NAPQI, which is immediately conjugated with glutathione to form a harmless mercapturic acid conjugate.
- When hepatic stores of glutathione are depleted to <70% of normal, the NAPQI metabolite can combine with hepatic macromolecules to produce hepatocellular damage.
- The acute toxic dose of acetaminophen is generally considered to be ***>200 mg/kg in children younger than 12 yr of age***; a single ingestion of >7.5 g is considered a minimum toxic dose in adolescents and adults.
- ***Adolescents have a higher incidence of toxic plasma concentrations after ingestion than do children***, and their exposures are often associated with intentional overdose.
- If untreated, patients with an acute overdose may pass through the 4 stages of acetaminophen toxicity
- After a large acute oral overdose, and when the need for antidotal treatment is determined, treatment should be started as soon as possible, including within 1–2 hr of the ingestion.
- The antidote for acetaminophen poisoning is NAC, which serves as a precursor for hepatic glutathione synthesis, replenishing glutathione stores and preventing the reaction of NAPQI with hepatocytes. ***NAC therapy is most effective when initiated early in the course of intoxication (within 8 hr), but may have value even if started 24–36 hr after the ingestion in severe cases.***
- N-acetylcysteine: Ingestion-treatment interval is critical; earlier the better. ***It is practically ineffective if started 16 hours or more after paracetamol ingestion***"- *KDT 7th/ 206-07*
- Oral NAC is unpalatable and can be irritating to the gastrointestinal tract, so it should be diluted to a 5% solution with soda or fruit juice to minimize vomiting. Antiemetics (ondansetron) may be used to control vomiting and/or NAC may be administered directly into the stomach or upper intestine by tube.
- ***An IV preparation of NAC is also available (Acetadote)***
- N-acetyl cysteine can cause ***nausea, vomiting, and diarrhea or constipation.*** Rarely, it can cause ***rashes, fever, headache, drowsiness, low blood pressure, and liver problems.***When inhaled (breathed into the lungs), it can also cause swelling in the mouth, runny nose, drowsiness, clamminess, and chest tightness.N-acetyl cysteine has an unpleasant odor that may make it hard to take

Paracetamol: Adverse Effects

◈ *Katzung 13th/1006-07*

- In therapeutic doses, a mild increase in hepatic enzymes may occasionally occur in the absence of jaundice; this is reversible when the drug is withdrawn. With larger doses, dizziness, excitement, and disorientation can be seen. Ingestion of 15 g of acetaminophen may be fatal, death being caused by ***severe hepatotoxicity with centrilobular necrosis, sometimes associated with acute renal tubular necrosis.***
- Doses greater than 4–6 g/d are not recommended and a history of alcoholism contraindicates even this dose. Early symptoms of hepatic damage include nausea, vomiting, diarrhea, and abdominal pain. ***Cases of renal damage without hepatic damage have occurred***, even after usual doses of acetaminophen.
- Hemolytic anemia and methemoglobinemia are very rare adverse events. I***nterstitial nephritis and papillary necrosis***— serious complications of phenacetin—have not occurred nor has gastrointestinal bleeding.

Table *(Nelson 20th/453)*: **Common antidotes for poisoning**

Antidote	Poisoning	Dose	Route	Adverse Effects
N-Acetylcysteine (Mucomyst)	Acetaminophen; carbon tetrachloride and chloroform	140 mg/kg loading, followed by 70 mg/kg q4h for 17 doses	PO	Vomiting
N-Acetylcysteine (Acetodote)	Acetaminophen	150 mg/kg over 30–60 min, followed by 50 mg/kg over 4 hrs, followed by 100 mg/kg over 16 hrs.	IV	Anaphylactoid reaction

ORTHOPAEDICS

213. Ans. (c) Rarely associated with meniscal injury

[Ref: Maheshwari 5th/148-49; Apley 9th/876; www.mayoclinic.org]

"Bony fragment from the lateral tibial condyle on the AP view represents a **Segond fracture due to avulsion at the anterolateral capsular attachment.** ***Segond fractures have a very high association with ACL tears*** and meniscal injuries and should prompt further evaluation with an MRI"- radiopaedia. org

Anterior Cruciate Ligament

◈ *Maheshwari 5th/148-49*

- *This ligament is most commonly ruptured, **often in association with tears of medial or lateral collateral ligaments***
- *Commonly, it occurs as a result of twisting force on a semi-flexed knee*
- *Often the injury to medial collateral ligament, medial meniscus and anterior cruciate ligament occur together. This is called O' Donoghue triad*

"*Approximately* **50 percent of ACL injuries** *occur in combination with **damage to the meniscus**, articular cartilage, or other ligaments*"- *orthoinfo.aaos.org*

Anterior Cruciate Ligament (ACL)

◈ *emedicine.medscape.com*

- Anterior cruciate ligament (ACL) injuries are most often a result of low-velocity, noncontact, deceleration injuries and contact injuries with a rotational component. Contact sports also may produce injury to the ACL secondary to ***twisting, valgus stress, or hyperextension*** all directly related to contact or collision.
- The ***Lachman test is the most sensitive test for acute ACL rupture***. It is performed with the knee in 30° of flexion, with the patient lying supine.
- Other tests for ACL injury:**Anterior drawer test** and **pivot shift test**

Table *(Maheshwari 5th/149)*: **Essential features of knee ligament injury**

Name of the ligament	Mechanism of injury	Clinical features			
		Pain	Swelling	Tenderness	Tests
• Medial collateral	Valgus force	Medial side	Medial side	Medially, on the femoral condyle	Valgue stress + at 30° knee flexion
• Lateral collateral	Varus force	Lateral side	Lateral side	Laterally, on fibular head	Varus stress + at 30° knee flexion
• Anterior cruciate	Twisting extension	Diffuse	Haemarthrosis	Vague	Anterior drawer test + Lachmann test +
• Posterior cruciate	Backward force on tibia	Diffuse	Haemarthrosis	Vague	Posterior drawer test +

214. Ans. (a) Curvature of the medial border of the foot

[Ref: Apley 9th/591-95;www.bjj.boneandjoint.org.uk]

Club Foot (CTEV) Scoring Systems

◈ *www.bjj.boneandjoint.org.uk*

- There is no agreed method of grading the severity of deformity or monitoring the natural history, but there is a reported need for such a classification, which should be reliable, reproducible, feasible in a clinical setting, and predict appropriate treatment.
- Pirani et al devised a simple scoring system based on **six clinical signs** of contracture.
- Each is scored according to the following principle:
  0, no abnormality;
  0.5, moderate abnormality;
  1, severe abnormality.
- The six signs are separated into ***three related to the hindfoot (severity of the posterior crease, emptiness of the heel and rigidity of the equinus), and three related to the midfoot (curvature of the lateral border of the foot, severity of the medial crease and position of the lateral part of the head of the talus).***
- Thus, each foot can receive a hindfoot score between 0 and 3, a midfoot score between 0 and 3 and a total score between 0 and 6.

Table: Pirani scoring

Paramaters	Normal	Moderate	Severe
Midfoot			
Curved lateral border	0	0.5	1
Medial crease	0	0.5	1
Talar Head coverage	0	0.5	1
Hindfoot			
Posterior crease	0	0.5	1
Rigid equines	0	0.5	1
Empty heel	0	0.5	1

215. Ans. (a) Middle path regimen is used..., (c) Commonly spread by hematogenous..., (e) Lower thoracic and upper lumbar is ...

[Ref: Maheshwari 5th/185-94; Apley 9th/472-74,8th/44,387-89;Children Orthopaedics and Fracture by Michael 2nd/159; Danhert Radiology 7th/231]

The spine is the most common (30% to 50%) site of osseous involvement. A primary accompanying lesion may be discovered from the pulmonary or urogenital system or from an unknown source. ***Lymphogenous and hematogenous spread has been implicated in thoracolumbar lesions***, but less often in cervical or sacral lesions. A peridiscal presentation occurs in approximately 80% of patients, with the ***anterior vertebral body affected*** and contiguous progression through subligamentous burrowing (anterior longitudinal ligament) and eventual extension to the adjacent vertebrae"-*Campbell's Orthopaedics 11th/Chap 18*

"Spinal involvement is usually a result of hematogenous spread of* M. tuberculosis *into the dense vasculature of cancellous bone of the vertebral bodies"- *www.ncbi.nlm.nih.gov*

Tuberculosis of the Spine (Pott's Disease)

◈ *Maheshwari 5th/185-94*

- "Dorso-lumbar region being the one affected most frequently"
- "Like T.B of the bones and joints elsewhere in the body, TB of the spine is always secondary. The bacteria reach the spine via the hematogenous route, from the lungs or lymph nodes"
- "While the ***upper thoracic spine is the most common site of spinal TB in children,*** the ***lower thoracic and upper lumbar vertebrae*** are usually affected in adults. From the ***anterior superior or inferior angle of the vertebral body, the lesion slowly reaches the adjacent body, later affecting the intervertebral disk.*** With advanced disease, collapse of vertebral bodies results in kyphosis (*gibbus*). A paravertebral "cold" abscess may also form"- *Harrison 19th/1110*
- ***"Paradiscal is the commonest type.*** *In this, the contiguous areas of two adjacent vertebrae along with the intervening disc are affected"*
- "**Site affected in Pott's spine:** *Vertebral body (82%) with predilection for anterior part adjacent to superior/inferior endplate>> posterior elements (18%)"-Danhert Radiology 7th/231*
- "**Location of Pott's spine:** ***Upper lumbar+lower thoracic spine (L1 most common),*** *typically more than one(upto 5-10) vertebrae affected"- Danhert Radiology 7th/231*
- ***Acute onset paraplegia has a better prognosis"***- *Maheshwari 5th/194*
- "Conservative treatment: ATT forms the mainstay of treatment. All patients are started on 4-drugs ATT as soon as diagnosis is made"
- Operative procedures: Costo-transversectomy, antero-lateral decompression(ALD), radical debridement and arthrodesis(Hongkong operation) and laminectomy

Different Regime for Tuberculosis of Spine

◈ *dnborthopaedics.wordpress.com*

- ***Middle Path regime (By Dr. Tully):*** **a.** Rest, **b.** Drugs- Intensive Phase: HRO (5-6 months); Continuation Phase: HZ (3-4 months) + HR (4-5 months); Prophylactic Phase: HE (4-5 months), **c.** Radioogical Follow-up (X-ray, MRI), **d. Gradual** Mobilisation +/- Spinal braces,**e.** Management of Abscess/Sinuses, **f. Management of Neurological complications, g.** Surgey(Excisional surgery; Definitive Surgery: Indication of Surgery in Pott's spine), **h.**Post-operative care
- **$HRZE_4$ + HRE/HRZ_3 + HR_{11}**

"The 'middle path' regime for treatment of spinal tuberculosis in the 1970s by Tuli: In the management of spinal tuberculosis, at one extreme is the thought that the non-operative (conservative) management is unjustifiable in all cases because of a slow response time. The disease may progress and cause deficits. At the other extreme is to perfom surgical extirpation of the abscess-bone-granulation tissue, which allows for a speedy recovery but seems to be unnecessary in a lot of cases. The **'middle path'** is when surgery is performed only if there is no improvement using conservative treatment, or if the patients develops progressive neurological deficits or has a symptomatic prevertebral abscess"-www.neurologyindia.com

216. Ans. (b) Radial nerve involvement after manipulation, (c) Pathological fractures, (d) Vascular injury, (e) Multiple fractures

[Ref: Apley 9th/748-51; orthobullets.com/trauma; Campbell's Operative Orthopaedics, 11th ed./chap 54]

Fractured Shaft of Humerus: Operative Treatment –Indications

◈ *Apley 9th/748-49*

- ***Severe multiple injuries***
- *An open fracture*
- *Segmental fractures*
- *Displaced intra-articular extension of the fracture*
- ***A pathological fracture***
- *A floating elbow(simultaneous unstable humeral and forearm fractures)*
- ***Radial nerve palsy after manipulation***
- *Non-union*
- *Problems with nursing care in a dependent person*

Operative Treatment

◈ *Campbell's Operative Orthopaedics, 11th ed./chap 54*

- The choice of operative treatment for a humeral shaft fracture depends on multiple factors. McKee divided the indications for operative treatment into three categories: (1) fracture indications, (2) associated injuries, and (3) patient indications.
- Some indications are more absolute than others. Failure of conservative treatment, ***pathological fracture***, displaced intraarticular extension, ***vascular injury, and brachial plexus injury*** almost always require surgery.
- Other conditions, such as minimally displaced segmental fractures and obesity, are only relative indications. Our most common indication for operative treatment is early mobilization of patients with polytrauma. Treatment decisions must take all factors into consideration, tailoring the treatment to the specific patient.

Table *(Campbell's Operative Orthopaedics, 11th ed./chap 54)*

Indications for primary operative treatment of humeral shaft fractures
Fracture Indications
Failure to obtain and maintain adequate closed reduction
Shortening >3 cm
Rotation >30 degrees
Angulation >20 degrees
Segmental fracture
Pathological fracture
Intraarticular extension
Shoulder joint
Elbow joint
Associated Injuries
Open wound
Vascular injury
Brachial plexus injury
Ipsilateral forearm fracture
Ipsilateral shoulder or elbow fracture
Bilateral humeral fractures
Lower extremity fracture requiring upper extremity weight bearing
Burns
High-velocity gunshot injury
Chronic associated joint stiffness of elbow or shoulder
Patient Indications
Multiple injuries, polytrauma
Head injury (Glasgow Coma Scale score = 8)
Chest trauma
Poor patient tolerance, compliance
Unfavorable body habitus
Morbid obesity
Large breasts

217. Ans. (b) Ewing's sarcoma is second most common ..., (d) Fever and weight loss may be present...

[Ref: Maheshwari 5th/243; Apley 9th/212-13;Robbins 9th/1203;Harrison 19th/119e-4;Nelson 20th(SAE)/2473]

Vascular tumours *are: Hemangioma, glomangioma, angiosarcoma"- Maheshwari 5th/236*

"**Marrow tumours** *are:* ***Ewing sarcoma***, *multiple myeloma, plasma cell tumour etc"- Maheshwari 5th/236*

"Ewing's sarcoma, which ***constitutes ~10–15% of all bone sarcomas***, is common in adolescence and has a peak incidence in the second decade of life. It typically involves the ***diaphyseal region*** of long bones and also has an affinity for flat bones"- *Harrison 19th/119e-4*

Osteosarcoma is the most common primary malignant bone tumour in children and adolescents, followed by Ewing's sarcoma. In children younger than 10 year of age, Ewing's sarcoma is more common than osteosarcoma"- *Nelson 20th(SAE)/2470*

"Ewing sarcoma often is associated with ***systemic manifestations, such as fever and weight loss****"- Nelson 20th(SAE)/2473*

Ewing Sarcoma

◈ *Maheshwari 5th/243*

- This is highly malignant tumour occurring b/w the age of ***10-20 years***, sometimes up to 30 years
- **Site:** The tumour may benign anywhere, but ***diaphysis of the long bone*** is the ***most common site***
- ***Often there is associated fever***, in which case it may be confused with osteomyelitis
- This ***a highly radiosensitive tumour***, melts quickly but recurs.
- Treatment consists of ***control of local tumour by radiotherapy*** and control of metastasis by chemotherapy

Ewing Sarcoma

◈ *Apley 9th/212-13*

- It occurs most ***commonly b/w the ages of 10 and 20 years***
- It is believed to arise from ***endothelial cells in the bone marrow***
- The prognosis is always poor and ***surgery alone does little to improve it.***
- ***Radiotherapy has a dramatic effect on the tumour*** but overall survival is not much enhanced

"**Ewing sarcoma family tumors** account for approximately 6% to 10% of primary malignant bone tumors and follow osteosarcoma as the second most common group of bone sarcomas in children of all bone sarcomas, ESFT have the youngest average age at presentation, since ***approximately 80% are younger than 20 years***. Boys are affected slightly more frequently than girls"- *Robbins 9th/1203*

218. Ans. (a) Most common age..., (c) Pulmonary metastasis..., (d) A locally aggressive tumour, (e) May involve sacrum

[Ref: Maheshwari 5th/237-39; Apley 9th/ 202-03;Robbins 9th/1203-04;Sabiston 19th/786-87]

"Although benign, giant cell tumors can be locally aggressive. GCT is more common in females, and typically occurs in the epiphysis of long bones after the physis has closed. The ***knee, vertebra, distal radius, and sacrum*** are common sites"-CSDT 14th/1143

GCT: It perhaps represents the ***most aggressive benign tumor*** and threatens the true definition of a benign cancer because benign pulmonary ***metastases develop in approximately 1% to 2% of giant cell tumors.*** This tumor typically develops in the epiphysis of long bones, although it may occur in the ***flat bones of the pelvis,*** **often between the ages of 20 and 40.**Giant cell tumors in the ***spine, sacrum, and pelvis*** present greater surgical challenges"- *Sabiston 19th/786-87*

Giant cell Tumor

◈ *Robbins 9th/1203-04*

- It is a relatively ***uncommon benign,*** but ***locally aggressive,*** neoplasm. It usually arises in individuals in their ***20s to 40s.***
- Giant cell tumors arise in the epiphysis but may extend into the metaphysis. The majority arise around the knee (***distal femur and proximal tibia***), but virtually any bone can be involved. The typical location of these tumors near joints frequently causes arthritis-like symptoms.
- Occasionally, they present with pathologic fractures. Most are solitary; however, multicentric tumors do occur, especially in the distal extremities.
- Although GCTs are considered benign, roughly half recur after simple curettage, and as ***many as 2% spread to the lungs as localized lesions*** that are cured by local excision.

"*The bone affected commonly are those around knee i,e, the* ***lower end of femur*** *and the upper end of the tibia"- Maheshwari 5th/237-39*

219. Ans. (c) Acetabulum fracture of pelvis

[Ref: Campbell's Operative Orthopaedics, 11th/Chap 33; www.orthobullets.com/trauma/1034/ acetabular-fractures; emedicine.medscape.com/article/385838-overview]

"Although several of the associated fracture types involve both columns of the acetabulum, the designation ***both-column fracture*** denotes that none of the articular fracture fragments of the acetabulum maintain bony continuity with the axial skeleton: a fracture line divides the ilium, so the sacroiliac joint is not connected to any articular segment. The **spur sign**, shown on the obturator oblique view, is pathognomonic of a both-column fracture. It represents the remaining portion of the ilium still attached to the sacrum and is seen projected lateral to the medially displaced acetabulum"- *Campbell's Operative Orthopaedics, 11th/Chap 33*

The **spur sign** is seen on transverse computed tomographic (CT) images or conventional ***obturator oblique radiographs of the pelvis.*** The appearance is the result of an inferiorly directed apex of a triangular fragment of bone (the spur) and is suggestive of ***fracture of both anterior and posterior acetabular columns.*** www.orthobullets.com/trauma/1034/acetabular-fractures

"**Special radiographic signs** to look for include the **Gull Sign** (lateral spike protruding from acetabulum) which signifies a posterior wall fracture and the **Spur Sign** (lateral continuation of the ilium that is seen as a spike above the acetabulum on an obturator view) which signifies an associated both column fracture"- *www.orthopaedicsone.com*

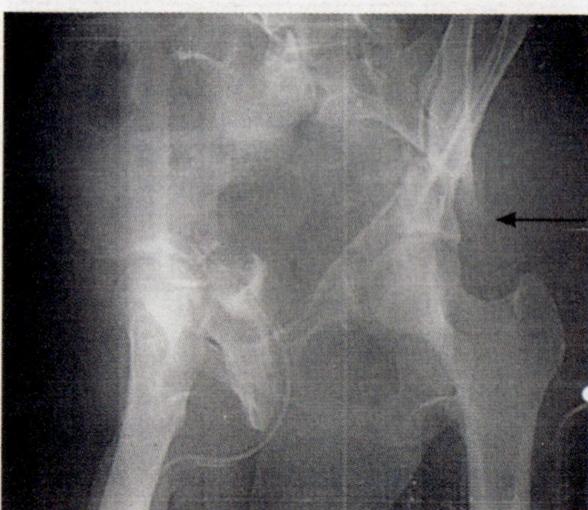

Fig: 53-18 *(Campbell 11th):* Spur sign in both-column fracture of acetabulum

Both-column fractures are the most common ***acetabular injury.*** As the name implies, the anterior and posterior columns are involved. On AP radiographs, a disruption of the iliopectineal and ilioischial lines, as well as the obturator ring, may be seen (see the first image below). An iliac wing fracture may be seen on the AP view, but often, it is appreciated only on the iliac oblique radiograph. The **pathognomonic spur sign** is present on the obturator oblique view and confirmed on a CT scan"- emedicine.medscape.com/article/385838-overview

220. Ans. a. Fracture of..., b. Steroid..., c. Alcohol... d. Sickle cell disease, e. Caisson disease

[Ref: Maheshwari 5th/318-19; Dahnert Radiology Review manual 7th/51-56; Apley 9th/103-06;orthopedics.about. com]

"**AVN of femoral head** *occurs in fracture of the femoral neck- Maheshwari 5th/318*

Table *(Maheshwari 5th/318-19):* **Cause of avascular necrosis of femoral head**

- Idiopathic-commonest
- Alcoholism
- Steroid therapy
- Sickle cell disease
- Patient of renal dialysis
- Patient on anticancer drug
- Post-partum necrosis
- Goucher's disease
- Caisson's disease

Avascular Necrosis or Osteonecrosis or Aseptic Necrosis

◈ *Orthopedics.about.com*

- *Avascular necrosis is common in fracture of- femoral neck (including slipped capital femoral epiphysis, posterior dislocation of hip), neck talus, waist scaphoid and lunate (dislocation) (Apley 8th/570)*
- *Although it can occur in any bone, osteonecrosis most often affects the hip.*

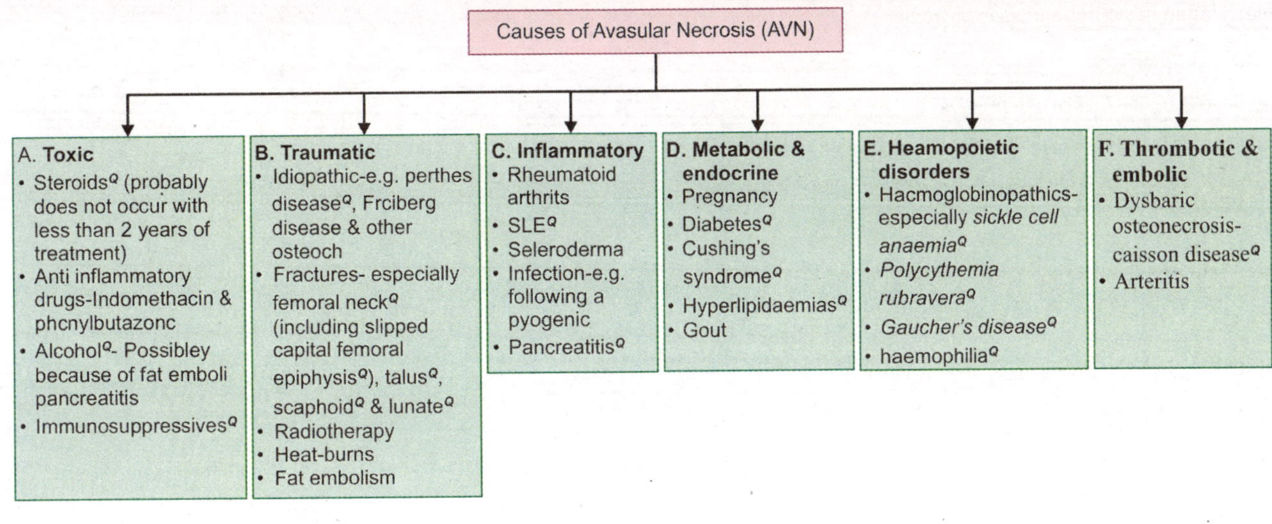

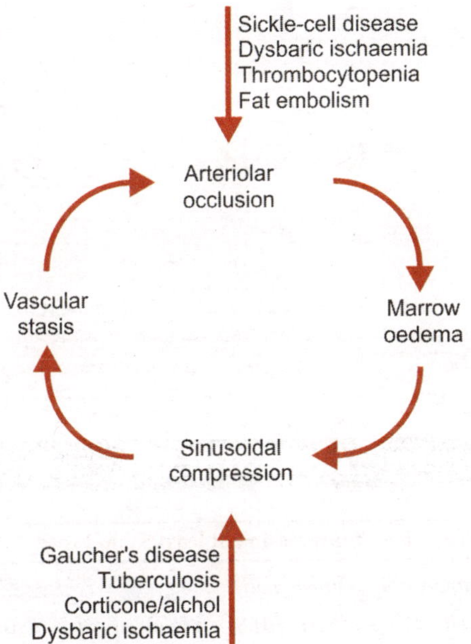

Fig: *(Apley 9th/104):* Algorithim showing how various disorders may enters the vicious cycle of capillary stasis and marrow engorgement

221. Ans. (c) Deep vein thrombosis

[Ref: Maheshwari 5th/43-44; Apley 9th/681; www.openanesthesia.org/fat_embolism/]

Fat embolism

◈ *www.openanesthesia.org*

- Diagnosis is usually made on the basis of clinical findings but biochemical changes may be of value.
- The most commonly used set of major and minor diagnostic criteria are those published by Gurd The major criteria are based on the classic triad and clinical diagnosis is made by the presence of respiratory insufficiency, neurological impairment, and a petechial rash. In the appropriate setting, the rash is considered pathognomonic, although it is present in only 20–50% of cases. For the diagnosis of fat embolism syndrome, at least one major and four minor criteria must be present.
- The reliability of these parameters in Gurd's criteria have been questioned and other schemes based more on respiratory features alone (**Lindeque's criteria**) have been proposed.
- More recently, a fat embolism index has been proposed as a semi-quantitative means of diagnosing fat embolism syndrome, in which there are seven clinical features (**Schonfeld's criteria**); each one is given a particular score. A score of >5 is required for a positive diagnosis.

Table: Gurd's criteria *academic.oup.com*

Major criteria
Axillary or subconjunctival petechiae
Hypoxaemia Pa_{O_2} <60 mm Hg; Fi_{O2} = 0.4)
Central nervous system depression disproportionate to hypoxaemia
Pulmonary oedema
Minor criteria
Tachycardia <110 bpm
Pyrexia <38.5°C
Emboli present in the retina on fundoscopy
Fat present in urine
A sudden inexplicable drop in haematocrit or platelet values
Increasing ESR
Fat globules present in the sputum

Table: Lindeque's criteria *academic.oup.com*

Lindeque's criteria
Sustained Pa_{o2} <8 kPa
Sustained Pco_2 of >7.3 kPa or a pH <7.3
Sustained respiratory rate >35 breaths min^{-1}, despite sedation
Increased work of breathing: dyspnoea, accessory muscle use, tachycardia, and anxiety

Table: Schonfeld's criteria *academic.oup.com/bjaed*

Criterion	Score
Petechiae	5
Chest X-ray changes (diffuse alveolar infiltrates)	4
Hypoxaemia (Pa_{o2} < 9.3 kPa)	3
Fever (>38°C)	1
Tachycardia (>120 beats min^{-1})	1
Tachypnoea (>30 bpm)	1
Cumulative score >5 required for diagnosis	

222. Ans. (c) Apical subungual infection- V-shaped piece is removed..., (d) When the pus extends beneath the nail, it is necessary...

[Ref: Maheshwari 5th/205-07; BDC 7th/ Vol. I 132-34; Apley 9th]

"In **apical subungual infection:** For drainage, a ***small V-shaped piece is removed from the center of the free edge*** of the nail along with a little wedge of the full thickness of the skin overlying the abscess"- Maheshwari 5th/206

"In **acute paronychia**: When the pus extends beneath the nail, it is necessary to ***remove the proximal one-third of the nail for adequate drainage***"- Maheshwari 5th/2056

Terminal Pulp Infection (Whitlow or Felon)

◈ *Maheshwari 5th/206; emedicine.medscape.com*

- The index and the thumb are affected most often
- When suppuration has occurred, drainage is required
- **DO NOT perform a "fishmouth" incision** since this may results in: ***Unstable finger pad, neuroma, and/or loss of sensation***"- www.wikem.org/wiki/Felon
- The ***felon should be incised in the area of maximum swelling and tenderness***. The incision should not cross the distal interphalangeal (DIP) joint to prevent formation of a flexion contracture at the DIP flexion crease. Probing is not carried out proximally to avoid extension of infection into the flexor tendon sheath.
- Lateral or transverse incisions frequently cause ischemia and anesthesia by ***injuring one or both neurovascular bundles.***
- Fish-mouth incision can lead to an ***unstable painful fingertip***"emedicine.medscape.com

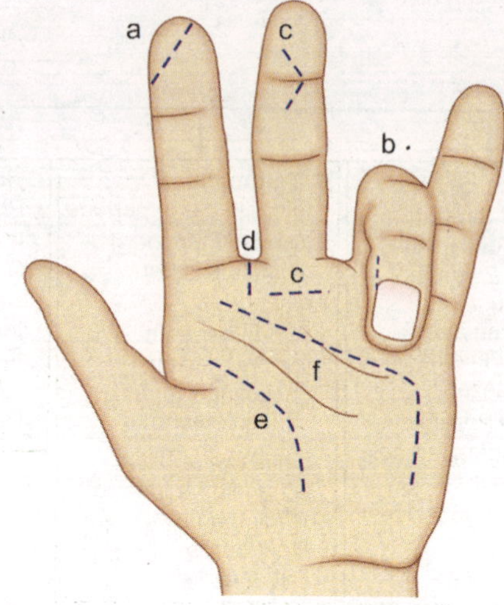

Fig: *(Apley 9th/16):* Incision for surgical drainage: a. pulp space (directly over abscess), b.nail-fold(it may be necessary to excise the edge of the nail, c. tendon sheath, d. web space, e. thenar space, f. mid-palmar space

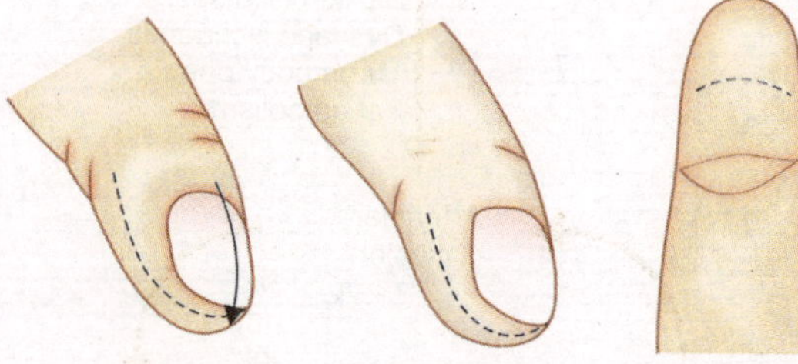

Fig: *(www.slideshare.net):* Incision used in Felon(from left to right) – Fish mouth incision,Hockey stick incision/J-shaped incision and transverse palmar incision

ANAESTHESIA

223. Ans. (b) Chest compression at least 5 cm/2 inch

[Ref: http://circ.ahajournals.org/]

- ***Basic life support (BLS), advanced cardiovascular life support (ACLS), and post-cardiac arrest care*** are labels of convenience that each describe a set of skills and knowledge that are applied sequentially during the treatment of patients who have a cardiac arrest.
- There is overlap as each stage of care progresses to the next, but generally ***ACLS comprises the level of care between BLS and post-cardiac arrest care***

Update recommendations for advanced cardiac life support 2015:

- ***The combined use of vasopressin and epinephrine offers no advantage to using standard-dose epinephrine*** in cardiac arrest.

- Also, vasopressin does not offer an advantage over the use of epinephrine alone. Therefore, to simplify the algorithm, ***vasopressin has been removed from the Adult Cardiac Arrest Algorithm–2015 Update.***

Advanced Cardiac Life Support

◈ *www.ijncollege.edu.my*

- Once an advanced airway is in place, the 2 providers should no longer deliver cycles of CPR (ie, compressions interrupted by pauses for ventilation) unless ventilation is inadequate when compressions are not paused.
- Instead the compressing provider should give continuous chest compressions at a rate ***of 100/min to 120/min***, without pauses for ventilation. The provider delivering ventilation should provide ***1 breath every 6 seconds*** (***10 breaths per minute***).

Hemodynamic Goals After Resuscitation

◈ *www.ijncollege.edu.my*

- 2015 (New): ***It may be reasonable to avoid and immediately correct hypotension (SBP < 90 mm Hg, MAP < 65 mm Hg) during post–cardiac arrest care.***

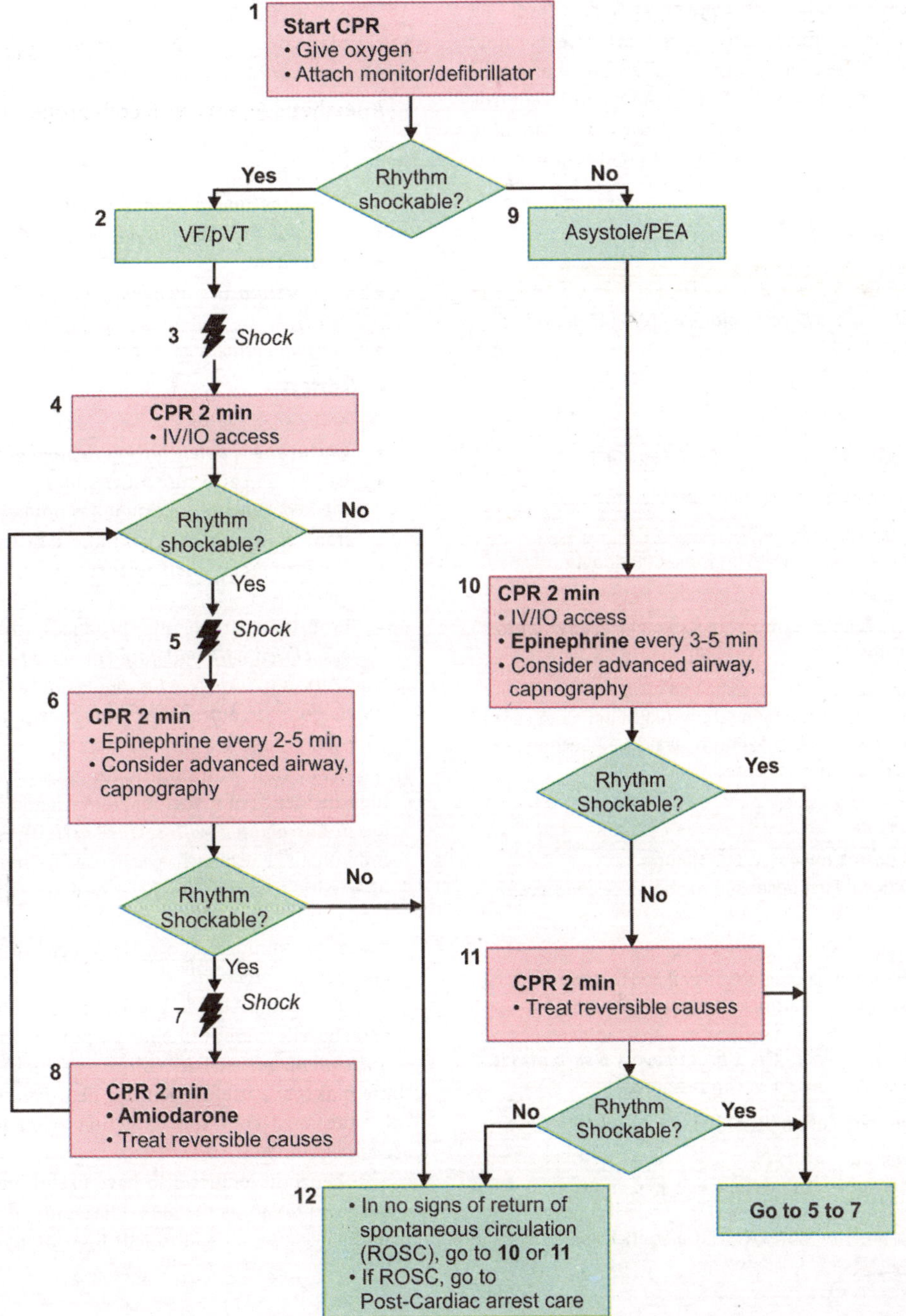

Fig: Adult Cardiac arrest algorithm-2015

- ***2010(Earlier):*** Once the patient achieves ROSC, one of the priorities highlighted in the 2010 guidelines was to optimize the patient's hemodynamic status. Although the 2010 cardiac arrest algorithm lists a target of 90 mm Hg, the actual recommendation at the time was to achieve a ***mean arterial pressure (MAP) of at least 65 mm Hg.***
- Reason for change in 2015: Studies of patients after cardiac arrest have found that a SBP < 90 mm Hg or a MAP < 65 mm Hg is associated with higher mortality and diminished functional recovery, while systolic arterial pressures of greater than 100 mm Hg are associated with better recovery. While higher pressures appear superior, specific systolic or mean arterial pressure targets could not be identified, because trials typically studied a bundle of many interventions, including hemodynamic control. Also, because baseline blood pressure varies from patient to patient, different patients may have different requirements to maintain optimal organ perfusion

Table: Adult cardiac arrest -2015

CPR Quality
• Push hard ***(at least 2 inches [5 cm]) and fast (100-120/min)*** and allow complete chest recoil.
• Minimize interruptions in compressions.
• Avoid excessive ventilation
• Rotate compressor every 2 minutes, or sooner if fatigued.
• If no advanced airway, 30:2 compression-ventilation ratio.
• Quantitative waveform capnography ▪ If $PETCO_2$ <10 mm Hg, attempt to improve CPR quality
• Intra-arterial pressure ▪ If relaxation phase (diastolic) pressure <20 mm Hg, attempt to improve CPR quality.
Shock Energy of Defibrillation • **Biphasic:** Manufacturer recommendation (e.g., initial dose of 120-200 J); if unknown, use maximum available. Second and subsequent doses should be considered. • **Monophasic**: 360 J
Drug Therapy • **Epinephrine IV/IO dose:**1 mg every 3–5 minutes • **Amiodarone IV/IO dose:** First dose: 300 mg bolus. Second dose: 150 mg.
Advanced Airway • Endotracheal intubation or supraglottic advanced airway • Waveform capnography to confirm and monitor ET tube placement • Once advanced airway in place, give ***1 breath every 6 seconds (10 breaths/min)*** with continuous chest compresions
Return of Spontaneous circulation (ROSC)
• Pulse and blood pressure
• Abrupt sustained increase in $PETCO_2$ (typically ≥40 mm Hg)
• Spontaneous arterial pressure waves with intra-arterial monitoring

224. Ans. (a) Atracurium, (c) Enflurane (d) Pethidine

[Ref: Ajay Yadav 5th/131; Morgan 5th/165,216,583-84;Lee 13th/18]

Etomidate does not have epileptogenic potential(according to Morgan and Miller)

*"**Enflurane**: At high doses it produces spike and wave pattern in EEG which culminates into **frank tonic-clonic seizure**"- Ajay Yadav 5th/83*

"**Atracurium: Laudanosine Toxicity**-Laudanosine, a tertiary amine, is a breakdown product of atracurium's Hofmann elimination and has been associated with central nervous system excitation, resulting in elevation of the minimum alveolar concentration and ***even precipitation of seizures***"- *Morgan 5th/216*

Anesthetic Agents with Epileptogenic Potential

◈ *Ajay Yadav 3rd/68*

- Methohexital
- Ketamine(due to its preservative)
- *Propofol (opisthotonus has been reported)*
- ***Enflurane***
- ***Atracurium*** *(its metabolic product laudanosine is epileptogenic)*
- *Local anaesthetic toxicity*

CNS Effect

◈ *Miller Anestheia 7th*

- **Enflurane** is ***potentially epileptogenic*** in the clinical setting
- Isoflurane can cause EEG spiking and myoclonus, but in the experimental setting it has not been associated with the frank epileptoid activity induced by enflurane.
- **Ketamine** can ***elicit seizures*** in patients with an epileptic diathesis
- **Etomidate** frequently produces myoclonus that is ***not associated with epileptiform activity on the EEG***

*"Patient with a history of fits should not be exposed to epileptogenic agents such as **enflurane, methohexitone or ketamine**" (Lee 13th/18)*

"Induction with **etomidate** is associated with a relatively high incidence of myoclonic movements, but these movements are ***not associated with seizure activity on the EEG*** in normal individuals. The drug has ***been used to treat seizures***, but reports of seizure activity following etomidate suggest that the drug is best avoided in patients with a history of epilepsy. In fact, small doses of etomidate can activate seizure foci in patients with epilepsy"- *Morgan 5th/584*

"**Propofol**: Although it has been associated with dystonic and choreiform movements, propofol seems to ***have significant anticonvulsant activity***. Moreover, its short elimination half-life makes it a useful agent for neuroanesthesia. Propofol is by far the most common induction agent for neuroanesthesia"- *Morgan 5th/584*

"Benzodiazepines also have useful ***anticonvulsant*** properties. Midazolam is the benzodiazepine of choice in neuroanesthesia because of its short half-life"- *Morgan 5th/584*

"**Opioids** generally have minimal effects on CBF, CMR, and ICP. Small doses of **alfentanil** (<50 mg/kg) can ***activate seizure foci in patients with epilepsy***. **Morphine** is generally not considered optimal as a component of anesthesia for intracranial surgery. **Normeperidine**, a metabolite of meperidine, ***can induce seizures***, particularly in patients with renal failure"-*Morgan 5th/583*

"Meperidine (pethidine)–pethidine is metabolized to norpethdine. Which has half the analgesic potency of the parent compound but is twice as active as convulsout"-*www.medmerits.com*

Table *(Morgan 5th/165)*: **Clinical pharmacology of inhalational anesthetics.**

	Nitrous Oxide	Halothane	Isoflurane	Desflurane	Sevoflurane
Seizures	↓	↓	↓	↓	↓

225. Ans. (a) Environment friendly, (c) Low blood solubility, (d) Inert, (e) Stable

[Ref: Ajay Yadav 5th/78-79; Morgan 5th/164,173; Miller's Anesthesia 6th/626,649; Wiley 7th/527-532]

Table *(Morgan 5th/164)* **Advantages and disadvantages of xenon (Xe) anesthesia**

Advantages
Inert (probably nontoxic with no metabolism)
Minimal cardiovascular effects
Low blood solubility
Rapid induction and recovery
Does not trigger malignant hyperthermia
Environmentally friendly
Nonexplosive
Disadvantages
High cost
Low potency (MAC=70%)

XENON

◈ *Morgan 5th/173*

- Xenon is a "noble" gas that has long been known to have anesthetic properties.
- It is an **inert element** that does not form chemical bonds.
- Xenon is scavenged from the atmosphere through a costly distillation process. It is an odorless, nonexplosive, naturally occurring gas with a MAC of.71 and a blood/gas coefficient of 0.115, giving it very fast onset and emergence parameters.
- Xenon seems to have little effect on cardiovascular, hepatic, or renal systems and has been found to be protective against neuronal ischemia.
- As a natural element, it has no effect upon the ozone layer compared with another NMDA antagonist, nitrous oxide.
- ***Cost and limited availability*** have prevented its widespread use.
- "Xenon is a heavy (i.e. *4.5 times heavier than air) gas*"-*(nobel. scas.bcit.ca/resource/ ptable/xe.htm)*

Xenon

◈ *Miller's Anesthesia 6th/ 626,649*

- It has received considerable interest in the last few years because it has many characteristics approaching those of an "ideal" inhaled anesthetic
- Its ***blood:gas partition coefficient is 0.14***, and unlike the other potent volatile anesthetics (except methoxyflurane), xenon provides some degree of analgesia.
- *The MAC of xenon in humans is 71%(i.e high MAC), which might prove to be a limitation. It is nonexplosive,* nonpungent, and odorless, and thus can be inhaled with ease
- Because of its ***scarcity and high cost***, new anesthetic systems need to be developed to provide for recycling of xenon.
- *"It has no effects on cardiac output or cardiac rhythm and is not thought to have a significant effect on systemic vascular resistance. It also does not affect pulmonary function and is not known to have any hepatic or renal toxicity"- (G and G 11th/chap 13)*

226. Ans. (b) Pressure gradient, (e) Density of gas

[Ref: Ajay Yadav 5th/ 11; Morgan 5th/55; Lee Synopsis 13th/86]

"When **flow is laminar**, the flow rate is directly proportional to the ***pressure gradient*** causing it. When flow is **turbulent**, the flow rate is proportional - to the ***square root of the pressure gradient***. In terms of the physical properties of the flowing gas, laminar flow depends on viscosity, and ***turbulent flow depends on density***"- *Lee Synopsis 13th/86*

"Flowmeters are calibrated for specific gases, as the flow rate across a constriction depends on the gas viscosity at low laminar flows (Poiseuille's law) and its density at high turbulent flows. To minimize the effect of friction between them and the tube's wall, floats are designed to rotate constantly, which keeps them centered in the tube"-*Morgan 5th/55*

Flow of Gases: Laminar or Turbulent

◈ *Ajay Yadav 5th/ 11*

Laminar

- It is produced when the gas pass through straight tube. Flow is smooth
- Laminar flow is ***more dependent on viscosity***

Turbulent

- Turbulent flow is produced if flow rate is very high or if gas passes through bends, constrictions. Flow is rough
- Reynold's number must exceed to 2000 for turbulence
- Turbulent flow is ***more dependent on density***

227. Ans. (c) CO_2, (d) Cyclopropane, (e) Nitrous oxide

[Ref: Ajay Yadav 5th/ 90-91, 77; Morgan 5th/164; Lee Synopsis 13th/83, 85]

*"**Oxygen, nitrogen, air and helium** are stored in **cylinders as gases. Nitrous oxide, carbon dioxide and cycloproprane are stored in as liquid** in equilibrium with saturated vapour"- Lee Synopsis 13th/85*

"**Nitrous oxide**: Stored as liquid in ***blue colour cylinders***(cylinder pressure 760 psi)"- *Ajay Yadav 5th/77*

Table: Physical properties medical gases in cylinders

	Oxygen	Nitrous oxide	Entonox	Air	Carbon dioxide
Physical state in cylinder	Gas	Liquid	Gas	Gas	Liquid

Table: Gradestack.com

Colour of Cylinders	Pressure	Filled as
a. O_2–Black body with white shoulders	2000 psi	Gas
b. N_2O– Blue	760 psi	Liquid
c. CO_2–Grey	750 psi	Liquid
d. **Cyclopropane**–orange	75 psi	Liquid
e. **Helium**–Brown	1400 psi	Gas
f. **Air**–Grey body with black and white shoulders	2000 psi	Gas
g. **Entonox**–Blue body with blue and white shoulders (50% O_2 + 50% N_2O)	2000 psi	Gas

Pressure and Filling

◈ *www.ncbi.nlm.nih.gov/pmc*

- The majority of the gases are stored in cylinders as compressed gases (***oxygen, air, nitrogen, helium, heliox***). These ***gases do not liquefy at ordinary ambient temperature*** regardless of pressure applied as their critical temperature is low.
- ***Nitrous oxide and carbon-dioxide liquefy at pressures*** to which cylinders are filled (at ambient temperature) and are therefore stored as liquids.

228. Ans. (a) Average distance from…, (c) Beyond 6–7 years of…, (d) 2-3 cm of epidural catheter…, (e) Distance from the upper …

[Ref: Ajay Yadav 5th/ 165-67; Morgan 5th/964-66; Lee Synopsis 13th/501-04; Cousins and Bridenbaugh's Neural Blockade in Clinical Anesthesia and Pain 4th/608]

"The **distance from the skin to the anterior wall of the sacral canal** *varies from* ***10 to 39 mm (mean 21 mm)*** *in children ranging in age from 2 month to 7 years, which means that the epidural space can usually be entered through sacrococcygeal membrane at a distance less than 20 mm from the covering skin. The* **distance from the upper border of the sacral hiatus to the dural sac** *in children aged 10 month to 18 years equal* ***30 ± 10.4 mm*** *(range 13.6 to 54.7 mm)"- Cousins and Bridenbaugh's Neural Blockade in Clinical Anesthesia and Pain* 4th/608

"Palpating sacral hiatus in children is easier. **In infants** –the sacral canal is ***filled with fluid fat and loose areolar connective tissue*** *which allows* ***easy spread of anesthethetic solutions up to age of 6 or 7 years****, also this fluidity of epidural fat* ***allows catheter insertion easier****"- resident-anesthesiology. blogspot.in*

*"****Identification of sacral hiatus become more difficult above age of 6-8 yr****. It cause increased failure rate" ratewww.slideshare. net*

"After general anaesthesia, ultrasonography was performed at the sacral hiatus in 130 children aged 2–84 months positioned in the lateral position. The median [range] values for the ***intercornual, caudal space depth and the distance from skin to the posterior sacral bony surface were 17.0 [9.6–24] mm, 3.5 [1–8] mm and 21.0 [10–39] mm,*** respectively. The optimal angle showed no significant correlation with age, weight, height or body surface area. The median [range] calculated optimal angle for the needle was 21.0 [10–38]. -onlinelibrary.wiley.com/ doi

Caudal Anesthesia

◈ *Miller 7th*

- Caudal anesthesia is basically a single-shot technique. Occasionally, placement of an epidural catheter for repeat/ continuous infusion is contemplated. The ***"normal" length of catheter to be introduced into the epidural space is 2 to 3 cm***, as for any epidural block.
- The dosage prescription scheme of Armitage that was published many years ago still remains the most dependable
  - With 0.5 mL/kg, ***all sacral dermatomes are blocked.***
  - With 1.0 mL/kg, ***all sacral and lumba****r* dermatomes are blocked.
  - With 1.25 mL/kg, the upper limit of anesthesia is at least midthoracic.
  - However, when 1.25 mL/kg is injected there is a danger of excessive rostral spread, it is therefore preferable not to administer more than 1.0 mL/kg of local anesthetic.
- Block failure is not unusual (3% to 5%), especially in children older than 7 years of age, but even in younger patients the failure rate can be rather high.

Caudal Anaesthesia

◈ *Lee Synopsis 13th/501-04*

- *A 5 cm needle is inserted through the sacrococcygeal membrane at 45°. After aspiration tests for blood and CSF have proved negative, injection is performed*
- *The dose of 0.25%* ***bupivacaine is 0.5-0.75 ml/kg***
- *The* **extradural space** *below sacral hiatus may range from being deep to excessively shallow-its* ***average length is 10-15 cm***

"**Caudal block**: For single-dose administration (outpatient surgeries) bupivacaine, 0.25 to 0.175% solution, or ropivacaine, 0.2 to 0.175%, at a ***dose of 1 mL/kg*** is commonly used. Postoperative analgesia typically lasts 4 to 6 hours and is not associated with a motor paralysis at these concentrations. This route can be used for either a single-dose injection or for catheter advancement for continuous infusion"-Barash Anesthesia 6th/ chap 45

Caudal Epidural

◈ *Morgan 5th/964-66*

- Its anatomy is more easily appreciated in ***infants and children***
- A ***dosage of 0.5–1.0 mL/kg of 0.125–0.25% bupivacaine*** (or ropivacaine), with or without epinephrine, can be used.

Caudal Block

◈ *www.dvcipm.org*

- **Indications**: ***Use for patients < 8 years old to provide intraoperative and postoperative analgesia*** for abdominal and lower extremity surgery.

- Technique. A pop will be felt as the needle passes through the sacrococcygeal membrane. Once the sacrococcygeal membrane is pierced, drop the needle angle to 20° to 40° from the skin and ***advance the needle and the catheter 2 to 4 mm.***

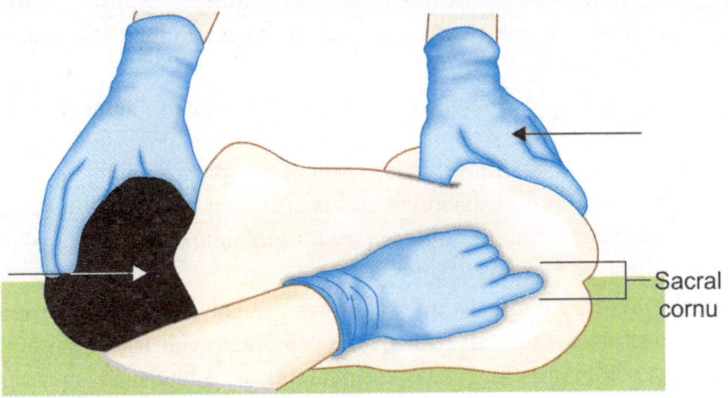

Fig: *(Morgan 5th/964):* Positioning an anesthetized child for caudal block and palpation for the sacral hiatus.

SKIN

229. Ans. **(a) Lichen planus, (b) Bullous pemphigoid, (c) Dermatitis herpetiformis**

[Ref: Neena Khanna 5th/77-79; Harrison 19th/370; Roxburg 17th/92; Pathology of Skin by Farmer and Hood 2nd/222; Robbins 9th/1169-70]

*"Familial benign pemphigus(**Hailey-Hailey disease**): Extensive areas of **acantholysis** giving a dilapidated brick wall appearance"- Neena Khanna 5th/84*

*"**Acantholytic disorders** includes **Pemphigus family** (including paraneoplastic pemphigus), eosinophilic spongiosis, Darier's disease , **Hailey-Hailey diaease** (Familial benign chronic pemphigus)and transient acantholytic dermatosis (Grover's disease), as well as specific histological pattern such as focal acantholytic dyskeratosis and epidermolytic hyperkeratosis" (Pathology of Skin by Farmer and Hood 2nd/222)*

Acantholysis

- Acantholysis is separation of *epidermal cells* from each other *(Neena Khanna 5th/79)*
- The common denominator, histologically in all forms of *pemphigus is acantholysis*
- This term implies dissolution or lysis of the intercellular adhesion sites within a squamous epithelial surface.
- Acantholytic disorders are of two types –Immunologic (includes pemphigus) and Nonimmunogenic

"The common histologic denominator in all forms of pemphigus is **acantholysis,** lysis of the intercellular adhesive junctions between neighboring squamous epithelial cells that results in the rounding up of detached cells. In ***pemphigus vulgaris, acantholysis selectively involves the layer of cells immediately above the basal cell layer***, giving rise to a **suprabasal acantholytic blister**. - *Robbins 9th/1169-70*

Table *(Harrison 19th/370):* **Immunologically mediated blistering diseases**

Disease	Clinical	Histology
Pemphigus foliaceus	Crusts and shallow erosions on scalp, central face, upper chest, and back	***Acantholytic blister*** formed in superficial layer of epidermis
Pemphigus vulgaris	Flaccid blisters, denuded skin, oromucosal lesions	***Acantholytic blister*** formed in suprabasal layer of epidermis
Paraneoplastic pemphigus	Painful stomatitis with papulosquamous or lichenoid eruptions that progress to blisters	***Acantholysis,*** keratinocyte necrosis and vacuolar interface dermatitis
Bullous pemphigoid	Large tense blisters on flexor surfaces and trunk	Subepidermal blister with eosinophil-rich infiltrate
Dermatitis herpetiformis	Extremely pruritic small papules and vesicles on elbows, knees, buttocks, and posterior neck	Subepidermal blister with neutrophils in dermal papillae

Table *(Neena Khanna 5th/77):* **Tzanck smear finding in bullous disorders**

Findings	Disorders
Acantholytic cells	Pemphigus group
Multinucleated giant cells	Varicella-zoster infection, herpes simplex infection
Necrotic keratinocytes	Epidermal necrolysis
Predominantly eosinophils	Bullous pemphigoid
Predominantly neutrophils	Bullous impetigo, chronic bullous disease of childhood

230. Ans. **(e) Seborrheic patch at back**

[Ref: Neena Khanna 5th/423-24;Roxburg 17th/281-285]

"Seborrheic dermatitis: *Aetiology- overgrowth of yeast, malassezia furfur may play an important pathogenic* **role"**- *Roxburg 17th/107*

Cutaneous Markers of Internal Malignancies Due to

◈ *Neena Khanna 5th/423*

- Metastases: To skin
- Genodermatoses: With an increased predisposition to internal neoplasia
- Exposure to carcinogens: Which result in skin changes as well as internal neoplasia
- Paraneoplastic syndromes: Are cutaneous reaction patterns associated with internal neoplasia

Paraneoplastic Diseases

◈ *Neena Khanna 5th/424*

- **Malignant acanthosis nigricans.** Associated with malignancies of gut, especially gastric adenocarcinoma.
- **Dermatomyositis:** Associated with bronchogenic carcinoma (males), carcinoma of breast and ovaries (females).
- **Paraneoplastic pemphigus**: Associated internal malignancies, e.g. thvmoma, lymphoma and Castleman's disease.
- **Migratory thromhophlebitis:** Associated with malignancies of pancreas and lung.
- **Necrolytic migratory erythema**

Genodermatoses

◈ *www.dermnetnz.org*

- Birt–Hogg–Dubé syndrome
- Cowden disease
- Gardner syndrome
- Gorlin syndrome (basal cell naevus syndrome)
- Multiple endocrine neoplasm type 2B
- Neurofibromatosis
- Peutz-Jeghers syndrome
- Torre-Muir syndrome
- Progeria (premature aging syndromes)

Cutaneous Paraneoplastic Syndromes

◈ *www.dermnetnz.org*

Papulosquamous	Erythematous
• Acanthosis nigricans • Acquired ichthyosis • Acrokeratosis paraneoplastica • Extramammary Paget disease • Florid cutaneous papillomatosis • Palmoplantar keratoderma • Pityriasis rotunda • *Sign of Leser-Trelat* • *Tripe palms*	• Dermatomyositis • Erythema gyratum repens (see erythema annulare centrifugum) • Hypertrophic osteoarthropathy and digital clubbing • Multicentric reticulohistiocytosis • Necrolytic migratory erythema • Sweet disease • Eosinophilic dermatosis of haematologic malignancy
Bullous	**Miscellaneous**
• Paraneoplastic pemphigus	• Generalised granuloma annulare (rarely) • Granulomatous dermatitis • Carcinoid syndrome • Hypertrichosis lanuginosa acquisita • Trousseau syndrome • Paraneoplastic pruritus (cancer itch)

231. Ans. (b) Hailey-Hailey disease, (e) Grover disease

[Ref: Neena Khanna 5th/79; Harrison 19th/131, 134, 370]

"**Pemphigus vulgaris**: Application of tangential pressure on normal skin(usually on pretibial area) results in formation of new bulla(***Nikolsky's sign***). Nikolsky's sign is also elicitable in ***staphylococcal scalded skin syndrome and epidermal necrolysis***"- *Neena Khanna 5th/79*

"**Staphylococcal scalded-skin syndrome**: Diffuse tender erythema, often with bullae and desquamation and ***Nikolsky's sign***"- *Harrison 19th/131*

"**Pemphigus**: Manual pressure to the skin of these patients may elicit the separation of the epidermis (***Nikolsky's sign***). This finding, while characteristic of pemphigus, is not specific to this group of disorders and is also seen in ***toxic epidermal necrolysis, Stevens-Johnson syndrome***, and a few other skin diseases"-*Harrison 19th/370*

"**Nikolsky's sign** is almost always present in toxic epidermal necrolysis and is associated with pemphigus vulgaris. It is useful in differentiating between pemphigus vulgaris or mucous membrane pemphigoid (where it is present) and ***bullous pemphigoid (where it is absent).*** Also present in Staphylococcal scalded skin syndrome caused by the exfoliative toxin of *Staphylococcus aureus*"-*wikipedia*

"**Grover's disease** (transient acantholytic dermatosis) is a condition that appears suddenly as itchy red spots on the trunk, most often in older men. Minor cases of Grover's disease may be rather common"- *www.aocd.org*

232. Ans. (a) Pus under nail bed, (b) Pus may extend to base of nail, (c) Swelling of nail fold

[Ref: Neena Khanna 5th/152-54; Maheshwari 5th/204-05; Roxburg 17th/277]

Acute Paronychia

◈ *Neena Khanna 5th/152*

- Paronychia is inflammation of ***nail folds***
- **Etiology:** ***Staphylococcus*** enter the nail fold (through breaks in the skin of nail fold or cuticle)
- Predisposing factors: including chronic paronychia, nail biting and hang nails
- **Clinical feature:** Nail fold is swollen, red and tender. ***Pus may be visible under the nail fold or on the nail bed.*** May be associated with lymadenopathy and constitutional symptoms
- **Treatment:** Systemic antistaphylococcal antibiotics (erythromycin and cloxacillin). If needed, surgical drainage

"Acute paronychia: There is pain, tenderness, redness and swelling at one or both sides of the nail fold and ***at the base of the nail*** if suppuration has extended deep to nail"- *Maheshwari 5th/204-05*

Chronic Paronychia

◈ *Neena Khanna 5th/153-54*

- *It is an inflammatory dermatosis of nail folds with secondary effects on the nail matrix and nail growth*
- *Etiology: Microbial colonization: the space b/w nail plate and proximal nail fold is colonized by* ***candida***, Staphylococcus and gram negative bacteria

- *Predisposing factor: wet work, finger sucking, DM, candidal vulvovaginitis*
- *Clinical features: Nail fold is swollen and rolled. Adjacent nail plate becomes riged and disclored. Sometime a bead of pus can be expressed fromunder the nail fold*
- *Treatment: Topical antibiotics (gentamycin, ciprofloxacin) and antifungal (clotrimazole); Systemic antibiotics (may help in more inflamed lesions) and weekly fluconazole (in recurrent disease)*

PSYCHIATRY

233. Ans. (a) Undoing, (b) Reaction formation, (d) Isolation of affect

[Ref: Ahuja 7th/95-98,208-210; Synopsis of Psychiatry by Kaplan and Sadock 11th/161-62,418-27]

Defense Mechanisms

◈ *Synopsis of Psychiatry by Kaplan and Sadock 11th/160*

- At each phase of libidinal development, specific drive components evoke characteristic ego defenses.
- The **anal phase**, for example, is associated with ***reaction formation***, as manifested by the development of shame and disgust in relation to anal impulses and pleasures.
- Defenses can be grouped hierarchically according to the relative degree of maturity associated with them. Narcissistic defenses are the most primitive and appear in children and persons who are psychotically disturbed. **Immature** defenses are seen in *adolescents and some nonpsychotic patients*.
- **Neurotic defenses** are encountered in ***obsessive-compulsive*** and hysterical patients as well as in adults under stress.
- Narcissistic-Psychotic Defenses are ***Projection, Denial and Distortion***.
- "**Projection** is Perceiving and reacting to unacceptable inner impulses and their derivatives as though they were outside the self. On a psychotic level, this takes the form of frank delusions about external reality, usually persecutory, includes both perception of one's own feelings and those of another with subsequent acting on the perception (psychotic paranoid delusions). Impulses may derive from id or superego (hallucinated recriminations)". *Kaplan and Sadock 11th/161*

"**Suppression** is mature defence. Suppression is conscious or semiconscious decision to postpone attention to a conscious impulse or conflict"- *Kaplan and Sadock 11th/162*

Table *(Ahuja 7th/208-210;6th/ 221-22):* **Ego defense mechanisms**

Defense mechanism	Illustration(s) from clinical situations
Displacement	• *Phobia(Especially in children)* • *OCD*
Reaction formation	• *Obscessive compulsive personality traits and disorder* • *OCD*
Undoing	• *Compulsive acts in OCD* • *Compulsive rituals*
Inhibition	• *OCD* • *Phobias*
Isolation	*Obsessional thoughts*
Dissociation	*Dissociative disorders e.g Psychogenic amnesia, sychogenic fugue, multiple personality etc.*

Contd...

Table *(Kaplan and Sadock 11th/162):* **Classification of neurotic defense mechanisms**

Controlling	The excessive attempt to manage or regulate events or objects in the environment in the interest of minimizing anxiety and solving internal conflicts.
Displacement	Involves a purposeful, unconscious shifting of impulses or affective investment from one object to another in the interest of solving a conflict.
Dissociation	A temporary but drastic modification of character or sense of personal identify to avoid emotional distress; it includes fugue states and hysterical conversion reactions.
Externalization	A general term, correlative to intermalization, referring to the tendency to perceive in the external world and attitudes, and styles of thinking.
Inhibition	The unconsciously determined limitation or renunciation of specific ego functions, singly or in combination, to avoid anxiety arising out of conflict with instinctual impulses, superego, or environmental forces or figures.
Intellectualization	The control of affects and impulses by way of thinking about them instead of experiencing them.
Isolation	The intrapsychic splitting or separation of affect from content resulting in repression of either idea or affect or the displacement of affect to a different or substitute content.
Rationalization	A justification of attitudes, beliefs, or behavior that might other wisebe unacceptable by an incorrect application of justifying reasons or the invention of a convincing fallacy.
Reaction formation	The management of unacceptable impulses by permitting expression of the impulse in antithetical form. This is equivalently an expression of the impuse in the negative. Where instinctual conflict is persistent, reaction formation can become a character trait on a permanent basis, usually as an aspect of obsessional character.
Repression	Consists of the expelling and withholding from conscious awareness of an idea or feeling.
Sexualization	The endowing of an object or function with sexual significance that it did not previously have, or possesses to a lesser degree, to ward off anxieties connected with prohibited impulses.

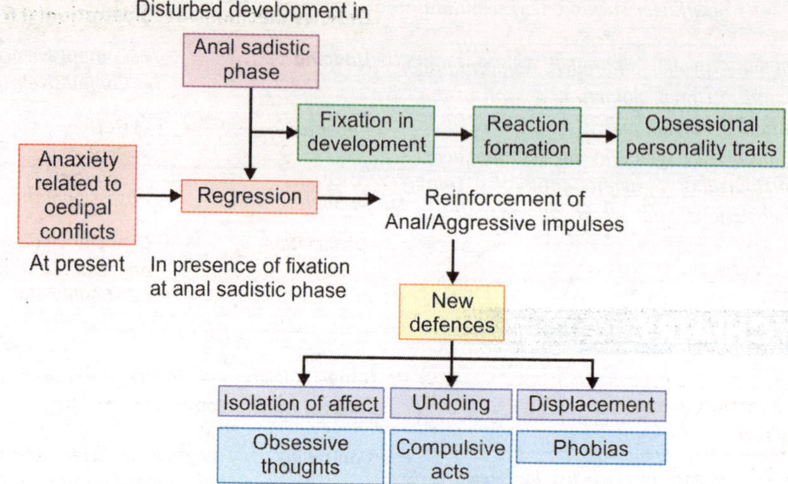

Fig: (Ahuja 7th/97): Psychodynamic theory of OCD: A brief summary

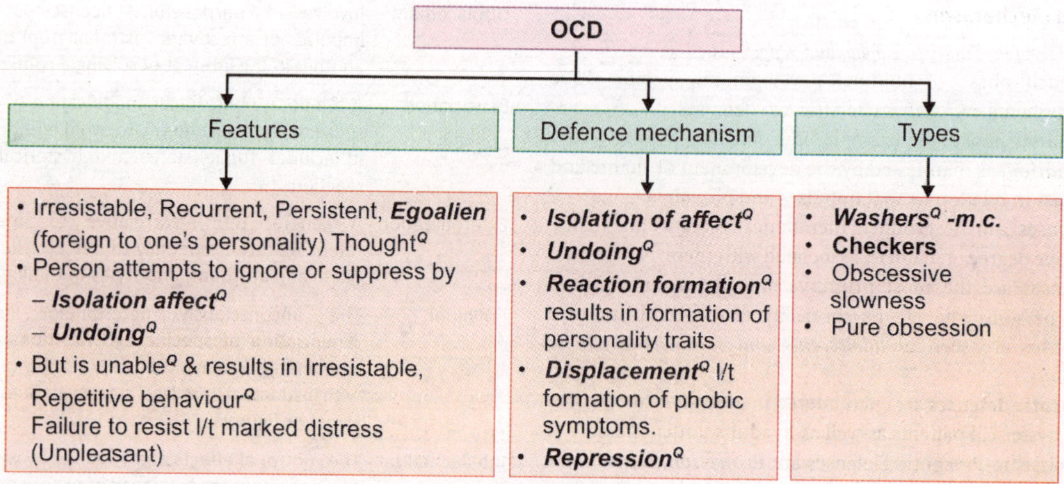

Fig: OCD

234. Ans. (a) Self, (b) Future, (d) World and environment

[Ref: Synopsis of Psychiatry by Kaplan and Sadock 11th/355; www.tutor2u.net/psychology]

"**Cognitive Theory**. According to cognitive theory, depression results from specific cognitive distortions present in persons susceptible to depression. These distortions, referred to as depressogenic schemata, are cognitive templates that perceive both internal and external data in ways that are altered by early experiences. Aaron Beck postulated a **cognitive triad of depression** that consists of ***(1) views about the self-a negative self precept, (2) about the environment-a tendency to experience the world as hostile and demanding, and (3) about the future-the expectation of suffering and failure. Therapy consists of modifying these distortions.*** **Cognitive triad**: Beliefs about oneself, the world, and the future"- *Kaplan and Sadock 11th/355*

Beck's Cognitive Triad *www.tutor2u.net/psychology*

- Also known as the **negative triad,** is an irrational and pessimistic view of the three key elements of a person's belief system present in depression.
- It was proposed byAaron Beck in 1976. The triad forms part of his cognitive theory of depression and the concept is used as part of CBT, particularly in Beck›s «Treatment of Negative Automatic Thoughts» (TNAT) approach.
- The triad involves «automatic, spontaneous and seemingly uncontrollable negative thoughts about:The *self,* The *world or environment and* The *future*
- Examples of this negative thinking include:
  - The self - "I'm worthless and ugly" or "I wish I was different"
  - The world - "No one values me" or "people ignore me all the time"

- The future - "I'm hopeless because things will never change" or "things can only get worse!"

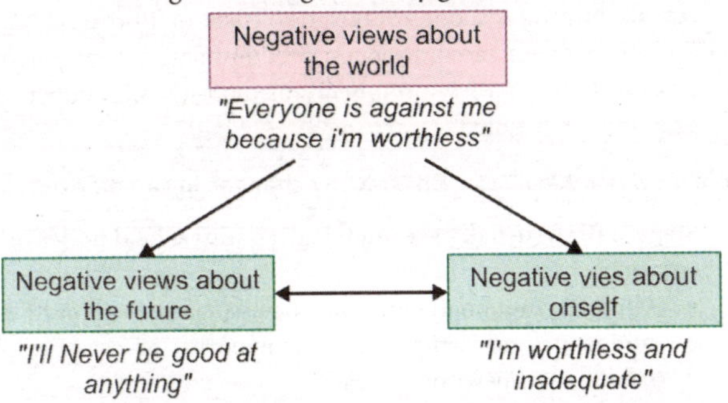

Fig: Beck's cognitive triad

235. Ans. (e) Cognitive therapy

[Ref: Synopsis of Psychiatry by Kaplan and Sadock 11th/1065-81; www.nimh.nih.gov]

Brain Stimulation Technique

◈ *Synopsis of Psychiatry by Kaplan and Sadock 11th/1065-81*

- Brain stimulation in psychiatric practice and research uses ***electrical currents or magnetic fields to alter neuronal firing. There*** is a growing list of tools capable of eliciting such neuromodulation, each with a different spectrum of action. These tools either apply electrical or magnetic fields transcranially or involve the surgical implantation of electrodes to deliver electrical currents to a cranial nerve or to the brain directly.
- The transcranial techniques include ***cranial electrical stimulation (CES), electroconvulsive therapy (ECT), transcranial direct current stimulation (tDCS, also called direct current polarization), transcranial magnetic stimulation (TMS), and magnetic seizure therapy (MST). The surgical techniques include cortical brain stimulation (CBS), deep brain stimulation (DBS), and vagus nerve stimulation (VNS).***
- **TMS** is the application of a rapidly changing magnetic field to the superficial layers of the cerebral cortex, which locally induces small electric currents, also referred to as eddy currents
- Transcranial direct current stimulation is a noninvasive form of treatment that uses very weak (1 to 3 mA) direct electrical current applied to the scalp.
- CBS is a novel neurosurgical approach in which electrodes are implanted over the surface of the cortex to provide electrical brain stimulation in a targeted superficial region.

Kinds of Brain-Stimulating Techniques

◈ *www.psychcentral.com*

- **Electroconvulsive therapy (ECT)** is the oldest and the best known and, in fact, is still recognized as the most effective treatment for severe depression.
- Another technique, **rapid transcranial magnetic stimulation (rTMS)**, involves the placement of an electromagnetic coil on the scalp.
- Yet another approach, **magnetic seizure therapy**, is a combination of ECT and rTMS.
- Finally, **vagus nerve stimulation (VNS)** involves the implantation of a small device about the size of a pocket watch in the upper left area of the chest. The devise is connected via an electrical lead to the vagus nerve in the left side of the neck. (The vagus is one of the 12 pairs of nerves that originate in the brain.)

236. Ans. (b) Auditory hallucination may occur, (c) Visual hallucination may be present, (d) Predominantly low-voltage fast activity on EEG, (e) Most severe alcohol withdrawal syndrome

[Ref: Ahuja 7th/38; Synopsis of Psychiatry by Kaplan and Sadock 11th/631-32,88]

Electroencephalography (EEG)- Alterations associated with ***Alcohol withdrawal***:May be normal in patients who are not delirious; ***excessive fast activity*** in patients with delirium"- *Kaplan and Sadock 11th/88(Table)*

Delirium tremens is associated with ***predominantly low-voltage fast activity***, making it an important exception. EEG characteristics in delirium include slowing or dropout of the dominant posterior rhythm, diffuse theta or delta waves (i.e., slowing), poor organization of background rhythm, and loss of reactivity of the EEG to eye opening and closing"-*Book.google.co.in*

EEG in Early or Impending DT

◈ *ournals.sagepub.com*

- ***Extremely low-voltage background*** activity particularly over the posterior temporal, central, and occipital regions.
- *Paucity or absence of alpha rhythm*, even during the resting state with eyes closed.
- Relative non-reactivity of background faster frequencies, particularly over the posterior regions.

Delirium Tremens

◈ *Ahuja 7th/38*

- Delirium tremens (DT) is the ***most severe alcohol withdrawal syndrome***. It occurs usually within 2-4 days of complete or significant abstinence from heavy alcohol drinking in about ***5% of patients,*** as compared to ***acute tremulousness which occurs in about 34% of patients.***
- The course is short, with recovery occurring within 3-7 days. This is an acute organic brain syndrome (delirium) with characteristic features of:
    - Clouding of consciousness with disorientation in time and place.
    - Poor attention span and distractibility.
    - **Visual (and also auditory) hallucinations** and illusions, which are often vivid and very frightening. Tactile hallucinations of insects crawling over the body may occur.
    - Marked autonomic disturbance with tachycardia, fever, hypertension, sweating and pupillary dilatation.
    - Psychomotor agitation and ataxia.
    - Insomnia, with a reversal of sleep-wake pattern.
    - Dehydration with electrolyte imbalance.

- Death can occur in 5–10% of patients with delirium tremens and is often due to cardiovascular collapse, infection, hyperthermia or self-inflicted injury.

Alcohol Withdrawal

◈ *Kaplan and Sadock 11th/631*

- The ***classic sign of alcohol withdrawal is tremulousness***, although the spectrum of symptoms can expand to include psychotic and perceptual symptoms (e.g., delusions and hallucinations), seizures, and the symptoms of delirium tremens (DTs), called alcohol delirium in DSM-5.
- **Tremulousness** (commonly called the "shakes" or the "jitters") develops 6 to 8 hours after the cessation of drinking, the psychotic and perceptual symptoms begin in 8 to 12 hours, seizures in 12 to 24 hours, and **DTs** anytime during the first 72 hours, although physicians should watch for the development of DTs for the first week of withdrawal.
- **Other symptoms of withdrawal** include general irritability, gastrointestinal symptoms (e.g., nausea and vomiting), and sympathetic autonomic hyperactivity, including anxiety, arousal, sweating, facial flushing, mydriasis, tachycardia, and mild hypertension. Patients experiencing alcohol withdrawal are generally alert but may startle easily.

237. Ans. (a) A

[Ref: Robbins 9th/494]

"**Other factors for Atherosclerosis**. Factors associated with a less pronounced and/or difficult-to-quantitate risk include lack of exercise; competitive, stressful life style (***"type A" personality***); and obesity (the latter also being complicated by hypertension, diabetes, hypertriglyceridemia, and decreased HDL)"-*Robbins 9th/494*

"Psychosocial factors, including ***type A personality***, anger, hostility, and anxiety, have been implicated in the ***pathogenesis of cardiovascular disease***. Abnormal sympathetic responses to stress may help explain the link between certain behavior patterns and cardiovascular disease. We tested the hypothesis that in normal humans, type A personality characteristics are associated with exaggerated heart rate, pressor, and sympathetic nerve responses to mental and physical stress"- *hyper.ahajournals.org*

RADIOLOGY

238. Ans. (a) Bilateral hilar lymphadenopathy, (c) Upper lobe parenchymal infiltrates

[Ref: Harrison 19th/2206-07;Danhert Radiology Review Manual 7th/540; Davidson 22nd/711]

"Although the CT scan is more sensitive, the **standard scoring system described by Scadding in 1961 for chest roentgenograms** remains the preferred method of characterizing the chest involvement. **Stage1** is hilar adenopathy alone, often with right paratracheal involvement. **Stage 2** is a combination of adenopathy plus infiltrates, whereas **stage 3** reveals infiltrates alone. **Stage 4** consists of fibrosis. Usually the infiltrates in sarcoidosis are predominantly an ***upper lobe process***. Only in a few noninfectious diseases is an upper lobe predominance noted"- *Harrison 19th/2206-07*

Table *(Davidson 22nd/711)*: **Chest X-ray changes in sarcoidosis**

Stage I: BHL (usually symmetrical); paratracheal nodes often enlarged

- Often asymptomatic, but may be associated with erythema nodosum and arthralgia. The majority of cases resolve spontaneously within 1 year

Stage II: BHL and parenchymal infiltrates

- Patients may present with breathlessness or cough. The majority of cases resolve spontaneously

Stage III: parenchymal infiltrates without BHL

- Disease less likely to resolve spontaneously

Stage IV: pulmonary fibrosis

- Can cause progression to ventilatory failure, pulmonary hypertension and cor pulmonale

Note: (BHL = bilateral hilar lymphadenopathy)

Table: *(Danhert Radiology Review Manual 7th/540)*

Satge	Presentation	%
0	Normal chest radiograph	5
I	Hilar + mediastinal lymphadenopathy	50
II	Lymphadenopathy +parenchymal disease	30
III	Diffuse parenchymal disease only	15
IV	Pulmonary fibrosis	20

239. Ans. (b) 30 grays (Gy) in 10 fractions

[Ref: Sumer Sethi 6th/181; Harrison 19th/605]

"***Whole-brain radiotherapy (WBRT) to 30 grays (Gy) in 10 fractions*** is the standard treatment in patients with multiple brain metastases in the majority of treatment centers worldwide. The current study investigated the potential benefit of dose ***escalation beyond 30 Gy***"- onlinelibrary.wiley.com

"The **standard treatment for brain metastases** has been whole-brain radiotherapy (WBRT) usually administered to a total dose of ***3000 cGy in 10 fractions***. This affords rapid palliation, and approximately 80% of patients improve with glucocorticoids and RT. However, it is not curative. Median survival is only 4–6 months. More recently, SRS delivered through a variety of techniques including the gamma knife, linear accelerator, proton beam, and CyberKnife all can deliver highly focused doses of RT, usually in a single fraction. SRS can effectively sterilize the visible lesions and afford local disease control in 80–90% of patients"-*Harrison 19th/605*

ANSWER SHEET

1 – 50						51 – 100						101 – 150						151 – 200						201 – 250					
1	A	B	C	D	E	51	A	B	C	D	E	101	A	B	C	D	E	151	A	B	C	D	E	201	A	B	C	D	E
2	A	B	C	D	E	52	A	B	C	D	E	102	A	B	C	D	E	152	A	B	C	D	E	202	A	B	C	D	E
3	A	B	C	D	E	53	A	B	C	D	E	103	A	B	C	D	E	153	A	B	C	D	E	203	A	B	C	D	E
4	A	B	C	D	E	54	A	B	C	D	E	104	A	B	C	D	E	154	A	B	C	D	E	204	A	B	C	D	E
5	A	B	C	D	E	55	A	B	C	D	E	105	A	B	C	D	E	155	A	B	C	D	E	205	A	B	C	D	E
6	A	B	C	D	E	56	A	B	C	D	E	106	A	B	C	D	E	156	A	B	C	D	E	206	A	B	C	D	E
7	A	B	C	D	E	57	A	B	C	D	E	107	A	B	C	D	E	157	A	B	C	D	E	207	A	B	C	D	E
8	A	B	C	D	E	58	A	B	C	D	E	108	A	B	C	D	E	158	A	B	C	D	E	208	A	B	C	D	E
9	A	B	C	D	E	59	A	B	C	D	E	109	A	B	C	D	E	159	A	B	C	D	E	209	A	B	C	D	E
10	A	B	C	D	E	60	A	B	C	D	E	110	A	B	C	D	E	160	A	B	C	D	E	210	A	B	C	D	E
11	A	B	C	D	E	61	A	B	C	D	E	111	A	B	C	D	E	161	A	B	C	D	E	211	A	B	C	D	E
12	A	B	C	D	E	62	A	B	C	D	E	112	A	B	C	D	E	162	A	B	C	D	E	212	A	B	C	D	E
13	A	B	C	D	E	63	A	B	C	D	E	113	A	B	C	D	E	163	A	B	C	D	E	213	A	B	C	D	E
14	A	B	C	D	E	64	A	B	C	D	E	114	A	B	C	D	E	164	A	B	C	D	E	214	A	B	C	D	E
15	A	B	C	D	E	65	A	B	C	D	E	115	A	B	C	D	E	165	A	B	C	D	E	215	A	B	C	D	E
16	A	B	C	D	E	66	A	B	C	D	E	116	A	B	C	D	E	166	A	B	C	D	E	216	A	B	C	D	E
17	A	B	C	D	E	67	A	B	C	D	E	117	A	B	C	D	E	167	A	B	C	D	E	217	A	B	C	D	E
18	A	B	C	D	E	68	A	B	C	D	E	118	A	B	C	D	E	168	A	B	C	D	E	218	A	B	C	D	E
19	A	B	C	D	E	69	A	B	C	D	E	119	A	B	C	D	E	169	A	B	C	D	E	219	A	B	C	D	E
20	A	B	C	D	E	70	A	B	C	D	E	120	A	B	C	D	E	170	A	B	C	D	E	220	A	B	C	D	E
21	A	B	C	D	E	71	A	B	C	D	E	121	A	B	C	D	E	171	A	B	C	D	E	221	A	B	C	D	E
22	A	B	C	D	E	72	A	B	C	D	E	122	A	B	C	D	E	172	A	B	C	D	E	222	A	B	C	D	E
23	A	B	C	D	E	73	A	B	C	D	E	123	A	B	C	D	E	173	A	B	C	D	E	223	A	B	C	D	E
24	A	B	C	D	E	74	A	B	C	D	E	124	A	B	C	D	E	174	A	B	C	D	E	224	A	B	C	D	E
25	A	B	C	D	E	75	A	B	C	D	E	125	A	B	C	D	E	175	A	B	C	D	E	225	A	B	C	D	E
26	A	B	C	D	E	76	A	B	C	D	E	126	A	B	C	D	E	176	A	B	C	D	E	226	A	B	C	D	E
27	A	B	C	D	E	77	A	B	C	D	E	127	A	B	C	D	E	177	A	B	C	D	E	227	A	B	C	D	E
28	A	B	C	D	E	78	A	B	C	D	E	128	A	B	C	D	E	178	A	B	C	D	E	228	A	B	C	D	E
29	A	B	C	D	E	79	A	B	C	D	E	129	A	B	C	D	E	179	A	B	C	D	E	229	A	B	C	D	E
30	A	B	C	D	E	80	A	B	C	D	E	130	A	B	C	D	E	180	A	B	C	D	E	230	A	B	C	D	E
31	A	B	C	D	E	81	A	B	C	D	E	131	A	B	C	D	E	181	A	B	C	D	E	231	A	B	C	D	E
32	A	B	C	D	E	82	A	B	C	D	E	132	A	B	C	D	E	182	A	B	C	D	E	232	A	B	C	D	E
33	A	B	C	D	E	83	A	B	C	D	E	133	A	B	C	D	E	183	A	B	C	D	E	233	A	B	C	D	E
34	A	B	C	D	E	84	A	B	C	D	E	134	A	B	C	D	E	184	A	B	C	D	E	234	A	B	C	D	E
35	A	B	C	D	E	85	A	B	C	D	E	135	A	B	C	D	E	185	A	B	C	D	E	235	A	B	C	D	E
36	A	B	C	D	E	86	A	B	C	D	E	136	A	B	C	D	E	186	A	B	C	D	E	236	A	B	C	D	E
37	A	B	C	D	E	87	A	B	C	D	E	137	A	B	C	D	E	187	A	B	C	D	E	237	A	B	C	D	E
38	A	B	C	D	E	88	A	B	C	D	E	138	A	B	C	D	E	188	A	B	C	D	E	238	A	B	C	D	E
39	A	B	C	D	E	89	A	B	C	D	E	139	A	B	C	D	E	189	A	B	C	D	E	239	A	B	C	D	E
40	A	B	C	D	E	90	A	B	C	D	E	140	A	B	C	D	E	190	A	B	C	D	E	240	A	B	C	D	E
41	A	B	C	D	E	91	A	B	C	D	E	141	A	B	C	D	E	191	A	B	C	D	E	241	A	B	C	D	E
42	A	B	C	D	E	92	A	B	C	D	E	142	A	B	C	D	E	192	A	B	C	D	E	242	A	B	C	D	E
43	A	B	C	D	E	93	A	B	C	D	E	143	A	B	C	D	E	193	A	B	C	D	E	243	A	B	C	D	E
44	A	B	C	D	E	94	A	B	C	D	E	144	A	B	C	D	E	194	A	B	C	D	E	244	A	B	C	D	E
45	A	B	C	D	E	95	A	B	C	D	E	145	A	B	C	D	E	195	A	B	C	D	E	245	A	B	C	D	E
46	A	B	C	D	E	96	A	B	C	D	E	146	A	B	C	D	E	196	A	B	C	D	E	246	A	B	C	D	E
47	A	B	C	D	E	97	A	B	C	D	E	147	A	B	C	D	E	197	A	B	C	D	E	247	A	B	C	D	E
48	A	B	C	D	E	98	A	B	C	D	E	148	A	B	C	D	E	198	A	B	C	D	E	248	A	B	C	D	E
49	A	B	C	D	E	99	A	B	C	D	E	149	A	B	C	D	E	199	A	B	C	D	E	249	A	B	C	D	E
50	A	B	C	D	E	100	A	B	C	D	E	150	A	B	C	D	E	200	A	B	C	D	E	250	A	B	C	D	E

NAME OF THE CANDIDATE	ROLL NO.					CENTRE NO.		QUESTION BOOKLET NO.					BOOKLET CODE
CATEGORY	0	0	0	0	0	0	0	0	0	0	0	0	A
	1	1	1	1	1	1	1	1	1	1	1	1	B
SC ○	2	2	2	2	2	2	2	2	2	2	2	2	C
ST ○	3	3	3	3	3	3	3	3	3	3	3	3	D
OBC ○	4	4	4	4	4	4	4	4	4	4	4	4	
GEN ○	5	5	5	5	5	5	5	5	5	5	5	5	
CW ○	6	6	6	6	6	6	6	6	6	6	6	6	
PH ○	7	7	7	7	7	7	7	7	7	7	7	7	
	8	8	8	8	8	8	8	8	8	8	8	8	
	9	9	9	9	9	9	9	9	9	9	9	9	

INSTRUCTIONS FOR FILLING THE SHEET

1. This sheet should not be folded or crushed.
2. Use only blue/black ball pen to fill the circles.
3. Use of pencil is strictly prohibited.
4. Circles should be darkened properly and completely.
5. Cutting & erasing on this sheet is not allowed.
6. Do not use any stray marks on the sheet.
7. Do not use marker, white fluid or any other device to hide the shading already done.

WRONG METHOD

× ● ✓ ●

CORRECT METHOD

●

CANDIDATE'S SIGNATURE

(in ball - point pen)

INVIGILATOR'S SIGNATURE

(in ball - point pen)

MAY

2016

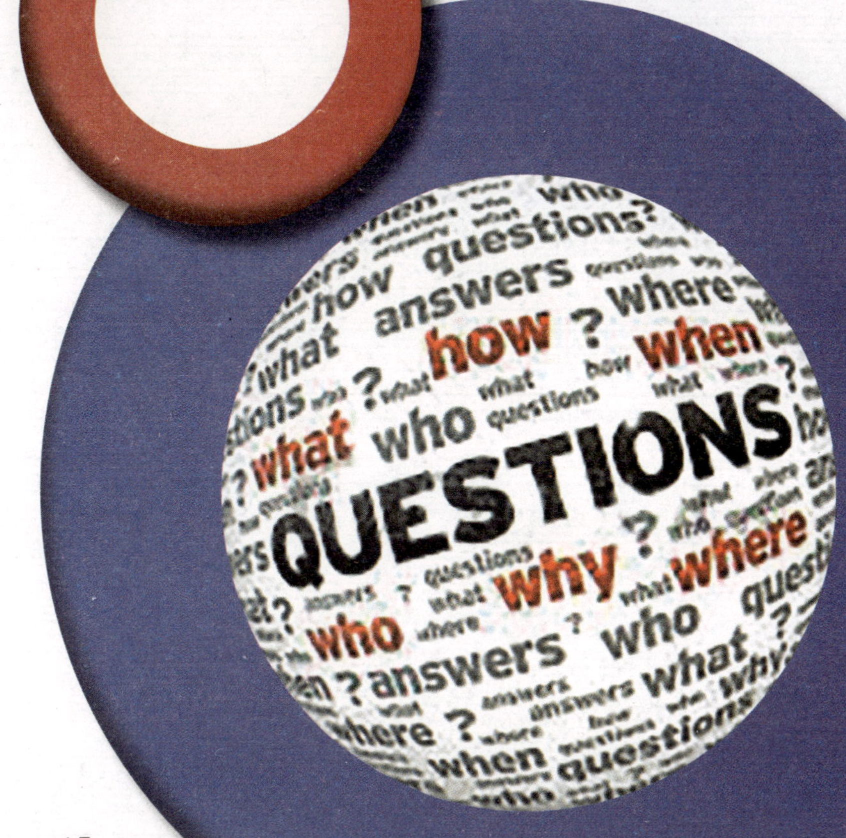

Multiple Choice Questions
Answers & Explanations

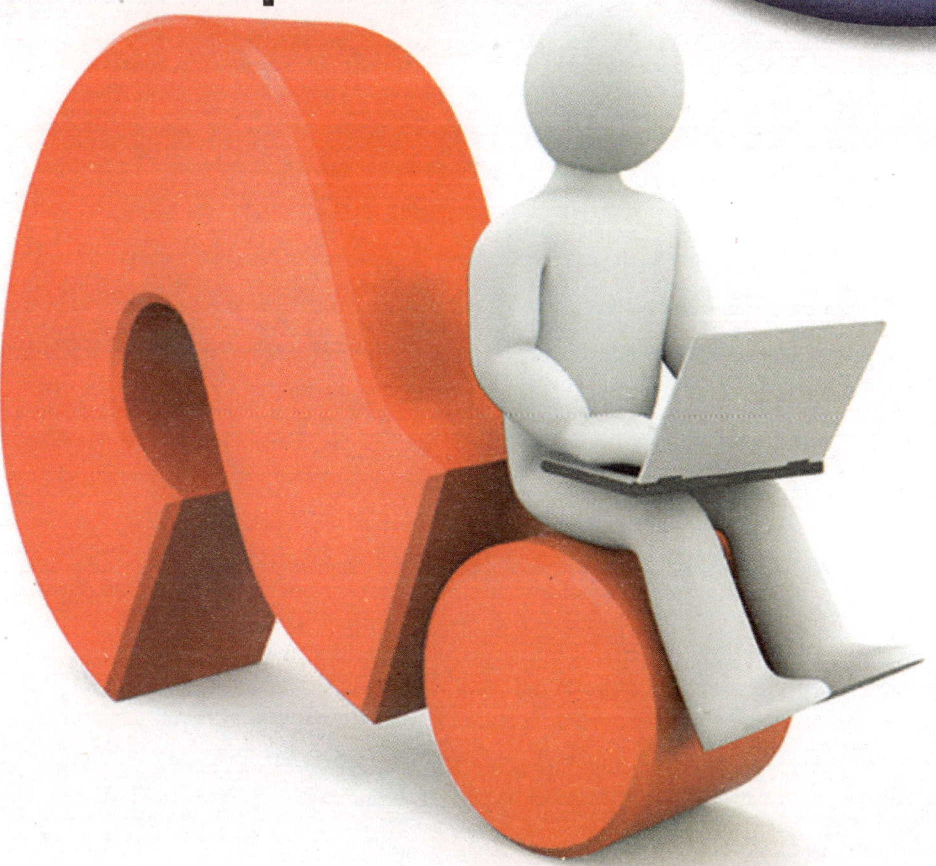

MAY 2016 MULTIPLE CHOICE QUESTIONS

ANATOMY

1. **True about inferior oblique muscle:**
   a. Supplied by inferior division of 3rd CN
   b. Primary eye action—Extorsion, abduction & depression
   c. The muscle pass below inferior rectus
   d. Origin from lacrimal bone
   e. Nerve enters the muscle from ocular surface
2. **True about Submandibular gland duct obstruction by stone:**
   a. Presents as a mass below body of mandible
   b. Stone in Wharton duct can be palpated below mucous membrane of floor of mouth
   c. Starts pain just after starting a meal
   d. Pain carried by glossopharyngeal nerve
3. **True about palatine tonsil:**
   a. Crypts is lined by squamous epithelium
   b. Supplied by IX CN
   c. Tongue depressor is used for examination
   d. Arterial supply is by tonsillar ascending branch of grater palatine artery
   e. Present in oropharynx
4. **True about articular cartilage:**
   a. In zone 1 chondrocytes are smaller
   b. Zone 2 contains articular cartilage progenitor cells
   c. Zone 3 contains calcified cartilage
   d. Zone 4 contain calcified cartilage
   e. Chondrocytes are active cell
5. **True about innervation of parotid gland:**
   a. Postganglionic parasympathetic fibre—secretomotor
   b. Preganglionic parasympathetic fibre relay in Otic ganglion
   c. Preganglionic parasympathetic nerve begin in inferior petrosal nucleus
   d. Sympathetic nerve are vasomotor
   e. Postganglionic parasympathetic fibres pass through the glossopharyngeal nerve
6. **Which of the following muscle is supplied by median nerve:**
   a. Oppenens pollocis
   b. Adductor pollicis
   c. Lateral half of the Flexor digitorum profundus
   d. Superficial head of flexor pollicis brevis
   e. Deep part of flexor pollicis brevis
7. **True about abduction at shoulder joint:**
   a. Supraspinatus initiates abduction
   b. Serratus anterior & trapezius also help in abduction
   c. Multipinnate deltoid clavicular fiber is main abductor
   d. Axillary nerve injury has no effect on abduction
   e. Musculotendinous cuff stabilizes shoulder joint
8. **Organ which have no lymphatic supply:**
   a. Eyeball b. Brain
   c. Liver d. Kidney
   e. Spinal cord
9. **Which of the following statement(s) is/are true about sphincters of body:**
   a. Lower 5 cm of esophageal act as esophageal sphincter & it is not morphologically different from other portion of oesophagus
   b. Esophageal & pyloric sphinter remains in tonically contracted state
   c. Pre-capillary sphincter is present in b/w meta-arteriole & capillary
   d. Pudendal nerve supplies the sphincter urethrae
   e. Sphincter of oddi lies at junction of duodenum & CBD
10. **Muscle(s), which form the floor of Pelvis:**
    a. Obturator internus b. Piriformis
    c. Puborectalis d. Pubococcygeus
    e. Ischiococcygeus
11. **True about Atlanto-axial joint:**
    a. Vertebral artery pass through grove on arch of atlas vertebrae to foramen magnum
    b. Permits flexion & extension
    c. Permit side to side movement of head
    d. Permits flexion only
    e. Permits rotation
12. **All are true about CSF except:**
    a. Total volume is 250 ml
    b. Pressure is 60-180 mm of H_2O
    c. Formed from choroid plexus of 3rd ventricle
    d. Formed from choroid plexus of lateral ventricle

PHYSIOLOGY

13. **Which of the following play most important role in memory:**
    a. Synaptic network
    b. Electric conduction network
    c. Conductivity circuit
    d. Conductivity network
14. **Cyanide poisoning block K influx & Na efflux. But ATP reverse this effect. So true statement(s) related to mechanism of action of cyanide is/are:**
    a. K influx & Na efflux is regulated by Na-K ATPase enzyme
    b. K influx & Na efflux is regulated by Na-K pump
    c. ATP provide energy for this channel
    d. Na-K ATPase channel is ATP independent

Answer

1. a, c.	2. a, b, c, d.	3. a, b, c, e.	4. a, d, e.	5. a, b, d.	6. a, c, d.	7. a, b, e.
8. a, b, e.	9. b, c, d, e.	10. c, d, e.	11. a, c, e.	12. a.	13. a.	14. a, b, c.

15. True about Carbon monoxide poisoning:
- a. CO has 100 times more affinity than O_2 for Hb
- b. Cause right side shifting of O_2 dissociation curve
- c. Oxygen-haemoglobin saturation curve becomes hyperbolic shape
- d. Pulse oximetry can accurately detect level of CO
- e. 10-15% level of CO normally may occur in healthy non-smoker

16. Dead space is increased in:
- a. Positive pressure ventilation
- b. Extension of neck
- c. Anticholinergic drug
- d. Endotracheal tube intubation
- e. Emphysema

17. Which of the following is true about cardiac innervation:
- a. T1-T5 is sympathetic supply
- b. Inferior & superior cervical ganglia not involve in innervation
- c. Parasympathetic supply is from vagus nerve
- d. Great cardiac nerve arise from superior cervical ganglia
- e. Inferior cervical ganglia gives off Inferior cardiac nerve

18. True about cortisol level in blood plasma:
- a. Morning concentration is 17-18nmol/dL
- b. Morning concentration is 5-23 µg/dL
- c. Evening concentration is almost half of morning concentration
- d. Evening concentration is 5-23 µg/dL

19. Saccadicc eye movement is controlled by:
- a. Parietal lobe
- b. Prefrontal lobe
- c. Temporal lobe
- d. Frontal cortex
- e. Occipital lobe

20. True about normal ECG:
- a. Normal PR interval is 0.12-0.20 s
- b. PR internal correspondence initiation of P wave to initiation of R wave
- c. QT internal correspondence initiation of Q wave to initiation of T wave
- d. Normal QRS interval < 0.12 s
- e. Normal QTc interval <0.47 s

21. Which of the following is/are true about SIADH:
- a. Desmopressin is used for treatment
- b. Vasopressin level is inappropriately high
- c. Plasma osmolality is higher than urine osmolality
- d. ↑ed Osmolality of urine
- e. ↑ed Osmolality of plasma

22. Which of the following feature(s) is/are suggestive of nephrogenic DI in comparison to central DI:
- a. Desmopressin nasal spray restore urine output to normal level
- b. Basal vasopressin level > 1 pg/ml
- c. Normal posterior pituitary bright spot is not visible on MRI scan
- d. Change in water loss during fluid deprivation test

BIOCHEMISTRY

23. All are Urea cycle enzymes except:
- a. Ornithine transcarbamoylase
- b. Carbamoyl-phosphate synthetase I
- c. Argininosuccinase
- d. Citrulline synthase
- e. Arginosuccinnic acid synthetase

24. Non-polar amino acids are:
- a. Proline
- b. Lysine
- c. Isoleucine
- d. Arginine
- e. Asparginine

25. True about squalene:
- a. Present in subhuman primate only
- b. It is one of the major carbohydrate of body
- c. It involves in synthesis of cholesterol
- d. It involves in synthesis of steroids

26. Molecular weight of protein can be determined/estimated by:
- a. SDS-PAGE
- b. Gel filtration chromatography
- c. Agarose gel electrophosis
- d. Ultracentrifugation
- e. FRET microscopy

27. Gel used in RNA electrophoresis:
- a. Agarose gel
- b. Polyacrylamide plain gel
- c. Polyacrylamide SDS (Sodium dodecyl sulphate) impregnated Polyacrylamide gel

28. Which of following releases/provide energy:
- a. Conversion of ADP to ATP
- b. Breaking of high energy bond to low energy bond
- c. Conversion of pyruvate to lactate
- d. Electrical gradient across inner & outer side of mitochondrial membrane
- e. Passage of e- through FAD in electron transport chain

Answer

15. c.	16. a, b, c, e.	17. a, e.	18. b, c.	19. d.	20. a, d.	21. b, d.
22. b.	23. d.	24. a, c.	25. c, d.	26. a, b, d.	27. a.	28. b, d, e.

29. Which of the following is feature(s) of diabetic ketoacidosis:
a. Decreased triglyceride level
b. Increased fatty acid level
c. ↑Lipoprotein
d. Decreased ketone bodies
e. High Anion gap acidosis

30. Which of the following is/are true about pH of solution:
a. Absolute concentration of acid & salt
b. Relative concentration of acid & salt in solution
c. Increase of temperature increases pH
d. A rise in H^+ concentration decreases pH

31. True statement(s) about Magnetic-activated cell sorting:
a. It is a method to separate specific cell from complex mixture
b. Fluorescent dyes are uses
c. Antibody-coated magnetic nanoparticles are used
d. Antibodies used are specific for certain cell surface markers
e. Magnetic field is applied

32. Silver staining is done for:
a. DNA b. RNA
c. Karyotyping analysis d. Protein
e. Collagen

IMMUNOGENETICS & MOLECULAR BIOLOGY

33. Non-coding RNA is/are:
a. miRNA b. Si RNA
c. tRNA d. mRNA
e. rRNA

34. Polymerase III synthesizes:
a. Fragment 28S of rRNA b. Fragment 23S of rRNA
c. Fragment 5 S of rRNA d. tRNA
e. mRNA

35. Two strands of DNA is/are held by:
a. Glycosidic bond b. Hydrogen bond
c. Covalent bond d. Ionic bond
e. Van der waal force

36. Which of the following is/are true about Translation:
a. N-formyl methionine is first amino acid in prokaryotes
b. Uses energy in form of GMP
c. Elongation factor EF-1 & EF-2 used in prokaryotes
d. Elongation factor P is used in eukaryotic organism
e. Three initiation factors are required in prokaryotes

37. Nucleic acid amplification techniques are:
a. PCR
b. Real time PCR
c. DNA Cloning
d. Next generation DNA sequencing
e. ELISA

38. Second messenger is/are:
a. Ca^{2+} b. DNA
c. Histone d. cDNA

39. True about genetic code:
a. Follow Mendelian law
b. It is total number of chromosome in the body
c. It is nucleotide sequence which codes for amino acids
d. It codes for DNA
e. None

40. Restriction endonuclease cleaves:
a. dsDNA b. RNA
c. Histone d. Protein
e. ssDNA

41. Phospholipase A2 act on:
a. Phosphoglyceric acid b. Phosphate
c. Ca^+ d. Phosphatidyl-inositol

42. Enzyme used in DNA repair is/are:
a. DNA gyrase
b. DNA polymerase
c. Restriction endonuclease
d. DNA ligase

43. Nucleosome contains:
a. DNA b. RNA
c. Chromatin d. Histone

PATHOLOGY

44. Serotonin, a mediator of inflammation in our body, is secreted/released by:
a. Leukocytes b. Endothelial cell
c. Mast cell d. Platelet
e. Macrophage

45. Autosomal recessive disease(s) is/are:
a. Sickle cell anaemia b. Phenylketonuria
c. Tuberous sclerosis d. Familial polyposis coli
e. Marfan syndrome

46. Which of the following is/are features(s) of lewy body dementia:
a. Plaque containing beta-amyloid peptide
b. Deposition of α-synuclein protein
c. Often resistant to standard treatment
d. Common in elderly
e. Risk of falling may present

47. True about Alzheimer's disease:
a. More common in older age
b. Impairment of the ability to remember new information
c. Mainly affects long term memory
d. General cognitive behavior impaired in prodromal phase
e. Atrophy of frontal & parietal lobe

Answer

29. b, c, e.	30. b, d.	31. a, c, d, e.	32. All.	33. a, b, c, e.	34. c, d.	35. b.
36. a, e.	37. a. b.	38. a.	39. c.	40. a.	41. d.	42. b, d.
43. a, d.	44. d.	45. a, b.	46. b, c, d, e.	47. a, b, d, e.		

48. All are true about hypersensitivity pneumonitis except:
a. Type IV Hypersensitivity reaction
b. More common in smoker
c. Bronchoalveolar lavage shows CD4+ and CD8+ T lymphocytes
d. May presents with cough, dyspnea & breathlessness

49. RS cell having same immunophenotyping are present in which subtypes of Hodgkin's lymphoma:
a. Nodular sclerosis
b. Lymphocyte predominant
c. Lymphocyte rich
d. Mixed cellularity
e. Lymphocyte depletion

50. True about Lyonisation of X chromosome:
a. Inactivation of X chromosome only in somatic cell
b. Inactivation of X chromosome only in germ cell
c. Inactivation of X chromosome in somatic & germ cell both
d. Maximun number of Barr body is equal to X chromosome

51. Two most common cancer in Indian woman are:
a. Carcinoma breast
b. Carcinoma cervix
c. Carcinoma colon
d. Carcinoma stomach
e. Carcinoma lung

52. Which of the following is paraganglioma:
a. Adrenal Pheochromocytoma
b. Extra-adrenal Pheochromocytoma
c. Carotid body tumour
d. Carcinoid tumour
e. Glomus tympanicum

53. Feature(s) of XIII factor deficiency is/are:
a. Delayed wound closure
b. Clot solubility tests are abnormal
c. ↑aPTT
d. ↑PT
e. ↑ BT

54. Which of the following statement(s) is/are correct except:
a. Increased PT in extrinsic pathways
b. Increased aPTT in instrinsic pathways
c. If platelet count is > 1.5 lac/microL, then normal homeostasis present
d. BT is decreased in platelet abnormality

55. True about Dentigerous cyst:
a. Arises in relation to unerupted teeth
b. It most commonly encroaches maxillary antrum
c. Mandibular third molar is common site
d. Common in mandible

56. Prognostic factors for carcinoma esophagus is/are:
a. Depth of invasion
b. Lymph node status
c. Tumour grading
d. Stage of the disease

57. True about surgical jaundice:
a. Increase of serum bilirubin
b. Increase acid phosphatase
c. Increase alkaline phosphatase
d. Urine bilirubin is absent
e. Stool sterocobilinogen absent

58. Which of the following marker favours diagnosis of preinvasive & invasive cervical cancer:
a. Ki67
b. Oncoprotein E6
c. p16INK4, cyclin E, and Ki-67
d. Oncoprotein E8

59. Which of the following marker/mutation is/are seen in papillary carcinoma of thyroid:
a. Synaptophysin
b. RET/PTC
c. P53
d. NTRK1
e. RAS

PHARMACOLOGY

60. Which of the following is/are true about pregabalin:
a. Approved drug for diabetic neuropathy
b. Approved for treatment of generalized tonic clonic seizure
c. Peripheral edema is side effect
d. Somnolence is side effect
e. Approved for use in partial seizure

61. Drug(s) used for overactive bladder:
a. Oxybutinin
b. Tolterodine
c. Mirabegron
d. Onabotulinum toxin A
e. Pirenzepine

62. All are true about warfarin except:
a. Act through inhibition of coagulation factor IX
b. Protamine sulphate reverses its action
c. Monitoring is done through INR
d. Target of INR with warfarin is generally 2-3
e. Skin necrosis is usually occur in 3-10 days of initiation of warfarin

63. True about M/A of doxorubicin:
a. Intercalate b/w DNA strands
b. Inhibition of DNA polymerase
c. Inhibition of RNA polymerase
d. Inhibition of topoisomerase II
e. Inhibition of protein synthesis

64. Anticholinergic drug side-effect includes:
a. Constipation
b. Urinary retention
c. Mydriasis
d. Hypothermia
e. Blurring of vision

Answer

48. b.	49. a, c, d, e.	50. a.	51. a, b.	52. b, c, e.	53. a, b.	54. d.
55. a, c, d.	56. All	57. a, c, e.	58. a, b, c.	59. b, d, e.	60. a, c, d, e.	61. a, b, c, d.
62. b.	63. a, d.	64. a, b, c, e.				

65. Which of the following is/are true about benefits of Sustained release formulation of drugs:
- a. Decreased incidence and/or intensity of undesired effects
- b. Increases potency of the drug
- c. Release of drug is less influenced by pH
- d. Prolong drug effect
- e. Decreased frequency of administration

66. True about drug-response curve (DRC):
- a. Steepest in middle portion of the DRC
- b. Inverted U shaped curve may be for some drug
- c. Rectangular hyperbola- when plotted in logarithmic scale
- d. Sigmoid shape- when plotted in logarithm is used
- e. Enables comparison of potency of drugs

67. True about organophosphorus poisoning:
- a. Atropine is best for early treatment & maintenance
- b. Pralidoxime is important for restoring neuromuscular transmission
- c. Phenytoin is the primary drug used for seizure control
- d. Mydriasis present
- e. Pralidoxime & atropine works synergistically

68. Which of the following drug(s) act by inhibiting protein synthesis by attaching to 50 S ribosome:
- a. Tetracycline
- b. Aminoglycoside
- c. Rifampicin
- d. Chloramphenicol
- e. Trimethoprim

69. OCP efficacy decreases with concurrent administration of which of the following drug(s):
- a. Phenytoin
- b. Ampicillin
- c. Isoniazid
- d. Imipramine
- e. Ethionamide

70. Which of following true regarding acetylcholine receptors:
- a. M2 receptor- heart
- b. M1 receptor- smooth muscle
- c. NM receptor is present on neuromuscular junction
- d. Synaptic junction-Ach is transmitter
- e. NN located on adrenal medulla

71. All are true about tamoxifene except:
- a. Used as adjuvant therapy in estrogen receptor positive breast cancer
- b. Approved for the primary prophylaxis of breast cancer in high risk woman
- c. No effect on uterus
- d. Pro-estrogen effect on bone
- e. Cause endometrial Ca

72. Which of the following drug(s) comes in risk category B of FDA teratogenic risk categories for pregnancy:
- a. Phenytoin
- b. Resperidone
- c. Olanazapine
- d. Clozapine
- e. Arpirazole

73. Which of the following is true regarding ropinirole wrt L-dopa:
- a. Cognitive symptom improves
- b. Lower incidence of hallucination
- c. Cause excessive sleepiness
- d. More effective in the treatment of patients who have developed on/off phenomena
- e. Provide neuroprotective effect

74. True about methanol poisoning:
- a. Gastric decontamination is helpful
- b. Formate & formaldehyde are active metabolite
- c. Taking with Ethanol cause more toxicity
- d. Fomipezole a specific antagonist, is given for treatment
- e. Cause high anion gap acidosis

75. S/E of Bevacizumab includes:
- a. Hypertension
- b. Hemoptysis
- c. Malena
- d. Cerebellar stroke
- e. Not cause gastrointestinal perforation

76. TNF-α Inhibitors are used for:
- a. Ulcerative colitis
- b. Crohn's disease
- c. Rheumatoid arthritis
- d. Psoariasis
- e. Lichen planus

77. Antibiotic of choice for Stenotrophomonas maltophilia infection is:
- a. Ampicillin
- b. Trimethoprim-sulfamethoxazole (TMP-SMX)
- c. Penicillin
- d. Ciprofloxacin

MICROBIOLOGY

78. In which of the following condition(s), children are prone to fungal & viral infection:
- a. Thymic aplasia
- b. Agammaglobulinemia
- c. Lymphocytopenia
- d. Severe combined immune deficiencies (SCID)
- e. Chediak–Higashi syndrome

79. Which of the following is type 3 hypersensitivity reaction (immune complex disease):
- a. SLE
- b. Diabetes Mellitus I
- c. Goodpasteur syndrome
- d. Multiple sclerosis
- e. Bronchial asthma

80. Which of the following infection has incubation period <4 week:
- a. Brucella
- b. Gonorrhoea
- c. Syphilis
- d. HBV
- e. Leishmaniasis

Answer

65. a, c, d, e. 66. a, b, d, e. 67. a, b, e. 68. b, d. 69. a, b. 70. a, c, d, e. 71. c.
72. d. 73. c, d, e. 74. a, b, d, e. 75. a, b, c, d. 76. a, b, c, d. 77. b. 78. a, c, d.
79. a. 80. a, b, c.

81. Stain used for Mycobacterium tuberculosis is/are:
a. Ziehl-Neelsen technique of staining
b. Auramine-rhodamine stain
c. Gomori methenamine silver stain
d. Kinyoun stain
e. Gram staining

82. Food borne diseases are:
a. Japanese encephalitis
b. Hemophilia
c. HBV
d. Botulism
e. Typhoidfever

83. Which of the following is NOT lysine positive non-fermentor:
a. Burkholderia pseudomallei
b. Burkhomelia mallei
c. Burkholderia cepacia
d. Stenotrophomonas maltophilia
e. Pseudomonas aeruginosa

84. A person is suffering from acquired immunodeficiency disease (AIDS) & visited zoo. After somedays, he is complaining of headache & cough. He has also have some neurological symptom. On staining of CSF sample, it shows capsulated yeast. Likely infection is:
a. Histoplasma
b. Aspergillus
c. Cryptococcus
d. Blastomycosis
e. Coccidioidomycosis

85. Normal flora of Oral cavity is/are:
a. Veillonella
b. Anerobic micrococci
c. Geotrichum
d. Gemella
e. Yersinia

86. Gold standard diagnostic test for babeiosis is:
a. Peripheral blood smear examination
b. Blood Culture
c. PCR
d. ELISA
e. Indirect fluorescent antibody (IFA) test

87. True about listeria monocytogens infection:
a. Common in pregnant women
b. Common in elderly
c. Common in children
d. Common in newborns
e. Ampicillin is drug of choice

88. True about Japanese encephalitis:
a. Most severe epidemic spread occured in 2006
b. Main vector in India is culex tritaeniorhynchus
c. Spread by aedes mosquito
d. India still not able to develop vaccine indigenously
e. Pigs are amplifier host

89. Not AIDS defining cancer:
a. Anal carcioma
b. Hodgkin's lymphoma
c. Cervial cancer
d. Non –Hodgkins lymphoma
e. Kaposi carcinoma

90. True about Plasmodium falciparum:
a. Increased size of infected RBC
b. Crescentric shaped gametocyte
c. Delicate ring present
d. Small & multiple rings common
e. Erythrocyte preference- old cells

91. Which of the following statement is/are true about Giardia:
a. Cause bloody diarrhorea
b. Invasive to GI mucosa
c. More common in hypogammaglobulinemic person
d. Less common in achlorohydria
e. Metronidazole is effective in treatment

92. In which organism can be isolated:
a. CSF specimen of tetanus infection
b. CSF specimen of listeria monocytogenes
c. From valves in rheumatic valvulitis
d. From myocardium in diphtheric myocarditis
e. Meningococcal rash

93. True about cytomegalovirus:
a. Characteristic owl eye appearance
b. Type 5 Human herpesvirus type
c. Lymphocyte enlargement
d. Cause congenital infection
e. Lymphoproliferative

94. Which of the following is/are true about Mycoplasma pneumonia infection except:
a. Causes many extrapulmonary manifestations
b. Cold agglutinin titer is not increased
c. Cause atypical pneumonia
d. Paucity of respiratory signs on physical examination
e. Cough is typically productive

95. True about enteroviruses:
a. In 1999, wild polio virus 2 was eradicated from world
b. Vaccine associated paralytic poliomyelitis(VAPP) most frequently caused by serotype 1 vaccine
c. Bivalent OPV contains type 1 & type 3 strain
d. Primary course of OPV consists of only 1 dose
e. Coxasackie A7 & enterovirus type 71 causes aseptic meningitis

96. True about chickengunya fever:
a. Caused by single stranded RNA arbovirus
b. Excruiting arthralgia in peripheral joints
c. Antiviral therapy is very effective
d. Absolute lymphocytosis is present
e. Vector is aedes mosquitoes

97. True about Zika virus:
a. Sexually transmitted
b. 50% infected person develop symptoms
c. Effective therapy available
d. Transmitted by Aedes vector
e. Transmission in utero

Answer

81. a, b, d.	82. d, e.	83. a, b, e.	84. c.	85. a, b, c, d.	86. a.	87. a, b, d, e.
88. b, e.	89. a, b.	90. b, c, d.	91. c, e.	92. b, e.	93. a, b, d.	94. b, e.
95. a, c, d, e.	96. a, b, e.	97. a, d, e.				

98. **Biosafety level 4 infection includes:**
 a. Hantavirus b. Nile virus
 c. Ebola virus d. Crimean-Congo HF
 e. Lyssa Fever

99. **Serological test is/are useful in diagnosis of which of the following disease:**
 a. Typhoid
 b. Q fever
 c. Acanthamoeba infection
 d. Scrub typhus
 e. Brucellosis

100. **All are true about gas gangrene except:**
 a. Type 1 gangrene is fournier's gangrene
 b. Devitalized tissue predispose to gas gangrene
 c. High O_2 tension in tissue is important precondition
 d. α -toxin is main cause of the toxaemia associated with gas gangrene
 e. Mainly caused by C. perfringens

101. **Which are transmitted by Dog:**
 a. Echinococcus granulosus
 b. Toxocara canis
 c. Echinococcus multiocularis
 d. Toxoplasma Gondii

FORENSIC MEDICINE

102. **Which of the following is/are paraphilia:**
 a. Pedophilia
 b. Sodomy
 c. Frotteurism
 d. Voyeurism
 e. Exhibitionism

103. **Which of the following joint is best predictor of age of 16-17 year by X-ray:**
 a. Knee b. Elbow
 c. Hip d. Wrist
 e. Ankle

104. **Which of the following is/are feature(s) of human hair:**
 a. Medullary index: <0.3
 b. Cortex is thin
 c. Cortex is thick
 d. Medulla-narrow
 e. Medulla-wider

105. **Which of the following is true statement(s) about exhumation:**
 a. Police can order for exhumation
 b. Executive magistrate can order for exhumation
 c. Postmortem can not be done on exhumated body
 d. Cr PC 176(4) is related to enquiry of exhumated body
 e. CrPC 174 is related to enquiry of exhumated body

106. **True about cadaveric spasm:**
 a. Same mechanism as rigor mortis
 b. Mechanism is unknown
 c. Also k/a instantaneous rigor
 d. Occur only in cold environment
 e. Can be seen in some drowning case

107. **Cause(s) of Ophisthotonus is/are:**
 a. Cocaine b. Strychnos Nux Vomica seed
 c. Strychnine d. Codeine
 e. Curare

108. **Which of the following is not rape:**
 a. Sexual intercourse with wife, of age below 15 year, with consent
 b. Sexual intercourse with wife, of age below 16 year, with consent
 c. Sexual intercourse with a girl below 18 years of age, with consent
 d. Sexual intercourse with a girl of 18 year with consent
 e. Sexual intercourse with wife who is living separately from him under a decree of separation, or any custom or usage with her consent

PREVENTIVE & SOCIAL MEDICINE

109. **Follow up is not required in which of the following study:**
 a. Prospective study b. Retrospective study
 c. Cross-sectional study d. Longitudinal study
 e. Cohort study

110. **Special protection includes:**
 a. Personality development
 b. Immunization against specific disease
 c. Specific nutritional diet
 d. Protection from occupational hazard
 e. Environmental modification

111. **True about Civil registration system in India:**
 a. Dual record system
 b. Deficient
 c. Head of institution or officer-in charge is responsible for registration
 d. Birth & Death both are registered
 e. Cause of death is recorded

112. **True about silicosis:**
 a. Caused by exposure of silica oxide
 b. Severe exposure- whole lung lavage may helpful in alleviating symptoms
 c. Fibrosis of upper lung
 d. Fibrotic change can be reversed after stopping exposure
 e. More risk of TB & lung cancer

Answer

98. c, d, e.	99. a, b, d.	100. c.	101. a, c.	102. a, c, d, e.	103. e.	104. a, c, d.
105. b, d.	106. b, c, e.	107. b, c.	108. b, d, e.	109. b, c.	110. b, c, d.	111. b, c, d, e.
112. a, b, c, e.						

113. Which of the following is/are true about use of Bar diagram:

a. Comparison of 2 categorial data which are not-additive
b. Comparison of 2 categorial data which are proportional percentage contribution of categories
c. Pie chart is used for comparison of 2 categorial data which are proportional percentage contribution of categories
d. Comparison of magnitude of different frequencies in discrete data
e. Comparison of continuous data

114. Benefit of vertical health programme includes:

a. More focus on efficiency
b. More rapid results
c. Dedicated worker always available
d. Many programme can run at one time
e. Effective way of maximizing the impact of the available resources

OPHTHALMOLOGY

115. Cause(s) of mydriasis:

a. Organophosphorus poisoning
b. Horner syndrome
c. Oculomotor nerve palsy
d. Parasympathetic stimulation

116. True about primary open angle glaucoma:

a. Also k/a Chronic simple glaucoma
b. Hypermeteropeas are more predisposed
c. Polygenic inheritance
d. Laser iridotomy is used for treatment
e. Fundus examination reveals large cup

117. Cloudy cornea is/are seen:

a. Klinefelter syndrome
b. Turner syndrome
c. Megalocornea
d. Mucopolysaccharidosis

118. Which of the following combination is/are true about ectopia lentis:

a. Superior temporal displacement- Marfan syndrome
b. Inferior temporal displacement- Homocystinuria
c. Inferior nasal displacement- Homocystinuria
d. Downwards and temporal sublaxaion- Weil-Marchesani syndrome

119. Not feature of Fuchs' heterochromiciridocyclitis:

a. White nodules on the anterior surface of the iris
b. Koppeprecipitates present at back of cornea
c. Granulomatous type of low grade anterior uveitis
d. Topical corticosteroids are used for treatment

120. True about iris:

a. Eye colour is due to relative number of melanocytes
b. Stroma is responsible for pigmentation
c. Sphincter pupillae is supplied by parasympathetic fibres
d. Dilator pupillae is supplied by sympathetic fibres
e. Stroma is covered on its anterior surface by two layers of pigmented epithelium

121. Which of the following is/are not the feature(s) of corneal ulcer due to herpes virus:

a. Rose Bengal staining of margin of ulcer
b. Decreased corneal sensitivity
c. Fluorescein staining of floor of the ulcer
d. Ring infiltration

ENT

122. True about Reinke's oedema:

a. Usually unilateral
b. Common in smoker
c. Corticosteroid is mainstay of treatment
d. Involve whole of membranous part of the vocal cords
e. Patient has low pitch voice

123. Feature(s) of Scheibe's syndromeis/are:

a. Semicircular canal fistula
b. Abnormality in bony labyrinth
c. Dysplasia of cochlea
d. Middle ear anaomaly

124. True about nasopharyngeal carcinoma:

a. Level 4 cervical lymph node not involved
b. Radiotherapy is treatment of choice
c. Also k/a Guangdong tumour
d. May associated with U/L otitis media
e. Associated with EBV

125. True about tubercular otitis media:

a. Multiple hole in tympanic membrane
b. Pale granulation mass seen in middle ear
c. No extra-auricular complication
d. Corticosteriod is used in treatment
e. Painless

126. Evidence-based therapy of Bell's palsy include(s):

a. Facial nerve massage
b. Facial nerve stimulation
c. Steroid
d. Acyclovir

127. A person has vertigo without CNS involvement. Causes is/are:

a. Perilymph fistula
b. Otolithiasis
c. Vestibular neuritis
d. Meniere's disease
e. Multiple sclerosis

MCQs

Answer

113. a, c, d. 114. a, b, c, e. 115. c. 116. a, c, e. 117. d. 118. a, b. 119. c.
120. a, b, c, e. 121. a, b, c. 122. b, d, e. 123. c. 124. All 125. a, b, e. 126. c.
127. a, b, c, d.

MEDICINE

128. All are true about chronic fatigue syndrome except:

a. For diagnosis, duration of fatigue should be atleast 6 month
b. Impaired memory and concentration may present
c. Fatigue relieved by rest
d. Physical examination shows no abnormalities
e. Cognitive behavioral therapy is useful for treatment

129. All are true about primary aldosteronism except:

a. One of the most common cause of secondary hypertension
b. Hyperkalemia
c. Sodium retention
d. Ratio of plasma aldosterone to plasma renin activity (PA/PRA) is a useful screening test
e. Tetany may occur

130. All are true about acute pericarditis except:

a. Pain radiate to left shoulder & arm
b. Widespread elevation of the ST segments, often with upward concavity & then return to baseline
c. Pain relieved by lying supine & intensified by sitting up and leaning forward
d. Corticosteroid relieves symptoms
e. High-pitched scratching or crunching noise may heard in auscultation

131. Hypercalcemia is/are associated with paraneoplastic syndrome of which of the following cancer:

a. Ovary cancer
b. Cervical cancer
c. Squamous cell carcinoma of lung
d. Renal cancer
e. Malignant melanoma

132. Which of the following markers suggest likely primary cancer in carcinoma of unknown primary(CUP):

a. CK7 is found in tumors of the lung, ovary, endometrium & breast
b. CK20+/CDX-2+/CK7–, suggestive of lower gastrointestinal cancer
c. Calretin & WT-1 for melanoma
d. Chromogranin, synaptophysin & CD56 are marker of neuroendocrine prrimary

133. Which is true about thrombolysis in acute ischemic stroke:

a. Most effective if used within 3 hour
b. Contraindicated in h/o prior intracranial haemorrahage
c. Use of heparin within 48 hr is not a contraindication
d. Contraindicated if platelets <100, 000 per microliter

134. High anion gap metabolic acidosis is/are present in:

a. Asthma
b. COPD with CO_2 retention
c. Poorly controlled diabetes
d. Renal tubular acidosis

135. True about McCune-Albright syndrome:

a. Occur in children & during puberty
b. Precocious puberty in female
c. Involve long bone of limb
d. Associated with hypothyroidism

136. Increased portal vein pressure & normal hepatic vein pressure can be seen in all except:

a. Alcoholic cirhhosis
b. Alcholoic hepatitis
c. Budd Chairi syndrome
d. Portal vein thrombosis
e. Inferior vena cava obstruction

137. Which of the following statement(s) is/are regarding American Heart Association (AHA) Guideline-2015 for cardiopulmonary resuscitation (CPR) & Emergency cardiovascular care (ECC):

a. Chest compression: ventilation Compression ventilation ratio without advanced airway – rate 30:2 irrespective of rescuer & age of patient
b. Compression rate- at least 100/min
c. Failure to achieve an ETCO2 of 10 mm Hg by waveform capnography after 20 minutes of resuscitation has been associated with an extremely poor chance of return of spontaneous circulation (ROSC)
d. Limit interruptions in chest compressions to less than 10 seconds

138. True about multiple sclerosis:

a. Corticosteroids are used in acute attack
b. Intravenous Immunoglobulin is effective mode of treatment
c. IFN α- used in recurrence
d. IFN-β- used in recurrence
e. Plasmapheresis may be used in severe relapses

139. Extrathyroid feature of hypothyroidism includes:

a. Pretibial myxedema
b. Carpal tunnel syndrome
c. Bradycardia
d. Thyroid acropathy
e. Peripheral edema

140. Which of the following is true about medication overuse headache:

a. Not associated with triptanuse
b. Restriction of analgesics should be done
c. Opioid is mainly responsible
d. Preventive therapy should be encouraged after stopping/reducing analgesic

141. Which of the following is/are feature(s) of acute interstitial nephritis:

a. Eosinophiluria
b. Peripheral eosinophilia
c. WBC cast
d. Gross haematuria
e. Significant proteinuria

Answer

128. c.	129. b.	130. c.	131. a, c, d.	132. a, b, d.	133. a, b, d.	134. c.
135. a, b, c.	136. c, e.	137. c, d.	138. a, d, e.	139. b, c, e.	140. b, c, d.	141. a, b, c.

142. Feature(s) of Bulbar palsy is/are:
a. Dysphagia
b. Absent jaw jerk
c. Absent gag reflex
d. Tongue atrophy
e. Tongue wasting & fasciculations

143. All are true about hepatorenal syndrome except:
a. Creatinine level raised
b. Albumin infusion given
c. Liver transplantation improves renal functions
d. May occur in cirrhoss
e. Low dose dopamine infusion is very effective

144. Which of the following is/are used for assessment of carbohydrate malabsorption:
a. Schilling test
b. Steatorrhoea
c. D-xylose test

145. True about Swan-Ganz catheter:
a. Measures right atrial pressure
b. Measures left ventricular filling pressure
c. Measure PCWP
d. Inserted through left subclavian vein
e. Inserted directly in Right atrium

146. Treatment of acute Hyperleukocytosis includes:
a. Hydroxyurea
b. Isotretinoin
c. Leukapheresis
d. Vincristine

SURGERY

147. Feature(s) of 3rd degree burn is/are:
a. Blister formation
b. Very painful
c. No spontaneous healing
d. Dry eschar formation
e. Thrombosed vessels can be seen under the skin

148. True about Babcock forcep:
a. Teeth at end
b. Serration at end
c. Triangular orifice in blades
d. Used for soft delicate tubular structure
e. Curved forcep

149. Gas used in creating pneumoperitonem:
a. Water
b. CO_2
c. O_2
d. Air
e. CO

150. Carbon dioxide is used in laproscopy for creating pneumoperitoneum in place of air because:
a. Less absorption from peritoneal surface
b. Fast clearance from body
c. Less solubility in blood
d. Electrocautery is safe to use
e. Less risk of gas embolism

151. Acute haemorrhagic pancreatitis produce which of the following sign:
a. Cullen sign
b. Rovsing sign
c. Psoas sign
d. Grey Turner sign
e. Kehr sign

152. True regarding urinary catheterization with 16 French size:
a. It is the suitable size to use in adult female
b. It can cause UTI in long term use
c. Used in management of urethral obstruction
d. Diameter is 4 mm
e. Sterile technique must be used for insertion

153. Which of the following is/are true about obstructive uropathy:
a. Stricture in ureter is cause
b. Stone in ureter is cause
c. RTA type 4 can occur
d. Absence of hydronephrosis on USG rule out obstructive uropathy
e. When obstruction is above the level of the bladder, bilateralhydroureter and hydronephrosis occurs

154. True about brachial fistula:
a. External opening near the anterior border of sternocleido-mastoid
b. External opening at junction of upper & middle third of sternocleidomastoid muscle
c. Develop due to persistence of 2nd branchial cleft
d. Open in oropharynx
e. Move with swallowing

155. True about 1st degree haemorrhoid:
a. Painless bleeding
b. Malaenae occur
c. Constipation may be present
d. Prolapse on defaecation
e. Never prolapse

156. Which of the following examination is done in supine position:
a. Tredelenburg position
b. ReverseTredelenburg position
c. Sims position
d. Jack knife position
e. Lloyd-Davies position

157. True about lip carcinoma:
a. Common in smoker
b. More common in lower lip
c. More common in upper lip
d. Always painful to touch
e. Distant metastasis is late

Answer

142. All	143. e.	144. c.	145. a, b, c, d.	146. a, c, d.	147. c, d, e.	148. c, d.
149. b. c. d.	150. b, d, e.	151. a, d.	152. a, b, c, e.	153. a, b, c.	154. a, c, d.	155. a, c, e.
156. a, b, e.	157. a, b, e.					

158. True about mediastinal teratoma:
a. Most common tumour of anterior mediastinum
b. Most common germ cell tumour of mediastinum
c. More commonly occurs in anterior mediastinum
d. Contain teeth, skin, hair, cartilage and bone
e. Histologically graded as differentiated & undifferentiated

159. True about inguinal hernia in children:
a. Occur due to persistence of processus vaginalis
b. Defect in abdominal may present
c. Most common variety is direct type
d. Difficult to reduce non-operatively
e. More common in girls

160. True regarding testicular tumour:
a. For stage I seminoma- orchidectomy alone used for treatment
b. For stage I seminoma- orchidectomy + radiotherapy used for treatment
c. Stage I non-seminomatous germ cell tumour-orchidectmy +radiotherapy used for treatment
d. Staging is important for planning management
e. βHCG & AFP may be used as marker the response of treatment

161. Feature(s) of Fournier's gangrene:
a. Necrotizing fasciitis of the male genitalia and perineum
b. Diabetes is risk factor
c. Urgent wide surgical excision of the dead and infected tissue is essential
d. Testis need to be removed in all cases

162. Which of the following is/are feature(s) of enlarged kidney:
a. Ballotable
b. Upper border can be reached
c. Shift to paracolic gutter on compression
d. Do not move with respiration
e. Dull on percussion on renal angle

163. Hypoparathyoidism can occur in:
a. After thyroid surgery b. DiGeorge syndrome
c. Radical resection of head & neck cancer
d. MEN I

164. True about breast cyst:
a. Mostly seen in premenopausal period
b. Most common in young woman
c. Usually unilateral
d. Yellowish-greenish discharge
e. Adhere to underlying skin

165. Fibrocystic disease differ from fibroadenoma by having:
a. Pain shift with cycle b. Freely mobile
c. Usually bilateral d. Firm & rubbery
e. Well demarcated border

166. Test for incompetent valve done by:
a. Cough impulse test b. Trendelenburg I test
c. Percussion wave travel in retrograde direction along varicose vein
d. Percussion wave travel in orthograde direction along varicose vein

167. Which of the following is/are true about renal carcinoma of T3a stage:
a. Involve Gerota fascia
b. Involve perinephric fat
c. Renal vein involvement
d. Inferior vena cava involvement
e. Size >10 cm

168. True about extracorporeal shock wave lithotripsy (ECWL):
a. C/I in pregnancy
b. Less satisfactory for hard stones
c. Stone is breaked into small pieces which comes out with urine
d. Safer in coagulopathy
e. Endoscopic retrieval is sometimes used for impacted stone fragment produced by lithotripsy

169. True about carcinoma gall bladder:
a. Increased bilirubin level is contraindication for surgery
b. Palliative treatment is for advanced disease
c. Metastatic recurrence is common in liver
d. When gallbladder wall is involved, extended cholecystectomy is done
e. Surgery should be done in all cases

170. True about paramedian incision:
a. It is made below umbilicus
b. Better in obese person
c. Cause abdominal hernia
d. Cut anterior surface of rectus sheath
e. Cut posterior surface of rectus sheath

171. All are true about full thickness rectal prolapse except:
a. Elderly are at risk
b. Common in children
c. More common in female
d. Sensation of incomplete evacuation
e. May associated with a weak pelvic floor

172. Which of the following is/are feature(s) of Keloid:
a. Collagen fibers are randomly arranged
b. Type IV collagen dominates
c. Lesion with healthy margin removed
d. Steroid is very useful
e. Goes beyond margin of wound

173. True about Congenital hypertrophic pyloric stenosis:
a. Shortening of pyloric canal on barium contrast imaging
b. Elongation of pyloric canal on barium contrast imaging
c. Narrowing of pyloric canal on barium contrast imaging
d. Thickened pyloric muscle on USG
e. Child should be given normal saline with KCl

Answer

158. b, c, d, e. 159. a, b, d. 160. b, d, e. 161. a, b, c. 162. a, e. 163. a, c. 164. a, c, d.
165. a, c. 166. a, b, c. 167. b, c, e. 168. a, b, c, e. 169. b, c, d. 170. c, d, e. 171. b.
172. b, d, e. 173. b, c, d, e.

174. In comparison to ulcerative colitis, which of the following is/are feature(s) of crohn's disease:
a. Transmural inflammation
b. More common in smoker
c. More pANCA positivity
d. TNF-alpha inhibitor role only in CD

175. True about paralytic ileus:
a. Postoperative ileus primarily affects the stomach and colon
b. Mostly resolve after 24-72 hours
c. Return of function occurs in the following order: stomach, large bowel and small bowel.
d. If opioid is used as postoperative analgesia, then chance increases
e. Is an anticipated complications of abdominal operations

176. Acinic cell carcinoma is/are found in:
a. Breast
b. Parotid
c. Lacrimal gland
d. Pancrease
e. Minor salivary gland

177. Which are Radio-opaque stones:
a. Pure uric acid
b. Cysteine
c. Phosphate
d. Oxalate
e. Impure uric acid

178. True about lymphangioma circumscriptum:
a. Compressible swelling
b. Often contain clear fluid
c. Groups of vesicles are found on skin
d. May present at birth or shortly after birth

179. A child has sacrococcygeal teratoma. Following are true about this condition:
a. Diagnosis of this condition can be done antenatally
b. β-hCG level is increased in maternal serum
c. AFP is elevated in maternal serum
d. Most are benign
e. More common in girls

180. True about central venous catheterization:
a. Catheter may be placed through subclavian vein
b. If the CVP is low in the presence of a low MAP or cardiac output, then fluid resuscitation is necessary
c. Can be used for gaining venous access in patient with poor peripheral veins
d. Subclavian vein route is safest in term of complications

181. True about care of polytrauma patient:
a. CT scan of whole body can be done to exclude injuries
b. Long spinal cord injury support is given if spinal cord injury is suspected
c. Triage of injuries with colour coding like red, yellow, green & black can be done in case of mass casualty
d. Initial fluid management is done as early as possible

182. Which of the following is true about suture technique:
a. Subcuticular suture is used where cosmetic appearance is important
b. Vertical mattress causes cause prominent stitch mark scars
c. Horizontal mattress is used for fragile skin
d. Vertical mattress is used for fragile skin

OBSTETRICS & GYNECOLOGY

183. True about placenta accreta:
a. Incidence is about 1 in 2500 pregnancy
b. Incidence increased in last decade
c. Absence of decidua basalis
d. Fibrinoid layer deficient
e. More common in primi

184. True about low grade squamous intraepithelial lesions:
a. Confined to the lower 1/3 of the epithelium of cervix
b. All cases are treated by cryotherapy
c. 30% progress to invasive cancer in 10 years
d. It is kept under observation with PAP smear or HPV DNA tests

185. True about endometriosis:
a. Laparoscopy is gold standard for diagnosis
b. COC is used to relieve mild pain
c. GnRH antagonist is used to relieve severe pain
d. Can be managed expectantly in asymtomatic cases

186. Which is true regarding premenstrual dysphoric disorder (PMDD):
a. Severe depressed mood
b. Pain ceases at onset of menses
c. Depression may continue after menstrual period
d. Antidepressant is given for treatment
e. Pain ceases after menses is over

187. True about diagnosis of gestational diabetes mellitus (GDM):
a. If post prandial sugar >200 mg/dl, then overt diabetes
b. If fasting sugar is 100-120 mg/dl, then overt diabetes
c. If fasting sugar is ≥126 mg/dl, then overt diabetes
d. If Postprandial sugar is <140 mg/dl, then IGT
e. If fasting sugar is 110-125 mg/dl, then IGT

188. True about primary amenorrhoea:
a. In Rokitansky-Kuster-Hauser syndrome, FSH is normal
b. In Turner syndrome, FSH is decreased
c. In Kallman syndrome, FSH is increased
d. In Kallman syndrome, LH is reduced

189. In assisted breech delivery, after coming head is delivered by:
a. Head delivered spontaneously
b. Pinard manaeuvre
c. Modified Mauriceau-Smellie-Veit technique
d. Special forcep for delivering head is used
e. Prague maneuver

Answer

174. a, b, d. 175. a, b, d, e. 176. b, d, e. 177. b, d, e. 178. b, c, d. 179. a, c, d, e. 180. a, b, c.
181. All 182. a, b, c. 183. b, c, d. 184. a, d. 185. a, b, d. 186. a, d, e. 187. a, c, e.
188. a, d. 189. c, d, e.

190. Which of the following is/are ultrasonographic finding of twins:

a. Type of twin pregnancy can be diagnosed in first trimester
b. Lambda sign indicates dichorionicity
c. T sign suggests monochorionic diamniotic pregnancy
d. Monozygotic twins are more common

191. Markers of malignant ovaria tumour is/are:

a. Inhibin
b. Beta human chorionic gonadotropin
c. Alphafetoprotein (AFP)
d. Pax 7
e. NB/70K

192. Which of the following indicates high risk choriocarcinoma-:

a. Initial serum hCG> 40, 000 mIU/mL
b. Prior chemotherapy failure
c. Following term pregnancy
d. Metastasis limited to lung and vagina
e. Long duration of disease

193. True about mature ovarian teratoma:

a. Recurrence is common after excision
b. Contain hair Teeth, bone & cartilage
c. Mostly benign
d. May be bilateral
e. Torsion is common complication

194. Poor prognostic factors for heart disease in pregnancy is/are:

a. EF <50%
b. Prior cardiac failure, arrhythmia or transient ischemic attack
c. Aortic valve area <1.5 cm^2
d. Class III & IV NYHA patient
e. Peak LV out flow tract gradient > 30 mm Hg by echocardiography

195. True about abdominal hysterectomy:

a. Preferred for prolapse in postmenopausal woman
b. Ureter injury can be avoided by opening the retroperitoneum & identifying ureter
c. Postoperative complications are less than vaginal hysterectomy
d. Preferred in obese patient
e. Enables wide exploration of abdomen

196. True about Copper containing IUCD:

a. Increased copper level in milk
b. Increased risk of ectopic pregnancy
c. Increased bleeding in menstruation with pain
d. Provide protection against PID
e. Irregular menses

197. True about Progestogen only pill (POP):

a. It is taken daily on the same time
b. Higher failure rate than COC
c. Fertility return to normal after discontinuation without any delay
d. Suited for lactating women lactating women
e. Ectopic pregnancy risk are same as COC

198. A 30 year lady delivered a baby. Which of the following statement(s) is not true about postpartum contraception:

a. OCP is not given because it can causes venous thrombosis & have adverse impact on milk production
b. POP is contraceptive of choice for lactating women
c. POP should be started after 6 week
d. LNG-IUD is good in lactating women
e. For non-lactating women, ovulation not occurs until 12 week

PEDIATRICS

199. Corticosteroids are useful in which of the following paediatrics disease:

a. TB meningitis
b. Endobronchial TB
c. Spinaventosa
d. Acute tuberculous pericardial effusion
e. Severe miliary tuberculosis

200. Eosinophilia in children is/are present in:

a. Allergic rhinitis
b. Echinococcosis
c. Rheumatoid arthritis
d. Infectious mononucleosis
e. Wiskott-Aldrich syndrome

201. Syndrome not associated with childhood leukemia:

a. Edward syndrome
b. Fanconi syndrome
c. Diamond-Blackfan anemia
d. Patau syndrome
e. Kostmann syndrome

202. A child has vitamin D deficiency rickets. Which of the following is/are correct regarding biochemical changes:

a. ↑ Alkaline phosphatase
b. ↑ serum calcium
c. ↑ parathyroid hormone
d. ↑ phosphate
e. ↑ 25-(OH)D3

203. True about fetal alcohol syndrome:

a. Increased birth weight
b. Normal fine motor development
c. Normal social skill development
d. Facial abnormalities
e. Intelligence subnormal

204. Feature(s) of congenital rubella syndrome include:

a. Cataract
b. ASD
c. Deafness
d. Patent ductus arteriosus

Answer

190. a, b, c. 191. a, b, c, e. 192. a, b, c, e. 193. b, c, d, e. 194. b, c, d, e. 195. b, e. 196. b, c, e.
197. a, b, d. 198. e. 199. a, b, d, e. 200. a, b, c, e. 201. a, d. 202. a, c. 203. d, e.
204. a, c, d.

205. A 4.2 kg baby born to uncontrolled diabetic mother. The following condition will not occur in the baby:
- a. Hypercalcemia
- b. Hypoglycemia
- c. Hyperbilirubinemia
- d. Polycythemia
- e. Cardiovascular defects

206. True about caput succedaneum
- a. Edematous swelling of scalp
- b. Margins are clearly defined
- c. Swelling resolve spontaneously after few days of birth
- d. Swelling remains for three months
- e. Maximum size at birth

207. A child has fever with redness of cheek. The causative organism for this condition is:
- a. Herpes virus
- b. Parvo virus B-19
- c. Adenovirus
- d. Rubella
- e. Roseola

208. Which of the following is/are true about minimal change disease:
- a. Not same as lipoid nephrosis
- b. Corticosteroids are not used for treatment
- c. Effacement of the epithelial cell foot processes
- d. Onset may be preceded by an upper respiratory tract infection
- e. Steroid is given for treatment

209. Which of the following true about newborn & children:
- a. Erythropoeitin level is more in preterm than term
- b. Erythropoeitin given to preterm only in some special cases
- c. Erythropoeitin given to preterm can cause complication

210. In which condition(s), urethral opening is never at tip of glans penis:
- a. Epispadias
- b. Hypospadias
- c. Urethral stricture
- d. Bladder exstrophy

211. Ingestion of which of the following mimics scurvy in child:
- a. Magnesium
- b. Potassium iodide
- c. Arsenic
- d. Iron
- e. Copper

ORTHOPEDICS

212. True about Butonnaire deformity:
- a. Flexion of proximal interphalangeal joint & hyperextension of distal interphalangeal joint
- b. Hyperextension of proximal interphalangeal joint & flexion of distal interphalangeal joint
- c. Flexion at proximal interphalangeal & extension at metacarpophalangeal joint
- d. Flexion deformity of the proximal interphalangeal joint occur due to tear in central slip of extensor tendon
- e. May occur in rheumatoid arthritis

213. True about ankylosing spondylitis:
- a. Romanus lesion may be found
- b. If left untreated, spine fusion may occur
- c. Predilection of the joints of the axial skeleton
- d. Bony erosions do not occur

214. Which of the following is/are true about Giant cell tumour:
- a. Commonly occurs in bones around knee joint
- b. Radiotherapy is given for treatment
- c. Cause cortical thinning by expansion
- d. Most commonly occur during puberty

215. Which of the following is/are true about simple bone cyst:
- a. Most commonly occur in adult
- b. Commonest site is the upper end of the humerus
- c. Cortex may be thin
- d. Cause pathological fracture
- e. No risk of recurrence after removal

216. True about Colle's fracture:
- a. Occur at distal end of radius, about 2 cm from distal articular surface
- b. Fracture also involves radiocarpal joint
- c. Fracture also involves proximal radioulnar joint
- d. Cause ulnar deviation
- e. Common in women

217. For assessing the injury of meniscus of knee joint, which of the following test is/are done:
- a. Apley's test
- b. Lachmann test
- c. McMurray's test
- d. Thessaly test
- e. Hamilton ruler test

218. A 70 year old lady got compression fracture of L1 vertebra. There is no neurological deficit to this patient. What advise will you give for this patient:
- a. Vitamin D supplementation
- b. Do MRI scan
- c. Go for screw fixation of L1 vertebra
- d. To take Dexamethasone
- e. To take Alendronate

ANESTHESIA

219. True about tracheostomy:
- a. Tracheostomy tube may closed by mucous secretion & crust formation
- b. Copious secretion from tube is always due pulmonary infection
- c. X-ray chest should be done for confirmation in every case
- d. Improper positioning may lead to fatal haemorrhage
- e. Displacing of tube after 2 week is medical emergency

Answer

205. a. 206. a, c, e. 207. b. 208. c, d, e. 209. b, c. 210. a, b, d. 211. a.
212. a, d, e. 213. a, b, c. 214. a, b, c. 215. b, c, d. 216. a, e. 217. a, c, d. 218. a, e.
219. a, d.

220. True about desflurane:
a. Boiling point is <23°C
b. Chemically it is Flourinated methyl ethylether
c. It increases the effect of muscle relaxant
d. Can be given safely to patient susceptible to malignant hyperthermia
e. More potent than isoflurane

221. Drug(s) not given as transdermal patch:
a. Fentanyl
b. Diclofenac
c. Morphine
d. Clonidine
e. Buprenorphine

222. Endotracheal intubation is/are assessed by:
a. Mallampati grading
b. ASA physical status grading
c. Thyromental distance
d. Teeth arrangement

SKIN

223. Which of the following is/are used in psoriasis:
a. High dose oral dexamethasone
b. Methotrexate
c. TNF-alpha inhibitor
d. Acitretin
e. Narrow band UVB

224. True about skin:
a. Epidermis is highly vascular
b. Melanocyte is derived from neural crest
c. Sebaecous gland- holocrine & absent in palm
d. Apocrine gland presents in axilla & groin
e. Hiraadenitis suppurita is infection of apocrine gland

225. Acneiform eruption is/are side effect of:
a. Tetracycline
b. Phenytoin
c. Isoniazid
d. Steroid
e. Potassium iodide

226. Cicatrical alopecia is/are seen in:
a. Lichen planopilaris
b. Discoid lupus erythematous
c. Andogen efflvum
d. Lichen planus
e. Trichotillomania

227. Wavelength of UVB is:
a. 250-280 nm
b. 280-320 nm
c. 320-400 nm
d. 400-700 nm
e. 100-200 nm

228. Which of the following statement(s) is/are true about physical urticaria
a. Cholinergic urticarial is precipitated by cold
b. Solar urticaria is skin sign of erythropoietic protoporphyria
c. Dermatographism is an example
d. Cold urticaria is precipitated by emotion

PSYCHIATRY

229. True about schizophrenia:
a. Q-EEG finding is one of diagnostic criteria for schizophrenia
b. Psychosurgery can be done for some resistant cases
c. Family history of schizophrenia is poor prognosis
d. Depression may be found
e. Onset only after 40 year of age

230. Which of the following is/are not side-effect of lithium:
a. Seizure
b. Hyporeflexia
c. Nephrogenic diabetes insipidus
d. Alopecia
e. Tremor

RADIOLOGY

231. True about photodynamic therapy of head & neck cancer:
a. Tumour sensitizer is used
b. Singlet oxygen is produced in tumour cell
c. After therapy, radiosensitizer may remain with tumour cell
d. Hemoporphyrin given as radiosensitizer
e. Photosensitivity is a side-effect after therapy

232. Which of the following cell(s) are less radiosensitive:
a. Osteocyte
b. Erythroblasts
c. Chondrocyte
d. Spermatogonia
e. Lymphocyte

233. All are true about gamma knife except:
a. Focussed radiation is delivered to tumor
b. Provide equal exposure to surrounding healthy tissue
c. It is a type of stereotactic surgery
d. Primarily used for small brain tumours
e. Uses Co-60 as source of radiation

234. Gamma radiation is/are produced by:
a. Co-60
b. Caesium-137
c. P-32
d. Iridium-192
e. Strontium-90

Answer

220. a, b, c. 221. b, c. 222. a, c, d, 223. b, c, d. 224. b, c, d, e. 225. b, c, d, e. 226. a, b, d.
227. b. 228. b, c. 229. b, c, d. 230. b. 231. a, b, c, e. 232. a, c. 233. b.
234. a, b, d.

235. Precise FNAC can be obtained by using:

a. USG
b. CT
c. Endoscopic USG
d. MRI
e. Plain-Xray

236. True about signal characteristic of CSF on MRI & FLAIR:

a. Hyperintense on T1WI
b. Hypointense on T1WI
c. Hyperintense on T2WI
d. FLAIR reduces CSF signal
e. FLAIR increases CSF signal

237. Contrast agent which are not used for CT scan:

a. Water
b. CO_2
c. Barium compounds
d. Iodinated high-osmolality contrast media
e. Polyethylene glycol

238. True about USG:

a. Uses most commonly frequency of 20-50 MHz for diagnostic ultrasound
b. Work on principle of piezoelectric effect
c. Ultrasonic waves only penetrates gas , not liquid
d. Gas filled microbubbles are used as contrast media

239. True about finding of pleural effusion:

a. CT scan can distinguish between a pleural effusion and a pleural empyema
b. USG can detect very small amount of fluid
c. X-ray- homogenous opacity with obliteration of CP angle
d. MRI cannot differentiate malignant from benign pleural disease
e. MRI can differentiate malignant from benign pleural disease

MCQs

Answer

235. a. 236. b, c, d. 237. b. 238. b, d. 239. a, b, c, e.

MAY 2016 ANSWERS & EXPLANATIONS

ANATOMY

1. **Ans. a. Supplied by..... c. The muscle pass...**

[Ref: BDC 6th/ Vol. III 208-11; Snell 9th/556-57; Essential Anatomy by Moore 2nd/539]

*"Occulomotor nerve in orbit: The **larger, lower division** divides into 3 branches for the medial rectus, the inferior rectus & the **inferior oblique**. The **smaller, upper division** supplies the superior rectus & part of the levator palpebrae superioris. **All branches enter the muscle on their ocular surfaces except that for the IO which enters its posterior border**" (BDC 6th/ Vol. III 362)*

*"**Origin:** IO arises from the orbital surface of the maxilla, lateral to the lacrimal groove. The muscle is situated near the **anterior margin of the orbit**"(BDC 6th/ Vol. III 208)*

*"**Insertion:** The IO is fleshly throughout. It passes laterally, upwards & backwards **below the inferior rectus** & then deep to the lateral rectus. The IO inserted close to the superior oblique a little below & posterior to the latter" (BDC 6th/ Vol. III 208)*

*"**IO:** Origin- floor of orbit cavity & insertion- lateral surface of eyeball deep to lateral rectus" (Snell 9th/551)*

Table *(BDC 6th/ Vol. III 211)*: **Actions of Individual Muscles**

Muscle	Vertical axis	Main action horizontal axis	Anteroposterior axis
Superior rectus	Elevates	Adducts	Rotates medially (Intorsion)
Inferior rectus	Depresses	Adducts	Rotates Laterally (Extorsion)
Superior oblique	Depresses	Abducts	Rotates medially(Intorsion)
Inferior oblique	**Elevates**	**Abducts**	**Rotates Laterally (Extorsion)**
Medial rectus	-	Adducts	-
Lateral rectus	-	Abducts	-

Table: Extraocular Muscles of Orbit

Muscle	Origin	Insertion	Innervation	Main Action
Inferior oblique (IO)	Anterior part of floor of orbit	Sclera deep to lateral rectus muscle	Oculomotor nerve (CN III)	**Abducts, elevates, and laterally rotates eyeball**

2. **Ans. a. Presents as a mass... b. Stone in Wharton duct... c. Starts pain just after... d. Pain carried by...**

[Ref: BDC 6th/ Vol. III 133-36; Snell 9th/ 633-34; Essential Anatomy by Moore 2nd/568; Gray's 40th/520-21]

"The submandibular salivary gland is a common site of calculus formation. The presence of a tense swelling below the body of the mandible, which is greatest before or during ameal and is reduced in size or absent between meals, is diagnostic of the condition. Examination of the floor of the mouth will reveal absence of ejection of saliva from the orifice of the duct of the affected gland. Frequently, the stone can be palpated in the duct, which lies below the mucous membrane of the floor of the mouth" *(Snell 9th/ 633-34)*

Table *(A. K. Jain 6th/204)*: **Salivary Gland –main differentiating features**

Gland	Secretory duct	Parasympathetic supply (Secretomotor)
Parotid	Stensen's duct	IX (Glossopharyngeal n.)
Submandibular	Wharton duct	VII (Facial n.)
Sublingual	Duct of Rivinus	VII (Facial n.)

"All the 3 pairs of salivary glands are supplied by efferent (Parasympathetic & sympathetic) & afferent nerves (chorda tympani- br. of VII nerve & ***IX nerve***). Afferent fibers carry ***pain impulse*** from salivary glands" *(A. K. Jain 6th/204)*

Sialolithiasis

◈ *Radiopaedia. org/articles*

- It refers to formation of concrements (sialoliths) inside the ducts or parenchyma of salivary glands, and most commonly occurs in the submandibular glands and their ducts.
- Sialolithiasis is most common disease of salivary glands, accounting for approximately 50% of all major salivary gland pathology. The submandibular salivary gland is most commonly affected (80-90% of cases) with almost all the remaining cases located in the parotid duct. This is primarily believed to be due to the increased viscosity of the secretions from the submandibular gland
- It is a disease of adults, typically between 30 and 60 years of age. There is a male predilection
- Typically patient presents with a history of recurrent swelling and ***pain in the involved gland*** usually associated with eating due to obstructions of the draining duct.
- Patients most often present with a ***colicky postprandial swelling of the gland.***

What are the Symptoms of Salivary Gland Stones

◈ *http://patient. info/health/salivary-gland-stones*

- When spit (saliva) cannot exit a blocked tube (duct), it backs up into the gland, causing pain and swelling of the gland.
- The most common symptoms are pain and swelling of the affected gland at mealtimes. This occurs if the stone completely blocks a duct. The saliva cannot pass into your mouth if the duct is blocked by a stone.
- ***The pain can be sudden and intense just after starting a meal. Swelling soon follows. The pain and swelling ease over about 1-2 hours after a meal.***

3. **Ans. a. Crypts is lined..., b. Supplied by IX CN, c. Tongue depressor..., e. Present in oropharynx**

[Ref: BDC 6th/ Vol. III 229-30; Gray's 40th/566-67;Dhingra 6th/ 257-58; Snell's 9th/636]

Examination of oropharynx: *First examine the oropharynx by asking the patient to open the mouth widely.* ***Tongue depressor*** *is used when this preliminary examination is unsatisfactory, or when it is required to displace tongue to one side to examine tonsillolingual sulcus, or to* ***press on the tonsils to look for the contents of tonsillar crypts****" (Dhingra 6th/ 383)*

Palatine Tonsil

◈ *BDC 6th/ Vol. III 229-30; Dhingra 6th/ 257-58*

- It occupies the tonsillar sinus or fossa b/w the palatoglossal & palatopharyngeal arches
- It can be seen through the mouth
- Medial surface of the tonsil is covered by ***nonkeratinizing stratified squamous*** epithelium which dips into the substance of tonsil in form of crypts
- **Nerve supply:** Lesser palatine branches of sphenopalatine ganglion(CN V) & **glossopharyngeal nerve** provide sensory nerve supply
- **Blood supply:** 5 arteries 1) ***Tonsillar branch of facial artery***. This is main artery 2) Ascending pharyngeal artery from external carotid 3) Ascending palatine, a branch of facial artery 4) Dorsal linguae branches of lingual artery 5) Descending palatine branch of maxillary artery
- Palatine tonsil is situated at the ***oropharyngeal isthmus*** *(BDC 6th/ Vol. III 230)*

Palatine Tonsil

◈ *Gray's 40th/566-67*

- Each palatine tonsil is situated in the **lateral wall of the oropharynx**
- It is covered on its oropharyngeal aspect by ***nonkeratinized stratified squamous*** epithelium. The ***epithelium lining the cypts is mostly similar to that of oropharyngeal surface, i.e., stratified squamous***, but there are also patches of reticulated epithelium, which is much thinner
- ***The largest artery supplying tonsil is Tonsillar artery, which is a branch of facial or sometimes the ascending palatine artery***

4. **Ans. a. In zone 1 chondrocytes... d. Zone 4 contain... e. Chondrocytes...**

[Ref: Guyton 40th/82-83]

Articular Hyaline Cartilage

◈ *Guyton 40th/82-83*

- Articular hyaline cartilage covers articular surfaces in synovial joints. It provides an extremely smooth, resistant surface bathed by synovial fluid, which allows almost frictionless movement.
- ***Adult articular cartilage shows a structural zonation with increasing depth from the surface.***
- **Zone 1** is the superficial or tangential layer. The free articular surfaceis a thin, cell-free layer, which contains ***fine collagen type II fibrils*** covered superficially by a protein coating. The cells are ***small, oval*** or elongated and ***parallel to the surface***, relatively inactive, and surrounded by fine tangential fibres. The collagen fibres deeper within this zone are regularly tangential, their diameters and density increase with depth.
- **Zone 2** is the transitional or intermediate layer. The cells are larger, rounder, and are either single or in isogenous groups. ***Mostare typical active chondrocytes,*** surrounded by oblique collagen fibres.
- **Zone 3** (radiate layer)- cells are large, round and often disposed in vertical columns, with intervening radial collagen fibres. As elsewhere, the cells, either singly or in groups, are encapsulated in pericellular matrix which has fine fibrils and ***contains fibronectin and type II, IX and XI collagen.***
- The ***deepest layer or calcified layer*** (**zone 4**) lies adjacent to the subchondral bone (hypochondral osseouslamina) of the epiphysis. The adjacent surfaces show reciprocal fine ridges, grooves and interdigitations, which, with the confluence of their fibrous arrays, resist shearing stresses produced by postural changes and muscle action. ***The junction between zones 3 and 4 is called the tide mark.*** With age, articular cartilage thins and degenerates by advancement of the tide mark zone, and the replacement of ***calcified cartilage*** by bone.

Zones of Articular Cartilage

◈ *www. orthobullets. com/basic-science*

Superficial zone (tangential zone)	• Type II collagen orientation is parallel to joint. • Has flattened chondrocytes, condensed collagen fibers, and sparse proteoglycans. • ***Only zone where articular cartilage progenitor cells have been found***
Intermediate zone	• Type II collagen has an oblique or random organization • Is the thickest layer with round chondrocytes, and abundant proteoglycan content
Deep layer (basal layer)	• **Type II** collagen is perpendicular to joint and crosses tidemark; has the highest concentration of proteoglycans • Round chondrocytes arranged in columns
Tidemark	• Is deep to the basal layer and separates the true articular cartilage from the deeper cartilage that is A remnant of the cartilage anlage

Articular Cartilage

◈ *http://www. lab. anhb. uwa. edu. au*

- It is a specialised form of hyaline cartilage.
- It is not surrounded by a perichondrium and is partly vascularised.
- It is, depending on the arrangement of chondrocytes and collagenous fibres, divided into several zones:

Tangential Layer (Zone 1)

- ***Chondrocytes are rather small*** and flattened parallel to the surface. The most superficial part (lamina splendens) is devoid of cells. Collagen fibres in the matrix of the tangential layer are very fine. They run parallel to the surface of the cartilage.

Transitional Zone (Zone 2)

- The chondrocytes are slightly larger, are round and occur both singly and in isogenous groups.
- Collagen fibres take an oblique course through the matrix of the transitional zone.

Radial Zone (Zone 3)

- Fairly large chondrocytes form radial columns, i.e.. the stacks of cells are oriented perpendicular to the articulating surface.
- The course of the collagen fibres follows the orientation of the chondrocyte columns.

Calcified Cartilage Layer (Zone 4)

- It rests on the underlying cortex of the bone.
- The matrix of the ***calcified cartilage*** layer stains slightly darker (H&E) than the matrix of the other layers.

5. **Ans. a. Postganglionic parasympathetic fibre-secretomotor. b. Preganglionic parasympathetic fibre relay in Otic ganglion. d. Sympathetic nerve are vasomotor.**

[Ref: BDC 6th/ Vol. III 106-12; Snell 9th/630-32; Essential Anatomy by Moore 2nd/513-14; Gray's 40th/497]

"**Preganglionic nerves** *travel in the lesser petrosal branch of the glossopharyngeal nerve & synapse in otic ganglion.* **Postganglionic** *secretomotor fibres reach the gland via the auricuotemporal nerve" (Gray's 40th/497)*

Nerve Supply of Parotid Gland

◈ *BDC 6th/ Vol. III 110-11*

- ***Parasympathetic nerves are secretomotor****: They reach the gland through the auriculotemporal nerve (br. of V CN). The* ***preganglionic fibres begin in the inferior salivatory nucleus****; pass through the glossopharyngeal nerve, its tympanic branch, the tympanic plexus & the lesser petrosal nerve & relay in the* ***otic ganglion****. The postganglionic fibres pass through the auriculotemporal nerve & reach the gland*
- ***Sympathetic nerves are vasomotor*** *& are derived from the plexus around the middle meningeal artery*
- **Sensory nerves** *to the gland come from the auriculotemporal nerve but the parotid fascia is innervated by the sensory fibres of the great auricular nerve (C2, C3)*

Parotid Gland

◈ *Essential Anatomy by Moore 2nd/513-14*

- It is the largest of three paired salivary glands.
- ***The parasympathetic component of the glossopharyngeal nerve (CN IX) supplies presynpatic secretory fibers to the otic ganglion.***
- ***The postsynaptic parasympathetic fibers are conveyed from the ganglion to the gland by the auriculotemporal nerve.***
- Stimulation of the **parasympathetic fibers** produces a thin, watery saliva.
- **Sympathetic fibers** are derived from the cervical ganglia through the external carotid nerve plexus on the external carotid artery. The vasomotor activity of these fibers may reduce secretion from the gland.
- **Sensory nerve fibers** pass to the gland through ***the great auricular and auriculotemporal nerves.***

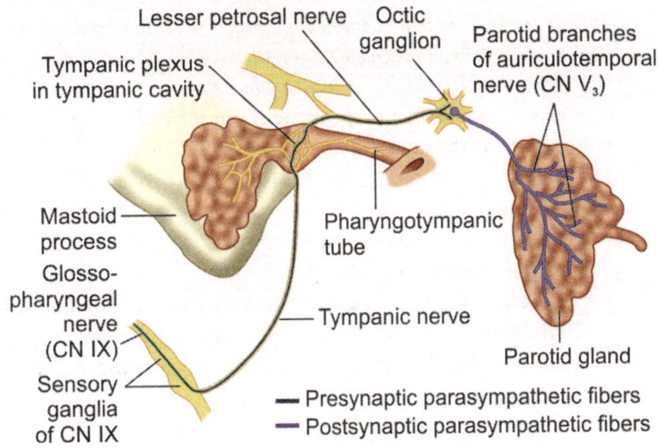

Fig: Innervation of parotid gland

6. **Ans. a. Oppenens pollocis, c. Lateral half of..., d. Superficial head....**

[Ref: BDC 6th/ Vol. I 110; Snell 9th/ 431-32; Essential Anatomy by Moore 2nd/454, 458-59; Gray's 40th/883]

"**Flexor pollicis brevis:** The **superficial head** is usually innervated by the lateral terminal branch of the ***median nerve.*** The **deep part** is often innervated by the deep branch of the ***ulnar nerve*** (C8, T1)" *(Gray's 40th/883)*

Muscles of thenar eminence (Abductor pollicis brevis, flexor pollicis brevis & opponens pollicis) is supplied by median nerve" *(BDC 6th/ Vol. I 120)*

Muscles of hypothenar eminence(abductor digiti minimi, flexor digiti minimi & oppnens digiti minimi) & adductor of thumb (adductor pollicis) are supplied by deep branch of ulnar nerve" *(BDC 6th/ Vol. I 120)*

Median Nerve

◈ *BDC 6th/ Vol. I 110*

- **Muscular branch**: ***Flexor carpi radialis, palmaris longus & flexor digitorum superficialis***
- **Anterior interosseus branch:** ***Flexor pollicis longus, the lateral half of the flexor digitorum profundus & pronator quadratus***

Ulnar Nerve

◈ *BDC 6th/ Vol. I 111*

Muscular branch: ***Flexor carpi ulnaris & the medial half of the flexor digitorum profundus***

7. **Ans. a. Supraspinatus initiates... b. Serratus anterior... e. Musculotendinous cuff...**

[Ref: BDC 6th/ Vol. I 67-70, 146; Snell 9th/364-65; Essential Anatomy by Moore 2nd/484; Gray's 40th/812]

"The conventional view is that **supraspinatus** *initiates abduction of shoulder & assists deltoid in abduction thereafter. However,*

there is evidence that both supraspinatus & deltoid are involved throughout the range of abduction, including the initiation of the movement" (Gray's 40th/812)

*"The **multipennate acromial fibres** are **powerful abductors** of arm at the shoulder joint from beginning to 900. A multipennate arrangement allows a large number of muscle fibres to be packed into a relatively small volume. As the strength of contraction of a muscle is proportional to the number of muscle fibres present in it(And not on their length), **a multipennate muscle is much stronger than other muscles having the same volume**" (BDC 6th/ Vol. I 67)*

The deltoid originates in **three distinct sets of fibers,** often referred to as "heads"

- The **anterior or clavicular** fibers assist Pectoralis Major to flex the shoulder.
- The **lateral fibers** or **acromial fibers** perform basic ***shoulder abduction*** when the shoulder is internally rotated, and perform shoulder transverse abduction when the shoulder is externally rotated
- The **posterior fibers** or **spinal fibers** assist Latissimus Dorsi to extend the shoulder

"**Axillary nerve damage**: ***Deltoid is paralyzed, with loss of the power of abduction up to 900 at the shoulder, rounded contour of shoulder is lost*** *& there is sensory loss over the lower half of the deltoid in a badge-like area called regimental badge" (BDC 6th/ Vol. I 68)*

"**Musculotendinous cuff of the shoulder or rotator cuff** *gives strength to the capsule of shoulder joint all around except inferiorly" (BDC 6th/ Vol. I 69)*

*"**Trapezius** upper & lower fibres act with **serratus anterior** & rotate the scapula forwards round the chest wall thus playing an **important role in abduction of the arm beyond 900**" (BDC 6th/ Vol. I 62)*

8. Ans. a. Eyeball. b. Brain. e. Spinal cord.

[Ref: Handbook of General Anatomy by BDC 5th/ 189; Snell 9th/19]

*"Lymph capillaries are absent from the cellular structures like **brain, spinal cord, splenic pulp, bone marrow, articular cartilage, epidermis, hair, nail & cornea**" (Handbook of General Anatomy by BDC 5th/ 189)*

*"Lymphatic vessel are found in all tissue & organ of body except the **central nervous system, eyeball, internal ear, epidermis of the skin, cartilage & bone**" (Snell 9th/19)*

"Lymphatic vessels (lymphatics), a nearly bodywide network of thin-walled vessels that have abundant lymphatic valves. Lymphatic capillaries and vessels occur almost everywhere blood capillaries are found, except for example, ***teeth, bone, bone marrow, and the entire central nervous system.*** (Excess tissue fluid here drains into the cerebrospinal fluid.)"

"Lymphatics of the kidney drain into the lateral aortic nodes" *(BDC 6th/Vol. II 316)*

9. Ans. b. Esophageal..., c. Pre-capillary sphin..., d. Pudendal ner.... e. Sphincter of oddi....

[Ref: BDC 6th/ Vol. II 249, 375; Guyton 12th/226; Essential Anatomy by Moore 2nd/ 168; Gray's 40th/ 953, 1178]

*"**The common bile duct enters the duodenum** at duodenum papilla. **Its orifice is surrounded by the sphincter of Oddi** & it usually unites with the main pancreatic duct just before entering the duodenum" (Ganong 25th/508)*

*"At the lower end of the esophagus, extending upward about **3 cm** above its junction with stomach, it is broad lower esophageal sphincter, also called gasteroesophageal sphincter. This sphincter comprising of circular muscle normally remains **tonically constricted** with an intraluminal pressure of about 30 mm Hg, in contrast to the midportion of the esophagus, which normally remain relaxed" (Guyton 12th/445)*

"**Lower oesophageal sphincter**, a ***specialized zone of circular smooth muscle*** surrounding the oesophagus at its transit through the diaphragm and for much of its short abdominal course. ***This region of the oesophagus is maintained under tonic contraction***"*(Gray's 40th/ 953) "At the point where each true capillary originates from a metaarteriole, a smooth muscle fiber usually encircles the capillary. This is called the* **precapillary sphincter**. *This sphincter can open & close the entrance to the capillary" (Guyton 12th/226)*

"**Pyloric sphincter** *remain slightly **tonically contracted** almost all the time. Despite normal tonic contraction of the pyloric sphincter, the pylorus usually is open enough for water & other fluids to empty from the stomach into the duodenum with ease" (Guyton 12th/447)*

*"The **somatic, pudendal nerve supplies the sphincter urethrae** which is voluntary & situated within the wall of urethra" (BDC 6th/ Vol. II 375)*

10. Ans. c. Puborec..., d. Pubococc....,e. Ischiococcy....

[Ref: BDC 6th/ Vol. II 369; Snell 9th/252; Essential Anatomy by Moore 2nd/210, 17]

Pelvic Floor

◈ *BDC 6th/ Vol. II 369, 425*

- The pelvic floor is formed by the pelvic diaphragm which consists of the ***levator ani & the coccygeus***
- **Levator ani** is divisible into a ***pubococcygeus part, an iliococcygeus part & an ischiococcygeus part***
- **Pubococcygeus middle fibers constitute Puborectalis**

Table *(Moore)*: **Muscles of Pelvic Walls and Floor**

Boundary	Muscle	Proximal Attachment	Distal Attachment	Innervation	Main Action
Lateral wall	Obturator internus	Pelvic surfaces of ilium and ischium; obturator membrane	Greater trochanter of femur	Nerve to obturator internus (L5, S1, S2)	Rotates thigh laterally; assists in holding head of femur in acetabulum

Contd...

Boundary	Muscle	Proximal Attachment	Distal Attachment	Innervation	Main Action
Posterolateral wall	Piriformis	Pelvic surface of S2-S4 segments; superior margin of greater sciatic notch and sacrotuberous ligament	Greater trochanter of femur	Anterior rami of S1 and S2	Rotates thigh laterally; abducts thigh; assists in holding head of femur in acetabulum
Floor	Coccygeus (ischiococcygeus)	Ischial spine	Inferior end of sacrum and coccyx	Branches of S4 and S5 spinal nerves	Forms small part of pelvic diaphragm that supports pelvic viscera; flexes coccyx
	Levator ani (***puborectalis, pubococcygeus, and iliococcygeus***)	Body of pubis; tendinous arch of obturator fascia; ischial spine	Perineal body; coccyx; anococcygeal ligament; walls of prostate or vagina, rectum, and anal canal	Nerve to levator ani (branches of S4), inferior anal (rectal) nerve, and coccygeal plexus	Forms most of pelvic diaphragm that helps support pelvic viscera and resists increases in intra-abdominal press

11. Ans. a. Vertebral artery..., c. Permit side to side..., e. Permits rota....

[Ref: BDC 6th/ Vol. III 172-74; Snell 9th/688-89;Essential Anatomy by Moore 2nd/288-89; Gray's 40th/734-35]

The vertebral artery has a characteristic anatomical course through six (C6-C1) foramina transversaria of the cervical vertebrae (2nd part), passing through the groove on the surface of the arch of the atlas(3rd part) & through foramen magnum in cranial cavity (4th part)" *(Stroke. ahajournals. org & BDC 6th/ Vol. III 174)*

"**Atlanto-occipital joint** *permit* ***flexion, extension & lateral bending****" (BDC 6th/ Vol. III 172)*

"**Atlanto-axial joints**: *Movement is simultaneous at* ***all three joint****& consists almost exclusively of rotation around the axis. Rotation is limited mainly by the alar ligaments, with a minor contribution from the accessory atlanto-axial ligament. The normal range of atlano-axial rotation is about 400" (Gray's 40th/735)*

Atlantoaxial Joints

- *BDC 6th/ Vol. III 172-74; Essential Anatomy by Moore 2nd/288-89*
- It is b/w C1 & C2 vertebrae
- *There are* ***3 atlantoaxial articulations****- two lateral atlantoaxial joints b/w the lateral masses of C1 & C2 vertebrae & one median atlantoaxial joint b/w the dens of C2 & the anterior arch & transverse ligament of the atlas*
- *Movement(mainly rotation) at all three atlantoaxial joints permits the head to be turned* ***from side to side,*** *as occurs when rotating the head to indicate disapproval(the 'NO' movement)*
- *The most important factors maintaining stability are the ligaments, of which the transverse atlantal ligament is the stongest. The alar ligaments are weaker*

Atlantoaxial joints

- *Snell 9th/688-89*

There can be ***extensive rotation*** of the atlas & thus of the head on the axis

12. Ans. a. Total volume is....,

[Ref: Ganong 25th/603;BDC 6th/ Vol. III 331-33; Snell 9th/707; Essential Anatomy by Essential Anatomy by Moore 2nd/516]

Cerebrospinal Fluid (CSF)

- *Ganong 25th/603*
- ***Volume is 150 ml***
- ***Rate of CSF production is 550 ml/day****. Thus the CSF turns over about 3. 7 times a day*
- ***Lumbar pressure is normally 70-180 mm H_2O***

Cerebrospinal Fluid (CSF)

- *BDC 6th/ Vol. III 331-33*
- *The* ***total quantity of CSF is about 150 ml.***
- *It is formed at the rate of about 200 ml per hour or 5000 ml per day(It may be incorrect!!!!)*
- *CSF is secreted @0. 35-0. 40 ml per minute, which mean that normally about 50% of the total volume of CSF is replaced every 5 to 6 hours- Gray's 40th/243*
- *The* ***normal pressure of CSF is 60 to 100 mm of water***
- *Formation: The bulk of CSF is formed by the* ***choroid plexuses of lateral ventricles****& lesser amount by the choroid plexuses of the third & fourth ventricles. Possibly, it is also formed by the capillaries on the surface of the brain & spinal cord*
- *Absorption: CSF is absorbed chiefly through the arachnoid villi & granulations & is thus drained into the cranial venous sinuses. It is also absorbed partly by the perineural lymphatics around the first, second & eight cranial nerves. It is also absorbed by veins related to spinal nerves*

PHYSIOLOGY

13. Ans. a. Synaptic Net....

[Ref: Ganong 25th/283-88; Guyton 12th/ 673; A K Jain 6th/1039-40]

Synaptic network s single best answer (No idea about other options)

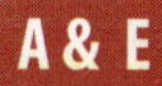

"Long-term memory involves changes in the structure of neurons including ***growth of new processes and synapses***. So, to the extent that you remember anything about this material on memory tomorrow, or next week, or next year, it will be ***because structural changes in synapses are beginning in your brains***. An enduring form of synaptic plasticity called long-term potentiation (LTP) is believed to be involved in many examples of declarative memory"-neuroscience. uth. tmc

Memory

◈ *http://www. human-memory. net/processes_consolidation. html*

- **Encoding:** The persistent spiking in working memory can enhance the synaptic and cellular changes in the encoding of episodic memory
- **Consolidation and reconsolidation:** Short-term memory (STM) is temporary and subject to disruption, while long-term memory (LTM), once consolidated, is persistent and stable. Consolidation of STM into LTM at the molecular level presumably involves two processes: synaptic consolidation and system consolidation. The former involves a protein synthesis process in the medial temporal lobe (MTL), whereas the latter transforms the MTL-dependent memory into an MTL-independent memory over months to years
- It should be remembered that each neuron makes thousands of connections with other neurons, and memories and neural connections are mutually interconnected in extremely complex ways. Unlike the functioning of a computer, each memory is embedded in many connections, and each connection is involved in several memories. Thus, ***multiple memories may be encoded within a single neural network, by different patterns of synaptic connections.*** Conversely, a single memory may involve simultaneously activating several different groups of neurons in completely different parts of the brain.

*"The key to memory is alteration in the strength of **selected synaptic connections.** Second messenger systems contribute to the changes in neural **circuitary required** for learning & memory. Alternation in cellular membrane channels are often correlated to learning & memory. In all but the simplest of cases, the alternation involves the **synthesis of proteins & the activation of genes.** This occurs during the change from short-term working memory to long-term memory" (Ganong 25th/286)*

*Discharge of neuron during learning session could lead to changes which increases mRNA synthesis & hence increase synthesis of particular proteins. These proteins could **modify synaptic transmission** by affecting- transmitter synthesis, membrane permeability & some other neural process" (A K Jain 6th/1039)*

Storage of Information-Memory

◈ *Guyton 12th/ 673*

- Only a small fraction of even the most important sensory information usually causes immediate motor response. But much of the information is stored for future control of motor activities and for use in the thinking processes. Most storage occurs in the cerebral cortex, but even the basal regions of the brain and the spinal cord can store small amounts of information.
- The storage of information is the process we call memory, and this, too, is a ***function of the synapses***. Each time certain types of sensory signals pass through sequences of synapses, these synapses become more capable of transmitting the same type of signal the next time, a process called facilitation.

14. Ans. a. K influx... b. K influx... c. ATP provide.

[Ref: Reddy 32nd/595; Katzung 13th/1010; Guyton 12th/.357; A K Jain 6th/459]

"In *Complex IV* (cytochrome *c* oxidase), sometimes called cytochrome A3, four electrons are removed from four molecules of cytochrome *c* and transferred to molecular oxygen (O_2), producing two molecules of water. At the same time, eight protons are removed from the mitochondrial matrix (although only four are translocated across the membrane), contributing to the ***proton gradient which helps in ATP synthesis***. The ***activity of cytochrome c oxidase is inhibited by cyanide***"

Na^+/K^+–ATPase

- **Na^+/K^+–ATPase** (sodium-potassium adenosine triphosphatase, also known as the **Na^+ /K^+ pump** or **sodium-potassium pump**) is an ***enzyme*** (an electrogenic transmembrane ATPase) found in the plasma membrane of all animal cells. The Na+ /K+-ATPase enzyme is a solute pump that pumps sodium out of cells while pumping potassium into cells, both against their concentration gradients. This pumping is active (i.e. ***it uses energy from ATP***) and is important for cell physiology. An example application is nerve conduction.
- The process of moving sodium and potassium ions across the cell membrane is an active transport process involving the hydrolysis of ATP to provide the necessary energy. It involves an enzyme referred to as Na^+/K+-ATPase. This process is responsible for maintaining the large excess of Na^+ outside the cell and the large excess of K^+ ions on the inside
- It accomplishes the transport of ***three Na^+ to the outside of the cell and the transport of two K^+ ions to the inside.***

Cyanide

◈ *Harrison 19th/262e-7*

- Cyanide directly poisons the last step in the mitochondrial electron transport chain, ***cytochrome a3***, which results in a ***shutdown of cellular energy production***. Tissues are poisoned in direct proportion to their metabolic rate, with the carotid baroreceptors and the brain—the most metabolically active tissues in the body—affected fastest and most severely.
- This *poisoning results from cyanide's high affinity for certain metals, notably Co and Fe+++. Cytochrome a3 contains Fe+++, to which CN– binds.*

Cyanide Poisoning

◈ *Reddy 32nd/595*

- It inhibits the action of cytochrome oxidase, carbonic anhydrase & probably of other enzyme system
- *It blocks the final step of oxidative phosphorylation & **prevents the formation of ATP** & its use as energy source*

15. Ans. c. Oxygen-haemoglobin saturation...

[Ref: Ganong 25th/650-51; Guyton 12th/352; A K Jain 6th/ 431; https://pedclerk. bsd. uchicago. edu/page/carbon-monoxide-poisoning]

"Carbon monoxide shifts the oxygen-haemoglobin saturation curve to the left and changes it to a more hyperbolic shape. Less oxygen is available for the tissues" *(www. ncbi. nlm. nih. gov)*

"The plasma level of carboxyhemoglobin is normally quite low. ***At baseline, levels up to 3 percent may be seen in nonsmokers, while smokers may have levels up to 10-15 percent***" *(pedclerk. bsd. uchicago. edu)*

*"**Left shift of O_2-Hb dissociation curve** occur in – **CO poisoning**, HbF, myoglobin & decrease in body temperature" (A K Jain 6th/ 431)*

Detection in Biological Specimens

- Carboxyhemoglobin blood saturations may range up to ***8–10% in heavy smokers*** or persons extensively exposed to automotive exhaust gases. In symptomatic poisoned people they are often in the 10–30% range, while persons who succumb may have postmortem blood levels of 30–90%.
- A ***CO-oximeter*** is used to determine carboxyhemoglobin levels. ***Pulse CO-oximeters*** estimate ***carboxyhemoglobin with a non-invasive finger clip similar to a pulse oximeter.***
- The ***use of a regular pulse oximeter*** is not effective in the diagnosis of carbon monoxide poisoning as people suffering from carbon monoxide poisoning may have a normal oxygen saturation level on a pulse oximeter. This is due to the carboxyhemoglobin being misrepresented as oxyhemoglobin.

Carbon Monoxide Poisoning

◈ *Ganong 25th/651*

- ***The affinity of hemoglobin for CO is 210 times its affinity for O_2***, and COHb liberates CO very slowly.
- An additional difficulty is that when COHb is present the ***dissociation curve of the remaining HbO_2 shifts to the left***, decreasing the amount of O_2 released.
- Death results when about 70–80% of the circulating hemoglobin is converted to COHb.

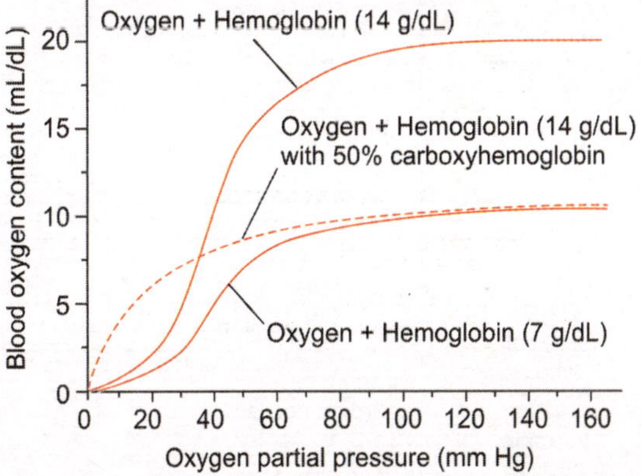

Fig: *(Ganong 25th/650):* Effects of anemia and CO on hemoglobin binding of O_2. Normal oxyhemoglobin (14 g/dL hemoglobin) dissociation curve compared with anemia (7 g/dL hemoglobin) and with oxyhemoglobin dissociation curves in CO poisoning (50% carboxyhemoglobin).

Note: That the CO-poisoning curve is shifted to the left of the anemia curve.

Respiratory Physiology-The Essentials, 8th Edition: Writes

- Carbon monoxide interferes with the O_2 transport function of blood by combining with Hb to form carboxyhemoglobin (COHb). ***CO has about 240 times the affinity of O_2 for Hb***; this means that CO will combine with the same amount of Hb as O_2 when the CO partial pressure is 240 times lower.
- In fact, the ***CO dissociation curve is almost identical in shape to the O_2 dissociation curve***, except that the PCO axis is greatly compressed.
- ***The presence of COHb also shifts the O_2 dissociation curve to the left***, thus interfering with the unloading of O_2. This is an additional feature of the toxicity of CO.
- ***The normal level of COHb is 1%-2% in non-smokers. Tobacco combustion produces CO so smokers have COHb levels of 5%-10%.***

16. Ans. a. Positive pres..., b. Extension..., c. Anticholine..., e. Emphy...,.

[Ref: Ajay Yadav 5th/4-5; Ganong 25th/632-33; Guyton 12th/323; A K Jain 6th/421]

Physiological dead space or total dead space: *It includes anatomical dead space plus volume of air in alveoli which does not take part in exchange of gases(i.e. wasted alveolar ventilation) (A K Jain 6th/421)*

Emphysema *increases dead space (A K Jain 6th/422)*

Anatomical Dead Space Increased in

◈ *Ajay Yadav 5th/5*

- *Old age*
- ***Neck extension***
- *Jaw protrusion*
- *Bronchodilators*
- *Increasing lung volume(like it is more in inspiration)*
- ***Atropine(cause bronchodilation)***
- *Anaesthesia mask, circuits*
- ***Intermittent positive pressure ventilation (IPPV) & positive end expiratory pressure (PEEP)***

Factors that Increase Dead Space

◈ *www. openanesthesia. org*

- **General anesthesia:** Multifactorial, including loss of skeletal muscle tone and bronchoconstrictor tone
- Anesthesia apparatus/circuit
- Artificial airway
- ***Neck extension and jaw protrusion (can increase it twofold)***
- ***Positive pressure ventilation (i.e. increased airway pressure)***
- Upright posture as opposed to supine (because of decreased perfusion to the uppermost alveoli)
- Pulmonary embolus, PA thrombosis, hemorrhage, hypotension, surgical manipulation of pulmonary artery tree – anything that decreases perfusion to well-ventilated alveoli

- ***Emphysema*** (blebs, loss of alveolar septa and vasculature)
- Age
- ***Anticholinergic drugs***

Alveolar Dead Space

◈ *Increased by Ajay Yadav 5th/5*

- *Lung pathologies affecting diffusion at capillary membrane like interstitial lung disease, pulmonary embolism, pulmonary edema & ARDS*
- *General anaesthesia*
- *IPPV*
- *PEEP*
- *Hypotension*

Anatomical Dead Space

◈ *Decreased in Ajay Yadav 5th/5*

- ***Intubation*** *(nasal cavity is bypassed & diameter of tube is less than airway diameter*
- *Tracheostomy (upper airways & nasal cavity bypassed)*
- *Hyperventilation (decreasing lung volume)*
- *Neck flexion*
- *Bronchoconstrictors*

17. Ans. a. T1-T5 is sympathetic..., e. Inferior cervical ganglia...

[Ref: BDC 6th/ Vol. I 267;Gray's 40th/982; Guyton 12th/178; A K Jain 6th/ 324]

Cardiac Innervation

- The **cervical ganglia** are paravertebral ganglia of the sympathetic nervous system. Preganglionic nerves from the thoracic spinal cord enter into the cervical ganglions and synapses with its postganglionic fibers or nerves.
- The cervical ganglion has **three paravertebral ganglia:**
- **Superior cervical ganglion** (largest) - adjacent to C2 & C3; postganglionic axon projects to target: (***heart***, head, neck) via "hitchhiking" on the carotid arteries
- **Middle cervical ganglion** (the smallest) - adjacent to C6; target: ***heart***, neck
- **Inferior cervical ganglion.** The inferior ganglion may be fused with the first thoracic ganglion to form a single structure, the stellate ganglion. –adjacent to C7; target: ***heart,*** lower neck, arm, posterior cranial arteries
- The inferior cervical ganglion gives off Inferior cardiac nerve
- The **middle cardiac nerve** (***great cardiac nerve***), the largest of the three cardiac nerves, arises from the middle cervical ganglion
- ***Nerves emerging from cervical sympathetic ganglia contribute to the cardiac plexus,*** among other things. Unlike all other ganglia, the medial branches of the cervical ganglia are 95% postganglionic axons.
- **Sympathetic stimulation** causes increased heart rate, impulse conduction, force of contraction, and, at the same time, increased blood flow through the coronary vessels to support the increased activity.
- **Parasympathetic stimulation** slows the heart rate, reduces the force of the contraction, and constricts the coronary arteries, saving energy between periods of increased demand.

Cardiac Innervation

◈ *A K Jain 6th/ 324*

- ***Sympathetic supply: T1 to T5 spinal segments.***
- *Sympathetic preganglionic fibres pass into the sympathetic trunk to* ***superior, middle & inferior cardiac ganglion***
- *Sympathetic postganglionic fibres passes via superior, middle & inferior cardiac sympathetic nerves*
- *Parasympathetic supply to heart is via* ***two vagus nerves*** *with their cell bodies located in medulla in the nucleus ambigus*

Nerve Supply of Heart

◈ *BDC 6th/ Vol. I 267*

- **Sympathetic nerves** are derived from the **upper 4 to 5 thoracic segments of spinal cord**. These are cardio-acceleratory & on stimulation they increases the heart rate & also dilate the coronary arteries
- Parasympathetic nerves reach the heart via the vagus. These are cardioinhibitory; on stimulation they slow down the heart rate
- Both parasympathetic & sympathetic nerves from the ***superficial & deep cardiac plexuses,*** the branches of which run along the coronary arteries to reach the myocardium
- Superficial cardiac plexus is situated below the arch of the aorta in front of the right pulmonary artery. It is formed by
  - The superficial cervical cardiac branch of the left sympathetic chain
  - The inferior cervical cardiac branch of the left vagus nerve

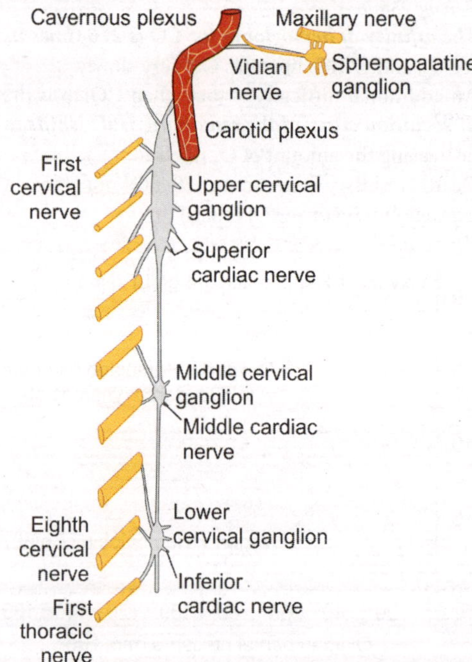

Fig: Cervical sympathetic system

18. Ans. b. Morning concent..., c. Evening concentrati...,

[Ref: Ganong 25th/ 367; Guyton 12th/600; A K Jain 6th/716;CMDT 2016/1716;webmed. com]

Evening concentration is almost half of morning concentration (a/c below reference values)

"Cortisol concentration at 8. 00 am in morning 5–20 mcg/dL (140-550 nmol/L)" *(CMDT 2016/1716)*

Table: Reference Ranges for Blood Plasma Content of free Cortisol

Time	Lower limit	Upper limit	Unit
09:00 am	140	700	nmol/L
	5	25	μg/dL
Midnight	80	350	nmol/L
	2. 9	13	μg/dL

Cortisol

Adult/Child	Morning	5-23 micrograms per deciliter (μg/dL) or 138-635 nanomoles per liter (nmol/L)
	Afternoon	3–16 μg/dL or 83–441 nmol/L
Newborn		2–11 μg/dL or 55–304 nmol/L

Reference ranges for serum cortisol:

- Morning - 7–28 μg/dL
- Afternoon - 2–18 μg/dL
- Stimulated - ≥ 18 μg/dL
- Suppressed - < 2 μg/dL

"The ***concentration of cortisol in the blood averages 12*** μg/***100 ml***, and the ***secretory rate averages 15 mg/day.*** However, blood concentration and secretion rate of cortisol fluctuate throughout the day, rising in the early morning and declining in the evening" *(Guyton 12th/594)*

Circadian Rhythm of Glucocorticoid Secretion

- The secretory rates of CRF, ACTH, and cortisol are ***high in the early morning but low in the late evening***; the plasma cortisol level ranges between a ***high of about 20*** μg/***dl an hour before arising in the morning and a low of about 5*** μg/***dl around midnight.***

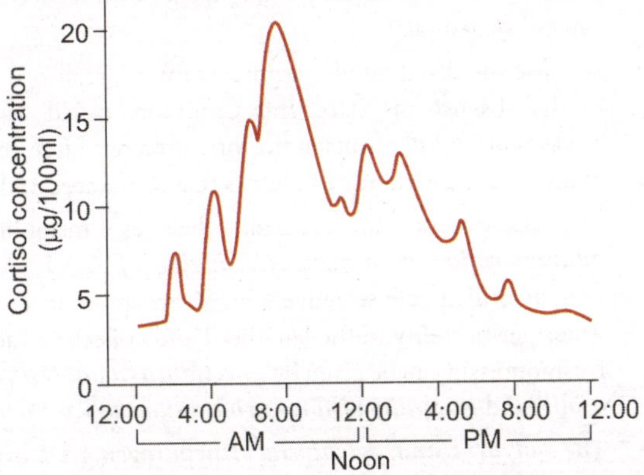

Fig. *(Guyton 12th/600)*: Typical pattern of cortisol concentration during the day. Note the oscillations in secretion as well as a daily secretory surge an hour or so after awaking in the morning

- This effect results from a 24-hour cyclical alteration in the signals from the hypothalamus that cause cortisol secretion. When a person changes daily sleeping habits, the cycle changes correspondingly. Therefore, measurements of blood cortisol levels are meaningful only when expressed in terms of the time in the cycle at which the measurements are made.

19. Ans. d. Frontal cortex

[Ref: Ganong 25th/189, 195-96; Guyton 12th/786; A K Jain 6th/1115-16]

"Normally saccadic movements are voluntary but can be aroused by peripheral visual or auditory stimuli by stimulation of ***frontal eye fields(area 8).*** *Thus these movements are programmed in the* ***frontal cortex****"* *(A K Jain 6th/1115-16)*

Prefrontal lobe: *It lies anterior to the* ***motor areas 4, 6 & 8.*** *The major areas of the prefrontal lobes are: Broadmann's areas 9 to 13, 24, 32& 44 to 47" (A K Jain 6th/1118)*

"***Saccades are programmed in the frontal cortex*** and the superior colliculi and pursuit movements in the cerebellum" *(Ganong 25th/196)*

Neural Pathways

◈ *Ganong 25th/189*

- Saccades, sudden jerky movements, occur as the gaze shifts from one object to another *(Ganong 25th/195)*
- The frontal cortex is also concerned with eye movement, and especially its refinement. The bilateral **frontal eye fields** in this part of the cortex are concerned with control of ***saccades***, and an area just anterior to these fields is concerned with vergence and the near response. The frontal areas concerned with vision probably project to the nucleus reticularis tegmentalis pontinus, and from there to the other brain stem nuclei mentioned above.

20. Ans. a. Normal PR interval... d. Normal QRS interval...

[Ref: Ganong 25th/524; Guyton 12th/179-80; ECG made Easy by Hampton 4th/6-7]

"The PR interval is measured from beginning of P wave to the beginning of QRS complex" (ECG made Easy by Hampton 4th/6)

A QTc interval longer than 0.45 s is likely to be abnormal *(ECG Made Easy by Hampton 4th/157)*

"Normal QRS interval duration is no greater than 0. 12s" (ECG made Easy by Hampton 4th/87)

"**QT interval** is a measure of the time between the ***start of the Q wave and the end of the T wave*** in the heart's electrical cycle"

ECG Waveforms and Intervals

- There are four major ECG intervals: RR, PR, QRS, and QT
- The ***PR interval measures the time (normally 120–200 ms)*** between atrial and ventricular depolarization, which includes the physiologic delay imposed by stimulation of cells in the AV junction area.
- ***The QRS interval (normally 100–110 ms or less)*** reflects the duration of ventricular depolarization.
- The QT interval includes both ventricular depolarization and repolarization times and varies inversely with the heart rate.

- A rate-related ("corrected") QT interval, **QTc,** can be calculated as QT/√RR and ***normally is ≤0. 44 s.*** (Some references give QTc upper normal limits as 0. 43 s in men and 0. 45 s in women. Also, a number of different formulas have been proposed, without consensus, for calculating the QTc.)

Table *(Ganong 25th/524)*: **ECG Intervals**

	Normal Durations		
Intervals	**Average**	**Range**	**Events in the. Heart during Interval**
PR interva	0.18	0.12–0.20	Atrial depolarization and conduction through AV node
QRS duration	0.08	to 0.10	Ventrizular depolarization and atrial reprivatization
QT interval	0.40	to 0.43	Ventricular depolariztion plus ventricular repolarization
ST interval (QT minus QRS)	0.32	...	Ventricular repolarization (during T wave)

Contd...

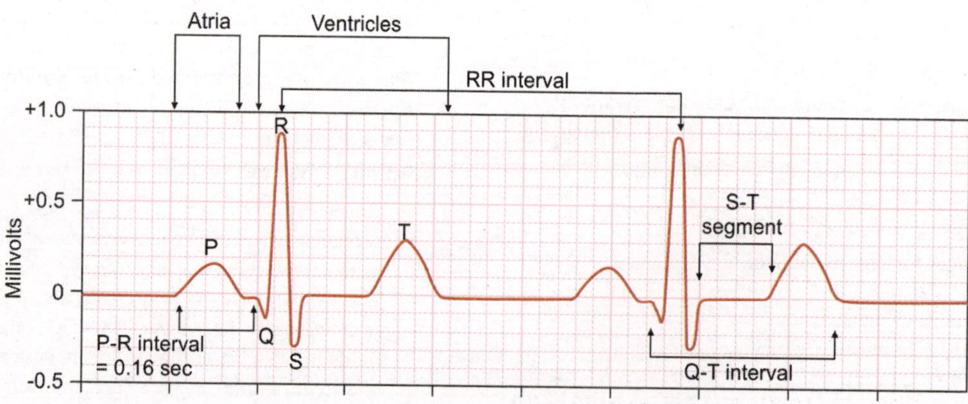

Fig: *(Guyton 12th/ 179)*: Normal electrocardiogram

21. Ans. b. Vasopressin level... d. ↑ed Osmolality of...

[Ref:Harrison 19th/2280; Ganong 25th/698; A K Jain 6th/ 673-74]

Desmopressin is very useful in ***management of diabetes insipidus"*** *(A K Jain 6th/ 673)*

Syndrome of Inappropriate Antidiurectic Hormone

◈ *Ganong 25th/698*

- The syndrome of "inappropriate" hypersecretion of antidiuretic hormone (SIADH) occurs when ***vasopressin is inappropriately high relative to serum osmolality.***
- Vasopressin is responsible not only for ***dilutional hyponatremia*** (serum sodium < 135 mmol/L) but also for ***loss of salt in the urine*** when water retention is sufficient to expand the ECF volume, reducing aldosterone secretion

Syndrome of Inappropriate Antidiurectic Hormone Secretion

◈ *A K Jain 6th/ 673-74*

- *Hyposmolality*
- *↑ed urine osmolality*
- *Urine osmolality becomes higher than plasma osmolality*
- *Urinary Na+ exceeds 20 mEq/L*

22. Ans. b. Basal vasopressin level...

[Ref: Ganong 25th/698; Guyton 12th/488-89; A K Jain 6th/674]

Failure to Produce ADH: "Central" Diabetes Insipidus

◈ *Guyton 12th/488*

- An inability to produce or release ADH from the posterior pituitary can be caused by head injuries or infections, or it can be congenital.
- Because the distal tubular segments cannot reabsorb water in the absence of ADH, this condition, called *"central" diabetes insipidus*, results in the formation of a large volume of dilute urine with urine volumes that can exceed 15 L/day.
- The **treatment** for central diabetes insipidus is ***administration of a synthetic analog of ADH, desmopressin,*** which acts selectively on V_2 receptors to increase water permeability in the late distal and collecting tubules. Desmopressin can be given by ***injection, as a nasal spray, or orally,*** and ***it rapidly restores urine output toward normal.***
- The ***polyuria and polydipsia of nephrogenic DI are not affected by treatment with standard doses of DDAVP***

Inability of the Kidneys to Respond to ADH: "Nephrogenic" Diabetes Insipidus

◈ *Guyton 12th/488-89*

- In some circumstances normal or elevated levels of ADH are present but the renal tubular segments cannot respond appropriately. This condition is referred to as *"nephrogenic" diabetes insipidus* because the abnormality resides in the kidneys.
- This abnormality can be due to either failure of the ***counter current mechanism*** to form a hyperosmotic renal medullary interstitium or failure of the distal and collecting tubules and collecting ducts to respond to ADH.
- The treatment is to correct, if possible, the underlying renal disorder. The hypernatremia can also be attenuated by a low-sodium diet and administration of a diuretic that enhances renal sodium excretion, such as a thiazide diuretic.

Distinction b/w Central DI & Nephrogenic DI

◈ *H19 2277-78*

- Nephrogenic diabetes insipidus can be distinguished from central diabetes insipidus by ***administration of desmopressin***. Lack of a prompt decrease in urine volume and an increase in urine osmolarity within 2 hours after injection of desmopressin is strongly suggestive of nephrogenic diabetes insipidus.
- A simpler but equally reliable way to differentiate between pituitary DI, nephrogenic DI, and primary polydipsia is to **measure basal plasma AVP**. If plasma AVP *on ad libitum fluid intake* is normal or elevated (>1 pg/mL) when measured by a sensitive and specific assay, both primary polydipsia and pituitary DI are excluded and the diagnosis of nephrogenic DI can be confirmed, if desired, by a 1- to 2-day outpatient trial of desmopressin therapy. If, however, basal plasma AVP is low or undetectable (<1 pg/ mL), nephrogenic DI is very unlikely and MRI of the brain can be used to differentiate pituitary DI from primary polydipsia.
- A **fluid** or **water deprivation test** is used to determine whether the patient has diabetes insipidus as opposed to other causes of polydipsia (a condition of excessive thirst that causes an excessive intake of water). The patient is required, for a prolonged period, to forgo intake of water completely, to determine the cause of the thirst. If there is no change in the water loss despite fluid deprivation, desmopressin may be administered to distinguish between the two types of diabetes insipidus which are central & nephrogenic diabetes insipidus.
- ***If MRI and/or AVP assays with the requisite sensitivity and specificity are unavailable and a fluid deprivation test*** is impractical or undesirable, a third way to differentiate between pituitary DI, nephrogenic DI, and primary polydipsia is a ***trial of desmopressin therapy***.

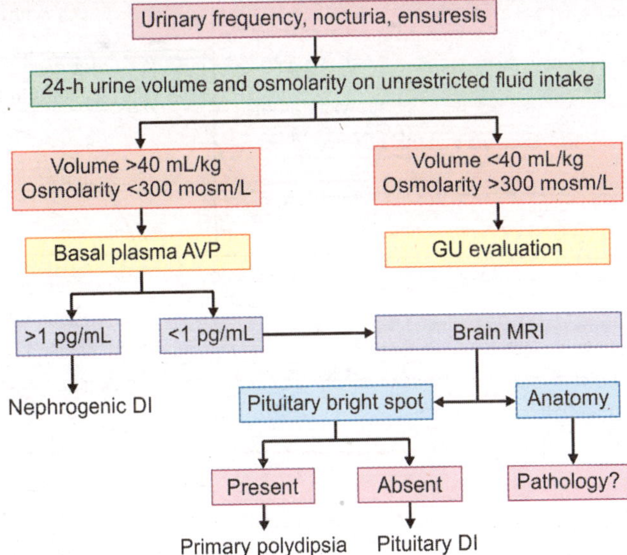

Fig: *(Harrison 19th/ 2278):* Simplified approach to the differential diagnosis of diabetes insipidus. When symptoms suggest diabetes insipidus (DI), the syndrome should be differentiated from a genitourinary (GU) abnormality by measuring the 24-h urine volume and osmolarity on unrestricted fluid intake. If DI is confirmed, basal plasma arginine vasopressin (AVP) should be measured on unrestricted fluid intake. If AVP is normal or elevated (>1 pg/mL), the patient probably has nephrogenic DI. However, if plasma AVP is low or undetectable, the patient has either pituitary DI or primary polydipsia. In that case, magnetic resonance imaging (MRI) of the brain can be performed to differentiate between these two conditions by determining whether or not the normal posterior pituitary bright spot is visible on T1-weighted midsagittal images. In addition, the MRI anatomy of the pituitary hypothalamic area can be examined to look for evidence of pathology that sometimes causes pituitary DI or the dipsogenic form of primary polydipsia. MRI is not reliable for differential diagnosis unless nephrogenic DI has been excluded because the bright spot is also absent, small, or faint in this condition

BIOCHEMISTRY

23. Ans. d. Citrulline synthase

[Ref: Harper 30th/290-96, 29th/274-88; Lippincott 6th/ 253-55; Shinde 7th/450-51; Vasudevan 5th/180-81]

Urea Cycle: 5 Steps *(Shown in Figure)*

- Synthesis of carbamoyl-phosphate
- Synthesis of citrulline
- Synthesis of argininosuccinate
- Cleavage of argininosuccinate
- Cleavage of arginine to form ornithine & urea

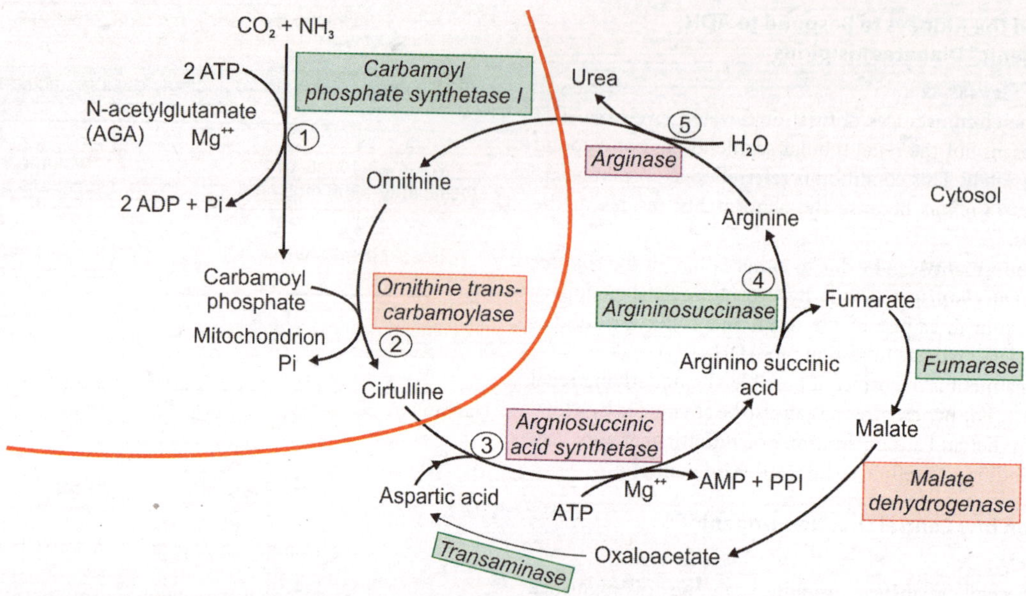

Fig: Biosynthesis of urea or Ornithine—Urea cycle

Note: **"Rate-limiting enzyme (pacemaker enzyme) of Urea cycle:** *Carbamoyl phosphate synthetase I (CPS II is involved in pyrimidine synthesis)" (Harper 29th/274, 28th/245)*

24. Ans. a. Proline c. Isoleucine

[Ref: Harper 30th/16-22; Lippincott 6th/1-9; Satyanarayan 4th/ 48]

Polar Amino Acids with Polar Side Chains

Acidic and Polar Side Chains

- Aspartic Acid
- Glutamic Acid

Basic and Polar Side Chains

- ***Arginine***
- ***Lysine***
- *Histidine*

Uncharged & Polar Side Chains

- ***Asparginine***
- Glutamine
- Serine
- Threonine
- Tyrosine

Note: Carboxyl side chains are associated with Acidic amino acids while Amino side chains are associated with Basic Amino acids, both of which are 'Polar' molecules.

Non Polar Amino Acids with Non Polar Side Chains

- Glycine
- *Alanine*
- *Valine*
- *Leucine*
- ***Isoleucine***
- ***Proline***
- *Phenylalanine*
- *Methionine*
- *Tryptoplan*
- Cystine

Note: Methyl side chains and Methylene side chains are non polar side chains associated with non polar Amino acids.

25. Ans. c. It involves in synthesis of cholesterol, d. It involves in synthesis of steroids.

[Ref: Harper 30th/267-69; Lippincott 6th/221-22; Satyanarayan 4th/310]

Squalene

- It is a natural 30-carbon organic compound originally obtained for commercial purposes primarily from ***shark liver oil*** (hence its name), although plant sources (primarily vegetable oils) are now used as well, including amaranth seed, rice bran, wheat germ, and olives.
- It is also found in high concentrations in the stomach oil of ***birds*** in the order Procellariiformes.
- All plants and animals produce squalene as a biochemical intermediate, including humans.
- Squalene is a hydrocarbon and a triterpene, and is a natural and ***vital part of the synthesis of all plant and animal sterols, including cholesterol, steroid hormones, and vitamin D in the human body.***
- Squalene is used in cosmetics, and more recently as an immunologic adjuvant in vaccines.
- In animals, squalene is the biochemical precursor to the whole family of steroids. Oxidation (via squalene mono oxygenase) of one of the terminal double bonds of squalene yields 2, 3-squalene oxide, which undergoes enzyme-catalyzed cyclization to afford lanosterol, which is then elaborated into ***cholesterol*** and other steroids.

Squalene: Main Properties

◈ *www. scienceforlife*

- ***Squalene an omega 2 fatty acid*** has unlike omega 3 fish oils more complete and effective chemical groups.
- The biochemical structure of squalene is C30 H50 (C30: 6n-omega 2) all trans isoprenoid, that means a C30 polyprenyl compound hold 6 prenyl (better known as isoprenoid or isoprene).

Application of Squalene

- Anti-oxidation—powerful Anti-oxidant
- Oxygen generator—vast recuperation
- Immune stimulator—good immune response
- Fat regulator/energy modulator—natural vitality

Squalene

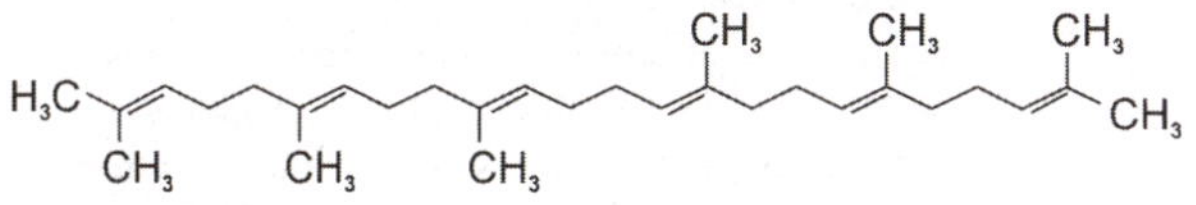

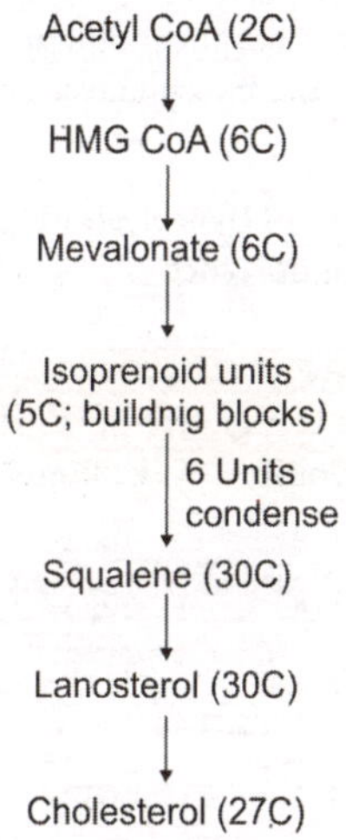

H_3C CH_3 CH_3 CH_3 CH_3 CH_3 CH_3 CH_3 CH_3

Acetyl CoA (2C)
↓
HMG CoA (6C)
↓
Mevalonate (6C)
↓
Isoprenoid units (5C; buildnig blocks)
↓ 6 Units condense
Squalene (30C)
↓
Lanosterol (30C)
↓
Cholesterol (27C)

Fig: *(Satyanarayan):* Outline of cholesterol biosynthesis

26. Ans. a. SDS-...., b. Gel filtration..., d. Ultracentrifugation

[Ref: Harper 30th/28; Shinde 7th/772-74; Satyanarayan 4th/ 725, 60; Vasudevan 5th/482-85]

"**SDS-PAGE** *is commonly used for* ***molecular weight determination of proteins***" *(Vasudevan 5th/482)*

"**SDS-PAGE** *is a* ***popular technique for determination of molecular weight of proteins***" *(Satyanarayan 4th/ 725)*

"***Sodium dodecyl sulfate-polyacrylamide gel electrophoresis (SDS-PAGE) is a reliable method for determining the molecular weight (MW) of an unknown protein***" *(net)*

"*The* **gel filtration chromatography technique** *is used for-separation of protein molecules, purification of proteins &* ***molecular weight determinations***" *(Vasudevan 5th/485)*

"**Ultra centrifugation** *is an indispensable tool for the isolation of subcellular organelles, proteins, & nucleic acids. In addition, this technique is also employed in* ***determination of molecular weight of macromolecules***" *(Satyanarayan 4th/727)*

"In order to understand the physical interactions between protein partners involved in a typical biomolecular process, the relative proximity of the molecules must be determined more precisely than diffraction-limited traditional optical imaging methods permit. The technique of **fluorescence resonance energy transfer** (more commonly referred to by the acronym **FRET**), when applied to optical microscopy, permits determination of the approach between two molecules within several nanometers, a distance sufficiently close for molecular interactions to occur" *(http://www. olympusmicro. com/)*

Table *(Shinde 7th/774)*: **Types of Electrophoresis and their Applications**

Type	Support	Applications
Paper electrophoresis	Whatsman No. 3 or Cellulose acetate membrane	Detection of gross abnormalities in plasma proteins in certain diseases, e. g. Multiple myeloma, Cirrhosis, Nephrotic syndrome, etc
PAGE/SDS PAGE	Polyacrylamide plain or SDS (Sodium dodecyl sulphate) impregnated gels	Separation and purification of individual proteins, determination of molecular weight of purified polypeptides
Starch	Hydrolyzed Starch	Isozyme analysis
Agarose	Agarose gel	Separation of nucleic acids, Nucleotide sequencing
Immunoelectrophoresis 1. Rocket 2. Crossed 3. Immunofixation	Agarose, Acrylamide, preformed microscopic slides	Detection and characterization of antigens (e.g. Plasma proteins, enzymes, cell membrane Ag) or antibodies
Isoelectric focusing	Laboratory made or preformed pH Gradient gels of Polyacrylamide or agarose	Phenotyping of α1-antitrypsin, Genetic variants of enzymes, hemoglobins and other proteins

27. Ans. a. Agarose gel

[Ref: www. lonza. com/go/literature/2043; Shinde 7th/774]

Refer explanation (Table) of above

"Separation of RNA in agarose gels is used for a number of different purposes, including Northern blots to monitor RNA expression levels, checking RNA integrity and size selection of RNA for cloning experiments. Separation of RNA based on fragment length requires conditions that are different from DNA analysis. These include sample preparation, the use of sample and gel denaturants, electrophoresis buffers, and visualization. The purpose of the experiment and the size of the RNA being separated are the primary drivers in determining which denaturing system to use. The most frequently used denaturants for RNA agarose gel electrophoresis are formaldehyde, formaldehyde/formamide, and glyoxal plus DMSO. In each system, the denatured RNA migrates through the agarose gel in a linear relation to the log of its molecular weight (similar to DNA). The most efficient RNA denaturant is methylmercury hydroxide. Because of the hazards associated with this denaturant, it is the least used system for RNA analysis" *(www. lonza. com/go/literature/2043)*

28. Ans. b. Breaking of high... d. Electrical gradient across... e. Passage of e- through FAD....

[Ref: Harper 30th/115-16; Lippincott 6th/72-77;Shinde 7th/313; Satyanarayan 4th/222-25]

*"In absence of O_2 pyruvate is reduced to lactic acid (**without producing ATP**). In anaerobic glycolysis, pyruvate acts as a temporary H-store. It dehydrogenates (oxidizes), the reduced NADH + H+ back to oxidized NAD^+, so that glycolysis can continue even in absence of O_2. In presence of O_2, lactic acid can be oxidized to pyruvic acid again" (Shinde 7th/313, 311)*

***"FAD accepts 2 electrons & 2 H^+ in the dehydrogenases reaction in ETC forming FADH2"** (Harper 30th/121)*

***"FADH2 produces 2 ATP during the ETC** because it gives up its electron to Complex II, bypassing Complex I. By bypassing Complex I, we missed a chance to pump protons across the membrane, so less protons have been pumped by the time we get to Complex IV. Protons still have been pumped, enough to fuel 2 ATP created by ATP synthase" *(http://www. life. illinois. edu/)*

Table *(Satyanarayan 4th/222-25)*: **Standard free Energy of Hydrolysis of Some Important Compounds**

Compounds	Δ (Cal/mol)
High-energy phosphates	
Phosphenol pyruvate	– 14. 8
Carbamoyl phosphate	– 12. 3
1, 3-Bisphosphoglycerate	– 11. 8
Phosphocreatine	– 10. 3
Acetyl phosphate	– 10. 3
S-Adenosylmethionine	– 10. 0
Pyrophosphate	– 8. 0
Acetyl CoA	– 7. 7
ATP→ADP +Pi	– 7. 3
Low-energy phosphates	
ADP→ AMP + PI	– 6. 6
Glucose 1-phosphate	– 5. 0
Fructose 6-phosphate	– 3. 8
Glucose 6-phosphate	– 3. 3
Glycerol 3-phosphate	– 2. 2

"Proton pump: Electron transport is coupled to the phosphorylation of ADP by the transport ("pumping") of protons (H^+) across the inner mitochondrial membrane from the matrix to the inter membrane space at Complexes I, III, and IV. This process creates an ***electrical gradient (with more positive charges on the outside of the membrane than on the inside***) and a pH gradient (the outside of the membrane is at a lower pH than the inside). ***The energy generated by this proton gradient is sufficient to drive ATP synthesis.*** Thus, the proton gradient serves as the common intermediate that couples oxidation to phosphorylation. *(Lippincott 6th/77-78)*

The Intermediate Value for the Free Energy of Hydrolysis of ATP Has Important Bioenergetic Significance

◈ *Harper 30th/115-16*

- An estimate of the comparative tendency of each of the phosphate groups to transfer to a suitable acceptor may be obtained from the ΔG0' of hydrolysis at 37 °C. The value for the hydrolysis of the terminal phosphate of ATP divides the list into two groups.
- **Low-energy phosphates,** exemplified by the ester phosphates found in the intermediates of glycolysis, have ΔG0' values smaller than that of ATP, while in **high-energy phosphates** the value is higher than that of ATP.
- The components of this latter group, including ATP, are usually anhydrides (e.g., the 1-phosphate of 1, 3-bisphosphoglycerate), enolphosphates (e.g., phosphoenolpyruvate), and phosphoguanidines (e.g., creatine phosphate, arginine phosphate).

Table *(Harper 30th/116)*: **Standard free Energy of Hydrolysis of Some Organophosphates of Biochemical Importance**

	Δ G0'	
Compound	**kJ/mol**	**kcal/mol**
Phosphoenolpyruvate	-61. 9	-14. 8
Carbamoyl phosphate	-51. 4	-12. 3
1, 3-Bisphosphoglycerate (to 3-phosphoglycerate)	-49. 3	-11. 8
Creatine phosphate	-43. 1	-10. 3
ATP → AMP + PP_i	-32. 2	-7. 7
ATP → ADP + P_i	-30. 5	-7. 3
Glucose 1-phosphate	-20. 9	-5. 0
PP_i	-19. 2	-4. 6
Fructose 6-phosphate	-15. 9	-3. 8
Glucose 6-phosphate	-13. 8	-3. 3
Glycerol 3-phosphate	-9. 2	-2. 2

29. Ans. b. Increased fatty... c. ↑Lipopro..., e. High An....

[Ref: Harper 30th/ 231; Lippincott 6th/339, 345; Satyanarayan 4th/481, 682; Harrison 19th/ 2417-18]

Diabetic Ketoacidosis (DKA)

◈ *Harrison 19th/ 2417-18*

- DKA is characterized by hyperglycemia, ***ketosis, and metabolic acidosis (increased anion gap)*** along with a number of secondary metabolic derangements

- Leukocytosis, ***hypertriglyceridemia***, and ***hyperlipoproteinemia*** are commonly found as well
- Ketosis results from a marked ***increase in free fatty acid release from adipocytes***, with a resulting shift toward ketone body synthesis in the liver.
- Reduced insulin levels, in combination with elevations in catecholamines and growth hormone, ***increase lipolysis and the release of free fatty acids. Normally, these free fatty acids are converted to triglycerides or very-low-density lipoprotein (VLDL) in the liver.***
- Increased lactic acid production also contributes to the acidosis. The ***increased free fatty acids increase triglyceride and VLDL production.*** VLDL clearance is also reduced because the activity of insulin-sensitive lipoprotein lipase in muscle and fat is decreased. Hypertriglyceridemia may be severe enough to cause pancreatitis.

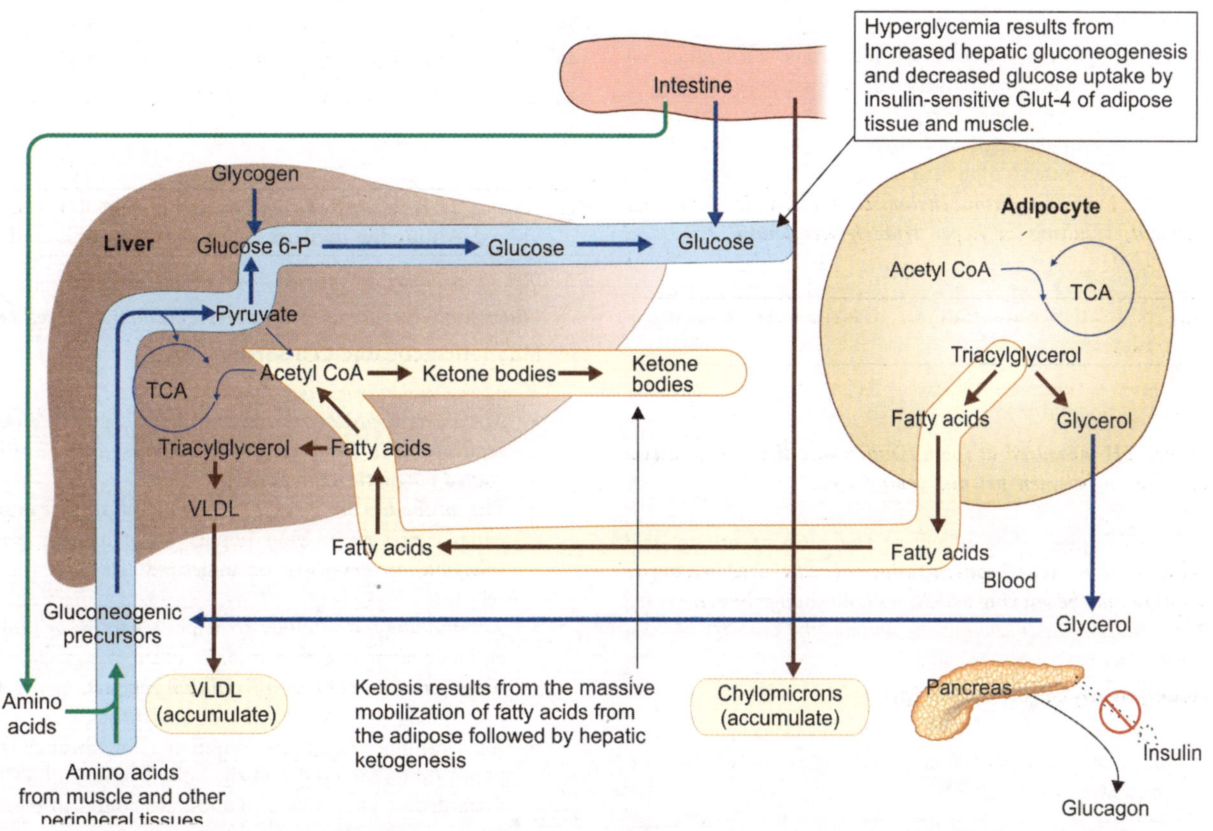

Fig: *(Lippincott)*: Intertissue relationships in type 1 diabetes

Table *(Harrison 19th/2417)*: **Laboratory Values in Diabetic Ketoacidosis (DKA) and Hyperglycemic Hyperosmolar State (HHS) (Representative Ranges at Presentation)**

	DKA	HHS
Glucose, mmol/L (mg/dL)	13. 9–33. 3 (250–600)	33. 3–66. 6 (600–1200)
Sodium, meq/L	125–135	135–145
Potassium	Normal to ↑	Normal
Magnesium	Normal	Normal
Chloride	Normal	Normal
Phosphate	Normal	Normal
Creatinine	Slightly ↑	Moderately ↑
Osmolality (mOsm/mL)	300–320	330–380
Plasma ketones	++++	+/–
Serum bicarbonate, meq/L	<15 meq/L	Normal to slightly ↓
Arterial pH	6. 8–7. 3	>7. 3

Contd...

	DKA	HHS
Arterial PCO_2,mmHg	20–30	Normal
Anion gap [Na – (Cl + HCO_3)]	↑	Normal to slightly ↑

- *Large changes occur during treatment of DKA.*
- *Although plasma levels may be normal or high at presentation, total-body stores are usually depleted.*

"**Hyper triacylglycerolemia:** Not all the fatty acids flooding the liver can be disposed of through oxidation or ketone body synthesis. These excess fatty acids are converted to triacylglycerol, which is packaged and secreted in very-low-density lipoproteins (VLDL). Chylomicrons are synthesized from dietary lipids by the intestinal mucosal cells following a meal. Because lipoprotein degradation catalyzed by lipoprotein lipase in the capillary beds of muscle and adipose tissue is low in diabetics (synthesis of the enzyme is decreased when insulin levels are low), the ***plasma chylomicron and VLDL levels are elevated, resulting in hyper triacylglycerolemia***" *(Lippincott 6th/339-40)*

30. Ans. b. Relative concentration..., d. A rise in H⁺ concentration....

[Ref: Harper 30th/10-13; Vasudevan 5th/362; Lippincott 6th/6; Satyanarayan 4th/710]

"***When pH measured at room temperature there is no direct correlation between pH and temperature***" *(www. researchgate. net)*

"Factor affecting pH of a buffer: ***The ratio of salt to acid concentration- Actual concentrations of salt & acid in a buffer solution may be varying widely, with no change in pH,*** *so long as the ratio of the concentrations remains the same" (Vasudevan 5th/362)*

Hydogen Ion Concentration (pH)

◈ *Satyanarayan 4th/710*

- pH is defined as the negative logarithm of H+ ion concentration
- The pH is a narrow scale, ranging from 0 to 14 which correspondences to 1M solution to 10-14 M solution of [H+] concentration
- Pure water has an equal concentration of H^+& OH^- ion i.e., 10-7 M each. ***Thus pure water has a pH 7 which is neutral***
- Solution with pH less than 7 are said to be acidic while those with pH greater than 7 are alkaline
- It must be remembered that the ***term acidic or alkaline are not absolute but only relative***
- A rise in H^+ concentration decreases pH while a fall in H^+ concentration increases pH. The reverse is true for OH^- concentration

"**Temperature coefficient of variation of pH buffers**: *Although the temperature coefficient variation of pH buffers may vary only minimally over a wide span of temperatures in the acid region, it may be quite dramatic in the alkaline region. The consequential error can be substantial in the alkaline region" (http://reagecon. com/pdf/technical papers)*

Table: Temperature Effects on the Value of pH Buffers

Temperature °C	pH 4.00 + 0.01 @ 25°C[10]	pH 7.00 + 0.01 @ 25 °C [10]	pH 10.00 + 0.01 @ 25°C[10]
10	4.00	7.07	10.18
15	4.00	7.04	10.14
20	4.00	7.02	10.06
25	4.00	7.00	10.00
30	4.01	6.99	9.95
35	4.02	6.98	9.91
40	4.03	6.97	9.85
50	4.05	6.96	9.78
60	4.08	6.96	9.75

31. Ans. a. It is a method..., c. Antibody-coated magnetic..., d. Antibodies used are..., e. Magnetic field is appli...

[Ref: www. sepmag. eu/blog/bid/. stackexchange. com]

Fluorescent dyes are used in fluorescence-activated cell sorting

Magnetic-activated Cell Sorting (MACS)

◈ *biology. stackexchange. com*

- MACS, is a procedure developed by Miltenyi Biotec to ***separate cells from complex mixtures*** using ***antibody-coated magnetic nano particles.***
- The ***antibodies are specific for certain cell surface markers,*** either expressed on your population of interest (***positive selection***), or expressed on undesired cell types (negative selection).
- After adding the antibody-coated beads to the cell mixture and incubating, the suspension is added to a ***special single-use separation column affixed to a magnet,*** to which the beads stick, while unlabeled cells flow through.
- If performing a negative selection, the flow-through is your population of interest and the bound beads and cells are discarded. If your cells of interest are bound to the beads (positive selection), the column is washed several times to make sure unbound or weakly-bound cells are washed through, then the column is removed from the ***magnet*** and the cell-bead complexes are eluted.

Magnetic-activated Cell Sorting (MACS)

◈ *http://www. biocompare. com/Bench-Tips/*

- **Three major techniques** have emerged as most widely used for separation of specific cells within a complex cell mixture: ***centrifugation-based, fluorescence-activated cell sorting (FACS), and magnetic cell separation.***
- FACS and magnetic cell separation are far more specific than centrifugation, as the methodologies utilize conjugated antibodies that specifically recognize the target cells. Using FACS, cells are separated based on the expression of several antigens simultaneously.
- Magnetic separation is limited to one or two antigens, but has multiple advantages over FACS, including a much shorter

processing time, a simpler platform, and significantly lower cost. As magnetic separation is becoming a more widely adopted technique, here are four important points to consider when performing this method.

"In **fluorescence-activated cell sorting or FACS,** the initial complex cell mixture is first labeled with one or more cell surface marker-specific antibodies that have been conjugated to ***fluorescent dyes***. Cells can also be analyzed that express one or more recombinant fluorescent proteins in conjunction with a gene of interest, allowing for selection of cells without using antibodies. After incubation and wash steps, red blood cells are lysed, if analyzing whole blood. "

32. Ans. All (a. b. c. d. e.)

[Ref: www. gelifesciences. com/gehcls_images; https://en. wikipedia. org]

"Silver staining is a highly sensitive method for ***detecting proteins*** and ***nucleic acids (dsDNA & RNA)*** in polyacrylamide slab gels" *(http://www. bio-rad. com)*

"**Silver staining** is the use of silver to selectively alter the appearance of a target in microscopy of histological sections; in temperature gradient gel electrophoresis; and in poly acrylamide gels" *(wiki)*

"Silver staining is the most sensitive method for permanent ***staining of proteins or nucleic acids*** in poly acrylamide gels"- *(www. gelifesciences. com)*

Silver Staining: Application

◈ *wiki*

- **Histological characterization:** Silver staining aids the visualization of targets of interest, namely intracellular and extracellular cellular components such as ***DNA*** and ***proteins, such as type III collagen*** and ***reticulin*** fibres by the deposition of metallic silver particles on the targets of interest.
- **Diagnostic microbiology:** *Pseudomonas*, *Legionella*, *Leptospira*, *H. pylori*, and fungi such as *Pneumocystis* and *Candida* are organisms that are stained with silver
- **Karyotype analysis:** Silver staining is used in karyotyping. Silver nitrate stains the nucleolar organization region (NOR)-associated protein, producing a dark region wherein the silver is deposited and denoting the activity of rRNA genes within the NOR. Human chromosomes 13, 14, 15, 21, and 22 have NORs, which increase the silver stain activity by at least 50 times
- **Genomic and proteomic analysis:** Silver staining is used to stain gels

"**Silver staining** is used to ***detect proteins*** after electrophoretic separation on poly acrylamide gels. It combines excellent sensitivity (in the low nanogram range) whilst using very simple and cheap equipment and chemicals" *(http://www. ncbi. nlm. nih. gov)*

IMMUNOGENETICS & MOLECULAR BIOLOGY

33. Ans. a. miRN A, b. Si RNA, c. tRNA, e. rRNA

[Ref: Harper 30th/394-95, 368; en. wikipedia. org; Lippincott 6th/417]

RNA Exists in two Major Classes

◈ *Harper 30th/394*

- All eukaryotic cells have two major classes of RNA, the **protein coding RNAs**, or messenger RNAs (**mRNAs**), and two forms of abundant **non-protein coding RNAs** delineated on the basis of size: the large ribosomal RNAs (**rRNA**) and long noncoding RNAs (**lncRNAs**) and small noncoding RNAs transfer RNAs (**tRNA**), the small nuclear RNAs (**snRNAs**) and the micro and silencing RNAs (**miRNAs** and **siRNAs**).
- The mRNAs, rRNAs and tRNAs are directly involved in protein synthesis while the other RNAs are participate in either mRNA splicing (SnRNAs) or modulation of gene expression by altering mRNA function (mi/SiRNAs) and/or expression (lncRNAs). These RNA differ in their diversity, stability, and abundance in cells.

Table *(Harper 30th/395)*: **Classes of Eukaryotic RNA**

RNA	Types	Abundance	Stability
Protein coding RNA			
Messenger (mRNA)	$\geq 10^5$ Different species	2 – 5% of total	Unstable to very stable
Nonprotein coding RNAs (ncRNAs)			
Large ncRNAs			
Ribosomal (rRNA)	28S, 18S, 5.8S, 5S	80% of total	very stable
IncRNAs	~1000s	~1 – 2%	Unstable to very stable
Small ncRNAs			
Transfer RNAs	~60 Different species	~15% of total	very stable
Small nuclear (mi/SiRNAs)	~ 30 Different Species	≤1% of total	very stable
Micro/ Silencing (mi/ SiRNAs)	100s - 1000	<1% of total	Stable

34. Ans. c. Fragment 5 S..., d. tRNA

[Ref: Harper 30th/395-98; Lippincott 428]

"**RNA polymerase III:** This enzyme synthesizes tRNA, 5S rRNA, and some snRNA and snoRNA" *(Lippincott 428)*

Table *(Harper 30th/398)*: **Mammalian Nuclear DNA-Dependent RNA Polymerases.**

Form of RNA Polymerase	Major Products
I	rRNA
II	mRNA, IncRNA, miRNA, SnRNA
III	tRNA, 5S rRNA

35. Ans. b. Hydrogen...

[Ref: Harper 30th/359; Lippincott 6th/396-97; Satyanarayan 4th/75]

"The two strands are held together by ***hydrogen bond*** formed by ***complementary base pairs***" *(Satyanarayan 4th/75)*

"The ***base pairs are held together by hydrogen bonds***: two between A and T and three between G and C. These ***hydrogen bonds***, plus the hydrophobic interactions between the stacked bases, ***stabilize the structure of the double helix***" *(Lippincott 6th/397)*

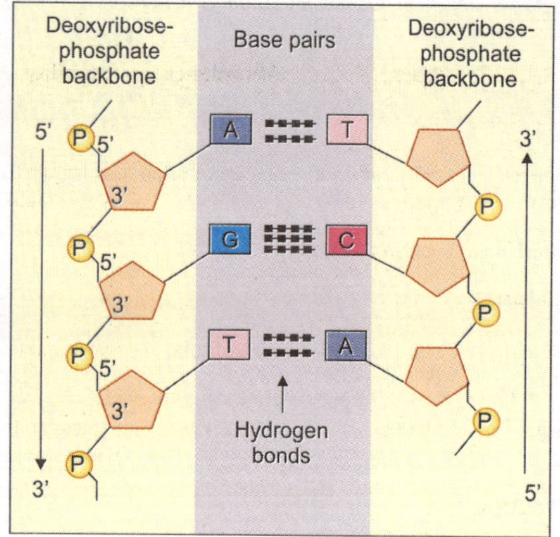

Fig: *(Lippincott 6th/ 397)*: Two complementary DNA sequences

36. Ans. a. N-formyl methionin..., e. Three initiation...

[Ref: Harper 30th/419-23; Lippincott 6th/438-42; Satyanarayan 4th/554-60]

"In eukaryotes, the first amino acid incorporated is methionine (AUG codon). But in prokaryotes, the same codon attracts N-formyl methionine, which is the first amino acid" *(Vasudevan 5th/432)*

"**Elongation factor P** is a ***prokaryotic protein translation factor*** required for efficient peptide bond synthesis on 70S ribosomes from fMet-tRNAf Met. It probably functions indirectly by altering the affinity of the ribosome for aminoacyl-tRNA, thus increasing their reactivity as acceptors for peptidyl transferase" *(nature. com/nrmicro)*

Table *(Shinde 7th/435)*: **Comparison of Translation in Eukaryotes and Prokaryotes. Mitochondria are Similar to Prokaryotes**

Features	Eukaryotes (mammalian cells)	Prokaryotes (bacteria)	Mitochondria
DNA	Open	Circular	Circular
Ribosomes	80S	70S	70S
tRNA (No.)	31	22	22
Initiating amino acid	Methionine	**Formyl Methionine**	Formyl Methionine
Effect of tetracycline	Not affected	Inhibited	Inhibited
Initiation factors	**10**	**3**	
Elongation factors	**EF-1 alpha, EF-1 beta, EF-1 gamma EF-2**	**EF-Tu; EF-Ts**	

Steps in Protein Synthesis

Lippincott 6th/438-42

- The process of protein synthesis translates the three-letter alphabet of nucleotide sequences on mRNA into the 20-letter alphabet of amino acids that constitute proteins. The mRNA is translated from its 5'-end to its 3'-end, producing a protein synthesized from its amino-terminal end to its carboxyl-terminal end.
- **Prokaryotic mRNAs** often have several coding regions, that is, they are polycistronic. Each coding region has its own initiation and termination codon and produces a separate species of polypeptide.
- In contrast, each **eukaryotic mRNA** has only one coding region, that is, it is monocistronic. The process of translation is divided into three separate steps: ***initiation, elongation, and termination.***
- Eukaryotic protein synthesis resembles that of prokaryotes in most aspects. ***One important difference is that translation and transcription are coupled in prokaryotes,*** with translation starting before transcription is completed. Coupling is a consequence of the lack of a nuclear membrane in prokaryotes.

Initiation

- Initiation of protein synthesis involves the assembly of the components of the translation system before peptide bond formation occurs. These components include the two ribosomal subunits, the mRNA to be translated, the aminoacyl-tRNA specified by the first codon in the message, ***GTP*** (which provides energy for the process), and initiation factors that facilitate the assembly of this initiation complex
- In prokaryotes, ***three initiation factors are known (IF-1, IF-2, and IF-3***), whereas in ***eukaryotes, there are over ten (designated eIF to indicate eukaryotic origin)***. Eukaryotes also require ATP for initiation.

Translocation

- The now deacylated tRNA is attached by its anticodon to the P site at one end and by the open CCA tail to an **exit (E) site** on the large ribosomal subunit. At this point, **elongation factor 2 (EF2)** binds to and displaces the peptidyl tRNA from the A site to the P site. In turn, the deacylated tRNA is on the E site, from which it leaves the ribosome.
- The EF2-GTP complex is hydrolyzed to EF2-GDP, effectively moving the mRNA forward by one codon and leaving the A site open for occupancy by another ternary complex of amino acid tRNA-EF1A-GTP and another cycle of elongation.

Materials Required for Protein Synthesis

◈ *(Shinde)*

- Amino acids
- DNA & 3 RNAs (m-RNA, t-RNA, r-RNA)
- Polyribosomes (polysomes)
- ***Enzymes**: Aminoacyl-t-RNA synthetase, peptidyl transferase*
- ***Factors***
  - ***Initiation facors**- IF1 to 3 (For prokaryotes)*
  - *10 initiation factors **for eukaryotes** (elF-1, elF-2, elF-3, elF-4A, elF-4B, elF-4G, elF- 4E, elf-5)*
  - ***Elongation factors**-EF1 & EF2 (**for eukaryotes**)*
  - ***Release factors** R1 & R2*
    - Coenzymes & cofactors; FH4 Mg^{2+}
- Energy
  - ATP, GTP

Steps of Translation (Protein synthesis)

- Activation of amino acids
- Initiation
- Elongation
- Termination
- Post-translational processing

37. Ans. a. PCR, b. Real time....

[Ref: Harper 30th/458; Robbins 9th/180; Lippincott 6th/479;Harrison 19th/ 150e-7; http://link. springer. com]

"Introduction of a ***foreign DNA*** molecule into a replication cell permits the ***cloning or amplification of DNA***" *(Lippincott 6th/467)*

"**ELISA**: *Detects proteins(antigens) or antibodies" (Lippincott 6th/485)*

"**Real-time PCR** *automates the laborious process of **amplification by quantitating reaction** products for each sample in every cycle" (Shinde 7th/269)*

Nucleic Acid Amplification Test (NAAT) Strategies

◈ *Harrison 19th/ 150e-7*

- There are several methods for amplification (copying) of small numbers of molecules of nucleic acid to readily detectable levels. ***These NAATs include PCR, LCR, strand displacement amplification, and self-sustaining sequence replication.***
- In each case, exponential amplification of a pathogen-specific DNA or RNA sequence depends on primers that anneal to the target sequence. The amplified nucleic acid can be detected after the reaction is complete or (in real-time detection) as amplification proceeds. The sensitivity of NAATs is far greater than that of traditional assay methods such as culture.

Table *(Harrison 18th/)*: **Techniques Commonly Used for Mutation Detection**

Method	Principle	Type of Mutation Detected
Polymerase chain reaction (PCR)	**Amplification of DNA segment**	Expansion of triplet repeats, variable number of tandem repeats (VNTR), gene rearrangements, translocations; prepare DNA for other mutation methods
Reverse transcriptase PCR (RT-PCR)	Reverse transcription, ***amplification of DNA segment*** → absence or reduction of mRNA transcription	Analyze expressed mRNA (cDNA) sequence; detect loss of expression
Traditional DNA sequencing	Direct sequencing of PCR products Sequencing of DNA segments cloned into plasmId vectors	Point mutations, small deletions and insertions
Next-generation DNA sequencing	Sequencing of large contiguous genomic regions, exome of single or all chromosomes.	Deep sequencing for detection of mutations and SNPs. Sequencing of whole genomes of microorganisms

Table: Nucleic Acid Amplification Methods

Amplification method	Amplification category	Manufacturer/license (trade mark)	Enzymes used	Temperature requirement	Nucleic acid target
Polymerase chain reaction (PCR)	Target	Roche Molecular System, Inc., Branchburg, NJ, USA (A mplicor)	Taq DNA polymerase	Thermal cycler	DNA or RNA
Transcription-mediated amplification (TMA)	Target	Gen-Probe, Inc., San Diego. CA, USA (APTIMA)	Reverse transcriptase, RNA polymerase. RNase H	Isothermal	RNA or DNA

Contd...

Amplification method	Amplification category	Manufacturer/license (trade mark)	Enzymes used	Temperature requirement	Nucleic acid target
Nucleic acid sequence—based amplification (NASBA)	Target	Organon-Teknika. Corp., Durham, NC, USA (Nuclisens)	Reverse transcriptase, RNA polymerase, RNase H	Isothermal	RNA or DNA
Strand displacement amplification (SDA)	Target	Becton-Dickinson, Sparks, MD, USA (ProbTec)	Restrictive endonucleonase, DNA polymerase	Isothermal	DNA or RNA
Invader technology	Probe	Third Wave. Madison. WI, USA	Cleavage	Isothermal	DNA
Cycling probe technology (CPT)	Probe	ID Biomedical Corp., Vancouver, Canada	RNase H	Isothermal	DNA or RNA
Ligase chain reaction (LCR)	Probe	Abbott Laboratories, Abbott Park, IL, USA (LCx)	DNA ligase	Thermal cycler	DNA or RNA
Hybrid capture system	Signal	Digene Diagnostics, Inc., Silver Spring, MD. USA	None	Isothermal	DNA
Branched DNA (bDNA)	Signal	Chiron Corp., Emeryville. CA, USA	None	Isothermal	DNA or RNA

38. Ans. a. Ca^{2+}

[Ref: Harper 30th/501, 91-92, 179, 343; Lippincott 6th/94-95]

Second Messenger

Lippincott 6th/91

- Nucleotides, such as ***cyclic adenosine mono-phosphate (cAMP) and cyclic guanosine monophosphate (cGMP), serve as second messengers*** in signal transduction pathways.
- "Second messenger" molecules—so named because they intervene between the original messenger (the neurotransmitter or hormone) and the ultimate effect on the cell—are part of the cascade of events that translates hormone or neurotransmitter binding into a cellular response. Two of the most widely recognized ***second messenger systems are the calcium/phosphatidy linositol system, and the adenylyl cyclase system***, which is particularly important in regulating the pathways of intermediary metabolism.

Table *(Harper 30th/501)*: **Classification of Hormones by Mechanism of Action**

I. Hormones that bind to intracellular receptors

Androgens
Calcitriol (1,25[OH],-D3).
Estrogens
Glucocorticoids
Mineralocorticoids
Progestins
Retinoic acid
Thyroid hormones (T3 and T4)

Contd...

II. Hormones that bind to cell surface receptors

A. The second messenger is cAMP

α2 Adrenergic catecholamines
β-Adrenergic catecholamines
Adrenocorticotropic hormone (ACTH)
Antidiuretic hormone (vasopressin)
Calcitonin
Chorionic gonadotropin hormone (CGH)
Corticotropin-releasing hormone
Follicle-stimulating hormone (FSH)
Glucagon
Lipotropin (LPH)
Luteinizing hormone (LH)
Melanocyte-stimulating hormone (MSH)
Parathyroid hormone (PTH)
Somatostatin
Thyroid-stimulating hormone (TSH)

B. The second messenger is cGMP

Atrial natriuretic factor
Nitric oxide

C. The second messenger is calcium or phosphatidylinositols (or both)

Acetylcholine (muscuranic)
α1 -Adrenergic catecholamines
Angiotensin II
Antidiuretic hormone (vasopressin)
Cholecystokinin
Gastrin
Gonadotropin-releasing hormone
Oxytocin
Platelet-derived growth factor (PDGF)
Substance P
Thyrotropin-releasing hormone (TRH)

Contd...

D. The second messenger is a kinase or phosphatase cascade
Adiponectin
Chorionic somatomammotropin
Epidermal growth factor (EGF)
Erythropoietin (EPO)
Fibroblast growth factor (FGF)
Growth hormone (GH)
Insulin
Insulin-like growth factors I and II
Leptin
Nerve growth factor (NGF)
Platelet-derived growth factor
Prolactin

39. Ans. c. It is nucleotide sequence which...,

[Ref: Harper 30th/413-15; Lippincott 6th/431-34]

"**Mendelian genetics** (or Mendelian inheritance or Mendelism) is a theory of genetic inheritance which was developed by *Gregor Mendel. Mendelian Genetics* is widely regarded as the corner stone of classical genetics. It is a set of primary beliefs relating to the transmission of hereditary characteristic from parent organisms to their offspring; it underlies much of genetics" *(www. innovateus. net/science)*

Mendelian Genetics

◈ *anthro. palomar. edu/mendel*

Inheritance patterns which can be explained by simple rules of dominance and recessiveness of genes.

Genetic Code

◈ *Lippincott 6th/431-34*

- The genetic code is a dictionary that identifies the ***correspondence between a sequence of nucleotide bases and a sequence of amino acids***. Each individual "word" in the code is composed of three nucleotide bases. These genetic words are called codons.
- The process of translation requires a genetic code, through which the information contained in the nucleic acid sequence is expressed to produce a ***specific sequence of amino acids.***

The Nucleotide Sequence of an mRNA Molecule Consists of a Series of Codons that Specify the Amino Acid Sequence of the Encoded Protein

◈ *Harper 30th/414*

- There are 64 (43) specific codons.
- It is now known that each codon consists of a sequence of three nucleotides; i.e, **it is a triplet code**. The deciphering of the genetic code depended heavily on the chemical synthesis of nucleotide polymers, particularly triplets in repeated sequence. These synthetic triplet ribonucleotides were used to program protein synthesis, allowing investigators to deduce the genetic code.

Table *(Harper 30th/ 415)*: **Features of the Genetic Code**

Degenerate
Unambiguous
Nonoverlapping
Not punctuated
Universal

Contd...

40. Ans. a. dsDNA

[Ref: Lippincott 6th/465-66; Harper 30th/ 452-54;Satyanarayana 3rd / 580]

"**Restriction endonucleases** (restriction enzymes), which cleave ***double-stranded (ds) DNA*** into smaller, more manageable fragments, has opened the way for DNA analysis" *(Lippincott 6th/465)*

Restriction Enzyme (RE or Restriction Endonuclease)

- It is an enzyme that ***cleave double-stranded DNA***[Q] ***at specific recognition nucleotide known as restriction sites***[Q].
- To cut the DNA, a restriction enzyme makes two incisions, one through each ***sugar-phosphate backbone***[Q] (i.e.. each strand) of the DNA double helix. This ***enzyme can restrict viral replication so called restriction enzymes.***
- The cut DNA fragments by RE may have ***sticky ends (cohesive ends)***[Q] or ***blunts ends***[Q] depending on the mechanism used by enzyme
- DNA fragments with **sticky ends** are particularly useful for recombinant DNA experiments (hybrid or chimeric DNA molecules)
- Restriction enzyme is ***named according to the organism from which it was isolated.***

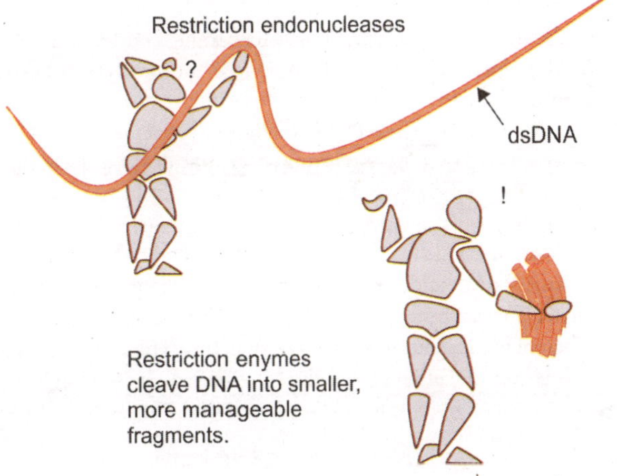

Fig: *(Lippincott 6th/465)*

41. Ans. d. Phosphati....

[Ref: Harper 30th/501, 91-92, 179, 343; Lippincott 6th/207-08]

Phosphatidyl-inositol is a Type of Phospholipid

◈ *Shinde 7th/45 Lippincott 6th/207-08: Writes*

- Phospholipases hydrolyze the phosphodiester bonds of phosphoglycerides, with each enzyme cleaving the phospholipid at a specific site.
- Phospholipases release molecules that can serve as messengers (for example, DAG and IP3), or that are the substrates for synthesis of messengers (for example, arachidonic acid).

[Note: Phospholipases are responsible not only for degrading phospholipids, but also for "remodeling" them. For example, ***phospholipases A1 and A2 remove specific fatty acids from membrane-bound phospholipids****; these can be replaced with alternative fatty acids using fatty acyl CoA transferase]*

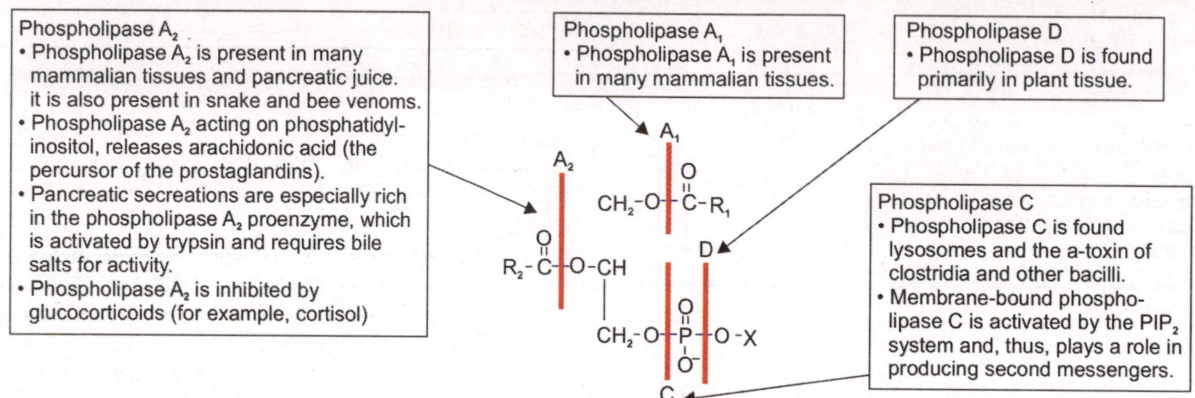

Fig: *(Lippincott 6th/207):* Degradation of glycerophospholipids by phospholipases

42. Ans. b. DNA polymerase, d. DNA ligase

[Ref: Harper 30th/382, 389-92; Lippincott 6th/ 411-13]

"**Repair of damaged DNA:** When the strand containing the mismatch is identified, an endonuclease nicks the strand and the mismatched nucleotide(s) is/are removed by an exonuclease. Additional nucleotides at the 5'- and 3'-ends of the mismatch are also removed. The gap left by removal of the nucleotides is filled, using the sister strand as a template, by a ***DNA polymerase.*** The 3'-hydroxyl of the newly synthesized DNA is joined to the 5'-phosphate of the remaining stretch of the original DNA strand by ***DNA ligase***" *(Lippincott 6th/ 411)*

Damage to DNA by environmental, physical, and chemical agents may be classified into four types. Abnormal regions of DNA, either from copying errors or DNA damage, are replaced by four mechanisms: (1) mismatch repair, (2) base excision-repair, (3) nucleotide excision-repair, and (4) double-strand break repair. These mechanisms exploit the redundancy of information inherent in the double helical DNA structure. The defective region in one strand can be returned to its original form by relying on the complementary information stored in the unaffected strand.

Table *(Harper 30th/382)*: **Mechanism of DNA Repair**

Mechanism	Problem	Solution
Mismatch repair	Copying errors (single base or two- to five-base unpaired loops)	Methyl-directed strand cutting, exonuclease digestion, and replacement
Base excision–repair	Spontaneous, chemical, or radiation damage to a single base	Base removal by *N*-glycosylase, a basic sugar removal, replacement
Nucleotide excision–repair	Spontaneous, chemical, or radiation damage to a DNA segment	Removal of an approximately 30-nucleotide oligomer and replacement
Double-strand break repair	Ionizing radiation, chemotherapy, oxidative free radicals	Synapsis, unwinding, alignment, ligation

Contd...

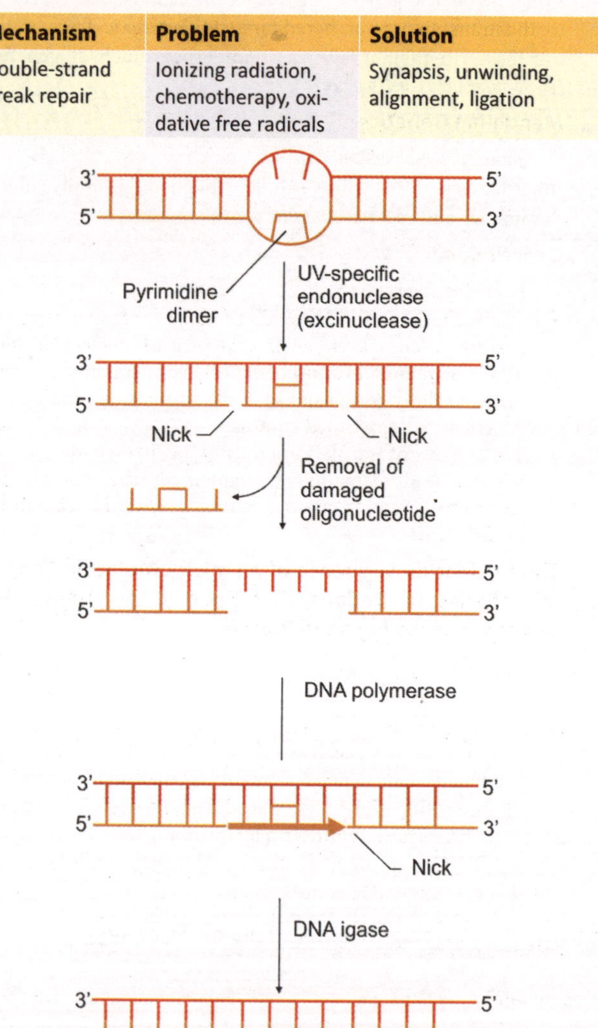

Fig: *(Lippincott 6th/ 412):* Nucleotide excision repair of pyrimidine dimers in E. coli DNA

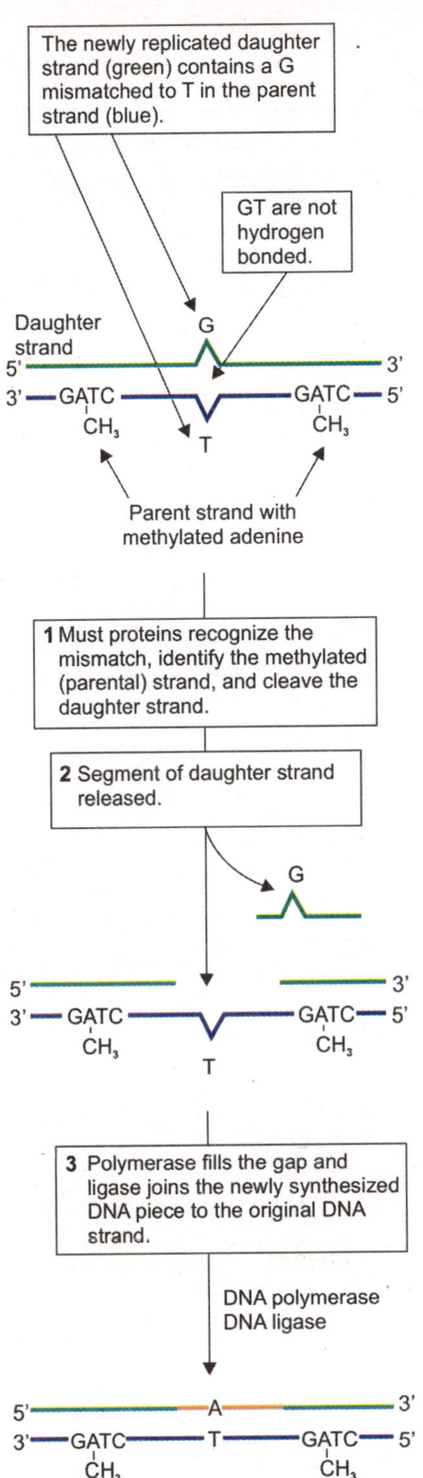

Fig: *(Lippincott 6th/ 411):* Methyl-directed mismatch repair

Table *(Harper 30th/382)*: **Classes of Proteins Involved in Replication**

Protein	Function
DNA polymerases	Deoxynucleotide polymerization
Helicases	Processive unwinding of DNA
Topoisomerases	Relieve torsional strain that results from helicase-induced unwinding
DNA primase	Initiates synthesis of RNA primers
Single-strand binding proteins	Prevent premature reannealing of dsDNA
DNA ligase	Seals the single strand nick between the nascent chain and Okazaki fragments on lagging strand

43. Ans. a. DNA d. Histone

[Ref: Harper 30th/371-72; Lippincott 6th/ 409]

"**Histones** are highly alkaline proteins found in eukaryotic cell nuclei that package and order the DNA into structural units called ***nucleosomes***. They are the ***chief protein components of chromatin,*** acting as spools around which DNA winds, and playing a role in gene regulation. Without histones, the unwound DNA in chromosomes would be very long (a length to width ratio of more than 10 million to 1 in human DNA)"

The Nucleosome Contains Histone & DNA

◈ *Harper 30th/371-72*

- When the histone octamer is mixed with purified dsDNA under appropriate ionic conditions, the same x-ray diffraction pattern is formed as that observed in freshly isolated chromatin. Biochemical and electron microscopic studies confirm the existence of reconstituted nucleosomes. Furthermore, the reconstitution of nucleosomes from DNA and histones
- H2A, H2B, H3, and H4 is independent of the cor cellular origin of the various components. Neither the histone H1 nor the nonhistone proteins are necessary for the reconstitution of the nucleosome core.
- In the ***nucleosome, the DNA is super coiled in a left handed helix over the surface of the disk-shaped histone*** octamer. The majority of core histone proteins interact with the DNA on the inside of the super coil without protruding, although the amino terminal tails of all the histones are thought to extend outside of this structure and are available for regulatory PTMs

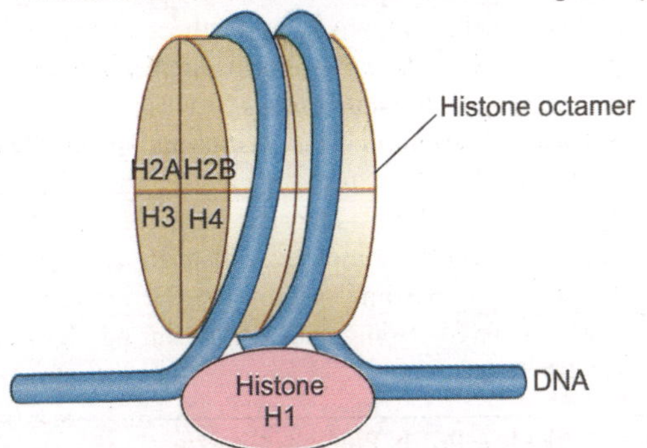

Fig: *(Harper 30th/371)*

Model for the structure of the nucleosome, in which DNA is wrapped around the surface of a protein cylinder consisting of two each of histones H2A, H2B, H3, and H4 that form the histone octamer. The ~145 bp of DNA, consisting of 1. 75 superhelical turns, are in contact with the histone octamer. The position of histone H1, when it is present, is indicated by the dashed outline at the bottom of the figure. Histone H1 interacts with DNA as it enters and exits the nucleosome.

PATHOLOGY

44. Ans. d. Platelet

[Ref: Robbins 9th/83; Harshmohan 7th/123; A. K. Jain 6th/762; Ananthanarayan 9th/164]

Mast cell secretes serotonin only in rodents (not in human)

"**Serotonin**: *It is found in the* ***intestinal mucosa, brain tissue & platelets***" *(Ananthanarayan 9th/ 164)*

"*About 90% of body's content of serotonin is localized in the* ***intestine****; most of the* ***rest is in platelets & brain****. Platelets do not synthesize serotonin but acquire it by uptake during passage through intestinal blood vessels*" *(KDT 7th/170)*

"**Serotonin:** *It is present in tissue like chromaffin cells of GIT, spleen, nervous tissue, mast cells & plateles*" *(Harshmohan 7th/123)*

"**Serotonin:** It carries signals along and between nerves - a neurotransmitter. It is mainly found in the ***brain, bowels and blood platelets***" *(http://www. medicalnewstoday. com/articles/232248. php)*

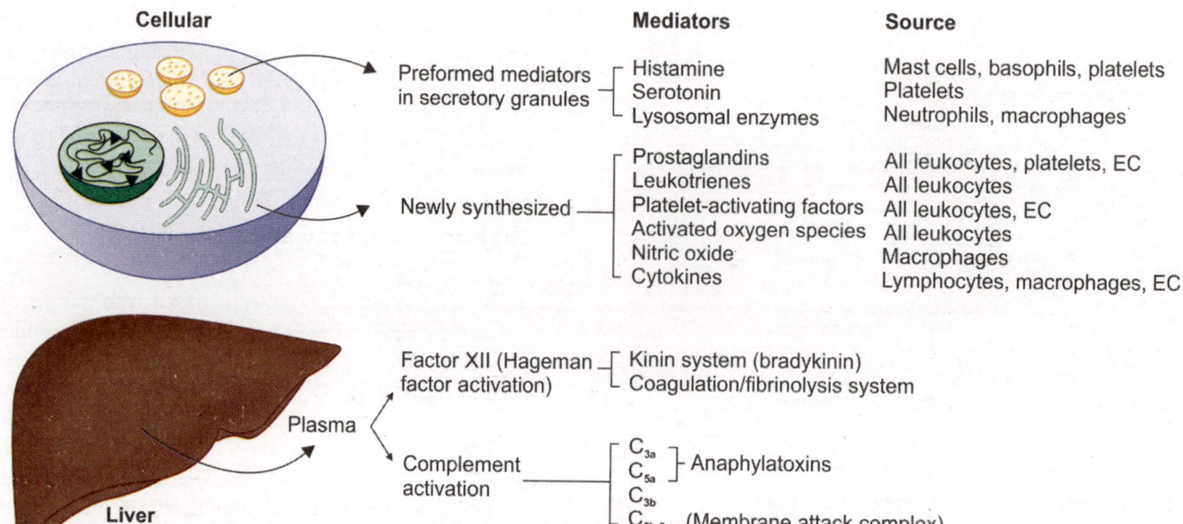

Fig: *(Robbins):* Chemical mediators of inflammation

Abbreviation: EC, endothelial cells.

Serotonin

◈ *Robbins 9th/83*

- *Serotonin* (5-hydroxytryptamine) is a preformed vasoactive mediator with actions similar to those of histamine. It is present in ***platelets and enterochromaffin cells, and in mast cells in rodents but not humans.***
- ***Release of serotonin (and histamine) from platelets*** is stimulated when platelets aggregate after contact with collagen, thrombin, adenosine diphosphate (ADP), and antigen-antibody complexes. Platelet aggregation and release are also stimulated by platelet activating factors (PAF) derived from mast cells during IgE-mediated reactions.

45. Ans. a. Sickle cell..., b. Phenylketonuria

[Ref: Robbins 9th/141; Harshmohan 7th/255; Davidson 22nd/53]

Table *(Robbins 9th/141)*: **Autosomal Recessive Disorders**

System	Disorder
Metabolic	Cystic fibrosis
	Phenylketonuria
	Galactosemia
	Homocystinuria
	Lysosomal storage diseases
	α_1-Antitrypsin deficiency
	Wilson disease
	Hemochromatosis
	Glycogen storage diseases
Hematopoietic	**Sickle cell anemia**

System	Disorder
	Thalassemias
Endocrine	Congenital adrenal hyperplasia
Skeletal	Ehlers-Danlos syndrome (some variants)
	Alkaptonuria
Nervous	Neurogenic muscular atrophies
	Friedreich ataxia
	Spinal muscular atrophy

Table *(Robbins 9th/141)*: **Autosomal Dominant Disorders**

System	Disorder
Nervous	Huntington disease Neurofibromatosis Myotonic dystrophy **Tuberous sclerosis**
Urinary	Polycystic kidney disease
Gastrointestinal	**Familial polyposis coli**
Hematopoietic	Hereditary spherocytosis von Willebrand disease
Skeletal	**Marfan syndrome**
	Ehlers-Danlos syndrome (some variants) Osteogenesis imperfecta Achondroplasia
Metabolic	Familial hyper cholesterolemia Acute intermittent porphyria

46. Ans. b. Deposition of..., c. Often resistant..., d. Common in elderly, e. Risk of falling....

[Ref: Davidson 22nd/252, 1195;Robbins 9th/1295-96; Harrison 19th/170-74, 2605-06; Harshmohan 7th/877; CMDT 2016/1003]

"Around half of people with DLB experience freezing while they are moving & this put them at ***risk of falling****" (www. lewybody. org/node)*

Table *(CMDT 2016/1003)*: **Common Causes of Age-related Dementia**

Disorder	Pathology	Clinical Features
Alzheimer disease	Plaques containing beta-amyloid peptide, and neurofibrillary tangles containing tau protein, occur throughout the neocortex	• Most common age-related neurode generative disease; incidence doubles every 5 years after age 60 • Short-term memory impairment is early and prominent in most cases • Uriable deficits of executive function, visuospatial function, and language
Vascular dementia	Multifocal ischemic change	• Stepwise or progressive accumulation of cognitive deficits in association with repeated strokes • Symptoms depend on localization of strokes
Dementia with Lewy bodies	Histologically indistinguishable from Parkinson disease: alpha-synuclein-containing Lewy bodies occur in the brainstem, midbrain, olfactory bulb, and neocortex. Alzheimer pathology may coexist.	• Cognitive dysfunction, with prominent visuospatial and executive deficits • Psychiatric disturbance, with anxiety, visual hallucinations, and fluctuating delirium • Parkinsonian motor deficits with or after other features • Cholinesterase inhibitors lessen delirium; poor tolerance of many psychoactive medications, including neuroleptics and dopaminergics

Contd...

Dementia with Lewy Body

◈ *Robbins 9th/1295-96*

- *About 10% to 15% of individuals with PD develop dementia, particularly with* ***advancing age***
- *Characteristic features of this disorder include a fluctuating course, hallucinations & prominent frontal signs*

Lewy Body Dementia

◈ *Davidson 22nd/252*

- This is a neuro degenerative disorder clinically characterized by dementia and signs of Parkinson's disease.
- The cognitive state often fluctuates and there is a high incidence of visual hallucinations.
- Affected individuals are particularly sensitive to the side-effects of anti-Parkinsonian medication and also to antipsychotic drugs.
- The condition is associated with accumulation of abnormal protein aggregates in neurons that contain the protein α-synuclein in association with other proteins including ubiquitin.
- The condition is often inherited and mutations in the α-synuclein and β-synuclein genes have been identified in affected patients.
- There is no specific treatment but anticholinesterase agents may well be helpful.

Dementia with Lewy Bodies (DLB)

◈ *Harrison 19th/2605-06*

- The DLB clinical syndrome is characterized by visual hallucinations, parkinsonism, fluctuating alertness, ***falls etc***
- In DLB, dementia and neuropsychiatric syndrome precede the parkinsonism
- The key neuropathologic feature in DLB is the presence of ***Lewy bodies and Lewy neurites***

47. Ans. a. More common..., b. Impairment of the ability..., d. General cognitive..., e. Atrophy of frontal...

[Ref: Robbins 9th/1287-92; Harrison 19th/2598-2602; Harshmohan 7th/876-77; CMDT 2016/1003]

- "**Alzheimer disease:** The key clinical feature is ***impairment of the ability to remember new information.*** Hence, patients present with gradual impairment of memory, usually in association with disorders of other cortical functions. ***Short-term & long-term memory are both affected, but the defects in former are usually more obvious*** *(Davidson 22nd/252)*
- "Alzheimer disease (AD):Short-term memory impairment is early and prominent in most cases." *(CMDT 2016/1003)*

"Alzheimer disease (AD) is the most common cause of dementia in the elderly. The disease usually becomes clinically apparent as ***insidious impairment of higher intellectual function,*** with alterations in ***mood and behavior.*** Later, progressive disorientation, memory loss, and aphasia indicate severe cortical dysfunction, and eventually, in 5 to 10 years, the patient becomes profoundly disabled, mute, and immobile" *(Robbins 9th/1287)*

"Macroscopic examination of the brain shows a variable degree of **cortical atrophy** with widening of the cerebral sulci that is most pronounced in the ***frontal, temporal, and parietal lobes.*** With significant atrophy, there is compensatory ventricular enlargement (hydrocephalus ex vacuo) secondary to loss of parenchyma. The major microscopic abnormalities of Alzheimer disease are **neuritic (senile) plaques, neurofibrillary tangles, and amyloid angiopathy**" *(Robbins 9th/1288)*

Alzheimer's Disease

◈ *Harrison 19th/2598-2602*

- Approximately 10% of all persons over the age of 70 years have significant memory loss, and in more than half, the cause is Alzheimer's disease (AD).AD can manifest as young as the third decade, but it is the most common cause of dementia in the elderly.
- In the early stages of typical amnestic AD, the memory loss may go unrecognized or be ascribed to benign forgetfulness of aging. Once the memory loss becomes noticeable to the patient and spouse and falls 1. 5 standard deviations below normal on standardized memory tests, the term ***mild cognitive impairment*** (MCI) is applied. This construct provides useful prognostic information, because approximately 50% of patients with MCI (roughly 12% per year) will progress to AD over 4 years.

48. Ans. b. More common...,

[Ref: Robbins 9th/694-95;Davidson 22nd/719-20; Harrison 19th/ 1681-83]

*"The pathology of HP is consistent with **both type III & type IV immunological mechanism.** For reasons that remain uncertain, there is a **lower incidence of HP in smoker than non-smoker.** Clinical features includes influenza like symptoms accompanied by **cough, breathlessness & wheeze**"- Davidson 22nd/719*

Hypersensitivity Pneumonitis

◈ *Robbins 9th/694-95*

- The term *hypersensitivity pneumonitis* describes a spectrum of immunologically mediated, predominantly interstitial, lung disorders caused by intense, often prolonged exposure to inhaled organic antigens.
- Most commonly, hypersensitivity results from the inhalation of organic dust containing antigens made up of the spores of thermophilic bacteria, fungi, animal proteins, or bacterial products.
- Bronchoalveolar lavage specimens from the acute phase show increased levels of proinflammatory chemokines such as macrophage inflammatory protein 1α and IL-8.
- ***Bronchoalveolar lavage specimens also consistently demonstrate increased numbers of both CD4+ and CD8+ T lymphocytes.***
- ***The presence of noncaseating granulomas in two thirds of the patients suggests that T-cell-mediated (type IV) hypersensitivity reactions against the implicated antigens are also common and have a pathogenic role.***
- The clinical manifestations are varied. Acute attacks, which follow inhalation of antigenic dust in sensitized patients, consist of ***recurring episodes of fever, dyspnea, cough, and leukocytosis.***

Hypersensitivity Pneumonitis (HP)

◈ *Harrison 19th/ 1681-83*

- HP has been traditionally categorized as having **acute, subacute, and chronic forms.**
- **Acute HP** usually manifests itself 4–8 h following exposure to the inciting antigen, often intense in nature. Systemic symptoms, including ***fevers, chills, and malaise, are prominent and are accompanied by dyspnea.*** Symptoms resolve within hours to days if no further exposure to the offending antigen occurs.
- In **subacute HP** resulting from ongoing antigen exposure, the onset of respiratory and systemic symptoms is typically more gradual over the course of weeks.
- **Chronic HP** can present with an even more gradual onset of symptoms than subacute HP, with progressive dyspnea, cough, fatigue, weight loss, and clubbing of the digits.

49. Ans. a. Nodular sclero..., c. Lymphocyte..., d. Mixed cellula..., e. Lymphocyte deple....

[Ref: Robbins 9th/ 606-10; Harrison 19th/ 708-09; Harshmohan 7th/349-51]

"In the **first four subtypes**—nodular sclerosis, mixed cellularity, lymphocyte-rich, and lymphocyte depletion—the Reed-Sternberg cells have ***a similar immunophenotype***; as a result, these subtypes are often lumped together as *classical* forms of HL. In **lymphocyte predominance HL**, the Reed-Sternberg cells have a ***characteristic B-cell immunophenotype distinct from that of the classical HL subtypes***" *(Robbins 9th/ 607)*

Table *(Robbins 9th/ 609)*: **Classification of Hodgkin Lymphoma**

Subtype	Morphology and Immunophenotype	Typical Clinical Features
Nodular sclerosis	Frequent lacunar cells and occasional diagnostic R-S cells; background infiltrate composed of T lymphocytes, eosinophils, macrophages and plasma cells; fibrous bands dividing cellular areas into nodules. ***R-S cells CD15+, CD30+; EBV-.***	Most common subtype;Usually Stage 1 or 2 disease; Frequent mediastinal involvement. F = M, most patients young adults
Mixed cellularity	Frequent mononuclear and diagnostic R-S cells; background infiltrate rich in T lymphocytes, eosinophils, macrophages, plasma cells. ***R-S cells CD15+, CD30+; 70% EBV+.***	More than 50% present as stage 3 or 4 disease. M > F. Biphasic incidence, peaking in young adults and again in adults older than 55.
Lymphocyte-rich	Frequent mononuclear and diagnostic R-S cells; background infiltrate rich in T lymphocytes. ***R-S cells CD15+, CD30+; 40% EBV+.***	Uncommon. M > F. Tends to be seen in older adults.
Lymphocyte depletion	Reticular variant: Frequent diagnostic R-S cells and variants with a paucity of background reactive cells; diffuse fibrosis variant; hypocellular fibrillar background with scattered diagnostic R-S cells and variants and few reactive cells. ***R-S cells CD15+, CD30+; most EBV+.***	Uncommon. More common in older males, HIV-infected individuals, and in developing countries. More likely to present with advanced disease.
Lymphocyte predominance	Frequent L&H (popcorn cell) variants in a background of follicular dendritic cells and reactive B cells. ***R-S cells CD20+, CD15-, C30-; EBV-.***	Uncommon. Young males with cervical or axillary lymphadenopathy. Mediastinal.

50. Ans. a. Inactivation of X chromosome...,

[Ref: Robbins 9th/ 164-65; Genetics in Medicine by Thompson 8th/91;Harrison 19th/735; Harshmohan 7th/252]

Lyonization or Inactivation of X-chromosome

Harshmohan

◈ *7th/252, 896*

- *In female, one of two X-chromosome (either paternal or maternal) is inactivated during embryogenesis as stated in Lyon hypothesis*
- ***This inactivation is passed to all the somatic cells while the germ cells in the female remain unaffected*** *i.e.. ovary will always have active X chromosome*
- *Such an inactive X-chromosome in the somatic cells in female lies condensed in the nucleus & is called as sex chromatin seen specifically in the somatic cells in female*
- ***Males have a Barr body count of less than 2%***
- ***A minimum of 30% cells positive for sex chromatin is indicative of genetically female composition***

"*The principle of X inactivation is that in somatic cells in normal females (but not in normal males), one X chromosome is inactivated early in development, thus equalizing the expression of X-linked genes in the two sexes*" *(Genetics in Medicine by Thompson 8th/91)*

"In humans with more than one X chromosome, the number of Barr bodies visible at interphase is always ***one fewer than the total number of X chromosomes***. For example, men with Klinefelter syndrome (47, XXY karyotype) have a single Barr body, whereas women with a 47, XXX karyotype have two Barr bodies. Barr bodies can be seen on the nucleus of neutrophils"- http://biology. tutorvista. com/

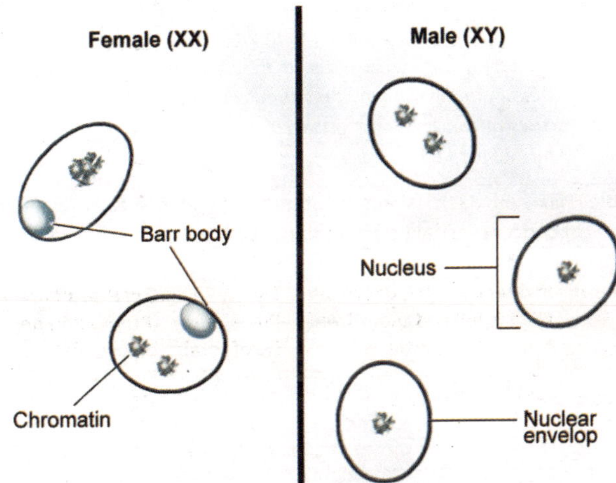

Cytogenetic Disorders Involving Sex Chromosomes

◈ *Robbins 9th/ 164-65*

- There are two factors that are peculiar to the sex chromosomes: (1) lyonization or inactivation of all but one X chromosome and (2) the modest amount of genetic material carried by the Y chromosome.
- Lyon outlined the X-inactivation, or what is commonly known as the **Lyon hypothesis**. It states that (1) *only one of the X chromosomes is genetically active*, (2) *the other X of either maternal or paternal origin undergoes heteropyknosis and is rendered inactive*, (3) *inactivation of either the maternal or paternal X occurs at random among all the cells of the blastocyst on or about the 16th day of embryonic life*, and (4) *inactivation of the same X chromosome persists in all the cells derived from each precursor cell.*

- The inactive X can be seen in the interphase nucleus as a darkly staining small mass in contact with the nuclear membrane known as the ***Barr body*, or *X chromatin*.**

51. Ans. a. Carcinoma..., b. Carcinoma....

[Ref: Park 23rd/ 382-83; Harshmohan 7th/198]

"The **five most frequent** cancers (2012) in **men** were cancer lung, lip & oral cavity, stomach, colorectum & pharynx & in **women,** cancer breast, cervix uteri, colorectum, ovary, lip & oral cavity"- *Park 23rd/ 383*

Cancer

◈ *Park 23rd/ 382-84*

- *In India, the national cancer registry programme of the ICMR provides data on incidence, mortality & distribution of cancer from 25 population-based registries & 5 hospitals based registries*
- *"Breast cancer: It is the most common cancer both in developed & developing countries. It is estimated that during the year 2012, about 144937 new cases of breast cancer in women occurred, which accounts for 27 % of malignant cases in women(an incidence of 25. 8 per lac)"- 23rd/ 389*
- *According to park (ICMR 2012 data) breast cancer is most common cancer in women in India.*
- *Cancer of cervix: In india, it is second most common killer cancer among women. It is estimated during 2012, 122644 new cases of cancer cervix occurred in the country (an incidence rate 22 per lac)" (23rd/ 388)*

Table *(Park 23rd/ 384)*: **Women: Estimated Incidence & Prevalence of cancer (Partial list) in India, 2012**

Cancer	Incidence (%of total)	Incidence (age standardized rate)	5 yr Prevalence (% of total)	5 yr Prevalence (Proportion per-lac population)
Breast	27.0	25.8	35.3	92.6
Cervix-uteri	22.9	22.0	27.4	72.0

Table *(Park 23rd/ 384)*: **Men: Estimated Incidence & Prevalence of cancer (Partial list) in India 2012**

Cancer	Incidence (% of total)	Incidence (age standardized rate)	5 yr Prevalence (% of total)	5 yr Prevalence (Proportion per lac population)
Lung	11. 3	11. 0	3. 7	5. 4
Lip & oral cavity	11. 3	10. 1	12. 6	18. 5

52. Ans. b. Extra-adrenal... c. Carotid body tumour... e. Glomus tympanicum.

[Ref: Robbins 9th/ 741-42; Harrison 19th/ 2329-35;Davidson 22nd/ 781; CMDT 2016/ 1158; Danhert Radiology Review Manual 7th/401]

Pheochromocytoma is a chromaffin-cell neoplasm that can arise as an adrenal (adrenal medulla) or extraadrenal tumor. ***Extraadrenal pheochromocytoma is also referred to as paraganglioma***" *(Anderson Manual of Medical Oncology/Chap 31)*

Glenner Classification of Extraadrenal Paragangliomas

◈ *Danhert Radiology Review Manual 7th/401*

A. Branchiomeric distribution
   1. Associated with great vessels of chest+neck including carotid body, glomus jugulare, glomus tympanicum

B. Parasympathetic distribution
   2. Associated with vagal nerve
   3. Associated with aorticosympathetic chain in thoracolumbar region from aortic arch to urinary bladder, including organ of Zuckerkandl
   4. Associated with visceral organ

Location of Functioning Paragangliomas

◈ *Danhert Radiology Review Manual 7th/401*

a. Adrenal medulla (>80%)
b. Extra adrenal intra abdominal (8-16%)
c. Extra adrenal in head & neck (2-4%)

Four common sites in head & neck & chest- carotid body, jugular foramen, path of vagus nerve & middle ear

Danhert Radiology Review Manual 7th/401-02: Writes

- ***Carotid body tumour***: Painless pulsatile firm neck mass below the angle of jaw
- ***Glomus tympanicum***: Most common tumour in middle ear
- ***Glomus jugulare tumour***: Most common tumour in jugular fossa
- ***Glomus vagale tumour***: *Paraganglioma of vagus nerve*
- ***Inferior nodose paraganglion***: *Compression of internal jugular vein*
- ***Superior jugular paraganglion***: *Dumbbell shaped mass*

Paraganglioma (Carotid Body Tumor)

◈ *Robbins 9th/ 741-42*

- *Paraganglia are clusters of neuroendocrine cells dispersed throughout the body, some connected with the sympathetic nervous system and others with the parasympathetic nervous system. The largest collection of these cells is found in the adrenal medulla, where they give rise to pheochromocytomas.*
- *Tumors arising in* **extra-adrenal paraganglia** *are not surprisingly referred to as paragangliomas.*
- *Paragangliomas develop in two general locations:*
  - ***Paravertebral paraganglia*** (e.g., organs of Zuckerkandl and, rarely, bladder). Such tumors have sympathetic connections and are chromaffin positive; about half elaborate catecholamines, as do pheochromocytomas.
  - ***Paraganglia related to the great vessels*** of the head and neck, the so-called aorticopulmonary chain, including the carotid bodies; aortic bodies; jugulotympanic ganglia; ganglion nodosum of the vagus nerve; and clusters located about the oral cavity, nose, nasopharynx, larynx, and orbit. These are innervated by the parasympathetic nervous system, and their tumors are referred to as ***nonchromaffin paragangliomas***. These tumors infrequently release catecholamines

- ***Carotid body tumors (and paragangliomas in general)*** are rare. They usually arise in the sixth decade of life. The **carotid body tumor** is a prototype of a parasympathetic paraganglioma.

53. Ans. a. Delayed wound... b. Clot solubility...

[Ref: Davidson 22nd/998, 1007, 1054; Harrison 19th/ 733, 736; CMDT 2016/ 556-57]

Deficiency of Factor XIII

◈ *CMDT 2016/ 556-57*

It characteristically leads to delayed bleeding that occurs hours to days after a hemostatic challenge (such as surgery or trauma). The condition is usually life-long, and spontaneous intracranial hemorrhages as well as recurrent pregnancy loss appear to occur with increased frequency in these patients compared with other congenital deficiencies.

Cryoprecipitate or infusion of a plasma-derived factor XIII concentrate (available through a research study; appropriate for patients with A-subunit deficiency only) is the treatment of choice for bleeding or surgical prophylaxis.

- Severe deficiencies of factor VII, X and XIII occur as autosomal recessive disorders. They are rare but are associated with severe bleeding. Typical features include haemorrhage from the umbilical stump and intracranial haemorrhage. Factor XIII deficiency is typically associated with female infertility *(Davidson 22nd/1054)*

Factor XIII Deficiency

◈ *Wintrobe's Clinical Hematology 12th/Chap 57*

- The initial hemostatic plug is not sufficient to prevent blood loss unless it is stabilized by the action of plasma factor XIII (fibrin-stabilizing factor). A complex set of reactions among thrombin, fibrin, and plasma factor XIII is necessary for clot stabilization
- Rebleeding at circumcision is also common. Other bleeding manifestations in these patients include ***soft tissue hemorrhage, hemarthrosis, hematomas, and the development of large pseudocysts.*** The most life-threatening complication of factor XIII deficiency is ***spontaneous intracranial hemorrhage***. Intracranial hemorrhage is more prevalent in factor XIII deficiency than in other inherited bleeding disorders.
- ***Surgery in these patients is often complicated by abnormal wound healing and excessive postoperative bleeding,*** which can occur either immediately or later.

Table *(Harrison 19th/ 733)*: **Laboratory Characteristics of Inherited Coagulation Disorders**

Clotting Factor Deficiency	Laboratory Abnormality[a]		
	aPTT	PT	TT
Factor XIII	–	–	+/–

a-Value within normal range(-) or prolonged(+)

Table *(Wintrobe's Clinical Hematology 12th/Chap 57)*: **Laboratory Findings in Common Inherited Coagulation Disorders**

Disorder	Partial Thromboplastin Time	Prothrombin Time	Thrombin Time	Ancillary Tests
Factor XIII deficiency	N	N	N	***Clot solubility tests are abnormal.***

A, abnormal; N, normal; v, variable

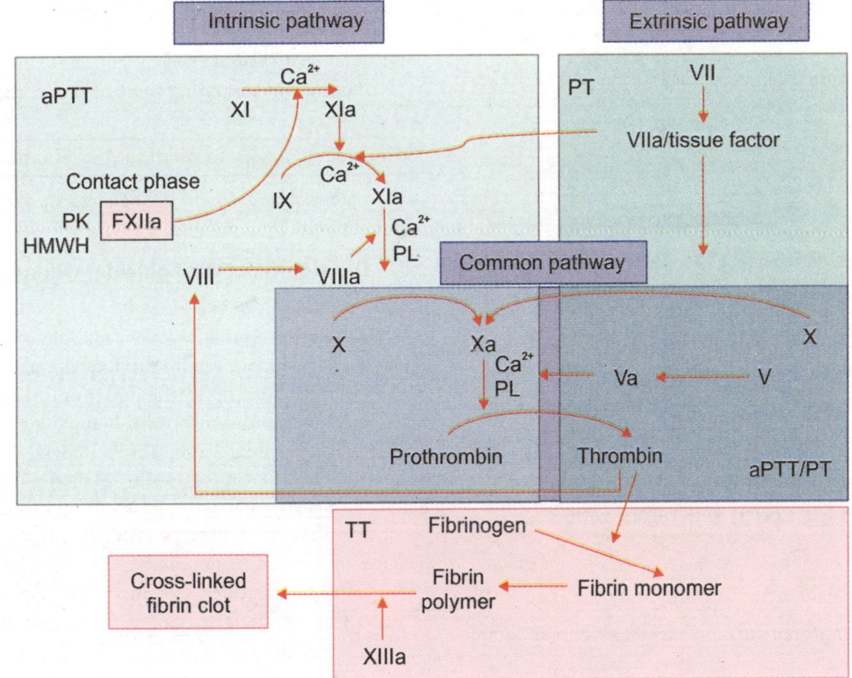

Fig: *(Harrison 19th/ 733)*: Coagulation cascade and laboratory assessment of clotting factor deficiency by activated partial prothrombin time (aPTT), prothrombin time (PT), and thrombin time (TT)

54. Ans. d. BT is decreased in...,

[Ref: Robbins 9th/118-119; Harrison 19th/406; Harshmohan 7th/307-10]

"Hemostasis is spontaneous arrest of bleeding by physiological process. Platelet plays very important role in hemostasis. Normal platelet count is 1.5-4. 0 lacs/microL. Thrombocytopenia is platelet count less than 1.5 lacs/microL. Spontaneous bleeding occurs when platelet count become less than 20, 000/microL" (A. K. Jain 6th/93; Harshmohan 7th/310)

Coagulation Cascade

◈ *Robbins 9th/118-119*

- **Prothrombin time (PT):** This assay tests the ***extrinsic and common coagulation pathways***. A prolonged PT can result from deficiency or dysfunction of factor V, factor VII, factor X, prothrombin, or fibrinogen.
- **Partial thromboplastin time (PTT)**: This assay tests the ***intrinsic and common clotting pathways***. Prolongation of the PTT can be due to deficiency or dysfunction of factor V, VIII, IX, X, XI, or XII, prothrombin, or fibrinogen.
- **Bleeding time**: This measures the time taken for a standardized skin puncture to stop bleeding and provides ***an in vivo assessment of platelet response*** to limited vascular injury. The reference range depends on the actual method employed and varies from 2 to 9 minutes. Prolongation generally indicates a ***defect in platelet numbers or function***.
- **Platelet counts:** The reference range is ***150 to 300 × $10^3/\mu L$***.

Table *(Harrison 19th/406)*: **Hemostatic Disorders and Coagulation Test Abnormalities**

Prolonged Activated Partial Thromboplastin Time (aPTT)
No clinical bleeding—↓ factors XII, high-molecular-weight kininogen, prekallikrein
Variable, but usually mild, bleeding—↓factor XI, mild↓FVIII and FIX
Frequent, severe bleeding—severe deficiencies of FVIII and FIX
Heparin
Prolonged Prothrombin Time (PT)
Factor VII deficiency
Vitamin K deficiency—early
Warfarin anticoagulation
Prolonged aPTT and PT
Factor II, V, X, or fibrinogen deficiency
Vitamin K deficiency—late
Direct thrombin inhibitors
Prolonged Thrombin Time
Heparin or heparin-like inhibitors
Mild or no bleeding—dysfibrinogenemia
Frequent, severe bleeding—afibrinogenemia
Prolonged PT and/or aPTT Not Correct with Mixing with Normal Plasma
Bleeding—specific factor inhibitor
No symptoms, or clotting and/or pregnancy loss—lupus anticoagulant
Disseminated intravascular coagulation
Heparin or direct thrombin inhibitor
Abnormal Clot Solubility
Factor XIII deficiency
Inhibitors or defective cross-linking
Rapid Clot Lysis
Deficiency of α_2-antiplasmin or plasminogen activator inhibitor 1
Treatment with fibrinolytic therapy

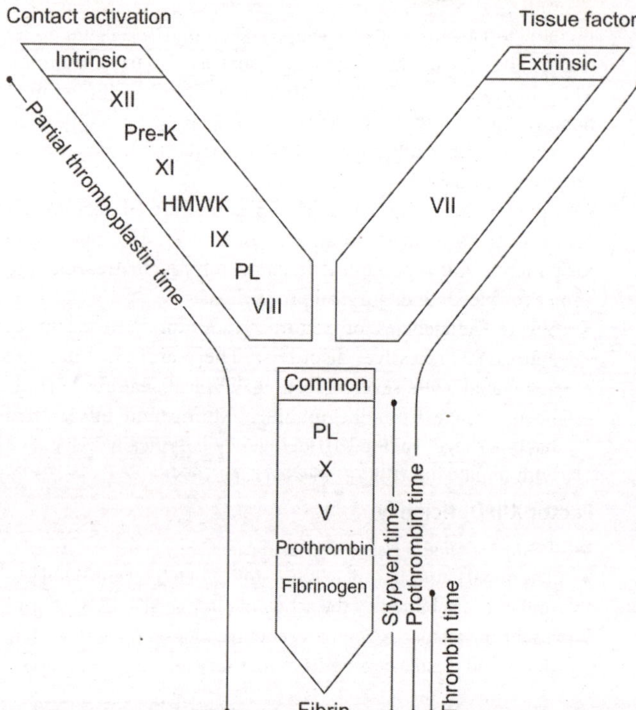

Fig: *(Wintrobe's Clinical Hematology 12th/Chap 49)*: **The interpretation of common screening tests of blood coagulation**

55. Ans. a. Arises in relation..., c. Mandibular..., d. Common....

[Ref: Robbins 9th/ 734; Manipal Surgery 4th/292-93;Harshmohan 7th/511-12]

Dentigerous Cyst: Follicular Odontome

◈ *Manipal Surgery 4th/293*

- Common in lower jaw (mandible) in women 30-40 years
- It occurs in relation to unerupted, permanent, molar tooth, most commonly the upper or lower third molar
- Most commonly occur in maxillary premolar or mandibular third molar *(Logan Turner 10th/49)*
- This unerupted tooth constantly irritates the cells, produce degeneration of cells resulting in a dentigerous cyst
- Absence of molar tooth
- Expansion of mandible- since the inner table of the mandible is strong, the expansion mainly occurs in the outer aspect of mandible. The bone gets thinned out resulting in egg-shell crackling

Dentigerous Cyst (Follicular cyst)

◈ *Harshmohan 7th/512*

- Arise from enamel of an unerupted tooth
- Mandibular 3rd molar & maxillary canines are most often involved
- Less common than radicular cyst
- More commonly occur in children & young individuals
- These cysts are more significant because of reported occurrence of ameloblastoma & carcinoma in them

Dental Cyst: Radicular Cyst/Periapical Cyst

◈ *Manipal Surgery 4th/292*

- *This arise from normally erupted, chronically infected, pulp-less caries tooth*
- *Common in women in around 3rd-4th decades*
- *Commonly affects the upper jaw(maxilla)*
- *It represents as a slow-growing swelling in the maxillary region resulting in deformity of the face*
- ***Diagnosis:** Presence of caries tooth with expansion of maxilla*

Radicular Cyst or Apical or Periodontal or Dental Cyst

◈ *Harshmohan 7th/511-12*

Most often it observed at apex of an erupted tooth & sometime contain thick pultaceous material

Odontogenic Cysts and Tumors

◈ *Robbins 9th/ 734*

- The overwhelming majority of odontogenic cysts are derived from remnants of odontogenic epithelium present within the jaws. In contrast to the rest of the skeleton, epithelial-lined cysts are quite common in the jaws. In general, these cysts are subclassified as either inflammatory or developmental.
- The **dentigerous cyst** is defined as a cyst that originates around the crown of an ***unerupted tooth*** and is thought to be the result of fluid accumulation between the developing tooth and the dental follicle. Radiographically, these are unilocular lesions most often associated with ***impacted third molar*** (wisdom) teeth.

Table *(Robbins 9th/ 734)*: **Histologic Classification of Odontogenic Cysts**

1. *Inflammatory*
  a. Periapical cyst
  b. Residual cyst
  c. Paradental cyst

2. *Developmental*
  a. Dentigerous cyst
  b. Odontogenic keratocyst
  c. Gingival cyst of newborn
  d. Gingival cyst of adult
  e. Eruption cyst
  f. Lateral periodontal cyst
  g. Glandular odontogenic cyst
  h. Calcifying epithelial odontogenic cyst (Gorlin cyst)

56. Ans. All (a. b. c. d.)

[Ref: Robbins 9th/ 760; Harshmohan 7th/524; Harrison 19th/ 533; Davidson 22nd/870-71]

"***Ca esophagus: Lymph node metastasis,*** *which are common, are associated with poor prognosis" (Robbins 9th/ 760)*

"***Lymph node involvement*** *is a bad prognostic factor" (L & B 26th/1004)*

The ***stage of the disease*** is the most important prognostic factor. Overall 5-year survival for esophageal cancer remains around 25% *(CSDT)*

Ca Esophagus

◈ *Sabiston 19th/1054-55*

- The **location of the tumor** also directs the management of esophageal cancer. Eight percent of all esophageal tumors present in the cervical esophagus and are almost always squamous cell cancers. These tumors may be locally aggressive and are managed with chemoradiotherapy followed by segmental resection of the cervical esophagus.
- The **depth of invasion** of a tumor, the T status, is ***another important variable*** in determining stage and treatment of esophageal cancer.

"***Tumor size, grade of differentiation, lymphadenopathy, stage of cancer, and family history*** of esophageal cancer were identified as prognostic factors after esophagectomy. Family history of esophageal cancer is an important prognostic factor that surgeons should take into consideration when selecting a treatment method" *(ncbi. nlm. nih. gov)*

"***Tumor length, the number of involved lymph nodes, and the ratio of positive lymph nodes are important prognostic factors*** for survival in patients with esophageal carcinoma. A revised TNM classification system for patients with esophageal carcinoma might consider adding tumor length and number of positive lymph nodes as two important prognostic factors" (*http://onlinelibrary. wiley. com)*

Prognostic Factors for Esophageal Cancer

◈ *http://www. cancer. ca/en/cancer-information*

- **Stage:** The ***most reliable prognostic factor*** for esophageal cancer is the stage of the tumour at the time of diagnosis. As with most cancers, the lower the stage, the better the outcome. Tumours that are only in the lining of the esophagus have a more favourable prognosis than those that have grown through the muscle wall or that have spread to other organs.
- **Tumour size**: Small tumours have a more favourable prognosis than large tumours.
- **Lymph nodes status**: The fewer lymph nodes that have cancer, the better the prognosis.
- **Cancer has spread to distant organs**: Esophageal cancer that has spread to distant organs has a less favourable prognosis.
- **Cancer that remains after surgery**: The amount of cancer that remains after surgery is called residual disease. No residual disease has a better prognosis than if there is cancer remaining after surgery.
- **Cancer that responds to neoadjuvant therapy**: Esophageal cancer that responds to neoadjuvant therapy is more likely to be completely removed by surgery. As a result, cancer that responds to neoadjuvant therapy has a better prognosis than cancer that doesn't respond to it.
- **Tumour grade**: A low-grade, or well-differentiated, tumour (G1) often grows slower and is less likely to spread than a high-grade tumour (G3 or G4).

57. **Ans.** **a. Increase..., c. Increase alkaline... e. Stool stero....**

[Ref: PJM 20th/20;Harrison 19th/281; CMDT 2016/665]

Table *(CMDT 2016/665)*: **Liver Biochemical Tests: Normal values and changes in hepatocellular and obstructive jaundice**

Tests	Normal Values	Hepatocellular Jaundice	Obstructive Jaundice
Bilurubin			
Direct	0.1-0.3 mg/dL (1.71-5.13 mcmol/L)	Increased	Increased
Indirect	0.2-0.7 mg/dL (3.42-11.97 mcmol/L)	Increased	Increased
Urine bilirubin	None	Increased	Increased
Serum albumin	3.5-5.5 g/dL (35-55 g/L)	Decreased	Generally unchanged
Alkaline phosphatase	30-115 units/L (0.6-2.3 inkat/L)	Mildly increased (+)	Markedly increased (++++)
Prothrombin time	INRof 1.0-1.4. After vitamin K, 10% decrease in 24 hours	Prolonged if damage is severe; does not respond to parenteral vitamin K	Prolonged & obstruction is marked; generally responds to parenteral vitamin K
ALT, AST	ALT < 30 units/L (0.6 mkat/L) (men), ≤ 19 units/L (0.38 mkat/L) (women); AST 5-40 units/L (0.1-0.8 mkat/L)	Increased, as in viral hepatitis	Minimally increased

Table *(PJM 20th/20)*: **Differential Diagnosis of Jaundice**

	Hepatocellular	Obstructive	Hemolytic
I. HISTORY			
1. Abdominal pain	Absent	Present	Present in crisis
2. Pruritus	Transient	Marked	Absent
3. Past history	(a) Contact with jaundice patient (b) Drugs	(a) Pain (**Stones**)	(a) Of crisis (b) Drugs, blood transfusion, etc.
II. EXAMINATION			
1. Tender liver	May be present	Absent	Absent
2. Spleen	May be present	Absent	Present
3. Gallbladder	Not palpable	Palpable if due to neoplasm	Not palpable
4. Pallor	Absent	Present	Present
III. INVESTIGATIONS			
1. Urine:			
Bilirubin	Present	Present	Absent
Urobilinogen	Present	Absent	Present
2. Stools: Sterocobilinogen	Present	Absent	Present
3. Peripheral smear	Leucopenia in infective hepatitis	Normal	Reticulocytosis Spherocytosis
4. LFT			
(a) Bilirubin	++	++	+
(b) Alkaline phosphate	Raised	Markedly raised	Normal
(c) SGOT	Markedly raised	Raised	Normal
5. Barium meal and cholangiography	Normal	May reveal pancreatic growth	Normal
6. RBC Survival	Normal	Normal	Decreased

58. **Ans.** **a. Ki67..., b. Oncoprotein..., c. p16INK4...,**

[Ref: Robbins 9th/1002-04; Harrison 19th/595; Harshmohan 7th/716]

"Continuous expression of the ***HPV oncoproteins E6, E7 and E5*** of the high risk HPV subtypes also appears to be necessary for maintaining the malignant phenotype of cervical cancer patients" *(nature. com/bjc)*

"The functional inactivation of p53 and pRb oncosuppressors by ***E6 and E7 oncoproteins*** determines the alteration of several cellular pathways relevant for cell transformation and cancer development. The expression of E7 determines the inactivation of pRb with a consequent increase of free E2F in the cell, leading to both an increase of ***cyclin-dependent kinase inhibitor p16 (p16INK4a)*** and aberrant proliferation (marked by increased levels of ***Ki-67 expression***). Therefore, p16 overexpression, identified by immunostaining or enzyme-linked immunosorbent assay (ELISA), can be considered as a marker of HPV infection and of activated expression of viral oncogenes and virus-induced cell cycle deregulation" *(hindawi. com/journals/bmri)*

"The immunohistochemical identification of increased expression of host cell biomarkers (such as ***p16INK4, cyclin E, and Ki-67***) are expressed in a greater proportion of cells in precancerous lesions (due to cell cycle disturbances) and will frequently distinguish these from non-neoplastic epithelial changes in cervix"

Molecular Studies

◈ *Harshmohan 7th/716*

Upon integration, protein product of HPV 16 & 18, E7 &E6 protein respectively, inactivate tumour suppressor genes, p53 & RB-1 genes, thus permitting uncontrolled cellular proliferation

Preinvasive & invasive Cervical Cancer

◈ *Robbins 9th/1002-04*

- Experimental data indicate that viral (*E6* and *E7*) genes of high risk HPVs can disrupt the cell cycle via binding to RB with up-regulation of ***Cyclin E (E7)*** and ***p16INK4***; interrupt cell death pathways by binding to ***p53 (E6)***; induce centrosome duplication and genomic instability (E6, E7); and prevent replicative senescence by up-regulation of telomerase (E6).
- HPV E6 induces rapid degradation of p53 via ubiquitin-dependent proteolysis, reducing p53 levels by two- to three-fold. E7 complexes with the hypophosphorylated (active) form of RB, promoting its proteolysis via the proteosome pathway. The viral oncogenes are critical in extending the life span of genital epithelial cells-a necessary component of tumor development.

59. Ans. b. RET..., d. NTRK1, e. RAS

[Ref: Robbins 9th/1095; Harrison 19th/2305; L & B 26th/764]

"**Synaptophysin** is an immunohistochemical markers for ***neuroendocrine tumors***. Synaptophysin was consistently present in the tumor cells of pheochromocytomas, ***thyroid medullary carcinomas***, and pancreatic islet cell tumor"

Papillary Thyroid Carcinomas

◈ *Robbins 9th/1095*

- Molecular pathways involves rearrangements of the tyrosine kinase receptors ***RET or NTRK1*** (neurotrophic tyrosine kinase receptor 1) and another involves activating mutations in the ***BRAF* oncogene.**
- A third pathway involves ***RAS* mutations** (10% to 20% of papillary carcinomas), suggesting that some of these cancers are related to follicular adenomas.
- *RET*, located on chromosome 10q11, and *NTRK1*, located on chromosome 1q21, belong to the family of receptor tyrosine kinases that transduce extracellular signals for cell growth and differentiation and exert many of their downstream effects through the ubiquitous MAP kinase signaling pathway
- Neither receptor is normally expressed on the surface of thyroid follicular cells. In papillary thyroid cancers, either a paracentric inversion of chromosome 10 or a reciprocal translocation between chromosomes 10 and 17 places the tyrosine kinase domain of *RET* under the transcriptional control of constitutively active genes on these two chromosomes. The novel fusion genes that are so formed are known as ***ret/PTC*** (ret/papillary thyroid carcinoma) and are present in approximately one-fifth of papillary thyroid cancers.

Table *(341-12 Harrison 19th/2305)*: **Genetic Alterations in Thyroid Neoplasia**

Gene/Protein	Type of Gene	Chromosomal Location	Genetic Abnormality	Tumor
TSH receptor	GPCR receptor	14q31	Point mutations	Toxic adenoma, differentiated carcinomas
$G_{S\alpha}$	G protein	20q13. 2	Point mutations	Toxic adenoma, differentiated carcinomas
RET/PTC	Receptor tyrosine kinase	10q11. 2	Rearrangements PTC1: (inv(10)q11. 2q21)PTC2: (t(10;17)(q11. 2;q23)) PTC3: ELE1/TK	PTC
RET	Receptor tyrosine kinase	10q11. 2	Point mutations	MEN 2, medullary thyroid cancer
BRAF	MEK kinase	7q24	Point mutations, rearrangements	PTC, ATC
TRK	Receptor tyrosine kinase	1q23-24	Rearrangements	Multinodular goiter, papillary thyroid cancer

Contd...

Gene/Protein	Type of Gene	Chromosomal Location	Genetic Abnormality	Tumor
RAS	Signal transducing p21	Hras 11p15. 5Kras 12p12. 1; Nras 1p13. 2	Point mutations	FTC, PTC follicular variant, adenomas
p53	Tumor suppressor, cell cycle control, apoptosis	17p13	Point mutations Deletion, insertion	Anaplastic cancer
APC	Tumor suppressor, adenomatous polyposis coli gene	5q21-q22	Point mutations	Anaplastic cancer, also associated with familial polyposis coli
p16 (MTS1, CDKN2A)	Tumor suppressor, cell cycle control	9p21	Deletions	Differentiated carcinomas
p21/WAF	Tumor suppressor, cell cycle control	6p21. 2	Over expression	Anaplastic cancer
MET	Receptor tyrosine kinase	7q31	Over expression	Follicular thyroid cancer
c-MYC	Receptor tyrosine kinase	8q24. 12. -13	Over expression	Differentiated carcinoma
PTEN	Phosphatase	10q23	Point mutations	PTC in Cowden's syndrome (multiple hamartomas, breast tumors, gastrointestinal polyps, thyroid tumors)
CTNNB1	β-Catenin	3p22	Point mutations	Anaplastic cancer
Loss of heterozygosity (LOH)	?Tumor suppressors	3p; 11q13, other loci	Deletions	Differentiated thyroid carcinomas, anaplastic cancer
PAX8-PPARγ1	Transcription factor Nuclear receptor fusion	t(2;3)(q13;p25)	Translocation	Follicular adenoma or carcinoma, rare PTC follicular variant

PHARMACOLOGY

60. Ans. a. Appro..., c. Peripheral..., d. Somn..., e. Approved...

[Ref: KDT 7th/419; Katzung 13th/406, 419; Harrison 19th/2682; Pharmacology by Satoskar 24th/ 139]

*"**Pregabalin side-effect includes:** Cognitive changes, sedation & **peripheral edema**"- Harrison 19th/2682(Table)*

Pregabalin

◈ *KDT 7th/419; Katzung 13th/406, 419*

- Pregabalin is another GABA analog, closely related to gabapentin. This drug has been approved for both ***antiseizure activity and for its analgesic properties.***
- In spite of their close structural resemblance to GABA, gabapentin and pregabalin do not act directly on GABA receptors. They may, however, modify the synaptic or nonsynaptic release of GABA.
- Pregabalin is approved for the adjunctive ***treatment of partial seizures***, with or without secondary generalization; controlled clinical trials have documented its effectiveness.
- It is available only in oral form, and the daily dose ranges from 150 to 600 mg/d, usually in two or three divided administrations.
- Pregabalin is also approved for use in ***neuropathic pain, including painful diabetic peripheral neuropathy, post herpetic neuralgia & complex regional pain syndrome etc.***
- Pregabalin, like gabapentin, is not metabolized and is almost entirely excreted unchanged in the urine. It is not bound to plasma proteins and has virtually no drug-drug interactions, again resembling the characteristics of gabapentin.
- Sedative side effects are less prominent, but poor concentration, allergic reactions & rash have been complained
- Toxicity includes- ***Somnolence***, dizziness, ataxia

61. Ans. a. Oxybut..., b. Toltero..., c. Mirabeg..., d. Onabotuli...

[Ref: KDT 7th/117-18; Katzung 13th/ 127-28; Rang & Dale 8th/366; Pharmacology by Satoskar 24th/305-07]

Overactive Bladder

◈ *Pharmacology by Satoskar 24th/305-07; Katzung 13th/ 127-28*

- It is a symptom complex that includes urinary urgency with or without urge incontinence, urinary frequency & nocturia (Awakening more than once at night to void urine)
- *"Antimuscuranic drugs such as **oxybutynin, flavoxate, tolterodine & trospium** are used for both neurogenic & non-neurogenic overactive bladder. **Solifenacin & darifenacin** are the new drugs(M3 antagonist) for use in overactive bladder"*

- "Mirabegron is beta-3 adrenergic agoinst used for overactive bladder"
- "Onabotulinum toxin A is used as single intradetrusor injection, to treat overactive bladder"

62. Ans. b. Protamine sulphate....

[Ref: KDT 7th/620-24; Katzung 13th/ 590-92; Rang & Dale 8th/ 300; Pharmacology by Satoskar 24th/ 300-301]

*"Warfarin induced **skin necrosis** is a rare complication characterized by the appearance of skin lesion **3 to 10 days** after initiation of treatment" (G & G 11th/1478)*

***"The dose of warfarin is adjusted to give an INR of 2-4**, the precise target depending on the clinical situation" (Rang & Dale 8th/300)*

*"The dose of warfarin is adjusted by measuring INR, which is generally maintained **b/w 2. 0 & 3. 5**" (Pharmacology by Satoskar 24th/ 301)*

"The reference range for **prothrombin time** is usually around **12–13 seconds** and the **INR** in absence of anticoagulation therapy is **0. 8-1. 2**. The target range for INR in anticoagulant use (e.g. warfarin) is 2 to 3. In some cases, if more intense anticoagulation is thought to be required, the target range may be as high as 2. 5-3. 5 depending on the indication for anticoagulation"

"Warfarin causes necrosis of soft tissue(e. g breast or buttock) owing to thrombosis in venules is a rare but serious effect that occurs shortly after starting treatment"- Rang & Dale 8th/ 300

Warfarin

◈ *KDT 7th/620-24; Katzung 13th/ 590-92*

- ***It block the γ -carboxylation of several glutamate residues in prothrombin and factors VII, IX, and X as well as the endogenous anticoagulant proteins C and S***
- The blockade results in incomplete coagulation factor molecules that are biologically inactive. The protein carboxylation reaction is coupled to the oxidation of vitamin K. The vitamin must then be reduced to reactivate it.
- Warfarin prevents reductive metabolism of the inactive vitamin K epoxide back to its active hydroquinone form.
- ***Dose regulation is done by prothrombin time & INR(c. f Heparin-aPTT/clotting time)***
- **Antagonist is Vit K** (c. f Heparin- Protamine sulphate)
- Side effect- bledding, alopecia, dermatitis, diarrhea etc.
- Warfarin used clinically is a racemic mixture composed of equal amounts of two enantiomorphs. The Levorotatory S warfarin is four times more potent than the dextrorotatory R -warfarin.

63. Ans. a. Intercalate b/w..., d. Inhibition of protein...

[Ref: KDT 7th/867; Katzung 13th/932-35; G & G 11th/1358; Pharmacology by Satoskar 24th/835]

*"**Doxorubicin:** It acts as non-specific **inhibitor** of **topoisomerase-II, thus interfering with DNA replication"** (Pharmacology by Satoskar 24th/835)*

***"Doxorubicin:** It **intercalate b/w DNA strands & block DNA as well as RNA synthesis. They are capable of causing breaks in DNA strands by activating(wrong!!, see other references) topoisomerase-II & generating quinone type free radical**"- (KDT 7th/867)*

Doxorubicin & other Anthracycline Antibiotics

◈ *G & G 11th/1358*

- *These compounds can **intercalate with DNA,** directly affecting **transcription and replication.***
- *A more important action is the ability of these drugs to form a **tripartite complex with topoisomerase II** and DNA. Formation of the tripartite complex with anthracyclines and with etoposide **inhibits the religation of the broken DNA strands, leading to apoptosis.***
- *Defects in DNA double-strand break repair sensitize cells to damage by these drugs, while over expression of transcription-linked DNA repair may contribute to resistance.*

Table *(Katzung 13th/932)*: **Cancer Chemotherapy drug (Partial list)**

Drug	Mechanism of action	Clinical application	Acute toxicity	Delayed toxicity
Doxorubicin	**Oxygen free radicals bind to DNA causing single- and double strand DNA breaks; inhibits topoisomerase II; intercalates into DNA**	Breast cancer, Hodgkin's and non-Hodgkin's lymphoma, soft tissue sarcoma, ovarian cancer, non-small cell and small cell lung cancer, thyroid cancer, Wilms' tumor, neuroblastoma	Nausea, red urine (not hematuria)	Cardiotoxicity, alopecia, myelosuppression, stomatitis

64. Ans. a. Constipa..., b. Urinary..., c. Mydrias..., e. Blurring...

[Ref: KDT 7th/120;G & G 11th/194; Katzung 13th/ 129; Rang & Dale 8th/ 164-65; Pharmacology by Satoskar 24th/301]

*"**Body temperature is frequently elevated.** Unfortunately, children, especially infants, are very sensitive to hyperthermic effects of atropine" (Katzung 13th/ 129)*

*"**Constipation & urinary retention**(precipitation especially in elderly) can occur with atropine": Pharmacology by Satoskar 24th/301*

Adverse Effects & Toxicity of Anticholinergic Drugs

◈ *Katzung 13th/ 129; KDT 7th/120*

- Treatment with atropine or its congeners directed at one organ system almost always induces undesirable effects in other organ systems.
- **Side-effects includes:** *Difficulty in swallowing & talking, dry mouth, **fever**, dry-flushed & hot skin, difficulty in micturition, **mydriasis**, photophobia, **blurring of near vision,** palpitation, dreadful visual hallucination, ataxia, delirium, psychotic behavior, weak & rapid pulse, hypotension, cardiovascular collapse with respiratory depression, convulsion & coma*

- **C/I:** In individual with narrow iridocorneal angle-may precipitate acute congestive glaucoma & use cautiously in elderly male with ***prostatic hypertrophy-urinary retention*** can occur

65. Ans. a. Decrea..., c. Release..., d. Prolong..., e. Decreased...,

[Ref: KDT 7th/35; G & G 11th/5; Pharmacology by Satoskar 24th/7; http://www. pharmatutor. org/articles/review-sustained-release-dosage-forms]

Sustained Release Formulation

- It is defined as the type of dosage form in which a portion i.e., (initial dose) of the drug is released immediately, in order to achieve desired therapeutic response more promptly, & the remaining(maintenance dose) is then released slowly there by achieving a therapeutic level which is prolonged but not maintained constant
- Sustained release implies slow release of the drug over a time period. ***It may or may not be controlled release***

Controlled-Release Preparations

◈ *G & G 11th/5*

- *A slow rate of dissolution of a drug in GI fluids is the basis for controlled-release, extended release, sustained-release, and prolonged-action preparations that are designed to produce slow, uniform absorption of the drug for 8 hours or longer. Such preparations are offered for medications in all major drug categories.*
- *Potential advantages are reduction in the frequency of administration of the drug as compared with conventional dosage forms (possibly with improved compliance by the patient), maintenance of a therapeutic effect overnight, and decreased incidence and/or intensity of both undesired effects (by elimination of the peaks in drug concentration) and non therapeutic blood levels of the drug (by elimination of troughs in concentration) that occur after administration of immediate-release dosage forms.*
- *Controlled-release dosage forms, while more expensive, are most appropriate for drugs with short t1/2 (<4 hours) where patient noncompliance becomes a determinant of therapeutic failure.*

Sustained Release Concept

- Sustained release, sustained action, prolong action, controlled release, extended action, depot are terms used to identify drug delivery systems that are designed to achieve ***prolong therapeutic effect by continuously releasing medication over an extended period of time after administration of single dose.***
- In the case of orally administer this period is measured in hours while in the case of injectables this period varies from days to months.

Advantages of sustained release dosage forms

- Control of drug therapy is achieved.
- Rate and extent of drug absorption can be is modified
- ***Frequency of drug administration is reduced.***
- Patient compliance can be improved.
- Drug administration can be made convenient
- Maximizing the availability of drug with minimum dose.
- The safety margin of high potency drug can be increased.

Disadvantages of sustained release dosage forms:

- It not permits prompt termination of therapy.
- Less flexibility in dose adjustment.
- These dosage forms are designed on the basis of average biological half life.
- They are costly.

Parameters for Drug to be Formulated in Sustained Release Dosage form

Physicochemical parameters for drug selection.

- Molecular weight/size < 1000 Daltons.
- Solubility > 0. 1 mg/ml for pH 1 to pH 7. 8.
- Apparent partition coefficient High.
- Absorption mechanism Diffusion.
- General absorbability from all GI segments.
- ***Release should not be influenced by pH and enzymes.***

Pharmacokinetic parameters for drug selection

- Elimination half-life preferably between 2 to 8 hrs
- Total clearance should not be dose dependent
- Elimination rate constant required for design
- Absolute bioavailability should be 75% or more
- Intrinsic absorption rate must be greater than release rate

Controlled Drug Release

- It deliver drug the drug at a pre determined rate for a specific period of time
- Controlled release is perfectly zero order that is the drug release over time irrespective of concentration

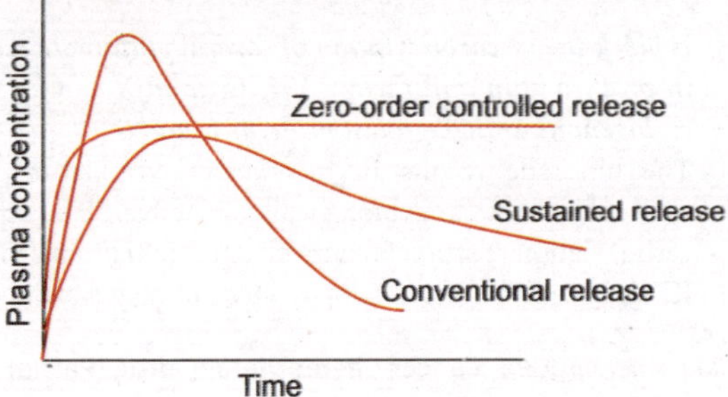

Fig: Plasma drug concentration profile for conventional release, a sustained release and zero order controlled release formulation

66. Ans. a. Steepest..., b. Inverted..., d. Sigmoid..., e. Enables...

[Ref: KDT 7th/53-54; Katzung 13th/35-36; Rang & Dale 8th/9, 94; Pharmacology by Satoskar 24th/37-38]

Dose-Response Relationship

◈ *KDT 7th/53-54*

- Generally, the intensity of response increases with increase in dose (or more precisely concentration at the receptor) & the dose-response curve is a ***rectangular hyperbola***
- If the dose is plotted on a logarithmic scale, the curve become sigmoid
- ***Sigmoidal curve in dose –response relationship: the steepest portion in the middle***-wiki
- DRC is used to measure- drug potency, drug efficacy & drug safety- slideshare. (net)

Dose-Response Relationship

◈ *G & G 11th/34*

- *Some drugs cause low-dose stimulation and high-dose inhibition of response. These* **U-shaped relationships** *for some receptor systems are said to display* hormesis.
- *Several drug–receptor systems can display this property (e.g., prostaglandins, endothelin, and purinergic and serotonergic agonists, among others), which is likely to be at the root of drug toxicity.*

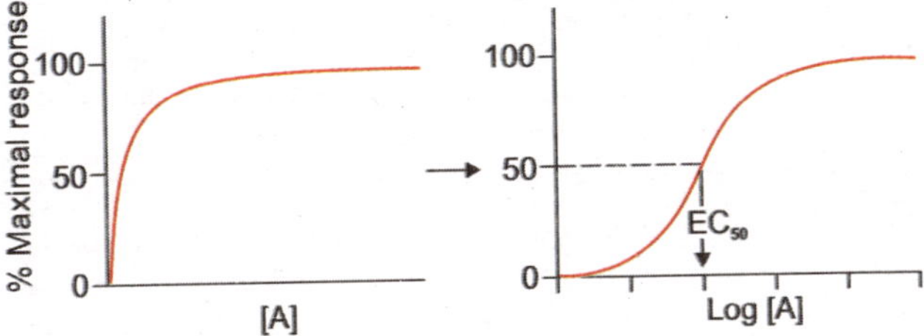

Fig: *(G & G 11th/34):* Graded responses expressed as a function of the concentration of drug A present at the receptor.

The hyperbolic shape of the curve in panel A becomes sigmoid when plotted semi-logarithmically, as in panel B. The concentration of drug that produces 50% of the maximal response quantifies drug activity and is referred to as the EC50 (effective concentration for 50% response).

Dose-Response Relationship

◈ *Pharmacology by Satoskar 24th/37-38*

- Two basic type of dose effect relationship have been observed: (1) Graded or Quantitative dose-response relationship & (2) Quantal or all or none dose-response relationship
- **Graded or Quantitative dose-response relationship: rectangular hyperbola & Sigmoid curve(on logarithmic scale)**
- Quantal or all or none dose-response relationship: A Gaussian (normal distribution curve)

67. Ans. a. Atropine..., b. Pralidoxime..., e. Pralidoxi....

[Ref: Reddy 32nd/495-97;G & G 11th/210;KDT 7th/111; Katzung 13th/979-80; Pharmacology by Satoskar 24th/297]

Organophosphorus

◈ *Katzung 13th/979-80*

- The ***use of oximes in organophosphate poisoning is secondary to that of atropine***. Moreover, the clinical benefit of oxime therapy is highly variable depending upon the compound involved(different organophosphate 'age' at different rates), the amount of poison that has entered the body, time lapsed before therapy is started & dose of oxime
- Atropine is highly effective in counter-acting the muscuranic symptoms, but higher doses are required to antagonize the central effects. It does not reverse peripheral muscular paralysis which is a nicotinic action

Organophosphorus Poisoning

◈ *Reddy 32nd/495-97*

- **Pupil:** Miosis, occasionally unequal or dilated
- Pralidoxime & atropine work synergistically & should be used together
- Convulsion can be controlled with i.v diazepam, repeated if necessary. This may be followed by i.v infusion over 24 hr. If convulsion persists, use phenobarbital or phenytoin

Organophosphorus Poisoning

◈ *KDT 7th/111*

- *All case of Anti-ChE poisoning must be must be promptly given atropine 2 mg i. v repeated every 10 min till dryness of mouth or other signs of atropinization appear. Continued treatment with maintenance doses may be required for 1-2 weeks*
- *The use of oximes in organophosphate poisoning id secondary to that of atropine. Morever, the clinical benefit of oximes is highly variables*
- *Control of convulsion with judicious use of diazepam*

Organophosphorus Poisoning

◈ *G & G 11th/210*

- *Ocular manifestations include marked miosis, ocular pain, conjunctival congestion, diminished vision, ciliary spasm, and brow ache.*
- *Atropine in sufficient dosage effectively antagonizes the actions at muscarinic receptor sites, and to a moderate extent, at peripheral ganglionic and central sites*
- *A mild degree of atropine block should then be maintained for as long as symptoms are evident. Atropine is virtually without effect against the peripheral neuromuscular compromise, which may be reversed by pralidoxime (2-PAM), a cholinesterase reactivator. AChE reactivators are beneficial in the therapy of organophosphorus anti-ChE intoxication, but their use is supplemental to the administration of atropine*
- *Alleviation of persistent convulsions with diazepam (5–10 mg, intravenously)*

68. Ans. b. Aminoglyc..., d. Chloram....

[Ref: KDT 7th/734, 768; Katzung 13th/789]

"Rifampin: It interrupts ***RNA synthesis*** *by binding to β subunit of mycobacterial DNA-dependent RNA polymerase" (KDT 7th/768)*

Trimethoprim Selectively Inhibit Bacterial Dihydrofolate Reductase (DHFRase)"

◈ *KDT 7th/706*

Action of Antibiotics on Bacterial Protein Synthesis

◈ *(KDT 7th/734)*

- Tetracyclines bind to 30S ribosome & inhibit aminoacyl tRNA attachment to the A site
- Erythromycin & clindamycin bind to 50S ribosome & hinder translocation of the elongated peptide chain back from A site to P site. Peptide synthesis may be prematurely terminated
- Chloramphenicol binds to 50S subunit. It interfere with peptide bond formation & transfer of peptide chain from P site
- Aminoglycosides bind to several sites at 30S & 50S subunits-freeze initiation, interfere with polysome formation & cause misreading of mRNA code

69. Ans. a. Phenytoin, b. Ampicillin

[Ref: KDT 7th/ 326; Katzung 13th/712; Rang & Dale 8th/ 434; Pharmacology by Satoskar 24th/ 967]

Contraceptive Failure may Occur with Concurrent Administration of

◈ *KDT 7th/ 326*

- *Enzyme inducer: **Phenytoin**, phenobarbitone, primidone, carbamazepine, rifampin, ritonavir. Metabolism of estrogenic & progestational component is increased*
- *Suppression of intestinal flora: tetracyclines, **ampicillin** etc. Deconjugation of estrogens excreted in bile fails to occur → their enterohepatic circulation is interrupted → blood level falls*

Drug Causing Decreased Efficacy of OC Pills

◈ *Rang & Dale 8th/ 434)*

"Rifampicin, Rifabutin, carbamazepine, Phenytoin & others"

Drug Causing Decreased Efficacy of OC Pills

◈ *Pharmacology by (Satoskar 24th/ 967)*

*"Barbiturates, Antiepileptics drugs, Rifampicin, Griseofulvin, **Ampicillin**, Tetracyclines"*

"Women using oral contraceptives must be made aware of an important interaction that occurs with antimicrobial drugs. Because the normal gastrointestinal flora increase the enterohepatic cycling (and bioavailability) of estrogens, antimicrobial drugs that interfere with these organisms may reduce the efficacy of oral contraceptives. Additionally, coadministration with potent inducers of the hepatic microsomal metabolizing enzymes, such as ***rifampin***, may increase liver catabolism of estrogens or progestins and diminish the efficacy of oral contraceptives" *(Katzung 13th/712)*

70. Ans. a. M2 rec..., c. NM..., d. Synaptic..., e. NN

[Ref: KDT 7th/101-02; Katzung 13th/ 106]

NM: *Located in neuromuscular junction & cause depolarization of muscle end plate (KDT 7th/102)*

*NN located on autonomic ganglia, **adrenal medulla** & CNS (KDT 7th/102)*

"Most smooth muscles & glands have M2 & M3 subtypes; M3 predominates" (KDT 7th/102)

Ach is a major neurotransmitter at autonomic, somatic as well as central sites. Release of Ach from nerve terminal help in synaptic transmission (KDT 7th/99 & Ganong 25th/122)

Table *(Katzung 13th/ 106)*: **Muscarinic Receptor Subgroups and their Antagonists**

Property	M_1	M_2	M_3
Primary locations	Nerves	Heart, nerves, smooth muscle	Glands, smooth muscle, endothelium
Dominant effector system	↑IP_3, ↑DAG	↓ cAMP, ↑ K^+ channel current	↑ IP_3, ↑ DAG
Antagonists	Pirenzepine, telenzepine, decyclomine	Gallamine, methoctramine	4-DAMP, darrifenacin, solifenacin, oxybutynin

Table *(Katzung 13th/97)*: **Major Autonomic Receptor Types**

Receptor Name	Typical Locations	Result of Ligand Binding
Cholinoceptors		
Muscarinic M_1	CNS neurons, sympathetic postaganglionic neurons, some presynaptic sites	Formation of IP_3 and DAG, increased intracellular calcium
Muscarinic M_2	Myocardium, smooth muscle, some presynaptic sites; CNS neurons	Opening of potassium channels, inhibition of adenylyl cyclase
Muscarinic M_3	Exocrine glands, vessels (smooth muscle and endothelium); CNS neurons	Like M_1 receptor-ligand binding
Muscarinic M_4	CNS neurons; possibly vagal nerve endings	Like M_2 receptor-ligand binding
Muscarinic M_5	Vascular endothelium, especially cerebral vessels; CNS neurons	Like M_1 receptor-ligand binding
Nicotinic N_N	Postganglionic neurons, some presynaptic cholinergic terminals	Opening of Na^+, K^+ channels, depolarization
Nicotinic N_M	Skeletal muscle neuromuscular end plates	Opening of Na^+, K^+ channels, depolarization

71. Ans. c. No effect on uterus

[Ref: KDT 7th/ 312-15; Katzung 13th/713;Pharmacology by Satoskar 24th/ 837-38]

Tamoxifen

- Tamoxifen use as adjuvant therapy in estrogen receptor positive breast cancer
- ***Tamoxifen is associated with reduced risk of cancer in the contralateral breast***
- The response, rate on tamoxifen is higher in patient with positive receptor but some estrogen receptor negative patient also responds suggesting additional non hormonal mechanism of action
- It is ***also approved for the primary prophylaxis of breast cancer in high risk woman***
- ***It reduces the recurrence rate of breast cancer in ipsilateral as well contralateral breast*** *(KDT)*
- Studies of patients treated with tamoxifen as adjuvant therapy for early breast cancer have shown a 35% decrease in contralateral breast cancer- *(Katzung 10th/671)*
- Tamoxifen also decreases total and LDL cholesterol without any change in HDL and triglyceride level.

- It also improve the bone mass due to antiresorptive effect
- Tamoxifen is effective orally
- It has biphasis plasma t½ (10 hrs. and 7 days) and long duration of action.
- Hot flushes and nausea and vomiting occur in 25% of patients, and many other minor adverse effects are observed.
- *Tamoxifen increases the risk of thromboembolic events*[Q'] - *(Goodman Gillman 10th/1441)*
- *"Tamoxifen causes retinal deposits, decreased visual acuity and cataracts in occasional patients" (Goodman Gillman 10th /1441)*

Tamoxifen Citrate

◈ *KDT 7th/ 312-15*

- Acts as potent estrogen antagonist in breast carcinoma cells, blood vessels & at some peripheral sites
- ***Partial agonist in uterus, bone,*** liver & pituitary
- Inhibition of human breast cancer cells & hot flushes reflect antiestrogenic action
- ***Weak estrogenic action*** manifests as stimulation of endometrial proliferation, lowering Gn & prolactin levels in postmenopausal women as well as improvement in their bone density

Tamoxifen May Lead To Endometrial Hyperplasia and Endometrial Cancer

- *While tamoxifen blocks estrogen receptors on the breast, it stimulates these receptors in the uterus (because tamoxifen is a partial against of ER)*[Q].
- ***Stimulation of estrogen receptors in the uterus may predispose the patients to endometrial hyperplasia and for endometrial cancer***

72. Ans. d. Clozapine

[Ref: KDT 7th/90; Katzung 13th/1018; Rang & Dale 8th/700; Pharmacology by Satoskar 24th/ 1122; http://schizophrenia bulletin. oxford journal]

Antipsychotic Therapy in pregnancy & FDA Category

◈ *http://schizophrenia bulletin. oxford journals*

- **Aripiprazole** is rated FDA Pregnancy ***Category C:*** this means that there is positive evidence of human fetal risk, but the benefits from use in pregnant women may be acceptable despite the risk
- **Clozapine** is rated FDA Pregnancy ***Category B***, despite paucity of data. Reproductive studies performed in rats and rabbits at doses of approximately 2–4 times the human dose revealed no harm to the fetus. 34In humans, information on the safety of clozapine in human pregnancies has been available since the early 1990s
- **Olanzapine** is rated FDA Pregnancy Category C. Reproductive studies show no evidence of fetal harm in animals.
- **Risperidone** is rated FDA Pregnancy Category C, and the drug has shown no direct teratogenic effects in animal studies
- **Ziprasidone** is rated FDA Pregnancy Category C. In animal studies, ziprasidone demonstrated developmental toxicity, including possible teratogenic effects
- **Haloperidol** is rated FDA Pregnancy Category C
- **Sertindole** is rated FDA Pregnancy Category C
- **Quetiapine** is rated FDA Pregnancy Category C

Risk Category of Drugs During Pregnancy

◈ *KDT 7th/90*

- **Category D:** Phenytoin, carbamazepine, valproate
- **Category C:** Thiopentone
- **Category B:** Penicillin V, amoxicillin, cefaclor, erythromycin, paracetamol, lidocaine

Table *(Katzung 13th/1018)*: **FDA teratogenic risk categories**

Category	Description
A	Controlled studies in women fail to demonstrate a risk to the fetus in the first trimester (and there is no evidence of a risk in late trimesters), and the possibility of fetal harm appears remote.
B	Either animal-reproduction studies have not demonstrated a fetal risk, but there are no controlled studies in pregnant women, or animal-reproduction studies have shown an adverse effect (other than a decrease in fertility) that was not confirmed in controlled studies in women in the first trimester (and there is no evidence of a risk in later trimesters).
C	Either studies in animals have revealed adverse effects on the fetus (teratogenic or embryocidal or other) and there are no controlled studies in women or studies in women and animal are not available. Drugs should be given only if the potential benefit justifies the potential risk to the fetus.
D	There is positive evidence of human fetal risk, but the benefits from use in pregnant women may be acceptable despite the risk (e.g., if the drug is needed in a life-threatening situation or for a serious disease for which safer drugs cannot be used or are ineffective).
E	Studies in animals or human beings have demonstrated fetal abnormalities or there is evidence of fetal risk based on human experience or both, and the risk of the use of the drug in pregnant women clearly outweighs any possible benefit. There drug is contraindicated in women who are or may become pregnant.

Table: Pregnancy Drug Categories

Categories	Significance	Examples
Category A	No risk to fetus in human studies	• Levothyroxine • Potassium • Supplementation • MgSO4
Category B	• Animal studies show no risk • Human studies are lacking	• Penicillins • Cephalosporins • Macrolides • Brimonidine
Category C	• Animal studies show positive teratogenic risk • Human studies are not available	• Albuterol • Zidovudine • CCB • Morphine • Atropine

Contd...

Categories	Significance	Examples
Category D	• Human and animal studies show positive teratogenic risk • Can be used in pregnancy because of benefits greater than risk might be acceptable.	• Corticosteroids • Azathioprine • Carbamazepine • Valproate • Methotrexate • Lithium
Category X	Human and animal studies show positive teratogenic risk Absolutely contraindicated in pregnancy because of risk greater than benefits.	• Thalidomide • Isotretinoin • Fluoroquinolones • Tetracyclines • Chloramphenicol • Warfarin • ACE inhibitors

73. Ans. c. Cause exc..., d. More effective..., e. Provide...

[Ref: KDT 7th/430-31; G & G 10th/535-38;Katzung 13th/478; Rang & Dale 8th/494-95; Pharmacology by Satoskar 24th/237]

"All the dopamine agonists in larger doses can cause severe neuropsychiatric adverse effects" *(Pharmacology by Satoskar 24th/237)*

Ropinirole & Pramipexole

◈ *G & G 10th/535-38*

- The duration of action of the dopamine agonists (8–24 hours) often is longer than that of levodopa (6–8 hours), and they are particularly effective in the treatment of patients who ***have developed on/off phenomena.***
- The ***somnolence can be quite severe;*** and it is prudent to advise patients of this possibility and to switch to another treatment if sleepiness interferes with daily life or poses a hazard
- These selective agonists are well tolerated and are used increasingly as ***initial treatment for PD rather than as adjuncts to levodopa.***
- This change has been driven by two factors: (1) the belief that because of their longer duration of action, dopamine agonists may be less likely than levodopa to induce on/off effects and dyskinesias and (2) the concern that levodopa may contribute to oxidative stress, thereby accelerating loss of dopaminergic neurons.
- Many experts favor *dopamine agonists as initial therapy in younger patients with PD* and *levodopa as the initial treatment in older patients* who ***may be more vulnerable to the adverse cognitive effects of the agonists***
- ***They provide neuroprotective effect by reducing endogenous dopamine production & release & thereby diminish oxidative stress***

Ropinirole & Pramipexole

◈ *Rang & Dale 8th/494-95*

- *Selective D2/D3 receptor agonists*
- *Better tolerated & do not show the fluctuations in efficacy associated with levodopa*
- ***They do, however, cause somnolence*** *& sometimes hallucinations & recent evidence suggests that they may predispose to compulsive behaviours, such as excessive gambling, over-eating & sexual excess, related to the reward functions of dopamine*
- *A disadvantage of current dopamine agonists is their short plasma half-life(6-8 hr), requiring 3 times daily dosage, though slow release once daily formulations are now available*

Ropinirole & Pramipexole

◈ *KDT 7th/430-31*

- *Trial have found them to **afford symptom relief comparable to levodopa**. Some trials have noted lower incidence of dyskinesias & motor fluctuations among patients treated with these drugs than dose treated with levodopa*
- *It is longer acting than levodopa*
- ***Higher incidence of hallucination & sleepiness***

Ropinirole

◈ *Katzung 13th/478*

Another non-ergoline derivative, ropinirole is a relatively pure D² receptor agonist that is ***effective as monotherapy in patients with mild disease and as a means of smoothing the response to levodopa in patients with more advanced disease and response fluctuations.***

74. Ans. a. Gastric..., b. Formate..., d. Fomi..., e. Cause....

[Ref: KDT 7th/ 394-96; Katzung 13th/393; Pharmacology by Satoskar 24th/ 95-96]

Methanol

◈ *Katzung 13th/393*

- Methanol concentrations higher than 50 mg/dL are thought to be an absolute indication for hemodialysis and treatment with ***fomepizole or ethanol,*** although formate blood levels are a better indication of clinical pathology.
- Additional laboratory evidence includes ***metabolic acidosis with an elevated anion gap*** and osmolar gap. A decrease in serum bicarbonate is a uniform feature of severe methanol poisoning.
- The enzyme chiefly responsible for methanol oxidation in the liver is alcohol dehydrogenase. ***Ethanol has a higher affinity than methanol for alcohol dehydrogenase; thus, saturation of the enzyme with ethanol reduces formate production.***
- ***Ethanol is used intravenously as treatment for methanol poisoning.*** The dose-dependent characteristics of ethanol metabolism and the variability of ethanol metabolism require frequent monitoring of blood ethanol levels to ensure appropriate alcohol concentration.
- **Fomepizole,** an alcohol dehydrogenase inhibitor, is approved for the treatment of ethylene glycol poisoning and methanol poisoning.

Treatment of Methyl Alcohol

◈ *Pharmacology by Satoskar 24th/ 95-96, KDT 7th/ 394-96*

- *Hospitalisation, nursing care*
- ***Gastric lavage, activated charcoal***
- *Treatment of acidosis/hypoglycemia*
- *Inhibition of methanol metabolism- Giving ethyl alcohol & **fomepizole** (a specific inhibitor of alcohol dehydrogenase & drug of choice for methanol poisoning)*

- *Promote metabolic degradation of formate: folinic acid together with folic acid*
- *Diuretics, urine alkalinisation*
- *Hemodialysis in severe case*
- *Maintenance of nutrition*

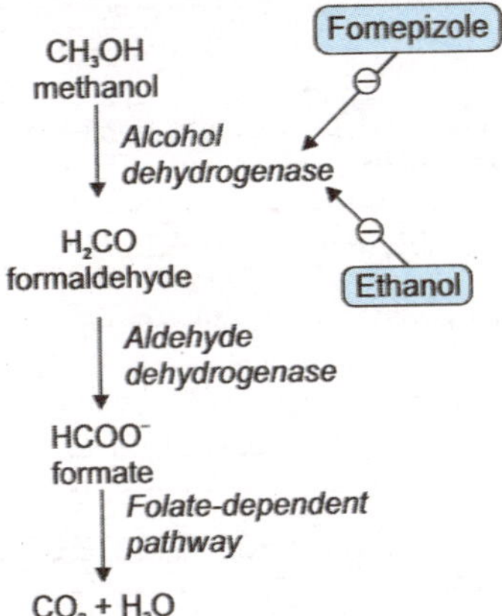

Fig: *(Katzung 13th/393):* Methanol is converted to the toxic metabolites formaldehyde and formate by alcohol dehydrogenase and aldehyde dehydrogenase. By inhibiting alcohol dehydrogenase, ethanol and fomepizole reduce the formation of toxic metabolites.

75. Ans. a. Hyperten..., b. Hemo..., c. Malena..., d. Cerebell....

[Ref: KDT 7th/871; Katzung 13th/ 937-38; Rang & Dale 8th/; Pharmacology by Satoskar 24th/840]

S/E of Bevacizumab: Hypertension; pulmonary hemorrhage (*Hemoptysis*); neovascularization progression gastrointestinal perforation; proteinuria; congestive heart failure"- *(G & G 11th/1377)*

"S/E of Bevacizumab:blood in urine or stools(*malena*), vomit that looks like blood or coffee grounds" *(www. rxlist. com/avastin-side-effect)*

S/E of Bevacizumab

◈ *KDT 7th/871*

- *Hypertension*
- *Arterial thromboembolism-heart attack & stroke*
- *Vessel injury & haemorrhages*
- *Heart failure*
- *Proteinuria*
- *Gastrointestinal perforation*
- *Healing defect*

Bevacizumab

◈ *Katzung 13th/937-38*

- It is a recombinant humanized monoclonal antibody that targets all forms of VEGF-A. This antibody binds to and prevents VEGF-A from interacting with the target VEGF receptors. Bevacizumab can be safely and effectively combined with 5-FU-, irinotecan-based chemotherapy, and oxaliplatin-based chemotherapy in the treatment of metastatic colorectal cancer.
- One potential advantage of this antibody is that it does not appear to exacerbate the toxicities typically observed with cytotoxic chemotherapy.
- The main safety concerns associated with bevacizumab include *hypertension, an increased incidence of arterial thromboembolic events (transient ischemic attack, stroke, angina, and myocardial infarction), wound healing complications and gastrointestinal perforations, and proteinuria.*

Table *(Katzung 13th/937)*

Bevacizumab	Inhibits binding of VEGF to VEGFR leading to inhibition of VEGF signaling; inhibits tumor vascular permeability but enhances tumor blood flow and drug delivery	Colorectal cancer, breast cancer, non-small cell lung cancer, renal cell cancer	Hypertension, infusion reaction	Arterial thromboembolic events, gastrointestinal perforations, wound healing complications, proteinuria

76. Ans. a. Ulcer..., b. Crohn's..., c. Rheum..., d. Psoari....

[Ref: Harrison 19th/1961;Neena Khanna 5th/58, 68;CMDT 2016/641; KDT 7th/883-84]

TNF-α Inhibitors are not given in Drug List of Lichen Planus Treatment *(Neena Khanna 5th/68)*

TNF-α Inhibitors: Use

◈ *KDT 7th/883-84 & Harrison 19th/1961*

- *Etanercept-Rheumatoid arthritis, severe/refractory ankylosing spondylitis, plaque psoriasis, polyarticular idiopathic juvenile arthritis*
- *Infliximab- refractory rheumatoid arthritis, ankylosing spondylitis, psoriasis, fistulating Crohn's disease, ulcerative colitis*
- *Adalimumab- Use as like infliximab*
- Certolizumab- *Crohn's disease(Harrison)*
- Golimumab - *ulcerative colitis (Harrison)*

"Psoriasis: Treatment includes TNF blockers like etanercept, infliximab, etc" (Neena Khanna 5th/58)

77. Ans. b. Trimethoprim....

[Ref:Harrison 19th/1045, 1048; Katzung 13th/ 876-77]

Stenotrophomonas maltophilia: Drug of first choice is trimethoprim-sulfamethoxazole. Alternative drugs are- *minocycline, ticarcillin-clavulanate, tigecycline, ceftazidime, quinolones" (Katzung 13th/ 876-77(Table))*

"The intrinsic resistance of *S. maltophilia* to most antibiotics renders infection difficult to treat. The antibiotics to which it is most often (although not uniformly) susceptible are *trimethoprim-sulfamethoxazole (TMP-SMX),* ticarcillin/

clavulanate, levofloxacin, and tigecycline. Consequently, a combination of TMPSMX and ticarcillin/clavulanate is recommended for initial therapy"-Harrison 19th/1048

MICROBIOLOGY

78. Ans. a. Thymic ap..., c. Lymphocyto..., d. Lymphocytopenia...

[Ref: Harrison 19th/2104-08; Ananthanarayan 9th/171-76; Jawetz 27th/146-47; Greenwood 16th/148]

"**T cell disorders** affect both cell-mediated and humoral immunity making the patient susceptible to ***viral, protozoal and fungal infections***. Viral infections such as those by cytomegalovirus and attenuated *measles* in the vaccine can be fatal in these patients" *(www. microbiologybook. org)*

"Lymphocytopenia is most often due to AIDS or undernutrition, but it also may be inherited or caused by various infections, drugs, or autoimmune disorders. ***Patients have recurrent viral, fungal, or parasitic infections***" *(www. merckmanuals.com)*

"**Hypogammaglobulinemia** leads to ***recurrent bacterial infections***. Viral & fungal infections are controlled by cell-mediated immunity, which is normal in hypogammaglobulinemic individual" *(https://books.google.co.in/books)*

Diagnosis of Primary Immunodeficiencies (PID)

Harrison 19th/2104

- The most frequent symptom prompting the diagnosis of a PID is the presence of recurrent or unusually severe infections.
- Infections of the respiratory tract (bronchi, sinuses) mostly suggest a defective antibody response. In general, invasive **bacterial infections** can result from ***complement deficiencies, signaling defects of innate immune responses, asplenia, or defective antibody responses.***
- **Viral infections, recurrent *Candida* infections, and opportunistic infections are generally suggestive of impaired T cell immunity**. Skin infections and deep-seated abscesses primarily reflect innate immune defects (such as chronic granulomatous disease); however, they may also appear in the autosomal dominant hyper-IgE syndrome.

Table *(Harrison 19th/2104)*: **Classification of Primary Immune Deficiency Diseases**

Deficiencies of the Adaptive Immune System	
T lymphocytes	
• Impaired development	Severe combined immune deficiencies (SCIDs) DiGeorge syndrome
• Impaired survival, migration, function	Severe combined immunodeficiencies Hyper-IgE syndrome (autosomal dominant) DOCK8 deficiency CD40 ligand deficiency Wiskott-Aldrich syndrome Ataxia-telangiectasia and other DNA repair deficiencies
B lymphocytes	
• Impaired development	XL and AR agammaglobulinemia
• Impaired function	Hyper-IgM syndrome Common variable immunodeficiency (CVID) IgA deficiency

Contd...

Table *(Ananthanarayan 9th/172)*: **Classification of Primary Immunodeficiency Syndromes**

A. Disorders of specific immunity

I. Humoral immunodeficiencies (B cell defects)

a. X-linked agammaglbulinemia
b. Transient hypogammaglobulinemia of infancy
c. Common variable immunodeficiency (late onset hypogammaglobulinemia)
d. Selective immunoglobulin deficiencies (IgA, IgM or IgG subclasses)
e. Immunodeficiencies with hyper-IgM
f. Trascobalamin II deficiency

II. Cellular immunodeficiencies (T cell defects)

a. Thymic hypoplalsia (Digeorge syndrome)
b Chronic mucocutaneous candidiasis
c. Purine nucleoside phosphorylase (PNP) deficiency

III. Combined immunodeficiencies (B and T cell defects)

a. Cellular immunodeficiency with abnormal immunoglobulin synthesis (Nezel of syndrome)
b. Ataxia telangiectasia
c. Wiskott–Aldrich syndrome
d. Immunodeficiency with thymoma
e. Immunodeficiency with short-limbed dwarfism
f. Episodic lymphopenia with lymphocytotoxin
g. Severe combined immunodeficiencies
   1. 'Swiss type' agammaglobulinemia
   2. Reticular dysgenesis of de vaal
   3. Adenosine deaminase (ADA) deficiency

B. Disorders of complement

a. Complement component deficiencies
b. Complement inhibitor deficiencies

C. Disorders of phagocytosis

a. Chronic granulomatous disease
b. Myeloperoxidase deficiency
c. Chediak–Higashi syndrome
d. Leukocyte G6PD deficiency
e. Job's syndrome
f. Tuftsin deficiency
g. Lazy leukocyte syndrome
h. Hyper-IgE syndrome
i. Actin binding protein deficiency
j. Shwachman's disease

79. Ans. a. SLE

[Ref: Ananthanarayan 9th/162-67; Robbins 9th/201; Jawetz 27th/145-46; Greenwood 16th/144]

Type 3 Hypersensitivity Reaction (Immune Complex Disease)

- *Ananthanarayan 9th/162*
- *It is two types-arthus reaction & serum sickness*
- *Here the damage is caused by antigen-antibody complexes. These may precipitate in & around small blood vessels causing damage to cells secondarily, or on membranes, interfering with their function*

Table *(Robbins 9th/201)*: **Mechanisms of Hypersensitivity Reactions**

Type	Immune Mechanisms	Histopathologic Lesions	Prototypical Disorders
Immediate (type I) hypersensitivity	Production of IgE → antibody immediate release of vasoactive amines and other mediators from mast cells; later recruitment of inflammatory cells	Vascular dilation, edema, smooth muscle contraction, mucus production, tissue injury, inflammation	Anaphylaxis: allergies; bronchial asthma (atopic forms)
Antibody-mediated type(II) hypersensitivity	Production of IgG, IgM → binds to antigen on target cell or tissue → phagocytosis or lysis of target cell by activated complement or Fc receptors; recruitment of leukocytes	Phagocytosis and lysis of cells: inflammation; in some diseases, functional derangements without cell or tissue injury	Autoimmune hemolytic anemia; Goodpasture syndrome
Immune complex-mediated (type III) hypersensitivity	Deposition of antigen-antibody complexes → complement activation →recruitment of leukocytes by complement products and Fc receptors → release of enzymes and other toxic molecules	Inflammation, necrotizing vasculitis (fibrinoid necrosis)	Systemic lupus erythematosus; some forms of glomerulonephritis; serum sickness; Arthus reaction
Cell-mediated (type IV) hypersensitivity	Activated T lymphocytes → (1) release of cytokines, inflammation and macrophage activation: (2) T: cell-mediated cytotoxicity	Perivascular cellular infiltrates: edema: granuloma formation: cell destruction	Contact dermatitis: multiple sclerosis: type 1 diabetes tuberculosis

Table *(Ananthanarayan 9th/162)*: **Types of Hypersensitivity Reactions and their Features**

Type of Reaction	Clinical syndrome	Time required for manifestation	Mediators
Type I: IgE type	1. Anaphylaxis 2. Atopy	Minutes	IgE: histamine and other pharmacological agents IgG: IgM, C
Type II: Cytolytic and cytotoxic	Antibody mediated damage-thrombocytopania, agranulocytosis, hemolytic anemia, etc.	Variable: hours to days	
Type III: Immune complex	1. Arthus reaction 2. Serum sickness	Variable: hours to days	IgG: IgM, C, leucocytes
Type IV: Delayed hypersensitivity	1. Tuberculin 2. Contact dermatitis	Hours to days	T cells; Lymphokines; macrophages

80. Ans. a. Brucella, b. Gonorrhoea, c. Syphilis

[Ref: Harrison 19th/1134, 194e-2, 1005; Ananthanarayan 9th/341]

"**Brucella:** The incubation period is usually ***about 10-30 days***, but may be sometimes be very prolonged" *(Ananthanarayan 9th/341)*

"**Brucella**: The incubation period varies from 1 week to several months, and the onset of fever and other symptoms may be abrupt or insidious" *(Harrison 19th/194e-2)*

"**Syphilis:** *Clinical disease sets in after an incubation period of about a month(range 10-90 days)" (Ananthanarayan 9th/372)*

"**Syphilis***:* The median incubation period in humans (~21 days) suggests an average inoculum of 500–1000 infectious organisms for naturally acquired disease; the incubation period rarely exceeds 6 weeks" *(Harrison 19th/1134)*

Primary syphilis*: Incubation period 3 weeks(10-90 days)- (Jawetz 27th/795)*

Hepatitis B*: The incubation is long, about* ***1-6 months"*** *(Ananthanarayan 9th/542)*

Leishmaniasis*: Incubation period is usually* ***2-6 months,*** *occasionally it may be short as 10 days or as long as 2 years" (Panikar Parasitology 7th/52)*

Gonococcal infection ***in men:*** *Acute urethritis is the most common clinical manifestation of gonorrhea in male patients. The* ***usual incubation period after exposure is 2-7 days,*** *although the interval can be longer & some men remain asymptomatic (Harrison 19th/1005)*

81. Ans. a. Ziehl-Neelsen techni..., b. Auramine-rhodamine sta..., d. Kinyoun stain.....

[Ref: Harrison 19th/1113; Ananthanarayan 9th/346-48; Lippincott Microbiology 3rd/ 21; Jawetz 27th/38; Text Book of Diagnostic microbiology by Connie R. Mohan 3rd/691;Greenwood 16th/15]

"When stained with ***carbol fuchsin by Ziehl-Neelsen method*** *or by fluorescent dyes (****Auramine O, Rhodamine****), mycobacterium tuberculosis reist decolourisation by 20% sulphuric acid & are therefore called acid fast" (Ananthanarayan 9th/346)*

"Ziehl-Neelsen method & phenol-auramine procedures are methods of great practical importance in diagnosis of mycobacterial diseases" *(Greenwood 16th/15)*

Some Acid Fast Staining Techniques

- Ziehl–Neelsen stain (Classic and modified bleach types)
- Kinyoun stain
- For color blind people (or in backgrounds where detecting red bacteria is difficult) Victoria Blue can be substituted for carbol fuchsin and Picric acid can be used as the counter stain instead of methylene blue, and rest of Kinyoun technique can be used.
- Various bacterial spore staining techniques using Kenyon e. g.
    - Moeller's method
    - Dorners method (acid alcohol decolorizer) without the Schaeffer–Fulton modification (decolorize by water)
    - Detergent method, using Tergitol 7, nonionic polyglycol ether surfactants type NP-7
    - Fite stain
        - Fite-Faraco Staining
        - Wade Fite staining
- Ellis and Zabrowarny stain (no Phenol/carbolic acid)
- Auramine-rhodamine stain
- Auramine phenol stain

"In pathology, the **Grocott-Gomori's (or Gömöri) methenamine silver stain,** is a popular staining method in histology. It is used widely as a screen for fungal organisms. Particularly useful in staining carbohydrates. It can be used to identify the yeast-like fungus *Pneumocystis jiroveci* which causes a form of pneumonia called Pneumocystis Pneumonia (PCP) or Pneumocystosis. The cell walls of these organisms are outlined by the brown to black stain"- wikipedia. org

"**Gram-indeterminate bacteria** do not respond predictably to Gram staining and, therefore, cannot be determined as either gram-positive or gram-negative; they tend to stain unevenly, appearing partially gram-positive and partially gram-negative, or unstained by either crystal violet or safranin. Examples include many species of ***Mycobacterium***, including *M. tuberculosis* and *M. leprae*. Gram-indeterminate bacteria are best stained using acid-fast staining techniques. Staining older cultures (over 48 hours) can lead to false gram-variable results, probably due to changes in the cell wall with ageing" *(wiki)*

"The **Kinyoun method**, or **Kinyoun stain**, is an acid-fast procedure used to stain any species of the genus *Mycobacterium* and *Nocardia* species. It involves the application of a primary stain (carbol fuchsin), a decolorizer (acid-alcohol), and a counter stain (methylene blue)" *(en. wikipedia. org)*

AFB Kinyoun Kit (Cold Method): Method of staining acid-fast microorganisms, specifically mycobacterium. Procedure is similar to Ziehl-Neelson stain, but does not involve heating the slides" *(http://www. polysciences. com/ Catalog/)*

"The traditional method—light microscopy of specimens stained with ***Ziehl-Neelsen basic*** fuchsin dyes—is nevertheless satisfactory, although time-consuming. Most modern laboratories processing large numbers of diagnostic specimens use ***auramine-rhodamine*** staining and fluorescence microscopy"*(Harrison 19th/1113)*

"Mycobacteria cannot be classified as ***either gram-positive or gram-negative***. The **Ziehl-Neelsen technique** of staining is employed for identification of acid-fast bacteria. In smears of sputum or sections of tissue, mycobacteria can be demonstrated by yellow-orange fluorescence after staining with fluorochrome stains (eg, ***auramine, rhodamine***)" *(Jawetz 27th/38)*

82. Ans. d. Botulism, e. Typhoid...

[Ref: Park 23rd/657]

Food-Borne Diseases *(Park 23rd/657)*

The term" food-borne disease" is defined as: "A disease, usually either infectious or toxic in nature, caused by agents that enter the body through the ingestion of food. " With the catering systems, food-borne diseases are on the increase throughout the world. Food-borne diseases may be classified as:

A. Food-borne intoxications

1. Due to naturally occurring toxins in some foods
    a. Lathyrism (beta oxallyl amino-alanine)
    b. Endemic ascitis (Pyrrolizidine alkaloids)
2. Due to toxins produced by certain bacteria
    a. Botulism
    b. Staphyloccus poisons
3. Due to toxins produced by some fungi
    a. Aflatoxin
    b. Ergot
    c. Fusarium toxins
4. Food-borne chemical poisoning
    a. Heavy metals, e.g., mercury (usually in fish), cadmium (in certain shellfish) and lead (in canned food)
    b. Oils, petroleum derivatives and solvents (e.g., Trycresyn phosphate or TCP)
    c. Migrant chemicals from package materials
    d. Asbestos
    e. Pesticide residues (DDT, BHC)

B. Food–borne infections

Group	Examples of illness in each group
1. Bacterial diseases	***Typhoid fever***, Paratyphoid fever, salmonellosis, staphylococcal intoxication, *C. Perfringens* illness, ***botulism***, B. cereus food poisoning, E. coli diarrhoes, non-cholera vibrio illness, V. parahaemolyticus infection, streptococcal infection. Shigellosis brucellosis

Contd...

2. Viral diseases	Viral hepatitis, gastroenteritis
3. Parasites	Taeniasis hydatidosis, trichinosis, ascariasis, amoebiasis, oxyuriasis

83. Ans. a. Burkholderia..., b. Burkhomelia..., e. Pseudomonas Aeru......

[Ref: Harrison 19th/1048; Ananthanarayan 9th/316-17; Jawetz 27th/248, Greenwood 16th/ 286; medind. nic. in]

"The ***Burkholderia cepacia complex (BCC) and Stenotrophomonas maltophilia*** are closely related groups of ***non-fermenting gram-negative bacilli*** (NFGNBs) having a similar spectrum of infections ranging from superficial to deep-seated and disseminated infections. Identification of these ***lysine decarboxylase-positive NFGNBs*** lags behind in most Indian laboratories. A simplified identification scheme was devised for these two pathogens that allowed us to isolate them with an increasing frequency at our tertiary care institute" *(www. ncbi. nlm. nih. gov)*

"Non-fermenting Gram negative bacilli (NFGNB) includs *Pseudomonas* spp., *Acinetobacter* spp., *Stenotrophomonas maltophilia, Burkholderia cepacia* complex (BCC)" *(www. ijpmonline. org)*

"***Burkholderia cepacia* complex (BCC)**, or simply ***Burkholderia cepacia*** is a group of catalase-producing, lactose-nonfermenting, Gram-negative bacteria composed of at least 18 different species, including *B. cepacia, B. multivorans, B. cenocepacia, B. vietnamiensis, B. stabilis, B. ambifaria, B. dolosa, B. anthina, B. pyrrocinia* and *B. ubonensis*"*(wiki)*

Burkholderia cepacia is oxidase positive & lysine decarboxylase positive and produce acid from glucose *(Jawetz 27th/248)*

"Stenotrophomonas maltophilia is oxidase negative & positive for lysine decarboxylase" *(Jawetz 27th/249)*

"The *Burkholderia cepacia* complex (BCC) and *Stenotrophomonas maltophilia* are a closely related group of ***non-fermenting gram-negative bacilli*** (NFGNBs) found in many niches of both natural and clinical environments" *(medind. nic. in)*

84. Ans. c. Cryptococcus

[Ref: Harrison 19th/1339-42; Ananthanarayan 9th/613-14; Jawetz 27th/ 687-89]

Cryptococcus

◈ *Harrison 19th/1339-42*

- *Cryptococcus*, a genus of ***yeast-like fungi***, is the etiologic agent of cryptococcosis. There are two species, *C. neoformans* and *C. gattii*, each of which can cause cryptococcosis in humans.
- Cryptococcosis should be included in the differential diagnosis when any patient presents with findings suggestive of chronic meningitis. Concern about cryptococcosis is heightened by a ***history of headache and neurologic symptoms in a patient with an underlying immunosuppressive disorder or state that is associated with an increased incidence of cryptococcosis, such as advanced HIV infection or solid organ transplantation.***
- The clinical manifestations of cryptococcosis reflect the site of fungal infection. Although infection can affect any tissue or organ, the majority of cases that come to clinical attention involve the CNS and/or the lungs. CNS involvement usually presents as signs and symptoms of chronic meningitis, such as ***headache, fever, lethargy, sensory deficits, memory deficits, cranial nerve paresis, vision deficits, and meningismus.***
- Cryptococcal meningitis differs from bacterial meningitis in that many *Cryptococcus*-infected patients present with ***symptoms of several weeks' duration***. In addition, classic characteristics of meningeal irritation, such as meningismus, may be absent in cryptococcal meningitis. Indolent cases can present as subacute dementia. Meningeal cryptococcosis can lead to sudden catastrophic vision loss.
- Pulmonary cryptococcosis usually presents as ***cough***, increased sputum production, and chest pain. Patients infected with *C. gattii* can present with granulomatous pulmonary masses known as *cryptococcomas*. Fever develops in a minority of cases.
- Like CNS disease, pulmonary cryptococcosis can follow an indolent course, and the majority of cases probably do not come to clinical attention. In fact, many cases are discovered incidentally during the workup of an abnormal chest radiograph obtained for other diagnostic purposes.
- Pulmonary cryptococcosis can be associated with antecedent diseases such as malignancy, diabetes, and tuberculosis.

Cryptococcus

◈ *Ananthanarayan 9th/613-14*

- *Infection can be acquired by inhalation of desiccated yeasts(or basidiospores)* ***from feces of pigeon & other birds***
- *Microscopy: Direct microscopic examination of India ink-stained wet films of material from lesions reveals capsulated, budding yeast cells; the capsule are prominent in the India ink preparation*
- *C. meningitis is often seen in* ***AIDS***

85. Ans. a. Veillonella b. Anerobic microc..., c. Geotrichum d. Gemella

[Ref: Ananthanarayan 9th/622; Lippincott Microbiology 3rd/ 8-9; Jawetz 27th/171-73]

"More than 700 bacterial species or phylotypes, of which over 50% have not been cultivated, have been detected in the oral cavity. Thirteen new phylotypes were identified. Species common to all sites belonged to the genera **Gemella, Granulicatella, Streptococcus, and Veillonella**" *(http://www. ncbi. nlm. nih. gov/pmc)*

Normal Flora of Mouth & Upper Respiratory Tract

◈ *Ananthanarayan 9th/622*

- The mouth contains a plethora of organisms- pigmented & non-pigmented micrococci; some of which are aerobic, gram positive, aerobic, spore bearing bacilli, coliforms, proteus & lactobacilli
- The gum pocket b/w the teeths, & the crypts of the nostrils have a wide spectrum of ***anaerobic flora- anerobic micro-***

cocci, microaerophilic & anaerobic streptococci, vibrios, fusiform bacilli, corynebactrium species, actinomyces, leptothrix, mycoplasma, Neisseria & bacteriodes are all found in varying extents. Among fungi, candida & geotrichum have been reported

"**Veillonella** are gram-negative anaerobic cocci. It is thought that this species thrives in the acidic environment of caries and is thought to slow the development of ***dental caries***. It converts the acidic products of other species to less acidic products"

Normal Flora of the Mouth & Upper Respiratory Tract

◈ *Jawetz 27th/171-73*

- The mucous membranes of the mouth and pharynx are often sterile at birth but may be contaminated by passage through the birth canal. Within 4–12 hours after birth, ***viridans streptococci*** become established as the most prominent members of the resident flora and remain so for life.
- Early in life, aerobic and anaerobic staphylococci, gram-negative diplococci (neisseriae, *Moraxella catarrhalis*), diphtheroids, and occasional lactobacilli are added. When teeth begin to erupt, the anaerobic spirochetes, *Prevotella* species (especially *P melaninogenica*), *Fusobacterium* species, *Rothia* species, and *Capnocytophaga* species establish themselves, along with some anaerobic vibrios and lactobacilli.
- *Actinomyces* species are normally present in tonsillar tissue and on the gingivae in adults, and various protozoa may also be present. Yeasts (*Candida* species) occur in the mouth.
- Infections of the mouth and respiratory tract are usually caused by mixed oronasal flora, including anaerobes. Periodontal infections, perioral abscesses, sinusitis, and mastoiditis may involve predominantly *Prevotella melaninogenica*, fusobacteria, and peptostreptococci.

86. Ans. a. Peripheral blood smear...

[Ref: Harrison 19th/1385-86; Paniker Parasitology 7th/85;Chatterjee Parasitology 13th/137; Lippincott Microbiology 3rd/225; Jawetz 27th/708; Greenwood 16th/599]

"***Microscopic examination of stained blood smear is gold standard test for babesiosis***" *(www. cdc. gov)*

"**Diagnosis of babesiosis** *is primarily done by* ***examination of blood films stained with Leishman or Giemsa stain***" *(Paniker Parasitology 7th/85)*

Serology: ***It is useful to confirm the diagnosis***" *(Paniker Parasitology 7th/85)*

"***Babesiosis diagnosis by blood smears, tetrad forms(Maltese cross) inside RBCs***" *(Jawetz 27th/708)*

"**Laboratory Findings of babeiosis:** ***Identification of the intraerythrocytic parasite on Giemsa stained blood smears establishes the diagnosis***. These can be confused with malaria parasites, but the morphology is distinctive. An indirect immunofluorescent antibody test for B microti is available from the CDC; antibody is detectable within 2–4 weeks after the onset of symptoms and persists for months. Diagnosis can also be made by PCR or by inoculation of hamsters or gerbils" *(CMDT 2016/1497)*

Diagnosis of Babesiosis

◈ *Harrison 19th/1385-86*

- ***A specific diagnosis usually is established by microscopic examination of Giemsa-stained thin blood smears***. *Babesia* trophozoites appear round, pear-shaped, or ameboid. The ring form is most common and lacks the central brownish deposit (hemozoin) typical of *Plasmodium falciparum* trophozoites. Other distinguishing features are the absence of schizonts and gametocytes and the occasional presence of tetrads ("Maltese cross").
- If parasites cannot be identified by microscopy and the disease is still suspected, amplification of the babesial 18S rRNA gene by polymerase chain reaction (PCR) is recommended. Quantitative PCR has greatly lowered the threshold for detection of *B. microti* DNA.
- ***Serology can suggest or confirm the diagnosis of babesiosis.*** An indirect immunofluorescent antibody test for *B. microti* is most commonly used.

Diagnostic Tests

◈ *(wiki)*

- ***As a protozoan parasite, the most effective way to identify Babesia*** infection is through blood sample testing. It is important to pay specific attention to particular morphologies of *Babesia* in blood smears because its substantial similarity to the malarial parasite*Plasmodium falciparum* results in many patients suffering from babesiosis being misdiagnosed.
- To supplement a blood smear, diagnoses should be made with an indirect fluorescent antibody (IFA) test.

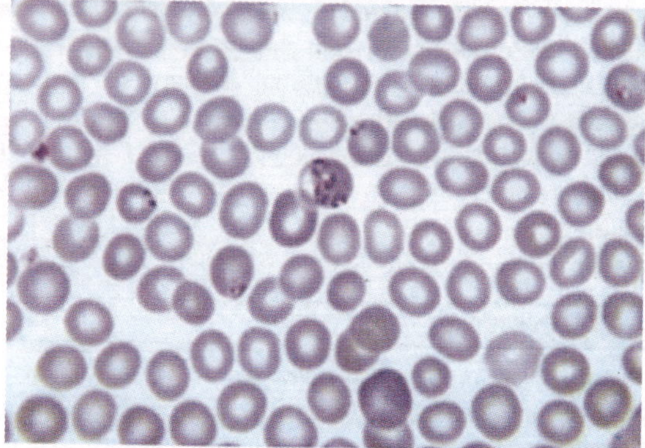

Fig: *(CMDT 2016/1497):* Blood smear showing Babesia spp. rings with basophilic stippling

87. Ans. a. Common in pregnant..., b. Common in elderly..., d. Common in newborns, e. Ampicillin....

[Ref: Harrison 19th/982-84; Ananthanarayan 9th/395-96; Lippincott Microbiology 3rd/ 98; Jawetz 27th/ 197-98; Greenwood 16th/195-96]

"Listeria infections are ***most common in pregnant women, fetuses and newborns***, and in immunocompromised ***individuals, such as older adults*** and patients receiving corticosteroids" *(Lippincott Microbiology 3rd/ 98)*

"The disease affects pregnant women, newborns, adults with weakened immune systems, and the elderly" *(wiki)*

"**Listeria infections**: *Ampicillin, cotrimoxazole & gentamicin are effective. Meningitis can be treated with penicillin*" *(Ananthanarayan 9th/395-96)*

Listeria Monocytogenes

◈ *Harrison 19th/982-84*

- "*Listeria monocytogenes* is a food-borne pathogen that can cause serious infections, particularly in pregnant women and immunocompromised individuals"
- Timely diagnosis requires that the illness be considered in groups at risk: ***pregnant women; elderly persons; neonates; individuals immunocompromised by organ transplantation, cancer, or treatment with tumor necrosis factor antagonists or glucocorticoids; and patients with a variety of chronic medical conditions, including alcoholism, diabetes, renal disease, and rheumatologic and hepatic illnesses.***
- Meningitis in older adults (especially with parenchymal brain involvement or subcortical brain abscess) should trigger consideration of *L. monocytogenes* infection and treatment. Listeriosis occasionally affects healthy, young, nonpregnant individuals.
- Infection in Pregnant Women: Listeriosis in pregnancy is a severe and important infection. The usual presentation is a nonspecific acute or subacute febrile illness with myalgias, arthralgias, backache, and headache. Pregnant women with listeriosis are usually bacteremic.
- ***Ampicillin is the drug of choice***, although penicillin also is highly active. TMP-SMX, given IV, is the best alternative for the penicillin allergic patient

88. Ans. b. Main vector in India..., e. Pigs are amplifier host....

[Ref: Park 23rd/284-87;Harrison 19th/1315; Ananthanarayan 9th/520-22, 519]

In 2006, epidemic spread was of chikungunya (not JE), in India

"During 2006, there was a large outbreak of **chikungunya** in India, with 1. 39 million officially reported cases spread over 16 states; attack rates were estimated at 45% in some areas" *(Park 23rd/289)*

"***Central Research Institute, Kasuali, has developed Japanese encephalitis vaccine indigenously***. It is a mouse brain killed vaccine and 3 doses are required to produce primary immunization. Two doses are administered sub-cutaneously within a gap of 7-14 days followed by third dose any time after one month and before one year of the second dose. A booster is required after 3 years" *(http://www. nvbdcp. gov. in/je7. html)*

"India on Friday (Oct 4, 2013) ***launched its first indigenous vaccine*** to protect children from Japanese encephalitis. Until now, the country has been importing the vaccine from China. The Vero cell-derived purified inactivated JE vaccine–JENVAC, which received manufacturing and marketing approvals from the Drug Controller General of India, is the first vaccine to be manufactured in the public-private partnership mode between the Indian Council of Medical Research and Bharat Biotech" *(http://www. thehindu. com/news)*

Japanese Encephalitis

◈ *Park 23rd/284-87; Ananthanarayan 9th/520-22*

- *Culicine mosquitoes, notably C. tritaeniorhynchus(principal vector), C. Vishnui & C. gelidus along with some anophelines have been incriminated as vector of JE*
- *In India, JE was first recognized in 1955 in Tamil Nadu. JE remained confined to southeastern parts of India till 1973, when it caused a large outbreak in West Bengal. From 1976, there have been periodic outbreaks of the disease in various parts of India*
- ***Pigs are amplifier host***

Japanese Encephalitis

◈ *Harrison 19th/1315*

- The virus is particularly common in areas where irrigated rice fields attract the natural avian vertebrate hosts and provide abundant breeding sites for mosquitoes such as ***Culex tritaeniorhynchus***, which transmit the virus to humans.
- ***Additional amplification by pigs***, which suffer abortion, and horses, which develop encephalitis, may be significant as well. Vaccination of these additional amplifying hosts may reduce the transmission of the virus.
- Effective vaccines are available.

89. Ans. a. Anal carcioma, b. Hodgkin's lymphoma

[Ref: Harrison 19th/1268; Ananthanarayan 9th/576-77; Lippincott Microbiology 3rd/ 302]

Neoplastic Diseases

◈ *Harrison 19th/1268*

- The neoplastic diseases considered to be AIDS defining conditions are ***Kaposi's sarcoma, non-Hodgkin's lymphoma, and invasive cervical carcinoma.***
- In addition, there is also an increase in the incidence of a variety of **non-AIDS-defining malignancies** including ***Hodgkin's disease; multiple myeloma; leukemia; melanoma;and cervical, brain, testicular, oral, lung, gastric, liver, renal, and anal cancers.***

90. Ans. b. Crescentric shaped..., c. Delicate ring present..., d. Small & multiple....

[Ref: Harrison 19th/1369; Parasitology by Chatterjee 13th/103; Parasitolgy by Paniker 7th/75]

P. falciparum

◈ *Parasitolgy by Paniker 7th/75, 67*

- *Ring stage-* ***delicate, small****, double chromatin, multiple rings common, Accole forms found*
- *Macrogametocyte- Crescentric, deep blue cytoplasm, large diffuse nucleus*
- *The mature gametocytes are round in shape, except in P. falciparum, in which they are crescent-shaped*
- *Schizont: Fills two-third of* ***red blood cell which is not enlarged****-* Chatterjee 13th/103

- *Infected erythrocyte- **Normal size,** Maurer's cleft, sometimes basophilic stippling*
- *Erythrocyte preference- young erythrocyte, but can infect all stages*

Table *(Harrison 19th/1369)*: **Characteristics of *Plasmodium* Species Infecting Humans**

	Finding for Indicated Species			
Characteristic	***P. falciparum***	***P. vivax***	***P. ovale***	***P. malariae***
Duration of intrahepatic phase (days)	5. 5	8	9	15
Number of merozoites released per infected hepatocyte	30, 000	10, 000	15, 000	15, 000
Duration of erythrocytic cycle (hours)	48	48	50	72
Red cell preference	Younger cells (but can invade cells of all ages)	Reticulocytes and cells up to 2 weeks old	Reticulocytes	Older cells
Morphology	***Usually only ring*** forms; banana-shaped gametocytes	Irregularly shaped large rings and trophozoites; enlarged erythrocytes; Schüffner's dots	Infected erythrocytes, enlarged and oval with tufted ends; Schüffner's dots	Band or rectangular forms of trophozoites common
Pigment color	Black	Yellow-brown	Dark brown	Brown-black
Ability to cause relapses	No	Yes	Yes	No

91. Ans. c. More common in.... e. Metronidazole is effective...

[Ref: Parasitology by Chatterjee 13th/47-48;Parasitolgy by Paniker 7th/32-33;Harrison 19th/1406]

Giardiasis

❖ *Parasitology by Chatterjee 13th/47-48*

- *The person having **hypo- & agammaglobulinemia** & malnourished persons are **more susceptible to giardiasis***
- *Metronidazole, trimidazole, furazoilidone have been found to be effective for giardiasis*
- *G. lamblia is typically seen within the crypts of duodenal & jejunal mucosa. **It does not invade the tissue,** but remains tightly adhered to intestinal epithelium by means of the sucking disc (Parasitology by Paniker 7th/32)*
- *Often they are asymptomatic, but in some cases, Giardia may lead to **mucus diarrhea,** fat malabsorption (steatorrhea), dull epigastric pain & flatulence. The stool contains excess mucus & fat but **no blood** (Parasitolgy by Paniker 7th/32)*
- ***Increased susceptibility:** Achlorohydia, use of cannabis, blood group A, chronic pancreatitis, malnutrition & **immune deficiency as hypogammaglobulinemia***

Giardiasis

❖ *Harrison 19th/1406*

- Because patients with ***hypogammaglobulinemia*** suffer from prolonged, severe infections that are poorly responsive to treatment, humoral immune responses appear to be important.
- Prominent early symptoms include ***diarrhea***, abdominal pain, bloating, belching, flatus, nausea, and vomiting. Although diarrhea is common, upper intestinal manifestations such as nausea, vomiting, bloating, and abdominal pain may predominate.
- Fever, the ***presence of blood*** and/or mucus in the stools, and other signs and symptoms of colitis are uncommon and suggest a different diagnosis or a concomitant illness.
- Cure rates with ***metronidazole*** are usually >90%. Tinidazole may be more effective than metronidazole. Albendazole is as effective as metronidazole and is associated with fewer side effects.

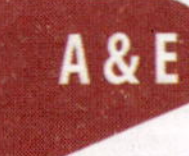

92. Ans. b. CSF specimen of.... e. Meningococcal rash.

[Ref: Harrison 19th/985; Robbins 9th/365; Ananthanarayan 9th/230, 396, 229, 261;Greenwood 16th/236-37]

*"Diphtheria: **Although the bacterial invasion remains localized,** with **entry of exotoxin into the blood** & its systemic distribution, there may fatty change in the myocardium with isolated myofiber necrosis" (Robbins 9th/365)*

*"In case of diphthitic myocarditis, the myocardial injury is a consequence of **diphtheria toxin** released by causal organism, C. diphtheriae" (Robbins 9th/571)*

*"When tetanus occurs naturally, the tetanus bacilli stay at the site of initial infection & are not generally invasive. **Toxin diffuses** to affect the relevant level of the spinal cord(local tetanus) & then to affect the entire system(generalized tetanus). Gram smears of the **wound exudate & any necrotic material** may show the typical drumstick bacilli"- Greenwood 16th/236-37*

Tetanus: *Laboratory diagnosis may be demonstration of C. tetani by microscopy, culture or toxigenicity- Ananthanarayan 9th/261*

"Culture of C. tetani from a wound provide supportive evidence" *(Harrison 19th/985)*

Listeria monocytogenes: Laboratory diagnosis is established by the ***isolation of the bacillus*** from appropriate clinical material such as cervical & vaginal secretions, lochia, meconium, cord blood, blood & ***cerebrospinal fluid*** by incubating under 5% CO_2 environment on blood agar" *(Ananthanarayan 9th/396)*

"***L. monocytogenes*:** The diagnosis is typically made by culture of blood, **cerebrospinal fluid (CSF),** or amniotic fluid. *L. monocytogenes* may be confused with "diphtheroids" or pneumococci in gram-stained CSF or may be gram-variable and confused with *Haemophilus* spp. Serologic tests and polymerase chain reaction assays are not clinically useful diagnostic tools at present" *(Harrison 19th/983)*

"***Petechial lesion*: *Meningococci*** *may sometimes be demonstrated in petechial lesions by microscopy & culture" (Ananthanarayan 9th/230)*

"**Rheumatic valvulitis** is manifestation of rheumatic heart disease. Rheumatic fever is an acute, ***immunologically mediated, multisystem inflammatory disease*** classically occurring a few week after an episode of group A streptococcal infection" *(Robbins 9th/557-59)*

"**Acute rheumatic fever**: This occur after 1-3 week after acute infection of S. pyogens so that ***organism may not be detectable*** when sequelae set in. Essential lesion is characterized by Aschoff nodules" *(Ananthanarayan 9th/214)*

93. Ans. a. Characteristic..., b. Type 5 Human..., d. Cause congenital....

[Ref: Harrison 19th/1190-91; Ananthanarayan 9th/473-74; Jawetz 27th/470-74]

Cytomegalovirus (Human Herpesvirus type 5)

- It is cytomegalic (***not lymphoproliferative***, which occur in HHV4, 6 & 7)
- Characterized by ***enlargement of infected cells***
- Congenital infection- Intrauterine infection leads to fetal death or cytomegalic inclusion disease of newborn which is often fatal

Cytomegalovirus (Human Herpesvirus Type 5)

◈ *Harrison 19th/1190-91*

- Human CMV is one of several related species-specific viruses that cause similar diseases in various animals. All are associated with the production of ***characteristic enlarged cells***—hence the name *cytomegalovirus*.
- **Cytomegalic cells** in vivo (presumed to be ***infected epithelial cells***) are two to four times larger than surrounding cells and often contain an 8- to 10-μm intranuclear inclusion that is eccentrically placed and is surrounded by a clear halo, producing an "***owl's eye" appearance.***
- In addition to inducing ***severe birth defects***, CMV causes a wide spectrum of disorders in older children and adults, ranging from an asymptomatic subclinical infection to a *mononucleosis syndrome* in healthy individuals to disseminated disease in immunocompromised patients.
- Primary infection with CMV in late childhood or adulthood is often associated with a vigorous T lymphocyte response that may contribute to the development of a mononucleosis syndrome similar to that which follows infection with Epstein-Barr virus. The hallmark of such infection is the appearance of ***atypical lymphocytes in the peripheral blood; these cells are predominantly activated CD8+ T lymphocytes.***
- Polyclonal activation of B cells by CMV contributes to the development of rheumatoid factors and other autoantibodies during mononucleosis.

94. Ans. b. Cold agglutinin..., e. Cough is typically....

[Ref: Harrison 19th/1163-64; Ananthanarayan 9th/388-89; Lippincott Microbiology 3rd/173; Jawetz 27th/337-38 Greenwood 16th/ 385]

"Cold hemagglutinins for group O human erythrocyte appear in about 50% of untreated patients, in rising titer, with the maximum reached in the third or fourth week after onset. A titer of 1:64 or more supports the diagnosis of M. pneumoniae infection" *(Jawetz 27th/338)*

Mycoplasma Pneumonia

◈ *Lippincott Microbiology 3rd/173; Jawetz 27th/337-38; Greenwood 16th/ 385*

Extrapulmonary manifestations- hemolytic anaemia, Stevens-Johnson syndrome, erythema multiforme & other rashes, meningitis or encephalitis (& other neurological sequelae), arthralgia, myocarditis, pericarditis, pancreatitis, polyneuritis etc.

Mycoplasma Pneumonia (Primary Atypical Pneumonia)

◈ *Ananthanarayan 9th/388-89*

- The disease is typically tracheobronchitis. Acute pharyngitis is uncommon & only a third of the patients develop pneumonia
- The disease is characterized by ***paucity of respiratory signs*** on physical examination but radiological evidence of consolidation, which is usually patchy, involving one of the lower lobes, starting at the hilum & fanning out to the periphery is seen
- The disease is usually self-limiting, recovery occurring in 1-2 weeks, but can be prolonged
- The disease is found worldwide & at all ages
- Transmisson is by droplets of nasopharyngeal secretions

Upper Respiratory Tract Infections and Pneumonia

◈ *Harrison 19th/1163-64*

- Acute *M. pneumonia* infections generally manifest as pharyngitis, tracheobronchitis, reactive airway disease/wheezing, or a *nonspecific upper respiratory syndrome.*
- Pneumonia develops in 3–13% of infected individuals; its onset is usually gradual, occurring over several days, but may be more abrupt.
- The ***cough is typically nonproductive***, but some patients produce sputum. Headache, malaise, chills, and fever are noted in the majority of patients.
- 'On physical examination, wheezes or rales are detected in ~80% of patients with *M. pneumoniae* pneumonia. In many patients, however, pneumonia can be diagnosed only by chest radiography.
- The most common radiographic pattern is that of peribronchial pneumonia with thickened bronchial markings, streaks of interstitial infiltration, and areas of subsegmental atelectasis.
- Hematologic manifestations of *M. pneumoniae* infection include hemolytic anemia, aplastic anemia, **cold**

agglutinins, disseminated intravascular coagulation, and hypercoagulopathy. When anemia does occur, it generally develops in the second or third week of illness

- ***Although of historical interest, the measurement of cold agglutinin titers is no longer recommended for the diagnosis of M. pneumonia infection because the findings are nonspecific*** and assays specific for *M. pneumoniae* are now available.

95. Ans. a. In 1999..., c. Bivalent... d. Primary..., e. Coxasackie...

[Ref: Park 23rd/ 202-09; Harrison 19th/1289-91; Ananthanarayan 9th/485]

Polio

◈ *Park 23rd/ 202-09*

- Vaccine associated paralytic poliomyelitis(VAPP) occurs in both OPV recipients & their unimmunized contacts; it is frequently associated with ***Sabin 3*** (60% cases), followed by Sabin 2 & Sabin 1
- Of the 3 strains of wild poliovirus, ***wild poliovirus type 2 was eradicated in 1999*** & case numbers of type 3 are down to the lowest-ever levels with the last case reported in Nov 2012 from Nigeria
- ***Bivalent OPV contains type 1 & type 3 strain***
- The WHO programme on immunization(EPI) & the national immunization programme in India recommended a ***primary course of 3 doses*** of OPV at one-month intervals, commencing the first dose when infant is 6 weeks old. It is recommended that a dose of OPV(zero-dose) is required to be given to all children delivered in health institution before their discharge from hospital

"**Poliovirus type 1** *is responsible for* ***most epidemics of paralytic poliomyelitis.*** *Type 3 also causes epidemics to a lesser extent.. Type 2 usually causes inapparent infections in western countries but in India paralysis due to type 2 is quite common" (Ananthanarayan 9th/485 & Park 23rd/205)*

Table *(Ananthanarayan 9th/485)*: **Enterovirus serotypes**

Group	Serotypes
Poliovirus	1-3
Coxsackie virus A	1-22, 24
Coxsackie virus B	1-6
Echovirus	1-9, 11-27, 29-34
Numbered enterovirus	(EV) 68-78

Table *(Harrison 19th/1291)*: **Manifestations Commonly Associated With Enterovirus Serotypes**

	Serotype(s) of Indicated Virus	
Manifestation	**Coxsackie virus**	**Echovirus (E) and Enterovirus (Ent)**
Acute hemorrhagic conjunctivitis	A24	E70
Aseptic meningitis	A2, 4, 7, 9, 10; B1–5	E4, 6, 7, 9, 11, 13, 16, 18, 19, 30, 33; Ent70, 71
Encephalitis	A9; B1–5	E3, 4, 6, 7, 9, 11, 18, 25, 30; Ent71
Exanthem	A4, 5, 9, 10, 16; B1, 3–5	E4–7, 9, 11, 16–19, 25, 30; Ent71
Generalized disease of the newborn	B1–5	E4–6, 7, 9, 11, 14, 16, 18, 19
Hand-foot-and-mouth disease	A5, 7, 9, 10, 16; B1, 2, 5	Ent71
Herpangina	A1–10, 16, 22; B1–5	E6, 9, 11, 16, 17, 25, 30; Ent71
Myocarditis, pericarditis	A4, 9, 16; B1–5	E6, 9, 11, 22
Paralysis	A4, 7, 9; B1–5	E2–4, 6, 7, 9, 11, 18, 30; Ent70, 71
Pleurodynia	A1, 2, 4, 6, 9, 10, 16; B1–6	E1–3, 6, 7, 9, 11, 12, 14, 16, 19, 24, 25, 30
Pneumonia	A9, 16; B1–5	E6, 7, 9, 11, 12, 19, 20, 30; Ent-D68, 71

96. Ans. a. Caused by..., b. Excruiting..., e. Vector....

[Ref: Harrison 19th/1313; Park 23rd/289; Ananthanarayan 9th/440, 519; Jawetz 27th/ 548]

"**Chickengunya**: Blood counts may be normal, or patients may have leukopenia with ***relative lymphocytosis***" *(www. ncbi. nlm. nih. gov)*

"**Chickengunya**: Mild leukopenia occurs as does thrombocytopenia, which is seldom severe" *(CMDT 2016/1385)*

Chikungunya Fever

◈ *Ananthanarayan 9th/519*

- The vector is ***Aedes aegypti***
- It is caused by ***arbovirus*** (Family- Togaviridae, Genus- Alphavirus) *(Ananthanarayan 9th/517)*
- The Chikungunya virus by ***single stranded RNA virus***- *(Ananthanarayan 9th/440)*

Chikungunya Fever

◈ *Park 23rd/289*

- Chikungunya is a local word meaning doubling up owing to ***excruciating joint pains***
- There is ***no specific treatment*** & ***usually self limiting.*** Analgesics & antipyretics along with fluid supplementation are recommended to manage infection & relieve fever, joint pains & swelling. Drugs like aspirin & steroids should be avoided

Chikungunya Virus Disease

◈ *Harrison 19th/1313*

- ***Aedes aegypti*** mosquitoes are the usual vectors for the disease in urban areas.

- Fever (often severe) with a saddleback pattern and severe arthralgia are accompanied by chills and constitutional symptoms and signs, such as abdominal pain, anorexia, conjunctival injection, headache, nausea, and photophobia.
- Migratory polyarthritis mainly affects the small joints of the ankles, feet, hands, and wrists, but the larger joints are not necessarily spared.
- Rash may appear at the outset or several days into the illness
- Recovery may require weeks, and some elderly patients may continue to ***experience joint pain***, recurrent effusions, or stiffness for several years.
- In addition to arthritis, petechiae are occasionally seen and epistaxis is not uncommon, but chikungunya virus should not be considered a VHF agent.
- ***A few patients develop leukopenia***. Elevated concentrations of aspartate aminotransferase (AST) and C-reactive protein have been described, as have mildly decreased platelet counts.
- Treatment of chikungunya virus disease relies on ***nonsteroidal anti-inflammatory drugs*** and sometimes chloroquine for refractory arthritis.

97. Ans. a. Sexually..., d. Transmitted..., e. Transmission....

[Ref: Harrison 19th/1314; www. cdc. gov; http://www. nytimes. com]

Zika Virus Infection

◈ *www. cdc. gov & other sites*

- It is spread mostly by the bite of an infected *Aedes* species mosquito (*A. aegypti* and *A. albopictus*). These mosquitoes are aggressive daytime biters. They can also bite at night.
- It can be ***passed from a pregnant woman to her fetus.*** Infection during pregnancy can cause certain birth defects.
- It can be ***passed through sex*** from a person who has Zika to his or her partners. It can be passed through sex, even if the infected person does not have symptoms at the time.
- ***The majority of people infected with Zika virus do not display any symptoms***
- According to the Pan American Health Organization (PAHO), **only 1 in 4 people infected with Zika virus develop symptoms.** In contrast, the CDC state the figure is **1 in 5.** According to the Pan American Health Organization (PAHO), **only 1 in 4 people infected with Zika virus develop symptoms.** In contrast, the CDC state the figure is **1 in 5.**
- The infections in adults may result rarely in Guillain–Barré syndrome
- A blood or urine test can confirm Zika infection diagnosis.
- Real-time reverse transcription-polymerase chain reaction (rRT-PCR) testing should be performed on serum collected during the first two weeks after symptom onset.
- A negative rRT-PCR result does not exclude Zika virus infection and serum should be analyzed by IgM antibody (serological) testing.
- Zika virus-specific IgM and neutralizing antibodies typically develop toward the end of the first week of illness.
- ***There's no vaccine or specific treatment for the disease.*** Treatment instead focuses on relieving symptoms and includes rest, rehydration and medications for fever and pain.

Zika Virus Infection

◈ *Harrison 19th/1314*

- Zika virus is an emerging pathogen that is transmitted among nonhuman primates and humans by ***Aedes mosquitoes.***
- Human infections are usually benign and are most likely misdiagnosed as dengue or influenza. Zika virus infection is characterized by influenza-like clinical signs, including fever, headaches, and malaise.
- A maculopapular rash, conjunctivitis, myalgia, and arthralgia usually accompany or follow those manifestations.

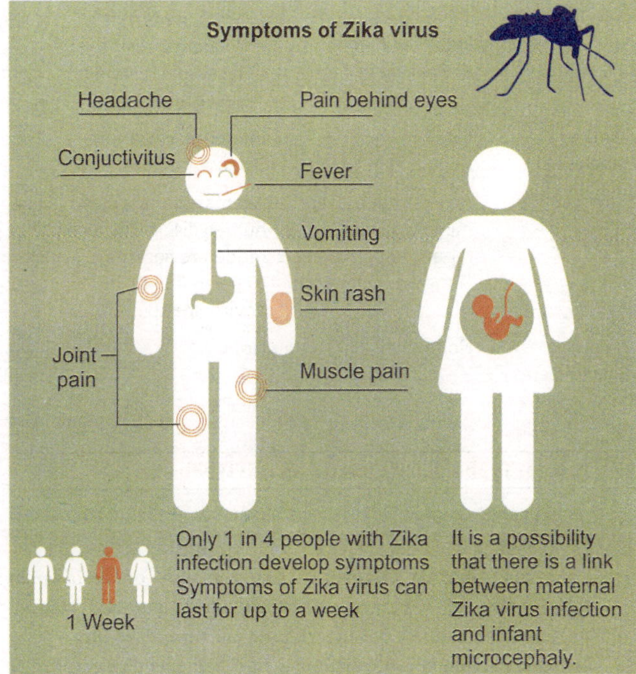

98. Ans. c. Ebola..., d. Crimean..., e. Lyssa....

[Ref: Harrison 19th/1323, 1328; consteril. com/biosafety-levels; thecerebrallounge. wordpress. com]

"If EVD (Ebola virus disease) or MVD (Marburg virus disease) is suspected on the basis of epidemiologic history, exposure history, and/or clinical manifestations, infectious disease specialists and the proper public health authorities, including the WHO, should be notified immediately. Laboratory diagnosis of EVD and MVD is relatively straightforward but requires maximal containment (***biosafety level 4)"*** *(Harrison 19th/1328)*

"**Filoviruses (includes three genera:** *Cueva virus, Ebola virus,* and *Marburg virus)* are categorized as World Health Organization (WHO) Risk Group 4 Pathogens. Consequently, all work with material suspected of containing filoviruses should be conducted only in maximal containment (***biosafety level 4***) laboratories. Experienced personnel handling these viruses must wear appropriate personal protective gear and follow rigorous standard operating procedures. The proper authorities and

WHO reference laboratories should be contacted immediately when filovirus infections are suspected" *(Harrison 19th/1323)*

Biosafety Level 4

- *the cerebrallounge.wordpress.com*
- Hemorrhagic fevers
- Marburg virus
- Ebola virus
- Lassa virus
- Smallpox

"**Biosafety Level 4**: This level is required for work with dangerous and exotic agents that pose a high individual risk of aerosol-transmitted laboratory infections, agents which cause severe to fatal disease in humans for which vaccines or other treatments are *not* available, such as Bolivian and Argentine hemorrhagic fevers, Marburg virus, ***Ebola virus, Lassa fever, Crimean-Congo hemorrhagic fever, smallpox***, and various other hemorrhagic diseases.

When dealing with biological hazards at this level the use of a positive pressure personnel suit, with a segregated air supply, is mandatory" *(wiki)*

Biosafelty Level	BSL-1	BSL-2	BSL-3	BSL-4
Description	• No Containment • Defined organisms • Unlikely to cause disease	• Containment • Moderate Risk • Disease of varying severity	• High Containment • Aerosol • Transmission • Serious/Potentially lethal disease	• Max Containment • "Exotic", High-Risk Agents • Life-threatening disease
Sample Organisms	E.coli	Influenza, HIV, Lyme Disease	Tuberculosis	Ebola Virus
Pathogen Type	Agents that present minimal potential hazard to personnel & the environment	Agents associated with human disease & pose moderate hazards to personnel & the environment	Indigenous or exotic agents, agents that present a potential For aerosol transmission, & agents causing serious or potentially lethal disease.	Dangerous & exotic agents that pose a high risk of aerosol-transmitted laboratory infections & life-threatening disease.
Autoclave Requirements	None	None	Pass-thru autoclave with bioseal required in Laboratory room.	Pass-thru autoclave with Bioseal required in Laboratory room.

99. Ans. a. Typhoid, b. Q fever, d. Scrub typhus

[Ref: Ananthanarayan 9th/103-118; Panikar Parasitology 7th/28; Jawetz 27th/347]

"The **diagnosis of Q fever** is based mainly on ***serological tests***, such as microagglutination, complement fixation, immunofluorescence & ELISA *(Ananthanarayan 9th/412)*

"**Q fever:** Serology is the diagnostic method of choice & indirect immunofluorescence is considered the best method" *(Jawetz 27th/347)*

*"**Serological tests:** There are not used for early diagnosis of rickettsial diseases(including Q fever, scrub typhus), from a treatment perspective, but to **confirm the diagnosis for epidemiological investigations**" (Ananthanarayan 9th/410)*

"**Scrub typhus:** Serological assay (indirect fluorescent antibody, indirect immunoperoxidae & enzyme immunoassays), are mainstays of laboratory diagnosis" *(Harrison 19th/1159)*

Tube agglutination is routinely used for serological diagnosis of ***typhoid, brucellosis & typhus fever***" *(Ananthanarayan 9th/109)*

"As culture of often unsuccessful, serological methods are important in diagnosis. Several serological tests have been developed, including agglutination, complement fixation & ELISA" (Ananthanarayan 9th/342)

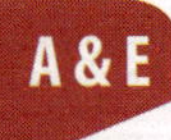

Laboratory Diagnosis of Acanthamoeba

- *Panikar Parasitology 7th/28*

"Early diagnosis is essential for effective treatment of *Acanthamoeba* keratitis. The infection is usually diagnosed by an eye specialist based on symptoms, growth of the ameba from a scraping of the eye, and/or seeing the amoeba by a process called confocal microscopy"

"**Granulomatous Amebic Encephalitis** (GAE) and **disseminated infection** are more difficult to diagnose and are often at advanced stages when they are diagnosed. Tests useful in the diagnosis of GAE include brain scans, biopsies, or spinal taps. In disseminated disease, biopsy of the involved sites *e.g.*, skin, sinuses) can be useful in diagnosis" *(cdc. gov/parasites/acanthamoeba)*

Antigen-antibody reactions in vitro are known as serological reaction. Two important parameters of serologicals test are sensitivity & specificity *(Ananthanarayan 9th/103-04)*

Serological Reactions

- *Ananthanarayan 9th/103*
- Precipitation raction
- Agglutination reaction
- Complement fixation test
- Neutralisation test
- Opsonisation
- Radioimmunoassa
- Enzyme immunoassay (ELISA)
- Chemiluminescence immmunoassay
- Immunoelectroblot/Western blot technique
- Immunochromatographic test
- Immunoelectronmicroscopic tests
- Immunofluoresence

100. Ans. e. Mainly caused by.....

[Ref: Harrison 19th/990-95; Ananthanarayan 9th/257-59; Jawetz 27th/186-87;Greenwood 16th /231-35]

"*C. perfringens* in association with mixed aerobic and anaerobic microbes can cause aggressive life-threatening ***type I necrotizing fasciitis or Fournier's gangrene***" *(Harrison 19th/991)*

Gas Gangrene

◈ *Greenwood 16th /232-33*

- *The presence of **devitalized or dead tissue**, blood clot, extravasated fluid, foreign bodies & co-incident pyogenic infection are all that promote the occurrence of gas gangrene in a wound*
- *Predisposing host factors include debility, old age & diabetes*
- When clostridial infection has been initiated in a focus of devitalized anaerobic tissue, the organism multiply rapidly & produce a range of toxins & aggression. These damage tissue by various necrotizing effects. They spread into adjacent viable tissue, particularly muscle, kill it & render it anaerobic & vulnerable to further colonization, with production of more toxins & aggressins
- α –toxin is generally considered to be the main cause of the toxaemia associated with gas gangrene

"**α–toxin:** *This is the most important toxin biologically & is responsible for profound toxaemia of gas gangrene" (Ananthanarayan 9th/ 254)*

Gas Gangrene

◈ *Ananthanarayan 9th/ 257-59*

- *Gas gangrene results only if the condition favourable for clostridium multiplication exist in wound*
- *The most important of these is **low oxygen tension***
- *The ionized calcium salts & silicic acid in soil cause necrosis*
- *Crushing tissue or tearing of arteries produce anoxia of muscle*
- *The Eh & pH of the damaged tissue fall & these change along with the chemical change that occur in damaged & anoxic muscle, provide ideal pabulum for the proliferation of anaerobes*
- *Clostridium multiply & elaborate toxins which cause further damage. These include- lecithinase, collagenase, α –toxin etc*
- *Drug of choice is metronidazole given i.v before surgery*

Gas Gangrene (Clostridial Myonecrosis)

- Gas gangrene is characterized by ***rapid and extensive necrosis of muscle***[Q] accompanied by gas formation and systemic toxicity and occurs when bacteria invade healthy muscle from adjacent traumatized muscle or soft tissue
- The incubation period of gas gangrene is usually short: almost always <3 days and frequently <24 h. ***Some 80% of cases are caused by C. perfringens, while C. novyi, C. septicum, and C. histolyticum cause most of the remaining cases***
- An essential factor in the genesis of gas gangrene appears to be ***trauma***
- C. Perferingens has ***at least 17 possible virulence factors including 12 active tissue toxin and enterotoxin***[Q].
- The α toxin is a phospholipase C (lecithinase) that splits lecithin into phosphorylcholine and diglyceride. It has been associated with ***gas gangrene and is known to be hemolytic***[Q] to destroy platelets and polymorphonuclear leukocytes (PMNs), and to cause widespread capillary damage.
- The α toxin may be important in the initiation of muscle infections that can progress to gas gangrene.

Table *(Harrison 19th/991)*: **Treatment of Gas Gangrene**

Condition	Antibiotic Treatment	Adjunctive Treatment/Note
Gas gangrene	*Penicillin G plus Clindamycin*	Emergent surgical exploration and thorough debridement are extremely important. Hyperbaric oxygen therapy may be considered after surgery and antibiotics have been initiated.

101. Ans. a. Echinococcus..., c. Echinococcus multiocularis

[Ref: Park 23rd/304;Harrison 19th/1432, 167e-1; Chatterjee Parasitology 13th/159; CMDT 2016/1280]

"Echinococcus granulosus (Dog tapeworm): Human infection follows ingestion of the eggs due to intimae handling of infected dogs or by eating raw vegetables or other food items contaminated with dog feces" *(Panikar Parasitology 7th/128 & Chatterjee Parasitology 13th/159)*

"Alveolar echinococcosis (AE) is caused by infection with the larval stage of *Echinococcus multilocularis*. The adult tapeworm is normally found in foxes, coyotes, and ***dogs.*** Infection with the larval stages is transmitted to people through ingestion of food or water contaminated with tapeworm eggs" *(cdc. gov/parasites)*

*"**Toxocara canis:** Human infection is by ingestion of eggs, which are shed in feces of dog (Panikar Parasitology 7th/201)*

"***Toxoplasma gondii:*** Man acquires infection by ingestion of contaminated food and water containing sporulated oocyst (from cat) or by ingestion of undercooked meat containing tissue cyst" *(Panikar 7th/89)*

FORENSIC MEDICINE

102. Ans. a. Pedoph..., c. Frotteur..., d. Voyeurism..., e. Exhib....

[Ref: Synopsis of Psychiatry by Kaplon & Saddock 11th/593-97; Reddy 32nd/ 411; Neeraj Ahuja 7th/124-26; Parikh 7th/ 411-12]

Paraphilic Disorders

◈ *Kaplon&Saddock 11th/593-97*

- Paraphilias or perversions are sexual stimuli or acts that are deviations from normal sexual behaviors, but are necessary for some persons to experience arousal and orgasm.
- According to the **Diagnostic and Statistical Manual of Mental Disorders, fifth edition (DSM-5),** the term paraphilic disorder is reserved for those cases in which a sexually deviant fantasy or impulse has been expressed behaviorally.
- Individuals with paraphilic interests can experience sexual pleasure, but they are inhibited from responding to stimuli that are normally considered erotic. The paraphiliac person's sexuality is mainly restricted to specific deviant stimuli or acts.

- Persons that occasionally experiment with paraphilic behavior (e.g., infrequent episode of bondage or dressing in costumes), but are capable of responding to more typical erotic stimuli, are not seen as having paraphilic disorders.
- DSM-5 lists ***pedophilia, frotteurism, voyeurism, exhibitionism, sexual sadism, sexual masochism, fetishism, and transvestism*** with explicit diagnostic criteria because of their threat to others and/or because they are **relatively common paraphilias**. There are ***many other paraphilias that may be diagnosed***.
- **Exhibitionism** is the recurrent urge to expose the genitals to a stranger or to an unsuspecting person
- **Frotteurism** is usually characterized by a man's rubbing his penis against the buttocks or other body parts of a fully clothed woman to achieve orgasm. At other times, he may use his hands to rub an unsuspecting victim
- **Pedophilia** involves recurrent intense sexual urges toward, or arousal by, children 13 years of age or younger, over a period of at least 6 months. Persons with pedophilia are at least 16 years of age and at least 5 years older than the victims. When a perpetrator is a late adolescent involved in an ongoing sexual relationship with a 12- or 13-year-old, the diagnosis is not warranted
- **Voyeurism,** also known as ***scopophilia***, is the recurrent preoccupation with fantasies and acts that involve observing unsuspecting persons who are naked or engaged in grooming or sexual activity
- **Transvestism,** formerly called ***transvestic fetishism***, is described as fantasies and sexual urges to dress in opposite gender clothing as a means of arousal and as an adjunct to masturbation or coitus.
- In **DSM-5,** the criteria for paraphilic disorder requires the patient to have experienced intense and recurrent arousal from their deviant fantasy for ***at least 6 months*** and to have acted on the paraphilic impulse.

Special Note: Homosexuality (gay and lesbianism) was previously listed as a paraphilia in the DSM-I and DSM-II, but this was declassified from DSM-III, DSM-IV & DSM-V, consistent with the change of attitude among psychiatrists and psychologists. ***Homosexuality is no longer considered a paraphilia.***

Paraphilias: *Abnormal & unorthodox sexplay by using objects or parts of body are known as paraphilias (Reddy 32nd/ 411)*

Sodomy is unnatural sex (S 377, IPC) *(Reddy 32nd/ 408)*

103. Ans. e. Ankle....

[Ref: Reddy 32nd/78, 77, 74; Parikh 7th/ 61-63]

Fusion of Bones/Joints

◈ *Reddy 32nd/78*

16 years: elbow joint

16 to 17 years: Ankle joint

17 to 18 years: Hip joint

18 to 19 years: Knee, shoulder & wrist joint

20 to 21 years: Fusion of iliac crest, ischial tuberosity & inner end of clavicle

The opinion about the age should be given based on the findings of ***physical, dental & radiological examination****. Multiple criteria of skeletal age should be used*

For estimation of Age: Take X-ray

◈ *Reddy 32nd/78 (A for appearance)*

6-12 years

- Elbow joint
- Wrist joint
- (6 yr- center for lower end of ulna (A); medial epicondyle of the humerus (A)

9 years: *Olecranon (A)*

9 to 11 years: *Trochela of humerus (A)*

10th to 11th year: *Pisiform (A)*

11th year: *Lateral epicondyle of humerus (A)*

13 to 16 years: *X-ray of pelvis elbow joint &pelvis (13thyr – separate centers in triradiate cartilage of acetabulum (A)*

12 to 14 years: *Lesser trochanter of femur (A)*

14th year: *Crest of ilium (A), fusion of medial epicondyle of humerus, lateral epicondyle with trochlea*

15th year: *fusion of triradiate cartilage of acetabulum*

16th year: Ischial tuberosity (A), Fusion of lower end of humerus; Olecranon of ulna & upper end of radius

104. Ans. a. Medullary index..., c. Cortex is thick, d. Medullanar row

[Ref: Reddy 32nd/91; Parikh 7th/ 499]

Table *(Reddy 32nd/91; Parikh 7th/ 499)*: **Difference b/w Human & Animal Hair**

Trait	Human Hair	Animal hair
Character	Fine & thin	Coarse & thick
Cuticle	Cuticular scales are short, broad, thin & irregularly annular	Cuticular scales are very large & have step-like or wavy projections
Cortex	***Thick***, well –striated & 4 to 10 times as broad as medulla	***Thin***, rarely more than twice as broad as medulla
Medulla	Varies considerably, usually ***narrow***, discontinuous, fragmented or entirely absent	Continuous & ***wider***
Pigment	Evenly distributed	Mostly present in the medulla
Precipitin	Specific for human	Specific for different animals
Medullary index (Diameter of medulla/Diameter of shaft)	Below 0.3	Above 0.5

105. Ans. b. Executive magistrate..., d. CrPC 176 (4) is related...

[Ref: Reddy 32nd/ 128-29; Parikh 7th/133-34]

Exhumation

◈ *Parikh 7th/133-34; Reddy 32nd/ 128-29*

- *It is digging out of an already buried body legally from the grave*
- *There is no time limit for exhumation in India*
- ***Autopsies are performed on exhumed bodies:*** *(1) In criminal cases, such as homicide, suspected homicide disguised as suicide or other types of death, suspicious poisoning, death as a result of criminal abortion & criminal negligence; (2) In civil cases, such as accidental death claim, insurance, workmen's compensation claim, liability for professional negligence, survivorship & inheritance claims or disputed identity*
- **Authorisation**: *The body is exhumated only when, there is a* ***written order from the executive magistrate. The body can be exhumated by any government doctor***
- *The body is exhumated under the supervision of a medical officer & magistrate in the presence of a police officer*
- *Whenever practicable, the magistrate should inform the relatives of the deceased & allow them to remain present at the enquiry (176 (4) Cr. P.C)*
- *If the body has been buried recently, the postmortem examination is conducted in the usual manner*
- *In much putrefied bodies, an attempt should be made to establish the identity. All viscera should be preserved for chemical analysis*

CrPC 176 (4): Where an inquiry is to be held under this section, the Magistrate shall, wherever practicable, inform the relatives of the deceased whose names and addresses are known, and shall allow them to remain present at the inquiry. Explanation- In this section, expression" relative" means parents, children, brothers, sisters and spouse-*indiankanoon.org*

"**CrPC 174**- ***Police to enquire and report on suicide***, etc." *(indiankanoon.org)*

106. Ans. b. Mechanism..., c. Also k/a..., e. Can be seen.....

[Ref: Reddy 32nd/156; Parikh 7th/ 147-50]

"**Cadaveric spasm**: *It may indicate the nature of death viz suicide, homicide or accident. E.g. certain case of* ***drowning*** *when grass, weeds, or other objects in the fluid medium are clutched by the deceased" (Parikh 7th/ 151)*

Cadaveric Spasm (Cataleptic Rigidity or Instantaneous Rigor)

- It is a rare condition. In this, the muscles that were contracted during life become stiff and rigid ***immediately after death*** without passing into the stage of primary relaxation.
- As such, the change preserves the exact attitude of the person at the time of death for several hours afterwards.
- It occurs especially in *cases of sudden death, excitement, fear, severe pain, exhaustion, cerebral haemorrhage, injury to the nervous system, firearm wound of the head,* ***drowning,*** *convulsant poisons (such as strychnine) etc.*
- *No other condition simulates cadaveric spasm* and *it cannot be produced by any method after death*

Table: Difference b/w Rigor mortis & Cadaveric spasm

Feature	Cadaveric Spasm	Rigor Mortis
Definition	This is continuation after death, of the state of contraction in ***which muscles were at the instant of death***. The stage of primary relaxation is absent. The stiffening is therefore instantaneous at the time of death	This is d/t changes in muscles after molecular death of their cells and is preceded by general relaxation of the muscles. A 2-3 hour lapse is therefore necessary before stiffening occurs
Mechanism	Not known	Known
Predisposing factors	Sudden death Emotional tension (excitement, fear, exhaustion) Physical activity at the time of death	None
Preceded By	Primary relaxation is absent	**Stage of primary relaxation**
Time of onset	**Instantaneous**	2-3 hours after death
Muscles Involved	Certain groups of voluntary muscles	All muscles, both voluntary & involuntary
Muscles stiffening	Is quite marked and considerable force is required to break it	Is less marked & only moderate force required to break it
Molecular Death	Does not occur	Occurs
Electrical stimuli	Muscle respond	Does not respond
Produced	Can not be produced by any method after death. It is impossible to simulate it	Cold stiffening (<4°C) & heat coagulation (>70°C) simulate rigor mortis
Medicolegal Importance	**Indicates time since death**[Q]	Indicates circumstances & mode of death[Q] e.g suicide, homicide or accident
Body heat	Warm	Cold

107. Ans. b. Strychnos Nux..., c. Strychnine

[Ref: Reddy 32nd/581; Parikh 7th/639-40]

Strychnine *(**alkaloid from seeds of strychnosnux-vomica**) cause* ***opisthotonus*** *(Parikh 7th/639-40)*

"**Strychnine:** *The convulsions are most marked in antigravity muscles, so that the body typically arches in hyperextension (**opisthotonus**)" (Reddy 32nd/581)*

Causes of Opisthotonus

- *www.nytimes.com/health/guides*
- *Arnold-Chiari syndrome*
- *Meningitis*
- *Brain tumor*
- *Gaucher disease*
- *Growth hormone deficiency (occasionally)*
- *Glutaricaciduria and organic acidemias (forms of chemical poisoning)*
- *Krabbe Disease*
- *Seizures*
- *Severe electrolyte imbalance*
- *Severe head injury*
- *Stiff-person syndrome (a condition that makes a person rigid and have spasms)*
- *Subarachnoid hemorrhage (bleeding in the brain)*
- *Tetanus*
- *Drugs such as phenothiazines and other antipsychotic medications, can cause a side effect called acute dystonic reaction. Opisthotonos may be part of this reaction.*

108. Ans. b. Sexual intercourse with..., d. Sexual intercourse with a girl..., e. Sexual intercourse with wife who is living......

[Ref: Reddy 32nd/ 392-95; Parikh 7th/389-91]

*There is controversial reference regarding age of wife, either 16 or 15 year in Reddy (old & new ed.) & Parikh. But, **best reliable source is*** **Gazette Notification of GOI regarding Criminal Law (amendendment) Act, 2013** *released on 2 april, 2013.It is age 15 year (Also confirmed from Mr Himanshu Pansaria IIT, LLB, LLM)*

"Exception to S. 375, I.P.C: Sexual intercourse or sexual acts by a man with his own wife, ***the wife not being under 15 years of age, is not sexual assault"*** *(Gazette Notification of GOI regarding Criminal Law (amendendment) Act, 2013)*

Exception to S. 375, I.P.C: Sexual intercourse or sexual acts by a man with his own wife, ***the wife not being under 16 years of age, is not sexual assault*** *(Reddy 32nd/ 392)*

(New edition, in accordance with New Criminal Law amendment Bill, 2013)

Exception to S. 375, I.P.C: Sexual intercourse or sexual acts by a man with his own wife, ***the wife not being under 15 years of age, is not sexual assault*** *(Reddy 27th/351 (old edition))*

"**Under S 375 IPC**, rape is defined as unlawful sexual intercourse by a man with ***his wife under the age of 15 years***, with any other woman ***under the age of 18 years***, or above that age, against her will, without her consent, or with her consent when it has been obtained by unlawful means" *(Parikh 7th/390)*

Statutory rape: It is sexual intercourse with a girl below 18 years of age even with her consent. It is neither violent **nor physically coerced** *(Reddy 32nd/ 395)*

Marital rape: *It is forceful sexual intercourse with wife who is living separately from him under a decree of separation, or any custom or usage without her consent (Reddy 32nd/ 395)*

PREVENTIVE & SOCIAL MEDICINE

109. Ans. b. Retrospective study, c. Cross-sectional study

[Ref: Park 23rd/ 62, 69; Community Medicine by Piyush Gupta 1st/588]

Cohort (Known by a variety of names- ***prospective study, longitudinal study***, incidence study & forward looking study) is ***follow up study*** with individual as unit of study *(Park 23rd/ 62, 75)*

Case control studies, often called retrospective studies: *No attrition problems, because case control studies **do not require follow-up** of individual into the future (Park 23rd/74)*

Cross-sectional studies *(Also k/a prevalence study) is **single examination (so no follow up)** of a cross-section of population at one point in time- the results of which can be projected on the whole population (Park 23rd/ 69)*

Longitudinal studies: *Observations are repeated in the same population over a prolonged period of time by means of **follow-up examinations** (Park 23rd/ 69)*

110. Ans. b. Immunization against..., c. Specific nutritional diet..., d. Protection from occupational....

[Ref: Park 23rd/42-43; Community Medicine by Piyush Gupta 1st/ 6; Community Medicine with Recent Advances by Suryakantha 4th/18]

Specific Protection

- Park 23rd/43
- ***Immunization***
- ***Use of specific nutrients***
- ***Chemoprophylaxis***
- ***Protection against occupational hazards***
- Protection against accident
- Protection from carcinogens
- Avoidance of allergens
- The control of specific hazards in the general environment e.g., air pollution, noise control
- Control of consumer product quality & safety of foods, drugs, cosmetics etc

Health Promotion

- *Park 23rd/43*
- *Health education*
- ***Environmental modification*** *such as provision of safe water, installation of sanitary latrines, control of insects & rodents, improvement of housing etc*
- ***Nutritional intervention:*** *Food distribution & nutritional improvement of vulnerable groups, child feeding programmes, food fortification, nutrition education*
- ***Lifestyle & behavioural changes***

Modes of Intervention

- *Park 23rd/42*
- *Health promotion*
- *Specific protection*
- *Early diagnosis & treatment*
- *Disability limitation*
- *Rehabilitation*

Table *(Suryakantha 4th/18)*: **Natural History of a Communicable Disease and Application of Preventive Measures**

Levels of prevention	**Primary prevention**		**Secondary prevention**	**Tertiary prevention**	
Modes of intervention	Health promotion	**Specific promotion**	Early diagnosis and treatment	Disability limitation	Rehabilitation
Nature or measures	Promotion	Preventive	Curative	Restorative	Rehabilitative
Examples	• Health education • Sex education • Adequate nutrition • Improvement of sanitation • Promotion of breastfeeding • Family planning • Genetic counseling • Recreation facilities • Yoga exercises	• **Immunization** • Condom against AIDS • **Vitamin A against nutritional blindness** • Helmet against head injury • **Lead apron against radiation hazards** • Avoidance of allergens and carcinogens • Pasteurization of milk	***Screening procedures for early diagnosis*** • Recording weight to diagnose malnutrition • Investigations in a pregnant mother • Contact tracing and cluster testing for STDs • Blood and urine exam for diabetes • Periodical examination of industrial workers • Pap smear for Ca Cx ***Modalities of Treatment*** • Chemotherapy • Surgery • Immunotherapy • Radiotherapy • Psychotherapy • Oral rehydration therapy	Intensive or aggressive treatment ***E.g.,*** Treatment of corneal xerosis to prevent blindness	**Types** • Physical • Vocational • Social • Psychological **Examples:** School for the blind Braile for the blind, Artificial limb, crutches, wheel chair, hearing aid, Graded exercises, intraocular lens for cataract patients Reconstructive surgery in leprosy

111. Ans. b. Deficient, c. Head of institution..., d. Birth & Death both..., e. Cause of death...

[Ref: Park 23rd/ 840-41; Community Medicine by Piyush Gupta 1st/606; http: //www.advocatekhoj.com; Community Medicine with Recent Advances by Suryakantha 4th/1012-13]

Registration of Vital Events/Civil Registration System

◈ *Park 23rd/ 840-41; Community Medicine by Piyush Gupta 1st/606*

- The registration system in India tended to be ***very unreliable, the data being grossly deficient in regards to accuracy, timeliness, completeness & coverage***. This is because of illiteracy, ignorance, lack of concern, & motivation
- The central births & Death Registration Act, 1969 fixes the responsibility for reporting births & deaths. While the public (e.g, parents, relatives) are to report events occurring in their households, the ***heads of hospital, nursing homes, hotels, jails or dharmashalas*** are to report events ***occurring in such institutions*** to be concerning registrar
- The time limit for registering the events of birth & that of deaths is 21 days uniformly all over India. In case of default a late fee can be imposed

Registration of Births and Deaths Act, 1969

◈ *http: //www.advocatekhoj.com/*

- *Duty of certain persons to notify or death births and deaths and to certify cause of death*

Table *(Suryakantha 4th/1013)*: **Limitations in Civil Registration**

- Wide scattering of villages
- Illiteracy and ignorance about registration among the people
- Lack of proper maintenance of records
- Negligence by village *chowkidars*
- Deaths among those, who do not possess any property are often not registered
- False registration can take place
- Public health department has no powers to deal with the defaulters. Even if defaulters are prosecuted, punishment is nominal
- Lack of medical personnel in interior areas.

Sample Registration System (SRS)

- Since *civil registration system is deficient* in India, SRS was initiate in the mid-1960s to provide reliable estimates of birth & death rates at the national & state level
- *SRS is dual record system,* consisting of continuous enumeration of births & deaths by an enumerator & an independent survey every 6 month by an investigator-supervisor
- Since the introduction of this system, more reliable information on birth & death rates, age-specific fertility & mortality rates, infant, under-five & adult mortality etc have become available

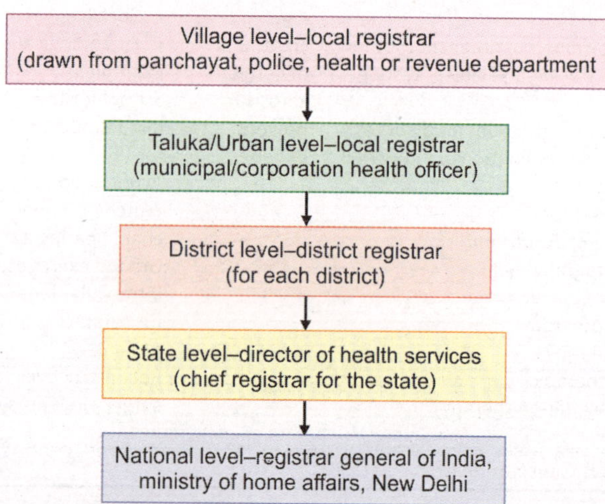

Fig: *(Suryakantha 4th/1012):* The channel of collection & sending information

112. Ans. a. Caused by..., b. Severe exposure..., c. Fibrosis of upper..., e. More risk....

[Ref: Park 23rd/806; Community Medicine by Piyush Gupta 1st/746; Community Medicine with Recent Advances by Suryakantha 4th/222-25]

"*Tubercular infection is common in silica-affected workers. There are indications of an association b/w silica & lung cancer*" *(Community Medicine by Piyush Gupta 1st/746)*

Silicosis

◈ *Park 23rd/806*

- It is caused by inhalation of dust containing *free silica or silicon dioxide (SiO_2)*
- The incidence of silicosis depends upon the chemical composition of the dust, size of particles, duration of exposure & individual susceptibility
- The *higher the concentration of free silica in the dust, the greater the hazard*
- The incubation period may vary from a few months upto 6 years of exposure
- Pathologically, silicosis is characterized by a *dense nodular fibrosis,* the nodule ranging from 3 to 4 mm in diameter.
- A X-ray of chest shows snow storm appearance in the lung
- Silicosis is progressive & what is more important is that *silicotics are prone to tuberculosis*
- There is *no effective treatment for silicosis.* Fibrotic changes that have already taken place cannot be reversed
- The only way that silicosis can be controlled (if not altogether eliminated) is by (a) rigorous dust control measures, e.g., substitution, complete enclosure, isolation, hydroblasting, good house-keeping, personal protection measures & (b) regular physical examination of workers

Silicosis

◈ *Community Medicine with Recent Advances by Suryakantha 4th/222-2*

- Inhalation of *free silica (i.e. SiO_2)* over prolonged period cause major fibrogenic damage in lung
- Nodular fibrosis, more frequent in apex & posterior border (*upper part of lung*) (*c.f in asbestosis-fibrosis in lower half of lung)*
- Silicotics are more prone to develop pulmonary tuberculosis (but in recent year there is doubt whether silicotics really develop T.B.)
- The *fibrotic change can not be reversed*
- There is no treatment for silicosis

"**Whole lung lavage** may be *useful in some cases of acute silicosis.* Whole lung lavage can reduce the total mineral dust load in the lungs of patients with chronic silicosis. Some studies have shown short-term reduction in symptoms after lavage, but controlled trials have not been done. Anecdotal evidence supports the use of oral corticosteroids in acute and accelerated silicosis. Lung transplantation is a last resort" *(www.merckmanuals.com)*

"For acute silicosis, *bronchoalveolar lavage* may alleviate symptoms, but does not decrease overall mortality" *(wikipedia.org)*

113. Ans. a. Comparison..., c. Pie chart is..., d. Comparison of magnitude....

[Ref: Biostatistics by Mahajan 7th/28-30; Biostatistics by KV Rao 2nd/31; Park 23rd/844-45; Community Medicine by Piyush Gupta 1st/ 650-52]

Table *(Piyush Gupta 1st/ 650):* **Conditions under which Various Types of Diagrams are Appropriate**

Categories on x-axis	Quantity to be represented on y-axis*	Appropriate diagram
Continuous	Additive (frequency or percentage)	Pie if proportional contribution of the categories is to be represented, otherwise histogram
	Non-additive (number, rate or ratio)	Line for depiction of trend, otherwise bar
Discrete or categorical	Additive (frequency or percentage)	Pie if proportional percentage contribution of the categories is to be represented, otherwise bar
	Non-additive (number, rate or ratio)	Bar

** No x- or y-axis in case of pie diagram*

Bar Diagram

- *Length of bar represents frequency of a character*
- *Popular & easy method*
- *Used for comparison of magnitude of different frequencies in* ***discrete data***
- *Spacing b/w any two bars should be nearly equal to half of the width of the bar*
- *3 Types- simple, proportionate & multiple*

Bar Chart or Bar Graph

A **bar chart or bar graph** is a chart that presents grouped data with rectangular bars with lengths proportional to the values that they represent. The bars can be plotted vertically or horizontally. A vertical bar chart is sometimes called a **column bar chart.**

A bar graph is a chart that uses either horizontal or vertical bars to show comparisons among categories.

One axis of the chart shows the specific categories being compared, and the other axis represents a discrete value. Some bar graphs present bars clustered in groups of more than one (***grouped bar graphs***), and others show the bars divided into subparts to show cumulative effect (***stacked bar graphs***).

Bar charts have a discrete range. Bar charts are usually scaled so that all the data can fit on the chart.

Bars on the chart may be arranged in any order. Bar charts arranged from highest to lowest incidence are called Pareto charts. Normally, bars showing frequency will be arranged in chronological (time) sequence.

Bar graphs/charts provide a visual presentation of categorical data. Categorical data is a grouping of data into discrete groups, such as months of the year, age group, shoe sizes, and animals. These categories are usually qualitative. In a column bar chart, the categories appear along the horizontal axis; the height of the bar corresponds to the value of each category.

114. Ans. a. More focus..., b. More rapid..., c. Dedicated worker..., e. Effective way of...

[Ref: Community Medicine by Piyush Gupta 1st/803-04; Community Medicine with Recent Advances by Suryakantha 4th/896; www.who.int/management/district/services]

What is Meant by Vertical Versus Integrated Programmes

- **Vertical programmes** are "so called because they are ***directed, supervised, and executed, either wholly or to a great extent, by a specialized service using dedicated health workers***"
- In contrast, an **integrated programme** is "the process of bringing together common functions within and between organizations to solve common problems, developing a commitment to shared vision and goals and using common technologies and resources to achieve these goals"
- **Vertical programmes** (also known as stand-alone, categorical or free-standing programmes or the vertical approach) refer to instances where "the solution of a given health problem [is addressed] through the application of specific measures ***through single-purpose machinery***"
- In contrast, **integrated programmes** (also known as horizontal programmes, integrated health services or horizontal approaches) seek to "*tackle the overall health problems on a wide front and on a long-term basis through the creation of a system of permanent institutions commonly* known as '**general health services**'" and include "a variety of managerial or operational changes to health systems to bring together inputs, delivery, management and organization of particular service functions" or described as "a process where disease control activities are functionally merged or ***tightly coordinated with multifunctional health care delivery***"

Arguments for Vertical Programmes

- **Greater service specialization and concentration:** The most important rationale for vertical programmes is driven by the assumption that concentrating on a few well-focused interventions is an ***effective way of maximizing the impact and time response of the available resources.*** Waiting for changes in the health system to occur so that the delivery of better services would be viable (such as staff training and efficient supply systems) would simply be unacceptable for some. From this perspective, a call for systemic or multifactor approaches would introduce unnecessary delays in obtaining the desired results.
- **Increased profile for a high-priority disease or service:** The support galvanized by the United Nations Children's Fund (UNICEF) and other partners around universal childhood immunization in the 1980s and 1990s has been replicated more recently for HIV, tuberculosis and malaria – leading to the establishment of the Global Fund as well as disease-specific initiatives such as Roll Back Malaria – and for neglected diseases such as schistosomiasis.
- **Better accountability:** By making clear who is responsible for delivering what and what budget is available, vertical programmes ***promote a more transparent environment for accountability.***
- **More rapid results in weak health systems:** Vertical programmes are likely to lead to ***more rapid results*** than strategies that attempt to strengthen broader systems as a platform for service delivery, especially in weak health systems. Although effective public health interventions must be underpinned by **strong health systems** and especially stronger primary health care if they are to be ***sustained in the medium and long term,*** time-limited programmes with focused efforts that avoid negative spillover effects can be beneficial.
- **Better chance of success in weak states:** In weak states or states in conflict where health systems are already disintegrated, vertical programmes might be the ***only means of ensuring the delivery of at least selected priority services.***

Arguments against Vertical Programmes

- **Value driven:** Vertical programmes have been criticized for being value driven, lacking an empirical foundation and ***excessively focusing on efficiency gains.*** Many vertical programmes are ***externally driven and top-down in their approach,*** leading to ***inadequate engagement of local populations*** in planning or implementation. Hence, they can distort priorities and undermine local ownership and the responsiveness of local health services to the needs of service users.

- **Negative spillover effects:** Many critics have argued that vertical programmes create negative spillover effects for the non-participant or non-targeted population. In particular, vertical programmes are criticized as they lead to service fragmentation, ***create barriers to access, cause waste and inefficiency***, promote clinical, social and cultural iatrogenesis and crowd out prevention and access to general services for the majority of the population
- **Reduced chance of sustainability:** It is argued that vertical programmes waste resources as they ***encourage duplication and inefficiency and may overburden staff***, such as through multiple reporting channels. By creating unjustifiable differences of pay and status – that lead to employee dissatisfaction – and consuming scarce resources that could be used elsewhere, they ***reduce health system effectiveness*** while reducing the chances of being sustainable once the additional resources from external donors cease
- **Groups opposing health system reform:** Vertical programmes can create vested interest groups that may obstruct later reforms designed to integrate services, which are unlikely to serve the personal interests of stakeholders in the vertical programme.
- **Discouraging comprehensive approaches:** Vertical programmes hinder the development of comprehensive approaches needed to tackle social inequity and the wider determinants of health, thereby negatively affecting the health development process
- **Responsive to diseases and not to the users of services:** By their nature, vertical programmes are robust if the conditions they are designed to address have a single specific cause and less likely to be effective in responding to conditions that have multiple causes or comorbidity, such as cardiovascular diseases, cancer, tuberculosis, HIV and disability.

Table: Impact of vertical programmes on health system

Level	Positive Impact	Negative impact
Community and household	Programme aimed at eradication of dracunculiasis (Guinea worm) led to community mobilization with a focus on disadvantaged groups and the establishment of a surveillance system	***High dropout rate of volunteers***, limited use of community for other health problems and inefficiency due to the use of single-community workers
	The Global Polio Eradication Initiative promoted social mobilization in the middle-income countries of Latin America and India, with increased confidence in health systems and a rise in demand	Constrained interaction between the Expanded programme on Immunization and Global Polio Eradication Initiative in Benin and Niger due to lack of social mobilization
		Conflicts between local demand and immunization targets as well as high opportunity costs for communities and health services
Health services delivery	Smallpox eradication programme was able to use existing workforce rather than establish a parallel structure	***Inefficient use of health workers who make repeated visits to communities for a single purpose***
	Geographic mapping and numbering households for regular visiting (from the malaria eradication programme), organizing and delivering effective immunization services establishing active surveillance systems, quality control within laboratory network (from the yaws eradication programme)	
	Distribution of vitamin A during national immunization days	
Health sector policy and strategic management	Strengthened managerial, surveillance and laboratory capacity and promoting leadership	***Inefficient distribution of resources for routine Expanded Programme on Immunization services and other health services***

OPHTHALMOLOGY

115. Ans. c. Oculomotor nerve palsy

[Ref: Khurana 6th/504; Parson 22nd/32]

"Organophosphorus poisoning: Miosis, occasionally unequal or dilated" *(Reddy 32nd/495)*

"Organophosphorus poisoning: *Ocular manifestations include marked miosis" (G & G 11th/210)*

Causes of Mydriasis

Khurana 6th/504

- Effect of topical ***sympathomimetic drugs*** (*e.g.*, adrenaline and phenylephrine)
- Effect of topical ***parasympatholytic drugs*** (*e.g.*, atopine, homatropine, tropicamide and cyclopentolate)
- Acute congestive glaucoma (vertically oval large immobile pupil)
- Absolute glaucoma

- Optic atrophy
- Retinal detachment
- Internal ophthalmoplegia
- ***3rd nerve paralysis (Oculomotor nerve palsy)***
- Belladonna poisoning

Normal pupil size varies from 3 to 4 mm depending upon the illumination. But it may be abnormally small (*miosis*) or large (*mydriasis*)

Causes of Miosis

◈ *Khurana 6th/504*

- Effect of local miotic drugs (***parasympathomimetic drugs***)
- Effect of systemic morphine
- Iridocyclitis (narrow, irregular, non-reacting pupil)
- ***Horner's syndrome***
- Head injury (pontine haemorrhage)
- Senile rigid miotic pupil.
- Due to effect of strong light
- During sleep pupil is pinpoint.

116. Ans. a. Also k/a Chronic... c. Laser iridotomy.... e. Fundus examination.

[Ref: Khurana 6th/ 228-32; Parson 22nd/ 290-96]

Hypermetropic eyes with shallow anterior chamber & short axial length are predisposed to primary angle closure glaucoma *(Khurana 6th/240)*

Laser iridotomy is used for treatment *of primary angle closure glaucoma* *(Khurana 6th/ 247)*

Primary Open Angle Glaucoma

- It is a type of primary glaucoma, where there is no obvious systemic or ocular cause of rise in the intraocular pressure. It occurs in eyes with open angle of the anterior chamber.
- T is ***also known as chronic simple glaucoma*** of adult onset and is typically characterized by slowly progressive raised intraocular pressure (>21 mmHg recorded on at least a few occasions) associated with ***characteristic optic disc cupping and specific visual field defects.***
- **Pathogenesis:** The rise in intraocular pressure in POAG is related to an increased resistance to the outflow of aqueous at the trabecular mesh work, especially at the juxtacanalicular region. In part, this is due to age-related changes in this tissue.
- ***Heredity:*** POAG has a polygenic inheritance. The approximate risk of getting disease is 10% in the siblings, and 4% in the offspring of patients with POAG
- ***Age:*** The risk increases with increasing age. The POAG is more commonly seen in elderly between 5th and 7th decades.
- ***Myopes are more predisposed*** than the normals.
- *Diabetics* have a higher prevalence of POAG than non-diabetics.
- *Cigarette smoking* is also thought to increase its risk.
- *High blood pressure* is not the cause of rise in IOP, however the prevalence of POAG is more in hypertensives than the normotensives.
- *Thyrotoxicosis* is also not the cause of rise in IOP, but the prevalence of POAG is more inpatients suffering from Graves' ophthalmic disease than the normals.
- Patients may experience mild headache and eyeache.
- Reading and close work often present increasing difficulties owing to accommodative failure due to constant pressure on the ciliary muscle and its nerve supply. Therefore, patients usually complain of *frequent changes in presbyopic glasses.*
- Patients develop *delayed dark adaptation,* a disability which becomes increasingly disturbing in the later stages.
- ***Anterior segment signs.*** Ocular examination including slit-lamp biomicroscopy may ***reveal normal anterior segment.*** In late stages pupil reflex becomes sluggish and cornea may show slight haze.
- ***Fundus examination show large cup,*** **i.e. 0.6 or more (normal cup size is 0.3 to 0.4)**

117. Ans. d. Mucopolysaccharidosis

[Ref: Khurana 6th/97-98; Parson 22nd/221]

"**Megalocornea**: *Cornea is **usually clear** with normal thickness & vision" (Khurana 6th/97)*

Congenital Cloudy Cornea

◈ *Khurana 6th/97-98*

The acronym **'STUMPED'** helps to remember the common conditions to be included in differential diagnosis of neonatal cloudy cornea. The conditions are as follows:

- Sclerocornea
- Tears in Descemet's membrane
- Ulcer
- ***Metabolic conditions***
- Posterior corneal defect
- Endothelial dystrophy
- Dermoid

Congenital Opacity of Cornea (STUMPED)

◈ *Parson 22nd/221*

- **S**-Sclerocornea
- T-Trauma
- U-Ulcer
- ***M- Mucopolysaccharidosis***
- P-Peter anomaly
- ED- Congenital hereditary endothelial dystrophy

"**Mucopolysaccharidoses (MPS)** can manifest with corneal clouding, including *Hurler, Scheie, and Hurler-Scheie syndromes (all MPS I); Morquio syndrome (MPS IV); and Maroteaux-Lamy syndrome (MPS VI). Corneal clouding is not present in Hunter syndrome (MPS II) and Sanfilippo syndrome (MPS III)" (emedicine.medscape.com)*

118. Ans. a. Superior temporal displacement..., b. Inferior temporal displacement.........

[Ref: Khurana 6th/215-16; Parson 22nd/275]

Marfan syndrome: Usually superotemporal displacement *(Parson 22nd/275)*

Homocystinuria: Usually inferotemporal displacement *(Parson 22nd/275)*

Ectopia Lentis

◈ *Parson 22nd/275*

- This is a congenital dislocation or subluxation of the lens, usually upwards and bilateral. Lens displacement from its normal position is described as *subluxation of the lens* if there is a partial displacement and *dislocation* of the lens if there is a complete displacement of the lens from its normal position. The condition is often hereditary.

- The lens is small, but the edge is generally invisible until the pupil is dilated.

Ectopia Lentis with Systemic Anomalies

◈ *Khurana 6th/215-16*

1. ***Marfan's syndrome:*** In this condition lens is displaced upwards and temporally (bilaterally symmetrical)
2. ***Homocystinuria:*** In it the lens is usually subluxated downwards and nasally.
3. ***Weil-Marchesani syndrome:*** forward subluxation of lens which may cause pupil block glaucoma.
4. ***Ehlers-Danlos syndrome.*** In it the *ocular features* are subluxation of lens and blue sclera.
5. ***Hyperlysinaemia***: It is an extremely rare condition occasionally associated with ectopialentis.
6. ***Stickler syndrome.*** Ectopialentis is occasionally associated in this condition
7. ***Sulphite oxidase deficiency:*** Ectopialentis is a universal *ocular feature.*

Table *(Parson 22nd/275)*: **Causes of Ectopia Lentis**

A. Familial
Autosomal dominant form
Autosomal recessive form (associated with iris coloboma, aniridia, microspherophakia, ectopiapupillae)

B. Other systemic diseases
Marfan, Ehlers-Danlos, Weil-Marchesani, Homocystinuria, Sulphite oxidase deficiency, Hyperlysinaemia

C. Secondary to eye diseases
Uveitis, hypermature cataract, pseudoexfoliation syndrome, ciliary body tumour

D. Secondary to trauma
(May or may not be associated with underlying defective zonules due to syphilis)

119. Ans. c. Granulomatous type of low...

[Ref: Khurana 6th/169; Parson 22nd/ 300]

Fuchs' Uveitis Syndrom E (FUS)

◈ *Khurana 6th/169*

- Fuchs' heterochromiciridocyclitis is a chronic ***nongranulomatous type*** of low grade anterior uveitis. It typically occurs unilaterally in middle-aged persons
- The disease is characterised by:
  - Heterochromia of iris,
  - Diffuse stromal iris atrophy,
  - *Fine KPs at back of cornea,*
  - *Faint aqueous flare,*
  - Absence of posterior synechiae,
  - A fairly common rubeosisiridis, sometimes associated with neovascularization of the angle of anterior chamber, and
  - Comparatively early development of complicated cataract and secondary glaucoma (usually open angle type).
- ***Treatment:*** Topical corticosteroids are all that is required. Cycloplegics are not required as usually there are no posterior synechiae.

Fuchs Heterochromiciridocyclitis

◈ *Parson 22nd/ 300*

- It consists of a chronic, low-grade iritis with posterior subcapsular cataract and secondary glaucoma.
- It is rare, unilateral in 90%of cases, occurs between the third and fourth decades of life and is associated with a change in colour of the iris.
- The inflammation consists of low-grade flare and cells, with stellate ***keratic precipitates*** and fine filaments scattered over the entire endothelium.
- "This is a low-grade chronic cyclitis, the only apparent features of which are a lightening of the colour of the affected iris and the ***presence of a few keratic precipitates on the cornea.*** The latter distinguish the condition from congenital heterochromia" *(Parson 22nd/ 251)*
- Anterior vitreous opacities may be present and occasionally small ***white nodules on the anterior surface of the iris.***
- Secondary glaucoma has been reported in 15% of patients at presentation. Vision decreases as the cataract progresses.
- Control of the uveitis with ***topical corticosteroids*** and non-steroidal anti-inflammatory drugs (NSAIDs) is apriority. The intraocular pressure is initially reduced below 20 mmHg by medical means. Glaucoma therapy is re-evaluated once the inflammation subsides completely, as in POAG.

120. Ans. a. Eye colour is due... b. Stroma is responsible... c. Sphincter pupillae, e. Stroma is covered on

[Ref: Khurana 6th/146-47; Parson 22nd/ 8]

From anterior (front) to posterior (back), the layers of the iris are:

- *Anterior limiting layer*
- *Stroma of iris*
- *Iris sphincter muscle*
- *Iris dilator muscle (myopeithelium)*
- *Anterior pigment epithelium*
- *Posterior pigment epithelium*

"***Eye color is determined by the relative number of melanocytes in the stroma*** and of course the density of melanin granules produced. Few cells give a blue color, whereas many melanin-containing cells produce a dark brown color; gray and green are the intermediate colors"

Iris

◈ *Parson 22nd/8*

- The *iris* is thinnest at its attachment to the ciliary body, so that if torn it tends to give way in this region. It is composed of a ***stroma containing branched connective tissue cells, usually pigmented but largely unpigmented in blue irides,*** with a rich supply of blood vessels which run in a general radial direction.
- The tissue spaces communicate directly with the anterior-chamber through crypts found mainly near the ciliary border; this allows the easy transfer of fluid between the iris and the anterior chamber.

- ***The stroma is covered on its posterior surface by two layers of pigmented epithelium***, which developmentally are derived from theretina and are continuous with each other at the pupillary margin.
- The anterior layer consists of flattened cells and the posterior of cuboidal cells. From the epithelial cells of the former, two unstriped muscles are developed which control the movements of the pupil, the ***sphincter pupillae***, a circular bundle running round the pupillary margin, and the ***dilator pupillae***, arranged radially near the root of the iris.
- The anterior surface of the iris is covered with a single layer of endothelium, except at some minute depressions or crypts which are found mainly at the ciliary border; it usually atrophies in adult life.
- The iris is richly supplied by sensory nerve fibres derived from the trigeminal nerve. The ***sphincter pupillae is supplied by parasympathetic autonomous secretomotor nerve fibres derived from the oculomotor nerve, while the motor fibres of the dilator muscle are derived from the cervical sympathetic chain.***

IRIS Consists of Four Layers which from Anterior to Posterior are

◈ *Khurana 6th/146-47*

- **Anterior limiting layer**: It is the ***anterior most condensed part of the stroma***. It consists of ***melanocytes*** and fibroblasts. Previously this layer was called endothelial layer of iris which was a misnomer. This layer is deficient in the areas of crypts. The ***definitive colour of the iris depends on this layer***. *In blue iris this layer is thin and contains few pigment cells. While in brown iris it is thick and densely pigmented.*
- **Iris stroma**: It consists of loosely arranged collagenous network in which are embedded the ***sphincter pupillae muscle, dilator pupillae muscle***, vessels, nerves, ***pigment cells*** and other cells which include lymphocytes, fibroblasts, macrophages and mast cells.
  The **sphincter pupillae muscle** forms one millimetre broad circular band in the pupillary part of the iris. It is ***supplied by parasympathetic fibres*** through third nerve. It constricts the pupil.
  The **dilator pupillae muscle** lies in the posterior part of stroma of the ciliary zone of iris. Its myofilaments are located in the outer part of the cells of anterior pigment epithelial layer. It is ***supplied by cervical sympathetic nerves*** and dilates the pupil.
- **Anterior epithelial layer**: It is ***anterior continuation of the pigment epithelium of retina and ciliary body***. This layer gives rise to the dilator pupillae muscle.
- **The posterior pigmented epithelial layer**: It is anterior continuation of the ***non-pigmented epithelium of ciliary*** body. At the pupillary margin it forms the pigmented frill and becomes continuous with the anterior pigmented epithelial layer.

121. Ans. a. Rose Bengal staining..., b. Decreased corneal..., c. Fluorescein staining....

[Ref: Khurana 6th/107-09; Parson 22nd/205-07]

"**Acanthamoeb keratitis: *Ring infiltartes***, *central or paracentral, with overlying epithelial defects & underlying keratic precipitate*" *(Khurana 6th/113)*

"Dendritic ulcer base stains with fluorescein & the margins with rose Bengal" *(Parson 22nd/206)*

"Fluorescein installation illuminated by blue light shows up corneal ulceration at an early stage" *(L & B 26th/626)*

Dendritic Ulcer

◈ *Khurana 6th/108*

- Dendritic ulcer is a typical lesion of recurrent epithelial keratitis.
- The ulcer is of an irregular, zigzag linear branching shape. The branches are generally knobbed at the ends. ***Floor of the ulcer stains with fluoresce in*** and the ***virus-laden cells at the margin take up rose bengal***.
- There is ***an associated marked diminution of corneal sensations.***

Herpes Simplex

◈ *Parson 22nd/205-07*

- Ocular involvement with the herpes simplex virus has varied manifestations which include blepharitis, conjunctivitis, keratitis and iridocyclitis. The corneal involvement can be epithelial (dendritic or geographic keratitis), stromal (necrotizing and non-necrotizing stromal keratitis) and endothelial.
- The herpesvirus has a widespread distribution. It can be grown in tissue culture and elementary bodies can be found by ***suitable staining methods*** in the vesicular fluid.
- In all cases the ***cornea is relatively insensitive***. In severe forms, **dendritic ulcers** develop.
- *The infiltrates, spreading in all directions, coalesce and form a large shallow ulcer with crenated edges.* More often grey striae extend in one or more directions, increase in length, and send out lateral branches which are generally knobbed at the ends so that a dendritic figure, not unlike a liverwort, is formed. This resembles no other condition and is pathognomonic. The surface over the infiltrates breaks down and an extremely irritating and chronic ulcer is produced, persisting with exacerbations for weeks or months, sending out fresh branches but never extending in depth.
- ***Generally only one or two of the infiltrates stain with fluorescein at any given time, but fresh spots are continually being formed and the disease frequency recurs; alternatively, a large confluent ulcer may be formed.***
- ***Diagnostic tests are limited to immunofluorescence and culture of epithelial scrapings or tissue biopsies***

ENT

122. Ans. b. Common in smoker, d. Involve whole..., e. Patient has low pitch voice

[Ref: Dhingra 6th/292; L & T 10 th/168; ENT by P.Hazarika 3rd/609]

Reinke's oedema (Polypoid degeneration of vocal cords) *(Dhingra 6th/292)*

- It is ***bilateral symmetrical swelling*** of the ***whole of membranous part of the vocal cords***, most often seen in middle-aged men & women

- This is due to ***oedema of the subepithelial space*** (Reinke's space) of the vocal cords
- Chronic irritation of vocal cords due to misuse of voice, ***heavy smoking***, chronic sinusitis & laryngopharyngeal reflex are the probable etiological factors. It can also occur in myxoedema
- Hoarseness is the common symptoms.
- Patient uses false cords for voice production & this gives him a ***low-pitched & rough voice***
- **Treatment includes:**
  - Decortication of the vocal cords *i.e.,* removal of strip of epithelium, is done first on one side & 3-4 weeks alter on the other;
  - Voice rest &
  - Speech therapy for proper voice production

123. Ans. c. Dysplasia of cochlea

[Ref: Dhingra 6th/115; ENT by P.Hazarika 3rd/81]

Scheibe's Syndrome or Dysplasia

◈ *Dhingra 6th/115*

- *It is most common inner ear anomaly*
- *Bony labyrinth is normal*
- *Superior part of membranous labyrinth (utricle & semicircular canal ducts) is also normal*
- *Dysplasia is seen in the cochlea & saccule; hence also called cochleosaccular dysplasia*
- *It is inherited as an autosomal recessive nonsyndromic trait*

Scheibe's syndrome: Cochleosaccular aplasia with normal bony labyrinth" *(ENT by P.Hazarika 3rd/81)*

124. Ans. All (a, b, c, d, e.)

[Ref: Dhingra 6th/250-53; L & T 10 th/109-11; ENT by P.Hazarika 3rd/521-29]

There are three main etiological factors in etiology of NPC- ***Epstein-Barr virus****, genetically determined susceptibility& environmental factors" (ENT by P.Hazarika 3rd/ 522)*

"**NPC**: *Due to obstruction of Eustachian tube, there is conductive hearing loss,* ***serous or suppurative otitis media****. Presence of unilateral serous otitis media should raise suspicion of nasopharyngeal growth" (Dhingra 6th/251)*

Nasopharyngeal Carcinoma (NPC, Guangdong Tumor)

◈ *Dhingra 6th/250-53; L & T 10 th/109-11)*

- *It is uncommon in India & most common in China*
- *It is mostly seen in fifth to seventh decades but may involve younger age groups*
- *Males are three times more prone than female*
- ***Epstein-Barr virus*** *is closely associated with nasopharyngeal carcinoma*
- *Squamous cell carcinoma in various grades of its differentiation or its variant as transitional cell carcinoma & lymphoepithelioma is the most common (85%)*
- *There* ***may be evidence of fluid in middle ear*** *or the eardrum may be drawn*
- ***Radiotherapy: It is treatment of choice for nasopharyngeal carcinoma.*** *Stage I & II are treated by radiotherapy alone while stage III & IV require concomitant radiation & chemotherapy or radiation followed by chemotherapy*
- *Enlarged palpable cervical lymph nodes are frequently found affecting the* ***level II, III & Va nodes***

125. Ans. a. Multiple hole in..., b. Pale granulation mass..., e. Painless....

[Ref: Dhingra 6th/74; L & T 10th/292-93; ENT by P.Hazarika 3rd/161]

"Treatment of **Tubercular otitis media: This consists of intensive chemotherapy with antituberculous drugs, but surgical treatment may be also be required"** *(L & T 10th/293)*
"Extensive granulation tissue in middle ear & mastoid can lead to early facial nerve palsy" (P.Hazarika 3rd/161)

Tubercular Otitis Media

◈ *Dhingra 6th/74*

- Disease is mostly seen in children & young adults
- There is ***painless necrosis of tympanic membrane. Earache is characteristically absent*** in cases of tubercular otitis media
- ***Multiple perforation*** may form which coalesces to form a single large perforation
- Middle ear & mastoid get filled with ***pale granulations***
- ***Mastoiditis, facial paralysis, postauricular fistula, osteomyelitis*** with formation of bony sequestra& profound hearing loss are often seen in these cases
- There is severe hearing loss, out of proportion to symptoms
- **Facial paralysis**: It is a common complication & may come unexpectedly
- Systemic antitubercular therapy is given for primary disease. Local treatment in the form of aural toilet & control of secondary pyogenic infection
- ***Mastoid surgery indicated for complication.***

126. Ans. c. Steroid

[Ref: CMDT 2016/1024; Harrison 19th/2648, Dhingra 6th/95; L & T 10 th/359; ENT by P.Hazarika 3rd/ 186-87]

Bell's Palsy: Treatment

◈ *Harrison 19th/2648*

- Symptomatic measures include
  - The use of paper tape to depress the upper eyelid during sleep and prevent corneal drying, and
  - ***Massage of the weakened muscles***.
- A ***course of glucocorticoids***, given as prednisone 60–80 mg daily during the first 5 days and then tapered over the next 5 days, modestly shortens the recovery period and improves the functional outcome.
- Although large and well controlled randomized trials found ***no added benefit*** of the **antiviral agents** valacyclovir (1000 mg daily for 5–7 days) or acyclovir (400 mg five times daily for 10 days) ***compared to glucocorticoids alone***, some earlier data suggested that combination therapy with prednisone plus valacyclovir might be marginally better than prednisolone alone, especially in patients with severe clinical presentations.

- For patients with permanent paralysis from Bell's palsy, a number of ***cosmetic surgical procedures*** have been used to restore a relatively symmetric appearance to the face.

Bell's Palsy: Treatment

◈ *CMDT 2016/1024*

- The ***only medical treatment that may influence the outcome is administration of corticosteroids***, but this must be commenced within 5 days of onset. Treatment with prednisone, 60–80 mg orally daily for 4 or 5 days, followed by tapering of the dose over the next 7–10 days, is a satisfactory regimen; prednisolone (50 mg daily orally) for 10 days is another acceptable alternative. It is helpful to protect the eye with lubricating drops (or lubricating ointment at night) and a patch if eye closure is not possible.
- ***Acyclovir does not confer any additional benefit.*** There is ***no evidence that surgical procedures to decompress the facial nerve are of benefit.*** Physical therapy may improve facial function.

Medical Management of Bell's Palsy

◈ *Dhingra 6th/95*

- **Steroids:** Their utility has not been proved beyond doubt in carefully controlled studies. Prednisolone is the drug of choice
- **Other drugs:** Vasodilators, vitamins, mast cell inhibitors & antihistaminics have not been found useful

Surgical Management of Bell's Palsy

◈ *Dhingra 6th/95*

- ***Nerve decompression relieves pressure on the nerve fibres***& thus improves the microcirculation of the nerve. Vertical & tympanic segments of nerve are decompressed

Treatment of Bell's Palsy

◈ *L & T 10 th/359*

- Treatment of the condition is similarly confused. The standard treatment is steroids in various forms (ACTH, prednisolone, cortisone), ***although no valid trials have confirmed the usefulness of this method.*** They make the patient feel better but have not been shown to have any effect on the prognosis of the palsy
- ***Surgical decompression of the nerve is contentious.*** The decision to do this to avoid a poor end-result relies on the results of the prognostic electrophysiological tests

Treatment of Bell's Palsy

◈ *http//www.bellspalsy.ws/treatment.htm*

In a study released by the Quality Standards Subcommittee of the American Academy of Neurology (May 2001), Drs. Patrick Grogan and Gary Gronseth pooled the data of existing studies published from 1996 through 2000 regarding the effectiveness of steroids, anti-virals, and decompression surgery as treatment for Bell's palsy. Their conclusions are:

- **Regarding the use of steroids:** ***Steroids are "safe and probably effective in improving facial functional outcomes*** in patients with Bell's palsy." Results show significantly better outcomes with steroids. However, they do not find any difference in the time frame for recovery.
- **Regarding the use of antivirals used in combination with steroids:** Based on the limited data available, "**acyclovir** (combined with prednisone) is safe and possibly effective in improving facial functional outcomes in patients with Bell's palsy."
- **Regarding decompression surgery:** "The **risk of bias** in all studies describing facial outcomes in surgically treated Bell's palsy patients was ***too high to support evidence-based conclusions.*** Additionally, serious complications, including permanent hearing loss, were reported from surgical facial nerve decompression."

Empiric Therapy Regimens

◈ *http: //emedicine.medscape.com/article/2018337-overview*

Empiric therapeutic regimens for Bell palsy are outlined below, including those for corticosteroid treatment and eye care.

- The ***most widely accepted treatment for Bell palsy is corticosteroids. Multiple randomized controlled trials show benefit with the use of corticosteroids.*** The ***revised 2012 guidelines for Bell palsy issued by the American Academy of Neurology support the use of corticosteroids and rate them as "highly effective."***

Antiviral agents have also been studied in this setting and may be used in conjunction with corticosteroids. ***Evidence suggests antivirals have no benefit by themselves.*** Two meta-analyses showed conflicting conclusions for the value of combining antiviral agents and corticosteroids. However, more recent evidence suggests that a combination of antivirals and corticosteroids is more effective than corticosteroids alone. *If antivirals are used, they should be used in combination with corticosteroids.*

The following guidelines from the American Academy of Otolaryngology–Head and Neck Surgery Foundation were issued in November 2013 and support the use of corticosteroids and the optional use of antiviral agents

- **Oral corticosteroids** should be given within 72 hours of symptom onset in patients aged 16 years or older
- **Antiviral monotherapy** should not be given in new-onset disease; *antiviral agents may be offered in combination with corticosteroids*

127. Ans. a. Perilymph..., b. Otolithiasis, c. Vestibular..., d. Meniere's disease

[Ref: Dhingra 6th/45-46; L & T 10 th/334; ENT by P.Hazarika 3rd/98-103]

*"Vestibular neuronitis: It is characterized by **severe vertigo** of sudden onset with no cochlear symptoms"- Dhingra 6th/45*

"Otolithiasis is an inner ear problem that causes ***repeated episodes of vertigo*** lasting for seconds. It occurs with position changes. Commonly occurs when rolling over in bed, bending over, or looking upward. This problem occurs when inner ear calcium particles fall into an inner ear semicircular canal. The problem may occur with or without a history of head trauma" *(http: //www.lubbocksinusdoctor.com/)*

Disorder of Vestibular System

◈ *Dhingra 6th/45-46*

- *This cause vertigo & divided into peripheral & central disorder*

- *Peripheral: It involves vestibular end organs & their 1st order neuron (i.e. the vestibular nerve). The cause lies in the internal ear or the VIIIth nerve. They are responsible for 85% of all cases*
- *Central: It involves **central nervous system** after the entrance of vestibular nerve in the brainstem & involve vestibilo-ocular, vestibulospinal & other central nervous system pathways*

Meniere's Disease (Endolymphatic Hydrops)

◈ *Dhingra 6th/45*

- It is characterized by vertigo, fluctuating hearing loss, tinnitus & sense of pressure in the involved ear
- Vertigo is of sudden onset, lasts for a few minutes to 24 hr or so

Table *(Dhingra 6th/46)*: **Vestibular disorders**

Peripheral (Lesions of end organs vestibular nerve)	Central (Lesions of brainstem & central connection)
• Meniere's disease • Benign paroxysmal positional vertigo • Vestibular neronitis • Labyrinthitis • Vestibulotoxic drugs • Head trauma • Perilymph fistula • Syphilis • Acoustic neuroma	• Vertebrobasilar insufficiency • Posterior inferior cerebellar artery syndrome • Basilar migraine • Cerebellar diseases • Multiple sclerosis • Tumours of brainstem & fourth ventricle • Epilepsy • Cervical vertigo

MEDICINE

128. Ans. c. Fatigue relieved by rest

[Ref: Harrison 19th/ 464e1-3; CMDT 2016/37-38; Davidson 22nd/246; Synopsis of Psychiatry by Kaplon 11th/504-07]

*"The **physical examination** in patients with CFS characteristically **shows no abnormalities**" (Kaplon 11th/506)*

"The diagnosis of CFS is primarily one of exclusion of alternate conditions" (Kaplon 11th/506)

"**Characteristic symptoms** of chronic fatigue syndrome (CFS) include fatigue, myalgia, arthralgia, ***impaired memory and concentration***, and unrefreshing sleep" *(Kaplon 11th/506)*

Chronic Fatigue Syndrome (A/K Neurasthenia)

◈ *Davidson 22nd/246*

- It is characterized by excessive fatigue after minimal physical or mental exertion, poor concentration, dizziness, muscular aches and sleep disturbance.
- This pattern of symptoms may follow a viral infection such as infectious mononucleosis, influenza or hepatitis.
- Symptoms overlap with those of depression and anxiety.
- There is good evidence that many patients improve with carefully graded exercise and with **Cognitive behavioral therapy** (CBT), as long as the benefits of such treatment are carefully explained.

Chronic Fatigue Syndrome

◈ *Harrison 19th/ 464e1-3*

- Chronic fatigue syndrome (CFS) is a disorder characterized by persistent and unexplained fatigue resulting in severe impairment in daily functioning.
- Besides intense fatigue, most patients with CFS report concomitant symptoms such as pain, cognitive dysfunction, and unrefreshing sleep.
- Additional symptoms can include headache, sorethroat, tender lymph nodes, muscle aches, joint aches, feverishness, difficulty sleeping, psychiatric problems, allergies, and abdominal cramps. Criteria for the diagnosis of CFS have been developed by the U.S. Centers for Disease Control and Prevention
- ***The mean age of onset is between 29 and 35 years.*** Many patients probably go undiagnosed and/or do not seek help.
- There are numerous hypotheses about the etiology of CFS; there is no definitively identified cause.
- The pathophysiology of CFS is unclear. ***Neuro physiologic studies have shown altered CNS activation patterns during muscle contraction.***
- Evidence for immunologic dysfunction is inconsistent.
- In addition to a thorough history, a systematic physical examination is warranted to exclude disorders causing fatigue (e.g., endocrine disorders, neoplasms, heart failure).
- Laboratory tests serve primarily to exclude other diagnoses; ***no test can diagnose CFS.***
- Serology for viral or bacterial infections usually is not helpful. ***No specific abnormalities have been identified on MRI or CT scans.***
- CFS is a constellation of symptoms with no pathognomonic features and ***remains a diagnosis of exclusion.***
- Concurrent psychiatric disorders, especially anxiety and mood disorders, are present in 30–60% of cases.
- For patients with headache, diffuse pain, and feverishness, nonsteroidal anti-inflammatory drugs may be helpful.
- The patient should be encouraged to maintain regular sleep patterns, to remain as active as possible, and to gradually return to previous levels of exercise and other activity (work).
- ***CBT and graded exercise therapy (GET) have been found to be the only beneficial interventions in CFS.***

Table *(Harrison 19th/464e-1)*: **Diagnostic Criteria for Chronic Fatigue Syndrome**

A. Characteristic Persistent or Relapsing Unexplained Chronic Fatigue

- *Fatigue lasts for **a least 6 months***
- Fatigue is of new or definite onset
- Fatigue is not the result of an organic disease or of continuing exertion
- *Fatigue is **not alleviated by rest***
- Fatigue results in a substantial reduction in previous occupational, educational, social, and personal activities.

Contd...

- **Four or more of the following symptoms are concurrently present for 6 months:** ***impaired memory or concentration,*** *sore throat, tender cervical or axillary lymph nodes, muscle pain, pain in several joints, new headaches, unrefreshing sleep, or malaise after exertion*

B. Exclusion criteria
- Medical condition explaining fatigue
- Major depressive disorder (psychotic features) or bipolar disorder
- Schizophrenia, dementia, or delusional disorder
- Anorexia nervosa, bulimia nervosa
- Alcohol or substance abuse
- Severe obesity (body mass index >40)

129. Ans. b. Hyperkalemia

[Ref: Harrison 19th/ 16118-19, 2318-19; CMDT 2016/ 437-38; Davidson 22nd/ 780-81; Robbins 9th/1126-27, 490]

"**Primary hyperaldosteronism** *is* ***one of the most common cause of secondary hypertension***" *(Robbins 9th/490)*

"The most important clinical consequence of hyperaldosteronism is hypertension. With an estimated prevalence rate of 5% to 10% among non-selected hypertensive patients, ***primary hyperaldosteronism may be most common cause of secondary hypertension*** *(i.e, hypertension secondary to an identifiable cause) - Robbins 9th/1126*

Primary Hyperaldosteronism

◈ *Robbins 9th/1126-27*

- *Hyperaldosteronism* is the generic term for a small group of closely related, uncommon syndromes, all characterized by chronic excess aldosterone secretion. *Excessive levels of* ***aldosterone cause sodium retention and potassium excretion,*** *with resultant hypertension and hypokalemia.*
- *The* ***clinical manifestations of primary hyperaldosteronism are hypertension and hypokalemia.Serum renin,*** is low.
- Hypokalemia results from renal potassium wasting and can cause a variety of neuromuscular manifestations, including ***weakness, paresthesias, visual disturbances, and occasionally frank tetany.***
- ***Sodium retention increases the total body sodium*** and expands the extracellular fluid volume, leading to ***elevation of the serum sodium concentration*** and an increase in intracellular sodium with increased vascular reactivity.
- ***The diagnosis of primary hyperaldosteronism is confirmed by the elevated levels of aldosterone and depressed levels of renin in the circulation.*** Even when the diagnosis of primary hyperaldosteronism is made, it is necessary to distinguish among the various causes, particularly the differentiation of an adenoma, which is amenable to surgical excision.

Primary Aldosteronism

◈ *Harrison 19th/ 1618-19; 19th/2319*

- Excess aldosterone production due to primary aldosteronism is a potentially curable form of hypertension. In patients with primary aldosteronism, increased aldosterone production is independent of the renin-angiotensin system, and the consequences are ***sodium retention, hypertension, hypokalemia, and low PRA.***
- Hypertension is usually mild to moderate but occasionally may be severe. Most patients are asymptomatic, although, infrequently, ***polyuria, polydipsia, paresthesias,*** or ***muscle weakness*** may be present as a consequence of hypokalemic alkalosis.
- The ***ratio of plasma aldosterone to plasma renin activity (PA/PRA) is a useful screening test.***
- ***Some 60–70% of patients have an aldosterone-producing adrenal adenoma.*** The tumor is almost always unilateral, and most often measures <3 cm in diameter. ***Most of the remainder of these patients have bilateral adrenocortical hyperplasia (idiopathic hyperaldosteronism).***
- Excess activation of the mineralocorticoid receptor leads to ***potassium depletion and increased sodium retention,*** with the latter causing an expansion of extracellular and plasma volume. Increased ENaC activity also results in hydrogen depletion thatcan cause ***metabolic alkalosis.***
- ***Severe alkalosis contributes to muscle cramps and, in severe cases, can cause tetany.***

Primary Hyperaldosteronism

◈ *Davidson 22nd/780-81*

- ***Occasionally tetany*** may present (because of associated metabolic alkalosis and low ionised calcium).
- Routine blood tests may show a hypokalaemic alkalosis. ***Sodium is usually at the upper end of the reference range in primary hyperaldosteronism, but is characteristically low in secondary hyperaldosteronism*** (because low plasma volume stimulates antidiuretic hormone (ADH) release and high angiotensin II levels stimulatethirst).
- The ***key measurements are plasma renin andaldosterone,*** and in many centres, ***the aldosterone: renin ratio (ARR)*** is employed as a screening test for primary hyperaldosteronism in hypertensive patients.

130. Ans. c. Pain relieved by lying supine...

[Ref: Harrison 19th/ 1571-72; Davidson 22nd/639-41; CMDT 2016/422-23; Robbins 9th/573-74]

Sound Characteristic

◈ *depts.washington.edu*

Pleural friction rub	Pericardial friction rub
High frequency (hear best with diaphragm of stethoscope)	High frequency (hear best with diaphragm of stethoscope)
Grating or creaking sound	**Scratchy, gratin or squeaking**

"ECG may manifest a characteristic progression beginning with ***diffuse ST elevation, followed by a return to baseline & then to T-wave inversion****" (CMDT 2016/423)*

Acute Pericarditis

◈ *Harrison 19th/1571-72*

- *Chest pain* is usually present in acute infectious pericarditis and in many of the forms presumed to be related to hypersensitivity or autoimmunity. The pain of acute pericarditis is often severe, ***retrosternal, and left precordial, and referred to the neck, arms, or left shoulder.***

- Frequently the pain is pleuritic, consequent toaccompanying pleural inflammation (*i.e.*, sharp and aggravated byinspiration and coughing), but sometimes it is steady, constricting, radiates into either arm or both arms
- Characteristically, however, ***pericardial pain may be relieved by sitting up and leaning forward and is intensified by lying supine.***
- A ***pericardial friction rub*** is audible at some point in about 85% of patients with acute pericarditis, may have up to three components per cardiac cycle, is high-pitched, and is described as ***rasping, scratching, or grating.*** It is heard most frequently at end expiration with the patient upright and leaning forward.
- The **electrocardiogram (ECG)** in acute pericarditis without massive effusion usually displays changes secondary to acute subepicardial inflammation. It typically evolves through four stages.
- In stage 1, there is ***widespread elevation of the ST segments, often with upward concavity,*** involving two or three standard limb leads and V2 to V6, with ***reciprocal depressions only in aVR and sometimes V1.*** Also, there is depression of the PR segment below the TP segment, reflecting atrial involvement. Usually there are ***no significant changes in QRS complexes. After several days, the ST segments return to normal*** (stage 2), and only then, or even later, ***do the T waves become inverted*** (stage 3). Weeks or months after the onset of acute pericarditis, the ECG returns to normal (stage 4). In contrast, in AMI, ***ST elevations are convex, and reciprocal depression is usually more prominent***; these changes may return to normal within a day or two. Q waves may develop, with loss of R-wave amplitude, and T-wave inversions are usually seen within hours *before* the ST segments have become isoelectric

Acute Pericarditis

◈ *Davidson 22nd/639-41*

- The ***characteristic pain of pericarditis is retrosternal, radiates to the shoulders and neck,*** and is typically aggravated by deep breathing, movement, a change of position, exercise and swallowing.
- A pericardial friction rub is a ***high-pitchedsuperficial scratching or crunching noise,*** produced by movement of the inflamed pericardium, and is diagnostic of pericarditis; it is usually heard in systole but may also be audible in diastole and frequently has a 'to-and - fro' quality.
- ***The ECG shows ST elevation with upward concavity*** over the affected area, which may be wide spread. ***PR interval depression is a very specific indicator of acute pericarditis. Later, there may be T-wave inversion, particularly if there is a degree of myocarditis.***
- The pain is usually relieved by ***aspirin*** (600 mg6 times daily) but a more potent anti-inflammatory agent, such as indomethacin (25 mg 3 times daily), may be required. ***Colchicine or corticosteroids*** may ***suppress symptoms*** but there is no evidence that they accelerate cure.
- "***Systemic corticosteroid can be used in patients with severe symptoms,*** in refractory cases or in patients with immune-mediated immunologies" *(CMDT 2016/423)*

Pericardial friction rubs are characterized by
(depts.washington.edu)

- One systolic sound and two diastolic sounds (3 component rub) (systolic sound between $S_1$and S_2)
- One diastolic sound in early diastole and one at end diastole (2 component rub)

131. Ans. a. Ovary cancer, c. Squamous cell..., d. Renal cancer

[Ref: Harrison 19th/608-09; CMDT 2016/ 1586-88; Robbins 9th/330-31]

"Hypercalcemia is probably the most common paraneoplastic syndrome; overtly symptomatic hypercalcemia is most often related to some form of cancer rather than to hyperparathyroidism. Two general processes are involved in cancer-associated hypercalcemia: osteolysis induced by cancer, whether primary in bone, such as multiple myeloma, or metastatic to bone from any primary lesion, and, the production of calcemic humoral substances by extraosseous neoplasms. *Hypercalcemia owing to skeletal metastases is not a paraneoplastic syndrome" (Robbins 9th/330)*

Table *(Robbins 9th/330)*: **Paraneoplastic Syndromes**

Clinical Syndromes	Major Forms of Underlying Cancer	Causal Mechanism
Hypercalcemia	***Squamous cell carcinoma of lung, Breast carcinoma, Ovarian carcinoma, Renal carcinoma, Adult T-cell leukemia/lymphoma***	Parathyroid hormone-related protein (PTHRP), TGF-α, TNF, IL-1

Table *(Harrison 19th/609)*: **Paraneoplastic Syndromes Caused by Ectopic Hormone Production**

Paraneoplastic Syndrome	Ectopic Hormone	Typical Tumor Types
Common		
Hypercalcemia of malignancy	Parathyroid hormone-related protein (PTHrP)	Squamous cell (head and neck, lung, skin), breast, genitourinary, gastrointestinal
	1, 25 dihydroxyvitamin D	Lymphomas
	Parathyroid hormone (PTH) (rare)	Lung, ovary
	Prostaglandin E2 (PGE2) (rare)	Renal, lung

Table *(CMDT 2016/ 1588)*: **Paraneoplastic Syndromes Associated with Cancer**

Hormone Excess or Syndrome	Non-Small Cell Lung Cancer	Small Cell Lung Cancer	Breast Cancer	Renal Cell Carcinoma	Adrenal Cancer	Hepalo cellular Carcinoma	Gastro intestinal Cancers	Multiple Myeloma	Lymphoma	Thymoma	Prostatic Cancer	Ovarian Cancer	Choriocarcinoma	Germ Cell Cancers
Endocrine														
Hypercalcemia	++		++	++	++			++	+		++			
Cushing syndrome	+	++		+	++					++	+			
SIADH	++	++												
Hypoglycemia					+	++	+							
Gonadotropin secretion	+	++		+	+	+	+						++	++
Hyperthyroidism													++	+

+, reported associated; ++, strong association.

132. Ans. a. CK7 is found..., b. CK20+/CDX-2+/CK7... d. Chromogranin...

[Ref: Harrison 19th/ 120e; Davidson 22nd/ 282]

Table *(Harrison (19th/ 120e-2)*: **Select Immunohistochemical Stains Useful in the Diagnosis of Carcinoma of Unknown Primary (CUP)**

Likely Primary Profile	Commonly Considered IHC to Assist in Differential Diagnosis of CUP[a]
Breast	Estrogen receptor (ER), gross cystic disease fibrous protein-15 (GCDFP-15), mammaglobin, Her-2/neu
Ovarian/mullerian	Estrogen receptor (ER), Wilms'tumor gene (WF-1), PAX8, PAX2
Lung adenocarcinoma	Thyroid transcription factor (TTF-1; nuclear staining), napsin A, surfactant protein A precursor (S P-Al)
Germ cell	β-hCG, , AFP OCT3/4, CKIT, CD30 (embryonal), SALL4
Prostate	PSA, α-methylacyl CoA racemase/P504S(AMACR/P501S (prostein), and prostate-specific membrane antigen (PSMA)
Intestinal	CK7, CK20, CDX-2, carcinoembryonic antigen (CEA)
Neuroendocrine	Chromogranin, synaptophysin, CD56
Sarcoma	Desmin (desmoid tumors), factor VIII (angiosarcomas), CD31, smooth muscle actin (leiomyosarcoma), MyoD1 (rhabdomyosarcoma)
Renal	RCC, CD10, PAX8
Hepatocellular carcinoma	Hep par-1, arginase-1 (Arg-1), TTF-1 (granular cytoplasmic staining)
Melanoma	S100, vimentin, HMB-45, tyrosinase and melan-A
Urothelial	CK7, CK20, thrombomodulin
Mesothelioma	Calretinin, WT-1
Lymphoma	Leukocyte common antigen (LCA), CD3 CD4, CD5, CD20, CD45
Squamous cell carcinoma (SCC)	P63, p40 (lung SCC), CK5/6

Carcinoma of unknown Primary (CUP)

◈ *Davidson 22nd/ 282*

- Some patients are found to have evidence of metastatic disease at their initial presentation prior to diagnosis of a primary site. In many cases, a subsequent biopsy reveals adenocarcinoma but the primary site is not always clear.

CUP Evaluation

◈ *Harrison 19th/ 120e*

- Initial CUP evaluation has two goals: search for the primary tumor based on pathologic evaluation of the metastases and determine the extent of disease. Obtaining a thorough medical history from CUP patients is essential, including paying particular attention to previous surgeries, removed lesions, and family medical history to assess potential hereditary cancers.
- Adequate physical examination, including a digital rectal examination in men and breast and pelvic examinations in women, should be performed based on clinical presentation.
- ***Role of Serum Tumor Markers and Cytogenetics*** Most tumor markers, including ***CEA, CA-125, CA 19-9, and CA 15-3, when elevated, are nonspecific and not helpful in determining the primary tumor site. Men who present with adenocarcinoma and osteoblastic metastasis should undergo a prostate-specific antigen (PSA) test. In patients with undifferentiated or poorly differentiated carcinoma (especially with a midline tumor), elevated β-human chorionic gonadotropin (β-hCG) and α fetoprotein (AFP) levels suggest the possibility of anextragonadal germ cell (testicular) tumor.*** With the availability of IHC, cytogenetic studies are rarely needed.

Role of Immunohistochemical Analysis

- There are >20 subtypes of ***cytokeratin (CK)*** intermediate filaments with different molecular weights and differential expression in various cell types and cancers. Monoclonal antibodies to specific CK subtypes have been used to help classify tumors according to their site of origin; commonly used CK stains in adenocarcinoma CUP are CK7 and CK20. ***CK7 is found in tumors of the lung, ovary, endometrium, breast, and upper gastrointestinal tract including pancreaticobiliary cancers,*** whereas ***CK20 is normally expressed in the gastrointestinal epithelium, urothelium, and Merkel cells.***
- ***Thyroid transcription factor 1 (TTF-1)*** nuclear staining is typically positive in lung and thyroid cancers. Approximately 68% of adenocarcinomas and 25% of squamous cell lung cancers stain positive for TTF-1, which helps differentiate a lung primary tumor from metastatic adenocarcinoma in a pleural effusion, the mediastinum, or the lung parenchyma.
- IHC performs the best when used in groups that give rise to patterns that are strongly indicative of certain profiles. For example, the ***TTF-1/CK7+ and CK20+/CDX-2+/CK7– phenotypes have been reported as very suggestive of lung and lower gastrointestinal cancer*** profiles, respectively, although these patterns have not been validated

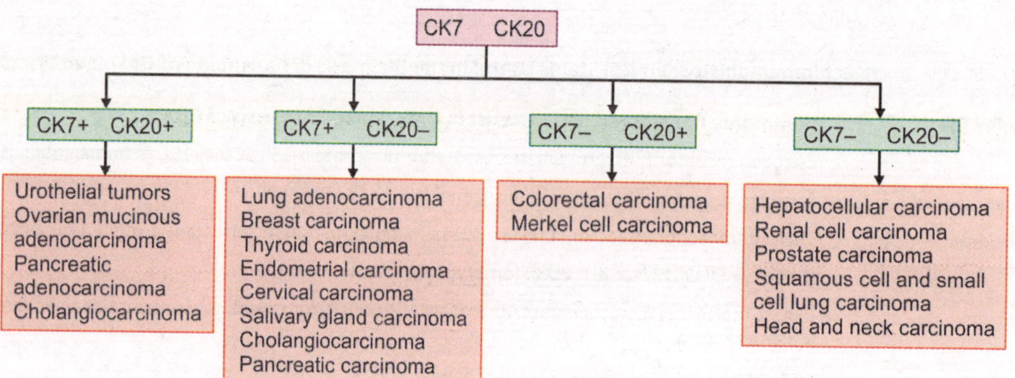

Fig: Approach to cytokeratin (CK7 and CK20) markers used in CUP

133. Ans. a. Most effective..., b. Contraindicated..., d. Contraindicated if platelets...,

[Ref: Harrison 19th/ 2561-62; CMDT 2016/981; Davidson 22nd/1244]

Table *(Harrison)*: **Administration of Intravenous Recombinant Tissue Plasminogen Activator (RTPA) for Acute Ischemic Stroke**

Indication	Contraindication
Clinical diagnosis of stroke	Sustained BP >185/110 mm Hg despite treatment
Onset of symptoms to time of drug administration ≤4.5 h(3h-Harrison 18th)	Platelets <100,000; HCT <25%; glucose <50 or >400 mg/dL
CT scan showing no hemorrhage or edema of >1/3 of the MCA territory	Use of heparin within 48 h and prolonged PTT, or elevated INR
Age ≥18 years	Rapidly improving symptoms
Consent by patient or surrogate	***Prior stroke or head injury within 3 months; prior intracranial hemorr***hage
	Major surgery in preceding 14 days
	Minor stroke symptoms
	Gastrointestinal bleeding in preceding 21 days
	Recent myocardial infarction
	Coma or stupor

Intravenous Thrombolysis

◈ *Harrison 19th/ 2561-62*

- ***Despite an increased incidence of symptomatic intracranial hemorrhage, treatment with IV rtPA within 3 h of the onset of ischemic stroke improved clinical outcome.***
- ***Based on these data, rtPA is approved in the 3- to 4.5-h window in Europe and Canada, but is still only approved for 0–3 h in the United States and Canada.***

Thrombolysis

◈ *Davidson 22nd/1244*

- Intravenous thrombolysis with recombinant tissue plasminogen activator (rt-PA) increases the risk of haemorrhagic transformation of the cerebral infarct with potentially fatal results. ***However, if it is given within 4.5 hours of symptom onset to carefully selected patients, the haemorrhagic risk is offset by an improvement in overall outcome***

Thrombolysis

◈ *CMDT 2016/ 981*

- ***Prophylactic measures were considered earlier in discussing transient ischemic attacks. The management of acute stroke should be in a stroke care unit, when feasible. Intravenous thrombolytic therapy with recombinant tissue plasminogen activator (rtPA; 0.9 mg/kg to a maximum of 90 mg, with 10% given as a bolus over 1 minute and the remainder over 1 hour) is effective in reducing the neurologic deficit in selected patients without CT evidence of intracranial hemorrhage.***
- ***Patients should receive tPA within 1 hour after arriving to the hospital but not more than 4.5 hours after the onset of ischemic symptoms. Recent data for treatment with tPA up to 4.5 hours after the onset of symptoms show reduced disability at 90 days.***

134. Ans. c. Poorly controlled......

[Ref: Harrison 19th/318, 322-23; CMDT 2016/890-96; Davidson 22nd/445]

Asthma & COPD presents with respiratory acidosis

Respiratory acidosis- hypercapnia; *CMDT 2016/895*

Respiratory alkalosis- hypocapia; *CMDT 2016/895*

Respiratory acidosis *Harrison 19th/322-23*

- Acute hypercapnia follows sudden occlusion of the upper airway or generalized bronchospasm as in ***severe asthma***, anaphylaxis, inhalational burn, or toxin injury. ***Chronic hypercapnia and respiratory acidosis occur in end-stage obstructive lung disease.*** Restrictive disorders involving both the chest wall and the lungs can cause respiratory acidosis because the high metabolic cost of respiration causes ventilatory muscle fatigue.

Table *(Harrison 19th/318)*: **Causes of High Anion–Gap Metabolic Acidosis**

Lactic acidosis	Toxins
Ketoacidosis	Ethylene glycol
Diabetic	Methanol
Alcoholic	Salicylates
Starvation	Propylene glycol
	Pyroglutamic acid
	Renal failure (acute and chronic)

Table *(Davidson 22nd/445)*: **Causes of Metabolic Acidosis**

Disorder	Mechanism
A. Normal anion gap	
Ingestion or infusion of inorganic acid	Therapeutic infusion of or poisoning with NH_4Cl, HCl
Gastrointestinal HCO_3 loss	Loss of HCO_3 in diarrhoea, small bowel fistula, urinary diversion procedure
Renal tubular acidosis (RTA)	Urinary loss of HCO_3 in proximal RTA; impaired tubular acid secretion in distal RTA
B. Increased anion gap	
Endogenous acid load	
Diabetic ketoacidosis	Accumulation of ketones with hyperglycaemia
Starvation ketosis	Accumulation of ketones without hyperglycaemia
Lactic acidosis	Shock, liver disease, drugs
Renal failure	Accumulation of organic acids
Exogenous acid load	
Aspirin poisoning	Accumulation of salicylate
Methanol poisoning	Accumulation of formate
Ethylene glycol poisoning	Accumulation of glycolate, oxalate

Table *(CMDT2016/890)*: **Anion Gap in Metabolic Acidosis**

Decreased (<6 mEq)
Hypoalbuminemia (decreased unmeasured anion)
Plasma cell dyscrasias
Monoclonal protein (cationic paraprotein) (accompanied by chloride and bicarbonate)
Bromide intoxication

Contd...

Increased (> 12 mEq)

A. Metabolic anion

Diabetic ketoacidosis

Alcoholic ketoacidosis

Lactic acidosis

Chronic kidney disease (advanced stages) (PO_4^{3-}, SO_4^{2-})

Starvation

Metabolic alkalosis (increased number of negative charges on protein)

5–oxoproline acidosis from acetaminophen toxicity

B. Drug or chemical anion

Salicylate intoxication

Sodium carbenicillin therapy

Methanol (formic acid)

Ethylene glycol (oxalic acid)

Normal (6–12 mEq)

A. Loss of HCO_3

Diarrhea

Recovery from diabetic ketoacidosis

Pancreatic fluid loss, ileostomy (unadapted)

Carbonic anhydrase inhibitors

B. Chloride retention

Renal tubular acidosis

Ileal loop bladder

C. Administration of HCl equivalent or NH_4Cl

Arginine and lysine in parenteral nutrition

135. Ans. a. Occur in children..., b. Precocious puberty..., c. Involve long....

[Ref: Harrison 19th/ 2344; Nelson 20th/2660-61; CMDT 2016/1167; Davidson 22nd/ 1131, 59; Robbins 9th/1206-07: Maheshwari 5th/249]

*"The **hyperthyroidism** that occur is differ from that characteristic of Graves disease. Clinical hyperthyroidism is uncommon in children, but goiters, mildly elevated tri-iodothyronine levels, suppressed TSH levels & abnormalities on ultrasound have been reported. Thyroidectomy is rarely necessary"-Nelson 20th/2661*

*"Precocious puberty has been described predominantly in girls. The **average age at onset in affected girls is about 3** yr, but vaginal bleeding has occurred as early as 4 month of age. In boys, precocious puberty is less common" (Nelson 20th/2660)*

McCune-Albright Syndrome

◈ *Robbins 9th/1206-07*

- The most common clinical presentation of McCune-Albright syndrome is ***precocious sexual development***, which occurs ***most often in girls.*** The syndrome can include other endocrinopathies such as ***hyperthyroidism***, pituitary adenomas that secrete growth hormone, and primary adrenal hyperplasia.
- The ***bone lesions*** are often unilateral, and the skin pigmentation is usually limited to the same side of the body. The cutaneous macules are classically large; dark to café-au-lait in color; have irregular serpiginous borders; and are found primarily on the neck, chest, back, shoulder, and pelvic region. The skeletal manifestations are managed as for other polyostotic fibrous dysplasia while the endocrinopathies are treated medically, for example with aromatase inhibitors for precocious puberty.

McCune-Albright Syndrome

◈ *Harrison 19th/ 2344*

- *McCune-Albright syndrome* consists of ***polyostotic fibrous dysplasia***, pigmented skin patches, and a variety of endocrine disorders, including acromegaly, adrenal adenomas, and autonomous ovarian function. Hormonal hypersecretion results from constitutive cyclic AMP production caused by inactivation of the GTPase activity of Gsα.
- McCune-Albright syndrome (MAS) is characterized by the triad of polyostotic fibrous dysplasia, which may be associated with hypophosphatemic rickets; cafe au lait skin pigmentation; and peripheral ***precocious puberty***; other endocrine abnormalities include thyrotoxicosis, which may be associated with a multinodular goiter, somatotrope tumors, and Cushing's syndrome (due to adrenal tumors).
- Often in Polyostotic fibrous dysplasia, the ***bones of a single limb (i.e. long bone)*** are affected-*Maheshwari 5th/249*
- Investigation and treatment for each endocrinopathy are similar to those used in patients without MAS.

136. Ans. c. Alcholoic hepatitis, e. Inferior vena cava...

[Ref: Kundu 4th/120; Harshmohan 7th/615-16; Harrison 19th/ 2063; PJM 20th/84-85; Davidson 22nd/ 945-46; Robbins 9th/829]

Increased portal vein pressure is seen in any cause of portal hypertension, but increase in hepatic vein pressure is seen in obstruction of hepatic vein & beyond (i.e. post hepatic obstruction)

"Budd-Chiari syndrome (Obstruction of hepatic veins at any site from efferent vein of the lobule to the entry of the IVC into right atrium) *(Kundu 4th/120)*

Table *(Harrison 19th/2063)*: **Classification of Portal Hypertension**

Prehepatic

- Portal vein thrombosis; Splenic vein thrombosis: Massive splenomegaly (Banti's syndrome)

Hepatic

A. **Presinusoidal:** Schistosomiasis & Congenital hepatic fibrosis
B. **Sinusoidal:** Cirrhosis—many causes& Alcoholic hepatitis
C. **Postsinusoidal:** Hepatic sinusoidal obstruction (venoocclusive syndrome)

Posthepatic

- Budd-Chiari syndrome, Inferior vena caval webs& Cardiac causes (Restrictive cardiomyopathy, Constrictive pericarditis& Severe congestive heart failure)

Table: *(PJM 20th/85)*

Feature	Cirrhosis of liver	Non-cirrhotic portal fibrosis	Extra-hepatic portal vein obstruction
Site of obstruction	Intrahepatic, sinusoidal & post sinusoidal	Intrahepatic, sinusoidal & post sinusoidal	Extrahepatic
Portal vein pressure	High	High	Normal
Hepatic wedge pressure	High	High/Normal	Normal

137. Ans. c. Failure to achieve an... d. Limit interruptions.

[Ref: https: //eccguidelines. heart.org/wp-content/uploads/2015/10/2015-AHA-Guidelines-Highlights-English.pdf*]*

$ETCO_2$ for Prediction of Failed Resuscitation

2015 (New): In intubated patients, failure to achieve an ETCO2 of greater than 10 mm Hg by waveform capnography after 20 minutes of CPR may be considered as one component of a multimodal approach to decide when to end resuscitative efforts but should not be used in isolation.

Why: Failure to achieve an ***$ETCO_2$ of 10 mm*** Hg by waveform capnography after 20 minutes of resuscitation has been associated with an extremely poor chance of ROSC and survival.

However, the studies to date are limited in that they have potential confounders and have included relatively small numbers of patients, so it is inadvisable to rely solely on $ETCO_2$ in determining when to terminate resuscitation

Table: Summary of High-Quality CPR Components for BLS providers

Component	Adults and adolescents	Children (Age 1 year to puberty)	Infants (Age less than 1 year, excluding newborns)
Scene safety	Make sure the environment is safe for rescuers and victim		
Recognition of cardiac arrest	Check for responsiveness No breathing only gasping (i.e., no normal breathing) No definite pulse felt within 10 seconds (Breathing and pulse check can be performed simultaneously in less than 10 seconds)		
Activity of emergency response system	If you are alone with no mobile phone, leave the victim to activate the emergency response system and get the AED before beginning CPR Otherwise, send someone and begin CPR immediately, use the AED as soon as it is available	**Witnessed collapse** Follow steps for adults and adolescents on the left **Unwitnessed collapse** Give 2 minutes of CPR Leave the victim to activate the emergency response system and get the AED Return to the child or infant and resume CPR; use the AED as soon as it is available	
Compression ventilation ratio without advanced airway	1 or 2 rescuers 30: 2	***1 rescuer*** 30: 2 ***2 or more rescuers*** 15: 2	
Compression ventilation ratio with advanced airway	Continuous compressions at a rate of 100-120/min Give 1 breath every 6 seconds (10 breaths/min)		
Compression rate	100-1200/min		
Compression depth	At least 2 inches (5 cm) *	At least one third AP diameter of chest About 2 inches (5 cm)	At least one third AP diameter of chest About 1½ inches (4 cm)
Hand placement	2 hands on the lower half of the breastbone (sternum)	2 hands or 1 hand (optional for very small child) on the lower half of the breastbone (sternum)	**1 rescuer** 2 fingers in the centre of the chest, just below the nipple line **2 or more rescuers** 2 thumb-encircling hand in the center of the chest, just below the nipple line
Chest recoil	Allow full recoil of chest after each compression; do not lean on the chest after each compression		
Minimizing interruptions	Limit interruption in chest compression to less than 10 seconds		

** Compression depth should be no more than 2.4 inches (6 cm). Abbreviations: AED, automated external defibrillator; AP, anteroposterior; CPR, anteroposterior; CPR, cardiopulmonary resuscitation*

Adult Basic Life Support and CPR Quality

Lay Rescuer CPR

Summary of Key Issues and Major Changes in the 2015 Guidelines Update recommendations for adult CPR by lay rescuers include the following:

- The crucial links in the out-of-hospital adult Chain of Survival are unchanged from 2010, with continued emphasis on the simplified universal Adult Basic Life Support (BLS) Algorithm.
- The Adult BLS Algorithm has been modified to reflect the fact that rescuers can activate an emergency response (i.e., through use of a mobile telephone) without leaving the victim's side.
- It is recommended that communities with people at risk for cardiac arrest implement PAD programs.
- Recommendations have been strengthened to encourage immediate recognition of unresponsiveness, activation of the emergency response system, and initiation of CPR if the lay rescuer finds an unresponsive victim is not breathing or not breathing normally (e.g., gasping).
- Emphasis has been increased about the rapid identification of potential cardiac arrest by dispatchers, with immediate provision of CPR instructions to the caller (ie, dispatch-guided CPR).
- The recommended sequence for a single rescuer has been confirmed: the single rescuer is to initiate chest compressions before giving rescue breaths (***C-A-B rather than A-B-C***) to reduce delay to first compression. The single rescuer should begin CPR with 30 chest compressions followed by 2 breaths.
- There is ***continued emphasis on the characteristics of high-quality CPR***: compressing the chest at an adequate rate and depth, allowing complete chest recoil after each compression, minimizing interruptions in compressions, and avoiding excessive ventilation.
- ***The recommended chest compression rate is 100 to 120/min (updated from at least 100/min)***.
- The clarified recommendation for chest compression depth for adults is at ***least 2 inches (5 cm) but not greater than 2.4 inches (6 cm).***
- Bystander-administered naloxone may be considered for suspected life-threatening opioid-associated emergencies.

Adult Basic Life Support and CPR Quality: HCP BLS

Key Issues & Major Changes in the 2015 Guidelines Update recommendations for HCPs include the following:

- These recommendations allow flexibility for activation of the emergency response system to better match the HCP's clinical setting.
- Trained rescuers are encouraged to simultaneously perform some steps (*i.e.,* checking for breathing and pulse at the same time), in an effort to reduce the time to first chest compression.
- Integrated teams of highly trained rescuers may use a choreographed approach that accomplishes multiple steps and assessments simultaneously rather than the sequential manner used by individual rescuers (e.g., one rescuer activates the emergency response system while another begins chest compressions, a third either provides ventilation or retrieves the bag-mask device for rescue breaths, and a fourth retrieves and sets up a defibrillator).
- Increased emphasis has been placed on high-quality CPR using performance targets (compressions of adequate rate and depth, allowing complete chest recoil between compressions, minimizing interruptions in compressions, and avoiding excessive ventilation).
- ***Compression rate is modified to a range of 100 to 120/min.***
    - Compression depth for adults is modified to ***at least 2 inches*** (5 cm) but should not exceed 2.4 inches (6 cm).
    - To allow full chest wall recoil after each compression, rescuers must avoid leaning on the chest between compressions.
    - Criteria for minimizing interruptions is clarified with a goal of chest compression fraction as high as possible, with a target of at least 60%.
    - Where EMS systems have adopted bundles of care involving continuous chest compressions, the use of passive ventilation techniques may be considered as part of that bundle for victims of OHCA.
    - For patients with ongoing CPR and an advanced airway in place, a simplified ventilation rate of 1 breath every 6 seconds (10 breaths per minute) is recommended.

138. Ans. a. Corticosteroids, d. IFN-β- used..., e. Plasmaphere...

[Ref: Harrison 19th/ 2661-70, 2656; CMDT 2016/1007-09; Davidson 22nd/1188-92]

Harrison, Davidson & CMDT do not mentioned IV immunoglobulin in treatment list

Multiple Sclerosis

◈ *Harrison 19th/ 2667-70*

- Therapy for MS can be divided into several categories: (1) Treatment of acute attacks, (2) treatment with disease-modifying agents that reduce the biologic activity of MS, and (3) symptomatic therapy.

Acute Attacks or Initial Demyelinating Episodes

- ***Glucocorticoids*** are used to manage either first attacks or acute exacerbations. They provide short-term clinical benefit by reducing the severity and shortening the duration of attacks. Whether treatment provides any long-term benefit on the course of the illness is less clear. Therefore, mild attacks are often not treated.
- ***Plasma exchange*** (five to seven exchanges: 40–60 mL/kg per exchange, every other day for 14 days) may benefit patients with fulminant attacks of demyelination that are unresponsive to glucocorticoids.

Disease-Modifying Therapies for Relapsing Forms of MS (RRMS, SPMS With Exacerbations)

- Ten such agents are approved by the US Food and Drug Administration (FDA): (1) IFN-β-1a (Avonex), (2) IFN-β-1a (Rebif), (3) ***IFN-β-1b*** (Betaseron or Extavia),

(4) glatiramer acetate (Copaxone), (5) natalizumab (Tysabri), (6) fingolimod (Gilenya), (7) dimethyl fumarate (Tecfidera), (8) teriflunomide (Aubagio), (9) mitoxantrone (Novantrone), and (10) alemtuzumab (Lemtrada).

- **Interferon-β:** IFN-β reduces the attack rate and improves disease severity measures such as EDSS progression and MRI-documented disease burden. IFN-β should be considered in patients with either RRMS or SPMS with superimposed relapses. In patients with SPMS but without relapses, efficacy has not been established.

Promising Experimental Therapies

Numerous clinical trials are currently under way. These include studies on (1) monoclonal antibodies against CD20 to deplete B cells and against the IL-2 receptor; (2) selective oral sphingosine-1-phosphate receptor antagonists to sequester lymphocytes in secondary lymphoid organs; (3) estriol to induce apregnancy-like state; (4) molecules to promote remyelination; and (4) bone marrow transplantation.

Corticosteroids in Multiple Sclerosis

◈ *Davidson 22nd/1191*

- '***There is evidence favouring corticosteroids (methylprednisolone) for acute exacerbations of multiple sclerosis***, but there areinsufficient data to estimate reliably the effect of corticosteroidson prevention of new exacerbations and reduction of long-termdisability.'
- 'There is currently no evidence that long-term corticosteroid treatment delays progression of long-term disability in multiple sclerosis.'

Disease-modifying Therapies in Multiple Sclerosis

◈ *Davidson 22nd/1191*

- '**Beta-interferons** have a modest effect on exacerbations anddisease progression in relapsing–remitting MS but do notprevent the development of permanent physical disability onslowly progressive multiple sclerosis.'
- '**Natalizumab** reduces relapses and disability at 2 years in relapsing–remitting multiple sclerosis

Treatment Multiple Sclerosis

◈ *CMDT 2016/1008*

- ***Recovery from acute relapses may be hastened by treatment with corticosteroids, but the extent of recovery is unchanged***. Long-term treatment with corticosteroids provides no benefit and does not prevent further relapses.
- In patients with relapsing disease, numerous injectable medications have well-established efficacy at reducing the frequency of attacks, including ***beta-interferon*** and glatirameracetate
- ***Pegylated interferon*** 1a allows less frequent administration
- Natalizumab reduces the relapse rate when given intravenously once monthly but increases the risk of developing progressive multifocal leukoencephalopathy
- ***Alemtuzumab*** is a lymphocyte inhibitor that similarly reduces relapse rate when given in a short course of infusions once yearly, but its association with autoimmune disease, infusion reactions, and malignancy limits its use to patients in whom two or more other therapies have failed.
- Oral therapies are less well-established, but offer excellent efficacy (at reducing the relapse rate), convenience, and tolerability; these include dimethyl fumarate and fingolimod. Teriflunomide is another effective oral therapy, limited by liver toxicity in some patients. For patients with severe or progressive disease, limited evidence supports immuno suppressive therapy with rituximab, cyclophosphamide, azathioprine, methotrexate, ormitoxantrone.
- ***Plasmapheresis is sometimes helpful inpatients with severe relapses unresponsive to corticosteroids***.

139. Ans. b. Carpal tunnel..., c. Bradycardia, e. Peripheral edema

[Ref: Harrison 19th/2290; CMDT 2016/ 1100; Davidson 22nd/741-45]

"**Thyroid acropachy** is an extreme and unusual manifestation of ***Graves disease.*** It represents with digital clubbing, swelling of fingers and toes, and a periosteal reaction of extremity bones. It is ordinarily associated with ophthalopathy and thyroid dermopathy. Most patients are smokers" *(CMDT 2016/ 1107)*

"***Graves dermopathy (pretibial myxedema) occurs in about 3% of patients with Graves disease usually in the pretibial region. It is more common in patients with high levels of serum TSI in those with severe Graves ophthalmopathy. Glycosaminoglycans accumulation and lymphoid infiltration occur in affected skin, which becomes erythematous with a thickened, rough texture. Elephantiasis of the legs is a rare complication***"*(CMDT 2016/ 1107)*

Table *(Harrison 19th/2290)*: **Signs and Symptoms of Hypothyroidism (Descending Order of Frequency)**

Symptoms	Signs
Tiredness, weakness	Dry coarse skin; cool peripheral extremities
Dry skin	Puffy face, hands, and feet (myxedema)
Feeling cold	Diffuse alopecia
Hair loss	Bradycardia
Difficulty concentrating and poor memory	Peripheral edema
Constipation	Delayed tendon reflex relaxation
Weight gain with poor appetite	Carpal tunnel syndrome
Dyspnea	Serous cavity effusions
Hoarse voice	
Menorrhagia (later oligomenorrhea or amenorrhea)	
Paresthesia	
Impaired hearing	

Table *(Davidson 22nd/741)*: **Clinical Features of Thyroid Dysfunction**

Thyrotoxicosis		Hypothyroidism	
Symptoms	**Signs**	**Symptoms**	**Signs**
Common			
Weight loss despite normal or increased appetite Heat intolerance, sweating Palpitations, tremor Dyspnoea, fatigue Irritability, emotional lability	Weight loss Tremor Palmar erythema Sinus tachycardia Lid retraction, lid lag	Weight gain Cold intolerance Fatigue, somnolence Dry skin Dry hair Menorrhagia	Weight gain
Less common			
Osteoporosis (fracture, loss of height) Diarrhoea, steatorrhoea Angina Ankle swelling Anxiety, psychosis Muscle weakness Periodic paralysis (predominantly in Chinese) Pruritus, alopecia Amenorrhoea/oligomenorrhoea Infertility, spontaneous abortion Loss of libido, impotence Excessive lacrimation	Goitre with bruit[1] Atrial fibrillation[2] Systolic hypertension/increased pulse pressure cardiac failure[2] Hyperreflexia Ill–sustained clonus Proximal myopathy Bulbar myopathy[2] Hyperreflexia Ill-sustained clonus Proximal myopathy Bulbar myopathy[2]	Constipation Hoarseness Carpal tunnel syndrome Alopecia Aches and pains Muscle stiffness Depression Infertility	Hoarse voice Facial features: Purplish lips Malar flush Periorbital oedema Loss of lateral eyebrows Anaemia Carotenaemia Erythema abigne Bradycardia hypertension Delayed relaxation of reflexes Dermal myxoedema
Rare			
Vomiting Apathy Anorexia Exacerbation of asthma	Gynaecomastia Spider naevi Onycholysis Pigmentation	Psychosis (myxoedema madness) Galactorrhoea Impotence	Ileus, ascites Pericardial and pleural effusions Cerebellar ataxia Myotonia

[1]In Graves' diseases only.
[2]Features found particularly in elderly patients

140. Ans. b. Restriction of analgesics..., c. Opioid is mainly..., d. Preventive therapy....

[Ref: Harrison 19th/109; CMDT 2016/965; Davidson 22nd/ 1177]

Medication Overuse Headache (MOH)

◈ *Davidson 22nd/ 1177*

- With increasing availability of over-the-counter medication, headache syndromes perpetuated by analgesia intake are becoming much more common. MOH can complicate any other headache syndrome, but is especially associated with migraine and tension headache.
- The medications that are the ***most common culprits are compound analgesia (particularly codeine and other opiate-containing preparations) and triptans***, and MOH is usually associated with use on more than 10–15 days per month.
- ***Management is by withdrawal of the responsible analgesics***; patients should be warned that the initial effect will be to exacerbate the headache.
- ***Migraine prophylactics*** may be helpful in reducing the rebound headaches. In severe cases, hospital admission with or without a course of corticosteroids may be helpful.

Medication-Overuse Headache

◈ *Harrison 19th/109*

- ***Overuse of analgesic medication*** for headache can aggravate headache frequency, markedly impair the effect of preventive medicines, and induce a state of refractory daily or near-daily headache called *medication-overuse headache.*
- A proportion of patients ***who stop taking analgesics will experience substantial improvement*** in the severity and frequency of their headache. However, even after cessation of analgesic use, many patients continue to have headache, although they *may feel clinically improved in some way, especially if they have been using opioids or barbiturates regularly*. The residual symptoms probably represent the underlying primary headache disorder, and most commonly, this issue occurs in patients prone to migraine.
- For patients who overuse medications, it is essential ***that analgesic use be reduced and eliminated***. One approach is to reduce the medication dose by 10% every 1–2 weeks. Immediate cessation of analgesic use is possible for some patients, provided there is no contraindication. Both approaches are facilitated by the use of a medication diary maintained during the month or two before cessation; this

helps to identify the scope of the problem. A small dose of a nonsteroidal anti-inflammatory drug (NSAID) such as naproxen, 500 mg bid, if tolerated, will help relieve residual pain as analgesic use is reduced.

- ***Once the patient has substantially reduced analgesic use, a preventive medication should be introduced.*** It must be emphasized that ***preventives generally do not work in the presence of analgesic overuse.***
- The most common cause of **unresponsiveness to treatment** is the ***use of a preventive when analgesics continue to be used regularly.*** For some patients, discontinuing analgesics is very difficult; often the best approach is to directly inform the patient that some degree of pain is inevitable during this initial period.

Medication Overuse (Analgesic Rebound Headache)

◈ *CMDT 2016/965*

- In approximately half of all patients with chronic daily headaches, medication overuse is responsible. Patients have chronic pain or severe headache unresponsive tomedication.
- Early initiation of a migraine preventive therapy permits withdrawal of analgesics and eventual relief of headache.

Medication Overuse Headache

◈ *patient.info/health*

- Medication-induced (medication-overuse) headache is a cause of frequent or daily headaches. It is caused by taking ***pain killers or triptan medicines*** very regularly for headaches or migraine.
- The treatment is to stop the ***painkillers or triptan.*** This is ***vital to cure the problem.***

141. Ans. a. Eosinophiluria, b. Peripheral..., c. WBC

[Ref: Harrison 19th/ 1806, 290; Nelson 20th/2536; CMDT 2016/907; Davidson 22nd/481, 503]

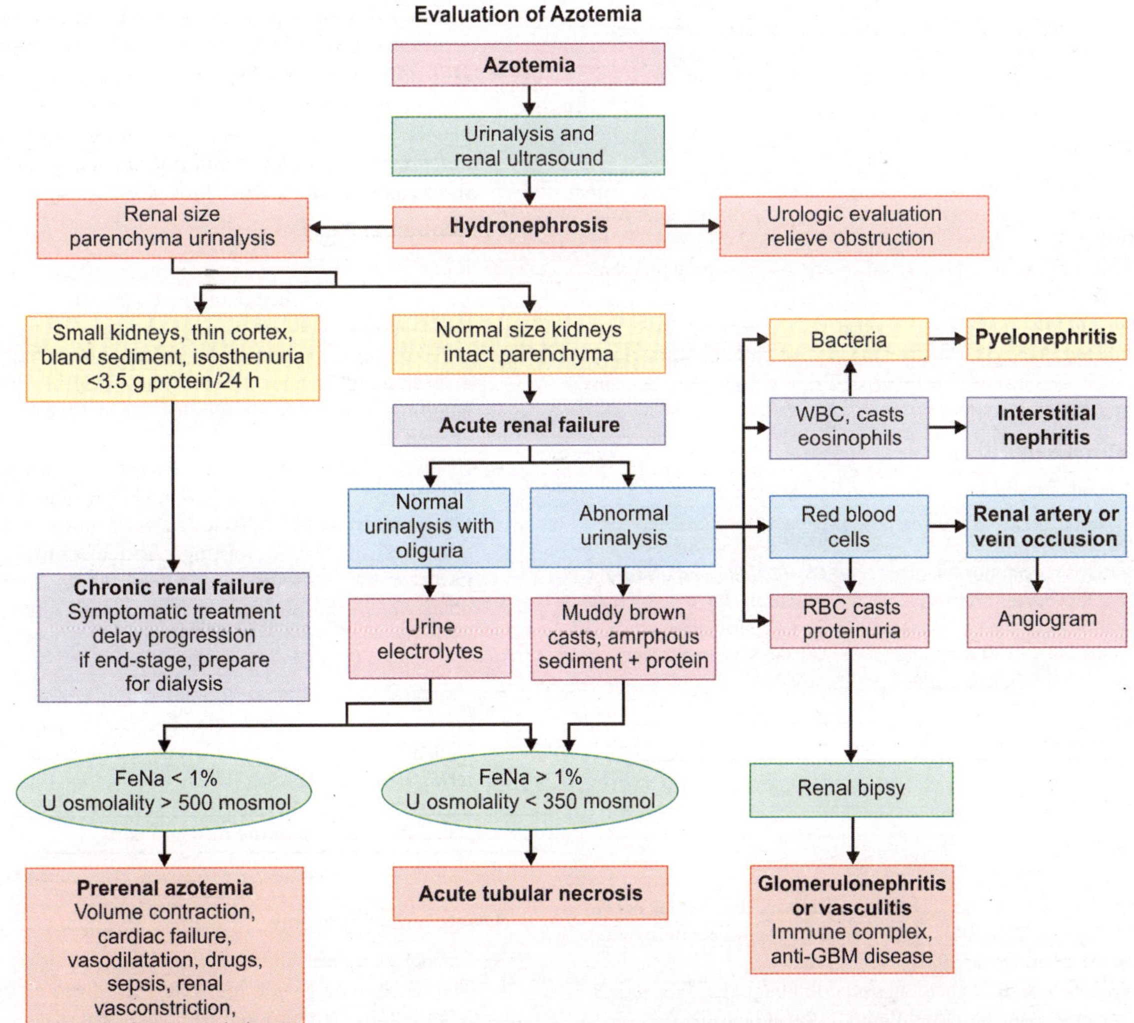

*"**Tubulointerstitial nephritis (TIN, also called interstitial nephritis):** **Peripheral eosinophilia** can occur, especially with drug induced TIN. Some degree of **microscopic hematuria is invariably present, but significant hematuria or proteinuria >1.5 g/day is uncommon**. Urinalysis can reveal **white blood cell, granular or hyaline cast**, but red blood cell cast (a characteristic of glomerular disease) are absent. The presence of **urine eosinophils** is neither sensitive or specific. Because of **pyuria**, the initial diagnosis may be a urinary tract infection" (Nelson 20th/2536)*

*"**Proteinuria** can be a feature, particularly in NSAIDS-induced interstitial nephritis, but it is usually modest (less than 2g/24 hr). Eosinophiluria is neither very sensitive nor specific but can be detected by Wright or Hensel stain" (CMDT 2016/907)*

Table *(Harrison 19th/ 1806)*: **Major Causes, Clinical Features, and Diagnostic Studies for Acute Kidney Injury**

Etiology	Clinical Features	Laboratory Features	Comments
Interstitial nephritis	Nondrug-related causes include tubulointerstitial nephritis-uveitis (TINU) syndrome, Legionella infection	***Eosinophilia, sterile pyuria;*** often nonoliguric	Urine eosinophils have limited diagnostic accuracy; kidney biopsy may be necessary

Investigations

❖ *Davidson 22nd/503*

- **Renal biopsy** is usually required to confirm the diagnosis. This typically shows evidence of intense inflammation, with infiltration of the tubules and interstitium by ***polymorphonuclear leucocytes, and lymphocytes.***
- ***Eosinophils*** may also be observed, especially in drug-induced AIN. The degree of chronic inflammation in a biopsy is a useful predictor of the eventual outcome for renal function.

Interstitial Nephritis

❖ *Davidson 22nd/481*

Possibility	Consider
• Consider if urinary abnormalities minor but ***leucocytes present.*** • Usually non-oliguric in early stages. Take detailed history of exposure to drugs and other possible causes	• ***Eosinophilia and urinary eosinophils*** • Renal biopsy • Uric acid if tumour lysis possible

142. Ans. All (a. b. c. d. e.)

[Ref: Kundu 4th/273-75; Harrison 19th/ 154; PJM 20th/321-22; CMDT 2016/1016]

Bulbar Palsy

❖ *Kundu 4th/273-75*

- Paralysis or loss of function supplied by cranial nerve arising from bulb (old name of medulla oblongata). Affected CN are 9, 10, 11 & 12th.
- **Jaw jerk absent** (c.f brisk in psuedobulbar palsy). Jaw jerk is very important sign for differentiation at bedside
- **Tongue**- ***flaccid, wasted, fasciculation may be present*** (c.f spastic in psuedobulbar palsy)
- Major symptom- Dysarthria, dysphonia, dysphagia & nasal regurgitation

Bulbar Palsy

❖ *PJM 20th/321-22*

- It refers to weakness of the lower cranial nerve with or without affection of pyramidal, spinothalmic, proprioceptive & sympathetic fibers due to lesion in the medulla oblongata
- Clinical features occurs due to lesions of cranial nerve nuclei & damage to fiber tracts
- **Involvement of IX & X CN:** Nasal twang, nasal regurgitation, hoarse voice, ***dysphagia,*** loss of sensation over P1/3 tongue, weak cough, ***absent gag reflex***& weak cough reflex. In u/l lesion, there is never a complete paralysis of ***deglutition*** or of articulation, but in extensive or bilateral lesions there may be profound impairment of these functions
- **XII CN:** ***Dysarthria, wasting & weakness of tongue*** muscles & sometimes ***fibrillations over the tongue***

Bulbar Palsy

❖ *CMDT 2016/2016*

- Bulbar involvement predominates owing to disease processes affecting primarily the motor nuclei of the cranial nerves.
- ***Difficulty in swallowing, chewing, coughing, breathing, and talking (dysarthria) occur with bulbar involvement.*** In **progressive bulbar palsy**, there is ***drooping of the palate; a depressed gag reflex; pooling of saliva in the pharynx; a weak cough; and a wasted, fasciculating tongue.***

Pseudobulbar Palsy

❖ *CMDT 2016/1016*

- Bulbar involvement predominates in this variety also, but it is due to bilateral corticobulbar disease and thus reflects upper motor neuron dysfunction. There may be a "pseudobulbar affect, " with uncontrollable episodes of laughing or crying to stimuli that would not normally have elicited such marked reactions.
- In pseudobulbar palsy, the ***tongue is contracted and spastic*** and cannot be moved rapidly from side to side. **Limb involvement** is characterized by motor disturbances (weakness, stiffness, wasting, fasciculations) reflecting lower or upper motor neuron dysfunction; there are no objective changes on sensory examination, although there may be vague sensory complaints. The sphincters are generally spared.
- "Bilateral corticobulbar lesions produce a *pseudobulbar palsy*: dysarthria, ***dysphagi***a, dysphonia, and emotional lability accompany bilateral facial weakness and a ***brisk jaw jerk***" (Harrison 19th/ 154)

143. Ans. e. Low dose dopamine infusion is....

[Ref: Harrison 19th/2066; CMDT 2016/690-91; Davidson 22nd/940-41]

Hepatorenal Syndrome

❖ *Harrison 19th/2066*

- The hepatorenal syndrome (HRS) is a form of functional renal failure without renal pathology that occurs in ***about 10% of patients with advanced cirrhosis or acute liver failure.***

- There are ***marked disturbances in the arterial renal circulation*** in patients with HRS; these include an ***increase in vascular resistance accompanied by a reduction in systemic vascular resistance.***
- The **diagnosis** is made usually in the presence of a large amount of ascites in patients who have a stepwise ***progressive increase in creatinine.***
- **Type 1 HRS** is characterized by a progressive impairment in renal function and a ***significant reduction in creatinine clearance*** within 1–2 weeks of presentation.
- **Type 2 HRS** is characterized by a reduction in glomerular filtration rate with ***an elevation of serum creatinine level***, but it is fairly stable and is associated with a better outcome than that of Type 1 HRS.
- HRS is ***often seen in patients with refractory ascites*** and requires exclusion of other causes of acute renal failure.
- Treatment has, unfortunately, been difficult, and in the past, ***dopamine or prostaglandin analogues*** were used as renal vasodilating medications. Carefully performed studies have ***failed*** to show clear-cut benefit from these therapeutic approaches.
- Currently, patients are treated with ***midodrine***, an α-agonist, along with ***octreotide and intravenous albumin.***
- The ***best therapy*** for HRS is **liver transplantation;** ***recovery of renal function is typical in this setting.*** In patients with either type 1 or type 2 HRS, the ***prognosis is poor unless transplant can be achieved within a short period of time.***

Hepatorenal Syndrome

◈ *Davidson 22nd/940-41*

- This occurs in ***10% of patients with advanced cirrhosiscomplicated by ascites.*** There are two clinical types; bothare mediated by ***renal vasoconstriction due to under filling of the arterial circulation.***
- **Type 1 hepatorenal syndrome**is characterised byprogressive oliguria, ***a rapid rise of the serum creatinine*** and a very poor prognosis (without treatment, median survival is less than 1 month).There is usually no proteinuria, a urine sodium excretion of less than 10 mmol/day and a urine plasma osmolarity ratio of more than 1.5. Treatment consists of ***albumin infusions in combination with terlipressin*** and is effective in about two-thirds of patients. Haemodialysis should not be used routinely because it does not improve the outcome.Patients who survive should be considered for **liver transplantation.**
- **Type 2 hepatorenal syndrome** usually occurs inpatients with refractory ascites, is characterised by a moderate and ***stable increase in serum creatinine***, and has a better prognosis.

Hepatorenal Syndrome

◈ *CMDT 2016/690-91*

- Hepatorenal syndrome occurs in up to 10% of patients with advanced cirrhosis and ascites and is characterized by azotemia (serum creatinine>1.5 mg/dL in the absence of parenchymal kidney disease or shock and by failure of kidney function to improve following 2 days of diuretic withdrawal and volume expansion with albumin, 1 g/kg up to a maximum of 100 g/d. Oliguria, hyponatremia, and a low urinary sodium concentration are typical features.
- Urinary neutrophil gelatinase-associated lipocalin levels (normal, 20 ng/mL) and ther biomarkers may help distinguish hepatorenal syndrome (105 ng/mL) from chronic kidney disease (50 ng/mL) and acute kidney injury (325 ng/mL).
- ***Hepatorenal syndrome is diagnosed only when other causes of acute kidney injury (including prerenal azotemia and acute tubular necrosis) have been excluded.***
- ***Type 1 Hepatorenal syndrome is characterized by doubling of the serum creatinine to a level >2.5 mg/dLor by halving of the creatinine clearance to <20 mL/min in < 2 weeks.***
- *Type II hepatorenal syndrome is more slowly progressive and chronic. An acute decrease in cardiac output is often the precipitating event. In addition to discontinuation of diuretics, clinical improvement and an increase in short-term survival may follow intravenous infusion of albumin in combination with one of the following vasoconstrictor regimens for 7–14 days: oral midodrine, an alpha-adrenergic drug, plus the somatostatin analog octreotide, subcutaneously or intravenously; intravenous terlipressin (a long-acting vasopressin analog) or intravenous norepinephrine.*
- *Prolongation of survival has been associated with use of MARS, a modified dialysis method that selectively removes albumin-bound substances. Improvement and sometimes normalization of kidney function may also follow placement of a TIPS*
- *Continuous venovenous hemofiltration and hemodialysis are of uncertain value in hepatorenal syndrome. Liver transplantation is the treatment of choice*

---

144. Ans. c. D-xylose.....

[Ref: Harrison 19th/1938; CMDT 2016/623]

The Schilling Test

◈ *Harrison 19th/1938*

- This test is performed to determine the cause of ***cobalamin malabsorption***. An understanding of the physiology and pathophysiology of cobalamin absorption is very valuable, enhancing comprehension of aspects of gastric, pancreatic, and ileal function.

Urinary D-Xylose Test

◈ *Harrison 19th/1938*

- The urinary d-xylose ***test for carbohydrate absorption*** providesan assessment of proximal small-intestinal mucosal function. d-Xylose, a pentose, is absorbed almost exclusively in the proximal small intestine. The d-xylose test is usually performed by administering 25 g of d-xylose and collecting urine for 5 h. An abnormal test (excretion of <4.5 g) primarily reflects ***duodenal/jejunal mucosal disease.***
- The d-xylose test can also be abnormal in patients with ***blind loop syndrome*** (as a consequence primarily of an abnormal intestinal mucosa) and, as a false-positive study, in patients with large collections of fluid in a third space (i.e., ascites, pleural fluid).

Table *(CMDT 2016/623)*: **Clinical Manifestations and Laboratory Findings in Malabsorption of Various Nutrients**

Manifestations	Laboratory Findings	Malabsorbed Nutrients
Steatorrhea (bulky, light-colored stools)	Increased fecal fat; decreased serum cholesterol; decreased serum carotene, vitamin A, vitamin D	Triglycerides, fatty acids, phospholipids, cholesterol. Fat soluble vitamins: A, D, E, K
Diarrhea (increased fecal water)	Increased stool volume and weight; increased fecal fat; increased stool osmolality gap	Fats, carbohydrates
Weight loss; muscle wasting	Increased fecal fat; decreased carbohydrate (D-xylose) absorption	Fat, protein, carbohydrates
Macrocytic anemia	Low serum iron	Iron
Macrocytic anemia	Decreased serum vitamin B_{12} or red blood cell folate	Vitamin B12, or folic acid
Paresthesia; tetany; positive Trousseau and Chvostek signs	Decreased serum calcium or magnesium	Calcium, vitamin D, magnesium
Bone pain; pathologic fractures; skeletal deformities	Osteopenia on radiograph; osteoporosis (adults); osteomalacia (children)	Calcium, vitamin D
Bleeding tendency (ecchymoses, epistaxis)	Prolonged prothrombin time or INR	Vitamin K
Edema	Decreased serum total protein and albumin; increased fecal loss of alpha-1 -antitrypsin	Protein
Milk intolerance (cramps, bloating, diarrhea)	Abnormal lactose tolerance test	Lactose

Table *(Harrison 19th/1941)*: **Results of Diagnostic Studies in Steatorrhea of Various Etiologies**

	D-Xylose Test	Schilling Test	Duodenal mucosal biopsy
Chronic pancreatitis	Normal	50% abnormal; if abnormal, normal with pancreatic enzyme treatment	Normal
Bacterial overgrowth syndromes	Normal or only modestly abnormal	Abnormal	Usually normal
Ileal disease	Normal	Normal	Normal
Celiac disease	Decreased	Normal	Abnormal: probably flat
Intestinal lymphangiectasia	Normal		Abnormal: dilated lymphatics

145. Ans. a. Measures right..., b. Measures left..., c. Measure PCWP, d. Inserted through...

[Ref: Harrison 19th/ 1607; Davidson 22nd/ 185-86; lifeinthefastlane.com]

USES of Swan-Ganz Catheter

- *http: //lifeinthefastlane.com*
- ***Continuous cardiac output monitoring***
- *Central temperature monitoring*
- ***Measurement of pulmonary artery pressure (can also measure RA and RV pressures during insertion)***
- *Measurement of **mixed venous saturations***
- *Estimation of **diastolic filling of left heart** (normal PCWP 2-12 mmHg)*

Pulmonary Artery Catheterisation and Pulmonary Artery 'Wedge' Pressure

- *Davidson 22nd/ 185-86*
- The CVP is usually an adequate guide to the filling pressures of both sides of the heart. However, certain conditions, such as pulmonary hypertension or right ventricular dysfunction, may lead to raised CVP level seven in the presence of hypovolaemia. In these circumstances, it may be appropriate to insert a ***pulmonary artery flotation catheter*** so that ***pulmonary artery pressure and pulmonary artery 'wedge' pressure (PAWP),*** which approximates to ***left atrial pressure,*** can be measured.
- ***Pulmonary artery catheters*** also allow ***measurement of cardiac output and sampling of blood from the pulmonary artery ('mixed venous' samples), permitting continuous monitoring of the mixed venous oxygen saturation (SvO2) by oximetry.*** Measurement of SvO2 gives an indication of the adequacy of cardiac output (and hence DO2) in relation to the body's metabolic requirements. It is especially useful in low cardiac output states.

Hemodynamic Assessment

- *Harrison 19th/ 1607*
- Positioning of a balloon flotation **(Swan-Ganz) catheter** in the pulmonary artery ***permits monitoring of LV filling pressure***; this technique is useful in patients who exhibit hypotension and/or clinical evidence of CHF.
- ***Cardiac output can also be determined with a pulmonary artery catheter. With the addition of intra-arterial pressure***

monitoring, systemic vascular resistance can be calculated as a guide to adjusting vasopressor and vasodilator therapy.

Pulmonary Artery Catheterization

Harrison 19th/ 1760

- The use of **pulmonary artery (Swan-Ganz)** catheters in patients with established or suspected cardiogenic shock (CS) is controversial. Their use is generally recommended for ***measurement of filling pressures and cardiac output*** to confirm the diagnosis and to optimize the use of IV fluids, inotropic agents, and vasopressors in persistent shock.

Pulmonary Artery Catheterization

http: //emedicine.medscape.com/

The PAC is inserted percutaneously into a major vein (jugular, subclavian, femoral) via an introducer sheath.

- **Right internal jugular vein (RIJ):** Shortest and straightest path to the heart
- **Left subclavian:** Does not require the PAC to pass and course at an acute angle to enter the SVC (compared to the right subclavian or left internal jugular [LIJ])
- **Femoral veins:** These access points are distant sites, from which passing a PAC into the heart can be difficult, especially if the right-sided cardiac chambers are enlarged. Often, fluoroscopic assistance is necessary. Nevertheless, these sites are compressible and may be preferable if the risk of hemorrhage is high.

Use of Pulmonary Artery Catheterization

http: //emedicine.medscape.com

- Important information provided by a PAC catheter includes the ***PCWP, assessment of left ventricular (LV) filling pressure, CO, mixed venous oxygen saturation (SaO_2), and oxygen saturations*** in the right heart chambers to assess for the presence of an intracardiac shunt.
- Using these measurements, other variables can be derived, including pulmonary or systemic vascular resistance and the difference between arterial and venous oxygen content (see images below). Obtaining CO and PCWP measurements is the primary reason for inserting most PACs; therefore, understanding how they are obtained and what factors alter their values is of prime importance.

Swan-Ganz Catheterization

(http//www.healthline.com/)

- A Swan-Ganz catheterization is a type of pulmonary artery catheterization procedure.
- The procedure involves the insertion of a pulmonary artery catheter (PAC), also known as a **Swan-Ganz catheter or right heart catheter,** into the right side of the heart and into the arteries that lead to the lungs.
- The procedure itself is sometimes called "right heart catheterization." This is because it can measure the pressure of blood as it flows through the right side of your heart. It measures the pressure at three different places: ***right atrium, pulmonary artery, and pulmonary capillaries***.
- These measurements can be used to figure out the amount of oxygen in the blood of the right portion of heart.

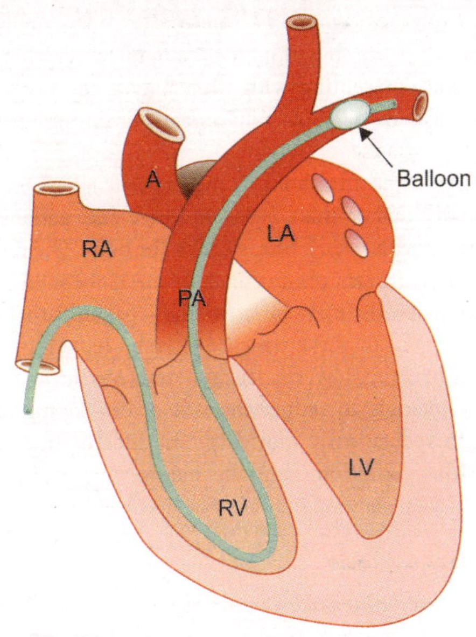

146. Ans. a. Hydroxyurea, c. Leukapheresis, d. Vincristine

[Ref: Harrison 19th/413-23, 1793; Davidson 22nd/1005]

Isotretinoin (13-cis retinoic acid) is used in treatment of acne *(KDT 7th/911)*

Tretinoin (all trans-retinoic acid) *is used in* ***acute promyelocytic leukaemia*** *(KDT 7th/869)*

"The cytoreduction in **hyperleukocytosis**can be achieved by either ***leukapheresis and/or hydroxyurea"*** *(www.bloodreviews.com)*

Hyperleukocytosis

link. springer.com

- It refers to a laboratory abnormality that has been variably defined as a total leukemia blood cell count greater than 100 × 10^9/L (100, 000/microL). In contrast, leukostasis (also called symptomatic hyperleukocytosis) is a medical emergency most commonly seen in patients with acute myeloid leukemia (AML) or chronic myeloid leukemia (CML) in blast crisis. Acute leukemia is the most common etiology in pediatric practice. It is characterized by an extremely elevated blast cell count and symptoms of decreased tissue perfusion.
- **Leukostasis** is a pathologic diagnosis in which white cell plugs are seen in the microvasculature. Clinically, leukostasis is typically diagnosed empirically when a patient with leukemia and hyperleukocytosis presents with respiratory or neurological distress. Prompt treatment is indicated since, if left untreated, the one-week mortality rate is approximately 20 to 40 percent.
- ***"Leukapheresis is the treatment of choice*** for a very high count, or in patients with symptomatic hyperleukocytosis"- *(www.ncbi.nlm.nih.gov)*
- "The management of hyperleukocytosis and leukostasis is centered on cytoreduction and maximizing vascular flow through supportive measures. In patients with AML,

hydroxyurea should be started, 1 to 3 g orally every 6 hours, in combination with emergent leukapheresis for patients presenting with white blood cell (WBC) counts higher than 100, 000/mm^3 or signs or symptoms indicative of leukostasis.

- In ALL, the threshold to initiate leukapheresis is higher, usually higher than 200, 000/mm^3, and patients may be treated with ***vincristine,*** steroids, or both. The replacement of fresh-frozen plasma that occurs in conjunction with leukapheresis may improve the coagulopathy that may be present in these patients, thereby reducing the risk of hemorrhage. However, leukapheresis has never been shown convincingly to reduce the risk of developing leukostasis or to reduce early mortality. The most definitive therapy for this condition, naturally, involves urgent institution of induction chemotherapy" *(www.clevelandclinicmeded)*

Hyperleukocytosis

- *emedicine.medscape.com/article/956278-treatment*
- In extreme instances of hyperleukocytosis syndrome (*e.g.*, acute leukemia), ***leukapheresis, hydration, and urine alkalinization*** to facilitate uric acid excretion are indicated; however, perform these treatments only in consultation with a hematologist, oncologist, or both. Direct treatment toward the underlying etiology.
- Leukemic hyperleukocytosis may cause clinically significant complications when the WBC count exceeds 100, 000/μ L in acute myelogenous leukemia and 300, 000/μ L in acute lymphoblastic leukemia. Therefore, in patients with these findings, measures to reduce the WBC count are advisable. However, a decrease in leukocyte count that is too rapid carries a risk of severe tumor lysis syndrome and should be avoided.
- Leukapheresis or exchange blood transfusion is a treatment of choice for this purpose, with hydration, urine alkalinization, and administration of ***allopurinol or rasburicase*** (uric acid oxydase) to reduce serum uric acid and minimize tumor lysis syndrome. When rasburicase is used, urine alkalinization is not recommended.

SURGERY

147. Ans. c. No spontaneous..., d. Dry eschar..., e. Thrombosed...

[Ref: Manipal Surgery 4th/187; Reddy 32nd/304-05; Sabiston 19th/522-35; L & B 26th/390; Schwartz 9th/199-200]

Table *(Manipal Surgery 4th/187)*: **Various Degree of Burn**

	Involved area	Pain	Adnexa	Appearance	Healing
I° Burn	Only epidermis	+	+	Erythema/oedema	3–5 days without scar
II° Burn	Varying depth of dermis	++/–	+	Blister, soft waxy, white, elastic, pain sensation to needle prick present	10–20 days, with hypertrophic scar
III° Burn	Involvement of entire depth of epidermis and dermis	--	Lost	**Tough & dryeschar, thrombosed subcutaneous vein. Pain sensation to needle prick absent**	3–5 weeks, eschar separates. Always needs split skin graft

Full-Thickness Burns (3°BURN)

- *L&B 26th/390*
- The ***whole of the dermisis destroyed in these burns.***
- Clinically, they ***have a hard, leathery feel.*** The appearance can vary from that similar to the patient's normal skin to charred black, depending upon the intensity of the heat.
- The reis*nocapillary return.* Often, ***thrombosed vessels can be seen under the skin.***
- These burns are ***completely anesthetized:*** a needle can be stuck deep into the dermis without any pain or bleeding.

Burn

- *CSDT 11th/267-72*
- Traditionally, burns have been classified as ***first-, second-, and third-degree,*** but the current emphasis on burn healing has led to classification as ***partial-thickness burns, which can heal spontaneously, and full thickness burns,*** which requires in grafting,although deep partial-thickness burns are usually excised and grafted as well.
- A **first-degree burn** involves only the epidermis and is characterized by erythema and minor microscopic changes; tissue damage is minimal, protective functions of the skin are intact, skin edema is minimal, and systemic effects are rare. Pain, the chief symptom, usually resolves in 48–72 hours, and healing takes place uneventfully.
- **Second-degree or partial-thickness burns** are deeper, involving all of the epidermis and some of the corium or dermis. The systemic severity of the burn and the quality of subsequent healing are directly related to the amount of undamaged dermis. Superficial burns are often characterized by ***blister formation,*** while deeper partial thickness burns have a ***reddish appearance*** or a layer of whitish nonviable dermis firmly adherent to the remaining viable tissue. Blisters, when present, continue to increase in size in the post burn period as the *osmotically active particles in the blister fluid attract water.*
- **Deep dermal burns** heal over a period of 25–35 days with a fragile epithelial covering that arises from the residual uninjured epithelium of the deep dermal sweat glands and hair follicles. Severe hypertrophics carrying occurs when such an injury heals; the resulting epithelial covering is prone to ***blistering and breakdown. Evaporative losses*** after healing remain high compared with losses in normal skin.

Full-thickness (third-degree) burns have a characteristic white, waxy appearance and may appear to the untrained eye as unburned skin. Burns caused by prolonged exposure, with involvement of fat and underlying tissue, may be brown, darkred, or black. The diagnostic findings of full thickness burns are ***lack of sensation in the burned skin, lack of capillary refill, and a leathery texture*** that is unlike normal skin. All epithelial elements are destroyed, ***leaving no potential for reepithelialization.***

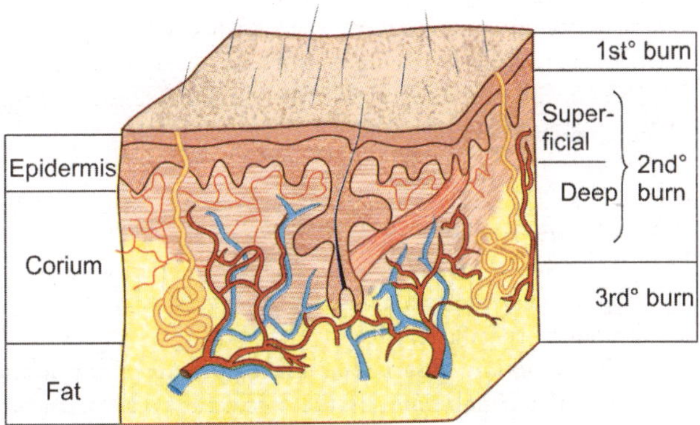

Fig: Layers of the skin showing depth off first-degree, second-degree, and third-degree burns

148. Ans. c. Triangular orifice..., d. Used for soft...

[Ref: surgicalunits.com; quizlet.com/65378451/instruments-clamps-forceps-scissors-scalpel-handle-flash-cards; Manipal Surgery 4th/ 1130; Dutta Gynae 6th/639; Obstetrics by J B Sharma 1st/743]

Babcock's Forcep

◈ *Manipal Surgery 4th/ 1130*

- An instrument with a ratchet & a ***triangular expansion*** with ***fenestrations at the operating end***
- ***It does not have any teeth***
- This instrument can be used to hold intestine, thyroid gland, mesoappendix, uterine tube etc.

◈ *surgicalunits.com*

- Rachet mechanism
- Ring handles
- Blades have triangular orifice, along with a horizontal groove at the terminal in one blade & ridge in the other blade
- Non-traumatic instrument

Babcock's Forcep

◈ *Obstetrics by J B Sharma 1st/743*

- It is a non-traumatic instrument with ***fenestrated triangular blades*** & grooved jaws.
- It is about 10 cm long & has small blades

"**Sklar Black™ Babcock Forceps** are finger ring, ratcheted, non-perforating forceps used to ***grasp delicate tissue*** in laser procedures. They are frequently used with intestinal and laparotomy procedures. Babcock Forceps are similar to Allis forceps; however, may be considered ***less traumatic*** due to their wider, ***rounded grasping surface***. The jaws are circumferential and the ***tips are triangular and fenestrated***. They are particularly useful for ***grasping tube-shaped structures***" *(quizlet.com/65378451)*

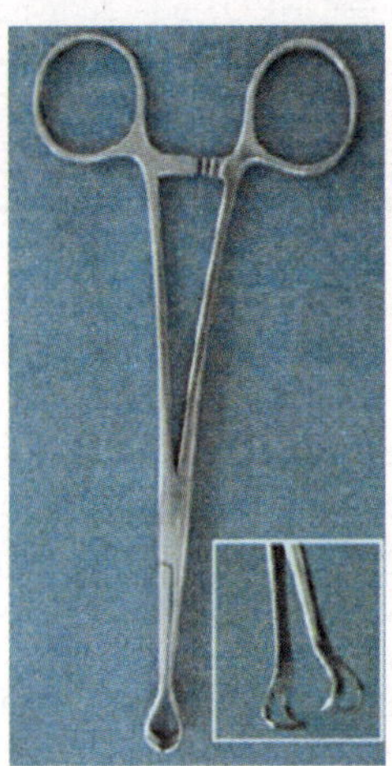

149. Ans. b. CO_2, c. O_2 d. Air

[Ref: Manipal Surgery 4th/1175; L & B 26th/98; Schwartz 9th/361]

N_2O, CO_2 & air *are used for creating pneumoperitoneum- Schwartz 9th/361*

Table *(Manipal Surgery 4th/1175)*: **Gases used for Pneumoperitoneum**

Gases	Advantages	Disadvantages
Air	Historical importance	***Poorly insoluble in blood***, *so slower absorption, More painful*
CO_2	Inert	**Rapidly absorbable, Respiratory acidosis**
N_2O	Inert, Less painful, Reduced intraoperative end tidal CO_2	Rapidly absorbable, Danger of combustion, Not safe in pregnancy

"Factors that determine the most appropriate gas for pneumoperitoneum are type of anesthesia, physiologic compatibility, toxicity, ease of use, safety, delivery method, cost, and non-combustibility. Gases used for pneumoperitoneum include ***carbon dioxide (CO_2), air, oxygen, nitrous oxide (N_2O), argon, helium and mixtures of these gases***" *(http: //laparoscopy.blogs.com)*

150. Ans. b. Fast clearance..., d. Electrocautery is..., e. Less risk of gas...

[Ref: Above Q reference; Manipal Surgery 4th/1175; Schwartz 9th/361-62]

Pneumoperitoneum

◈ *http: //laparoscopy.blogs.com/*

- CO_2 gas insufflation is preferred by most laparoscopists because it has a ***high diffusion coefficient and is a normal metabolic end product rapidly cleared from the body***.
- Also, ***CO_2 is highly soluble in blood*** and tissues and ***does not support combustion. The risk of gas embolism is lowest***

with CO_2. Cardiac arrhythmias can occur with CO_2 pneumoperitoneum.

- Because of possible CO_2 induced hypercarbia, ***N_2O may be preferred in patients with cardiac disease***. With prolonged procedures, ***CO_2 retention is possible*** as evidenced by tachycardia and acidosis.
- *CO_2 is Noncombustible = safe to use with electrosurgical devices*
- *Systemic absorption thought to be facilitated by CO_2 specific widening of inter-cellular junctions in peritoneum → buffering of CO_2 as above → Systemic Acidification*

Pneumoperitoneum

◈ *http: //laparoscopy.blogs.com; www.ncbi.nlm.nih.gov*

- The ideal gas for pneumoperitoneum insufflation should be non-toxic, colorless, ***readily soluble in blood,*** easily expelled from the body or expired through the lungs, ***non-flammable and inexpensive***. CO_2 best satisfies these characteristics.
- ***Oxygen and air are not readily absorbed through the peritoneum and can result in air embolism. Nitrous oxide (N_2O) has unpredictable absorption***. Helium is relatively insoluble in blood compared to CO_2.
- Argon has a more significant depressant effect on hemodynamics than CO_2.
- ***Oxygen and N_2O, if mixed with methane, support combustion and are dangerous***. The ***best compromise of factors of safety, utility and cost dictates using CO_2***.
- Carbon dioxide, which still stays in the abdomen after laparoscopic surgery, ***may cause postoperative pain***. Thus, other gases, such as nitrous oxide and helium, have been suggested as alternatives to carbon dioxide for establishing pneumoperitoneum.

In conclusion, **nitrous oxide** pneumoperitoneum during laparoscopic abdominal surgery appears to ***decrease postoperative pain*** in patients with low anaesthetic risk. ***Helium pneumoperitoneum decreases cardiopulmonary changes associated with laparoscopic abdominal surgery***. However, this did not translate into any clinical benefit over carbon dioxide pneumoperitoneum. The safety of nitrous oxide and helium pneumoperitoneum has yet to be established. http: //www.ncbi.nlm.nih.gov/

"We conclude that ***CO_2 pneumoperitoneum has a better outcome than Air*** especially for day-case diagnostic laparoscopy. However, ***room Air pneumoperitoneum is safe, cheap, and available and may be recommended for low resource settings***" *(http: //www.ncbi.nlm.nih.gov)*

Laparoscopy

◈ *Schwartz 9th/361-62*

- The physiologic effects of CO_2pneumoperitoneum can be divided into two areas: (1) gas-specific effects and (2) pressure-specific effects.
- ***CO_2 is rapidly absorbed across the peritoneal membrane into the circulation***. In the circulation, CO_2 creates a respiratory acidosis by the generation of carbonic acid. Body buffers, the largest reserve of which lies in bone, absorb CO_2 (up to 120 L) and minimize the development of ***hypercarbia or respiratory acidosis*** during brief endoscopic procedures. Once the body buffers are saturated, respiratory acidosis develops rapidly, and the respiratory system assumes the burden of keeping up with the absorption of CO_2 and its release from these buffers

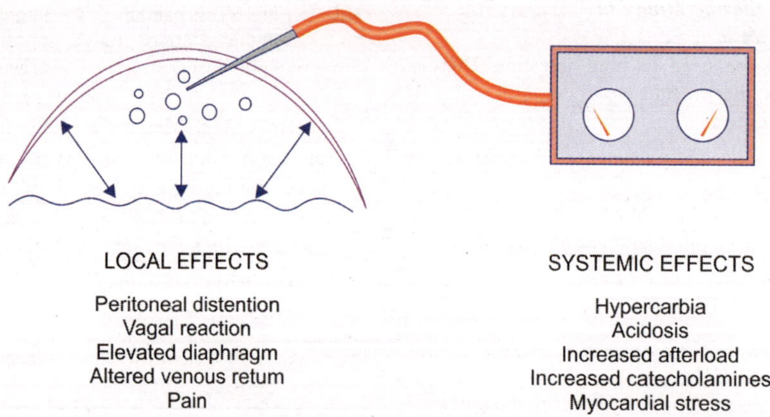

Fig: ***(Schwartz 9th/361):*** Carbon dioxide gas insufflated into the peritoneal cavity has both local and systemic effects that cause a complex set of hemodynamic and metabolic alterations

151. Ans. a. Cullen..., d. Grey Turner.....

[Ref: Manipal Surgery 4th/601; L & B 26th/1128; Schwartz 9th/ 1181]

"**Acute pancreatitis**: With increasing severity of disease, the intravascular fluid loss may become life-threatening as a result of sequestration of edematous fluid in the retroperitoneum. Hemoconcentration then results in an elevated hematocrit. However, there also may be bleeding into the retroperitoneum or the peritoneal cavity. In some patients (about 1%), the blood from necrotizing pancreatitis may dissect through the soft tissues and manifest as a blueish discoloration around the umbilicus (***Cullen's sign***) or in the flanks (***Grey Turner sign***). The severe fluid loss may lead to prerenal azotemia with elevated blood urea nitrogen and creatinine levels. There also may be hyperglycemia, hypoalbuminemia, and hypocalcemia sufficient in some cases to produce tetany" *(Schwartz 9th/ 1181)*

"***Rovsing sign:*** *Palpation of left iliac region of abdomen produces pain in the right iliac region. It is found in* ***acute appendicitis***" *(Manipal Surgery 4th/828)*

"**Kehr's sign** is the occurrence of acute pain in the tip of the shoulder due to the presence of blood or other irritants in the peritoneal cavity when a person is lying down and the legs are elevated. **Kehr's sign** in the left shoulder is considered a classic symptom of a ruptured spleen" *(S.Das Textbook of Surgery 5th/941)*

"Bleeding into the fascial planes can produce bluish discolouration of the flanks (***Grey Turner's sign)*** or umbilicus (Cullen's sign). ***Neither sign is pathognomonic of acute pancreatitis;*** Cullen's sign was first described in association with rupture of an ectopic pregnancy. Subcutaneous fat necrosis may produce small, red, tender nodules on the skin of the legs"- *L &B26th/ 1128*

Cullen sign: Bluish ecchymotic discolouration seen around umbilicus- *Manipal Surgery 4th/601*

Acute Pancreatitis

◈ *L & B 26th/1128*

- ***Bleeding into the fascial plane scan produce bluish discolouration of the flanks (Grey Turner's sign) or umbilicus (Cullen's sign).***
- Neither sign is pathognomonic of acute pancreatitis; Cullen's sign was first described in association with rupture of an ectopic pregnancy. Subcutaneous fat necrosis may produce small, red, tender nodules on the skin of the legs.

Table *(Harrison 19th/1987)*: **Classic Signs of Appendicitis in Patients with Abdominal Pain**

Maneuver	Findings
Rovsing's sign	Palpating in the left lower quadrant causes pain in the right lower quadrant
Obturator sign	Internal rotation of the hip causes pain, suggesting the possibility of an inflamed appendix located in the pelvis
Iliopsoas sign	Extending the right hip causes pain along posterolateral back and hip, suggesting retrocecal appendicitis

152. Ans. a. It is the suitable..., b. It can cause UTI..., c. Used in management..., e. Sterile technique must...

[Ref: http: //www.med.uottawa.ca/procedures/ucath; L& B 26TH/1313; Obstetrics by JB Sharma 1st/737; Manipal Surgery 4th/ 1139; Schwartz 9th/ 1468-69]

"Usually No. 14 or 16 F (French size) catheter is used for catheterization of a female urethra" *(Obstetrics by JB Sharma 1st/737)*

Urinary Catheter (Foley's Catheter)

◈ *med.uottawa.ca/procedures/ucath*

- A Foley catheter is a thin, ***sterile tube*** inserted into the bladder to drain urine. It is held in place with a balloon at the end, which is filled with sterile water to prevent the catheter from being removed from the bladder. The urine drains through the catheter tube into a bag, which is emptied when full. The procedure to insert a catheter is called ***catheterization.***
- **Sterile technique must be used for insertion to prevent spread of infection.**
- **Following a thorough hand wash, sterile gloves are donned. The genitalia are cleaned using soapy antiseptic**
- By inserting a Foley catheter, you are gaining access to the bladder and its contents. Thus enabling you to drain bladder contents, decompress the bladder, obtain a specimen, and introduce a passage into the GU tract. ***This will allow you to treat urinary retention, and bladder outlet obstruction.***
- In the emergency department, catheters can be used to aid in the diagnosis of GU bleeding.
- ***In some cases, as in urethral stricture or prostatic hypertrophy, insertion will be difficult*** and early consultation with urology is essential.
- Foley catheters are contraindicated in the presence of ***urethral trauma.*** Urethral injuries may occur in patients with multisystem injuries and pelvic factures, as well as straddle impacts. If this is suspected, one must perform a genital and rectal exam first. *If one finds blood at the meatus of the urethra, a scrotal hematoma, a pelvic fracture, or a high riding prostate then a high suspicion of urethral tear is present.* One must then perform retrograde urethrography (injecting 20 cc of contrast into the urethra).
- ***Internal catheters usually have their outside diameters measured in French sizes.*** *The French catheter scale or "French units" (Fr) is commonly used to measure the outside diameter of needles as well as catheters. 1 "French" or "Fr" is equivalent to 0.33 mm = .013" = 1/77" of diameter. The size in French units is roughly equal to the circumference of the catheter in millimeters. A 14 to 16 French is used on most adults.*
- *Larger catheters of 22 French are recommended for patients with hematuria or clots.* ***Pediatric French sizes range from 3 to 14.*** *A catheter that is too big can lead to urethral irritation and difficult placement. A catheter that is too small can lead to kinking and urinary leakage.*

French Gauge	Diameter (mm)
12	4
13	4.3
14	4.7

Contd...

French Gauge	Diameter (mm)
15	5
16	5.3
17	5.7
18	6

A Foley Catheter is used with Many Disorders, Procedures, or Problems Such as these

◈ *http: //www.emedicinehealth.com/*

- Retention of urine leading to urinary hesitancy, straining to urinate, decrease in size and force of the urinary stream, interruption of urinary stream, and sensation of incomplete emptying
- ***Obstruction of the urethra by an anatomical condition that makes it difficult for one to urinate:*** prostate hypertrophy, prostate cancer, or narrowing of the urethra.
- Urine output monitoring in a critically ill or injured person
- Collection of a sterile urine specimen for diagnostic purposes
- Nerve-related bladder dysfunction, such as after spinal trauma (A catheter can be inserted regularly to assist with urination.)
- Imaging study of the lower urinary tract
- After surgery

Foley Catheter Risks

◈ *http: //www.emedicinehealth.com*

- The Foley catheter may introduce an infection into the bladder. The risk of infection in the urine increases with the number of days the catheter is in place.
- If the balloon is opened before the Foley catheter is completely inserted into the bladder, bleeding, damage and even rupture of the urethra can occur. In some individuals, long-term permanent scarring and strictures of the urethra could occur.

153. Ans. a. Stricture in ureter..., b. Stone in ureter..., c. RTA type 4...

[Ref: CSDT 11th/1029-32; Harrison 19th/320, 1871-73; Schwartz 9th/1471-72]

"In **generalized distal nephron dysfunction (type 4 RTA)**, hyperkalemia is disproportionate to the reduction in GFR because of coexisting dysfunction of potassium and acid secretion. Urinary ammonium excretion is invariably depressed, and renal function may be compromised, for example, due to diabetic nephropathy, ***obstructive uropathy***, or chronic tubulointerstitial disease" *(Harrison 19th/320)*

*"The **hallmark of partial or complete upper urinary tract obstruction is hydronephrosis,** with the ureteral dilation extending to the level of obstruction. HN may be seen on CT imaging or USG. In acute setting, the degree of HN does not necessarily correlate with degree of obstruction, as it may take time for severe HN to develop" (Schwartz 9th/1470-71)*

Urinary Tract Obstruction

◈ *Harrison 19th/1871-73*

- Obstruction to the flow of urine, with attendant stasis and elevation in urinary tract pressure, impairs renal and urinary conduit functions and is a common cause of **acute and chronic kidney disease** ***(obstructive nephropathy).***
- With early relief of obstruction, the defects in function usually disappear completely. However, chronic obstruction may produce permanent loss of renal mass (renal atrophy) and excretory capability, as well as enhanced susceptibility to local infection and stone formation.
- Early diagnosis and prompt therapy are, therefore, essential to minimize the otherwise devastating effects of obstruction on kidney structure and function
- Mechanical obstruction can occur at any level of the urinary tract, from the renal calyces to the external urethral meatus. Normal points of narrowing, such as the ureteropelvic and ureterovesical junctions, bladder neck, and urethral meatus, are common sites of obstruction. In adults, urinary tract obstruction (UTO) is due mainly to *acquired defects*. Pelvic tumors, calculi, and urethral stricture predominate.
- ***When obstruction is above the level of the bladder, unilateral dilatation of the ureter (hydroureter) and renal pyelocalyceal system (hydronephrosis) occurs; lesions at or below the level of the bladder cause bilateral involvement***
- Partial bilateral UTO often results in ***acquired distal renal tubular acidosis***, *hyperkalemia*, and *renal salt wasting.*

Table *(Harrison 19th/1871)*: **Common Mechanical Causes of Urinary Tract Obstruction**

Ureter	Bladder Outlet	Urethra
Congenital		
Ureteropelvic junction narrowing or obstruction Ureterovesical junction narrowing or obstruction and reflux Ureterocele Retrocaval ureter	Bladder neck obstruction Ureterocele	Posterior urethral valves Anterior urethral valves Stricture Meatal stenosis Phimosis
Acquired Intrinsic Defects		
Calculi Inflammation Infection Trauma Sloughed papillae Tumor Blood clots	Benign prostatic hyperplasia Cancer of prostate Cancer of bladder Calculi Diabetic neuropathy Spinal cord disease Anticholinergic drugs and α-adrenergic antagonists	***Stricture*** Tumor Calculi Trauma Phimosis

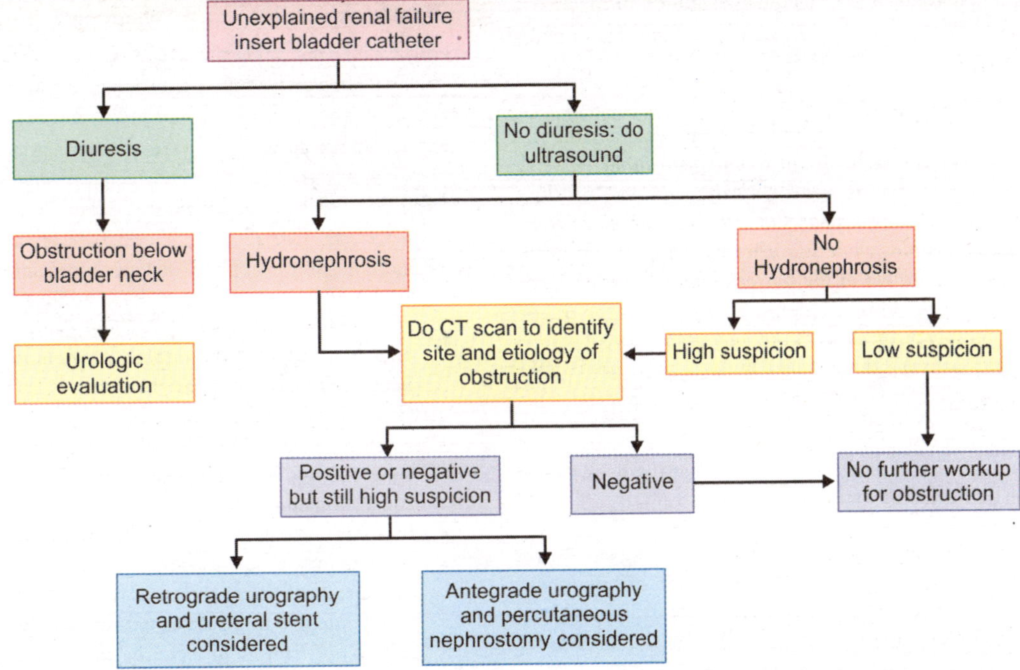

Fig: *(Harrison 19th/320):* Diagnostic approach for urinary tract obstruction in unexplained renal failure.

Obstructive Uropathy

◈ *CSDT 11th/1029-32*

- Obstruction is one of the most important abnormalities of the urinary tract, since it eventually leads to decompensation of the muscular conduits and reservoirs, back pressure, and ***atrophy of renal parenchyma***. It also ***invites infection and stone formation***
- Both the level and the degree of obstruction are important to an understanding of the pathologic consequences. Any ***obstruction at or distal to the bladder neck may lead to back pressure*** affecting both kidneys. ***Obstruction at or proximal to the ureteral orifice leads to unilateral damage*** unless the lesion involves both ureters simultaneously. Complete obstruction leads to rapid decompensation of the system proximal to the site of obstruction. **Partial obstruction** leads to gradual progressive muscular hypertrophy followed by dilation, decompensation, and ***hydronephrotic changes.***
- Acquired urinary tract obstruction may be due to inflammatory or ***traumatic urethral strictures***, bladder outlet obstruction (benign prostatic hyperplasia or cancer of the prostate), vesical tumors, neuropathic bladder, extrinsic ureteral compression (tumor, retroperitoneal fibrosis, or enlarged lymph nodes), ***ureteral or pelvic stones, ureteral strictures,*** or ureteral or pelvic tumors.
- *Regardless of its cause, acquired obstruction leads to similar changes in the urinary tract, which vary depending on the severity and duration of obstruction.*
- With continued pelvicaliceal distention, there is parenchymal compression against the renal capsule and, more importantly, compression of the arcuate vessels results in a marked drop in renal blood flow leading to parenchymal ischemic atrophy. *With increased intrapelvic pressure, there is progressive dilation of the collecting and distal tubules, with compression and atrophy of tubular cells.*
- **Ultrasonography**: This will reveal the degree of dilation of the renal pelvis and calices and allows for ***diagnosis of hydronephrosis*** even in the prenatal period. Color Doppler ultrasound can reveal blood flow and restrictive indices to help determine functional impairment.

154. Ans. a. External opening..., c. Develop due to persistence..., d. Open in oropharynx

[Ref: Manipal Surgery 4th/253; Schwartz 9th/1414-15; Dhingra 6th/392, 240]

"**B.fistula:** ***Pierces the pharyngeal wall & ends in the tonsillar-fossa (which is part of oropharynx)*** *(Dhingra 6th/392, 240)*

"Swelling which moves with deglutination (swallowing) - ***thyroid swelling, thyroglossalcyst, prelaryngeal & pretracheal lymph node, subhyoid bursitis*** *(S.Das Clinical Surgery 11th/371)*

Branchial Fistula

◈ *Manipal Surgery 4th/253*

- This is always congenital &***occurs due to persistent 2nd branchial cleft***
- **External opening** is situated at the ***junction of middle 1/3 & lower 1/3 of sternomastoid***
- The tract from the skin passes through the fork of common carotid artery deep to the accessory & hypoglossal nerve & opens in the anterior aspect of posterior pillars of tonsil
- The patient may complain of a ***dimple***, discharging mucus & the dimple becomes ***more obvious when the patient is asked to swallow***

- Can be unilateral or bilateral, equally common in males & females

Branchial Fistula

◈ *L & B 26th/700*

- A branchial fistula may be unilateral or bilateral and is thought to ***represent a persistent second branchial cleft.***
- The **external orifice** ***is nearly always situated in the lower third of the neck near the anterior border of the sternocleidomastoid***, while the **internal orifice** is located on the ***anterior aspect of the posterior faucial pillar just behind the tonsil***. However, the internal aspect of the tract may end blindly at or close to the *lateral pharyngeal wall*, constituting a sinus rather than a fistula.

Branchial Fistula

◈ *S.Das Clinical Surgery 11th/371*

- External orifice is situated in lower third of the neck near the anterior border of sternocleidomastoid
- Fistula represent persistent 2nd branchial cleft
- This fistula is congenital & should not be confused with an acquired sinus which results from incision of inflamed branchial cyst (sinus will be situated in upper 3rd of neck)
- Internal orifice-anterior aspect of the posterior pillar of fauces.

"Paired branchial clefts and arches develop early in the fourth gestational week. The first cleft and the first, second, third, and fourth pouches give rise to adult organs. ***The embryologic communication between the pharynx and the external surface may persist as a fistula.*** A fistula is seen most commonly with the second branchial cleft, which normally disappears, and extends from the ***anterior border of the sternocleidomastoid muscle superiorly***, inward through the bifurcation of the carotid artery, and enters the ***posterolateral pharynx just below the tonsillar fossa***. The branchial cleft remnants may contain small pieces of cartilage and cysts, but internal fistulas are rare. A second branchial cleft sinus is suspected when clear fluid is noted ***draining from the external opening of the tract at the anterior border of the lower third of the sternocleidomastoid muscle***" *(Schwartz 9th/1414-15)*

155. Ans. a. Painless bleeding, c. Constipation..., e. Never prolapse

[Ref: Manipal Surgery 4th/ 793-95; L & B 26th/ 1251-52; Schwartz 9th/ 1058]

Haemorrhoids

◈ *Manipal Surgery 4th/ 793*

- Painless bleeding- fresh bleeding occurs after defaecation (splash in the pan). This cause chronic anaemia. Haemorrhoids which bleed are called ***Grade I haemorrhoids***
- ***Most of patient complains of constipation***

Table *(Manipal Surgery 4th/ 793)*: **Grades of Haemorrhoids**

Grade features	Symptoms
I. Never prolapse	*Bleeding per rectum*
II. Prolapse on defaecation, spontaneous reduction	Something coming down & going back
III. Prolapse on defaecation, require manual reduction	Something coming down, bleeding, mucus discharge, pruritus
VI. Permanent prolapse	Acute pain, throbbing discomfort

Haemorrhoids

◈ *L & B 26th/ 1251-52*

- Patients may complain of true 'piles', lumps that appear at the anal orifice during defaecation and which ***return spontaneously after wards (second-degree haemorrhoids)***, piles that have to be ***replaced manually (third-degree haemorrhoids)*** or piles that lie permanently outside (fourth-degree haemorrhoids).
- By this stage, there is often a significant cutaneous component to the pile masses, which arise through repeated congestion and oedema.
- In addition to the main symptoms of pain and prolapse, patients may complain of anal irritation, which may occur as a result of mucus secretion from the caudally displaced rectal mucosa, minor leakage through a now imperfect anal seal or ***difficulties in cleaning after defaecation because ofthe irregularity of the anal***

Four Degrees of Haemorrhoids

◈ *L & B 26th/ 1252*

- **First degree:** ***bleed only, no prolapse***
- **Second degree:** prolapse, but reduce spontaneously
- **Third degree:** prolapse and have to be manually reduced
- **Fourth degree:** permanently prolapsed

Haemorrhoids: Clinical Features

◈ *L & B 26th/ 1251*

- Haemorrhoids or piles are symptomatic anal cushions
- They are more common when intra-abdominal pressure is raised, e.g. in obesity, constipation and pregnancy
- Classically, they occur in the 3, 7 and 11 o'clock positions with the patient in the lithotomy position
- **Symptoms of haemorrhoids:** ***bright-red, painless bleeding mucous discharge prolapse pain only on prolapse***

156. Ans. a. Tredelenburg, b. Reverse Tredelenburg, e. Lloyd-Davies

[Ref: L & B 26th/1239, 760, 1232, 890]

"**Tredelenburg position:** Lithotomy with head down" *(L& B 26th/1232, 890)*

"**Reverse Tredelenburg position**: The patient is ***supine on*** the operating table with the table tilted up 15° at the head end to reduce venous engorgement" *(L & B 26th/760)*

"Most commonly, the patient is examined in the ***left lateral (Sims) position*** with the buttocks overlying the edge of the examination couch and with the axis of the torso crossing, rather than parallel with, the edge of the couch. Alternatively, in younger patients, the ***prone jackknife or knee–elbow*** positions may be used" *(L & B 26th/1239)*

"**Lloyd-Davies position** is a medical term referring to a common position for surgical procedures involving the pelvis and lower abdomen. The majority of colorectal and pelvic surgery is conducted with the patient in the Lloyd-Davis position"

"**Lloyd-Davies Position:** It is also known as the Trendelenburg position with legs apart. The basic angle is a 30-degree Trendelenburg with the hips flexed at 15 degrees; this can be adjusted with leg supports"

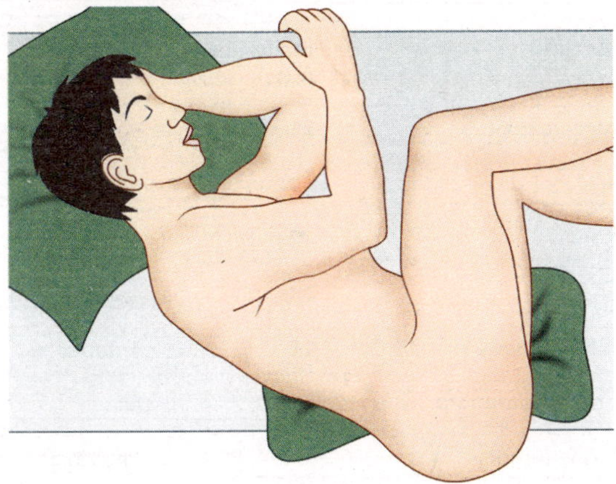

Fig: *(L & B 26th/1239)*: Positions for digital rectal examination- Left lateral (Sims).

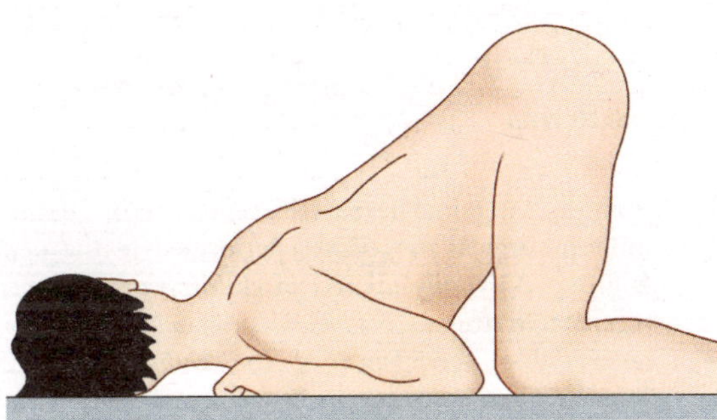

Fig: *(L & B 26th/1239)*: ***Jackknife or knee–elbow***

157. Ans. a. Common..., b. More common...; e. Distant metastasis....

[Ref: Dhingra 6th/226; Manipal Surgery 4th/286-90; L & B 26th/710-12]

Carcinoma Lip

◈ *Devita 7th/673-78*

- The most common neoplasms are squamous cell carcinomas. Basal cell carcinomas start on the skin of the lip and may secondarily invade the vermilion.
- *Persons with light-colored skin or with prolonged exposure to sunlight are most prone to develop lip carcinoma*
- The ***vermilion is the most common site of origin.***
- Squamous cell carcinoma may present as an ***enlarging discrete lesion that is not tender until it ulcerates***.
- Some lesions develop very slowly on a background of leukoplakia or carcinoma in situ and present as *superficially ulcerated lesions with little or no bulk.*
- Erythema of the adjacent skin suggests *dermal lymphatic invasion*. Palpation of the lip will reveal the extent of induration. Paresthesia of the skin of the lip indicate nerve invasion.
- Squamous cell carcinoma starts on the vermilion of the lip and invades adjacent skin and the orbicular muscle. Advanced lesions invade the *adjacent commissures of the lip, the buccal mucosa, the skin and wet mucosa of the lip, the adjacent mandible, and eventually the mental nerve.*
- Lymphatic spread moves to the submental and submandibular lymph nodes and then to the jugular chain. The risk for lymph node metastases is approximately 5% at diagnosis and is increased by high-grade histology, large lesions, invasion of the wet mucosa of the lip and buccal mucosa, and for patients with recurrent disease

Carcinoma Lip

◈ *Dhingra 6th/226*

- ***Lower lip is more often involved***
- ***Incidence of oral cancer is six times more in smoker than non-smoker***
- Site of predilection is b/w the midline & commissure of the lip
- Mostly, it is squamous cell carcinoma, often seen in males in the age group of 40-70 years
- ***L.N metastases develop late.***Submental& submandibular nodes are the first to be involved; other deep cervical nodes may also get involved later

Lip Cancer

◈ *L & B 26th/710-12; Manipal Surgery 4th/286-90*

- Lip cancer presents early as it is readily visible to the patient. It usually arises as an ulcer on the vermilion border.
- ***In total, 95 per cent of carcinomas of the lip arise on the lower lip and 15 per cent arise in the central one-third and commissures.***
- Tumours tend to spread laterally over the mucosal surface. Lymph node metastases, usually to the submental or submandibular nodes, occur late.
- ***Blood spread is uncommon***

158. Ans. b. Most common..., c. More commonly..., d. Contain teeth..., e. Histologically

[Ref: Manipal Surgery 4th/1021; CSDT 11th/1346-47; L & B 26th/868; Schwartz 9th/575-76]

"**Thymoma** is the ***most frequently encountered*** neoplasm (25% of total mediastinal mass, c.f germ cell tumour-13%) of anterior mediastinum of adult"-Schwartz 9th/573&L & B 26th/868

Mediastinal Germ Cell Tumors

◈ *Schwartz 9th/575-76*

- Germ cell tumors are uncommon neoplasms. However, they are the most common malignancy in young men between age 15 and 35 years.
- Most germ cell tumors are gonadal in origin. Those with the mediastinum as the primary site are rare, constituting less than 5% of all germ cell tumors, and less than 1% of all mediastinal tumors (usually occurring in the ***anterior compartment***).

- If a malignant mediastinal germ cell tumor is found, it is important to exclude a gonadal primary tumor.
- **Primary mediastinal germ cell tumors** (including ***teratomas, seminomas, and nonseminomatous*** malignant germ cell tumors) are a heterogeneous group of ***benign and malignant neoplasms*** thought to originate from primitive pluripotent germ cells "misplaced" in the mediastinum during embryonic development.
- Previously, most mediastinal germ cell tumors were thought to be metastatic. However, evidence suggested that many mediastinal germ cell tumors are primary, developing from pluripotent primordial germ cells in the mediastinum
- **Mature teratomas** are ***benign*** and can generally be diagnosed by the characteristic CT findings of ***multilocular cystic tumors, encapsulated with combinations of fluid, soft tissue, calcium, and/or fat attenuation in the anterior compartment.***

Teratoma

◈ *Schwartz 9th/576*

- Teratomas are the ***most common type of mediastinal germ cell tumors,*** accounting for 60 to 70% of mediastinal germ cell tumors.
- They contain two or three embryonic layers that may include ***teeth, skin, hair (ectodermal), cartilage and bone (mesodermal), or bronchial, intestinal, or pancreatic tissue (endodermal).***
- Therapy for mature, benign teratomas is ***surgical resection,*** which confers an excellent prognosis.
- *Rarely, teratomas may contain a focus of carcinoma*; these malignant teratomas (or teratocarcinomas) are locally aggressive. Often diagnosed at an unresectable stage, they respond poorly to chemotherapy and in a limited manner to radiotherapy; the prognosis is uniformly poor.

Germ Cell Tumour

◈ *L & B 26th/868*

- The anterior mediastinum is the ***most common site of extra gonadal germ cell tumours.*** They account for 13 per cent of all mediastinal masses and cysts and contain elements from ***all three cell types (mesoderm, endoderm and ectoderm).***
- They tend to present in young adults and75 per cent are benign and cystic, although they may cause compression of neighbouring structures; hence, dermoid cysts are best excised.
- Malignancy is suspected if elevated levels of serum alpha-fetoprotein, human chorionic gonadotrophin and carcinoembryonic antigen are detected.
- After initial treatment with chemotherapy, a patient with tumour marker normalisation and a persistent mass on CT may be considered

Mediastinal Teratomas may either be: *(http: //radiopaedia.org)*

- **Mature:** Well differentiated
- **Immature:** Poorly differentiated
- With malignant transformation

Generally, ***cystic lesions tend to be benign whereas solid lesions tend to be malignant however the final diagnosis is made histologically.***

"Mature teratomas and most immature teratomas are benign tumours, but still carry a risk of malignancy despite being indolent initially and require close clinical, serological, and radiological follow-up, or surgical excision.There is also a low incidence of malignant transformation of somatic cells (i.e. non germ cell components) within these tumours, e.g. carcinoma, sarcoma, leukaemia"

Table *(Schwartz 9th/570)*: **Mediastinal Tumors in Adults**

Tumor type	Incidence (%)	Location
Neurogenic tumors	21	Posterior
Cysts	20	All
Thymomas	19	Anterior
Lymphoma	13	Anterior/middle
Germ cell tumors	11	Anterior
Mesenchymal tumors	7	All
Endocrine tumors	6	Anterior/middle

159. Ans. a. Occur due..., b. Defect in abdominal..., d. Difficult to reduce...

[Ref: Manipal Surgery 4th/845-46; Sabiston 19th/1856, 1114; Schwartz 9th/ 144-45, 1340-41]

Inguinal Hernia

◈ *Sabiston 19th/1856*

- Repair of an inguinal hernia (IH) represents one of the most common surgical procedures performed in the pediatric age group. ***Virtually all IHs in children are indirect and congenital in origin.***
- The variable ***persistence of the embryonic processus vaginalis*** offers a spectrum of abnormalities, including a scrotal hernia, communicating hydrocele, hydrocele of the cord, or simple hydrocele
- In preterm infants, the incidence may be as high as 30%. About one third of children with IH are younger than 6 months, and ***males are affected about six times more often than females.***
- The ***right side is involved in 60% and the left in 30% of patients***; bilateral hernias are seen in 10%. The higher incidence on the right side compared with the left is probably related to the later descent and ***obliteration of the processus vaginalis of the right testis.***
- Most IHs present as a bulge in the region of the external ring extending downward for varying distances to the scrotum or labia. Inguinal pain may also be a presenting complaint.
- Incarceration and possible strangulation are the most feared consequences of IH and occur more frequently in premature infants. Because of the risk for these complications, ***all IHs in children need to be repaired.***
- A communicating hydrocele is basically a small IH in which fluid, but not peritoneal structures, traverses the processus vaginalis.

Inguinal Hernia

◈ *Schwartz 9th/1444-45*

- *The presence of an inguinal hernia in a child is an indication for **surgical repair**.* The operation is termed a ***herniorrhaphy*** because it involves *closing off the patent processusvaginalis.*
- This is to be contrasted with the ***hernioplasty that is performed in adults***, which requires a reconstruction of the inguinal floor.
- Inguinal hernia results from a failure of closure of the processusvaginalis
- High incidence of inguinal hernias occurs in premature infants.
- When the processusvaginalis remains completely patent, a ***communication persists between the peritoneal cavity and the groin***, resulting in a hernia.
- Partial closure can result in entrapped fluid, which is known as a hydrocele.
- Using the classification system that is typically applied to adult hernias, ***all congenital hernias in children are by definition indirect inguinal hernias***. Children also present with direct inguinal and femoral hernias, although these are much less common.
- Inguinal hernias occur more commonly in males than females (10: 1) and are more common on the right side than the left.
- Infants are at high risk for incarceration of an inguinal hernia because of the narrow inguinal ring.
- ***Spontaneous resolution does not occur, and therefore, a nonoperative approach cannot ever be justified.***
- An inguinal hernia in a female infant or child frequently contains an ovary rather than intestine.

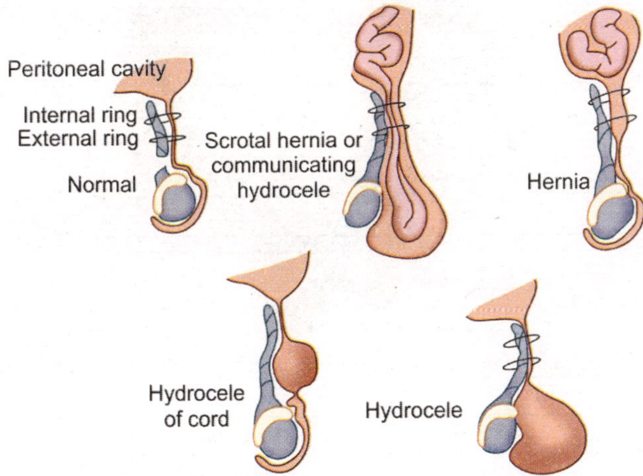

Fig: Anatomic variants of inguinal hernia and hydrocele

160. Ans. b. For stage I seminoma- orchidectomy + radiotherapy used..., d. Staging is important..., e. βHCG & AFP may be...

[Ref: Manipal Surgery 4th/994-98; L & B 26th/ 185-88; Schwartz 9th/1462]

"***Radical inguinal orchidectomy** is the treatment of choice in all testicular tumour irrespective of the histological type & stage" (Manipal Surgery 4th/997)*

"**Testicular tumour: *In confirmed cases, staging is an essential step in planning treatment.*** Blood is taken prior to orchidectomy to measure the levels of tumour markers which are raised in around 50 per cent of cases. A rise in AFP is seen in around 50–70 per cent of NSGCTs and a rise in ***HCG is seen in 40–60 per cent of NSGCTs and around 30 per cent of seminomas.*** When raised, these markers are used to monitor the response to treatment. The mean serum half-lives of AFP and HCG are 5–7 days and 2–3 days, respectively, and reassessment of the markers following orchidectomy can indicate whether all the tumour tissue has been removed"-L & B 26th/ 186-87

Testicular Tumour: Treatment

◈ *L & B 26th/1387-88*

- *Scrotal exploration and orchidectomy for suspected testicular tumour*
- ***Management by staging and histological diagnosis** (after orchidectomy):* The treatment of patients with testicular tumours is usually successful, even in cases that are advanced at presentation. This largely reflects the excellent response of these tumours to ***platinum-based chemotherapy and (for seminomatous tumours) to radiotherapy.***
- **Stage I tumours**: **Seminomas *are radio sensitive*** and for many years ***adjuvant radiotherapy to the para-aortic nodes was the mainstay of treatment for stage I disease.*** Some years ago, the excellent response to ***platinum-based chemotherapy led to chemotherapy being introduced for most men with stage 1 seminoma.*** However, current practice uses CT and tumour marker-based surveillance protocols with ***chemotherapy being reserved for men who demonstrate relapse.*** **NSGCTs** are ***not radiosensitive***, but they are ***highly sensitive to combination chemotherapy*** with bleomycin, etoposide andcis-platinum (so called BEP chemotherapy). Some good prognosis NSGCTs can be managed by surveillance protocols (using regular CT scanning and tumour marker measurement) with the more high risk cases receiving chemotherapy.
- **Stage II–IV tumours**: ***Combination BEP chemotherapy is the mainstay of treatment for stages II–IV seminoma and NSGCT.*** *Retroperitoneal lymph node dissection* is sometimes needed in some cases of NSGCT when retroperitoneal masses remain after chemotherapy.

Testicular Tumour: Staging

◈ *L & B 26th/ 1387*

- **Stage I:** The tumour is confined to the testis;
- **Stage II:** Nodal disease is present but is confined to nodes below the diaphragm;
- **Stage III:** Nodal disease is present above the diaphragm;
- **Stage IV:** Nonlymphatic metastatic disease (most typically within the lungs)

161. Ans. a. Necrotizing fasciitis..., b. Diabetes..., c. Urgent wide...

[Ref: Manipal Surgery 4th/998-99; L & B 26th/ 1388; Schwartz 9th/ 1469-70]

Fournier's Gangrene

◈ *Schwartz 9th/ 1469*

- Fournier's gangrene is a ***necrotizing fasciitis of the male genitalia and perineum that can be rapidly progressing and fatal if not treated promptly***. The mortality rate has been reported to be as high as 30% to 40%.
- **Risk factors** for Fournier's gangrene include urethral strictures, perirectal abscesses, poor perineal hygiene, ***diabetes***, cancer, human immunodeficiency virus (HIV), and other immunocompromised states.
- The infection spreads along the *dartos, Scarpa's, and Colles' fascias.*
- Clinical signs include fevers, perineal and scrotal pain, and associated indurated tissue. ***Cellulitis, eschars, necrosis, flaking skin, and crepitus*** may all be observed.
- The diagnosis is largely made on clinical suspicion, and significantly less often made on laboratory or radiographic findings. Classically, the patient describes pain out of proportion to the physical findings.
- Prompt debridement of nonviable tissue and broad spectrum antibiotics are necessary to prevent further spread.
- If there is damage to the external anal sphincter, patients may require a colostomy.
- Because the ***testes have aseparate blood supply, they are usually not threatened and do not need to be removed.*** They may be tucked subcutaneously into the thigh ("thigh pouch") to ease postoperative management.
- Patients frequently require return trips to the operating room for further debridement. Tight glucose control and adequate nutrition are necessary to facilitate wound healing. The large tissue defect should be initially treated with frequent dressing changes.
- Reconstructive strategies involving skin ngrafting are needed when large tissue defects result from extensive tissue damage.

Fournier's Gangrene

◈ *L & B 26th/ 1388*

- Fournier's gangrene is an uncommon and nasty condition of infective origin that is characterised by ***sudden scrotal inflammation, with rapid onset of gangrene leading to exposure of the scrotal contents.***
- Although it can occur inconjunction with sepsis of the testis, epididymis or perianal region, an obvious cause is absent in over half the cases.
- It can arise following minor injuries or procedures in the perineal area, such as a bruise, scratch, urethral dilatation, injection of haemorrhoids or opening of a periurethral abscess. Many patients have concurrent illnesses that diminish their defences, most notably ***diabetes mellitus and alcoholism.***
- There is a mixed infection of aerobic and anaerobic bacteria in a fulminating inflammation of the subcutaneous tissues, which results in an obliterative arteritis of the arterioles to the scrotal skin which in turn results in gangrene. The condition can spread rapidly to involve the fascia and skin of the penis, perineum and abdominal wall.
- There is sudden pain in the scrotum associated with prostration, pallor and pyrexia. Cellulitis spreads rapidly (within hours) and progresses to necrosis until the entire scrotal and penile coverings slough, leaving the testes exposed but healthy.
- **Treatment** of a case of Fournier's gangrene is a *surgical emergency*. ***Urgent wide surgical excision of the dead and infected tissue is essential.*** This should be accompanied by intravenous antibiotics.
- Supportive care is essential, because the patients often become severely septic. Early review of the wounds is helpful to confirm that all dead tissue has been removed, and if the patient survives the acute episode, skin grafting is often necessary. Despite best therapy, mortality rates as high as 50 per cent are often reported

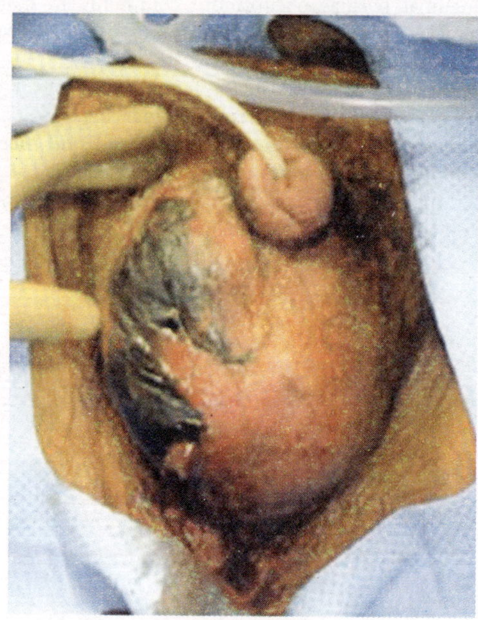

Fig: *(Schwartz 9th/ 1470)*: Necrotic scrotal skin from Fournier's gangrene

162. Ans. a. Ballotable, e. Dull on percussion...

[Ref: Manual on Clinical Surgery 11th/526, 561-62; Manipal Surgery 4th/905-08]

"The **paracolic gutters (paracolic sulci, paracolic recesses)** are spaces between the ***colon and the abdominal wall.***

These gutters are clinically important because they allow a passage for infectious fluids from different compartments of the abdomen. For example; ***fluid from an infected appendix can track up the right paracolic gutter to the hepatorenal recess***" *(www.wisegeek.com)*

A & E

Exammination of Abdominal Mass

◈ *Manipal Surgery 4th/905-08*

- Renal swelling moves with respiration because kidney is enclosed by fascia of Gerota which is attached above the diaphragm
- Liver, stomach, spleen, gall bladder move very well with respiration
- Finger insulation test- Liver and spleen are under right & left coastal margin respectively. Hence, it is not possible to get the upper margins or upper border of these organs
- Upper border cannot be made out in liver, spleen & renal swelling
- Lower border is not appreciated in pelvic masses e.g. uterine fibroid, ovarian cyst (pelvic)
- Reniform swelling suggest renal swelling
- Renal mass comes down during inspiration. As it comes down, it can beheld back & can be pushed back to the renal pouch
- Grossly enlarged swelling may be bimanually palpable such as liver, spleen, kidney
- Typically kidney swelling are ballottable. Ballottabilty is due to perirenal pad of fat& due to pedicle
- Renal angle percussion: ***In case of enlargement of kidney, there will be a band of resonance anteriorly due to colon but posteriorly it gives a dull note***
- ***Dull note- liver, spleen, renal angle***
- ***Resonant note- Bowel anterior to mass***

Features of Kidney Swelling

◈ *Manual on Clinical Surgery 11th/526*

- It is a reniform swelling
- It ***moves very slightly with respiration*** as it comes down a little at the height of inspiration
- It is ***ballottable***
- A sickening sensation is often felt during manipulation
- A ***hand can be easily insinuated b/w the upper pole of swelling & the costal margin***
- ***Percussion will reveal resonant note in front of a kidney swelling*** as coils of intestine & colon will always be in front of the kidney

163. Ans. a. After thyroid..., c. Radical resection...

[Ref: Manipal Surgery 4th/363; Sabiston 19th/ 113-14, 928; L & B 26th/776-77, 762; Schwartz 9th/1388]

MEN I cause Hyperparathyroidism (Manipal Surgery 4th/363)

Hypoparathyroidism: Causes

◈ *Sabiston 19th/ 113-14*

- Surgery in central neck (such as *radical resection of head & neck cancer*)
- ***1-2% of patients after total thyroidectomy***
- ***Hypoplasia or aplasia like DiGeorge syndrome***

Parathyroid Insufficiency after Thyroid Surgery

◈ *L & B 26th/762*

- This is due to removal of the parathyroid glands or infarction through damage to the parathyroid end artery; often, both factors occur together.
- Vascular injury is probably far more important Important than inadvertent removal.
- The incidence of permanent hypoparathyroidism should be less than 1 per cent and most cases present dramatically 2–5 days after operation but, very rarely, the onset is delayed for 2–3 weeks or if a patient with marked hypocalcaemia is asymptomatic.

Hypoparathyroidism

◈ *L& B 26th/776-77*

- While there are rare congenital (**DiGeorge**) and medical (***autoimmune polyglandular and Wilson)*** syndromes causing hypoparathyroidism, for practical purposes postoperative hypoparathyroidism is the dominant management issue in surgical practice. This results from removal, trauma or devascularisation of the parathyroid glands which may be deliberate but is more often inadvertent.

Hypoparathyroidism

◈ *Schwartz 9th/1388*

- The parathyroid glands may be congenitally absent in the ***DiGeorge syndrome***, which also is characterized by lack of thymic development, and, therefore, a thymus-dependent lymphoid system.
- Hyperparathyroidism in pregnant women can lead to hypoparathyroidism in neonates from suppression of fetal parathyroid tissue.
- ***By far, the most common cause of hypoparathyroidism is thyroid surgery, particularly total thyroidectomy*** with a concomitant central neck dissection.
- Hypoparathyroidism may also occur after parathyroid surgery, which is more likely if patients have parathyroid hyperplasia and undergo a subtotal resection or total parathyroidectomy with parathyroid autotransplantation.

164. Ans. a. Mostly seen..., c. Usually unilateral, d. Yellowish-greenish...

[Ref: Manipal Surgery 4th/ 385-90; S.Das textbook 5th/702-03; Sabiston 19th/838-39; L & B 26th/807]

Breast Cysts

◈ *S.Das textbook 5th/702-03*

- Classically seen in perimenopausal women mostly in last decade of reproductive life
- Smooth & dent on palpation. The have ***degree of mobility***
- Cyst fluid varies in colour ranging from pale yellow to almost black. The aspirate is ***usually translucent,*** though it may be thick & turgid

Breast Cysts

◈ *Sabiston 19th/838-39*

- Cysts within the breast are fluid-filled, epithelium-lined cavities that may vary in size from microscopic to large, palpable masses containing as much as 20 to 30 mL of fluid.
- A palpable cyst develops in at least 1 in every 14 women, and ***50% of cysts are multiple or recurrent.*** The pathogenesis of cyst formation is not well understood; however, cysts

appear to arise from destruction and dilation of lobules and terminal ductules.

- Microscopic studies have shown that fibrosis at or near the lobule, combined with continued secretion, results in unfolding of the lobule and expansion of an epithelium-lined cavity containing fluid.
- Cysts are influenced by ovarian hormones, a fact that explains their variation with the menstrual cycle. ***Most cysts occur in women older than 35.*** The ***incidence of cyst development steadily increases until menopause and sharply declines thereafter.*** New cyst formation in older women is generally associated with exogenous hormone replacement.
- There is no evidence of increased risk for breast cancer associated with cyst formation.
- A palpable mass can be confirmed to be a cyst by aspiration or ultrasound.
- **Cyst fluid** can be ***straw colored, opaque, or dark green and may contain flecks of debris.***
- Given the low risk for malignancy within a cyst, if the palpable mass disappears completely after aspiration and the ***cyst contents are not grossly bloody,*** the fluid need not be sent for cytologic analysis.
- If the cyst recurs multiple times (more than two times is a reasonable rule), cytology is justified.
- Surgical removal of a cyst is usually indicated if the cytologic findings are suspicious or the cyst recurs multiple times.

Breast Cysts

◈ *L & B 26th/807*

- These occur most commonly in the ***last decade of reproductive life*** as a result of a non-integrated involution of stroma and epithelium.
- They are ***often multiple, may be bilateral*** and can mimic malignancy.
- Diagnosis can be confirmed by aspiration and/or ultrasound. They typically present suddenly and cause great alarm; prompt diagnosis and drainage provides immediate relief.
- A solitary cyst or small collection of cysts can be aspirated.
- If they resolve completely, and if the ***fluid is not blood-stained,*** no further treatment is required.
- However, 30 per cent will recur and require reaspiration.
- Cytological examination of cyst fluid is no longer practised routinely.
- If there is a residual lump or if the fluid is blood-stained, a core biopsy or local excision for histological diagnosis is advisable, which is also the case if the cyst reforms repeatedly. This will exclude cyst adenocarcinoma, which is more common in elderly women.

165. Ans. a. Pain shift with..., c. Usually bilateral

[Ref: Manipal Surgery 4th/385-88; CSDT 11th/340-42; L & B 26th/802-08]

Fibrocystic Disease (Mammary Dysplasia)

◈ *CSDT 11th/340-42*

Essentials of Diagnosis

- Painful, often multiple, usually bilateral masses in the breast.
- ***Rapid fluctuation in the size of the masses is common.***
- ***Frequently, pain occurs or increases and size increases during premenstrual phase of cycle.***
- Most common age is 30–50 years. Rare in postmenopausal women not receiving hormonal replacement.

General Considerations

- Fibrocystic condition is the most frequent lesion of the breast. Although commonly referred to as "fibrocystic disease," it does not, in fact, represent a pathologic or anatomic disorder.
- It is common in women 30–50 years of age but rare in postmenopausal women who are not taking hormonal replacement medications. Estrogen hormone is considered a causative factor.
- There may be an increased risk in women who drink alcohol, especially women between 18 and 22 years of age. Fibrocystic condition encompasses a wide variety of histologic changes. These lesions are always associated with benign changes in the breast epithelium, some of which are found so commonly in normal breasts that they are probably variants of normal breast histology but have nonetheless been termed a "condition."
- The microscopic findings of fibrocystic condition include ***cysts*** (gross and microscopic), papillomatosis, adenosis, fibrosis, and ductal epithelial hyperplasia. Although fibrocystic condition has generally been considered to increase the risk of subsequent breast cancer, only the variants in which proliferation (especially with atypia) of epithelial components is demonstrated represent true risk factors.

Symptoms and Signs

- Fibrocystic condition may produce an asymptomatic lump in the breast that is discovered by accident, but ***pain or tenderness often calls attention to the mass.*** There may be ***discharge from the nipple.*** In many cases, ***discomfort occurs or is increased during the premenstrual phase of the cycle,*** at which time the cysts tend to enlarge. Fluctuation in size and rapid appearance or disappearance of a breast mass are common with this condition. ***Multiple or bilateral masses are common,*** and many patients will give a history of a ***transient lump in the breast or cyclic breast pain.***

Differential Diagnosis

- ***Pain, fluctuation in size, and multiplicity of lesions*** are the features most helpful in differentiating fibrocystic condition from carcinoma. If a dominant mass is present, the diagnosis of cancer should be assumed until disproved by biopsy.

Fibroadenoma

◈ *L & B 26th/807*

- These usually arise in the fully developed breast between the ages of 15 and 25 years, although occasionally they occur in much older women. They arise from hyperplasia of a single lobule and usually grow up to 2–3 cm in size. They are surrounded by a ***well-marked capsule*** and can thus be enucleated through a cosmetically appropriate incision.
- A fibroadenoma does not require excision unless associated with suspicious cytology, it becomes very large or the patient expressly desires the lump to be removed.

- Giant fibroadenomas occasionally occur during puberty. They are over 5 cm in diameter and are often rapidly growing but, in other respects, are similar to smaller fibroadenomas and can be enucleated through a submammary incision. They are more common in the Afro-Caribbean population.

Fibroadenoma

◈ *Manipal Surgery 4th/388*
- Peak age of incidence is at 20 year
- Present with painless lump
- It is smooth, round bordered, firm to hard in consistency & freely mobile within the breast (so called breast mouse)

Table *(Manipal Surgery 4th/385)*: **Difference b/w fibroadenoma & fibroadenosis**

	Fibroadenoma	Fibroadenosis
Incidence	Less common	More common
Nature	Benign tumour of one lobule	Aberration of normal changes in breast
Pain in the breast	Not a feature	Very common, premenstrual
Location	Unilateral	Usually bilateral
Lump	**Well-defined, firm, mobile**	Irregular, ill-defined, tender lump
Capsule	**Well-defined**	No capsule
Discharge	No	Serous or green coloured
Malignancy	Rarely-sarcoma	Carcinoma (if epitheliosis is present)
Treatment	Excision	Excision or drugs

166. Ans. a. Cough impulse..., b. Trendelenburg..., c. Percussation wave...

[Ref: S.Das Clinical Surgery 11th/102-04; Manipal Surgery 4th/131-33; L & B 26th/904]

"**Percussion**: If the most prominent parts of the varicose veins are tapped, an impulse can be felt by the finger at the saphenous opening. This is known as **Schwartz test**. Sometimes the percussion wave can be ***transmitted from above downwards (i.e. retrograde direction)*** & this will imply absent or incompetent valves"-S.Das Clinical Surgery 11th/104

"**Brodie-Trendelenburg test:** This test is performed to determine the incompetency of the sapheno-femoral valve"-*S. Das Clinical Surgery 11th/102*

Cough impulse test (Morrissey's test): Fluid thrill, an impulse felt by the fingers, is indicative of ***saphenofemoral incompetence***"- Manipal Surgery 4th/131

Tests for Varicose Vein & Inference

◈ *Manipal Surgery 4th/131*
- **Cough impulse test:** ***saphenofemoral incompetence***
- **Trendelenburg I:** ***saphenofemoral incompetence***
- **Trendelenburg II:** Perforator incompetence
- **Multiple tourniquet test:** Site of perforator incompetence
- **Schwartz test:** Superficial column of blood
- **Modified Perthe's test:** Deep vein thrombosis
- **Fegan's test:** To locate the ***perforators in the deep fascia***

167. Ans. b. Involve..., c. Renal vein involvement, e. Size >10 cm.

[Ref: Harrison 19th/579; Manipal Surgery 4th/947-950; Sabiston 19th/2071; L & B 26th/1304-06]

Staging is different in different textbooks (Harrison, Sabiston, Manipal Surgery)

According to Harrison: Answer is B, C& E

According to Sabiston: Answer is B & E

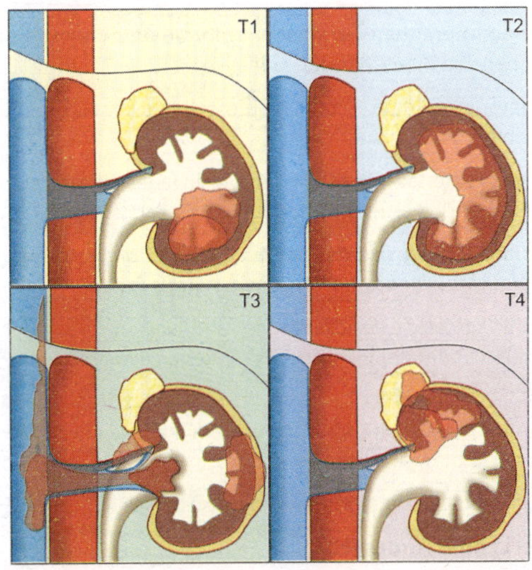

Fig: *(Harrison 19th/579)*: Renal cell carcinoma staging

TNM	Involvement	Extent of Disease
TX	Primary not involved	
T1 T1a T1b	≤ 7 cm ≤ 4 cm ≤ 4 cm	Limited to kidney
T2 T2a T2b	> 7 cm > 7 cm to ≤ 10 cm > 10 cm	Limited to kidney
T3 T3a T3b T3c	into major veins or perinephric tissues in renal vein or renal sinus fat into vena cava into vena cava	not beyond Gerota's Fascia not beyond Gerota's Fascia below diaphragm above diaphragm
T4	invasion beyond Gerota's Fascia	including contiguous extentions & into ipsilateral adrenal gland
Regional		
NX	Regional lymph not assessed	
NO	No lymph involvement	
N1	Regional lymph involvement	
Distant Metastases		
M0	No distant metastases	
M1	Distant metastases	

Table *(Sabiston 19th/ 2071)*: **TNM Classification for Renal Cell Carcinoma**

Primary Tumor (T)	
TX	Primary tumor cannot be assessed
T0	No evidence of primary tumor
T1	Tumor 7 cm or less in greatest dimension, limited to the kidney
T1a	Tumor 4 cm or less in greatest dimension, limited to the kidney
T1b	Tumor more than 4 cm but not more than 7 cm in greatest dimension, limited to the kidney
T2	Tumor more than 7 cm in greatest dimension, limited to the kidney
T3	Tumor extends into major veins or invades adrenal gland or perinephric tissues but not beyond Gerota's fascia
T3a	***Tumor directly invades adrenal gland or perirenal and/or renal sinus fat but not beyond Gerota's fasica***
T3b	Tumor grossly extends into the ***renal vein*** or its segmental (muscle-containing) branches, or ***vena cava*** below the diaphragm
T3c	Tumor grossly extends into ***vena cava*** above diaphragm or invades the wall of the vena cava
T4	Tumor invades beyond Gerota's fascia
Regional Lymph Nodes (N)	
NX	Regional lymph nodes cannot be assessed
N0	No regional lymph node metastases
N1	Metastases in a single regional lymph node
N2	Metastases in more than one regional lymph node
Distant Metastasis (M)	
MX	Distant metastasis cannot be assessed
M0	No distant metastasis
M1	Distant metastasis

168. Ans. a. C/I in..., b. Less..., c. Stone is breaked..., e. Endoscopic retrieval....

[Ref: Manipal Surgery 4th/938; Sabiston 19th/ 2059, 236; L & B 26th/1294, 1296]

Smith General Urology 17th: Writes

- "***Pregnant women*** and patients with large abdominal aortic aneurysms or ***uncorrectable bleeding disorders*** should ***not be treated with ESWL***"
- Patients with large renal pelvic calculi (>1.5 cm) have a stone-free rate at 3 months approximating 75%, in comparison with those with a similar stone in a lower calyx, which approximates only 50%. Patients with small renal pelvic stones (<1.5 cm) have approximately a 90% stone free rate in comparison to those with similar stones in a middle calyx (approximately 75%) or lower calyx (approximately 70%). Lower calyceal stone-free rates are increased with a small stone burden, a short and wide infundibulum, and a nonacute infundibulo-pelvic angle. Overall, approximately 75% of patients with renal calculi treated with ESWL become stone-free in 3 months. ***As stones increase in size, stone-free rates decrease, more so in the lower and middle calyces than in superior calyceal and renal pelvic locations.***
- Large-volume stones (>3 cm, stone surface >500 mm2) (e.g., staghorn stones). These stones can be treated by several sessions of ESWL, but only about 30% of patients become stone free. However, problems associated with passing large quantities of gravel (e.g., ureteral obstruction, pain, fever, sepsis) can be prevented by first percutaneously debulking the stone and then performing ESWL for endoscopically inaccessible stones.
- For ***extraction of distal ureteral stones that are unresponsiveto ESWL, short rigid ureterorenoscopes*** and alligator-forceps or Dormia baskets are most helpful. Ureteroscop-icclearance rates for distal ureteral stones reach 93–100%.
- Impacted proximal ureteral stones that did not respond toin situ ESWL and could not be dislodged with a ureteral catheter usually can be repositioned into the renal pelvis under direct vision for subsequent ESWL using a small semirigid or rigid ureterorenoscope. If the stones are too large or impacted, intraureteral lithotripsy for stone disintegration may be necessary in a few cases.
- Ureteroscopic stone extraction is highly efficacious for lower ureteral calculi.

Extracorporeal Shock Wave Lithotripsy

◈ *L & B 26th/1294*

- Crystalline stones disintegrate under the impact of shock waves produced by the ESWL machine. The shocks may be aimed by ultrasound or x-ray imaging. The devices also differ in the disruptive force that they can develop. Less powerful machines break stones less effectively and several treatments may be necessary. Weaker shocks hurt less and treatment can be given without general anaesthesia.
- Ureteric colic is common after ESWL, and the patient needs analgesia, usually in the form of a non-steroidal anti-inflammatory drug. ***Bulky stone fragments may impact in the ureter***, causing obstruction. To avoid this, a stent should be placedin the ureter to drain the kidney while stone fragments pass.
- ***Occasionally, impacted fragments have to be removed ureteroscopically*** The principal complication of ESWL is infection. Many calculi contain bacteria, which are released from the broken stone.
- It is wise to give prophylactic antibiotics before ESWL, and an obstructed system should be decompressed by a ureteric stent or percutaneous nephrostomy before treatment.
- The clearance of stone from the kidney will depend up on the ***consistency of the stone*** and its site. Most oxalate and phosphate stones fragment well and, if lying in the renal pelvis, will clear within days. The results with harder stones, especially ***cystine stones, are less satisfactory***. When treating calyceal stones, the patients should be warned that the clearance may take months.

Ureteroscopic Stone Removal

◈ *L & B 26th/1297-98*

A ureteroscope is introduced transurethrally across the bladder into the ureter to ***remove stones impacted in the ureter***. Stones that cannot be caught in baskets or endoscopic forceps under direct vision are fragmented using an electrohydraulic, percussive or laser lithotripter.

169. Ans. b. Palliative treatment..., c. Metastatic recurrence..., d. When gallbladder...

[Ref: Manipal Surgery 4th/ 589-90; Sabiston 19th/1505-08; L & B 26th/1116-17; Schwartz 9th/ 1161-62]

Obstructive jaundice (increased bilirubin level) is common presentation *(Manipal Surgery 4th/ 589)*

Treatment of Gall Bladder Cancer

◈ *Manipal Surgery 4th/ 589-90*

- If GB cancer is found at cholecystectomy & if mucosa alone is involved, then cholecystectomy is sufficient
- If GB wall is involved, then ***extended cholecystectomy is done***
- Radiation has very small benefit. Chemotherapy also has been tried. 5-FU, mitomycin C, doxorubicin are drugs used
- Prognosis is very poor. Aggressive surgery & complete clearance give best results

Treatment and Prognosis of Gall Bladder Cancer

◈ *L & B 26th/1117*

- The majority of patients have **advanced disease** at presentation, and are ***not candidates for surgical therapy. Surgery is indicated in only very selected cases.***
- **Radical en-bloc resections** which may include ***segmental or extended hepatectomy, bile duct resection*** and regional lymphadenectomy should be considered in selected patients.
- ***For early stage disease confined to the mucosa or muscle of the gall bladder, no further treatment is indicated.***
- However, for **transmural disease**, ***a radical en-bloc resection of the gall bladder fossa and surrounding liver along with the regional lymph nodes*** should be performed. If the initial procedure was performed laparoscopically, the surgeon should examine the laparoscopic port sites. Routine resection of port sites is no longer recommended. However, it is recognized that the finding of disease at the port sites is a sign of generalized peritoneal disease and portends a very poor prognosis.
- ***For the majority of patients, a non-operative approach to palliation is best.*** Obstructive jaundice can be relieved by endoscopic and/or percutaneous methods. *The value of adjuvant therapy is unproven.*
- ***Gallbladder cancer for most patients is a lethal disease with agrim prognosis.*** The median survival is less than six months and a five-year survival figure of 5 per cent reported.

Treatment and Prognosis of Gall Bladder Cancer

◈ *Schwartz 9th/ 1161-62*

- ***Surgery remains the only curative option for gallbladder cancer***
- However, palliative procedures for patients with unresectable cancer and jaundice or duodenal obstruction remain the most frequently performed surgery for gallbladder cancers.
- Today, patients with obstructive jaundice can frequently be managed with either endoscopic or percutaneously-placed biliary stents.
- ***There are no proven effective options for adjuvant radiation or chemotherapy for patients with gallbladder cancer.***
- The **pathologic stage of gallbladder** cancer determines the operative treatment for patients with localized gallbladder cancer. *Patients without evidence of distant metastasis warrant exploration for tissue diagnosis, pathologic staging, and possible curative resection.*
- Tumors limited to the muscular layer of the gallbladder (T1), are usually identified incidentally, after cholecystectomy for gallstone disease. There is near-universal agreement that ***simple cholecystectomy is an adequate treatment for T1 lesions*** and results in a near 100% overall 5-year survival rate.
- When the tumor invades the perimuscular connective tissue without extension beyond the serosa or into the liver (T2 tumors), an **extended cholecystectomy** should be performed. That includes *resection of liver segments IVB and V, and lymphadenectomy of the cystic duct, and pericholedochal, portal, right celiac, and posterior pancreatoduodenal lymph nodes.*
- An ***aggressive approach*** in patients who will tolerate surgery has resulted in an increased survival for T3 and T4 lesions.
- **Most patients with gallbladder cance**r have ***unresectable disease*** at the time of diagnosis. The 5-year survival rate of all patients with gallbladder cancer is less than 5%, with a median survival of 6 months.
- **Recurrence after resection of gallbladder cancer** occurs ***most commonly in the liver or the celiac or retropancreatic nodes.*** The ***prognosis for recurrent disease is very poor.*** Death occurs most commonly secondary to biliary sepsis or liver failure. The ***main goal of follow-up is to provide palliative care.*** The most common problems are pruritus and cholangitis associated with obstructive jaundice, bowel obstruction secondary to carcinomatosis, and pain.

170. Ans. c. Cause abdominal..., d. Cut anterior..., e. Cut posterior...

[Ref: Manipal Surgery 4th/866-67; Sabiston 19th/1129; L & B 26th/34; Schwartz 9th/ 1269-70]

"**Nerve supply of abdominal wall:** Lower six thoracic & first lumbar nerve. They enter the rectus sheath laterally. In case **of paramedian incisions**, ***after opening the anterior rectus sheath***, rectus should be retracted laterally to define &***incise the posterior rectus sheath***"

"***Lumbar incision, lower midline incision & large transverse incision often give rise to incisional hernia*** *(Manipal Surgery 4th/866)*

"Whether the type of initial abdominal incision influences the **incisional hernia** rate remains controversial. As noted, the incidence of incisional herniation after midline laparotomy ranges from 3% to 20% & doubles if the operation is associated with a surgical site infection. A meta-analysis of 11 studies examining the incidence of incisional hernia formation after various types of abdominal incisions has concluded that the risk is ***10.5% for midline, 7.5% for transverse & 2.5% for paramedian incisions***" *(Sabiston19th/1129)*

Paramedian Incision

◈ *http: //www.fastbleep.com*

Use: provides laterality to the midline incision, allowing lateral structures such as the kidney, adrenals and spleen to be accessed.

Location: about 2-5 cm to the left or right of the midline incision. Incision is over the medial aspect of the transverse convexity of the rectus.

Layers of the abdominal wall: skin, fascia (camper's and scarpa's) and the anterior rectus sheath are incised. The anterior rectus muscle is freed from the anterior sheath and retracted laterally. The posterior rectus sheath (if above the arcuate line) or transversalis fascia (if below the arcuate line), extraperitoneal fat and peritoneum are then excised allowing entry to the abdominal cavity.

Advantages

- Provides access to lateral structures
- Rectus muscle is not divided
- ***Incisions in anterior and posterior sheath*** is seperated by muscle which acts as a buttress, therefore closure is more secure
- Can be extended by a curvilinear incision towards the xiphoid process if required

Disadvantages

- Takes longer to make and close
- Incision needs to be closed in layers
- Difficult extension superiorly as limited by the costal margin
- Tends to strip the muscles of their lateral blood and nerve supply resulting in atrophy of the muscle medial to the incision

Midline Incision

◈ *http: //www.fastbleep.com*

Use: Virtually all abdominal procedures may be performed through this incision.

Location: in the midline of the abdomen, and can extend from the xiphoid process to just above the umbilicus. It can be continued to below the umbilicus by curving the incision around the umbilicus.

Layers of the abdominal wall: skin, fascia (camper's and scarpa's), linea alba, transversalis fascia, extraperitoneal fat and peritoneum.

Advantages

- Adequate exposure of most if not all of the abdominal viscera
- Minimal blood loss as the incision is through the linea alba
- Minimal nerve injury
- Minimal muscle injury
- Can be quickly made, such as in an emergency and quickly closed with a mass closure technique

Disadvantages

- Care needs to be taken just above the umbilicus where the falciform ligament is
- Midline scar

Transverse Incision

◈ *http: //www.fastbleep.com*

Use: right or left colon, duodenum, pancreas, subhepatic space.

Location: This incision is made just above the umbilicus, dividing one or both of the rectus muscles.

Layers of the abdomen: skin, fascia, anterior rectus sheath, rectus muscle (+/- internal oblique, depending on the length of the incision), transversus abdominus, transversalis fascia, extraperitoneal fat and peritoneum. The medial aspect of this incision will be through the layers just like as in the midline incision.

Advantages

- Less pain than a midline incision
- Good access to midline upper GI structures
- Transverse incisions cause the least amount of damage
- As the recti have a segmental nerve supply, it can be cut transversely without weakening a denervated segment
- Muscular segments can be rejoined
- Commonly used in children and the ***obese*** as greater abdominal exposure is gained in comparison with the vertical midline. This is due to the longer transverse length of the abdomen in children and the obese.

Disadvantages

- Limited lateral access in comparison with midline incisions that can then be extended
- More wound infections compared to midline thought to be due to greater difficulty in controlling bleeding and haematoma formation.

Abdominal Incisions

◈ *L & B 26th/34*

- In the ***past, traditionally vertical midline or paramedian incisions*** were used for the majority of abdominal procedures, but there is a ***current trend to utilise transverse incisions*** wherever possible as this minimises postoperative complications.

"The rectus sheath is composed of the aponeuroses of transversus abdominis, external oblique and internal oblique muscles, which form an anterior and posterior sheath that fuse laterally at the linea semilunaris and in the midline at linea alba. Only the middle segment of the rectus abdominis is completely enclosed, with the posterior sheath lacking in parts of the superior and inferior segments" *(Manipal Surgery 4th/866)*

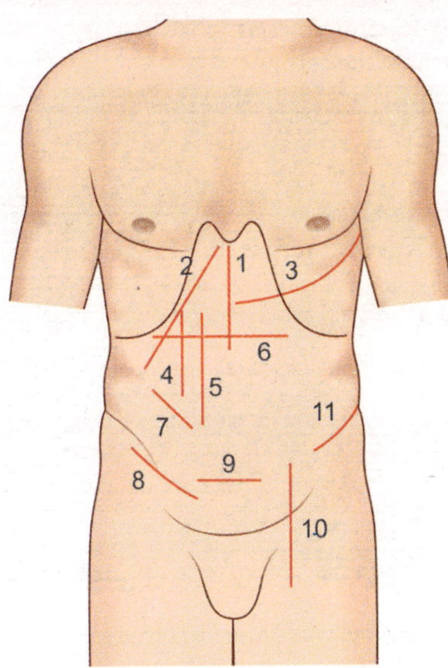

Fig: *(L & B 26th/34):* Abdominal incisions. 1. Midline; 2. Kocher's; 3. thoracoabdominal; 4. rectus split; 5. paramedian; 6. transverse; 7. McBurney's gridiron; 8. inguinal; 9. pfannenstiel; 10. McEvedy; 11. Rutherford Morison.

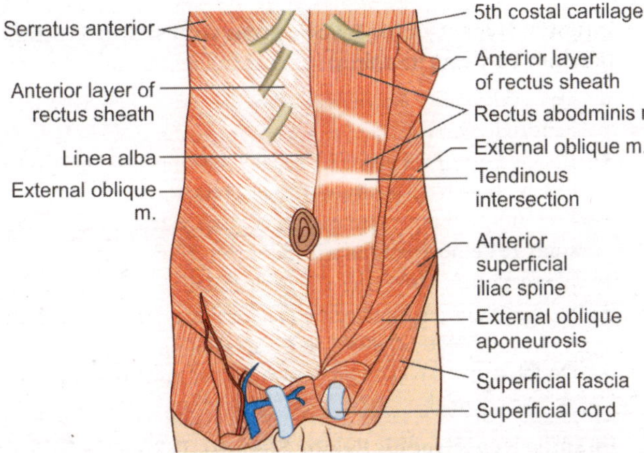

Fig: *(Schwartz):* Anterior abdominal wall. Linea albais the midline aponeurotic demarcation between the bellies of the rectus abdominis muscles. The rectus abdominis muscleand its tendinous intersections on the left are shown deep to the reflected anterior rectus sheath.

171. Ans. b. Common in children

[Ref: Manipal Surgery 4th/788-90; L & B 26th/1220-21; Schwartz 9th/1054]

Complete/Total Rectal Prolapse

◈ *Manipal Surgery 4th/788-90*

- ***F:M ratio is 6: 1***
- ***Common in elderly women who are multipara***
- ***Constipation is important feature***
- ***Tenesmus common***
- ***Some degree of incontinence of faeces& flatus is always present***

Full-thickness Prolapse

◈ *L & B 26th/1220-21*

- Full-thickness prolapse (synonym: procidentia) is less common than the mucosal variety. The protrusion consists of all layers of the rectal wall and is usually ***associated with a weak pelvic floor***.
- The prolapse is thought to commence as an intussusception of the rectum, which descends to protrude outside the anus.
- The process starts with the anterior wall of the rectum, where the supporting tissues are weakest, especially in ***women***. It is more than 4 cm and commonly as much as 10–15 cm in length.
- ***On palpation between the finger and thumb, the prolapse feels much thicker than a mucosal prolapse***, and obviously consists of a double thickness of the entire wall of the rectum.
- ***Complete prolapse is uncommon in children.***
- In adults, it can occur at any age, but it is ***more common in the elderly. Women are affected six times more often than men, and it is commonly associated with prolapse of the uterus.***
- In ***approximately 50 per cent of adults, faecal incontinence is also a feature.***

Rectal Prolapse

◈ *Schwartz 9th/1054*

- In adults, this condition is ***far more common among women***, with a ***female:male ratio of 6:1***. Prolapse becomes more prevalent with age in women and ***peaks in the seventh decade of life***. In men, prevalence is unrelated to age.
- ***Symptoms include tenesmus***, a sensation of tissue protruding from the anus that may or may not spontaneously reduce, and a ***sensation of incomplete evacuation***.

172. Ans. b. Type IV collagen... d. Steroid is very... e. Goes beyond...

[Ref: Manipal Surgery 4th/8-9; L & B 26th/ 30; Schwartz 9th/ 225-27]

"***Injection of steroid preparation such as triamcinolone acetate has been found very useful***. It flatten the keloids. Intrakeloidal excision & skin grafting is to be tried last. ***Recurrence is common. Care should be taken not to extend the excision on to the normal surrounding tissues***" *(Manipal Surgery 4th/9)*

Scars

◈ *L & B 26th/30*

- The maturation phase of wound healing has been discussed above and represents the formation of what is described as a scar. The immature scar becomes mature over a period lasting a year or more, but it is at first pink, hard, raised and often itchy. ***The disorganised collagen fibres become aligned along stress lines*** with their strength being in their weave rather than in their amount. As the collagen matures and becomes denser, the scar becomes almost acellular as the fibroblasts and blood vessels reduce.
- Scars are often described as being atrophic, hypertrophic and keloid.

- A **hypertrophic scar** is defined as excessive scar tissue that d*oes not extend beyond the boundary of the original incision or wound.* It results from a prolonged inflammatory phase of wound healing and from unfavourable scar siting (i.e. across the lines of skin tension). In the face, these are known as the lines of facial expression.
- A **keloid scar** is defined as excessive scar tissue that ***extends beyond the boundaries of the original incision*** or wound. Its aetiology is unknown, but it is associated with elevated levels of growth factor, deeply pigmented skin, an inherited tendency and certain areas of the body (e.g. a triangle whose points are the xiphisternum and each shoulder tip).
- The **histology of both hypertrophic and keloid scars** shows ***excess collagen with hypervascularity,*** but this is more marked in ***keloids where there is more type III collagen***.
- ***Hypertrophic scars improve spontaneously*** with time, ***whereas keloid scars do not.***

Table *(Manipal Surgery 4th/8)*: **Aetiology of Keloid**

- **Key factors:** Surgery, burns, vaccinations
- Elevated levels of growth factor (more of type 'B' collagen)
- Laceration or abrasion
- Over the sternum (incision)
- Inheritance and injection
- Deep pigmented skin

Treatment of Hypertrophic and Keloid Scars

◈ *L & B 26th/30*

- Pressure – local moulds or elasticated garments
- Silicone gel sheeting (mechanism unknown)
- ***Intralesional steroid injection*** (triamcinolone)
- Excision and steroid injections
- Excision and postoperative radiation (external beam or brachytherapy)
- Intralesional excision (keloids only)
- Laser – to reduce redness (which may resolve in any event)
- Vitamin E or palm oil massage (unproven)

Hypertrophic Scars and Keloids

◈ *schwartz*

- Both keloids and hypertrophic scars are characterized by ***excessive collagen deposition*** versus collagen degradation.
- *Keloids* are defined as scars that ***grow beyond the borders of the original wounds,*** and these ***scars rarely regress with time.*** Keloids are more prevalent in patients with more darkly pigmented skin
- Keloids appear to have a genetic predisposition.
- ***Keloids and hypertrophic scars have stretched collagen bundles aligned in the same plane as the epidermis, as opposed to normal scar tissue, where the collagen bundles are randomly arrayed and relaxed.***
- In addition, ***keloid scars have thicker, more abundant collagen bundles*** that form acellular node like structures in the deep dermal portion of the keloid lesion. The center of keloid lesions also contains a paucity of cells in comparison to hypertrophic scars, which have islands composed of aggregates of fibroblasts, small vessels, and collagen fibers throughout the dermis

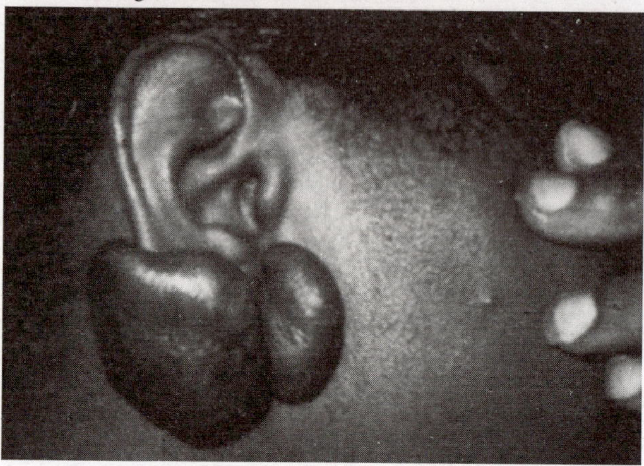

Fig: Keloids caused by ear piercing

173. Ans. b. Elongation of pyloric..., c. Narrowing of pyloric... d. Thickened pyloric... e. Child should be given...

[Ref: Dahnert Radiology Review Manual 7th/858-59; Sabiston 19th/1841; L & B 26th/113-14; Robbins 9th/751]

Infantile Hypertrophic Pyloric Stenosis (IHPS)-UGI Study (Barium Contrast Imaging)

◈ *Dahnert Radiology Review Manual 7th/859*

- Sensitivity 95%
- Imaging confirmation is sought by most clinician to differentiate from gastroesophageal reflex
- Precaution: Empty stomach via nasogastric tube before study & Remove contrast at end
- Elongation & narrowing of pyloric canal
- String sign=passing of small barium streak through elongated pyloric channel (most specific sign)
- Double/triple track sign: crowding of mucosal folds in pyloric channel

Infantile Hypertrophic Pyloric Stenosis (IHPS)

◈ *Ultrasound Dahnert Radiology Review Manual 7th/859*

- Method of choice due to direct visualization of HPS
- Target sign= hypoechoic ring of ***hypertrophized pyloric muscle*** around echogenic mucosa centrally on cross-section
- Elongated pylorus with thickened muscle
- Pyloric muscle wall thickness≥3.0-3.2 mm
- Elongated pyloric canal ≥ 16-17 mm in length

Adult form of Hypertrophic Pyloric Stenosis

◈ *Dahnert Radiology Review Manual 7th/859*

- Persistent elongation (2-4cm) + concentric narrowing of pyloric channel
- Parallel + preserved mucosal fold

Infantile Hypertrophic Pyloric Stenosis

◈ *L & B 26th/113-14*

- The diagnosis can be confirmed by an **ultrasound**, which shows the ***thickened pyloric muscle.***

- IHPS is readily treated by surgery but the infant must be adequately rehydrated and the ***hypochloraemic-hypokalaemic alkalosis corrected;*** this may take 48 hours.
- In most babies, the dehydration and alkalosis can be corrected by ***giving 150–180 mL/kg per day of 0.45 per cent saline with 0.15 percent KCl in 5 per cent glucose.***
- Oral feeding is discontinued and the stomach emptied with an 8–10 Fr nasogastric tube; ongoing gastric losses should be replaced with ***normal saline containing potassium chloride.***
- Ramstedt's pyloromyotomy is performed through an incision around the umbilicus.

Hypertrophic Pyloric Stenosis

◈ *Sabiston 19th/ 1841*

- This condition is most common between the ages of 2 and 8 weeks.
- In HPS, ***hypertrophy of the circular muscle of the pylorus*** results in c***onstriction and obstruction of the gastric outlet.***
- Palpation of the pyloric tumor (also called the *olive*) in the epigastrium or right upper quadrant by a skilled examiner is pathognomonic for the diagnosis of HPS. If the olive is palpated, no additional diagnostic testing is necessary.
- When the olive cannot be palpated, the diagnosis of HPS can be made with an ultrasound exam or fluoroscopic UGI series. These imaging tests are similar in terms of sensitivity and specificity for the diagnosis of HPS. The
- UGI is useful for the evaluation of other causes of vomiting, whereas the absence of radiation exposure and cost make the ultrasound the usual preferred study. A ***persistent pyloric muscle thickness*** of more than 3 to 4 mm or ***pyloric length of more than 15 to 18 mm*** in the presence of functional gastric outlet obstruction is generally considered diagnostic.
- Treatment of HPS is by a pyloromyotomy.

174. Ans. a. Transmu..., b. More com..., d. TNF-alpha inhibitor...

[Ref: Harrison 19th/1955; CMDT 2016/642-50; Davidson 22nd/905; Manipal Surgery 4th/ 683-86; L & B 26th/1145-52; Schwartz 9th/995]

"***pANCA positivity is found in about 60-70% of UC patients & 5-10% of CD***" *(Harrison 19th/1955)*

"Two most commonly tested antibodies are- pANCA & anti-Saccharomyces cerevisiae antibody (ASCA). ***ASCA+/pANCA, is associated with diagnosis of Crohn's disease, while ASCA-/pANCA+ is correlated with UC***" *(Schwartz 9th/995)*

"**Anti-TNF therapies**: The first biologic therapy approved for Crohn's disease was infliximab, a chimeric IgG1 antibody against TNF-alpha, which is now also approved for treatment of moderately to severely active ulcerative colitis" *(Harrison 19th/1961)*

Crohn's Disease

◈ *Manipal Surgery 4th/ 683-86*

"Smoking increases the risk of Crohn's disease three-fold unlike its protective effect against ulcerative colitis"

Crohn's Disease (Regional Enteritis)

◈ *L & B 26th/1145-52*

- ***Smoking increases the relative risk of CD*** three fold and is certainly an exacerbating factor after diagnosis, contrary to the protective effect seen in UC.
- ***CD is characterised by a chronic full thickness*** inflammatory process that can affect any part of the gastrointestinal tract from the lips to the anal margin.
- The ***terminal ileum is most commonly involved (60 per cent),*** either in isolation or in combination with colonic disease.

Table *(Davidson 22nd/905)*: **Biological Therapy in the Management of Inflammatory Bowel Disease**

- Infliximab or adalimumab is recommended for patients with severely active Crohn's disease not responding to conventional immunosuppressive therapy, including corticosteroids, or where such therapies are contraindicated.
- Infliximab is also licensed for use in children and for fistulating Crohn's disease, and is an effective rescue therapy for patients with acute severe ulcerative colitis not responding to intravenous corticosteroids.
- Infliximab and adalimumab are also both effective for moderately active ulcerative colitis.

Table *(L&B)*: **Distinguishing Ulcerative Colitis and Crohn's Disease**

	Ulcerative colitis	Crohn's disease
Macroscopic		
Distribution	Colon/rectum	Anywhere in the gastrointestinal tract
Rectum	Always involved	Often spared
Perianal disease	Rare	Common
Fistula formation	Rare	Common
Stricture	Rare	Common
Microscopic		
Layers involved	Mucosa/submucosa	Full thickness
Granulomas	No	Common
Fissuring	No	Common
Crypt abscesses	Common	Rare

175. Ans. a. Postoperative ileus..., b. Mostly resolve..., d. If opioid is used..., e. Is an anticipated....

[Ref: CSDT 11th/677; Manipal Surgery 4th/765; Sabiston 19th/307-08; L & B 26th/1197, 276; Schwartz 9th/ 992-93]

"***Following most abdominal operations or injuries***, the motility of the gastrointestinal tract is transiently impaired. The return of normal motility generally follows a characteristic temporal sequence, with ***small-intestinal motility returning to normal within the first 24 hours*** after laparotomy and ***gastric and colonic motility returning to normal by 48 hours and 3 to 5 days, respectively***. Resolution of ileus may be delayed in the presence of other factors capable of inciting ileus such as the presence of intra-abdominal abscesses or electrolyte abnormalities. Patient medication lists should be reviewed for the presence of drugs, ***especially opiates***, known to be associated with impaired intestinal motility. ***Routine postoperative ileus***

should be expected and requires no diagnostic evaluation. If ileus persists beyond 3 to 5 days postoperatively or occurs in the absence of abdominal surgery, diagnostic evaluation to detect specific underlying factors capable of inciting ileus and to rule out the presence of mechanical obstruction is warranted" *(Schwartz 9th/ 992-93)*

"In the immediate postoperative period, restricted oral intake and ***postoperative narcotic analgesia*** also contribute to altered small bowel motility. ***Opiates and opioid peptides in the enteric nervous system suppress neuronal excitability. Postoperative ileus affects the stomach and colon primarily***. After laparotomy, small bowel motility returns within several hours, gastric motility within 24 to 48 hours, and colonic motility in 48 to 72 hours. Secretions and swallowed air are not emptied from the stomach, and gastric dilation and vomiting may occur. Return of bowel activity is heralded by the presence of bowel sounds, flatus, and bowel movements" *(Sabiston 19th/308)*

Paralytic ileus

◈ *L & B 26th/276*

- Paralytic ileus may present with nausea, vomiting, loss of appetite, ***bowel distension*** and absence of flatus or bowel movements.
- Following laparotomy, gastrointestinal motility temporarily decreases. Treatment is usually supportive with maintenance of adequate hydration and electrolyte levels. However, intestinal complications may present as prolonged ileus and so should be actively sought and treated.
- **Return of function of the intestine occurs in the following order**: small bowel, large bowel and then stomach. This pattern allows the passage of faeces despite continuing lack of stomach emptying and, therefore, vomiting may continue even when the lower bowel has already started functioning normally.

Paralytic Ileus

◈ *L & B 26th/1197*

- This may be defined as a state in which there is failure of transmission of peristaltic waves secondary to neuromuscular failure (i.e. in the myenteric (Auerbach's) and submucous (Meissner's) plexuses). The resultant stasis leads to accumulation of fluid and gas within the bowel, with associated distension, vomiting, absence of bowel sounds and absolute constipation.
- The following varieties are recognised: **Postoperative, Infection, Reflex ileus &Metabolic**
- **Postoperative**. A degree of ileus usually occurs after any abdominal procedure and is ***self-limiting***, with a variable ***duration of 24–72 hours.*** Postoperative ileus may be prolonged in the presence of hypoproteinaemia or metabolic abnormality
- Paralytic ileus takes on a clinical significance if, ***72 hours*** after laparotomy: there has been no return of bowel sounds on auscultation & there has been no passage of flatus.
- Colicky pain is not a feature.

176. Ans. b. Breast..., d. Pancrse..., e. Minor salivary...

[Ref: Manipal Surgery 4th/519; Devita 8th/723, 727; L & B 26th/733]

"**Major Salivary Glands (including parotid)**: Acinic cell tumors typically are indolent low-grade neoplasms appearing in all age groups and are most common in women. Metastases occur in a small percentage of cases and cannot be predicted by the histologic picture" *(Devita 8th/727)*

Minor Salivary Glands: Approximately one half of minor salivary gland tumors are malignant. The histologic varieties of malignant tumors include adenoid cystic carcinoma, mucoepidermoid carcinoma, adenocarcinoma, malignant mixed, acinic cell, and oncocytic carcinomas" *(Devita 8th/723)*

"Lung tumour classificaion: Carcinomas of Salivary Gland Type-These carcinomas include mucoepidermoid carcinomas (low and high grade), recognized by their characteristic intermediate or transitional cells, adenoid-cystic carcinoma, which shares the aggressiveness of its salivary gland counterpart, and the low-grade, acinic cell carcinoma. All are predominantly found in ***large bronchi*** and thought to arise from submucosal gland epithelium" *(Devita 8th/761)*

"Acinar cell caricinoma are malignant epithelial neoplasm (***of pancrease)*** that show evidence of exocrine enzyme production" *(Devita 8th/949)*

177. Ans. b. Cysteine..., d. Oxalate..., e. Impure uric...

[Ref: Danhert Radiology Review Manual 7th/1005; Harshmohan 7th/672; L & B 26th/ 1292-96]

Renal Calculus

◈ *L & B 26th/ 1292*

- Oxalate stones are irregular with sharp projections. A calcium oxalate monohydrate stone is hard and ***radiodense.***
- A **phosphate calculus** (calcium phosphate often with ammonium magnesium phosphate (struvite)) is smooth and dirty white. It grows in alkaline urine, especially when urea-splitting *Proteus* organisms are present. The calculus may enlarge to fill most of the collecting system, forming a stag-horn calculus. Even a large stag-horn calculus may be asymptomatic for years until it presents with haematuria, urinary infection or renal failure.
- *Uric acid and urate calculi* are hard, smooth and often multiple and multifaceted. Pure uric acid stones are radiolucent. CT will distinguish them from other causes of filling defects including tumours of the ureter. Most uric acid stones contain some calcium, so they cast against radiological shadow.
- *Cystine calculus* An uncommon congenital error of metabolism leads to cystinuria. Cystine stones are often multiple and may grow to form a cast of the collecting system. Cystine stones are radio-opaque and very hard.

Table *(Danhert Radiology Review Manual 7th/1005)*: **Frequency and Radiographic opacity of Urolithiasis**

Mineral Composition	Frequency (%)	Opacity
A. Calcium stones	70–80	+++
1. Calcium oxalate	20–30	+++
a. Calcium oxalate monohydrate (= whewellite) ▪ Small highly opaque		
b. Calcium oxalate dihydrate (= wedellite) ▪ may be speculated/mamillate ("mulberry stone")		
2. Calcium oxalate-phosphate (calcium oxalate plus apatite)	30–40	+++
3. Calcium phosphate (= apatite) ▪ Rarely pure (= laminated), occasionally forms in infected alkaline urine	5–10	+++
4. Calcium hydrogen phosphate (= brushite)		+++
B. Struvite stone	15-20	++
1. Magnesium ammonium phosphate (= struvite)		
laminated, result of urea-splitting organism (usually proteus) ▪ most common constituent of staghorn calculus	1	++
2. Struvite plus calcium phosphate ▪ associated with infection	15-20	++
C. Cystine mildly opaque	1–3	+
D. Uric acid radiolucent	5–10	–
E. Xanthine nonopaque	Extremely rare	–
F. Matrix (mucoprotein/ mucopolysaccharide) nonopaque	rare	–

178. Ans. b. Often contain..., c. Groups of..., d. May present...

[Ref: Manual of Clinical Surgery by S.Das 11th/ 51; Sabiston 19th/ 1825; L & B 26th/927; Schwartz 9th/1667-69; Neena Khanna 5th/182-83]

Simple or Capillary Lymphangioma (Also k/a Lymphangioma Circumscriptum)

◈ *Manual of Clinical Surgery by S.Das 11th/ 51*

- *This type presents as circumscribed lesion which appears as small vesicle or small blister or slightly elevated skin patch*
- *The size varies from 0.5 to 4 mm in diameter*
- *A large area of skin may be involved on the* ***inner side of the thigh, buttock, on the shoulder or in the axilla***
- *The* ***whole lesion is soft & spongy***
- ***Fluctuation, fluid thrill & translucency test are always positive****. The* ***swelling is not compressible***
- *The* ***margins of the swelling are indistinct***
- *The skin vesicles* ***contain clear fluid*** *which looks watery & yellow but blood in the vesicles turn them brown or dark red*
- *The regional L.N are usually not enlarged unless the cysts become infected*

"**Lymphangioma circumscriptum:** This is a microcytic lymphatic malformation unlike Cystic Lymphangioma and is manifested by a ***cluster of tiny firm abscesses filled with lymph fluid***, identical to frogspawn. The color of these blisters may range from clear to pink, dark red, brown or black and may turn warty while affecting the palm or sole. It is most commonly found to arise on the shoulders, neck, armpits, limbs and the mouth. It is usually prominent at puberty and may often start bleeding" *(http: //www.hxbenefit.com)*

Lymphangioma Circumscriptum

◈ *http: //www.aocd.org/?page=Lymphangioma Circums*

- It is a congenital malformation of the superficial lymphatics. The lymphatic vessels become blocked causing a ***backup of lymph into small pockets***.
- They are often noted to have a ***frogspawn appearance***. These ***groups of vesicles are found*** most commonly on the abdomen, axillae (armpit), and mouth.

These malformations cause cyst-like lesions due to lymph backup into small pockets, giving them a yellow appearance. If blood is present in the lesion it will appear red or pink. The papules can look like **warts**, especially when located on the palms and soles.

The diagnosis is made by inspection. This condition can be associated with deeper lymphatic malformations in the subcutaneous tissues and muscles. The deeper malformations should be evaluated with an MRI or other radiologic imaging.

It is a benign condition so treatment is not required. However, it is often bothersome so the vesicles are surgically removed.

Drainage of the cysts is a possible treatment but does not have lasting effects. Several procedures can be used to remove the lesions such as dermabrasion and **laser therapy**. If there is no deeper malformation, then these treatments provide an excellent prognosis.

Lymphangioma Circumscriptum

◈ *emedicine.medscape.com/*

The typical ***history*** involves a ***small number of vesicles*** on the skin ***at birth or shortly after***. In subsequent years, they tend to increase in number, and the area of skin involved continues to expand.

Usually, lesions are asymptomatic, but, occasionally, patients may have spontaneous episodes of ***minor bleeding and copious drainage of clear fluid from ruptured vesicles.***

It the common form of cutaneous lymphangioma, is characterized by persistent, ***multiple clusters of translucent vesicles that usually contain clear lymph fluid*** (often compared with frog spawn).

These vesicles represent ***superficial saccular dilations*** from underlying lymphatic vessels that occupy the papilla and push upward against the overlying epidermis.

Each skin lesion may range from a minute vesicle to a small bulla-sized lesion.

These vesicles can be clear or vary from pink to dark red because of serosanguineous fluid and hemorrhage. These vesicles often are associated with verrucous changes, which give them a warty appearance.

It has a high recurrence rate after excision because of its deep component

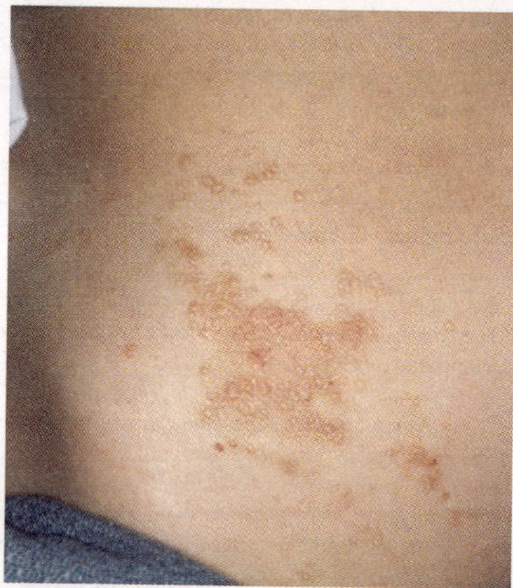

Fig: Lymphangioma circumscriptum

"Lymphangiomas are dilated dermal lymphatics that 'blister' onto the skin surface. The fluid is usually clear but may be blood-stained. In the long term, lymphangiomas thrombose and fibrose, forming hard nodules that may raise concerns about malignancy. If ***lymphangiomas are <5 cm across***, they are termed ***lymphangioma circumscriptum***, and if they are more widespread, they are termed lymphangioma diffusum" *(L & B 26th/927)*

179. Ans. a. Diagnosis of this condition..., c. AFP is elevated..., d. Most are beni..., e. More common....

[Ref: Manipal Surgery 4th/ 806; Nelson 20th/2478-79; CSDT 11th/1347; Sabiston 19th/1865-66; Schwartz 9th/1450-51]

"Maternal serum AFP is elevated in sacrococcygeal teratoma" *(William's Obs 23rd/291)*

"**Teratoma:** The serum alpha-fetoprotein (AFP) level is elevated in tumors containing malignant endodermal sinus (yolk sac) elements. Serial AFP levels are markers for recurrence. Beta-human chorionic gonadotropin (β-hCG) is produced from those containing malignant choriocarcinoma tissue. Rarely, enough β-hCG is produced to cause precocious puberty. Elevated AFP and β-hCG levels in histologically benign tumors indicate an increased risk of recurrence and malignant transformation, particularly with "immature" benign teratomas" *(CSDT 11th/1347)*

Sacrococcygeal Teratoma

◈ *CSDT 11th/1347*

- The majority of sacrococcygeal teratomas present in the newborn period and can be detected by prenatal ultrasound. Females predominate; a history of twins is common.
- Pregnancy may be complicated by fetal high-output cardiac failure via arteriovenous shunting within the tumor, maternal polyhydramnios, and hydrops fetalis leading to fetal demise. Fetal surgery has been utilized successfully in those with hydrops.
- Treatment is excision of the tumor and coccyx
- The majority (97%) of newborn sacrococcygeal teratomas are benign and do not require adjuvant therapy.
- ***Follow-up requires serial AFP levels and physical examinations***, including digital rectal examination. Recurrent tumors are excised. The greatest risk factor for malignancy is age at diagnosis. The malignancy rate is approximately 50–60% after 2 months of age. Malignant tumors are often treated with surgery and chemotherapy.

Sacrococcygeal Teratoma

◈ *Schwartz 9th/1450*

- Sacrococcygeal teratoma usually presents as a ***large mass extending from the sacrum*** in the newborn period.
- ***Diagnosis may be established by prenatal ultrasound***. In fetuses with evidence of hydrops and a large sacrococcygeal teratoma, prognosis is poor; thus prenatal intervention has been advocated in such patients.
- The mass may be as small as a few centimeters in diameter or as massive as the size of the infant.
- The tumor has been classified based on the location and degree of intrapelvic extension. Lesions with growth predominantly into the presacral space often present later in childhood. The differential diagnosis consists of neural tumors, lipoma, and myelomeningoceles
- ***Most tumors are identified at birth and are benign***. Malignant yolk sac tumor histology occurs in a minority of these tumors.
- Complete resection of the tumor as early as possible is essential. The rectum and genital structures are often distorted by the tumor, but usually can be preserved in the course of resection.
- Perioperative complications of hypothermia and hemorrhage can occur with massive tumors and may prove lethal. This is of particular concern in small preterm infants with large tumors.
- The cure rate is excellent if the tumor is excised completely. The majority of patients who develop recurrent disease are salvageable with subsequent platinum-based chemotherapy

Sacrococcygeal Teratoma

◈ *Sabiston 19th/1865-66*

- SCT accounts for 60% of all teratomas & can present as large exophytic masses in utero. In such cases, ***they are detected on prenatal USG***
- Teratomas occur most frequently in the neonatal period, and the ***sacrococcygeal region is the most common*** site.
- It is ***four times more common in females*** and is most often an obvious external presacral mass
- Although most of the tumor is usually external, with a minimal intrapelvic presacral component, there is a spectrum of tumor distribution, to the extent of being entirely presacral, with no visible external component. As such, a *digital rectal examination of a neonate with care to feel the normal presacral space may be an important screening technique.*

- *Most neonatal SCTs are benign.*
- *Treatment of SCT is complete surgical excision*

180. Ans. a. Catheter may..., b. If the CVP is low... c. Can be used for...

[Ref: Morgan 5th/100-103;Harrison 19th/1443,1748,1757; CMDT 2016/492; Davidson 22nd/18283,185]

Central Venous Pressure

◈ *Morgan 5th/100-103*

- *Used for monitoring of CVP, administration of fluid to treat hypovolemia & shock, infusion of caustic drug & total parenteral nutrition, aspiration of emboli, insertion of transcutaneous pacing leads & **gaining venous access in patient with poor peripheral veins***
- **Relative contraindication** *includes tumour, clots or tricuspid valve vegetations that could be dislodged or embolized during cannulation*
- ***Subclavian vein cannulation is relatively contraindicated*** *in receiving anticoagulants(due to inability to provide direct compression in the event of an accidental arterial puncture)*

Table *(Morgan 5th/100)*: **Relative rating of central venous access**

	Basilic	External Jugular	Internal jugular	Subclavian	Femoral
Ease of cannulation	1	3	2	5	3
Long term use	4	3	2	1	5
Success rate (Pulmonary artery catheter placement)	4	5	1	2	3
Complication (Technique related)	1	2	4	5	3

Central Venous Pressure

◈ *Davidson 22nd/185*

- CVP or right atrial pressure (RAP) is monitored using a catheter inserted via either the ***internal jugular or the subclavian vein***, with the distal end sited in the upper right atrium.
- The CVP may help in assessing the need for ***intravascular fluid replacement*** and the rate at which this should be given
- ***If the CVP is low in the presence of a low MAP or cardiac output, fluid resuscitation is necessary***.
- However, a raised level does not necessarily mean that the patient is adequately volume-resuscitated. Right heart function, pulmonary artery pressure, intrathoracic pressure and venous 'tone' also influence CVP, and may lead to a raised CVP even when the patient is hypovolaemic. In addition, positive pressure ventilation raises intrathoracic pressure and causes marked swings in atrial pressures and systemic BP in time with respiration.
- Pressure measurements should be recorded at end-expiration. In severe hypovolaemia, the RAP may be sustained by peripheral venoconstriction, and transfusion may initially produce little or no change in the CVP

Central Venous Pressure

◈ *CMDT 2016/492*

- Early consideration is given to placement of a central venous catheter (CVC) for infusion of fluids and medications and for hemodynamic pressure measurements. A CVC can provide measurements of the central venous pressure (CVP) and the central venous oxygen saturation ($ScvO_2$), both of which can be used to manage sepsis.
- ***A CVP < 5 mm Hg suggests hypovolemia, and a CVP over 18 mm Hg suggests volume overload, cardiac failure, tamponade, or pulmonary hypertension.*** A cardiac index< ***2 L/min/m2 indicates a need for inotropic support.***

181. Ans. All (a, b, c, d.)

[Ref: CSDT 11th/230-40; Park 23rd/796; L & B 26th/296-297, 301-07]

"**Because of CT**, an increasing amount of both blunt &penetrating trauma has been safely managed non-operatively" *(Washington Manual of Surgery 5th/371)*

'The availability of high resolution multislice scanners, promoting the development of protocols in some centers that call for ***early intergration of complete body*** (i.e. head, cervical spine, chest, abdomen & pelvis) CT scanning of selected trauma patient"-Washington Manual of Surgery 5th/371

"Immediate measures at scene of an accident-If there is any question of injury to spine? If so, protect the neck & spine before moving the patient" *(CSDT 11th/230)*

"Intravenous line are critical for intravenous volume resuscitation. The infusion should be started after the patient is en route whenever possible" *(CSDT 11th/230)*

"This advanced triage system involves a color-coding scheme using red, yellow, green, white, and black tags: Red indicates high priority treatment or transfer, yellow signals medium priority, green indicates ambulatory patients & black for dead or moribund" *(Park 23rd/796)*

Initial Management

◈ *L & B 26th/296-297*

- Anticipating and dealing with **potential rate-limiting steps** in the patient's journey will allow delays to be avoided and further reduce the response time. The component of the response that will be the rate-limiting step will depend on local, as well as general circumstances. Examples of *causes of delay are obtaining a CT scan, getting the patient into an operating theatre or obtaining a necessary specialist opinion.* Such steps that can potentially bring the progress of the patient to a halt need to be addressed early and sometimes in a way that may seem out of the normal sequence. This is one of the major roles of the team leader who should have an overview and be able to foresee and pre-empt problems. Whenever a system is protocol driven, someone should be in a position to take the responsibility to break protocol if required to keep the overall process flowing.
- Having a practised common pathway can be disadvantageous; a patient with the wrong 'label' may go along the

wrong pathway. We all have to be wary of labelling. Should two patients with identical histories and injuries arrive in an emergency department with one on a spine board and the other in a chair, the former will be treated as if more severely injured when in fact that may not be the case. We must make our own judgements on reasonable evidence and not just rely on the labels (in this case, the cervical collars) applied by others.

- ***Labelling*** is most frequently a dangerous problem in the elderly. A patient with an obviously short externally rotated leg may be quickly given the label 'NOF' (fracture neck of femur).
- There are a number of problems with this practice. The focus is now on the orthopaedic label rather than the whole patient.
- The incorrect label may mask the fact that the patient could be dying. The patient may have fallen as a consequence of a cardiac arrhythmia or other comorbidity; the early labelling may therefore send the patient off on entirely the wrong pathway. ***All vulnerable patients should have a physiological triage to avoid such problems.*** This means assessing the airway, respiratory rate, blood pressure, pulse rate and consciousness. All of these assessments are more important, even in the elderly, than the presence of a fractured hip.

Local Protocols and Guidelines

◈ *L & B 26th/297*

- A general guideline, such as ATLS, deals with some aspects of patient management and is used in many institutions. However, hospitals generally have individual policies to guide or direct decision making in smaller areas of practice. Examples are prophylaxis against infection and thromboembolism, the use of steroids in spinal injury and clearance of the cervical spine.
- These represent the efforts of individuals within an institution to plan for common and foreseeable circumstances. These protocols allow for easier and quicker decision making. Their application should protect the patient and, in an increasingly litigious world, the doctor as well.
- ***'Clearing' of the spine is a practice that has particular relevance to trauma.*** The early policy for managing the spine in polytrauma patients is straightforward; it can be summarised as ***'suspect and protect'.*** This approach is widely employed, and so very many patients have their spine protected. However, this is a precautionary approach and at some stage one has to have a strategy for discontinuing protection, or 'clearing' the spine in those patients in whom protection is not required. In the event that it is not possible to exclude spinal injury on clinical grounds, ***the managing clinicians may request clearance on radiological grounds.***

182. Ans. a. Subcuticular suture..., b. Vertical mattress..., c. Horizontal mattress...

[Ref: Sabiston 19th/233; L & B 26th/ 39]

"The **horizontal mattress stitch** is a suture technique used to close wounds. It everts skin well and spreads tension along the wound edge. ***This makes it ideal for holding together fragile skin*** as well as skin under high tension such as the distant edges of a large laceration or as the initial holding suture in complicated repairs" *(www.aafp.org)*

"The advantages of the **vertical mattress suture** are that it provides closure for both deep and superficial layers, and also allows perfect eversion and vertical opposition of the superficial skin edges. Its disadvantage is a relatively high propensity to dig into skin and ***cause prominent stitch mark scars.*** The vertical mattress stitch is most commonly used in anatomic locations which tend to invert, such as the posterior aspect of the neck, and sites of greater skin laxity such as closure of lax skin after removing a dermoid cyst. It is useful for deep lacerations, where it can replace two layers of deep and superficial sutures. It can help bring the deep layers together alone, allowing several simple interrupted or running stitches to close the remaining superficial skin. ***Vertical mattress sutures are not recommended for sites such as the palm of the hand,*** where important structures lie fairly superficial to the epidermis. *(www.aafp.org)*

Mattress Sutures

◈ *L & B 26th/39*

- Mattress sutures may be either vertical or horizontal and tend to be used to produce either eversion or inversion of a wound edge. The initial suture is inserted as for an interrupted suture, but then the needle either moves horizontally or vertically and traverses both edges of the wound once again.
- Such sutures are very useful in producing ***accurate approximation of wound edges***, especially when the edges to be anastomosed are irregular in depth or disposition.

Subcuticular Suture

◈ *L & B 26th/39*

- This technique is used in skin where a ***cosmetic appearance is important*** and where the skin edges may be approximated easily. The suture material used may be either absorbable or non-absorbable.
- For non-absorbable sutures, the ends may be secured by means of a collar and bead, or tied loosely over the wound. When absorbable sutures are used, the ends may be secured using a buried knot. Small bites of the sub cuticular tissues are taken on alternate sites of the wound and then gently pulled together thus approximating the wound edges without the risk of the cross-hatched markings of interrupted sutures.

OBSTETRICS & GYNECOLOGY

183. Ans. b. Incidence increased..., c. Absence of decidua..., d. Fibrinoid...

[Ref: Dutta Obs 8th/ 486; William's Obs 23rd/776-80; Obs by JB Sharma 1st/344-45; Normal & Problem Pregnancy by Gabbe 6th/ 423]

"Incidence: ***It is rising from 1:2500 deliveries in 1980s to 1 in 210 deliveries*** *in 2006 mainly due to rising caesarean section" (Obs by JB Sharma 1st/344)*

"The placenta is firmly adherent to the uterine wall due to partial or ***total absence of decidua basalis & fibrinoid layer (Nitabuch layer)"*** *(Obs by JB Sharma 1st/344)*

Placenta Accreta (Morbid Adherent Placenta)

- The American college of Obstetricians & Gynecologists (**2002**) estimated that placenta accrete complicates **1 in 2500 deliveries** *(William's Obs 23rd/777)*
- Overall incidence is ***1 in 550 delveries*** *(Dutta Obs 8th/ 486)*
- It is an extremely rare form in which the placenta is directly anchored to the myometrium partially or completely without any intervening decidua. The probable cause is ***due to absence of decidua basalis & poor development of fibrinoid layer***
- ***Pathological confirmation includes: absence of decidua basalis, absence of Nitabuch's fibrinoid layer, varying degree of penetration of the villi into muscle bundle (increta) or uptoserosal layer (percreta)***
- ***Risk includes-Haemorrhage, shock, infection & rarely inversion of uterus***
- Most important risk factor are ***placenta previa & prior caesarean delivery***
- ***Increasing maternal age & parity (grand multipara) is risk factor***

184. Ans. a. Confined to the..., d. It is kept under....

[Ref: Shaw's Gynae 16th/485-94; Dutta Gynae 6th/320-30]

Cervical Intraepithelial Neoplasia (CIN) or Pre-Invasive Cervical Cancer (Stage 0)

Shaw's Gynae 16th/485-94; Dutta Gynae 6th/320-30)

- CIN refers to the histopathological description in which a part or the full thickness of the stratified squamous epithelium is replaced by cells showing varying degree of dysplasia, however the basement membrane is intact
- These lesions progress with time & ultimately ends up as frank invasive cancers. While 4% reach the invasive stage by the end of 1 year & 11% by end of 3 years, as much as 22% become invasive by 5 years & 30% by 10 years
- CIN-I (**Low grade squamous intraepithelial lesions): It is often seen with inflammatory conditions like trichomoniasis & HP & is reversible following treatment**
- **Severe dysplasia** (**CIN III**) progress to invasive cancer in about ***10-30% in 5-10 years time***
- **Women with CIN I**, confirmed on biopsy is ***kept under observation with pap smear follow up at 6 months or HPV DNA tests at 12 month.*** If both tests are negative routine recall (screening) is done.If these tests are persistent then treat it as HSIL *(Dutta Gynae 6th/327 & Shaw's Gynae 16th/494)*
- "**CIN II:** The fact that over a prolonged follow-up, about 10-15% of CIN I & CIN II progress to CIS. The again, it is quite impossible to predict which one will remain stationary & which one will progress to severe dysplasia or CIS. ***As such, CIN II is commonly treated with LLETZ***" *(Dutta Gynae. 6th/327)*

Mild dysplasia (CIN-I, Low grade squamous intraepithelial lesions)	Moderate dyspalsia (CIN-II)	Severe dysplasia & Ca in situ (CIN-III)	High-grade squamous intraepithelial lesions (HSIL)
The undifferentiated cells are confined to the lower 1/3 of the epithelium	The undifferentiated cells occupy the lower 50-75% of the epithelium thickness (lower 2/3)	In this grade of dysplasia, the entire thickness of the epithelium is replaced by abnormal cells	CIN II + CIN III

Table *(Shaw's Gynae 16th/486)*: **Course of CIN Diseases**

	Regression	Persistence	Progresses	Age
CIN I	80-90%	10-20%	1-4%	<30 yr
CIN II	30-40%	40%	20%	30-35 yrs
CIN II	20-30%	50-60%	Almost all	35-45 yrs

Treatment Options for CIN-II & CIN-III (HSIL)

Shaw's 16th/491

- Local destructive methods- ***cryosurgery***, fulgration/electro coagulation & laser abalation
- Excision of abnormal tissue: Cold-knife conization, laser conization, LLETZ, LEEP & NETZ
- Surgery: Therapeutic conization, hysterectomy, hysterectomy with removal of vaginal cuff if carcinoma in situ extends to the vaginal vault
- Follow up with coloposcopy & /or cytology

185. Ans. a. Laparoscopy..., b. COC is used..., d. Can be managed....

[Ref: Shaw's Gynae 16th/ 409-19; Dutta Gynae 6th/304-09; Novak'sgynae 15th/532-40; Robert Shaw's Gynae 4th/ 500-506]

Pain Management of Endometriosis: *The American College of Obstetricians and Gynecologists Guidelines*

www.acog.org

- Endometriosis is a leading cause of ***chronic pelvic pain*** and a common cause of infertility, the two main symptoms. Some women with endometriosis have no symptoms, but for those that do, ***pain can range from mild to severe.***
- "We recommend starting with conservative approaches to treating women with endometriosis-associated pain". For instance, **continuous oral contraceptives and nonsteroidal anti-inflammatory drugs** are effective. ***If these fail and further medical management is needed***, then **gonadotropin-releasing hormone agonists or progestins** can help by suppressing the disease." Medical therapy, however, will not improve fertility for women trying to get pregnant since most of these drugs suppress ovulation.
- Medical therapy is effective while using it, but recurrence of pain symptoms is common after discontinuing the drugs.
- Laparoscopy also can remove visible endometriosis lesions, but it is not 100% effective in helping pain. As with medical therapy, there is a high recurrence of symptoms in patients after laparoscopic surgery. ***Both laparoscopic surgery and long-term hormone suppression—typically with an oral contraceptive—will likely be needed to control pain.***

"Endometriosis: Treatment for 3 month with ***GnRH agonist*** is effective in improving pain for 6 moth" *(Novak's 15th/539)*

"If the patient desires treatment of pain symptoms that are suggestive of endometriosis in the absence of a definitive diagnosis, empirical treatment is appropriate and includes counseling, analgesia, nutritional therapy, progestins, or combined oral contraceptives. It is unclear whether oral contraceptives should be taken in a conventional, continuous, or tricycle regimen. A GnRH agonist may be taken, but is not recommended, because this class of drug is more expensive and associated with more side effects and concerns about bone density" *(Novak's 15th/532)*

"Using **hormonal contraceptives**-especially continuous cycle regimens, may reduce or eliminate the pain of mild to moderate endometriosis" *(www.mayoclinic.org)*

"GnRH agonists: The goal of add-back is to effectively treat endometriosis and endometriosis-associated pain, while preventing vasomotor symptoms and bone loss" *(guidelines.endometriosis.org)*

Endometriosis

◈ *Shaw's Gynae 16th/ 409-19*

- ***"Laparoscopy is the gold standard in the diagnosis of endometriosis"Laproscopy is the gold standard in diagnosis of endometriosis.*** *It is both diagnostic & therapeutic" (Shaws Gynaecology 16th/ 415)*
- ***Combined oral contraceptives: administered intermittently or continuously, may alleviate the disease***
- GnRH is administered continuously to down regulate & suppress pituitary gonadotropins; it cause atrophy of the endometriotic tissue in 90% cases
- ***Minimal asymptomatic case should be observed over 6-8 months.*** Infertility should be investigated & treated as necessary. All symptomatic women need treatment *(Shaws Gynaecology 16th/ 416)*
- **Treatment options**: ***Expectant management (observation only);*** *Medical therapy (Hormones & other), Surgery (Conservative & Definitive) & Combined (Medical & Surgical) (Dutta Gynae 6th/310)*

Endometriosis

◈ *Jeffcoate 7th/ 369-370*

- Occurrence of functioning endometrial tissue (both glands + stroma) outside the cavity of uterus.
- ***Age group:30 -40 years (Most common)***
- Seen in high socioeconomic status because of late marriage & late child bearing.
- Most common in nulliparous females
- Familial predisposition (risk is seven times higher if a ***first degree relative has diseases***. Risk is further increased in homozygous twins).
- It is a hormone dependant condition (Estrogen dependant)
- **Site:** Itcan occur anywhere in the body. Most common site is ovary (30-40%, 2nd most common site is pouch of Douglas
- Patients present with a characteristic triad of: ***infertility, Progressively increasing dysmenorrhea & Dyspareunia***

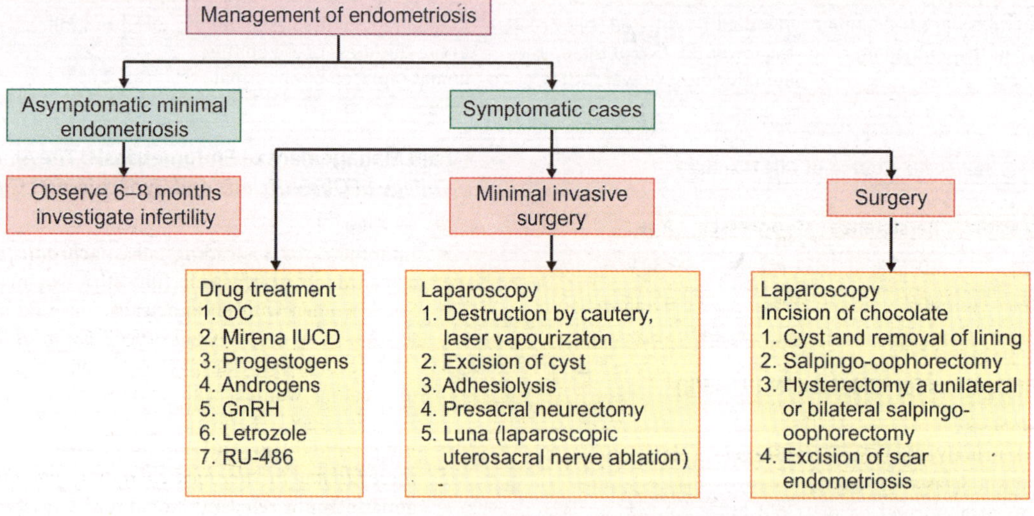

Fig: *(Shaw's Gynae 16th/409)*: Management of Endometriosis

186. Ans. a. Severe... d. Antidepressant... e. Pain ceases....

[Ref: Shaw's Gynae 16th/ 473-74; Synopsis of Psychiatry by Kaplon 11th/841-42; DuttaGynae 6th/182-83; Novak's gynae 15th/311-13; Robert Shaw's Gynae 4th/391-94]

A & E

Premenstrual syndrome (PMS) & Premenstrual dysphoric disorder (PMDD)

◈ *Shaw's Gynae 16th/ 473-74; Dutta Gynae 6th/182-83*

- PMS is a pyscho-neuroendocrine disorder of unknown etioloy, often noticed just prior to menstruation (last 7-10 days of the menstrual cycle)
- It should fulfil the following criteria
  - No related to any organic lesion
  - Regularly occurring during the luteal phase of each cycle
  - Symptom must be severe enough to disturb the life style of women or she requires medical help
  - Symptom free period during rest of the cycle

- ***When these symptoms disrupt daily functioning they are grouped under the name premenstrual dysphoric disorder (PMDD)***
- More common in women aged 30-35 yr. It may related to childbirth or a disturbing life event
- There are no pelvic findings except features of pelvic congestion
- "5% suffer from severe symptoms which influence daily activities"
- ***SSRI & Noradrenaline Reuptake inhibitos (SNRI)*** are found to be very effective *(Dutta Gynae 6th/183)*

Table *(Kaplon 11th/841)*: **DSM-5 Criteria for Premenstrual Dysphoric Disorder**

A. In the majority of menstrual cycles, at least five symptoms must be present in the final week before the onset of menses, start to improve within a few days after the onset of menses, and become minimal or absent in the week postmenses.

B. One (or more) of the following symptoms must be present:
1. Market affective lability (e.g., mood swings; feeling suddenly sad or tearful, or increased sensitivity to rejection).
2. Marked irritability or anger or increased interpersonal conflicts.
3. Marked depressed mood, feelings of hopelessness, or self-deprecating thoughts.
4. Marked anxiety, tension, and/or feelings of being keyed up or on edge.

C. One (or more) of the following symptoms must additionally be present, to reach a total of five symptoms when combined with symptoms from Criterion B above.
1. Decreased interest in usual activities (e.g., work, school, fiends, hobbies)
2. Subjective difficulty in concentration.
3. Lethargy, easy fatigability, or marked lack or energy
4. Marked change in appetite; overeating; or specific food cravings
5. Hypersomnia or insomnia.
6. A sense of being overwhelmed or out of control
7. Physical symptoms such as breast tenderness or swelling, joint or muscle pain, a sensation of "bloating" or weight gain.

Note: The symptoms in Criteria A-C must have been met for most menstrual cycles that occurred in the preceding year.

D. The symptoms are associated with clinically significant distress or interference with work, school, usual social activities, or relationship with others (e.g., avoidance of social activities; decreased productivity and efficiency at work, school, or home).

E. The disturbance is not merely an exacerbation of the symptoms or another disorder, such as major depressive disorder, panic disorder, persistent depressive disorder (dysthymia), or a personality disorder (although it may co-occur with any of these disorders).

F. Criterion A should be confirmed by prospective daily ratings during at least two symptomatic cycles. (Note: The diagnosis may be made provisionally prior to this confirmation.)

G. The symptoms are not attributable to the physiological effects of a substance (e.g., a drug of abuse, a medication, other treatment) or another medical condition (e.g., hyperthyroidism).

Table *(Dutta Gynae 6th/182)*: **Symtomatology of PMS & PMDD**

Related to water retention	• Abdominal bloating • Breast tenderness • Swelling of the extremities • Weight gain	
Neuropsychiatric symptoms	• Irritability • Depression • Mood swings • Forgetfulness • Restlessness • Increased appetite	• Tearfulness • Anxiety • Tension • Confusion • Headache • Anger
Behavioral symptoms	• Fatigue • Dyspareunia	• Tiredness • Insomnia

Table *(Shaw's Gynae 16th/ 474)*: **Management of PMS**

Psychosomatic	Vitamins B1, B6, E selective serotonin reuptake Inhibitor, sertraline, citalopram anxiolytics
Breast pain	Danazol, bromocryptine GnRh
Pelvic pain and bloatedness	Yasmin, primrose Prostaglandin inhibitors OC, progestogen Mirena IUCD

187. Ans. a. If post prandial..., c. If fasting sugar..., e. If fasting sugar....

[Ref: Dutta Obs 8th/ 326-27; William's Obs 23rd/1104-08; Obs by JB Sharma 1st/508; Normal & Problem Pregnancy by Gabbe 6th/ 906]

Overt Diabetes

◈ *Dutta Obs 8th/ 326-28*

"According to American diabetic Association **diagnosis is positive** if a) ***the fasting plasma glucose exceeds 126*** mg/dl; b) the ***2 hr post glucose (75 gm) value exceeds 200 mg/dl***; c) HbA1C≥6.5%"

Criteria for diagnosis of impaired glucose tolerance & diabetes with 75 gm oral glucose (American diabetic association) *(Dutta Obs 8th/328)*

Time	Normal tolerance	Impaired glucose tolerance	Diabetes
Fasting	<100	≥100 & <126	≥ 126
2 hour post glucose	<140	≥ 140 & <200	≥ 200

Table *(Obs by JB Sharma 1st/508)*: **Criteria for Diagnosis of Impaired Glucose Tolerance & Diabetes with 75 gm Oral Glucose (WHO)**

Time	Normal tolerance	Impaired glucose tolerance	Diabetes
Fasting	<110	110-126	≥ 126
2 hour post glucose	<140	140-199	≥ 200

188. Ans. a. In Rokitansky..., d. In Kallman syndrome...,

[Ref: Shaw's Gynae 16th/322-23; Dutta Gynae 6th/ 450-54]

Primary Amenorrhoea

◈ *Shaw's Gynae 16th/322*

- The spectrum of diagnosis presenting clinically as primary amenorrhoea can be conventionally **classified** according to the status of her serum FSH levels into ***hypergonadotropic (FSH>40 mIU/mL), eugonadotropic or hypogonadotropic***
- "**Kallmann's syndrome**-*inadequate GnRH pulse secretion-* ***reduced FSH & LH***" *(Dutta Gynae 6th/ 450-54)*

Hypergonadotropic Primary Amenorrhoea *(Shaw's)*	**Eugonadotropic primary amenorrhoea** *(Shaw's)*
• Gonadal dysgenesis: 45 OX (***Turner's syndrome*** mosaics, abnormal X.) • 46 XX pure gonadal dysgenesis • 46 XY gonadal dysgenesis–Swyer syndrome, testicular feminizing syndrome • Gonadotropin-resistant ovary syndrome-***Savage syndrome***	A. **Absence of Mullerian development** ▪ Androgen insensitivity syndrome (testicular feminization) ▪ Mullerian agenesis–absence of uterus/vagina. Rokitansky-Kuster-Hauser syndrome B. **Norma Mullerian development** ▪ Female or true intersex ▪ Polycystic ovary syndrome ▪ Adrenal or thyroid diseases C. Cryptomenorrhoea-imperforate hymen, vaginal septum, cervical atresia. D. Tubercularendometritis E. Constitutional delay-Nutrition

Hypogonadotropic Primary Amenorrhoea *(Shaw's)*
A. **Hypothalamic causes:** ▪ Delayed menarche and puberty ▪ Hypothalamic hypogonadism (***Kallmann syndrome***). GnRh deficiency syndrome. ▪ Psychogenic causes, weight loss. Stress anorexia nervosa and malnutrition. B. **Pituitary causes:** ▪ Pituitarism causes short stature, obesity genital dystrophy, mental retardation, polydactyly and retinitis pigmentosa. ▪ Neoplasma-prolactinomas, craniopharyngiomas, adenomas and empty sellaturcica. ▪ Hypopituitary states-Simmond's disease, Chiari-Frommel syndrome, Forbes-Albright syndrome and pineal gland tumour. C. Severe systemic disease like tuberculosis, syphilis D. Other endocrinal disorders-thyroid or adrenal gland.

189. Ans. c. Modified..., d. Special forcep..., e. Prague maneuver.

[Ref: Dutta Obs 8th/444-46;Obs by JB Sharma 1st/310-11]

Pinard'smaneuver *for* ***Frank breech extraction****: It is done to convert a frank breech to a footling breech (Obs by JB Sharma 1st/312)*

Delivery of the Aftercoming head of Breech

◈ *Dutta Obs 8th/444-46; Obs by JB Sharma 1st/310-11*

- This is most important stage of delivery. Not more than 10 minutes (preferably 5 minutes) should elapse b/w the delivery of umbilicus & head to reduce chance of fetal asphyxia
- **Various method of safe delivery of after coming head**
  - *Burns-Marshall method*
  - *Forcep delivery (Piper forcep, Das forcep, Neville Barne's forcep)*
  - *Malar flexion & shoulder traction (modified Mauriceau-Smellie-Veit technique)*

Arrest of After Coming Head (Difficulty with After-Coming Head): *Managed*

◈ *Obs by JB Sharma 1st/312*

- ***Burns-Marshall method***
- ***Modified Mauriceau-Smellie-Veit technique***
- ***Brachtmaneuver***
- ***Wigand-Martin maneuver***
- ***Prague maneuver***
- ***Forcep application***
- ***Duhrssen's incision***
- ***Craniotomy***

Second Stage of Labour: *3 Methods of Vaginal Breech Delivery*

◈ *Obs by JB Sharma 1st/308-09*

- **Spontaneous breech delivery (10%)** -The whole of the fetus is expelled spontaneously without any traction or manipulation other than support of newborn & perineum
- **Assisted breech delivery** (Partial breech extraction, 80-90%)
- **Breech extraction**-Entire body of fetus expelled by obstetrician without any effort on the part of the patient

190. Ans. a. Type of twin..., b. Lambda sign..., c. T sign suggest...

[Ref: Dutta Obs 8th/233-37; William's Obs 23rd/ 859-65; Obs by JB Sharma 1st/446-50]

"Presence of ***lambda or twin peak sign*** indicates ***dichorionic placenta*** *(Dutta Obs 8th/237)*

Twins

- Sonography done to obtain following information: ***Confirmation of diagnosis as early as tenth week of pregnancy***; chorionicity (***lambda or twin peak sign***); viability of foetuses, vanishing twin in the second trimester; twin transfusion (Doppler studies) etc
- Presence of one gestational sac with a thin dividing membrane & two foetuses (**T sign**) suggests ***monochorionic diamniotic pregnancy***
- ***Dizygotic twins (80%): It is most common & result from fertilisation of 2 ova***
- ***Monozygotic twins (20%) fertilization of single ovum***

Table *(Obs by JB Sharma 1st/447)*: **Differences b/w Monozygotic & Dizygotic Twins**

Features	Monozygotic twin pregnancy	Dizygotic twin pregnancy
Ovum	Single	Two
Sperm	Single	Two
Sex	Same	Opposite or same

Contd...

Features	Monozygotic twin pregnancy	Dizygotic twin pregnancy
Similarity	Identical	Fraternal resemblance only (similarity like b/w two brothers or sisters)
Placenta a) Communicating vessel b) Intervening membrane c) Thickness of intervening membrane d) Twin peak sign	Single (43%) or double a) Present b) Absent in monochorionic & monoamniotic twin c) <2 mm (82-89%) d) Usually absent (44%)	Usually double occasionally fused at margin a) Absent b) Present c) >2 mm (95%) usually d) Usually present (97.3%)
Genetic features	Same	Different
DNA microprobe technique (Most definite)	Same	Different
Skin grafting from one to another	Accepted	Rejected

Table *(Obs by Gabbe 6th/675)*: **Determination of Chorinicity & Amnionicity in First Trimester Pregnancies**

Placentation	No. of gestational sac	No. of yolk sac	No. of amniotic cavity
Dichorionic, Diamniotic	2	2	2 (thick dividing membrane)
Monochorionic, Diamniotic	1	2	2 (thin dividing membrane)
Monoorionic, Monoamniotic	1	2	1

191. Ans. a. Inhibin, b. Beta human..., c. Alphafeto..., e. NB/70K.

[Ref: Shaw'sGynae 16th/521; Dutta Gynae 6th/377]

"**PAX7 (Paired Box 7)** is a protein coding gene. Diseases associated with PAX7 is ***alveolar rhabdomyosarcoma***" *(www.genecards.org)*

Tumour Marker in Epithelial Ovarian Cancer

◈ *Dutta Gynae 6th/377, 371*

- **CA-125:** Used for screening of epithelial cancer of ovary
- Other tumour of value are-macrophage colony stimulating factor (M-CSF), OVXI, HER-2/Neu & inhibin
- hCG is used as marker for diagnosis of ovarian choriocarcinoma
- BRCA1 & BRCA2 (Serous carcinoma)
- MLH1, MSH2 & MSH6 (HNPCC associated ovarian cancer)
- AFP, hCG & CEA-Germ cell tumour- *Shaw's Gynae 16th/521*
- Tumour marker- for embryonal carcinoma (AFP, hCG), endodermal sinus tumour (AFP) & choriocarcinoma (hCG) *(Shaw's Gynae 16th/523)*
- Germ cell tumor-AFP, hCG, NB/70K, placental alkaline phosphatase & lactate dehydrogenase are tissue tumour marker for germ cell tumour *(Shaw's Gynae 16th/527)*
- NB/70K raised in 60% of epithelial tumour

Table *(researchgate.net)*: **Clinically Applicable Tumor Markers of Cancer Ovary**

Tumor Market	Type of Ovarian Malignancy
Cancer Antigen CA 125 (CA 125)	Marker of first choice for epithelial ovarian malignancy
Human chorionic Gonadotrophin (hCG)	Marker of 1st choice for Choriocarcinoma ovary
Alpha fetoprotein (AFP)	Marker of 1st choice for endodermal sinus tumor of ovary
HCG and/or AFP	Mixed germ cell tumor of ovary

Tumor markers used in ovarian cancer include

◈ *www.oncolink.org*

CA-125

- Used to help in diagnosis, assessment of response to treatment, and monitoring for recurrence.

Alpha-fetoprotein (AFP)

- Used in ovarian germ cell tumors.
- Used to assess stage, prognosis, and response to treatment.

Beta-hCG (Beta Human Chorionic Gonadotropin)

- Used in ovarian germ cell tumors.
- Used to assess stage, prognosis, and response to treatment.

HE4

- HE4 can be used to help diagnose ovarian cancer in a woman with symptoms and may be more sensitive than CA125.
- It can also be used to assess response to treatment and monitor for recurrence.

Inhibin A & B

- A hormone that is normally produced by ovarian tissue, but may be elevated in certain types of ovarian cancer (mucinous epithelial carcinoma, granulosa cell tumors).
- Can be used to assess response to treatment and monitor for recurrence.

CEA (Carcinoembryonic Antigen)

- Can be elevated in ovarian tumors and may be used to evaluate response to treatment.

192. Ans. a. Initial serum..., b. Prior chemotherapy..., c. Following term..., e. Long duration...

[Ref: Obs by JB Sharma 1st/143-50; Dutta Obs 8th/ 222-26;Shaw's Gynae 16th/517; Dutta Gynae 6th/361]

Table: *(Obs by JB Sharma 1st/143-50)*

Choriocarcinoma: (a) Non metastatic disease & (b) Metastatic disease:

Contd...

A. Low risk (good prognosis)
- Disease is present < 4 months duration
- Initial serum hCG level < 40, 000 mIU/mL
- **Metastasis limited to lung and vagina**
- **No prior chemotherapy**
- **No preceding term delivery**

B. High risk (poor prognosis)
- Long duration of disease (> 4 months)
- Initial serum hCG> 40, 000 mIU/mL
- **Brain or liver metastasis**
- Failure of prior chemotherapy
- **Following term pregnancy**
- WHO score > 7

Risk factors for malignant change *(Dutta Obs 8th/ 222)*
- **Patient's age** ≥ 40 or < 20 years irrespective of parity
- **Parity** ≥3. Age is more important than the parity
- **Serum hCG**> 100, 000 mIU/mL
- **Uterine size** > 20 weeks
- **Previous history** of molar pregnancy
- **Theca lutein cysts:** large (>6 cm diameter)

Classification of GTD
- Hydatidiform mole: Complete & Partial
- Invasive mole
- Placental site trophoblastic tumor
- Choriocarcinoma

193. Ans. b. Contain hair..., c. Mostly benign..., d. May be bilateral..., e. Torsion is common...

[Ref: Shaw's Gynae 16th/439-40; Dutta Gynae 6th/ 293-96]

"**Teratoma** are divided into three categories- ***mature (benign) e.g. dermoid cyst***; immature (essentially malignant), e.g. solid teratoma & monodermal or highly specialized e.g. struma ovarii" *(Shaw's)*

Dermoid Cyst

◈ *Shaw's Gynae 16th/439-40; Dutta Gynae 6th/ 293-96*

- Of all cystic tumours of the ovary, 5-10% are dermoids
- It constitute 97% of all ovarian teratoma
- It contains sebaceous material & ***hair, & the wall is lined in part by squamous epithelium which contains hair follicle & sebaceous glands***
- ***Teeth, bone, cartilage, thyroid tissue & bronchial*** mucus membrane are often found in the wall
- Dermoid cysts are innocent ovarian tumours but epidermoid carcinoma occur in 1.7% & sarcomatous change have been described
- Dermoids are bilateral in 12-15%
- Torsion is most common (15-20%) & rupture is an uncommon (1%) complication

194. Ans. b. Prior cardiac..., c. Aortic valve..., d. Class III & IV..., e. Peak LV out...

[Ref: Dutta Obs 8th/ 323; Obs by JB Sharma 1st/498-500; Normal & Problem Pregnancy by Gabbe 6th/828-32]

Ejection Fraction

◈ *www.heart.org*

- A ***normal heart's ejection fraction may be between 50 and 70.***
- A measurement under 40 may be evidence of heart failure or cardiomyopathy.
- An EF from 41 to 49 may be considered "borderline" but does not always indicate that a person is developing heart failure. It may indicate damage, perhaps from a previous heart attack.
- In severe cases, EF can be very low.

Predictor of Adverse Maternal Outcome

◈ *Dutta Obs 8th/ 323*

- Prior ***cardiac failure, arrhythmia or transient ischemic attack***
- Baseline NYHA class > 2 or associated cyanosis
- Left heart obstruction: ***Mitral valve area<2 cm^2, aortic valve area <1.5 cm^2***, or peak ventricular outflow gradient >30 mm Hg by echocardiography
- ***Left ventricular ejection fraction<40%***

Table *(Obs by JB Sharma 1st/498)*: **Risk Wise Categorization of Cardiac Disease During Pregnancy**

Cardiac Disorder	Mortality
Group 1 – Minimal Risk Atrial septal defect Ventricular septal defect Patent ductus arteriosus Pulmonic or tricuspid disease Fallot tetralogy, corrected Bioprosthetic valve Mitral stenosis, NYHA class I and II	**0–1%**
Group 2 – Moderate Risk	**5–15%**
2A: Mitral stenosis, NYHA class III and IV Aortic stenosis Aortic coarctation without valvular involvement Fallot tetralogy, uncorrected Previous myocardial infarction Marfan syndrome, normal aorta	
2B: Mitral stenosis with atrial fibrillation Artificial valve	
Group 3 – Major Risk Pulmonary hypertension Aortic coarctation with valvular involvement Marfan syndrome with aortic involvement	**25–50%**

Table *(Obs by JB Sharma 1st/499)*: **Risk factors for maternal cardiovascular events during pregnancy**

1. Past history of cardiac event like Heart failure, TIA, stroke before pregnancy or arrhythmias
2. ***Baseline NYHA class III or IV*** or cyanosis in current pregnancy
3. Left heart obstruction (MVA <2 cm^2, aortic valve area < 1.5 cm^2, ***peak LV out flow tract gradient > 30 mm Hg by echocardiography***)

Contd...

4. Reduced systemic ventricular systolic function, i.e. ***ejection fraction < 40%.***

No risk factors – 5% risk of complications;1 risk factor- 27% risk of complications; > 1 risk factor- 75% risk of complication

TIA: Transient ischemic attack; NYHA: New York Heart Association; MVA: Mitral valve area;

Table *(Dutta Obs. 8th/202)*: **Risks of Maternal Mortality with Heart Disease (NYHA, 1992)**

Cardiac Disease
Group 1 (minimal risk): ASD, VSD, PDA, Fallot tetralogy (corrected), Mitral stenosis (NYHA–Grade I and II), bioprosthetic valve
Group 2 (moderate risk): MS (NYHA—III and IV) AS, Marfan syndrome (Normal aorta), Fallot tetralogy (uncorrected), MS with atrial fibrillation, artificial valve
Group 3 (major risk): ***Pulmonary hypertension, Marfan syndrome (aortic involvement), aortic coarctation with valvular involvement***

"**Eisenmenger's syndrome**: Maternal mortality is about 50% & so also the perinatal loss (50%). ***Termination of pregnancy should be seriously considered"*** *(Dutta's Obstetrics 7th/280)*

"**Therapeutic or medical termination of pregnancy**: Cardiac diseases (***Grade III & IV***) ***with history of decompensation in the previous pregnancy or in b/w the pregnancies***" *(Dutta's Obstetrics 7th/173)*

195. Ans. b. Ureter injury..., e. Enables wide...

[Ref: Shaw's Gynae 16th/356, 359; Dutta Gynae 6th/ 593-400; Novak's gynae 15th/809-20, 1370-71]

"**Management of genital prolapse** (of women beyond 40 yr & multipara) - ***Vaginal hysterectomy*** & pelvic floor repair" *(Shaw's Gynae 16th/356)*

"**Injury to ureter** *is one of the most formidable complication of hysterectomy. Most ureteral injuries can be avoided by* ***opening the retroperitoneum & directly identifying the ureter***" *(Novak's gynae 15th/816)*

Table *(Dutta Gynae 6th/593)*: **Indication of Abdominal Hysterectomy**

Benign	• Dysfunctional uterine bleeding • Fibroid uterus • Tubo-ovarian mass • Endometriosis • Adenomyosis • CIN • Endometrial hyperplasia • Benign ovarian tumor in perimenopausal age
Malignancy	• Carcinoma cervix • Carcinoma ovary • Carcinoma endometrium • Uterine sarcoma • Choriocarcinoma
Traumatic	• Uterine perforation • Cervical tear • Rupture uterus
Obstetrical	• Atonic PPH • Morbid adherent placenta • Hydatidiform mole >35 years • Septic abortion

Contd...

Table *(Dutta Gynae 6th/ 598)*: **Vaginal hysterectomy**

Advantage	Disadvantages
1. Can be effectively done in obese patients	1. More skill and experience are needed on the part of the surgeon
2. Postoperative complications are less	2. Exploration of abdominal and pelvic organs cannot be done
3. Less morbidity and mortality	3. Difficult in cases with restricted uterine mobility, limited vaginal space and associated adnexal pathology
4. Less postoperative pain and less need of analgesia	4. Limitation in cases with: uterus >12 weeks of size, presence of pelvic adhesion or, previous history of laparotomy with adhesions
5. Less hospital stay	
6. Early resumption of day-to day activities	
7. No abdominal incision and scar	

Table *(Dutta Gynae 6th/ 598)*: **Abdominal hysterectomy**

Advantages	Disadvantages
1. Scope of wide exploration of the abdominal and pelvic organs (ovaries, appendix, gallbladder, etc.)	1. Difficult to perform in too obese patients
2. Tubo-ovarian pathology can be tackled effectively and simultaneously	2. Postoperative complications are slightly high. There is increased incidence of peritonitis, fever, pulmonary and vascular complications
3. Concurrent surgical procedures (appendicectomy may be performed when need)	3. More postoperative pain and more need of analgesia
4. Operation can be done by a relatively less experienced surgeon	4. More hospital stay
	5. Delayed resumption in day-to-day activities
	6. Morbidity and mortality are more compared to a vaginal hysterectomy
	7. Presence of abdominal scar

196. Ans. b. Increased risk..., c. Increased bleeding..., e. Irregular menses.

[Ref: Shaw's Gynae 16th/269; Obs by JB Sharma 1st/678-84;Dutta Obs 8th/618-20]

Copper containing IUCD acts locally in uterus, so not affects Cu level in milk

Cu Containing Devices

- *Shaw's Gynae 16th/269*
- Cu wire of surface area 200 to 250 mm is wrapped round the vertical stem of a polypropylene frame
- Cu devices are more expensive than inert devices but are reported to exert a better contraceptive effect, with fewer side effects
- They have an effective life of about 3–5 years
- It is estimated that about 50 mcg of copper is eluted daily in the uterus
- CuT 380A, known as paraguard, has a lifespan of 10 years. NovaT has silver wire added to the copper wire, thereby increasing lifespan to 5 yr

Complication of IUCD

- *Obs by JB Sharma 1st/682-83; Dutta Obs 8th/618-20*
- Dysmenorrhoea: Painful pèriods can occur with IUD
- Menstrual dysfunction: IUD use is associated with increased bleeding problems like prolonged & heavy bleeding
- PID: Risk of developing PID is 2-10 times greater among IUD users
- Should pregnancy occur with a device in situ, there is risk of ectopic pregnancy (0.02%). IUD thus prevent pregnancy but not ectopic pregnancy. Third generation IUDs like CuT 380A & LNG-IUS give some amount of protection against ectopic pregnancy.

Advantage of Newer IUCD

- *Obs by JB Sharma 1st/678-84*
- Ectopic pregnancy is highly unlikely with LNG-IUCD & CuT 380A (<0.02/HWY)
- Incidence of PID is very less with LNG-IUCD due to protective effect of progesterone against infection

197. Ans. a. It is taken daily..., b. Higher failure..., d. Suited for lactating....

[Ref: Shaw's Gynae 16th/275-76; Obs by JB Sharma 1st/694-95;Novak's gynae 15th/226; Robert Shaw's Gynae 4th/ 527]

"**Ectopic pregnancy:** These are ***more likely to occur in women taking progesterone***-only pills, but not in those taking combined pills" *(Park 23rd/502)*

"**Subsequent fertility**: In general, oral contraceptives use seems to be followed by a ***slight delay in conception***" *(Park 23rd/502s)*

Progestogen Only Pill/Minipill

- *Shaw's Gynae 16th/275-76; Obs by JB Sharma 1st/694-95*
- The low dose POP (norethisterone 350 mcg, desogestrel 75 mcg, norgestrel 30/75 mcg or LNG 30/75 mcg) have been introduced to avoid the side effect of estrogen in combined pills.
- The pill should be started within 5-7 days of the menstruation & taken at the same time with a leeway of 3 hr on either side of fixed time each day
- It is well suited for lactating women
- **Desogestrel containing POP:** No ectopic pregnancy
- Easy to take as there is no "On & Off regime"
- It may be prescribed in patients having (medical disorders) hypertension, fibroid, diabetes, epilepsy, smoking & history of thromboembolism
- Side effects- weight gain, irregular menstrual bleeding, depression, breast cancer & thromboembolism *(Shaw's Gynae 16th/276)*
- *Higher failure rate (1/HWY) than COC (0.1/HWY)*
- "It is to be noted that POP is less effective & more expensive than COC & even one tablet cannot be missed. Hence it is only used where COCs are contraindicated as COCs are drug of first choice for contraception" *(Obs by JB Sharma 1st/695)*

Progestogen Only Pill (POP)/Minipil

- *Shaws Gynaecology 16th/275-76*
- *Minipill does not have some of the major side effects of the combined pills & it is well suited for lactating women; Some progestogens, in fact, increases milk secretion*
- *Side-effect:* ***Weight gain****, irregular menstrual bleeding, depression,* ***breast cancer****, thromboembolism*
- *Advantage: They can be recommended to–lactating women, women over 35 years, those with focal migraine, those intolerant to estrogen or oestrogen contraindicated, diabetic, hypertensive & sickle cell anemia*
- ***As regards to return of fertility, it is faster than in COC users because ovulation is not suppressed in all cases (suppressed in 40%)***
- **Contraindication:** *C/I to POP are previous are previous ectopic pregnancy, ovarian cyst, breast & genital cancer, abnormal vaginal bleeding, active liver & arterial disease, porphyria, liver tumor*
- *Because of osteopenia, it is contraindicated in adolescents & young women*

"Progestin-only pill is started 21 day postpartum[Q] & soon after abortion. The tablet is taken daily without a break"- Shaw's Gynecology 14th/210

"Progestin-only pill can be started 2 to 3 days postpartum[Q], whereas depot medroxyprogesterone acetate (Depoprovera) injections or implants can begin at 6 weeks" *(Novak's Gynecology 14th/254)*

COC

- *Shaw's Gynae 16th/275*
- Reduced incidence of ectopic pregnancy is due to suppression of ovulation & reduction in PID
- Ninety percent ovulate within 3 month of stopping the drug. 90% of women will have normal menstrual cycles within 6 months of stopping OC

198. Ans. e. For non-lactating women, ovulation not...

[Ref: Shaw's Gynae 16th/285, 270; Dutta Gynae 6th/480-81, 500-501; Park 23rd/497-98]

*"**Non-lactating (Postpartum):** Contraceptive practice should be started after 3 week. Pill is good; IUD is equally effective alternative" (Dutta Gynae 6th/500)*

"POP is safe in lactating women & can be started 6 weeks onwards. LNG is safer than desogestrel & gestagen from thrombosis point of view" (Shaw's Gynae 16th/285)

"Intramuscular & progestogen implant can be prescribed 6 week after deliver" (Shaw's Gynae 16th/285)

"IUCD insertion within 10 min of expulsion of placenta or within 24 hr of delivery is proved safe & effective" (Shaw's Gynae 16th/285)

*"**COC** are contraindicated in the puerperium, both because of its adverse on milk secretion in a lactating women & **increased risk of thromboembolic episode**. COC can be prescribed to a non-lactating woman 3 weeks after delivery"- Shaw's Gynae 16th/285*

*"**Regular lactation with one feed at night delays ovulation & pregnancy for upto 6 months**, provided she remains amenohoeic. After 6 months, lactation has no bearing on ovulation & pregnancy can occur, despite amenorrhoea. Thereafter, the women needs some form of contraceptive precautions" (Shaw's Gynae 16th/285)*

"In a non-lactating woman, ***COC can be started after 3 weeks of delivery***, but can be given soon after an abortion, MTP or an ectopic pregnancy"

*"**Use of COC generally is not advised during lactation** because they reduce the amount & quality of breast milk. It can be used after 6 weeks, once milk production is established. Progestin-only pills, implants & injectable contraception do not affect milk quality or quantity" (Novak's 14th/254)*

Timing of Insertion of IUCD

◈ *Shaws Gynaecology 16th/270*

- It is advisable to insert IUCD ***during or soon after menstruation & after abortion or MTP***
- Lately, **immediate postpartum** insertion within 10 min of placental expulsion or within 24 hr of delivery is practiced & is found effective. This save the woman second visit to the clinic. There is no clinical evidence of increase in perforation, expulsion etc.

PEDIATRICS

199. Ans. a. TB meningitis, b. Endobronchial TB, d. Acute tuber..., e. Severe miliary...

[Ref: O.P.Ghai 8th/568; Nelson (SAE) 20th/1459]

"**Tubercular meningitis:** *Steroid reduce the intensity of cerebral edema, risk of development of arachnoiditis, fibrosis & spinal shock" (O.P.Ghai 8th/568)*

"Spina ventosa: This is a name given to T.B of phalanges of hand" *(Maheshwari 5th/203)*

Tuberculous infection of metacarpals, metatarsals and phalanges is known as tuberculous dactylitis. There is a spindle shaped expansion of the short tubular bones due to tuberculous granuloma. Hence it is also known as ***spinaventosa***. In general tuberculous dactylitis is **treated with ATT**" *(ncbi.nlm.nih.gov)*

Corticosteroids use in Tuberculosis

◈ *Nelson (SAE) 20th/1459*

- These are useful in the treatment of some children with tuberculosis disease. They are most beneficial when the host inflammatory reaction contributes significantly to tissue damage or impairment of organ function. There is convincing evidence that corticosteroids decrease mortality rates and long-term neurologic sequelae in some patients with **tuberculous meningitis** by reducing vasculitis, inflammation, and, ultimately, intracranial pressure. Lowering the intracranial pressure limits tissue damage and favors circulation of antituberculosis drugs through the brain and meninges.
- Short courses of corticosteroids also may be effective for children with **endobronchial tuberculosis** that causes respiratory distress, localized emphysema, or segmental pulmonary lesions.
- Several randomized clinical trials have shown that corticosteroids can help relieve symptoms and constriction associated with acute tuberculous **pericardial effusion.**
- Corticosteroids may cause dramatic improvement in symptoms in some patients with ***tuberculous pleural effusion*** and shift of the mediastinum. However, the long-term course of disease is probably unaffected.
- Some children with severe **miliary tuberculosis** have dramatic improvement with corticosteroid therapy if the inflammatory reaction is so severe that alveolocapillary block is present. There is no convincing evidence that 1 corticosteroid preparation is better than another. The most commonly prescribed regimen is prednisone, 1–2 mg/kg/day in 1–2 divided doses orally for 4–6 wk, followed by gradual tapering.

200. Ans. a. Allergic rhinitis, b. Echinococcosis, c. Rheumatoid..., e. Wiskott-Aldrich...

[Ref: Nelson (SAE) 20th / 1039;O.P.Ghai 8th/358-59]

"Infectious mononucleosis-cause lymphocytosis" *(O.P.Ghai 8th/358)*

Table *(O.P.Ghai 8th/358)*: **Common causes of eosinophilia**

Acute
Allergic disorders: Asthma, atopic dermatitis, urticaria, drug hypersensitivity, pemphigoid
Parasitic infestations: Toxocara, ascaris, amebiasis, strongyloidiasis, filarial, toxoplasmosis, trichinosia, schistosomiasis, malaria, scabies
Fungal infections: Bronchopulmonary aspergillosis, coccidiomycosis
Malignancy: Hodgkin lymphoma, T cell lymphoma, acute myelogenous leukemia, myeloproliferative syndrome
Hypereosinophilic syndrome

Contd...

Chronic
Allergic disorders: Pemphigus, dermatitis herpetiformis ***Autoimmune disorders:*** Inflammatory bowel disease, rheumatoid arthritis Myeloproliferative syndrome, hypereosinophilic syndrome Loeffler syndrome Loeffler syndrome **Immunodeficiency syndromes:** Hyper IgE, Wiskott Aldrich syndrome; Omenn syndrome; graft versus host reaction ***Miscellaneous:*** Thrombocytopenia with absent radii; renal allograft rejection; Addison disease

Table *(O.P.Ghai 8th/357)*: **Common causes of Neutrophilia**

Acute
Acute bacterial infections
Epinephrine, corticosteroids, granulocyte colony stimulating factor
Hemorrhage; hemolysis
Hypoxia
Trauma, burns, exercise, heat stroke
Renal failure, diabetic ketoacidosis, hepatic failure
Hodgkin lymphoma
Chronic
Chronic myeloid leukemia
Rheumatological and inflammatory diseases
Hemolytic anemias; sickle cell anemia
Post-splenectomy
Chronic blood loss
Thyrotoxicosis
Chronic idiopathic neutrophilia
Genetic Causes or Syndromes
Down syndrome
Asplenia
Leukocyte adhesion defects

201. Ans. a. Edward..., d. Patau syndrome

[Ref: O.P.Ghai 8th/ 599; Nelson (SAE) 20th/ 2437]

Table *(Nelson (O.P.Ghai 8th/ 599)*: **Risk factors for Childhood Leukemia**

Genetic	Environmental
Down syndrome	Ionizing radiation
Fanconi anemia Shwachman-Diamond syndrome	Alkylating agents (cyclophosphamide, ifosfamide, carboplatin, procarbazine)
Blood syndrome Ataxia telangiectasia	Epipodophyllotoxins (etoposide, tenoposide)
Diamond-Blackfananemia	Nitrosourea (nitrogen mustard) Benzene
Kostmann syndrome	
Li-Fraumeni syndrome	
Severe combined immune deficiency	
Paroxysmal nocturnal hemoglobinuria	
Neurofibromatosis type 1	

Contd...

Table *(Nelson (SAE) 20th/ 2437)*: **Factors Predisposing to Childhood Leukemia**

Genetic Conditions

- Down syndrome
- Fanconi syndrome
- Bloom syndrome
- Diamond-Blackfan anemia
- Schwachman syndrome
- Klinefelter syndrome
- Turner syndrome
- Neurofibromatosis type 1
- Ataxia-telangiectasia
- Severe combined immune deficiency
- Paroxysmal nocturnal hemoglobinuria
- Li-Fraumeni syndrome

202. Ans. a. ↑ Alkaline phosphatase, c. ↑ parathyroid...

[Ref: O.P.Ghai 8th/ 113-15; Nelson (SAE) 20th/333-36]

"**Vitamin D deficiency rickets:** ***Laboratory diagnosis of Vit D deficiency rickets are based onlow circulating 25- (OH) D3. An increased 1, 25- (OH) $_2$D3 indicates deficient intake of calcium or phosphorus. Blood level of alkaline phosphate are elevated; calcium & phosphate levels may be normal or low***" *(O.P.Ghai 8th/ 113)*

"The **initial laboratory** tests in a child with rickets should include serum calcium; phosphorus; alkaline phosphatase; parathyroid hormone (PTH); 25-hydroxy vitamin D; 1, 25-dihydroxyvitamin D_3; creatinine; and electrolytes. Urinalysis is useful for detecting the glycosuria and amino aciduria (positive dipstick for protein) seen with Fanconi syndrome. Evaluation of urinary excretion of calcium (24 hr collection for calcium or calcium-creatinine ratio) is helpful if hereditary hypophosphatemic rickets with hypercalciuria or Fanconi syndrome is suspected. Direct measurement of other fat-soluble vitamins (A, E, and K) or indirect assessment of deficiency (prothrombin time for vitamin K deficiency) is appropriate if malabsorption is a consideration" *(Nelson (SAE) 20th/334)*

Table *(Nelson)*: **Laboratory Findings in Disorders Causing Rickets**

Disorder	Ca	Pi	PTH	25-OHD	1, 25- (OH) $_2$D	ALK PHOS	URINE Ca	URINE Pi
Vitamin D deficiency	N, ↓	↓	↑	↓	↓, N, ↑	↑	↓	↑
VDDR, type 1	N, ↓	↓	↑	N	↓	↑	↓	↑
VDDR, type 2	N, ↓	↓	↑	N	↑↑	↑	↓	↑
Chronic renal failure	N, ↓	↑	↑	N	↓	↑	N, ↓	↓
Dietary Pi deficiency	N	↓	N, ↓	N	↑	↑	↑	↓
XLH	N	↓	N	N	RD	↑	↓	↑
ADHR	N	↓	N	N	RD	↑	↓	↑
HHRH	N	↓	N, ↓	N	RD	↑	↑	↑
Tumor-induced rickets	N	↓	N	N	RD	↑	↓	↑
Fanconi syndrome	N	↓	N	N	RD or ↑	↑	↓ or ↑	↑
Dietary Ca deficiency	N, ↓	↓	↑	N	↑	↑	↓	↑

Note: ADHR, autosomal dominant hypophosphatemic rickets; AlkPhos, alkaline phosphatase; Ca, calcium; HHRH, hereditary hypophosphatemic rickets with hypercalicuria; N, normal; Pi, phosphorus; PTH, parathyroid hormone; RD, relatively decreased (because it should be increased given the concurrent hypophosphatemia); VDDR, vitamin D–dependent rickets; XLH, X-linked hypophosphatemic rickets; 1, 25- (OH) $_2$D, 1, 25-dihydroxy vitamin D; 25-OHD, 25-hydroxy vitamin D; ↓, decreased; ↑, increased; ↑↑, extremely increased.

203. Ans. d. Facial abnormalities, e. Intelligence subnormal

[Ref:CMDT 2016/785;Harrison 19th/2725; Nelson (SAE) 20th/895-96]

In fetal alcohol syndrome, birth weight is less (IUGR) (*Nelson (SAE) 20th/895*)

"Heavy drinking during pregnancy results in the rapid placental transfer of both ethanol and acetaldehyde, which may have serious consequences for fetal development. One severe result is the *fetal alcohol syndrome* (FAS), seen in ~5% of children born to heavy-drinking mothers, which can include any of the following: ***facial changes with epicanthal eye folds; poorly formed ear concha; small teeth with faulty enamel; cardiac atrial or ventricular septal defects; an aberrant palmar crease and limitation in joint movement; and microcephaly with mental retardation***. A less severe condition is the *fetal alcohol spectrum disorder* (FASD), which can include ***low birth weight, a lower IQ, hyperactive behavior, and some modest cognitive deficits***. The amount of ethanol required and the time of vulnerability during pregnancy have not been defined, making it advisable for pregnant women to abstain completely" (*Harrison 19th/2725*)

"**Fetal alcohol syndrome**, manifestation includes ***growth restriction;*** facial, skeletal, and cardiac abnormalities; and serious central nervous system dysfunction" (*CMDT 2016/785*)

Fetal Alcohol Syndrome Manifestations

- Short palpebral fissure
- Thin vermillion of upper lip

Contd...

Fetal Alcohol Syndrome Manifestations

- Flattened phitrum
- Microcephaly
- Partial or complete agenesis of the callosum
- Optic nerve hypoplasia
- Hypotonia, poor feeding
- VSD

Fetal Alcohol Syndrome

Nelson (SAE) 20th/895-96

- High levels of alcohol ingestion during pregnancy can be damaging to embryonic and fetal development. A specific pattern of malformation identified as *fetal alcohol syndrome* has been documented, and major and minor components of the syndrome are expressed in 1–2 infants/1, 000 live births.
- Both moderate and high levels of alcohol intake during early pregnancy may result in alterations in growth and morphogenesis of the fetus; the greater the intake, the more severe the signs.
- Characteristics of fetal alcohol syndrome include
  - Prenatal onset and persistence of ***growth deficiency for length, weight, and head circumference***;
  - ***Facial abnormalities, including short palpebral fissures, epicanthal folds, maxillary hypoplasia, micrognathia, smooth philtrum, and a thin, smooth upper lip***;
  - **Cardiac defects**, ***primarily septal defects***;
  - ***Minor joint and limb abnormalities***, including some restriction of movement and altered palmar crease patterns; and
  - ***Delayed development and mental deficiency*** varying from borderline to severe.
- Fetal alcohol syndrome is a common identifiable cause of ***mental retardation***. The severity of dysmorphogenesis may range from severely affected infants with full manifestations of fetal alcohol syndrome to those mildly affected with only a few manifestations.

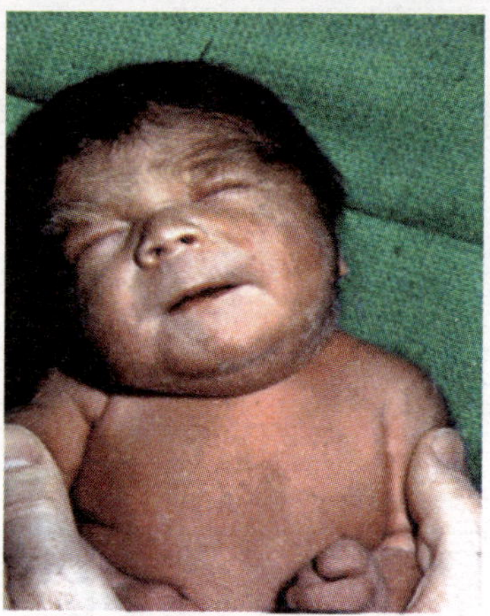

Fig: *(Nelson (SAE) 20th/896):* Fetal alcohol syndrome

204. Ans. a. Cataract, c. Deafness, d. Patent ductus arteriosus.

[Ref: O.P. Ghai 8th/ 272; Nelson (SAE) 20th/1550-51]

"Classical triad of **congenital rubella syndrome consists of deafness, cataract & congenital heart disease"** *(O.P. Ghai 8th/ 272)*

Congenital Rubella Syndrome

Nelson (SAE) 20th/1549-51

- Nerve deafness is the single most common finding among infants with CRS. Most infants have some degree of intrauterine growth restriction. Retinal findings described as **salt-and-pepper retinopathy** are the most common ocular abnormality, but it has little early effect on vision.
- ***Unilateral or bilateral cataracts*** are the most serious eye finding, occurring in about ⅓ of infants.
- **Cardiac abnormalities** occur in half of the children infected during the 1st 8 wk of gestation. ***Patent ductus arteriosus*** is the most frequently reported cardiac defect, followed by lesions of the pulmonary arteries and valvular disease. Interstitial pneumonitis leading to death in some cases has been reported.
- **Neurologic abnormalities** are common and may progress following birth. ***Meningoencephalitis*** is present in 10–20% of infants with CRS and may persist for up to 12 mo. Longitudinal follow-up through 9–12 yr of infants without initial retardation revealed progressive development of additional sensory, motor, and behavioral abnormalities, including hearing loss and autism. PRP has also been recognized rarely following CRS. Subsequent postnatal growth retardation and ultimate short stature has been reported in a minority of cases. Rare reports of immunologic deficiency syndromes have also been described.
- A variety of late-onset manifestations of CRS have been recognized. In addition to PRP, these include diabetes mellitus (20%), thyroid dysfunction (5%), and glaucoma and visual abnormalities associated with the retinopathy, which had previously been considered benign.

Table *(Nelson (SAE) 20th/1549)*: **Pathologic Findings of Congenital Rubella Syndrome**

System	Pathologic Findings
Cardiovascular	Patent ductus arteriosus Pulmonary artery stenosis Ventriculo septal defect Myocarditis
Central nervous system	Chronic meningitis Parenchymal necrosis Vasculitis with calcification
Eye	Microphthalmia Cataract Iridocyclitis Ciliary body necrosis Glaucoma Retinopathy
Ear	Cochlear hemorrhage Endothelial necrosis
Lung	Chronic mononuclear interstitial pneumonitis
Liver	Hepatic giant cell transformation Fibrosis Lobular disarray Bile stasis
Kidneys	Interstitial nephritis
Andrenal glands	Cortical cytomegaly
Bone	Malformed osteoid Poor mineralization of osteoid Thinning cartilage
Spleen, lymph nodes	Extramedullary hematopoiesis
Thymus	Histiocytic reaction Absence of germinal centers
Skin	Erythropoiesis in dermis

205. Ans. a. Hypercalcemia

[Ref: O.P.Ghai 8th/ 181; Nelson (SAE) 20th/897-99;Dutta Obs 8th/330]

Neonatal Complication

Dutta Obs 8th/330

- ***Hypoglycemia***
- ***Respiratory distress syndrome***
- **Hyperbilirubinemia**
- **Hypocalcemia**
- **Hypomagnesemia**
- **Polycythemia**
- **Cardiomyopathy**

Table *(Dutta Obs 8th/330)*: **Major Birth Defect in Infant of Diabetic Mother (6-10%)**

CNS and Skeletal	Cardiovascular	Renal	Gastrointestinal	Others
Neural tube defects	VSD, ASD	Renal agenesis	Duodenal atresia	Single umbilical artery
Anencephaly	Coarctation of aorta	Hydronephrosis	Anorectal atresia	
Microcephaly	Transposition of great vessels	Double ureter	Omphalocele	
Caudal regression syndrome	Situs inversus	Polycystic kidneys	Tracheoesophageal fistula	
Sacral agenesis	Fallot's tetralogy			

Clinical Manifestations

◈ *Nelson (SAE) 20th/897-99*

- ***Hypoglycemia*** *develops in about 25–50% of infants of diabetic mothers and 15–25% of infants of mothers with gestational diabetes*, but only a small percentage of these infants become symptomatic.
- The incidence of **congenital anomalies** is increased threefold in infants of diabetic mothers; cardiac malformations *(ventricular or atrial septal defect, transposition of the great vessels, truncus arteriosus, double-outlet right ventricle, tricuspid atresia, coarctation of the aorta) and lumbosacral agenesis are most common.*
- Additional anomalies include neural tube defects, hydronephrosis, renal agenesis and dysplasia, duodenal or anorectal atresia, situs inversus, double ureter, and holoprosencephaly. These infants may also develop abdominal distention caused by a transient delay in development of the left side of the colon, the small left colon syndrome.

Effect of Maternal Diabetes on Fetus

◈ *O.P.Ghai 8th/ 181*

- ***Macrosomia or large of the body*** & its attending risks during pregnancy such as birth trauma, asphyxia & increased possibilities of caesarean section
- Neonatal respiratory distress
- Metabolic problems such as ***hypogycemia & hypocalcemia***
- ***Polycythemia***, increased viscosity of blood & hyperbilirubinemia
- Higher risk of congenital anomalies (Infants of mothers with diabetes are 20 times more at risk to develop cardiovascular defects)
- Fetus may die suddenly during the last trimester of pregnancy

206. Ans. a. Edematous..., c. Swelling resolve..., e. Maximum size.

[Ref: O.P.Ghai 8th/138, 141; Nelson (SAE) 20th/ 834]

Caput succedaneum is a diffuse, sometimes ecchymotic, ***edematous swelling of the soft tissues of the scalp*** involving the area presenting during vertex delivery. ***It may extend across the midline and across suture lines.*** The ***edema disappears within the 1st few days of life.*** Molding of the head and overriding of the parietal bones are frequently associated with caput succedaneum and become more evident after the caput has receded; they disappear during the 1st weeks of life. Rarely, a hemorrhagic caput may result in shock and require blood transfusion. Analogous swelling, discoloration, and distortion of the face are seen in face presentations. No specific treatment is needed, but if extensive ecchymoses are present, hyperbilirubinemia may develop"-*Nelson (SAE) 20th/ 834*

Table *(O.P.Ghai 8th/14)*: **Difference b/w Caput Succedaneum & Cephalohematoma**

Characteristic	Caput succedaneum	Cephalohematoma
Incidence	Common	Less common
Location	Subcutaneous plane	Over parietal bones, b/w skull & periosteum
Time of presentation	**Maximum size & firmness at birth**	Increasing size for 12-24 hr & then stable
Time course	**Softens progressively from birth & resolves within 2-3 days**	Takes 3-6 weeks to resolve
Characteristic findings	**Diffuse; cross suture line**	**Does not cross suture line; has distinct margins**
Association	None	Linear skull fracture (5-25%); hyperbilirubinemia

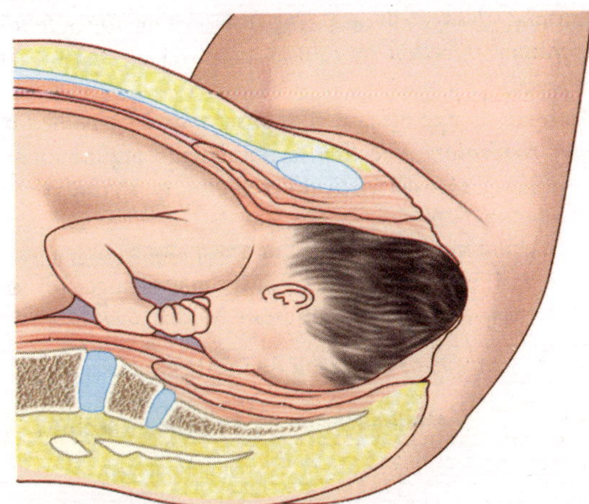

Fig: *(William's Obs)*: Formation of caput succedaneum and head molding

207. Ans. b. Parvo virus B-19

[Ref: O.P.Ghai 8th/ 216; Nelson (SAE) 20th/1570]

"**Erythema infectiosum**: *The characteristic rash first appears as erythematous flushing on the face in a* ***slapped cheek appearance (red cheek)***" *(O.P.Ghai 8th/ 216)*

Erythema Infectiosum (Fifth Disease)

◈ *Nelson (SAE) 20th/1570*

- The ***most common manifestation of parvovirus B19 is erythema infectiosum***, also known as fifth disease, which is a benign, self-limited exanthematous illness of childhood.
- It was the 5th in a classification scheme of common childhood exanthems. The **preceding 4 exanthems** were measles, scarlet fever, rubella, and Filatov-Dukes disease (an atypical scarlet fever), with roseola infantum as the "sixth disease."
- The incubation period for erythema infectiosum is 4–28 days (average 16–17 days).
- The prodromal phase is mild and consists of low-grade fever, headache, and symptoms of mild upper respiratory tract infection.
- The hallmark of erythema infectiosum is the **characteristic rash,** which occurs in 3 stages that are not always distinguishable. The initial stage is an erythematous facial flushing, often described as a **"slapped-cheek" appearance**. The rash spreads rapidly or concurrently to the trunk and proximal extremities as a diffuse macular erythema in the 2nd stage.
- Central clearing of macular lesions occurs promptly, giving the rash a **lacy, reticulated appearance**

Table: Red rashes in children

Condition	Prodrome	Rash	Comments, Other Diagnostic Features
Adenovirus	URI; cough; fever	Morbilliform (may be petechial)	Respiratory symptoms are prominent. No koplik spots. No desquamation
Measles	Cough, rhinitis, conjunctivitis	Maculopapular; face to trunk; lasts 7–10 d; Koplik spots in mouth	Toxic. Bright red rash becomes confluent, may desquamate. Fever falls after rash appears.
Rubella	Usually none	Mild maculopapular, rapid spread face to extremities; gone by day 4	Postauricular, occipital adenopathy common. Polyarthralgia in some older girls. Mild clinical illness.
Roseola (exanthema subitum)	Fever (3–4 days)	Pink, macular rash occurs at end of illness; transient	Fever often high; disappears when rash develops; child appears well. Usually occurs in children 6 month to 2 yr of age. Seizures may complicate.
Erythema infectiosum	None	Erythematous *"slapped" cheeks;* then reticular rash on extremities, trunk	Rash may reappear over weeks, especially with exposure to heat, sunlight. May cause arthralgia/arthritis, usually in older children or adults. Red cell maturation arrest in children with chronic hemolysis can cause aplastic crisis.

208. Ans. c. Effacement of the..., d. Onset may be preceded..., e. Steroid is given...

[Ref: O.P.Ghai 8th/477-78; Nelson (SAE) 20th/2521-26]

"**Minimal change disease-** also k/a ***lipoid nephrosis,*** foot process disease & Nil deposit disease" *(Harshmohan 7th/656)*

"**Minimal change disease**: The disease ***sometimes follows a respiratory infection*** or routine prophylactic immunization" *(Robbins 9th/917)*

"**Minimal change disease**: The ***onset may be preceded by an upper respiratory infection***, atopic allergy or immunisation. The disease ***characteristically respond to steroid therapy***" *(Harshmohan 7th/656)*

"NS in children can be divided into two groups based on renal histological characteristics: (1) Minimal change NS & (2) Nephrotic syndrome with significant lesions" *(O.P. Ghai 8th/477)*

Table *(Ghai)*: **Features of idiopathic nephritic syndrome**

Features	Minimal lesion	Significant lesions
Age at onset	2–6 yr	Older children
Sex incidence	Higher in boys	Equal
Hematuria	Rare	Usual
Blood pressure	Normal	Normal or increased
GFR	Normal	Normal or decreased
Renal biopsy	Normal glomeruli; mild mesangial proliferation; often. IgM deposits	Changes of varying severity; C3, immunoglobulin deposits
Serum C3	Normal	Low in MPGN
Selectivity of proteinuria	High	Low
Response to steroids	Remission in >95%	Unsatisfactory
Prognosis	Good; relapses stop by second decade	Variable progression of renal damage

Contd...

Nephrotic Syndrome

◈ *Nelson (SAE) 20th/2523*

- Approx. 90% of children with nephrotic syndrome have a form of the idiopathic nephrotic syndrome. Causes of idiopathic nephrotic syndrome include ***minimal change***

disease (85%), mesangial proliferation (5%), and focal segmental glomerulo sclerosis (10%). The remaining 10% of children with nephrotic syndrome have secondary nephrotic syndrome related to systemic

Minimal Change NS

◈ *Nelson (SAE) 20th/2523*

- Glomeruli appear normal or show a minimal increase in mesangial cells & matrix
- Finding on immunofluorescence microscopy are typically negative & electron microscopy simply reveals ***effacement of the epithelial cell foot processes***
- ***More than 95% of children with minimal change disease respond to corticosteroid therapy***

Table *(Nelson 20th/2523)*: **Minimal Change Nephrotic Syndrome**

Clinical Manifestations	
Age (Yr)	2–6, some adults
Sex	2:1 male
Nephrotic syndrome	100%
Asymptomatic proteinuria	0
Hematuria	10–20%
Hypertension	10%
Rate of progression to renal failure	Does not progress
Renal Pathology	
Light microscopy	Normal
Immunofluorescence	Negative
Electron microscopy	Foot process fusion
Response to steroids	90%

209. Ans. b. Erythropoeitin given..., c. Erythropoeitin given....

[Ref: Nelson (SAE) 20th/2305-09, 2372-74; Chloherty Manual of Neonatal Care 7th/568-70]

RBC & Erythropoietin

◈ *Nelson (SAE) 20th/2372-74*

- During the first few wk of life, all neonates experience a decline in circulating RBC mass caused both by physiologic factors and, in sick premature infants, by phlebotomy blood losses.
- In healthy term infants, the nadir hemoglobin value rarely falls to <11 g/dL at an age of 10–12 wk. This ***"physiologic" drop in RBCs*** does not require transfusions.
- In contrast, the decline occurs earlier and is more pronounced in **premature infants**, even in those without complicating illnesses, in which the mean hemoglobin concentration falls to approximately 8 g/dL in infants of 1.0–1.5 kg birthweight and to 7 g/dL in infants weighing <1.0 kg at birth.
- Most infants with birthweight of <1.0 kg need RBC transfusions. A key reason why the nadir hemoglobin values of **premature infants** are lower than those of term infants is the former group's relatively ***diminished plasma EPO level in response to anemia***
- The mechanisms responsible for **low plasma EPO** levels are only partially defined. One factor is the reliance of preterm infants on the liver as the primary site of EPO production during the first few wk of life. The liver is less responsive than the kidneys to anemia and tissue hypoxia.
- Preterm infants exhibit a sluggish EPO response to falling hematocrit values. ***Low plasma EPO levels provide a rationale for the use of recombinant EPO in the treatment of anemia of prematurity***. Proper doses of EPO and iron effectively stimulate neonatal erythropoiesis. ***However, the efficacy of EPO therapy to substantially diminish the need for RBC transfusions has not been convincingly demonstrated, particularly for sick, extremely premature neonates, and recombinant EPO has not been widely accepted as a treatment for anemia of prematurity.***
- ***In rare cases, some preparations of EPO have been associated with the development of anti-EPO antibodies that result in severe anemia.***

Table *(Nelson)*: **Guidelines for Pediatric Red Blood Cell Transfusions**

Children and Adolescents
• Acute loss of >25% at circulating blood volume • Hemoglobin of <8.0 g/dLin the perioperative period • Hemoglobin of <13.0 g/dL and *severe* cardiopulmonary disease • Hemoglobin of <8.0 g/dL and *symptomatic* chronic anemia • Hemoglobin of <8.0 g/dL and *marrow failure*
Infants Within the First 4 Month of Life
• Hemoglobin of <13.0 g/dL and *severe* pulmonary disease • Hemoglobin of <10.0 g/dL and *moderate* pulmonary disease • Hemoglobin of <13.0 g/dL and *severe* cardiac disease • Hemoglobin of <10.0 g/dL and *major* surgery • Hemoglobin of <8.0 g/dL and *symptomatic* anemia

210. Ans. a. Epispadias, b. Hypospadias, d. Bladder exstrophy.

[Ref: Manipal Surgery 4th/967; CSDT 11th/1028; S.Das Clinical Manual 11th/583; L & B 26th/1360]

"The male **external urethral orifice** is the external opening or urinary meatus, normally located at the tip of the ***glans penis. Congenital disorders*** of the meatus include ***epispadias*** – the misplacement to the upper aspect and ***hypospadias*** – the misplacement to the underside of the penis."

"**Ectopia vesicae or exstrophy of bladder**: Urine constantly dribbles through the ureteric orifices. Penis is ill-developed & its dorsal surface is split open (**epispadias**)" *(S.Das Clinical Manual 11th/583)*

"**Urethral stricture** causes ***obstruction along some part of the length of the urethra***. It almost always occurs in boys, is usually acquired, and typically results from a crush injury after straddle trauma. Congenital urethral stricture ***may manifest similarly to urethral valves*** and may be diagnosed by prenatal ultrasonography, or postnatally by symptoms and ***signs of outlet obstruction or patent urachus*** and is confirmed by retrograde urethrography. Initial management is often with endoscopic urethrotomy, although open urethroplasty may be necessary" *(merckmanuals.com)*

Hypospadias

◈ *CSDT 11th/1028*

- ***The urethral meatus is ventrally displaced on the glans on the shaft of the penis or more proximal at the level of the scrotum or perineum.***
- In hypospadias with the meatus positioned proximal to the corona, the prepuce is abnormal—not forming a complete cylinder due to a ventral defect.
- ***If the opening is glandular or coronal (85% of patients),*** the penis is usually functional both for micturition and procreation, and repair is done primarily for cosmetic reasons. Openings that are more proximal on the shaft require correction to allow voiding while standing, normal erection, and proper sperm deposition during intercourse.

Epispadias

◈ *CSDT 11th/1028*

- Epispadias is a rare congenital anomaly that is commonly associated with ***bladder exstrophy***. When it occurs alone, it is considered a milder degree of the exstrophy complex.
- The ***urethra opens on the dorsum of the penis***, with deficient corpus spongiosum and loosely attached corpora cavernosa. If the defect is extensive, it may extend to the bladder neck, causing incontinence.

Urethral Strictures

◈ *CSDT 11th/1028*

- Congenital urethral strictures are rare but when present are most common in the ***fossa navicularis (just proximal to the meatus)*** and in the ***bulbomembranous urethra.***
- Commonly, these strictures are thin diaphragms that may respond to simple dilation or to direct vision internal urethrotomy.

Urethral Diverticulum

◈ *CSDT 11th/1028*

- In males, urethral diverticula are nearly always in the ***pendulous or bulbous urethra***. They are often associated with an obstructive flap of the urethral mucosa (anterior urethral valve) —thought to represent incomplete closure of the urethral folds.

Hypospadias

◈ *L & B 26th/1360*

- Hypospadias occurs in around one in 200–300 male live births and is the most common congenital abnormality of the urethra.
- There are three characteristic features. Firstly the ***external meatus opens on the underside of the penis*** or the perineum, secondly the ventral aspect of the prepuce is poorly developed ('hooded prepuce') and thirdly there is a ventral deformity of the erect penis (chordee).

Epispadias

◈ *L & B 26th/1360*

- Epispadias is very rare. In penile epispadias, the ***urethral opening is on the dorsum of the penis*** and is associated with an upwardcurvature of the penis
- ***Epispadias often coexists with bladder exstrophy*** and other severe developmental defects

211. Ans. a. Magnesium

[Ref: O.P.Ghai 8th/121 -22; Nelson (SAE) 20th/365, 330-31:Harrison 19th/2462-63]

Hypermagnesemia is most probable answer because it also cause paralysis (c. f. pseudoparalysis in scurvy)

Clinical Manifestations of Vit C Deficiency

◈ *Nelson (SAE) 20th/330*

- Very low intake of vitamin C over time may lead to the deficiency disease **scurvy.** In infants and young children, the usual age of onset of clinical manifestations of scurvy is 6–24 mo. The early symptoms are rather general and include low-grade fever, irritability, tachypnea, digestive disturbances, loss of appetite, and generalized tenderness, particularly in the legs, which is noticeable when the diaper is changed.
- The pain results in ***pseudoparalysis***, with the hips and knees semi-flexed and the feet rotated outward. Edematous swelling along the shafts of the legs may be present; in some cases, there is subperiosteal hemorrhage at the end of the femur
- A "rosary" at the costochondral junctions and depression of the sternum are other typical features. The angulation of scorbutic beads is usually sharper than that of a rachitic rosary.
- Changes in the gums are most noticeable after **teeth** have erupted and are manifested as bluish purple, spongy swellings of the mucous membrane, especially over the upper incisors
- Anemia, which is seen primarily in infants and young children, may be related to ***impaired ability to use iron or folate***. Patients may present with the sicca syndrome of Sjögren, consisting of xerostomia, kerato conjunctivitis sicca, and enlarged salivary glands. Other clinical manifestations seen in infants as well as in older children and adolescents include swollen joints, purpura and ecchymoses, poor wound and fracture healing, petechiae, perifollicular hemorrhages, hyperkeratosis of hair follicles, arthralgia, and muscle weakness.
- Endochondral bone formation may not proceed because osteoblasts cannot form osteoid. Bony trabeculae that have been formed become brittle and fracture easily. Irritability and other psychologic manifestations are likely due to impaired neurotransmitter metabolism. Severe vitamin C deficiency may result in degeneration of skeletal muscles, cardiac hypertrophy, bone marrow depletion, and adrenal atrophy.

"Scurvy is often misdiagnosed as arthritis or osteomyelitis, nonaccidental trauma (child abuse) or ***acrodynia (Mercury toxicity)***. The early irritability & the bone pain are sometimes attributed to nonspecific pains or other nutritional deficiencies. ***Copper deficiency also results in a radiographic picture that is very similar to that of scurvy***. Henoch-Schönlein purpura, thrombocytopenic purpura, leukemia, meningitis, or nephritis may also be suspected" *(Nelson (SAE) 20th/330-31)*

Hypermagnesemia

◈ *Nelson*

- Symptoms usually do not appear until the plasma magnesium level is >4.5 mg/dL.
- Hypermagnesemia inhibits acetylcholine release at the ***neuromuscular junction, producing hypotonia, hyporeflexia, and weakness; paralysis occurs at high concentrations***. The neuromuscular effects may be exacerbated by aminoglycoside antibiotics.
- Direct central nervous system depression causes lethargy and sleepiness; infants have a poor suck.
- Elevated magnesium levels are associated with hypotension because of vascular dilation, which also causes flushing. Hypotension can be profound at higher concentrations due to a direct effect on cardiac function.
- ECG changes include prolonged P-R, QRS, and Q-T intervals. Severe hypermagnesemia (>15 mg/dL) causes complete heart block and cardiac arrest.
- Other manifestations of *hypermagnesemia include nausea, vomiting, and hypocalcemia.*

ORTHOPEDICS

212. Ans. a. Flexion of proximal..., d. Flexion deformity..., e. May occur...

[Ref: Maheshwari 5th/288; Apley 9th/ 61; BDC 6th/Vol. I 159]

Boutonniere Deformity

- It is a deformed position of the ***fingers*** or toes, in which the joint nearest the knuckle (the proximal interphalangeal joint, or PIP) is permanently bent toward the palm while the farthest joint (the distal interphalangeal joint, or DIP) is bent back away (***PIP flexion with DIP hyperextension***).
- It is commonly caused by injuryor by an inflammatory condition like ***rheumatoid arthritis***, or genetic conditions like Ehlers Danlos Syndrome.
- This **flexion deformity of the proximal interphalangeal joint** is due to ***interruption of the central slip of the extensor tendon*** *such that the lateral slips* separate and the head of thc proximal phalanx pops through the gap like a finger through a button hole (thus the name, from French *boutonnière* "button hole").
- The distal joint is subsequently drawn into **hyperextension** because the ***two peripheral slips of the extensor tendon are stretched by the head of the proximal phalanx*** (note that the two peripheral slips are inserted into the distal phalanx, while the proximal slip is inserted into the middle phalanx). *This deformity makes it difficult or impossible to extend the proximal interphalangeal joint.*
- A boutonnière (buttonhole) deformity (BD) may develop either in the acute setting (secondary to trauma) or progressively (secondary to arthritis).
- **2nd to 5th digit:** Flexion (flexor digitorum superficialis at PIP & flexor digitorum profundus at DIP) & extension (Interossei & lumbricals) *(BDC 6th/Vol. I 159)*

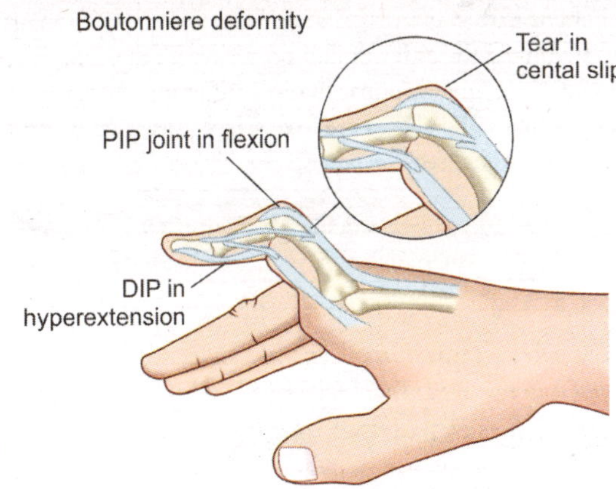

Fig: *(dynasplint.com)*: Boutonniere deformity

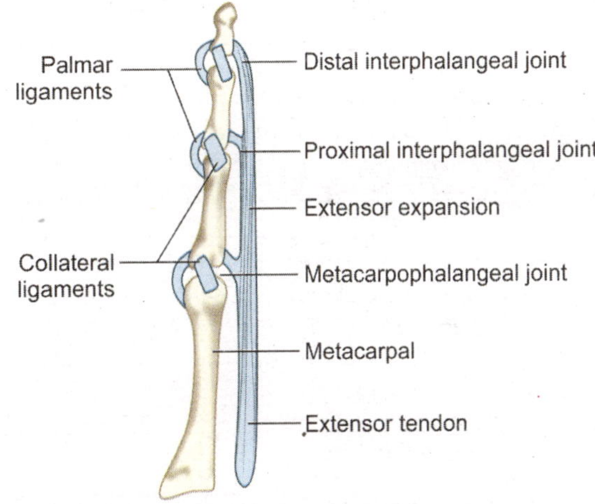

Fig: *(BDC 6th/Vol. I 159)*: Joints of finger

213. Ans. a. Romanus lesion..., b. If left untreated..., c. Predilection of the joints

[Ref: Maheshwari 5th/290-94; Apley 9th/ 66-69;http://radiopaedia.org/articles/romanus-lesion]

Ankylosingspondylitis

◈ *Maheshwari 5th/290-94*

- AS is a chronic disease characterized by a progressive inflammatory stiffening of the joints, with a predilection for the ***joints of the axial skeleton, especially the sacro-iliac joints***
- Sacro-iliac joints are usually the first to get involved, followed by the spine from the lumbar region upwards
- The hip, the knee & the manubrio-sternal joints are also involved frequently
- Initially synovitis occurs, followed later by ***cartilage destruction & bony erosion***
- ***After bony fusion occurs***, the pain may subside, leaving the spine permanently stiff (***burnt out disease***)
- Gaenslen test is done

"The **Romanus lesion** ***represents an early finding in inflammatory spondyloarthropathies, such as ankylosing spondylitis*** and enteropathic arthritis, and appears as irregularity and erosion involving the anterior and posterior edges of the vertebral endplates. Healing response to these inflammatory erosions appears radiographically as ***reactive sclerosis***, which is known as the shiny corner sign" *(radiopaedia.org/articles/romanus-lesion)*

214. Ans. a. Commonly occurs in..., b. Radiotherapy is..., c. Cause cortical....

[Ref: Maheshwari 5th/237-39; Apley 9th/ 202-03;Robbins 9th/1203-04]

"**GCT**: *The* ***cortex is thin*** *& sometime ballooned; aggressive lesion extend into the soft tissue" (Apley 9th/ 203)*

Osteoclastoma (Giant Cell Tumour)

- The tumour is seen commonly in the ***age group of 20-40 years i.e., after epiphyseal fusion***
- The ***bones affected commonly are those around the knee*** i.e., lower end of femur & upper end of the tibia. Lower end of the radius is another common site
- The tumour is located at the epiphysis. It often reaches almost up to the joint surface
- Aggressive lesions have a ***poorly defined edge & extend well into the surrounding bone***
- Whenever possible, ***excision of the tumour*** is the best treatment.
- For sites like the spine, where excision is sometimes technically not possible, ***radiotherapy is done***
- ***"GCT often destroys the overlying cortex, producing a bulging soft tissue mass delinated by a thin shell of reactive bone"*** *(Robbins 9th/1203-04)*

215. Ans. b. Commonest site..., c. Cortex may..., d. Cause pathological...

[Ref: Maheshwari 5th/248-49; Apley 9th/200-01]

Simple Bone Cyst

◈ *Maheshwari 5th/248-49*

- This is the only true cyst of the bone
- It ***occurs in children & adolescents***
- The ends of long bones are the favourite sites, the ***commonest being the upper end of the humerus***
- The cyst is known to undergo spontaneous healing, particularly after a fracture

Simple Bone Cyst (Also k/a Solitary or Unicameral Cyst)

◈ *Apley 9th/200-01*

- It ***appear during childhood***, typically in metaphysis in one of the long bones & ***most commonly in proximal humerus or femur***
- It is ***not a tumour***, it tend to heal spontaneously
- It is ***seldom seen in adults***
- This condition is usually discovered after a pathological fracture or as an incidental finding on X-ray
- X-ray shows a well demarcated radiolucent area in the ***metaphysis***, often extending up to the physeal plate; the ***cortex may be thinned & the bone expanded***
- Treatment depends on whether the cyst is symptomatic, actively growing or involved in a fracture
- **Surgery:** The cavity should be ***thoroughly cleaned by curettage*** & then packed with bone chips
- There is ***always risk that cyst will recur*** & more than one operation needed

Bone Cyst

◈ *orthoinfo.aaos.org*

3 type- ***Unicameral Bone Cyst (Simple bone cyst), Aneurysmal bone cyst & Traumatic bone cyst***

- A **unicameral**, or simple, bone cyst is a common, benign (noncancerous) bone tumor that primarily occurs in children and adolescents.
- **UBC** are cavities within bone that are filled with fluid. Although they can develop in any bone, UBCs usually affect the long bones – most often the upper arm bone (humerus) and the thighbone (femur).
- In most cases, **unicameral bone cysts** are not painful, and are often discovered incidentally when an X-ray is obtained for another reason. Because these cysts can weaken the surrounding bone, fractures through UBCs do occur.
- Treatment for a **UBC** is based on several factors, including the size and location of the cyst, and the risk for fracture. In some cases, surgery may be recommended.

216. Ans. a. Occur at distal end..., e. Common in women

[Ref: Maheshwari 5th/111-14; Apley 9th/ 772-75]

*"****Colle's fracture complication:*** *Wrist movements especially ulnar deviation & forearm rotations are painful & restricted" (Maheshwari 5th/114)*

Colle's Fracture

◈ *Maheshwari 5th/111-14*

- *This is a fracture at the distal end of the radius, at its cortico-cancellous junction (****about 2 cm from the distal articular surface****), in adults, with typical displacement*
- *It nearly always results from a fall on an out-stretched hand*
- *It is commonest fracture in people above forty years*
- ***Particularly common in women*** *because of postmenopausal osteoporosis*
- *Displacement- dorsal displacement, dorsal tilt (most characteristic), lateral displacement, dorsal tilt, supination & impaction of fragments*
- *Complication:* ***Dinner fork deformity & Sublaxation of the inferior radio-ulnar joint (distal radio-carpal joint)***
- *It is most common of all fracture in older people (Apley 9th/ 772)*

ALSO KNOW

- **Barton fracture**: *This is an intra-articular fracture of the distal radius (Maheshwari 5th/114)*
- **Galeazzi fracture dislocation**: *It is fracture of the* ***lower third of radius with dislocation or sublaxation of the distal radio-ulnar joint*** *(Maheshwari 5th/111)*
- **Monteggia fracture dislocation-** *This is a fracture of the upper-third of the ulna with dislocation of the head of the radius (Maheshwari 5th/110)*

217. Ans. a. Apley's test..., c. McMurray's test..., d. Thessaly test.

[Ref: Maheshwari 5th/150-52, 367-68; Apley 9th/ 552]

"The manoeuvres carried out to detect a hidden meniscus tear are ***McMurray's & Apley's test***" *(Maheshwari 5th/151)*

Tests for Meniscal Injuries

◈ *Apley 9th/ 552*

- **McMurray's test**- This classic test for a torn meniscus is seldom used now that the diagnosis can easily be made by MRI. A positive test is helpful but not pathognomonic, a negative test does not exclude a tear
- **Thessaly test:** This test has shown a high diagnostic accuracy rate at the level of 95% in detecting meniscal tears

Table *(Maheshwari 5th/368)*: **Signs and Tests**

- **Adson's test:** For thoracic outlet syndrome
- **Allen's test:** for testing patency of radial and ulnar arteries
- **Alli's test:** for CDH
- **Anvil test:** for testing tenderness of the spine
- **Ape thumb:** for median nerve injury
- **Apley's grinding test:** for meniscus injury
- **Apprehension test:** for recurrent dislocation of the shoulder
- **Barlow's test:** for CDH
- **Blue sclera:** Osteogenesis imperfecta
- **Bryant's test:** for anterior dislocation of the shoulder
- **Callaways' test:** for anterior dislocation of the shoulder
- **Chvostek's sign:** for tetany
- **Claw hand:** for ulnar nerve injury
- **Coin test:** for dorsoumbar tuberculosis of spine
- **Cozen's test:** for tennis elbow
- **Drawer test:** for ACL and PCL injuries
  - **Anterior:** for ACL injury
  - **Posterior:** for PCL injury
- **Finkelstein's test:** for de Quervain'stenovaginitis
- **Foot drop:** for common peroneal nerve injury
- **Froment's sign:** nerve injury
- **Gaenslen's test:** for SI joint involvement
- **Gallezzi sign:** for CDH
- **Gower's sign:** for muscular dystrophy
- **Hamilton ruler test:** for anterior dislocation of shoulder
- **Kanavel's sign:** for infection in ulnar bursa
- **Lasegue's test:** for disc prolapsed
- **Lachmann test:** for ACL injury
- **Ludloff sign:** for avulsion of lesser trochanter
- **McMurray's test:** for meniscus injury
- **Nagffziger test:** for disc prolapsed
- **Ober's test:** for tight ilio-tibial band (e.g., in polio)
- **O'Donoghue triad:** triad of MCL, ACL & medial meniscus injuries occurring together
- **Ortolani's test:** for CDH
- **Pivot shift test:** for ACL injury
- **Policeman tip:** for Erb's palsy
- **Runner's knee:** patellar tendinitis
- **Sulcus sign:** for inferior dislocation of the shoulder
- **Thomas' test:** for hip flexion deformity
- **Trendelenburg's test:** for unstable hip due to any reason (e.g., CDH)
- **Tinel's sign:** for detecting improving nerve injury
- **Volkmann's sign:** for ischaemic contracture of forearm muscles
- **Wrist drop:** for radial nerve injury

218. Ans. a. Vitamin D..., e. To take Alendronate.

[Ref: Maheshwari 5th/ 308-10, 274; Apley 9th/131-34, 809-15, 821-25]

It is a case of osteoporotic fracture of lumbar spine

Osteoporosis

◈ *Maheshwari 5th/ 308-10*

- It is an asymptomatic disorders unless complications (predominantly fractures) occur.

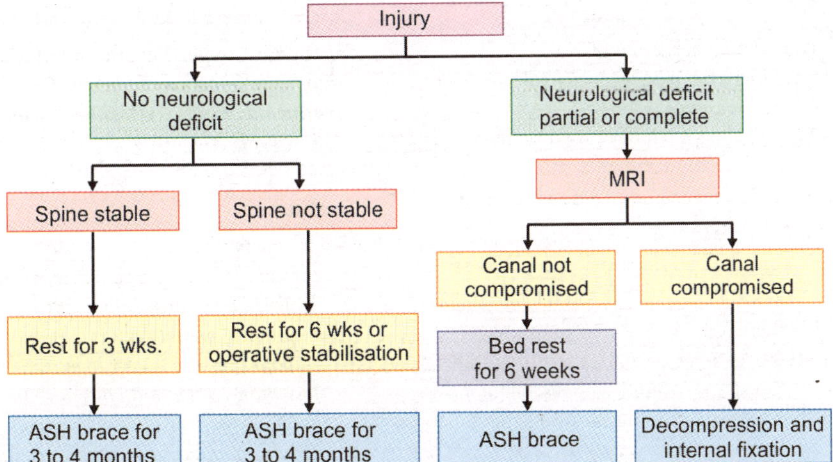

Fig: *(Maheshwari 5th/ 274):* Treatment plan of Dorso-lumbar spine injury

- Loss of bone mass lead to loss of strength so that a trivial trauma is sufficient to cause a fracture. ***Dorso-lumbar spine is the most frequent site.*** Pain from these fracture is usually the reason for a person to consult a physician. Other fractures whose etiology has been linked to underlying osteoporosis are Colle's fracture & fracture of neck of femur
- Treatment can be divided into medical & preventive
- **Medical:** ***High protein diet, androgen, estrogen, Vitamin D, fluoride, alendronate, calcitonin, teripratide, denosumab & strontium (both are antiresorptive agent)***
- Orthopaedic treatment: Exercise & Bracing (ASH brace or Taylor brace)

ANESTHESIA

219. Ans. a. Tacheostomy tube may..., d. Improper positioning...

[Ref: Schwartz 9th/59-10;http://www.nurses.com/;P.L.Dhingra 6th/316-20;Ajay Yadav 5th/48-49; Miller Anaesthesia 7th/2378, 1871-72]

"**Changing the tube:** *Tracheostomy tube should not be disturbed for the first 48-72 hr, but thereafter the tube is* ***changed daily & cleaned at regular interval.*** *On insertion, the tube it is essential to check that it is in trachea & not* ***lying anterior to it in the mediastinum.*** *If this happen respiration will not be heard through the tube &* ***vascular erosion may occur, which may fatal***" *(L & T 10th/195-96)*

"***Recent study do not support obtaining a routine post tracheostomy chest X-ray.*** *The most dramatic complication is* **racheo-innonimate artery fistula (TIAF).***Should a TIAF be suspected, the patient should be transported immediately to operating room for* ***fiberoptic evaluation.*** *If needed remove tracheostomy & place finger to apply direct pressure anteriorly for compression of the innominate artery*" *(Schwartz 9th/328-29)*

"**Tracheal deviation** may signal ***abnormal bleeding.*** A misaligned tube puts pressure on the tracheal wall increasing risk for wall necrosis and erosion. ***Palpable tube pulsations suggest impending erosion of an artery***" *(hopkinsmedicine.org)*

Secretions

◈ *www.rch.org.au*
- What is the color, consistency, and amount?
- Expect secretions to ***increase due to tracheal mucosa irritation from the tube's presence.***
- Bloody secretions beyond the fourth day post-tracheotomy are abnormal.
- Dry secretions can signal dehydration; ***copious secretions can signal fluid volume overload.***

Stoma

◈ *www.rch.org.au*
- Is it clean and dry? Is there redness or purulent drainage?
- Note that 60% to 100% of long-term tracheostomy sites have colonization of the stoma wound with *Pseudomonas* or other gram-negative bacteria. Colonization sets the stage for infection.
- ***Reintubation in the first 36 hours after tracheotomy is an emergency.*** The stoma may collapse. If reintubation is unsuccessful, call for emergency personnel and provide assisted ventilation. Use a bag-valve-mask device and oxygen placed over the patient's mouth and nose.

"**Decanulation**: The surgeons will monitor the healing for several days after the tracheostomy. Usually, the initial tube that was placed at the time of surgery will be changed to a new tube sometime ***between 10 and 14 days*** following surgery, depending on the specific circumstances. Subsequent tube changes are usually managed by the treating physician or ***nursing*** staff. ***Bronchoscopy*** evaluation is usually performed prior to planned decannulation to evaluate airway stability, assess possible granulation or suprastomal collapse, to assess whether the child can maintain their airway and ventilation adequately without the tracheostomy tube".

Immediate Post-Operative Complications Include

◈ *www.rch.org.au*
- Blocked tube
- Bleeding from the airway/tracheostomy tube
- Pneumothorax
- Subcutaneous and/or mediastinal emphysema
- Respiratory and/or cardiovascular collapse
- Dislodged tube
- Granulation tissue
- Tracheo-oesophageal fistula

Long Term Complications Include

◈ *www.rch.org.au*
- Acute airway obstruction
- Blocked tube
- Infection (localised to stoma or tracheo-bronchial)
- Aspiration
- Tracheal trauma
- Dislodged tube
- Stoma or tracheal granulation tissue
- Tracheal stenosis

220. Ans. a. Boiling point..., b. Chemically it..., c. It increases....

[Ref: Ajay Yadav 5th/ 82; Morgan 5th/170-71]

"**Malignant hyperthermia:** ***Inhalational agent causing MH – Halothane (most common), isoflurane, enflurane, desflurane, sevoflurane, methoxyflurane, cyclopropane, ether & nitrous oxide (weak triggering agent). Xenon does not trigger MH***" *(Ajay Yadav 5th/ 133)*

Desflurane

◈ *Ajay Yadav 5th/ 82;*
- *It is similar to isoflurane except chlorine atom of isoflurane is replaced by fluorine atom which produces significant changes in physical properties*
- *Vapour pressure is very high (681 mm Hg) &* ***boiling point is less than 23 °C,*** *so it boils at room temperature that is why a special vaporizer (TEC 6) is required for its delivery*
- ***Produces maximum muscle relaxation among the agents*** *which are used now a days*
- ***5 times less potent than isoflurane*** *(KDT 7th/380)*

Desflurane

◈ *Barash Anaesthsia 6th*

- Desflurane is a ***fluorinated methyl ethyl ether*** that differs from isoflurane by just one atom: a fluorine atom is substituted for a chlorine atom on the α-ethyl component of isoflurane
- The process of complete fluorination of the ether molecule has several effects. It decreases blood and tissue solubility (the blood:gas solubility of desflurane equals that of nitrous oxide), and ***it results in a loss of potency (the MAC of desflurane is 5 times higher than isoflurane).***
- Moreover, fluorination of the methyl ether molecule results in a high vapor pressure owing to decreased intermolecular attraction. Thus, a new vaporizer technology was developed to deliver a regulated concentration of desflurane as agas. It is a heated, pressurized vaporizer requiring electrical power and more frequent servicing.
- One of the advantages of desflurane is the near-absent metabolism to serum trifluoroacetate. This makes ***immune-mediated hepatitis a rare occurrence.***
- Desflurane is the ***most pungent of the volatile anesthetics,*** and if administered via the face mask results in coughing, salivation, breath holding, and laryngospasm. In extremely dry CO_2 absorbers, desflurane (and to a lesser extent isoflurane, enflurane, and sevoflurane) degrades to form carbon monoxide.
- ***Desflurane has the lowest blood: gas solubility of the potent*** volatile anesthetics
- Desflurane has been associated with *tachycardia, hypertension,* and, in select cases, myocardial ischemia when used in high concentrations or rapidly increasing the inspired concentration (without using opioid adjuvants to prevent such a response).

221. Ans. b. Diclofenac... c. Morphine.

[Ref: KDT 7th/476, Ajay Yadav 5th/231]

"***Transdermal fentanyl (Durogesic)*** *has become available for use in cancer/terminal illness" (KDT 7th/476)*

"**Butrans** skin patches contain ***buprenorphine***, an opioid pain medication"-www.drugs.com

"**Clonidine transdermal system** USP 0.1 mg/day, 0.2 mg/day or 0.3 mg/day are available as 4 pouched systems and 4 adhesive covers per carton. Each system is a round corner, rectangular flexible transdermal system with a tan matte backing and clear membrane" *(www.drugs.com)*

"**Clonidine transdermal delivery** (patch) systems have been available since the 1980s and pharmacokinetic studies of these products demonstrate a linear relationship between the size of the patch and the steady-state serum concentrations achieved. The amount of drug administered, therefore, *depends on the contact surface area of the patch rather than the size of the system reservoir" (ncbi.nlm.nih.gov)*

222. Ans. a. Mallampati..., c. Thyromental..., d. Teeth....

[Ref: Manipal Surgery 4th/ 1072-73; Ajay Yadav 5th/53, 124; Morgan 5th/ 312-13]

ASA physical status grading is for general health status of patient (not for assessing intubation)

Assessment of Difficult Intubation

◈ *Ajay Yadav 5th/124*

- **Mallampati grading**: It is done to assess mouth opening
- **Thyromental distance** (distance b/w thyroid notch to mental prominence with fully extended neck)
- **Mentohyoid distance**: normal > 5 cm
- Assessment of TM joint function: **Inter incisor gap** (mouth opening) should be at least 5 cm (2 finger breadth)
- **Neck movement**

Table: ASA Physical Status Classification System

ASA PS Classification	Definition
ASA I	A normal healthy patient
ASA II	A patient with mild systemic disease
ASA III	A patient with severe systemic disease
ASA IV	A patient with severe systemic disease that is a constant threat to life
ASA V	A moribund patient who is not expected to survive without the operation
ASA VI	A declared brain-dead patient whose organs are being removed for donor purposes

SKIN

223. Ans. b. Methotrexate... c. TNF-alpha..., d. Acitretin.

[Ref: Neena Khanna 5th/54-59; Harrison 19th/348; Roxburg 17th/138-42]

"Various systemic agents can be used for severe, widespread psoriatic disease. ***Oral glucocorticoids should not be*** used for the treatment of **psoriasis** due to the potential for developing life-threatening pustular psoriasis when therapy is discontinued. Methotrexate is an effective agent, especially in patients with psoriatic arthritis. The synthetic ***retinoid acitretin*** is useful, especially when immunosuppression must be avoided; however, teratogenicity limits its use" *(Harrison 19th/348)*

"Most patients with localized, plaque-type psoriasis can be managed with ***midpotency topical glucocorticoids***, although their long-term use is often accompanied by loss of effectiveness (tachyphylaxis) and atrophy of the skin. A topical vitamin D analogue (***calcipotriene***) and a retinoid (**tazarotene**) are also efficacious in the treatment of limited psoriasis and have largely replaced other topical agents such as coal tar, salicylic acid, and anthralin" *(Harrison 19th/348)*

"Ultraviolet light, natural or artificial, is an effective therapy for many patients with widespread psoriasis. ***Ultraviolet B (UV-B) light, narrowband UV-B, and ultraviolet A (UV-A)*** spectrum with either oral or topical **psoralens** (**PUVA**) are also extremely effective. The long-term use of UV light may be associated with an increased incidence of nonmelanoma and melanoma skin cancer. UV-light therapy is contraindicated in patients receiving cyclosporine and should be used with great care in all immunocompromised patients due to an increased risk of developing skin cancers" *(Harrison 19th/348)*

Biological response modifiers used to treat psoriasis include: ***T cell inhibitors (alefacept, adalimumab, itolizumab), TNF α-blockers (etanercept, infliximab) & Anti IL 12/23 (ustekinumab)*** *(Neena Khanna 5th/58)*

Psoriasis: ***Corticosteriods (only topical!!)*** *are used routinely especially in combination" (Neena Khanna 5th/55)*

Psoriasis: *Systemic corticosteroids are only indicated for generalized pustular psoriasis in pregnancy (impetigo herpetiformis)" (Neena Khanna 5th/55)*

Table *(Neena Khanna 5th/59)*: **Treatment Strategies in Psoriasis**

	Treatment of Choice	**Alternatives**
A. Psoriasis Vulgaris		
▪ Localized (<10% BSA)	• Topical coal for salicylic acid • Topical dithranol (short contact)	• Topical steroids + salicylic acid
▪ Medically extensive (10-30% ESA)	• NB UVB, FUVA/FUVA sol	• Methotrexate
▪ Extensive (>30% BSA)	• Methotrexate	• NB UVB, PUVA/PUVA sol, Cyclosporine
▪ Facial lesions	• Topical, low-mid potency steroids	• Tacrolimus/pimecrolimus
▪ Palmoplantar psoriasis	• Topical, high (even ultra high in resistant cases) potency steroid combined with salicylic acid	• Methotrexate (low-dose) in debilitating cases
B. Erythrodermic psoriasis	Methotrexate+ emollients, Acitretin + emollients	• Cyclosporine
C. Guttate psoriasis	• Antibiotics+ emollients, PUVA/PUVA sol/NB UBB	• Coal tar, Tacrolimus & Mild topical steroids
D. Flexural psoriasis	• Topical low-medium potency steroids + antifungal agents	
E. Pustular psoriasis		
Hands & feet	• Topical high potency steroids + salicylic acid; Topical PUVA/PUVA sol	• Methotrexate (low-dose)
Generalizes	• Methotrexate + emollients	• Acitretin;Cyclosporine • Oral steroids, but only in pregnant women

BSA: Body surface area; NBUVB: Narrow band UVB, 311 um; PVA/PUVA sol: Psoralens + UVA/Psoralents+sunlight

224. Ans. b. Melanocyte..., c. Sebaecous gland..., d. Apocrine gland..., e. Hiraadenitis...

[Ref: Neena Khanna 5th/ 119, 451-53; Harrison 19th/1099; Roxburg 17th/ 4-11; General Anatomy by BD Chaurasia 5th/254-60]

"**Hidradenitis suppurativa** (Synonym- apocrine acne): ***Axillary apocrine sweat gland infection*** *(Harrison 19th/1099; Neena Khanna 5th/ 139)*

"**Sweat glands are two types**- *eccrine & apocrine.* **Eccrine glands** *are merocrine in nature & are large in the axilla & groin, most numerous in the palms & soles, & least numerous in the neck & back. Eccrine glands are supplied & controlled by cholinergic sympathetic nerves.* **Apocrine glands** *are confined to axilla, eyelids (Moll's gland), nipple & areola of the breast,* ***perianal region*** *& the* ***external genitalia****" (General Anatomy by BD Chaurasia 5th/256-57)*

"**Sebaceous glands** *are* ***holocrine in nature,*** *i.e. they produce their secretion by complete fatty degeneration of the central cells of the alveolus, which are replaced by the proliferating peripheral cells. They are widely distributed all over the dermis of the skin* ***except for the palms & soles.*** *The secretion is under hormonal control, especially the androgen" (General Anatomy by BD Chaurasia 5th/258-59)*

The ***pigment cells (melanocyte) of the skin are derived from neural crest*** *(Human Embryology by I B Singh 10th/324 & ncbi.nlm.nih.go)*

A & E

Structure of Skin

◈ *Roxburg 17th/ 4-11*

- The epidermis contains keratinocytes mainly, but also non-keratinocytes- melanocytes & Langerhans cells
- There are ***no blood vessels in the epidermis*** & the necessary oxygen & nutrients diffuse from the capillaries in the dermal papillae. These capillaries arise from horizontally arranged plexuses in the dermis
- The ***apocrine sweat glands drains directly into hair follicles in the axillae & groins***
- The **eccrine sweat glands** are an extremely important part of the body's mesothermic mechanism. Apart from heat, eccrine sweat secretion may also be stimulated by emotional factors & by fear & anxiety. Certain body sites, such as the plams, soles, forehead, axillae & inguinal regions, secrete sweat selectively during emotional stimulation

Structure of Skin

◈ *Neena Khanna 5th/ 119, 451-53*

- The skin has three layers: Epidermis, dermis & subcutis
- Skin contains appendages- hair, sebaceous glands, sweat gland & nails
- **Sebaceous gland** are located throughout the skin except on palms & soles. Glands made up of acini of lipid containing cells, which secrete sebum as a ***holocrine secretion***
- **Eccrine sweat glands** present all over body, especially on palms, soles & in axillae. Human have 2-24 million eccrine sweat glands

225. Ans. **b. Phenytoin..., c. Isoniazid..., d. Steroid..., e. Potassium....**

[Ref: Neena Khanna 5th/125; Harrison 19th/356; Harrison 14th/425; Roxburg 17th/154-55]

Tetracycline-Acneiform eruption is not mentioned as side effect *(KDT 7th/735-37)*

Drug-Induced Acneiform Eruptions

- *Neena Khanna 5th/125*
- *Steroids (corticosteroids, androgens, anabolic steroids), oral contraceptives,* ***antitubercular drugs, anticonvulsants*** *& halides (**iodides**, bromides)*
- *Trunk especially back, face may be involved*
- *Lesions are monomorphic, consisting of papules & sometimes pustules*

Acne

- *Harrison 14th/425 (Table of adverse reaction to drugs, Not given in newer editions)*
- *Anabolic & androgenic steroids*
- *Bromides*
- *Glucocorticoids*
- *Iodides*
- *Isoniazid*
- *Oral contraceptives*
- *Troxidone*

Table *(Harrison 19th/356)*: **Causes of Acneiform Eruptions**

I. Primary cutaneous disorders
- A. Acne vulgaris
- B. Acne rosacea

II. Drugs, e.g., ***anabolic steroids, glucocorticoids, lithium, EGFR[a] inhibitors, iodides***

III. Systemic diseases
- A. Increased androgen production
  1. Adrenal origin, e.g., Cushing's disease, 21-hydroxylase deficiency
  2. Ovarian origin, e.g., polycystic ovary syndrome
- B. Cryptococcosis, disseminated
- C. Dimorphic fungi
- D. Behçet's disease

Drug-Induced Acne and Acneiform Eruptions

- *www.the-dermatologist.com*
- **Aromatic Anticonvulsants**: Aromatic anticonvulsant medications have been associated with the induction of acne. This is particularly the case with ***phenytoin***. It is likely that **carbamazepine** can also induce acne
- **Calcineurin Blockers:** Oral cyclosporine is associated with drug-induced acne. Sirolimus plus cyclosporine caused more acne than sirolimus plus tacrolimus in high-risk renal allograft recipients
- **Psychotropic Medications**: trazodone, haloperidol & aripiprazole have been linked to the induction of acne.
- **Epidermal Growth Factor Blockers**: cetuximab is commonly linked to an acne-like eruption
- **Isoniazid** is an uncommon inducer of acne
- In addition, it should be noted that gram-negative folliculitis can arise against a background of antibiotic use, but it is ***not an actual side effect of antibiotics such as minocycline or doxycycline.***

226. Ans. **a. Lichen..., b. Discoid lupus..., d. Lichen...**

[Ref: Neena Khanna 5th/141; Harrison 19th/355; Roxburg 17th/ 270]

"Trichotillomania (compulsive hair-pulling) *is characterized by noticeable hair loss caused by person's persistent & recurrent failure to resist impulses to pullout hairs"-Ahuja 7th/119*

Cicatrical (Scarring) Alopecia

- *Neena Khanna 5th/141*
- *Aplasia cutis*
- ***Lichen planopilaris, Discoid lupus erythematous***
- *Favus, kerion*
- *Naevus sebaceous*
- *Physical, chemical*
- *Basal cell carcinoma*
- *Pseudopelade of Brocq*

Table *(Harrison 19th/355)*: **Causes of Alopecia**

I. Nonscarring alopecia
- A. Primary cutaneous disorders
  1. ***Telogen effluvium***
  2. Androgenetic alopecia
  3. Alopecia areata
  4. Tinea capitis
  5. Traumatic alopecia
- B. Drugs
- C. Systemic diseases
  1. Systemic lupus erythematosus
  2. Secondary syphilis
  3. Hypothyroidism
  4. Hyperthyroidism
  5. Hypopituitarism
  6. Deficiencies of protein, iron, biotin, and zinc

II. Scarring alopecia
- A. Primary cutaneous disorders
  1. Cutaneous lupus (chronic discoid lesions)
  2. ***Lichen planus***
  3. Central centrifugal cicatricial alopecia
  4. Folliculitis decalvans
  5. Linear scleroderma (morphea)
- B. Systemic diseases
  1. Discoid lesions in the setting of ***systemic lupus erythematosus***
  2. Sarcoidosis
  3. Cutaneous metastases

227. Ans. **b. 280-320 nm**

[Ref: Neena Khanna 5th/ 433; Roxburg 17th/27]

"The wavelength found most effective in treating skin disease with phototherapy is UVB with ***wavelength of 311± 2nm*** (narrow band UVB, NBUVB)"*(Neena Khanna 5th/ 433)*

"Three segments of UV radiation (UVR) are recognized: UVA (320-400) or long-wave UVR; ***UVB (280-320nm)*** *or medium wave UVR; & UVC (250-280 nm) or short wave UVR"* *(Roxburg 17th/27)*

Phototherapy/Photochemotherapy: Indications

◈ *Neena Khanna 5th/ 433*
- *Psoriasis*
- *Vitiligo*
- *Atopic dermatitis*
- *Alopecia totalis & universalis*
- *Others: Pityriasis lichenoides chronica, pitriasis rosea & patch stage of mycosis fungoides*

"The **UV spectrum** reaching the earth represents <10% of total incident solar energy and is arbitrarily divided into two major segments, UV-B and UV-A, constituting the wavelengths from 290–400 nm. ***UV-B consists of wavelengths between 290 and 320 nm.*** This portion of the photobiologic action spectrum is the most efficient in producing redness or erythema in human skin and hence sometimes is known as the "sunburn spectrum." UV-A includes wavelengths between 320 and 400 nm and is ~1000-fold less efficient in producing skin redness than is UV-B"

"The wavelengths between ***400 and 700 nm are visible to the human eye.*** The photon energy in the visible spectrum is not capable of damaging human skin in the absence of a photosensitizing chemical"

228. Ans. b. Solar urticaria..., c. Dermatographism....

[Ref: Neena Khanna 5th/189; Harrison 19th/363; Roxburg 17th/74-74]

Inducible Urticaria (Earlier Labelled Physical Urticaria)

◈ *Neena Khanna 5th/189*
- *Demographic urticaria*
- *Cholinergic urticaria*
- *Cold urticaria*
- *Heat urticaria*
- *Solar urticaria*
- *Delayed pressure urticaria*

Physical Urticarias

◈ *Harrison 19th/363*
- The common *physical urticarias* include dermatographism, solar urticaria, cold urticaria, and cholinergic urticaria.
- Patients with **dermatographism** exhibit linear wheals following minor pressure or scratching of the skin. It is a common disorder, affecting ~5% of the population.
- **Solar urticaria** characteristically occurs within minutes of sun exposure and is a skin sign of one systemic disease—erythropoietic protoporphyria. In addition to the urticaria, these patients have subtle pitted scarring of the nose and hands.
- **Cold urticaria** is precipitated by exposure to the ***cold***, and therefore exposed areas are usually affected. In occasional patients, the disease is associated with abnormal circulating proteins—more commonly cryoglobulins and less commonly cryofibrinogens. Additional systemic symptoms include wheezing and syncope, thus explaining the need for these patients to avoid swimming in cold water.
- **Cholinergic urticaria** is precipitated by ***heat, exercise, or emotion*** and is characterized by small wheals with relatively large flares. It is occasionally associated with wheezing

Table *(Harrison 19th/363)*: **Causes of Urticaria and Angioedema**

I. Primary cutaneous disorders
A. Acute and chronic urticaria
B. Physical urticaria
1. Dermatographism
2. Solar urticaria
3. Cold urticaria
4. Cholinergic urticaria

C. Angioedema (hereditary and acquired)

II. Systemic diseases
A. Urticarial vasculitis
B. Hepatitis B or C infection
C. Serum sickness
D. Angioedema (hereditary and acquired)

PSYCHIATRY

229. Ans. b. Psychosurgery..., c. Family history..., d. Depression...

[Ref: Ahuja 7th/54-68; Synopsis of Psychiatry by Kaplan & Sadock 11th/300-325]

"**Psychosurgery** *is not routinely indicated. When used, the treatment of choice is limbic leucotomy in some cases with severe & very prominent depression, anxiety or obsessional symptoms" (Ahuja 7th/67)*

Schizophrenia

◈ *Synopsis of Psychiatry by Kaplan & Sadock 11th/300-325*
- Schizophrenia is ***equally prevalent in men and women.*** The two genders differ, however, in the onset and course of illness. Onset is earlier in men than in women. More than half of all male schizophrenia patients, but only one-third of all female schizophrenia patients, are first admitted to a psychiatric hospital ***before age 25 years***. The ***peak ages of onset are 10 to 25 years for men and 25 to 35 years for women.*** Unlike men, women display a bimodal age distribution, with a second peak occurring in middle age.
- Other feeling tones include perplexity, a sense of isolation, overwhelming ambivalence, and ***depression.***
- "**Electroencephalographic studies** indicate that many schizophrenia patients have abnormal records, increased sensitivity to activation procedures (e.g., frequent spike activity after sleep deprivation), ***decreased alpha activity, increased theta and delta activity***, possibly more epileptiform activity than usual, and possibly more left-sided abnormalities than usual"

EEG & Quantitative Electroencephalography (qEEG) in Schizophrenia

◈ *qeegsupport.com; neurofeedback.csusb.edu*
- Electroencephalography (EEG) is the measurement of electrical patterns at the surface of the scalp which reflect cortical activity, and are commonly referred to as "brainwaves".
- Quantitative EEG (qEEG) is the analysis of the digitized EEG, and in lay terms this sometimes is also called "**Brain Mapping**". The qEEG is an extension of the analysis of

the visual EEG interpretation which may assist and even augment our understanding of the EEG and brain function.

- Quantitative Electroencephalography (qEEG) is a procedure that processes the recorded EEG activity from a ***multi-electrode recording using a computer***. This multi-channel EEG data is processed with various algorithms, such as the "Fourier" classically, or in more modern applications "Wavelet" analysis). The digital data is statistically analyzed, sometimes comparing values with "normative" database reference values. The processed EEG is commonly converted into color maps of brain functioning called "Brain maps".
- EEG/QEEG Findings: In Schizophrenia Evaluation of EEG and QEEG literature on schizophrenia is complicated by the evident heterogeneity of the illness and the diversity of medication histories and dosage levels at the time of examination. In spite of these potential sources of difference among findings, considerable agreement nonetheless appears. There have been numerous studies conducted on the EEG and QEEG changes in schizophrenia. ***Abnormal conventional EEG findings are seen in 20-60% of schizophrenic patients.***
- ***Most often schizophrenic EEGs have also been characterized by decreased alpha activity and/or increased beta activity.*** Others have reported shifted alpha mean frequency or reduced alpha responsiveness and increased slow activities.
- In studies where symptoms were correlated with EEG changes, negative symptoms have been correlated with delta waves especially in temporal areas coupled with the decreased alpha and increased beta activity.
- Other studies have ***found heterogeneity in the QEEG findings,*** and these subgroups had different treatment response characteristics. In studies conducted by John et al., five subtypes were detected by a cluster analysis, with their ***QEEG profiles characterized by increased theta and decreased alpha and beta in anterior regions; excessive beta especially in anterior temporal regions; increased theta and alpha with decreased beta; increased alpha with a decrease in all other activities with a noticeable decrease in delta; and theta in frontal areas, and excessive theta with excessive delta in posterior areas.***
- Schizophrenic patients with QEEG profiles corresponding to some of the groups identified by this cluster analysis have been reported to *display differential responses to treatment* with haloperidol or risperidone. Additional evidence of heterogeneity in the schizophrenic population has been provided in QEEG studies by other groups. *Other studies conducted have shown greater values of coherence in schizophrenic patients as compared to healthy controls*

Table *(Kaplan & Sadock 11th/308)*: **DSM-5 Diagnostic Criteria for Schizophrenia**

A. Two (or more) of the following, each present for a significant portion of time during a 1-month period (or less if successfully treatment). At least one of these must be (1), (2), or (3):

1. Delusion
2. Hallucinations
3. Disorganized speech (*e.g.,* frequent derailment or incoherence)
4. Grossly disorganized or catatonic behavior
5. Negative symptoms (i.e., diminished emotional expression or avolition).

B. For a significant portion of the time since the onset of the disturbance, level of functioning in one or more major areas of functioning, such as work, interpersonal relations, or self-care, is markedly below the level achieved before the onset (or when the onset is in childhood or adolescence, there is failure to achieve expected level of interpersonal, academic, or occupational functioning).

C. Continuous signs of the disturbance persist for at least 6 months. This 6-month period must include at least 1 month of symptoms (or less if successfully treated) that meet Criterion A (i.e., active-phase symptoms) and may include periods of prodromal or residual symptoms. During these prodromal or residual periods, the signs of the disturbance may be manifested by only negative symptoms or by two or more symptoms listed in Criterion A present in an attenuated form (e.g., odd beliefs, unusual perceptual experiences).

D. Schizoaffective disorder and depressive or bipolar disorder with psychotic features have been ruled out because either (1) no major depressive or manic episodes have occurred concurrently with the active-phase symptoms, or (2) if mood episodes have occurred during active-phase symptoms, they have been present for a minority of the total duration of the active and residual periods of the illness.

E. The disturbance is not attributable to the physiological effects of a substance (e.g., a drug of abuse, a medication) or another medical condition.

F. If there is a history of autism spectrum disorder or a communication disorder of childhood onset, the additional diagnosis of schizophrenia is made only if prominent delusions or hallucinations, in addition to the other required symptoms of schizophrenia, are also present for at least 1 month (or less if successfully treated).

Table *(Kaplan & Sadock 11th/318 & Ahuja 7th/62)*: **Features Weighting Toward Good to Poor Prognosis in Schizophrenia**

Good Prognosis	Poor Prognosis
Late onset (Onset >35 yr) Short duration (<6months)	Young onset Early onset(<20 yr of age)
Obvious precipitating factors	No precipitating factors
Acute onset/ Abrupt onset	Insidious onset
Good premorbid social, sexual, and work histories	Poor premorbid social, sexual, and work histories
Mood disorder symptoms (especially depressive disorders)	Withdrawn, autistic behavior
Married Family history of mood disorders	Single, divorced, or widowed **Family history of schizophrenia**

Contd...

Good Prognosis	Poor Prognosis
Positive symptoms	Negative symptoms
Presence of precipitating stressor	Neurological signs and symptoms
Catatonic subtype (Paranoid-intermediate prognosis)	History of perinatal trauma
First episode	No remissions in 3 years
Pyknic (fat) body	Many relapses
Female sex	History of assaultiveness
Presence of confusion, perplexity or disorientation in the acute phase	Absence of stressor
	Disorganised, simple, undifferentiated or chronic catatonic subtypes
Normal cranial CT	Chronic course (> 2 yr)
Outpatient treatment	Absence of depression
Proper treatment & good response to treatment	Asthenic (thin) body
	Male sex
	Evidence of ventricular enlargement on cranial CT
	Absence of proper treatment
	Flat or blunted affect

230. Ans. b. Hyporeflexia

[Ref: Ahuja 7th/78, 188-91; Synopsis of Psychiatry by Kaplan & Sadock 11th/985-88; KDT 7th/449; Pharmacology by Satoskar 24th/225]

Lithium

Pharmacology by Satoskar 24th/225

- **Mild toxicity**: GI disturbances, drowsiness, muscular weakness, ***alopecia***, allergic reaction, blurred vision, glycosuria, *polyuria & weight gain*
- Large doses (level >1.5 mmol/L): sodium depletion, cerebellar ataxia, tremors, cardiac arrhythmias, seizures, hypotension & coma
- **Chronic administration**: goiter formation, hypothyroidism & ECG changes
- **Embryotoxicity**: Li is embryotoxic & increases the risk of Ebstein's anomaly
- **Hyper**-reflexia:KDT 7th/449

Table *(Kaplan & Sadock 11th/985)*: **Signs and Symptoms of Lithium Toxicity**

Mild to moderate intoxication (lithium level = 1.5 to 2.0 mEq/L)	
GI	Vomiting Abdominal pain Dryness of mouth
Neurologic	Ataxia Dizziness Slurred speech Nystagmus Lethargy or excitement Muscle weakness
Moderate to severe intoxication (lithium level = 2.0 to 2.5 mEq/L)	
GI	Anorexia Persistent nausea and vomiting
Neurologic	Blurred vision Muscle fasciculations Clonic limb movements Hyperactive deep tendon reflexes Choreoathetoid movements Convulsions Delirium Syncope Electroencephalographic changes Stupor Coma Circulatory failure (lowered BP, cardiac arrhythmias, and conduction abnormalities)
Severe lithium intoxication (lithium level >2.5 mEq/L)	
Generalized convulsions Oliguria and renal failure Death	

Contd...

RADIOLOGY

231. Ans. a. Tumour..., b. Singlet oxygen..., c. After therapy..., e. Photosensitivity....

[Ref: Sabiston 19th/236; Ballenger's Otorhinolaryngology 16th/1324]

"**Hematoporphyrin**: A dark red, almost purple, porphyrin resulting from the decomposition of hemoglobin;chemical composition is that of heme with the iron removed and the two vinyl groups hydrated to hydroxyethyl" *(www.medical-dictionary)*

Photodynamic Therapy

Sabiston 19th/236

- Photodynamic therapy is a new treatment that ***allows destruction of cancer cells*** and has recently been expanded to the ***eradication of metaplastic cells.***
- It begins with the administration of a ***target-specific photosensitizer*** that is eventually ***concentrated in the target tissue***.
- The photosensitizing agent is then activated with a ***wavelength-specific light energy source***, which leads to ***the generation of free radicals cytotoxic to the target tissue***.
- Photodynamic therapy has been used to treat different types of late-stage cancer, mainly in a palliative setting, but it has also been used in the treatment of some chemoresistant tumors.
- Applications reported in the literature include treating early radiographically detected *non-small cell lung cancer, pancreatic cancer, squamous cell and basal cell carcinoma of the skin, recurrent superficial bladder cancer, chest wall involvement from breast cancer, and even chest wall recurrence of breast cancer.* Its utility has recently expanded to include the treatment of noncancer conditions such as Barrett's esophagus and psoriasis

"Photosensitizers such as ***porfimer sodium*** (Photofrin) are used in photodynamic therapy. Given systemically, these drugs are ***preferentially taken up in tumor cells, rendering them more sensitive to light-mediated cell killing*** than their surrounding tissues. Although not approved specifically for HNC, these drugs have been used for palliation in ***advanced HNC or the treatment of early-stage HNC***" *(Ballenger's Otorhinolaryngology 16th/1324)*

Photodynamic Therapy

◈ *http://www.isla-laser.org*

- Penetration of light with wavelengths within the range of 630 - 700 nm, which are utilized in PDT for excitation of most of the preparations, seems to be the limiting factor as their penetration is up to 6 mm only. Therefore PDT is suitable for treatment of early stages of solid carcinomas and/or paliative treatment.
- The mechanisms of photodynamic therapy Photodynamic therapy is based on photooxidation of living matter involving three basic constituents: the photosensitizer (S), the radiation (with a wavelength appropriate to the maximum absorption of the substance in use), and oxygen.
- Oxygen species, in different toxic forms, represent the most important agents of the cellular death processes during the photodynamic therapy. Active oxygen species can be generated through a type II reaction mechanism between the photosensitizer molecule, (***being in an active triplet state - 3 S****) and the biologic environment (B).
- The sequence of the reactions is: $3\ S^* + 3\ O_2 \Rightarrow 1\ S + 1\ O_2{}^*$ & $1\ O_2{}^* + B \Rightarrow$ Box, ***where: 3 O_2 is the triplet excited state of oxygen, 1 O_2 is the singlet oxygen molecule***, and Box is the target substrate oxidated.
- *Molecular oxygen, as a singlet, (1 O_2) acts rapidly and no discriminatingly with electrophyle molecules (B) like unsaturated lipids, proteins, nucleic acids, etc. After transferring the energy to oxygen, the photosensitizer can restore its fundamental state (1 S) and the cycle repeats.*

Photodynamic Therapy

◈ *oswellpark.org/cancer/head-and-neck/treatment*

- Treatment begins when you receive the compound intravenously (through an IV). The compound, called a photosensitizer, is absorbed by the cells in your body. After a few days, however, the ***compound is shed by healthy cells but stays inside the cancerous cells.***
- ***Tumors are then exposed to light of a specific wavelength,*** delivered through very thin, *flexible fiberoptic cables.*
- The light goes through the tissue and ***activates the photosensitizer. Because the photosensitizer is inside the cancerous cells only, those cells are targeted for destruction, with little impact on healthy cells.***
- The ***photosensitizer causes no side effects other than sensitivity to light***. Depending on the type of photosensitizer you receive, for several weeks after treatment ***you will need to cover up, use sunscreen, and stay out of direct sunlight.***

PDT is FDA approved for the treatment of ***esophageal cancer and non-small cell lung cancer.***

PDT has three Effects

1. *It kills cancer cells directly.*
2. *It shuts down new blood vessels that are being created to feed the tumor. This helps cut off the tumor's oxygen supply.*
3. *It helps your immune system wake up, both in the area of the tumor and throughout your body, alerting it to destroy cancer cells.*

Photodynamic Therapy (PDT)

◈ *archotol.jamanetwork.com*

- Photodynamic therapy (PDT) is a minimally invasive treatment that ***involves localized photoactivation of a drug that generates cytotoxic reactive oxygen species, resulting in direct damage to tumor cells.***
- Tumor destruction following PDT is also accomplished by ***microvascular collapse within the tumor***, as well as ***intense stimulation of the innate and adaptive immune responses.***
- Photodynamic therapy using the photosensitizer ***porfimer sodium*** (Photofrin) is approved by the Food and Drug Administration for several clinical indications, including obstructing esophageal cancer, high-grade dysplasia in Barrett esophagus, and early-stage and advanced-stage endobronchial cancer.
- Clinical studies have also highlighted the potential usefulness of PDT in the management of head and neck cancer.
- While porfimer sodium–mediated PDT is effective, the ***persistence of the photosensitizer in skin necessitates protection of patients from sunlight and other sources*** of bright light for long periods (***up to 90 days***).
- Another limitation is that its longest absorption peak is 630 nm, and this ***interferes with tissue light penetration as a result of absorption by hemoglobin.***

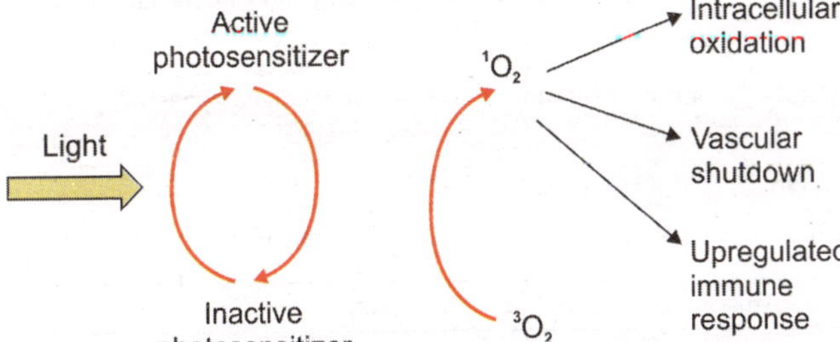

Photodynamic Therapy Illustrated by Process Layout

Photodynamic therapy requires the 3 elements of light, photosensitizer, and oxygen. Light of a specific wavelength activates a specific photosensitizer. ***This activation results in the creation of singlet oxygen, which in turn destroys tissue by intracellular oxidation, shutdown of the microvasculature, and concomitant upregulated immune response at the tumor site and humorally.***

Photodynamic Therapy

◈ *www.cancer.org/treatment/treatments and side effects*

It has some advantages, such as:

- It has no long-term side effects when used properly.
- It's less invasive than surgery.
- It usually takes only a short time and is most often done as an outpatient.
- It can be targeted very precisely.

- Unlike radiation, PDT can be repeated many times at the same site if needed.
- There's usually little or no scarring after the site heals.
- It often costs less than other cancer treatments.

But PDT has limits, too

- PDT can only treat areas where light can reach. This means it's mainly used to treat problems on or just under the skin, or in the lining of organs that can be reached with a light source. Because light can't travel very far through body tissues, PDT can't be used to treat large cancers or cancers that have grown deeply into the skin or other organs.
- PDT can't be used to treat cancers that have spread to many places.
- The drugs used for PDT leave people very sensitive to light for some time, so special precautions must be taken after the drugs are put in or on the body.
- PDT can't be used in people who have certain blood diseases, such as any of the porphyrias (a rare group of diseases that affect the skin or nervous system) or people who are allergic to porphyrins. This allergy is rare, but it may happen in those who have gotten porphyrins in the past.

Table: Current status of approved photodynamic therapy

Year	Photosensitizer	Disease
1993	Porfimer sodium	Early bladder tumors
1996	Porfimer sodium	Obstructive tumor of esophagus
1997	Porfimer sodium	Advance lung and esophageal tumors
1997	Porfimer sodium	Advance lung and esophageal tumors
1997	Porfimer sodium	Early lung cancer
1997	Porfimer sodium	Early esophageal, lung, gastric, cervical cancer
1998	Porfimer sodium	Endobronhial cancer
2000	Verteporfin	Age-related macular degeneration

232. Ans. a. Osteocyte.... c. Chondrocyte.

[Ref: Sumer Sethi 6th/174; Radiology & Imaging by Thayalan 1st/310]

***"Lymphoid tissue & rapidly proliferating tissue, such as spermatids & bone marrow stem cells** are relatively **radiosensitive. Nerve cells are least radiosensitive"** (Radiology & Imaging by Thayalan 1st/310)*

Note: (Sumer Sethi 6th/174)

Most radiosensitive blood cell- Lymphocyte

Least radiosensitive blood cell- Platelet

Most radiosensitive tissue of body- Bone marrow

Least radiosensitive tissue of body-Nervous tissue/brain

Human Cell Radiation Sensitivity

◈ *http://inpp.ohiou.edu/~massey*

- **High**: ***Lymphocytes*** (white blood cells) ***Spermatogonia*** (sperm-producing cells) ***Erythroblasts*** (immature red blood cells) ***Intestinal crypt cells*** (small intestine)
- **Mid: Spermatids** (non-dividing immature sperm) ***Osteoblasts*** (immature bone cells)
- **Low**: Muscle cells & Nerve cells
- **Radiosensitivity of cell (Decreasing order)** *quizlet.com/4498538/effects-of-radiation-exposure*
- White blood cells (lymphocytes) > Red Blood cells (erythrocytes) > Immature reproductive cells> Epithelial Cells >Endothelial cells> Connective tissue cells> Bone cells> Nerve cells> Brain cells> Muscle cells

Cell Radio Sensitivity

◈ *www.nde-ed.org*

- Radio sensitivity is the relative susceptibility of cells, tissues, organs, organisms, or other substances to the injurious action of radiation. In general, it has been found that cell radio sensitivity is directly proportional to the rate of cell division and inversely proportional to the degree of cell differentiation. In short, this means that actively dividing cells or those not fully mature are most at risk from radiation. The most radio-sensitive cells are those which have a high division rate, have a high metabolic rate, are of a non-specialized type & are well nourished

High Radiosensitive
Lymphoid organs, bone marrow, blood, testes, ovaries, intestines
Fairly High Radiosensitive
Skin and other organs with epithelial cell lining (cornea, oral cavity, esophagus, rectum, bladder, vagina, cervix, ureters)
Moderate Radiosensitive
Optic lens, stomach, growing cartilage, fine vasculature, growing bone
Fairly Low Radiosensitive
Mature cartilage or bones, salivary glands, respiratory organs, kidneys, liver, pancreas, thyroid, adrenal and pituitary glands
Low Radiosensitive
Muscle, brain, spinal cord

Extremely radiosensitive	Highly radiosensitive
Bone marrow Lymphoid tissues Testes Ovaries Intestines	Skin Cornea Oral cavity, Oesophagus Rectum Bladder, Ureters Vagina, Uterine cervix
Moderately radiosensitive	**Low radiosensitive**
Optic lens Stomach Growing cartilage/bone Fine vasculature	Mature cartilage/bones Salivary glands Respiratory organs Kidneys, adrenal, pancreas, liver Thyroid, pituitary gland
Least radiosensitive	
Muscle Brain, spinal cord	

233. Ans. b. Provide equal exposure...

[Ref: Sumer Sethi 6th/196-97]

Stereotactic Radiosurgery

◈ *Sumer Sethi 6th/196-97*

- Stereotactic radiosurgery may be performed using a ***linear accelerator or a gamma knife***
- The **goal of stereotactic radiosurgery** is to ***deliver enough radiation to destroy or stop the growth*** of a lesion previously defined by specialized imaging techniques ***without adversely affecting surrounding tissue***
- A **gamma knife** typically contains 201 cobalt-60 sources of approximately 30 curies. An ablative dose of radiation is thereby sent through the tumour in one treatment session, while surrounding brain tissues are relatively spared
- Indications of gamma knife– ***intracranial tumour, arterio-venous malformation & trigeminal neuralgia***

Gamma Knife Radio Surgery

◈ *www.mayoclinic.org*

- ***Gamma Knife radiosurgery is a type of radiation therapy used to treat tumors and other abnormalities in the brain.***
- In Gamma Knife radiosurgery, specialized equipment focuses close to **200 tiny beams** of radiation on a tumor or other target. Although each beam has very little effect on the brain tissue it passes through, a strong dose of radiation is delivered to the site where all the beams meet.
- The precision of Gamma Knife radiosurgery results in ***minimal damage to healthy tissues surrounding*** the target. In some cases, Gamma Knife radiosurgery may have a lower risk of side effects compared with other types of radiation therapy. Also, Gamma Knife radiosurgery is often a safer option than is traditional brain surgery.
- Gamma Knife radiosurgery is usually a one-time therapy completed in a single day.

Gamma Knife

◈ *www.ucsfhealth.org;irsa.org/gamma*

- The Gamma Knife is an advanced radiation treatment for adults and children with small to medium ***brain tumors, abnormal blood vessel formations called arteriovenous malformations, epilepsy, trigeminal neuralgia,*** a nerve condition that causes chronic pain, and other neurological conditions.
- Despite its name, the Gamma Knife isn't a knife but is a ***machine that delivers a single, finely focused, high dose of radiation to its target,*** while causing little or no damage to surrounding tissue. *Abnormalities measuring less than 3 centimeters, or 1 inch in diameter, can be treated with the Gamma Knife.*
- The same as neurosurgery, the Gamma Knife® allows noninvasive **cerebral surgery** to be performed in one session and with extreme precision, sparing tissues adjacent to the target.
- Based on preoperative radiological examinations, such as CT scans, MR scans and angiography, the unit provides ***highly accurate irradiation of deep-seated targets***, using a multitude of collimated beams of ionizing radiation with scalpel-like precision.
- Its development has enhanced neurosurgical treatments offered to patients with brain tumors and vascular malformations by providing a safe, accurate and reliable treatment option. Gamma Knife® enables patients to undergo a non-invasive form of brain surgery ***without surgical risks, a long hospital stay or subsequent rehabilitation.***
- Like other radiosurgery, Gamma Knife® surgery is unique in that no ***surgical incision is made to expose the inside of the brain***, thereby reducing the risk of surgical complications and eliminating the side effects and dangers of general anesthesia.
- ***The "blades" of the Gamma Knife® are the beams of gamma radiation programmed to target the lesion*** at the point where they intersect. In a single treatment session, 201 beams of gamma radiation focus precisely on the lesion. Over time, most lesions slowly decrease in size and dissolve. The exposure is brief and only the tissue being treated receives a significant radiation dose, while the surrounding tissue remains unharmed.
- With the Gamma Knife®, a ***surgical incision is not required;***

234. Ans. a. Co-60..., b. Caesium..., d. Iridium...

[Ref: Sumer Sethi 6th/177, 184; Radiology & Imaging by Thayalan 1st/17, 278

Table *(Sumer Sethi 6th/177, 184)*: **Radiation emitted by Radionuclides**

Radionuclide	Radiation emitted
Radium-226	Gamma rays
Caesium-137	Gamma rays
Cobalt-60	Gamma rays
Iridium-192	Gamma rays
Gold-198	Gamma rays
Samarium -153	Gamma rays
Rhenium-186	Gamma rays & Beta rays
Iodine-131	Gamma rays & Beta rays
Strontium-90	Beta rays
Yttrium-90	Beta rays
Phosphorus-32	Beta rays
Rhenium-188	Beta rays

235. Ans. a. USG

[Ref: Danhert Radiology Manual 7th/368;Harshmohan 7th/902-03;Robbins 9th/333]

Radiological Imaging Aids for FNAC

◈ *Harshmohan 7th/902-03*

- *Non-palpable lesion require some form of localization by radiological aids for FNAC to be carried out.*
- **Plain X-ray films** *are usually adequate for lesions within bones & for some lesions within the chest*
- *FNAC of chest may also be attempted under* **image amplified fluoroscopy** *which allows visualization of needle placement on the television monitor*

- **CT guidance** *is also used for lesions within the chest & abdomen*
- *The* ***most versatile radiological*** *aid is* **ultrasonograpicguidance (USG)** *which allow direct visualization of needle placement in real time & is free from radiation hazards. It is* ***an extremely valuable*** *aid for FNAC of thyroid nodules, soft tissue masses, intra-abdominal lesions & for intrathoracic which abut the chest wall, but no help in deep intrathoracic lesions or in bony lesions*

"**Precision of USG and CT scan** is comparable for guidance in FNAC from thoracic mass lesions" *(ncbi.nlm.nih.gov/pmc/articles)*

"***For biopsies in the breast,*** *ultrasound-guided* ***fine needle biopsy is the most common***"

"**CT-guided FNAC** using a 20-gauge spinal needle is a highly sensitive and specific technique with a good diagnostic accuracy and can be used safely as an outdoor procedure in the ***diagnosis of thoracic masses that are not approachable by ultrasound***" *(jri.org/article.asp)*

"**MRI-guided FNAC** is a cost-effective tool for establishing tissue diagnosis as a primary investigative modality. It is helpful and accurate in the diagnosis of deep lesions in the head and neck and in follow-up of patients, thereby avoiding further surgical intervention" *(ncbi.nlm.nih.gov)*

Fine-needle Aspiration Cytology (FNAC)

- **Fine-needle aspiration biopsy** (**FNAB, FNA** or **NAB**), or **fine-needle aspiration cytology** (**FNAC**), is a diagnostic procedure used to investigate lumps or masses.
- In this technique, a thin, hollow ***needle*** is inserted into the mass for ***sampling*** of cells that, after being stained, will be examined under a ***microscope***. There could be ***cytology*** exam of aspirate (cell specimen evaluation, FNAC) or ***histological*** (***biopsy*** - tissue specimen evaluation, FNAB). Fine-needle aspiration biopsies are very safe, minor ***surgical*** procedures. Often, a major surgical (excisional or open) biopsy can be avoided by performing a needle aspiration biopsy instead.
- Today, this procedure is widely used in the diagnosis of cancer and inflammatory conditions.
- A needle aspiration biopsy is ***safer and less traumatic than an open surgical biopsy***, and significant complications are usually rare, depending on the body site.
- Common complications include bruising and soreness. There is a risk, because the biopsy is very small (only a few cells), that the problematic cells will be missed, resulting in a false negative result. There is also a risk that the cells taken will not enable a definitive diagnosis.
- When the lump can be felt, the biopsy is usually performed by a ***cytopathologist*** or a ***surgeon***. In this case, the procedure is usually short and simple. Otherwise, it may be performed by an interventional ***radiologist***, a doctor with training in performing such biopsies ***under*** *x-ray* ***or*** *ultrasound* ***guidance***. In this case, the procedure may require more extensive preparation and take more time to perform.

236. Ans. b. Hypointense..., c. Hyperintense on..., d. FLAIR reduces...

[Ref: Sumer Sethi 6th/15; Radiology & Imaging by Thayalan 1st/386-89]

MRI Signal Characteristic

- *Sumer Sethi 6th/15*
- CSF: ***Hypointense on T1WI***, hyperintense on T2WI
- ***Grey/White matter:*** Grey matter is grey & white matter s white n T1WI & relationship is reversed on T2WI

"*The* fluid-attenuated inversion-recovery (**FLAIR**) uses longer T1 (2400ms) & TR (7000ms) to reduce the signal level of CSF & other tissue with long T1 relaxation constant. It ***reduces CSF signal*** & other water-bound anatomy in MR image by using a T1 detected at or near the bounce point of CSF"- *Radiology & Imaging by Thayalan 1st/388*

Fluid-attenuated Inversion-recovery (FLAIR)

- *http://www.ajronline.org*
- At many institutions, the ***FLAIR*** pulse sequence has become a routine part of ***MRI*** studies of the ***brain***.
- ***FLAIR MRI*** techniques consist of an inversion recovery pulse to null the signal from ***CSF*** and a long echo time to produce a heavily T2-weighted sequence.
- The ***FLAIR*** technique produces images highly sensitive to T2-weighted prolongation in tissue. In addition, factors that affect the T1-weighted relaxation time of ***CSF*** may interfere with its suppression and result ***in CSF hyperintensity***.
- Compared with conventional T2-weighted and proton density–weighted imaging, use of the ***FLAIR*** sequence improves detection of lesions within the ***subarachnoid space*** and ***brain*** parenchyma, particularly of lesions near the ***brain–CSF*** interface.
- When disease occurs within the ***subarachnoid space***, the relaxation time of ***CSF*** is altered. This change translates into lesser degrees of ***CSF*** signal nulling and ***resultant hyperintensity of the*** *CSF* or ***subarachnoid space*** during the ***FLAIR*** sequence. Such findings have been well described in a wide range of pathologic conditions, such as subarachnoid hemorrhage (SAH), meningitis, and leptomeningeal spread of malignant disease. Other, less common causes of subarachnoid ***FLAIR*** hyperintensity are artifacts. With increased routine use of the ***FLAIR*** sequence, radiologists need to be familiar with the causes of subarachnoid ***FLAIR*** hyperintensity.
- Analysis of the distribution of sulcal ***FLAIR*** hyperintensity and the associated imaging findings related to the primary pathologic condition (e.g., the presence of an adjacent mass) can help elucidate the cause. In many instances, however, particularly when there are no ancillary findings and the distribution is diffuse, the finding remains nonspecific, and clinical correlation alone or in combination with ***CSF*** analysis may be needed. This pictorial essay illustrates the known causes of ***FLAIR*** hyperintensity in the ***subarachnoid space*** and briefly outlines the mechanisms for each of the findings.

237. Ans. b. CO_2

[Ref: Sumer Sethi 6th/20; Radiology & Imaging by Thayalan 1st/159; Danhert Radiology Manual 7th/1147-48]

Radiocontrast Agents

◈ *radiologyinfo.org*

- **Radiocontrast agents** are a type of medical ***contrast medium*** used to improve the visibility of internal bodily structures in ***X-ray***-based imaging techniques such as ***computed tomography*** (CT), ***radiography***, and ***fluoroscopy***. Radiocontrast agents are typically ***iodine*** or ***barium*** compounds. When an agent improves visibility of an area, it is called "contrast enhancing".
- ***Magnetic resonance imaging*** (MRI) functions through different principles and thus utilizes ***different contrast agents***. These compounds work by altering the magnetic properties of nearby hydrogen nuclei.
- When iodine-based and barium-sulfate contrast materials are present in a specific area of the body, they block or limit the ability of x-rays to pass through. As a result, blood vessels, organs and other body tissue that temporarily contain ***iodine-based or barium compounds*** change their appearance on x-ray or CT images.
- **Gadolinium** is the key component of the contrast material most often used in magnetic resonance (MR) exams. When this substance is present in the body, it alters the magnetic properties of nearby water molecules, which enhances the quality of MR images.
- ***Saline (salt water) and air*** are also used as contrast materials in imaging exams. Microbubbles and microspheres have been administered for ultrasound imaging exams, particularly exams of the heart.
- ***Iodine***-based and ***barium-sulfate*** compounds are used in x-ray and computed tomography (CT) imaging exams.

American College of Radiology: 10th Edition (2016) of the ACR Manual on Contrast Media Replaces

- ***Oral, rectal, and intravenous contrast agents*** are utilized in a variety of ways for imaging of the gastrointestinal system. Oral contrast agents are used for fluoroscopic studies, such as dynamic pharyngography, esophagography, upper gastrointestinal (UGI) series, and small bowel follow-through (SBFT) examinations. They are also used to highlight the gastrointestinal tract in routine computed tomography (CT) of the abdomen and pelvis, CT enterography, magnetic resonance imaging (MRI), magnetic resonance enterography, CT colonography, CT positron emission tomography (PET), and MRI-PET.
- Oral agents are also occasionally used to opacify the biliary tree. Rectal contrast media is given for conventional fluoroscopic colon studies and colon cleansing. Rectal contrast media may also opacify the colonic lumen during CT imaging of the abdomen and pelvis. Intravenous contrast media of various types may be used to opacify the biliary tree during CT and MRI cholangiopancreatography, as well as for generalized enhancement of vascularized structures and organs in routine CT and MR of the abdomen and pelvis. Direct injection of contrast media into the biliary and pancreatic ductal systems is performed during endoscopic retrograde cholangiopancreatography (ERCP) and percutaneous antegrade studies of the biliary tree.
- **Barium sulfate contrast media** continue to be the preferred agents for opacification of the gastrointestinal tract for conventional fluoroscopic examinations
- The current use of **iodinated water-soluble** contrast media is primarily limited to select situations
- Two commercial **water-soluble iodinated high-osmolality contrast media (HOCMs)** specifically designed for enteric opacification are in common use. ***Gastrografin*** and ***Gastroview***
- Orally administered contrast media are used for gastrointestinal opacification during routine abdominopelvic **CT**. There is no significant difference in the diagnostic quality of the subsequently obtained CT examinations with ***barium agents, HOCM, or LOCM***, assuming appropriate dilution of contrast material. ***Barium products for oral use in CT*** are commercially available in appropriate concentrations.
- **Indications for CT enterography**: CT enterography is currently used for the CT diagnosis and assessment of inflammatory bowel disease, localizing sites of GI tract bleeding, and, less commonly, for detection of small bowel neoplasms. While small bowel distention can be achieved by the use of high attenuation oral contrast agents (e.g., ***dilute barium or water-soluble iodinated contrast media***), there is increasing use of neutral (low attenuation) contrast agents (e.g., 0.1% w/v ultra-low-dose barium with 2% sorbitol
- Other low attenuation oral contrast agents that have been utilized, albeit much less frequently, for **CT** enterography include ***water, lactulose solution, polyethylene glycol (PEG) electrolyte solution [84], Mucofalk, and methylcellulose.***

238. Ans. b. Work on principle..., d. Gas filled microbubbles...

[Ref: Sumer Sethi 6th/9-10; Radiology & Imaging by Thayalan 1st/334-40]

Contrast-enhanced Ultrasound (CEUS)

◈ *hpubs.rsna.org;en.wikipedia.org*

- It is the application of ***ultrasound contrast medium*** to traditional ***medical sonography***.
- Ultrasound contrast agents rely on the different ways in which sound waves are reflected from interfaces between substances. This may be the surface of a small air bubble or a more complex structure.
- Commercially available contrast media are ***gas-filled*** (air or ***perfluorocarbon)*** microbubbles that are administered intravenously to the ***systemic circulation***. ***Microbubbles have a high degree of echogenicity*** (the ability of an object to reflect ultrasound waves).
- There is a great difference in echogenicity between the gas in the microbubbles and the soft ***tissue*** surroundings of the body. Thus, ***ultrasonic imaging*** using microbubble contrast agents enhances the ultrasound ***backscatter*** (reflection)

of the ultrasound waves, to produce a ***sonogram*** with increased contrast due to the ***high echogenicity difference***.

- Contrast-enhanced ultrasound can be used to image blood ***perfusion*** in organs, measure ***blood flow*** rate in the ***heart*** and other organs, and for other applications.

Ultrasound Imaging

◈ *Radiology & Imaging by Thayalan 1st/334-40*

- ***Diagnostic ultrasound uses 1-20 MHz frequency*** *&* ***the velocity depend on the nature of medium*** *through which it travels & independent of frequency.*
- *It is not an electromagnetic radiation, but undergoes reflection & refraction at interfaces. The reflection from tissue is* ***called echo,*** *which forms the image*
- ***Sound wave travel faster in solids & slower in gases***

USG

◈ *Sumer Sethi 6th/9-10*

- *Ultrasonic image (sonographic/echographic) is based on mechanical oscillations of the crystal excited by electrical pulses* (**piezoelectric effect**)*. Numerous crystal are assembled to form the transducer*
- *Medical ultrasound transducer contains more than one operating frequency. For example, 3-5 Mhz for general abdominal imaging & 7-12 MHz for superficial imaging*
- ***Crystal:*** *PZT Lead ZircnateTitanate*
- *Best for solid vs cystic lesions, minimal fluid*
- *Modes in USG- A mode, B mode & M mode*
- *Advantage- No radiation & portability*
- *Disadvantage- operator dependence*

239. Ans. a. CT scan can..., b. USG can detect very..., c. X-ray-homogenous..., e. MRI can differentiate...

[Ref: Sumer Sethi 6th/49; Danhert Radiology Manual 7th/446; WHO Manual of Radiographic Interpretation 2002/41-42]

What are the Imaging Criteria for Pleural Effusion in CXR

◈ *www.stritch.luc.edu/lumen*

Imaging criteria are:

- **Homogenous density**
- **Density in dependent portion**
  - **Upright:** Costophrenic angle in PA view
  - **Lateral view:** Anterior and posterior portions of gutter
  - **Lateral decubitus position:** Along sides
  - **Supine position:** Along posteriorly, giving diffuse haziness on the side of effusion
- **Silhouette of upper limit of density**
  - Upper margin high in axilla in PA view (yellow arrows)
  - Upper margin high anteriorly and posteriorly in lateral view
  - This is just an illusion
- **Loss of silhouette:** In the images below note lack of identifiable left diaphragm before and visible diaphragm after clearance of fluid (Silhouette sign principle)
- **Mediastinal shift**

Pleural Effusion- X-ray Chest

◈ *WHO Manual of Radiographic Interpretation 2002/41-42*

- A small amount of fluid can difficult to detect
- It is not possible to differentiate b/w different types of pleural effusion e.g., transudate, exudate, blood (haemothorax), pus (empyema), by looking at the X-ray film
- It is very difficult to estimate the amount of fluid radiologically
- It is often difficult to differentiate pleural fluid from pleural thickening or scarring. A decubitus film can be very helpful

Pleural Effusion- X-Ray

◈ *Danhert Radiology Manual 7th/ 446*

- *First 300 ml not visualized on PA view*
- *Lateral decubitus views may detect as little as 25 ml*

Ultrasound

◈ *www.stritch.luc.edu/lumen*

- Ideal for localizing, loculated or small effusions for thoracentesis.
- This can be done at the bedside.
- Debris or septations may be seen in hemothorax or empyema.
- Pleural masses may be seen.
- *USG best investigation to detect minimal fluid*
- US can also guide thoracentesis and placement of tubes into pleural space for drainage.

Ultrasound

◈ *radiopaedia.org*

- Ultrasound allows the detection of small amounts of pleural locular fluid, with positive identification of amounts as small as 3 to 5 ml, that cannot be identified by x-rays, which is only capable of detecting volumes above 50 ml of liquid.
- Contrary to the radiological method, ultrasound allows an ***easy differentiation of pleural locular liquid and thickened pleura***. And it's efficient in pinpointing thoracocentesis, even in small fluid collections
- The ultrasound image of ***pleural effusion*** is characterized by an echo-free space between the visceral and parietal ***pleura***. Septations (if seen) in the pleural fluid may indicate tuberculous pathology.
- Ultrasound can also be used to enable percutaneous diagnostic or therapeutic drainage ***(thoracocentesis)***.

CT

◈ *radiopaedia.org*

- CT scanning is excellent at detecting small amounts of fluid and is also often able to identify the underlying ***intrathoracic causes*** (e.g. ***malignant pleural deposits*** or ***primary lung neoplasms***) as well as ***subdiaphragmatic diseases*** (e.g. ***subdiaphragmatic abscess***).
- In addition CT can also help ***distinguish between a*** *pleural effusion* ***and a*** *pleural empyema*
- CT can also guide placement of tubes into pleural space for drainage.

Pleural Effusion-CT Scan

◈ *Danhert Radiology Manual 7th/ 446*

- Fluid outside diaphragm
- Fluid elevating crus of diaphragm
- Indistinct fluid-liver interface
- Fluid posteromedial to liver (= bare area of liver)

Magnetic Resonance Imaging

◈ *emedicine.medscape*

- MRI can help in evaluating the ***etiology of the pleural effusion***. Nodularity and/or irregularity of the pleural contour, circumferential pleural thickening, mediastinal pleural involvement, and infiltration of the chest wall and/or diaphragm are suggestive of a malignant cause both on CT scans and MRIs.
- It has been suggested that MRI signal intensity is a valuable tool for differentiating ***malignant from benign pleural disease***.
- Malignant pleural lesions are typically enhancing on contrast-enhanced T1-weighted images and hyperintense on proton density– and T2-weighted images. A pleural lesion with low signal intensity on images obtained with a long repetition time is a reliable and predictive sign of benign disease. Pleural calcification likely indicates a benign cause.
- The **signal intensity of the pleural fluids depends** on their biochemical characteristics. In most cases of nonhemorrhagic or nonchylous effusions, the fluids have high signal intensity on T2-weighted images and low signal intensity on T1-weighted images.
- The combination of MRI signal intensity and morphologic features is more useful than, and superior to, CT scanning in differentiating malignant from benign pleural disease.

ANSWER SHEET

1 – 50	51 – 100	101 – 150	151 – 200	201 – 250
1 A B C D E	51 A B C D E	101 A B C D E	151 A B C D E	201 A B C D E
2 A B C D E	52 A B C D E	102 A B C D E	152 A B C D E	202 A B C D E
3 A B C D E	53 A B C D E	103 A B C D E	153 A B C D E	203 A B C D E
4 A B C D E	54 A B C D E	104 A B C D E	154 A B C D E	204 A B C D E
5 A B C D E	55 A B C D E	105 A B C D E	155 A B C D E	205 A B C D E
6 A B C D E	56 A B C D E	106 A B C D E	156 A B C D E	206 A B C D E
7 A B C D E	57 A B C D E	107 A B C D E	157 A B C D E	207 A B C D E
8 A B C D E	58 A B C D E	108 A B C D E	158 A B C D E	208 A B C D E
9 A B C D E	59 A B C D E	109 A B C D E	159 A B C D E	209 A B C D E
10 A B C D E	60 A B C D E	110 A B C D E	160 A B C D E	210 A B C D E
11 A B C D E	61 A B C D E	111 A B C D E	161 A B C D E	211 A B C D E
12 A B C D E	62 A B C D E	112 A B C D E	162 A B C D E	212 A B C D E
13 A B C D E	63 A B C D E	113 A B C D E	163 A B C D E	213 A B C D E
14 A B C D E	64 A B C D E	114 A B C D E	164 A B C D E	214 A B C D E
15 A B C D E	65 A B C D E	115 A B C D E	165 A B C D E	215 A B C D E
16 A B C D E	66 A B C D E	116 A B C D E	166 A B C D E	216 A B C D E
17 A B C D E	67 A B C D E	117 A B C D E	167 A B C D E	217 A B C D E
18 A B C D E	68 A B C D E	118 A B C D E	168 A B C D E	218 A B C D E
19 A B C D E	69 A B C D E	119 A B C D E	169 A B C D E	219 A B C D E
20 A B C D E	70 A B C D E	120 A B C D E	170 A B C D E	220 A B C D E
21 A B C D E	71 A B C D E	121 A B C D E	171 A B C D E	221 A B C D E
22 A B C D E	72 A B C D E	122 A B C D E	172 A B C D E	222 A B C D E
23 A B C D E	73 A B C D E	123 A B C D E	173 A B C D E	223 A B C D E
24 A B C D E	74 A B C D E	124 A B C D E	174 A B C D E	224 A B C D E
25 A B C D E	75 A B C D E	125 A B C D E	175 A B C D E	225 A B C D E
26 A B C D E	76 A B C D E	126 A B C D E	176 A B C D E	226 A B C D E
27 A B C D E	77 A B C D E	127 A B C D E	177 A B C D E	227 A B C D E
28 A B C D E	78 A B C D E	128 A B C D E	178 A B C D E	228 A B C D E
29 A B C D E	79 A B C D E	129 A B C D E	179 A B C D E	229 A B C D E
30 A B C D E	80 A B C D E	130 A B C D E	180 A B C D E	230 A B C D E
31 A B C D E	81 A B C D E	131 A B C D E	181 A B C D E	231 A B C D E
32 A B C D E	82 A B C D E	132 A B C D E	182 A B C D E	232 A B C D E
33 A B C D E	83 A B C D E	133 A B C D E	183 A B C D E	233 A B C D E
34 A B C D E	84 A B C D E	134 A B C D E	184 A B C D E	234 A B C D E
35 A B C D E	85 A B C D E	135 A B C D E	185 A B C D E	235 A B C D E
36 A B C D E	86 A B C D E	136 A B C D E	186 A B C D E	236 A B C D E
37 A B C D E	87 A B C D E	137 A B C D E	187 A B C D E	237 A B C D E
38 A B C D E	88 A B C D E	138 A B C D E	188 A B C D E	238 A B C D E
39 A B C D E	89 A B C D E	139 A B C D E	189 A B C D E	239 A B C D E
40 A B C D E	90 A B C D E	140 A B C D E	190 A B C D E	240 A B C D E
41 A B C D E	91 A B C D E	141 A B C D E	191 A B C D E	241 A B C D E
42 A B C D E	92 A B C D E	142 A B C D E	192 A B C D E	242 A B C D E
43 A B C D E	93 A B C D E	143 A B C D E	193 A B C D E	243 A B C D E
44 A B C D E	94 A B C D E	144 A B C D E	194 A B C D E	244 A B C D E
45 A B C D E	95 A B C D E	145 A B C D E	195 A B C D E	245 A B C D E
46 A B C D E	96 A B C D E	146 A B C D E	196 A B C D E	246 A B C D E
47 A B C D E	97 A B C D E	147 A B C D E	197 A B C D E	247 A B C D E
48 A B C D E	98 A B C D E	148 A B C D E	198 A B C D E	248 A B C D E
49 A B C D E	99 A B C D E	149 A B C D E	199 A B C D E	249 A B C D E
50 A B C D E	100 A B C D E	150 A B C D E	200 A B C D E	250 A B C D E

NAME OF THE CANDIDATE	ROLL NO.					CENTRE NO.		QUESTION BOOKLET NO.					BOOKLET CODE
CATEGORY	0	0	0	0	0	0	0	0	0	0	0	0	A
	1	1	1	1	1	1	1	1	1	1	1	1	B
SC ○	2	2	2	2	2	2	2	2	2	2	2	2	C
ST ○	3	3	3	3	3	3	3	3	3	3	3	3	D
OBC ○	4	4	4	4	4	4	4	4	4	4	4	4	
GEN ○	5	5	5	5	5	5	5	5	5	5	5	5	
CW ○	6	6	6	6	6	6	6	6	6	6	6	6	
PH ○	7	7	7	7	7	7	7	7	7	7	7	7	
	8	8	8	8	8	8	8	8	8	8	8	8	
	9	9	9	9	9	9	9	9	9	9	9	9	

INSTRUCTIONS FOR FILLING THE SHEET

1. This sheet should not be folded or crushed.
2. Use only blue/black ball pen to fill the circles.
3. Use of pencil is strictly prohibited.
4. Circles should be darkened properly and completely.
5. Cutting & erasing on this sheet is not allowed.
6. Do not use any stray marks on the sheet.
7. Do not use marker, white fluid or any other device to hide the shading already done.

WRONG METHOD

CORRECT METHOD

CANDIDATE'S SIGNATURE
(in ball - point pen)

INVIGILATOR'S SIGNATURE
(in ball - point pen)

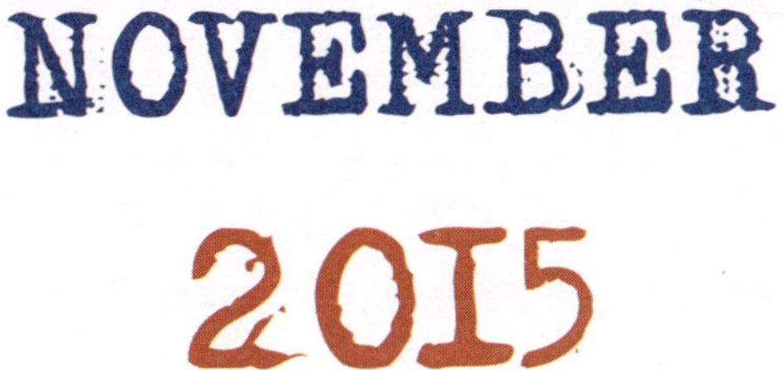

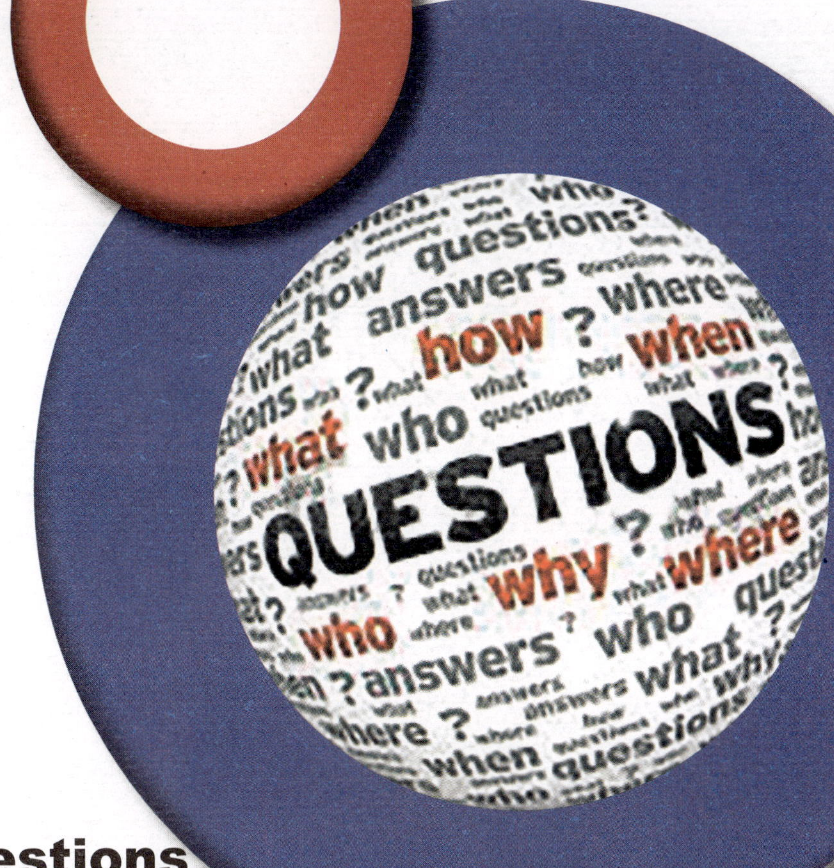

Multiple Choice Questions
Answers & Explanations

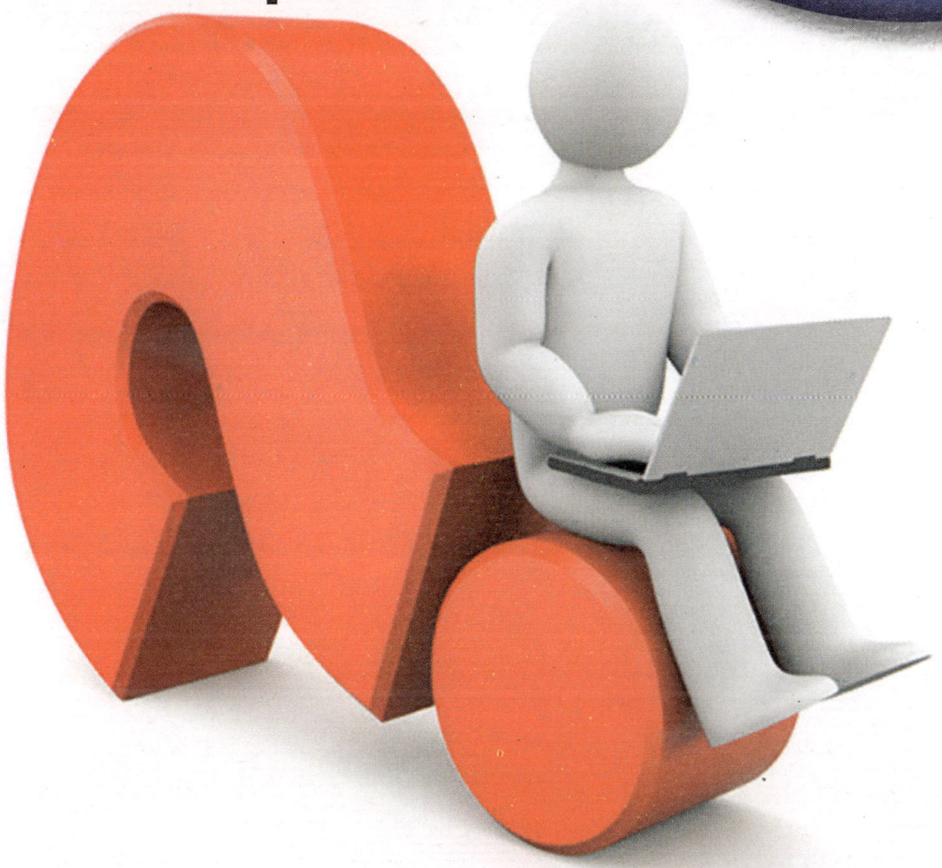

NOVEMBER 2015 MULTIPLE CHOICE QUESTIONS

ANATOMY

1. **True statement about development of pancreas:**
   a. Uncinate process from ventral bud
   b. Lower part of head from dorsal bud
   c. Duct of Wirsung develops from dorsal bud only
   d. Pancreatic divisum is due to abnormal development of ducts of pancreas
   e. Body is formed from dorsal bud
2. **Which of the following combination is/are true regarding epithelial lining of urinary system:**
   a. Urinary bladder- transitional epithelium
   b. Pre-prostatic urethra- stratified columnar
   c. Membranous urethra- transitional epithelium
   d. Distal part of penile urethra- non-keratinising stratified squamous epithelium
   e. Urethral meatus- keratinising stratified squamous epithelium
3. **Which of the following statement is/are true regarding lesion of IX CN:**
   a. Gag reflex-absent
   b. Deviation of tongue to one side
   c. Loss of taste sensation in the posterior 1/3 of the tongue
   d. Loss of taste sensation in the anterior 2/3 of the tongue
   e. May cause bulbar palsy
4. **Feature(s) of oculomotor nerve palsy is/are:**
   a. Ptosis
   b. Miosis
   c. Mydriasis
   d. Diplopia
   e. Loss of accomodation
5. **Cervix is/are drained by:**
   a. External iliac lymph node
   b. Internal iliac lymph node
   c. Aortic lymph node
   d. Inguinal lymph node
   e. Sacral lymph node
6. **Which of the following may occur in common peroneal nerve injury:**
   a. Dorsiflexion not possible
   b. Foot drop
   c. High stepping gait
   d. Loss of inversion of foot
   e. Eversion of foot affected
7. **O'Donoghue's triad comprises of:**
   a. Anterior cruciate ligament tear
   b. Posterior cruciate ligament tear
   c. Medial meniscus
   d. Lateral meniscus
   e. Medial collateral ligament
8. **Which of the following vein(s) is/are part of portal circulation:**
   a. Splenic vein
   b. Paraumbilical vein
   c. Superior rectal vein
   d. Left gastric vein
   e. Inferior rectal vein
9. **Thrombosis of anterior cerebral artery cause:**
   a. Left foot paralysis in right anterior cerebral artery thrombosis
   b. Urinary incontinence
   c. Paralysis of the contralateral face, arm, and leg
   d. Homonymous hemianopia
   e. Gegenhalten rigidity
10. **Fibrocartilage is/are found in:**
    a. Temporomandibular joint
    b. Sternoclavicular joint
    c. Hip joint
    d. Vertebral disc
    e. Inferior radioulnar joint

PHYSIOLOGY

11. **Parasympathetic nerve stimulation results in:**
    a. Sphincter closure of gallbladder
    b. Increased peristalsis
    c. Decreased GIT motility
    d. Detrusor muscle relaxation
    e. Gallbladder musculature contraction
12. **True about muscle spindle:**
    a. Group Ia fiber contain sensory afferent
    b. Nuclear bag & nuclear chain fibers present in intrafusal muscle fiber
    c. Motor supply by Aα fiber
    d. Motor supply by γ fiber
    e. Secondary ending is stimulated by nuclear bag fiber
13. **Hyperbaric oxygen therapy is/are used in:**
    a. Radiation induced proctitis
    b. Tension pneumothorax
    c. Bleomycin induced lung damage
    d. Gas gangrene
    e. Carbon mono-oxide poisoning
14. **Peripheral cyanosis is/are associated with:**
    a. SLE
    b. TAPVC
    c. Atrial septal defect
    d. Methemoglobinemia
    e. Cardiogenic shock

Answer

1. a, d, e.	2. a, d, e.	3. a, c, e.	4. a, b, d, e.	5. a, b, e.	6. a, b, c, e.	7. a, c, e.
8. a, b, c, d.	9. a, b, e.	10. a, b, d, e.	11. b, e.	12. a, b, d.	13. a, d, e.	14. e.

15. **Blood in foetus is/are formed by:**
    a. Liver
    b. Lymph nodes
    c. Spleen
    d. Bone marrow
    e. Yolk sac
16. **Important buffer system operating in blood:**
    a. Protein system buffer
    b. Phosphate buffer
    c. Carbonic acid- Bicarbonate system buffer
    d. Hemoglobin system buffer

BIOCHEMISTRY

17. **True about collagen:**
    a. Double helix structure
    b. Single helix structure
    c. Triple helix structure
    d. β-pleated structure
    e. Component of connective tissue of body
18. **At isoelectric point (pI) net charge of amino acis is:**
    a. –1
    b. +1
    c. –2
    d. +1
    e. 0
19. **Hexosaminidase A deficiency causes:**
    a. Niemann-pick
    b. Tay-Sachs disease
    c. Hurler syndrome
    d. Gaucher's disease
    e. Krabbe's disease
20. **Mitchondrial matrix contains enzymes of:**
    a. Pyruvate dehydrogenase
    b. TCA cycle enzyme
    c. Acyl CoA synthetase
    d. ATP synthase
    e. β-oxidation enzymes
21. **Which of the following group(s) are present in natural amino acids:**
    a. Imidazole group
    b. Tetrapyrrole group
    c. Indole group
    d. Guanidinium group
    e. Keto group
22. **Which of the following vitamin deficiency cause triad of mental confusion, ophthalmoplegia & ataxia:**
    a. Vit B2
    b. Vit B1
    c. Vit B6
    d. Vit C
    e. Vit. B12
23. **Which of the following enzyme(s) is/are involved in gluconeogenesis:**
    a. Pyruvate carboxylase
    b. Phosphoenolpyruvate carboxykinase
    c. Phosphofructokinase-1
    d. Glucose 6-phosphatase
    e. Pyruvate dehydrogenase
24. **Gel used in electrophoresis is/are:**
    a. Agarose gel
    b. Polyacrylamide plain gel
    c. Polyacrylamide SDS (Sodium dodecyl sulphate) impregnated Polyacrylamide gel

IMMUNOGENETICS & MOLECULAR BIOLOGY

25. **Which of the following method(s) is/are used for detection of nucleic acid:**
    a. Northern blotting
    b. Southern blotting
    c. Western blotting
    d. Microarray
    e. ELISA
26. **True regarding reverse transcriptase:**
    a. Help in synthesis of DNA from RNA
    b. Help in synthesis of RNA from DNA
    c. RNA-dependent DNA polymerase
    d. DNA-dependent RNA polymerase
    e. Involved in protein synthesis
27. **Which of the following is purine:**
    a. Adenine
    b. Cytosine
    c. Thymine
    d. Guanine
    e. Urracil
28. **True about restriction endonuclease:**
    a. Protects bacteria by cleaving the DNA of infecting viruses
    b. Protects bacteria by methylating the DNA of infecting viruses
    c. Present only in eukaryotes
    d. RE II has methylase activity
    e. Also known as molecular scissor

PATHOLOGY

29. **True about miliary tuberculosis:**
    a. Occur primarily due to hematogenous spread
    b. Miliary lesion is generally of size 1-2 mm
    c. Diffuse bilateral crepitation is always present
    d. Onset is generally acute
    e. Sputum smear microscopy is negative in 80% of cases
30. **Which of the following cancer spread primarily by hematogenous route:**
    a. Papillary carcinoma thyroid
    b. Renal cell carcinoma
    c. Pheochromocytoma
    d. Glioblastoma multiforme
    e. Follicular carcinoma of thyroid

Answer

15. All	16. a, c, d.	17. c, e.	18. e.	19. b.	20. a, b, d.	21. a, b, c, d.
22. b.	23. a, b, d.	24. All	25. a, b, d.	26. a, c.	27. a, d.	28. a, e.
29. a, b, e.	30. b, c, e.					

31. Presentation of Pierre-Robin syndrome includes:
a. Retrognathia
b. Low set ear
c. Prominent forehead
d. Isolated cleft palate
e. Glossoptosis

32. True about mammalian mitochondrial DNA:
a. Contains around 16500 nucleotide sequence
b. Makes up around 3% total cellular DNA
c. Makes up around 10% total cellular DNA
d. Makes up around 0.3% total cellular DNA
e. Makes up around 1% total cellular DNA

33. High level of β hCG is/are seen in all except:
a. Down syndrome
b. Neural tube defect
c. Germ cell tumor
d. Gestational trophoblastic disease
e. Multiple pregnancy

34. Human papilloma virus is/are associated with all except:
a. Oropharyngeal tumors
b. Carcinoma nasophraynx
c. Carcinoma anal canal
d. Carcinoma pancreas
e. Carcinoma cervix

35. True about Hodgkin's lymphoma :
a. Often localized to single axial group of lymph node
b. Hepatomegaly is always present
c. Contiguous spread of lymph node
d. Can be cured by chemotherapy & radiotherapy
e. Commonly resents with painless lymphadenopathy

36. CD 30 is/are marker for:
a. Anaplastic large cell lymphoma
b. Embryonal cell carcinoma
c. Squamous Cell Carcinoma
d. Seminoma
e. Hodgkin's lymphoma

37. All are true about intestinal polyp syndrome except:
a. Cowden disease- Hamartomatous polyps
b. Hereditary nonpolyposis colorectal carcinoma(HNPCC)- Multiple adenomatous polyps
c. Peutz-Jeghers syndrome-associated with colonic carcinoma
d. Colonic hyperplastic polyp has malignant potential
e. Cronkhite-Canada syndrome- may have associated breast tumour

38. Increased thickness of gastric mucosal fold is seen in:
a. Menetrier's disease
b. Gastritis cystica
c. Boerhaave syndrome
d. Zollinger-Ellison syndrome

39. Blood transfusion reaction can leads to:
a. Acute glomerulonephritis
b. Myoglobinuria
c. Hemoglobinuria
d. Transfusion-related acute lung injury
e. Acute renal tubular necrosis

40. Not seen in post streptococcal glomerulonephritis(PSGN):
a. Nephrotic range proteinuria
b. Neutrophilic infiltration of tubules
c. Subepithelial deposits
d. Linear deposits along glomerular basement membrane

41. True about fibrolamellar carcinoma of liver:
a. Better prognosis than typical hepatocellular carcinoma
b. Associated with cirrhosis
c. AFP-positive
d. Occur in younger adults
e. More common in females

42. Chromosomal abnormalities in Down syndrome is/are due to:
a. Nondisjunctional of maternal chromosome
b. Nondisjunctional of paternal chromosome
c. Translocations between chromosome 21 & 14
d. Disjunction of paternal chromosome
e. Disjuction of maternal chromosome

43. Schaumann bodies are not seen in :
a. Sarcoidosis
b. Histoplasmosis
c. Cryptococcosis
d. Hypersensitivity pneumonitis
e. Tuberculosis

44. Neuroendocrine cell tumour markers are:
a. Chromogranin A
b. CD56
c. Neuron-specific enolase
d. Synaptophysin
e. Cytokeratin 7

45. All are true about focal nodular hyperplasia except:
a. Multiple nodule may present
b. More common in male
c. May be associated with contraceptive pills use
d. Hypovascular on the arterial-phase and hypervascular on the delayed-phase CT images
e. CT is less sensitive than MRI in depicting the characteristic central scar

PHARMACOLOGY

46. All are true about tamoxifen except:
a. Used as adjuvant therapy in estrogen receptor positive breast cancer
b. No effect on uterus
c. Pro-estrogen effect on bone
d. Reduces chance of osteoporosis
e. Reduces coronary artery diseases

Answer

31. a, d, e.	32. a, e.	33. b.	34. b, d.	35. a, c, d, e.	36. a, b, e.	37. d.
38. a, b, d.	39. c, d, e.	40. a, b, d.	41. a, d, e.	42. a, b, c.	43. b, c.	44. a, b, c, d.
45. b.	46. b, e.					

47. True about Hyoscine:
a. Cause mydriasis
b. Cause miosis
c. Used for motion sickness
d. Better BBB penetration than atropine
e. Central nervous system depressant

48. True statement(s) about Rutin:
a. Has anti-fibrinolytic action
b. Has anti-platelet action
c. Antioxidant property
d. A citrus flavonoid glycoside found in many plants including buckwheat

49. Which of the following is/are 3rd generation cephalosprorin:
a. Cefotaxime b. Ceftazidime
c. Ceftabiprole d. Cefixime
e. Cefpirome

50. Side-effect(s) of Zoledronic acid is/are all except:
a. Flu-like symptoms b. Osteonecrosis of the jaw
c. Dizziness d. Constipation
e. Renal toxicity

51. Anti-microbial agents acting on nucleic acid are all except:
a. Acyclovir b. Linezolid
c. Fluroquinolones d. Streptomycin
e. Rifampin

52. Anti-metabolite drugs are:
a. Methotrexate b. Daunorubicin
c. Doxorubicin d. Gemcitabine
e. Bleomycin

53. Side-effect(s) of fluroquinolones include:
a. Aseptic meningitis
b. Hyperkeratosis of palm and sole
c. Tendinitis
d. Constipation e. Photosensitivity

54. Phosphodiesterase-5 inhibitor(s) is/are:
a. Sildenafil b. Tadalafil
c. Acomprostate d. Alprostadil
e. Vardenafil

55. CNS stimulants are:
a. Cocaine b. Amphetamine
c. Cannabis d. Dexamphetamine
e. MDMA (ecstasy)

56. Drug contraindicated in pregnancy:
a. Sulfonamide b. ACE inhibitors
c. Phenytoin d. Ciprofloxacin
e. Furosemide

57. In which of the following liver flukes, triclabendazole is/are used:
a. Clonorchis sinensis b. Opisthorchis viverrini
c. Fasciola hepatica d. Fasciola gigantica
e. Opisthorchis felineus

MICROBIOLOGY

58. Griffith conducted transformation experiment in:
a. Salmonella b. Streptococcus pneumoniae
c. E.coli d. Staphylococcus

59. True about Ebola virus:
a. Ribavirin is very useful
b. Spread by droplet contact
c. Transmitted by sexual contact
d. Spread by direct contact with the blood or other body fluid

60. True about chancroid:
a. Bacilli causing the disease shows School of fish appearance
b. Painful ulcer
c. Incubation period is 10-90 day
d. Presents as painless lymphadenopathy
e. Sharply demarcated & elevated edge

61. Which of the following spread by ingestion of eggs:
a. Strongyloides b. Trichinella
c. Trichuris d. Ascaris
e. Ancylostoma duodenale

62. To check the efficiency of the heat sterilization, which of the following microbe is/are used:
a. Geobacillus stearothermophilus
b. Bacillus subtilis
c. Salmonella
d. Pneumococcus
e. Bacillus stearothermophilus

63. Dimorphic fungi are all except:
a. Blastomycosis dermatitidis
b. Coccidioides immitis
c. Histoplasma capsulatum
d. Cryptococcus neoformans

64. Which of the following is/are true regarding disease caused by enterovirus:
a. Coxsackie virus B causes pleurodynia
b. Enterovirus 71 causes aseptic meningitis
c. Enterovirus 71 cause pericarditis
d. Coxsackie virus A encephalitis

65. All are true about cytomegalovirus except:
a. May be transmitted from pregnant mother to foetus
b. Type 5 Human herpes virus
c. Lymphocyte enlargement
d. Cause congenital diseases
e. May lead to fetal death

66. True about bacteriorhodopsin:
a. Present in the cell membrane
b. It acts as proton pump
c. Generate ATP
d. Use light energy
e. Same as rhodopsin found in human

Answer

47. a, c, d, e.	48. b, c, d.	49. a, b, d.	50. d.	51. b, d.	52. a, d.	53. c, e.
54. a, b, e.	55. a, b, d, e.	56. b, c.	57. c, d,	58. b.	59. c, d.	60. a, b, d.
61. c, d.	62. a, b, e.	63. d.	64. a, b, d.	65. c.	66. a, b, c, d.	

FORENSIC MEDICINE

67. True statement(s) regarding the power of chief judicial magistrate:

a. Can give imprisonment of <3 year only
b. Can give imprisonment of any duration
c. Can give imprisonment up to 5 year
d. Can give imprisonment up to 7 year
e. Can impose unlimited fine

68. Which of the following feature is/are related to mandible of male in comparison to female:

a. Ascending ramus- smaller breadth
b. Angle of ramus- More obtuse
c. Larger condyle
d. Mental tubercles- larger & prominent
e. Symphyseal height more

69. Which of the following statement is/are true about carbamate poisoning:

a. Cause pinpoint pupil
b. Atropine is antidote
c. Adrenergic action
d. Spontaneously hydrolyses from the cholinesterase enzymatic site
e. CNS toxicity is more as compared to organophosphorus

70. All are included in rape except:

a. Insertion of finger in urethra
b. Inserting object in cervix
c. Kissing
d. Oral sex
e. Rubbing finger on vagina

71. Which of the following is true about rigor mortis in comparison to cadaveric spasm:

a. Mechanism of rigor mortis is same as cadaveric spasm
b. Death clutch is seen in cadaveric spasm
c. Generally occurs 2-3 hours after death
d. Involves only certain groups of voluntary muscles

72. Post-mortem caloricity is/are seen in all except:

a. Strychnine poisoning
b. Septicaemic condition
c. Cholera
d. Barbiturate poisoning
e. Tetanus

73. Treatment of carbolic acid poisoning includes:

a. Repeated lavage should be done
b. Intubation may be required in case of respiratory compromise
c. Emetics is very beneficial
d. Saline containing sodium carbonate is given i.v

SPM

74. Which of the following is/are true about vasectomy:

a. May affects erection of penis after procedure
b. Additional contraceptive is generally needed for around 12 weeks
c. Highly effective method of family planning
d. Minor surgical procedure
e. Incidence of recanalization is around 10% after procedure

75. All are elements of primary health care except:

a. Adequate supply of safe water
b. Provision of free essential drugs only to poor
c. Promotion of food supply & proper nutrition
d. Prevention & control of locally endemic disease
e. Education concerning health problems

76. MMR (Measles, mumps, rubella) vaccine is an example of:

a. Live attenuated vaccine
b. Conjugated vaccine
c. Polysaccharide vaccine
d. Killed vaccine
e. Toxiod

77. All are steps of investigation of an epidemic except:

a. Verify the diagnosis
b. Before starting investigation, inform the media
c. Formulation of hypotheses
d. Confirmation of existence of an epidemic
e. Plan & implement control measures

78. Which of the following is/are method of health communication:

a. Lecture
b. Imitation
c. Group discussion
d. Panel discussion
e. Role play

79. All are true about lepromatous leprosy(LL) except:

a. Multibacillary(MB)- Multi drug therapy(MDT) is given for treatment
b. On split stain-multiple bacilli
c. Sensation present in lesions
d. Multiple symmetrical skin lesion present
e. Lepromin test positive

80. Which of the following is part of national health policy 2015 draft except:

a. Increase GDP share to health to 5%
b. Assure universal availability of free, comprehensive primary health care services, as an entitlement, for all aspects of reproductive, maternal, child and adolescent health
c. Provision of right to health
d. Engage private doctors
e. Enable universal access to free essential drugs & diagnostics in public health facilities

Answer

67. d, e.	68. c, d, e.	69. b, d.	70. c.	71. b, c.	72. d.	73. a, b, d.
74. b, c, d.	75. b.	76. a.	77. b.	78. a, c, d, e.	79. e.	80. a.

OPHTHALMOLOGY

81. Which of the following vitamin deficiency can cause centrocecal scotoma:
a. Vit A
b. Vit E
c. B6
d. B2
e. B12

82. True about electroretinogram:
a. a wave- arises from rods and cones
b. b wave - d/t activity of bipolar cells
c. b-wave response is subnormal in early cases of retinitis pigmentosa
d. c wave - representing metabolic activity of pigment epithelium
e. Best disease shows abnormal ERG

83. True about Ciliary body:
a. It forms aqueous humour
b. Anterior smooth part is called pars plana
c. Ciliary processes are finger-like projections from the pars plicata part
d. Ciliary muscles help in accommodation

84. Which of the following statement(s) is/are true about Jones dye test:
a. Done for assessment of epiphora
b. Positive test-1: primary hypersecretion
c. Negative test-1: partial obstruction or failure of lacrimal pump mechanism.
d. Positive test-2: failure of lacrimal pump mechanism
e. Negative test-2: partial obstruction

85. True about Kayser-Fleischer ring:
a. Deposition of copper
b. Deposition of iron
c. Found in Wilson disease
d. Deposition under Descemet's membrane of the cornea

86. Ectopia entis is/are associated with:
a. Homocystinuria
b. Alport syndrome
c. Lowe syndrome
d. Marfan syndrome
e. Sulphite oxidase deficiency

87. True about congenital esotropia:
a. Amblyopia may develops
b. Angle of deviation is usually fixed & large
c. Surgery should be done after 2 year
d. Onset only after 1 year of age
e. May be associated with inferior oblique overaction

ENT

88. Which is true about Tuning fork test in hearing loss:
a. Rinne test is negative in conductive deafness
b. Weber test- lateralized to the worst ear in sensorineural deafness
c. Lateralization of sound in Weber test with a tunning fork of 512 Hz implies a conductive loss of 15-20 dB in ipsilateral ear
d. Negative Rinne test indicates a minimum air-bone gap of 15-20 dB
e. A Rinne negative for all the three tunning forks of 256,512 & 1024 Hz indicates air-bone gap of 30-45

89. Which of the following causes lower motor neuron(LMN) type of facial nerve paralysis:
a. Bell palsy
b. Parotid tumor
c. Guillain-Barré syndrome
d. Middle cerebral artery infarct
e. Multiple sclerosis

90. True about tympanometry:
a. Flat in ossiccular discontinuity
b. As type in otosclerosis
c. Dome shaped indicates fluid in middle ear
d. Ad type in ossiccular discontinuity
e. C type in eustachian tube obstruction

91. True about bilateral abductor paralysis:
a. Voice is good
b. Stridor is present
c. Cords lie in abducted position
d. Urgent tracheostomy is needed

92. All are true about mandible fracture except:
a. Condylar neck is most common site
b. Malocclusion of teeth may occur
c. Anterior superior alveolar nerve is most commonly injured
d. Panorex radiographs are useful for diagnosis
e. Malunion& non-union are complications

93. True about chronic suppurative otitis media (CSOM):
a. Foul smelling discharge in atticoantral variety
b. Facial nerve involvement in tubotympanic variety
c. Atticoantral variety is associate with cholestetoma
d. May cause hearing loss

94. True about ranula:
a. Mucous retention cyst
b. Seen in floor of mouth
c. Marsupialization for large cyst
d. Parotid is most common site of origin
e. Arises from sublingual salivary gland

95. Not a premalignant lesion of oral cavity:
a. Leukoplakia
b. Erythroplakia
c. Lichen planus
d. Apthus ulcer
e. Submucosal fibrosis

MCQs

Answer

81. e.	82. a, b, c, d.	83. a, c, d.	84. a, b, c.	85. a, c, d.	86. a, d, e.	87. a, b, e.
88. a, c, d.	89. a, b, c.	90. b, c, d, e.	91. a, b, d.	92. c.	93. a, c, d.	94. a, b, c, e.
95. d.						

MEDICINE

96. Hain test is/are used for:

a. Detection of INH resistance only
b. Detection of rifampicin resistance only
c. Detection of both rifampicin & INH resistance
d. Detection of resistance of all drugs of first line ATT

97. True about Pulmonary artery catheterization (Swan-Ganz catheter placement):

a. Measures right atrial pressure
b. Measures left ventricular filling pressure
c. Measure PCWP
d. Inserted through left subclavian vein
e. Measures central venous pressure

98. Presentation of tabes dorsalis includes:

a. Lancinating pain in leg
b. Loss of proprioception
c. Sensory defect
d. No involvement of bladder & bowel
e. Sensory ataxia

99. True about Prinzmetal's angina:

a. May present at rest
b. Occurs due atherosclerotic obstruction of coronary arteries
c. Smoking is a risk factor
d. Nitrates are used for treatment
e. CCBs are used for treatment

100. Which of the following is/are true about Revised Jones Criteria 2015 of AHA for diagnosis of acute rheumatic fever:

a. Polyarthritis in low-risk populations is a major criteria
b. Polyarthralgia in moderate- and high-risk populations is a minor criteria
c. Monoarthritis in moderate- and high-risk populations is a major criteria
d. Echocardiography with Doppler study should be performed in all cases of confirmed and suspected ARF
e. Echocardiography/Doppler study should be performed to assess whether carditis is present in the absence of auscultatory findings

101. Feature(s) of increased ICP is/are:

a. Hypotension
b. Decrease HR
c. Increase HR
d. Hypertension
e. Decreased level of consciousness

102. All are true about Hepatitis E except:

a. May be fatal in pregnant women
b. May cause acute liver failure
c. Carrier state is common
d. Majority progress to chronicity
e. Feco-oral transmission

103. Which of the following feature favours diagnosis of chronic renal failure rather than acute renal failure:

a. Anaemia
b. Renal osteodystrophy
c. Raised creatinine level
d. Peripheral neuropathy
e. Small kidney

104. Which of the following is/are true about sarcoidosis:

a. Show cutaneous anergy
b. High CD4/CD8 ratio
c. Schauman bodies is pathognomic of sarcoidosis
d. May be associated with uveitis

105. Which of the following cranial nerve is/are involved in Gag reflex:

a. 9
b. 10
c. 11
d. 12
e. 7

106. Which of the following is/are true about Duchene muscular dystrophy:

a. Mental impairment may present
b. ↑Serum CK levels
c. Cardiomyopathy may be present
d. Autosomal recessive disorder
e. Onset during puberty

107. True about acute intermittent porphyria:

a. Occur due to deficiency of enzyme HMB-synthase
b. Uroporphyrin is present in urine
c. Abdominal pain is common symptom
d. ↑ Porphobilinogen in the urine
e. Leukocytosis is often present

108. Child Pugh A criteria for clinical severity of cirrhosis includes:

a. Bilirubin < 2.0 mg/dL
b. Prothrombin time >70 (% of control)
c. Serum albumin 2.0-3.0 g/dl
d. Presence of encephalopathy
e. Absence of ascites

109. All are true about Abdominal aneurysm except:

a. Atherosclerosis is the commonest cause
b. Most commonly arises from above the level of renal artery
c. For asymptomatic aneurysms, repair is indicated if the diameter is >5.5 cm
d. Endovascular placement of an aortic stent is use for repair
e. Mostly asymptomatic

Answer

96. c.	97. a, b, c, d.	98. a, b, c, e.	99. a, c, d, e.	100. a, c, d, e.	101. b, d, e.	102. c, d.
103. b, d, e.	104. a, b, d.	105. a, b.	106. a, b, c.	107. a, b, c, d.	108. a, b, e.	109. b.

110. A patient diagnosed with cushing's syndrome. Dexamathasone suppression test showed decrease in cortisol levels and corticotrophin-releasing hormone (CRH) administration causes increased cortisol levels. Treatment option(s) for this patient is/are:
a. Adrenalectomy
b. Pituitary irradiation
c. Adrenal gland removal
d. Stereotactic pituitary radiosurgery
e. Surgical removal of ectopic tissue producing ACTH in different organs

111. In which of the following vasculitis lung involvement does not occur:
a. Eosoniphilic granulomatosis with vasculitis
b. Polyarteritis nodosa (PAN)
c. Microscopic polyangitis
d. Granulomatosis with polyangitis
e. Bechet syndrome

112. Drug causing scleroderma is/are:
a. Bleomycin
b. Pentazocin
c. Polyinyl chloride
d. Steroid
e. Tetracycline

113. Which of the following is/are true regarding cardiac arrest management according to 2015 American Heart Association (AHA) Guidelines for Cardiopulmonary Resuscitation (CPR) and Emergency Cardiovascular Care (ECC):
a. Biphasic shock is given initially with 120-200 Joules
b. Monophasic shock is given with 360 Joules
c. IV cannula is secured for administration of drugs
d. Biphasic defibrillators are preferred over monophasic devices
e. After placing an advanced airway, ventilation rate of 18-20 breaths per minute is maintained

114. A patient of asthma was on inhaled short acting β-agonist. But there was no significant relief. After that he added low dose of inhaled steroid from last 5 day by MDI, but still not responding. What you will advise him for next line of treatment:
a. Continue inhaled short acting β-agonist
b. Add inhaled long acting β-agonist
c. Increase dose of inhaled corticosteroid
d. Start oral corticosteroid
e. Start parenteral corticosteroid

115. Which of the following clinical criteria belongs to HIV stage I:
a. Asymptomatic patient
b. Persistent generalised lymphadenopathy
c. Unexplained chronic diarrhoea for > 1 month
d. Unexplained persistent fever (> 37.5°C for > 1 month)
e. Neutropenia

SURGERY

116. Full form of SCIWORA is:
a. Spinal cord injury with radiographic abnormality
b. Spinal cord injury with radiographic aberration
c. Spinal cord injury without radiographic aberration
d. Spinal cord injury without radiographic abnormality
e. Spinal cord injury with vertebral fracture with radiographic abnormality

117. Which of the following is/are true about breast carcinoma in male except:
a. Often presented at advanced stage at the time of diagnosis
b. Associated with gynaecomastia
c. Staging is different than female
d. Tamoxifene is used in treatment
e. Associated with excess endogenous or exogenous oestrogen

118. All are true about medullary thyroid carcinoma except:
a. Involves the parafollicular cell
b. Radiosensitive
c. Amyloid stroma is present
d. Elevated level of calcitonin
e. High level of carcinoembryonic antigen

119. True about Caroli's disease:
a. Intrahepatic bile duct dilation
b. Jaundice may be seen
c. ↑ Serum alkaline phosphatase
d. Not associated with portal hypertension
e. Surgery is treatment of choice localized hepatic involvement

120. True about esophageal varices:
a. Left gastric vein is portal vessel involved
b. Occur at mid esophagus level
c. Occur at pharyngeal level
d. Epigastric vein is systemic vein involved
e. Occur at lower end of esophagus

121. Which of the following is/are feature of highly selective vagotomy in comparison to truncal vagotomy with drainage:
a. Better tolerated
b. Dumping is more common
c. Diarrhea is less
d. High recurrence rate
e. Operative mortality rate very less

122. Which of the following is/are true regarding parathyroid gland surgery in parathyroid adenoma/hyperplasia:
a. Superior parathyroid gland lies posterior to RLN
b. Gland can be differentiated from surrounding tissue due to its color
c. The presence of a normal parathyroid gland at operation indicates that the tumor removed is an adenoma rather than parathyroid hyperplasia
d. Intraoperative PTH estimation is done to check status of gland removal
e. 6% person have 5 parathyroid gland

Answer

110. a, b, c, d. 111. b. 112. a, b, c. 113. a, b, c, d. 114. a, b, c. 115. a, b. 116. d.
117. c. 118. b 119. a, b, c, e. 120. a, e. 121. a, c, d, e. 122. a, b, c, d.

123. Video assisted thoracotomy is/are commonly used for:
- a. Pneumonectomy
- b. Lung biopsy
- c. Hemothorax with active bleeding
- d. Repair of large vessel tear in thorax
- e. Diagnosis and staging of thoracic malignancies

124. Which of the following is included in management of traumatic brain injury:
- a. Mannitol infusion
- b. Decompressive craniectomy
- c. CT scan
- d. Pneumococcal vaccination
- e. Antiepileptics

125. True regarding urethral injury:
- a. Straddle injuries are often associated with posterior urethral injuries
- b. Pelvic injuries is frequently associated with anterior urethral injuries
- c. Problem in voiding
- d. Initial management is insertion of a suprapubic catheter
- e. Suspect if there is blood at the urethral meatus in case of pelvic fracture

126. Statement true about crush injury & syndrome:
- a. Often seen during earthquake
- b. Myoglobinuria occurs
- c. Presents as glomerulonephritis
- d. May cause compartment syndrome
- e. May be associated with rhabdomyolysis

127. True about gallbladder :
- a. Absent of submucosa
- b. Muscularis mucosa is present
- c. Brush border columnar epithelial lining on luminal surface
- d. Cholecystokinin contract gallbladder musculature
- e. Pain of gallbladder stone may radiates to between shoulder blades

128. High imperforate anus is/are associated with:
- a. Underdeveloped pelvic & gluteal musculature
- b. Associated with maldeveloped urinary system
- c. Associated with VACTERL syndrome
- d. Fistula formation with bladder
- e. Normal anal sphinter mechanism

129. True about Mallory-Weiss tear :
- a. Alcoholism is a predisposing factor
- b. Tear involves up to muscularis mucosa
- c. Tear involves gastric mucosa near gastro-esophageal junction
- d. Associated with hiatus hernia
- e. Important cause of upper GI bleeding

130. Which of the following is/are true about breast self-examination:
- a. Performed in different positions like standing, sitting, supine etc
- b. ↑ survival rate
- c. Done about 2-3 day before menstrual cycle in premenopausal women
- d. It should be start only after 35 year
- e. Monthly breast self-examination (BSE) is recommended

OBSTETRICS & GYNAECOLOGY

131. Failure rate of <2/100 women years is/are seen:
- a. Male condom
- b. Implanon
- c. COC
- d. Vaginal diaphragm
- e. IUCD

132. True about breech presentation:
- a. More common in primi
- b. Incidence is about 7% at term pregnancy
- c. More common in postdated pregnancy
- d. More in pelvic anomaly
- e. External cephalic version decreases incidence of breech presentation

133. True about treatment of bacterial vaginosis:
- a. Metronidazole is the drug of choice
- b. Metronidazole should take in dose of 500 mg, orally twice a day for 7 day
- c. Intravaginal clindamycin is used
- d. Male partner is also treated in all cases
- e. Clotrimazole 2% cream is used intravaginally

134. True about gestational hypertension:
- a. Return to normal BP within 12 week of postpartum
- b. BP > 140/90 mmHg
- c. Develop beyond the 20th week of pregnancy
- d. May continue even after 12 week of delivery
- e. Final diagnosis made only in postpartum

135. True about stage Ib cervix carcinoma management:
- a. Radiotherapy alone
- b. Simple hysterectomy alone
- c. Primary chemoradiation
- d. Wertheim hysterectomy + pelvic lymphadenectomy
- e. Simple hysterectomy + adjuvant chemotherapy

136. True about Mirena:
- a. Effective life is 5-10 yr
- b. Gives protection against HIV & STD
- c. Contraindicated in suspected pregnancy
- d. Contraindicated in breast carcinoma
- e. Useful in controlling menorrhagia in fibroid

137. Intracytoplasmic sperm injection (ICSI) is/are useful in condition of:
- a. Mullerian agenesis
- b. Unexplained infertility
- c. Hostile cervical mucus
- d. Oligospermia
- e. Presence of sperm antibodies

Answer

123. a, b, c, e. 124. All 125. c, d, e. 126. a, b, d, e. 127. a, c, d, e. 128. a, b, c, d. 129. a, c, d, e.
130. a. 131. b, c, e. 132. d, e. 133. a, b, c. 134. a, b, c, e. 135. c, d. 136. a, c, d, e.
137. b, d, e.

138. Indication of artificial insemination is/are:
a. Male factor infertility
b. Unexplained infertility
c. PCOD
d. Tubal factor infertility
e. Hostile cervical mucus

139. True about Ectopic pregnancy:
a. OCP use increase risk
b. IUCD failure increase chance of ectopic pregnancy
c. βhCG rise is not parallel to normal pregnancy
d. Trans vaginal USG is 100% diagnostic
e. More common in primi

140. Medical treatment of myoma includes:
a. Tamoxifen
b. Mifepristone
c. LNG-IUD
d. GnRH agonist
e. GnRH antagonist

141. True about Medical Termination of Pregnancy in India:
a. Can be done in any hospital by a trained obstetrician
b. Only women consent is needed, husband consent not mandatory
c. Opinion of two doctors are needed if carried after 20 weeks
d. Opinion of one doctors is needed if carried before 20 weeks
e. Both surgical & medical method for termination are available

142. True about emergency contraceptive:
a. Available as over the counter (OTC)
b. LNG alone, 0.75 initially followed by another 0.75mg 12 hours apart is emergency contraceptive method of choice
c. Ethinyl estradiol (EE) should be taken within 72 hours
d. Copper IUD is used within 5 days of unprotected sex
e. LNG-IUS is one of best method

143. Which of the following is true about changes during Pregnancy:
a. ↑Minute ventilation
b. ↓Tidal volume
c. ↑ Minimum alveolar concentration (MAC) of anaesthetic gases
d. ↑Blood volume & RBC volume
e. ↑Respiratory rate

144. Combined oral pills should not be given in:
a. Women of > 35 year who smoke heavily
b. Women > 40 year
c. Previous thromboembolic event or stroke
d. Severe hypertension
e. Menorrhagia

145. Most common cause of primary post-partum hemorrhage is:
a. Uterine atony
b. Uterine inertia
c. Uterine inversion
d. Retained placenta
e. Traumatic

146. Screening tests for cervical cancer includes:
a. HPV serology
b. Cervical biopsy
c. Colposcopy
d. Cytology
e. Conisation

147. True about endometriosis:
a. USG is very helpful in diagnosis
b. Severity of disease is based on pain complaint
c. Laparoscopy is gold standard for diagnosis
d. COC is used to relieve mild pain

PAEDITRICS

148. Vitamin K dependent coagulation factor(s) in children is/are:
a. Factor 2
b. Factor 7
c. Factor 8
d. Factor 9
e. Factor 10

149. Child can Swaps object from one hand to other in:
a. 2-3 month
b. 5-6 month
c. 6-12 Months
d. 12-18 Months
e. 20-24 Months

150. Congenital hyperbilirubinemia is/are seen in:
a. Prematurity
b. Hypoalbuminaemic state
c. Hepatitis
d. Sepsis
e. Polycythemia

151. Common cause of distal small intestinal obstruction in infants /child:
a. Meconium ileus
b. Jejunal atresia
c. Ileal atresia
d. Meckel's diverticulum
e. Duodenal atresia

ORTHOPAEDICS

152. Not an Intra-articular fracture:
a. Rolando fracture
b. March fracture
c. Bennett's fracture
d. Barton's fracture
e. Hoffa fracture

153. All are true about supracondylar fracture of humerus except:
a. Posterior shift of distal fragment
b. Median nerve is most common nerve damaged
c. Injury of brachial artery may occur
d. Common in elderly
e. Volkmann's ischemic contracture may occur

Answer

138. a, b, e.	139. b, c.	140. b, c, d, e.	141. b, e.	142. a, b, c, d.	143. a, b, d.	144. a, b, c, d.
145. a.	146. a, d.	147. c, d.	148. a, b, d, e.	149. b.	150. a, c, d, e.	151. a, b, c, d.
152. b.	153. d.					

154. All are true Volkmann ischemic contracture except:
- a. Ischemic muscle is replaced by fibrous
- b. Ulnar nerve palsy may be present
- c. Extention deformity of the wrist & fingers
- d. Flexion at the metacarpophalangeal
- e. Tendon transfer helps in restoring movements

155. True about Dupuytren's contracture:
- a. Commonly affect ring & small finger
- b. May involve penis
- c. Involves metacarpo-phalangeal joint
- d. Knee reflex diminished
- e. Involves neck flexors

156. True about complex regional pain syndrome:
- a. Sudeck's atrophy is an example
- b. Pain is out of proportion to precipitating cause
- c. Hyperaesthesia of skin may be present
- d. Adults are usual sufferer
- e. Parasympathetic mediated enhancement of pain

ANAESTHESIA

157. Which of the following statement(s) is/are correct regarding management of malignant hyperthermia except:
- a. Discontinue all anaesthetics immediately
- b. Dantrolene is mainstay of therapy for MH
- c. Hyperventilation with 100% oxygen is helpful
- d. Sodium bicarbonate is given to correct alkalosis
- e. Correct hyperkalemia by giving dextrose & insulin

158. Which of the following is/are true about pre-anaesthetic checkup (PAC):
- a. Not necessary in children
- b. Used to assess patient condition to tolerate anaesthesia & surgery
- c. Can be performed by surgical faculty
- d. Relieves anxiety of patient
- e. Help in planning anaesthesia technique

159. Which of the following statement is/are true regarding intravenous fluid:
- a. Ringer lactate is crystalloid of choice for blood loss replacement
- b. Colloid is fluid of choice in severe shock
- c. 5% Dextrose should be avoided in head injury
- d. 0.45% saline contains 154 mEq/L Na+ & 154 mEq/L Cl-
- e. Dextrose normal saline (DNS) is hypotonic

SKIN

160. Kobner's phenomenon can occur in:
- a. Lichen planus
- b. Vitiligo
- c. Psoriasis
- d. Bullous pemphigoid
- e. Dicoid lupus erythematosus

161. All are true about pompholyx except:
- a. It is a form of hand/foot eczema
- b. Also called as dyshidrotic eczema
- c. Vesicle & blisters are present
- d. Secondary bacterial infection are common
- e. Steroids should not be used as it can exacerbate the condition

PSYCHIATRY

162. Which of the following is/are true regarding use of Lithium in prophylaxis of bipolar disorder except:
- a. Effective for prevention of depressive episode
- b. Effective for prevention of manic episode
- c. It lengthens the interval between cycles of mania & depression
- d. It reduces the incidence of suicide in bipolar I disorder
- e. It has established role in prevention of acute mania but no role in prevention of depressive episode

163. Neologism is characteristic of:
- a. OCD
- b. Mania
- c. Bipolar disorder
- d. Schizophrenia
- e. Autism

164. Good prognosis in schizophrenia is/are seen in:
- a. Negative symptoms
- b. Early onset
- c. Acute onset
- d. Family history of schizophrenia
- e. Insidious onset

165. True about Alprazolam:
- a. Antidepressant
- b. Antipsychotic
- c. Anti-anxiety
- d. Hypnotic
- e. Benzodiazepine

166. Feature (s) of Delusion:
- a. Shakeable
- b. True belief
- c. False belief
- d. Bizarre
- e. Non-bizarre

167. Which of the following statement(s) is/are about α-wave of EEG:
- a. Frequency is 8-13 Hz
- b. Frequency is 4-8 Hz
- c. Originate during wakeful relaxation with closed eyes
- d. Occur most intensely in the occipital region
- e. Voltage is usually about 50 microvolts

Answer

154. c.	155. a, b, c.	156. a, b, c, d.	157. d.	158. b, d, e.	159. a, b, c.	160. a, b, c, e.
161. e.	162. e.	163. d.	164. c.	165. c. d. e.	166. c. d. e.	167. a. c. d. e.

RADIOLOGY

168. Which of the following is/are used in neuroendocrine tumor evaluation:
a. 68Ga-DOTA-TOC
b. MIBG
c. 68Ga-DOTA-NOC
d. F-18 Fluorodopa
e. 68Ga-DOTA-TATE

169. USG is/are based on:
a. Piezoelectric effect
b. Diamagnetic effect
c. Paramagnetic effect
d. Ferromagnetic effect
e. Electromagnetic effect

170. X-ray feature (s) of Left Atrial Hypertrophy:
a. Boot shaped heart
b. Widened carina
c. Straightened left border
d. Double atrial shadow
e. Money bag appearance

171. Contrast agent(s) which can be safely used in diabetic patients:
a. Ionic high-osmolar contrast media (HOCM)
b. Nonionic low-osmolar contrast media (LOCM)
c. Nonionic iso-osmolar contrast media (IOCM)
d. Gadolinium
e. Barium sulfate

172. Which of the following is/are common radiation induced cancers:
a. Breast cancer
b. Gonadal cancer
c. Leukaemia
d. Renal cell carcinoma
e. Prostate cancer

173. Which of the following is/are used for radiotherapy:
a. I-131
b. I-123
c. Gallium-68
d. Strontium-90
e. P-32

174. Contrast agent which are used for CT scan:
a. Water
b. Barium compounds
c. Iodinated high-osmolality contrast media
d. Polyethylene glycol
e. Microbubble

Answer

168. All 169. a. 170. b. c. d. 171. b. c. e. 172. a. b. c. 173. a. d. e. 174. a. b. c. d.

NOVEMBER 2015 ANSWERS & EXPLANATIONS

ANATOMY

1. **Ans. a. Uncinate process..., d. Pancreatic divisum..., e. Body is formed....,**

[Ref: Embryology by Inderbir Singh 10th/1207-10; Snell's 9th/204; Gray's 40th/1183-90]

"One important clinically important variation is **'pancreatic divisum'**, *where* ***entirely separate drainage occurs for different portions of pancreas*** *& which may allow some forms of pancreatitis to affect only one portion of the gland" (Gray's 40th/1185)*

"Pancreatic divisum is a congenital anomaly ***in the anatomy of the ducts of the pancreas*** in which a single pancreatic duct is not formed, but rather ***remains as two distinct dorsal and ventral ducts***" *(en.wikipedia.org)*

Development of Pancreas

◈ *Embryology by Inderbir Singh 10th/1207-10*

- The pancreas develops from two endodermal buds, ***dorsal & ventral***, which arise from the part of the gut that later forms the second part of the duodenum
- The **ventral bud** forms the ***lower part of the head & the uncinate process of the pancreas***, while the ***upper part of head, the body & the tail are formed from*** the **dorsal bud**
- The **main pancreatic duct (duct of Wirsung)** is formed, in its ***distal part by the duct of the dorsal bud*** and in ***its proximal part, by the duct of the ventral bud***
- The **secretory elements** of the pancreas are formed by proliferation of the *primitive ducts.* The islets of Langerhans are also derived from the primitive duct system

2. **Ans. a. Urinary bladder..., d. Distal part ..., e. Urethral meatus.....**

[Ref: Gray's 40th/1250-52; A.K.Jain Physiology 6th/573]

"**Urinary bladder** is lined by uroepithelium (***transitional epithelium***)" *(Gray's 40th/1250)*

"The lining of urethra varies from urothelium of the bladder to ***keratinized stratified squamous epithelium*** *of the glans" (medscape.com)*

Urethra

◈ *Gray's 40th/1252*

- *The epithelium lining the* **preprostatic urethra & the proximalpart of the prostatic urethra** *is a* ***typical uroepithelium***
- *The epithelium change below the opening of the ejaculatory ducts to a* ***pseudostratified or stratified columnar****, which lines the* **membranous urethra & the major part of the penile urethra**
- *Towards the* **distal end of penile urethra** *the epithelium changes once again, becoming* ***stratified squamous*** *.This epithelium also lines the navicular fossa & become* ***keratinized*** at **external meatus**

Region	Description	Epithelium
Pre-prostatic urethra	This is the intramural part of the urethra and varies between 0.5 and 1.5 cm in length depending on the fullness of the bladder.	*Transitional*
Prostatic urethra	Crosses through the prostate gland. There are several openings: (1) the ejaculatory duct receives sperm from the vas deferens and ejaculate fluid from the seminal vesicle, (2) several prostatic ducts where fluid from the prostate enters and contributes to the ejaculate, (3) the prostatic utricle	*Transitional*
Membranous urethra	A small (1 or 2 cm) portion passing through the external urethral sphincter. This is the narrowest part of the urethra. It is located in the deep perineal pouch. The bulbourethral glands (Cowper's gland) are found posterior to this region but open in the spongy urethra.	*Pseudostratified columnar*
Spongy urethra (or *penile urethra*)	Runs along the length of the penis on its ventral (underneath) surface. It is about 15–16 cm in length, and travels through the corpus spongiosum.	*Pseudostratified columnar – proximally, Stratified squamous – distally*

3. **Ans. a. Gag reflex..., c. Loss of taste..., e. May cause....**

[Ref: PJM 20th/ 320; Kundu 4th/273]

Glossopharyngeal Nerve Palsy

◈ *Kundu 4th/273*

- *Loss of sensation over the mucous membrane of pharynx*
- *Loss of taste sensation in the* ***posterior 1/3 of the tongue*** *(c.f A 2/3 by facial nerve)*
- ***Gag reflex****-Lost in lesion of IX & X CN*

Hypoglossal Nerve Palsy

◈ *Kundu 4th/273*

- ***Tongue deviation on protrusion (deviated to side of paralysis)***
- ***Wasting & fasciculation in tongue***

"Bulbar palsy: Lesion of CN 9-12" *(PJM 20th/321)*

4. **Ans. a. Ptos..., b. Mios..., d. Diplo..., e. Loss of....**

[Ref: B.D.C 6th/Vol.III 362; PJM 20th/310]

Oculomotor Nerve

◈ *B.D.C 6th/Vol.III 362*

- **Complete & total paralysis** – ***ptosis, lateral squint, dilation of pupil, loss of accommodation, slight proptosis & diplopia***
- *Pupillary light reflex in affected eye is absent*
- *Pupil dilates & becomes fixed to light*
- **Weber syndrome**: a midbrain lesion causing contralateral hemiplegia & ipsilateral paralysis of the third nerve

5. **Ans. a. External iliac..., b. Aortic lymph..., e. Sacral....**

[Ref: B.D.C 6th/Vol.II 390; Snell's 9th/287; Gray's 40th/1290;Dutta Obs 8th/8]

*"Cervix: On each side, the lymphatics drian into (1) **external iliac, obturator lymph nodes either directly or through paracervical lymph nodes**, (2) **internal iliac groups** & (3) **sacral groups**" (Dutta Obs 8th/8)*

Lymphatic Drainage of Uterus

◈ *B.D.C 6th/Vol.II 390*

Part of uterus	Draining L.N
Upper lymphatics from the fundus & upper part of the body	Mainly- Aortic nodes Partly- Superficial inguinal L.N
Middle lymphatics from lower part of body	External iliac node
Lower lymphatics from the cervix	***External iliac, internal iliac & sacral node***

6. **Ans. a. Dorsiflexion..., b. Foot drop, c. High stepping..., e. Eversion....**

[Ref: Maheshwari 5th/69; B.D.C. 6th/Vol. II 80,4th/Vol II 86, 174; Gray's 40th/1427;Snells' Anatomy 8th/660; Last's anatomy 11th/168-169; Moore's Anatomy 2nd/331]

"**Common peroneal nerve injury**: *It supplies the **extensors & evertors** of the foot. Paralysis of these muscle result in **foot drop**. The patient walks with a **'high step gait'**, i.e. while walking he has to lift the foot high in order to clear the ground. The **plantar flexors of the foot are normal**" (Maheshwari 5th/69)*

Common Peroneal Nerve Dysfunction Symptoms

◈ *medlineplus.gov*

When the nerve is injured and results in dysfunction, **symptoms** may include:

- *Decreased sensation, numbness, or tingling in the top of the foot or the outer part of the upper or lower leg*
- ***Foot that drops (unable to hold the foot up)***
- ***"Slapping" gait** (walking pattern in which each step makes a slapping noise)*
- *Toes drag while walking*
- *Walking problems*
- *Weakness of the ankles or feet*
- *Loss of muscle mass because the nerves aren't stimulating the muscles*

"***Common peroneal nerve***: It is commonly injured in fractures of the ***neck of the fibula***" *(Snells' Anatomy 8th/660)*

Common Peroneal Nerve Injury

◈ *B.D.C, Snell, Moore, Last's &Internet*

- **Mode of injury**- Lathi injury on lateral side of knee Jt, Plaster on leg & Fracture of neck of femur
- **Motor loss**
  - **Muscles of anterior compartment (tibialis anterior, extensor digitorum longus, peroneus tertius & extensor hallucis longus:** Deep peroneal nerve) & Lateral compart-ment (peroneus longus & brevis: superficial peroneal nerve) are paralysed & as a result there is **weakness of dorsiflexion & eversion of foot.** As a result the opposing muscle, the plantar flexors of ankle Jt & invertors of subtalar & transverse tarsal joint, cause the foot to be plantar flexed **(foot drop)** & inverted, an attitude referred to as **equinovarus**
  - ***Plantar flexion & inversion are normal***
  - The patient has a ***high stepping gait***
  - All **reflex are intact** (the ankle jerk is lost in sciatic nerve lesion)
- **Sensory loss**
  - Loss of sensation of anterior & **lateral sides of leg** & dorsum of the foot & toes including the medial **side of the big toe**
  - Lateral border of foot & lateral side of little toe are virtually unaffected (sural nerve mainly formed from tibial nerve)
  - The medial border of foot as far as the ball of the big toe is completely unaffected (saphenous nerve is branch of femoral N)

7. **Ans. a. Anterior..., c. Medial..., e. Medial collateral....**

[Ref: radiopaedia.org; Snell's 9th/ 502-03]

"**O'Donoghue's unhappy triad** results from valgus stress with rotation of the knee. ***It comprises ACL tear and medial collateral ligament injury (tear or sprain) with a medial meniscal tear***" *(radiopaedia.org)*

"An **unhappy triad** (or **terrible triad**, "horrible triangle", **O'Donoghue's triad** or a **"blown knee"**) is an injury to the ***anterior cruciate ligament, medial collateral ligament, and the medial meniscus***" *(wiki)*

8. Ans. a. Splenic..., b. Paraumbilical..., c. Superior rectal..., d. Left gastric...

[Ref: B.D.C 6th/Vol.II 283-85]

Table *(B.D.C 6th/Vol.II 285)*: **Sites of portocaval/portosystemic anastomoses**

S. No. Position	Portal vein	Systemic vein
1. Lower end of esophagus	Left gastric	Oesophageal veins
2. Lower end of rectum	Superior rectal	Middle and interior rectal veins
3. Umbilicus	Paraumbilical	Above–Superior epigastric, lateral thoracic Below–Superficial epigastric, inferior epigastric Sides–Posterior intercostals and lumber
4. Posterior abdominal wall	Splenic	Left renal vein
5. Bare area of liver	Portal radicles	Diaphragmatic
6. Falciform ligament	Paraumbilical	Diaphragmatic
7. Ligamentum venosum	Left branch of portal	Interior vena cava

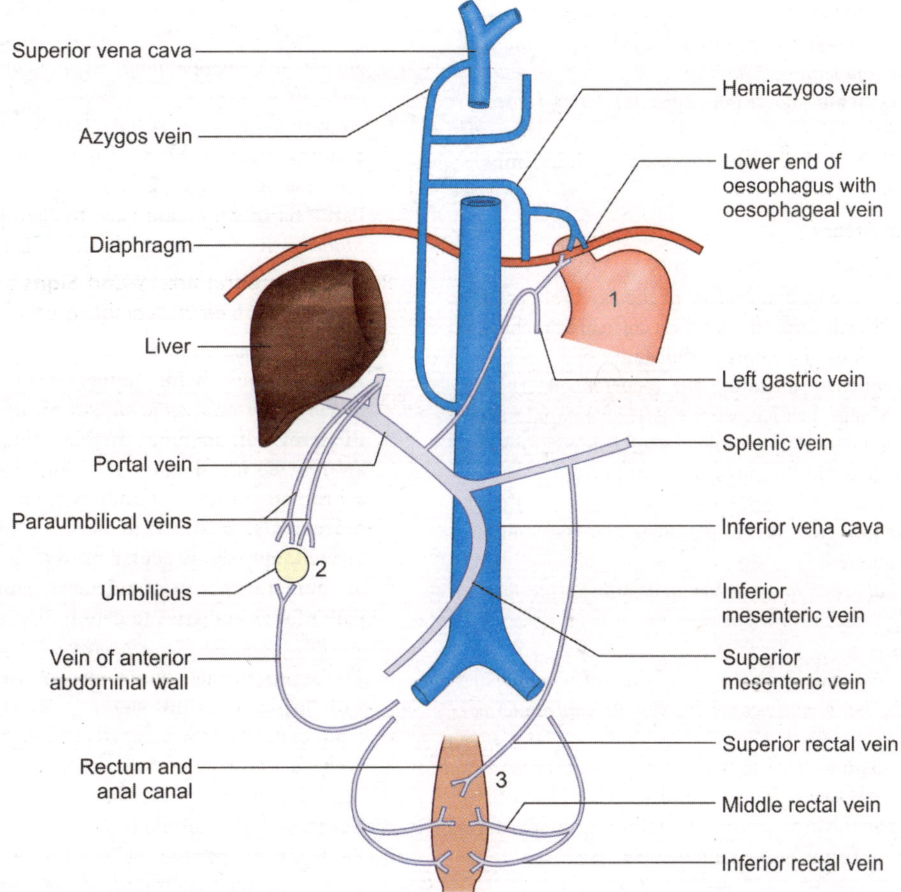

Fig: *(B.D.C 6th/Vol.II 284)*: Important sites of communication of portal & systemic veins: (1) Lower end of oesophagus, (2) Around umbilicus & (3) Anal canal

9. Ans. a. Left foot paralysis..., b. Urinary..., e. Gegenhalten....

[Ref: Harrison 19th/2573-74;B.D.C 6th/Vol.III 460-62,420-24]

"Thrombosis of **posterior cerebral artery** *results in* ***homonymous hemianopia*** *on the opposite side"* (B.D.C 6th/Vol.III 458)

"Thrombosis of lateral striate branches of **middle cerebral artery** *causes* ***motor & sensory loss to most of the opposite side of body except lower limb****"* (B.D.C 6th/Vol.III 460)

Anterior Cerebral Artery: Signs and Symptoms with Structures Involved

◈ *Harrison 19th/2574*

1. **Paralysis of opposite foot and leg**: *Motor leg area*
2. **A lesser degree of paresis of opposite arm**: *Arm area of cortex or fibers descending to corona radiate*
3. **Cortical sensory loss over toes, foot, and leg**: *Sensory area for foot and leg*
4. **Urinary incontinence**: *Sensorimotor area in paracentral lobule*
5. **Contralateral grasp reflex, sucking reflex, gegenhalten (paratonic rigidity)**: *Medial surface of the posterior frontal lobe; likely supplemental motor area*
6. **Abulia (akinetic mutism), slowness, delay, intermittent interruption, lack of spontaneity, whispering, reflex distraction to sights and sounds**: *Uncertain localization—probably cingulate gyrus and medial inferior portion of frontal, parietal, and temporal lobes*
7. **Impairment of gait and stance (gait apraxia):** *Frontal cortex near leg motor area*
8. **Dyspraxia of left limbs, tactile aphasia in left limbs**: *Corpus callosum*

Anterior Cerebral Artery

◈ *www.meddean.luc.edu*

- Supplies most of the medial surface of the cerebral cortex (anterior three fourths), frontal pole (via cortical branches), and anterior portions of the corpus callosum.
- **Perforating branches** (including the recurrent artery of Heubner and Medial Lenticulostriate Arteries) supply the anterior limb of the internal capsule, the inferior portions of head of the caudate and anterior globus pallidus.
- **Bilateral occlusion** of Anterior Cerebral Arteries at their stems results in infarction of the anteromedial surface of the cerebral hemispheres:
  - *Paraplegia affecting lower extremities and sparing face/hands.*
  - *Incontinence*
  - *Abulic and motor aphasia*
  - *Frontal lobe Symptoms: personality change, contralateral grasp reflex.*
- **Unilateral occlusion** (distal to Ant. Comm. origin) of Anterior Cerebral Artery produces contralateral sensorimotor deficits mainly involving the lower extremity with sparing of face and hands (think of the humunculus).

Middle Cerebral Artery- Signs and Symptoms with Structures Involved

◈ *Harrison 19th/2573*

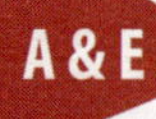

1. **Paralysis of the contralateral face, arm, and leg; sensory impairment over the same area (pinprick, cotton touch, vibration, position, two-point discrimination, stereognosis, tactile localization, barognosis, cutaneographia):** *Somatic motor area for face and arm and the fibers descending from the leg area to enter the corona radiata and corresponding somatic sensory system*
2. **Motor aphasia**: *Motor speech area of the dominant hemisphere*
3. **Central aphasia, word deafness, anomia, jargon speech, sensory agraphia, acalculia, alexia, finger agnosia, right-left confusion (the last four comprise the Gerstmann syndrome):** *Central, suprasylvian speech area and parietooccipital cortex of the dominant hemisphere*
4. **Conduction aphasia:** *Central speech area (parietal operculum)*
5. **Apractagnosia of the nondominant hemisphere, anosognosia, hemiasomatognosia, unilateral neglect, agnosia for the left half of external space, dressing "apraxia," constructional "apraxia," distortion of visual coordinates, inaccurate localization in the half field, impaired ability to judge distance, upside-down reading, visual illusions (e.g., it may appear that another person walks through a table):** *Nondominant parietal lobe (area corresponding to speech area in dominant hemisphere); loss of topographic memory is usually due to a nondominant lesion, occasionally to a dominant one*
6. **Homonymous hemianopia (often homonymous inferior quadrantanopia):** *Optic radiation deep to second temporal convolution*
7. **Paralysis of conjugate gaze to the opposite side:** *Frontal contraversive eye field or projecting fibers*

Posterior cerebral artery and Signs and symptoms with structures involved *(not complete list)*

◈ *Harrison 19th/2573*

1. **Homonymous hemianopia** (often upper quadrantic): *Calcarine cortex or optic radiation nearby.*
2. **Bilateral homonymous hemianopia, cortical blindness, awareness or denial of blindness; tactile naming, achromatopia (color blindness), failure to see to-and-fro movements, inability to perceive objects not centrally located, apraxia of ocular movements, inability to count or enumerate objects, tendency to run into things that the patient sees and tries to avoid:** *Bilateral occipital lobe with possibly the parietal lobe involved.*
3. **Thalamoperforate syndrome: crossed cerebellar ataxia with ipsilateral third nerve palsy (Claude's syndrome):** *Dentatothalamic tract and issuing third nerve.*
4. **Weber's syndrome: third nerve palsy and contralateral hemiplegia:** *Third nerve and cerebral peduncle.*
5. **Contralateral hemiplegia:** *Cerebral peduncle.*
6. **Paralysis or paresis of vertical eye movement, skew deviation, sluggish pupillary responses to light, slight miosis and ptosis (retraction nystagmus and "tucking" of the eyelids may be associated):** *Supranuclear fibers to third nerve, interstitial nucleus of Cajal, nucleus of Darkschewitsch, and posterior commissure.*
7. Contralateral rhythmic, ataxic action tremor; rhythmic postural or "holding" tremor (rubral tremor): *Dentatothalamic tract.*

10. Ans. a. Temporo..., b. Sternocla..., d. Vertebral..., e. Inferior....

[Ref: B.D.C 6th/Vol.III 121; Handbook of General Anatomy by BDC 5th/76; Snell's 9th/32; Gray's 40th/83-84]

There are 3 types of cartilage: *Hyaline cartilage,* ***fibrocartilage*** *& elastic cartilage (Handbook of General Anatomy by BDC 5th/75)*

Type of joints: *Fibrous joint (united by fibrous tissue), cartilaginous joint (united by cartilage or fibrocartilage) & synovial joint (covered with cartilage & united by a fibrous capsule) (Moore 2nd/17)*

Fibrocartilage

◈ *Snell's 9th/32*

- *It has many collagen fibers embedded in a small amount of matrix & is found in the discs within joints (e.g., the* ***temporomandibular joint, Sternoclavicular joint, the knee joint & on the articular surfaces of the clavicle & mandible***
- *Fibrocartilage, if damaged, repairs itself slowly in a manner similar to fibrous tissue elsewhere*
- *Joint discs have a poor blood supply & therefore do not repair themselves when damaged*

"Fibrocartilage: *In the* ***vertebral disc, interpubic disc of symphysis pubis, articular discs of temporomandibular joints (TMJ), sternoclavicular joint & inferior radioulnar joint****" (Handbook of General Anatomy by BDC 5th/76)*

TM joint- *This is a synovial joint of the condylar variety. Articular surfaces are* ***covered with fibrocartilage****" (B.D.C 6th/Vol.III 121)*

"Sternoclavicular joint *is a synovial joint. The articular surface of the clavicle is covered with* ***fibrocartilage****" (B.D.C 6th/Vol.I 141)*

PHYSIOLOGY

11. Ans. b. Increased... e. Gallbladder....

[Ref: Ganong 25th/257-60, 24th/265; Guyton 12th/804; Katzung 13th/110-11]

"**Parasympathetic nerves** are ***motor to musculature of the gallbladder*** & bile duct, but ***inhibitory to the sphincter.*** **Sympathetic nerves** from T7-9 are vasomotor & ***motor to sphincters***" *(BDC 6th/Vol. II 290)*

Parasympathetic Division

◈ *Ganong 24th/257-58*

The **cranial outflow of the parasympathetic division** supplies the visceral structures in the head via the oculomotor, facial, and glossopharyngeal nerves, and those in the ***thorax and upper abdomen via the vagus nerves.***

- The **sacral outflow** supplies the ***pelvic viscera via the pelvic branches*** of the second to fourth sacral spinal nerves. The preganglionic fibers in both outflows end on short postganglionic neurons located on or near the visceral structures
- *"Approx.* ***75% of all parasympathetic nerve fibers are in the vagus (X) nerve****" (A.K.Jain 6th/923)*

Table *(Guyton 12th/804)*: **Autonomic Effects on Various Organs of the Body**

Organ	Effect of Sympathetic Stimulation	Effect of Parasympathetic Stimulation
Eye		
Pupil	Dilated (Mydriasis)	Constricted (Miosis)
Ciliary muscle	Slight relaxation (far vision)	Constricted (near vision)
Glands (Nasal, Lacrimal, Parotid, Submandibular, Gastric Pancreatic)	Vasoconstriction and slight secretion	Stimulation of copious secretion (containing many enzymes for enzyme-secreting glands)
Sweat glands	Copious sweating (cholinergic)	Sweating on palms of hands
Apocrine glands	Thick, odoriferous secretion	None
Blood vessels	Most often constricted	Most often little or no effect
Heart		
Muscle	Increased rate	Slowed rate
	Increased force of contraction	Decreased force of contraction (especially of atria)
Coronaries	Dilated (β_2); constricted (α)	Dilated
Lungs		
Bronchial muscle	Relaxation	Contraction
Blood vessels	Mildly constricted	? Dilated
Gut		
Lumen	Decreased peristalsis and tone	Increased peristalsis and tone
Sphincter	Increased tone (most times)	Relaxed (most times)
Gallbladder and bile ducts	Relaxed	Contracted
Kidney	Decreased urine output and increased renin secretion	None
Bladder		
Detrusor	Relaxed (slight)	Contracted
Trigone	Contracted	Relaxed

12. Ans. a. Group Ia..., b. Nuclear bag..., d. Motor supply...

[Ref: A.K.Jain 6th/873-76; Guyton 12th/ 770-73]

Sensory supply: *2 types of sensory ending-* **primary (or annulospiral) ending** *with termination of* ***group Ia (or Aα) afferent fiber*** *&* **secondary ending** *with* ***termination of group II (or Aβ) afferent fiber"*** *(A.K.Jain 6th/875)*

*"**Motor supply** to the muscle spindle comes from ventral horn cells in the spinal cord by γ* efferent fibers*" (A.K.Jain 6th/875)*

*"**Intrafusal fiber** of two type-* ***nuclear bag fibers & nuclear chain fibers"*** *(A.K.Jain 6th/874)*

Division of the Intrafusal Fibers into Nuclear Bag and Nuclear Chain Fibers-Dynamic and Static Responses of the Muscle Spindle

- There are also **two types of muscle spindle intrafusal fibers**: (1) ***nuclear bag muscle fibers*** (one to three in each spindle), (2) ***nuclear chain fibers*** (three to nine).The **primary sensory** nerve ending (the 17-micrometer sensory fiber) is excited ***by both the nuclear bag intrafusal fibers and the nuclear chain*** fibers. Conversely, the **secondary ending** (the 8-micrometer sensory fiber) is usually excited only by ***nuclear chain fibers***.

Response of the Primary Ending (but Not the Secondary Ending) to Rate of Change of Receptor Length-"Dynamic" Response

- Control of Intensity of the Static and Dynamic Responses by the Gamma Motor Nerves

Muscle Sensory Receptors-Muscle Spindles and Golgi Tendon Organs & Their Roles in Muscle Control

◈ *Guyton 12th/ 770-73*

- The muscles and their tendons are supplied abundantly with **two special types of sensory receptors**: (1) **muscle spindles**, which are distributed throughout the belly of the muscle and send information to the nervous system about ***muscle length or rate of change of length***, and (2) ***Golgi tendon organs***, which are located in the muscle tendons and transmit information about ***tendon tension or rate of change of tension***.
- The signals from these two receptors are either entirely or almost entirely for the purpose of intrinsic muscle control. They operate almost completely at a subconscious level.

Receptor Function of the Muscle Spindle

A. Structure and Motor Innervation of the Muscle Spindle

- Each spindle is 3 to 10 millimeters long. It is built around 3 to 12 tiny ***intrafusal muscle fibers*** that are pointed at their ends and attached to the glycocalyx of the surrounding **large *extrafusal*** skeletal muscle fibers.
- Each **intrafusal muscle fiber** is a tiny skeletal muscle fiber. However, the central region of each of these fibers-that is, the area midway between its two ends-has few or no actin and myosin filaments. Therefore, this central portion does not contract when the ends do. Instead, it functions as a sensory receptor. The end portions that do contract are excited by small ***gamma motor nerve fibers*** that originate from ***small type A gamma motor neurons*** in the anterior horns of the spinal cord. These gamma motor nerve fibers are also called *gamma efferent fibers,* in contradistinction to the large ***alpha efferent fibers*** (type A alpha nerve fibers) that innervate the ***extrafusal skeletal muscle***.

B. Sensory Innervation of the Muscle Spindle

- The ***muscle spindle receptor can be excited in two ways:***
  1. **Lengthening the whole muscle stretches the midportion** of the spindle and, therefore, excites the receptor.
  2. Even if the length of the entire muscle does not change, contraction of the end portions of the spindle's intrafusal fibers stretches the midportion of the spindle and therefore excites the receptor.
- ***Two types of sensory endings are found in this central receptor area of the muscle spindle.*** They are the ***primary ending*** **and the *secondary ending*.**
- **Primary ending**: This nerve fiber is type Ia fiber
- **Secondary Ending**: This nerve fibers is type II fibers

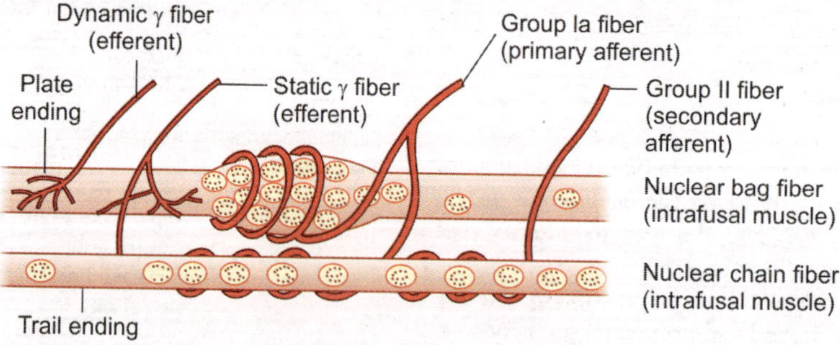

Fig: *(Guyton 12th/ 770):* Details of nerve connections from the nuclear bag and nuclear chain muscle spindle fibers.

A & E

13. Ans. a. Radiation..., d. Gasa angrene..., e. Carbon mono...

[Ref: Manipal Surgery 4th/176; A.K.Jain 6th/461;Ganong 25th/651-52; Guyton 12th/ 391-92]

"**Contraindication**- ***untreated pneumothorax***: Can expand with hyperbaric O_2 resulting in life-threatening tension pneumothorax" *(Manipal Surgery 4th/176)*

"The only **absolute contraindication** to hyperbaric oxygen therapy is ***untreated pneumothorax***. The reason is, concern that it can progress to tension pneumothorax, especially during the decompression phase of therapy, although treatment on oxygen-based tables may avoid that progression" *(en.wikipedia.org)*

"Bleomycin should be discontinued in all patients with documented or strongly suspected **bleomycin-induced lung injury.** Treatment with ***glucocorticoids*** is reserved for patients with symptomatic lung toxicity as spontaneous resolution of asymptomatic radiographic opacities has been described" *(www.hindawi.com)*

"Radiation proctitis *is a* ***known complication following radiation therapy for pelvic malignancy***"

Hyperbaric Oxygen Therapy

◈ *A.K.Jain 6th/461*

The main aim is to increase the amount of dissolved O_2 in plasma

It is useful in

- *Anaemic hypoxia (specially due to* ***carbon mono-oxide poisoning*** *or severe blood loss)*
- *Stagnant hypoxia*
- *Histotoxic hypoxia (****Radiation induced tissue injury & gas gangrene****)*

Hyperbaric Oxygen Therapy

◈ *Manipal Surgery 4th/176*

- ***CO poisoning***
- ***Infection such as gas gangrene***
- ***Cancer therapy to potentiate radiotherapy***
- *Arterial insufficiency*
- *Decompression sickness & air embolism*

Hyperbaric Oxygen Therapy

◈ *Ganong 25th/652*

- It is of demonstrated value in ***carbon monoxide poisoning, radiation-induced tissue injury, gas gangrene, very severe blood loss anemia, diabetic leg ulcers and other wounds that are slow to heal, and rescue of skin flaps and grafts in which the circulation is marginal. It is also the primary treatment for decompression sickness and air embolism.***
- In **hypercapnic patients in severe pulmonary failure**, the CO_2 level may be so high that it depresses rather than stimulates respiration. Some of these patients keep breathing only because the carotid and aortic chemoreceptors drive the respiratory center. If the hypoxic drive is withdrawn by administering O_2, breathing may stop. During the resultant apnea, the arterial PO_2 drops but breathing may not start again, as PCO_2 further depresses the respiratory center. Therefore, ***O_2 therapy in this situation must be started with care.***
- When 80–100% O_2 is administered to humans for periods of 8 h or more, the respiratory passages become irritated, causing substernal distress, nasal congestion, sore throat, and coughing.
- **Complication: bronchopulmonary dysplasia & retinopathy of prematurity (retrolental fibroplasia)**

Hyperbaric Oxygen Therapy

◈ *Guyton 12th/ 391-92*

- Probably the most successful use of hyperbaric oxygen has been for treatment of ***gas gangrene***.
- Other conditions in which hyperbaric oxygen therapy has been either valuable or possibly valuable include ***decompression sickness, arterial gas embolism, carbon monoxide poisoning, osteomyelitis, and myocardial infarction***.

The following Indications are Approved uses of Hyperbaric Oxygen Therapy as Defined by the UHMS

(United States the Undersea and Hyperbaric Medical Society, known as UHMS) *(Net)*

- Air or gas embolism;
- Carbon monoxide poisoning;
    - Carbon monoxide poisoning complicated by cyanide poisoning;
- Central retinal artery occlusion;
- Clostridal myositis and myonecrosis (gas gangrene);
- Crush injury, compartment syndrome, and other acute traumatic ischemias;
- Decompression sickness;
- Enhancement of healing in selected problem wounds;
    - Diabetically derived illness, such as diabetic foot, diabetic retinopathy, diabetic nephropathy;
- Exceptional blood loss (anemia)
- Idiopathic sudden sensorineural hearing loss
- Intracranial abscess
- Mucormycosis, especially rhinocerebral disease in the setting of diabetes mellitus;
- Necrotizing soft tissue infections (necrotizing fasciitis)
- Osteomyelitis (refractory)
- Delayed radiation injury (soft tissue and bony necrosis)
- Skin grafts and flaps (compromised)
- Thermal burns.

Patients should not Undergo HBO Therapy if they are Taking or have Recently Taken the following Drugs

- ***Doxorubicin (Adriamycin):*** *A chemotherapeutic drug. This drug has been shown to potentiate cytotoxicity during HBO therapy.*
- ***Cisplatin:*** *Also a chemotherapeutic drug.*
- ***Disulfiram (Antabuse):*** *Used in the treatment of alcoholism.*
- *Mafenide acetate (Sulfamylon): Suppresses bacterial infections in burn wounds*

---

14. Ans. e. Cardiogenic shock

[Ref: PJM 20th/16-19; Ganong 25th/642;Nelson 18th/2033;A.K.Jain 5th/482; Guyton 11th/531; Harrison 17th/230-31; Nelson 18th/2033]

"**Central cyanosis** due to severe pulmonary hypertension combined with pericarditis as the initial manifestation of ***systemic lupus erythematosus***" *(ncbi.nlm.nih.gov)*

Total anomalous pulmonary venous connection (TAPVC)- ***cause central cyanosis*** *(O.P.Ghai 8th/427)*

Atrial septal defect is ***acyanotic heart disease*** *(O.P.Ghai 8th/413)*

"The classical signs of carbon monoxide poisoning— described as cherry-red lips, peripheral cyanosis, and retinal haemorrhages are rarely seen"

"An methemoglobin **level of 15% (i.e. 1.5 g/dl)**[Q] is associated with ***visible cyanosis***[Q]; a level of 70% MHg level is fatal" *(Nelson 18th/2033)*

*"**Methemoglobinemia** in children usually results from exposure to: Oxidizing substances nitrates or nitrites, aniline dyes, or medications, indications, including lidocaine, prilocaine, and phenazopyridine hydrochloride"*

Cyanosis Occurs When

- ***Deoxygenated hemoglobin (usually in amounts >4 g/dL) or***
- ***Methemoglobin (>1.5 g/dL)***[Q] ***or***
- ***Sulfhemoglobin (>0.5 g/dL***[Q]***)***

CYANOSIS

Central Cyanosis	Peripheral Cyanosis
• Central cyanosis is caused by in adequate oxygenation of systemic arterial blood due to decreased arterial oxygen saturation or Hemoglobin abnormalities • It results from cardiac shunting, pulmonary diseases or hematological disorders (Hb abnormalities) • Central cyanosis is charachterized by cyanosis affective both mucous membranes and skin	• Peripheral cyanosis is caused by slowing of blood flow and increased extraction of oxygen from normally saturated blood • It results from vasoconstriction or decreased peripheral blood flow, reduced cardiac output or vascular occlusion • Peripheral cyanosis is characterized by cyanosis of skin alone and sparing of mucous membranes
Causes	**Causes**
Decreased arterial oxygen saturation • ***Decreased atmospheric pressure*** *– high altitude* • ***Impaired pulmonary function*** ▪ *Alveolar hyoventilation* ▪ *Uneven relationships between pulmonary ventilation and perfusion (perfusion of hypoventilated alveoli)* ▪ *Impaired oxygen diffusion* • ***Anatomic shunts*** ▪ ***Certain types of congenital heart disease*** ▪ *Pulmonary arteriovenous fistulas* ▪ *Multiple small intrapulmonary shunts* • ***Hemoglobin with low affinity for oxygen*** **Hemoglobin abnormalities** • Methemoglobinemia – hereditary, acquired • Sulfhemoglobinema – acquired • Carboxyhemoglobinemia (not true cyanosis)	• ***Vascular occlusion*** ▪ *Arterial obstruction* ▪ *Venous obstruction* • *Reduced cardiac output* • *Cold exposure* • *Redistribution of blood flow from extremities*

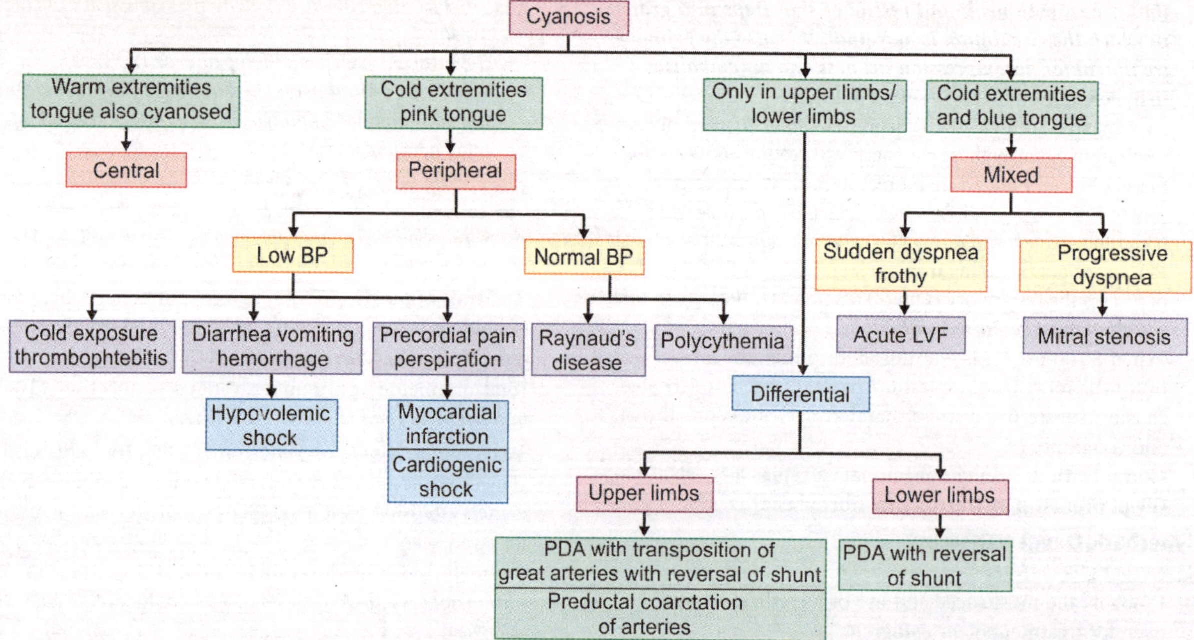

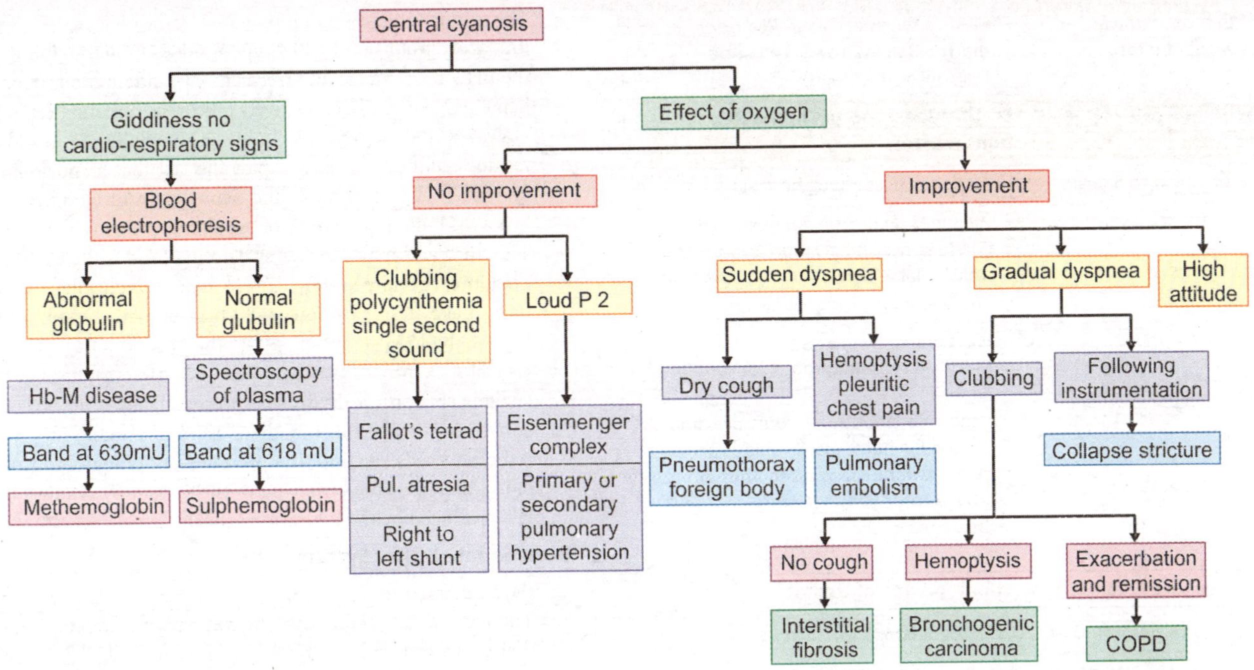

15. Ans. a. Liver, b. Lymph nodes, c. Spleen, d. Bone marrow & e. Yolk sac

[Ref: Ganong 25th/554; Guyton 12th/111,Guyton 11th/420; Chaudhuri Physiology 6th/32]

"**Blood formation** *occur later (5wk) throughout* **embryonic mesenchyme, then liver, then spleen/thymus, bone marrow, lymph node**" *(embryology.mrd.unsw.au)*

"*Formation of blood include* **formation of RBC, WBC & platelet**" *(A.K.Jain 6th/65)*

Production of Red Blood Cells

◈ *Guyton 12th/111*

- In the **early weeks of embryonic life**, primitive, nucleated red blood cells are produced in the ***yolk sac***. During the middle trimester of gestation, the ***liver*** is the main organ for production of red blood cells but reasonable numbers are also produced in the ***spleen*** **and** ***lymph nodes***. Then, during the last month or so of gestation and after birth, red blood cells are produced exclusively in the ***bone marrow***.
- ***The bone marrow of essentially all bones produces red blood cells until a person is 5 years old. The marrow of the long bones, except for the proximal portions of the humeri and tibiae, becomes quite fatty and produces no more red blood cells after about age 20 years. Beyond this age, most red cells continue to be produced in the marrow of the membranous bones, such as the vertebrae, sternum, ribs, and ilia. Even in these bones, the marrow becomes less productive as age increases.***

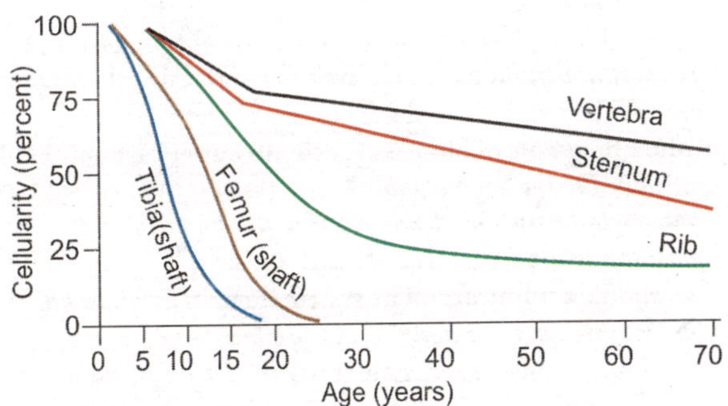

Fig: *(Guyton 12th/111):* Relative rates of red blood cell production in the bone marrow of different bones at different ages

"***Blood production starts from 3rd week of intrauterine life. B/W 3rd to 5th month of intrauterine life, erythropoiesis occur, principally in the liver & some extent in the spleen***" *(Chaudhuri Physiology 6th/32)*

Erythropoesis in Intrauterine Life	
• 3rd week to 3rd month (***Intravascular phase***) Q	• Erythropoesis occurs in the mesoderm of ***yolk sac*** • Only stage when erythropoesis occurs within the blood vessels (intravascular erythropoesis)
• 3rd month to 5th month (***Hepatic phase***)	• Erythropoesis occurs in ***liver & spleen***

Contd...

• 5th month onwards (***Myeloid phase***)	• Erythropoesis occurs in ***Red bone marrow*** (all marrow is red bone marrow at this stage)
Postnatal Erythropoesis	**Erythropoesis occurs in the Red bone marrow**
• From Birth to 5 years	• All bones (Flat + long bones)
• 5 years to 20 years	• All bones (Flat + long bones) (There is increasingly more production from flat bones & decreasing production from long bones)
• After 20 years	• Flat bones Most red cells are produced from flat bones Minor contribution from proximal portion of humerus & tibia marrow of other long bones becomes quiet fatty & produces no more red cells after age of 20

16. Ans. a. Protein..., c. Carbonic acid..., d. Hemoglobin...

[Ref: A.K.Jain 6th/559-60,55; Ganong 25th/643-44; Guyton 12th/504-08]

Phosphate Buffer System

◈ *Guyton 12th/507*

Although the phosphate buffer system is ***not important as an extracellular fluid buffer***, it plays a major role in buffering renal tubular fluid and intracellular fluids.

"**More than 90% of blood's capacity to buffer carbonic acid** *is attributed to the* ***haemoglobin buffer system****" (A.K.Jain 6th/559)*

"***Hemoglobin in blood has 6 times the buffering capacity of plasma proteins****" (A.K.Jain 6th/560)*

"**Carbonic acid-bicarbonate system** *is one of the* ***most effective buffer systems in the body****" (A.K.Jain 6th/560)*

"**Carbonic acid-bicarbonate system**: *There is no carbonic anhydrase in plasma, but there is an abundant supply in RBC, gastric acid secreting cells & renal tubular cells" (A.K.Jain 6th/560)*

"*In* ***plasma,*** *the* **phosphate concentration** *is too low for this system to be a quantitatively important buffer, but it is important intracellularily" (A.K.Jain 6th/560)*

Buffering in the Blood

◈ *Ganong 25th/643-44*

- Acid and base shifts in the blood are largely controlled by **three main buffers in blood**: ***(1) proteins, (2) hemoglobin, and (3) the carbonic acid–bicarbonate system.***
- Plasma **proteins** are effective buffers because both their free carboxyl and their free amino groups dissociate.
- The second buffer system is provided by the dissociation of the imidazole groups of the histidine residues in **hemoglobin.** In the pH 7.0–7.7 range, the free carboxyl and amino groups of hemoglobin contribute relatively little to its buffering capacity. However, the hemoglobin molecule contains 38 histidine residues, and on this basis—plus the fact that hemoglobin is present in large amounts—the hemoglobin in blood has six times the buffering capacity of the plasma proteins.
- The third and major buffer system in blood is the **carbonic acid–bicarbonate system.** There are two additional factors that make the carbonicacid- bicarbonate system such a good biological buffer. First, the reaction $CO_2 + H_2O \leftrightarrow H_2CO_3$ proceeds slowly in either direction unless the enzyme **carbonic anhydrase** is present.There is no carbonic anhydrase in plasma, but there is an abundant supply in red blood cells. Second, the presence of hemoglobin in the blood increases the buffering of the system by binding free H+ produced by the hydration of CO_2

Bicarbonate Buffer System

◈ *Guyton 12th/505*

- The bicarbonate buffer system consists of a water solution that contains two ingredients: (1) a weak acid, H_2CO_3, and (2) a bicarbonate salt, such as $NaHCO_3$.
- H_2CO_3 is formed in the body by the reaction of CO_2 with H_2O.

Proteins are Important Intracellular Buffers

◈ *Guyton 12th/507*

Proteins are among the most plentiful buffers in the body because of their high concentrations, especially within the cells

Defending Against Changes in H^+ Concentration: Buffers, Lungs, and Kidneys

◈ *Guyton 12th/504*

- Three primary systems regulate the H^+ concentration in the body fluids to prevent acidosis or alkalosis: (1) the *chemical acid-base buffer systems of the body fluids,* which immediately combine with acid or base to prevent excessive changes in H^+ concentration; (2) the *respiratory center,* which regulates the removal of CO_2 (and, therefore, H_2CO_3) from the extracellular fluid; and (3) the *kidneys,* which can excrete either acid or alkaline urine, thereby readjusting the extracellular fluid H^+ concentration toward normal during acidosis or alkalosis.
- When there is a change in H^+ concentration, the *buffer systems* of the body fluids react within seconds to minimize these changes. Buffer systems do not eliminate H^+ from or add them to the body but only keep them tied up until balance can be re-established.

Table *(A.K.Jain 6th/559)*: **The principal buffers in the body fluids i.e. 'Body Buffer Systems"**

1. Whole Blood	i. Haemoglobin system ($H Hb \rightleftharpoons H^+ + Hb^-$) ii. Protein system ($H Prot \rightleftharpoons H^+ + Prot^-$) iii. Carbonic Acid-Bicarbonate System ($H_2CO_3 \rightleftharpoons H^+ + HCO_3^-$)
2. Interstitial fluid	i. Carbonic Acid-Bicarbonate System ($H_2 CO_3 \rightleftharpoons H^+ + HCO_3^-$)
3. Intracellular fluid	i. Protein system ii. Phosphate system ($H_2PO_4^- \rightleftharpoons H + HPO_4^{2-}$)

A & E

BIOCHEMISTRY

17. Ans. c. Triple helix..., e. Component....

[Ref: Harper 30th/46-47,627-32; Lippincott 6th/43-48; Vasudevan 5th/254-55]

α *helix &* β-pleated **sheets are two types of regular structure of secondary structure of protein** *(Harper 30th/38)*

Collagen

Harper 30th/46-47,627-32; Lippincott 6th/43-48

- In collagen, the **collagen helix**, or type-2 helix, is a major shape in secondary structure
- All collagen have a ***triple helical*** structure.
- A striking characteristic of collagen is occurrence *of **glycine residue** at every third position* of triple helical portion of α chain. This repeating structure, represented as $(Gly\text{-}x\text{-}y)_n$, is an absolute requirement for the formation of the triple helix.
- Collagen the major component of most connective tissues, constitutes approximately 25% of the protein of mammals. At least 28 distincts types of collagen made up of over 30 distinct polypeptide chains have been identified in human tissues.
- The tropocollagen or collagen molecule is a subunit of larger collagen aggregates such as fibrils. At approximately 300 nm long and 1.5 nm in diameter, it is made up of three polypeptide strands (called ***alpha chains***), each possessing the conformation of ***a left-handed helix*** (its name is not to be confused with the commonly occurring alpha helix, a right-handed structure). These ***three left-handed helices are twisted together into a right-handed coiled coil, a triple helix or "super helix"***, a cooperative *quaternary* structure stabilized by numerous hydrogen bonds.

So far, 28 types of collagen have been identified and described. The five most common types are:

- *Collagen I: skin, tendon, vascular ligature, organs, bone (main component of bone)*
- *Collagen II: cartilage (main component of cartilage)*
- *Collagen III: reticulate (main component of reticular fibers), commonly found alongside type I.*
- *Collagen IV: forms bases of cell basement membrane*
- *Collagen V: cells surfaces, hair and placenta*

Collagen is the Most Abundant Protein in the Animal World

Harper 30th/627-32

- **Collagen,** the ***major component of most connective tissues,*** constitutes approximately 25% of the protein of mammals.
- It provides an extracellular framework for all metazoan animals and exists in virtually every animal tissue. At least 28 distinct types of collagen made up of over 30 distinct polypeptide chains (each encoded by a separate gene) have been identified in human tissues.

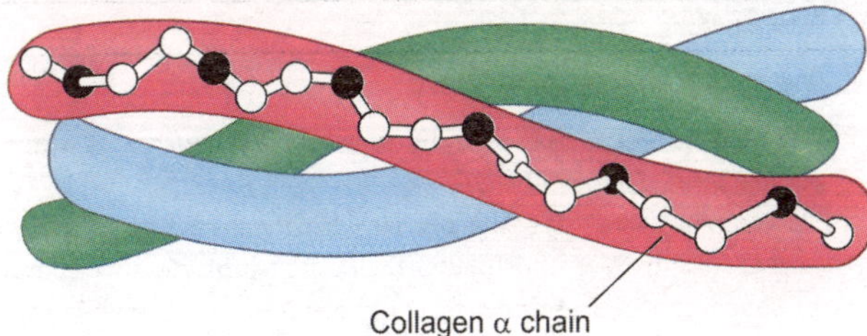

Fig: *(Lippincott 6th/43):* Triple-stranded helix of collagen

Type	Tissue Distribution
	Fibril-forming
I	Sikin, bone, tendon, blood vessels, cornea
II	Cartilage, intervertebral disk, vitreous body
III	Blood vessels, fetal skin
	Network-forming
IV	Basement membrane
VII	Beneath stratified squamous epithelia
	Fibril-associated
IX	Cartilage
XII	Tendon, ligaments, some other tissues.

Fig: *(Lippincott 6th/44):* The most common type of collagen

Table: Types of Collagen

Type	Tissue
I	Most connective tissues, including bone
II	Cartilage, vitreous humor
III	Extensible connective tissues such as skin, lung, and the vascular system
IV	Basement membranes
V	Minor component in tissues containing collagen I
VI	Most connective tissues
VII	Anchoring fibrils
VIII	Endothelium, other tissues
IX	Tissues containing collagen II
X	Hypertrophic cartilage
XI	Tissues containing collagen II
XII	Tissues containing collagen I
XIII	Many tissues
XIV	Tissues containing collagen I
XV	Many tissues
XVI	Many tissues
XVII	Skin hemidesmosomes
XVIII	Many tissues (e.g., liver, kidney)
XIX	Rhabdomyosarcoma cells

18. Ans. e. 0

[Ref: Harper 30th/20]

"**Isoelectric point (pI)** is *a pH in which* ***net charge of amino acid is zero***" *(Harper 30th/20)*

"Isoelectric point (pI) is ***a pH in which net charge of amino acid is zero.*** In case of proteins isoelectric point mostly depends on seven charged amino acids: glutamate (δ-carboxyl group), aspartate (ß-carboxyl group), cysteine (thiol group), tyrosine (phenol group), histidine (imidazole side chains), lysine (ε-ammonium group) and arginine (guanidinium group). Additonally, one should take into account charge of protein terminal groups.Each of them has its unique acid dissociation constant referred to as pK. Moreover, net charge of the protein is in tight relation with the solution (buffer) pH. Keeping in main this we can use Henderson-Hasselbach equation to calculate protein charge in certain pH"

19. Ans. b. Tay-Sachs....

[Ref: Harper 30th/251; Lippincott 6th/212; Harrison 19th/432e,433e]

What is Hexosaminidase A Deficiency

- Hexosaminidase A deficiency is an enzyme deficiency that causes brain and other nerve cells to die, which can lead to severe neurological and mental problems.
- Hexosaminidase A (HEX A) deficiency is caused by a deficiency in an enzyme called beta-hexosaminidase A. This enzyme helps break down a particular fatty acid called GM2 ganglioside. Without adequate amounts of functional enzymes, GM2 ganglioside will build up in nerve cells and cause them to die.
- There are several forms of HEX A deficiency, including ***acute infantile (Tay-Sachs disease), juvenile, chronic, or adult-onset forms.***

Table *(Harper 30th/251)*: **Examples of Sphingolipidoses**

Disease	Enzyme Deficiency	Clinical Symptoms
Tay-Sachs disease	Hexosaminidase A	Mental retardation, blindness, muscular weakness.
Fabry's disease	α-Galactosidase	Skin rash, kidney failure (full symptoms only in males; X-linked recessive).
Metachromatic leukodystrophy	Arylsulfatase A	Mental retardation and psychologic disturbances in adults; demyelination.
Krabbe's disease	β-Galactosidase	Mental retardation; myelin almost absent.
Gaucher's disease	β-Glucosidase	Enlarged liver and spleen, erosion of long bones, mental retardation in infants.
Niemann-Pick disease	Sphingomyelinase	Enlarged liver and spleen, mental retardation; fatal in early life.
Farber's disease	Ceramidase	Hoarseness, dermatitis, skeletal deformation, mental retardation; fatal in early life.

Table *(Harrison 19th/432e)*: **Selected Lysosomal Storage Diseases**

			Clinical Features					
Disorder	**Enzyme Deficiency [Specific Therapy]**	**Stored Material**	**Neurologic**	**Liver Spleen Enlargement**	**Skeletal Dysplasia**	**Ophthalmologic**	**Hematologic**	**Unique Features**
MPS I H, **Hurler** MPS I H/S, Hurler/Scheie MPS I S, Scheie	α-L-Iduronidase [ET, BMT]	Dermatan sulfate Heparan sulfate	Mental retardation Mental retardation None	+++	++++	Corneal clouding	Vacuolated lymphocytes	Coarse facies; cardiovascular involvement; joint stiffness
MPS II, Hunter	Iduronate sulfatase [ET]	Dermatan sulfate Heparan sulfate	Mental retardation, less in mild form	+++	++++	Retinal degeneration, no corneal clouding	Granulated lymphocytes	Coarse facies; cardiovascular involvement; joint stiffness; distinctive pebbly skin lesions

Table *(Harrison-Partial list)*: **Selected Lysosomal Storage Diseases**

Disorder	Enzyme Deficiency (Specific Therapy)	Stored Material	Clinical Features					
			Neurologic	Liver Spleen Enlargement	Skeletal Dysplasia	Ophthalmologic	Hematologic	Unique Features
Tay-Sachs disease	β Hexosaminidase A	GM_2 gangliosides	Mental retardation, seizures, later juvenile form	None	None	Cherry red spot in infantile form	None	Macrocephaly, hyperacusis in infantile form
Sandhoff disease	βHexosaminidases A and B	GM_2 gangliosides	Mental retardation, seizures	++	±	Cherry red spot	None	Macrocephaly, hyperacusis
Fabry disease	α-Galactosidase A (ET)	Globotriaosylceramide	Painful acroparesthesias	None	None	Corneal dystrophy, vascular lesions	None	Cutaneous angiokeratomas, hypohydrosis
Gaucher disease	Acid β-glucosidase (ET, SRT)	Glucosylceramide	None ++++ ++	++++ +++ ++++	++++ + ++++	None Eye movements Eye movements	Gaucher cells in bone marrow, cytopenias	Adult form highly variable
Niemann-Pick disease A and B	Sphingomye-linase	Sphingomyelin	Mental retardation and seizures	++++	None Osteoporosis	Macular degeneration	Foam cells in bone marrow	Pulmonary infiltrates Lung failure

20. Ans. a. Pyruvate..., b. TCA cycle..., d. ATP...

[Ref: Harper 30th/127,610-11; Lippincott 6th/74]

Matrix of the Mitochondrion

◈ *Lippincott 6th/74*

- This gel-like solution in the interior of mitochondria is 50% protein. These molecules include the ***enzymes responsible for the oxidation of pyruvate, amino acids, fatty acids (by β-oxidation), and those of the tricarboxylic acid (TCA) cycle.***
- The synthesis of glucose, urea, and heme occur partially in the matrix of mitochondria. In addition, the matrix contains NAD+ and FAD (the oxidized forms of the two coenzymes that are required as hydrogen acceptors) and ADP and Pi, which are used to produce ATP. [Note: The matrix also contains mitochondrial RNA and DNA (mtRNA and mtDNA) and mitochondrial ribosomes.]

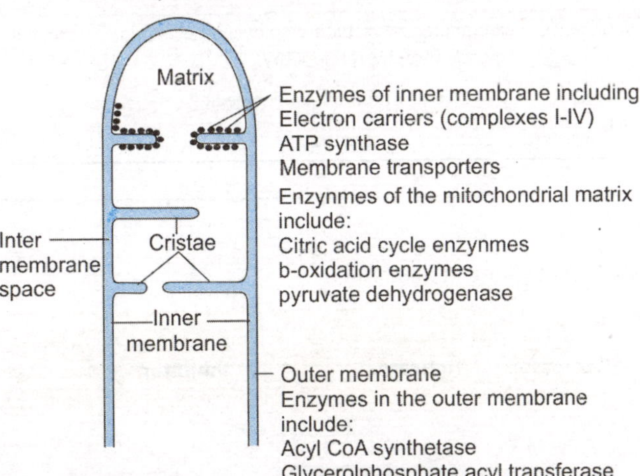

Fig: *(Harper 30th/127)*: Structure of the mitochondrial membranes. Note that the inner membrane contains many folds, or cristae

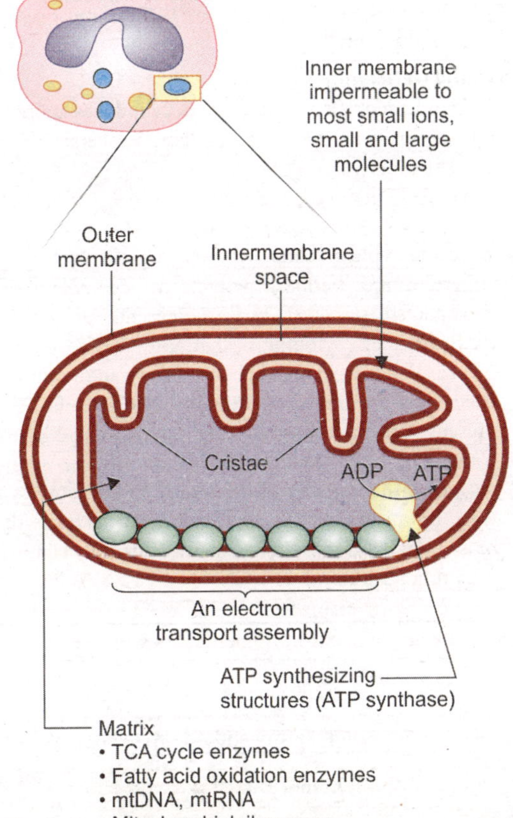

Fig: *(Lippincott 6th/74)*: Structure of mitochondria showing ETC & ATP synthesizing structure on inner membrane

21. **Ans.** **a. Imidazole..., b. Tetrapyrrole..., c. Indole..., d. Guanidinium....**

[Ref: Harper 30th/20-23; Lippincott 6th/1-11; Vasudevan 5th/19]

Imidazole group: *Histidine (Harper 30th/21, Vasudevan 5th/19)*
Sulfhydryl group: *Cysteine (Vasudevan 5th/19)*
Beta carboxyl group: *Aspartic acid (Vasudevan 5th/19)*
Gamma carboxyl group: *Glutamic acid (Vasudevan 5th/19)*
€-amino group: *Lysine (Vasudevan 5th/19)*

Special Groups in Amino Acids

Vasudevan 5th/17

Benzene group-*Phenylalanine*
Indole group in- *Tryptophan*
Pyrrolidine group - *Proline*
Guanidinium group- *Arginine*
Phenol group-*Tyrosine*

22. **Ans.** **b. Vit B1**

[Ref: Lippincott 6th/378-79; Harrison 19th/96e, 18th/594-96; Harper 30th/555-56, 28th/ 468]

"Classically, **Wernicke's encephalopathy** is characterized by the ***triad of ophthalmoplegia, ataxia, and mental confusion, but confusion & a staggering gait are perhaps most common***"- Synopsis of Psychaitry by *(Kaplon 11th/796-799)*

Thiamine Deficiency

- Thiamine deficiency in its early stage induces anorexia and nonspecific symptoms (e.g., irritability, decrease in short-term memory).
- Prolonged thiamine deficiency causes *beriberi*, which is classically categorized as wet or dry although there is considerable overlap between the two categories. In either form of beriberi, patients may complain of pain and paresthesia. *Wet beriberi* presents primarily with cardiovascular symptoms that are due to impaired myocardial energy metabolism and dysautonomia; it can occur after 3 months of a thiamine-deficient diet. Patients present with an enlarged heart, tachycardia, high-output congestive heart failure, peripheral edema, symmetric peripheral neuropathy of the motor and sensory systems, with diminished reflexes. The neuropathy affects the legs most markedly, and patients have difficulty rising from a squatting position.
- Alcoholic patients with chronic thiamine deficiency also may have central nervous system (CNS) manifestations known as ***Wernicke's encephalopathy***, which consists of horizontal nystagmus, ***ophthalmoplegia*** (due to weakness of one or more extraocular muscles), ***cerebellar ataxia***, and mental impairment
- When there is an additional loss of memory and a confabulatory psychosis, the syndrome is known as ***Wernicke-Korsakoff syndrome***. Despite the typical clinical picture and history, Wernicke-Korsakoff syndrome is underdiagnosed.

Table *(Harrison)*: **Principal clinical findings of vitamin malnutrition**

Nutrient	Clinical Finding
Thiamine	Beriberi: neuropathy, muscle weakness and wasting, cardiomegaly, edema, ophthalmoplegia, confabulation
Riboflavin	Magenta tongue, angular stomatitis, seborrhea, cheilosis
Niacin	Pellagra: pigmented rash of sun-exposed areas, bright red tongue, diarrhea, apathy, memory loss, disorientation
Vitamin B6	Seborrhea, glossitis, convulsions, neuropathy, depression, confusion, microcytic anemia
Folate	Megaloblastic anemia, atrophic glossitis, depression,↑ homocysteine
Vitamin B12	Megaloblastic anemia, loss of vibratory and position sense, abnormal gait, dementia, impotence, loss of bladder and bowel control, ↑homocysteine, ↑methylmalonic acid
Vitamin C	Scurvy: petechiae, ecchymosis, coiled hairs, inflamed and bleeding gums, joint effusion, poor wound healing, fatigue
Vitamin A	Xerophthalmia, night blindness, Bitot's spots, follicular hyperkeratosis, impaired embryonic development, immune dysfunction
Vitamin D	Rickets: skeletal deformation, rachitic rosary, bowed legs; osteomalacia
Vitamin E	Peripheral neuropathy, spinocerebellar ataxia, skeletal muscle atrophy, retinopathy
Vitamin K	Elevated prothrombin time, bleeding

23. **Ans.** **a. Pyruvate..., b. Phosphoeno..., d. Glucose 6...,**

[Ref: Harper 30th/188; Lippincott 6th/117-122; Harper 28th/ 165-68; Lippincott 4th/329]

Table *(Harper 30th/188)*: **Regulatory and Adaptive Enzymes Associated with Carbohydrate Metabolism.**

	Activity in					
	Carbohydrate Feeding	**Fasting and Diabetes**	**Inducer**	**Repressor**	**Activator**	**Inhibitor**
Glycogenolysis, glycolysis, and pyruvate oxidation						
Glycogen synthase	↑	↓			Insulin, glucose 6-phosphate	Glucagon
Hexokinase						Glucose 6-phosphate

Contd...

A & E

	Activity in					
	Carbohydrate Feeding	**Fasting and Diabetes**	**Inducer**	**Repressor**	**Activator**	**Inhibitor**
Glucokinase	↑	↓	Insulin	Glucagon		
Phosphofructokinase-1	↑	↓	Insulin	Glucagon	5'AMP, fructose 6-phosphate, fructose 2,6-bisphosphate, P_i	Citrate, ATP, glucagon
Pyruvate kinase	↑	↓	Insulin, fructose	Glucagon	Fructose 1,6-bisphosphate, insulin	ATP, alanine, glucagon, norepinephrine
Pyruvate dehydrogenase	↑	↓			CoA, NAD^+, insulin, ADP, pyruvate	Acetyl CoA, NADH, ATP (fatty acids, ketone bodies)
Gluconeogenesis						
Pyruvate carboxylase	↓	↑	Glucocorticoids, glucagon, epinephrine	Insulin	Acetyl CoA	ADP
Phosphoenolpyruvate carboxykinase	↓	↑	Glucocorticoids, glucagon, epinephrine	Insulin	Glucagon?	
Glucose 6-phosphatase	↓	↑	Glucocorticoids, glucagon, epinephrine	Insulin		

24. Ans. a. Agarose gel, b. Polyacrylamide plain gel & c. Polyacrylamide SDS (Sodium dodecyl sulphate) ...

[Ref: www.lonza.com/go/literature/2043; Shinde 7th/774]

"Separation of RNA in ***agarose gels*** is used for a number of different purposes, including Northern blots to monitor RNA expression levels, checking RNA integrity and size selection of RNA for cloning experiments. Separation of RNA based on fragment length requires conditions that are different from DNA analysis. These include sample preparation, the use of sample and *gel denaturants*, electrophoresis buffers, and visualization. The purpose of the experiment and the size of the RNA being separated are the primary drivers in determining which denaturing system to use. ***The most frequently used denaturants for RNA agarose gel electrophoresis are formaldehyde, formaldehyde/formamide, and glyoxal plus DMSO***. *(www.lonza.com/go/literature)*

Table *(Shinde 7th/774)*: **Types of electrophoresis and their applications**

Type	Support	Applications
Paper electrophoresis	Whatman No. 3 or Cellulose acetate membrane	Detection of gross abnormalities in plasma proteins in certain diseases, e.g. Multiple myeloma, Cirrhosis, Nephrotic syndrome, etc
PAGE/SDS PAGE	Polyacrylamide plain or SDS (Sodium dodecyl sulphate) impregnated gels	Separation and purification of individual proteins, determination of molecular weight of purified polypeptides
Starch	Hydrolyzed Starch	Isozyme analysis
Agarose	Agarose gel	Separation of nucleic acids, Nucleotide sequencing
Immunoelectrophoresis 1. Rocket 2. Crossed 3. Immunofixation	Agarose, Acrylamide, preformed microscopic slides	Detection and characterization of antigens (e.g. Plasma proteins, enzymes, cell membrane Ag) or antibodies
Isoelectric focusing	Laborator made or preformed pH Gradient gels of Polyacrylamide or agarose	Phenotyping of α_1-antitrypsin, Genetic variants of enzymes, hemoglobins and other proteins

IMMUNOGENETICS & MOLECULAR BIOLOGY

25. Ans. a. Northern..., b. Southern..., d. Microarray.

[Ref: Lippincott 6th/ 473; Harper 29th/483-85; Harrison 19th/83e,443-44,18th/ 508; Vasudevan 5th/454-56]

Table *(Lippincott's Biochemistry)*: **Techniques used to analyse DNA, RNA & proteins**

Technique	Sample Analysed	Gel Used	Purpose
Southern blot	*DNA*[Q]	Yes	Detect DNA changes
Northern blot	*RNA*[Q]	Yes	Measures mRNA amounts & size
Western blot	*Protein*[Q]	Yes	Measures *protein* amount
ASO	*DNA*[Q]	No	Detects *DNA* mutations[Q]
Microarray	*RNA or cDNA*	No	Measures many mRNA levels at one time
ELISA	*Proteins*[Q] *or antibodies*	No	Detects *proteins (antigens)or antibodies*[Q]
Proteomics	Proteins[Q]	Yes	Measures abundance, distribution, posttranslation modifications, functions & interactions of cellular *proteins*

ASO = Allele specific oligonucleotides

Table *(Harrison 18th/ 508)*: **Methods Used for the Detection of Mutations**

Method	Principle	Type of Mutation Detected
Fluorescent in situ hybridization (FISH)	Hybridization to chromosomes with fluorescently labeled probes	Numerical or structural abnormalities in chromosomes
Southern blot	Hybridization with genomic probe or cDNA probe after digestion of high molecular DNA	Large deletion, insertion, rearrangement, expansions of triplet repeat, amplification
Polymerase chain reaction (PCR)	Amplification of DNA segment	Expansion of triplet repeats, variable number of tandem repeats (VNTR), gene rearrangements, translocations; prepare DNA for other mutation methods
Reverse transcriptase PCR (RT-PCR)	Reverse transcription, amplification of DNA segment →absence or reduction of mRNA transcription	Analyze expressed mRNA (cDNA) sequence; detect loss of expression
DNA sequencing	Direct sequencing of PCR products Sequencing of DNA segments cloned into plasmid vectors	Point mutations, small deletions and insertions
Restriction fragment polymorphism (RFLP)	Detection of altered restriction pattern of genomic DNA (Southern blot) or PCR products	Point mutations, small deletions and insertions
Microarrays	Hybridization of PCR products to wild-type or mutated oligonucleotides	Point mutations, small deletions and insertions Genotyping of SNPs

26. Ans. a. Help in synthesis ..., c. RNA-dependent....

[Ref: Lippincott 6th /406; Harper 30th/364, 380, 470, 453]

"The genetic material for some animal and plant viruses is RNA rather than DNA. Although some RNA viruses never have their information transcribed into a DNA molecule, many animal RNA viruses-specifically, the retroviruses (the HIV virus, for example)-are transcribed by viral ***RNA-dependent DNA polymerase***, the so-called **reverse transcriptase,** to produce a double-stranded DNA copy of their RNA genome" *(Harper 30th/364)*

Reverse Transcriptases

◈ *Lippincott 6th /406*

- Reverse transcriptases, as seen with telomerase, are ***RNA-directed DNA polymerases.*** A reverse transcriptase is involved in the replication of retroviruses, such as human immunodeficiency virus (HIV).
- These viruses carry their genome in the form of ssRNA molecules. Following infection of a host cell, the viral enzyme, reverse transcriptase, ***uses the viral RNA as a template for the 5'→3' synthesis of viral DNA***, which then becomes integrated into host chromosomes.
- Reverse transcriptase activity is also seen with transposons, DNA elements that can move about the genome. In eukaryotes, such elements are transcribed to RNA, the RNA is used as a template for DNA synthesis by a reverse transcriptase encoded by the transposon, and the DNA is randomly inserted into the genome.

Note: Transposons that involve an RNA intermediate are called retrotransposons or retroposons.

Table *(Chatterjea & Shinde 7th/261; Harper 30th/453)*: **Enzymes used in recombinant DNA technology**

Name	Reaction	Function
Restriction endonuclease	Cut DNA at specific DNA sequence within the molecule	Chemical knife in recombinant DNA technology
Reverse transcriptase	Synthesizes DNA from RNA template	Synthesizes c-DNA from m-RNA
S_1 nuclease	Degrades ss-DNA	Removal of 'hairpin' in DNA synthesis of c-DNA

Contd...

Name	Reaction	Function
DNA Ligase	Catalyzes bond between DNA molecules	Joining of DNA molecules
DNA Polymerase I	Synthesizes ds-DNA from ss-DNA	Synthesis of ds c-DNA,; 'nick' translation[Q]
BAL3 1 nuclease	Degrades both 3' and 5' ends of DNA	Progressive shortening of DNA molecules
Alkaline phosphatase[Q]	Dephosphorylates 5' ends of RNA and DNA	Removal of 5' -PO_4 Groups to kinase labeling to prevent self ligation

27. Ans. a. Adenine, d. Guanine

[Ref: Harper 30th /360; Lippincott 6th /291-92]

"Both DNA and RNA contain the same **purine bases**: ***adenine (A) and guanine (G)***. Both DNA and RNA contain the pyrimidine cytosine (C), but they differ in their second pyrimidine base: DNA contains thymine (T), whereas RNA contains uracil (U). T and U differ in that only T has a methyl group" *(Lippincott 6th /291)*

DNA and RNA purines

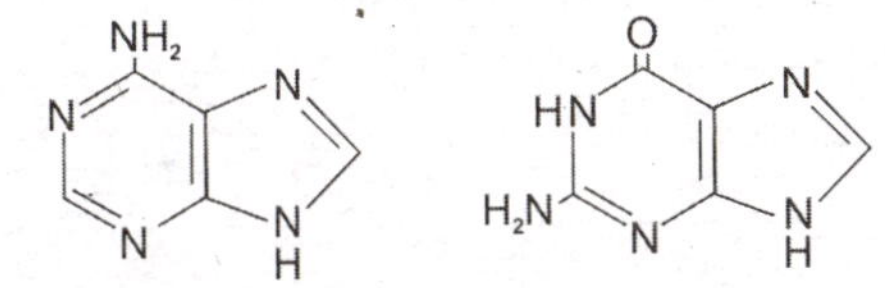

Adenine (A) Guanine (G)

RNA pyrimidines

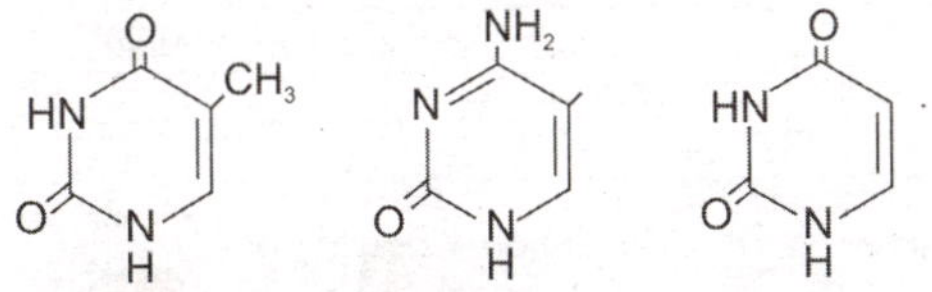

Thymine (T) Cytosine (C) Uracil (U)

DNA pyrimidines

Fig: *(Lippincott 6th /291)*: Purines and pyrimidines commonly found in DNA and RNA

28. Ans. a. Protects bacteria..., e. Also known....

[Ref: Harper 30th / 452-54,368; Lippincott 6th /465-67; Satyanarayana 3rd / 580]

RE *also known as molecular knives,* ***molecular scissor*** *& molecular scalpel" (mcqbiology.com)*

Table *(Chatterjea & Shinde7th/261;Harper 30th/453)*: **Enzymes used in recombinant DNA technology**

Name	Reaction	Function
Restriction endonuclease	Cut DNA at specific DNA sequence within the molecule	Chemical knife in recombinant DNA technology

"**RE** can specifically recognize DNA with particular sequence of 4-6 mucleotides and cleave. The recognition sequences are **palindromic** (i.e., twofold rotational symmetry" *(Lippincott 4th/466)* RE *restrict DNA replication" (Satyanarayana 3rd / 579)*

Restriction Enzyme (RE or Restriction Endonuclease)

- It is an enzyme that *cleave double-stranded DNA at specific recognition nucleotide known as restriction sites*
- To cut the DNA, a restriction enzyme makes two incisions,one through each *sugar-phosphate backbone* (i.e. each strand) of the DNA double helix. This enzyme can restrict viral replication so called restriction enzymes.
- The cut DNA fragments by RE may have *sticky ends (cohesive ends)*or blunts endsdepending on the mechanism used by enzyme
- DNA fragments with sticky ends are particularly useful for recombinant DNA experiments (hybrid or chimeric DNA molecules)
- Restriction enzyme is named according to the organism from which it was isolated

Types of RE

Type I: Multi-subunit, both endonuclease and ***methylase activities*** & cleaves at random, up to 1000 bp from recognition sequence

Type II: Mostly single subunit & cleave DNA within recognition sequence. It is commonly used in biotechnology and it does not require ATP, and are smaller and simpler.

Type III: Multi-subunit, endonuclease and ***methylase activity*** & cleaves about 25 bp from recognition sequence.

Restriction Endonuclease

- It is an enzyme that cuts DNA at specific recognition Nucleotide sequences (with Type II restriction enzymes cutting double-stranded DNA) known as restriction sites.
- Such enzymes, found in ***bacteria and archaea***, are thought to have evolved to provide a ***defense mechanism against invading viruses***.
- Inside a bacterial host, the restriction enzymes ***selectively cut up foreign DNA*** in a process called restriction; ***host DNA is methylated by a modification enzyme (a methylase)*** to protect it from the restriction enzyme's activity. Collectively, these two processes form the restriction modification system. To cut the DNA, a restriction enzyme makes two incisions, once through each sugar-phosphate backbone (i.e. each strand) of the DNA double helix.
- They are used to assist insertion of genes into plasmid vectors during gene cloning and protein expression experiments. For optimal use, plasmids that are commonly used for gene cloning are modified to include a short polylinker sequence
- In a similar manner, restriction enzymes are used to *digest genomic DNA for gene analysis by Southern blot.*

PATHOLOGY

29. Ans. a. Occur..., b. Miliary..., e. Sputum smear....

[Ref: Harrison 19th/1112; Robbins(SAE) 9th/371-76; Davidson 22nd/689-90; CMDT 2016/283; Park 23rd/188]

Miliary TB

◈ *Davidson 22nd/689-90*

- ***Blood-borne dissemination*** *gives rise to miliary TB, which* ***may be present acutely*** *but more frequently is characterized by 2-3 weeks of fever, night sweats, anorexia, weight loss & a dry cough*
- ***Auscultation is frequently normal, but in more advanced disease, widespread crackles are evident***

Miliary Pulmonary Disease

◈ *Robbins(SAE) 9th/376*

- Miliary pulmonary disease occurs when organisms draining through lymphatics enter the venous blood and circulate back to the lung.
- Individual lesions are either ***microscopic or small, visible (2-mm) foci*** of yellow-white consolidation scattered through the lung parenchyma (the adjective "miliary" is derived from the resemblance of these foci to millet seeds).
- Miliary lesions may expand and coalesce, resulting in consolidation of large regions or even whole lobes of the lung.
- **Systemic miliary tuberculosis** occurs when bacteria disseminate through the **systemic arterial system**.The upper parts of both lungs are riddled with gray-white areas of caseation and multiple areas of softening and cavitation. Tuberculosis is most prominent in the **liver, bone marrow, spleen, adrenals, meninges, kidneys, fallopian tubes, and epididymis**, but could involve any organ

Miliary or Disseminated TB

◈ *Harrison 19th/1112*

- Miliary TB is due to hematogenous spread (also by ***lymphatics***-*CMDT 2016/279*) of tubercle bacilli. Although in children it is often the consequence of primary infection, in adults it may be due to either recent infection or reactivation of old disseminated foci.
- The lesions are usually yellowish ***granulomas 1–2 mm*** in diameter that resemble millet seeds (thus the term *miliary*, coined by nineteenth-century pathologists).
- Clinical manifestations are nonspecific and protean, depending on the predominant site of involvement. ***Fever, night sweats, anorexia, weakness, and weight loss are presenting symptoms in the majority of cases***.
- At times, patients have a ***cough and other respiratory symptoms*** due to pulmonary involvement as well as abdominal symptoms.
- Physical findings include ***hepatomegaly, splenomegaly, and lymphadenopathy***.
- Eye examination may reveal choroidal tubercles, which are ***pathognomonic of miliary TB***, in up to 30% of cases. Meningismus occurs in <10% of cases.

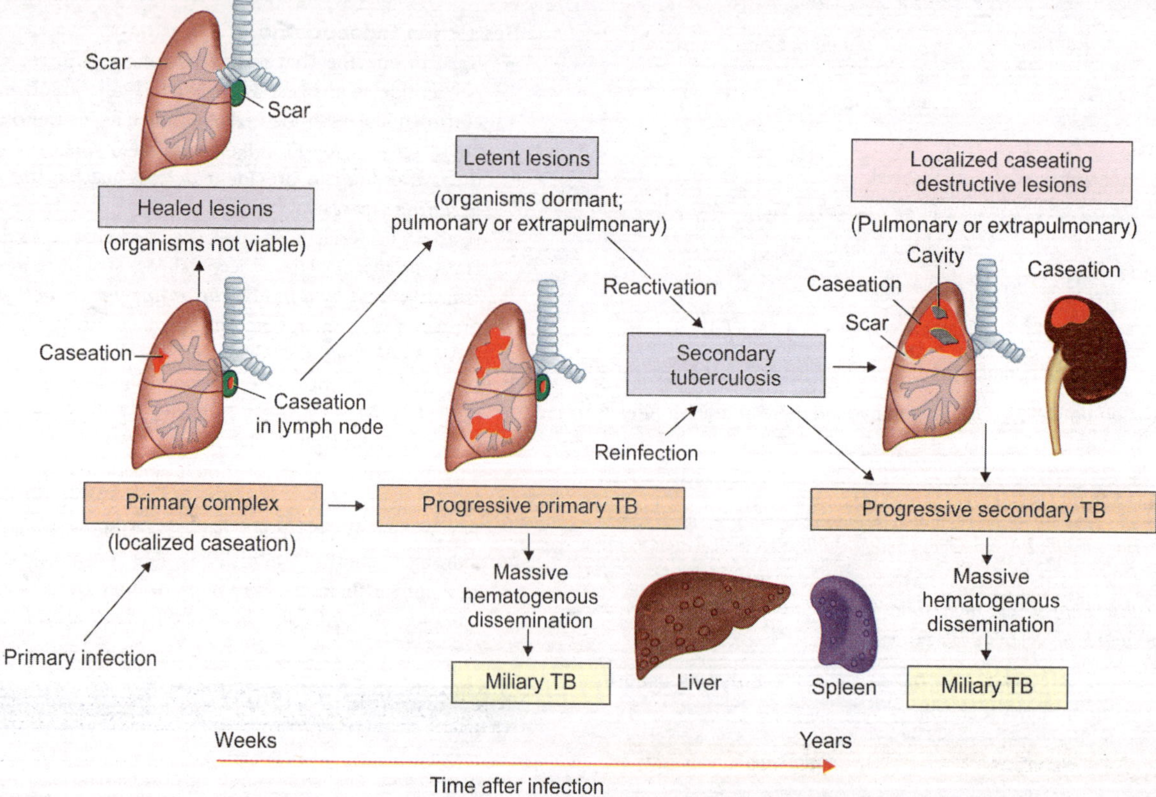

Fig: *(Robbins(SAE) 9th/374)*: The natural history and spectrum of tuberculosis

- A high index of suspicion is required for the diagnosis of miliary TB.
- Frequently, chest radiography reveals a miliary reticulonodular pattern (more easily seen on under penetrated film), although no radiographic abnormality may be evident early in the course and among HIV-infected patients.
- Other radiologic findings include large infiltrates, interstitial infiltrates (especially in HIV-infected patients), and pleural effusion.
- ***Sputum smear microscopy is negative in 80% of cases***. Various hematologic abnormalities may be seen, including anemia with leukopenia, lymphopenia, neutrophilic leukocytosis and leukemoid reactions, and polycythemia.
- The ***TST (Tuberculin skin test) may be negative*** in up to half of cases, but reactivity may be restored during chemotherapy.
- Bronchoalveolar lavage and transbronchial biopsy are more likely to provide bacteriologic confirmation, and granulomas are evident in liver or bone-marrow biopsy specimens from many patients.
- If it goes unrecognized, miliary TB is lethal; with proper early treatment, however, it is amenable to cure. Glucocorticoid therapy has not proved beneficial.
- *"In most cases, **regimens that are effective for treating pulmonary TB are also effective for treating extrapulmonary** disease. However, many expert recommended 9 months of therapy when **miliary**, meningeal or bone & joint disease is present" (CMDT 2016/283)*
- A rare presentation seen in the elderly is ***cryptic miliary TB*** that has a chronic course characterized by mild intermittent fever, anemia, and—ultimately—meningeal involvement preceding death.
- An acute septicemic form, *nonreactive miliary TB*, occurs very rarely and is due to massive hematogenous dissemination of tubercle bacilli.

30. Ans. b. Renal cell carcinoma, c. Pheochromocytoma, e. Follicular carcinoma of thyroid

[Ref: Robbins(SAE) 9th/ 1096,955,1135,273-74; Harrison 19th/91e]

*"Glioblastoma multiforme: **Malignant** cells carried in the CSF may spread (rarely) to the **spinal cord** or cause meningeal gliomatosis. However, **metastasis** of GBM beyond the **central nervous system** is extremely unusual"*

"A particularly troublesome feature of **renal cell carcinoma** is its tendency to metastasize widely before giving rise to any local symptoms or signs. In 25% of new patients with renal cell carcinoma, there is radiologic evidence of metastases at the time of presentation. The most common locations of ***metastasis are the lungs (more than 50%) and bones (33%),*** followed in frequency by the regional lymph nodes, liver, adrenal, and brain" *(Robbins 9th/ 955)*

"**Renal cell carcinoma**: *Tumour cells line the blood vessel which are responsible for* ***early blood spread*** *from RCC* ***(like follicular carcinoma of thyroid)*** *(Manipal Surgery 4th/948)*

"**Papillary carcinoma thyroid:** Foci of ***lymphatic invasion*** by tumor are often present, but ***involvement of blood vessels is relatively uncommon***, particularly in smaller lesions. Metastases to adjacent cervical lymph nodes occur in up to half of cases" *(Robbins 9th/ 1096)*

"**Follicular carcinoma of thyroid**: ***Blood borne metastases are more common*** *& lymph node involvement is much less common than papillary carcinoma" (L& B 26th/765)*

"Even capsular and ***vascular invasion*** may be encountered in benign lesions. Therefore, the definitive diagnosis of malignancy in **pheochromocytomas** is based exclusively on the presence of metastases. These may involve regional lymph nodes as well as more distant sites, including liver, lung, and bone" *(Robbins(SAE) 9th/ 1035)*

Pathways of Spread

◈ *Robbins 9th/ 273-74*

- Dissemination of cancers may occur through one of three pathways: (1) direct seeding of body cavities or surfaces, (2) lymphatic spread, and (3) hematogenous spread.
- **Seeding of body cavities and surfaces** may occur whenever a malignant neoplasm penetrates into a natural "open field." Most often involved is the peritoneal cavity, but any other cavity—pleural, pericardial, subarachnoid, and joint space—may be affected. Such seeding is particularly characteristic of carcinomas ***arising in the ovaries***, when, not infrequently, all peritoneal surfaces become coated with a heavy layer of cancerous glaze.
- **Transport through lymphatics** is the most common pathway for the initial dissemination of ***carcinomas, and sarcomas may also use this route****. The pattern of lymph node involvement follows the natural routes of lymphatic drainage.*
- **Hematogenous spread** is ***typical of sarcomas*** but is also seen with carcinomas. Understandably the ***liver and lungs are most frequently involved secondarily in such hematogenous dissemination.*** Cancers arising in close proximity to the vertebral column often embolize through the paravertebral plexus, and this pathway is probably involved in the frequent vertebral metastases of carcinomas of the ***thyroid and prostate.***

31. Ans. a. Retrogn..., d. Isolated..., e. Gloss...

[Ref: L & B 26th/634; P.L.Dhingra 6th/116-17,449; https://www.nlm.nih.gov/medlineplus]

"Although most clefts of the lip and palate occur as an isolated deformity, **Pierre Robin sequence** remains the most common syndrome. This syndrome comprises ***isolated cleft palate, retrognathia and a posteriorly displaced tongue (glossoptosis)***, which is associated with early respiratory and feeding difficulties" *(L & B 26th/634)*

Pierre Robin Sequence

◈ *P.L.Dhingra 6th/116-17,449*

- "A **triad** of ***micrognathia, glossoptosis & cleft palate***"
- *Often part of Sticker syndrome*
- *Conductive or SN hearing loss*
- *Autosomal dominant inheritance*

Pierre Robin Syndrome (or Sequence)

◈ *www.nlm.nih.gov/medlineplus*

- It is a condition present at birth, in which the infant has a *smaller-than-normal lower jaw, a tongue that falls back in the throat, and difficulty breathing.*

- The exact causes of Pierre Robin syndrome are unknown. It may be part of many genetic syndromes.
- The lower jaw develops slowly before birth, but may speed up during the first year of life.
- **Symptoms**
  - ***Cleft soft palate***
  - ***High-arched palate***
  - Jaw that is very small with small (receding) chin
  - Jaw that is far back in the throat
  - ***Repeated ear infections***

Small opening in the roof of the mouth, which may cause choking or regurgitation of liquids through the nose
Teeth that appear when the baby is born (natal teeth)
Tongue that is large compared to the jaw

Conditions are Associated with Low-set and Malformed Ears

◈ *www.healthcentral.com*

Common: Down syndrome & Turner syndrome
Rare: Treacher Collins syndrome, Potter syndrome, Trisomy 18, Beckwith-Wiedemann syndrome, Trisomy 13, Rubinstein-Taybi syndrome & *Smith-Lemli-Opitz syndrome*

32. Ans. a. Contains..., e. Makes up...

[Ref: Robbins 9th/ 171-72; Genetic Medicine by Thomson 8th/246; Molecular Biology of Cell by Alberts 6th/802]

"In mammalian cells, mitochondrial DNA makes up less than *1% of the total cellular DNA. However in other cells like leaves of higher plant & large egg cells of amphibian, a larger fraction of cellular DNA may present in mitochondria or chloroplast" (Molecular Biology of Cell by Alberts 6th/802)*

Mitochondria DNA

- Human mitochondria contain 2-10 copies of a small circular double-stranded DNA molecule that makes up *approximately **1% of total cellular DNA***
- A unique feature of mitochondrial DNA is ***maternal inheritance***
- The integrated activity of an estimated ***1500 gene products*** is required for normal mitochondrial biogenesis, function, and integrity. Most of these products are encoded by nuclear genes and thus follow the rules and patterns of nuclear genomic inheritance. These nuclear-encoded proteins are synthesized in the cell cytoplasm and imported to their location of activity in mitochondria through a complex biochemical process. In addition, the mitochondria have their own genome, which consists of numerous copies (polyploidy) per mitochondrion of a circular, double-strand mitochondrial DNA (mtDNA) molecule ***consisting of a 16,569-nucleotide sequence***.
- This mtDNA sequence contains a **total of 37 genes**, of which 13 encode mitochondrial protein components of the ETC. The remaining 22 tRNA- and 2 rRNA-encoding genes are dedicated to the process of translating the 13 mtDNA-encoded proteins.
- The accumulation of functional ***mtDNA deletions*** in a given tissue is expected to be associated with mitochondrial dysfunction, as reflected in an age-associated patchy and reduced cytochrome-c oxidase activity upon histochemical staining, especially in skeletal and cardiac muscle and brain.

Table *(Molecular Biology of Cell by Alberts 6th/802)*: **Relative amounts of organelle DAN in some cells and tissues**

Organism	Tissue or cell type	DNA molecules per organelle	Organelles per cell	Organelle DNA as percentage of total cellular DNA
Mitochondrial DNA				
Rat	Liver	5–10	1000	1
Yeast*	Vegetative	2–50	1–50	15
Frog	Egg	5–10	10^7	99
Chloroplast DNA				
Chlamydomonas	Vegetative	80	1	7
Maize	Leaves	0–300**	20–40	0–15**

* *The large variation in the number and size of mitochondria per cell in yeasts is due to mitochondrion fusion and fission*

** *In maize the amount of chloroplast DNA drops precipitously in mature leaves, after cell division ceases: the chloroplast DNA degraded and stable mRNAs persist to provide for protein synthesis.*

33. Ans. b. Neural...

[Ref: Robbins(SEA) 9th/337; Nelson 20th/979-80, 2477; Harrison 19th/473, 594,597, Dutta's Obstetrics 8th/ 66-67; Shaw's 15th/ 42; William's Obstetrics 22nd/70]

*"Amniotic fluid **AFP level** is high when the fetus suffers from **open neural tube defects**" (Dutta's Obstetrics 8th/ 130)*

*"**High level of hCG** could be detected in- **multiple pregnancy**, hydatiform mole or **choriocarcinoma** & relatively high in pregnancy with a trisomy fetus **(Down syndrome). Plasma lower levels are found in ectopic pregnancies & in spontaneous abortion**" (Dutta's Obstetrics 8th/ 67)*

***hCG** is produced by the syncytiotrophoblast of the placenta . Its value reach maximum levels ranging 100 IU & 200 IU/ml b/w 60-70 days of pregnancy. It can be detected in the maternal serum or urine as early as 8-9 days following ovulation. The rescue & maintenance of corpus luteum till 6 wk of pregnancy is the major biological function of hCG" (Dutta's Obstetrics 8th/ 67)*

"Human chorionic gonadotropin used as tumour marker in Gestational trophoblastic disease & gonadal germ cell tumour" *(Harrison 19th/473)*

Table *(Robbins(SEA) 9th/337)*: **Selected Tumor Markers**

Markers	Associated Cancers
Human chorionic gonadotropin	*Trophoblastic tumors, nonseminomatous testicular tumors*
Calcitonin	Medullary carcinoma of thyroid
Catecholamine and metabolites	Pheochromocytoma and related tumors
Ectopic hormones	Paraneoplastic Syndromes
α-Fetoprotein	*Liver cell cancer, nonseminomatous germ cell tumors of testis*
Carcinoembryonic antigen	Carcinomas of the colon, pancreas, lung, stomach, and heart

34. Ans. b. Oropharyngeal..., d. Carcinoma....

[Ref: Robbins(SEA) 9th/ 326-27; Harrison477,502; Ananthanarayan 9th/553]

Epstein-Barr virus *is closely associated with* ***nasopharyngeal cancer"*** *(P.L.Dhingra 6th/250)*

"In Western countries, the **human papilloma virus (HPV)** is associated with a rising incidence of tumors arising ***from the oropharynx***, i.e., the tonsillar bed and base of tongue. ***Over 50% of oropharyngeal tumors are caused by HPV*** in the United States. HPV 16 is the dominant viral subtype, although HPV 18 and other oncogenic subtypes are seen as well. **HPV-related oropharyngeal cancer occurs** in a younger patient population and is associated with increased numbers of sexual partners and oral sexual practices. It is associated with a better prognosis, especially for nonsmokers" *(Harrison 19th/502)*

Human Papillomavirus

◈ *Robbins(SEA) 9th/ 326*

- At least 70 genetically distinct types of HPV have been identified. Some types (e.g., 1, 2, 4, and 7) cause ***benign squamous papillomas (warts) in humans.***
- In contrast, high-risk HPVs (*e.g.,* types 16 and 18) have been implicated in the genesis of ***squamous cell carcinomas of the cervix, anogenital region, and head and neck (particularly tumors arising in the tonsillar mucosa).***

"HPV: Invasive cervical cancer & other squamous cell carcinoma & dysplasia such as anus, perianal region, vagina, vulva, penis & oral cavity" *(Harshmohan 7th/218)*

"**EBV,** a member of the herpes family, has been implicated in the pathogenesis of **several human tumors**: the African form of Burkitt lymphoma; B-cell lymphomas in immunosuppressed individuals (particularly in those with human immuno deficiency virus infection and those undergoing immuno-suppressive therapy after organ transplantation); some cases of ***Hodgkin lymphoma***; ***nasopharyngeal carcinomas*** & some gastric carcinoma & some rare form of T-cell lymphoma & NK cell lymphoma" *(Robbins(SEA) 9th/ 327)*

Table *(Harrison 19th/477)*: **Suspected Carcinogens** *(Incomplete list)*

Carcinogens	Associated Cancer or Neoplasm
Epstein-Barr virus	Burkitt's lymphoma, nasal T cell lymphoma
Helicobacter pylori	Gastric cancer, gastric MALT lymphoma
Hepatitis B or C virus	Liver cancer
Human immunodeficiency virus	Non-Hodgkin's lymphoma, Kaposi's sarcoma, squamous cell carcinomas (especially of the urogenital tract)
Human papilloma virus	***Cancer of cervix, anus, Oropharynx***
Human T cell lymphotropic virus type I (HTLV-I)	Adult T cell leukemia/lymphoma
Schistosomiasis	Bladder cancer (squamous cell)

35. Ans. a. Often localized..., c. Contiguous ..., d. Can be cured ..., e. Commonly...,

[Ref: Harrison 19th/708-09; Robbins(SAE) 9th/607,610-11; Oxford Textbook of Haematology 2nd/211; CMDT 2016/ 530-31]

"**Hepatosplenomegaly** ***may be present*** *but does not always indicate disease in those organs. Spread is contiguous from one node to next &* ***extranodal disease****, such as bone, brain or skin involvement,* ***is rare"*** *(Davidson 22nd/1042)*

"**HL:** Other ***uncommon sites of involvement include the gastrointestinal tract & skin***. Splenic involvement occurs in 30-40% cases" *(O.P.Ghai 8th/609)*

"***Patients with localized Hodgkin's lymphoma are cured >90% of the time.*** In patients with good prognostic factors, ***extended-field radiotherapy*** has a high cure rate. Increasingly, patients with **all stages of Hodgkin's** lymphoma are treated ***initially with chemotherapy***. Patients with localized or good-prognosis disease receive a brief course of chemotherapy followed by radiotherapy to sites of node involvement. Patients with **more extensive disease** or those with B symptoms receive a ***complete course of chemotherapy.*** The most popular chemotherapy regimen used in Hodgkin's lymphoma is a combination of doxorubicin, bleomycin, vinblastine, and dacarbazine **(ABVD).** Patients who relapse after primary therapy of Hodgkin's lymphoma can frequently still be cured. Patients who relapse after initial treatment with only radiotherapy have an excellent outcome when treated with chemotherapy" *(Harrison 19th/709)*

Table *(Robbins(SAE) 9th/607)*: **Differences between Hodgkin and Non-Hodgkin Lymphomas**

Hodgkin Lymphoma	Non-Hodgkin Lymphoma
More often localized to a ***single axial group of nodes*** (cervical, mediastinal, para-aortic)	More frequent involvement of multiple peripheral nodes
Orderly spread by ***contiguity***	Noncontiguous spread
Mesenteric nodes and waldeyer ring rarely involved	Waldeyer ring and mesenteric nodes commonly involved
Extranodal presentation rare	Extranodal presentation common

Hodgkin's lymphoma (HL)

◈ *Oxford Textbook of Haematology 2nd/211; Robbins (SAE) 9th/610-11*

- HL ***most commonly present as painless lymphadenopathy.*** Patients with the nodular sclerosis or lymphocyte predominance types tend to have stage I-II disease and are usually free of systemic manifestations.
- Patients with disseminated disease (stages III-IV) or the mixed-cellularity or lymphocyte depletion subtypes are more likely to have constitutional symptoms, such as *fever, night sweats, and weight loss.*
- The **spread of HL is remarkably stereotyped**: ***nodal disease first, then splenic disease, hepatic disease, and finally involvement of the marrow and other tissues.***
- Staging involves physical examination, radiologic imaging of the abdomen, pelvis, and chest, and biopsy of the bone marrow.

- With current treatment protocols, ***tumor stage rather than histologic type is the most important prognostic variable.*** The ***cure rate of patients with stages I and IIA is close to 90%.*** Even with advanced disease (stages IVA and IVB), disease-free survival at 5 years is 60% to 70%.
- Low-stage localized HL can be cured with ***involved field radiotherapy***, and indeed cure of such patients was one of the early success stories in oncology.
- Patients treated with early **chemotherapy regimens** containing *alkylating agents* also had a high
- incidence of secondary tumors, particularly acute myeloid leukemia. These sobering results spurred the development of current treatment regimens, which ***minimize the use of radiotherapy*** and employ ***less genotoxic chemotherapeutic agents***; as a result, the incidence of secondary tumors appears to have been reduced markedly, without any loss of therapeutic efficacy.
- Anti-CD30 antibodies have produced excellent responses

Treatment of Hodgkin Lymphoma

- Patient with localized Hodgkin's disease are cured >90% cases at time.
- Patient with localized or good prognosis disease received a ***complete course of chemotherapy followed by radiation at the site of involvement.***
- Patient with more extensive disease or B symptoms received a complete course of chemotherapy.
- The ***most common regimen for HD is ABVD regimen*** (Doxorubicin, Bleomycin, vinblastin Dacarbazine).
- Another commonly used regimen is ***MOOP*** (Mechlorethamine, Vincristin, Procarbazine and prednisone)

36. Ans. a. Anaplastic..., b. Embryonal..., e. Hodgkin's....

[Ref: Robbins (SAE) 9th/590,605]

"CD30 is positive in anaplastic large cell lymphoma & Hodgkin's lymphoma" *(Robbins(SAE) 9th/605)*

"**Embryonal carcinomas** *share some markers with* **seminoma** *such as OCT 3/4 & PLAP, but differ by being* **positive for cytokeratin & CD 30** *& negative for KIT" (Robbins(SAE) 9th/977)*

"CD30 is associated with ***anaplastic large cell lymphoma***. It is expressed in ***embryonal carcinoma*** but ***not in seminoma*** and is thus a useful marker in distinguishing between these germ cell tumors. ***CD30 and CD15 are also expressed on classical Hodgkin Lymphoma Reed-Sternberg cells***" *(pathologyoutlines.com)*

Table *(Robbins 9th/590)*: **Some Immune Cell Antigens Detected by Monoclonal Antibodies**

Antigen Designation	Normal Cellular Distribution
Primarily T-Cell Associated	
CD1	Thymocytes and Langerhans cells
CD3	Thymocytes, MatureT cells
CD4	Helper T cells, Subset of thymocytes
CD5	T cells and a small subset of B cells
CD8	Cytotoxic T cells, Subset of thymocytes, and some NK cells
Primarily B-Cell Associated	
CD10	Marrow pre-B cells and germinal center B cells
CD19	Marrow pre-B cells and mature B cells but not plasma cells
CD20	Marrow pre-B cells after CD19 and mature B cells but not plasma cells
CD21	EBV receptor; present on mature B cells and follicular dendritic cells
CD23	Activated mature B cells
CD79a	Marrow pre-B cells and mature B cells.
Primarily Monocyte or Macrophage Associated	
CD11c	Granulocytes, monocytes, and macrophages; also expressed by hairy cell leukemias
CD13	Immature and mature monocytes and granulocytes
CD14	Monocytes
CD15	Granulocytes; also expressed by Reed-Sternberg cells and variants in classical Hodgkin lymphoma
CD33	Myeloid progenitors and monocytes
CD64	Mature myeloid cells
Primarily NK-Cell Associated	
CD16	NK cells and granulocytes
CD56	NK cells and a subset of T cells
Primarily Stem Cell and Progenitor Cell Associated	
CD34	Pluripotent hematopoietic stem cells and progenitor cells of many lineages
Activation Markers	
CD30	Activated B cells, T cells, and monocytes; also expressed by Reed-Sternberg cells and variants in classical Hodgkin lymphoma
Present on All Leukocytes	
CD45	All leukocytes; also known as leukocyte common antigen (LCA)

37. Ans. d. Colonic hyperplastic....

[Ref: Robbins(SEA) 9th/806; Harrison 19th/538; Harshmohan 7th/566-70]

"**Colonic hyperplastic polyps** *are* **benign epithelial proliferation.** *Their chief significance is that they must be distinguished from sessile serrated* **adenomas**, *that are histologically similar but have* **malignant potential**" *(Robbins (SEA) 9th/804)*

Table *(Robbins(SEA) 9th/806)*: **Gastrointestinal Polyposis Syndromes**

Syndrome	Mean age at presentation (yr)	Mutated gene(s); Pathway	Gastrointestinal Lesions	Selected Extra-Gastrointestinal Manifestations
Juvenile polyposis	<5	*SMAD4, BMPR1 A; TGF-β signaling pathway*	Juvenile polyps; risk of gastric, small intestinal, colonic, and pancreatic adenocarcinoma	Congenital malformations, digital clubbing
Peutz-Jeghers syndrome	10–15	*STK 11*; AMP kinase-related pathways	Arborizing polyps; small intestine > colon > stomach; colonic adenocarcinoma	Pigmented macules; risk of colon, breast, lung, pancreatic, and thyroid cancer
Cowden syndrome. Bannayan-Ruvalcaba-Riley syndrome	<15	*PTEN:* PI3K/AKT pathway	Hamartomatous/inflammatory intestinal polyps, lipomas, ganglioneuromas	Benign skin tumors, benign and malignant thyroid and breast lesion: no increase in GI cancers
Cronkhite-canada syndrome	>50	Nonhereditary, unknown cause	Hamartomatous polyps of stomach small intestine, colon; abnormalities in nonpolypoid mucous	Nail atrophy, hair loss, abnormal skin pigmentation, cachexia, and anemia. Fatal in up to 50%
Tuberous sclerosis		*TSC1* (hamartin), *TSC2* (tuberin); mTOR pathway	Hamartomatous polyps	Mental retardation, epilepsy, facial angiofibroma, cortical (CNS) tubers, renal angiomyolipoma
Familial adenomatous polyposis (FAP)				
Classic FAP	10–15	*APC*	Multiple adenomas	Congenital RPE hypertrophy
Attenuated FAP	40–50	*APC*	Multiple adenomas	
Gardner syndrome	10–15	*APC*	Multiple adenomas	Osteomas, thyroid and desmoid tumor, skin cysts
Turcot syndrome	10–15	*APC*	Multiple adenomas	Medulloblastoma, glioblastoma
MYH-associated polyposis	30–50	*MYH*	Multiple adenomas	

Table: Tumors of the Small Intestine and Colon

Non-neoplastic (Benign) Polyps
Hyperplastic polyps
Hamartomatous polyps
• Juvenile polyps
• Peutz-Jeghers polyps
Inflammatory polyps
Lymphoid polyps
Neoplastic Epithelial Lesions
Benign
• Adenoma
Malignant
• Adenocarcinoma
• Carcinoid tumor
• Anal zone carcinoma
Mesenchymal Lesions
Gastrointestinal stromal tumor (GIST) (gradation from benign to malignant)

Contd...

Other benign lesions
• Lipoma
• Neuroma
• Angioma
• Kaposi sarcoma
• Lymphoma

38. Ans. a. Menetrier.., b. Gastritis.., d. Zollinger...

[Ref: Robbins(SEA) 9th/768-69; Harrison 19th/1932,1910,1927]

Hypertrophic Gastropathies

◈ *Robbins(SEA) 9th/768-69*

- Hypertrophic Gastropathies are uncommon diseases characterized by giant cerebriform enlargement of the rugal folds due to epithelial hyperplasia without inflammation. Two well defined examples ***are Ménétrier disease & Zollinger-Ellison syndrome***
- **Ménétrier disease**, resulting from profound ***hyperplasia of the surface mucous cells*** with accompanying glandular atrophy
- ***Gastric gland hyperplasia*** *secondary to excessive gastrin secretion*, in the setting of a gastrinoma ***(Zollinger-Ellison syndrome).***

- ***Hypertrophic-hypersecretory gastropathy***, associated with hyperplasia of the parietal and chief cells within gastric glands

"**Zollinger-Ellison syndrome (Gastrinomas):** Severe peptic ulcer diathesis secondary to gastric acid hypersecretion due to unregulated gastrin release from a non-β cell endocrine tumor (gastrinoma) defines the components of ZES" *(Harrison 19th/1932)*

"Most cases of esophageal perforation are from instrumentation of the esophagus or trauma. Alternatively, forceful vomiting or retching can lead to spontaneous rupture at the gastroesophageal junction (**Boerhaave's syndrome**) *(Harrison 19th/1932)*

MéNéTrier's Disease

◈ *Harrison 19th/1932*

- Ménétrier's disease is a rare entity characterized by large, ***tortuous gastric mucosal folds***. The differential diagnosis of **large gastric folds** includes ***ZES, malignancy, infectious etiologies (CMV, histoplasmosis, syphilis), and infiltrative disorders such as sarcoidosis***.
- The ***mucosal folds in Ménétrier's disease are often most prominent in the body and fundus***. Histologically, massive foveolar hyperplasia (hyperplasia of surface and glandular mucous cells) is noted, which replaces most of the chief and parietal cells. This hyperplasia produces the prominent folds observed. The pits of the gastric glands elongate and may become extremely tortuous. Although the lamina propria may contain a mild chronic inflammatory infiltrate, Ménétrier's disease is not considered a form of gastritis.

Table *(Robbins 9th/769)*: **Hypertrophic Gastropathies and Gastric Polyps**

Parameter	Menetrier Disease (adult)	Zollinger-Ellison Syndrome	Inflammatory & Hyperplastic polyps	Gastritis Cystica	Fundic Gland polyps	Gastric Adenomas
Mean patient age (yr)	30–60	50	50–60	Variable	50	50–60
Location	Body and fundus	Fundus	Antrum > body	Body	Body and funds	Antrum > body
Predominant cell type	Mucous	Parietal > mucous, endocrine	Mucous	Mucous cyst-lining	Parietal and chief	Dysplastic, intestinal
Inflammatory infiltrate	Limited lymphocytes	Neutrophils	Neutrophil and lymphocytes	Neutrophil and lymphocytes	None	Variable
Symptoms	Hypoproteinemia, weight loss, diarrhea	Peptic ulcers	Similar to chronic gastritis	Similar to chronic gastritis	None, nausea	Similar to chronic gastritis
Risk factors	None	Multiple endocrine neoplasia	Chronic gastritis, *H. pylori*	Trauma, prior surgery	PPIs, FAP	Chronic gastritis, atrophy, intestinal metaplasia
Association with adenocarcinoma	Yes	No	Occasional	No	Syndromic (FAP) only	Frequent

39. Ans. c. Hemogl..., d. Transfusion..., e. Acute renal...

[Ref: Robbins(SEA) 9th/665-66; Manipal Surgey 4th/179; Harshmohan 7th/318-19; Harrison 19th/ 138e5-6]

Transfusion Reactions

◈ *Harshmohan 7th/318*

- *2 types- Immunogenic transfusion reaction & Non-immune transfusion reactions*
- **Immunogenic transfusion reaction** *may be against red blood cells(hemolytic reactions), leucocytes, platelets or immunoglobulins*
- **Non-immune transfusion** *reactions include circulatory overload, massive transfusion or transmission of an infectious agent*

Immunogenic Transfusion Reaction

◈ *Harshmohan 7th/318*

- *Hemolytic transfusion reaction: may be immediate or delayed or intravascular or extravascular*
- *Intravascular hemolysis-very rapid cell destruction. Symptom includes restlessness, flushing, tachypnea, tachycardia, shock,* ***renal failure***
- *Transfusion-related acute lung injury* (**TRALI): Acute pulmonary oedema & signs & symptoms of respiratory failure**
- *Febrile reactions*
- *Anaphylactic shock*
- *Allergic reactions such as urticarial*
- Transfusion related graft-versus host disease

Hemolytic Reaction: Major (ABO) Incompatibility Reaction

◈ *Manipal Surgey 4th/179*

- *This is result from mismatched blood transfusion. This cause* ***intravascular hemolysis***
- *Clinical feature-* ***Hematuria****, pain in loins (bilateral), fever with chills & rigors*
- *Oliguria is due to products of mismatched blood transfusion* ***blocking the renal tubules.*** *It results in* ***acute renal tubular necrosis***

Hemolytic Reactions

◈ *Robbins (SEA) 9th/665-66*

- ***Acute hemolytic reactions* are usually caused by preformed IgM antibodies against donor red cells that fix complement.** Pre-existing high affinity "natural" IgM antibodies, usually against polysaccharide blood group antigens A or B, bind to red cells and rapidly induce complement mediated lysis, intravascular hemolysis, and ***hemoglobinuria.*** Fever, shaking chills, and flank pain appear rapidly.
- The direct Coombs test is typically positive, unless all of the donor red cells have lysed. The signs and symptoms are due to complement activation rather than intravascular hemolysis *per se*, as osmotic lysis of red cells (e.g., by mistakenly infusing red cells and 5% dextrose in water simultaneously) ***produces hemoglobinuria*** without any of the other symptoms of a hemolytic reaction. In severe cases the process may rapidly progress to DIC, shock, ***acute renal failure,*** and occasionally death.
- ***Delayed hemolytic reactions* are caused by antibodies that recognize red cell antigens that the recipient was sensitized to previously, for example, through a prior blood transfusion.** These are typically caused by IgG antibodies to foreign protein antigens

"*Transfusion-Related Acute Lung Injury* **(TRALI)** ***is a severe, frequently fatal complication in which factors in a transfused blood product trigger the activation of neutrophils in the lung microvasculature.*** The incidence of TRALI is low, probably less than 1 per 10,000 transfusions, but it may occur more frequently in patients with preexisting lung disease"- *(Robbins (SEA) 9th/665)*

40. Ans. a. Nephrotic..., b. Neutrophilic ..., d. Linear deposits...

[Ref: Robbins(SEA) 9th/ 909-12; Harshmohan 7th/652-54,6th/665]

"**Linear deposits along GBM** *are seen in* ***RPGN*** *(Type-I: anti-GBM type)" (Harshmohan 7th/663)*

"**PSGN**: *Typically, the patient is a young child, presenting with acute nephritic syndrome" (Harshmohan 7th/654)*

Light microscopic finding of tubules (PSGN): *Tubular changes are not very striking. There may swelling & hyaline droplets in tubular cells & tubular lamina may contain red cell mass" (Harshmohan 7th/653)*

"**PSGN**: *Immunofluorescence microscopy reveals that the* ***irregular deposits*** *along the globular basement membrane consists primarily of IgG & complement C3" (Harshmohan 7th/653)*

Post Streptococcal Glomerulonephritis (PSGN): *Morphology*

◈ *Robbins(SEA) 9th/ 910-11*

- The classic diagnostic picture is one of **enlarged, hypercellular glomeruli**.The hypercellularity is caused by (1) ***infiltration by leukocytes, both neutrophils and monocytes***; (2) proliferation of endothelial and mesangial cells; and (3) in severe cases by ***crescent formation.***
- The proliferation and **leukocyte infiltration** are diffuse, that is, involving ***all lobules of all glomeruli***. There is also swelling of endothelial cells, and the combination of proliferation, swelling, and leukocyte infiltration obliterates the capillary lumens. There may be interstitial edema and inflammation, and the ***tubules often contain red cell casts.***
- By **immunofluorescence microscopy,** there are granular deposits of IgG, IgM, and C3 in the mesangium and along the basement membrane. Although almost universally present, they are often focal and sparse.
- The characteristic **electron microscopic findings** are ***discrete, amorphous,*** electrondense deposits on the ***epithelial side of the membrane,*** often having the appearance of "**humps**", presumably representing the antigen-antibody complexes at the epithelial cell surface.
- ***Subendothelial and intramembranous deposits*** are also commonly seen, and mesangial deposits may be present. There is often swelling of endothelial and mesangial cells.

Poststreptococcal Glomerulonephritis (PSGN)

◈ *Harrison 17th / 1786-87*

- It typically affects children between the ages of 2 and 14 years, but 10% of cases are patients older than 40.
- It is more common in males
- Skin and throat infections with particular M types of streptococci (nephritogenic strains) antedate glomerular disease; M types 47, 49, 55, 2, 60, and 57 are seen following impetigo and M types 1, 2, 4, 3, 25, 49, and 12 with pharyngitis.
- Poststreptococcal glomerulonephritis due to impetigo develops 2–6 weeks after skin infection and 1–3 weeks after streptococcal pharyngitis.
- Hypercellularity of mesangial and endothelial cells, glomerular infiltrates of polymorphonuclear leukocytes, granular subendothelial immune deposits of IgG, IgM, C_3, C_4, and C_{5-9}, and ***subepithelial deposits (which appear as "humps")***
- The classic presentation is an acute ***nephritic picture with hematuria, pyuria, red blood cell casts, edema, hypertension, and oliguric renal failure,*** which may be severe enough to appear as RPGN
- In the first week of symptoms, 90% of patients will have a ***depressed*** CH_{50} ***and decreased levels of*** C_3 ***with normal levels of*** C_4
- Five percent of children and 20% of adults ***have proteinuria in the nephrotic range***[Q]. The prognosis is good, with permanent renal failure being very uncommon (1–3%).
- Complete resolution of the hematuria and proteinuria in children occurs within 3–6 weeks of the onset of nephritis.

Antibodies in streptococcal infection: ***ASO, Anti-DNAase B, Anti-Streptokinase, anti-Nicotinyl adenine dinucleotidase & Anti-Hyaluronidase*** *(Harshmohan 6th/665)*

Table *(Robbins(SEA) 9th/ 910)*: **Summary of Major Primary Glomerulonephritis**

Disease	Presentation	Pathogenesis	Glomerular Pathology Light Microscopy	Fluorescence Microscopy	Electron Microscopy
Poststreptococcal glomerulonephritis	Acute nephritis	Antibody mediated; circulating or planted antigen	Diffuse proliferation; leukocytic infiltration	Granular IgG and C3 in GBM and mesangium	***Subepithelial humps***

41. Ans. a. Better ..., d. Occur in ..., e. More common....

[Ref: Robbins(SEA) 9th/873; Harshmohan 7th/620; Harrison 19th/552]

"A distinctive variant of HCC is **fibrolamellar carcinoma**, constituting less than 5% of HCCs. 85% occur under the age of 35 years and ***without gender predilection or identifiable predisposing conditions.*** It usually presents as single large, hard "scirrhous" tumor with fibrous bands coursing through it. Microscopically, they are composed of well-differentiated cells rich in mitochondria (oncocytes) growing in nests or cords separated by parallel lamellae of dense collagen bundles (hence the name)" *(Robbins(SEA) 9th/873)*

"**FL-HCC:** *Found in young people of both sexes. The tumour forms a single large mass which may be encapsulated &* ***occurs in the absence of cirrhosis. Prognosis is better*** *than other forms of HCC" (Harshmohan 7th/620)*

Fibrolamellar HCC (FL-HCC)

◈ *Harrison 19th/552*

- This rarer variant of HCC has a quite different biology than adult-type HCC. None of the known HCC causative factors seem important here.
- It is typically a disease of younger adults, often teenagers and ***predominantly females.***
- It is ***AFP-negative***, but patients typically have ***elevated blood neurotensin levels,*** normal liver function tests, and ***no cirrhosis.***
- Radiology is similar for HCC, except that characteristic adult-type portal vein invasion is less common.
- Although it is ***often multifocal in the liver***, and therefore not resectable, metastases are common, especially to lungs and loco-regional lymph nodes, but ***survival is often much better than with adult-type HCC.***
- Resectable tumors are associated with 5-year survival ≥50%. Patients often present with a huge liver or unexplained weight loss, fever, or elevated liver function tests on routine evaluations. Surgical resection is the best management option, even for metastases, as these tumors respond much less well to chemotherapy than adult-type HCC.
- Although several series of OLTX for FL-HCC have been reported, the patients seem to die from tumor recurrences, with a 2- to 5-year lag compared with OLTX for adult-type HCC. Ancedotal responses to gemcitabine plus cisplatin-TACE are reported

A & E

42. Ans. a. Nondisjunctional..., b. Nondisjunctional..., c. Translocations...,

[Ref: Robbins (SEA) 9th/ 161-63; O.P.Ghai 8th/637-38; Harrison 19th/83e1-4]

Trisomy 21 (Down Syndrome)

◈ *O.P.Ghai 8th/637-38*

- *Chromosome no. 21 is present in triplicate, the origin of extra chromosome 21 being* ***either maternal or paternal***
- *In* ***most cases the extrachromosome from the mother***
- *Trisomy is found in 94% cases.*
- *Approx. 1% of cases are mosaic &* ***rest (5%) are due to translocations, most commonly involving chromosome 21 & 14***

Trisomy 21 (Down Syndrome)

◈ *Robbins (SEA) 9th/ 161*

- Down syndrome is the most common of the chromosomal disorders and is a major cause of mental retardation.
- Approximately 95% of affected ***individuals have trisomy 21,*** so their chromosome count is 47. Most others have normal chromosome numbers, but the extra chromosomal material is present as a ***translocation.*** The most common cause of trisomy and therefore of ***Down syndrome is meiotic nondisjunction.*** The parents of such children have a normal karyotype and are normal in all respects.
- Maternal age has a strong influence on the incidence of trisomy 21. It occurs once in 1550 live births in women under age 20, in contrast to 1 in 25 live births for mothers older than age 45. The correlation with **maternal age** suggested that ***most cases the meiotic nondisjunction of chromosome 21 occurs in the ovum.***
- Indeed, studies in which DNA polymorphisms were used to trace the parental origin of chromosome 21 have revealed that in ***95% of the cases with trisomy 21 the extra chromosome is of maternal origin.*** Although many hypotheses have been advanced, the reason for the increased ***susceptibility of the ovum to nondisjunction*** remains unknown.
- In about 4% of cases of Down syndrome, the extra chromosomal material derives from the presence of a **robertsonian translocation of the long arm of chromosome 21** to another ***acrocentric chromosome (e.g., 22 or 14).***
- Because the fertilized ovum already possesses two normal autosomes 21, the translocated material provides the same triple gene dosage as in trisomy 21. Such cases are frequently (but not always) familial, and the translocated chromosome is inherited from one of the parents (usually the mother), who is a carrier of a robertsonian translocation, for example, a mother with ***karyotype 45, XX, der (14; 21)*** (q10; q10). In cells with robertsonian translocations, the genetic material normally found on two pairs of chromosomes is distributed among only three chromosomes. This affects chromosome pairing during meiosis, and as a result the gametes have a high probability of being aneuploid.

- ***Approximately 1% of Down syndrome patients are mosaics, having a mixture of cells with 46 or 47 chromosomes.*** This mosaicism results from mitotic nondisjunction of chromosome 21 during an early stage of embryogenesis. Symptoms in such cases are variable and milder, depending on the proportion of abnormal cells.
- Clearly, in cases of translocation or mosaic Down syndrome, maternal age is of no importance.

43. Ans. b. Histoplasm..., c. Tubercu....

[Ref: Harshmohan 7th/155; Robbins (SEA) 9th/ 693]

"**Schaumann's bodies** *or conchoids (conch like) bodies which are concentric laminations of calcium & of iron salts, complexed with proteins,* ***found in sarcoidosis****" (Harshmohan 7th/155)*

"**Sarcoidosis:** Regardless of the tissue, involved tissues contain well-formed nonnecrotizing granulomas composed of aggregates of tightly clustered epithelioid macrophages, often with giant cells. Laminated concretions composed of calcium and proteins known as ***Schaumann bodies*** and stellate inclusions known as **asteroid bodies** are found within giant cells in approximately 60% of the granulomas. Though characteristic, these microscopic features are not pathognomonic of sarcoidosis, because asteroid and Schaumann bodies may be encountered in other ***granulomatous diseases*** (e.g., tuberculosis)" *(Robbins(SEA) 9th/ 693)*

"When cellular, non-necrotic granulomas are present in **tuberculosis**, the epithelioid cells and giant cells sometimes have inclusions, which were found in this case. These inclusions, the **Schaumann body** and the asteroid body, are ***not specific for tuberculosis***. They also occur in most other types of non-necrotic granulomas" *(pathhsw5m54.ucsf.edu)*

Schaumann Bodies

◈ *wikipedia.org*

These are calcium and protein inclusions inside of Langhans giant cells as part of a granuloma.

Many conditions can cause Schaumann bodies, including:

- *Sarcoidosis,*
- *Hypersensitivity pneumonitis, and*
- *Berylliosis.*
- *Uncommonly Crohn's disease & tuberculosis*

Table *(Harshmohan 7th/138)*: **Principal granulomatous conditions** *(Partial list)*

Condition	Special Characteristics
Sarcoidosis	Asteriod & ***Schaumann bodies*** in giant cells
Beryllioisis	Inclusions in giant cells(asteroids, ***Schaumann bodies*** & crystal)
Tuberculosis	Granuloma with central caseation, AFB
Cryptococcosis	Organism yeast-like with clear capsule

44. Ans. a. Chromogra..., b. CD5..., c. Neuron-sp..., d. Cytokeratin 7....

[Ref: Harrison 19th/558,2337,120e-2t]

Neuroendocrine Tumors: Synaptophysin, Chromogranins & CD 56 are markers" *(Harrison 19th/120e-2t)*

Table *(Harrison 19th/558)*: **General Characteristics of Gastrointestinal Neuroendocrine Tumors (GI-NETs [Carcinoids], Pancreatic Neuroendocrine Tumors [pNETs])**

Share general neuroendocrine cell markers (identification used for diagnosis)

1. Chromogranins (A, B, C) are acidic monomeric soluble proteins found in the large secretory granules. Chromogranin A is the most widely used.
2. Neuron-specific enolase (NSE) is the γ-γ dimer of the enzyme enolase and is a cytosolic marker of neuroendocrine differentiation.
3. Synaptophysin is an integral membrane glycoprotein of 38,000 molecular weight found in small vesicles of neurons and neuroendocrine tumors.

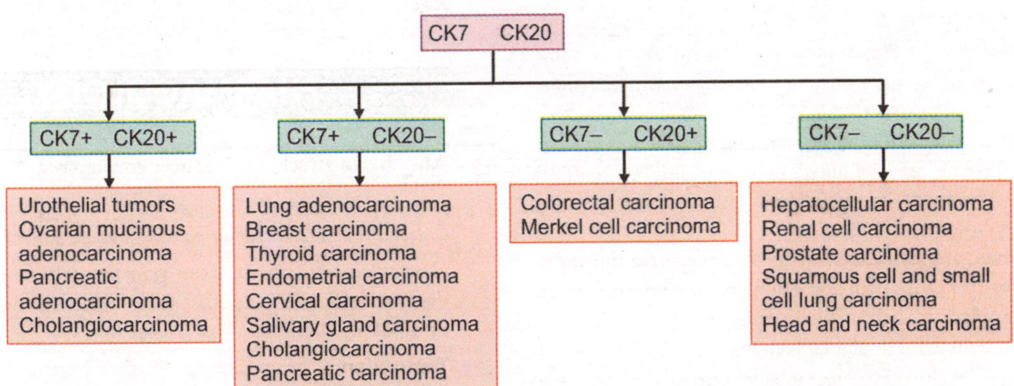

Fig: *(Harrison 19th/120e2):* Approach to cytokeratin (CK7 and CK20) markers used in CUP

45. Ans. **b. More common.....**

[Ref: Robbins(SEA) 9th/867; Harshmohan 7th/618; Harrison 19th/553-54]

"**FNH**: *The etiology is not known but these lesions are* ***more common in women taking oral contraceptives. Nodules may be single or multiple****, measuring about 5 cm in diameter"-Harshmohan 7th/618*

Focal Nodular Hyperplasia

◈ *Robbins(SEA) 9th/867*

- Solitary or multiple hyperplastic hepatocellular nodules may develop in the ***noncirrhotic liver.*** Two such conditions are *focal nodular hyperplasia* and *nodular regenerative hyperplasia.*
- The common factor in both types of nodules seems to be ***either focal or diffuse alterations in hepatic blood supply,*** arising from obliteration of portal vein radicles and ***compensatory augmentation of arterial blood supply.***
- **Focal nodular hyperplasia** appears as a well-demarcated but poorly encapsulated nodule, ranging up to many centimeters in diameter. It presents as a spontaneous mass lesion in an otherwise normal liver, most frequently in ***young to middle-aged adults.*** The lesion is generally lighter than the surrounding liver and is sometimes yellow indicating steatosis.
- Typically, there is a central gray-white, depressed stellate scar from which fibrous septa radiate to the periphery. The central scar contains large vessels, usually arterial, that typically show fibromuscular hyperplasia with eccentric or concentric narrowing of the lumen. The radiating septa show variable ductular reactions along septal margins.
- The parenchyma between septa is comprised of normal hepatocytes separated by thickened sinusoidal plate
- The vascular lesion, congenital or acquired, is probably the initiating insult. Resulting areas of hypoperfused parenchyma collapse to become the septa, while hypoperfused regions undergo hyperplasia

Benign Liver Tumors

◈ *Harrison 19th/553-54*

- Three common benign tumors occur and all are found predominantly in women. They are *hemangiomas, adenomas,* and *focal nodular hyperplasia* (FNH).
- **FNH** is typically benign, and usually no treatment is needed.
- **Hemangiomas** are the most common and are entirely benign. Treatment is unnecessary unless their expansion causes symptoms.
- **Adenomas** are associated with ***contraceptive hormone use.*** They can cause pain and can bleed or rupture, causing acute problems. Their main interest for the physician is a low potential for malignant change and a 30% risk of bleeding. For this reason, considerable effort has gone into differentiating these three entities radiologically. On discovery of a liver mass, patients are usually advised to ***stop taking sex steroids,*** because adenoma regression may then occasionally occur.
- **Adenomas** can often be large masses ranging from 8–15 cm. Due to their size and definite, but low, malignant potential and potential for bleeding, adenomas are typically resected.
- The **most useful diagnostic differentiating** tool is a **triphasic CT scan** performed with HCC fast bolus protocol for arterial-phase imaging, together with subsequent delayed venous-phase imaging.
- **Adenomas** usually do not appear on the basis of cirrhosis, although both adenomas and HCCs are intensely vascular on the CT arterial phase and both can exhibit hemorrhage (40% of adenomas). However, adenomas have smooth, well-defined edges, and enhance homogeneously, especially in the portal venous phase on delayed images, when HCCs no longer enhance.
- **FNHs** exhibit a characteristic central scar that ***is hypovascular on the arterial-phase and hypervascular on the delayed-phase CT images. MRI is even more sensitive in depicting the characteristic central scar of FNH.***

"Although the use of **contraceptive agents** has not been implicated in the pathogenesis of FNH, their use is associated with an ***increase in the risk of complications for patients with FNH***, and they may be a factor in the development of FNH. In symptomatic females, hemorrhagic foci or infarctions may occur within the FNH; these are aggravated by administration of contraceptive agents. The rare complication of a spontaneous rupture into the peritoneum has also been associated with ***contraceptive use***"-emedicine.medscape.com/

"**FNH** is most frequently found in young to middle-aged adults, with a strong ***female predilection***; ~15% (range 10-20%) occur in men. Although exogenous oestrogens do not cause FNH, they have been ***shown to increase the size of these masses***"-*radiopaedia.org*

"Histologically the lesion is ***multinodular***, composed of nearly normal hepatocytes arranged in 1-2 cell thick plates. Bile ductules are usually found at the interface between hepatocytes and fibrous regions. ***Kupffer cells*** are present. It should be noted that ***up to 20% of patients with an FNH will have multiple lesions*** " *(radiopaedia.org)*

PHARMACOLOGY

46. Ans. **b. No effect..., e. Reduces coronary...,**

[Ref: KDT 7th/ 312-15; Katzung 13th/713; Harrison 19th/2498,103e-15; CMDT 2016/1142,1181,Pharmacology by Satoskar 24th/ 837-38]

"***Hypertglyceridaemia, deep vein thrombosis, ischemic heart disease,*** *retinopathy & other complications to watch for, during* **tamoxifene therapy**" *(Shaw's Gynae 16th/554)*

Tamoxifen

- Tamoxifen use as adjuvant therapy in estrogen receptor positive breast cancer
- ***Tamoxifen is associated with reduced risk of cancer in the contralateral breast***

- The response, rate on tamoxifen is higher in patient with positive receptor but some estrogen receptor negative patient also responds suggesting additional non hormonal mechanism of action
- It is ***also approved for the primary prophylaxis of breast cancer in high risk woman***
- ***It reduces the recurrence rate of breast cancer in ipsilateral as well contralateral breast*** *(KDT)*
- Studies of patients treated with tamoxifen as adjuvant therapy for early breast cancer have shown a 35% decrease in contralateral breast cancer *(Katzung 10th/671)*
- Tamoxifen also decreases total and LDL cholesterol without any change in HDL and triglyceride level.
- It also ***improve the bone mass due to antiresorptive effect***
- Tamoxifen is effective orally
- It has biphasis plasma t½ (10 hrs. and 7 days) and long duration of action.
- Hot flushes and nausea and vomiting occur in 25% of patients, and many other minor adverse effects are observed.
- ***Tamoxifen increases the risk of thromboembolic events*** *(Goodman Gillman 10th/1441)*
- *"Tamoxifen causes retinal deposits, decreased visual acuity and cataracts in occasional patients" (Goodman Gillman 10th /1441)*

Tamoxifen Citrate

◈ *KDT 7th/ 312-15*

- Acts as potent estrogen antagonist in breast carcinoma cells, blood vessels & at some peripheral sites
- ***Partial agonist in uterus, bone,*** liver & pituitary
- Inhibition of human breast cancer cells & hot flushes reflect antiestrogenic action
- ***Weak estrogenic action*** manifests as stimulation of endometrial proliferation, lowering Gn & prolactin levels in postmenopausal women as well as improvement in their bone density

Tamoxifen may Lead to Endometrial Hyperplasia and Endometrial Cancer

- *While tamoxifen blocks estrogen receptors on the breast, it stimulates these receptors in the uterus (because tamoxifen is a partial against of ER)* [Q].
- ***Stimulation of estrogen receptors in the uterus may predispose the patients to endometrial hyperplasia and for endometrial cancer***

Pharmacological Therapy for Osteoporosis: SERM

◈ *Harrison 19th/2498*

- Two SERMs are used currently in postmenopausal women: **raloxifene,** which is approved for the ***prevention and treatment of osteoporosis*** as well as the prevention of breast cancer, ***and* tamoxifen, *which is approved for the prevention and treatment of breast cancer***
- A third SERM, bazedoxifene, has been complexed with conjugated estrogen, creating a tissue selective estrogen complex (TSEC). This agent has been approved for prevention of osteoporosis.
- ***Tamoxifen reduces bone turnover and bone loss*** in postmenopausal women compared with placebo groups. These findings support the concept that tamoxifen acts as an estrogenic agent in bone. There are limited data on the effect of tamoxifen on fracture risk, but the Breast Cancer Prevention Study indicated a ***possible reduction in clinical vertebral, hip, and Colles' fractures***
- The major benefit of **tamoxifen** is on breast cancer occurrence. The breast cancer prevention trial indicated that tamoxifen administration over 4–5 years reduced the incidence of new invasive and noninvasive breast cancer by ~45% in women at increased risk of breast cancer. The incidence of ER-positive breast cancers was reduced by 65%
- **Tamoxifen** increases the risk of uterine cancer and ***increases risk of venous thrombosis***, cataracts, and possibly stroke in postmenopausal women, limiting its use for breast cancer prevention in women at low or moderate risk

47. Ans. a. Cause..., c. Used for..., d. Better BBB..., e. Central nervous....

[Ref:KDT 7th/116; Katzung 13th/121-22; G & G 11th/189-99]

"Coventional systemic dose of atropine (0.6 mg) have little ocular effect, in contrast to equal dose of ***scopolamine, which cause definite mydriasis*** *& loss of accommodation" (G & G 11th/192)*

"Atropine is a central nervous system stimulant while ***hyoscine (scopolamine) is central depressant****" (Pharmacology by Satoskar 24th/300)*

Hyoscine

◈ *KDT 6th/109,113*

- *Applied to eyes they freely penetrate cornea*
- ***Has better BBB penetration***
- Shorter duration of action than atropine
- Chief source: Hyoscyamys niger

"**Motion sickness: *Hyoscine is the most effective drug for motion sickness*.** It is particularly valuable in highly susceptible individuals and for vigorous motions. The drug should be given prophylactically (0.2 mg oral), because administration after symptoms have setin is less effective, ***action lasts 4-6 hours***. A transdermal preparation applied behind the pinna 4 hours before journey has been shown to protect for 3 days. Side effects with low oral doses and transdermal medication are few, but *sedation and dry mouth may occur*. Hyoscine and other anticholinergics are not effective in other types of vomiting."

"Hyoscine has been used to produce ***sedation and amnesia*** during labour (twilight sleep) and to control maniacal states. It had earned a reputation as a ***'lie detector' during world war II***: its amnesic and depressant action was believed to put the subject 'off guard' in the face of sustained interrogation and sleep deprivation, so that he came out with the truth".

Table *(KDT 7th/116)*: **Comparative features of atropine & hyoscine**

	Atropine	Hyoscine
1. *Chief source*	Atropa belladona, Datura stramonium	Hyoscyamus
2. *Alkaloid ester of tropic acid with*	Tropine (base)	Scopine (base)

Contd...

	Atropine	Hyoscine
3. CNS effect Low dose High dose	***Excitatory*** *Excitation (mild)* *Excitation (mild)*	***Depressant** (amnesia, fatigue, drowsiness, N-REM sleep), Excitation*
4. Anticholinergic property	More potent on heart, bronchial muscle & intestine	More potent on eye & secretory glands
5. Duration of action	Longer	Shorter
6. Anti-motion sickness	++	+++

48. Ans. b. Has anti-..., c. Antioxidant..., d. A citrus flavonoid....

[Ref:KDT 7th/ 616; http://www.webmd.com/vitamins-supplements]

Rutin

- *KDT 7th/ 616*
- *It is **a plant glycoside** claimed to **reduce capillary bleeding***
- It has been used in a dose of 60mg oral BD-TDS along with Vit. C which is believed to facilitate its action

"**Bioflavonoids (Rutins)** are found in the rind of green citrus fruits and in rose hips and black currants. Bioflavonoids have been used in alternative medicine as an aid ***to enhance the action of vitamin C, to support blood circulation, as an antioxidant, and to treat allergies, viruses, or arthritis and other inflammatory conditions***" *(www.drugs.com)*

"The ***richest source is buckwheat.*** Rutin is also found in citrus fruits, noni, black tea, apple peel" *(phytochemicals.info)*

Rutin

- *jonbarron.org/herbal-library*
- One key benefit of rutin is its ability to ***strengthen the lining of the blood vessels throughout*** the body to reduce bleeding and prevent them from collapsing. It can be used for treating and preventing ***varicose veins and leg ulcers.*** Because rutin strengthens arteries and veins, it is also used to help ***treat hemorrhoids, internal bleeding, and to help prevent hemorrhagic strokes.***
- Rutin may also be able to ***stop the formation of blood clots (thrombosis)*** altogether. Not only can blood clots cause heart attacks and strokes, but deep venous thrombosis (DVT) and pulmonary embolisms as well. ***Rutin is proving to be very effective with blood clots because it helps treat and prevent clots in both arteries and veins.***
- Clots in arteries are platelet-rich and clots in veins are fibrin-rich. It could be a safe alternative to aspirin, Plavix, and warfarin (Coumadin). "Rutin proved to be the ***most potently anti-thrombotic*** compound that we ever tested
- In addition to these health benefits, ***rutin is also considered an antioxidant,*** meaning that it binds to free radicals in the body and neutralizes them. This ability to protect the body from disease as well as fight off any free radicals that accumulate offers other benefits as well. Since free radicals turn LDL cholesterol into plaques, blocking arteries and preventing normal blood flow (atherosclerosis), rutin may help ***reduce arterial blockage and high blood pressure, possibly decreasing the risk of heart disease and stroke.***
- **Other benefits include:**
  - *Increases the elasticity of the arterial walls, which, in turn, promotes greater blood flow and improved vascular health.*
  - *Works as an anti-inflammatory.*
  - *Used to prevent a side effect of cancer treatment called mucositis (a painful condition marked by swelling and ulcer formation in the mouth or lining of the digestive tract).*
  - *Used to treat Meniere's disease (a condition that causes ringing in the ears, dizziness and intermittent hearing loss).*
  - *In combination with the proteins trypsin and bromelain, rutin is also used to help treat osteoarthritis.*

Rutin Benefits

- *http://www.raysahelian.com/*
- ***Rutin inhibits platelet aggregation***, making the blood thinner and improve circulation.
- Has ***anti-inflammatory activity.***
- Rutin inhibits ***aldose reductase activity.*** Aldose reductase inhibitors prevent the accumulation of intracellular sorbitol.

Rutin

- *www.webmd.com/vitamins-supplements*
- Rutin is a ***plant pigment (flavonoid) that is found in certain fruits and vegetables.*** Rutin is used to make medicine. The major sources of rutin for medical use include **buckwheat,** Japanese pagoda tree, and Eucalyptus macrorhyncha. Other sources of rutin include the leaves of several species of eucalyptus, ***lime*** tree flowers, elder flowers, hawthorn leaves and flowers, rue, St. John's Wort, Ginkgo biloba, apples, and other fruits and vegetables.
- Some people believe that rutin can ***strengthen blood*** vessels, so they use it for varicose veins, internal bleeding, hemorrhoids, and to prevent strokes due to broken veins or arteries (hemorrhagic strokes).
- Rutin is also used to prevent a side effect of cancer treatment called ***mucositis.*** This is a painful condition marked by swelling and ulcer formation in the mouth or lining of the digestive tract.
- In combination with the proteins trypsin and bromelain, rutin is also used for osteoarthritis.
- Rutin has chemicals that might offer ***some protection against cancer.***

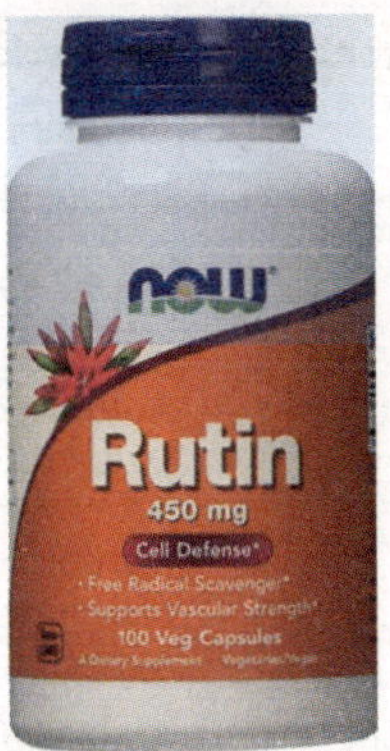

49. Ans. a. Cefotaxime..., b. Ceftazidi..., d. Cefixime...,

[Ref:KDT 7th/ 726; Katzung 13th/776-79]

Table *(KDT 7th/ 726)*: **Cephalosprorins**

Generation	Parenteral	Oral
1st generation	Cefazolin	Cephalexin, Cefadroxil
2nd generation	Cefuroxime, Cefoxitin	Cefaclor, Cefuroxime axetil, Cefprozil
3rd generation	***Cefotaxime***, Ceftizoxime, Ceftriaxone, ***Ceftazidime***, Cefoperazone	***Cefixime***, Cefpodoxime proxetil, Cefdinir, Ceftibuten, Ceftamet pivoxil
4th generation	Cefepime, ***Cefpirome***	
5th generation	Ceftaroline, ***Ceftabiprole***	

50. Ans. d. Constipation...

[Ref: KDT 7th/ 345; Katzung 13th/754-55; Harrison 19th/2499-2501,416e4; CMDT 2016/1141-42; Davidson 22nd/1123; Pharmacology by Satoskar 24th/ 1007]

"**Zoledronic acid (Zolendronate):** It is a ***type of bisphosphonates***. It is effective in the treatment of post-menopausal osteoporosis, corticosteroid induced osteoporosis & osteoporosis in men. It reduces the risk of vertebral fracture by about 75%" *(Davidson 22nd/1123)*

Zoledronate

◈ *KDT 7th/ 345*

- ***Flu-like symptoms*** *due to cytokine release attend the i.v infusion*
- *Nausea, vomiting, bodyache, dizziness are also common*
- ***Renal toxicity*** *has been encountered*
- ***Osteonecrosis of jaw*** *is a rare complication of i.v high dose*

Bisphosphonate Therapy (Zoledronic Acid)

◈ *CMDT 2016/1141-42*

- Bisphosphonate therapy can cause several side effects that are collectively known as the acute-phase response. Such a response occurs in 42% of patients following the first infusion of zoledronic acid and usually starts within the first few days following the infusion.
- Among patients receiving their first infusion of zoledronic acid, these adverse side effects have included ***fever, chills, or flushing (20%); musculoskeletal pain (20%); nausea, vomiting, or diarrhea (8%); nonspecific symptoms, such as fatigue, dyspnea, edema, headache, or dizziness (22%); and eye inflammation (0.6%).***
- ***Osteonecrosis of the jaw*** is a rare complication of bisphosphonate therapy for osteoporosis. A painful, necrotic, nonhealing lesion of the jaw occurs, particularly after tooth extraction. About 95% of jaw osteonecrosis cases have occurred with high-dose therapy with zoledronic acid or pamidronate
- ***Atypical "chalkstick" fractures of the femur*** occur rarely in patients taking bisphosphonates.
- Patients taking oral bisphosphonates have an increased risk of ***developing esophageal cancer***. In patients taking bisphosphonates, ***hypercalcemia*** is seen in 20% and serum PTH levels increase above normal in 10%, mimicking primary hyperparathyroidism. Hypocalcemia occurs frequently, resulting in secondary hyperparathyroidism; therefore, patients taking bisphosphonates are frequently prescribed prophylactic oral calcium supplements

Zoledronic Acid

◈ *Harrison 19th/2499-2501*

- In the treated population, there was an increased risk of transient postdose symptoms (acute-phase reaction) manifested by fever, arthralgia, myalgias, and headache.
- Recently there has been concern about two potential side effects associated with bisphosphonate use. The first is ***osteonecrosis of the jaw (ONJ)***. The second side effect is called ***atypical femur fracture***

51. Ans. b. Linezolid..., d. Streptom...

[Ref:KDT 7th/ 689-90; Katzung 12th/803]

Mechanism of Action of Drugs

◈ *KDT 7th/ 689-90*

1. *Inhibit cell wall synthesis: Penicillins, Cephalosporins, Cycloserine, Vancomycin, Bacitracin.*
2. *Cause leakage from cell membranes:* Polypeptides-Polymyxins, Colistin, Bacitracin. Polyenes-Amphotericin B, Nystatin, Hamycin
3. *Inhibit protein synthesis:* Tetracyclines, Chloramphenicol, Erythromycin, Clindamycin, ***Linezolid.***
4. *Cause misreading of m-RNA code and affect permeability:* **Aminoglycosides**-Streptomycin, Gentamicin, etc.
5. *Inhibit* **DNA gyrase**: ***Fluoroquinolones*** - Ciprofloxacin and others
6. *Interfere with* **DNA function**: ***Rifampin***
7. *Interfere with* **DNA synthesis**: ***Acyclovir***, Zidovudine
8. *Interfere with intermediary metabolism:* Sulfonamides, Sulfones, PAS, Trimethoprim, Pyrimethamine, Metronidazole

52. **Ans.** **a. Methotr..., d. Gemcitabi....**

[Ref: KDT 7th/858; Katzung 13th/928]

Table *(Katzung 13th/921)*: **Cell cycle effects of major classes of anticancer drugs**

Cell Cycle- Specific Agents	Cell Cycle–Nonspecific Agents
Antimetabolites (S phase) Capecitabine Cladribine Clofarabine Cytarabine (ara-C) Fludarabine 5-Fluorouracil (5-FU) Gemcitabine 6-Mercaptopurine (6-MP) Methotrexate (MTX) 6-Thioguanine (6-TG)	**Alkylating agents** Altretamine Bendamustine Busulfan Carmustine Chlorambucil Cyclophosphamide Dacarbazine Lomustine Mechlorethamine Melphalan Temozolomide Thiotepa

Contd...

Cell Cycle- Specific Agents	Cell Cycle–Nonspecific Agents
Epipodophylloxtoxin (toposiomerase II inlibitor) (G_1 – S phase) Etoposide	**Platinum analogs** Carboplatin Cisplatin Oxaliplatin
Txanes (M phase) Albumin-bound paclitaxel Docetaxel Paclitaxel	**Anthracyclines** Daunorubicin Doxorubicin Epirubicin Idarubicin Mitoxantrone
Vinca alkaloids (M phase) Vinblastine vincristine Vinorelbine	**Antitumor antibiotics** Dactinomycin Mitomycin
Antimicrotubule inhibitor (M phase) Ixabepilone	**Camptothecins (topoisomerase I inhibitors)** Irinotecan Topotecan
Antitumor antibiotics (G_2 – M phase) Bleomycin	

Table *(Katzung 13th/928)*: **Antimetabolites: Clinical spectrum of activity and toxicities**

Drug	Mechanism of Action	Clinical Applications	Toxicity
Capecitabine	Inhibits, TS; incorporation of FUTP into RNA resulting in alteration in RNA pro-cessing; incorporation of FdUPT into DNA resulting in inhibition of DNA synthesis and function	Breast cancer, colorectal cancer, gastro-esophageal cancer, hepatocellular cancer, pancreatic cancer	Diarrhea, hand-foot syndrome, myelosuppression nausea and vomiting
5-Fluorouracil	Inhibits TS; incorporation of FUTP into RNA resulting in alteration in RNA pro-cessing; incorporation of FdUTP into DNA resulting in inhibition of DNA syn-thesis and function	Colorectal cancer, and cancer, breast cancer, gastroesophageal cancer, head and neck cancer, hepatocellular cancer	Nausea, mucositis, diarrhea, bone marrow depression, neurotoxicity
Methotrexate	Inhibits DHFR, and purine nucleotide sunthesis	Breast cancer, head and neck cancer, osteogenic sarcoma, primary central nervous system lymphoma, non-Hodgkin's lymphoma, bladder cancer, choriocarcinoma	Mucositis, diarrhea, myelosuppression with neutropenia and thrombocytopenia
Pemetrexed	Inhibits TS, inhibits de novo purine nucleotide synthesis	Mesothelioma, non-small cell lung cancer	Myelosupression, skin rash, mucositis, diarrhea, fatigue
Cytarabine	Inhibits DNA synthesis and repair, inhibit ribonucleotide reductase with reduced formation of dNTPs, incorporation of cytarabine triphosphate into DNA	AML, ALL, CNL in blast crisis	Nausea and vomiting, myelosup-pression with neutropenia and thrombocytopenia, cerebellar ataxia
Gemcitabine	Inhibits DNA synthesis and repair; inhibits ribonucleotide reductase with reduced formation of dNTPs; incorporation of gemcitabine triphosphate into DNA resulting in inhibition of DNA synthesis and function	Pancreatic cancer, bladder cancer, breast cancer, non-small cell lung cancer, ovarian cancer, Non-Hodgkin's lymphoma, soft tissue sarcoma	Nausea, vomiting, diarrhea, myelosuppression
Fludarabine	Inhibits DNA synthesis and repair, inhibits ribonucleotide reductase; incorporation of fludarabine triphosphaste into DNA, induction of apoptosis	Non-Hodgkin's lymphoma, CLL	Myelosuppression, immunosuppression, fever, myalgias, arthralgias

Contd...

Drug	Mechanism of Action	Clinical Applications	Toxicity
Fludarabine	Inhibits DNA synthesis and repair; inhibits ribonucleotide reductase, incorporation of fludarabine triphosphate into DNA, induction of apoptosis	Non-Hodgkin's lymphoma, CLL	Myelosuppression, immunosuppression, fever, myalgias, arthralgias
Cladribine	Inhibits DNA synthesis and repair, inhibits ribonucleotide reductase; incorporation of cladribine triphosphate into DNA; induction of apoptosis	Hairy cell leukemia, CLL, non-Hodgkin's lymphoma	Myelosuppression, nausea and vomiting, and immunosuppression
6-Mercaptopurine	Inhibits de novo purine nucleotide synthesis; incorporation of triphosphate into RNA; incorporation of triphosphate into DNA	AML	Myelosuppression, immunosuppression, and hepatotoxicity
6-Thioguanine	Same as above	ALL, AML	Same as above

53. Ans. c. Tendi..., e. Photosens...

[Ref: KDT 7th/ 710-11; Katzung 13th/812-13; G & G 11th/1122]

"**Chronic arsenic poisoning: *Hyperkeratosis of palm*" *(Reddy 32nd/512)*

"**Hyperkeratosis:** It can be caused by ***vitamin A deficiency or chronic exposure to arsenic.*** *Hyperkeratosis can also be caused by B-Raf inhibitor drugs such as* ***Vemurafenib and Dabrafenib***" *(wikipedia)*

"**FQ gastrointestinal toxicity**: *Anorexia, nausea, vomiting, abdominal discomfort &* ***diarrhea*** *are the commonest side effects*" *(Pharmacology by Satoskar 24th/658)*

"**Aseptic meningitis**: ***Intravenous immunoglobulin*** *(Harrison 15th/428-Table, not mentioned FQ)*

Fluroquinolones (Ciprofloxacin)

◈ *KDT 7th/ 710-11*

- **Gastrointestinal:** Nausea, vomiting, bad taste& anorexia
- **CNS:** Dizziness, headache, restlessness, anxiety, insomnia, impairment of concentration & dexterity. Tremor & seizures are rare
- Skin hypersensitivity
- ***Tendinitis & tendon rupture***
- C/I during pregnancy

Fluoroquinolones (FQ): Adverse Effects

◈ *Katzung 13th/812-13*

- FQ are extremely well tolerated. The most common effects are ***nausea, vomiting, and diarrhea.***
- Occasionally, ***headache, dizziness, insomnia, skin rash, or abnormal liver function*** tests develop. **Photosensitivity** has been reported with lomefloxacin and pefloxacin. ***QTc prolongation*** may occur with gatifloxacin, levofloxacin, gemifloxacin, and moxifloxacin
- Fluoroquinolones may ***damage growing cartilage and cause an arthropathy.*** Thus, these drugs are not routinely recommended for patients under 18 years of age. However, the arthropathy is reversible, and there is a growing consensus that fluoroquinolones may be used in children in some cases (e.g., for treatment of pseudomonal infections in patients with cystic fibrosis).
- **Tendinitis**, a rare complication that has been reported in adults, is potentially more serious because of the risk of tendon rupture. Risk factors for tendonitis include advanced age, renal insufficiency, and concurrent steroid use.
- Fluoroquinolones should be *avoided during pregnancy in* the absence of specific data documenting their safety.

Adverse Effects of FQ

◈ *G & G 11th/1122*

- *The most common adverse reactions involve the GI tract, with 3–17% of patients reporting mostly mild nausea, vomiting, and/or abdominal discomfort.* ***Diarrhea and antibiotic-associated colitis*** *have been unusual.*
- **CNS side effects**, *predominately mild headache and dizziness, have been seen in 1–10% of patients. Rarely, hallucinations, delirium, and seizures have occurred, predominantly in patients who also were receiving* theophylline *or a nonsteroidal anti-inflammatory drug.*
- *Rashes, including* ***photosensitivity reactions****, also can occur.*
- ***Achilles tendon rupture or tendinitis has occurred rarely.*** *Renal disease, hemodialysis, and glucocorticoid use may be predisposing factors. Traditionally, the use of quinolones in children has been contraindicated because they have produced arthropathy in animal models. However, children with cystic fibrosis given ciprofloxacin, norfloxacin, and nalidixic acid have had few, and reversible, joint symptoms. Therefore, the benefits may outweigh the risks in some children.*
- *Leukopenia, eosinophilia, and mild elevations in serum transaminases occur rarely.*
- ***Prolongation of the QTc interval*** *has been observed with sparfloxacin and to a lesser extent with gatifloxacin and moxifloxacin. Quinolones probably should be used only with caution in patients who are taking certain antiarrhythmics, including* amiodarone, quinidine, *and* procainamide
- *The prescribing information for* ***gatifloxacin*** *includes a contraindication in diabetic patients due to serious reports of hypoglycemia and hyperglycemia. Risk factors for this adverse effect include older age, renal insufficiency, and concomitant therapy with glucose-altering medications.*

Drugs that can cause aseptic meningitis include the following: *(emedicine.medscape.com; wikipedia)*

- *Nonsteroidal anti-inflammatory drugs (NSAIDs)*
- *Antimicrobials (e.g., trimethoprim-sulfamethoxazole, amoxicillin, isoniazid)*

- *Muromonab-CD3 (Orthoclone OKT3)*
- *Azathioprine*
- *Intravenous immunoglobulin*
- *Intrathecal methotrexate*
- *Intrathecal cystine arabinoside*
- *Vaccines*
- *Allopurinol*

54. Ans. a. Silde..., b. Tadala..., e. Vardena...

[Ref: KDT 7th/303-04; Katzung 13th/197; Pharmacology by Satoskar 24th/985]

Acomprostate: *It is a weak NMDA-receptor antagonist with modest GABA$_A$ receptor agonistic activity being used for maintenance of alcohol abstinence*" *(KDT 7th/393)*

Phosphodiesterase-5 Inhibitors

◈ *KDT 7th/303-04; Katzung 13th/197*
- ***Sildenafil***
- ***Tadalafil***
- ***Vardenafil***

Drug used in Erectile Dysfunction

◈ *Katzung 13th/197*
- **Sildenafil** (Viagra) acts to increase cGMP by inhibiting its breakdown by phosphodiesterase isoform 5 (PDE-5). The drug has been very successful in the marketplace because it can be taken orally. Sildenafil has effects on *color vision, causing difficulty in blue-green discrimination.*
- Two similar PDE-5 inhibitors, **tadalafil** and **vardenafil,** are available.
- The drug most commonly used in patients who do not respond to sildenafil is **alprostadil,** a ***PGE1 analog*** that can be injected directly into the cavernosa or placed in the urethra as a minisuppository, from which it diffuses into the cavernosal tissue. Phentolamine can be used by injection into the cavernosa. These drugs will cause erection in most men who do not respond to sildenafil.

55. Ans. a. Cocai..., b. Amphet..., d. Dexamphe..., e. MDMA...

[Ref:KDT 7th/ 486,452; Pharmacology by Satoskar 24th/9227-30]

"**Psychotogenic (Hallucinogens) drugs** *are- **Cannabis,** LSD,-mescaline, endocannabinoid*" *(Pharmacology by Satoskar 24th/9227-30)*

CNS Stimulant

◈ *KDT 7th/ 486*

1. **Convulsants:** Strychnine, picrotoxin, bicuculline, pentylenetetrazol
2. **Analeptics:** Doxapram
3. *Psychostimulants: **Amphetamine,** Methylphenidate, atomoxetine, modafinil, armodafinil, pemoline, **cocaine** & caffeine*

"CNS stimulants: *Amphetamine, methamphetamine & dexamphetamine*" *(KDT 7th/ 134)*

"Methylene dioxy methamphetamine (MDMA): It is an amphetamine like ***synthetic compound stimulant*** & hallucinogenic properties, that has been abused as a recreational & euphoriant drug, especially by college students under the name **"Ecstasy"**. Fear of neurotoxicity has reduced its popularity" *(KDT 7th/ 452)*

56. Ans. b. ACE..., c. Phenyto...

[Ref:Katzung 10th/975; KDT 6th /484,405]

Furosemide can be used in pregnancy. No fetal anomalies are mentioned

"Phenytoin produces ***fetal hydantoin syndrome*** which is characterised by *hypoplastic plalanges, cleft palate, hare lip and microcephaly* when used in pregnancy" *(KDT 6th /405)*

Table *(Katzung 10th/975)*: **Drugs with significant adverse effects on the fetus**

Drug	Trimester	Effect
ACE inhibitors	All, especially second and third	***Renal damage***
Aminopterin	First	Multiple gross anomalies
Amphetamines	All	Suspected abnormal developmental patterns, decreased school performance
Androgens	Second and third	Masculinization of female fetus
Antidepressants, tricyclic	Third	Neonatal withdrawal symptoms have been reported in a few cases with clomipramine, desipramine, and imipramine
Barbiturates	All	Chronic use can lead to neonatal dependence.
Busulfan	All	Various congenital malformations; low birth weight
Carbamazepine	First	Neural tube defects
Chlorpropamide	All	Prolonged symptomatic neonatal hypoglycemia
Clomipramine	Third	Neonatal lethargy, hypotonia, cyanosis, hypothermia
Cocaine	All	Increased risk of spontaneous abortion, abruptio placentae, and premature labor; neonatal cerebral infarction, abnormal development, and decreased school performance
Cyclophosphamide	First	Various congenital malformations
Cytarabine	First, second	Various congenital malformations

Contd...

Drug	Trimester	Effect
Diazepam	All	Chronic use may lead to neonatal dependence
Diethylstilbestrol	All	Vaginal adenosis, clear cell vaginal adenocarcinoma
Ethanol	All	Risk of fetal alcohol syndrome and alcohol-related neurodevelopmental defects
Etretinate	All	High risk of multiple congenital malformations
Heroin	All	Chronic use leads to neonatal dependence
Iodide	All	Congenital goiter, hypothyroidism
Isotretinoin	All	Extremely high risk of CNS, face, ear, and other malformations
Lithium	First	Ebstein's anomaly
Methadone	All	Chronic use leads to neonatal dependence
Methotrexate	First	Multiple congenital malformations
Methylthiouracil	All	Hypothyroidism
Metronidazole	First	May be mutagenic (from animal studies; there is no evidence for mutagenic or teratogenic effects in humans)
Organic solvents	First	Multiple malformations
Misoprostol	First	Mobius sequence
Penicillamine	First	Cutis laxa, other congenital malformations
Phencyclidine	All	Abnormal neurologic examination, poor suck reflex and feeding
Phenytoin	***All***	***Fetal hydantoin syndrome***
Propylthiouracil	All	Congenital goiter
Streptomycin	All	Eighth nerve toxicity
Smoking (constituents of tobacco smoke)	All	Intrauterine growth retardation; prematurity; sudden infant death syndrome; perinatal complications
Tamoxifen	All	Increased risk of spontaneous abortion or fetal damage
Tetracycline	All	Discoloration and defects of teeth and altered bone growth
Thalidomide	First	Phocomelia (shortened or absent long bones of the limbs) and many internal malformations
Trimethadione	All	Multiple congenital anomalies
Valproic acid	All	Neural tube defects, cardiac and limb malformations
Warfarin	First	Hypoplastic nasal bridge, chondrodysplasia
	Second	CNS malformations
	Third	Risk of bleeding. Discontinue use 1 month before delivery

57. Ans. c. Fasciola he..., d. Fasciola....

[Ref: Harrison 19th/1428; KDT 7th/851; G & G 11th/1078; Panikar Parasitology 6th/127-29]

"**Fasciola hepatica**: ***Triclabendazole,*** *now is the drug of choice for human fascioliasis"* *(G & G 11th/1078)*

"Triclabendazole is highly effective against **adults of the common liver fluke** (***Fasciola hepatica***) as well as **all immature stages**, i.e. *early immature larvae* (1 to 6 weeks old) and *immature larvae* (6 to 9 weeks old). In fact, it is the only flukicide effective against all early immature liver fluke larvae. Triclabendazole is also effective against ***Fasciola gigantica*** and ***Fascioloides magna***. In contrast with most other benzimidazoles, triclabendazole has **no efficacy** against roundworms or tapeworms" *(parasitipedia.net)*

Table *(Harrison 19th/1428)*: **Drug Therapy for Human Trematode Infections**

Infection	Drug of choice	Adult does and duration
Blood Flukes		
S. mansoni, S. intercalatum, S. haematobium	Praziquantel	20 mg/kg, 2 does in 1day
S.japoincum, S.mekongi	Praziquantel	20 mg/kg, 3 does in 1 day
Biliary (Hepatic) Flukes		
Clonorchis sinensis, opisthorchis viverrin, O. felineus	Praziquantel	25 mg/kg, 3 does in 1 day
Fasciola hepatica, F. gigantica	**Triclabendazole**	10 mg/kg once
Intestinal Flukes		
Fasciolopsis buski, Heterophyes heterophyes	Praziquantel[a]	25 mg/kg, 3 does in 1 day
Lung Flukes		
Paragonimus westermani	Praziquantel[a]	25 mg/kg, 3 does per day for 2 day

[a]Not approved by the U.S. Food and Drug administration for this indication

Paragonimus westermani ***and Other*** **Paragonimus** ***Species*** *Called* ***lung flukes****, a number of* Paragonimus *species, of which* P. westermani *is the most common, are pathogenic for humans. Although these flukes are rather refractory to praziquantel, the drug is effective when used clinically.* Bithionol *is considered a second-line agent.* **Triclabendazole** ***also recently was shown to be efficacious****."* *(G & G 11th/1078)*

MICROBIOLOGY

58. Ans. **b. Streptococcus...**

[Ref: Ananthanarayan 9th/59]

Transformation

- *Ananthanarayan 9th/59*
- It is transfer of genetic information through the agency of free DNA.
- It was the first example of genetic exchange in bacteria to be discovered by ***Griffith in 1928.*** He found that mice died when injected with a mixture of live ***non-capsulated (R) Streptococcus pneumoniae*** & heat killed ***capsulated (S) S. pneumoniae,*** neither of which separately proved fatal

59. Ans. **c. Transmitte. ..., d. Spread by direct....**

[Ref: Park 23rd/356;Ananthanarayan 9th/ 559; Harrison 19th/1323-29]

Ebola Virus

- *Park 23rd/356*
- Incubation period is 2-21 days & is not infective during this period
- Case fatality rate may be as high as 70%
- The virus is transmitted through ***direct contact with blood, organs, body secretions or other body fluids*** of infected animals like chimpanzees, gorillas, monkeys, fruit bats etc.
- Human to human transmission is through blood or body fluids of an infected symptomatic person or through exposure to objects (such as needle) that have been contaminated with infected secretions
- It is ***not transmitted through air, water, or food***
- The illness is characterized by sudden onset of fever, intense weakness, muscle pain, headache, sorethroat, vomiting, diarrhea, rash, impaired kidney & liver function & in some both internal & external bleeding
- Currently there is ***no specific treatment for this disease***
- There is ***no vaccine against ebola***

"Human infections typically occur through ***direct exposure of skin lesions or mucosal surfaces to contaminated bodily fluids or material or by parenteral inoculation (e.g., via accidental needle sticks or reuse of needles in poorly equipped hospitals)***" *(Harrison 19th/1326-27)*

"Treatment of ebola is ***entirely supportive because no accepted/ approved, efficacious, specific antiviral agents or vaccines are yet available.*** The one exception is hyperimmune equine immunoglobulin, which has been approved in Russia—in the absence of convincing efficacy data—for emergency treatment of laboratory infections. Measures to stabilize patients include those generally recommended for severe septicemia/sepsis/ shock. Countermeasures should address hypotension and hypoperfusion, vascular leakage in the systemic and pulmonary circulatory system, disseminated intravascular coagulation and overt hemorrhaging, acute kidney failure, and electrolyte (especially potassium) imbalances. ***Pain management and administration of antipyretics and antiemetics should always be considered***" *(Harrison 19th/1328)*

Ebola Virus

- *www.cdc.gov*
- The length of time between exposure to the virus and the development of symptoms ***(incubation period)*** is between 2 to 21 days. Most often this is between 4 to 10 days.
- Between people, Ebola disease spreads only by ***direct contact with the blood or body fluids*** of a person who has developed symptoms of the disease. Body fluids that may contain ebola viruses include saliva, mucus, vomit, feces, sweat, tears, breast milk, urine and ***semen***.

- The WHO states that only people who are very sick are able to spread Ebola disease in ***saliva***, and whole virus has not been reported to be transmitted through sweat. Most people spread the virus through ***blood, feces and vomit***.
- Entry points for the virus include the ***nose, mouth, eyes, open wounds, cuts and abrasions***.
- The Ebola virus may be able to persist for up to ***8 weeks in the semen*** of survivors after they recovered, which could lead to ***infections via sexual intercourse***.
- **Dead bodies** remain infectious; thus, *people handling human remains in practices such as traditional burial rituals or more modern processes such as embalming are at risk*.
- The ***natural reservoir*** for Ebola has yet to be confirmed; however, ***bats*** are considered to be the most likely candidate species.
- The disease has a high risk of death, killing between 25 percent and 90 percent of those infected with the virus, averaging out at 50 percent. This is often due to ***low blood pressure from fluid loss***, and typically follows six to sixteen days after symptoms appear.

60. Ans. a. Bacilli causing..., b. Painful..., d. Presents....

[Ref: Ananthanarayan 9th/ 331; Harrison 19th/880, 1012-13]

Haemophilus Ducreyi

◈ *Ananthanarayan 9th/ 331*

- *Chancroid or soft sore is a venereal disease characterized by* ***tender non-indurated irregular ulcers on the genitalia***
- *The bacilli may be arranged in small groups or whorls or in parallel chains, giving a* ***'school of fish' or 'rail road track' appearance***
- *The infection remains localized, spreading only to the regional* ***lymph nodes which are enlarged & painful***

Haemophilus Ducreyi

◈ *Harrison 19th/1012-13*

- Infection is acquired as the result of a break in the epithelium during sexual contact with an infected individual.
- ***After an incubation period of 4–7 days***, the initial lesion-a papule with surrounding erythema, appears. In 2 or 3 days, the papule evolves into a pustule, which spontaneously ruptures and forms a sharply circumscribed ulcer that generally is not indurated
- The ***ulcers are painful and bleed easily***; little or no inflammation of the surrounding skin is evident.
- Approximately half of patients develop ***enlarged, tender inguinal lymph nodes***, which frequently become fluctuant and spontaneously rupture.
- Patients usually seek medical care after 1–3 weeks of painful symptoms.
- Multiple ulcers can coalesce to ***form giant ulcers***. Ulcers can appear and then resolve, with inguinal adenitis and suppuration following 1–3 weeks later; this clinical picture can be *confused with that of lymphogranuloma venereum*
- *Clinical diagnosis of chancroid is often inaccurate, and laboratory confirmation should be attempted in suspected cases.*
- An **accurate diagnosis** of chancroid relies on ***culture of H. ducreyi*** from the lesion or from an aspirate of suppurative lymph nodes.
- A **probable diagnosis** of chancroid can be made when the following criteria are met: *(1) one or more painful genital ulcers; (2) no evidence of Treponema pallidum infection by dark-field examination of ulcer exudate or by a negative serologic test for syphilis performed at least 7 days after ulcer onset; (3) a typical clinical presentation for chancroid; and (4) a negative test for herpes simplex virus in the ulcer exudate*

Table *(Harrison 19th/880)*: **Clinical Features of Genital Ulcer**

Feature	Syphilis	Herpes	Chancroid	Lymphogranuloma Venereum	Donovanosis
Incubation period	9–90 day	2–7 days	***1–14 days***	3 day–6 weeks	1–4 weeks (up to 6 months)
Early primary lesion	Papule	Vesicle	Pustule	Papule, pustule, or vesicle	Papule
No. of lesion	Usually one	Multiple	Usually multiple, may coalesce	Usually one; often not detected, despite lymphadenopathy	Variable
Diameter	5–15 mm	1–2 mm	Variable	2–10 mm	Variable
Edges	Sharply demarcated, elevated, round, or oval	Erythematous	***Undermined, ragged, irregular***	Elevated, round or oval	Elevated irregular
Depth	Superficial or deep	Superficial	Excavated	Superficial or deep	Elevated
Base	Smooth, non-purulent, relatively nonvascular	Serous, erythematous nonvascular	Purulent, bleeds easily	Variable, nonvascular	Red and velvety bleeds readily
Induration	Firm	None	Soft	Occasionally firm	Firm
Pain	Uncommon	Frequent tender	***Usually very tender***	Variable	Uncommon
Lymphadenopathy	Firm, nontender, bilateral	Firm, tender, often bilateral with initial episode	***Tender, may suppurate, loculated, usually unilateral***	Tender, may suppurate, loculated, usually unilateral	None; pseudobuboes

61. Ans. c. Trichu..., d. Ascar...

[Ref: Panikar Parasitology 7th/162]

Strongyloides: Infective form is ***filariform larva*** *(Panikar 7th/178)*

"**Trichinella**: Infective form is ***encysted larva*** found in muscles of pigs & other animals" *(Panikar 7th/168)*

"**Ancylostoma duodenale- Infective form is third stage filariform larva**" *(Panikar 7th/168)*

Mode of Infection

- *Panikar Parasitology7th/162*
- *By ingestion*
  - **Eggs: *Ascaris, enterobius, Trichuris***
  - Larva within intermediate host: Dracunculus
  - Encysted larvae in muscle: Trichinella
- By penetration of skin: ***Ancylostoma, Necator, Strongyloides***
- By blood sucking insects: Filariae
- By inhalation of dust containing eggs: ***Ascaris,*** enterobius

62. Ans. a. Geobacillus..., b. Pneumococc..., e. Bacillus...,

[Ref: Ananthanarayan 9th/30,32; Greenwood 16th/77]

Sterilisation Control (Dry Heat)

- *Biological Ananthanarayan 9th/30*
- *The spores of a non-toxigenic strain of* ***clostridium tetani or Bacillus subtilis subspecies niger*** *are used as a* **microbial test of dry heat efficiency**

Sterilisation Control (Moist Heat)

- *Biological Ananthanarayan 9th/32*
- *For determining the* **efficacy of moist heat sterilization,** ***spores of Bacillus stearothermophilus*** *are used as the test organism*

"**Geobacillus stearothermophilus** (or ***Bacillus stearothermophilus***) is constantly used in the biotech industry to test the success of sterilization cycles of equipment. Due to the bacteria's high resistance to heat, it is a ***suitable biological Indicator of microbe life after a sterilization cycle***" *(microbewiki.kenyon.edu)*

63. Ans. d. cryptococcus....

[Ref: Harrison 19th/ 1329; Ananthanarayan 9th/589-90; Jawetz 27th/853]

Cryptococcus is a yeast *(Ananthanarayan 9th/589)*

Dimorphic Fungi are

- *Jawetz 27th/853*
- ***Blastomycosis dermatitidis***
- Paracoccidioides brasiliensis
- Coccidioides posadasii & ***Coccidioides immitis***
- ***Histoplasma capsulatum***
- Sporotrix schenckii
- Penicillium marneffei

Fungus Classification

- *Harrison 19th/ 1329*
- Three terms frequently used in clinical discussions of fungal infections are ***yeast, mold, and dimorphic fungus.***
- ***Yeasts*** are seen as rounded single cells or as budding organisms. *Candida* and *Cryptococcus* are traditionally classified as yeasts.
- **Molds** grow as filamentous forms called *hyphae* both at room temperature and in invaded tissue. *Aspergillus, Rhizopus* (the genus that causes mucormycosis, also known as zygomycosis), and fungi commonly infecting the skin to cause ringworm and related cutaneous conditions are classified as molds.
- Variations occur within this classification of yeasts and molds. For instance, when *Candida* infects tissue, both yeasts and filamentous forms may be present (except with *C. glabrata*, which forms only yeasts in tissue); in contrast, *Cryptococcus* exists only in yeast form.
- **Dimorphic** is the term used to describe fungi that grow as yeasts or large spherical structures in tissue but as filamentous forms at room temperature in the environment. Classified in this group are the organisms causing ***blastomycosis, paracoccidioidomycosis, coccidioidomycosis, histoplasmosis, and sporotrichosis.***

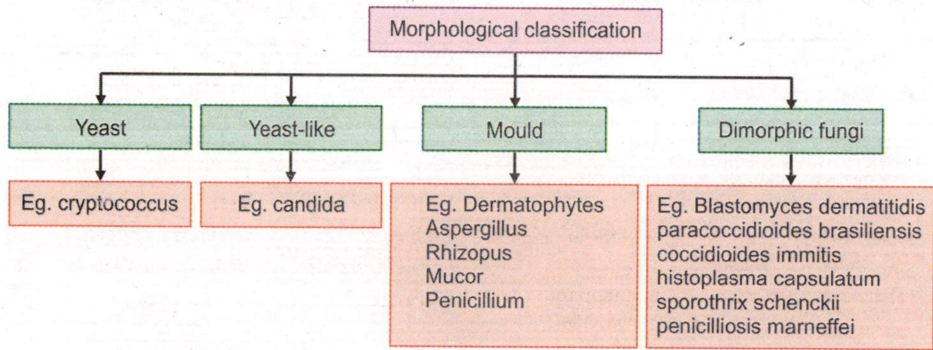

Fig: *(Ananthanarayan 9th/589):* Morphological Classification of fungus

64. Ans. a. Coxsackie..., b. Enterovirus..., d. Coxsackie...

[Ref: Ananthanarayan 9th/485; Harrison 19th/1291]

Table *(Anathanarayan 9th/485)*: **Enterovirus serotype**

Group	Serotype
Poliovirus	1–3
Coxsackie virus A	1–22, 24
Coxsackie virus B	1-6
Echovirus	1–9, 11-27, 29–34
Numbered echovirus	(EV) 68-78

Table *(Harrison 19th/1291)*: **Manifestations Commonly Associated With Enterovirus Serotypes**

Manifestation	Coxsackievirus	Echovirus (E) and Enterovirus (Ent)
Acute hemorrhagic conjunctivitis	A24	E70
Aseptic meningitis	A2, 4, 7, 9, 10; B1–5	E4, 6, 7, 9, 11, 13, 16, 18, 19, 30, 33; Ent 70, 71
Encephalitis	A9; B1–5	E3, 4, 6, 7, 9, 11, 18, 25, 30; Ent71
Exanthem	A4, 5, 9, 10, 16; B1, 3–5	E4–7, 9, 11, 16–19, 25, 30; Ent71
Generalized disease of the newborn	B1–5	E4–6, 7, 9, 11, 14, 16, 18, 19
Hand-foot-and-mouth disease	A5, 7, 9, 10, 16; B1, 2, 5	Ent71
Herpangina	A1–10, 16, 22; B1–5	E6, 9, 11, 16, 17, 25, 30; Ent71
Myocarditis, **pericarditis**	A4, 9, 16; B1–5	E6, 9, 11, 22
Paralysis	A4, 7, 9; B1–5	E2–4, 6, 7, 9, 11, 18, 30; Ent70, 71
Pleurodynia	A1, 2, 4, 6, 9, 10, 16; B1–6	E1–3, 6, 7, 9, 11, 12, 14, 16, 19, 24, 25, 30
Pneumonia	A9, 16; B1–5	E6, 7, 9, 11, 12, 19, 20, 30; Ent-D68, 71

Table *(Ananthanarayan 9th/485)*: **Clinical syndromes commonly caused by enterovirus**

Syndrome	Poliovirus	Coxsackie A	Coxsackie B	ECHO virus	New enterovirus types
Paralysis	1, 2, 3	7	–	–	–
Aseptic meningitis	1, 2, 3	7, 9, 23	1–6	Several (2, 3, 4, 6, 7, 9, 11, 14, 16, 17, 18, 19, 25, 33)	71
Encephalitis	1, 2, 3	9	3–6	6, 9, 17, 19	71
Fever with rash	–	9, 16, 23	–	4, 6, 9, 16	–
Hand, foot and mouth disease	–	5, 10, 16	–	–	71
Herpangina	–	1–6, 8, 10	–	–	–
Upper respiratory infection	–	21	–	11, 20	–
Penumonitis, bronchiolitis	–	–	–	–	68
Bornholm disease	–	–	1-5	–	–
Myocarditis, **pericarditis**	–	–	1-5	–	–
Acute hemorrhagic conjunctivitis	–	24	–	–	70

65. Ans. c. Lymphocyte...

[Ref: Harrison 19th/1190-91; Ananthanarayan 9th/473-74; Jawetz 27th/470-74]

Cytomegalovirus (Human Herpes Virus Type 5)

- It is cytomegalic (*not lymphoproliferative*, which occur in HHV4, 6 & 7)
- Characterized by *enlargement of infected cells*
- Congenital infection- Intrauterine infection leads to *fetal death or cytomegalic inclusion disease of newborn which is often fatal*

Cytomegalovirus (Human Herpesvirus Type 5)

◈ *Harrison 19th/1190-91*

- Human CMV is one of several related species-specific viruses that cause similar diseases in various animals. All are associated with the production of *characteristic enlarged cells*—hence the name *cytomegalovirus*.
- **Cytomegalic cells** in vivo (presumed to be *infected epithelial cells*) are two to four times larger than surrounding cells and often contain an 8- to 10-μm intranuclear inclusion that is eccentrically placed and is surrounded by a clear halo, producing an *"owl's eye" appearance.*
- In addition to inducing *severe birth defects*, CMV causes a wide spectrum of disorders in older children and adults, ranging from an asymptomatic subclinical infection to a *mononucleosis syndrome* in healthy individuals to disseminated disease in immunocompromised patients.
- Primary infection with CMV in late childhood or adulthood is often associated with a vigorous T lymphocyte response that may contribute to the development of a mononucleosis syndrome similar to that which follows infection with Epstein-Barr virus. The hallmark of such infection is the appearance of *atypical lymphocytes in the peripheral blood; these cells are predominantly activated CD8+ T lymphocytes.*
- Polyclonal activation of B cells by CMV contributes to the development of rheumatoid factors and other autoantibodies during mononucleosis.

66. Ans. a. Present..., b. It acts as..., c. Generate..., d. Same as rho....

[Ref:www.ks.uiuc.edu/Research/newbr/]

"**Bacteriorhodopsin** is a protein used by ***Archaea***, most notably by ***Halobacteria***, a ***class*** of the ***Euryarchaeota***. It ***acts as a proton pump***; that is, it ***captures light energy*** and uses it to move ***protons*** across the membrane out of the cell. The resulting ***proton gradient*** is subsequently ***converted into chemical energy***"

"**Rhodopsin** is a ***biological pigment found in the rods of the retina*** and is a ***G-protein-coupled receptor*** (GPCR). Rhodopsin is extremely sensitive to light, and thus enables vision in low-light conditions. When rhodopsin is exposed to light, it immediately ***photobleaches***. In ***humans***, it is regenerated fully in about 45 minutes"

Bacteriorhodopsin

◈ *cpclab.uni-duesseldorf*

- It is a ***light-driven proton pump*** that was first found in halophilic archaea. Recently it was shown that a homologous group of proteins called proteorhodopsins are widely distributed in aquatic bacteria. It allows the cells to ***harvest the energy of the sun light for phototrophic growth.***
- In contrast to the photosynthesis of endosymbiontic chloroplasts in plants and previously known groups of photosynthetic bacteria ***no electron transport*** is involved. Therefore bacterio- and proteorhodopsin-mediated phototrophic growth results in "proton transport phosphorylation, in contrast to the "electron transport phosphorylation" of the classical photosynthesis. However, both processes involve ***integral membrane proteins and result in an electrochemical gradient across a membrane which powers the ATPsynthase.***

"**Bacteriorhodopsin (BR)** is a relatively ***small membrane protein***. As all membrane proteins, it has been particularly challenging to structural analysis, due to difficulties in the process of purification. Membrane proteins, contrary to non-membrane proteins, expose their non-polar (hydrophobic) residues to the exterior. BR functions as a ***pump of protons from the cytoplasm to the extracelullar*** space, in order to create a proton gradient. Afterwards, protons enter the cell again favourably, and the cell takes advantage of that by coupling to a reaction that ***synthesizes ATP***. The energy required by BR is provided by green light. At the end of the process, the outcome is that ***the cell transformed energy from light into ATP, the energetic currency of the cell***" *(cpclab.uni-duesseldorf.de)*

"**Bacteriorhodopsin** is a ***trans-membrane protein found in the cellular membrane*** of *Halobacterium salinarium*, which functions as a ***light-driven proton pump.*** With the recent determination of the structure of bR by ***electron cryo-microscopy***, simulation of the proton pump cycle has become feasible" *(www.ks.uiuc.edu/)*

"**Bacteriorhodopsin** is a ***proton pump*** found in Archaea, it takes ***light energy and coverts it into chemical energy i.e. ATP***, that can be used by the cell for cellular functions" *(www.boundless.com)*

FORENSIC MEDICINE

67. Ans. d. Can give imprisonment..., e. Can impose....

[Ref: Reddy 34th/7; Reddy 27th/6 indiankanoon.org]

*In **new edition of Reddy (34th)**, amount regarding fine imposed by 1st & 2nd class magistrate is given wrong (!!!).*

But in old edition (27th), it is correctly given

Table *(Reddy 34nd/7)*: **Powers of magistrate**

Class of magistrate	Imprisonment	Fine
Chief judicial magistrate	***Up to seven years***	***Unlimited***
I class judicial magistrate	Up to three years	10,000 rupees
II class judicial magistrate	Up to one year	5000 rupees

Table *(Reddy 27th/6)*: **Powers of magistrate**

Class of magistrate	Imprisonment	Fine
Chief judicial magistrate	Up to seven years	Unlimited
I class judicial magistrate	Up to three years	5000 rupees
II class judicial magistrate	Up to one year	1000 rupees

Section 29 in the Code of Criminal Procedure, 1973

indiankanoon.org, Also confirmed by lawyers

Sentences which Magistrates may pass

- The Court of a **Chief Judicial Magistrate** may pass any sentence authorised by law ***except*** a sentence of death or of imprisonment for life or of imprisonment for a ***term exceeding seven years.***
- The Court of a **Magistrate of the first class** may pass a sentence of imprisonment for a term not exceeding three years, or of fine not exceeding five thousand rupees, or of both.
- The Court of a **Magistrate of the second class** may pass a sentence of imprisonment for a term not exceeding one year, or of fine not exceeding one thousand rupees, or of both.
- The Court of a **Chief Metropolitan Magistrate** shall have the powers of the Court of a Chief Judicial Magistrate and that of a Metropolitan Magistrate, the powers of the Court of a Magistrate of the first class.

68. Ans. c. Larger..., d. Mental tubercles..., e. Symphyseal....

[Ref: Reddy 32nd/60; Parikh 7th/ 79]

Symphyseal height is more in males *(Parikh 7th/79)*

Table *(Reddy 32nd/60)*: **Trait diagnostic of sex from skeleton (Mandible)**

Trait	Male	Female
General size	Larger & thicker	Smaller & thinner
Chin	Square (U-shaped)	Rounded
Body height	At symphysis greater	At symphysis smaller
Ascending ramus	Greater breadth	Smaller breadth
Angle of body & ramus (Gonion)	Less obtuse(under 125^0); Prominent & averted	More obtuse & not prominent
Condyles	Larger	Smaller
Mental tubercles	Large & prominent	Insignificant

69. Ans. b. Atropine.., d. Spontaneously...

[Ref: Reddy 32nd/495-98; Parikh 7th/625-28; G & G 11th/210;KDT 7th/111; Katzung 13th/979-80; Pharmacology by Satoskar 24th/297]

"Opiate overdose, pontine hemorrhage & organophosphate causes pin-point pupil"- *theemtspot.com*

Carbamates (Derivative of Carbonic Acid)

- They are ***anticholinergic***
- Symptoms begin in 15 minutes to 2 hr
- It **differs toxicologically from organophosphate:**
  - ***They will spontaneously hydrolyse from the cholinesterase enzymatic site within 24 to 48 hours, whereas organophosphates will not;***
  - ***They do not effectively penetrate into the CNS, & as such CNS toxicity is limited***
- All other clinical manifestations are *similar to organophosphates*
- **Treatment:** ***Atropine is the specific antidote. Pralidoxime*** may diminish the severity of symptoms & help prevent some morbidity. It improves respiratory functions & patients well being

Organophosphorus Poisoning

Reddy 32nd/495-97; KDT 7th/111

- Pupil: ***Miosis, occasionally unequal or dilated***
- Pralidoxime & atropine work synergistically & should be used together
- *All case of Anti-ChE poisoning must be must be promptly given* ***atropine*** *2 mg i.v repeated every 10 min till dryness of mouth or other signs of atropinisation appear. Continued treatment with maintenance doses may be required for 1-2 weeks*
- The use of oximes in organophosphate poisoning is secondary to that of atropine. Moreover, the clinical benefit of oximes is highly variables

70. Ans. c. Kissing

[Ref: Reddy 32nd/ 392; Parikh 7th/389-90]

Rape: The Criminal Law (Amendment) Bill, 2013 (S.375, I.P.C)

A person is said to ***commit sexual assault*** if that person *(Reddy 32nd/ 392)*

- **Penetrates his penis,** to any ***extent, into the vagina, mouth, urethra or anus of another person or makes the person to do so with him or any other person***
- **Inserts,** to any extent, **any object or a part of the body,** not being the ***penis, into the vagina, the urethra or anus*** of another person or makes the person to do so with him or any other person
- **Manipulates** any part of the body of another person so as to cause penetration into the ***vagina, urethra, anus or any part of body*** of such person to do so with him or any other person
- **Applies his mouth** to the penis, vagina, anus, urethra, of another person or makes such person to do so with him or any other person
- **Touches** the ***vagina, penis, anus or breast*** of the person or makes the person touch the vagina, penis, anus or breast of that person or any other person, except where such penetration or touching is carried out for proper hygienic or medical purposes under the circumstances falling under any of the **following seven descriptions**
  - *Against her will.*
  - *Without her consent.*
  - *With her consent, when her consent has been obtained by putting her or any person in whom she is interested, in fear of death or of hurt.*

- *With her consent, when the man knows that he is not her husband and that her consent is given because she believes that he is another man to whom she is or believes herself to be lawfully married.*
- *With her consent when, at the time of giving such consent, by reason of unsoundness of mind or intoxication or the administration by him personally or through another of any stupefying or unwholesome Substance, she is unable to understand the nature and consequences of that to which she gives consent.*
- *With or without her consent, when she is under eighteen years of age.*
- *When she is unable to communicate consent.*

71. Ans. b. Death clutch is seen..., c. Generally occurs....

[Ref: Reddy 32nd/153-55; Parikh 7th/ 147-50; Modi 22nd/231]

"***Cadaveric spasm is also known as death clutch***"-*Textbook of Forensic Medicine by NG Rao 1st/127*

Table: Difference Between Rigor mortis & Cadaveric spasm

Feature	Cadaveric Spasm	Rigor mortis
Definition	This is continuation after death, of the state of contraction in ***which muscles were at the instant of death***. The stage of primary relaxation is absent. The stiffening is therefore instantaneous at the time of death	This is d/t changes in muscles after molecular death of their cells and is preceded by general relaxation of the muscles. A ***2-3 hour lapse*** is therefore necessary before stiffening occurs.
Mechanism	Not known	Known
Predisposing factors	Sudden death Emotional tension (excitement, fear, exhaustion) Physical activity at the time of death	None
Preceded By	Primary relaxation is absent	Stage of primary relaxation
Time of onset	Instantaneous	2-3 hours after death
Muscles Involved	Certain groups of voluntary muscles	All muscles, both voluntary & involuntary
Muscles stiffening	Is quite marked and considerable force is required to break it	Is less marked & only moderate force required to break it
Molecular Death	Does not occur	Occurs
Electrical stimuli	Muscle respond	Does not respond
Produed	Can not be produced by any method after death. It is impossible to simulate it	Cold stiffening (<4°C) & heat coagulation (>70°C) simulate rigor mortis
Medicolegal Importance	***Indicates time since death***	Indicates circumstances & mode of death[Q] e.g. suicide, homicide or accident

Contd...

Conditions Simulating Rigor Mortis

1. Cold stiffening
2. *Heat stiffening or coagulation (Pugilistic attitude)*
3. *Cadaveric spasm or Instantaneous Rigor*
4. *Putrefaction* (only written in Parikh)

Table: Rigor Mortis

According to Reddy	According to Parikh
• **Time of onset:** ▪ ***In India (tropical countries) it starts 1-2 hours after death & takes further 1-2 hours to develop*** ▪ In temperate countries, it begins in 3-6 hours & takes further 2-3 hours to develop	• ***In India rigor mortis commences in 2-3 hours, takes about 12 develop form had to foot, persists for another 12 hours & takes about 12 hours to pass off***. So if rigor mortis has not set in the time since death would be within 2 hours & if it has affected the whole body, the time since death would be 12-24 hours.
• **Duration:** ▪ In tropical countries (India) it lasts 18-36 hours in summer & 24-48 hours in winter ▪ In temperate countries it lasts for 2-3 days	• ***It does not starts in all muscles simultaneously*** (Nysten's rule) • Order of appearance & disappearance ▪ Heart (left chamber in 1 hour) → Eyelids[Q] (3-4 hrs) → Face muscles → Neck & trunk → Upper extremities → legs → Small muscle of finger & toes (last to be affected, 11 -12 hours) ▪ It passes off in same order of appearance ▪ ***It usually lasts for 18-36 hours in summer & 24-28 hours in winter.***

72. Ans. d. Barbiturate....

[Ref: Reddy 33rd/155, 32rd/149; Parikh 7th/143,6th/ 3.8-3.9]

Post-Mortem Caloricity

◈ Reddy 33rd/155

- *In this condition, the temperature of the body remains raised for the first two hours or so after death*
- *This occur*
  - *When the regulation of heat production has been severely disturbed before death, as in sunstroke & in some nervous disorder*
  - *When there has been a great increase in heat production in the muscle due to convulsions, as in tetanus & strychnine poisoning etc*
  - *When there has been excessive bacterial activity, as in septicaemic condition, cholera & other fevers*

Post-Mortem Caloricity: Seen in

- *Parikh 6th/ 3.8-3.9*
  - *Pontine haemorrhage & sunstroke*
  - ***Tetanus & strychnine poisoning***
  - *Acute viral or viral infections such as lobar pneumonia, typhoid fever, encephalitis & encephalomyelitis*

Post-Mortem Caloricity

- *ourforensicmedicine. blogspot.in/2010/02/23-causes-of-post-mortem-caloricity.html*
- ***Septicaemia**: Infectious diseases, Bacteremia, **Tetanus**, Rabies, yellow fever*
- *Asphyxial Conditions*
- *Severe convulsions: **Tetanus & Strychnine***
- *Hyperpyrexia at death: Heat Stroke (sun stroke) & Pontine Haemorrhage*
- High Atmospheric Temperature
- Peritonitis, Meningitis, Nephritis
- Alcohol poisoning

*"**Factor affecting cooling of body (Algor mortis)**: Build of cadaver: Children & **old people cool more** rapidly than adult" (Reddy 33rd/155)*

73. Ans. a. Repeated..., b. Intubation..., d. Saline containing...

[Ref: Reddy 32nd/507; Parikh 7th/535-37]

Carbolic Acid

- *Reddy 32nd/507*
- An ***emetic often fails due to the anaesthetic effect***
- **Lavage:** The stomach should be ***washed repeatedly***, carefully with plenty of lukewarm water containing activated charcoal, olive oil, castor oil etc. Washing continued until the washings are clear & odourless
- When lavage is completed, 30 9ram of magnesium sulphate or a quantity of medicinal liquid paraffin should left in the stomach
- Demulcent
- ***Saline containing sodium carbonate*** is given i.v to combat circulatory depression, to dilute carbolic acid content of blood & to encourage excretion by producing diuresis
- Haemodialysis, if there is renal failure
- Methylene blue, i.v, if there is severe methaemoglobinaemia

"**Carbolic acid management:** Evaluate and ***support airway, breathing, and circulation***. ***Children*** may be more vulnerable to corrosive agents than adults because of the relatively smaller diameter of their airways. In cases of respiratory compromise secure airway and respiration via ***endotracheal intubation***. If not possible, surgically create an airway" *(www.atsdr.cdc.go)*

PSM

74. Ans. b. Additional contrace..., c. Highly effective..., d. Incidence of....

[Ref: Park 23rd/509;Cummunity Medicine with recent Advances by Suryakantha 4th/686; Dutta Obs 8th/ 631-32]

Vasectomy

- *Park 23rd/509; Suryakantha 4th/686*
- It is a permanent sterilization operation done in the male where a ***segment of vas deferens*** of both the sides are resected & the cut ends are ligated
- It is a simple, cheap, safe, very effective, permanent & quick surgical method of family planning
- **Failure rate** is generally low, ***0.15 pregnancies per 100 persons*** in the first year after the procedure
- ***Additional contraceptive protection is needed for about 2-3 months or at least 20-30 ejaculation***(whichever comes first) following operations, i.e. till the semen becomes free of sperm
- It is ***not castration, it does not affect the testes & it does not affect sexual ability***. Some men may complain of diminution of sexual vigour, impotence, headache, fatigue etc. Such adverse psychological effects are seen in men who have undergone vasectomy under emotional pressure
- Autoimmune response: Normally, 2% of fertile men have circulating antibodies against their own sperm. In men who have had vasectomies, the Fig: can be as high as 54%. There is no reason to believe that such antibodies are harmful to physical health
- The ***incidence of recanalization is 0-6% after procedure***
- In no-scalpel vasectomy(NSV): In this instead of incision, small puncture is made & require no suturing of punctured site, just a small bandage is sufficient

75. Ans. b. Provision of free....

[Ref: Park 23rd/ 891; Community Medicine with recent Advances by Suryakantha 4th/816]

Elements of primary health care: *8 Essential component* oulined in Alma- *(Ata declaration (1978) Park 23rd/ 891)*

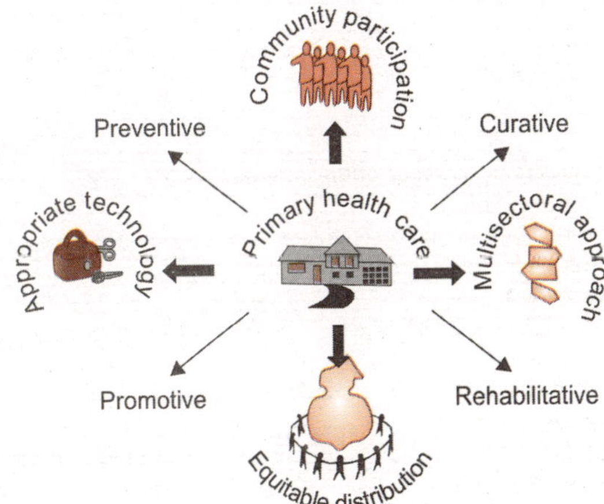

Fig: *(Suryakantha 4th/817)*: Principles & component of primary health care

1. ***Education concerning prevailing health problems & the methods of preventing & controlling them***
2. ***Promotion of food supply & proper nutrition***
3. ***An adequate supply of safe water & basic sanitation***

4. Maternal & child health care including family planning
5. Immunization against major infectious diseases
6. ***Prevention & control of locally endemic disease***
7. Appropriate treatment of common diseases & injuries
8. ***Provision of essential drug***

"**Definition of primary health care** *(Alma-Ata declaration1978)*: *Primary health care is essential health care made universally accessible to individuals & acceptable to them, through their full participation & at a cost the community & country can afford" (Park 23rd/ 891)*

76. Ans. a. Live attenuated...

[Ref: Park 23rd/103; O.P.Ghai 8th/195-96; Community Medicine with recent Advances by Suryakantha 3rd/320]

Table *(Park 23rd/ 103)*: **Vaccine currently in Use**

Live attenuated	Killed whole organism	Toxoid/ Protein	Polysaccharide	Glycoconjugate	Recombinant
BCG, Yellow fever,OPV, ***Measles, Mumps, Rubella***, Typhoid, Varicella, Rotavirus, Cholera, Cold-adopted influenza, Rotavirus reassortants, Zoster	Typhoid, Cholera, Plague, Pertussis, Influenza, Typhus, IPV, Rabies, JE,Tick borne encephailitis, HAV	Diphtheria, Tetanus, Acellular pertussis, Anthrax, Influenza subunit	Pneumococcus, Meningococcus, Hib, Typhoid(Vi)	Hib, Pneumococ-cus, MenACWY (Meningococcus)	HBV, Lyme disease, Cholera Toxin B, HPV

77. Ans. b. Before starting....

[Ref: Park 23rd/131-33; Community Medicine by Piyush Gupta 1st/598-603]

Investigation of an Epidemic

◈ *Steps Park 23rd/ 131-33*

- *Verification of diagnosis*
- *Confirmation of existence of an epidemic*
- *Defining the population at-risk*
- *Rapid search for all cases & their characteristic*
- *Data analysis*
- *Formulation of hypotheses*
- *Testing of hypotheses*
- *Evaluation of ecological factors*
- *Further investigation of population at risk*
- *Writing the report*

Table *(Piyush Gupta 1st/598)*: **Ten steps of a field investigation of epidemic**

1. Establish the existence of the outbreak.
2. Confirm the diagnosis.
3. Create a case definition and determine the number of cases.
4. Describe the case according to time (onset), place and person (age, sex, etc.)
5. Formulate a hypothesis to explain the exposure and mode of transmission.
6. Test the hypothesis by appropriate study (case control or cohort).
7. Compare the hypothesis with established facts and plan a more systematic study.
8. Plan and implement control measures.
9. Evaluate the effectiveness of control measures (establish a surveillance system).
10. Prepare a written report

78. Ans. a. Lectu... c. Group..., d. Panel..., e. Role play...

[Ref: Park 23rd/863-65; Cummunity Medicine with recent Advances by Suryakantha 4th/763;Community Medicine by Piyush Gupta 1st/756-65]

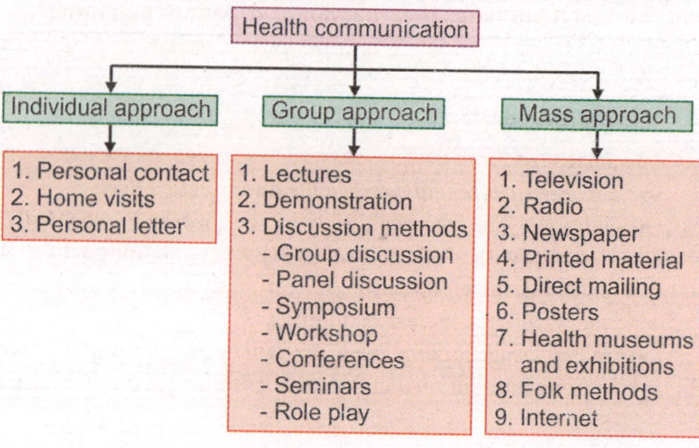

Fig: *(Park 23rd/863)*: Methods in Health communication

79. Ans. e. Lepromin test....

[Ref:Neena Khanna 5th/ 272-83; Roxburg 17th/;Park 23rd/314-29]

Slit smear: *All patients who are AFB positive should be given multibacillary treatment*, irrespective of the clinical presentation- *Neena Khanna 5th/ 281, 283*

"**Skin lesion in Lepromatous leprosy(LL): *Normoaesthetic/ minimally hypoaesthetic***"- *Neena Khanna 5th/ 276*

Multi Drug Therapy (MDT) Blister Packs are Available in 4 Colors

◈ *Neena Khanna 5th/ 284*

1. *Adult multibacillary(MB) pack: Pink-red color*
2. *Child multibacillary(MB) pack: Yellow color*
3. *Adult paucibacillary(PB) pack: Green color*
4. *Child paucibacillary(PB) pack: Blue color*

Table *(Neena Khanna 5th/ 283)*: **Profile of different types of leprosy**

	TT	BT	BB	BL	LL
Skin lesions					
Number	Single/few	Few	Several	Numerous	Innumerable
Size	Variable	May be large	Variable	Small	Small
Sensations	Anesthetic	Hypoesthetic	Hypoesthetic	Hypoesthetic	***Normoesthetic***
Symmetry	Asymmetrical	Asymmetrical	Bilateral, but Asymmetrical	Tendency to symmetry	***Symmetrical***
Morphology	Macule/plaque; well-defined	Plaques; well-defined with satellite lesions	Plaques; with sloping edge (inverted saucer appearance)	Macules/papules; nodules/plaques, ill-defined	Macules/papules; nodules/plaques, ill-defined
Nerves					
Number/symmetry	Single trunk	Few nerves, asymmetrical involvement	Several nerves, asymmetrical involvement	Several nerves, almost symmetrical involvement	***Several nerves, symmetrical involvement***
Character of nerve involvement	Early involvement. Related to lesion, may be nodular	Thickened, with anaesthesia in distribution of nerve	Thickened	Glove and stocking anaesthesia	Late involvement. Glove and stocking anaesthesia
Reactions	Stable	Type I	Type I	Type I/Type II	Type II
Lepromin	+	+/–	–	–	–
Histology					
Granuloma	Well-defined (compact), epithelioid cell granuloma	Epithelioid cell granuloma	Ill-defined macrophage granuloma	Ill-defined macrophage granuloma with many lymphocytes	Ill-defined (loose), foamy macrophage granuloma
Gernz zone	–	+	++	++	++
AFB	–	–	+/–	+	++

80. Ans. a. Increase GDP...

[Ref: http://www.mohfw.nic.in/showfile.php?lid=3014; www.mohfw.nic.in/showfile.php?lid=3014*]*

"The Union Ministry of Health and Family Welfare has suggested ***making health a fundamental right***, similar to education. ***This key proposal in the draft National Health Policy, 2015***, suggests making denial of health an offence"-*the hindu paper*

"The **National Health Policy** accepts and endorses the understanding that a full achievement of the goals and principles as defined would require an increased ***public health expenditure to 4 to 5% of the GDP***. However, given that the NHP, 2002 target of 2% was not met, and taking into account the financial capacity of the country to provide this amount and the institutional capacity to utilize the increased funding in an effective manner, this **policy proposes** a potentially achievable target of ***raising public health expenditure to 2.5 % of the GDP***. It also notes that 40% of this would need to come from Central expenditures. At current prices, a target of 2.5% of GDP translates to Rs. 3800 per capita, representing an almost four fold increase in five years. Thus a longer time frame may be appropriate to even reach this modest target"-*www.mohfw.nic.in*

National Health Policy 2015 Draft: Objectives

1. Improve population health status through concerted policy action in all sectors and expand preventive, promotive, curative, palliative and rehabilitative services provided by the public health sector.
2. Achieve a significant reduction in out of pocket expenditure due to health care costs and reduction in proportion of households experiencing catastrophic health expenditures and consequent impoverishment.
3. Assure universal availability of free, comprehensive primary health care services, as an entitlement, for all ***aspects of reproductive, maternal, child and adolescent health*** and for the most prevalent communicable and non-communicable diseases in the population.
4. *Enable universal access to free essential drugs*, diagnostics, emergency ambulance services, and emergency medical and surgical care services in public health facilities, so as to enhance the financial protection role of public facilities for all sections of the population.
5. Ensure improved access and affordability of secondary and tertiary care services through a combination of public hospitals and ***strategic purchasing of services from the private health sector***.

6. ***Influence the growth of the private health care industry*** and medical technologies to ensure alignment with public health goals, and enable contribution to making health care systems more effective, efficient, rational, safe, affordable and ethical.

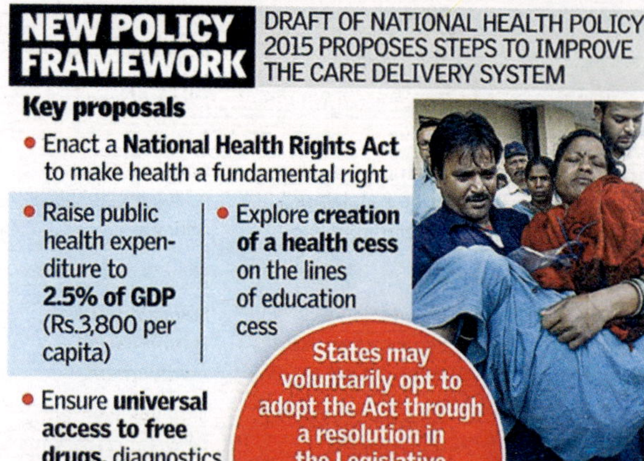

Fig: *(Newspaper):* Draft of national health policy

National Health Policy 2015 Draft: Goals & Principles

- **Goal**: The attainment of the highest possible level of good health and well-being, through a preventive and promotive health care orientation in all developmental policies, and universal access to good quality health care services without anyone having to face financial hardship as a consequence.
- **Key policy principles**:
  - **Equity:** Public expenditure in health care, prioritizing the needs of the most vulnerable, who suffer the largest burden of disease, would imply greater investment in access and financial protection measures for the poor. Reducing inequity would also mean affirmative action to reach the poorest and minimizing disparity on account of gender, poverty, caste, disability, other forms of social exclusion and geographical barriers.
  - **Universality:** Systems and services are designed to ***cater to the entire population***- not only a targeted sub-group. Care to be taken to prevent exclusions on social or economic grounds. Patient Centered & Quality of Care: Health Care services would be effective, safe, and convenient, provided with dignity and confidentiality with all facilities across all sectors being assessed, certified and incentivized to maintain quality of care.
  - **Inclusive Partnerships**: The task of providing health care for ***all cannot be undertaken by Government, acting alone***. It would also require the ***participation of communities*** – who view this participation as a means and a goal, as a right and as a duty. It would also require the widest level of partnerships with academic institutions, not for profit agencies and with the ***commercial private sector and health care industry to achieve these goals.***
  - **Pluralism:** Patients who so choose and when appropriate, would have access to AYUSH care providers based on validated local health traditions.
  - **Accountability:** Financial and performance accountability, transparency in decision making, and elimination of corruption in health care systems, both in the public systems and in the private health care industry, would be essential.
  - **Professionalism, Integrity and Ethics**: Health workers and managers shall perform their work with the highest level of professionalism, integrity and trust and be supported by a systems and regulatory environment that enables this.
  - **Learning and Adaptive System**: constantly improving dynamic organization of health care which is knowledge and evidence based, reflective and learning from the communities they serve, the experience of implementation itself, and from national and international knowledge partners.
  - **Affordability:** As costs of care rise, affordability, as distinct from equity, requires emphasis. Health care costs of a household exceeding 10% of its total monthly consumption expenditures or 40% of its non-food consumption expenditure- is designated catastrophic health expenditures- and is declared as an unacceptable level of health care costs. Impoverishment due to health care costs is of course, even more unacceptable.

OPHTHALMOLOGY

81. Ans. e. B12

[Ref: Harrison 19th/197 www.medmerits.com/index.php; http://doctors-junction.blogspot.in]

"**Centrocecal or cecocentral scotoma**: Field defect involving both the macula and the blind spot; seen in optic nerve disease, such as Leber's hereditary optic neuropathy, toxic or ***nutritional optic neuropathies*** (said to be typical of ***vitamin B12 deficiency optic neuropathy***), sometimes in optic neuritis" *(doctorsjunction.blogspot.in)*

Ophthalmologic Manifestations

◈ *www.medmerits.com/index*

- An unusual but well-documented manifestation of ***cobalamin deficiency is optic neuropathy***. This may present as a subacutely progressive decrease in visual acuity with a ***cecocentral scotoma*** (i.e., a scotoma obscuring central vision and enlarging the blind spot).
- The condition known as tobacco-ethanol amblyopia is similar, and may, at least in part, depend on cobalamin deficiency.

"Damage to papillomacular fibers causes a **cecocentral scotoma** that encompasses the blind spot and macula. If the damage is irreversible, pallor eventually appears in the temporal portion of the optic disc. Temporal pallor from a **cecocentral scotoma** may develop in optic neuritis, ***nutritional optic neuropathy***, toxic optic neuropathy, Leber's hereditary optic neuropathy, and compressive optic neuropathy" *(Harrison 19th/197)*

82. Ans. a. a wave- arises..., b. b wave - d/t..., c. b-wave... d. c wave - representing....

[Ref: A.K.Khurana 6th/518-19; Parson 22nd/109-10]

"Electrophysiology is an essential adjunct in distinguishing macular diseases and generalized retinal dysfunction . For example, **Best disease** and adult onset vitelliform macular dystrophy, both characterized by a similar fundus appearance and ***normal electroretinogram (ERG), can be distinguished by the electro-oculogram (EOG).*** We present a patient with vitelliform lesions in the macula and unexpected ERG results"- www.ncbi.nlm.nih.gov

Electroretinogram

◈ *A.K.Khurana 6th/518-19*

- ***Normal record of ERG*** consists of the following waves
  - *a-wave.* It is a negative wave possibly arising from the ***rods and cones.***
  - *b-wave.* It is a large positive wave which is generated by Muller cells, but represents the ***activity of the bipolar cells***
  - *c-wave.* It is also a positive wave representing ***metabolic activity of pigment epithelium.***
- Both scotopic and photopic responses can be elicited in ERG. Foveal ERG can provide information about the macula.
- ***Uses***: ERG is very useful in detecting functional abnormalities of the ***outer retina*** (up to bipolar cell layer), much before the ophthalmoscopic signs appear. However, ERG is normal in diseases involving ganglion cells and the higher visual pathway, such as ***optic atrophy.***
- ***Clinical applications of ERG***
  - Diagnosis and prognosis of retinal disorders such as retinitis pigmentosa, Leber's congenital amaurosis, retinal ischaemia and other chorioretinal degenerations.
  - To assess retinal function when fundus examination is not possible, e.g., in the presence of dense cataract and corneal opacity.
  - To assess the retinal function of the babies where possibilities of impaired vision is considered.
- ***Abnormal ERG response.*** It is graded as follows:
  - *Subnormal response.* ***b-wave response is subnormal in early cases of retinitis pigmentosa*** even before the appearance of ophthalmoscopic signs. A subnormal ERG indicates that a large area of retina is not functioning.
  - *Extinguished response* is seen when there is complete failure of rods and cones function e.g., advanced retinitis pigmentosa, complete retinal detachment, central retinal artery occlusion and advanced siderosis.
  - *A negative response* indicates gross disturbances of the retinal circulation.

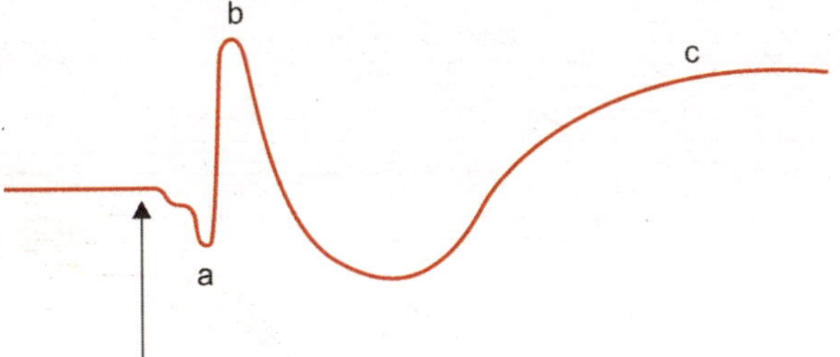

Fig: *(A.K.Khurana 6th/519):* Components of normal electroretinogram (ERG)

"The **EOG** indirectly measures the standing potential of the eye. A normal light peak/dark trough ratio (Arden ratio) is greater than 1.8. In **Best vitelliform macular dystrophy**, the EOG is abnormal with a reduced light peak/dark trough ratio almost always less than 1.5, typically between 1.0 and 1.3. The Arden ratio stays constant with age for these individuals"

83. Ans. a. It forms aqueous...., c. Ciliary processes..., d. Ciliary muscles....

[Ref: A.K.Khurana 6th/147-48; Parson 22nd/8-9]

Ciliary Body

◈ *A.K.Khurana 6th/147-48*

- Ciliary body is forward continuation of the choroid at ora serrata. In cut-section, it is *triangular in shape.*
- The inner side of the triangle is divided into two parts: The **anterior part** (about 2 mm) having finger-like ciliary processes is called ***pars plicata*** and the **posterior *smooth part*** (about 4 mm) is called ***pars plana***
- ***Microscopic structure***: From without inwards ciliary body consists of following **five layers:**
  - ***Supraciliary lamina***: It is the outermost condensed part of the stroma and consists of pigmented collagen fibres.
  - ***Stroma of the ciliary body.*** It consists of connective tissue of collagen and fibroblasts. Embedded in the stroma are ciliary muscle, vessels, nerves, pigment and other cells.*Ciliary muscle* occupies most of the outer part of ciliary body. Ciliary muscle is supplied by parasympathetic fibres through the short ciliary nerves.
  - ***Layer of pigmented epithelium.*** It is the forward continuation of the retinal pigment epithelium.
  - ***Layer of non-pigmented epithelium.***
  - ***Internal limiting membrane.***
- ***Ciliary processes***: These are finger-like projections from the pars plicata part of the ciliary body. These are about 70-80 in number. Each process is about2-mm long and 0.5-mm in diameter. These are white in color.
- *Structure:* Each process is lined by two layers of epithelial cells. The core of the ciliary process contains blood vessels and loose connective tissue. These processes are the site of aqueous production.
- ***Functions of ciliary body.*** (i) ***Formation of aqueous humour.*** (ii) ***Ciliary muscles help in accommodation.***

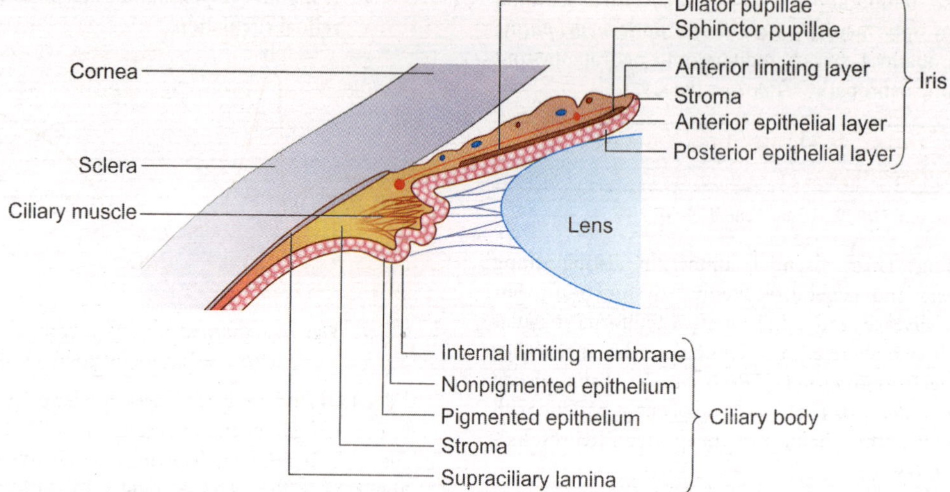

Fig: *(A.K.Khurana 6th/147):* Microscopic structure of the iris and ciliary body

84. Ans. a. Done for as..., b. Positive test-1..., c. Negative...

[Ref: A.K.Khurana 6th/392; Parson 22nd/478]

Jones Dye Tests

◈ *A.K.Khurana 6th/392*

- These are performed ***when partial obstruction is suspected.*** Jones dye tests are of ***no value in the presence of total obstruction.***
- **Jones primary test (Jones test I):** It is performed to *differentiate between watering due to partial obstruction of the lacrimal passages from that due to primary hypersecretion of tears.* Two drops of 2 percent fluorescein dye are instilled in the conjunctival sac and a cotton bud dipped in 1 percent xylocaine is placed in the inferior meatus at the opening of nasolacrimal duct. After 5 minutes the cotton bud is removed and inspected. A **dye-stained cotton bud** indicates ***adequate drainage*** through the lacrimal passages and the cause of watering is primary hypersecretion (further investigations should aim at finding the cause of primary hypersecretion). While the **unstained cotton bud** (negative test) indicates either a ***partial obstruction or failure of lacrimal pump mechanism.*** To differentiate between these conditions, Jones dye test-II is performed.
- **Jones secondary test (Jones test II):** When primary test is negative, the cotton bud is again placed in the inferior meatus and lacrimal syringing is performed. A **positive test** suggests that dye was present in the sac but could not reach the nose due to partial obstruction. A **negative test** indicates presence of ***lacrimal pump failure.***

85. Ans. a. Deposition..., c. Found in Wilson..., d. Deposition under...

[Ref: A.K.Khurana 6th/434; Parson 22nd/220]

"**Kayser-Fleischer ring:** It is a golden brown ring which occurs due to ***deposition of copper*** under peripheral parts of the Descemet's membrane of the cornea" *(A.K.Khurana 6th/434)*

86. Ans. a. Homocys..., d. Marfan..., e. Sulphite oxidase....

[Ref: A.K.Khurana 6th/215-16; Parson 22nd/275]

Ectopia Lentis with Systemic Anomalies

◈ *A.K.Khurana 6th/215-16*

1. ***Marfan's syndrome:*** In this condition lens is displaced upwards and temporally (bilaterally symmetrical)
2. ***Homocystinuria.*** It is an autosomal recessive, inborn error of metabolism. In it the lens is usually subluxated downwards and nasally.
3. ***Weil-Marchesani syndrome:*** *Ocular features* are spherophakia, and forward subluxation of lens which may cause pupil block glaucoma.
4. ***Ehlers-Danlos syndrome.*** In it the *ocular features* are subluxation of lens and blue sclera.
5. ***Hyperlysinaemia:*** It is an extremely rare condition occasionally associated with ectopia lentis.
6. ***Stickler syndrome.*** Ectopia lentis is occasionally associated in this condition
7. ***Sulphite oxidase deficiency:*** Ectopia lentis is a universal *ocular feature*

Table: Ectopia Lentis

Congenital lesion with Systemic anomalies	Spontaneous
• Marfan's syndrome (displaced upwards and temporally) [Q]	• Hypermature cataract
• ***Homocystinuria (subluxated downwards and nasally)*** [Q]	• Buphthalmos
• ***Weil-Marchesani syndrome (forward subluxation)*** [Q]	• High myopia
• ***Ehler ' Danlos syndrome (subluxation of lens and blue sclera)*** [Q]	• Staphyloma
• Hyperlysinaemia	• Intra-ocular tumors
• Stickler syndrome	• Uveitis .
• ***Sulphite oxidase deficiency***	

87. Ans. a. Amblyopia..., b. Angle of deviation..., e. May be associated....

[Ref: A.K.Khurana 6th/348; Parson 22nd/ 428-29; Kanski 5th/ 543]

Infantile Esotropia (Previously Called Congenital Esotropia)

◈ *A.K.Khurana 6th/348*

- Age of onset, is usually 1-2 months of age, but occur any time in first 6 months of life.
- **Angle of deviation is usually constant & fairly large (> 30°),**
- **Fixation pattern:** Binocular vision does not develop & there is alternate fixation in primary gaze and crossed fixation in lateral gaze.
- Amblyopia develops in 25-40% of cases
- Associations include ***inferior oblique overaction*** (usually developing after 1 year of age), dissociated vertical deviation (DVD) in about 70-90% cases & latent horizontal nystagmus
- **Treatment:** Surgery is treatment of choice
    - **Time of surgery:** Surgery should be *done b/w 6 months to 2 years* (preferably before 1 yr of age)
    - Amblyopia treatment by patching the normal eye should always be done before performing the surgery
    - Recession of both medial recti is preferred over unilateral recess-resect procedure

ENT

88. Ans. a. Rinne test is negative..., c. Lateralization of sound...., d. Negative Rinne...

[Ref: P.L.Dhingra 6th/22; L & T 10th/247-48]

Rinne Test

◈ *P.L.Dhingra 6th/22*

- *A negative test(BC>AC) is seen in conductive deafness. A negative Rinne indicates a minimum air-bone gap of* ***15-20 dB***
- *A prediction of air-bone gap can be made if tuning forks of 256, 512 & 1024 Hz are used*
- *A Rinne test equal or negative for 256 Hz but positive for 512 Hz indicates air-bone gap of 20-30 dB*
- *A Rinne test negative for 256 & 512 Hz but positive for 1024 Hz indicates air-bone gap of 30-45 dB*
- **A Rinne negative for all the three tunning forks** *of 256,512 & 1024 Hz indicates air-bone gap of* ***45-60 dB***

Weber Test

◈ *P.L.Dhingra 6th/22*

- *It is* ***lateralized to the worst ear in conductive deafness*** *& to the better ear in sensorineural deafness*
- *Lateralization of sound in Weber test with a tunning fork of 512 Hz implies a conductive loss of 15-20 dB in ipsilateral ear or a sensorineural loss in the contralateral ear*

Table *(P.L.Dhingra 6th/22)*: **Tuning Fork Tests & Their Interpretation**

Test	Normal	Conductive deafness	SN deafness
Rinne	*AC>BC (Rinne positive)*	*BC>AC (Rinne negative)*	*AC>BC*
Weber	*Not lateralized*	*Lateralized to poorer ear*	*Lateralized to better ear*
ABC	*Same as examiner's*	*Same asexaminer's*	*Reduced*
Schwabach	*Equal*	*Lengthened*	*Shortened*

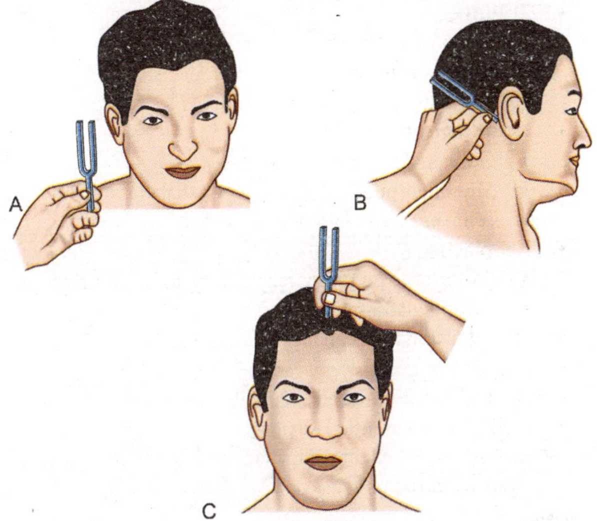

Fig: *(P.L.Dingra 6th/22):* Tuning fork test. (A) Testing for air conduction. (B) Testing for bone conduction. (C) Weber test

89. Ans. a. Bell palsy..., b. Parotid tu..., c. Guillain-Barré....

[Ref: P.L.Dhingra 6th/94-96; L & T 10th/356-60 BDC 4th/Vol.III 54; Harrison 19th/2577]

"**Facial paralysis** occur in occlusion of ***anterior inferior cerebellar artery*** (lateral inferior pontine syndrome *(Harrison 19th/2577)*

"**Bell's palsy:** It is *the* ***most common cause of acute LMN facial palsy***"

Facial Paralysis

◈ *patient.info/in/doctor*

In an LMN lesion, the patient can't wrinkle their forehead - the final common pathway to the muscles is destroyed. The lesion must be ***either in the pons, or outside the brainstem*** (posterior fossa, bony canal, middle ear or outside skull).

Aetiology

LMN

- Idiopathic (Bell's palsy):
    - Pregnancy - 3x more common.
    - Diabetes mellitus.

- Cerebrovascular disease (e.g., brainstem stroke).
- **Iatrogenic:**
  - Local anaesthetic for dental treatment.
  - Linezolid
- **Infective:**
  - Herpesvirus (type 1)
  - Herpes zoster (Ramsay Hunt syndrome) - see below.
  - HIV
  - Epstein-Barr virus.
  - Cytomegalovirus.
  - Lyme disease (more likely if bilateral when responsible for 36% of cases)
  - Otitis media or cholesteatoma
- **Trauma:**
  - Fractures of the skull base.
  - Forceps delivery
  - Haematoma after acupuncture
- **Neurological:**
  - Guillain-Barré syndrome.
  - Mononeuropathy- ***e.g.,*** due to diabetes mellitus, sarcoidosis or amyloidosis.
- **Neoplastic:**
  - Posterior fossa tumours, primary and secondary.
  - Parotid gland tumours.
- Hypertension in pregnancy and eclampsia.
- Sarcoidosis
- Sjögren's syndrome and rheumatoid arthritis
- Melkersson-Rosenthal syndrome (recurrent facial palsy, chronic facial oedema of the face and lips, and hypertrophy/fissuring of the tongue)

UMN

- Cerebrovascular disease.
- Intracranial tumours, primary and secondary.
- Multiple sclerosis.
- Syphilis.
- HIV
- Vasculitides

90. Ans. b. As type in..., c. Dome shaped..., d. Ad type in..., e. C type in eusta....

[Ref: P.L.Dhingra 6th/25; L & T 10th/ 251]

A — Normal

As — Reduced compliance at ambient pressure (otosclerosis). 's' stands for shallow tympanogram but remember for stiffness.

AD — Increased compliance at ambient pressure (ossicular discontinuity). 'd' stands for deep tympanogram. Remember disruption of ossicular chain.

B — Flat or dome-shaped (fluid in middle ear).

C — Maximum compliance at pressures more than –200 mm H_2O (negative pressure in middle ear), e.g. eustachian tube obstruction or early stage of otitis media with effusion.

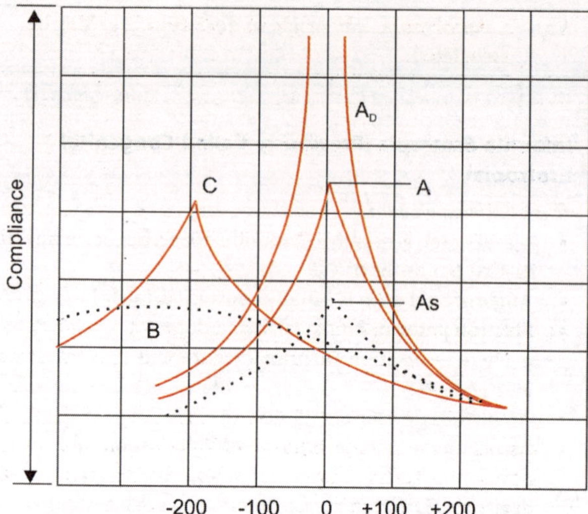

Fig: *(P.L.Dhingra 6th/25)*: Types of tympanograms

91. Ans. a. Voice..., b. Stridor..., d. Urgent tracheo...

[Ref: P.L.Dhingra 6th/300; Logan & Turner 10th/182-83]

Bilateral Abductor Paralysis

◈ *P.L.Dhingra 6th/300*

- *As both the cords lie in median or paramedian position, the airway is inadequate causing dyspnea & stridor but the voice is good*
- ***Tracheostomy:*** *Many cases require tracheostomy as an emergency procedure or when they develop upper respiratory tract infection*
- *Transverse cordotomy*
- *Partial arytenoidectomy*
- *Reinnervation procedures*
- *Thyroplasty II*

"Woodman's operation *(External arytenoidectomy) is done in* ***b/l abductor paralysis*** *(Logan & Turner 10th/183)*

"Endoscopic laser arytenoidectomy & Isshiki type II thyroplasty *is done for* ***lateralization of cord (in bilateral abductor paralysis)"*** *(Dhingra 5th/318-19, 362)*

92. Ans. c. Anterior superior....

[Ref: P.L. Dhingra 6th/185-86; 5th/199-200; L & B 25th/331-32; CSDT 11th/1256; Washington Manual of Surgery 5th/481; Sabiston 18th/494-95, 2143]

"The ***condylar neck*** is the ***weakest part of the mandible*** and is the ***most frequent site of fracture"*** *(L & B 25th/331)*

"Many patients with mandibular fractures experience trauma to the ***inferior alveolar nerve*** (a branch of the trigeminal nerve), which runs through a canal within the body of the mandible and terminates in the lower lip as the mental nerve. These patients may experience permanent numbness of the lower lip and teeth on the affected side. Fractures of the coronoid process of the mandible can result in ***trismus*** (inability to open the mouth) because the coronoid process normally passes beneath the zygomatic arch with mouth opening" *(Sabiston 18th/2143)*

Fracture of Mandible

◈ *P.L. Dhingra 6th/185-86*

- ***Condylar fractures are the most common:*** They are followed in frequency, by fracture of angle, body & symphysis (Mnemonics CABS). Fractures of the ramus, coronoid & alveolar processes are uncommon.
- In fracture of condyle, if fragments are not displaced, pain & trismus are the main features & tenderness is elicited at the site of fracture. If fragments are displaced, there is in addition, ***malocclusion of teeth*** & deviation of jaw to the opposite side on opening the mouth.
- X-rays useful in mandibular fractures are PA view of the skull (for condyle), right & left oblique view of mandible & ***panorex view***
- Both closed & open methods are used for reduction & fixation of the mandibular fractures

Fracture of Mandible

◈ *Washington Manual of Surgery 5th/481*

- ***Panorex radiographs*** are usually ***sufficient to diagnose mandible fracture*** & visualize postreduction
- Mandibualr fractures are not surgical emergencies & should be addressed after stabilization of patient. Fixation within 3 days has been shown to be result in more favourable outcome
- Complications includes *wound infection, malocculusion,* ***non-union,*** *tooth loss, temporomandibular joint ankylosis & paresthesis*

Fracture of Mandible

◈ *Sabiston 18th/494-95*

- Imaging techniques frequently used to identify and classify mandibular fractures include plain films, ***panoramic tomography (Panorex),*** and helical CT. A recent report has demonstrated the overall superiority of ***helical CT over Panorex*** in identifying and decreasing interpretation error in patients with mandibular fractures
- ***Reduction and fixation of mandibular fractures*** should be accomplished as precisely and expeditiously as possible because malocclusion is a major long-term complication.
- Condylar and subcondylar mandible fractures are most often treated by IMF alone. Surgical exposure of the temporomandibular joint places the facial nerve at risk and exposes the joint to possible injury and dysfunction.

Mandibular Fracture: Delayed Union and Nonunion

◈ *emedicine.medscape.com*

- *Delayed union and nonunion occur in approximately 3% of fractures.*
- *Delayed union is a temporary condition in which adequate reduction and immobilization eventually produce bony union.*
- *Nonunion indicates a lack of bony healing between the segments that persists indefinitely without evidence of bone healing unless surgical treatment is undertaken to repair the fracture.*
- *Nonunion is characterized by pain and abnormal mobility following treatment.*
- *Radiographs demonstrate no evidence of healing and in later stages show rounding off of the bone ends.*
- *The most likely cause for delayed union and nonunion is poor reduction and immobilization.*
- *Infection is often an underlying cause. Carefully assess teeth in the line of fractures for possible extraction or they may be a nidus for infection.*

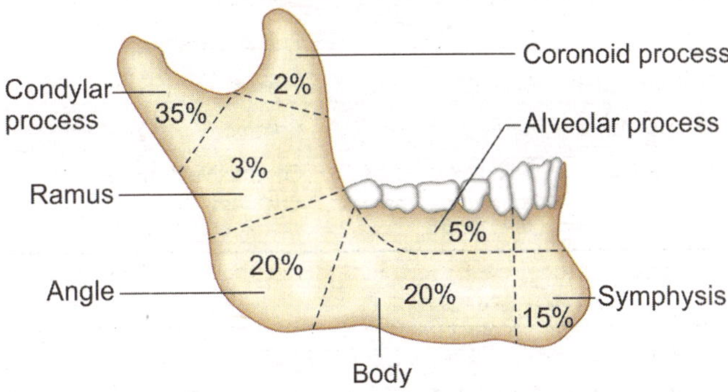

Fig: Fracture of mandible (Dingman's classification). Condylar fracture are the most common, followed by those of angle, body & symphysis of mandible

---

93. Ans. a. Foul smelling..., c. Facial nerve involve..., d. May cause hearing....

[Ref: Dhingra 6th/67-74; 5th/77,4th/68; L & T 10th/283-88]

CSOM

◈ *Dhingra 6th/67-74*

- Atticoantral variety: Facial weakness indicates erosion of facial canal *(Dhingra 6th/73)*
- Fallopian canal containing the facial nerve is at risk of erosion in Atticoantral variety *(L & T 10th/287)*

Cholesteatoma is commonly a/w atticontral or unsafe of CSOM

Cholesteatoma

- *Cholesteatoma,* stratified squamous epithelium in the middle ear or mastoid, occurs frequently in adults. This is a benign, slowly growing lesion that destroys bone and normal ear tissue.
- Theories of pathogenesis include traumatic implantation and invasion, immigration and invasion through a perforation, and metaplasia following chronic infection and irritation.
- On examination, there is often a perforation of the tympanic membrane filled with ***cheesy white squamous debris.*** A chronically draining ear that fails to respond to appropriate antibiotic therapy should raise suspicion of a cholesteatoma.
- *Conductive hearing loss* secondary to ossicular erosion is common. Surgery is required to remove this destructive process.

Table *(Dhingra 6th/69, 5th/77)*: **Differences b/w Atticoantral and Tubotympanic type of CSOM**

Feature	Tubotympanic or Safe type	Atticoantral or Unsafe type
Discharge	Profuse, mucoid	Scanty, purulent, foul-smelling
Perforation	Central	Attic or marginal
Granulations	Uncommon	Common
Polyp	Pale	Red and fleshy
Cholesteatoma	Absent	Present
Complications	Rare	Common
Audiogram	Mild to moderate conductive deafness	Conductive or mixed deafness

94. Ans. a. Mucous..., b. Seen in floor..., c. Marsupialization..., e. Arises from....

[Ref: P.L.Dhingra 6th/224-25; L & T 10th/127]

Ranula

◈ *P.L.Dhingra 6th/224*

- *It is cystic translucent lesion **seen in the floor of mouth** on one side of frenulum & pushing the tongue tip*
- *It arises from the **sublingual salivary gland** due to obstruction of its duct*
- *It can be either simple or cavernous. The simple variety is a true retention cyst of one of the **minor salivary glands** (L & T 10th/127)*
- *Some ranulae extend into the **neck(plunging type)***
- *"Plunging ranula presents as a neck selling in submandibular region as the cyst extends into the neck posterior to the mylohyoid muscle" (ENT by Hazarika 4th/712)*
- **Treatment** *is **complete surgical excision if small or marsupialization, if large**. Often it is not possible to excise the ranual completely because of its thin wall or ramifications in various tissue planes*

95. Ans. d. Apthus ulcer....

[Ref: Dhingra 6th/224-25,5th/238,233; Logan & Turner 10th /126]

Premalignant Lesion for Oral Cavity Cancer

◈ *Dhingra 6th/224-25, 5th/238,233*

- ***Leukoplakia*** ("white patch") is induced by the same factors (tobacco, alcohol) that cause carcinomas. The ***malignant potential of leukoplakia corresponds to the degree of cellular dysplasia seen on biopsy.***
- ***Erythroplakia*** ("red patch") usually shows severe cellular dysplasia and carries a ***50% risk of malignant degeneration***
- ***Melanosis & mucosal hyperpigmentation:*** *may transform into malignant melanoma*

Premalignant Conditions Associated with Oral Cancer

◈ *L & B 25th/735*

High Risk Lesions

- ***Erythroplakia***
- ***Speckled erythroplakia***
- ***Chronic hyperplastic candidiasis***

Medium Risk Lesions

- ***Oral submucous fibrosis***
- ***Syphilitic glossitis***
- ***Sideropenic dysphagia (Paterson-Kelly syndrome)***

Low Risk Lesions

- ***Oral lichen planus***
- ***Discoid lupus erythematous***
- ***Discoid keratosis congenita***

"**Aphthous ulcer:** It is a ***benign disease with unknown etiology***" *(Logan & Turner 10th /125)*

"**Ca oral tongue: It may also develop on a *pre-existing leukoplakia*, long standing dental ulcer or syphilitic glossitis. Vast majority are squamous cell type**" *(Dhingra 5th/ 240)*

"**Lichen planus: It has *no malignant potential***" *(Logan & Turner 10th /126)*

"*Chronic ulcerative* **Lichen planus of oral mucosa can undergo *malignant change(but this is decidedly rare!)***" *(Neena Khanna 3rd/54)*

"**Papillomas** *occur most usually on the soft palate, anterior pillar & buccal mucosa.* **They have *no malignant potential***" *(Logan & Turner 10th /126)*

"**Fordyce's spot** are aberrant sebaceous glands present under the buccal or labial mucosa & are ***considered normal***" *(Dhingra 5th/233)*

"**Keratoacanthoma (KA)** is a common low grade (unlikely to metastasize or invade) ***skin cancer*** that is believed to originate from the neck of the hair follicle. Many pathologists consider it to be a form of ***squamous cell carcinoma*** (SCC). KA is commonly found on sun exposed skin, and often is seen on the ***face, forearms and hands***" *(Neena Khanna 3rd/309)*

MEDICINE

96. Ans. c. Detection of both rif...

[Ref: www.cdc.gov/tb/topic/laboratory; www.tbcontrollers.org: www.slideshare.ne]

What Tests are Being used for Molecular Detection of Drug Resistance

- **Laboratory developed tests (LDT)** – (1) DNA sequencing & (2) Real-time PCR assays
- **Non-FDA approved tests** (Research Use Only [RUO]) -(1) ***Genotype® MTBDRplus*** and ***MTBDRsl- Hain Lifescience*** (2)Cepheid GeneXpert® Xpert MTB/RIF

"**Genotype MTBDR plus ("HAIN test") qNAA** and hybridization-based test use immobilized DNA probes on nitrocellulose membranes (line probe assay [LPA]) & Colorimetric change indicates hybridization & "Read" the bands to determine MTBC or not and to ***detect resistance-associated mutations for RMP and INH***" *(www.tbcontrollers.org)*

"Comparison of Xpert MTB/RIF with Line Probe Assay for Detection of Rifampin monoresistant ***M. tuberculosis***"

"The **MTBDR *plus* line probe assay (LPA)** and Xpert MTB/RIF have been endorsed by the World Health Organization for the rapid diagnosis of ***drug-resistant tuberculosis***. However, there is no clarity regarding the superiority of one over the other"

HAINs test: MTB DR plus: Line probe assay

- Based on PCR line probe assay
- Identifies M.tuberculosis and detects Rif & INH resistance in a day

Fig: *(www.slideshare.ne)*: Hain Test

Background on Molecular Drug-Resistance (DR) Tests

◈ *www.cdc.gov/tb/topic/laboratory*

- Recent advances in the understanding of the molecular basis or genetics of drug resistance have enabled development of rapid, DNA-based, molecular tests to ***detect mutations associated with drug resistance.***
- For hybridization assays such as the INNO-LiPA® Rif. TB (Innogenetics) and GenoType® MTBDR(*plus*) **(Hain LifeScience GmbH) line-probe assays,** the region of a gene associated with resistance is PCR amplified, and the labeled PCR products hybridized to oligonucleotide probes immobilized on a nitrocellulose strip. Mutations are detected by lack of binding to wild-type probes or by binding to probes specific for commonly occurring mutations.
- Compared to culture-based DS tests, the MTBDR(*plus*) line probe assay displays a pooled sensitivity of 0.98 and a pooled specificity of 0.99 for detecting ***rifampin resistance in isolates or directly from clinical specimens***

Hain/Line Probe Assays

◈ *www.tbcontrollers.org*

Advantages

- Works on processed specimens
- Rapid Assay
- Improved instrumentation for analysis and documentation of results
- Used in laboratories now

Disadvantages

- Multiple beacons needed to cover overlapping regions
- Silent mutations may result in false predication of resistance
- Not customizable by user

97. Ans. a. Measures right..., b. Measures left ventricular..., c. Measure..., d. Inserted through...,

[Ref: Harrison 19th/ 1607; Davidson 22nd/ 185-86; Manipal Surgery 4th/176; lifeinthefastlane.com]

USES of Swan-Ganz Catheter

◈ *lifeinthefastlane.com*

- ***Continuous cardiac output monitoring***
- *Central temperature monitoring*
- ***Measurement of pulmonary artery pressure** (can also* ***measure RA and RV pressures during insertion)***
- *Measurement of **mixed venous saturations***
- *Estimation of **diastolic filling of left heart** (normal PCWP 2-12mmHg)*

Use of Pulmonary Artery Catheterization

◈ *emedicine.medscape.com*

- Important information provided by a PAC catheter includes the ***PCWP, assessment of left ventricular (LV) filling pressure, CO, mixed venous oxygen saturation (SaO_2), and oxygen saturations*** in the right heart chambers to assess for the presence of an intracardiac shunt.
- Using these measurements, other variables can be derived, including pulmonary or systemic vascular resistance and the difference between arterial and venous oxygen content (see images below). Obtaining ***CO and PCWP measurements*** is the primary reason for inserting most PACs; therefore, understanding how they are obtained and what factors alter their values is of prime importance.

Pulmonary Artery Catheterisation and Pulmonary Artery 'Wedge' Pressure

◈ *Davidson 22nd/ 185-86*

- The CVP is usually an adequate guide to the filling pressures of both sides of the heart. However, certain conditions, such as pulmonary hypertension or right ventricular dysfunction, may lead to raised CVP levels even in the presence of hypovolaemia. In these circumstances, it may be appropriate to insert a ***pulmonary artery flotation catheter*** so that ***pulmonary artery pressure and pulmonary artery 'wedge' pressure (PAWP),*** which approximates to ***left atrial pressure,*** can be measured.
- **Pulmonary artery catheters** also allow ***measurement of cardiac output and sampling of blood from the pulmonary artery ('mixed venous' samples), permitting continuous monitoring of the mixed venous oxygen saturation (SvO2) by oximetry.*** Measurement of *Sv*O2 gives an indication of the adequacy of cardiac output (and hence *D*O2) in relation to the body's metabolic requirements. It is especially useful in low cardiac output states.

Hemodynamic Assessment

◈ *Harrison 19th/ 1607*

- Positioning of a balloon flotation **(Swan-Ganz) catheter** in the pulmonary artery ***permits monitoring of LV filling pressure***; this technique is useful in patients who exhibit hypotension and/or clinical evidence of CHF.
- ***Cardiac output can also be determined with a pulmonary artery catheter. With the addition of intra-arterial pressure monitoring, systemic vascular resistance can be calculated*** as a guide to adjusting vasopressor and vasodilator therapy.

Pulmonary Artery Catheterization

◈ *Harrison 19th/ 1760*

- The use of **pulmonary artery (Swan-Ganz)** catheters in patients with established or suspected cardiogenic shock(CS) is controversial. Their use is generally recommended for ***measurement of filling pressures and cardiac output*** to confirm the diagnosis and to optimize the use of IV fluids, inotropic agents, and vasopressors in persistent shock.

Pulmonary Artery Catheterization

◈ *emedicine.medscape.com*

The PAC is inserted percutaneously into a major vein (***jugular, subclavian, femoral***) via an introducer sheath.

- **Right internal jugular vein** (RIJ): Shortest and straightest path to the heart
- **Left subclavian**: Does not require the PAC to pass and course at an acute angle to enter the SVC (compared to the right subclavian or left internal jugular
- **Femoral veins**: These access points are distant sites, from which passing a PAC into the heart can be difficult, especially if the right-sided cardiac chambers are enlarged. Often, fluoroscopic assistance is necessary. Nevertheless, these sites are compressible and may be preferable if the risk of hemorrhage is high.

Swan-Ganz Catheterization

◈ *www.healthline.com*

- A Swan-Ganz catheterization is a type of pulmonary artery catheterization procedure.
- The procedure involves the insertion of a pulmonary artery catheter (PAC), also known as a Swan-Ganz catheter or right heart catheter, into the right side of the heart and into the arteries that lead to the lungs.
- The procedure itself is sometimes called "right heart catheterization." This is because it can measure the pressure of blood as it flows through the right side of your heart. It measures the pressure at three different places: ***right atrium, pulmonary artery, and pulmonary capillaries***.

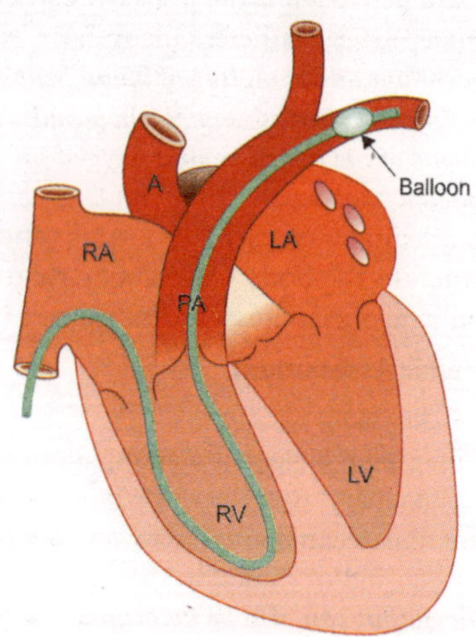

98. Ans. a. Lancinating..., b. Loss of proprio...., c. Sensory..., | e. Sensory ataxia...

[Ref: Harrison 19th/2659;P J Mehta 20th/371-73]

Tabes Dorsalis

◈ *Harrison 19th/2659*

- The classic syphilitic syndromes of tabes dorsalis and meningovascular inflammation of the spinal cord are now less frequent than in the past but must be considered in the differential diagnosis of spinal cord disorders.
- The characteristic symptoms of tabes are ***fleeting and repetitive lancinating pains, primarily in the legs*** or less often in the back, thorax, abdomen, arms, and face. ***Ataxia of the legs and gait due to loss of position sense occurs in half of patients.***
- ***Paresthesias, bladder disturbances, and acute abdominal pain with vomiting*** (visceral crisis) occur in 15–30% of patients.
- The cardinal signs of tabes are loss of reflexes in the legs; ***impaired position and vibratory sense***; ***Romberg's sign***; and, in almost all cases, bilateral Argyll Robertson pupils, which fail to constrict to light but accommodate. Diabetic polyradiculopathy may simulate tabes.

99. Ans. a. May present..., c. Smoking..., d. Nitrates are used..., e. CCBs are used for....

[Ref: Harrison 19th/1598;CMDT 2016/363; Braunwald's Heart Diasease 8th/478]

Prinzmetal's Variant Angina (PVA)

◈ *Harrison 19th/1598,CMDT06/347 Braunwald's Heart Diasease 8th/478*

- This syndrome is due to ***focal spasm*** of ***an epicardial coronary*** artery, leading to severe myocardial ischemia. The exact cause of the spasm is not well defined, but it may be related to hypercontractility of vascular smooth muscle due to vasoconstrictor
- The vasospastic process almost always involves large segments of the epicardial vessels at a single site, but at different times other sites may be involved. The ***right coronary artery*** is the most frequent site, followed by the left anterior descending coronary artery
- Patients with ***no or mild fixed coronary obstruction*** tend to experience a more benign course than patients with associated severe obstructive lesions
- When the endothelium is dysfunctional, stimulation with acetylcholine will fail to produce, or produce very little, nitric oxide. Thus, ***acetylcholine released by the parasympathetic system at rest will simply cause contraction of the vascular smooth muscle***. It is potentially by this mechanism that Prinzmetal's angina occurs.
- ***It usually occurs at rest*** and is associated with transient ST-segment elevation.
- Patients with variant angina are generally younger and have fewer coronary risk factors (with the exception of ***cigarette smoking***) than patients with UA secondary to coronary atherosclerosis.
- Many do not exhibit classic coronary risk factors except that they are often heavy cigarette smokers patients with PVA should be urged strongly to stop smoking
- "Attacks of PVA tend to cluster ***between midnight and 8 am***, and sometimes occur in clusters of two or three within 30 to 60 minutes"- *Braunwald's Heart Disease 8th/478*
- ECG finding will more often show ***ST segment elevation than ST depression***. Elevation ST-segment in II, III and aVf.
- ***Nitrates and calcium channel blockers are the main treatments for patients with variant angina. Aspirin may***

actually increase the severity of ischemic episodes, possibly as a result of the sensitivity of coronary tone to modest changes in the synthesis of prostacyclin. The response to beta blockers is variable. Coronary revascularization may be helpful in patients who also have discrete, flow-limiting, proximal fixed obstructive lesions

100. Ans. a. Polyarthritis..., c. Monoarthritis in ...., d. Echocardiography..., e. Echocardiography....

[Ref: http://www.acc.org; http://www.dnbpediatrics.com]

Revision of the Jones Criteria for the Diagnosis of Acute Rheumatic Fever in the Era of Doppler Echocardiography

◈ *http://www.acc.org*

- **Revised Jones criteria, low-risk populations**: Major and minor criteria are as follows:
    - Major criteria: carditis (clinical and/or subclinical), arthritis (polyarthritis), chorea, *Erythema marginatum*, and subcutaneous nodules
    - ***Minor criteria:*** olyarthralgia, fever (≥38.5° F), sedimentation rate ≥60 mm and/or C-reactive protein (CRP) ≥3.0 mg/dl, and prolonged PR interval (unless carditis is a major criterion)
- **Revised Jones criteria, moderate- and high-risk populations**: Major and minor criteria are as follows:
    - **Major criteria:** Carditis (clinical and/or subclinical), arthritis (monoarthritis or polyarthritis, or polyarthralgia), chorea, *Erythema marginatum*, and subcutaneous nodules
    - Minor criteria: fever (≥38.5° F), sedimentation rate ≥30 mm and/or CRP ≥3.0 mg/dl, and prolonged PR interval (unless carditis is a major criterion)
- **ARF diagnosis (initial episode):** The diagnosis of an initial episode of ARF requires two major criteria, or one major plus two minor criteria.

Carditis: Diagnosis in the Era of Widely Available Echocardiography:

- Echocardiography with Doppler should be performed in ***all cases of confirmed and suspected ARF*** (Class I; Level of Evidence B).
- It is reasonable to consider performing serial echocardiography/ Doppler studies in any patient with diagnosed or suspected ARF even if ***documented carditis*** is not present on diagnosis (Class IIa; Level of Evidence C).
- Echocardiography/Doppler testing should be performed to assess whether carditis is present in the ***absence of auscultatory findings***, particularly in ***moderate- to high-risk populations*** and when ARF is considered likely (Class I; Level of Evidence B).
- Echocardiography/Doppler findings not consistent with carditis should exclude that diagnosis in patients with a heart murmur otherwise thought to indicate rheumatic carditis (Class I; Level of Evidence B).

Revision of the Jones Criteria for the Diagnosis of Acute Rheumatic Fever: 2015

- The famous Jones criteria for diagnosis of Acure Rhemaric Fever are recently revised in 2015 by AHA with emphasis on doppler echocardiogarpghy for involvement of heart.
- It is the first substantial revision to the Jones Criteria by the American Heart Association since 1992.
- It is technology driven (ECHO) and focuses on epidemiological differences in high-risk and low-risk populations.
- As per epidemiological data, cases are divided into:
    - Low risk should be defined as having an ARF incidence <2 per 100 000 school-aged children (usually 5–14 years old) per year. Or an allege prevalence of RHD of ≤1 per 1000 population per year.
    - **Children not clearly from a low-risk population are at moderate to high risk depending on their reference population.**

Revised Jones Criteria (2015)

A. Diagnosis

For all patient populations with evidence of preceding GAS infection

Initial ARF-2 Major **or** 1 major plus 2 minor

Recurrent ARF-2 Major **or** 1 major and 2 minor or 3 minor

B. Major Criteria

Low-risk populations	Moderate-and high-risk population
1. Carditis ▪ Clinical and/or subclinical carditis	**1. Carditis** ▪ Clinical and/or subclinical carditis
2. Arthritis ▪ Polyarthritis	**2. Arthritis** ▪ Monoarthritis or polyarthritis ▪ Polyarthralgia
3. Chorea	**3. Chorea**
4. Erythema marginatum	**4. Erythema marginatum**
5. Subcutaneous nodules	**5. Subcutaneous nodules**

C. Minor criteria

Low-risk populations	Moderate-and high-risk populations
1. Polyarthralgia	1. Monoarthralgia
2. Fever (>38.5°)	2. Fever (≥38°C)
3. ESR ≥60 mm in 1st hour and/ or CRP≥3.0 mg/dl	3. ESR ≥30 mm/h and/or CRP ≥3.0 mg/dL
4. Prolonged PR interval, after accounting for age variability (unless carditis is a major criterion) in all population.	

Diagnostic strategy of rheumatic fever

A. Chorea

Clinical → Yes → ARF diagnosed

Clinical → No → Echo doppler - subclinical carditis → Yes → ARF diagnosed

Echo doppler - subclinical carditis → No → Rule out all else → ARF diagnosed

B. Arthritis

Arthritis → Clinical carditis or subclinical carditis on Echo doppler → ARF diagnosis

Arthritis → No carditis and negative Echo doppler → No criteria — Consider at diagnosis

No carditis and negative Echo doppler → Another major criteria or Two minor criteria → ARF diagnosed

C. Carditis

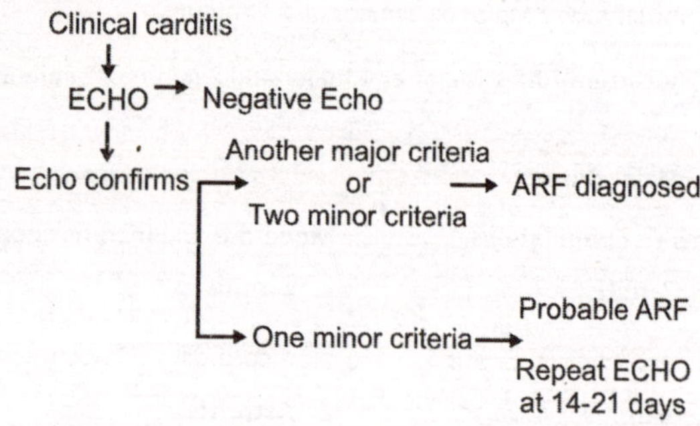

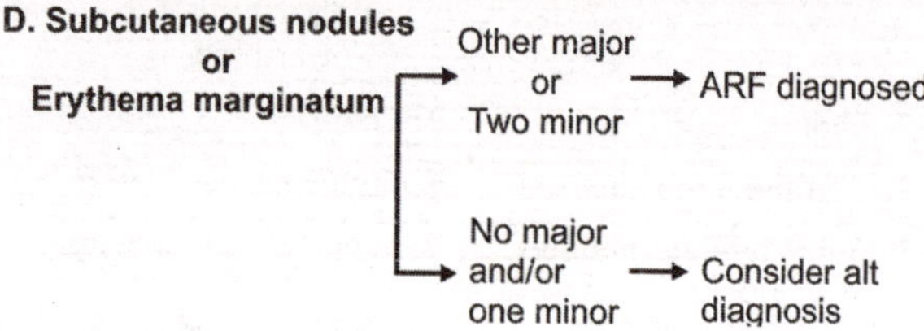

101. Ans. b. Decrease..., d. Hyperte..., e. Decreased....

[Ref: Guyton 11th/213;CSDT 11th/890; Harrison 19th/1778-79;Manipal Surgery 4th/1038]

"**Cushing triad of increased ICP**: ***Bradycardia, hypertension & irregular respiration***" *(Manipal Surgery 4th/1038)*

"**Blood pressure elevation** accompanied by ***bradycardia and respiratory slowing*** classically results from raised intracranial pressure. This "Cushing response," however, usually appears only when intracranial hypertension is severe" *(CSDT 11th/890)*

Features of Increased ICT

Loss of the normal autoregulation of blood pressure and pulse, called the ***Cushing's reflex, is a hallmark of severe brain injury or imminent crisis.*** This generally results in a *sudden rise in blood pressure and a slowing of the pulse.*

Signs of increased ICP include ***decreasing level of consciousness***, paralysis or weakness on one side of the body, and ***a blown pupil, one that fails to constrict in response to light or is slow to do so.***

Cushing's triad, a slow heart rate with high blood pressure and respiratory depression is a classic manifestation of significantly raised ICP.

Anisocoria, unequal pupil size, is another sign of serious traumatic brain injury

Abnormal posturing, a characteristic positioning of the limbs caused by severe diffuse injury or high ICP, is an ominous

Cushing Reaction

- *Guyton 11th/213*
- The so-called *Cushing reaction* is a special type of CNS ischemic response that results from ***increased pressure of the cerebrospinal fluid***[Q] around the brain in the cranial vault. For instance, when the cerebrospinal fluid pressure rises to equal the arterial pressure, it compresses the whole brain as well as the arteries in the brain and cuts off the blood supply to the brain. This initiates a CNS ischemic response that ***causes the arterial pressure to rise. When the arterial pressure has risen to a level higher than the cerebrospinal fluid pressure, blood will flow once again into the vessels of the brain to relieve the brain ischemia.***
- Ordinarily, the blood pressure comes to a new equilibrium level slightly higher than the cerebrospinal fluid pressure, thus allowing blood to begin again to flow through the brain. The ***Cushing reaction*** helps ***protect the vital centers of the brain from loss of nutrition if ever the cerebrospinal fluid pressure raise*** high enough to compress the cerebral arteries.

"Cushing's triad is the ***triad*** of ***widening pulse pressure (rising systolic, declining diastolic), change in respiratory pattern (irregular respirations), and bradycardia.*** It is **sign** of ***increased intracranial pressure***, and it *occurs as a result of the* ***Cushing reflex***" *(wikipedia)*

102. Ans. c. Carrier state..., d. Majority progress....

[Ref: Harrison 19th/2013,2018; Robbins(SAE) 9th/835-36;CMDT 2016/673]

"*Hepatitis A & E **never cause chronic hepatitis** except HEV in immunocompromised hosts & pregnant females*" *(Robbins(SAE) 9th/835)*

"Reported **extrahepatic manifestations** include arthritis, pancreatitis, and a variety of neurologic complications. In endemic regions, the ***mortality rate is high (10–20%) in pregnant women*** and correlates with high levels of HEV RNA in serum and gene mutations that lead to reduced expression of progesterone receptors, and the risk of hepatic decompensation is increased in patients with underlying chronic liver disease" *(CMDT 2016/673)*

Illness generally is self-limited (no carrier state)"- *(CMDT 2016/673)*

A & E

"The most feared complication of viral hepatitis is **fulminant hepatitis** (massive hepatic necrosis); fortunately, this is a rare event. Fulminant hepatitis is seen primarily in hepatitis B, D, and E, but rare fulminant cases of hepatitis A

Fulminant hepatitis is hardly ever seen in hepatitis C, but **hepatitis E,** can be complicated by ***fatal fulminant hepatitis in 1-2% of all cases*** and in ***up to 20% of cases in pregnant women***. Patients usually present with signs and symptoms of encephalopathy that may evolve to deep coma. ***The liver is usually small and the PT excessively prolonged.*** The combination of rapidly shrinking liver size, rapidly rising bilirubin level, and marked prolongation of the PT, even as aminotransferase levels fall, together with clinical signs of confusion, disorientation, somnolence, ascites, and edema, indicates that the patient has hepatic failure with encephalopathy" *(Harrison 19th/2018)*

Table *(Harrison 19th/2013)*: **Clinical and Epidemiologic Features of Viral Hepatitis**

Feature	HAV	HBV	HCV	HDV	HEV
Incubation (days)	15–45, mean 30	30–180, mean 60–90	15–160, mean 50	30–180, mean 60–90	14–60, mean 40
Onset	Acute	Insidious or acute	Insidious	Insidious or acute	Acute
Age preference	Children, young adults	Young adults (sexual and percutaneous), babies, toddlers	Any age, but more common in adults	Any age (similar to HBV)	Young adults (20–40 years)
Transmission					
Fecal-oral +++		–	–	–	+++
Percutaneous	Unusual	+++	+++	+++	–
Perinatal	–	+++	±	+	–
Sexual	±	++	±	++	–
Clinical					
Severity	Mild	Occasionally severe	Moderate	Occasionally severe	Mild
Fulminant	0.1%	0.1–1%	0.1%	5–20%	1–2%
Progression to chronicity	None	Occasional (1–10%) (90% of neonates)	Common (85%)	Common	None
Carrier	None	0.1–30%	1.5–3.2%	Variable	None
Cancer	None	+(Neonatal infection)	+	±	None
Prognosis	Excellent	Worse with age, debility	Moderate	Acute, good Chronic, poor	Good
Prophylaxis	Ig, inactivated vaccine	HBIG, recombinant vaccine	None	HBV vaccine (none for HBV carriers)	Vaccine
Therapy	None	Interferon Lamivudine Adefovir Pegylated interferon Entecavir Telbivudine Tenofovir	Pegylated interferon plus ribavirin, telaprevir, boceprevir	Interferon ±	None

103. Ans. b. Renal osteodys..., d. Peripheral..., e. Small....

[Ref: Harrison 19th/ 1808-20, 18th/ 2310-20; CMDT 09 / 797-807]

Anaemia & Raised Creatinine are also Found in ARF

The term ***chronic renal failure*** applies to the process of continuing significant irreversible reduction in nephron number, and typically corresponds to CKD stages 3–5

"The first step in evaluating a patient with **renal failure** is to determine if the disease is ***acute or chronic. If review of laboratory records demonstrates that the rise in blood urea nitrogen and creatinine is recent, this suggests that the process is acute***. However, previous measurements are not always available. **Findings that suggest chronic kidney disease** include ***anemia, evidence of renal osteodystrophy (radiologic or laboratory), and small scarred kidneys***. However, ***anemia may also complicate ARF***, and renal size may be normal or increased in several chronic renal diseases (*e.g.*, diabetic nephropathy, amyloidosis, polycystic kidney disease, HIV associated nephropathy)" *(Harrison 19th/1805)*

"***Anemia develops rapidly in ARF*** and is usually multifactorial in origin. Contributing factors include impaired erythropoiesis, hemolysis, bleeding, hemodilution, and reduced red cell survival time" *(Harrison 19th/1810)*

Cardiopulmonary complications of **ARF** include arrhythmias, ***pericarditis and pericardial effusion***, and pulmonary edema" *(Harrison 19th/1809)*

CRF: CMDT 09/797-807: States

- Pericardial effusions can occur with azotemia, and a ***pericardial friction rub*** can be present. Effusions may result in ***cardiac tamponade***
- **Elevated BUN and creatinine** are present, though ***these elevations do not in themselves distinguish acute from chronic renal failure***. Anemia can occur as a result of decreased erythropoietin production.
- Progressive azotemia over months to years.
- Symptoms and signs of uremia when nearing end-stage disease.
- Hypertension in the majority.
- Isosthenuria and ***broad casts*** in urinary sediment are common.
- ***Bilateral small kidneys in ultrasound are diagnostic***
- With uremia, ***pericarditis*** may develop.
- The anemia of chronic renal failure is characteristically ***normochromic and normocytic***
- **Peripheral neuropathies** manifest themselves as *sensorimotor polyneuropathies (stocking and glove distribution)* and isolated or multiple isolated mononeuropathies.

CRF

◈ *Harrison 19th/ 1818-19*

- A ***normocytic, normochromic anemia*** is observed as early as stage 3 CKD and is almost universal by stage 4. The primary cause in patients with CKD is insufficient production of erythropoietin (EPO) by the diseased kidneys and urine chemistry, abnormal imaging studies).
- Peripheral neuropathy usually becomes clinically evident after the patient reaches stage 4 CKD

"*Anaemia, metabolic acidosis, **hyperphosphatemia**, hypocalcemia & hyperkalemia can occur with both acute & chronic renal failure*" *(CMDT 06 / 908)*

104. Ans. a. Show cutaneous..., b. High CD4..., d. May be associated...

[Ref: Harrison 19th/ 2205-12; Robbins(SAE) 9th/693-94;CMDT 2016/292-93]

"**Sarcoidosis** is linked with ***clinical anergy*** and other evidence of diminished cellular immunity *(www.ncbi.nlm.nih.gov)*

"Regarding the **tuberculin skin test**, patients with sarcoidosis have impaired delayed-type immune reactions. Two thirds of patients with systemic sarcoidosis have ***cutaneous anergy*** to the tuberculin and other skin tests. It is not known if cutaneous anergy is frequent in patients with cutaneous lesions of sarcoidosis with little or no systemic involvement" *(emedicine.medscape.com)*

"***Bronchoalveolar lavage fluid in sarcoidosis is usually characterized by an increase in lymphocyte & a high CD4/CD8 ratio***" *(CMDT 2016/293)*

"The use of the lymphocyte markers CD4 and CD8 can be used to determine the CD4/CD8 ratio of these increased lymphocytes in the **BAL fluid**. A ***ratio of >. 3.5 is strongly supportive of sarcoidosis*** but is less sensitive than an increase in lymphocytes alone" *(Harrison 17th/2140)*

"**Sarcoidosis**: *Intra-alveolar & interstitial accumulation of CD4+ T cells, resulting in* CD4: CD8 *ratios ranging from* **5:1 to 15:1**" *(Robbins 9th/693)*

"**Schauman & asteroid bodies:*Although characteristic, these cells are not pathognomic of sarcoidosis*** because they may be ***encountered in other granulomatous diseases (e.g., tuberculosis)***" *(Robbins 9th/693)*

Sarcoidosis

- The ***granuloma is the pathologic hallmark of sarcoidosis***
- Sarcoidosis is an inflammatory disease characterized by the presence of ***noncaseating granulomas.***The disease is often multisystem and requires the presence of involvement in two or more organs for a specific diagnosis.
- Either direct vascular involvement or the consequence of fibrotic changes in the lung can lead to pulmonary arterial hypertension. In sarcoidosis patients with end-stage fibrosis awaiting lung transplant, 70% will have pulmonary arterial hypertension.
- The ***peribronchial thickening*** seen on CT scan seems to explain the high yield of ***granulomas*** from bronchial biopsies performed for diagnosis.
- A positive gallium scan can support the diagnosis if increased activity is noted in the parotids and lacrimal glands (*Panda sign*) or in the right paratracheal and left hilar area (*lambda sign*)
- The *Kviem-Siltzbach procedure* is a specific diagnostic test for sarcoidosis

105. Ans. a. 9... b. 10....

[Ref: Hutchison's clinical Method 21th/249; P.J. Mehta 16th/230]

Reflex	Afferent	Efferent
Light Reflex	Optic Nerve	Occulomotor nerve
Accomodation Reflex	Optic Nerve	Occulomotor nerve
Gag Reflex	Glossopharyngeal nerve	Vagus
Ciliospinal Reflex	Cervical nerve	Cervical portion of spinal cord

106. Ans. a. Mental impairmen... b. ↑Serum..., c. Cardiomy...

[Ref: Harrison 19th/ 462-e; Robbins 8th/1268-69; Nelson 18th/ 2540, 2554, 2565]

"**DMD:** ***Serum CK levels are invariably elevated*** to between 20 and 100 times normal. The levels are abnormal at birth but decline late in the disease because of inactivity and loss of muscle mass" *(Harrison 18th/ 3491)*

"**Duchenne Muscular Dystrophy**: This *X-linked recessive disorder*, sometimes also called pseudohypertrophic muscular dystrophy, has an incidence of ~30 per 100,000 live-born males"

Duchenne Muscular Dystrophy (DMD)

- DMD is the most severe and the most common form of muscular dystrophy
- DMD becomes ***clinically manifest by the age of 5 years***, with weakness leading to wheelchair dependence by 10 to 12 years of age, and progresses relentlessly until death by the early twenties.
- Histopathologic abnormalities common to DMD and BMD include (1) *variation in fiber size* (diameter) due to the presence of both small and enlarged fibers, sometimes with fiber splitting; (2) *increased numbers of internalized nuclei* (beyond the normal range of 3% to 5%); (3) *degeneration necrosis, and phagocytosis of muscle fibers;* (4) *regeneration of muscle fibers*; and (5) *proliferation of endomysial connective tissue*
- Histochemical reactions sometimes fail to identify distinct fiber types in DMD. In later stages, *the muscles eventually become almost totally replaced by fat and connective tissue.*
- **Cardiac involvement**, when present, consists of interstitial fibrosis, more prominent in the subendocardial layers. Despite the clinical evidence of CNS dysfunction in DMD, no consistent neuropathologic abnormalities have been described.

Table *(Harrison 19th/ 462-e)*: **Progressive Muscular Dystrophies**

Type	Inheritance	Defective Gene/Protein	Onset Age	Clinical Features	Other Organ Systems Involved
Duchenne's	XR	Dystrophin	***Before 5 years***	Progressive weakness of girdle muscles Unable to walk after age 12 Progressive kyphoscoliosis Respiratory failure in 2d or 3d decade	***Cardiomyopathy*** Mental impairment
Becker's	XR	Dystrophin	Early childhood to adult	Progressive weakness of girdle muscles Able to walk after age 15 Respiratory failure may develop by 4th decade	Cardiomyopathy

107. Ans. a. Occur..., b. Uroporp..., c. Abdominal..., d. ↑ Porpho

[Ref: Harrison 19th/ 2521-30, 18th/ 3167-74; CMDT 2016/1655-56; Nelson 18th/645-46]

"**AIP**: *Patients show* ***intermittent abdominal pain*** *of varying severity,* and in some instances it may so simulate acute abdomen as to lead to exploratory laparotomy. Because the origin of the ***abdominal pain is neurologic***, there is an absence of ***fever and leukocytosis***" *(CMDT 2016/1655)*

"The **diagnosis can be confirmed** by demonstrating an *increased amount of* ***porphobilinogen in the urine*** *during an acute attack*" *(CMDT 2016/1655)*

Acute Intermittent Porphyria (AIP)

◈ *Harrison 19th/ 2526*

- Because the neurovisceral symptoms rarely occur before puberty and are often nonspecific, a high index of suspicion is required to make the diagnosis.
- Abdominal pain, the ***most common symptom,*** is usually steady and poorly localized but may be ***cramping. Ileus, abdominal distention,*** and decreased bowel sounds are common.
- The ***peripheral neuropathy*** is due to axonal degeneration (rather than demyelinization) and primarily affects motor neurons. Motor neuropathy affects the proximal muscles initially, more often in the shoulders and arms. The course and degree of involvement are variable and sometimes may be focal and involve cranial nerves.
- ***Abdominal tenderness***, fever, and leukocytosis are usually absent or mild because the symptoms are neurologic rather than inflammatory.
- Nausea; vomiting; ***constipation; tachycardia; hypertension; mental symptoms***; pain in the limbs, head, neck, or chest; muscle weakness; ***sensory loss;*** dysuria; and urinary retention are characteristic. ***Tachycardia, hypertension, restlessness, tremors, and excess sweating are due to sympathetic overactivity.***
- Mental symptoms such as anxiety, insomnia, depression, ***disorientation, hallucinations, and paranoia*** can occur in acute attacks. Seizures can be due to neurologic effects or to hyponatremia.

Table *(Harrisonn 19th/2522)*: **Human Porphyrias-Major Clinical and Laboratory Features**

Porphyria	Deficient Enzyme	Inheri-tance	Prin-cipal Symp-toms	En-zyme Acti-vity % of Normal	Increased Porphyrin Precursors and/or Porphyrins		
			NV or CP		Erythrocytes	Urine	Stool
Hepatic Porphyrias							
5-ALA dehydratase-deficient porphyria (ADP)	ALA-dehydratase	AR	NV	~5	Zn-proto-porphyrin	ALA, Coproporphyrin III	—
Acute intermittent porphyria (AIP)	***HMB-synthase***	***AD***	NV	~50	—	ALA, ***PBG***, Uroporphyrin	—
Porphyria cutanea tarda (PCT)	URO-decarboxylase	AD	CP	~20	—	Uroporphyrin, 7-carboxylate porphyrin	Isocoproporphyrin
Hereditary coproporphyria (HCP)	COPRO-oxidase	AD	NV & CP	~50	—	ALA, PBG, Coproporphyrin III	Coproporphyrin III
Variegate porphyria (VP)	PROTO-oxidase	AD	NV & CP	~50	—	ALA, PBG, Coproporphyrin III	Coproporphyrin III Protoporphyrin
Erythropoietic Porphyrias							
Congenital erythropoietic porphyria (CEP)	URO-synthase	AR	CP	1–5	Uropor phyrin I Coproporphyrin I	Uroporphyrin I Coproporphyrin I	Coproporphyrin I
Erythropoietic protoporphyria (EPP)	Ferrochelatase	AD[a]	CP	~20–30	Proto-porphyrin	—	Protoporphyrin

Abbreviations: *AD, autosomal dominant; ALA, 5'-aminolevulinic acid; AR, autosomal recessive; CP, cutaneous photosensitivity; COPRO, coproporphyrinogen; HMB, hydroxymethylbilane; ISOCOPRO, isocoproporphyrin; NV, neurovisceral; PBG, porphobilinogen; PROTO, protoporphyrinogen; URO, uroporphyrinogen.*

108. Ans. a. Bilirubin..., b. Prothrombi..., e. Absence...

[Ref: Harrison 19th/1994-95;;CMDT 2016/693; L&B 25th/1083]

Table *(Schwartz)*: **Revised Child Classification of Clinical Severity of Cirrhosis**

Factor	A	B	C
Nutritional status[Q]	Excellent	Good	Poor
Ascites[Q]	None	Minimal, controlled	Moderate to severe
Encephalopathy[Q]	None	Minimal, controlled	Moderate to severe
Serum bilirubin (mg/dL)[Q]	<2	2–3	>3
Serum albumin (g/dL)[Q]	>3.5	2.8–3.5	<2.8
Prothrombin time (% of control)[Q]	>70	40–70	<40

Table *(Harrison 19th/1995)*: **Child-Pugh Classification of Cirrhosis**

Factor	Units	1	2	3
Serum bilirubin	μmol/L mg/dL	<34 <2.0	34–51 2.0–3.0	>51 >3.0
Serum albumin	g/L g/dL	>35 >3.5	30–35 3.0–3.5	<30 <3.0
Prothrombin time	seconds prolonged INR	0–4 <1.7	4–6 1.7–2.3	>6 >2.3
Ascites	None		Easily controlled	Poorly controlled
Hepatic encephalopathy[Q]	None		Minimal	Advanced

Note: The Child-Pugh score is calculated by adding the scores of the five factors and can range from 5–15. Child-Pugh class is either A (a score of 5–6), B (7–9), or C (10 or above). Decompensation indicates cirrhosis with a Child-Pugh score of 7 or more (class B). This level has been the accepted criterion for listing for liver transplantation

109. Ans. **b. Most common...**

[Ref: Harrison 19th/ 1639-40; CMDT 2016/476-78; Robbins 7th/531-32]

"Operative repair of the aneurysm with insertion of a ***prosthetic graft or endovascular placement of an aortic stent*** graft is indicated for abdominal aortic aneurysms of any size that are expanding rapidly or are associated with symptoms. For **asymptomatic aneurysms,** abdominal aortic aneurysm ***repair is indicated if the diameter is >5.5 cm***. In randomized trials of patients with abdominal aortic aneurysms <5.5 cm, there was no difference in the long-term (5- to 8-year) mortality rate between those followed with ultrasound surveillance and those undergoing elective surgical repair. Thus, ***serial noninvasive follow-up of smaller aneurysms*** (<5 cm) is an alternative to immediate repair. The decision to perform an open surgical operation or endovascular repair is based in part on the vascular anatomy and comorbid conditions. ***Endovascular repair of abdominal aortic aneurysms*** has a lower short-term morbidity rate but a comparable long-term mortality rate with open surgical reconstruction. Long-term surveillance with CT or MR aortography is indicated after endovascular repair to detect leaks and possible aneurysm expansion" *(Harrison 19th/1640)*

"***Majority are asymptomatic*** & often diagnosed incidently. Many have pulsatile epigastric mass. Rupture cause severe central abdominal & lumbar back pain, variable psoas spasm, sometime pain in lower limb d/t compression of lumbar or sciatic nerve root" *(Oxfore Textbook of Surgery/379-80)*

"Obstruction of a vessel, particularly of the iliac, renal, mesenteric, or vertebral branches that supply the spinal cord leading to ischemic tissue injury. The ***treatment*** of abdominal and thoracic aortic aneurysms is evolving toward ***endoluminal approaches using stent grafts*** (expandable wire frames covered by a cloth sleeve) rather than surgery for some patients" *(Robbins 7th/532)*

"Approx. 40-60% pt. have suitable anatomy & are candidate for ***endoluminal repair with stent placement***" *(Fisher Mastery of Surgery 5th/2052)*

Abdominal Aortic Aneurysm (AAA)

◈ *Harrison 19th/ 1639-40*

- 90% of abdominal aortic aneurysm (AAA) of ***size > 4cm*** in diameter is due to ***atherosclerosis.***
- ***Male*** are more frequently affected than female.
- An abdominal aortic aneurysm *commonly produces no symptoms*. It is usually detected on routine examination as a palpable, pulsatile, expansile, and nontender mass, or it is an incidental finding during an abdominal X-ray or ultrasound study performed for other reasons.
- As abdominal aortic aneurysms expand, however, they may become painful. Some patients complain of strong pulsations in the abdomen; others experience pain in the chest, lower back, or scrotum. Aneurysmal pain is usually a harbinger of rupture and represents a medical emergency
- The aneurysm **most commonly** arises ***below the level of renal artery.***
- Prognosis of abdominal aortic aneurysm is depends on size of the aneurysm and the severity of co-existing coronary artery and cerebrovascular disease. Most of the time they are asymptomatic
- Beta blocker decreases the perioperative cardiovascular morality.

110. Ans. **a. Adrenalec..., b. Pituitary... c. Stereotactic pit..., d. Surgical removal....**

[Ref: Harrison 19th/2271-73,2313-16; Davidson 22nd/775;CMDT 2016/1152-56]

*It is a case of **cushing's disease***

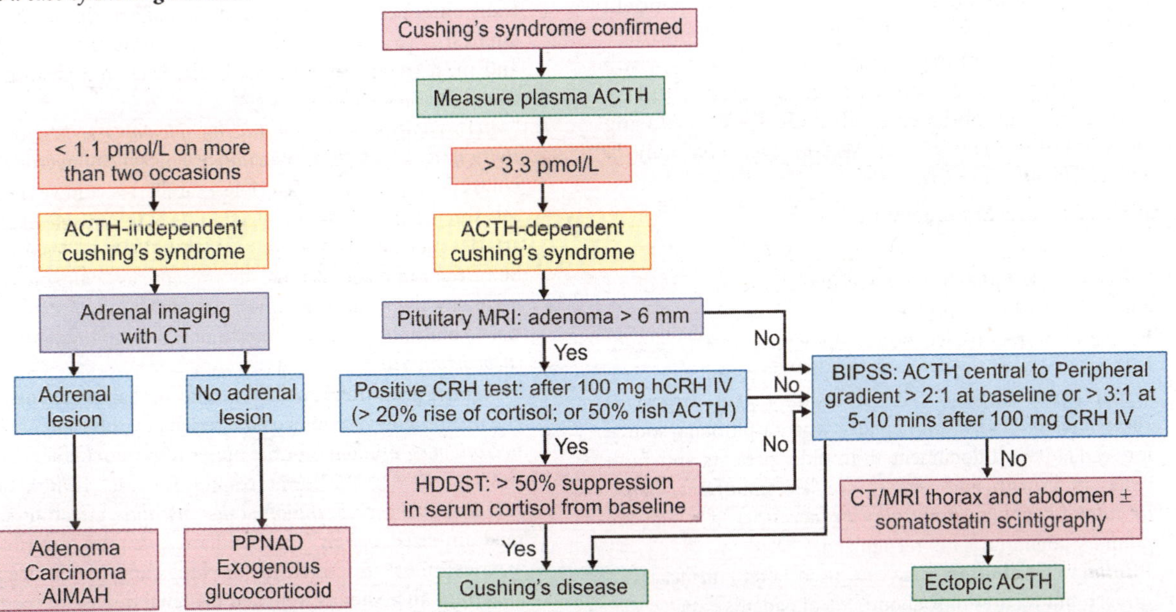

Fig: *(Davidson 22nd/775):* Determining the cause of confirmed Cushing's syndrome.(ACTH = adrenocorticotrophic hormone; AIMAH = ACTH-independent macronodular adrenal hyperplasia; BIPSS = bilateral inferior petrosal sinus sampling; CRH = corticotrophin-releasing hormone; HDDST = high-dose dexamethasone suppression test; PPNAD = primary pigmented nodular adrenal disease)

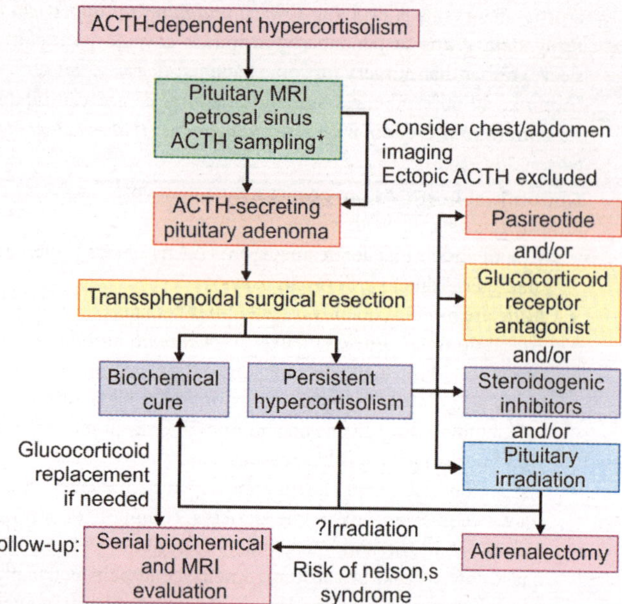

Fig: *(Harrison 19th/2273):* Management of Cushing's syndrome. ACTH, adrenocorticotropin hormone; MRI, magnetic resonance imaging.*, Not usually required

Cushing's Disease: Management

Davidson 22nd/775

- ***Trans-sphenoidal surgery*** carried out by an experienced surgeon with selective ***removal of the adenoma*** is the treatment of choice, with approximately 70% of patients going into immediate remission. Around 20% of patients suffer a recurrence, often years later, emphasising the need for life-long follow-up.
- **Laparoscopic bilateral adrenalectomy** performed by an expert surgeon effectively cures ACTH-dependent Cushing's syndrome, but in patients with pituitary dependent Cushing's syndrome, this can result in Nelson's syndrome, with an invasive pituitary macroadenoma and very high ACTH levels causing pigmentation. The ***risk of Nelson's syndrome may be reduced by pituitary irradiation***

Cushing's Disease: Management

Harrison 19th/2272

- ***Selective transsphenoidal resection*** is the treatment of choice for Cushing's disease
- Biochemical recurrence occurs in approximately 5% of patients in whom surgery was initially successful.
- When initial surgery is unsuccessful, ***repeat surgery is sometimes indicated***, particularly when a pituitary source for ACTH is well documented. In older patients, in whom issues of growth and fertility are less important, ***hemi- or total hypophysectomy may be necessary*** if a discrete pituitary adenoma is not recognized.
- ***Pituitary irradiation*** may be used after unsuccessful surgery, but it cures only about 15% of patients.
- The use of steroidogenic inhibitors has ***decreased the need for bilateral adrenalectomy***.
- **Prophylactic radiation therapy** may be indicated to prevent the development of Nelson's syndrome after adrenalectomy

Cushing Disease

CMDT 2016/1154

- It is best treated by ***transsphenoidal selective resection of the pituitary adenoma***. After pituitary surgery, the rest of the pituitary usually returns to normal function; however, the pituitary corticotrophs remain suppressed and require 6–36 months to recover normal function.
- ***Hydrocortisone or prednisone replacement therapy*** is necessary in the meantime. Patients who do not have a remission(or who have a recurrence) may be considered for treatment with cabergoline 0.5–3.5 mg orally twice weekly, which was successful in 40% of patients in one small study.
- ***Laparoscopic adrenalectomy*** should be offered to unresponsive patients.
- Another treatment option for patients with ACTH-secreting pituitary tumors is ***stereotactic pituitary radiosurgery (gamma knife or cyberknife),*** which normalizes urine free cortisol in two-thirds of patients within 12 months.
- **Pituitary radiosurgery** can also be used to treat Nelson syndrome, the progressive enlargement of ACTH-secreting pituitary tumors following bilateral adrenalectomy.

111. Ans. b. Polyarteritis....

[Ref: Harrison 17th/2118-2121; Robbins 9th/506; 7th/537;Davidson 22nd/713]

"**PAN** is a systemic vasculitis of small or medium-sized muscular arteries (but not arterioles, capillaries, or venules), typically involving renal and visceral vessels but ***sparing the pulmonary circulation***. Classic PAN occurs as segmental transmural necrotizing inflammation of **arteries of medium to small size, in any organ** with the possible exception of the lung, and most frequently kidneys, heart, liver, and gastrointestinal tract." *(Robbins 9th/509)*

"***Microscopic polyangiitis*** *(microscopic polyarteritis, hypersensitivity, or leukocytoclastic vasculitis)*: This type of necrotizing vasculitis generally affects arterioles, capillaries, and venules—vessels smaller than those involved in PAN.In unusual cases larger arteries may be involved. In contrast to PAN, all lesions tend to be of the same age. It typically presents as "palpable purpura" involving the skin, or involvement of the mucous membranes, lungs, brain, heart, gastrointestinal tract, kidneys, and muscle" *(Robbins 9th/510)*

"**Wegener granulomatosis (Granulomatosis with polyangitis)** is a necrotizing vasculitis characterized by the triad of (1) *acute necrotizing granulomas* of the upper respiratory tract (ear, nose, sinuses, throat), the lower respiratory tract (***lung***), or both; (2) *necrotizing or granulomatous vasculitis* affecting small to medium-sized vessels (e.g., capillaries, venules, arterioles, and arteries), most prominent in the lungs and upper airways but affecting other sites as well; and (3) renal disease in the form of *focal necrotizing, often crescentic, glomerulitis*" *(Robbins 9th/511)*

"**Churg- Strauss syndrome(allergic granulomatosis and angiitis)** is a multisystem diseases with cutaneous involvement (palpable purpura), gastrointestinal tract bleeding, and renal disease (primarily as focal and segmental glomerulosclerosis)" *(Robbins 9th/511)*

Eosinophilic granulomatosis with polyangiitis (Churg-Strauss): It can occur in any organ in the body; ***lung*** involvement is predominant, with skin, cardiovascular system, kidney, peripheral nervous system,and gastrointestinal tract also commonly involved" *(Harrison 17th/2186)*

112. Ans. a.Bleom..., b. Pentazo..., c. Polyinyl....

[Ref: Harrison 19th/2154-55]

"**Drug implicated in SSc-like illness** *includes* ***bleomycin, pentazocin & cocaine*** *and appetite suppressant linked with pulmonary hypertension" (Harrison 19th/2155)*

"Occupational exposure tentatively linked with ***SSc*** *include silica dust in miners,* ***polyvinyl chloride,*** *epoxy resins & aromatic hydrocarbons including toluene & trichloroethylene" (Harrison 19th/2155)*

Scleroderma *is thickening of skin that is characteristically found in* ***systemic sclerosis***

Table *(Harrison 19th/2218)*: **Drug-Induced Musculoskeletal Conditions**

Scleroderma
Vinyl chloride, bleomycin[Q], pentazocine[Q], organic solvents, carbidopa, tryptophan, rapeseed oil
Arthralgias
Quinidine, cimetidine, quinolones, chronic acyclovir, interferon, IL-2, nicardipine, vaccines, rifabutin, aromatase and HIV protease inhibitors
Myalgias/myopathy
Glucocorticoids, penicillamine, hydroxychloroquine, AZT, lovastatin, simvastatin, pravastatin, clofibrate, interferon, IL-2, alcohol, cocaine, taxol, docetaxel, colchicine, quinolones, cyclosporine
Tendon rupture
Quinolones, glucocorticoids
Gout
Diuretics, aspirin, cytotoxics, cyclosporine, alcohol, moonshine, ethambutol
Drug-induced lupus
Hydralazine[Q] procainamide[Q], quinidine[Q], phenytoin[Q], carbemazepine, methyldopa, isoniazid, chlorpromazine, lithium, penicillamine, tetracyclines, TNF inhibitors, ACE inhibitors, ticlopidine
Drug-induced subacute lupus
Proton pump inhibitors, calcium channel blockers (diltiazem), ACE inhibitors, TNF inhibitors, terbinafine, interferons (α and β-1a), paclitaxel, docetaxel, HCTZ (Hydrochlorothiazide)
Osteonecrosis
Glucocorticoids, alcohol, radiation, bisphosphonates
Osteopenia
Glucocorticoids, chronic heparin, phenytoin, methotrexate
Vasculitis
Allopurinol, amphetamines, cocaine, thiazides, penicillamine, propylthiouracil, montelukast, TNF inhibitors, hepatitis B vaccine, trimethoprim/sulfamethoxazole

Contd...

Table *(Harrison 19th/2154)*: **Conditions Associated with Scleroderma-Like Induration**

Chemically induced scleroderma-like conditions
Vinyl chloride–induced disease
Pentazocine-induced skin fibrosis
Paraneoplastic syndrome

113. Ans. a. Biphasic..., b. Monophasic..., c. IV cannula..., d. After placing.....

[Ref: ahaguidelines.heart.org; circ.ahajournals.org/]

"**2010 AHA guideline for CPR (No change in 2015 Guideline)**: *Contrary to previous recommendation of 3 successive shocks (200,300, 360 J) nowadays* ***1st & all subsequent shocks are of 360 Joules with monophasic & 120-200 Joules with biphasic"*** *(Ajay Yadav 5th/ 259)*

2015 American Heart Association (AHA) Guidelines Update for Cardiopulmonary Resuscitation (CPR) and Emergency Cardiovascular Care (ECC)

Defibrillation

At the advanced level, the ***cardiac arrest algorithm remains almost completely unchanged from the 2010 version.*** Recommendations for defibrillation remain unchanged. ***Biphasic defibrillators are still preferred over monophasic*** devices. Single shocks are still preferred over multiple or stacked shocks.

- The AHA continues to ***recommend that EMS providers deliver the manufacturer's recommended first energy dose.*** If that dose is unknown, ***deliver the maximum energy dose*** allowed by the machine. It is also reasonable to follow the defibrillator manufacturer's recommendations on energy levels for subsequent defibrillation attempts

Ventilation Rate

- After placing an advanced airway, the AHA continues to recommend a ***ventilation rate of 10 breaths per minute*** (one every six seconds) while providing continuous chest compressions.

Post-cardiac Arrest Care

- With a few notable exceptions, changes to recommendations for the post-cardiac arrest phase are minor, especially for those that could directly affect out-of-hospital care. Once the patient achieves ROSC, one of the priorities highlighted in the 2010 guidelines was to optimize the patient's hemodynamic status. Although the 2010 cardiac arrest algorithm lists a target of ***90 mm Hg, the actual recommendation at the time was to achieve a mean arterial pressure (MAP) of at least 65 mm Hg.***
- In preparing for the 2015 guidelines, the research review team could find no evidence of an optimal blood pressure

target. Therefore, the AHA believes it is reasonable to avoid and correct any hypotension (defined as a systolic blood pressure less than 90 mm Hg or a MAP less than 65 mm Hg) present during the post-resuscitation phase.

Summary of Key Issues and Major Changes

Key issues and major changes in the 2015 Guidelines Update recommendations for advanced cardiac life support include the following:

- The combined use of vasopressin and epinephrine offers no advantage to using standard-dose epinephrine in cardiac arrest. Also, vasopressin does not offer an advantage over the use of epinephrine alone. Therefore, to simplify the algorithm, vasopressin has been removed from the Adult Cardiac Arrest Algorithm–2015 Update.
- Low end-tidal carbon dioxide ($ETCO_2$) in intubated patients after 20 minutes of CPR is associated with a very low likelihood of resuscitation. While this parameter should not be used in isolation for decision making, providers may consider low $ETCO_2$ after 20 minutes of CPR in combination with other factors to help determine when to terminate resuscitation.
- Steroids may provide some benefit when bundled with vasopressin and epinephrine in treating IHCA. While routine use is not recommended pending follow-up studies, it would be reasonable for a provider to administer the bundle for IHCA.
- When rapidly implemented, ECPR can prolong viability, as it may provide time to treat potentially reversible conditions or arrange for cardiac transplantation for patients who are not resuscitated by conventional CPR.
- In cardiac arrest patients with nonshockable rhythm and who are otherwise receiving epinephrine, the early provision of epinephrine is suggested.
- Studies about the use of lidocaine after ROSC are conflicting, and routine lidocaine use is not recommended. However, the initiation or continuation of lidocaine may be considered immediately after ROSC from VF/pulseless ventricular tachycardia (pVT) cardiac arrest.
- One observational study suggests that ß-blocker use after cardiac arrest may be associated with better outcomes than when ß-blockers are not used. Although this observational study is not strong-enough evidence to recommend routine use, the initiation or continuation of an oral or intravenous (IV) ß-blocker may be considered early after hospitalization from cardiac arrest due to VF/pVT.

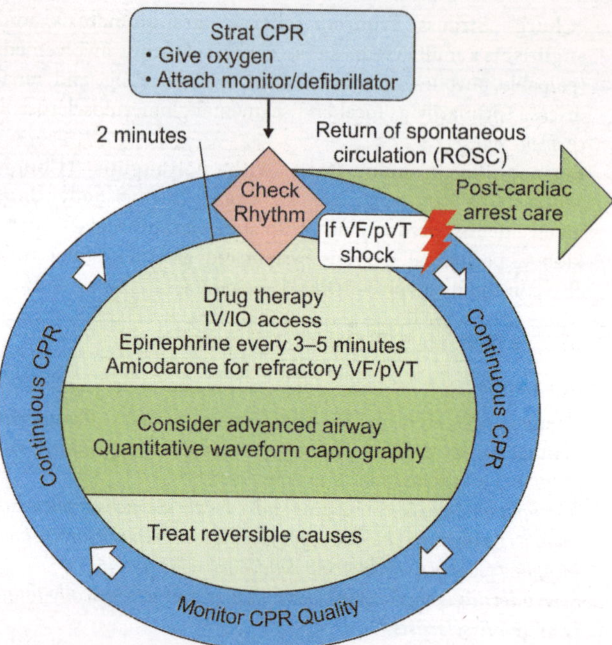

Fig: Adult cardiac arrest algorithm

CPR Quality

- Push hard (at least 2 inches [5 cm] and fast (100-120/min) and allow complete chest recoil.
- Minimize interruptions in compressions.
- Avoid excessive ventilation.
- Rotate compressor every 2 minutes, or sooner if fatigued.
- If no advanced airway, 30:2 compression-ventilation ratio.
- Quantitative waveform capnography
  - If ETCO2 <10mm Hg, attempt to improve CPR quality
- Intra arterial pressure.
  - If relaxation phase (diastolic) pressure <20 mm Hg, attempt to improve CPR quality.

Shock Energy for Defibrillation

- **Biphasic:** Manufacturer recommendation (e.g., initial dose of 120-200J); if unknown, use maximum available, Second and subsequent doses should be equivalent, and higher closes may be considered.
- **Monophasic:** 360 J

Drug Therapy

- **Epinephrine IV/IO dose:** 1 mg every 3-5 minutes
- **Amiodarone IV/IO dose:** First dose: 300 mg bolus, Second dose: 150 mg.

Contd...

Advanced Airway

- Endotracheal intubation or supraglottic advanced airway
- Waveform capnography or capnometry to confirm and monitor ET tube placement
- Once advanced airway in place, give 1 breath every 6 seconds (10 breaths/min) with continuous chest compressions

Return of Spontaneous Circulation (ROSC)

- Pulse and blood pressure
- Abrupt sustained increase in ETCO2 (typically ≥ 40 mm Hg)
- Spontaneous arterial pressure waves with intra-arterial monitoring

Reversible Causes

• Hypovolemia	• Tension pneumothorax
• Hypoxia	• Tamponade, cardiac
• Hydrogen ion (acidosis)	• Toxins
• Hypo-/hyperkalemia	• Thrombosis, pulmonary
• Hypothermia	• Thrombosis, coronary

114. Ans. a. Continue inh..., b. Add inhaled..., c. Increase dose...

[Ref: Davidson 22nd/669-71;Harrison 19th/1676-80; CMDT 06/231-36;KDT 6th/226; Emergency Medicine-American College of Physician 6th/289]

The Stepwise Approach to the Management of Asthma

Davidson 22nd/669-71

Step 1: Occasional use of inhaled short-acting β2-adreno-receptor agonist bronchodilators

- For patients with mild intermittent asthma (symptoms less than once a week for 3 months and fewer than two nocturnal episodes per month), it is usually sufficient to prescribe an ***inhaled short-acting*** **β2-*agonist***, such as salbutamol or terbutaline, to be used as required.
- A history of a severe exacerbation should lead to a step-up in treatment.
- The metered-dose inhaler remains the most widely prescribed inhaled devices

Step 2: Introduction of regular preventer therapy

- Regular anti-inflammatory therapy ***(preferably inhaled corticosteroids (ICS), such as beclometasone, budesonide (BUD), fluticasone or ciclesonide) should be started in addition to inhaled β2-agonists*** *taken on an as-required basis for any patient* who:
  - Has experienced an exacerbation of asthma in the last 2 years
  - Uses inhaled β2-agonists three times a week or more
  - Reports symptoms three times a week or more
  - Is awakened by asthma one night per week.
- Alternative but much less effective preventive agents include chromones, leukotriene receptor antagonists, and theophyllines.

Step 3: Add-on therapy

- If a patient remains poorly controlled, ***despite regular use of ICS,*** a thorough review should be undertaken of adherence, inhaler technique and ongoing exposure to modifiable aggravating factors.
- A further increase in the dose of ICS may benefit some patients but, in general, ***add-on therapy should be considered*** in adults taking 800 µg/day BDP (or equivalent).
- Long-acting β2-agonists (LABAs), such as salmeterol and formoterol (duration of action of at least 12 hours), represent the first choice of add-on therapy. They have consistently been demonstrated to improve asthma control and to reduce the frequency and severity of exacerbations when compared to increasing the dose of ICS alone. Fixed combination inhalers of ICS and LABAs have been developed; these are more convenient, increase compliance and prevent patients using a LABA as monotherapy – the latter may be accompanied by an increased risk of life-threatening attacks or asthma death. The onset of action of formoterol is similar to that of salbutamol such that, in carefully selected patients, a fixed combination of budesonide and formoterol may be used as both rescue and maintenance therapy. Oral leukotriene receptor antagonists (e.g. montelukast 10 mg daily) are generally less effective than LABA as add-on therapy, but may facilitate a reduction in the dose of ICS and control exacerbations. Oral theophyllines may be considered in some patients but their unpredictable metabolism, propensity for drug interactions and prominent side-effects limit their widespread use.

Step 4: Poor control on moderate dose of inhaled steroid and add-on therapy: addition of a fourth drug

- In adults, the dose of ICS may be increased to 2000 µg BDP/BUD (or equivalent) daily. A nasal corticosteroid preparation should be used in patients with prominent upper airway symptoms. Oral therapy with leukotriene receptor antagonists, theophyllines or a slow-release β2-agonist may be considered. If the trial of add-on therapy is ineffective, it should be discontinued. Oral itraconazole may be contemplated in patients with allergic bronchopulmonary aspergillosis

Step 5: Continuous or frequent use of oral steroids

- At this stage, prednisolone therapy (usually administered as a single daily dose in the morning) should be prescribed in the lowest amount necessary to control symptoms. Patients on long-term corticosteroid tablets (> 3 months) or receiving more than three or four courses per year will be at risk of systemic side-effects

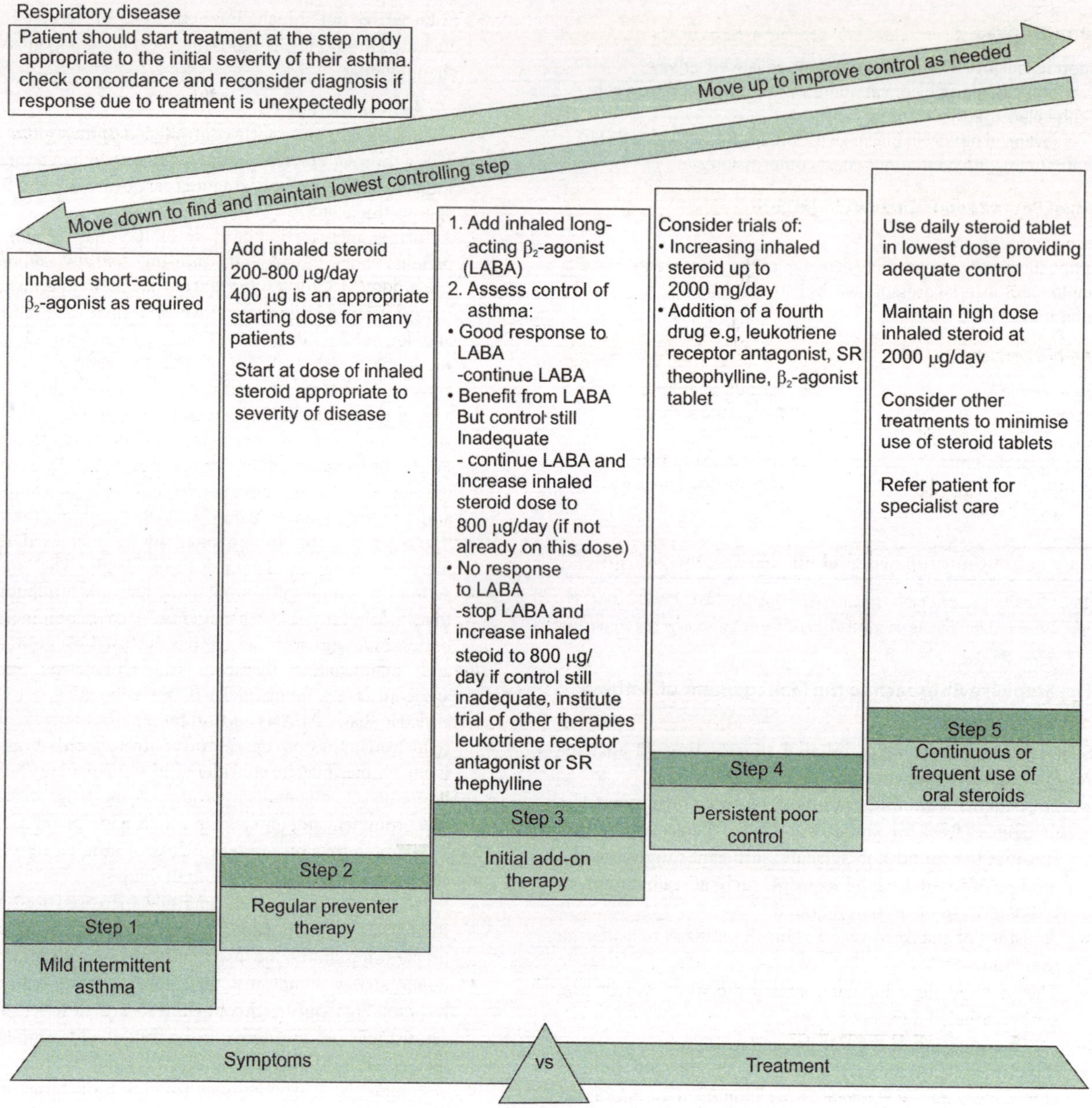

Respiratory disease
Patient should start treatment at the step mody appropriate to the initial severity of their asthma. check concordance and reconsider diagnosis if response due to treatment is unexpectedly poor
Move up to improve control as needed
Move down to find and maintain lowest controlling step
Inhaled short-acting β_2-agonist as required
Step 1
Mild intermittent asthma
Add inhaled steroid 200-800 µg/day
400 µg is an appropriate starting dose for many patients
Start at dose of inhaled steroid appropriate to severity of disease
Step 2
Regular preventer therapy
1. Add inhaled long-acting β_2-agonist (LABA)
2. Assess control of asthma:
• Good response to LABA -continue LABA
• Benefit from LABA But control still Inadequate - continue LABA and Increase inhaled steroid dose to 800 µg/day (if not already on this dose)
• No response to LABA -stop LABA and increase inhaled steoid to 800 µg/ day if control still inadequate, institute trial of other therapies leukotriene receptor antagonist or SR thephylline
Step 3
Initial add-on therapy
Consider trials of:
• Increasing inhaled steroid up to 2000 mg/day
• Addition of a fourth drug e.g, leukotriene receptor antagonist, SR theophylline, β_2-agonist tablet
Step 4
Persistent poor control
Use daily steroid tablet in lowest dose providing adequate control
Maintain high dose inhaled steroid at 2000 µg/day
Consider other treatments to minimise use of steroid tablets
Refer patient for specialist care
Step 5
Continuous or frequent use of oral steroids
Symptoms
vs
Treatment

Fig: *(Davidson 22nd/670):* Stepwise approach for asthma

OCS
LABA
LABA
LABA
ICS High dose
ICS High dose
ICS Low dose
ICS Low dose
Short-acting β_2-agonist as required for symptom relief
Mild intermittent
Mild perisistent
Moderate persistent
Severe persistent
Very severe persistent

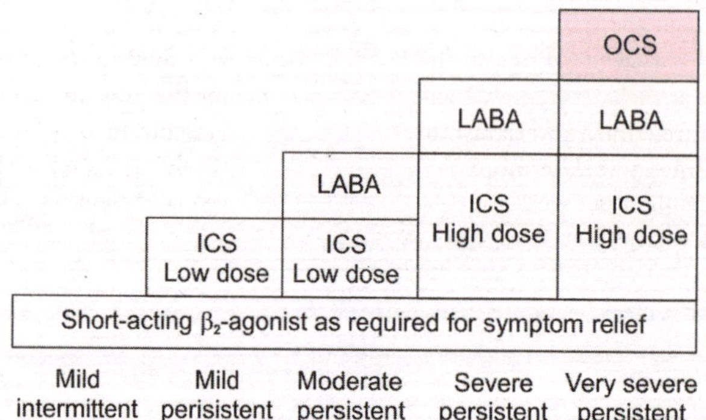

Fig: *(Harrison 19th/1679):* Stepwise approach to asthma therapy according to the severity of asthma and ability to control symptoms. ICS, inhaled corticosteroids; LABA, long-acting β2-agonist; OCS, oral corticosteroid.

"**MDI (Metered dose inhaler)** deliver a specified dose of the drug in spray form per actuation. A ***spacer*** (chamber imposed b/w the inhaler & the patients mouth) can be ***used to improve drug delivery. Nebulizers*** produces a mist of drug solution generated by pressurized air or oxygen which can be inhaled through mouth piece, face mask or in a tent" *(KDT 6th/226)*

Inhaled steroids are used in two form: *(KDT 6th/226)*

- **Use drug in solution:** metered dose inhaler, ***nebulizer***
- **Use drug as dry powder:** ***spinhaler, rotahaler***

"***Inhaled Corticosteroids*** (ICSs) are by far the most effective controllers for asthma, and their early use has revolutionized asthma therapy"*(Harrison 18th/ 2111)*

115. Ans. a. Asymptomatic...., b. Persistent generalised....

[Ref: Harrison 19th/ 1215-25; Davidson 22nd/394; Park 23rd/349]

Natural History & Clinical Staging of HIV

◈ *Davidson 22nd/394*

- Clinical staging of patients should be done at the initial medical examination, as it provides prognostic information and is a key criterion for initiating ART and prophylaxis against opportunistic infections. ***Two clinical staging systems*** are used internationally are- WHO system & CDC system
- In both systems, patients are staged according to the most severe manifestation and do not improve their classification. For example, a patient who is asymptomatic following a major opportunistic disease (AIDS) remains at stage 4 or category C of the **WHO and CDC systems** respectively, and never reverts to earlier stages.
- Finally, patients do not always progress steadily through all stages and may present with AIDS, having previously been asymptomatic.

Table *(Davidson 22nd/394)*: **HIV Clinical Staging Classifications**

World Health Organization (WHO) clinical stage {used in low- and middle-income countries}	Centers for Disease Control (CDC) clinical categories (used in high-income countries)
Stage 1 Asymptomatic Persistent generalised lymphadenopathy	**Category A** Primary HIV infection Asymptomatic Persistent generalised lymphadenopathy
Stage 2 Unexplained moderate weight loss (< 10% of body weight) Recurrent upper respiratory tract infections Herpes zoster Angular cheilitis Recurrent oral ulceration Papular pruritic eruptions Seborrhoeic dermatitis Fungal nail infections	**Category B** Bacillary angiomatosis Candidiasis, oropharyngeal (thrush) Candidiasis, vulvovaginal; persistent, frequent or poorly responsive to therapy Cervical dysplasia (moderate or severe) / cervical carcinoma in situ
Stage 3 Unexplained severe weight loss (> 10% of body weight) Unexplained chronic diarrhoea for > 1 mth Unexplained persistent fever (> 37.5°C for > 1 mth) Persistent oral candidiasis Oral hairy leucoplakia Pulmonary tuberculosis Severe bacterial infections Acute necrotising ulcerative stomatitis, gingivitis or periodontitis Unexplained anaemia (< 80 g/L (8 g/L)), neutropenia (< 0.5 × 10^9/L) and/ or chronic thrombocytopenia (< 50 × 10^9/L	Constitutional symptoms, such as fever (38.5°C) or diarrhoea lasting.> 1 mth Oral hairy leucoplakia Herpes zoster, involving two distinct episodes or more than one dermatome Idiopathic thrombocytopenic purpura Listeriosis Pelvic inflammatory, disease, particularly if complicated by tubo-ovarian abscess Peripheral neuropathy
Stage 4	**Category C** Candidiasis of oesophagus, trachea, bronchi or lungs Cervical carcinoma - invasive Cryptococcosis - exlrapulmonary Cryptosporilosis, chronic (> 1 mth) Cytomegalovirus disease (outside liver, spleen and nodes) Herpes simplex chronic (> 1 mth) ulcers or visceral HIV encephalopathy HIV wasting syndrome Isosporiasis, chronic (> 1 mth) Kaposi's sarcoma Lymphoma (cerebral or B-cell non-Hodgkin) Mycobacterial infection, non-tuberculous, extrapulmonary or disseminated Mycosis - disseminated endemic (coccidiodomycosis or histoplasmosis) Pneumocystis pneumonia Pneumonia, recurrent bacterial Progressive multioflocal leucoencephalopathy Toxoplasmosis – cerebral Tuberculosis - extrapulmonary (CDC includes pulmonary) Septicaemia, recurrent (including non-typhoidal Salmonella) (CDC only includes Salmonella)
Symptomatic HIV-associated nephropathy* Symptomatic HIV-associated cardiomyopathy* Leishmaniasis, atypical disseminated*	

*These conditions are in WHO stage 4 but not in CDC category C.

WHO Clinical Staging System for HIV Infection and HIV Related Disease

◈ *Park 23rd/349*

- WHO has developed a clinical staging system based on clinical criteria
- Clinical condition or performance score, which is the higher, determines whether a patient is at clinical stage 1, 2, 3 or 4
- Clinical stage is important as a criteria for starting antiretroviral therapy (ART)

Table *(Park 23rd/349)*: **WHO HIV Staging**

Clinical Stage 1
Asymptomatic
Persistent generalized lymphadenopathy
Clinical Stage 2
Moderate unexplained weight loss (under 10% of presumed or measured body weight)
Recurrent respiratory tract infections (sinusitis, tonsillitis, otitis media, pharyngitis)
Herpes zoster
Angular cheilitis
Recurrent oral ulcerations
Papular pruritic eruptions
Seborrhoeic dermatitis
Fungal nail infections
Clinical Stage 3
Unexplained severe weight loss (over 10% of presumed or measured body weight)
Unexplained chronic diarrhea for longer than 1 month
Unexplained persistent fever (intermittent or constant for longer than 1 month)
Persistent oral candidiasis
Oral hairy leukoplakia
Pulmonary tuberculosis
Severe bacterial infections (e.g. Pneumonia, Empyema, meningitis, pyomyositis, bone or joint infection bacteremia, Severe pelvic inflammatory disease)
Acute necrotizing ulcerative stomatitis, gingivitis or periodontitis
Unexplained anaemia (below 8 g/dl), neutropenia (below $0.5 \times 10^9/1$ and/or chronic thrombocytopenia (below $50 \times 10^9/1$)
Clinical Stage 4
HIV wasting syndrome
Pneumocystis jiroveci pneumonia
Recurrent severe bacterial pneumonia
Chronic herpes simplex infection (orolabial, genital or anorectal of more than 1 month's duration or visceral at any site)
Oesophageal candidiasis (or candidiasis of trachea, bronchi or lungs)
Extrapulmonary tuberculosis
Kaposi sarcoma
Cytomegalovirus disease (retinitis or infection of other organs, excluding liver, spleen and lymph nodes)
Central nervous system toxoplasmosis
HIV encephalopathy"
Extrapulmonary cryptococcosis including meningitis
Disseminated non-tuberculous mycobacteria infection
Progressive multifocal leukoencephalopathy

SURGERY

116. Ans. d. Spinal cord injury without....

[Ref: Sabiston 19th / 441]

"Vertebral & spinal cord injury in trauma patient: A small group of patients will have ***spinal cord injury without radiographic abnormality (SCIWORA)***. Originally described in pediatric patients, SCIWORA is now seen more frequently in adults. The use of magnetic resonance imaging (MRI) in these patients will reveal the cause of the injury in many patients"-*Sabiston 19th/441*

"The acronym **SCIWORA (Spinal Cord Injury Without Radiographic Abnormality)** was first developed and introduced by Pang and Wilberger who used it to define "***clinical symptoms of traumatic myelopathy with no radiographic or computed tomographic features of spinal fracture or instability***". SCIWORA is a clinical-radiological condition that mostly affects children. SCIWORA lesions are found mainly in the cervical spine but can also be seen, although much less frequently, in the thoracic or lumbar spine.. With recent advances in neuroimaging techniques, especially in magnetic resonance imaging, and with increasing availability of MRI as a diagnostic tool, the overall detection rate of SCIWORA has significantly improved"

117. Ans. c. Staging is different...

[Ref: L & B 26th/819; Manipal Surgery 4th/419;Schwartz 9th/468]

"Male breast cancers tends to ***more advanced at time of presentation*** *because of less subcutaneous fat" (Manipal Surgery 4th/419)*

Carcinoma of the Male Breast

◈ *L & B 26th/819*

- Carcinoma of the male breast accounts for less than 0.5 per cent of all cases of breast cancer. The known predisposing causes include ***gynaecomastia and excess endogenous or exogenous oestrogen***.
- As in the female, it tends to present as a lump and is ***most commonly an infiltrating ductal carcinoma.***
- ***Stage for stage the treatment is the same as for carcinoma in the female breast*** and prognosis depends upon stage at presentation.
- Adequate local excision, because of the small size of the breast, should always be with a 'mastectomy'.

Male Breast Cancer

◈ *Schwartz 9th/468*

- Less than 1% of all breast cancers occur in men. Male breast cancer is preceded by gynecomastia in 20% of men.
- It is associated with ***radiation exposure, estrogen therapy, testicular feminizing syndromes, and with Klinefelter's syndrome (XXY).***
- Breast cancer is rarely seen in young males and has a peak incidence in the sixth decade of life.
- A firm, nontender mass in the male breast requires investigation. Skin or chest wall fixation is particularly worrisome.

- DCIS makes up less than 15% of male breast cancer, while infiltrating NST makes up more than 85%. Special-type cancers, including infiltrating lobular carcinoma, have occasionally been reported.
- Male breast cancer is ***staged in an identical fashion to female breast cancer***, and, stage by stage, men with breast cancer have the same survival rate as women.
- Overall, men do worse because of the ***advanced stage of their cancer (stage III or IV) at the time of diagnosis***.
- The treatment of male breast cancer is surgical, with the most common procedure being a ***modified radical mastectomy***. Adjuvant radiation therapy is appropriate in cases where there is a high risk for local recurrence.
- Eighty percent of male breast cancers are hormone receptor–positive, and ***adjuvant tamoxifen is considered***.
- ***Systemic chemotherapy*** is considered for men with hormone receptor–negative cancers and for men with large primary tumours, positive nodes & locally advanced disease

118. Ans. b. Radiosen....

[Ref: L & B 26th/768-69; Sabiston 19th/1005-06]

Medullary Carcinoma

◈ *Sabiston 19th/1005-06*

- MCT accounts for 3% to 9% of thyroid cancers & arises from ***parafollicular cell, or C cell***, derived from the neural crest.
- MCT is associated with the ***secretion of a biologic marker, calcitonin***. Excess secretion of calcitonin has been demonstrated to be an effective marker for the presence of MCT. Calcitonin excess is not associated with hypocalcemia.
- Medullary carcinoma can occur in a sporadic form or as part of MEN 2A or 2B. MEN 2A usually has a more favorable long-term outcome than MEN 2B or sporadic MCT does
- In sporadic MCT, the tumors are usually single and have no familial predisposition. The presence of both a mass and an ***elevated calcitonin level*** is virtually diagnostic of MCT, whereas the finding of an elevated basal calcitonin level in the absence of a thyroid mass might require further workup, including repeat basal calcitonin measurement and a calcium-stimulated or gastrin-stimulated test.
- If MCT is suspected, ***serum calcium and urinary catecholamines*** must be determined to evaluate for hyperparathyroidism and possible pheochromocytoma.
- Recommended surgical treatment of MTC is influenced by several factors. First, the clinical course of MTC is usually more aggressive than that of differentiated thyroid cancer, with higher recurrence and mortality rates. Second, ***MTC cells do not take up radioactive iodine, and radiation therapy and chemotherapy are ineffective.*** Third, MTC is multicentric in 90% of patients with the hereditary forms of the disease. Fourth, in patients with palpable disease, more than 70% have nodal metastases. Lastly, the ability to measure postoperative stimulated calcitonin levels has allowed assessment of the adequacy of surgical extirpation. Screening for pheochromocytoma is done before performing thyroid surgery. If patients are found to have evidence of pheochromocytoma, adrenal surgery with perioperative α-blockade precedes other procedures

Medullary Carcinoma

◈ *L & B 26th/768-69*

- These are ***tumours of the parafollicular (C cells)*** derived from the neural crest and not from the cells of the thyroid follicle as are other primary thyroid carcinomas.
- The cells are not unlike those of a carcinoid tumour and there ***is a characteristic amyloid stroma. High levels of serum calcitonin and carcinoembryonic antigen*** are produced by many medullary tumours.
- ***Calcitonin levels fall after resection and rise again with recurrence making it a valuable tumour marker in the follow up of patients with this disease.***
- Diarrhoea is a feature in 30 per cent of cases and this may be due to ***5-hydroxytryptamine or prostaglandins*** produced by the tumour cells.
- Involvement of lymph nodes occurs in 50–60 per cent of cases of medullary carcinoma and blood-borne metastases are common. As would be expected, ***tumours are not TSH dependent and do not take up radioactive iodine.***

119. Ans. a. Intrahepatic..., b. Jaundice..., c. ↑ Serum... e. Surgery...

[Ref: L & B 26th/ 1105-06; Sabiston 19th/1465;Manipal Surgery 4th/582;Schwartz 9th/1119,1440;CSDT 11th/621]

"**Caroli's disease**: *Approx. 33% of affected patients develop* **biliary lithiasis** *& 7% develop cholangiocarcinoma.* ***Rarely, patients can present later in life with complication secondary to portal hypertension.*** *If disease is limited to a single lobe of liver,* ***hepatic resection*** *can be beneficial. Liver resection can be considered in the patients with hepatic decompensation or unresponsive recurrent cholangitis possibly in the patient with a small T1 or T2 cholangiocarcinoma*" (Schwartz 9th/1119)

Caroli's Disease

◈ *CSDT 11th/621*

- It consists of saccular intrahepatic dilatation of the ducts. In some cases, the biliary abnormality is an isolated finding, but more often it is associated with congenital hepatic fibrosis and medullary sponge kidney.
- The latter patients often present in childhood or as young adults ***with complications of portal hypertension***. Others have cholangitis and ***obstructive jaundice(So increased alkaline phosphatase) as initial manifestations***.
- There is no definitive surgical solution to the problem except in rare cases with isolated involvement of one hepatic lobe, where lobectomy is curative. Intermittent antibiotic therapy for cholangitis is the usual regimen.

Caroli's Disease

◈ *L & B 26th/ 1105-06*

- This is ***congenital dilatation of the intrahepatic biliary tree***, which is often complicated by the ***presence of intrahepatic stone formation.*** Presentation may be with abdominal pain or sepsis.
- ***Imaging is usually diagnostic***, with the finding on ultrasound or CT of intrahepatic biliary lakes containing

stones. Biliary stasis and stone formation combine to predispose to biliary sepsis, which may be life-threatening.

- Another well-recognised complication is the ***development of carcinoma.***
- ***No specific treatment is available. Acute infective episodes are treated with antibiotics.***
- Obstructed and septic bile ducts may be ***drained either radiologically or surgically.*** Malignant change within the ductal system results in cholangiocarcinoma, which may be amenable to resection.
- Segmental involvement of the liver by Caroli's disease may be treated by resection of the affected part, although the ductal dilatation is usually diffuse. ***Liver transplantation is a radical but definitive treatment.***

Caroli's Disease (Type V Choledochal Cyst)

Sabiston 19th/1465

- Caroli's disease is ***multifocal dilation of the segmental bile ducts*** that are separated by portions of normal-caliber bile ducts.
- When intrahepatic bile duct cysts are localized, ***hepatic resection with or without biliary reconstruction is the treatment of choice.***
- Treatment of diffuse hepatic involvement is poor, and probably the only effective treatment is **transplantation** in complicated cases

120. Ans. a. Left gastric..., e. Occur at lower....

[Ref: L & B 26th/ 1074-75; Manipal Surgery 4th/538; Harrison 19th/277]

"The **pharynx** extends from the base of the skull down to the inferior border of the cricoid cartilage (around the C6 vertebral level), ***where it becomes continuous with the esophagus***"

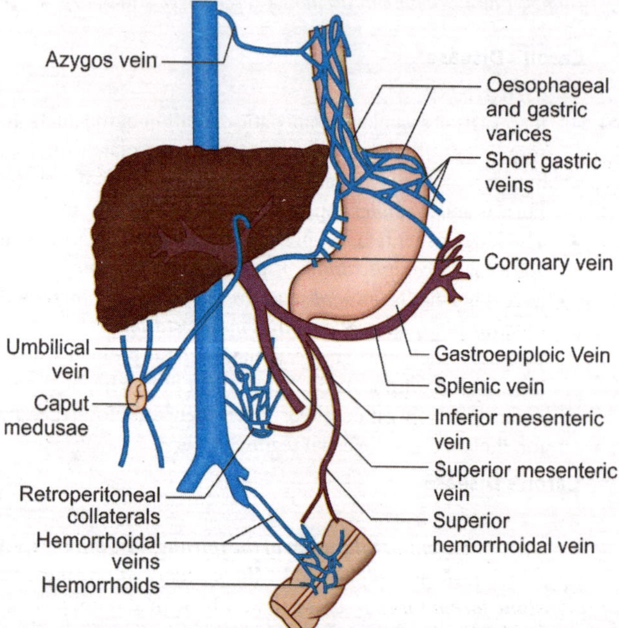

Fig: *(Manipal Surgery 4th/538):* Collaterals

Table *(Manipal Surgery 4th/538)*: **Anastomosis b/w the portal & systemic venous system**

Site	Portal vessels	Systemic vessels	Effect
1. Lower end of oesophagus	Branches of left gastric vein and short gastric vein	Branches from azygos vein	Oesophageal varices
2. Falciform ligament of liver (paraumbilical vein)	Veins which run in the falciform ligament	Anterior abdominal wall veins	Caput medusa*
3. Lower end of rectum	Superior haemorrhoidal vein	Inferior and middle haemorrhoidal vein	Piles (very rare), rectal varices
4. Retroperitoneum mesenteric veins	Branches of superior and inferior subdiaphragmatic veins	Retroperitoneal veins	Retroperitoneal varices (silent)

**Most often, veins which run in the falciform ligament are obliterated from birth. Hence, it is not commonly seen.*

Table *(B.D.C 6th/Vol.II 285)*: **Sites of portocaval/portosystemic anastomoses**

	Portal vein	Systemic vein
Lower end of esophagus	Left gastric	Oesophageal veins

121. Ans. a. Better tole..., c. Diarrhea..., d. High recurr..., e. Operative....

[Ref: L & B 26th/1036-38; Manipal Surgery 4th/473; Schwartz 9th/914-15]

Highly selective vagotomy *(Also called parietal cell vagotomy)*

Manipal Surgery 4th/473

- *In this, vagi are not divided at the trunk. The branch of nerves of Latarjet supplying parietal cell mass are divided.*
- ***Advantage***
  - *More physiological, with minimal disturbances*
  - *No drainage procedure is required because pyloric functions are preserved*
  - *Nerve supply to gallbladder & liver is not disturbed*
  - ***No diarrhea*** *as that can occur in 5-8% of cases of truncal vagotomy which can be morbid*
- ***Disadvantage***
  - *This is not the procedure for prepyloric ulcer as there is a high recurrence rate*

- *Complicated procedure- needs an experienced surgeon*
- ***Recurrence rate: 10-15%***
- *Rare chance of lesser curvature necrosis*

Table *(Schwartz 9th/915)*: **Clinical Results of Surgery for Duodenal Ulcer**

	Parietal Cell Vagotomy	Truncal Vagotomy and Pyloroplasty	Truncal Vagotomy and Antrectomy
Operative mortality rate (%)	0	<1	1
Ulcer recurrence rate (%)	5–15	5–15	<2
Dumping (%)			
Mild	<5	10	10–15
Severe	0	1	1–2
Diarrhea (%)			
Mild	<5	25	20
Severe	0	2	1–2

Table *(L & B 26th/1037)*: **Operative mortality, side effects and incidence of recurrence following duodenal ulcer operations**

Operation	Operative mortality (%)	Significant side-effects (%)	Recurrent ulceration (%)
Gastrectomy	1–2	20–40	1–4
Gastroenterostomy alone	<1	10–20	50
Truncal vagotomy and drainage	<1	10–20	2–7
Selective vagotomy and drainage	<1	10–20	5–10
Highly selective vagotomy	<0.2	< 5	2–10
Truncal vagotomy and antrectomy	1	10–20	1

Highly Selective Vagotomy

◈ *Schwartz 9th/914-15*

- Highly selective vagotomy (HSV), also called ***parietal cell vagotomy or proximal gastric vagotomy***, is safe (*mortality risk <0.5%*) and ***causes minimal side effects.***
- It preserves the vagal innervation to the antrum and pylorus, and the remaining abdominal viscera.
- HSV decreases total gastric acid secretion by about 65 to 75%, which is quite comparable to the reduction seen with truncal vagotomy and acid-suppressive medication. ***Gastric emptying of solids is typically normal*** in patients after parietal cell vagotomy; ***liquid emptying may be normal or increased*** due to decreased compliance associated with loss of receptive relaxation and accommodation.
- When applied to uncomplicated duodenal ulcer, the ***recurrence rate is higher with HSV than with vagotomy*** and antrectomy.
- HSV has not performed particularly well as a treatment for type II (gastric and duodenal) and III (prepyloric) gastric ulcer, perhaps ***because of hypergastrinemia caused by gastric outlet obstruction and persistent antral stasis.***

Highly Selective Vagotomy

◈ *L & B 26th/1037*

- In this only the parietal cell mass of the stomach was denervated. This proved to be the ***most satisfactory operation for duodenal ulceration,*** with a ***low incidence of side-effects and acceptable recurrence rates*** when performed to a high technical standard.
- The ***operative mortality rate was lower than any other definitive operation for duodenal ulceration***, in all probability because the gastrointestinal tract was not opened during this procedure.
- The unpleasant effects of surgery were largely avoided, although ***loss of receptive relaxation of the stomach did occur, leading to epigastric fullness and sometimes mild dumping***. However, ***the severe symptoms that are seen after other more destructive gastric operations did not occur.***
- It is often said that recurrent ulceration was the Achilles heel of this operation although, when performed well, ***recurrence was no more common than after truncal vagotomy.*** The *operation disappeared from routine use with the advent of anti-secretory agents and eradication therapy.*

Truncal Vagotomy and Drainage

◈ *L & B 26th/1036-38*

- The principle of the operation is that section of the vagus nerves, which are critically involved in the secretion of gastric acid, reduces the maximal acid output by approximately 50 per cent. Because the vagal nerves are motor to the stomach, denervation of the antropyloroduodenal segment results in ***gastric stasis in a sub- stantial proportion of patients*** on whom truncal vagotomy alone is performed. The most popular **drainage procedure** is the ***Heineke– Mikulicz pyloroplasty***
- The operation of truncal vagotomy and drainage is substantially safer than gastrectomy However, the side effects of surgery are, in fact, little different from those that follow gastrectomy.

122. Ans. a. Superior..., b. Gland can..., c. The presence..., d. Intraoperative...

[Ref: L & B 26th/774; Sabiston 19th/925-934;Nelon 20th/2691;Schwartz 9th/1381-83;CSDT 11th/307-08;Manipal Surgery 4th/363-64]

"There are usually ***four parathyroid glands***, which lie on the posterior surface of the thyroid. Common sites for **ectopic parathyroids** are the ***thyrothymic ligament, superior thyroid poles, tracheoesophageal groove, retroesophageal space, and carotid sheath. The percentage of individuals with supernumerary glands varies in published series from 2.5% to 22%***" *(Sabiston 19th/925)*

Anatomy of Parathyroid Gland

◈ *CSDT 11th/307-08*

- Four parathyroid glands are present in 85% of the population, and ***about 15% have more than four glands.*** Occasionally, one or more may be incorporated into the thyroid gland or thymus and hence are intrathyroidal or mediastinal in location
- The normal parathyroid gland has a ***distinct yellowish-brown color***, is ovoid, tongue-shaped, polypoid, or spherical, and averages 2 × 3 × 7 mm.

Primary Hyperparathyroidism: Operation

◈ *CSDT 11th/313*

- ***At operation, a normal and abnormal parathyroid should be identified on the side of the localized tumor.*** A focal operation can be done in similar patients and the **operation completed** when the ***intraoperative PTH level decreases by more than 50% from the highest pre-removed value 10 minutes after the parathyroid tumor is removed.***
- In over 80% of cases, the parathyroid tumor is found attached to the posterior capsule of the thyroid gland. The parathyroid glands are usually symmetrically placed, and ***lower parathyroid glands are situated anterior to the recurrent laryngeal nerve***, whereas the ***upper parathyroid glands lie posterior to the recurrent laryngeal nerve***
- Care must be taken to avoid bleeding and not to traumatize the parathyroid gland or tumors, ***since color is useful in distinguishing them from surrounding thyroid, thymus, lymph node, and fat.***
- One should attempt to identify four parathyroid glands when a bilateral approach is elected, though there may be more than four or fewer than four.
- ***If a probable parathyroid adenoma is found, it is removed and the diagnosis confirmed by frozen section or by a greater than 50% decrease in PTH.***
- ***The presence of a normal parathyroid gland at operation indicates that the tumor removed is an adenoma rather than parathyroid hyperplasia, since in hyperplasia all the parathyroid glands are involved.*** A compressed rim of ***normal parathyroid tissue is also suggestive of an adenoma.***
- When all parathyroid glands are hyperplastic, the most normal gland should be subtotally resected, leaving a 50 mg remnant, and confirmed histologically before removal of the remaining glands. The upper thymus and perithymic tract should be removed in patients with hyperplasia, because a ***fifth parathyroid gland is present in 15% of cases.***
- The **recurrence rate** of hyperparathyroidism after the removal of a single adenoma in patients with sporadic hyperparathyroidism is ***2% or less.***
- Following removal of a parathyroid adenoma or hyperplastic glands, the ***serum calcium concentration falls to normal or below normal in 24–48 hours.***

Parathyroid Gland

◈ *L & B 26th/774*

- The normal parathyroid gland weighs up to 50 mg with a ***characteristic orange/brown color and mobility*** within the surrounding fat and thymic tissue.
- Most adults have four parathyroid glands but supernumerary glands occur and nests of parathyroid tissue are commonly found in the thymus.

Operation for Primary Hyperparathyroidism

◈ *L & B 26th/774*

- A gamma probe can be used to guide exploration following preoperative injection of technetium-labeled sestamibi. The ***short serum half-life of PTH means that intraoperative measurement can be used to confirm that the source of excess PTH production has been excised.*** This is a more physiological approach than surgical opinion supported by frozen section and is routine in many centres but is not infallible or inexpensive.
- ***Serum levels of PTH are measured pre-incision, pre-removal, 5 minutes after removal and 10 minutes after removal. The assay takes 30 minutes and if the percentage drop is not >50 per cent then further exploration is indicated.***

---

123. Ans. a. Pneumone..., b. Lung..., c. Hemothorax..., e. Diagnosis....

[Ref: L & B 26th/857;CSDT 11th /245;Schwartz 9th/364,562,537,1423]

"**Throracoscopy**: *Used for esophageal & tracheoesophageal fistula repair (Schwartz 9th/1423)*

"**Thoracoscopy or video-assisted thoracoscopic surgery**: ***Pneumonectomy, lobectomy and empyema drainage*** are all possible. ***However, lung biopsy and the treatment of recurrent pneumothorax are the most frequent indications.*** The principal advantage is that a large incision is avoided resulting in less postoperative pain and a more rapid recovery" *(L & B 26th/857)*

"**Hemothorax:** Tube thoracostomy should be performed expeditiously for all hemo- or pneumothoraces. In 85% of cases, tube thoracostomy is the only treatment required. If bleeding is persistent, as noted by continued output from the chest tubes, it is more likely to be from a ***systemic (e.g., intercostal) rather than a pulmonary artery.*** When the rate of bleeding shows a steady trend of greater than 200 mL/h or the total hemorrhagic output exceeds 1500 mL, ***thoracoscopy*** or thoracotomy should usually be performed. The ***trend and rate of thoracic bleeding is probably more important than the absolute numbers in deciding to perform surgical intervention. Thoracoscopy has been shown to be effective in controlling chest tube bleeding in 82% of cases.*** This technique has also been shown to be 90% effective in evacuating retained hemothoraces. In most of these cases, the chest wall is the source of hemorrhage. ***Thoracotomy is required for management of injuries to the lungs, heart, pericardium, and great vessels***" *(CSDT 11th/245)*

Video-Assisted Thoracoscopic Surgery (VATS)

◈ *CSDT 11th/350*

- VATS plays an important role in the ***diagnosis and staging of thoracic malignancies*** (lung cancer, mesothelioma, etc) as well as in the resection of isolated peripheral pulmonary nodules and bullous lung disease. Furthermore, it has been an ***advance in lung biopsy and pleurodesis procedures.***
- However, despite gaining popularity, many thoracic surgeons consider the approach suboptimal for lung cancers.

- Full mediastinal lymph node dissections are not generally obtainable with standard VATS.
- At present VATS is most commonly applied to benign processes, including ***spontaneous pneumothoraces and pleural effusions, as well as for thoracic sympathectomy and thoracic vertebral discectomy.***

124. Ans. a. Mannitol infusion, b. Decompressive craniectomy, c. CT scan, d. Pneumococcal vaccination & e. Antiepileptics

[Ref: L & B 26th/314; Sabiston 19th/1892-95;Schwartz 9th/1522-26; Manipal Surgery 4th/1035-40]

Indications for pneumococcal vaccination: Individuals with ***cerebrospinal fluid leaks*** (trauma or major skull surgery)" *(patient.info/in)*

Measures to reduce the raised ICP: Hyperventilation, use of ***diuretics (furosemide, mannitol), seizure control*** etc" *(Manipal Surgery 4th/1040)*

"**Intracranial hematoma (in head injury)**: *CT scan of head has made the diagnosis easier & more specific" (Manipal Surgery 4th/1038)*

Management of Minor and Mild Head Injury

◈ *L & B 26th/314-15*

- In general, patients without on-going deficits can safely be discharged from the emergency department, provided they meet the certain criteria listed.
- Patients who do not meet all the discharge criteria will need admission for a further period of observation, and in this case it may be more economical to ***perform a CT to allow safe early discharge*** in this group. In the UK, the National Institute for Health and Clinical Excellence (NICE) also recommends CT imaging in patients with a persistent reduced conscious level, focal deficits, suspected fractures or risk factors for intracranial bleed

Management of Head Injuries

◈ *L & B 26th/315*

- Early discharge if NICE criteria are met
- Scalp wounds need closure
- Significant depressed fractures need ***elevating, antibiotics and antiepileptics***
- ***Skull base fractures may be associated with CSF leak.***
- ***Pneumococcus vaccination is valuable,*** but prophylactic antibiotics are not usually indicated

Intracranial Pressure Management

◈ *L & B 26th/318-19*

- Where initial measures fail adequately to control ICP, sedation may be escalated and supplemented with paralysis. External ventricular CSF drainage represents a useful adjunct to physiological compensation.
- ***Mannitol can be administered to control ICP temporarily.***
- ***Decompressive craniectomy*** involves removal of a portion of the skull vault and opening of the underlying dura, so that brain swelling can occur without the pressure increases predicted by the Monro Kellie doctrine. Generally, a ***unilateral or bifrontal decompressive craniectomy*** is performed, with the bone flap placed subcutaneously in the abdomen, then replaced (cranioplasty) weeks or months later.

- An alternative strategy for managing uncontrolled intracranial hypertension is induction of thiopentone coma.

Stage	Measures
Initial	• Head up • Loosen collar • Optimise ventilation (pO_2>11, pCO_2-4.5kPa) • Optimise electrolyte balance (hypertonic fluids if necessary), treat hyperglycemia • Sedation • Seizure control
Intermediate	• (Mannito/furosemide/hyperventilations temporising measures) • Heavy sedation • Paralysis • CSF drainage by insertion of EVD • Cooling (controversial)
Final	• Induction of thiopentone coma • Decompressive craniectoy

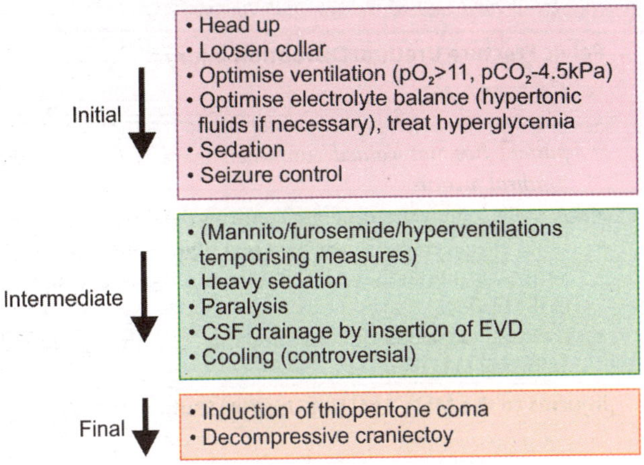

Fig: *(L & B 26th/319):* A hierarchy of intracranial pressure management strategies in ventilated head injury patients. EVD, external ventricular drainage.

Traumatic Brain Injury

◈ *Sabiston 19th/1892-95*

- Traumatic brain injury can be classified into ***primary and secondary injuries.*** Primary injury occurs at impact and is considered first. It includes bone ***fracture, intracranial hemorrhage, and diffuse axonal injury (DAI).*** Fractures of the cranial vault and skull base are indicative of the forces applied to the skull at the time of impact. Fractures of the skull base may be associated with cranial nerve deficit, arterial dissection, and CSF fistula formation.
- Fractures of the cranial vault are classified as follows: open/closed; depressed/nondepressed & linear/comminuted
- ***The CT scan is used to evaluate the presence or absence of fracture, epidural and subdural hematomas, intracerebral hematomas and contusions, shift of the midline structures, and the appearance of the basal and perimesencephalic cisterns.***
- If the ICP remains persistently elevated ***mannitol*** and other diuretic agents may be used.
- Second-tier therapeutic interventions (hypertonic saline, high-dose barbiturate therapy, ***decompressive craniectomy***) may be considered.
- ***Serial CT scans are critical throughout this treatment algorithm, and their use is tailored to the individual patient.***
- Prophylactic use of anticonvulsant drugs (phenytoin, carbamazepine, phenobarbital) is not indicated for the prevention of late post-traumatic seizures. ***Anticonvulsants may, however, be used to prevent early post-traumatic seizures***, primarily in patients at high risk for early seizures who may suffer adverse effects if they were to seize early in their hospital course.

125. Ans. c. Problem..., d. Initial management..., e. Suspect if there...

[Ref: L & B 26th/ 1361-63; Sabiston 19th/2065-66]

Pelvic Fracture Urethral Disruption Injury

◈ *L & B 26th/ 1363*

- Suspect the diagnosis in cases of pelvic fracture, when the ***patient has not voided*** and when there is ***blood at the urethral meatus***
- A water soluble urethrogram confirms the diagnosis
- Initial management is ***insertion of a suprapubic catheter***
- Surgical exploration is needed if there is coexistent rupture of the bladder
- Delayed anastomotic urethroplasty is the preferred definitive Management

Injuries to the Male Anterior Urethra (Bubar Urethra)

◈ *L & B 26th/ 1361-63*

- There is a history of a blow to the perineum, usually due to a ***fall astride injury***. The bulbar urethra is crushed upwards onto the pubic bone, typically with significant bruising.
- In the days of sailing ships, the common cause was ***falling astride a spar***
- The signs of a ruptured bulbar urethra are perineal bruising and haematoma, typically with a butterfly distribution. There is usually ***bleeding from the urethral meatus and retention of urine*** is also typically present.

Urethral Injuries

◈ *Sabiston 19th/2065-66*

- Urethral injuries are associated with 4% to 14% of all pelvic fractures and are more common in cases of bilateral pelvic injuries.
- Diagnosis of urethral injury is made by a ***high index of suspicion in the presence of blood at the urethral meatus, inability to urinate,*** or a palpable full bladder on abdominal examination.
- ***When blood is present at the meatus, retrograde urethrography aids in the diagnosis*** of urethral injury. In the presence of **minor urethral injury**, a ***catheter can be placed*** by an experienced urologist with or without the aid of a cystoscope.
- **Urethral injuries are classified** as those confined to the ***posterior urethra (above the urogenital diaphragm) or the anterior urethra (below the urogenital diaphragm).***
- Realignment of the damaged urethra with a ***stented Foley catheter can lead to either complete healing of the urethral injury or need for future endoscopic treatment of developed urethral strictures.*** If realignment of the damaged urethra cannot be achieved, then ***suprapubic catheterization,*** followed by delayed combined antegrade and retrograde endoscopic repair or open surgical repair, is undertaken.
- In contrast to **posterior urethral injuries,** which are ***often associated with many other pelvic injuries,*** **anterior urethral injuries** are often isolated and associated with ***straddle injuries. The bulbar urethra is typically the site of injury.***
- The best **initial treatment** modality for **anterior urethral injuries** is not well defined; however, most would agree that primary realignment with a ***Foley catheter is the best initial treatment.***
- In cases of severe anterior urethral injury, ***a suprapubic catheter*** may be required, followed by delayed open surgical repair.

126. Ans. a. Often seen..., b. Myoglobin..., d. May cause..., e. May be associated...

[Ref: L & B 26th/ 430; Schwartz 9th/184-85]

Crush Syndrome (Summary Box)

◈ *L & B 26th/ 430*

- *Arises as a result of reperfusion*
- ***Renal failure from myoglobinuria is a complication***
- *A late fasciotomy may make things worse not better*

Crush Injury and Syndrome

◈ *L & B 26th/ 430*

- A crush injury occurs when a body part is subjected to a high degree of force or pressure, usually after being squeezed between two heavy or immobile objects.
- Damage related to a crush injury includes ***lacerations, fractures, bleeding, bruising, compartment syndrome and crush syndrome.***
- The association between ***crush injury, rhabdomyolysis and acute renal failure*** was first reported in victims trapped during the 'London Blitz'. It is seen in ***earthquake*** and mining accident survivors and in battlefield casualties.
- This ***releases myoglobin and vasoactive mediators into the circulation.*** It also sequesters many litres of fluid, reducing the effective intravascular volume and resulting in ***renal vasoconstriction and ischaemia.*** The ***myoglobinuria leads to renal failure from tubular obstruction***
- Alkalinisation of the urine increases the solubility of acid haematin in urine and aids its excretion. This should be continued until myoglobin is no longer detectable in the urine.
- Mannitol administration can reduce the reperfusion component of this injury.
- A **late fasciotomy** when it is obvious that the muscles of that compartment must be dead is only likely to cause a massive release of myoglobin, as well as potentially introducing infection into dead tissue. It therefore best ***not to perform a fasciotomy in cases where entrapment has occurred for over 12 hours.*** Intensive care is required with close attention to fluid balance and renal dialysis if required.

Compartment Syndrome

◈ *L & B 26th/ 430-31*

- A compartment syndrome develops when the pressure within a muscle compartment starts to rise as a result of trauma.
- This normally only occurs in muscles enclosed in a fascia, ***such as the muscles of the calf and forearm, and the intrinsic muscles of the hand and foot.***

- It is *less likely to occur in an open fracture*, as the integrity of the fascial compartment is breached. An overly tight bandage or plaster, haemorrhage from a closed fracture,or severe blunt trauma to the muscle leads to a rise in pressure in the compartment until it exceeds venous drainage pressure.

127. Ans. a. Absent of..., c. Brush border..., d. Cholecystokinin..., e. Pain of gall...

[Ref: L & B 26th/1097-99; Schwartz 9th/1136-40]

"**Gall stone colic:** *It is severe colicky upper abdominal pain felt in right hypochondrium, may shoot to* ***back or between shoulder***" *(Manipal Surgery 4th/556)*

Gallbladder

◈ *Schwartz 9th/1136*

- The gallbladder is lined by a single, highly-folded, tall ***columnar epithelium(covered by microvilli on their luminal surface)*** that contains cholesterol and fat globules. The mucus secreted into the gallbladder originates in the tubuloalveolar glands found in the mucosa lining the infundibulum and neck of the gallbladder, but are absent from the body and fundus.
- The epithelial lining of the gallbladder is supported by a lamina propria. The muscle layer has circular longitudinal and oblique fibers, but without well-developed layers.
- The perimuscular subserosa contains connective tissue, nerves, vessels, lymphatics, and adipocytes. It is covered by the serosa except where the gallbladder is embedded in the liver. ***The gallbladder differs histologically from the rest of the gastrointestinal tract in that it lacks a muscularis mucosa and submucosa***
- **Cholecystokinin (CCK)** is the major physiologic stimulus for ***postprandial gallbladder contraction and relaxation of the sphincter***, but vagal impulses facilitate its action.

Gallbladder

◈ *L & B 26th/1097-99*

- The ***mucous membrane contains indentations of the mucosa that sink into the muscle coat***; these are the crypts of Luschka.
- The gallbladder is a reservoir for bile. During fasting, resistance to flow through the sphincter of Oddi is high, and bile excreted by the liver is diverted to the gallbladder. After feeding, the resistance to flow through the sphincter is reduced, the gallbladder contracts and the bile enters the duodenum. ***These motor responses of the biliary tract are in part effected by the hormone cholecystokinin.***
- Gallstones may remain symptomatic, being detected incidentally as imaging is performed for other symptoms. If symptoms occur, patients typically complain of ***right upper quadrant or epigastric pain, which may radiate to the back.*** This may be described as colicky, but more often is dull and constant.
- **Biliary colic** is typically present in 10–25 per cent of patients. This is described as a severe right upper quadrant pain which ebbs and flows associated with nausea and vomiting. ***Pain may radiate to the chest.***

128. Ans. a. Underdeveloped..., b. Associated..., c. Associated with VACT..., d. Fistula forma.....

[Ref: L & B 26th/ 1242-43; Schwartz 9th/1437-38]

Imperforate Anus

◈ *L & B 26th/ 1242-43*

- Imperforate anus (strictly, it should be anal 'agenesis' or 'atresia') has historically been divided into two main groups – **high and low** – depending on the level of termination of the rectum in relation to the pelvic floor.
- **Treatment and prognosis** are influenced by any ***associated abnormalities of the sacrum and genitourinary systems.***
- In both sexes, ***low defects embrace rectoperineal fistula, covered anus and anal membrane.*** The most frequent defect in boys with imperforate anus is one in which the distal rectum is sited within the puborectalis sling, but terminates as a fistula into the bulbar urethra or prostatic urethra above the main anal sphincter complex.
- ***Boys with a fistula into the bladder neck (a* high defect*)*** have the poorest prognosis because of the ***underdevelopment of the sacrum and pelvic and anal musculature.***
- The most common defect in girls is a rectovestibular fistula, in which the fistula opens into the posterior vestibule (not the vagina)

Anorectal Anomalies (Imperforate Anus)

◈ *Schwartz 9th/1437-38*

- Anomalies of the rectum develop as a result of faulty division of the cloaca into the urogenital sinus and rectum by the urorectal septum. In these anomalies, the ***internal sphincter and striated muscle complex are hypoplastic.*** Therefore, surgical repair results in varying degrees of continence.
- Physical examination of the perineum and imaging studies determine the extent of malformation of the anus or rectum. ***When an orifice is evident at the perineum or distal vagina, the anomaly is referred to as a low imperforate anus***; the absence of an obvious orifice at the perineal level suggests a high imperforate anus.
- In **low anomalies,** the anus may be ectopically placed anterior to its normal position or it may be in the normal position with a narrow outlet due to stenosis or an anal membrane. There may be no opening in the perineum, but the skin at the anal area is heaped up and may extend as a band in the perineal raphe completely covering the anal opening. ***A small fistula*** usually extends from the anus anteriorly to open in the raphe of the perineum, scrotum, or penis in the male or the vulva in the female. These babies often have well-developed ***perineal and gluteal musculature and rarely have sacral vertebral anomalies.***
- In **high anomalies** the rectum may end blindly (10%), but more commonly there is a ***fistula to the urethra or bladder in the male or the upper vagina in the female.*** Patients with high imperforate anus often have ***deficient pelvic and gluteal innervation and musculature, a high incidence of sacral anomalies***, and a ***poor prognosis for continence after surgical repair.*** The most severe of the high deformities is a cloacal anomaly in which there is a common channel

between the poorly developed pelvic structures (urogenital sinus and rectum) with a single perineal opening.

- ***Anomalies of the vertebrae and the urinary tract occur in two-thirds of all patients with high anomalies and in one-third of male patients with low anomalies. Vertebral abnormalities in females invariably indicate a high imperforate anus.***
- ***Associated anomalies occur in up to 70% in those with a high anomaly***. Imperforate anus is associated with the **VACTERL syndrome**. The possible constellation of anomalies includes *esophageal atresia, anomalies of the gastrointestinal tract, hemivertebrae or agenesis of one or more sacral vertebrae (agenesis of S1, S2, or S3 is associated with corresponding neurologic deficits, resulting in neuropathic bladder and greatly impaired continence), genitourinary anomalies (up to 50% incidence with high imperforate anus), and anomalies of the heart and upper limbs/digits.*

129. Ans. a. Alcoholism..., c. Tear involves..., d. Associated..., e. Important....

[Ref: L & B 26th/ 994; Harrison 19th/1891;Sabiston 19th/1167;Schwartz 9th/875-76]

"**Mallory-Weiss syndrome**: This syndrome, characterized by acute upper GI bleeding following vomiting, is considered to be the cause of up to 15% of all severe upper GI bleeds. The mechanism is similar to spontaneous esophageal perforation: ***an acute increase in intra-abdominal pressure against a closed glottis in a patient with a hiatal hernia***" *(Schwartz 9th/876)*

"Esophageal perforation: ***When a hiatal hernia is present and the sphincter remains exposed to abdominal pressure, the lesion produced is usually a Mallory-Weiss mucosal tear***, and bleeding rather than perforation is the problem. This is due to the stretching of the supradiaphragmatic portion of the gastric wall. In this situation, the hernia sac represents an extension of the abdominal cavity, and the GEJ remains exposed to abdominal pressure" *(Schwartz 9th/875)*

Mallory-Weiss tear: Lacerations of the gastroesophageal junction cause 5–10% of cases of upper gastrointestinal bleeding. Many patients report a history of heavy alcohol use or retching. Less than 10% have continued or recurrent bleeding *(CMDT 2016/584)*

"**Mallory-Weiss tears** are mucosal and submucosal tears that occur near the gastroesophageal junction. Classically, these lesions develop in ***alcoholic patients*** after a period of intense retching and vomiting after binge drinking, but they can occur in any patient who has a history of repeated emesis. ***Mallory-Weiss tears account for 5% to 10% of cases of upper GI bleeding***" *(Sabiston 19th/1167)*

Mallory-Weiss Tear

◈ *Harrison 19th/1891*

- A Mallory-Weiss tear is a linear mucosal rent ***near or across the gastroesophageal junction*** that is often associated with retching or vomiting.
- When the tear disrupts a ***submucosal arteriole***, brisk hemorrhage may result.
- Endoscopy is the best method of diagnosis, and an actively bleeding tear can be treated endoscopically with epinephrine injection, coaptive coagulation, band ligation, or hemoclips. Unlike peptic ulcer, a Mallory-Weiss tear with a nonbleeding sentinel clot in its base rarely rebleeds and thus does not necessitate endoscopic therapy.

Mallory–Weiss Syndrome

◈ *L & B 26th/ 994*

- Forceful vomiting may produce a mucosal tear at the cardia rather than a full perforation. The mechanism of injury is different.
- In Mallory– Weiss syndrome, vigorous vomiting produces a ***vertical split in the gastric mucosa, immediately below the squamocolumnar junction at the cardia in 90 per cent of cases.***
- In ***only 10 per cent is the tear in the oesophagus.***
- The condition presents with haematemesis. Usually, the bleeding is not severe, but endoscopic injection therapy may be required for the occasional, severe case.
- Surgery is rarely required.

Mallory-Weiss Syndrome

◈ *CMDT 2016/584*

- It is characterized by a ***nonpenetrating mucosal tear at the gastroesophageal junction*** that is hypothesized to arise from ***events that suddenly raise transabdominal pressure, such as lifting, retching, or vomiting.***
- ***Alcoholism is a strong predisposing factor.***
- Mallory- Weiss tears are responsible for approximately 5% of cases of upper gastrointestinal bleeding.
- Patients usually present with hematemesis with or without melena. A history of retching, vomiting, or straining is obtained in about 50% of cases.
- As with other causes of upper gastrointestinal hemorrhage, upper endoscopy should be performed after the patient has been appropriately resuscitated. The diagnosis is established by identification of a ***0.5- to 4-cm linear mucosal tear usually located either at the gastroesophageal junction or, more commonly, just below the junction in the gastric mucosa.***

"The ***lamina muscularis mucosae*** (or **muscularis mucosae**) is a thin layer (lamina) of muscle of the gastrointestinal tract, located outside the lamina propria mucosae and separating it from the submucosa"

130. Ans. a. Performed in different....

[Ref: Harrison 19th/480-81; Novak's 15th/655-56,1483;CSDT 11th/322; Sabiston 19th/829-30;Schwartz 9th/446-47]

Self-Examination

◈ *CSDT 11th/322*

- Breast self-examination (BSE) has ***not been shown to improve survival.***
- Despite this and despite possible increased biopsy rates, it is a useful technique since many patients do detect their own cancer, and women often feel more in control and proactive by using the procedure.

- Because of the absence of strong evidence supporting the value of BSE, the ***American Cancer Society no longer recommends monthly BSE beginning at age 20 years.***
- The recommendation is that patients be made aware of the potential benefits, limitations, and harms (increased biopsies or false-positive results) associated with BSE. Women who chose to perform BSE should be advised regarding the proper technique.
- ***Premenopausal women should perform the examination 7–8 days after the menstrual period.***
- The breasts should be inspected initially while **standing before a mirror** with the ***hands at the sides, overhead, and pressed firmly on the hips to contract the pectoralis muscles.*** Masses, asymmetry of breasts, and slight dimpling of the skin may become apparent as a result of these maneuvers.
- **Next, in a supine position**, each breast should be ***carefully palpated with the fingers of the opposite hand.***

Breast Self-Examination

◈ *Novak's 15th/655-56*

- There is controversy about recommending breast self-examination (BSE). ***There is no evidence that doing BSE improves survival rates from breast cancer.*** Staunch opponents of BSE argue that it doubles a woman's risk of undergoing a breast biopsy for benign pathology. BSE increases breast health awareness and helps promote early detection of cancer
- Most breast cancers are detected by women themselves (48%), followed by breast imaging (41%), and by physician clinical examination in only 11% . ***Although young women have a low incidence of breast cancer, it is important to teach BSE early so it becomes habitual.***
- The woman should **inspect her breasts** while ***standing or sitting before a mirror***, looking for any asymmetry, skin dimpling, or nipple retraction. ***Elevating her arms over her head*** or pressing her hands against her hips to contract the pectoralis muscles will highlight any skin dimpling.
- Finally, the woman should examine her breasts while ***bending over and leaning forward.***
- While standing or sitting, she should carefully ***palpate her breasts with the fingers of the opposite hand.*** She should lie down and again palpate each quadrant of the breast as well as the axilla using the pads of the three middle fingers with three pressures—light, medium, and deep—covering the entire breast from the clavicle to the inframammary fold, from sternum to latissimus dorsi laterally.
- The area within the **perimeter of the breast** should be ***palpated, preferably using an up-and-down method called vertical stripe***, rather than the concentric circular or radial methods, in which the edges of the breast tissue often are omitted.
- **It is helpful for all women to examine their breasts at the same time each month to develop a routine. Premenopausal women should examine their breasts monthly 7 to 10 days after the onset of the menstrual cycle. For postmenopausal women, selection of a specific calendar date is a helpful way to remember to perform a monthly BSE.**
- Women should be instructed to report any abnormalities or changes to their physicians. If the physician cannot confirm the patient's findings, the examination should be repeated in 1 month or after her next menstrual period.
- ***Monthly breast self-examination (BSE) is no longer recommended*** because there is little evidence to show that BSE is superior to heightened breast awareness such that any new symptoms related to the breast in daily activities would be reported promptly when noticed. BSE was not shown to improve survival.
- Women should be informed about the ***benefits and limitations of*** monthly BSE, mainly the risk of a false-positive result. Women who would still prefer to perform BSE should be instructed in the technique and occasionally have their technique reviewed
- **The following seven "P"s represent the essential components of breast examination:**
  - **Positions**
  - **Palpation**
  - **Pads of fingers for palpation**
  - **Pressure**
  - **Perimeter**
  - **Pattern of search**
  - **Patient education**

Breast Cancer

◈ *Harrison 19th/480*

- Breast self-examination, clinical breast examination by a caregiver, mammography, and magnetic resonance imaging (MRI) have all been variably advocated as useful screening tools.
- ***No study of breast self-examination has shown it to decrease mortality.*** A randomized controlled trial of approximately 266,000 women in China demonstrated ***no difference in breast cancer mortality*** between a group that received intensive breast self-exam instruction and reinforcement/reminders and controls at 10 years of follow-up. However, ***more benign breast lesions were discovered and more breast biopsies were performed in the self-examination arm.***
- Genetic screening for ***BRCA1* and *BRCA2*** mutations and other markers of breast cancer risk has identified a group of women at high risk for breast cancer. Unfortunately, when to begin and the optimal frequency of screening have not been defined.

Table *(Novak's 15th/1483)*: **Screening recommendation for breast cancer**

Bilateral Mammograms
Beginning at age 40 yearly mammograms, which should continue as long as the patient is in good health.
Self-examination
Is an option for women starting in their 20s. Women should be counseled on the benefits and limitation of breast self-examination and should be told to report any changes in their breasts to their health professional right away.

Contd...

Clinical Breast Examination
Age 20-40 examination by physician every 3 years, annually if positive history (May do annually if there is a positive family history) **Age ≥ 40** examination by physician every year
Breast Magnetic Resonance Imaging (MRI)
High risk women (greater than 20% lifetime risk) should undergo MRI and mammography every year **Medium risk women (15%–20 lifetime risk)** should talk to their health care professional about the benefits and limitations of adding MRI to their yearly mammographic screening. **Low risk women (less than 15% lifetime risk)** are not recommended to undergo additional MRI screening.

Table *(Harrison 19th/481)*: **Screening Recommendations for Asymptomatic Subjects not known to be at Increased Risk for the Target Condition**[a]

Cancer Type	Test or Procedure	USPSTF	ACS
Breast	Self-examination	"D"	Women ≥ 20 years: Breast self-exam is an option
	Clinical examination	Women ≥ 40 years: "I" (as a standalone without mammography)	Women 20-39 years: Perform every 3 years Women ≥40 years: Perform annually
	Mammography	Women 40–49 years: The decision should be an individual one, and take patient context/values into account ("C") Women 50–74 years: Every 2 years ("B") Women ≥75 years: "I"	Women ≥40 years: Screen annually for as long as the woman is in good health
	Magnetic resonance imaging (MRI)	"I"	Women with > 20% lifetime risk of breast cancer: Screen with MRI plus mammography annually Women with 15–20% lifetime risk of breast cancer: Discuss option of MRI plus mammography annually Women with <15% lifetime risk of breast cancer: Do not screen annually with MRI

* "B": The USPSTF recommends the service, because there is high certainty that the net benefit is moderate or moderate certainty that the net benefit is moderate to substantial.

** "C": The USPSTF recommends selectively offering or providing this service to individual patients based on professional judgment and patient preferences; there is at least moderate certainty that the net benefit is small.

*** "D": The USPSTF recommends against the service because there is moderate or high certainty that the service has no net benefit or that the harms outweigh the benefits.

****"I": The USPSTF concludes that the current evidence is insufficient to assess the balance of benefits and harms of the service.

OBSTETRICS & GYNAECOLOGY

131. Ans. b. Implan..., c. COC..., e. IUCD....

[Ref: Dutta Obstetrics 8th/ 611; Dutta Gynae 6th/476]

Table *(Dutta Obstetrics 8th/ 611; Dutta Gynae 6th/476)*: **Failure rate of contraceptive methods in first 12 months of use**

Methods	Pregnancy rate per 100 women years (approx.)
No method	*85*
Natural (Calender, temperature, mucus)	*25*
Withdrawl	*27*
Lactational amenorrhoea	*2*
Condom (male)	*15*
Condom (female)	*21*
Diaphragm	*16*
CuT 380A	*0.8*
LNG 20 (IUCD)	*0.1*
Combined oral pills	*0.1*
Progestin only pills	*1*
DMPA & NET injectables	*0.3*
Norplant	*0.05*
Implanon	*0.01*
Vasectomy	*0.15*
Tubectomy	*0.15*

132. Ans. d. More in pelvic..., e. External cephalic...

[Ref: Dutta Obs 8th/434-48; Williams Obs 23rd/527; Normal & Problem Pregnancy by Stevens G. Gabes 6th/396-407]

External Cephalic Version

- *Dutta Obs 8th/440*
- *It has been considered from 36 weeks*
- *Success rate of version is about 65%*
- ***Benefit***
  - *Reduction in the incidence of breech presentation at term.*
  - ***Reduction in the incidence of breech delivery** & associated complication.*

- *Reduction in the incidence of caesarean section by 5%*

*"Breech: **The incidence is about 20% at 28th week & drops to 5% at 34 week & 3-4% at term.** The incidence is expected to be low in hospitals where high parity births are minimal & routine external cephalic version is done in antenatal period" (Dutta Obs 8th/434)*

*"**Breech presentation** occurs in 3% **to 4% of labour overall**, although it is found in 7% of pregnancies at 32 weeks & in 25% of pregnancies of less than 28 weeks duration." (Normal & Problem Pregnancy by Stevens G. Gabes 6th/396)*

Etiology of Breech Presentation

◈ *Dutta's Obstetrics 8th/435; Normal & Problem Pregnancy by Stevens G. Gabes 6th/396*

- ***Prematurity: MC cause***
- *Factor preventing spontaneous version: Breech with extended legs; Twins; Oligohydramnios; **Congenital malformation of uterus such as septate or bicornuate uterus**; Short cord & IUD of the fetus*
- *Favourable adaptation: Hydrocephalous; Placenta previa; **Contracted pelvis** & Cornu-fundal attachment of the placenta*
- *Undue mobility of fetus: Hydramnios & **Multiparae** with lax abdominal wall*
- *Fetal abnormalities: Trisomies 13, 18, 21; Anencephaly & myotonic dystrophy due to alternation of fetal muscular tone & mobility*

Causes of Breech Presentation

◈ *COGDT*

- Breech presentation occurs when spontaneous version to cephalic presentation is prevented as term approaches or if labor and delivery occur prematurely before cephalic version has taken place. Some causes include oligohydramnios, hydramnios, ***uterine anomalies such as bicornuate or septate uterus***, pelvic tumors obstructing the birth canal, abnormal placentation, ***advanced multiparity***, and a ***contracted maternal pelvis.***
- In multiple gestations, each fetus may prevent the other from turning, with a 25% incidence of breech in the first twin, nearly 50% for the second twin, and higher percentages with additional fetuses.
- Additionally, 6% of breech presentations are found to have **congenital malformations**, which include *congenital hip dislocation, hydrocephalus, anencephalus, familial dysautonomia, spina bifida, meningomyelocele, and chromosomal trisomies 13, 18, and 21.* Thus, those conditions that alter fetal muscular tone and mobility increase the likelihood of breech presentation.

133. Ans. a. Metronidazole...., b. Metronidazole..., c. Intravaginal....

[Ref: Harrison 19th/873-75;Shaw's Gynae 16th/385; Dutta Gynae 6th/166; Novak's Gynae 15th/559; William Obstetrics 23rd/226]

Bacterial Vaginosis: Treatment

◈ *Novak's Gynae 15th/559*

- Ideally, treatment of BV should inhibit anaerobes but not vaginal lactobacilli. The following treatments are effective: ***Metronidazole***, an antibiotic with excellent activity against anaerobes but poor activity against lactobacilli, ***is the drug of choice for the treatment of BV***. A dose of 500 mg administered orally twice a day for 7 days should be used.
- Patients should be advised to avoid using alcohol during treatment with oral metronidazole and for 24 hours thereafter. Metronidazole gel, 0.75%, one applicator (5 g) intravaginally once daily for 5 days, may also be prescribed. The overall cure rates range from 75% to 84% with the aforementioned regimens.
- **Clindamycin in** the following regimens is effective in treating BV: Clindamycin ovules, 100 mg, intravaginally once at bedtime for 3 days; Clindamycin bioadhesive cream, 2%, 100 mg intravaginally in a single dose; Clindamycin cream, 2%, one applicator full (5 g) intravaginally at bedtime for 7 days; Clindamycin, 300 mg, orally twice daily for 7 days. Many clinicians prefer intravaginal treatment to avoid systemic side effects such as mild to moderate gastrointestinal upset and unpleasant taste.
- Treatment of the **male sexual partner** does not improve therapeutic response and therefore ***is not recommended***

"The standard dosage of ***oral metronidazole*** for the treatment of bacterial vaginosis is 500 mg twice daily for 7 days. Intravaginal treatment with 2% clindamycin each night for 7 nights) or with 0.75% metronidazole gel twice daily for 5 days is also approved . Other alternatives include ***oral clindamycin*** (300 mg twice daily for 7 days), clindamycin ovules (100 g intravaginally once at bedtime for 3 days), and ***oral tinidazole*** (1 g daily for 5 days or 2 g daily for 3 days)"-Harrison 19th/875

Bacterial Vaginosis: Treatment

◈ *Shaw's Gynae 16th/385*

- *Metronidazole*
- *Ampicillin or cephalosporin is also effective*
- *Tetracycline, doxycycline & sulphafurazole are alternate antibiotics*
- *Clindamycin (cream & oral) & Ornidazole (vaginal)*
- *Lacteal (lactate gel)*

Table *(Harrison 19th/873)*: **Diagnostic Features and Management of Vaginal Infection**

Feature	Normal Vaginal Examination	Vulvovaginal Candidiasis	Trichomonal Vaginitis	Bacterial Vaginosis
Etiology	Uninfected; lactobacilli predominant	Candida albicans	Trichomonas vaginalis	Associated with *Gardnerella vaginalis*, various anaerobic and/or noncultured bacteria, and mycoplasmas
Discharge				

Contd...

Feature	Normal Vaginal Examination	Vulvovaginal Candidiasis	Trichomonal Vaginitis	Bacterial Vaginosis
Amount	Variable; usually scant	Scant	Often profuse	Moderate
Color	Clear or slightly white	White	White or yellow	White or gray
pH of vaginal fluid	Usuall≤4.5	Usually ≤ 4.5	Usually ≥5.0	Usually >4.5
Amine ("fishy") odor with 10% KOH	None	None	May be present	Present
Usual treatment	None	Azole cream, tablet, or suppository—e.g., miconazole 100-mg vaginal suppository or clotrimazole 100-mg vaginal tablet, once daily for 7 days Fluconazole, 150 mg orally (single dose)	Metronidazole or tinidazole, 2 g orally (single dose) Metronidazole, 500 mg PO bid for 7 days	Metronidazole, 500 mg PO bid for 7 days Metronidazole gel, 0.75% Clindamycin, 2% cream, one full applicator vaginally each night for 7 days
Usual management of sexual partner	None	None; topical treatment if candidal dermatitis of penis is detected	Examination for STD; treatment with metronidazole, 2g PO (single dose)	None

134. Ans. a. Return to normal..., b. BP >..., c. Develop beyond..., e. Final diagnosis...,

[Ref: Dutta Obs 8th/276-777; Williams Obs 23rd/707-08]

Gestational Hypertension

◆ *Dutta Obs 8th/276*

- *A **sustained rise of BP to 140/90 mm Hg or more at least two occasions** 4 or more hours apart beyond the 20th week of pregnancy or within the first 48 hours of delivery in a previously normotensive woman is called gestational hypertension*
- *B.P should come down to normal within 12 weeks following deliver*

Gestational Hypertension

◆ *Williams Obs 23rd/707-08*

The diagnosis of gestational hypertension is made in women whose blood pressure ***reaches 140/90 mm Hg or greater for the first time during pregnancy*** but in whom *proteinuria is not identified.*

Gestational hypertension is also called *transient hypertension* if preeclampsia does not develop and the blood pressure has returned to ***normal by 12 weeks' postpartum***.

The final diagnosis that the woman *does not* have gestational hypertension is not made until several weeks after delivery. Thus, ***gestational hypertension is a diagnosis of exclusion***. Importantly, some women with gestational hypertension may later develop other findings of preeclampsia, for example, symptoms such as headaches or epigastric pain, proteinuria, or thrombocytopenia, all of which influence management.

Table *(William's Obs. 23rd/707)*: **Diagnosis of Hypertensive Disorders Complicating Pregnancy (Excluding pre-eclapsia & Eclampsia)**

Gestational Hypertension
BP ≥140/90 mm Hg for first time during pregnancy
No proteinuria
BP returns to normal < 12 weeks' postpartum
Final diagnosis made only postpartum
May have other signs or symptoms of preeclampsia, for example, epigastric discomfort or thrombocytopenia
Superimposed Preeclampsia (on Chronic Hypertension)
New-onset proteinuria ≥300 mg/24 hours in hypertensive women but no proteinuria before 20 weeks' gestation
A sudden increase in proteinuria or blood pressure or platelet count < 100,000/mm3 in women with hypertension and proteinuria before 20 weeks' gestation
Chronic Hypertension
BP ≥140/90 mm Hg before pregnancy or diagnosed before 20 weeks› gestation not attributable to gestational trophoblastic disease OR
Hypertension first diagnosed after 20 weeks' gestation and persistent after 12 weeks' postpartum

135. Ans. c. Primary..., d. Wertheim hysterectomy...,

[Ref: Shaw's Gynae 16th/502; Dutta Gynae 6th/ 351; Novak's Gynae 15th/1317-18; COGDT 10th/848]

Stage Ib, IIA Cervical Cancer

◈ *Dutta Gynae 6th/ 351*

- **Radical hysterectomy,** *pelvic lymphadenectomy (type III) with paraaortic lymph node evaluation.*
- ***External radiation*** *if the nodes are positive OR primary radiation with concomitant platinum based chemotherapy*

Stage Ib, IIA Cervical Cancer

◈ *Shaws 16th/502*

- ***Wertheim's hysterectomy***
- *Schauta vaginal hysterectomy (k/a Mitra operation in India) & Taussig's or laparoscopic lymphadenectomy*
- *Primary radiotherapy*
- *Combined surgery & radiotherapy. Negative sentinel lymph node(obturator gland) avoids pelvic lymphadenectomy*

Concurrent Chemoradiation: Treatment of Choice for *(Dutta's Textbook of Gynaecology 6th/353)*

- Early stage (Ia_2,Ib,IIa) disease after radical hysterectomy
- As a primary treatment for patient with bulky (> 4cm) tumor (stage Ib or IIa)
- Locally advanced stage disease(IIb to IVa) as a primary therapy

Table *(Novak's Gynae 15th/1317)*: **Management of Invasive Cancer of the Cervix**

Stage IA1	≤3 mm invasion, no LVSI	Conization or type I hysterectomy
	≤3 mm invasion, with LVSI	Radical trachelectomy or type II radical hysterectomy with pelvic lymphadenectomy
IA2	>3–5 mm invasion	Radical trachelectomy or type II radical hysterectomy with pelvic lymphadenectomy
IB1	>5 mm invasion, <2cm	Radical trachelectomy or type III radical hysterectomy with pelvic lymphadenectomy
	>5 mm invasion, >2 cm	Type III radical hysterectomy with pelvic lymphadenectomy
IB2		Type III radical hysterectomy with pelvic and para-aortic lymphadenectomy or primary chemoradiation
Stage IIA1, IIA2		Type III radical hysterectomy with pelvic and para-aortic lymphadenectomy or primary chemoradiation
IIB, IIIA, IIIB		Primary chemoradiation
Stage IVA		Primary chemoradiation or primary exenteration
IVB		Primary chemotherapy ± radiation

Contd...

LVSI, lymphovascular space invasion

"**Radical trachelectomy** is a procedure that is ***gaining popularity*** as a surgical management option for women with stage 1A2 and **IB1** disease who desire uterine preservation and fertility. This procedure may be performed vaginally, abdominally, laparoscopically, or robotically, and it usually is accompanied by pelvic lymphadenectomy and cervical cerclage placement" *(Novak's Gynae 15th/1318)*

136. Ans. a. Effective life..., c. Contraindicated..., d. Contraindicated..., e. Useful in controlling...,

[Ref: Dutta Obs 8th/616; Shaw's Gynae 16th/269-70,344; Dutta Gynae 6th/480-,484; Novak's Gynae 15th/224]

"The levonorgestrel-releasing intrauterine system **(LNG-IUS)** may be reasonable treatment for selected women with ***fibroid-associated menorrhagia***" *(Novak's Gynae 15th/450)*
Protection against HIV & STD are provided by barrier method *of contraception(e.g condom, femidom) (Dutta Obs 8th/612)*
*"The **LNG-IUD has an effective life of 10 years**" (Park 23rd/496)*
"**Contraindication of IUD:** *pregnancy, puerperal sepsis, PID or STDs current or within the past 3 month. Infection with HIV is not considered a contraindication for IUD use"-Novak's 15h/224*
"**Mirena:** *It is approved in USA for 5 years of use, although studies through 7 year of use show no loss of efficacy" (Novak's Gynae 15th/222)*
Mirena: *It induces strong & uniform* ***suppression of endometrium.*** *Cervical mucous become very scanty" (Dutta Gynaecology 5th/459)*
Contraindication of LNG-IUS: *Current breast cancer,* severe arterial disease & hepatic tumour or hepatocellular disease" *(Dutta Obs 8th/616)*

MIRENA

◈ *Shaw's Gynae 16th/269, 15th/304-05*

- Total amount of LNG is 52 mg & it is released at the rate of 20 μg/day
- Low pregnancy rate (0.2 per 100women)
- The LNG IUD can be used for at ***least 7 years*** & probably 10 years *(Park 23rd/497)*
- *"LNG IUD device is to be **replaced every 5yr**" (Dutta obs 7th/538)*
- Mirena IUCD is employed to control menorrhagia
- It ***directly suppresses endometrium*** with minimal side effects
- ***It has no action on ovaries*** therefore, estrogen & progesterone level remain normal *(Shaws 15th/304)*
- Mirena IUS thickens the cervical mucus, thins the endometrial lining, and may also alter tubal transport. The Mirena IUS is approved for 5 years of use and can also be used to treat menorrhagia and other menstrual disorders
- **Advantages:** Highly effective at preventing pregnancy, immediately effective after insertion with prompt return of fertility after removal, offers long-term protection. Mirena

A & E

IUS may also reduce menstrual blood loss and ***may decrease risk for endometrial cancer.***

- **Disadvantage:** slightly difficult to insert, take 3 months before it become effective, ***amenorrhoea occur*** in 20-25% which is not desirable in younger women etc

Patient Selection for IUD

◈ *Shaw's 16th/269*

- Low risk of STD
- ***Multiparous women***
- Monogamous relationship

Absolute Contraindication of IUD: *Suspected pregnancy; PID; vaginal bleeding of undiagnosed etiology; cancer of cervix, uterus, adnexia & other pelvic tumour & previous ectopic pregnancy" (Park 23rd/497)*

Relative Contraindication of IUD: *Distortion of uterine cavity due to congenital malformation, fibroids" (Park 23rd/497)*

137. Ans. b. Unexplained..., d. Oligosper..., e. Presence....

[Ref: Shaw's Gynae 16th/260-61; Dutta Gynae 6th/254; Novak's Gynae 15th/1171]

Intracytoplasmic Sperm Injection

◈ *Indications Shaw's Gynae 16th/260-61; Dutta Gynae 6th/254*

- ***Severe oligospermia*** *(5 million sperm/mL)*
- *Asthenopermia, teratospermia*
- ***Presence of sperm antibodies***
- *Obstruction of efferent duct system (male)*
- *Congenital absence of vas (bilateral)*
- *Failure of fertilization in IVF*
- *Fertilisation of cryopreserved oocytes (with hardened zona pellucida)*
- ***Unexplained infertility***

"Müllerian agenesis, also called Mayer- Rokitansky-Küster-Hauser syndrome or **MRKH,** is a congenital malformation characterized by a failure of the Müllerian duct to develop, resulting in a ***missing uterus and variable degrees of vaginal hypoplasia of its upper portion.*** Müllerian agenesis (including absence of the uterus, cervix and/or vagina) is the etiology in ***15% of cases of primary amenorrhoea***"

138. Ans. a. Male factor..., b. Unexplained..., e. Hostile cervical...,

[Ref: Shaw's Gynae 16th/246-47; Dutta Gynae 6th/250; Novak's Gynae 15th/ 1144-45]

"Artificial Insemination **(Intrauterine insemination is the most widely used technique of artificial insemination)** ***has mainly been used to treat unexplained infertility (usually combined with superovulation) & male factor infertility"*** *(Novak's Gynae 15th/ 1144)*

"Artificial Insemination: Involves the placement of whole semen or processed sperm into the female reproductive tract (Vagina, Cervix, Uterus)"

Indication of Artificial Insemination (IUI & Fallopian Tube Sperm Transfer)

◈ *Dutta Gynae 6th/250; Shaw's Gynae 16th/246-47*

- ***Hostile cervical mucus***
- *Cervical stenosis*
- *Oligospermia or asthenospermia*
- *Immune factor (male and female)*
- ***Male factor-*** *impotency or anatomical defect (hypospadias) but normal ejaculate cab be obtained*
- *Unexplained infertility*
- *Chronic medical disorder*
- *HIV-positive male or female*

Intrauterine insemination (IUI)

◈ *Novak's*

- Is the best studied & most widely practiced of all insemination techniques
- It involves placement of about 0.3 to 0.5 ml of washed, processed & concentrated sperm into the intrauterine cavity by transcervical catheterization
- The success rate of IUI is greater than intracervical insemination for unexplained infertility
- The protocol for processing whole semen includes the washing of specimen to remove seminal factors & to isolate pure sperm
- Phosphodiesterase inhibitors such as pentoxyphylline, have been used during semen processing in an attempt to enhance sperm motility, fertilization capacity, & acrosome reactivity for IVF procedures
- ***The IUI pregnancy rates are generally lower in couples with male factor infertility than in couples with unexplained infertility (4.8% versus 11.6%)***[Q]

ALSO KNOW

Indications of in-vitro Fertilization (IVF)

◈ *Shaw's Gynaecology 14th/187*

- *Mild endometriosis*
- *Blocked fallopian tube*
- *Failed intrauterine or fallopian insemination*
- *Immunological factor in male & female*
- *Abnormal semen finding*
- *Idiopathic or unexplained male or female infertility*

139. Ans. b. IUCD failure increase..., c. βhCG rise is not para...

[Ref: Dutta Obs 8th/207-18; Williams Obs 23rd/239-44; Clinical Obstetrics byE. Albert & John C. 3th/162; Fundamentals of Diagnostic Radiology by William E. Brant 2nd /885]

Ectopic is not, more common in primi

"**Nondiagnostic transvaginal USG:** *In many cases, sonography is not diagnostic & subsequent management is based on serial serum* ***βhCG values & repeated sonographic examinations"*** *(Williams Obs 23rd/244)*

"**Ectopic pregnancy:** *The suspicious findings are(1)Lower concentration of βhCG compared to normal pregnancy &(2) doubling time in plasma fails to occur in 2 days" (Dutta Obs 8th/213)*

"Prior tubal damage, either from a ***previous ectopic pregnancy*** *or from tubal surgery to relieve infertility or for sterilization,* ***confers the highest risk for ectopic pregnancy"*** *(William's Obstetrics 23th/238)*

Combined Pills: ↓ Chance of Ectopic

◈ *(Short discussion below)*

"**Progestin only pills & high oestrogen** *preparation* ***increases the chance of tubal pregnancy***[Q]" *(Dutta's Obstetrics 6th/180 & William's Obstetrics 23th/239)*

"**Combined pills** ***reduces incidence of ectopic pregnancy***" *(Shaw's 16th/274)*

"In fact, ***absolute no. of ectopic pregnancy*** *is* ***reduced with any contraceptive****, but in selected* ***contraception failure****, there is increased incidence of ectopic pregnancy" (Dutta's Obstetrics 8th/208)*

Risk Factors of Ectopic Pregnancy

◈ *Dutta Obs 8th/207; Dutta Obstetrics 6th/180*

- ***H/O PID***
- ***History of tubal ligation***
- ***Contraceptive failure (IUCD/Sterilization operation/ progesterone only pills/High estrogen preparations)***
- ***Previous ectopic pregnancy***
- ***Tubal reconstructive surgery***
- ***H/O infertility***
- ***ART (artificial reproductive therapy) particularly if the tubes are patent but damaged.***
- ***IUCD use***
- ***Previous induced abortion***
- ***Tubal endometriosis***

Table *(Williams Obs 23rd/239)*: **Risk factor for Ectopic pregnancy**

Risk Factor	Relative Risk
Previous ectopic pregnancy	*3-13*
Tubal corrective surgery	*4*
Tubal sterilization	*9*
Intrauterine device	*1-4.2*
Documented tubal pathology	*3.8-21*
Infertility	*2.5-3*
Assisted reproductive technology	*2-8*
Previous genital infection	*2-4*
Chlamydia	*2*
Salpingitis	*1.5-6.2*
Smoking	*1.7-4*
Prior abortion	*0.6-3*
Multiple sexual partners	*1.6-3.5*
Prior cesarean delivery	*1-2.1*

Ectopic Pregnancy

- "Serum progesterone level greater than 25 ng/ml is suggestive of viable intrauterine pregnancy whereas level less than 5 ng/ml suggests an ectopic or abnormal intrauterine pregnancy" *(Dutta Obstetrics 7th/183)*
- *Pregnancy test is positive* in 95% of ectopic pregnancy- *(Dutta's Textbook of Obstetrics 6th/186)*
- *"Serial βhCG levels are usually required when the initial ultrasound performed fails to demonstrate either intra- or extrauterine pregnancy. At βhCG levels of approximately 2000 mIU/ml, a viable intrauterine pregnancy should be seen by vaginal ultrasound" (Clinical Obstetrics by E. Albert & John C. 3th/162)*
- *"A intrauterine sac should be visible by TVS when the βhCG levels of approximately 1000 mIU/ml" (COGDT 10th/268)*
- *"The lowest level of βhCG at which gestational sac is consistently visible by TVS is 1500 mIU/mL" (Dutta's Textbook of Obstetrics 6th/186)*
- *"Medical management of ectopics include: methotrexate, potassium chloride, PGF2α, hyperosmolar glucose or actinomycin" (Dutta Obstetrics 7th/186)*

Limitation of βhCG

- *Its inability to distinguish a failing intrauterine pregnancy* from an ectopic pregnancy & the inherent 48 hr delay
- As there is *no definite laboratory level of βhCG permitting distinction b/w an ectopic & intrauterine pregnancy,* a more conservative approach toward interventions in abnormal pregnancies is mandatory *βhCG enzyme immunoassay, with a sensitivity of 25mIU/mL, is an accurate screening test & is positive in virtually all cases of ectopic pregnancy*

---

140. Ans. b. Mifepr..., c. LNG..., d. GnRH..., e. GnRH...

[Ref: Shaw's Gynae 16th/ 399-401; Dutta Gynae 6th/279-81; Novak's Gynae 15th/448-51]

Mifepristone *(RU-486) 10-25 mg daily for 3 month* ***causes amenorrhoea & shrinkage of the tumor by 50%"*** *(Shaw's Gynaecology 14th /323)*

Medical Therapy

◈ *Novak's Gynae 15th/449-50*

- Nonsteroidal anti-inflammatory drugs (NSAIDs) were not shown to be effective for the treatment of menorrhagia in women with fibroids.
- **Treatment with GnRH**-a decreases uterine volume, fibroid volume, and bleeding. However, the benefits of GnRH-a are limited by side effects and risks associated with long-term use
- **Gonadotropin-Releasing Hormone Antagonist** The immediate suppression of endogenous GnRH by daily subcutaneous injection of the GnRH antagonist ganirelix results in a 29% reduction in fibroid volume within 3 weeks
- The **levonorgestrel-releasing intrauterine system (LNG-IUS)** may be reasonable treatment for selected women with fibroid-associated menorrhagia.
- Some studies show that LNG-IUS expulsion rates are higher in women with fibroids than in women without fibroids

Drug used to minimize blood loss in myoma
(Dutta Gynae 6th/280)

- ***Antiprogesterones (Mifepristone)***
- ***Danazol***
- ***GnRH analogs- Agonists (e.g goserelin, luporelin) & antagonists (e.g ganirelix & cetrorelix)***
- ***LNG-IUS***
- ***Prostaglandin synthetase inhibitors***

141. Ans. b. Only women..., e. Both surgical & medical...

[Ref: Reddy 32nd/382;Shaw's Gynae 16th/286-92; Park 23rd/506-07]

Medical Termination of Pregnancy

◈ *Shaw's Gynae 16th/286-92*

- *The Indian act permits the wilful termination of pregnancy before the age of fetal viability (20 weeks gestation) for well defined indication*
- *It has to be **performed by recognized medical practitioners in a recognized place approved by the competent authority under the act***
- *The identity of person is treated as a statutory personal matter*
- *Document to be maintained: Form I, Form II & admission register*
- ***Written consent of woman is needed.** Husband consent is not required. In case of minor girl or lunatic or mentally retarded woman, written consent of her parents or legal guardian I to be taken (Obs by JB Sharma 1st/124)*
- ***Both medical & surgical methods are used.***
- *Surgical methods include-mannual vaccum aspiration, suction evacuation, dilation & evacuation & dilation & curettage*
- *Medical method includes-Mifepristone alone, Mifepristone & misoprostol, methotrexate & misoprostol, Tamoxifen & misoprostol, misoprostol alone etc.*

Medical Termination of Pregnancy

◈ *Reddy 32nd/382*

- ***If the period of pregnancy is below 12 weeks, it can be terminated on opinion of a single doctor***
- ***If the period of pregnancy is between 12 & 20 weeks, two doctors must agree***

142. Ans. a. Available as over, b. LNG alone, 0.75 initially..., c. Ethinyl estradiol..., d. Copper IUD is used....

[Ref: Shaw's Gynae 16th/279; Dutta Gynae 6th/493;Shaw's Textbook of Gynaecology 14th /213; Dutta's Textbook of Obstetrics 6th/549-50; Novak's Gynaecology 14th /283-85; William's Obstetrics 23rd/694]

"*In 2009, US FDA has approved the use of* **progestin only emergency contraception***(called plan B) without a prescription* ***(over the counter)*** *to woman 17 years or older due to efficacy, safety & intent in preventing unwanted adolescent pregnancies" (Obs By JB Sharma 1st/698)*

"**Emergency contraception** *is **now available over the counter (OTC)** but should not be misused. Proper counselling is important. The women should be encouraged to take regular contraceptives & should not use emergency contraceptives too often" (Obs By JB Sharma 1st/698)*

"***Emergency contraception can be achieved by inserting an IUD(not LNG-IUS)*** *within 5 days of unprotected sex) (Obs By JB Sharma 1st/698)*

Levonorgestrel (LNG)

"***LNG alone***^{Q}*, 0.75 initially followed by another 0.75mg 12 hours apart, is more effective than the combination of Ethinyl estradiol (EE) & lower dose LNG & **clearly the emergency contraceptive method of choice at present***^{Q}***. Alternately 2 tablets (1.5 mg) can be taken as a single dose**" (Novak's Gynaecology 14th/ 284 & Shaw's Gynaecology 16th/ 278)*

"The *progestin-only* method uses the progestin **levonorgestrel** in a dose of 1.5 mg, either as two 750 μg doses 12 hours apart, or ***more recently as a single dose within 72 hours of unprotected sex***" *(www.wikipedia.org)*

Danazol

"*An androgen, **danazol (400-600 mg, 2 dose, 12 hr apart, within 72 hr)** has also been used for **emergency contraception**^{Q}. The pregnancy rate was 2% among 998 women" (Novak's Gynaecology 14th /285& Leon Speroff 7th/927)*

Mifepristone

"A ***single dose of oral mifepristone 10 mg within 5 days*** is effective in preventing pregnancy in ***95% cases***" *(Shaw's Gynaecology 14th/214 Novak's Gynaecology 16th /279)*

"***Mifepristone***: The usual **abortifacient dose** is ***200 mg,*** but a **dose of only 10 mg** is ***effective for emergency contraception***" *(Novak's Gynaecology 16th /279)*

"**Postcoital contraception**^{Q}: Recent studies suggest that 600 mg ***mifepristone***^{Q} (RU486), a progesterone receptor antagonist, may be equally as effective as or more effective than hormonal regimens, with fewer side effects. Mifepristone is now available in the United States as Mifeprex, to be used with or without ***misoprostol***^{Q} (synthetic prostaglandin E_1, an off-label indication for this use of misoprostol) *(Harrison 17th/2333-34(Old edition)*

"**Postcoital contraception**: ***mifepristone is available for medical termination of intrauterine pregnancy but is not approved for emergency contraception***" *(Harrison 18th/3039)*

Table: Methods of Emergency Contraception

Regimen	Dose	Time period
Estrogen alone^{Q}		
• Ethinyl estradiol (EE)	2.5 mg BD x 5 days	Within 72 hrs.
• Conjugated estrogen	15 mg BD x 5 days	-do-
Progestogen alone		
• Levonorgestrel (LNG) (Method of choice)	0.75 mg stat then 0.75 mg after 12 hrs or 1.5 mg stat	-do-
Estrogen + Progestogen (Yuzpe method)		
• Oral (EE 50 mg + LNG 0.25 mg)	2 tabs stat F/B 2 tabs after 12 hrs	-do-
• Low dose OCP's	4 tabs stat F/B 4 tabs after 12 hr	
Copper IUD	-	Within 5-7 days
Mifepristone^{Q}	***50-600 mg single dose (Now 10 mg)***	On day 27 of mens. Cycle

143. Ans. a. ↑Minute..., b. ↓Tidal..., d. ↑Blood...,

[Ref: Dutta Obs 8th/58-63; Ajay Yadav 5th/71; Williams Obs 23rd/120]

"**Pregnancy**: *There is **decrease in MAC** (minimum alveolar concentration) so inhalational anaesthetics should be used in lower concentration" (Ajay Yadav 5th/71)*

"Changes in pregnancy: Cardiac output increases by 40%, ***Stroke volume increase by 27%, heart rate increases by 17%, systemic vascular resistance decreases by 21% & pulmonary vascular resistance decreases by 34%***" *(Dutta's Obstetrics 8th/60)*

A & E

Table *(Dutta's Obstetrics 8th/58)*: **Principal blood Changes during pregnancy**

Parameters	Change
Blood Volume (ml)	*+30-40%*
Plasma volume (ml)	*+40-50%*
Red cell volume (ml)	*+20-30%*
Total Hb (g)	*+18-20%*
Hematocrit (whole body)	*Diminished*

Table *(Dutta's Obstetrics 8th/63)*: **Changes in Respiratory system during pregnancy**

Parameters	Changes
Respiration rate/min	Unaffected
Vital capacity	Almost unaltered
Tidal volume	+40%
Residual volume	-20%
Inspiratory capacity	+10%
Minute ventilation	+40%
Total lung capacity	-5%

Table *(William's Obstetrics 23rd/ 120)*: **Hemodyamics Changes during pregnancy**

Pregnant		Postpartum	Change
Mean arterial pressure (mm Hg)	90 ± 6	86 ± 8	No change
Pulmonary capillary wedge pressure (mm Hg)	8 ± 2	6 ± 2	No change
Central venous pressure (mm Hg)	4 ± 3	4 ± 3	No change
Heart rate (beats/min)	83 ± 10	71 ± 10	+ 17%
Cardiac output (L /min)	6.2 ± 1.0	4.3 ± 0.9	+ 43%
Systemic vascular resistance (dyne/sec/cm^{-5})	1210 ± 266	1530 ± 520	—21%
Pulmonary vascular resistance (dyne/sec/cm^{-5})	78 ± 22	119 ± 47	—34%
Serum colloid osmotic pressure (mm Hg)	18.0 ± 1.5	20.8 ± 1.0	—14%
COP–PCWP gradient (mm Hg)	10.5 ± 2.7	14.5 ± 2.5	—28%
Left ventricular stroke work index (g/m/m^2)	48 ± 6	41 ± 8	No change

144. Ans. a. Women of..., b. Women >..., c. Previous thro..., d. Severe hypert....

[Ref: Shaw's Gynae 16th/273-75;Harrison 19th/2391;Katzung 10th/668-670;Dutta's Obstetrics 8th/623]

"**OCP:** *As it cause regular & scanty menstruation, it is* ***useful in menorrhgia*** *& polymenorrhoea. By virtue of non-ovulation, it can* ***relieve dysmenorrhoea*** *& premenstrual tension" (Shaw's 16th/274)*

Table *(Harrison 19th/2391)*: **Oral Contraceptives - Contraindications and Disease Risk**

Contraindications
Absolute
Previous thromboembolic event or stroke
History of an estrogen-dependent tumor
Active liver disease
Pregnancy
Undiagnosed abnormal uterine bleeding
Hypertriglyceridemia
Women over age 35 who smoke heavily (>15 cigarettes per day)
Relative
Hypertension; Women following bariatric surgery
Women receiving anticonvulsant drug therapy
Disease Risks
Increased
Coronary heart disease—increased only in smokers > 35; no relation to progestin type
Hypertension—relative risk 1.8 (current users) and 1.2 (previous users)
Venous thrombosis—relative risk ~4; markedly increased with factor V Leiden or prothrombin-gene mutations
Stroke—increased only in combination with hypertension; unclear relation to migraine headache
Cerebral vein thrombosis—relative risk ~13–15; synergistic with prothrombin-gene mutation
Cervical cancer—relative risk 2–4 Breast cancer- may increase risk in carrier of BRCA1 & possibly BCRA2
Decreased
Ovarian cancer—50% reduction in risk
Endometrial cancer—40% reduction in risk

Table *(Dutta Obstetrics 8th/623)*: **Contraindication of Combined Oral Pills**

Absolute			**Relative**
• **Circulatory disease (past or present)**	• **Disease of the liver**	**Others**	
▪ Arterial or venous thrombosis ▪ Severe hypertension, stroke ▪ Valvular heart disease, Ischaemic heart disease, Angina ▪ Diabetics with vascular complications ▪ Severe hypercholesterolemia ▪ Smoker over age 35 ▪ Focal migraine	▪ ***Active liver disease*** ▪ **Liver adenoma, *carcinoma***	▪ Pregnancy ▪ Undiagnosed genital tract bleeding ▪ Oestrogen dependent neoplasm *e.g.,* breast cancer ▪ Breast feeding(within 6 weeks postpartum) ▪ Major surgery or prolonged immobilization	▪ Age>40 yr ▪ Smoker or <35 year ▪ History of jaundice ▪ Diabetes ▪ Gallbladder disease ▪ Hyperlipidemia ▪ Post breast cancer ▪ Breastfeeding(Postpartum 6wk to 6 month) ▪ Sickle cell disease ▪ CIN

◈ *Park 23th/503: Writes*

- **Absolute**: ***Cancer of the breast and genitals; liver disease; previous history of thromboembolism***; cardiac abnormalities; congenital hyperlipidaemia; undiagnosed abnormal uterine bleeding.
- **Special problems requiring medical surveillance**: Age over 40 years; smoking and age over 35 years; ***mild hypertension***; chronic renal disease; epilepsy; migraine nursing mothers in the first 6 month; diabetes mellitus; gallbladder disease; history of infrequent bleeding, amenorrhoea, etc.
- ***Moderate to severe hypertension is absolute C/I for OCP[Q]. Mild hypertension is relative C/I[Q]*** *(Leon Speroff 7th/906)*

145. Ans. a. Uterine atony.....

[Ref:Dutta Obstetrics 8th/475-76;Obs by JB Sharma 1st/335]

"**Atonic uterus(80%):** Atonicity of uterus is the ***commonest cause*** of postpartum hemorrhage" *(Dutta Obstetrics 8th/475)*

"**Atonic uterus: *Uterine atony* is *most common*** (80% cases) cause of postpartum hemorrhage" *(Obs by JB Sharma 1st/335)*

Primary Postpartum Hemorrhage: Atonic Cause

◈ *Dutta Obstetrics 8th/475-76*

- *Grand multipara*
- *Overdistension of the uterus as in multiple pregnancy, hydramnios & big baby*
- *Uterine fibroid*
- *Placenta: Morbidly adherent placenta (accrete, percreta)*
- *Antepartum haemorrhage (both placenta praevia & abruption)*
- *Prolong labour*
- *Mismanaged 3rd stage* labour

Primary Postpartum Hemorrhage: 2 Types

- Primary PPH- Third stage hemorrhage & true PPH
- Secondary PPH- retained bits of placenta (most common)

146. Ans. a. HPV..., d. Cytolo....

[Ref: Shaw's Gynae 16th/488-89, 89; Dutta Gynae. 6th/111:Harrison 19th/481]

Cervical Cancer Screening

◈ *Shaw's Gynae 16th/488, Dutta Gynae. 6th/111*

- ***All sexually active women should be screened starting from the age of 21 years or after 3 years of vaginal sex with no upper age limits***
- ***Screening should be yearly till the age of 30. Thereafter, it should be done at an interval of every 2-3 years after 3 consecutive yearly negative smears*** *(ACOG 2009)*
- The risk group should be screened with HPV DNA testing combined with cytology. The negative predictive value of one negative HPV DNA test & two negative cytology tests are almost 100%. When both the tests are negative, the screening interval may be increased to 6 years

"In all women with abnormal pap tests showing mild dysplasias, it is ***important to treat any accompanying inflammatory pathology*** & ***repeat the pap test.*** If it persists to be abnormal, consider colposcopic examination & selective biopsies" *(Shaws Gynaecology 16th/488)*

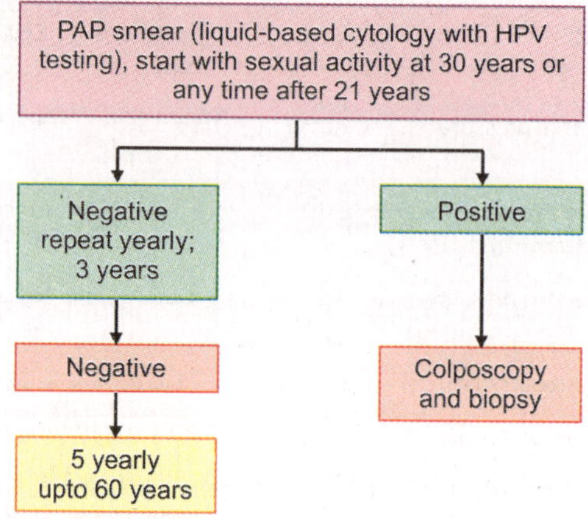

Fig: Cancer cervix screening

Cervical Cancer

◈ *Harrison 19th/480*

- Screening with **Papanicolaou (Pap) smears** decreases cervical cancer mortality. ***The cervical cancer mortality rate has fallen substantially since the widespread use of the Pap smear.***
- Screening guidelines recommend regular Pap testing for all women who have reached the age of 21 (prior to this age, even in individuals that have begun sexual activity, screening may cause more harm than benefit). The recommended interval for Pap screening is 3 years. Screening more frequently adds little benefit but leads to important harms, including unnecessary procedures and overtreatment of transient lesions.

- Beginning at age 30, guidelines also offer the alternative of ***combined Pap smear and HPV testing*** for women.

Table: Screening Recommendations for Asymptomatic Subjects not Known to be at Increased Risk for the Target Condition

Cancer Type	Test or Procedure	USPSTF	ACS
Cervical	Pap test (cytology	Women 21–65 years: Screen every 3 years ("A") Women <21 years: "D" Women >65 years, with adequate, normal prior Pap screenings: "D"	Women 21-29 years: Screen every 3 Years Women 30–65 years: Acceptable approach to screen with cytology every 3 years (see HPV test below) Women <21 years: No screening Women >65 years: No screening following adequate negative prior screening
		Women after total hysterectomy for noncancerous causes: "D"	Women after total hysterectomy for noncancerous causes: Do not screen
	HPV test	Women 30-65 years: Screen in combination with cytology every 5 years if woman desires to lengthen the screening interval (see Pap test, above) ("A")	Women 30–65 years: Preferred approach to screen with HPV and cytology co-testing every 5 years (see Pap test above)
		Women <30 years: "D" Women >65 years, with adequate, normal prior Pap screenings: "D" Women after total hysterectomy for noncancerous causes: "D"	Women <30 years: Do not use HPV testing Women >65 years: No screening following adequate negative prior screening Women after total hysterectomy for noncancerous causes: Do not screen

"A": The USPSTF recommends the service, because there is high certainty that the net benefit is substantial

"D": The USPSTF recommends against the service because there is moderate or high certainty that the service has no net benefit or that the harms outweigh the benefits;

147. Ans. c. Laparoscopy..., d. COC is used....

[Ref: Shaw's Gynae 16th/ 409-19; Dutta Gynae 6th/304-09;Novak's gynae 15th/532-40;Jeffcoate 7th/368-370; COGDT 10th/715]

*"**About 25% of patients with endometriosis have no symptom. Symptoms are not related with extent of lesion.** Even when the endometriosis is widespread, there may not be any symptom; **conversely, there may intense symptoms with minimal endometriosis.** Depth of penetration is more related to symptoms rather than the spread. Lesions penetrating more than 5 mm are responsible for pain, dysmenorrhea & dyspareunia"- (Dutta Gynae 6th/307)*

"USG is not Much Helpful to Diagnosis" *(Dutta Gynae 6th/308)*

Endometriosis

◈ *Shaw's Gynae 16th/ 409-19*

- ***"Laparoscopy is the gold standard in the diagnosis of endometriosis"Laproscopy is the gold standard in diagnosis of endometriosis.*** *It is both diagnostic & therapeutic" (Shaws Gynaecology 16th/ 415)*
- ***Combined oral contraceptives: administered intermittently or continuously, may alleviate the disease***
- GnRH is administered continuously to down regulate & suppress pituitary gonadotropins; it cause atrophy of the endometriotic tissue in 90% cases
- ***Minimal asymptomatic case should be observed over 6-8 months.*** Infertility should be investigated & treated as necessary. All symptomatic women need treatment *(Shaws Gynaecology 16th/ 416)*
- **Treatment options**: ***Expectant management (observation only);*** *Medical therapy (Hormones & other), Surgery (Conservative & Definitive) & Combined (Medical & Surgical)- (Dutta Gynae 6th/310)*

Endometriosis

◈ *Jeffcoate 7th/ 369-370*

- Occurrence of functioning endometrial tissue (both glands + stroma) outside the cavity of uterus.
- ***Age group: 30 -40 years (Most common)***
- Seen in high socio-economic status because of late marriage & late child bearing.
- Most common in nulliparous females
- Familial predisposition (risk is seven times higher if a ***first degree relative has diseases.*** Risk is further increased in homozygous twins).
- It is a hormlome dependant condition (Estrogen dependant)
- **Site:** It can occur anywhere in the body. Most common site is ovary (30-40%, 2nd most common site is pouch of Douglas
- Patients present with a characteristic triad of: ***infertility, Progressively increasing dysmenorrhea & Dyspareunia***

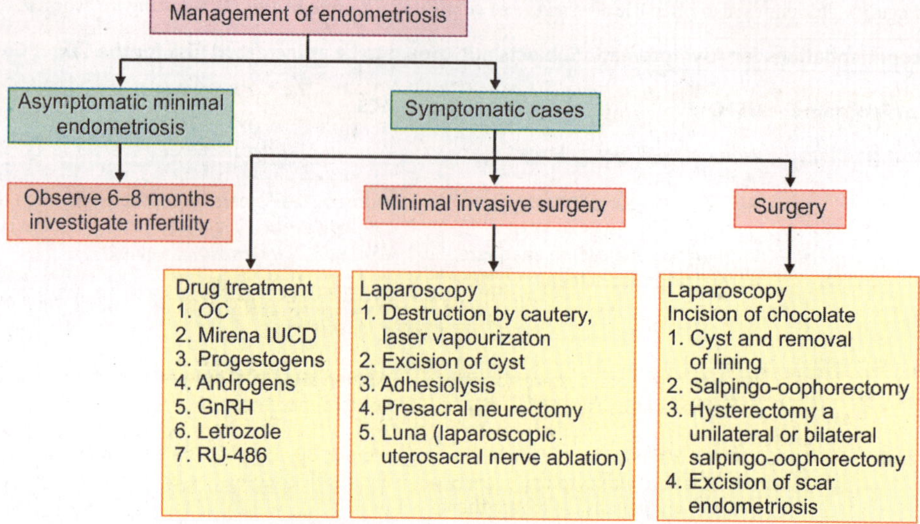

Fig: *(Shaw's Gynae 16th/409):* Management of Endometriosis

PAEDITRICS

148. Ans. a. Fact..., b. Fact..., d. Fact..., e. Fact....

[Ref: O.P.Ghai 8th/116]

"Vit. K carboxylates glutamic acids of translation products of vitamin K-dependent proteins, to produce ϒ-carboxyglutamate. ***Factor II, VII, IX & X are procoagulant proenzymes whereas*** *proteins C & S are anticoagulant proenzymes" (O.P.Ghai 8th/116)*

149. Ans. b. 5-6 mon...

[Ref: O.P.Ghai 8th/49; Nelson 20th/66]

"Child can transfer objects from one hand to other by 6-7 month" *(O.P.Ghai 8th/49)*

"Transfer objects hand to hand in 5.5 months" *(Nelson 20th/66)*

Table *(Nelson 20th/66):* **Developmental Milestones in the First 2 Yr of Life**

Milestone	Average Age of Attainment (Month)
GROSS MOTOR	
Holds head steady while sitting[Q]	2
Pulls to sit, with no head lag	3
Brings hands together in midline	3
Asymmetric tonic neck reflex gone[Q]	4
Sits without support[Q]	6
Rolls back to stomach	6.5
Walks alone[Q]	12
Runs[Q]	16

Contd...

Milestone	Average Age of Attainment (Month)
FINE MOTOR	
Grasps rattle[Q]	3.5
Reaches for objects	4
Palmar grasp gone	4
Transfers object hand to hand[Q]	5.5
Thumb-finger grasp	8
Turns pages of book	12
Scribbles	13
Builds tower of 2 cubes[Q]	15
Builds tower of 6 cubes	22
COMMUNICATION AND LANGUAGE	
Smiles in response to face, voice	1.5
Monosyllabic babble[Q]	6
Inhibits to "no"	7
Follows one-step command with gesture	7
Follows one-step command without gesture	10
Says "mama" or "dada"	10
Points to objects	10
Speaks first real word[Q]	12
Speaks 4-6 words	15
Speaks 10-15 words	18
Speaks 2 word sentences[Q] (e.g., "Mommy shoe")	19

Contd...

Milestone	Average Age of Attainment (Month)
COGNITIVE	
Stares momentarily at spot where object disappeared	2
Stares at own hand	4
Bangs 2 cubes	8
Uncovers toy (after seeing it hidden)	8
Egocentric symbolic play (e.g., pretends to drink from cup)	12
Uses stick to reach toy	17
Pretend play with doll (e.g., gives doll bottle)	17

150. Ans. a. Prem..., c. Hepati..., d. Seps..., e. Polyc...

[Ref: O.P.Ghai 8th/173; Nelson 20th/871-77;Cloherty Manual of Neonatal Care7th/308-11,323]

***Albumin less than 3.0 mg/dl is risk for* hyperbilirubinemia neurotoxicity** *(Cloherty Manual of Neonatal Care7th/322)*

"Hepatitis causes neonatal hyperbilirubinemia" *(Table)- Cloherty Manual of Neonatal Care 7th/309)*

Neonatal Jaundice: Important Cause

◈ *O.P.Ghai 8th/173*

- **Hemolytic**: Rh incompatibility, ABO incompatibility, G^PD deficiency, thalassemias, hereditary spherocytosis
- **Non-Hemolytic**: ***prematurity***, extravasated blood, inadequate feeding, polycythemia, idiopathic, breast milk jaundice

Risk Factor for Development of Severe Hyperbilirubinemia

◈ *O.P.Ghai 8th/173*

- Jaundice observed in the first 24 hr
- Blood group incompatibility with positive direct antiglobulin test, other known hemolytic diseases (*e.g.*, G6PD deficiency)
- ***Gestational age 35-36 week***
- Previous sibling received phototherapy
- Cephalohematoma or significant bruising
- If breastfeeding I inadequate with excessive weight loss

Risk Factor for Hyperbilirubinemia Neurotoxlclty

◈ *Cloherty Manual of Neonatal Care7th/322*

- G6PD deficiency
- Asphyxia
- Sepsis
- Acidosis
- ***Albumin less than 3.0 mg/dl***
- Isoimmune hemolytic disease

Risk Factors

◈ *http://patient.info/in/doctor/neonatal-jaundice-pro*

The risk of developing significant neonatal jaundice is increased in:

- ***Low birth weight: premature and small for dates.***
- Breast-fed babies.
- A previous sibling with neonatal jaundice requiring phototherapy.
- Visible jaundice in the first 24 hours.
- Infants of mothers who have diabetes.
- Male infants.
- East Asians.
- Populations living at high altitudes.

151. Ans. a. Mecon..., b. Jejunal..., c. Ileal..., d. Meckel's...

[Ref: CSDT 11th/1315-20; Nelson 20th/ 1801-02]

"The **primary etiologies of congenital small bowel obstruction** involves abnormalities in anatomic development (***jejunoileal stenosis & atresia***), mucus secretion (***meconium ileus***) & bowel wall innervation (***long-segment Hirschsprung disease***)" *(Nelson 20th/1802)*

"**Meconium ileus** occurs primarily in newborn infants with cystic fibrosis. In simple case, ***the distal 20-30 cm of ileum is collapsed*** & filled with pellets of pale stool" *(Nelson 20th/1802)*

"**Meckel diverticulum** is the ***most common congenital anomaly of GI tract*** & occur in 2-3% of all infants. A typical Meckel diverticulum is a 3-6 cm out pouching of the ileum along the antimesenteric border ***50-75 cm from ileocaecal valve***. Less often, it is ***associated with partial or complete bowel obstruction***" *(Nelson 20th/ 1804-05)*

Intestinal Obstruction in Newborn

◈ *CSDT 11th/1315-20*

- **Proximal GIT obstruction**: esophageal & ***duodenal obstruction***
- **Colonic obstruction:** Hirschrung's disease
- **Congenital duodenal obstruction:** *Atresia, mucosal web, annular pancreas, preduodenal portal vein, & peritoneal band (Ladd's band) from malrotation*
- Atresia of duodenum is twice as common as in jejunum or ileum
- **Meconium ileus-** This usually occur in the ***mid ileum*** buy may develop in the jejunum or colon

ORTHOPAEDICS

152. Ans. b. March...

[Ref: Essential Orthopaedics by Maheshwari 5th/166; Apley Orthopaedics 9th/789-90, 794; radiopaedia.org/articles/hoffa-fracture; http://www.eatonhand.com/dis/dis265.htm]

"March fracture: It is a ***fatigue fracture of shaft of second or third metatarsal***, resulting from long continued or often repeated stress, particularly from prolonged walking or running in those not accustomed to it" *(Essential Orthopaedics by Maheshwari 5th/3,166; Apley 9th/932)*

"***Rolando fracture*** is a three part or comminuted ***intra-articular fracture-dislocation*** of the base of thumb (proximal first metacarpal). It can be thought of as a comminuted *(radiopaedia.org)*

"**Pilon fracture**: *It is a communicated* ***intra-articular fracture*** *of the distal end of the tibia"* (Orthopaedics by Maheshwari 5th/3)

"**Bennett's fracture:** *It is an oblique* ***intra-articular fracture*** *of the base of the first metacarpal with sublaxation of the trapezio-metacarpal joint" (Orthopaedics by Maheshwari 5th/3)*

"***Barton's fracture*** *(Marginal fracture):* ***Intra-articular fractures*** *through the distal articular surface of the radius, taking a margin, anterior or posterior, of the distal radius with the carpals, displaced anteriorly or posteriorly" (Orthopaedics by Maheshwari 5th/3)*

Hoffa fracture is a type of supracondylar distal femoral fracture and is characterised by an associated fracture component in the coronal plane. Hoffa fractures are intra-articular and are characterised by a fracture in the coronal plane- *(radiopaedia.org/articles/hoffa-fracture)*

"**Intraarticular fractures** are those in which the ***break crosses into the surface of a joint***. They always result in *some degree of cartilage damage*. ***Some permanent loss of motion is to be expected and the joint may develop degenerative arthritis as a result of the injury"*** *(eatonhand.com/dis)*

Eponym	Fractures
Monteggai dislocation[Q]	***of the proximal third of ulna with radial head dislocation***[Q]
Galeazzi dislocation[Q]	***of the distal third of the radius with dislocation of the distal radio-ulnar joint***[Q]
Colle's[Q]	***at cortico-cancellous junction of the distal-end of radius with dorsal tilt***[Q]
Bumper[Q]	Comminuted, depressed of the lateral tibial condyle
Pott's[Q]	***Bimalleolar ankle***[Q]
Cotton's	Trimalleolar ankle
Pilon	Comminuted intra-articular of distal tibial end
March	Fatigue of the shaft of 2nd & 3rd metatarsal
Burst	Comminuted of the vertebral body[Q]
Jone's	Avulsion of the base of the 5th metatarsal
Bennet's [Q]	***Oblique intra-articular of the base of the 1***[st] metacarpal[Q]
Night stick fracture[Q]	Isolated fracture of the shaft of the ulna,[Q]
Smith's fracture [Q]	A fracture of distal end of radius at cortico-cancellous junction with ventral tilt and displacements (reverse Colle's)
Barton's fracture[Q]	A vertical, marginal intra-articular fracture of the distal end of radius occurring with volar or dorsal displacement.
Chauffeur fracture[Q]	An intra-articular oblique fracture of the styloid process of the radius[Q]
Boxer's fracture	A fracture through the neck of the 5th metacarpal.

Contd...

Eponym	Fractures
Maisonneuve's fracture [Q]	An ankle fracture associated with spiral fracture of neck of the fibula.
Pilon fracture (Explosion fracture)	A comminuted intra-articular fracture of the distal end of the tibia and fibula.
Aviator's fracture [Q]	Fracture of neck of the talus.
Lisfranc's fracture-dislocation	A fracture dislocation through tarso-metatarsal joints.
Chopart fracture-dislocation	A fracture dislocation through inter-tarsal joints.
Chance fracture (Car seat belt injury)	A horizontal of the vertebra extending from body to the posterior element, caused by a strong distraction force.
Clay-Shoveller fracture[Q]	An avulsion fracture of spinous process of the lower cervical or upper thoracic vertebrae.
Hangman's fracture[Q]	A fracture through the pedicle and lamina of C2 vertebra, with subluxation of C2 over C3-caused by hanging.
Jafferson fracture[Q]	Burst fracture of atlas vertebra.
Straddle fracture	Bilateral superior and inferior pubic rami fractures of the pelvis.
Malgaigne's fracture[Q]	A fracture of pelvis having a combination of ipsilateral fracture of pubic rami anteriorly and sacro-iliac joint disruption posteriorly.
Lefort's fracture	Facio-maxillary fracture.

153. Ans. d. Most.....

[Ref: Essential Orthopaedics by Maheshwari 5th/97-102; Apley Orthopaedics 9th/750, 761, 284; Campbell's Operative Orthopaedics, 11th ed./chap 44]

Supracondylar Fracture of the Humerus

- *Essential Orthopaedics by Maheshwari 5th/97-102*
- This is one of the most serious fracture in ***childhood*** as it is often associated with complications
- Complications are- immediate (occurring at time of fracture), early (occurring within first 2-3 days) & late(occurring weeks to months after the fracture)
- Immediate- ***injury to brachial artery*** & injury to nerve (***median nerve-most common,*** radial nerve-sometime affected)
- Early- *Volkmann's ischemia*
- Late complication- *Malunion (cubitus varus deformity), myositis ossificans & Volkmann's ischemic contracture*
- ***Displacement:*** *The distal fragment may be displaced in the following direction*
  - Posterior or backward shift
  - Posterior or backward tilt
  - Proximal shift
  - Medial or lateral shift
  - Medial tilt
  - Internal rotation

"The ***median nerve*** is the most commonly injured nerve. ***Radial nerve*** is also sometimes affected. Spontaneous recovery occurs in most cases" *(Maheswari 5th/ 101)*

"The ***radial nerve, median nerve (particularly the anterior interosseous branch) or the ulnar nerve*** may be injured" *(Apley 9th/ 761)*

154. Ans. c. Extention deformity.....

[Ref: Essential Orthopaedics by Maheshwari 5th/102-03; Apley Orthopaedics 9th/721-22,418,713]

"**VIC:** *Sometimes the picture is complicated by associated* ***damage to the ulnar or median nerve*** *(or both)*

Volkmann's Ischemic Contracture (VIC)

◈ *Maheshwari 5th/102-03*

- This is a sequel of Volkmann's ischemia
- The ischemic muscle is replaced by fibrous tissue, which contracts & draws the ***wrist & the finger into flexion***
- If peripheral nerves are also affected, there will be ***sensory loss & motor paralysis in the forearm & hand***
- There is marked ***atrophy of forearm with flexion deformity of the wrist & fingers***
- The skin over the forearm & hand is dry & scaly. The nails also show atrophic changes
- Volkmann's sign help in deciding the cause of flexion deformity of the fingers. In this sign, it is possible to extend the finger fully at interphalangeal joints only when the wrist is flexed

Volkmann's Ischemic Contracture (VIC)

◈ *Apley Orthopaedics 9th/721*

- Following arterial injury or compartment syndrome patient may develop ischemic contracture of affected muscle (*Volkmann's ischemic contracture)*
- The site most commonly affected are forearm, hand, leg & foot
- Nerve injured by ischaemia sometimes recover, at least partially; thus the patient presents with deformity & stiffness, but numbness is inconstant
- In a severe case affecting the forearm, there will be wasting of forearm & hand & clawing of the fingers
- The **intrinsic hand muscles fibrose** & shorten, pulling ***the finger into flexion at the metacarpophalangeal joints, but the interphalangeal joints remain straight***
- A pedicle nerve graft, using the proximal segments of the median & ulnar nerves may restore protective sensation in the hand & tendon transfer(wrist extensor to finger & thumb flexor) will allow active grasp

155. Ans. a. Commonly..., b. May involve..., c. Involves...

[Ref: Essential Orthopaedics by Maheshwari 5th/302; Apley Orthopaedics 9th/421-23,418; CSDT 11th/1284-85]

"It is frequently found in the plantar fascia of the instep and occasionally in the penis (***Peyronie's disease***). Dupuytren's contracture manifests itself most commonly in the palm by ***thickening, which may be nodular***, and therefore mistaken for a callosity. Dupuytren's fasciitis may involve any digit or web space, but it ***affects predominantly the ring and small fingers***. The hopelessly contracted ***little finger*** must sometimes be ***amputated***." *(CSDT 11th/1284-85)*

Dupuytren's Contracture

- This is a condition characterised by a flexion deformity of one or more fingers, ***nodular hypertrophy & contracture of superficial palmar fascia (palmar aponeurosis)***
- Occasionally the plantar aponeurosis is also affected
- The condition is inherited as an **autosomal dominant** pattern.
- It is more common in males than females. The prevalence increases with age, but onset at an early stage usually means aggressive disease.
- *"There is a high incidence in epileptics receiving phenytoin therapy; association with diabetes[Q], smoking[Q], alcoholic cirrhosis[Q], AIDS & pulmonary tuberculosis have also been described" - (Apley 8th/343)*
- Fingers are drawn into ***flexion at metacarpo-phalangeal & proximal interphalangeal joints***. The contracture is generally limited to the medial three fingers. *The* ***ring finger is the one affected most commonly.***
- The patient usually a middle aged man, complains of ***nodular thickening in the palm***. Pain may occur but is seldom a marked feature. Often both hands are involved, one more than other. Sometimes the dorsal knuckle pads are thickend **(Garrod's pads)**
- It may be associated with a thickening of plantar fascia or that of the penile fascia **(*Peyronie's disease)***
- Surgery does not cure the disease, it only partially corrects the deformity, & recurrence or extension is common. Surgery is indicated if the deformity is a nuisance or rapidly progressing. Only the thickened part of the fascia is excised (complete fascioctomy is usually unnecessary & fraught with complications)
- ***Amputation is occasionally advisable*** for severe, recurrent disease in the little finger.

156. Ans. a. Sudeck's..., b. Pain is out..., c. Hyperaesthesia..., d. Adults are....

[Ref: Essential Orthopaedics by Maheshwari 5th/51-52; Apley Orthopaedics 9th/261-62]

Complex Regional Pain Syndrome

◈ *Apley Orthopaedics 9th/261-62*

- A number of clinical syndromes appear under this heading, including ***Sudeck's atrophy, reflex sympathetic dystrophy, algodystrophy, shoulder–hand syndrome*** & particularly after a nerve injury-causalgia
- What they have in ***common is pain out of proportion*** (in both intensity & duration) to the precipitating cause, vasomotor instability, trophic skin changes, regional osteoporosis & functional impairment
- ***Precipitating causes are trauma*** (often trivial), ***operation or arthroscopy, a peripheral nerve lesion, myocardial infarction, stroke & hemiplegia***
- ***Adults are the usual sufferers but the condition occasionally occur in children***

- It is now recognized that **multiple mechanisms** are involved: abnormal cytokine release, neurogenic inflammation, ***sympathetic-mediated enhancement of pain responses*** & as yet poorly understood cortical reactions to noxious stimuli
- ***Reflex sympathetic dystrophy (Sudeck's dystrophy):*** *Clinical feature consists of pain, hyperaesthesia, tenderness & swelling. Skin become red, shiny & warm in early stage. Progressive atrophy of skin, muscles & nails occur in later stage. Joint deformities & stiffness ensues- Maheshwari 5th/52*

International Association for the Study of Pain (IASP) CRPS Clinical Diagnostic Criteria

◈ *emedicine.medscape.com*

A **clinical diagnosis of CRPS can be made when the following criteria are met:**

- *Continuing pain that is disproportionate to any inciting event*
- *At least 1 symptom reported in at least 3 of the following categories:*
    - *Sensory: Hyperesthesia or allodynia*
    - *Vasomotor: Temperature asymmetry, skin color changes, skin color asymmetry*
    - *Sudomotor/edema: Edema, sweating changes, or sweating asymmetry*
    - *Motor/trophic: Decreased range of motion, motor dysfunction (e.g., weakness, tremor, dystonia), or trophic changes (e.g., hair, nail, skin)*
- *At least 1 sign at time of evaluation in at least 2 of the following categories:*
    - *Sensory: Evidence of hyperalgesia (to pinprick), allodynia (to light touch, temperature sensation, deep somatic pressure, or joint movement)*
    - *Vasomotor: Evidence of temperature asymmetry (>1°C), skin color changes or asymmetry*
    - *Sudomotor/edema: Evidence of edema, sweating changes, or sweating asymmetry*
    - *Motor/trophic: Evidence of decreased range of motion, motor dysfunction (e.g., weakness, tremor, dystonia), or trophic changes (e.g., hair, nail, skin)*
- *No other diagnosis better explaining the signs and symptoms*

ANAESTHESIA

157. Ans. d. Sodium bicarbonate....

[Ref: Morgan Anaesthesia 5th/1187-90; Ajay Yadav 5th/133-35; Miller 7th/ 1187-89; Lee 13th/ 353; Wylie's Anaesthesia 7th/365, 367]

Malignant Hyperthermia

◈ *Ajay Yadav 5th/133-35*

- It is due to abnormality of ***type I Ryanodine receptor*** which is calcium releasing channel of sarcoplasmic reticulum
- The abnormality leads to excessive accumulation of calcium in sarcoplasmic reticulum which causes sustained contraction of muscle
- It is a genetic disease ***usually autosomal dominant*** but can be recessive also
- Screening/ evaluation of suspected individual: All high risk patient must undergo blood creatinine kinase level. Patients with elevated CK levels in normal resting conditions should be managed as susceptible & does not require further testing.
- Patient with normal CK levels should undergo muscle biopsy studies (where muscle is subjected to ***triggering factors like halothane & suxamethonium***).
- If the biopsy studies are negative then only the patient can be considered non susceptible
- **Treatment of MH**
    - Stop all anaesthetics immediately
    - Hyperventilation with 100% oxygen
    - Control temperature by: ice cooling, ice cold saline
    - Correct acidosis by giving sodium bicarbonate
    - Because ventricular fibrillation is most common cause of death therefore correction of hyperkalemia should be done on priority
    - Maintain urine output
    - **Dantrolene:** It is mainstay of therapy of MH. It directly binds to Ryanodine receptor inhibiting calcium release

Table *(Morgan Anaesthesia 5th/1187)*: **Protocol for immediate treatment of MH**

1. Discontinue volatile anesthetic and succinylcholine. Notify the surgeon. Call for help.
2. Mix dantrolene sodium with sterile distilled water and administer 2.5 mg/kg intravenously as soon as possible.
3. **Administer bicarbonate for metabolic acidosis**
4. Institute cooling measures (lavage, cooling blanket, cold intravenous solutions).
5. **Treat severe hyperkalemia with dextrose, 25-50 g intravenously & regular insulin 10-20 U (adult dose) intravenously**
6. Administer antiarrhythmic agents if needed despite correction of hyperkalemia and acidosis
7. Monitor end-tidal CO_2 tension, electrolytes blood gases, creatine kinase, serum myoglobin, core temperature, urinary output, and color, coagulation status

158. Ans. b. Used to assess..., d. Relieves anxiety..., e. Help in planning....

[Ref: Ajay Yadav 5th/53,194,225; Morgan Anaesthesia 5th/ 296-97; Lee13th/3; Miller Anaesthesia 7th/1001-10]

PAC is equally necessary in infant & children (in fact, even more than adult).

*"**Infants are at much greater risk of anesthetic morbidity & mortality** than older children; risk is generally inversely proportional to age. In addition, pediatric patients are prone to medical illness that require unique surgical & anesthetic strategies"-Morgan Anesthesia 5th/878*

Pre-anaesthetic Checkup (PAC): Goals

◈ *Ajay Yadav 5th/53*

- *To **reduce anxiety & educate the patient about anaesthesia***
- *To obtain information about patient's medical history*
- *To perform physical examination*
- *To determine which test are required*

- *To plan anaesthetic technique*
- To obtain informed consent
- To give any preoperative instructions

"Based on preoperative assessment, the patients are classified ***into six categories*** by American Society of Anesthesiologist(I-VI)" *(Ajay Yadav 5th/53)*

Table *(Miller Anaesthesia 7th/1001- Miller Anaesthesia 7th/1001)*: **Pre-anaesthetic checkup (PAC) or preoperative evaluation:**

1.	The **anesthesia preoperative evaluation** is the clinical foundation and framework of ***perioperative patient management and can potentially reduce operative morbidity and enhance patient outcome***s.
2.	The fundamental purpose of preoperative evaluation is to obtain pertinent information regarding the patient's current and past medical history and to formulate an assessment of the patient's intraoperative risk and requisite clinical optimization.
3.	***Basic and complex medical diseases and syndrome***s that can potentially affect anesthesia perioperative management require the anesthesiologist to be clinically knowledgeable and current in many aspects of internal medicine.
4.	***Patients require preoperative diagnostic and laboratory studie***s that are consistent with their medical history, the proposed surgical procedure, and the potential for intraoperative blood loss. Routine preoperative testing cannot be justified and is costly and clinically inappropriate.
5.	Preoperative patient education and individual discussion ***can significantly reduce patient anxiety and fears of the perioperative anesthesia process***.
6.	**Under the clinical directorship of an anesthesiologis**t, the anesthesia preoperative evaluation clinic can enhance operating room efficiency, decrease day-of-surgery cancellations and delays, reduce hospital costs, and enhance the quality of patient care.
7.	New and updated preoperative evaluation consensus and evidence-based guidelines published by multiple medical specialities have led to evaluation protocols for ***preparing patients for anesthesia and surgery***.
8.	Increasing regulatory and reporting requirements involving preoperative issues by agencies such as the Joint Commission on Accreditation of Healthcare Organizations require awareness and compliance by anesthesiologists.
9.	Information technology and decision support systems in preoperative evaluation can ***enhance the quality of patient care and clinical managemen***t through electronic integration and standardization of patient data.
10.	The anesthesiologist is the perioperative medical specialist and the ***only preoperative evaluation physician who can truly evaluate the risks associated with anesthesia, discuss these risks with the patient, and manage them intraoperativel***y.

Table: ASA Physical Status Classification

ASA PS Classification	Definition
ASA I	A normal healthy patient
ASA II	A patient with mild systemic disease
ASA III	A patient with severe systemic disease
ASA IV	A patient with severe systemic disease that is a constant threat to life
ASA V	A moribund patient who is not expected to survive without the operation
ASA VI	A declared brain-dead patient whose organs are being removed for donor purposes

"E" added to the classification indicates emergency surgery

159. Ans. a. Ringer lactate..., b. Colloid is fluid..., c. 5% Dextrose should...

[Ref: Morgan Anaesthesia 5th/1163-66; Ajay Yadav 5th/12-15; Lee Anaethesia 13th/232-33;Miller 7th/2799]

*"Mild to moderate shock should be treated with crystalloids. **Colloids are only reserved for severe shock** only where maintenance of intravascular volume is vital & where shock becomes moderate switch over to crystalloids as early as possible (as high dose colloids cause clotting inhibition)" (Ajay Yadav 5th/14-14)*

"Blood glucose control: *Hyperglycaemia is known to exacerbate cerebral lactic acidosis* and consequently ***aggravates cerebral ischaemia in head injury***. Therefore ***glucose solutions should be avoided,*** and initially hourly blood sugar monitoring/ insulin infusion implemented to keep blood glucose below 11mmol/L" *(www.nursingtimes.net)*

"Dextrose: Because of the hyperglycemic response associated with ***surgical stress,*** only infants and patients receiving insulin or drugs that interfere with glucose synthesis are at risk for hypoglycemia. Iatrogenic hyperglycemia can limit the effectiveness of fluid resuscitation by inducing an osmotic diuresis and, in animals, ***may aggravate ischemic neurologic injury***. Although associated with worsened outcome after subarachnoid hemorrhage and traumatic brain injury in humans, ***hyperglycemia may also constitute a hormonally mediated response to more severe injury***. In critically ill patients, some evidence suggests that ***tight control of plasma glucose*** (maintenance of plasma glucose between 80 and 110 mg/dL) is associated with ***reduced mortality and morbidity***, but other evidence does not. Evidence also suggests that ***tight glucose control improves outcome in surgical patients*** *(Barash Anaesthesia 6th/Chap 14)*

Normal saline (Iso - 308), Ringer Lactate (Iso – 273), ***DNS (Hyper)****, colloid (Iso) (Morgon 5th/1164)*

"5% dextrose is isotonic" (Ajay Yadav 5th/12)

Ringer Lactate Solution (RL, Hartman Solution)

- *Ajay Yadav 5th/12*
- *Lactate is metabolized to bicarbonate in liver*
- *"Ringer lactate is crystalloid of choice for blood loss replacement"*
- *RL is slightly hypotonic (Osmolality 273 mosmoles/L)*

Normal Saline

◈ *Ajay Yadav 5th/12*

- It is 0.9% NaCl ***isotonic solution***
- ***Na + & Cl⁻ each 154 mEq/L***
- It is preferred over RL for treating: hypochloremic metabolic alkalosis, brain injury (Ca^+ in lactate can increase the neuronal injury) & hyponatremia

Dextrose Normal Saline

◈ *Ajay Yadav 5th/12*

- DNS is ***hypertonic***
- It is best used as maintenance fluid

Hydroxyethyl Starch (Colloid)

◈ *Ajay Yadav 5th/12*

- Two kind of Hydroxyethyl Starches are available- Hexastarch & pentastarch
- Available as 6% & 10% solution. They have prolonged half life & expand plasma effectively for 4 hours
- These solution improve microcirculation & hence improve oxygen delivery to tissue

Table *(Morgan Anaesthesia 5th/1163)*: **Composition of crystalloid solutions**

Solution	Toxicity (mOsml/L)	Na^+ (mEq/L)	Cl^- (mEq/L)	K^+ (mEq/L)	Ca^{2+} (mEq/L)	Mg^{2+} (mEq/L)	Glucose (g/L)	Lactate (mEq/L)	HCO_3^- (mEq/L)	Acetate (mEq/L)	Gluconate (mEq/L)
5% dextrose in water (D_5W)	Hypo (253)						50				
Normal saline (NS)	Iso (308)	154	154								
D_5 ¼NS	Iso (355)	38.5	38.5				50				
D_5 ½ NS	Hyper (432)	77	77				50				
D_5NS	Hyper (586)	154	154				50				
Lactated Ringer's Injection (LR)	Iso (273)	130	109	4	3			28			
D_5LR	Hyper (525)	130	109	4	3		50	28			
½NS	Hypo (154)	77	77								
3%S	Hyper (1026)	513	513								
5%S	Hyper (1710)	855	855								
7.5% $NaHCO_3$	Hyper (1786)	893							893		
Plasmalyte	ISO(294)	140	98	5		3				27	23

SKIN

160. Ans. **a. Lichen..., b. Vitil..., c. Psoria..., e. Dicoid...**

[Ref: Neena Khanna 5th/45; Harrison 19th/347,1269; Roxburg 17th/ 130]

"***Kobner's phenomenon is characteristic of psoriasis,*** but it is also seen in ***lichen planus & dicoid lupus erythematosus***"- *(Roxburg 17th/ 130)*

Koebner's Phenomenon (Isomorphic Phenomenon)

◈ *Neena Khanna 5th/45*

- *New lesion of original disease develops at sites of trauma (scratches, surgical incisions & injury)*
- *This phenomenon is seen in* ***psoriasis, lichen planus, & vitiligo***
- *It indicates active disease*

Pseudo-isomorphic Phenomenon

◈ *Neena Khanna 5th/45*

- *It is due to auto-inoculation & is seen in infections (like* ***plane warts, molluscum contagiosum) & eczema***

"**Kaposi's sarcoma**: Lesions often appear in sun-exposed areas, particularly the tip of the nose, and have a ***propensity to occur in areas of trauma (Koebner phenomenon)***" *(Harriosn 19th/1269)*

Table *(www.dermnetnz.org)*: **Reported conditions exhibiting Koebner phenomenon**

True Koebner response	Psoriasis; Vitiligo; Lichen planus
Pseudo-Koebner response	• Molluscum contagiosum • Pyoderma gangrenosum • Warts
Occasional, localised traumatic lesions	• Behçet disease • Cancer • Darier disease • Erythema multiforme • Granuloma annulare • Hailey-Hailey disease • Kaposi sarcoma • Kyrle disease • Lichen sclerosus • Morphoea • Necrobiosis lipoidica • Pellagra • Perforating folliculitis • Reactive perforating collagenosis

161. Ans. e. Steroids should....

[Ref: Neena Khanna 5th/115-16; www.dermnetnz.org]

Pompholyx

◈ *Neena Khanna 5th/115-16*

Aetiology

- *Unknown*
- *Some patients with pompholyx develop a vesicular palmoplantar eruption on ingestion of minute amount of nickel*

Clinical Features

- *Summer aggravation*
- *Recurrent episodes of* **deep seated, bland (without inflammation) vesicles** *(sometimes blisters)*
- *Each episode self-limiting, but fresh crops of vesicles develop successively, leaving patient symptomatic for long periods*
- *Lesions occasionally get secondarily infected*
- ***Fingers & palms & sometimes soles***

Point for diagnosis: Based on

- Recurrent episode
- Presence of bland vesicles
- Presence on fingers, palms & soles

Treatment

- Saline soaked followed by ***topical steroids***
- *Appropriate antibiotics, if bacterial infection present*

Pompholyx (Dyshidrotic Eczema)

◈ *www.dermnetnz.org*

What is pompholyx?

Pompholyx is a form of ***hand/foot eczema characterised by vesicles or bullae*** **(blisters).** It is a form of vesicular dermatitis of hands and feet, also called vesicular endogenous eczema, and may be the same condition as ***dyshidrotic eczema***. It is sometimes subclassified as cheiropompholyx (***hands***) and pedopompholyx (***feet***).

Who gets pompholyx?

- Pompholyx most often affects young adults.
- It is more common in females than males.
- Many of them report palmoplantar hyperhidrosis.
- There is a personal or family history of atopic eczema in 50%.

What causes pompholyx?

Pompholyx is multifactorial. In many cases it appears to be related to sweating, as flares often occur during hot weather, humid conditions, or following emotional upset. Other contributing factors include:

- Genetics
- Contact with irritants such as water, detergents, solvents and friction
- Association with contact allergy to nickel and other allergens
- Inflammatory dermatophyte (tinea) infections (when it is known as a dermatophytid)
- Adverse reaction to drugs, most often immunoglobulin therapy

What are the clinical features of pompholyx?

Pompholyx presents as recurrent crops of deep-seated blisters on the palms and soles. They cause intense itch and/or a burning sensation. The blisters peel off and the skin then appears red, dry and has painful fissures (cracks).

When involving the distal finger adjacent or proximal to the nail fold, it can result in paronychia (nail fold swelling) and nail dystrophy with irregular pitting and ridges.

What are the complications of pompholyx?

Secondary bacterial infection with Staphylococcus aureus and/or Streptococcus pyogenes is common in pompholyx, and results in pain, swelling and pustules on the hands and feet.

How is pompholyx diagnosed?

- The clinical presentation is typical.
- Suspicious of a fungal infection (tinea pedis), skin scrapings should be taken for mycology.
- Patch testing is indicated in chronic or atypical cases.
- Skin biopsy is rarely necessary. It shows spongiotic eczema.

Aggravating Factors

As in other forms of hand dermatitis, pompholyx is aggravated by contact with irritants such as water, detergents and solvents. Contact with them must be avoided as much as possible and protective gloves worn to prevent additional irritant contact dermatitis.

People with pompholyx that are found to be allergic to nickel must try to avoid touching nickel items.

What is the treatment for pompholyx?

Pompholyx is challenging to treat. Topical therapy is relatively ineffective because of the thick horny layer of skin of palms and soles.

General Measures

- Wet dressings to dry up blisters, using dilute potassium permanganate, aluminium acetate or acetic acid
- Cold packs
- Soothing emollient lotions and creams
- Potent antiperspirants applied to palms and soles at night
- Protective gloves should be worn when doing wet or dirty work
- Well-fitting footwear, with 2 pairs of socks to absorb sweat and reduce friction

Prescription Medicines

- ***Ultrapotent topical corticosteroid creams*** applied to new blisters under occlusion, and ointments applied during the inflamed dry phase
- Short courses of ***systemic corticosteroids***, *e.g.*, prednisone or prednisolone, ***for flare-ups***
- Oral antistaphylococcal antibiotics for secondary infection
- Topical and oral antifungal agents for confirmed dermatophyte infection
- In patients with hyperhidrosis, probanthine or oxybutynin is worth trying.
- In severe cases, immune modulating medicines are indicated. These include: methotrexate, mycophenolate mofetil, azathioprine and ciclosporin.

- Where available, alitretinoin is used for resistant chronic disease.

Other Options

- Superficial radiotherapy
- Botulinum toxin injections (to prevent sweating)
- Phototherapy and photochemotherapy (PUVA) therapy

What is the outlook for pompholyx?

Pompholyx generally gradually subsides and resolves spontaneously. It may recur in hot weather or after a period of stress, and in some patients is recalcitrant.

PSYCHIATRY

162. Ans. e. It has established....

[Ref: Neeraj Ahuja 7th/78,188; Kaplan & Sadock's Synopsis of Psychiatry 11th/983-84; KDT 7th/450]

"Lithium in prophylaxis of bipolar disorder: *Li lengthens the interval between cycles of mood swings: episode of manias well as depression are attenuated, if not totally prevented*" *(KDT 7th/450)*

"Li:Continued treatment prevent cycic mood swing" (KDT 7th/447)

Lithium: Therapeutic indications

◈ *Kaplan & Sadock's Synopsis of Psychiatry 11th/983-84*

- **Manic episodes:** ***Lithium controls acute mania and prevents relapse in about 80 percent of persons with bipolar I disorder*** and in a somewhat smaller percentage of persons with mixed (mania and depression) episodes, rapid-cycling bipolar disorder, or mood changes in encephalopathy
- **Bipolar Depression:** Lithium has been shown to be ***effective in the treatment of depression*** associated with bipolar I disorder, as well as in the role of add-on therapy for patients with severe major depressive disorder
- **Maintenance**: Maintenance treatment with lithium markedly decreases the frequency, severity, and duration of manic and depressive episodes in persons with bipolar I disorder. ***Lithium provides relatively more effective prophylaxis for mania than for depression,*** and supplemental antidepressant strategies may be necessary either intermittently or continuously. Lithium maintenance is **almost always indicated** after ***the first episode of bipolar I disorder, depression or mania***, and should be considered after the first episode for adolescents or for persons who have a family history of bipolar I disorder. Others **who benefit** from lithium maintenance are those who have ***poor support systems, had no precipitating factors for the first episode, have a high suicide risk, had a sudden onset of the first episode, or had a first episode of mania***. Clinical studies have shown that lithium reduces the incidence of suicide in bipolar I disorder patients six fold or seven fold. Lithium is also an effective treatment for persons with severe cyclothymic disorder.
- **Major depressive disorder:** Lithium is effective in the long-term treatment of major depression, but it is not more effective than antidepressant drugs. The most common role for lithium in major depressive disorder is as an adjuvant to antidepressant use in persons who have failed to respond to the antidepressants alone

Lithium: Indications

◈ *Neeraj Ahuja 7th/78*

Established Indications

- ***Treatment of acute mania***
- ***Prophylaxis of bipolar mood disorder***

Possible Clinical Indication

- *Treatment of schizo-affective disorder*
- *Prophylaxis of unipolar mood disorder*
- *Treatment of cyclothymia*
- *Treatment of acute depression (as an adjuvant for refractory depression)*
- *Treatment of chronic alcoholism (in presence of significant depressive symptoms) & psychoactive use disorders (e.g cocaine dependence)*
- *Treatment of impulsive aggression*
- *Treatment of Kleine-Levin syndrome*

Table *(Kaplan11th/983)*: **Psychiatric use of Lithium**

- **Historical**
  - Gouty mania
- **Will established (FDA approved)**
  - Manic episode
  - Maintenance therapy
- **Reasonably well established**
  - Bipolar I disorder
  - Depressive episode
  - Bipolar II disorder
  - Rapid-cycling bipolar I disorder
  - Cyclothymic disorder
  - Major depressive disorder
  - Acute depression (as an augmenting agent)
  - Maintenance therapy
  - Schizoaffective disorder
- **Evidence of benefit in particular groups**
  - Schizophrenia
  - Aggression (episodic), explosive behavior, and self-mutilation
  - Conduct disorder in children and adolescents
  - Mental retardation
  - Cognitive disorders
  - Prisoners
- **Anecdotal, controversial, unresolved, or doubtful**
  - Alcohol and other substance-related disorders
  - Cocaine abuse
  - Substance-induced mood disorder with manic features
- Obsessive-compulsive disorder
- Phobias
- Posttraumatic stress disorder
- ADHD
- Eating disorders
- Kleine–Levin syndrome

Contd...

- Mental disorders caused by a general medical condition (*e.g.,* mood disorder caused by a general medical condition with manic features)
- Periodic catatonia
- Periodic hypersomnia
- Personality disorders (*e.g.,* antisocial, borderline, emotionally unstable, schizotpypal)
- Premenstrual dysphoric disorder
- Sexual disorders
- Transvestism
- Exhibitionism
- Pathological hypersexuality

163. Ans. d. Schizophre....

[Ref: Neeraj Ahuja 7th/56; Kaplan & Sadock's Synopsis of Psychiatry 11th/202]

Although it can be also found in mania (in mania with psychosis) & autism, but it is characteristic feature of schizophrenia only

"**Neologisms** refer to a new word or condensed combination of several words that is not a true word & is not readily understandable, although sometimes the intended meaning or partial meaning may be apparent" *(Kaplan 11th/202)*

Neologisms are feature of schizophrenia (thought & speech disorder) *(Neeraj Ahuja 7th/56)*

"**Formal thought disorder:** Disturbance in the form of thought rather than the content of thought; thinking characterized by loosened associations, ***neologisms,*** and illogical constructs; thought process is disordered, and the person is defined as psychotic. It is ***characteristic of schizophrenia***" *(Kaplan & Sadock's Synopsis of Psychiatry 11th/1412)*

"**Neologism**: New word or phrase whose derivation cannot be understood; ***often seen in schizophrenia***" *(Kaplan & Sadock's Synopsis of Psychiatry 11th/1415)*

"**Speech: Manic patients** cannot be interrupted while they are speaking, and they are often intrusive nuisances to those around them. Their speech is often disturbed. As the mania gets more intense, speech becomes louder, more rapid, and difficult to interpret. As the activated state increases, their speech is filled with puns, jokes, rhymes, plays on words, and irrelevancies. At a still greater activity level, associations become loosened, the ability to concentrate fades, and flight of ideas, clanging, and ***neologisms appear***. In acute manic excitement, speech can be totally incoherent and indistinguishable from that of a person with schizophrenia" *(Kaplan & Sadock's Synopsis of Psychiatry 11th/367)*

"**Thought:** Disturbances in thinking include ***neologisms***, word salad, circumstantiality, tangentiality, loosening of associations, flight of ideas, clang associations, and blocking. The loss of the ability to appreciate nuances of meaning (abstract thinking) may be an ***early sign of dementia***. Thinking is then described as concrete or literal" *(Kaplan & Sadock's Synopsis of Psychiatry 11th/1343)*

"In psychiatry, the term ***neologism*** is used to describe the use of words that have meaning only to the person who uses them, independent of their common meaning. This tendency is considered ***normal in children***, but in adults it can be a symptom of psychopathy or a thought disorder (indicative of a psychotic mental illness, such as ***schizophrenia***). People with ***autism*** also may create neologisms. Additionally, use of neologisms may be related to aphasia acquired after ***brain damage resulting from a stroke or head injury*** *(wikipedia)*

164. Ans. c. Acute ons...

[Ref: Neeraj Ahuja 7th/62; Kaplan & Sadock's Synopsis of Psychiatry 11th/318]

Table *(Kaplan & Sadock 11th/318 & Ahuja 7th/62)*: **Features Weighting Toward Good to Poor Prognosis in Schizophrenia**

Good Prognosis	Poor Prognosis
Late onset (Onset >35 yr)	Young onset
Short duration (<6months)	***Early onset (<20 yr of age)***
Obvious precipitating factors	No precipitating factors
Acute onset/ Abrupt onset	***Insidious onset***
Good premorbid social, sexual, and work histories	Poor premorbid social, sexual, and work histories
Mood disorder symptoms (especially depressive disorders)	Withdrawn, autistic behavior
Married	Single, divorced, or widowed
Family history of mood disorders	Family history of schizophrenia
Good social support systems	Poor support systems
Positive symptoms	***Negative symptoms***
Presence of precipitating stressor	Neurological signs and symptoms
Catatonic subtype (Paranoid-intermediate prognosis)	History of perinatal trauma
First episode	No remissions in 3 years
Pyknic (fat) body	Many relapses
Female sex	History of assaultiveness
Presence of confusion, perplexity or disorientation in the acute phase	Absence of stressor
Normal cranial CT	Disorganised, simple, undifferentiated or chronic catatonic subtypes
Outpatient treatment	Chronic course(> 2 yr)
Proper treatment & good response to treatment	Absence of depression
	Asthenic (thin) body
	Male sex
	Evidence of ventricular enlargement on cranial CT
	Absence of proper treatment
	Flat or blunted affect

165. Ans. c. Anti-an..., d. Hypno..., e. Benzodi...

[Ref: Neeraj Ahuja 7th/131;KDT 7th/465; Kaplan & Sadock's Synopsis of Psychiatry 11th/949]

Antianxiety Drugs

- *KDT 7th/465*
- *Benzodiazepine: Diazepam, Chlordiazepoxide, Oxazepam, Lorazepam, **Alprazolam***
- Azapirones: Buspirone, Gepirone, Ipsapirone
- Sedative antihistaminic: Hydroxyzine
- β blocker: Propranolol

Table(KDT 7th/465): Benzodiazepines

Hypnotic	Antianxiety	Anticonvulsant
• *Diazepam* • *Flurazepam* • *Nitrazepam* • ***Alprazolam*** • *Temazepam* • *Triazolam*	• *Diazepam* • *Chlordiazepoxide* • *Oxazepam* • *Lorazepam* • ***Alprazolam***	• Diazepam • Lorazepam • Clonazepam • Clobazam

166. Ans. c. False..., d. Bizar..., e. Non-bi....

[Ref: Neeraj Ahuja 7th/83-84; Kaplan & Sadock's Synopsis of Psychiatry 11th/ 202, 330-35]

*"Delusion are **false unshakable beliefs** which are not keeping with patients socio-cultural & educational background" (Neeraj Ahuja 7th/56)*

*"**Non-bizarre** type of delusion is found in delusion disorder whereas **bizarre** type of delusion is found in schizophrenia" (Neeraj Ahuja 7th/83)*

Delusion

- *Kaplan & Sadock's Synopsis of Psychiatry 11th/330-31*
- Delusions are ***false fixed beliefs not in keeping with the culture.***
- They are among the most interesting of psychiatric symptoms because of the great variety of false beliefs that can be held by so many people and because they are so ***difficult to treat.***
- The diagnosis of **delusional disorder** is made when a person exhibits ***nonbizarre delusions*** of at least 1 month's duration that cannot be attributed to other psychiatric disorders.
- **Nonbizarre** means that the delusions must be about situations that can occur in real life, such as being followed, infected, loved at a distance, and so on; that is, they usually have to do with phenomena that, although not real, are nonetheless possible. Several types of delusions may be present and the predominant type is specified when the diagnosis is made.

"Delusions are ***false, fixed ideas*** that are ***not shared by others*** and can be divided into ***bizarre and nonbizarre*** (nonbizarre delusions refer to thought content that is not true but is not out of the realm of possibility). **Common delusions** include ***grandiose, erotomanic, jealous, somatic, and persecutory.*** Paranoia can be closely related to delusional material and can range from "soft" paranoia, such as general suspiciousness, to more severe forms that impact daily functioning." *(Kaplan & Sadock's Synopsis of Psychiatry 11th/ 202)*

The psychiatrist and philosopher Karl Jaspers was the first to define the **three main criteria** for a belief to be considered delusional in his 1913 book *General Psychopathology*. **These criteria** are:

- ***Certainty (held with absolute conviction)***
- ***Incorrigibility (not changeable by compelling counterargument or proof to the contrary)***
- ***Impossibility or falsity of content (implausible, bizarre, or patently untrue)***

Delusions are categorized into **four different groups:** *(www.minddisorders.com)*

- **Bizarre delusion**
- **Non-bizarre delusion**
- **Mood-congruent delusion:** Any delusion with content consistent with either a depressive or manic state, e.g., a depressed person believes that news anchors on television highly disapprove of him, or a person in a manic state might believe she is a powerful deity
- **Mood-neutral delusion:** A delusion that does not relate to the sufferer's emotional state; for example, a belief that an extra limb is growing out of the back of one's head is neutral to either depression or mania

167. Ans. a. Frequency..., c. Originate..., d. Occur most..., e. Voltage is us....

[Ref: Guyton 12th/818-20;Neeraj Ahuja 7th/133-34;Kaplan & Sadock's Synopsis of Psychiatry 11th/ 533-35]

Alpha Waves

- *Guyton 12th/818*
- Alpha waves are ***rhythmical waves*** that occur at ***frequencies between 8 and 13 cycles*** per second and are ***found in the EEGs of almost all normal adults when they are awake and in a quiet, resting state of cerebration.***
- These waves ***occur most intensely in the occipital region*** but can also be recorded from the parietal and frontal regions of the scalp. Their ***voltage is usually about 50 microvolts.*** During deep sleep, the alpha waves disappear
- When the awake person's attention is directed to some specific type of mental activity, the alpha waves are replaced by ***asynchronous, higher-frequency but lower-voltage beta waves.***

"*Alpha waves* are one type of brain waves predominantly originate from the occipital lobe during ***wakeful relaxation with closed eyes.*** Alpha waves are reduced with open eyes, drowsiness and sleep"

Awake EEG

- *Kaplan 11th/ 86*
- The four basic wave forms are alpha, beta, delta, and theta.
- Highly rhythmic **alpha waves** with a ***frequency range of 8 to 1 3 Hz*** constitute the ***dominant brain wave frequency of the normal eyes-closed awake EEG.*** Alpha frequency can be ***increased or decreased by a wide variety of pharmacological, metabolic, or endocrine variables.***
- Frequencies that are faster than the upper 1 3 Hz limit of the alpha rhythm are termed **beta waves**, and they are

not uncommon in normal adult waking EEG studies, particularly over the frontal-central regions.

- **Delta waves (<3.5 Hz)** are not present in the normal waking EEG, but are a prominent feature of *deeper stages of sleep*. The presence of *significant generalized or focal delta waves in the awake EEG is strongly indicative of a pathophysiological process*.
- Waves with a frequency of *4.0 to 7.5 Hz* are collectively referred to as **theta waves.** A small amount of sporadic, arrhythmic, and isolated theta activity can be seen in many normal waking EEG studies, particularly in frontal-temporal regions. Although theta activity is limited in the waking EEG, it is a *prominent feature of the drowsy and sleep tracing*.

Table *(Kaplan 11th/534)*: **Stages of Sleep-Electrophysiological Criteria**

	Electroencephalogram	Electrooculogram	Electromyogram
Wakefulnes	Low-voltage, mixed frequency activity; Alpha (8–13 cps) activity with eyes closed	Eye movements and eye blinks	High tonic activity and voluntary movements
Nonrapid eye movement NREM sleep			
Stage I	Low-voltage, mixed frequency activity; Theta (3–7 cps) activity, vertex sharps waves	Slow eye movements	Tonic activity slightly decreased from wakefulness
Stage II	Low-voltage, mixed frequency background with sleep spindles (12–14 cps bursts) and K complexes (negative sharp wave followed by positive slow wave)	None	Low tonic activity
Stage III	High-amplitude (≥ 75 μV) slow waves (≤ 2 cps) occupying 20 to 50% of epoch	None	Low tonic activity
Stage IV	High-amplitude slow waves occupy >50% of epoch	None	Low tonic activity
REM sleep	Low-voltage, mixed frequency activity; saw-tooth waves, theta activity, and slow alpha activity	REMS	Tonic atonia with phasic twitches

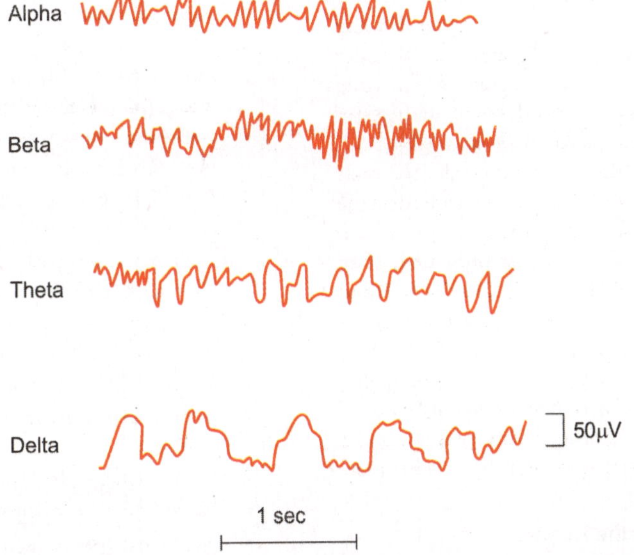

Fig: *(Guyton 12th/818)*: Different types of *brain waves* in the normal electroencephalogram

168. Ans. a. 68Ga-DOTA-TOC, b. MIBG, c. 68Ga-DOTA-NOC, d. F-18 Fluorodopa & e. 68Ga-DOTA-TATE

[Ref: Danhert Radiology Manual 7th/ 1141-42; Review of Radiology by Sumer Sethi 6th/ 34]

Gallium-68 DOTATOC/DOTANOC

- *(Dopamine receptor analogue) Sumer Sethi 6th/ 34*
- *Half life- 68 min*
- *Mode of production – Generator produced*
- *Parent molecule-Germanium 68*
- *Uses: For imaging of neuroendocrine tumors.* ***Higher sensitivity for GI neuroendocrine tumors***

MIBG Scanning useful in

- *Sumer Sethi 6th/ 32*
- ***Pheochromocytoma***
- *Neuroblastoma*
- *Ganglioneuroma*
- *Paraganglioma*

F-18 Fluorodopa: Dopamine analogue

- Uses: The most specific & sensitive agent for imaging of ***neuroendocrine tumors*** especially ***pheochromocytoma*** (adrenal & extra-adrenal) & neuroblastoma
- It has poor sensitivity in case of insulinomas & other G.I. neuroendocrine tumor

"**Somatostatin receptor PET tracers** such as ***[^{68}Ga-DOTA,1-Nal^{3}]-octreotide*** ***(^{68}Ga-DOTANOC)*** and ***[^{68}Ga-DOTA,Tyr^{3}]-octreotate (^{68}Ga-DOTATATE)*** have shown promising results in patients with ***neuroendocrine tumors***, with a higher lesion detection rate than is achieved with ***^{18}F-fluorodihydroxyphenyl-L-alanine*** PET, somatostatin receptor SPECT, CT, or MR imaging. **^{68}Ga-DOTANOC** has high affinity for somatostatin receptor subtypes 2, 3, and 5 ($sst_{2,3,5}$). It has a ***wider receptor binding profile than ^{68}Ga-DOTATATE***, which is sst_2-selective. The wider receptor binding profile ***might be advantageous*** for imaging because **neuroendocrine tumors** express different subtypes of somatostatin receptors" *(jnm.snmjournals.org/content/54/3/364.full)*

"Radiolabeled somatostatin analogs represent valuable tools for both in vivo diagnosis and therapy of **neuroendocrine tumors (NETs)** because of the frequent tumoral overexpression of somatostatin receptors (sst). The **2 compounds most** often used in functional imaging with PET are **^{68}Ga-DOTATATE and ^{68}Ga-DOTATOC**. Both ligands share a quite similar sst binding profile. However, the in vitro affinity of ^{68}Ga-DOTATATE in binding the sst subtype 2 (sst2) is approximately 10-fold higher than that of ^{68}Ga-DOTATOC. ***This difference may affect their efficiency in the detection of NET lesions*** because it is the sst2 that is predominantly overexpressed in NET." *(jnm.snmjournals.org/content/52/12/1864.full)*

Scintigraphy of Neuroendocrine Tumors

- *Danhert Radiology manual 7th/ 1141-42*
- Origin: embryonic neural crest tissue forming ***neuroendocrine cells + neuroendocrine tumors***
- **Location:** *hypothalamus, pituitary gland, thyroid gland, adrenal medulla, GI tract*
- Function: neuroendocrine cells synthesize amines from precursor molecules → decarboxylate amines → polypeptides (= neurotransmitters + hormones); former name: APUD (amine precursor uptake and decarboxylose) cells + APUDomas
- **Radiopharmaceuticals** similar in molecular structure to hormones that tumor synthesize/incorporate into metabolic + cellular processes
- **Somatostatin Analogs** = 14-amino acid peptide that inhibits peptide + hormone synthesis by neuroendocrine cells
- **Octreotide** = **Sandostatin**®= 8-amino acid analog of somatostatin
- **Indium-111 Pentetreotide** = Octreoscan®Indication: pituitary tumor, gastrinoma, paraganglioma, carcinoid, neuroblastoma, small cell lung cancer, pheochromocytoma
- **Guanethidine Analogs** Indications:catecholamine-producing adrenal medullary tumor (intrarenal pheochromocytoma + extraadrenal paraganglioma) and chromaffin cell tumor
- **I-131 Metaiodobenzylguanidine (MIBG)Sensitivity**: 77–100%
- **I-123 Metaiodobenzylguanidine (MIBG)**
- **Glucose Analogs2- (fluorine-18) fluoro-2-deoxy-D-glucose (FDG)**Uptake

169. Ans. a. Piezoelectric...

[Ref: Review of Radiology by Sumer Sethi 6th/ 9-11]

Ultrasonography

- *Sumer Sethi 6th/9-11*
- *Ultrasonic image (sonographic/echographic) is based on mechanical oscillations of the crystal excited by* ***electrical pulses (piezoelectric effect)***
- *Numerous crystals are assembled to form the transducer. A transducer converts one type of energy into another*
- *Based on the pulse-echo principle occurring with ultrasound piezoelectric crystals, ultrasound transducer convert electricity into sound*
- *Crystal- PZT lead zirconate titanate*
- *Frequency- 3-5 MHz (routine abdominal imaging) & 7-10 MHz (for superficial part)*
- *Modes in USG- A mode, B mode & M mode*
- *A mode (Amplitude mode): Opththalmology & orbital biometry*
- *B mode/Gray scale: For all routine application*
- *M mode: Echo cardiography*
- *Advantage: No radiation & portable*
- *Disadvantage: Operator dependence*

MRI: Proton(H+) acts as dipole with ***magnetic dipole movement & gyromagnetic property"*** *(Sumer Sethi 6th/14)*

170. Ans. b. Widened..., c. Straightened..., d. Double....

[Ref: PJM 20th/228; Danhert Radiology manual 5th/575,636-637;Review of Radiology by Sumer Sethi 6th/76-77,80]

***Flask-shaped/Pear-shaped/Leather bottle/Money-bag shaped heart* - Pericardial effusion"** *(Sumer Sethi 6th/76; www.netmedicos.com)*

"**Boot shaped heart** *is found in* ***tetralogy of Fallot*** *(Sumer Sethi 6th/80; Radiology by Samarjit Bhadury 2nd/38)*

Left Atrial Hypertrophy

◈ *PJM 20th/228*

- ***Double atrial shadow*** (Double density seen through right upper border)
- ***Straightened left border***
- ***Left bronchus lifted up with widened carina***
- ***Esophagus curving around the dilated left atrium***
- ***Splaying of mainstem bronchi*** (i.e. ↑ed cardinal angle)
- ***Small aorta (due to decrease of forward cardiac output)***
- Normal/Undersized LV

Left atrial Enlargement

◈ *Dahnert Radiology Review Manual 5th/575*

PA view chest X-ray

- ***Right retrocardiac double density***
- ***>75° splaying of carina with horizontal orientation of distal left mainstream bronchus***
- ***Enlargement of left atrial appendages***

Lateral View

- *Increased convexity of postero-superior cardiac margin*
- *Posterior displacement of left upper lobe bronchus*

X-Ray Findings - Chest

◈ *www.netmedicos.com/?xray_findings_chest*

Heart & Blood Vessels

- ***Flask-shaped/Pear-shaped/Leather bottle/Money-bag shaped heart*** - *Pericardial effusion*
- ***Boot-shaped heart/Coer-en-sabot*** - *Fallot's tetralogy*
- ***Box shaped appearance*** - *Tricuspid atresia*
- ***Jug Handle appearance*** - *Primary pulmonary artery hypertension*
- ***"3" like appearance*** - *Coarctation of Aorta*
- ***Egg on side appearance*** - *Transposition of great vessels*
- ***Egg in cup appearance*** - *Constrictive pericarditis*
- ***Snow-man heart*** - *TAPVC (total anomalous pulmonary venous connection)*
- ***Fig: of '8'*** - *TAPVC (total anomalous pulmonary venous connection)*
- ***Cottage Leaf appearance*** - *TAPVC*
- ***Pericardial calcification*** - *Constrictive pericarditis*
- ***Calcification in heart wall*** - *is seen in - Carcinoid syndrome*
- ***Calcification of ascending aorta*** - *Atherosclerosis, Syphilis*
- ***Hilar dance on fluoroscopy*** - *Atrial Septal Defect*
- *Xray finding in Ebstein's anomaly - Pulmonary oligemia*
- ***Posterior displacement of trachea*** - *seen in - aneurysm of aorta*
- ***Obliteration of left border of heart*** *(PA view of chest) is - suggestive of - Lingular pathology (left lung)*
- ***Bat's wings appearance*** - *Pulmonary oedema*
- ***Pruned tree appearance*** *(of pulmonary circulation) - Pulmonary artery hypertension*

Lungs

- ***Ground glass appearance*** - *Hyaline membrane disease*
- ***Solitary pulmonary mass lesion > 4cms*** - *is most commonly due to - Bronchial adenoma*
- ***Honey Comb appearance*** -
  - Sarcoidosis
  - Histiocytosis X
  - Interstitial lung disease
  - Tuberculosis
  - Collagen disorders
  - Pneumoconiosis
  - **Drugs:** bleomycin, busulphan, melphalan, cyclophosphamide
- ***Meniscus sign/Crescent sign*** *(mobile mass in pulmonary cavity) is most commonly seen in - Aspergilloma (fungal ball lesion)*
- ***Egg-Shell calcification*** - *Silicosis[Q] Sarcoidosis[Q] Coal miner's pneumoconiosis[Q], Lymphoma following radiotherapy[Q]*
- ***Pop-corn calcification/Craggy pop-corn calcification*** - *Pulmonary Hamartoma*
- ***Pleural calcification*** - *commonest cause is - Tuberculosis (Asbestosis)*
- ***Diaphragmatic Pleura calcification*** - *is due to - Asbestosis*
- ***Calcification in a pulmonary metastasis*** - *is most commonly due to - Osteosarcoma*
- ***Coin shadow*** *in the lung (single), with* ***calcification in the centre*** - *Epidermoid carcinoma*
- ***Plethoric lung fields*** - *seen in - L-R shunts (VSD, PDA, ASD)*
- ***Oligemic lung fields*** - *Pulmonary atreisa, Stenosis; Ebstein's anomaly*
- ***Perihilar fluffy opacities*** - *seen in - Pulmonary venous hypertension*

Ribs

- ***Superior surface notch*** *of ribs - seen in - Hyperparathyroidism, Neurofibromatosis, Connective tissue disorders*
- ***Inferior surface notch*** *of ribs - seen in - Coarctation of Aorta, SVC obstruction, Chest wall AV fistula, Aortic Thrombosis,*
- ***Unilateral notching*** *of ribs - Coarctation of Left subclavian artery, Subclavian artery block, Blalock-Taussig Operation*

Others

- ***Displacement of tracheal shadow*** - *most common cause is - Thyroid swelling*
- ***Water Lily sign*** - *Ruptured hydatid cyst*

171. Ans. b. Nonionic low ..., c. Nonionic iso..., e. Barium...

[Ref: Danhert Radiology manual 7th/1149; Review of Radiology by Sumer Sethi 6th/ 20-25 mriscans.cliniccompare.co.uk/ mri-scan-with-contrast-dye; Bhadury 2nd/177]

Diabetes & Contrast Agent

◈ *www.sfrnet.org*

Presentation

There is 3 problems with the diabetic patient: fasting, renal failure, and ongoing medication (insulin, oral antidiabetic, metformin).

- Fasting can cause hypoglycaemic accidents.
- Renal failure can be worsened by the injection of a contrast agent.
- Metformin exposes to the risk of lactic acidosis by diminution of renal clearance in case of ICM induced nephropathy

General Advice

- Have at hand a recent serum creatinine level test (less than 3 months old in the absence of intercurrent events).
- Use *low osmolality agents*.
- Keep the patient hydrated: orally = 2 litres of sodium rich water in the 24 hours preceding and following contrast medium injection; parenterally: 100ml per hour of saline isotonic serum or bicarbonated isotonic serum in the 12 hours to and after the injection of ICM.

Osmolality of contrast media compared with the osmolality of plasma seems to play an important role in nephrotoxicity. Contrast media usually have high viscosity and greater osmolality (more molecules per kilogram of water) than plasma. Ionicity is the characteristic of a molecule to break up into a cation and an anion, resulting in more molecules per kilogram of water and thus increasing osmolality. ***Nonionic agents not having this property are less osmolar.*** The osmotoxic effect of contrast agents is described in terms of the ratio of iodine atoms to dissolved particles: the higher the ratio, the better the attenuation of X-rays. ***Ionic high-osmolar contrast media*** (HOCM, e.g., diatrizoate, 1500 to 1800 mOsm/kg, i.e., 5–8 times the osmolality of plasma) have a ratio of 1.5 : 1, **nonionic low-osmolar contrast media** (LOCM, e.g., iohexol, 600 to 850 mOsm/kg, i.e., 2-3 times the osmolality of plasma) have a ratio of 3 : 1, and **nonionic iso-osmolar contrast media** (IOCM, e.g., iodixanol, approximately 290 mOsm/kg, i.e., the same osmolality as plasma) have a ratio of 6 : 1. ***Adverse reactions to contrast media range from 5% to 12% for HOCM and from 1% to 3% for LOCM. It has been shown that LOCM rather than HOCM are beneficial in the prevention of CIN to patients with preexisting renal failure.*** Iodixanol (IOCM) seems less nephrotoxic than iohexol (LOCM) at least in patients with intra-arterial administration of the drug and renal insufficiency"- *www.hindawi.com*

"**Diabetes and the administration of iodinated radiocontrast agents** are both associated with ***marked alterations of renal physiology***, including changes in GFR and renal hemodynamics, enhanced tubular transport activity and oxygen expenditure and intensification of medullary hypoxia, and ROS generation. Diabetes conceivably predisposes to CIN***(contrast induced nephropathy)*** principally through the amplification of these changes and the disruption of protective mechanisms, designed to maintain medullary oxygenation and to ameliorate oxidative stress. *www.ncbi.nlm.nih.gov*

"***Certain types of gadolinium contrast*** are now well known to be associated with a ***much lower risk of NSF*** in people with poor kidney function. If you need to have gadolinium contrast, ***the radiologist will use one of these lower risk types of gadolinium contrast.*** It is now thought that less than 1 in 100 people with severe kidney function impairment who have these lower-risk types of gadolinium contrast will develop NSF. It is often ***possible to carry out MRI without using any gadolinium contrast agents***, and this is preferred where possible for patients with very poor kidney function or who are on dialysis" *(www.insideradiology.com.au)*

- "**Contrast-induced nephropathy:** If you already have very poor kidney function, but are not on permanent dialysis due to kidney failure, there is a ***small risk that iodinated contrast will make your kidney function temporarily worse*** (20–40% of patients). This occurs mainly in people who have large amounts of iodine-containing contrast medium given into an artery (such as with coronary angiography or complex interventional procedures) or if they have more than one CT scan using intravenous contrast in a short period of time; that is, hours to 1–2 days"- *www.insideradiology.com.au*

*"**Nephrogenic systemic fibrosis or nephrogenic fibrosing dermopathy** is a rare & serious syndrome that involves fibrosis of skin, joints, eyes & internal organ. Its cause is not fully understood, but it seems to be associated with **exposure of gadolinium**(4 of 5 FDA-approved Gadolinium contrast agents have been principally implicated) in patients with **severe kidney failure**. As a result, **galolinium-containing contrast is now considered contraindicated in patients with an estimated GFR (a measure of renal function) under 60 & especially under 30**" (Sumer Sethi 6th/ 22)*

*"**Nephrogenic systemic fibrosis** caused by **galodinium based contrast**. Risk factor- Acute/chronic renal failure especially hepatorenal syndrome, perioperative transplantation period, renal transplant failure" (Danhert Radiology manual 7th/1151)*

"**Contrast induced nephropathy**: *Patients with pre-existing renal disease, particularly those with the renal complications of **DM,** multiple myeloma have an increased risk of an adverse reaction which **may precipitate renal failure**" (Sumer Sethi 6th/ 21)*

"**Acute renal failure in contrast reaction: *Diabetes mellitus with renal insufficiency(possibly related to dehydration/ hyperuricemia) is risk factor*.** Ratio **3 nonionic LOCM** appear to be 50% ***less nephrotoxic*** than ratio 1.5 ionic HOCM"- *Danhert Radiology manual 7th/1149*

"**Metformin** *should be discontinued for 48 hour after contrast medium administration (accumulation of metformin may result in lactic acidosis, which is fatal in 50%). It is **not necessary to stop metformin after galolinium administration because gadolinium is not nephrotoxic**"- (Danhert Radiology manual 7th/1149)*

Assessment of Patients before Contrast Injection

◈ *Danhert Radiology manual 7th/1150*

A. General status: Assess hemodynamic, neurologic, general nutritional, anxiety status
B. History of significant allergies1. Prior anaphylactic response to any allergen 2. Asthma
C. Renal disease 1. Renal dysfunction: obtain baseline BUN + creatinine 2. ***Diabetes mellitus 3.*** Multiple myeloma - Hydrate patients and limit contrast dose
D. Cardiac disease1. Angina 2. CHF with minimal exertion 3. Severe aortic stenosis4. Primary pulmonary hypertension5. Severe cardiomyopathy -Limit contrast dose

"The **contrast dye used in these MRI Scans** is generally ***gadolinium*** as ***complications are rarer in comparison to the Iodine origin dye used for x-rays and CT scans***"- *mriscans.cliniccompare.co.uk/ mri-scan-with-contrast-dye*

172. Ans. a. Breast..., b. Gonadal..., c. Leukae....

[Ref: Danhert Radiology manual 7th/ 574,154,408,313;Davidson 22nd/266; Review of Radiology by Sumer Sethi 6th/189,170-71; Harrison 19th/477, 193 e-4]

"Most commonly occurring radiation-induced cancer is: leukemia" *(www.flashcardmachine.com)*

"**Cancer induction** *is the largest risk of radiation exposure encountered in radiology.* ***Bone marrow, gastrointestinal tract mucosa, breast tissue, gonads & lymphatic tissue*** *are most susceptible to radiation induced malignancy. Cancer risk is higher for children than for adults"-Radiology & Imaging by K Thayalan 1st/311-12*

Table *(Harrison 19th/477)*: **Suspected Carcinogens**

Carcinogens	Associated Cancer or Neoplasm
Ionizing radiation (therapeutic or diagnostic)	Breast, bladder, thyroid, soft tissue, bone, hematopoietic, and many more

Table *(Sumer Sethi 6th/170)*: **Examples of radiation-induced cancers**

Types of Exposure	Types of Cancer Observed
Neck irradiation during infancy for benign conditions	Thyroid carcinoma
Radiation therapy for other malignant tumors	Thyroid carcinoma Breast cancer Gastric cancer Melanoma Lung cancer Sarcomas in the field
Cranial irradiation	Central nervous system tumors
Breast irradiation for postpartum mastitis	Breast cancer
Brush-licking by radium dial painters	Bone sarcomas
Uranium mining	Lung cancer
In utero exposure	Leukemia

"***A serious late toxicity is the development of second solid tumors in or adjacent to the radiation fields.*** Such tumors can develop in any organ or tissue and occur at a rate of about 1% per year beginning in the second decade after treatment. Some organs vary in susceptibility to radiation carcinogenesis. A woman who receives mantle field radiation therapy for Hodgkin's disease at age 25 years has a 30% risk of developing ***breast cancer*** by age 55 years" *(Harrison 19th/193 e-4)*

Table *(Davison 22nd/266)*: **Factor predisposing for cancer**

Radiation	Ultraviolet (UV) exposure	Basal cell carcinoma Melanoma Non-melanocytic skin cancer
	Nuclear fallout following explosion (e.g. Hiroshima)	Leukaemia Solid tumours, e.g. thyroid
	Diagnostic exposure (e.g. computed tomography (CT)	Cholangiocarcinoma following thorotrast usage
	Occupational exposure (e.g beryllium and strontium mining)	Lung cancer
	Therapeutic radiotherapy	Medullary thyroid cancer Sarcoma

173. Ans. a. I-131..., d. Strontium..., e. P-32...,

[Ref: Review of Radiology by Sumer Sethi 6th/ 177,184; Harrison 19th/; Grainger & Allison Radiology 6th/118;Dutta Gynaecology 5th/484, 4th/465; Merdith Radiation Physics & Nuclear Medicine/28]

"**Gallium-68** is a positron-emitting radioisotope that is produced from a ^{68}Ge/^{68}Ga generator. As such it is conveniently used, decoupling radiopharmacies from the need for a cyclotron on site. Gallium-68-labeled peptides have been recognized as a **new class of radiopharmaceuticals** showing fast target localization and blood clearance. ^{68}Ga-DOTATOC, ^{8}Ga-DOTATATE, ^{68}Ga-DOTANOC, are the most prominent radiopharmaceuticals currently in use for imaging and differentiating lesions of various somatostatin receptor subtypes, overexpressed in many ***neuroendocrine tumors***" *(www.ncbi.nlm.nih.gov)*

"***I-123:*** *It is agent of* ***choice for thyroid imaging***" *(Danhert Radiology manual 5th/1087)*

"For **radioactive iodine scanning *I-131 & I-123*** are used. ***For treatment of hyperthyroidism & thyroid cancer I-131 is used***" *(CMDT06/1127)*

Table: *(Dutta gynaecology 5th/484)*: **Radioisotopes commonly used in gynaecological malignancies (as brachytherapy)**

Isotope	Energy(MeV)	Half life
Cesium 137 (Cs137)	0.662	30 years
Radium 226 (Ra226)	0.8	1620 years
Cobalt 60 (Co60)	1.173	5.3 years
Iridium 192 (Ir 192) Q	0.47Q	74 days
Gold 198 (Au 198)	0.411	2.96 days
Iodine 125 (I-125)	0.027	60 days
Phosphorus 32 (P32)	0.698	14.3 days

Table *(Sumer Sethi 6th/ 177)*: **Brachytherapy Source**

Radionuclide	Radiation Emitted	Energy	Half-line	Form
Radium-226	Gamma rays	1 MeV	1620 years	Needles, tubes
Caesium-137	Gamma rays	0.66 MeV	30 years	Tubes, needles, pellets
Cobalt-60	Gamma rays	1.25 MeV	5.26 years	Rods
Iridium-192	Gamma rays	0.4 MeV	74 days	Wires
Gold-198	Gamma rays	0.41 MeV	2.7 days	Seeds
Strontium-90	Beta rays	2.27 MeV max	28.1 years	Plaques
Yttrium-90	Beta rays	2.27 MeV max	64 hours	Rods

Table *(Sumer Sethi 6th/ 177)*: **Radionucleotide suitable for unsealed use**

Radionuclide	Form in which used	Half-life	Radiation emitted	Method of administration
Iodine-131	Sodium iodide solution	8 days	Beta rays Gamma rays	Oral
Phosphorus- 32	Sodium orthophosphate solution	14.3 days	Beta rays	Intravenous injection
Yttrium-90	Colloidal liquid	64 hours	Beta rays	Intracavitary injection

Table *(Sumer Sethi 6th/ 177)*: **Systemic radionuceotide for treatment of bone metastases**

Radionuclide	Half-Life	Emission	Energy (MeV)	Status
Phosphorus 32 (32P)	14.2 days	Beta	1.71	Approved
Strontium 89 (89Sr)	50.6 days	Beta	1.492	Approved
Samarium 153 (153Sm)	46.3 hours	Gamma	0.81	Approved 0.10
Rhenium 186 (186Re)	90.6 hours	Beta Gamma	1.071 0.137	Investigational
Rhenium 188 (188Re)	16.7 hours	Beta	2.116	Investigational

174. Ans. a. Wate..., b. Barium..., c. Iodinated..., d. Polyethylene...

[Ref: Sumer Sethi 6th/20; Radiology & Imaging by Thayalan 1st/159;Danhert Radiology Manual 7th/1147-48]

A & E

Radiocontrast Agents

❖ *radiologyinfo.org*

- **Radiocontrast agents** are a type of medical contrast medium used to improve the visibility of internal bodily structures in X-ray-based imaging techniques such as computed tomography (CT), radiography, and fluoroscopy. Radiocontrast agents are typically iodine or barium compounds. When an agent improves visibility of an area, it is called "contrast enhancing".
- Magnetic resonance imaging (MRI) functions through different principles and thus utilizes different contrast agents. These compounds work by altering the magnetic properties of nearby hydrogen nuclei.
- When iodine-based and barium-sulfate contrast materials are present in a specific area of the body, they block or limit the ability of x-rays to pass through. As a result, blood vessels, organs and other body tissue that temporarily contain ***iodine-based or barium compounds*** change their appearance on x-ray or CT images.
- **Gadolinium** is the key component of the contrast material most often used in magnetic resonance (MR) exams. When this substance is present in the body, it alters the magnetic properties of nearby water molecules, which enhances the quality of MR images.
- ***Saline (salt water) and air*** are also used as contrast materials in imaging exams. ***Microbubbles and microspheres have been administered for ultrasound imaging exams***, particularly exams of the heart.
- Iodine-based and barium-sulfate compounds are used in x-ray and computed tomography (CT) imaging exams.

American College of Radiology: 10th Edition (2016) of the ACR Manual on Contrast Media replaces

- ***Oral, rectal, and intravenous contrast agents*** are utilized in a variety of ways for imaging of the gastrointestinal system. Oral contrast agents are used for fluoroscopic studies, such as dynamic pharyngography, esophagography, upper gastrointestinal (UGI) series, and small bowel follow-through (SBFT) examinations. They are also used to highlight the gastrointestinal tract in routine computed tomography (CT) of the abdomen and pelvis, CT enterography, magnetic resonance imaging (MRI), magnetic resonance enterography, CT colonography, CT positron emission tomography (PET), and MRI-PET.
- Oral agents are also occasionally used to opacify the biliary tree. Rectal contrast media is given for conventional fluoroscopic colon studies and colon cleansing. Rectal contrast media may also opacify the colonic lumen during CT imaging of the abdomen and pelvis. Intravenous contrast media of various types may be used to opacify the biliary tree during CT and MRI cholangiopancreatography, as well as for generalized enhancement of vascularized structures and organs in routine CT and MR of the abdomen and pelvis. Direct injection of contrast media into the biliary and pancreatic ductal systems is performed during endoscopic retrograde cholangiopancreatography (ERCP) and percutaneous antegrade studies of the biliary tree.
- **Barium sulfate contrast media** continue to be the preferred agents for opacification of the gastrointestinal tract for conventional fluoroscopic examinations
- The current use of **iodinated water-soluble** contrast media is primarily limited to select situations

- Two commercial **water-soluble iodinated high-osmolality contrast media (HOCMs)** specifically designed for enteric opacification are in common use. ***Gastrografin*** and ***Gastroview***
- Orally administered contrast media are used for gastrointestinal opacification during routine abdominopelvic **CT** . There is no significant difference in the diagnostic quality of the subsequently obtained CT examinations with ***barium agents, HOCM, or LOCM***, assuming appropriate dilution of contrast material. ***Barium products for oral use in CT*** are commercially available in appropriate concentrations.
- **Indications for CT enterography**: CT enterography is currently used for the CT diagnosis and assessment of inflammatory bowel disease, localizing sites of GI tract bleeding, and, less commonly, for detection of small bowel neoplasms . While small bowel distention can be achieved by the use of high attenuation oral contrast agents (*e.g.,* ***dilute barium or water-soluble iodinated contrast media***),there is increasing use of neutral (low attenuation) contrast agents (e.g., 0.1% w/v ultra-low-dose barium with 2% sorbitol
- Other low attenuation oral contrast agents that have been utilized, albeit much less frequently, for **CT** enterography include ***water, lactulose solution, polyethylene glycol (PEG) electrolyte solution, Mucofalk, and methylcellulose.***

ANSWER SHEET

1 – 50	51 – 100	101 – 150	151 – 200	201 – 250
1 A B C D E	51 A B C D E	101 A B C D E	151 A B C D E	201 A B C D E
2 A B C D E	52 A B C D E	102 A B C D E	152 A B C D E	202 A B C D E
3 A B C D E	53 A B C D E	103 A B C D E	153 A B C D E	203 A B C D E
4 A B C D E	54 A B C D E	104 A B C D E	154 A B C D E	204 A B C D E
5 A B C D E	55 A B C D E	105 A B C D E	155 A B C D E	205 A B C D E
6 A B C D E	56 A B C D E	106 A B C D E	156 A B C D E	206 A B C D E
7 A B C D E	57 A B C D E	107 A B C D E	157 A B C D E	207 A B C D E
8 A B C D E	58 A B C D E	108 A B C D E	158 A B C D E	208 A B C D E
9 A B C D E	59 A B C D E	109 A B C D E	159 A B C D E	209 A B C D E
10 A B C D E	60 A B C D E	110 A B C D E	160 A B C D E	210 A B C D E
11 A B C D E	61 A B C D E	111 A B C D E	161 A B C D E	211 A B C D E
12 A B C D E	62 A B C D E	112 A B C D E	162 A B C D E	212 A B C D E
13 A B C D E	63 A B C D E	113 A B C D E	163 A B C D E	213 A B C D E
14 A B C D E	64 A B C D E	114 A B C D E	164 A B C D E	214 A B C D E
15 A B C D E	65 A B C D E	115 A B C D E	165 A B C D E	215 A B C D E
16 A B C D E	66 A B C D E	116 A B C D E	166 A B C D E	216 A B C D E
17 A B C D E	67 A B C D E	117 A B C D E	167 A B C D E	217 A B C D E
18 A B C D E	68 A B C D E	118 A B C D E	168 A B C D E	218 A B C D E
19 A B C D E	69 A B C D E	119 A B C D E	169 A B C D E	219 A B C D E
20 A B C D E	70 A B C D E	120 A B C D E	170 A B C D E	220 A B C D E
21 A B C D E	71 A B C D E	121 A B C D E	171 A B C D E	221 A B C D E
22 A B C D E	72 A B C D E	122 A B C D E	172 A B C D E	222 A B C D E
23 A B C D E	73 A B C D E	123 A B C D E	173 A B C D E	223 A B C D E
24 A B C D E	74 A B C D E	124 A B C D E	174 A B C D E	224 A B C D E
25 A B C D E	75 A B C D E	125 A B C D E	175 A B C D E	225 A B C D E
26 A B C D E	76 A B C D E	126 A B C D E	176 A B C D E	226 A B C D E
27 A B C D E	77 A B C D E	127 A B C D E	177 A B C D E	227 A B C D E
28 A B C D E	78 A B C D E	128 A B C D E	178 A B C D E	228 A B C D E
29 A B C D E	79 A B C D E	129 A B C D E	179 A B C D E	229 A B C D E
30 A B C D E	80 A B C D E	130 A B C D E	180 A B C D E	230 A B C D E
31 A B C D E	81 A B C D E	131 A B C D E	181 A B C D E	231 A B C D E
32 A B C D E	82 A B C D E	132 A B C D E	182 A B C D E	232 A B C D E
33 A B C D E	83 A B C D E	133 A B C D E	183 A B C D E	233 A B C D E
34 A B C D E	84 A B C D E	134 A B C D E	184 A B C D E	234 A B C D E
35 A B C D E	85 A B C D E	135 A B C D E	185 A B C D E	235 A B C D E
36 A B C D E	86 A B C D E	136 A B C D E	186 A B C D E	236 A B C D E
37 A B C D E	87 A B C D E	137 A B C D E	187 A B C D E	237 A B C D E
38 A B C D E	88 A B C D E	138 A B C D E	188 A B C D E	238 A B C D E
39 A B C D E	89 A B C D E	139 A B C D E	189 A B C D E	239 A B C D E
40 A B C D E	90 A B C D E	140 A B C D E	190 A B C D E	240 A B C D E
41 A B C D E	91 A B C D E	141 A B C D E	191 A B C D E	241 A B C D E
42 A B C D E	92 A B C D E	142 A B C D E	192 A B C D E	242 A B C D E
43 A B C D E	93 A B C D E	143 A B C D E	193 A B C D E	243 A B C D E
44 A B C D E	94 A B C D E	144 A B C D E	194 A B C D E	244 A B C D E
45 A B C D E	95 A B C D E	145 A B C D E	195 A B C D E	245 A B C D E
46 A B C D E	96 A B C D E	146 A B C D E	196 A B C D E	246 A B C D E
47 A B C D E	97 A B C D E	147 A B C D E	197 A B C D E	247 A B C D E
48 A B C D E	98 A B C D E	148 A B C D E	198 A B C D E	248 A B C D E
49 A B C D E	99 A B C D E	149 A B C D E	199 A B C D E	249 A B C D E
50 A B C D E	100 A B C D E	150 A B C D E	200 A B C D E	250 A B C D E

NAME OF THE CANDIDATE	ROLL NO.	CENTRE NO.	QUESTION BOOKLET NO.	BOOKLET CODE

CATEGORY

- SC ○
- ST ○
- OBC ○
- GEN ○
- CW ○
- PH ○

ROLL NO.					CENTRE NO.		QUESTION BOOKLET NO.					BOOKLET CODE
0	0	0	0	0	0	0	0	0	0	0	0	A
1	1	1	1	1	1	1	1	1	1	1	1	B
2	2	2	2	2	2	2	2	2	2	2	2	C
3	3	3	3	3	3	3	3	3	3	3	3	D
4	4	4	4	4	4	4	4	4	4	4	4	
5	5	5	5	5	5	5	5	5	5	5	5	
6	6	6	6	6	6	6	6	6	6	6	6	
7	7	7	7	7	7	7	7	7	7	7	7	
8	8	8	8	8	8	8	8	8	8	8	8	
9	9	9	9	9	9	9	9	9	9	9	9	

INSTRUCTIONS FOR FILLING THE SHEET

1. This sheet should not be folded or crushed.
2. Use only blue/black ball pen to fill the circles.
3. Use of pencil is strictly prohibited.
4. Circles should be darkened properly and completely.
5. Cutting & erasing on this sheet is not allowed.
6. Do not use any stray marks on the sheet.
7. Do not use marker, white fluid or any other device to hide the shading already done.

WRONG METHOD

× ● ✓

CORRECT METHOD

CANDIDATE'S SIGNATURE
(in ball - point pen)

INVIGILATOR'S SIGNATURE
(in ball - point pen)

MAY

2015

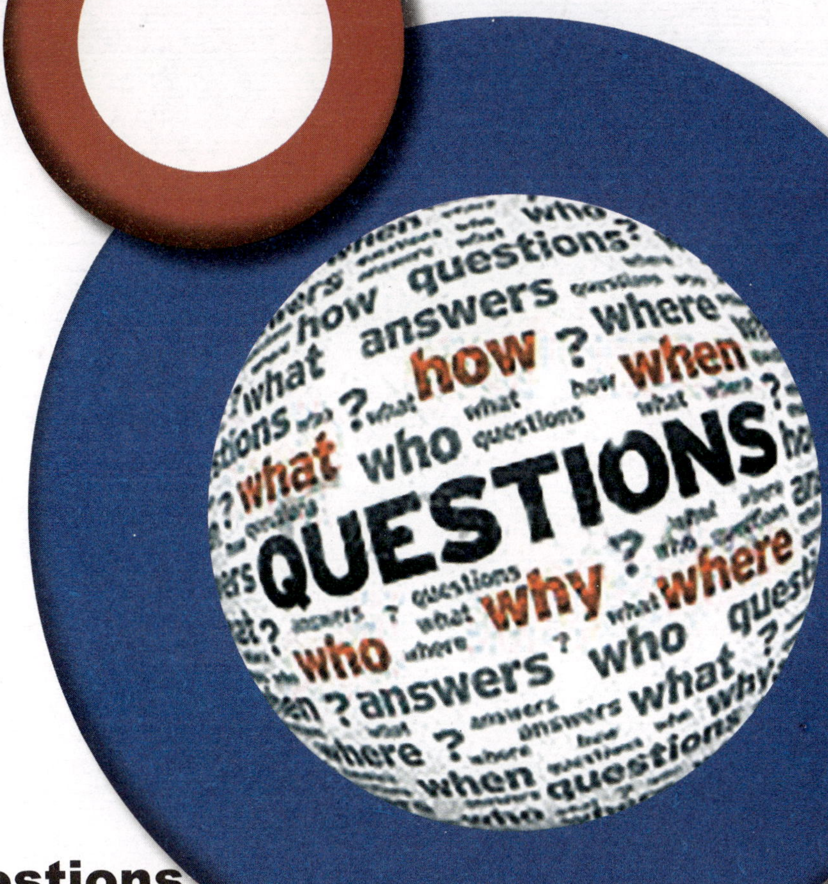

Multiple Choice Questions
Answers & Explanations

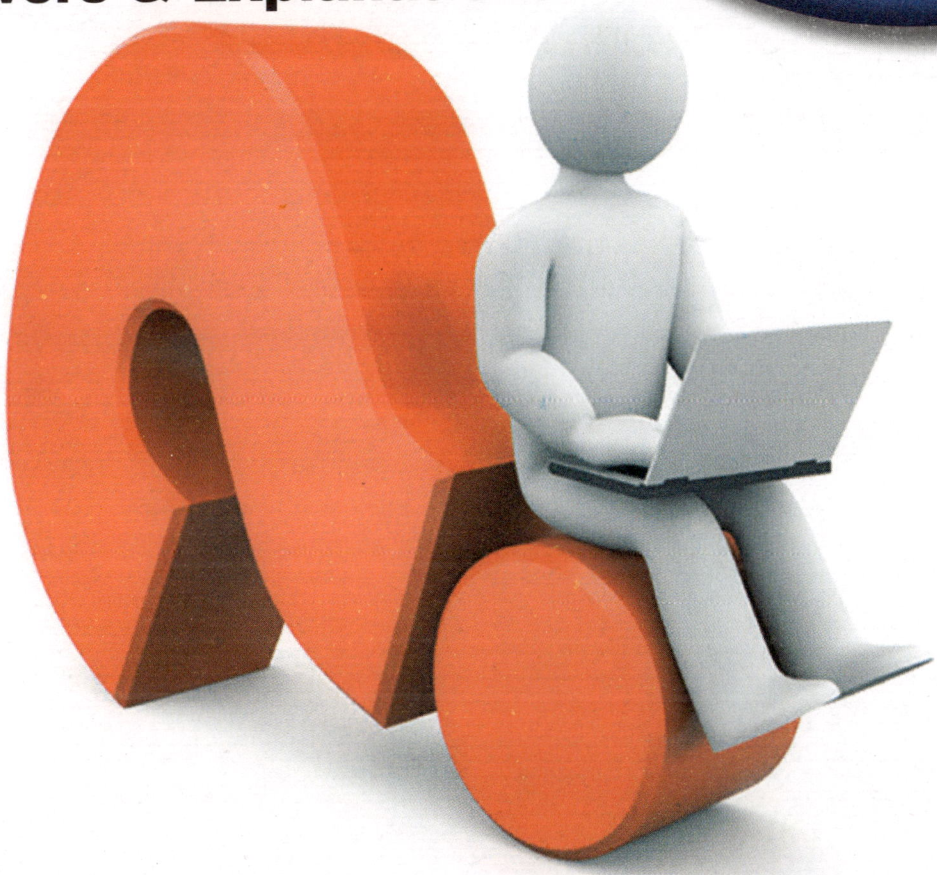

MAY 2015 MULTIPLE CHOICE QUESTIONS

ANATOMY

1. **Which of the following structure (s) pass through adductor magnus:**
   a. Femoral vessel
   b. Femoral nerve
   c. Femoral sheath
   d. Saphenous nerve
   e. Tibial nerve
2. **Which of the following statement(s) is true regarding axillay artery:**
   a. Start from upper border of clavicle
   b. Ulnar nerve lies medially to distal 1/3 of artery
   c. Radial nerve lies posteriorly distal 1/3 of artery
   d. Axillary vein lies laterally to proximal 1/3 of the artery
   e. End at lower border of pectoralis minor
3. **Facial development takes place b/w:**
   a. 4–8 week
   b. 8–10 week
   c. 12–14 week
   d. 18–20 week
   e. 6–10 week
4. **Muscle having double nerve supply:**
   a. Digastric muscle
   b. Omohyoid muscle
   c. Trapezius
   d. Thyrohyoid muscle
   e. Adductor magnus
5. **Which of the following is true regarding vertebral column curvature:**
   a. Primary curves are concave forward
   b. Lumbar curve is primary
   c. Thoracic curve develop when infant start walking
   d. Cervical appear when the infant starts supporting its head
   e. Lumbar curve appears when the child assumes the upright posture

PHYSIOLOGY

6. **Pepsinogen, the inactive form of pepsin, is secreted by:**
   a. Interstitial cell of Cajal
   b. Chief cell
   c. Paneth cell
   d. Goblet cell
   e. Zymogen Cells
7. **Type IIB muscle fibers are different from type I fiber with having:**
   a. Small diameter
   b. Calcium release by sarcoplasmic reticulum is low
   c. Fast fatigable
   d. Color pink
   e. Faster acting
8. **Which of the following is true regarding renal handling of substances:**
   a. Bicarbonate is completely reabsorbed
   b. Amount of Na^+ absorb is in excess than secreted
   c. Percentage reabsorption of Na^+ is more than K^+
   d. In absolute term (in meq) Na^+ is more excreted than K^+
   e. Total amount of urea filtered is completely excreted
9. **Vasomotor inputs to rostral nucleus of ventromedial medulla is/are from:**
   a. Inhibitory input from caudal ventrolateral medulla
   b. Excitatory inputs from cerebral cortex via hypothalamus
   c. Inhibitory inputs from cerebral cortex via hypothalamus
   d. Inhibitory inputs from brain stem reticular formation
   e. Inhibitory inputs pain pathway
10. **Parasympathetic stimulation results in:**
    a. Miosis
    b. Decreased GIT motility
    c. Detrusor muscle relaxation
    d. Mydriasis
    e. Contraction of bronchial muscle
11. **Which of the following are feature of blood-brain barrier:**
    a. Thick basement membrane
    b. Podocyte
    c. Closely associated layer of astrocyte
    d. Tight junction
    e. Decreased vesicles in endothelial cells
12. **For Growth hormone testing, which of the following stimulate the secretions of Growth hormone:**
    a. Glucagon
    b. Insulin
    c. Cortisol
    d. Water deprivation
    e. Arginine
13. **Which of the following is true about myoglobin:**
    a. Bind 1 mol of oxygen per mole of myoglobin
    b. Dissociation curve is a rectangular hyperbola
    c. Its curve lies right of the hemoglobin curve
    d. Bind oxygen at low PO2 pressure
    e. Show Bohr effect

BIOCHEMISTRY

14. **Mucopolysaccharidosis, which is a lysosomal storage disease, occurs due to abnormality in:**
    a. Hydrolase enzyme
    b. Dehydrogenase enzyme
    c. Lipase enzyme
    d. Phosphatase
    e. Acetyl-CoA carboxylase

Answer

1. a.	2. b, c.	3. a.	4. a, e.	5. a, d, e.	6. b, e.	7. c, e.
8. a, b, c, d.	9. a, b, c.	10. a, e.	11. a, c, d, e.	12. a, e.	13. a, b, d.	14. a.

15. **Sulphur of cystein are not used/ utilized in body for the following process/product:**
   a. Help in conversion of cyanide to thiocynate
   b. Thiosulphate formation
   c. Introduction of sulphur atom in methionine
   d. Disulfide bond formation b/w two adjacent peptide
16. **Which one of the following statements about protein structure is correct:**
   a. Proteins consisting of one polypeptide can have quaternary structure
   b. The formation of a disulfide bond in a protein requires that the two participating cysteine residues be adjacent to each other in the primary sequence of the protein
   c. The stability of quaternary structure in proteins is mainly a result of covalent bonds among the subunits
   d. The denaturation of proteins always leads to irreversible loss of secondary and tertiary structure
   e. The information required for the correct folding of a protein is contained in the specific sequence of amino acids along the polypeptide chain
17. **True about retinol:**
   a. Form part of rhodopsin
   b. Transported from intestine to liver by via chylomicrons
   c. Actively take part in visual cycle
   d. Implicated in growth & differentiation of tissue
   e. Not formed by retinoic acid
18. **In prolong fasting glycerol is formed from triglyceride. Which of the following statement (s) is/are true regarding glycerol:**
   a. Used in synthesis of chylomicron
   b. It is directly used by tissues for energy needs
   c. It is formed due to increased activity of lipoprotein lipase
   d. It is formed due to increased activity of hormone sensitive lipase
   e. Glycerol acts as a substrate for gluconeogenesis in the liver
19. **Pyruvate dehydrogenase complex uses following coenzymes/ cofactors:**
   a. Biotin
   b. Lipoic acid
   c. NAD
   d. FMN
   e. TPP
20. **In conversion of pyruvate to acetyl CoA & CO_2, which of the following coenzyme is used:**
   a. Biotin
   b. Lipoic acid
   c. TPP
   d. Pyridoxal phosphate
   e. Tetrahydrofolate
21. **True about urea cycle:**
   a. Nitrogen of the urea comes from alanine & ammonia
   b. Uses ATP during conversion of arginosuccinate to arginine
   c. On consumption of high amount of protein, excess of urea formed
   d. Occur mainly in cytoplasm
   e. Synthesis of arginosuccinate consumes energy
22. **Gangliosides contains:**
   a. Phosphate
   b. Galactose
   c. Sulphate
   d. Serine
   e. Sialic acid

IMMUNOGENETICS & MOLECULAR BIOLOGY

23. **All are true about structure of DNA except:**
   a. Right –handed helix
   b. Left-handed helix
   c. Phosphate form backbone
   d. Deoxyribose forms backbone
   e. Nitrogen bases form backbone
24. **Which of the following is false:**
   a. Ratio of A:T & G:C is approximately equal to 1:1
   b. Ratio of A:G & T:C is approximately equal to 1:1
   c. A+T=G+C
   d. A+C=G+T
   e. A+G= C+T
25. **True about restriction enzyme:**
   a. Also k/a restriction endonuclease
   b. Produce sticky ends
   c. Can detect mutations
   d. Obtained from virus
   e. Breaks at sugar-phosphate bond
26. **Which of the following is/are true about PCR except:**
   a. Uses heat labile DNA polymerase
   b. Uses heat stable DNA polymerase
   c. Is technique for DNA amplification
   d. Used to yield multiple copies of DNA
   e. Reverse transcriptase- PCR is used for quantification of RNA
27. **Which of the following techniques are used for detection of mutation:**
   a. RT-PCR
   b. Microarray
   c. Allele-specific oligonucleotide (ASO)
   d. Western blot
   e. DNA sequencing
28. **Which of the following is/are most severe/dangerous change in gene:**
   a. Deletion
   b. Insertion
   c. Mutation
   d. Translocation
   e. Duplication

MCQs

Answer

15. c	16. e	17. b, d, e	18. d, e	19. b, c, e	20. b, c	21. c, d, e
22. b, e	23. e	24. b, c	25. a, b, e	26. a	27. a, b, c, e	28. a, b

29. **Which of the following technique is/are used in quantification of viral nucleic acid:**
    a. MALDI-TOF MS
    b. Branched-chain DNA (bDNA)
    c. PCR
    d. Gas-Liquid Chromatography
    e. Biochemical phenotyping
30. **Genes in CpP island is inactivated by:**
    a. Methylation
    b. Metrylation
    c. Ubiquitisation
    d. Acetylation
31. **Which of the following is true regarding transcription except:**
    a. mRNA is formed
    b. DNA polymerase enzyme is used
    c. RNA Polymerase enzyme is used
    d. Eukaryotes possess 3 different types of RNA polymerase
32. **Which of the following RNA contains unusual bases:**
    a. mRNA
    b. rRNA
    c. tRNA
    d. 30 S RNA
    e. 50 S RNA

PATHOLOGY

33. **True about follicular lymphoma:**
    a. Lymphadenopathy is the most common presentation
    b. BCL-1 positive
    c. CD5 positive
    d. More common in males than females
34. **True about Chronic Lymphocytic Leukemia:**
    a. Most common leukemia in adult
    b. Proliferation center is pathognomonic
    c. Massive splenomegaly
    d. Radiotherapy & chemotherapy are given in treatment
35. **True about mitochondrial DNA:**
    a. Linear
    b. Circular
    c. Transmitted by mother only
    d. Transmitted by both parents
    e. Contains less gene than nuclear DNA
36. **True about autosomal dominant type of inheritance:**
    a. 25% affected & 50 % carrier, if one parent affected
    b. 50% affected & 75 % carrier, if both parent affected
    c. 75% affected, if both parent affected
    d. 50% affected, if one parent affected
    e. All carrier irrespective of either one parent affected or both parent affected
37. **In α-thalassemia, Hb Barts is said when number of gene loci affected is:**
    a. 1
    b. 2
    c. 3
    d. 4
    e. None
38. **Which of the following cellular component gives purplish blue color with H & E reagent:**
    a. Reticulum
    b. Elastin
    c. P-selectin
    d. Collagen
    e. Heterochromatin
39. **Which of the following is true about glutathione & glutathione peroxidase:**
    a. Act as scavenger of free radicle
    b. Glutathione has anti-oxidant property
    c. Reduced glutathione can chemically detoxify H_2O_2
    d. Oxidized glutathione can chemically detoxify H_2O_2
40. **Histological finding of hypertrophic cardiomyopathy includes:**
    a. Myocyte disarray
    b. Interstitial fibrosis
    c. Amyloid deposition in muscle
    d. Myocyte hypertrophy
    e. Myocardial fibers are arranged in parallel pattern
41. **True about bcl-2:**
    a. ↑ Apoptosis
    b. ↓ Apoptosis
    c. ↑ Resistance of tumour to treatment
    d. Only associated with follicular lymphoma
    e. Cause meningioma
42. **True about thrombus formation:**
    a. Arterial thrombus grow in direction toward heart
    b. Venous thrombus grow in direction toward heart
    c. Venous thrombus form chicken fat
    d. Line of Zahn is seen microscopically in red thrombi
43. **Red infarct occur in:**
    a. In tissues with dual circulations
    b. Occur only when both arterial & venous obstruction occurs simultaneously
    c. Organs which are previously congested
    d. Organs with loose tissue
44. **Spindle shaped cells is/are seen in which sarcoma:**
    a. Osteosarcoma
    b. Chondromyosarcoma
    c. Embryonal rhabdomyosarcoma
    d. Leiomyosarcoma
    e. Fibrosarcoma
45. **Which of the following dyads are correct:**
    a. WBC cast- Acute pyelonephritis
    b. Broad cast-CRF
    c. Eosinophilic cast-interstitial nephritis
    d. RBC cast- Glomerulonephritis
    e. Broad cast: chronic pyelonephritis
46. **Alpha feto protein is/are increased in:**
    a. Yolk sac tumour
    b. Seminoma
    c. Dysgerminoma
    d. Non-seminoma
    e. Hepatocellular carcinoma

Answer

29. b, c.	30. a.	31. b.	32. c.	33. a.	34. a, b, c.	35. b, c, e.
36. d.	37. d.	38. a, e.	39. a, b, c.	40. a, b, d.	41. b, c.	42. b, d.
43. a, c, d.	44. a, c, d, e.	45. a, b, d.	46. a, d, e.			

47. True about hemophilia B:
a. Factor 8 deficiency
b. Factor 9 deficiency
c. X-linked disorder
d. Clinically indistinguishable from hemophilia A
e. Fresh frozen plasma given for treatment

48. True about primary biliary cirrhosis:
a. More common in female
b. Periportal fibrosis
c. May be associated with Rheumatoid arthritis & crohn's disease
d. Jaundice may be present

49. Finding in histopathology of brain in rabies includes:
a. Negri body
b. Nodule
c. Neuronophagia
d. Vacuolar degenerative changes
e. Inflammatory cell

50. True about hyperacute rejection in renal transplant:
a. Occur within few days of transplant
b. T cell involvement
c. Blood vessel thrombosis
d. Eosinophilic infiltration
e. B cell infiltration

51. True about gluten sensitive enteropathy:
a. Diet should exclude barley, wheat & rye
b. Intestinal biopsy is diagnostic
c. Anti IgA endomycial antibody is specific
d. Mucosal hyperplasia

PHARMACOLOGY

52. Mechanism of action of gabapentin is/are:
a. Enhances GABA release
b. Agonist at GABAA receptor
c. Act on NMDA receptor
d. Prolongation of Na^+ Channel Inactivation
e. Inhibition of voltage-gated Ca^{2+} channels

53. Which of the following is/are true regarding muscarinic action except:
a. Miosis
b. Detrusor muscle contraction
c. Dicylomine is antimuscarinic drug used for smooth muscle relaxation
d. Cardiac muscuranic receptors are predominantly M 3 type
e. ↓salivary gland secretion

54. Disease modifying drug (s) used in treatment of rheumatoid arthritis:
a. Neproxen
b. Nabumetone
c. Abatacept
d. Monoclonal antibodies
e. Methotrexate

55. Levetiracetam is commonly used for:
a. Juvenile myoclonic epilepsy
b. Absence seizure
c. Generalised Tonic clonic seizure
d. Complex partial seizure
e. Act through GABA

56. Penicillinase resistant penicillin is/are:
a. Methicillin
b. Cloxacillin
c. Ampicillin
d. Dicloxacillin
e. Vancomycin

57. True about Jarisch - Hexheimer reaction:
a. Occur within hours after giving penicillin
b. Develop only after 1 week of Penicillin therapy
c. Aggravation of signs and symptoms of syphilis
d. It occur due to allergy to penicillin
e. Most common in secondary syphilis

58. For which of the following drug bacteria acquire drug resistance by inactivation or degradation by enzyme:
a. Quninolones
b. Aminoglycosides
c. Vancomycin
d. Ampicillin
e. Chloramphenicol

59. Which of the followings are feature of benzodiazepine withdrawal except:
a. Anxiety
b. Increased appetite
c. Hypersomnia
d. Bad dreams
e. Tremor

60. Which of the following drug is mainly excreted by kidney:
a. Tetracyclines
b. Doxycyclines
c. Ampicillin
d. Acyclovir
e. Rifampicin

61. All are true about acyclovir except:
a. Gunanosine analogue
b. Inhibit viral DNA gyrase
c. Inhibit viral DNA polymerase
d. Requires phosphorylation for activation
e. Excreted mainly in urine

62. S/E of clofaziamine includes:
a. Ichthyologist
b. Thrombocytosis
c. Skin pigmentation
d. Gastrointestinal disturbances
e. Weight gain

63. A person was on chemotherapy for 2 week for some mediastinal tumour. Now he develops high frequency hearing loss. Most probable cause of this condition is use of:
a. Cisplatin
b. Etoposide
c. Doxorubicin
d. Methotrexate

Answer

47. b, c, d. 48. a, b, d. 49. a, b, c, e. 50. c. 51. a, c. 52. a, e. 53. d, e.
54. c, d, e. 55. a, c, d, e. 56. a, b, d. 57. a, c, e. 58. b, e. 59. b, c. 60. a, c, d.
61. b. 62. a, c, d. 63. a.

64. **In comparison to haloperidol, clozapine causes:**
   a. Weight gain
   b. Agranulocytosis
   c. Sedation
   d. Severe extrapyramidal symptoms
   e. Less eliptogenic potential

65. **Which of the following condition increase chance of hyponatremia in patient treated with antidepressant:**
   a. Old age b. Low weight
   c. Cold climate d. Obesity
   e. Female sex

66. **Desmopressin is/are used in:**
   a. Diabetes insipidus b. Esophageal varices
   c. Haemophilia A d. Von Willebrand disease
   e. Hemophila B

67. **Which of the following is/are teratogens:**
   a. Artemisinin b. Aminoglycoside
   c. Carbamezapine d. Retinoic acid
   e. Phenytoin

68. **Which of the following is/are features of Triamcilone with respect to hydrocortisone:**
   a. Fluorinated at carbon atom 9
   b. Not used in oral form
   c. Mineralocorticoid activity present
   d. More potent than hydrocortisone
   e. Glucocorticoid activity is 5 times of hydrocortisone

MICROBIOLOGY

69. **Burkholderia cepacia infection is/are typically associated with:**
   a. Cystic fibrosis
   b. Chronic bronchitis
   c. Chronic granulomatous disease
   d. Multiple myeloma
   e. Myeloperoxidase deficiency

70. **T. saginata is differentiated from T. solium by presence of:**
   a. Hooks in scolex (head)
   b. 4 large pigmented sucker
   c. Uterus is thin & dichotomous
   d. Short neck
   e. Egg is not infective to man

71. **True about gas gangrene:**
   a. α –toxin is main cause of the toxaemia associated with gas gangrene
   b. Caused by mainly Clostridium intestinale
   c. Low oxygen tension in tissue is important precondition
   d. Devitalized tissue predisposes to gas gangrene
   e. Not occur if dead tissue is not present

72. **True about Botulinum toxin:**
   a. Interfere with adrenergic transmission
   b. Interfere with Cholinergic transmission
   c. Increase release of synaptic vesicles
   d. Inhibit release from synaptic vesicles
   e. Act also on CNS

73. **Which of the following is/are true about HIV-2:**
   a. HIV-2 first detected in West Africa in 1986
   b. Donated blood is only screened for HIV-1, not HIV-2
   c. More virulent than HIV 1
   d. More closely related to simian immunodeficiency virus than HIV 1
   e. Mode of transmission is like HIV1

74. **Features of stage III HIV infection is/are:**
   a. Fever > 38. 5°C
   b. Oral hairy leukoplakia
   c. Candidiasis
   d. Diarrhoea of >20 day duration
   e. > 26% CD4 count in adults

75. **Microbiological organism can be recovered from:**
   a. Sulphur granules of actinomycetes
   b. Streptococci from Valve leaflet lesion in rheumatic valvulilis
   c. Petechial purpura for Meningococci
   d. Corynebacterium in pseudomembrane in throat

76. **All are the feature (s) of chancorid except:**
   a. Ulcer bleed easily b. Painful
   c. Bubo formation d. Typically indurated
   e. Caused by H. ducreyi

77. **True about plague:**
   a. Seasonal spread
   b. No vaccine is available
   c. Tetracycline is used both for chemoprophylaxis & treatment
   d. Caused by gram negative motile bacteria
   e. All ages are equally affected

78. **Which of the following is picornaviridae:**
   a. Polio virus b. Coxasackie virus
   c. Rhinovirus d. Corona virus
   e. Reovirus

79. **All are true about severe combined immunodeficiency (SCID) except:**
   a. B & T cell deficiency
   b. Adenosine deaminase deficiency may occur
   c. Affected child can survives beyond adolescence without treatment
   d. Can transmit either as X-linked or autosomal recessive defect
   e. Person susceptible to recurrent & severe infections

Answer

64. a, b, c.	65. a.	66. a, c, d.	67. b, c, d, e.	68. d, e.	69. a, c.	70. b, c, e.
71. a, c, d.	72. b, d, e.	73. a, d, e.	74. b, c.	75. a, c, d.	76. d.	77. a, c, e.
78. a, b, c.	79. c.					

80. True statement regarding NK cells are all except:
a. Also called as Large granular lymphocyte
b. Can kill viral infected cell
c. Forms first line of defence
d. Can kill tumour cell
e. No role in cell mediated immunity

81. True about Swine flu:
a. Older bird influenza vaccine is equally effective in swine flu
b. Ostelmavir is effective in prevention
c. Zanamavir can be used for treatment
d. Influenza vaccine provides immunity just after vaccination

82. Laboratory finding (s) of a patient having chronic hepatitis B infection with low viral load:
a. HBsAg
b. Anti-HBs
c. Anti-HBe
d. Anti-HBc IgG
e. HBeAg

FORENSIC MEDICINE

83. Death in hanging occurs due to all except:
a. Asphyxia
b. Vagal inhibition
c. Vagal stimulation
d. Cerebral ischemia
e. Venous congestion

84. Grease collar is formed by:
a. Railway injury
b. Gutter fracture
c. Bullet exit wound
d. Bullet entry wound

85. Which of the following is/are type of abrasion:
a. Pattern
b. Imprint
c. Graze
d. Stretch
e. Scratch

86. I. P. C Section dealing with punishment for voluntary causing grievous injury:
a. 321 I. P. C
b. 322 I. P. C
c. 323 I. P. C
d. 324 I. P. C
e. 325 I. P. C

87. Post- mortem caloricity is/are seen in:
a. Drowning
b. Elderly
c. Strychnine poisoning
d. Sunstroke
e. Cholera

88. Mummification is/are favoured by:
a. Dry air
b. Humid air
c. Cold environment
d. Drowning
e. Warm air

89. Which of the following toxic agent is removed by hemodialysis, but not by gut detoxication through activated charcoal:
a. Theophylline
b. Benzodiazepines
c. Phenobarbitone
d. Ethylene glycol
e. Ethanol

90. All are true about eruption of teeth except:
a. First deciduous teeth erupt in 6 month
b. First permanent teeth erupt after 9 year
c. Canine teeth erupt earlier than molar teeth
d. Canine erupt after 2nd molar
e. Central incisor erupts earlier than lateral incisor

PSM

91. Which of the following vaccine is C/I in pregnancy:
a. BCG
b. Oral polio vaccine
c. Measles
d. Tetanus
e. Hepatitis B

92. Which of the following vaccine is C/I in symptomatic AIDS patient:
a. Measles
b. BCG
c. Rubella
d. Yellow fever
e. Hepatitis B

93. Which of the following is/are true regarding reference man & woman except:
a. Reference man is aged b/w 18-29 years & weighs 60kg
b. Reference man is aged b/w 18-29 years & weighs 55 kg
c. Reference man: he is engaged in 8 hours of occupation which usually involves moderate activity
d. Reference woman is aged b/w 18-29 years & weighs 50 kg
e. Reference woman: height of 1. 61 meter & a BMI of 21. 2

94. All of the following are true regarding water supply except:
a. Earlier recommended target of supply norm for rural area was 40 lpcd
b. 150-200 liters per capita is considered as an adequate supply to meet the needs for all urban domestic purpose
c. In 8th 5 –yr plan target set was 200 lpcd & accessibility of source of water < 200 meter for rural areas
d. For metro cities with population > 10 lakh, target is 150 lpcd
e. For municipality with population b/w 1-10 lakh, target is 100-135 lpcd

95. Deprivation index includes:
a. Education
b. Income
c. Working child
d. Drop out of child from school
e. Physical disability

96. Which of the most common cancer in Indian women according to latest data of ICMR:
a. Cervix
b. Vagina
c. Breast
d. Ovary
e. Oral cavity

MCQs

Answer

80. e.	81. b, c.	82. a, c, d.	83. c.	84. d.	85. a, b, c, e.	86. e.
87. c, d, e.	88. a, e.	89. e.	90. b, c, d.	91. a, b, c.	92. e.	93. b, d.
94. c.	95. a, b, e.	96. c.				

97. Which of the following dyads are corrects:
a. Child sex ratio is 914 according to 2011 census
b. CBR- 21. 3 in 2012
c. General fertility rate-88. 6 in 2012
d. CDR- 7 in 2012
e. 18yr- Legal age of marriage for female

98. Positive predictive value:
a. Numerator contains positive result by screening test
b. Denominator contains positive result by screening test
c. Numerator contains positive result by diagnostic test
d. Denominator contains positive result by diagnostic test
e. Numerator contains positive result by screening test & diagnostic test both

99. Incubatory carriers are:
a. Polio
b. Diphtheria
c. Anthrax
d. Pertussis
e. Hepatitis B

100. Which of the following disease have carrier stage:
a. Staph. aureus
b. Group B Streptococcus
c. Hepatitis B
d. Typhoid
e. Hemophilus influenza

101. True about Silicosis:
a. Birefringent particles are seen under polarized light in lung nodule
b. Fibrosis of lung
c. Stopping the exposure reverse the progression
d. Impairment of total lung capacity
e. Notifiable disease

102. Which of the following is not zoonosis:
a. Gonorrhoea
b. Pertussis
c. Anthrax
d. Brucella
e. Salmonella paratyphi B

OPHTHALMOLOGY

103. Periosteum of orbit is strongly attached to:
a. Medial wall of orbit
b. Lateral wall of orbit
c. Floor of orbit
d. Roof of orbit
e. Sutures lines

104. Poor prognostic factor for retinoblastoma includes:
a. > 4 mm size of tumour
b. > 2mm size of tumor
c. Associated glaucoma
d. Undifferentiated tumour cells
e. Sclera involvement

105. True about A-V pattern heterotropia squint:
a. The terms 'A' or 'V' pattern squint are labelled when the amount of deviation in squinting eye varies by more than 10° and 15°, respectively, between upward and downward gaze.
b. The terms 'A' or 'V' pattern squint are labelled when the amount of deviation in squinting eye varies by more than 20° and 25°, respectively, between upward and downward gaze.
c. Usually, over action of the inferior oblique or weakness of superior oblique leads to a A pattern & overaction of the superior oblique or weakness of inferior oblique to an V pattern
d. Usually, overaction of the inferior oblique or weakness of superior oblique leads to a V pattern & over action of the superior oblique or weakness of inferior oblique to an A pattern
e. Oblique muscle dysfunction is the commonest cause of AV pattern

106. True about congenital esotropia:
a. Onset is only after 1 year of age
b. Amblyopia may develop
c. Angle of deviation is usually fixed & large
d. Surgery should done after 2 years

107. True about lens of eye:
a. Avascular
b. Growth takes place throughout life
c. Derive its nutrition from aqueous humour
d. Transparent
e. Ectodermal in origin

108. Features of ocular ischemic syndrome includes all except:
a. Microaneurysm
b. Dot & blot haemorrhage
c. More common in elderly women than men
d. Disc edema
e. Amaurosis fugax

109. All are ocular emergency except:
a. Eye injury
b. Sympathetic ophthalmitis
c. Retinal artery occlusion
d. CRVO
e. Bacterial endophthalmitis

110. All are true regarding cornea except:
a. Endothelium help in maintaining dehydrated state
b. Oxygen is mostly derived by epithelium directly from the air through tear film
c. Glucose supply for corneal metabolism is mainly derived from the aqueous
d. Corneal thickness is more at center than periphery
e. Richly vascular

Answer

97. a, d, e.
98. b, d.
99. a, b, c, e.
100. a, c, d, e.
101. a, b, d, e.
102. a, b.
103. e.
104. a, c, d, e.
105. a, d, e.
106. b, c.
107. a, b, d, e.
108. c, d.
109. d.
110. d, e.

ENT

111. True about grommet insertion:
a. Small plastic tube aerating middle ear
b. Maximum duration of grommet insertion is 5 month
c. Healing occurs more quickly after extrusion than after removal
d. It is placed anteriorly on tympanic membrane
e. Surgery is always needed to remove it

112. True about Vasomotor rhinitis:
a. It is a type of allergic reaction
b. Clinically simulate nasal allergy
c. Nasal mucosa generally congested & hypertrophic
d. Hypertrophy of inferior turbinate is commonly present
e. Anti-histaminics & oral nasal decongestant are used in treatment

113. Structures preserved in radical neck dissection
a. Internal jugular vein
b. Carotid Artery
c. Accessory nerve
d. Brachial plexus
e. Sternocleidomastiod muscle

114. Feature of Granulomatosis with polyangitis:
a. Nasal polyp
b. Perforated Nasal septum
c. Persistant sinus
d. Crusting of nasal mucosa
e. Collapse of nasal bridge

115. True about vestibular schwanomma:
a. U/l hearing loss is common presentation
b. Mostly malignant
c. Most common tumour of CP angle
d. Sensorineural deafness
e. Uncapsulated

116. Tensor of vocal cord includes:
a. Arytenoid
b. Thyroarytenoid
c. Interarytenoid
d. Posterior cricoarytenoid
e. Cricothyroid

117. All are true about vocal cord nodule except:
a. Caused by phonotrauma
b. Commonly occur at Junction of middle & posterior 1/3
c. Common at junction of A 1/3 with P 2/3
d. Common in teachers
e. Treatment is speech therapy

118. True about allergic fungal sinusitis:
a. Fungal hyphae is present in allergic mucin which is pathological hallmark
b. Invasion of the sinus mucosa with fungus
c. Allergic reaction to fungus
d. Antifungal treatment lead to improvement of symptom
e. Surgical clearance is mainstay of treatment

119. True about conductive hearing loss:
a. Presbycusis
b. Cholestetoma
c. Acoustic neuroma
d. Perforation of tympanic membrane
e. Serous otitis media

120. True about Andy Gump deformity:
a. Occurs due to defects of the anterior mandibular arch
b. Hemimandibulectomy can cause
c. Marginal mandibulectomy can cause
d. Treatment is adequate reconstruction of anterior mandibular arch with plate & graft

121. Foreign body in trachea & bronchus can cause:
a. Bronchiectasis
b. Atelectasis
c. Subcutaneous emphysema
d. Pneumothorax

MEDICINE

122. Pulmonary blood flow increased in all except:
a. ASD
b. VSD
c. TOF
d. Transposition of great arteries (TGA)
e. PDA

123. Cauda equina is differentiated from conus medullaris by presence of:
a. Ankle jerk may lost
b. Knee jerk may lost
c. Motor changes
d. Bladder & bowel involvement as initial presentation
e. Root pain

124. Which of the following is/are the feature (s) of headache due to increase in intracranial pressure:
a. Increase on supine position
b. Most commonly presents as severe acute headache
c. Pulsatile in nature
d. Throbbing character
e. Analgesics are not very helpful

125. Early diastolic murmur is/are seen in:
a. VSD
b. ASD
c. Mitral stenosis
d. AR
e. PR

126. All are true about use of triptans in migraine except:
a. Used in prophylaxis of migraine
b. Efficacy increased with concomitant use of ergot
c. Can be given for long term where NSAIDS is not effective
d. Given when NSAIDS is not effective

MCQs

Answer

111. a, c, d.	112. b, c, d, e.	113. b, d.	114. b, c, d.	115. a, c, d.	116. b, e.	117. b.
118. a, c, e.	119. b, d, e.	120. a, b, d.	121. a, b, c, d.	122. c.	123. b, c, e.	124. a, e.
125. d, e.	126. a, b, c.					

127. All are true about renal artery stenosis except:
a. ACE inhibitors can be used in bilateral renal artery stenosis
b. ACE inhibitors can be used in unilateral renal artery stenosis
c. ACE inhibitors are best drug to control DM associated hypertension
d. Excision &Grafting is treatment of choice
e. Angioplasty with or without stenting, and surgical bypass used only in refractory cases

128. Which of the following causes glomerular proteinuria:
a. DM
b. Amyloidosis
c. Multiple myeloma
d. ACE inhibitors decreases proteinuria

129. All are true about Chylous pleural effusion except:
a. Stain positive with sudan III
b. Cutoff level of triglyceride for chylous effusion is > 150 mg/dl
c. Cutoff level of triglyceride for chylous effusion is > 50 mg/dl
d. Milky colour disappears with alkali
e. Milky colour disappears with ether

130. Chylous pleural effusion occur in:
a. T. B
b. Malignancy
c. SLE
d. Thoracic duct injury
e. Congestive heart failure

131. Feature of parkinsonism includes all except:
a. Mask face
b. Rigidity
c. Intention tremor
d. Resting tremor
e. Flaccidity

132. Which of the following causes massive splenomegaly:
a. CLL
b. Multiple myeloma
c. Follicular lymphangitis
d. Gaucher's disease
e. Sjogren's syndrome

133. ACTH dependent cushing syndrome is/are caused by:
a. Pituitary adenoma
b. Adrenal adenoma
c. Adrenocortical carcinoma
d. Pheochromocytoma

134. Hyperglycemic Hyperosmolar state (HHS) is characterized by:
a. Hyperglycemia
b. Acidosis
c. Dehydration
d. Coma

135. Which of the following is true about Pheochromocytoma:
a. Sestabimi scan is done before surgery
b. Mostly are malignant
c. Surgery is mainstay of treatment
d. Prior α blocker is given
e. Prior β blocker is given

136. Treatment of crohn's disease includes:
a. Steroid
b. 5-Aminosalicylic acid
c. Azathioprine
d. Daclizumab
e. Adalimumab

137. Energy selection in CPR according to AHA 2010 guideline is/are:
a. Monophasic 120-200J, Biphasic 360 J
b. Monophasic 200 J, Biphasic 360J
c. Monophasic 120 J, Biphasic 200J
d. Monophasic 360 J, Biphasic 120-200 J
e. Monophasic 360J, Biphasic 220J

138. Which of the following lesion represent tertiary syphilis:
a. Condylomata lata
b. Matted lymph node
c. Condylomata acuminata
d. Tabes dorsalis
e. Gumma formation

139. Which of the following statement (s) is/are correct regarding syphilis in pregnancy & congenital syphilis::
a. Foetus has more chance of infection in 3rd T. M
b. Syphilis can be prevented by giving penicillin in neonate
c. If infant showing signs of syphilis, he/she should be given single dose of crystalline penicillin
d. If infant does not have any signs of syphilis, he/she should be given benzathine penicillin
e. Foetus is most likely affected if mother is suffering from primary or secondary syphilis than late syphilis

140. Ascitic fluid with ↑ SAAG & ↑albumin is/are found in:
a. T. B
b. CHF
c. Cirrhosis
d. Pancreatitis
e. Nephrotic syndrome

141. Which of the following dyads are correct:
a. Pulsus paradoxus-Aortic regurgitation
b. Pulsus bisferiens- Aortic stenosis
c. Water-Hammer pulse- Aortic regurgitation
d. Pulsus parvus rt tardus -Aortic stenosis
e. Collapsing pulse- Aortic regurgitation

142. For cancer pain, ladder 2 step in WHO's pain step ladder includes:
a. Oral morphine
b. Injectable morphine
c. Codeine
d. Fentanyl
e. Tramadol

143. True about peptic ulcer:
a. H. pylori causes peptic ulcer
b. Eradication therapy better than PPI therapy
c. Eradication therapy also contain PPI
d. Duodenum ulcer is more commonly associated with H. pylori than gastric ulcer
e. Gastric ulcer is more commonly associated with H. pylori than duodenal ulcer

Answer

127. a, d.	128. a, b, d.	129. b, c.	130. a, b, d.	131. c.	132. a, d.	133. a, d.
134. a, c, d.	135. c, d, e.	136. a, b, c, e.	137. d.	138. d, e.	139. a, b, d, e.	140. b.
141. c, d, e.	142. c, e.	143. a, b, c, d.				

144. Features of Constrictive pericarditis which differentiate with restrictive cardiomyopathy:
a. Prominent y descent more common
b. Pericardial knock
c. Third heart sound
d. Thickened pericardium
e. Right ventricular hypertrophy

145. CURB-65 criteria for severe pneumonia includes:
a. Confusion
b. Uremia
c. Respiratory rate ≥30/min
d. Systolic Blood pressure ≤ 80 mmHg
e. Diastolic blood pressure ≤ 50 mmHg

146. Which of the following feature favours emphysema rather than interstitial fibrosis:
a. ↑FEV1
b. ↓FEV1/FEV6
c. ↑RV
d. ↑TLC
e. ↓Peak expiratory flow

147. True about Kaposi sarcoma:
a. Vascular tumor
b. Associated with HIV
c. Anti-retroviral therapy is given in AIDS associated KS
d. Associated with Human herpes virus-8
e. Radiotherapy may be used in treatment

148. Hypomagnesemia may lead to:
a. Hypotension
b. Bradycardia
c. Torsade de pointes
d. Tetany
e. Calcium should also be used in its treatment

149. Feature of unstable angina:
a. ↑ Troponin
b. Transient elevation of ST segment
c. Depression of ST segment
d. Pathological Q wave
e. T wave inversion

150. All are true about rheumatoid factor except:
a. Also found in Sjogren syndrome
b. May also present normally
c. It is basically IgM
d. Its presence is diagnostic of rheumatoid arthritis

SURGERY

151. Which of the following is the feature (s) of posterior cranial fossa fracture:
a. Bleeding from ear
b. Discolouration of skin & collection of blood occur in the region of mastoid process
c. Boggy swelling in the nape of the neck
d. Bleeding from nose
e. CSF rhinorrhoea

152. Symptom of overactive bladder are:
a. Increased day time frequency
b. Nocturia
c. Hesitancy
d. Dysuria
e. Urgency

153. All are true about undescended testis except:
a. Poses risk for malignancy
b. Treatment is manually repositioning testes into scrotum
c. At 1yr, about 1% children have undescended testis
d. Infertility may occur due to defect in spermatogenesis
e. Orchidectomy is treatment of choice

154. True about Psoas abscess:
a. Hip extension increases pain
b. Staphylococcus is most common cause
c. Presented with back pain
d. T. B can cause
e. Causes referred pain to the hip & groin

155. True about claudication:
a. Always B/l
b. Commonly present with pain in calf muscle
c. Pain increases with walking
d. Pain relieves with rest
e. Most commonly occurs due to neurological cause

156. True about abdominal aneurysm:
a. Size >4. 5 cm is indication for repair
b. Most common above renal artery
c. Typical triad of ruptured abdominal aneurysm is found in less than 50% case
d. Associated peripheral aneurysm is also commonly present
e. Treatment with shunt/graft

157. True about incisional hernia:
a. Incidence is about 10-15% of all abdominal wall hernia
b. Less chance in obese person
c. More common in woman
d. Commonly caused by lower abdominal surgery
e. May occur due to improper healing of abdominal incision

158. Which of following is/are true in accordance to revised gastric carcinoma staging:
a. All gastric tumours whose epicentre is within 5 cm of the gastroesophageal junction and extend into the oesophagus are now classified according to the revised gastric staging
b. 5 Node involvement- N2
c. T1N2M0- Stage II
d. Peritoneal spread is M0
e. Any tumour that perforates the serosa is now classified as T4 disease

159. All are true about dumping syndrome except:
a. Treatment consists of small meal at short interval
b. PPI is very useful in treatment
c. Watery & carbohydrate rich food are precipitating factors
d. May occur after gastrectomy or vagotomy and drainage operations
e. Rapid gastric emptying is common feature of both early & late dumping syndrome

Answer

144. a, b, d.	145. a, b, c.	146. b, c, d, e.	147. All	148. c, d, e.	149. b, c, e.	150. a, b, c.
151. b, c.	152. b, e.	153. e.	154. a, c, d, e.	155. b, c, d.	156. c, e.	157. a, c, d, e.
158. b, c, e.	159. b.					

160. Which of the following is/are true Boerhaave syndrome:
a. Occur due to increase in thoracic esophageal pressure
b. More common on left lateral wall of the esophagus
c. Caused by severe vomiting
d. Causes hydro-pnemothorax as complication
e. May be misdiagnosed as myocardial infarction

161. Features of Reidel thyroiditis are:
a. Presents as a goitre
b. Painful
c. Associated with IgG4 related systemic diseases
d. Fibrosis of interstitial thyroid stroma
e. Present with hypothyroidism

162. True about Sick euthyroid syndrome:
a. Normal TSH
b. T4 to T3 conversion impaired
c. High TSH
d. T4 high
e. Increased reverse T3

163. All are true about salivary gland tumor except:
a. Parotid gland is most common site of involvement
b. Warthin tumour almost always found in the parotid gland
c. Minor gland tumours are mostly malignant
d. Parotid tumours are mostly malignant
e. Superficial parotidectomy is done in pleomorphic adenoma

164. Which of the following is/are true regarding surgical shunt for esophageal varices in portal hypertension:
a. Prevention of esophageal bleed
b. Main indication of surgical shunt is a patient with Child's grade A cirrhosis, in whom the initial bleed has been controlled by sclerotherapy
c. Reduce the pressure in the portal circulation by diverting the blood into the low-pressure systemic circulation
d. Distal splenorenal shunt preserve blood flow to the liver

165. True about cleft lip:
a. Occurs d/t defect in fusion of frontal & nasal process
b. Only bilateral cases are associated with cleft palate
c. Repaired in neonatal period
d. Unilateral cases are more common in left side

166. Which of the following is/are true regarding management of a trauma presenting with shock:
a. Transfusion of PCV:FPP:Platelet should be in 1:1:1 ratio
b. First hemodynamic stabilize the patient, then go for CT scan
c. First go for CT scan, then stabilize the patient
d. CVP line should be placed

167. All are true about acute appendicitis except:
a. Clinically indifferent from Meckel diverticulum in children
b. Lymphoid hyperplasia may causes acute appendicitis
c. Pain shift to right iliac fossa
d. Ultrasound is more diagnostic than CT scan

168. Which of the following is true about esophageal adenocarcinoma:
a. Obesity is a risk factor
b. Most common in middle & lower 1/3
c. ↑Incidence in Barrett's oesophagus
d. Squamous metaplasia is a risk factor
e. Chronic gastroesophageal reflux an etiology of adenocarcinoma

169. True about intestinal pseudo-obstruction:
a. May be caused by hypokalemia
b. Bezoars can cause pseudo-obstruction
c. Neostigmine used in treatment
d. May be associated with diverticulosis
e. Colonoscopy is contraindicated

170. True about sigmoid volvulus:
a. Most common spontaneous type in adult
b. Less fiber diet is a risk factor
c. Treatment include resuscitation & decompression
d. Most common type of colonic volvulus
e. Low recurrence after conservative management

171. True about diverticular disease of colon:
a. Right side more common
b. Sign & symptoms indistinguishable from irritable bowel syndrome
c. Profuse & painless bleeding
d. Sigmoid is most common site

172. Which of the following is true about primary lymphoedema:
a. May be congenital
b. Lymphoedema congenita more commonly occur bilaterally
c. Condition improves with massage
d. Lymphatic hyperplasia

173. All are true about thymoma except:
a. MC tumor in anterior mediastinum
b. Treatment is thymectomy
c. Symptomatic cases present as endocrine abnormalities
d. May be associated with myasthenia gravis
e. Associated with thyroiditis

174. True about invasive thymoma:
a. Benign in nature
b. May be associated with EBV
c. Malignant in nature
d. Epithelial cells are most commonly of the cortical variety

175. True about cystosarcoma phylloides:
a. Usually bilateral
b. Usually occur in female over age of 40
c. Not involve nipple-areola complex
d. Treatment is mastectomy of malignant lesions
e. All are benign in nature

Answer

160. All
161. a, c, d.
162. a, b, e.
163. d.
164. a, b, c.
165. d.
166. b, d.
167. d.
168. a, c, e.
169. a, c.
170. a, c, d.
171. b, c, d.
172. a, b, c.
173. c.
174. a, b, d.
175. b, c, d.

176. True about anorectal abscess:
a. Ischiorectal is most common type
b. Primary modality of treatment is antibiotic without drain
c. Rupture can cause fistula formation
d. Common in diabetics
e. Drainage of pus with antibiotics is mainstay of treatment

177. Which of the following indicate poor prognosis in both Ranson & Glasgow scale of acute pancreatitis:
a. Albumin
b. Alanine aminotransferase
c. Aspartate aminotransferase
d. Lactate dehydrogenase
e. Base deficit

OBSTETRICS & GYNAECOLOGY

178. All are true about polycystic ovarian disease (PCOD) except:
a. Testosterone > 2 ng/ml
b. Infertility
c. High FSH/LH ratio
d. ↑ Insulin level
e. ↑ E2/oestrone (E1) ratio

179. Not true bout Endometriosis:
a. Sampson gave implantation theory
b. Cause infertility
c. Laproscopy is gold standard for diagnosis
d. Common in low socio-economic group

180. A young lady can be counseled for sterilization operation in all except:
a. A woman having no or few children may undergo sterilization
b. Woman with HIV either taking or not taking ART can go for sterilization
c. Husband consent is present
d. Young lactating women more than 25 years can go for sterilization
e. If the couple has 3 or more living children, the lower limit of age of the husband or wife may be relaxed at the discretion of the operating surgeon

181. Nulliparous women have high risk of following cancer:
a. Cervical cancer
b. Vaginal cancer
c. Breast cancer
d. Ovarian cancer
e. Endometrial Ca

182. Aneuplyid in 1st Trimester is detected by:
a. Nuchal translucency
b. MSAFP level
c. PAPP-A
d. Unconjugated estriol
e. β –hCG

183. True about testosterone in female:
a. > 50% testosterone secreted from ovary
b. > 80% testosterone secreted from ovary
c. ~ 0. 5 ng/ml is plasma concentration
d. Slight decrease in the secretion at time of ovulation
e. Daily production of testosterone is 0. 2-0. 3% mg

184. True about Nonoxynol-9:
a. Decrease risk of HIV
b. Prevent STD infection
c. Remain effective for 1-2 hr after application
d. Spermicidal action
e. Causes itching of vagina in female & itching of penis in male

185. Feature of false labor:
a. Steady intensity of pain
b. Cervical dilation
c. Discomfort is in the back and abdomen
d. Intervals remain long
e. Discomfort usually is relieved by sedation

186. Which of the following is true about Partial mole:
a. Karyotype is 69 XXY or 69XYY
b. High malignant potential
c. βHCG level is <50,000
d. Thecan lutein cysts common
e. Immunostaining (p57KIP2) positive

187. Which of the following is lower segment vertical incision:
a. Simon
b. Selheim
c. Kronig
d. Kerr
e. None

188. Appropriate time of IUCD insertion is/are:
a. Immediately after delivery
b. 1 week after delivery
c. Post-puerperal period
d. Before menstruation
e. Any time during lactation period

189. True about combined oral contraceptive (COC):
a. Pelvic examination is mandatory before prescribing COC
b. Pregnancy resumes soon after discontinuation of pill
c. Protect from endometrial cancer, cervical & ovarian cancer
d. HIV antiviral drugs reduce effectiveness of COC
e. Pregancy rate equal to non-hormonal contraceptive after discontinuation

190. True about implanon:
a. Releases > 67 μg/day of drug
b. Prevent STD
c. Life span is 3 years
d. Contains LNG
e. Has 6 implants

MCQs

Answer

176. c, d, e. 177. a, b, c, d. 178. c, e. 179. d. 180. a. 181. c, d, e. 182. b, d, e.
183. a, c, e. 184. c, d, e. 185. a, d. 186. a, c, e. 187. b, c. 188. a, b, c, e. 189. a, d.
190. c.

191. True about progestogen only pill:
a. Weight gain occurs
b. Cause irregular bleeding
c. It can be given to lactating mother
d. Should not be given to women over 35 years
e. Protect from breast cancer

192. True about Dysgerminoma:
a. Rare tumor in pregnancy
b. Always b/l
c. Total abdominal hysterectomy is usually done
d. Unilateral salpingo-oophorectomy is generally done
e. Constitute 30% of all malignant germ cell tumour

193. True about placental abruption:
a. Pre-eclampsia is a risk factor
b. Common in multigravida
c. Common in primigravida
d. Premature separation of normal implanted placentae
e. Character of bleeding is bright red blood

194. Diagnosis of Endometrial carcinoma can be made from:
a. Papanicolaou smear
b. Fractional curettage
c. Aspiration cytology from uterine
d. Hysteroscopy & biospy
e. Colposcopy

195. True about Klinefelter syndrome:
a. Legs are more in length than trunk
b. Intrauterine fertilization can not be successful even with TESA & ICSI
c. Gynaecomastia
d. FSH and luteinizing hormone (LH) are decreased

PAEDIATRICS

196. Which of the following causes neonatal jaundice:
a. Sickle cell anaemia
b. β-Thalassemia
c. Meningitis
d. G6PD deficiency
e. Rh incompatibility

197. Which of the following milestone is developed by child b/w 6 to 9 month:
a. Can point something with index finger
b. Swap some object from one palm to another
c. Can hold object with thumb & index finger
d. Can voluntary drop object
e. Can extend arm

198. True about osteum primum defect:
a. It is found in ASD
b. More commonly associated with ASD than VSD
c. May be associated with Down syndrome
d. Osteum primum ASD is more common than osteum secondum ASD

199. True about minimal change disease:
a. Peak incidence is between 2 and 4 years of age
b. Renal failure occur in adolescent
c. Steroid not very effective
d. Selective proteinuria

200. Vesico-ureteric reflex is commonly diagnosed by:
a. Micturating cystography
b. Radioisotope renography
c. IVU
d. CT scan

201. True about Tanner stage II:
a. Penis increases in length
b. Penis increases in width
c. Scanty hair at base of penis
d. Darkening of scrotum
e. More growth occur in boys than girls

ORTHOPAEDICS

202. True about Locking compression plate:
a. In osteoporotic patients, it should not be used
b. Can be used as buttress plate
c. Usually cause perosteal injury
d. Mechanically superior to a conventional plate
e. Can not be used as compression plate

203. Osteosclerotic metastases is/are common in cancer of:
a. Prostate
b. Breast
c. Lung
d. Malignant melanoma
e. Renal cell carcinoma

204. Following are immediate complications of fracture:
a. Vascular ischemia
b. Neuronal injury
c. Malunion
d. Compartment syndrome
e. Avascular necrosis

205. Which of the following cause malunion except:
a. Open #
b. Infection
c. Bone grafting
d. Soft tissue interposition
e. Proper alignment of fracture

206. True about Atypical CTEV:
a. Foot is flexed downward
b. Sole crease are not found
c. Difficult to treat than typical variety
d. May occur due to neurological disorder
e. May be associated with Meningomyelocele

207. In young person most common cancer among following is:
a. Giant cell
b. Osteosarcoma
c. Chondrosarcoma
d. Ewing sarcoma

Answer

191. a, b, c.	192. d, e.	193. a, b, d.	194. b, c, d.	195. a, c.	196. b, d, e.	197. b, c, d.
198. a, b, c.	199. a, d.	200. a, b.	201. a, c.	202. b, d.	203. a, b.	204. a, b.
205. c, e.	206. a, c, d, e.	207. b.				

208. All are true about septic arthritis except:
a. Staph. aureus is most common causative organism
b. Common in children
c. Affect growth plate
d. E. coli is the commonest causative organism
e. Aspiration of joint fluid is used for diagnosis

209. Features of fat embolism:
a. Bradycardia
b. Hypoxia
c. Hypotension
d. Tachypnoea
e. Petechial rash

210. Straight leg raising test is/are positive in:
a. Spinal stenosis
b. Spinal abscess
c. Also called as trendelenburg test
d. Prolapsed intervertebral disc
e. Sciatica

211. Which of the following is/are true about the gait in sensory deficit:
a. Antalgic gait
b. Apraxic
c. Trendelenburg
d. Positive Romberg sign
e. Apraxic gait

ANAESTHESIA

212. Which of the following is/are true regarding anaesthetic gas:
a. N2O- increases efficacy of other inhalational agents
b. Halothane- agent of choice in children
c. Sevoflurane is agent of choice in children
d. Isoflurane- smooth induction

213. All are true about malignant hyperthermia except:
a. Occurs due to defect in ryanodine receptor
b. Caffeine –halothane test on muscle fiber is used for diagnosis
c. Halothane precipitates
d. Thiopentone triggers
e. Usually AD in inheritance

214. True about Endotracheal tube:
a. Most common used size for adult male is 8-8. 5
b. Most common used size for adult female is 7-7. 5
c. PVC tube is reusable by cleaning
d. In children cuffed tube is not used
e. Cuff is for aspiration of secretions

215. True about subarachnoid block (spinal anesthesia):
a. Cannot be used in infant & children
b. Can be given by unskilled doctor
c. May be used when I. V access is not possible for intravenous drugs
d. Hypotension is most common side-effect

216. Indication of CVP line is/are:
a. CVP monitoring in shock patient
b. Prior to major surgery
c. For administering inotropics through CVP line in shock patients
d. In every case of caesarean section
e. For giving blood in patient with severe haemorrhage

SKIN

217. True about acute paronychia:
a. Fungal infection of nail pulp
b. Fungal infection of nail bed
c. Bacterial infection
d. Allergic reaction
e. Usually involve nail folds

218. True about Campbell de Morgan spots:
a. Benign
b. Malignant
c. Proliferation of blood vessel
d. Very painful
e. Cherry red in color

219. Which of the following disease is associated with hepatitis C infection:
a. Lichen planus
b. Psoariasis
c. Sjogren's syndrome
d. HUS
e. HSP

220. Which of the following statement is/are correct about Scabies:
a. Number of lesion correspondent to number of mite
b. Ivermectin not used for treatment
c. Itching worsen at night
d. Not involve face in children

221. All are true about Pitryiasis rosea except:
a. Usually self limiting
b. Drug induced
c. Herald patch precedes eruptions by 1-2 weeks
d. Caused by HHV 3 & 4

PSYCHIATRY

222. Exposure & response prevention technique is/are used in:
a. Schizophrenia
b. OCD
c. Phobia
d. Mania
e. Depression

Answer

208. d.	209. b, d, e.	210. d, e.	211. d.	212. a, c.	213. d.	214. a, b, d.
215. d.	216. a, b, c, e.	217. c, e.	218. a, c, e.	219. a, c.	220. c.	221. b, d.
222. b, c.						

223. Most common disorder (s) after trauma is:

a. Major depression
b. Mania
c. Schizophrenia
d. PTSD
e. Acute stress reaction

224. A woman has mild depression after few days of delivery & disappeared after 2 week in postpartum period. It may be due to:

a. Post-partum blue
b. Mania
c. Post-partum depression
d. Mild depression
e. Postpartum psychosis

RADIOLOGY

225. Water lily sign is seen in:

a. Hydatid cyst of lung
b. Aspergilloma lung
c. T. B
d. Silicosis
e. Hemartoma lung

226. Which of the following do not use radiation:

a. MRI
b. CT
c. USG
d. SPECT
e. PET

227. Which of the following is non-ionising radiation:

a. X-ray
b. β -rays
c. α -rays
d. Microwave
e. γ rays

228. On x-ray, small bowel can be differentiated by large bowel by having:

a. String of beads sign
b. Haustrations
c. Peripherally placed concave coil of intestine
d. Air fluid level
e. Valvulae conniventes

229. For radiotherapy an isotope is paced in or around canecr site. It is called as:

a. Brachytherapy
b. Teletherapy
c. External beam therapy
d. Intensity Medulated radiotherapy

230. Normal brain calcification is /are present in:

a. Pineal gland
b. Choroids plexus
c. Thalamus
d. Duramater
e. Hypothalamus

Answer

223. d, e. 224. a. 225. a. 226. a, c. 227. d. 228. a, d, e. 229. a.
230. a, b, d.

MAY 2015 ANSWERS & EXPLANATIONS

ANATOMY

1. Ans. a. Femoral Vessel

[Ref: B. D. C 6th/Vol. II 49, 56, 17, 59, 84: Snell's 9th/462; Gray's 40th/1376]

"The ***femoral vessels*** pass from the adductor canal into the popliteal fossa via the **adductor hiatus**, ***an opening in the tendon of adductor magnus*** adjacent to the femoral shaft, two-thirds of the way down the adductor canal" *(Gray's 40th/1376)*

Femoral artery pass through an ***opening in the adductor magnus*** to become continuous with the popliteal artery" *(B. D. C 6th/Vol. II 49)*

Femoral vein enters the thigh by passing through an ***opening in the adductor magnus*** as a continuation of the popliteal vein *(Snell's 9th/462)*

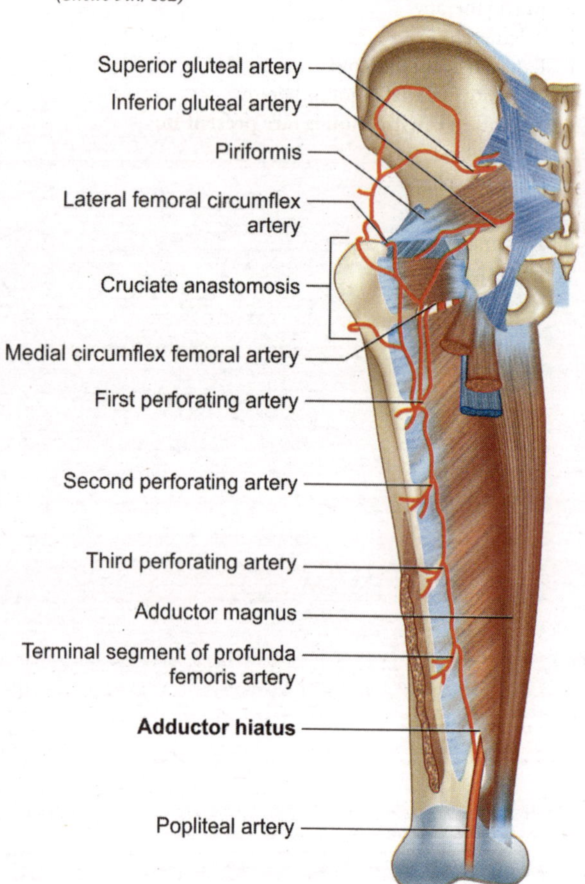

Fig: The arteries and muscles of the left gluteal and femoral regions (Posterior aspect)

ALSO KNOW

Adductor Canal

- *Gray's 40th/1376*
- *The adductor canal **(Hunter's canal[Q]; subsartorial canal)** is a trough shaped intermuscular tunnel occupying the distal two-thirds of the medial aspect of the thigh*
- *It is **triangul**ar in section, and is bounded anterolaterally by vastus medialis, posteromedially by adductor longus, and distal to adductor longus, by adductor magnus.*
- *The adductor canal **contains** the **femoral artery and vein[Q]**, the descending genicular and muscular branches of the femoral artery and their corresponding venous tributaries, the saphenous nerve, and the nerve to vastus medialis (until it enters its muscle).*

2. Ans. b. Ulnar nerve & c. Radial...

[Ref: B. D. C 6th/Vol. I 48-51: Gray's 40th/815-17; Snell's 9th/350-51]

Axillary Artery

- *B. D. C 6th/Vol. I 48-49*
- ***"It extends from the outer border of the first rib to the lower border of teres major*** where it continues as the brachial artery"*(B. D. C 6th/Vol. I 48-49)*
- ***The pectoralis minor muscle crosses the artery & divides it into three parts***
  - First part, superior (proximal) to the muscle
  - Second part, posterior (deep) to the muscle
  - Third part, inferior (distal) to the muscle
- **"3rd part posteriorly:** Axillary nerve & radial nerve lies behind the artery" *(Snell's 9th/351)*
- "**3rd part medially**: Ulnar nerve, axillary vein & medial cutaneous nerve of arm *(Snell's 9th/351)*

Axillary Artery

- *Gray's 40th/815*
- The axillary artery, a continuation of the subclavian artery, ***begins at the outer border of the first rib***, and ends nominally at the ***inferior border of teres major*** where it becomes the brachial artery.
- **Pectoralis minor** crosses it and so divides it into three parts which are proximal, posterior and distal to the muscle.
- ***Branches:*** The branches of the axillary artery are superior thoracic, thoracoacromial, lateral thoracic, subscapular, anterior and posterior circumflex humeral.

Table *(B. D. C 6th/Vol. I 48-51)*: **Important relation of the 3 parts of the axillary artery (Self drawn table from the text)**

Part/Relation	Anterior	Posterior	Lateral	Medial
1st Part (Proximal)	*Platysma; clavicular part of pectoralis major; Clavipectoral fascia with cephalic vein, lateral pectoral nerev & thoracoacromial artery*	*Medial cord of brachial plexus with its medial pectoral branch; 1st & 2nd digitations of serratous anterior with nerve to serratous anterior*	*Lateral & posterior cord of the brachial plexus*	*Axillary vein*

Contd...

Part/Relation	Anterior	Posterior	Lateral	Medial
2nd Part (deep to muscle)	*Pectoralis major; Pectoralis minor*	*Posterior cord of brachial plexus; subscapularis*	*Lateral cord of brachial plexus; Corachobrachialis*	*Medial cord of brachial plexus; Medial pectoral nerve; Axillary vein*
3rd Part (Distal)	*Pectoralis major; Medial root of the median nerve*	***Radial nerve**; Axillary nerve in the upper part; Subscapularis in the upper part; Tendon of the latissimus dorsi & the teres major in lower part*	*Corachobrachialis; Musculocutaneous nerve; Lateral root of the median nerve in the upper part; Trunk of median nerve*	*Axillary vein; Median cutaneous nerve of forearm & **ulnar nerve** b/w the axillary artery & axillary vein; Medial cutaneous nerve of arm, medial to axillary vein*

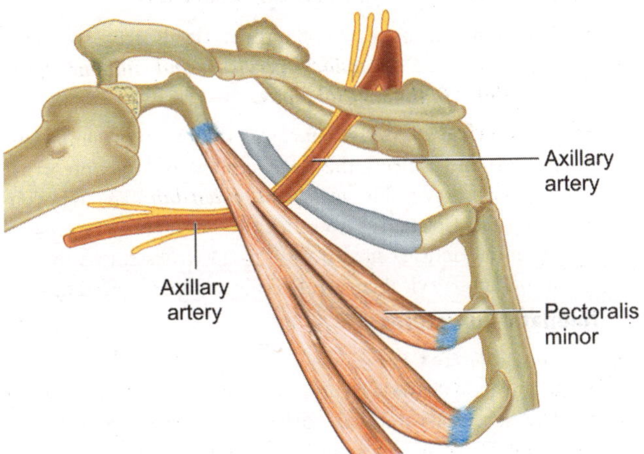

Fig: 3 Parts of axillary artery in relation with pectoralis minor muscle

3. Ans. a. 4-8 weeks

[Ref: Human Embryology by I. B. Singh 10th/166; Langman's Medical Embryology 9th/387; Snell's 9th/583-84; Gray's 40th/602]

"The ***period from 7 to 8 week is the final period of facial development***" *(Gray's 40th/602)*

"Early in development, face is represented by an area bounded cranially by the neural plate, caudally by the pericardium & laterally by the mandibular process of the first pharyngeal arch on each side. Buccopharyngeal membrane form the floor of the central depression of this area, the stomodeum. ***By the 4th week, Buccopharyngeal membrane breaks down so that the stomodeum communicate with the foregut***" *(Snell's 9th/583)*

Table *(I. B. Singh 10th/166):* **Human Embryology by**

Age	Developmental Events
4th week (28th day)	The frontonasal, maxillary and mandibular processes can be identified. The lens and nasal placodes are present.
5th week (31 to 35 days)	The nasal pits are established.
6th week	Tubercles for the development of pinna begins to be formed.
7th week	Eyelids are established. The maxillary process fuses with the medial nasal process.
8th week	Eyes shift from a lateral to a frontal position. Bucconasal membrane ruptures.
10th week	The palatal processes and nasal septum fuse with each other.

Face Development *(Langman's Medical Embryology 9th/387)*

- At the end of the **fourth week, facial prominences** consisting primarily of neural crest-derived mesenchyme and formed mainly by the first pair of pharyngeal arches appear. **Maxillary prominences** can be distinguished lateral to the stomodeum, and **mandibular prominences** can be distinguished caudal to this structure
- During the fifth week, the nasal placodes invaginate to form **nasal pits.** In so doing, they create a ridge of tissue that surrounds each pit and forms the **nasal prominences.** The prominences on the outer edge of the pits are the **lateral nasal prominences;** those on the inner edge are the **medial nasal prominences**
- **During the following 2 weeks,** the maxillary prominences continue to increase in size. Simultaneously, they grow medially, compressing the medial nasal prominences toward the midline.

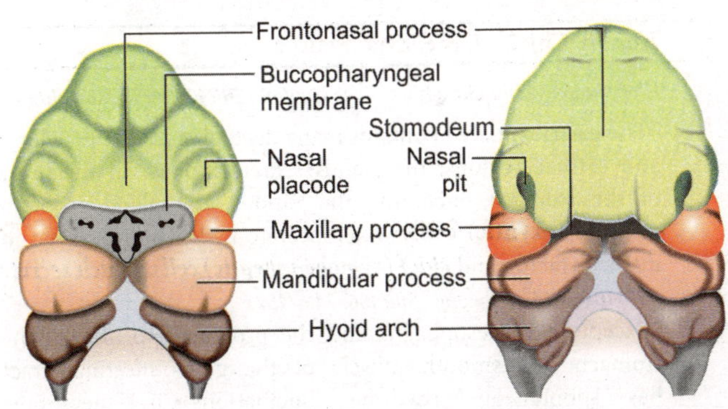

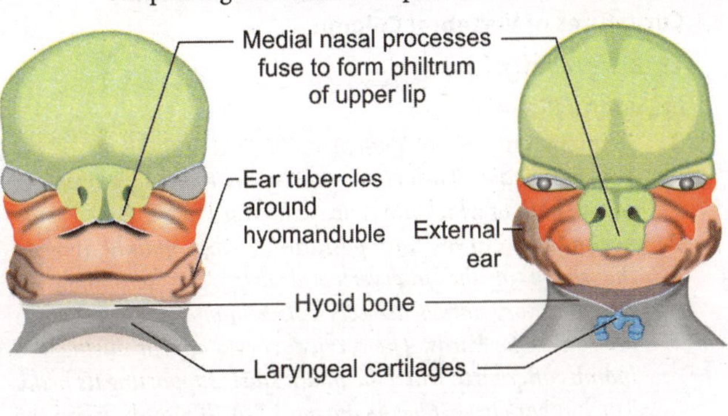

Fig: Development of the face. A, 4 weeks (3. 5 mm); B, 5 weeks (6. 5 mm); E, 7 weeks (19 mm); F, 8 weeks (28 mm).

Table *(Lang- man's Medical Embryology 9th/387)*: **Structures Contributing to Formation of the Face**

Prominence	Structure formed
Frontonasal	Forehead, bridge of nose, medial and lateral nasal prominences
Maxillary	Cheeks, lateral portion of upper lip
Medial Nasal	Philtrum of upper lip, crest and tip of nose
Lateral nasal	Alae of nose
Mandibular	Lowe lip

4. Ans. a. Digastric muscle & e. Adductor magnus

[Ref: B. D. C 6th/Vol. I 62, Vol. III 132, Vol. II 60]

"Adductor magnus: because of double nerve supply, it is called a hybrid muscle" *(B. D. C 6th/Vol. II 60)*

Digastric Muscle

◈ *B. D. C 6th/Vol. III 132*

- Anterior belly: nerve to mylohyoid
- Posterior belly by facial nerve

Trapezius Nerve Supply

◈ *B. D. C 6th/Vol. I 62)*

- Spinal part of accessory nerve is motor
- Branches from C3, C4 are proprioceptive

Muscle with Dual Nerve Supply

- *Brachialis*
- *Pectineus: obturator & femoral*
- *Digastric*
- *Adductor magnus: Pubic part by obturator nerve & ischial part by tibial part of sciatic nerve*
- *Flexor pollicis brevis*
- *Flexor digitorum profundus*
- *Bicep femoris: Long head by tibial part of sciatic nerve & short head by common peroneal part of sciatic nerve*
- *Tibialis anterior: Greater part by deep peroneal nerve & upper part by recurrent genicular nerve*

5. Ans. a. Primary...., d. Cervical... & e. Lumbar....

[Ref: B. D. C 6th/Vol. I 204: Snell's 9th/690-91; Gray's 40th/713-14]

Curvatures of Vertebral Column

◈ *B. D. C 6th/Vol. I 204*

In Sagittal Plane

1. **Primary curves** *are present at birth due to shape of the vertebral bodies. The primary curves are thoracic, thoracic & sacral, both of which are concave forward*
2. **Secondary curves** *are postural & are mainly due to the shape of the intervertebral disc. The secondary or compensatory curves are cervical & lumbar, both of which are convex forwards. The cervical curves appear during 4–5 months after birth when the infant starts supporting its head. The lumbar curve appears during 12 to 18 months when the child assumes the upright posture*

In Coronal Plane

6. *There is slight lateral curve in the thoracic region with its concavity towards the left. It is possible due to the greater use of the right upper limb & the pressure of the aorta*
7. *The curvature add to the elasticity of spine & the number of curves gives it a higher resistance to weight than would be afforded by a single curve*

Embryonic and Fetal Curvatures

◈ *Gray's 40th/713-14*

- The embryonic body appears flexed. It has ***primary thoracic and pelvic curves which are convex dorsally***.
- Functional muscle development leads to the early appearance of ***secondary cervical and lumbar spinal curvatures in the sagittal plane***.
- The **cervical curvature** appears at the end of the embryonic period, and reflects the development of function in the muscles responsible for ***head extension***, an important component of the 'grasp reflex'. Radiographic examination of human fetuses aged from 8 to 23 weeks shows that the secondary cervical curvature is almost always present.

Neonatal Curvatures

◈ *Gray's 40th/714*

- In the neonate the vertebral column has no fixed curvatures.
- The secondary lumbar curvature becomes important in maintaining the centre of gravity of the trunk over the legs when walking starts, and thus changes in body proportions exert a major influence on the subsequent shape of curvatures in the vertebral column.

Adult Curvatures

◈ *Gray's 40th/714*

- In adults, the cervical curve is a lordosis (convex forwards), and the least marked. It extends from the atlas to the second thoracic vertebra, with its apex between the fourth and fifth cervical vertebrae
- The lumbar curve is also a lordosis. It has a greater magnitude in females and extends from the 12th thoracic vertebra to the lumbosacral angle

PHYSIOLOGY

6. Ans. b. Chief cell & e. Zygometic. cells

[Ref: Ganong 25th/456, 24th/457-59; Guyton 12th/406; A. K. Jain 5th/202]

"The gastric mucosa contains many deep glands. In the pyloric and cardiac regions, the glands secrete mucus. In the body of the stomach, including the fundus, the glands contain **parietal (oxyntic) cells**, which secrete hydrochloric acid and intrinsic factor, and ***chief (zymogen, peptic) cells, which secrete pepsinogens***" *(Ganong 25th/456, 24th/457)*

"Except in the esophagus and the proximal portion of the stomach, the smooth muscle of the gastrointestinal tract has spontaneous rhythmic fluctuations in membrane potential between about -65 and -45 mV. This basic electrical rhythm (BER) is initiated by the ***interstitial cells of Cajal***" *(Ganong 25th/496, 24th/498)*

"**Paneth cells**—endocrine cells located in the depths of the crypts of Lieberkuhn—secrete defensins, naturally occurring peptide antibiotics that are also secreted elsewhere in the body. The migrating enterocytes are exposed to a high concentrate of the defensins, and this may protect them as they move to the tops of the villi. Paneth cells may also secret guanylin" *(A. K. Jain 5th/202)*

Table: Cells within Gastric Glands

Mucus Cell	Parietal/ Oxyntic Cells	Chief/ Zymogen Cells (Peptic Cell)	Enteroendocrine cells
Secrete Mucus Secrete HCO_3^-	Secrete HCl ***Secrete Intrinsic Factor***[Q]	Secrete Pepsinogen[Q]	Enterochromaffin Like Cells (ECL): Secrete Histamine[Q] **Gastrin G cells:** Secrete Gastrin[Q] 'D' Cells: Secrete Somatostatin[Q] Enterochromaffin cells (ECC): Secrete serotonin[Q]

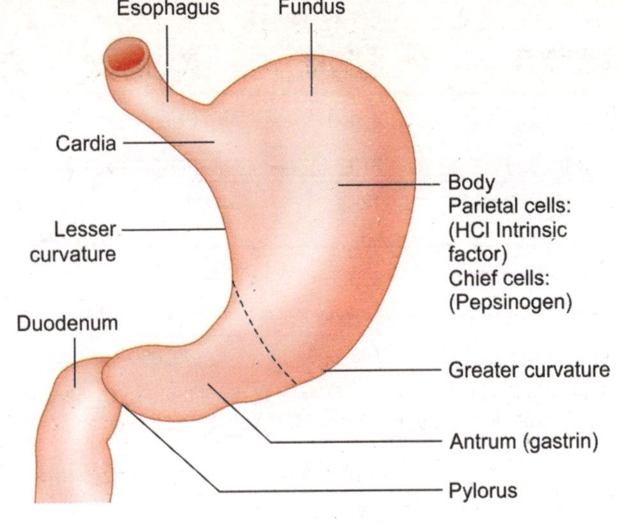

Fig: Anatomy of stomach

7. Ans. c. Fast fatigable & e. Faster acting ....

[Ref: Ganong 25th/108, 24th/107; 23rd/103; Guyton 12th/96; A. K. Jain 5th/173]

Table *(Ganong 25th/108, 24th/107, 23rd/103)*: **Classification of fiber type in skeletal muscle**

	Type I	Type IIA	Type IIB
Other names	Slow, oxidative (SO)	Fast, Oxidative, Glycolytic (FOG)	Fast, Glycolytic (FG)
Colour	Red	Red	White
Myosin ATPase activity	Slow	Fast	Fast
Ca2+ pumping capacity of sarcoplasmic reticulum	Moderate	High	High
Diameter	Small	Large	Large
Glycolytic capacity	Moderate	High	High
Oxidative capacity	High	Moderate	Low
Associated Motor Unit Type Membrane potential = -90mV	Slow (s)	Fast resistant to Fatigue (FR)	Fast Fatigable (FF)
Oxidative capacity	High	Moderate	Low

8. Ans. a. Bicarb....., b. Amo..., c. Percen... & d. In abso....

[Ref: Ganong 25th/688-90, 24th/681-85, 23rd/649; Guyton 12th/475-83]

Table *(Ganong 23rd/649)*: **Renal handling of various plasma constituents in a normal adult human on an average diet**

Substance	Per 24 Hours Filtered	Reabsorbed	Secreted	Excreted	Percentage Reabsorbed	Location[1]
Na^+ (meq)	26, 000	25, 850	–	150	99.4	P, L, D, C
K^+ (meq)	600	560[2]	50[2]	90	93.3	P, L, D, C
Cl^- (meq)	18, 000	17, 850	–	150	99.2	P, L, D, C

Contd...

Substance	Per 24 Hours Filtered	Reabsorbed	Secreted	Excreted	Percentage Reabsorbed	Location[1]
HCO_3^- (meq)	4, 900	4, 900	–	0	100	P, D
Urea (mmol)	870	460[3]	–	410	53	P, L, D, C
Creatinine (mmol)	12	1[4]	1[4]	12	–	–
Uric acid (mmol)	50	49	4	5	98	P
Glucose (mmol)	800	800	–	0	100	P
Total solute (mosm)	54, 000	53, 400	100	700	98. 9	P, L, D, C
Water (mL)	180, 000	179, 000	–	1000	99.4	P, L, D, C

[1] P, proximal tubules; L, loops of Henle; D, distal tubules; C, collecting ducts.; [2] K+ is both reabsorbed and secreted; [3] Urea moves into as well as out of some portions of the nephron. : [4] Variable secretion and probable reabsorption of creatinine in humans

Table *(Guyton 12th/476)*: **Filtration, Reabsorption, and Excretion Rates of Different Substances by the Kidneys**

	Amount Filtered	Amount Reabsorbed	Amount Excreted	% of Filtered Load Reabsorbed
Glucose (g/day)	180	180	0	100
Bicarbonate (mEq/day)	4, 320	4, 318	2	>99. 9
Sodium (mEq/day)	25, 560	25, 410	150	99.4
Chloride (mEq/day)	19, 440	19, 260	180	99. 1
Potassium (mEq/day)	756	664	92	87. 8
Urea (g/day)	46. 8	23.4	23.4	50
Creatinine (g/day)	1. 8	0	1. 8	0

9. Ans. a. Inhibitory.., b. Excitat.... & c. Inhibito....

[Ref: Ganong 25th/587-89, 24th/589-91, 265; Guyton 12th/248-50]

Medullary control of the cardiovascular system

Ganong 25th/587, 24th/589-91

- *One of the major source of excitatory input to sympathetic nerves controlling the vasculature is a group of neurons located near the pial surface of the medulla in the* ***Rostral Ventrolateral Medulla (RVLM)****. This region is sometimes called a* ***vasomotor area***
- Neurovascular compression of the RVLM has been linked to some cases of essential hypertension in humans
- The activity of RVLM neurons is determined by many factors

Table *(Ganong 25th/589, 24th/591)*: **Factors affecting the activity of RVLM**

Direct stimulation: CO_2, hypoxia
Excitatory inputs: ***cortex via hypothalamus***, mesencephalic periaqueductal gray, ***brain stem reticular formation, pain pathway***, somatic afferent (somatosympathetic reflex), Carotid & aortic chemoreceptors

Contd...

Direct stimulation: CO_2, hypoxia
Inhibitory inputs: ***cortex via hypothalamus***, ***caudal ventrolateral medulla***, caudal medullary raphe nuclei, lung inflation afferents; carotid, aortic & cardiopulmonary baroreceptors

10. Ans. a. Miosis & e. Contraction of...

[Ref: Ganong 25th/257, 24th/265; Guyton 12th/804]

Parasympathetic Division

Ganong 25th/257, 24th/257-58

- The cranial outflow of the parasympathetic division supplies the visceral structures in the head via the oculomotor, facial, and glossopharyngeal nerves, and those in the thorax and upper abdomen via the vagus nerves.
- The sacral outflow supplies the pelvic viscera via the pelvic branches of the second to fourth sacral spinal nerves. The preganglionic fibers in both outflows end on short postganglionic neurons located on or near the visceral structures

Table *(Guyton 12th/804)*: **Autonomic Effects on Various Organs of the Body**

Organ	Effect of Sympathetic Stimulation	Effect of Parasympathetic Stimulation
Eye		
Pupil	Dilated (Mydriasis)	Constricted (Miosis)
Ciliary muscle	Slight relaxation (far vision)	Constricted (near vision)
Glands (Nasal, Lacrimal, Parotid, Submandibular, Gastric Pancreatic)	Vasoconstriction and slight secretion	Stimulation of copious secretion (containing many enzymes for enzyme-secreting glands)
Sweat glands	Copious sweating (cholinergic)	Sweating on palms of hands
Apocrine glands	Thick, odoriferous secretion	None
Blood vessels	Most often constricted	Most often little or no effect
Heart		
Muscle	Increased rate	Slowed rate
	Increased force of contraction	Decreased force of contraction (especially of atria)
Coronaries	Dilated (β_2); constricted (α)	Dilated
Lungs		
Bronchial muscle	Relaxation	Contraction
Blood vessels	Mildly constricted	Dilated
Gut		
Lumen	Decreased peristalsis and tone	Increased peristalsis and tone
Sphincter	Increased tone (most times)	Relaxed (most times)
Gallbladder and bile ducts	Relaxed	Contracted
Kidney	Decreased urine output and increased renin secretion	None
Bladder		
Detrusor	Relaxed (slight)	Contracted
Trigone	Contracted	Relaxed

11. Ans. a. Thick…., c. Close…, d. Tig… & e. Decrea….

[Ref: Ganong 25th/671, 24th/604-06; Guyton 12th/816-17; Gray's 40th/48-49; BDC4th/Vol. III386-87; Robbins 9th/1252-54, 7th/1349-50]

Blood–brain Barrier (BBB)

◈ *Guyton 12th/817*

- Barriers exist both at the choroid plexus and at the tissue capillary membranes in essentially all areas of the brain parenchyma ***except in some areas of the hypothalamus, pineal gland, and area postrema,*** where substances diffuse with greater ease into the tissue spaces
- The cause of the low permeability of the blood-brain barriers is the manner in which the endothelial cells of the brain tissue capillaries are joined to one another. They are joined by so-called ***tight junctions.*** That is, the membranes of the adjacent endothelial cells are tightly fused rather than having large slit-pores between them, as is the case for most other capillaries of the body.

Glia *(Robbins 9th/1252-54, 7th/1349-50)*

- **Glial cells** are derived from ***neuroectoderm (macroglia: astrocytes, oligodendrocytes, ependyma) or from bone marrow (microglia).***
- **"Astrocyte cell projections called astrocytic feet (also known as "glia limitans") surround the endothelial cells of the BBB, providing biochemical support to those cells"**
- "**Glial cells (astrocytes)** form a layer around brain blood vessels and may important in the development of the **BBB**. Astrocytes may be also be responsible for transporting ions from the brain to the blood"

Functions of the BBB

- *Protects the brain from "foreign substances" in the blood that may injure the brain.*
- *Protects the brain from hormones and neurotransmitters in the rest of the body.*
- *Maintains a constant environment for the brain.*

"**Circumventricular Organs** include: ***Pineal body, Area postrema, Subfornical organ, Vascular organ of the lamina terminalis & Median eminence***"

12. Ans. a. Glucagon & e. Arginine

[Ref: Ganong 25th/328-29, 24th/330-32; Guyton 12th/555-56; A. K. Jain 5th/685]

GH Testing

◈ *http://labtestsonline. org/understanding/analytes/growth-hormone/tab/test*

- Because growth hormone is released in pulses, a single measurement of the blood level is not normally clinically useful. Therefore, testing for the suppression or stimulation of growth hormone release from the pituitary is usually done.
- **GH stimulation tests** help to ***diagnose GH deficiency and hypopituitarism.*** The most commonly used stimulant is ***arginine***, but others include ***clonidine and glucagon***
- **GH suppression tests** help to diagnose GH excess.

"The normal concentration of growth hormone in the plasma of an adult is between 1. 6 and 3 ng/ml. Growth hormone is secreted in a pulsatile pattern, increasing and decreasing"- *Guyton 12th/555-56*

Stimuli Affecting Growth Hormone Secretion

◈ *Ganong 25th/328-29, 24th/330-31*

- The basal plasma growth hormone concentration ranges from 0–3 ng/mL in normal adults. It is not significantly higher in children.
- However, secretory rates cannot be estimated from single values, because there are irregular "spikes" of secretion throughout the day

Table *(Ganong 25th/328, 24th/330)*: **Stimuli that affect growth hormone secretion in humans**

Stimuli that Increase secretion
Hypoglycemia, 2-Deoxyglucose
Exercise, Fasting
Increase in circulating levels of certain amino acids
Protein meal, Stressful stimuli, Pyrogen
Infusion of arginine and some other amino acids
Glucagon, Lysine vasopressin
Various psychologic stresses, Going to sleep
L-Dopa and α-adrenergic agonists that penetrate the brain
Apomorphine and other dopamine receptor agonists
Estrogens and androgens
Stimuli that decrease secretion
REM sleep, Glucose, ***Cortisol***, FFA
Medroxyprogesterone
Growth hormone & IGF-I

Table *(Guyton 12th/556)*: **Factors That Stimulate or Inhibit Secretion of Growth Hormone**

Stimulate Growth Hormone Secretion	Inhibit Growth Hormone Secretion
Decreased blood glucose Decreased blood free fatty acids Increased blood amino acids (***arginine***) Starvation or fasting, protein deficiency Trauma, stress, excitement Exercise Testosterone, estrogen Deep sleep (stages II and IV) Growth hormone-releasing hormone Ghrelin	Increased blood glucose Increased blood free fatty acids Aging Obesity Growth hormone inhibitory hormone (somatostatin) Growth hormone (exogenous) Somatomedins (***insulin-like growth factors***)

13. Ans. a. Bind 1 mol..., b. Dissociation curve... & d. Bind oxygen...

[Ref: Ganong 25th/641-42, 24th/643-44; Guyton 12th/96; A. K. Jain 5th/450]

Myoglobin

◈ *Ganong 25th/641-42, 24th/643*

- Myoglobin is an iron-containing pigment found in skeletal muscle. ***It resembles hemoglobin but binds 1 rather than 4 mol of O_2 per mole.***
- Its dissociation curve is a ***rectangular hyperbola rather than a sigmoid curve.***
- Because its ***curve is to the left of the hemoglobin curve***, it takes up O_2 from hemoglobin in the blood. It releases O_2 only at low PO_2 values, but the PO_2 in exercising muscle is close to zero.
- The myoglobin content is greatest in muscles specialized for sustained contraction. The muscle blood supply is compressed during such contractions, and myoglobin may provide O_2 when blood flow is cut off.
- There is also evidence that myoglobin facilitates the diffusion of O_2 from the blood to the mitochondria, where the oxidative reactions occur.

Role of Myoglobin

◈ *A. K. Jain 5th/450*

- It ***contain one heme group with one polypeptide chain***.
- It takes up oxygen at low pressure more readily than does blood. Thus, its ***dissociation curve is a rectangular hyperbola rather than sigmoid curve***
- It does ***not show Bohr effect***

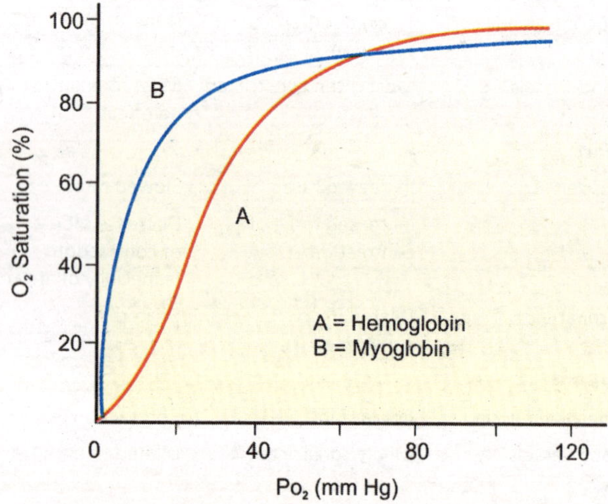

Fig: Dissociation curve of hemoglobin and myoglobin

BIOCHEMISTRY

14. Ans. a. Hydrolase enzyme

[Ref: Harper 30th/638-39, 29th/589, 599, 600; Lippincott 6th/163-64]

Mucopolysaccharidosis

◈ *Lippincott 6th/163-64, Harper 30th/638, 29th/599-600*

- The mucopolysaccharidoses are hereditary diseases caused by a deficiency of any one of the ***lysosomal hydrolases*** normally involved in the degradation of heparan sulfate and/or dermatan sulfate
- They are progressive disorders characterized by ***accumulation of glycosaminoglycans*** in various tissues, causing a range of symptoms, such as skeletal and extracellular matrix deformities, and mental retardation.
- Children who are homozygous for any one of these diseases are apparently normal at birth, then gradually deteriorate. In severe cases, death occurs in childhood.

- All are autosomal recessive diseases except Hunter syndrome, which is X-linked.
- Diagnosis is confirmed by measuring the ***patient's cellular level of the lysosomal hydrolases.*** Bone marrow and cord blood transplants have been used to treat Hurler and Hunter syndrome
- **Degradation** of GAGs is carried out by a battery of **lysosomal hydrolases.** These include certain endoglycosidases, various exoglycosidases, and sulfatases, generally acting in sequence to degrade the various GAGs.
- They are inherited in an **autosomal recessive** manner, with ***Hurler** and **Hunter syndromes*** being perhaps the most widely studied. None are common.

Table *(Harper 30th/639, 29th/599)*: **Biochemical Defects and Diagnostic Tests in Mucopolysaccharidoses (MPS)**

Name (Syndrome)	Enzymatic Defect
Syndrome Hurler-Scheie	α-L-Iduronidase
Hunter	Iduronate sulfatase
Sanfilippo A	Heparan sulfate N-sulfatase (sulfamidase)
Sanfilippo B	α-N-Acetylglucosaminidase
Sanfilippo C	Acetyltransferase
Sanfilippo D	N-Acetylglucosamine 6-sulfatase
Morquio A	Galactosamine 6-sulfatase
Morquio B	β-Galactosidase
Maroteaux-Lamy	N-Acetylgalactosamine 4-sulfatase (arylsulfatase B)
Sly	β-Glucuronidase
Natowicz syndrome	Hyaluronidase

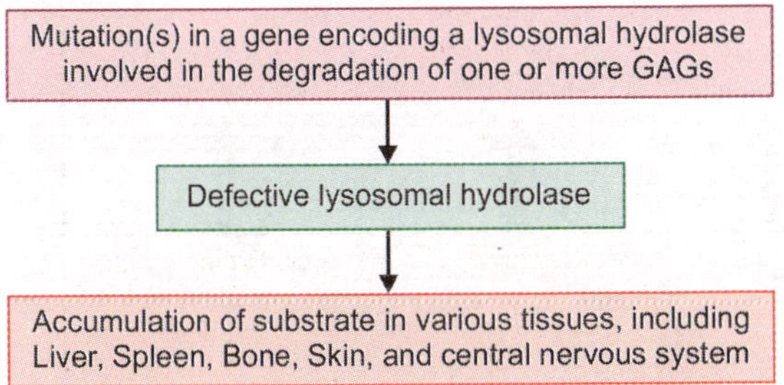

Fig: Simplified scheme of causation of a mucopolysaccharidosis, such as Hurler syndrome

15. Ans. c. Introduction of ......

[Ref: Harper 30th/301-02, 313-14, 29th/285-86; Lippincott 6th/263-68; Shinde 7th/471-73, 578; Vasudevan 5th/191; Satyanarayan 3rd/361]

*"The H_2S derived from the **cysteine** may be oxidized to **sulfites & thiosulfates & further oxidized to sulfate**"*- Vasudevan 5th/193

*"Two molecules of cysteine are joined together by **S-S bond** to form one molecule of cystine **(disulphide bond)**"* *(Shinde 7th/473)*

Degradation of Cysteine

◈ *Vasudevan 5th/191*

- *Transamination: **Cysteine transaminates** to form beta mercapto pyruvic acid & finally pyruvate. The beta mercapto pyruvate can transfer **S to CN to form thiocynate** (SCN)*
- *The sulphur may be removed either as H_2S or elemental sulphur or as sulfite*
- Cysteine on decarboxylation gives beta mercapto ethanolamine. This is used for synthesis of co-enzyme A

"**Formation of cysteine** *is by using the carbon skeleton contributed by serine & sulphur originating from* **methionine**"- *Vasudevan 5th*/191

"Sulphur containing amino acids in body are- methionine, cysteine & cystine. Other source of sulphur in body are sulphur containing amino acids: thiamine, lipoic acid & biotin" (Shinde 7th/471)

"**Cystine:** This amino acid is reduced to cysteine, using NADH + H^+ as a reductant. **Cysteine** undergoes desulfuration to yield can be oxidized to its disulfide derivative, cystine" *(Lippincott 6th/263)*

16. Ans. e. The information required for the correct...

[Ref: Harper 30th/36-41, 29th/36-40; Lippincott 6th/24, 13-20]

◈ *This Q is direct repeat from Lippincott Biochemistry- Q 2. 1 Lippincott 6th/24*

Lippincott 6th/24

◈ *(Direct quotes of Explanation given)*

"The correct folding of a protein is guided by specific interactions between the side chains of the amino acid residues of a polypeptide chain. The two cysteine residues that react to form the disulfide bond may be a great distance apart in the primary structure (or on separate polypeptides), but are brought into close proximity by the three-dimensional folding of the polypeptide chain. ***Denaturation may either be reversible or irreversible. Quaternary structure requires more than one polypeptide chain.*** These chains associate through ***noncovalent interactions***"

"The modular nature of protein synthesis and folding are embodied in the concept of orders of protein structure: **primary structure,** the sequence of the amino acids in a polypeptide chain; **secondary structure,** the folding of short (3- to 30-residue), contiguous segments of polypeptide into geometrically ordered units; **tertiary structure,** the assembly of secondary structural units into larger functional units such as the mature polypeptide and its component domains; and **quaternary structure,** the number and types of polypeptide units of oligomeric proteins and their spatial arrangement" *(Harper 30th/37, 29th/36)*

"**Primary structures** are stabilized by ***covalent peptide bonds.*** **Higher orders of structure** are stabilized by weak forces—***multiple hydrogen bonds, salt (electrostatic) bonds, and association of hydrophobic R groups***"

"**Higher orders of protein** structure are stabilized primarily—and often exclusively—by ***noncovalent interactions***" *(Harper 30th/41, 29th/40)*

"**Protein denaturation** results in the unfolding and disorganization of the protein's structure, which are not accompanied by hydrolysis of peptide bonds. Denaturation ***may be reversible or, more commonly, irreversible***" (*Lippincott 6th/22*)

17. Ans. b. Transported. from..., d. Implicate... & e. Not fo...

[Ref: Harper 30th/547-51, 29th/526-28; Lippincott 6th/381-83; Shinde 7th/152-56; Vasudevan 5th/284-86]

*"Retinoic acid is produced by oxidation of retinal. However, **retinoic acid cannot give rise to the formation of retinal or retinol**" (Satyanarayan 3rd/119)*

Vitamin A

- *Vasudevan 5th/284-86*
- ***"Retinal is the active form required for normal vision"***
- *Retinoic acid is implicated in growth & differentiation of tissue*
- ***Retinol is necessary for the reproductive system**. Retinol acts like a steroid hormone in controlling the expression of certain genes. This may account for the requirement of Vit A for normal reproduction*
- *Antioxidant property- attributed to carotenoids*
- *The retinal may reduced to retinol by retinal reductase (reversible reaction). Retinal is oxidized to retinoic acid, which can be converted back to other forms*

- *Lippincott 6th/381-83*

"**Retinoic acid**, derived from oxidation of dietary retinol, ***mediates most of the actions of the retinoids, except for vision, which depends on retinal, the aldehyde derivative of retinol.***

- **Retinol:** A primary alcohol containing a β-ionone ring with an unsaturated side chain, retinol is found in animal tissues as a retinyl ester with long-chain fatty acids.
- **Retinal:** This is the aldehyde derived from the oxidation of retinol. Retinal and retinol can readily be interconverted.
- **Retinoic acid:** This is the acid derived from the oxidation of retinal. Retinoic acid cannot be reduced in the body, and, therefore, cannot give rise to either retinal or retinol.
- **β -Carotene**

Absorption and Transport of Vitamin A

- **Transport to the liver:** Retinyl esters present in the diet are hydrolyzed in the intestinal mucosa, releasing retinol and free fatty acids. Retinol derived from esters and from the cleavage and reduction of carotenes is re-esterified to long-chain fatty acids in the intestinal mucosa and secreted as a component of chylomicrons into the lymphatic system. ***Retinyl esters contained in chylomicron remnants are taken up by, and stored in, the liver.***
- **Release from the liver:** When needed, retinol is ***released from the liver and transported to extrahepatic tissues by the plasma retinol binding protein (RBP).***

"**Visual cycle:** Vitamin A is a component of the visual pigments of rod and cone cells. ***Rhodopsin, the visual pigment of the rod cells in the retina, consists of 11-cis retinal specifically bound to the protein opsin.*** When rhodopsin is exposed to light, a series of photochemical isomerizations occurs, which results in the bleaching of the visual pigment and release of all-trans retinal and opsin"

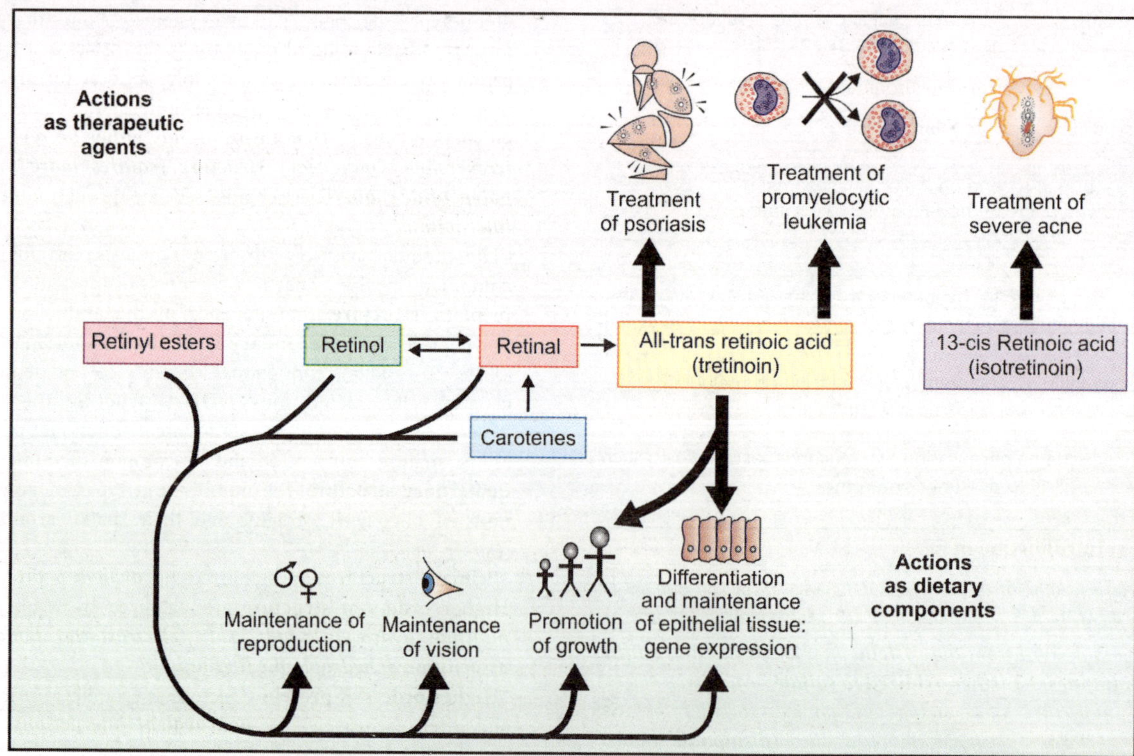

Fig: Summary of action of retinoids

18. Ans. d. It is... & e. Glycer...

[Ref: Harper 30th/262, 149, 29th/160-61; Lippincott 6th/331, 178, 190]

"Fasting: In adipose tissue the decrease in insulin and increase in glucagon results in inhibition of lipogenesis, ***inactivation of lipoprotein lipase, and activation of intracellular hormone-sensitive lipase***. This leads to release from adipose tissue of ***increased amounts of glycerol*** (which is a ***substrate for gluconeogenesis in the liver)*** and free fatty acids, which are used by liver, heart, and skeletal muscle as their preferred metabolic fuel, therefore sparing glucose. " *(Harper 30th/149, 29th/160-61)*

Fat Metabolism in Fasting

◈ *Lippincott 6th/331*

- **Increased degradation of TAG:** The ***activation of hormonesensitive*** lipase and subsequent hydrolysis of stored
- **Increased release of fatty acids:** ***The glycerol produced from TAG degradation is used as a gluconeogenic precursor by the liver.***
- **Decreased uptake of fatty acids:** In fasting, lipoprotein lipase activity of adipose tissue is low. Consequently, circulating TAG of lipoproteins is not available to adipose tissue.

Lipolysis Is Controlled by Hormone-Sensitive Lipase

◈ *Harper 30th/262, 28th/220*

- **Hormone-sensitive lipase is activated** by ***ACTH, TSH, glucagon, epinephrine, norepinephrine, and vasopressin and inhibited by insulin, prostaglandin*** E_1, ***and nicotinic acid***
- Activity of the hormone-sensitive lipase is ***increased by fasting and stress*** and decreased by feeding and insulin. Conversely, feeding increases and fasting and stress decrease the activity of lipoprotein lipase.

19. Ans. b. Lipoic. acid., c. NAD & e. TPP

[Ref: Harper 30th/172-74, 29th/174-75; Lippincott 6th/109-11; Satyanarayan 3rd/253-54]

FMN is cofactor for L-Amino Acid Oxidase

◈ *Satyanarayan 3rd/139)*

Pyruvate Dehydrogenase Complex (PDH)

◈ *Satyanarayan 3rd/253-54*

- It is found only in mitochondria
- High activity of PDH are found in cardiac muscle & kidney
- The enzyme PDH requires **five cofactors** (coenzymes) namely-***TPP, lipoamide (it contains lipoic acid linked to ε-amino group of lysine), FAD, coenzyme A & NAD+***
- PDH is inhibited by arsenite

Oxidative Decarboxylation of Pyruvate

◈ *Lippincott 6th/109-11*

- Oxidative decarboxylation of pyruvate by pyruvate dehydrogenase complex is an important pathway in tissues with a high oxidative capacity, such as cardiac muscle. Pyruvate dehydrogenase irreversibly ***converts pyruvate, the end product of glycolysis, into acetyl CoA***, a major fuel for the TCA cycle and the building block for fatty acid synthesis

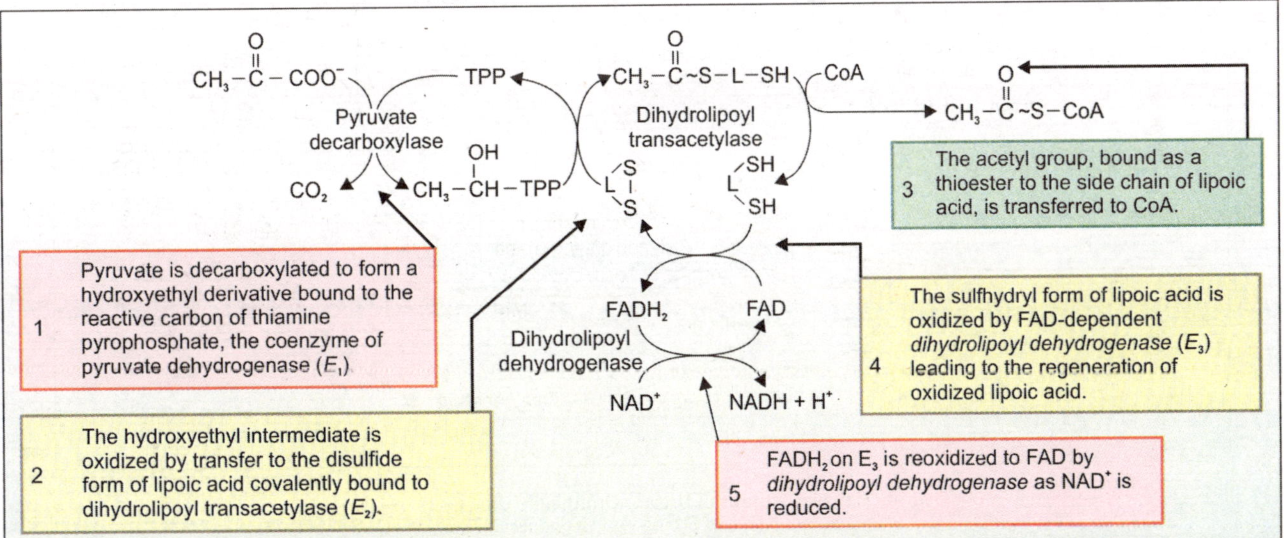

Fig: Mechanism of action of the pyruvate dehydrogenase complex. TPP = thiamine pyrophosphate; L = lipoic acid.

- **Component enzymes:** The pyruvate dehydrogenase complex (PDH complex) is a multimolecular aggregate of three enzymes, pyruvate dehydrogenase (PDH or E1, also called a decarboxylase), dihydrolipoyl transacetylase (E2), and dihydrolipoyl dehydrogenase (E3). Each catalyzes a part of the overall reaction.
- **Coenzymes:** The PDH complex contains ***five coenzymes that act as carriers or oxidants for the intermediates of the reactions.*** E1 requires thiamine pyrophosphate (TPP), E2 requires lipoic acid and CoA, and E3 requires FAD and NAD^+.

20. Ans. b. Lip... & c. TPP

[Ref: above Q; Harper 30th/172-74, 29th/174-75; Lippincott 6th/109-11; Satyanarayan 3rd/253-54]

"Pyruvate dehydrogenase irreversibly ***converts pyruvate, the end product of glycolysis, into acetyl CoA***, a major fuel for the TCA cycle and the building block for fatty acid synthesis" *(Lippincott 6th/109-10)*

21. Ans. c. On consumption of high..., d. Occur mainly in cytoplasm & e. Synthesis of argininosuccinate....

[Ref: Harper 30th/290-96, 29th/274-88; Lippincott 6th/253-55; Shinde 7th/450-51; Vasudevan 5th/180-81]

"In healthy people, the normal blood urea concentration is 10-40 mg/dl. Higher protein intake marginally increases blood urea level" *(Satyanarayan 3rd/340)*

"Citrulline Plus aspartate forms argininosuccinate, catalysed by enzyme **Argininosuccinate synthase**. The reaction requires ATP. Cleavage of argininosuccinate, catalyzed by **argininosuccinase,** proceeds with retention of nitrogen in arginine and release of the aspartate skeleton as fumarate (require no ATP)" *(Harper 30th/294, 29th/276-77)*

"***Major changes in diet can increase the concentrations of individual urea cycle enzymes 10- to 20-fold***. Starvation, for example, elevates enzyme levels, presumably to cope with the increased production of ammonia that accompanies enhanced protein degradation" *(Harper 30th/294, 29th/278)*

"***The excess nitrogen forms urea***" *(Harper 29th/271)*

"**Urea** *has two amino groups,* ***one derived from ammonia & other from aspartate***. *Carbon atom is supplied from carbon dioxide" (Satyanarayan 3rd/337)*

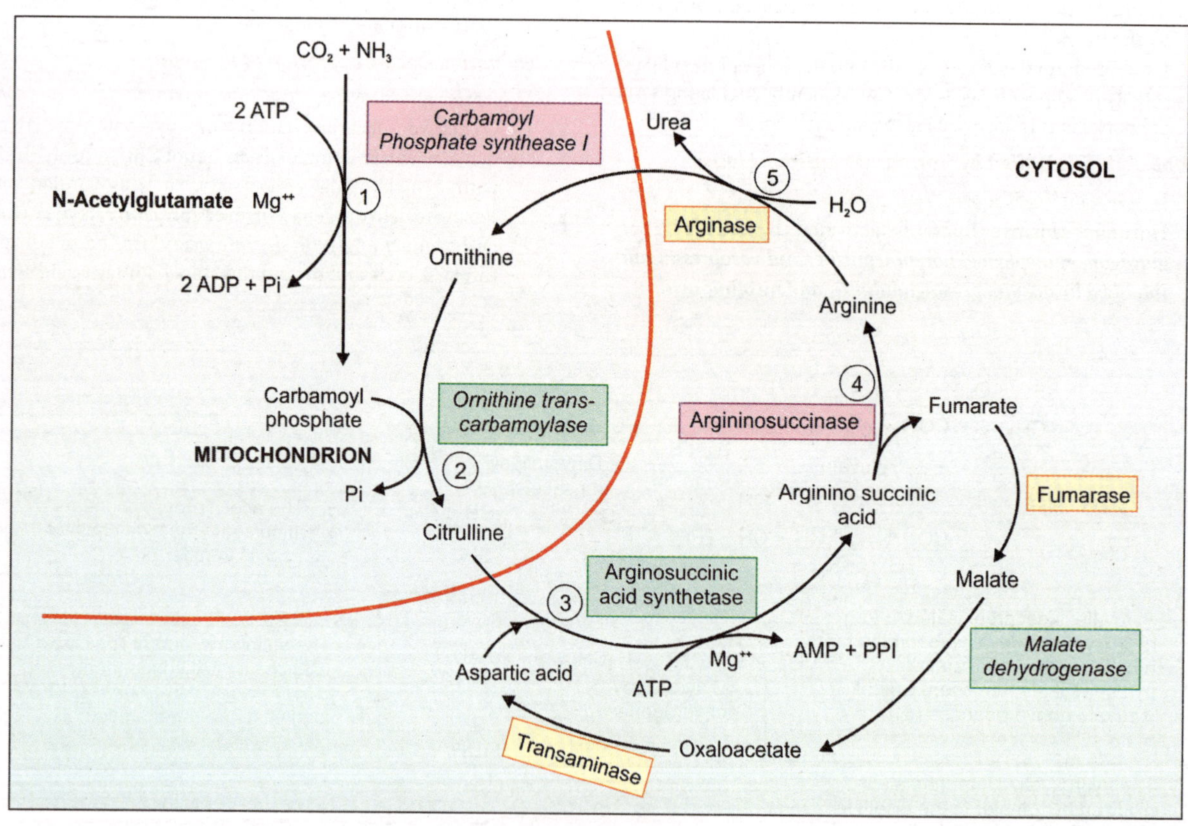

Fig: Biosynthesis of Urea or Ornithine – Urea Cycle

Urea cycle: ***NH_3 + CO_2 + Aspartate → Urea + Fumarate***

"Rate-limiting enzyme (pacemaker enzyme) of Urea cycle: ***Carbamoyl phosphate synthetase I*** (CPS II is involved in pyrimidine synthesis)" *(Harper 30th/293, 29th/274)*

"**Significance of urea cycle**: ***detoxication of ammonia to urea*** & biosynthesis of arginine (arginine is used in protein synthesis)" *(Shinde 7th/450)*

Synthesis of **1 mol of urea**[Q] requires ***3 mol of ATP plus 1 mol each of ammonium ion & of the α-amino nitrogen of aspartate***[Q] *(Harper 30th/292, 28th/243)*

Urea Cycle: 5 Steps *(Shown in Figure)*

- Synthesis of carbamoyl-phosphate
- Synthesis of citrulline
- Synthesis of argininosuccinate
- Cleavage of argininosuccinate
- Cleavage of arginine to form ornithine & urea

22. Ans. b. Galactose & e. Sailic acid.

[Ref: Harper 30th/218, 250-51, 29th/146, 136, 234; Lippincott 6th/209; Vasudevan 5th/78; Chatterjea & Shinde 7th/45, 58-61]

Gangliosides

- The highest concentration found in gray matter of brain
- On hydrolysis gangliosides yield the following
  - **A long chain fatty acid**[Q] (usually C_{18} to C_{24})
  - **Alcohol sphingosine**[Q]
  - A carbohydrate moiety[Q] which usually contains: Glucose &/or galactose
  - One molecule of N-acetyl galactosamine
  - At least one molecules of N-acetyl neuraminic acid (NANA) (also called, sailic acid[Q])
- As it is a type of glycolipid, it has no phosphoric acid or glycerol[Q]
- Over 30 types of gangliosides has been isolated from brain tissue. Four important types are: GM-1, GM-2, GM-3 & GD-3. GM 1 is known to be the receptor in human intestine, for cholera toxin[Q]
- **Tay-Sachs disease** (GM_2 gangliosidosis)- Accumulation of gangliosides in brain & nervous tissues takes place. The enzyme deficiency is hexosaminidase A[Q]. A cherry-red spot[Q] about the macula is pathognomonic.
- **GM_1 gangliosidosis** – It is due to deficiency of enzyme β galactosidase[Q].
- Gangliosides are mainly components of 'membranes'.

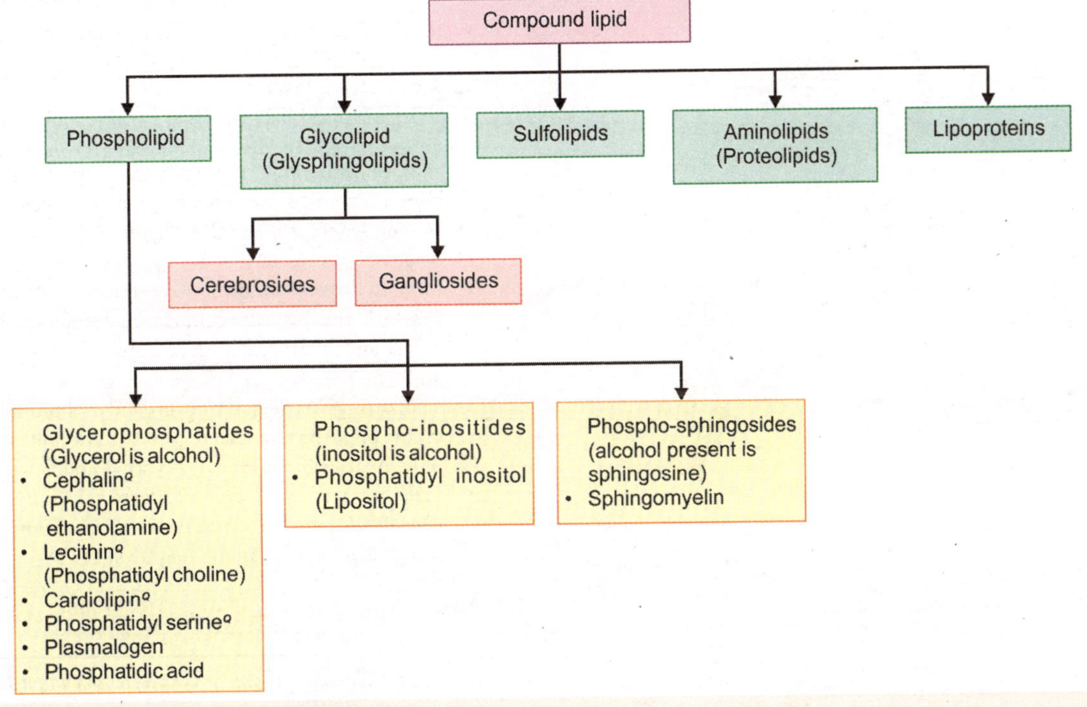

Note: *Gangliosides does not contain phosphate*

IMMUNOGENETICS & MOLECULAR BIOLOGY

23. Ans. e. Nitroge...

[Ref: Harper 30th/359-61, 29th/354-60; Lippincott 6th/395-400; Ananthanarayan 9th/54]

*"Each chain of double helix has a backbone of **deoxyribose & phosphate** residues arranged alternately. Attached to each deoxyribose is one of the 4 nitrogenous bases: A, G, C & T"- Ananthanarayan 9th/54*

*"The **common form of DNA is said to be right-handed**. In the test tube, double-stranded DNA can exist in **at least six forms** (A-E & Z)" (Harper 30th/360)*

Structure of DNA

◈ *Lippincott 6th/398)*

- DNA is a polymer of deoxyribonucleoside monophosphates covalently linked by 3'→5'–phosphodiester bonds.
- With the exception of a few viruses that contain single-stranded (ss) DNA, DNA exists as a doublestranded (ds) molecule, in which the two strands wind around each other, forming a ***double helix***.

- There are **three major structural forms of DNA**: the ***B form***, described by Watson and Crick in 1953, the ***A form***, and the ***Z form***. The ***B form is a right-handed helix*** with ten residues per 360° turn of the helix. Chromosomal DNA is thought to consist primarily of B-DNA.
- The **A form** is produced by moderately dehydrating the B form. It is also ***a right-handed helix***, but there are 11 base pairs per turn, and the planes of the base pairs are tilted 20° away from the perpendicular to the helical axis.
- **Z-DNA** is a ***left-handed helix*** that contains about 12 base pairs per turn (Note: The deoxyribose –phosphate backbone "zigzags," hence, the name "Z"-DNA)

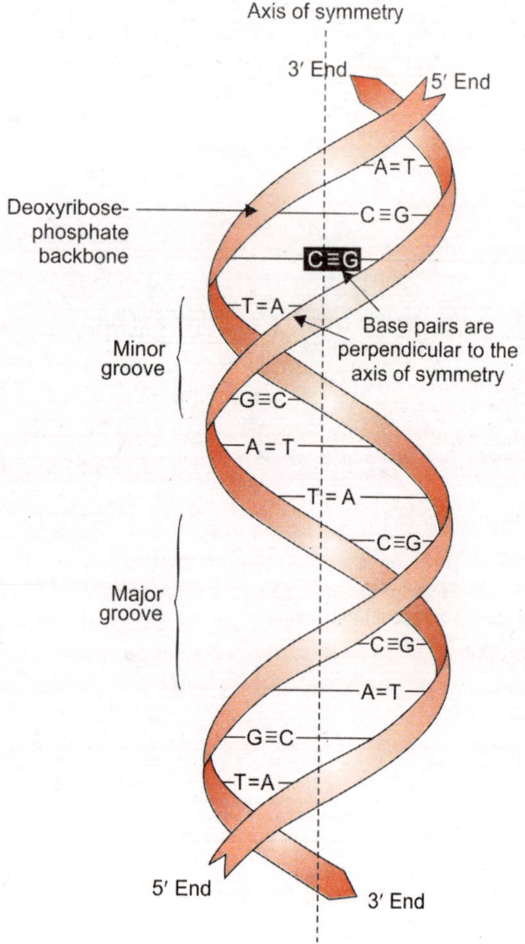

Fig: DNA double helix, illustrating some of its major structural features

24. Ans. b. Ratio of A: G… & c. A+T=G+C

[Ref: Harper 30th/360-61; Satyanarayan 3rd/73; Lippincott 4th/291; Ananthanarayan 9th/54-55]

Chargaff's Rule of Molar Equivalence between the Purine & Pyrimidine *(Satyanarayan 3rd/73; Harper 30th/360)*

- A=T & G=C
- Adenine & Guanine are purine whereas cytosine, thymine & uracil are pyrimidine

DNA Contains Four Deoxynucleotides *(Harper 30th/360-61)*

- There are four monomeric deoxynucleotide units in DNA—**deoxyadenylate, deoxyguanylate, deoxycytidylate,** and **thymidylate**.
- These monomeric units of DNA are held in polymeric form by ***3', 5'-phosphodiester bridges*** constituting a single strand.
- The informational content of DNA (the genetic code) resides in the sequence in which these monomers—purine and pyrimidine deoxyribonucleotides—are ordered.
- The polymer possesses a polarity; *one end has a 5'-hydroxyl or phosphate terminal while the other has a 3'-phosphate or hydroxyl terminal.*
- Chargaff rule stated that in DNA molecules the concentration of ***deoxyadenosine (A) nucleotides equals that of thymidine (T) nucleotides (A = T), while the concentration of deoxyguanosine (G) nucleotides equals that of deoxycytidine (C) nucleotides (G = C)***
- The two strands of this double-stranded helix are held by both, **hydrogen bonds** between the purine and pyrimidine bases of the respective linear molecules and by vander Waals and hydrophobic interactions between the stacked adjacent base pairs.
- The pairings between the purine and pyrimidine nucleotides on the opposite strands are very specific and are dependent upon hydrogen bonding of **A with T** and **G with C**
- *"The ratio of each pair of* ***bases (A+T)/(G+C) though constant for each species****, varies widely from one bacterial species to another"- Ananthanarayan 9th/54*

25. Ans. a. Also k/a. restriction…, b. Produce sticky ends & e. Breaks at sugar-phosphate bond.

[Ref: Harper 30th/452-54, 28th/388-90; Lippincott 4th/465-66; Satyanarayana 3rd/580]

"**RE** can ***specifically*** recognize DNA with particular sequence of 4-6 Mucleotides and cleave. The recognition sequences are ***palindromic***[Q] (*i.e.,* twofold rotational symmetry" *(Lippincott 4th/466)*

"RE *restrict DNA replication*Q" *(Satyanarayana 3rd/579)*

Restriction Enzyme (RE or Restriction Endonuclease)

- It is an enzyme that ***cleaves double-stranded DNA***Q ***at specific recognition nucleotide known as restriction sites***Q.
- To cut the DNA, a restriction enzyme makes two incisions, one through each ***sugar-phosphate backbone***Q (i.e. each strand) of the DNA double helix. This ***enzyme can restrict viral replication so called restriction enzymes.***
- The cut DNA fragments by RE may have ***sticky ends (cohesive ends)***Q or ***blunts ends***Q depending on the mechanism used by enzyme
- DNA fragments with **sticky ends** are particularly useful for recombinant DNA experiments (hybrid or chimeric DNA molecules)
- Restriction enzyme is ***named according to the organism from which it was isolated.***

Restriction Enzyme (or Restriction Endo-nuclease)

◈ *Lippincott 4th/465-66*

- It is an enzyme that cuts DNA at specific recognition nucleotide sequences (with Type II restriction enzymes cutting double-stranded DNA) known as restriction sites.
- Such enzymes, found in ***bacteria and archaea***, are thought to have evolved to provide a ***defense mechanism against invading viruses***. Inside a bacterial host, the restriction enzymes selectively cut up *foreign* DNA in a process called *restriction*; host DNA is methylated by a modification enzyme (a methylase) to protect it from the restriction enzyme's activity. Collectively, these two processes form the restriction modification system.
- To cut the DNA, a restriction enzyme makes ***two incisions, once through each sugar-phosphate backbone (i.e. each strand) of the DNA double helix.***
- Over 3000 restriction enzymes have been studied in detail, and more than 600 of these are available commercially and are routinely ***used for DNA modification*** and manipulation in laboratories
- Restriction enzymes can also be used to distinguish gene alleles by specifically recognizing single base changes in DNA known as single nucleotide ***polymorphisms (SNPs).***
- In a similar manner, restriction enzymes are used to ***digest genomic DNA for gene analysis by Southern blot***. This technique allows researchers to identify how many copies (or paralogues) of a gene are present in the genome of one individual, or how many gene mutations (polymorphisms) have occurred within a population. The latter example is called ***restriction fragment length polymorphism (RFLP)***

26. Ans. a. Uses….

[Ref: Harper 30th/458-59; Lippincott 6th/479-83, 5th/497-83; Chatterjea & Shinde7th/267-272]

"Reverse transcriptase- PCR is used for quantitification of RNA" *(Harper 30th/459, Lippincott 6th/483)*

Polymerase Chain Reaction

- PCR provides a sensitive, selective & extremely rapid means of amplifying a desired sequence of DNA. Twenty cycles provide an ***amplification***Q of 10^6 & 30 cycles of 10^9 *(Harper 30th/458, 27th/410-11)*
- ***Specificity***Q is based on the use of two oligonucleotide primers that hybridize to complementary sequence on opposite strands of DNA & flank the target sequence

Double stranded DNA can be disrupted by heat or high pH, giving rise to single stranded DNA. The single stranded DNA serves as a template for synthesis of a complementary strand by replicating enzymes, DNA polymerase

Early PCR reaction used an *E. coli* ***DNA polymerase*** that was destroyed by each heat denaturation cycle. Substitution of a heat-stable DNA polymerase (**Taq polymerase**)Q from Thermus aquaticus, obviates this problem & has made possible automation of the reaction, since the polymerase reactions can be run at 70°C

PCR is a cyclic process & cycle contains **three steps** that involves *(Chatterjea & Shinde)*

- *Denaturation* of DNA duplex (94-98°C)
- *Annealing* of primers (37-60°C)
- *Extension* of the primers with a polymerase in the presence of dNTP (about 72°C)

Use of PCRQ

- In detection of bacterial infections, retroviral infection & latent virus
- *Application in forensic medicine*Q
- *In prenatal diagnosis – in diagnosis of inherited disease*
- *In cancer detection*Q
- *In transplantation*
- *To study evolution*
- *In sex determination of embryos*
- *To determine viral load*
- *In DNA sequencing*Q

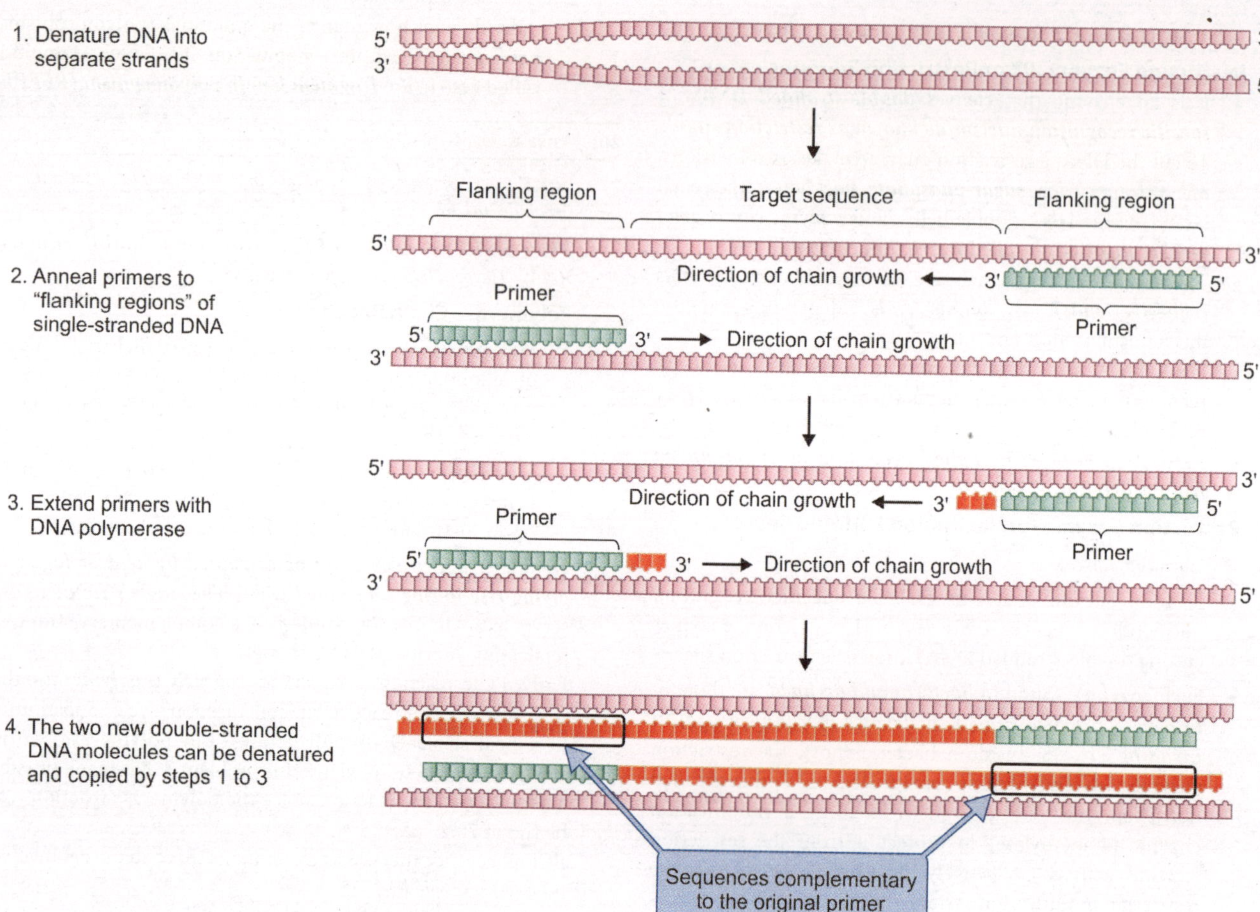

Fig: Steps in one cycle of the polymerase chain reaction

27. Ans. a. RT-PCR, b. Microarray, c. Allelle... & e. DNA...

[Ref: Lippincott 6th/473; Harper 30th/470, 29th/483-85; Harrison 19th/83e, 443-44, 18th/508, 17th/406; Vasudevan 5th/454-56]

"**Mutational analysis:** More discrete sequence alterations rely heavily on the use of PCR, which allows rapid gene amplification and analysis. Moreover, ***PCR makes it possible to perform genetic testing and mutational analysis with small amounts of DNA extracted*** from leukocytes or even from single cells, buccal cells, or hair roots. DNA sequencing can be performed directly on PCR products or on fragments cloned into plasmid vectors amplified in bacterial host cells" *(Harrison 19th/444)*

Detection of Mutations *(Lippincott 6th/473)*

- **Southern blotting** can detect DNA mutations such as the ***insertion or deletion*** of nucleotides.
- It can also detect point mutations that cause the loss or gain of restriction enzyme cleavage sites. Such mutations cause the pattern of bands to differ from those seen with a normal gene.

Table *(Lippincott's Biochemistry)*: **Techniques used to analyse DNA, RNA & proteins**

Technique	Sample Analysed	Gel Used	Purpose
Southern blot	DNA[Q]	Yes	Detect DNA changes
Northern blot	RNA[Q]	Yes	Measures mRNA amounts & size
Western blot	Protein[Q]	Yes	Measures protein amounts
ASO	DNA[Q]	No	Detects *DNA mutations*[Q]
Microarray	RNA or cDNA	No	Measures many mRNA levels at once

Table *(Harrison 17th/406, modified in 18th)*: **Methods Used for the Detection of Mutations**

Method	Principle	Type of Mutation Detected
Commonly Used Techniques		
Fluorescent in situ hybridization (FISH)	Hybridization to chromosomes with fluorescently labeled probes	Numerical or structural abnormalities in chromosomes
Southern blot	Hybridization with genomic probe or cDNA probe after digestion of high molecular DNA	Large deletion, insertion, rearrangement, expansions of triplet repeat, amplification
Polymerase chain reaction (PCR)	Amplification of DNA segment	Expansion of triplet repeats, variable number of tandem repeats (VNTR), gene rearrangements, translocations; prepare DNA for other mutation methods
Reverse transcriptase PCR (RT-PCR)	Reverse transcription, amplification of DNA segment →absence or reduction of mRNA transcription	Analyze expressed mRNA (cDNA) sequence; ***detect loss of expression***
DNA sequencing	Direct sequencing of PCR products	Point mutations, small deletions and insertions
	Sequencing of DNA segments cloned into plasmid vectors	
Restriction fragment polymorphism (RFLP)	Detection of altered restriction pattern of genomic DNA (Southern blot) or PCR products	Point mutations, small deletions and insertions
Other Techniques		
Single-strand conformational polymorphism (SSCP)	PCR of DNA segment: Mutations result in conformational change and altered mobility	Point mutations, small deletions and insertions
Denaturing gradient gel electrophoresis (DGGE)	PCR of DNA segment: Mutations result in conformational change and altered mobility	Point mutations, small deletions and insertions
RNAse cleavage	Cleavage of mismatch between mutated and wild-type sequence	Point mutations, small deletions and insertions
Oligonucleotide specific hybridization (OSH)	Hybridization of PCR products to wild-type or mutated oligonucleotides immobilized on chips or slides	Point mutations, small deletions and insertions
Microarrays	Hybridization of PCR products to wild-type or mutated oligonucleotides	***Point mutations***, small deletions and insertions Genotyping of SNPs

Contd...

Microarray Technology

- A comprehensive approach to ***genome-scale studies*** consists of *microarrays, or DNA chips.*
- *Used to determine the **gene expression pattern** of thousands of genes simultaneously*
- Microarrays allow the detection of variations in DNA sequence and are used for ***mutational analysis and genotyping.***

28. Ans. a. Deletion & b. Insertion -Most probably

[Ref: Harper 30th/416-19; Lippincott 6th/434; Harrison 19th/432-34; Robbins 9th/160-61; Harshmohan 7th/255]

Note: Deletion & Insertion could be possible answer (Please go through explanation given & other references for deciding appropriate answer)

Frameshift Mutations Result from Deletion or Insertion of Nucleotides in DNA That Generates Altered mRNAs

◈ *Harper 30th/417*

- The ***deletion of a single nucleotide*** from the coding strand of a gene results in ***an altered reading frame in the mRNA.*** Altering the reading frame results in a garbled translation of the mRNA distal to the single nucleotide deletion. Not only is the sequence of amino acids distal to this deletion garbled, but reading of the message can also result in the appearance of a ***nonsense codon*** and thus the production of a polypeptide both ***garbled and prematurely terminated***
- If **three nucleotides or a multiple of three** are deleted from a coding region, the corresponding mRNA when translated will provide a protein from which is ***missing the corresponding number of amino acids.*** Because the reading frame is a triplet, the reading phase will not be disturbed for those codons distal to the deletion.
- If, however, **deletion of one or two nucleotides** occurs just prior to or within the normal termination codon (nonsense codon), the reading of the normal termination signal is disturbed. Such a deletion might result in reading through a ***termination signal until another nonsense codon is encountered***
- **Insertions** of one or two or nonmultiples of three nucleotides into a gene result in an mRNA in which the reading frame is distorted upon translation, and the same effects that occur with deletions are reflected in the mRNA translation.

This may ***result in garbled amino acid*** sequences distal to the insertion and the generation of a **nonsense codon** at or distal to the insertion, or perhaps reading through the normal termination codon.

Mutation

◈ *Harper 30th/417*

Single base change in the mRNA may have one of the several effects when translated into protein

- Silent mutation
- *Missense mutation*
- *Non-sense*

◈ *Harrison 19th/432-34: Writes*

- Mutations can occur in all domains of a gene. A point mutation occurring within the coding region leads to an amino acid substitution if the codon is altered. Point mutations that introduce a premature stop codon result in a truncated protein.
- ***Large deletions may affect a portion of a gene or an entire gene, whereas small deletions and insertions alter the reading frame if they do not represent a multiple of three bases. These "frameshift" mutations lead to an entirely altered carboxy terminus.***
- Mutations in intronic sequences or in exon junctions may destroy or create splice donor or splice acceptor sites. Mutations may also be found in the regulatory sequences of genes, resulting in reduced or enhanced gene transcription.

Frame-shift Mutation

◈ *Lippincott 6th/434*

- If one or two nucleotides are either ***deleted from or added to the coding region of a message sequence, a frame-shift mutation occurs and the reading frame is altered***. This can result in a product with a radically different amino acid sequence, or a truncated product due to the creation of a termination codon.
- If three nucleotides are added, a new amino acid is added to the peptide or, if three nucleotides are deleted, an amino acid is lost. Loss of three nucleotides maintains the reading frame, but can result in serious pathology.

Consequences of Altering the Nucleotide Sequence

◈ *Lippincott 6th/433-34*

Changing a single nucleotide base on the mRNA chain (a "point mutation") can lead to any one of three results:

- ***Silent mutation:*** The codon containing the changed base may code for the same amino acid.
- ***Missense mutation:*** *The codon containing the changed base may code for a different amino acid.*
- ***Nonsense mutation:*** *The codon containing the changed base may become a termination codon.*
- ***Other mutations:*** *These can alter the amount or structure of the protein produced by translation.*
    - Trinucleotide repeat expansion
    - Splice site mutations
    - Frame-shift mutations

"**Deletion or insertion** of single base pairs, generally has a profound effect on the protein because the protein's synthesis, which is carried out by the reading of triplet codons in a linear fashion from one end of the gene to the other, is thrown off. This change leads to a ***frameshift*** in reading the gene such that all amino acids are incorrect from the mutation onward. More-complex combinations of base substitutions, insertions, and deletions can also be observed in some mutant genes"- *(http://www. britannica. com/science/mutation-genetics)*

"**Translocation** A break in at least two chromosomes with exchange of material. In a reciprocal translocation, there is no obvious loss of chromosomal material. Translocations are indicated by t; the chromosomes involved are noted in the first set of parentheses and the breakpoints in the second set of parentheses. For example, the Ph translocation is t (9; 22) (q34; q11.2)"

29. Ans. b. Branched... & c. PCR

[Ref: Harper 29th/26; Lippincott 6th/482, 485; Harrison 19th/150e-3-6, 183e-1, 194e-3; http://www. researchgate. net/profile/Ivo_Gut/ publication/8597456_DNA_ analysis_by_MALDI-TOF]

Quantitative Nucleic Acid Test (NAAT) Strategies

◈ *Harrison 19th/150e-6*

- With the advent of newer therapeutic regimens for HIV-associated disease, cytomegalovirus infection, and hepatitis B and C virus infections, the response to therapy has been monitored by determining both genotype and viral load at various times after treatment initiation.
- ***Quantitative NAATs are available for HIV (PCR), cytomegalovirus (PCR), hepatitis B virus (PCR), and hepatitis C virus (PCR and TMA)***.
- Many laboratories have validated and perform quantitative assays for these and other pathogens (*e.g.,* Epstein-Barr virus), using analyte specific reagents for NAATs.
- **Branched-chain DNA (bDNA)** testing is an ***alternative to NAAT (Nucleic acid amplification techniques)*** for ***quantitative nucleic acid testing.*** In such testing, bDNA attaches to a site different from the target-binding sequence of the original probe. Chemiluminescence-labeled oligonucleotides can then bind to multiple repeating sequences on the bDNA. The amplified bDNA signal is detected by chemiluminescence. bDNA assays for ***viral load of HIV***, hepatitis B virus, and hepatitis C virus have been approved by the FDA. The advantage of bDNA assays over PCR is that only a single heating/annealing step is required to hybridize the target-binding probe to the target sequence for amplification.

Identification Methods For Microbes

- Once bacteria are isolated, characteristics that are readily detectable after growth on agar media (colony size, color, hemolytic reactions, odor, microscopic appearance) may suggest a species, but definitive identification requires additional tests.
- Identification methods include ***classic biochemical phenotyping***, which is still the most common approach,

as well as more sophisticated methods such as ***mass spectrometry, gas chromatography, and nucleic acid tests.***

- **Biochemical Phenotyping** Classic biochemical identification of bacteria entails tests for protein or carbohydrate antigens, the production of specific enzymes, the ability to metabolize specific substrates and carbon sources (such as carbohydrates), or the production of certain metabolites.
- **Gas-Liquid Chromatography:** Gas-liquid chromatography often is used to detect metabolic end products of bacterial fermentation.
- **Matrix-Assisted Laser Desorption/Ionization/Time-of-Flight Mass Spectrometry (MALDI- TOF MS):** MALDI-TOF MS is a rapid and accurate method for ***identifying microorganisms*** by ***protein analysis***. The organism is mixed with a chemical matrix, dried on a target plate, and then pulsed with a laser. The laser ionizes and vaporizes the microbial proteins, which then travel through a charged vacuum chamber to a detector. The time of flight to the detector is measured for the individual proteins, and the resulting pattern (or fingerprint) is compared with a library of known patterns for various microorganisms to identify the test organism. The primary clinical advantage of MALDI-TOF is that it takes ***only minutes to identify an organism***, whereas several hours are needed for conventional phenotyping. MALDI-TOF is highly accurate for identification of most bacteria and yeasts grown on solid agar or in blood culture broth.

"**Isolation of a specific protein: Chromatographic separations** partition molecules between two phases, one mobile and the other stationary. For separation of amino acids or sugars, the stationary phase, or matrix, may be a sheet of filter paper (paper chromatography) or a thin layer of cellulose, silica, or alumina (thin-layer chromatography; TLC)" *(Harper 29th/26)*

"In biology, a **branched DNA assay** is a signal amplification assay (as opposed to a target amplification assay) that is used to detect nucleic acid molecules. The assay can be used to detect and quantify many types of RNA or DNA target"

"The bDNA assay is a sandwich nucleic acid hybridization method that uses bDNA molecules to amplify signal from captured target RNA. bDNA technology forms the basis of the FDA-approved ***clinical diagnostic VERSANT 3. 0 assays for HIV, HCV and HBV viral load"*** *(http://www. panomics. com/products/gene-expression/single-plex-assay/overview)*

"PCR offers a rapid and sensitive method for ***detecting viral DNA sequences*** even when only a small proportion of cells is harboring the virus"(Lippincott 6th/482)

30. Ans. a. Methylation

[Ref: Lippincott 6th/709; Harrison 19th/101e-4, 18th/668, 679; Robbins 9th/893; Satyanarayan 3rd/359, 572; Lippincott 4th/460-62; Chatterjea & Shinde 7th/346, 426; en. wikipedia. org/wiki/DNA_methylation]

"**CpG islands**: ***Methylation of cytosine by a methyltransferase*** *is associated with silencing of the activities of certain gene"-Lippincott 6th/709*

"**Cytosine** in the sequence CG of DNA gets ***methylated to form 5'-methylcytosine.*** A major portion of CG (about 20%) in human DNA exists in methylated form. In general, methylation leads to loss of transcriptional activity & thus inactivation of genes"-*Satyanarayan 3rd/572*

◈ *Harrison19th/101e-4, 18th/667-68: Writes*

- Gene silencing, **an epigenetic change** that leads to the ***loss of gene expression and occurs in conjunction with hypermethylation of the promoter and histone deacetylation,*** is another mechanism of tumor-suppressor gene inactivation.
- The role of **epigenetic control mechanisms** in the development of human cancer is unclear. However, a *general decrease in the level of DNA methylation has been noted as a common change in cancer. In addition, numerous genes, including some tumor-suppressor genes, appear to become hypermethylated and silenced during tumorigenesis.*

DNA Methylation Mechanism

◈ *en. wikipedia. org/wiki/DNA_methylation*

- After every cycle of DNA replication, several modifications occur in the DNA. *DNA methylation is one such post-synthesis modification.* DNA methylation has been proven by research to be manifested in a number of biological processes such as regulation of ***imprinted genes, X chromosome inactivation, and tumor suppressor gene silencing in cancerous cells.***
- It also acts as a protection mechanism adopted by the pathogen DNA (mainly bacterial against the endonuclease activity that destroys any foreign DNA).
- In ***DNA, methylation usually occurs in the CpG islands,*** a CG rich region, upstream of the promoter region. In humans, DNA methylation is carried out by a group of enzymes called ***DNA methyltransferases.***
- DNA methylation stably ***alters the gene expression pattern in cells*** such that cells can "remember where they have been" or decrease gene expression.

31. Ans. b. DNA...

[Ref: Harper 30th/395-98; Lippincott 6th/429]

Transcription

- There are three distinct classes of RNA polymerase in the nucleus of eukaryotic cells. **RNA polymerase I** synthesizes the precursor of large rRNA in the nucleolus. **RNA polymerase II** synthesizes the precursors for mRNA and some ncRNAs in the nucleoplasm, and **RNA polymerase III** produces the precursors of **tRNA** in the nucleoplasm. In both prokaryotes and eukaryotes, RNA polymerase does not require a primer, and has no proofreading activity.
- **A primary transcript** is a linear copy of a **transcription unit**—the segment of DNA between specific initiation and termination sequences. The primary transcripts of both prokaryotic and eukaryotic tRNA and rRNA are **post transcriptionally modified** by cleavage of the original transcripts by ribonucleases. **rRNA** of both prokaryotic and eukaryotic cells are synthesized from long precursor molecules called **preribosomal RNA.**
- Prokaryotic mRNA is generally identical to its primary transcript, whereas eukaryotic mRNA is extensively modified co- and posttranscriptionally. For example, a **7-methylguanosine "cap"** is attached to the 5'-terminal end of the mRNA through a 5'→5' linkage. A **long poly-A tail**—not transcribed from the DNA—is attached to the

3'-end of most mRNA. Most eukaryotic mRNAs also contain **intervening sequences (introns)** that must be removed to make the mRNA functional. Their removal, as well as the **joining of expressed sequences (exons)**, requires a **spliceosome** composed of **small, nuclear ribonucleoprotein particles** that mediate the process of **splicing**. Eukaryotic mRNA is monocistronic, containing information from just one gene.

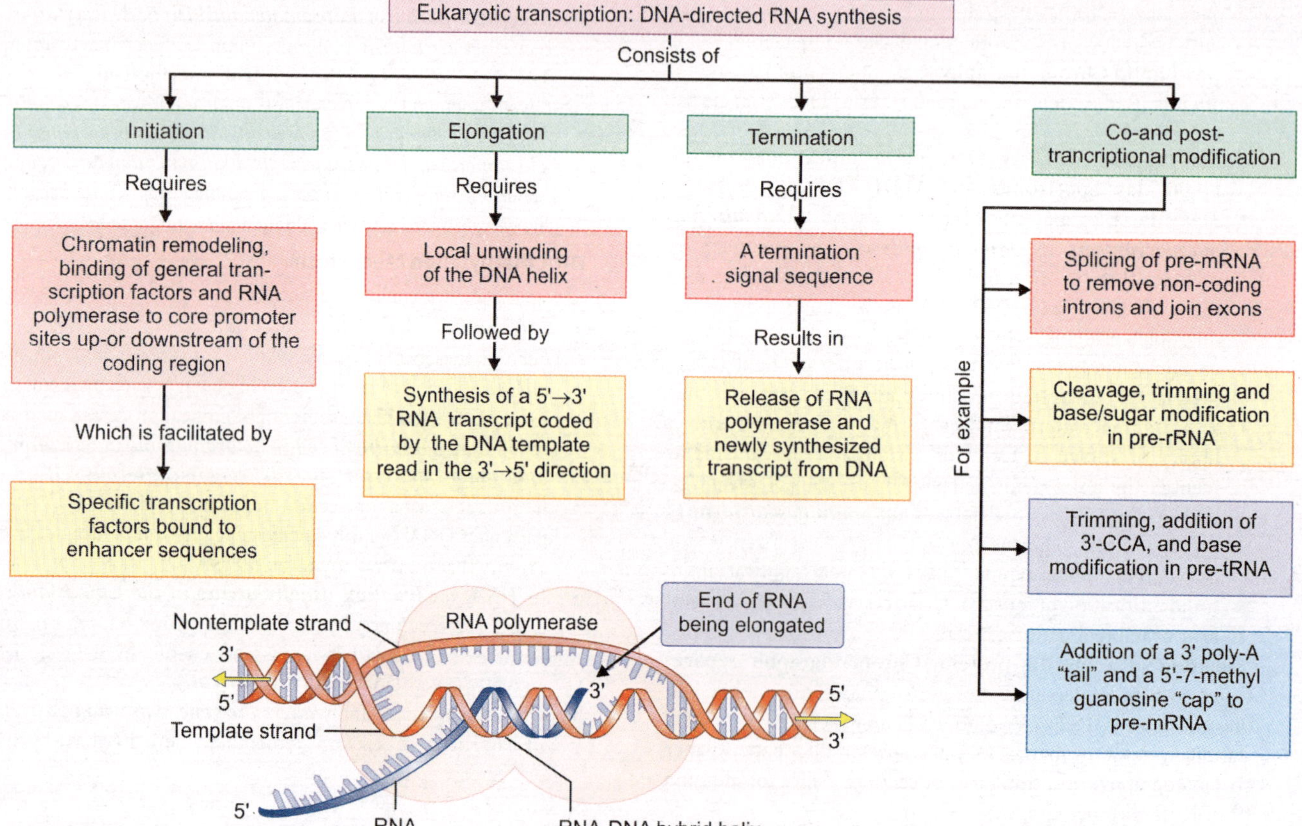

32. Ans. c. tRNA

[Ref: Harper 30th/394, 411; Lippincott 6th/418]

*"tRNA molecule contain a high percentage of **unusal bases**, for example, **dihydrouracil** & have extensive intra-chain base pairing that leads to characteristic secondary & tertiary structure"- Lippincott 6th/418*

Transfer RNA *(Lippincott 6th/418)*

- tRNAs are the smallest (4S) of the three major types of RNA molecules. There is at least one specific type of tRNA molecule for each of the 20 amino acids commonly found in proteins. Together, tRNAs make up about 15% of the total RNA in the cell.
- ***The tRNA molecules contain a high percentage of unusual bases (for example, dihydro uracil)*** and have extensive intrachain base-pairing that leads to characteristic secondary and tertiary structure.
- Each tRNA serves as an "adaptor" molecule that carries its specific amino acid—covalently attached to its 3'-end—to the site of protein synthesis. There it recognizes the genetic code sequence on an mRNA, which specifies the addition of its amino acid to the growing peptide chain

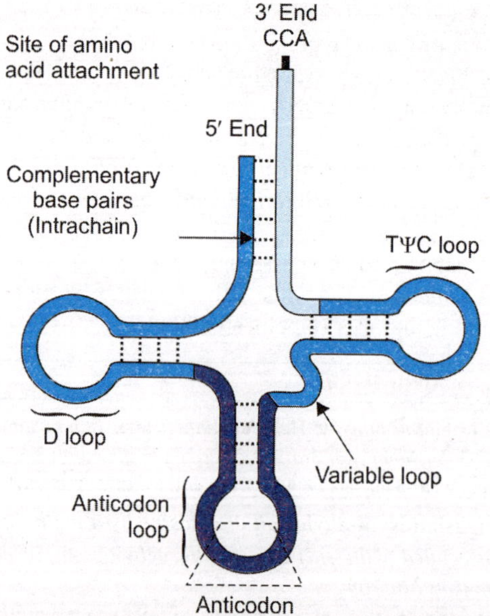

Fig: Characteristic tRNA secondary structure

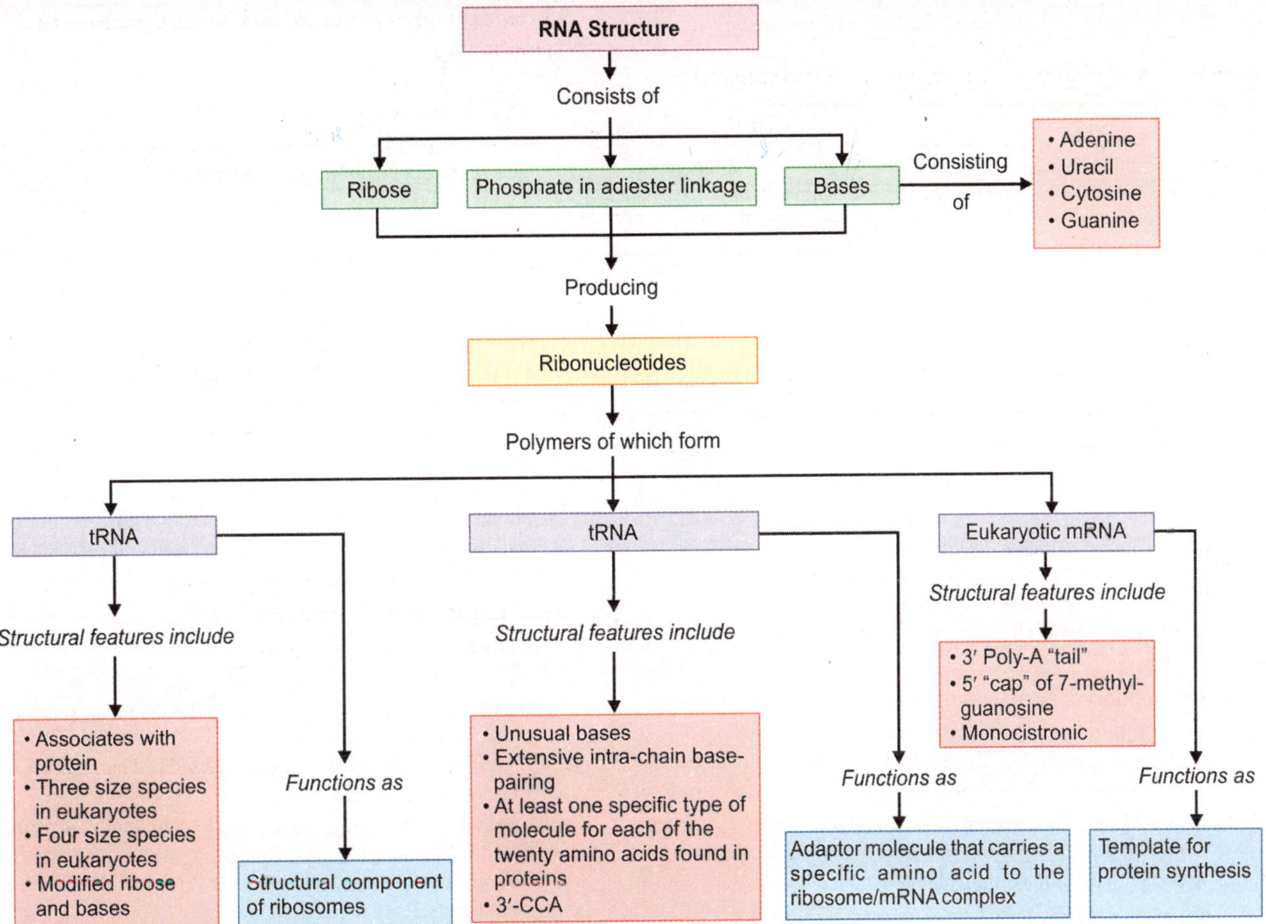

Fig: Chart depicting RNA structure

PATHOLOGY

33. Ans. a. Lymp...

[Ref: Robbins 9th/594-95; Harrison 19th/704-05, 702; Devita 7th/1975-77; Abeloff's Clinical Oncology 4th/74]

"The **most common presentation** for follicular lymphoma is with ***new painless lymphadenopathy***"- *Harrison 19th/704*

Follicular Lymphoma

◈ *Robbins 9th/594-95*

- Follicular lymphoma is the most common form of indolent NHL. It usually presents in middle age and ***affects males and females equally***. It is less common in Europe and rare in Asian populations.
- Follicular lymphoma likely arises from germinal center B cells and is strongly associated with chromosomal translocations involving ***BCL2***. Its hallmark is a (14; 18) translocation that juxtaposes the *IGH* locus on chromosome 14 and the *BCL2* locus on chromosome 18. The t (14; 18) is seen in up to 90% of follicular lymphomas, and leads to overexpression of BCL2.
- ***BCL2 antagonizes apoptosis*** and promotes the survival of follicular lymphoma cells.

Follicular Cell Lymphoma

◈ *Abeloff's Oncology 4th/74*

Positive for: CD 20 & CD 10[Q]

Negative for: CD 3 & CD 5[Q]

- The neoplastic cells resemble normal follicular centre B cells, exressing CD 19, **CD 20**[Q], CD 10 (CALLA) & surface immunoglobulin.
- Unlike in chronic lymphocytic leukemia & mantle cell lymphoma. **CD5** is ***not expressed***[Q]
- The *hallmark* of typical follicular lymphoma is a **(14: 18) translocation**[Q] that juxtaposes the IgH locus on chr 14 & the BCL 2 locus on chromosome 18- *(Robbins 9th/594)*
- Express **BCL 2 & BCL 6**[Q]
- Follicular lymphoma is one of the malignancies most resposive to chemotherapy & radio therapy *(Harrison 19th/704)*
- It makes 22% of NHL worldwide & at least 30% of NHL diagnosed in the United States *(Harrison 19th/704)*
- Most common presentation – Painless lymphadenopathy

Table *(Robbins 9th/591)*: **Summary of Follicular Lymphoma**

Diagnosis	Cell of Origin	Genotype	Salient Clinical Features
Follicular lymphoma	Germinal center B-cell; typically expresses CD10, BCL2, and BCL6	t (14; 18) involving the BCL2 gene	Older adults with generalized lymphadenopathy and marrow involvement; indolent

Key Concepts

◈ *Robbins 9th/598*

Common Forms of Lymphoid Leukemia and Lymphoma

Acute Lymphoblastic Leukemia/Lymphoblastic Lymphoma

- Most common type of cancer in children, may be derived from either precursor B or T cells
- Highly aggressive tumors manifest with signs and symptoms of bone marrow failure, or as rapidly growing masses.
- Tumor cells contain genetic lesions that block differentiation, leading to the accumulation of immature, nonfunctional blasts.

Small Lymphocytic Lymphoma/Chronic Lymphocytic Leukemia

- Most common leukemia of adults
- Tumor of mature B cells that usually manifests with bone marrow and lymph node involvement
- Indolent course, commonly associated with immune abnormalities, including an increased susceptibility to infection and autoimmune disorders

Follicular Lymphoma

- Most common indolent lymphoma of adults
- Tumor cells recapitulate the growth pattern of normal germinal center B cells; most cases are associated with a (14; 18) translocation that results in the overexpression of BCL2.

Diffuse Large B-Cell Lymphoma

- Most common lymphoma of adults
- Heterogeneous group of mature B-cell tumors that shares a large cell morphology and aggressive clinical behavior
- Rearrangements or mutations of *BCL6* gene are recognized associations; one third carry a (14; 18) translocation involving *BCL2* and may arise from follicular lymphomas.

Burkitt Lymphoma

- Very aggressive tumor of mature B cells that usually arises at extranodal sites.
- Strongly associated with translocations involving the *MYC* proto-oncogene
- Tumor cells often are latently infected by EBV.

34. Ans. a. Most..., b. Proli... & c. Mass...

[Ref: Robbins 9th/593-94; Harrison 19th/701-02; Robbins 7th/673- 74; Oxford Handbook of Clinical Hematology 2nd/170; CMDT 2015/519-20]

"CLL: Most common leukemia of adults"-*(Robbins 9th/598)*

"CLL causes massive splenomegaly"*(Harrison 19th/412 (Table))*

A & E

Chronic Lymphocytic Leukemia, Small Lymphocytic Lymphoma

◈ *Robbins 9th/593-94*

- **CLL is the most common leukemia of adults in the Western world.** The ***median age at diagnosis is 60 years***, and there is a ***2: 1 male predominance***.
- Lymph nodes are diffusely effaced by an infiltrate of predominantly small lymphocytes 6 to 12 μm in diameter with round to slightly irregular nuclei, condensed chromatin, and scant cytoplasm. Admixed are variable numbers of larger activated lymphocytes that often gather in loose aggregates referred to as ***proliferation centers***, which contain mitotically active cells. When present, **proliferation centers are pathognomonic for CLL/SLL**. The blood contains large numbers of small round lymphocytes with scant cytoplasm.
- Some of these cells are usually disrupted in the process of making smears, producing so-called **smudge cells**. The bone marrow is always involved by interstitial infiltrates or aggregates of tumor cells. Infiltrates are also virtually always seen in the splenic white and red pulp and the hepatic portal tracts.

B Cell Chronic Lymphoid Leukemia/SLL

◈ *Robbins 9th/593-94; Harrison 19th/701-02*

- CLL & SLL are morphologically, and genotypically indistinguishable, differing only in the degree of peripheral blood lymphocytosis- Robbins 9th/593, 7th/673
- B-cell CLL is the ***most common***[Q] ***lymphoid leukemia.***
- Presentation can be either as leukemia or lymphoma
- Typically B-cell CLL often found incidentally in routine blood test.
- It is the commonest leukemia in western adult (25-30% of all leukemia)
- Median age at diagnosis is ***65 yrs.*** [Q]
- Male: Female ratio is ***2: 1***[Q]
- CLL is often a symptomatic and leukocytosis (>5x109/L) on routine FBC.

"In approximately 2% to 6% of patients, CLL may evolve into a high-grade lymphoma of the diffuse large cell type ***(Richter's transformation)*** [Q]. Prolymphocytic leukemia develops in approximately 2% to 5% of CLL patients"- *Devita 7th/2141*

Diagnosis: The diagnosis of typical B cell CLL is made when an increased number of circulating lymphocytes (i.e., >4 x 109/L and usually >10 x 109/L) is found Lymphocytosis >4 x 109 and usually > 10 x 109/L

Blood Film: *shows lymphocytosis with nature appearance and shows* ***'Smudge 'or 'bucket cell***[Q]'

Treatment: The most common treatments for patients with typical B cell CLL/small lymphocytic lymphoma have been ***chlorambucil or fludarabine, alone or in combination.*** Young patients with this disease can be candidates for **bone marrow transplantation.** Allogeneic bone marrow transplantation can be curative but is associated with a significant treatment-related mortality rate. Mini-transplants using immunosuppressive rather than myeloablative doses of preparative drugs are being studied

35. Ans. b. Circular, c. Transmi... & e. Contains...

[Ref: Robbins 9th/171-72; 7th/185; Harrison 19th/Chap 85e1-8; Harper 30th/378, 27th/330-31]

Table: Some major features of the structure and function of human mitochondrial DNA

- Is circular[Q], double-stranded[Q], and composed of heavy (H) and light (L) chains or strands
- Contains 16, 569 bp
- Encodes ***13 protein***[Q] subunits of respiratory chain (of a total of about 67)
  - Seven subunits of Nochrome oxidase (complex IV)
  - Two subunits of ATP synthase
- Encodes large (16s) and small (12s) t ribosomal RNAs
- Encodes *22 mt tRNA* molecules
- Genetic code differs slightly from the standard code
  - ***UGA (standard stop codon) is read as Trp***
  - AGA and AGG (standard codons for Arg) are read as stop codons
- Contains ***very few untranslated sequences***[Q]
- High mutation rate (five to ten times that of nuclear DNA)
- Comparisons of mtDNA sequences provide evidence about evolutionary origins of primates and other species

- Human mitochondria contain 2-10 copies of a small circular double-stranded DNA molecule that makes up approximately **1% of total cellular DNA**[Q].
- A unique feature of mitochondrial DNA is **maternal inheritance**[Q]
- Disease associated with mitochondrial inheritance is rare.

Mitochondrial DNA

◈ *Harrison 19th/Chap 85e; 17th/Part 18 e-39*

- The DNA sequence of mtDNA has been determined from a large number of organisms and individuals (including some organisms that are extinct), and the comparison of those DNA sequences represents a mainstay of phylogenetics, in that it allows biologists to elucidate the evolutionary relationships among species.
- ***Mothers transmit their mtDNA to both their sons and daughters,*** only the daughters are able to transmit the inherited mtDNA to future generations ***(Maternal inheritance)***
- ***High somatic mtDNA mutation*** rate and the global effect on mitochondrial function counterbalance the reduced impact of the multiple copy number of each individual mtDNA mutation.
- This mtDNA sequence contains a total of ***37 genes, of which 13 encode mitochondrial protein components of the ETC. The remaining 22 tRNA- and 2 rRNA-encoding genes are dedicated to the process of translation of the 13 mtDNA-encoded proteins.***

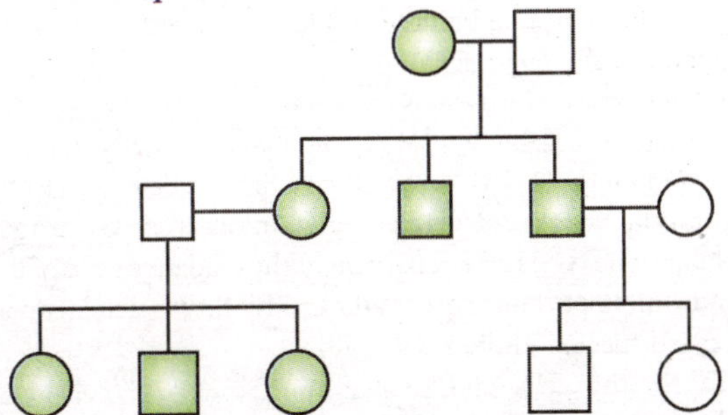

Fig: Mitochondrial inheritance

36. Ans. d. 50% affected if one parent affected.

[Ref: Robbins 9th/140-41; Harrison 19th/437-38]

Autosomal Dominant Disorders

◈ *Robbins 9th/140-41*

- Autosomal dominant disorders are manifested in the heterozygous state, so at least one parent of an index case is usually affected; both males and females are affected, and both can transmit the condition. ***When an affected person marries an unaffected one, every child has one chance in two of having the disease.***
- Clinical features can be modified by reduced penetrance and variable expressivity. Some individuals inherit the mutant gene but are ***phenotypically normal.*** This is referred to as ***reduced penetrance***. Penetrance is expressed in mathematical terms: Thus, 50% penetrance indicates that 50% of those who carry the gene express the trait.
- In contrast to penetrance, if a trait is seen in all individuals carrying the mutant gene but is expressed differently among individuals, the phenomenon is called ***variable expressivity.***

◈ *Harrison 19th/437-38*

- In autosomal dominant disorders, individuals are affected in successive generations; the disease does not occur in the offspring of unaffected individuals. ***Males and females are affected with equal frequency*** because the defective gene resides on one of the 22 autosomes.
- Autosomal dominant mutations alter one of the two alleles at a given locus. ***Because the alleles segregate randomly at meiosis, the probability that an offspring will be affected is 50%. Unless there is a new germline mutation, an affected individual has an affected parent.*** Children with a normal genotype do not transmit the disorder.

37. Ans. d. 4

[Ref: Robbins 9th/641-42; Harrison 19th/638]

[Thalassemia Syndromes] The four classic α thalassemias, most common in Asians, are α -thalassemia-2 trait, in which one of the four α -globin loci is deleted; α -thalassemia-1 trait, with two deleted loci; HbH disease, with three loci deleted; and hydrops fetalis with Hb Barts, with all four loci deleted. Nondeletion forms of α thalassemia also exist"- (Harrison 19th/638)

α-THALASSEMIAS

◈ *Robbins 9th/641-42*

- **The α-thalassemias are caused by inherited deletions that result in reduced or absent synthesis of α-globin chains.**
- Normally, ***there are four α-globin genes***, and the severity of α-thalassemia depends on how many α-globin genes are affected.
- In **newborns** with α-thalassemia, excess unpaired γ-globin chains ***form γ4 tetramers*** known as ***hemoglobin Barts,*** whereas in **older children and adults** excess β-globin chains form β4 tetramers known as ***HbH***.

Table: Clinical and Genetic Classification of α-Thalassemias

Clinical Nomenclature	Genotype	Disease	Molecular Genetics
Hydrops fetails	-/- -/-	Lethal in utero without transfusions	Mainly gene deletions
HbH disease	-/- -/α	Severe; resembles β-thalassemia intermedia	
α- Thalassemia trait	-/- α/α (Asian) -/α -/α (black African)	Asymptomatic, like β-thalassemia minor	
Silent carrier	-/α α/α	Asymptomatic; no red cell abnormality	

Hydrops Fetalis

◈ *Robbins 9th/642*

- Hydrops fetalis is the most severe form of α-thalassemia and is caused by ***deletion of all four α-globin genes.***
- In the ***fetus, excess γ-globin chains form tetramers (hemoglobin Barts)*** that have such a high affinity for oxygen that they deliver little to tissues.
- Survival in early development is due to the expression of ζ chains, an embryonic globin that pairs with γ chains to form a functional ζ2γ2 Hb tetramer.
- Signs of fetal distress usually become evident by the third trimester of pregnancy. In the past, severe tissue anoxia led to death in utero or shortly after birth; with intrauterine transfusion many such infants are now saved.

38. Ans. a. Reticulum & e. Heterochromatin

[Ref: Harshmohan 7th/899, 17, 72-73; http://histology. leeds. ac. uk/what-is-histology/H_and_E. php]

What Structures are Stained Purple (Basophilic)

DNA (heterochromatin and the nucleolus) in the nucleus, and RNA in ribosomes and in the rough endoplasmic reticulum are both acidic, and so hematoxylin binds to them and stains them *purple*. Some extracellular materials (i.e. carbohydrates in cartilage) are also basophilic.

What structures are stained pink (eosinophilic or acidophilic)

Most proteins in the cytoplasm are basic, and so eosin binds to these proteins and stains them pink. This includes cytoplasmic filaments in muscle cells, intracellular membranes, and extracellular fibres

H & E Staining

- The most commonly used staining system is called H&E (Haemotoxylin and Eosin). H&E contains the two dyes haemotoxylin and eosin.
- Eosin is an acidic dye: It is negatively charged. It stains basic (or acidophilic) structures red or pink. This is also sometimes termed 'eosinophilic'.
- "Eosin stains nearly everything that hematoxylin will not stain. When applied correctly, eosin produces three different hues which can be used to differentiate various tissue elements; red blood cells stain dark reddish orange, *collagen (acidophilic) stains a lighter pastel pink*, and smooth muscle stains bright pink"- *http://www. ispybio. com/search*
- Haematoxylin can be considered as a basic dye. It is used to stain acidic (or basophilic) structures a *purplish blue.* Nucleus is stained purple by H&E staining. This means that the nucleus, and parts of the cytoplasm that contain RNA stain up in one colour (purple), and the rest of the cytoplasm stains up a different colour (pink).

Hematoxylin and Eosin Stain (H&E Stain or HE Stain)

◈ *http://en. wikipedia. org/wiki/H%26E_stain*

- It is one of the principal stains in histology. It is the most widely used stain in medical diagnosis and is often the gold standard; for example when a pathologist looks at a biopsy of a suspected cancer, the histological section is likely to be stained with H&E .
- The staining method involves application of hemalum, a complex formed from aluminum ions and hematein (an oxidation product of haematoxylin). *Hemalum colors nuclei of cells (and a few other objects, such as keratohyalin granules and calcified material) blue.*
- The nuclear staining is followed by counterstaining with an aqueous or alcoholic solution of eosin Y, which colors eosinophilic structures in various shades of *red, pink and orange.*
- A mnemonic often used to remember the coloring process is Acidic Attaches Acidophilic Applying Auburn and Basic Binds Basophilic Becoming Blue.

What is H&E?

◈ *http://histology. leeds. ac. uk/what-is-histology/H_and_E. php*

- Acidic dyes react with cationic or basic components in cells. Proteins and other components in the cytoplasm are basic, and will bind to acidic dyes. Another way of saying this is that cytoplasmic proteins are acidophilic (acid liking - i.e. bind to acidic dyes).

Basic dyes react with anionic or acidic components in cells. Nucleic acids are acidic, and therefore bind to basic dyes. Another way of saying this is that nucleic acids are basophilic (basic liking).

39. Ans. a. Act as., b. Gluta… & c. Reduce…

[Ref: Robbins 9th/48, 80; Harshmohan 7th/15; Harper 30th/122; Lippincott Bio. 6th/148]

"*Reduced glutathione can chemically detoxify H_2O_2. This reaction is catalyzed by* glutathione peroxidase, forms, oxidized glutathione, which no longer has protective properties"- *Lippincott Bio. 6th/148*

"*Reduced glutathione removes H_2O_2 in a reaction catalysed by* glutathione peroxidase & it is converted to oxidized glutathione"- *Harper 30th/200, 122*

"*Glutathione peroxidase* also protects against injury by catalyzing free radical breakdown (H_2O_2 + 2 GSH → GSSG [glutathione homodimer] + 2 H_2O, or 2 OH + 2 GSH → GSSG + 2 H_2O). The intracellular ratio of oxidized glutathione (GSSG) to reduced glutathione (GSH) is a reflection of the oxidative state of the cell and is an important aspect of the cell's ability to detoxify reactive oxygen species"- Robbins 9th/48

"In healthy cells and tissue, more than 90% of the total glutathione pool is in the reduced form (GSH) and less than 10% exists in the disulfide form (GSSG). An increased GSSG-to-GSH ratio is considered indicative of oxidative stress"

Removal of Free Radicals: Nonenzymatic and Enzymatic Mechanisms to Remove Free Radicals

◈ *Robbins 9th/48*

- *Antioxidants* either block free radical formation or inactivate (*e.g., scavenge*) free radicals. Examples are the lipid-soluble vitamins E and A as well as ascorbic acid and *glutathione in the cytosol.*

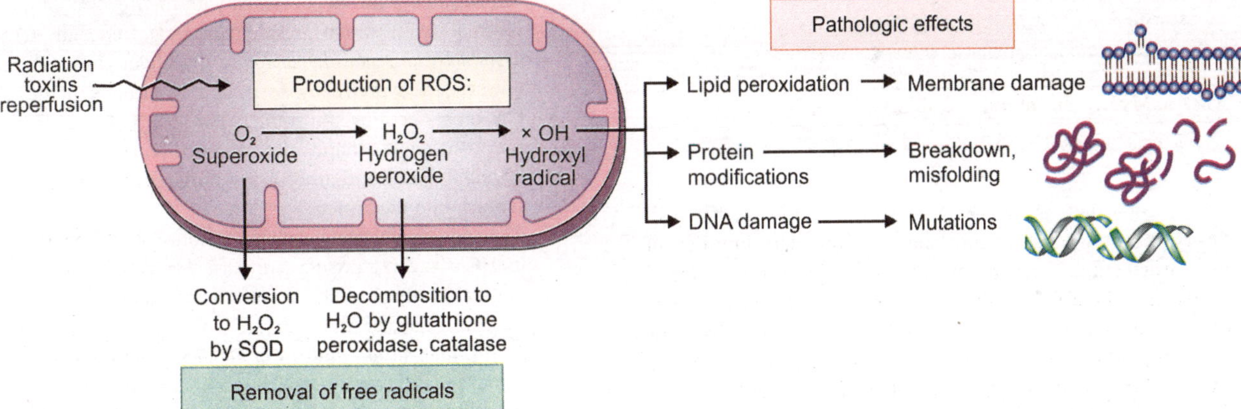

Fig: The generation, removal, and role of reactive oxygen species (ROS) in cell injury. The production of ROS is increased by many injurious stimuli. These free radicals are removed by spontaneous decay and by specialized enzymatic systems. Excessive production or inadequate removal leads to accumulation of free radicals in cells, which may damage lipids (by peroxidation), proteins, and deoxyribonucleic acid (DNA), resulting in cell injury.

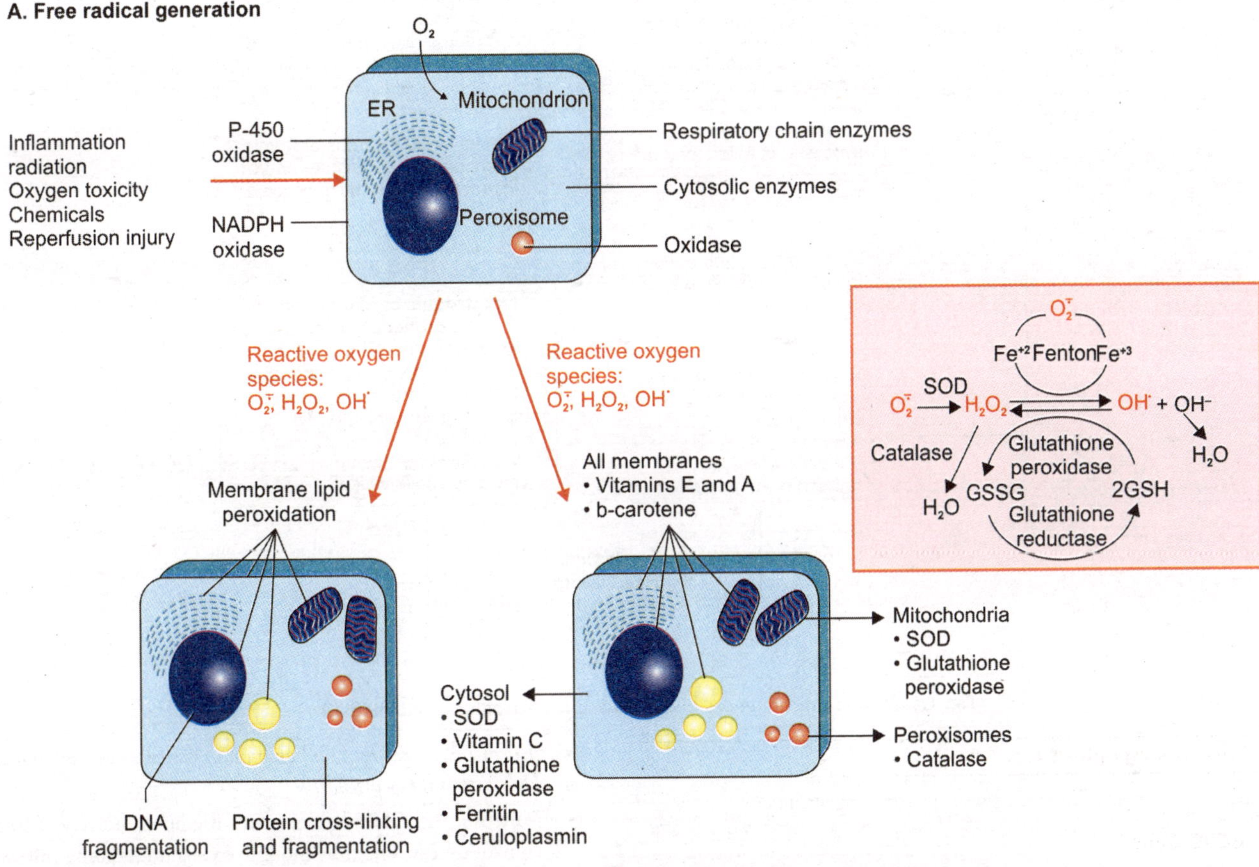

Fig: The role of reactive oxygen species in cell injury

- A series of *enzymes* acts as free radical-scavenging systems and breaks down H_2O_2 and O_2 –. These enzymes are located near the sites of generation of the oxidants and include the following:
  - Catalase,
  - *Superoxidase dismutases* (SODs)
  - *Glutathione peroxidase*

40. Ans. a. Myo…., b. Interst… & d. Myoc….

[Ref: Robbins 9th/568, 7th/605; Harrison 19th/1568-69, 1566; Harrison 18th/1967-69; Harshmohan 7th/435, 6th/455]

"Microscopically, the classical feature is myocardial cell disorganization in the ventricular septum. The bundles of myocardial fibers are irregularly & haphazardly arranged rather than the usual parallel pattern & are separated by bands of interstitial fibrous tissue. The individual muscle cells show hypertrophy & large prominent nuclei" *(Harshmohan 7th/435)*

"Amyloidosis is the major cause of restrictive cardiomyopathy" *(Harrison 19th/1566)*

Hypertrophic Cardiomyopathy-*Morphology* *Robbins 9th/568*

- The essential feature of HCM is massive *myocardial hypertrophy without ventricular dilation.*
- The classic pattern is disproportionate thickening of the ventricular septum as compared with the free wall of the left ventricle (with a ratio greater than 1: 3), frequently termed *asymmetrical septal hypertrophy.* In about 10% of cases, however, the hypertrophy is symmetrical throughout the heart.
- On cross-section, the ventricular cavity loses its usual round-to-ovoid shape and may be compressed into a "*banana-like*" configuration by bulging of the ventricular septum into the lumen.
- The most important histologic features of the myocardium in HCM are (1) *extensive myocyte hypertrophy* to a degree unusual in other conditions, with transverse myocyte diameters frequently greater than 40 μm (normal, approximately 15 μm); (2) *haphazard disarray of bundles of myocytes,* individual myocytes, and contractile elements in sarcomeres within cells (*myofiber disarray*)[Q]; and (3) interstitial and replacement fibrosis

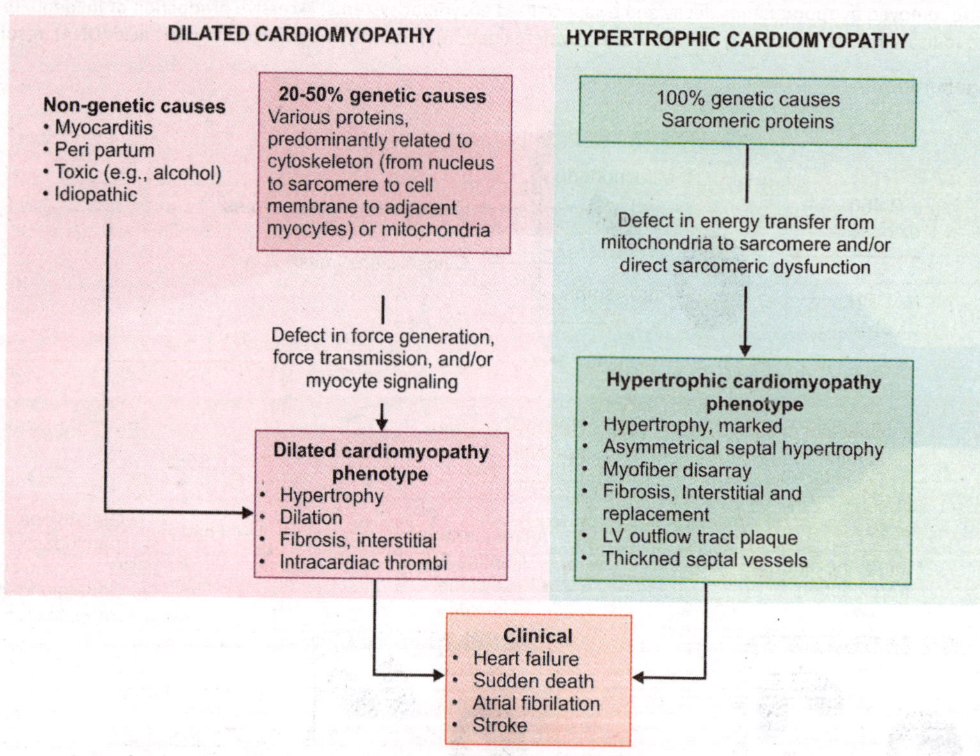

Fig: Causes and consequences of dilated and hypertrophic cardiomyopathy

41. Ans. b. ↓ Apoptosis & c. ↑ Resi…..

[Ref: Robbins 9th/55Harrison 19th/101e; Harshmohan 7th/208]

BCL 2 Gene

◈ *Harshmohan 7th/208*

- *It is seen in normal lymphocyte but its mutant form with characteristic translocation (t14; 18) (q32; q21) was first described in B-cell lymphoma & hence the name BCL.*
- *It is also seen in many other human cancers such as that of breast, thyroid & prostate*
- Mutation in BCL2 gene removes the apoptosis–Inhibitory control on cancers, thus more live cells undergoing mitosis contributing to tumour growth

"The evolution of tumor cells to a more malignant phenotype requires the acquisition of genetic changes that *subvert apoptosis pathways and promote cancer cell survival and resistance to anticancer therapies*. However, cancer cells may be more vulnerable than normal cells to therapeutic interventions that target the apoptosis pathways on which cancer cells depend on. For instance, overexpression of Bcl-2 as a result of the t (14; 18) translocation contributes to follicular lymphoma. Upregulation of Bcl-2 expression is also observed in *prostate, breast, and lung cancers and melanoma*"- *Harrison 19th/102e-10*

"Damage to the Bcl-2 gene has been identified as a cause of a number of cancers, including melanoma, breast, prostate, chronic lymphocytic leukemia, and lung cancer, and a possible cause of schizophrenia and autoimmunity. *It is also a cause of resistance to cancer treatments*" *(https://en. wikipedia. org/wiki/Bcl-2)*

Table *(Harrison 19th/101e-2)*: **Representative Oncogenes at Chromosomal Translocations**

Gene (Chromosome)	Translocation	Malignancy
ABL (9q34. 1)–BCR (22q11)	(9; 22) (q34; q11)	Chronic myeloid leukemia
ATF1 (12q13)–EWS (22q12)	(12; 22) (q13; q12)	Malignant melanoma of soft parts
BCL1 (11q13.3)–IgH (14q32)	(11; 14) (q13; q32)	Mantle cell lymphoma
BCL2 (18q21.3)–IgH (14q32)	(14; 18) (q32; q21)	***Follicular lymphoma***

The Intrinsic (Mitochondrial) Pathway

◈ *Robbins 9th/55*

- Growth factors and other survival signals stimulate the production of *anti-apoptotic members of the Bcl-2 family of proteins*.
- This family is named after Bcl-2, which was identified as *an oncogene in a B cell lymphoma* and is homologous to the *C. elegans* protein, Ced-9.
- There are more than 20 proteins in this family, all of which function to regulate apoptosis; the *two main anti-apoptotic ones are Bcl-2 and Bcl-x*. These anti-apoptotic proteins normally reside in mitochondrial membranes and the cytoplasm. When cells are deprived of survival signals or subjected to stress, *Bcl-2 and/or Bcl-x are lost from the mitochondrial membrane* and are replaced by pro-apoptotic members of the family, such as Bak, Bax, and Bim.
- When Bcl-2/Bcl-x levels decrease, the permeability of the mitochondrial membrane increases, and several proteins that can activate the caspase cascade leak out. The net result is the initiation of a caspase cascade.
- Thus, *the essence of this intrinsic pathway is a balance between pro-apoptotic and protective molecules that regulate mitochondrial permeability and the release of death inducers that are normally sequestered within the mitochondria*.

42. Ans. b. Venous....& d. Line...

[Ref: Robbins 9th/125-27; Harshmohan 7th/103-05]

"Microscopically, all types of thrombi (arterial & venous) show lines of Zahn formed by alternate layers of light-staining aggregated platelets & dark staining red cells" (Harshmohan 7th/105)

"Arterial thrombi tend to be white & mural while the venous thrombi (red thrombi) are red & occlusive" *(Harshmohan 7th/103)*

"Postmortem clot: *The surface is chicken fat yellow covering the underlying red currant jelly*" *(Harshmohan 7th/104)*

Morphology

◈ *Robbins 9th/125*

- Arterial or cardiac thrombi usually begin at a site of endothelial injury (*e.g.*, atherosclerotic plaque) or turbulence (vessel bifurcation); *venous thrombi characteristically occur in sites of stasis*.
- An area of attachment to the underlying vessel or heart wall, frequently firmest at the point of origin, is characteristic of all thrombosis.
- *Arterial thrombi tend to grow in a retrograde direction from the point of attachment, whereas venous thrombi extend in the direction of blood flow (i.e., toward the heart)*. The propagating tail may not be well attached and, particularly in veins, is prone to fragmentation, creating an embolus.
- When formed in the heart or aorta, thrombi may have grossly (and microscopically) apparent laminations, called lines of Zahn; these are produced by alternating pale layers of platelets admixed with some fibrin and darker layers containing more red cells.
- Lines of Zahn are significant only in that they imply thrombosis at a site of blood flow; in veins or in smaller arteries, the laminations are typically not as apparent
- When arterial thrombi arise in heart chambers or in the aortic lumen, they usually adhere to the wall of the underlying structure and are termed mural thrombi.
- Arterial thrombi are usually occlusive; the most common sites, in descending order, are coronary, cerebral, and femoral arteries.
- Venous thrombosis, or phlebothrombosis, is almost invariably occlusive; the thrombus often creates a long cast of the vein lumen. Because these thrombi form in a relatively static environment, they tend to contain more enmeshed erythrocytes and are therefore known as red, or stasis, thrombi.

43. Ans. a. In tissue..., c. Organ, d. Organ...

[Ref: Robbins 9th/129-30; Harshmohan 7th/112]

Red (Hemorrhagic) Infarcts Occur

◈ *Robbins 9th/129-30*

- With venous occlusions (such as in ovarian torsion);
- In loose tissues (such as lung), which allow blood to collect in the infarcted zone;
- In tissues with dual circulations (*e.g.*, lung and small intestine), permitting flow of blood from the unobstructed vessel into the necrotic zone (obviously such perfusion is not sufficient to rescue the ischemic tissues);

- In tissues that were previously congested because of sluggish venous outflow; and
- When flow is re-established to a site of previous arterial occlusion and necrosis (*e.g.*, following fragmentation of an occlusive embolus or angioplasty of a thrombotic lesion)

Types of Infarcts

◈ *Harshmohan 7th/112*

- **Pale or anaemic:** It occurs due to *arterial occlusion* & are seen in *compact organs* e. g in the kidney, heart, spleen etc
- **Red or haemorrhagic:** Seen in soft loose tissue & are caused either by pulmonary arterial obstruction (e. g in the lungs) or *by arterial or venous occlusion* (e. g in the intestine)

44. Ans. a. Osteosarcoma., c. Embr…, d. Leio… & e. Fibr…

[Ref: Robbins 9th/1224; Harshmohan 7th/855, 852]

Soft tissue tumor *consists of 3 type of cell (Spindle cell, small round cells & epitheloid cell- Harshmohan 7th/852)*

Table *(Robbins 8th)*: **Morphology of Cells in Soft Tissue Tumors**

Cell Type	Features	Tumor Type
Spindle cell	Rod-shaped, long axis twice as great as short axis	Fibrous, fibrohistiocytic, smooth muscle, Schwann cell
Small round cell	Size of a lymphocyte with little cytoplasm	***Rhabdomyosarcoma***, primitive neuroectodermal tumor
Epithelioid	Polyhedral with abundant cytoplasm, nucleus is centrally located	Smooth muscle, Schwann cell endothelial, epithelioid sarcoma

"Osteosarcoma: *The tumour cells may have various shapes such as spindled, round, oval, polygonal & bizarre tumour gaint cells" (Harshmohan 7th/833)*

"Leiomyosarcomas: They consist of eosinophilic *spindle cells* with blunt-ended, hyperchromatic nuclei arranged in interweaving fascicles"*(Robbins 9th/1223)*

"Fibrosarcoma: It is composed of malignant fibroblasts arranged in a herringbone pattern. Malignant fibrous histiocytoma consists of a background of *spindled fibroblasts* arranged in a storiform pattern admixed with large, ovoid, bizarre multinucleated tumor giant cells" *(Harshmohan 7th/855)*

"Embryonal rhabdomyosarcoma: The tumor cells mimic skeletal muscle at various stages of embryogenesis and consist of sheets of both primitive round and *spindled cells* in a myxoid stroma. Rhabdomyoblasts with visible cross-striations may be present"*(Robbins 9th/1222)*

"Synovial sarcomas are morphologically monophasic (spindle cell) & monophasic (spindle cell plus gland like structure composed of cuboidal or columnar epithelium cell)" (Robbins 9th/1224)

"Liposarcomas are histologically divided into three morphologic. Well-differentiated liposarcoma contains adipocytes with scattered *atypical spindle cells"(Robbins 9th/1220)*

Table *(Robbins 9th/1220)*: **Soft tissue sarcoma**

Category	Behaviour	Tumor type	Common locations	Age (yr)	Morphology
Adipose	Benign	Lipoma	Superficial extremity, trunk	40–60	Mature adipos tissue
	Malignant	Well-differentiated Liposarcoma	Deep extremity, retroperitoneum	50–60	Adpose tissue with scattered atypical spindle cells
		Myxoid liposarcoma	Thigh, leg	30s	Myxoid matrix, 'chicken wire' vessels, round cells, lipoblasts
Fibrous	Benign	Nodular fascilitis	Arm, forearm	20–30	Tissue culture growth, extravasated erythrocytes
		Deep fibromatosis	Abdominal wall	30–40	Dense collgen, long, unidirectional fascicles
Skeletal muscle	Benign	Rhabdomyosarcoma	Head and neck	0–60	Polygonal rhabdomyoblasts, "spider" cells
	Malignant	Alveolar rhabdomyosarcoma	Extremities, sunises	5–15	Uniform round discohesive cells between septae
		Embryonal rhabdomyosarcoma	Genitourinary tract	1–5	Primitice spindle cells : "strap" cells
Vascular	Benign	Hemangioma	Head and neck	0–10	Circumscribed mass of capillary or venous channels

Contd...

Category	Behaviour	Tumor type	Common locations	Age (yr)	Morphology
	Malignant	Angiosarcoma	Skin, deep lower extremity	50–80	Infiltrating capillary channels
Nerve sheath	Benign	Schwannoma	Head and neck	20–50	Encapsulated, fibrillar stroma, nuclear palisading
		Neurofibroma	Wide, cutaneous, subcutis	10–20+	Myxoid, ropy collagen, loose fascicles, mast cells
	Malignant	Malignant peripheral nerve sheath tumor	Extremities, shoulder girdle	20–50	Tight fascicles, atypia, mitotic activity, necrosis
Uncertain histotype	Benign	Solitary fibrous tumor	Pelvis, pleura	20–70	Branching ecstatic vessels
	Malignant	Synovial sarcoma	Thigh, leg	15–40	Tight fascicles of uniform basophilic spindle cells, Pseudoglandular structures
		Undifferentiated pleomorphic sarcoma	Thigh	40–70	High grade anaplastic polygonal, round or spindle cells
					Bizarre nuclei, atypical mitosis, necrosis
		Alveolar soft part sarcoma	Trunk, extremities	15–35	Multiple nodules of eosinophilic round cells, septae
		Clear cell sarcoma	Tendons, extremities	20–40	Sheets of pale of clear spindle cells, wreath-like giant cells

45. Ans. a. WB..., b. Broad... & d. RBC...

[Ref: Robbins 9th/929; Harrison 19th/294; CMDT 2015/891]

Table *(CMDT 2015/891)*: **Significance of specific urinary casts**

Type	Significance
Hyaline casts	Concentrated urine, febrile disease, after strenuous exercise, in the course of diuretic therapy (not indicative of renal disease)
Red cell casts	Glomerulonephritis
White cell casts	Pyelonephritis, interstitial nephritis (indicative of infection or inflammation)
Renal tubular cell casts	Acute tubular necrosis, interstitial nephritis
Coarse, granular casts	Nonspecific; can represent acute tubular necrosis
Broad, waxy casts	Chronic renal failure (indicative of stasis in enlarged collecting tubules)

"Eosinophilic hyaline casts, as well as pigmented granular casts, are common, particularly in distal tubules and collecting ducts. These casts consist principally of *Tamm-Horsfall protein* (a urinary glycoprotein normally secreted by the cells of ascending thick limb and distal tubules) in conjunction with other plasma proteins" *(Robbins 9th/929)*

"Acute pyelonephritis: The finding of leukocyte *casts*, typically rich in neutrophils (pus casts), indicates renal involvement, because casts are formed only in tubules. The diagnosis of infection is established by quantitative urine culture" *(Robbins 9th/933)*

Casts in CRD

◈ *Harrison 19th/294*

- In chronic renal disease, degenerated cellular casts called waxy casts[Q] can be seen in urine.
- Broad casts are thought to be arise in the dilated tubules of enlarged nephrons that have undergone compensatory hypertrophy in response to reduced renal mass (i.e., *chronic renal failure*[Q])
- WBC cast are seen in - *Pyelonephritis*[Q], *interstitial nephritis*[Q], SLE & transplant rejection.
- RBC cast are seen in - *Acute glomerulonephritis*[Q]

46. Ans. a. Yolk sac., d. Non-seminoma. & e. Hepat....

[Ref: Robbins 9th/663, 8th/672; Harrison 19th/732-34, 18th/974-977; CMDT 2016/553-54]

Alpha-fetoprotein (AFP)

◈ *CSDT 11th/572*

- *AFP, a glycoprotein* normally present only in the fetal circulation, is present in *high concentrations in the serum of many patients with primary hepatomas and testicular tumors.*
- Additionally, some patients may have normal AFP levels, despite the presence of advanced disease. *In general, AFP levels correlate with tumor size* and vascular invasion, and a number of studies have shown a *correlation between high AFP levels and recurrent cancer after resection.*

"About 95% of testicular tumors are germ cell tumors (seminomas or nonseminomas). *Seminomas do not produce α-fetoprotein,* but about 5–10% produce some hCG. *Nonseminomas,* on the other hand, produce increased serum levels of one or both of these markers in about 90% of cases. Men with liver disease may have misleadingly high levels of α-fetoprotein" *(CMDT 2016/1635)*

"The diagnosis of hepatocellular carcinoma is established (without the need for biopsy) for lesions > 2 cm when characteristic arterial hypervascularity is demonstrated on both helical CT and MRI (or on either CT or MRI if the *serum α -fetoprotein level is higher than 200 mg/L*). In a population of patients with cirrhosis, over 60% of nodules < 2 cm in diameter is detected on a screening ultrasound prove to be hepatocellular carcinoma" *(CMDT 2016/1596, 2006/682)*

Alpha-Fetoprotein in Maternal Serum

- This glycoprotein is synthesized early in gestation by the fetal yolk sac & later by fetal gastrointestinal tract & liver
- Highest level of AFP in fetal serum & amniotic fluid is reached around 13 weeks[Q] & thereafter it decreases. Maternal serum level reaches a peak around 32 weeks[Q].

Elevated AFP

◈ *Williams 22nd/321*

- Neural tube defect[Q]
- Esophageal or intestinal obstruction
- Cystic hygroma[Q]
- Abdominal wall defect-omphalocele[Q], gastrochisis[Q]
- Renal anomalies-polycystic or absent kidneys
- Osteogenesis imperfect; Cloacal exstrophy[Q]
- Placental abruption; Oligohydraminos
- Multifetal gestation; Fetal death[Q]
- Underestimated maternal age
- Pilonidal cysts[Q]; Liver necrosis
- Sacrococcygeal teratoma[Q]
- Urinary obstruction; Congenital nephrosis[Q]
- Congenital skin defects
- Chorioangioma of placenta[Q]
- Placenta accrete; Preeclampsia[Q]
- Low birth weight
- Improper adjustment for low maternal weight
- Maternal hepatoma or teratoma[Q]

Alphafetoprotein	Hepatocellular carcinoma, gonadal germ cell tumor	Cirrhosis, hepatitis[Q]

47. Ans. b. Factor 9, c. X-linked. & d. Clinica....

[Ref: Robbins 9th/663; Harrison 19th/732-34; Harrison 18th/974-977; CMDT06/526; Robbins 8th/672]

Hemophilia B (Christmas Disease, Factor IX Deficiency)

◈ *Robbins 9th/663*

- Severe factor IX deficiency produces a disorder *clinically indistinguishable from factor VIII deficiency (hemophilia A).* This should not be surprising, given that factors VIII and IX function together to activate factor X.
- Like hemophilia A, it is inherited as an *X-linked recessive trait* and shows variable clinical severity. In about 15% of these patients, factor IX protein is present but is nonfunctional.
- As with hemophilia A, the PTT is prolonged and the PT is normal.
- Diagnosis of Christmas disease (named after the first patient identified with this condition, and not the holiday) is possible only by assay of the factor levels.
- The disease is treated with *infusions of recombinant factor IX.*

Hemophilia

- Hemophilia is an X-linked recessive hemorrhagic disease due to mutations in the F8 gene (hemophilia A or classic hemophilia) or F9 gene (hemophilia B).
- Male subjects are clinically affected; women, who carry a single mutated gene, are generally asymptomatic. Clinically, hemophilia A and hemophilia B are indistinguishable.
- The disease phenotype correlates with the residual activity of FVIII or FIX and can be classified as severe (<1%), moderate (1–5%), or mild (6–30%).
- In the severe and moderate forms, the disease is characterized by bleeding into the joints (hemarthrosis), soft tissues, and muscles after minor trauma or even spontaneously.

Von-Willebrand Disease[Q]	↑Bleeding time (Despite a normal platelet count)
	↑PTT (Type 1 & 3)
Hemophilia A[Q]	Normal BT, platelet count & PT
	↑PTTQ
Hemophilia B[Q]	Normal BT & PT[Q]
	↑PTT
Henoch-schonlein purpura[Q]	Normal BT, PT, PTT & platelet count
Bernard –Sourlier syndrome[Q]	↑BT

48. Ans. a. More..., b. Peripor....& d. Jaun....

[Ref: Robbins 9th/858-59; Harshmohan 7th / 609-13; Harrison 19th/2060-61]

Primary Biliary Cirrhosis *(Harrison 19th/2060-61)*

- "PBC is primarily a disease of *middle-aged women*, with a *female predominance of 9: 1.* Occurring between the ages of *30 and 70 years*, its peak incidence is between 40 and 50 years of age. *Antimitochondrial antibodies are the most characteristic laboratory finding in PBC" (Robbins 9th/858)*
- "Primary biliary cirrhosis: Increased incidence of associated autoimmune diseases (*e. g.*, scleroderma, Sjogren's syndrome, CREST syndrome & autoimmune thyroiditis)" *(Harshmohan 7th/610)*
- PBC has a strong female preponderance and a median age of around 50 years at the time of diagnosis.
- The cause of PBC is unknown; it is characterized by *portal inflammation and necrosis* of cholangiocytes in small- and medium-sized bile ducts.

- Liver transplantation is the treatment of choice for patients with decompensated cirrhosis due to PBC.
- *Antimitochondrial antibodies (AMA) are present in about 90% of patients with PBC.*
- Histopathologic analyses of liver biopsies of patients with PBC have resulted in identifying four distinct stages of the disease as it progresses. The earliest lesion is termed *chronic nonsuppurative destructive cholangitis* and is a necrotizing inflammatory process of the portal tracts. Medium and small bile ducts are infiltrated with lymphocytes and undergo duct destruction. Mild fibrosis and sometimes bile stasis can occur. With progression, the inflammatory infiltrate becomes less prominent, but the number of bile ducts is reduced and there is proliferation of smaller bile ductules. Increased fibrosis ensues with the expansion of *periportal fibrosis to bridging fibrosis*. Finally, cirrhosis, which may be micronodular or macronodular, develops.
- *Pruritus that presents prior to the development of jaundice indicates severe disease and a poor prognosis.*
- Physical examination can show jaundice and other complications of chronic liver disease, including hepatomegaly, splenomegaly, ascites, and edema.
- Other features that are unique to PBC include hyperpigmentation, xanthelasma, and xanthomata, which are related to the altered cholesterol metabolism seen in this disease.

Clinical Features

◈ *Robbins 9th/859*

- Most cases are diagnosed when asymptomatic, with elevated serum alkaline phosphatase and γ-glutamyltransferase. Both of these are markers of cholestasis and indicate the need for a liver disease work-up.
- Hypercholesterolemia is common. Antimitochondrial antibodies are present in 90% to 95% of patients. They are highly characteristic of PBC, although other autoantibodies may be seen in a small number of cases.
- *The disease is confirmed by liver biopsy, which is considered diagnostic if a florid duct lesion is present.* When symptomatic, the onset is insidious, presenting with fatigue and pruritus, which increase slowly over time.

49. Ans. a. Negri Body, b. Nodule, c. Neuronophagia & e. Inflammatory cell

[Ref: Robbins 9th/1277-78; Harshmohan 7th/178; Harrison 19th/1301]

Vacuolar degenerative (hydropic changes) means accumulation of water within the cytoplasm of the cell. Variant Creutzfeldt-Jakob disease (vCJD) shows significant vacuolar degenerative alterations specifically affecting brain macrophages/microglia within the thalamus and, to a lesser extent"- *Harshmohan 7th/17; http://www. ncbi. nlm. nih. gov*

Rabies

◈ *Robbins 9th/1277-78*

- Rabies is a severe encephalitis transmitted to humans by the bite of a rabid animal, a dog or various wild animals that form natural reservoirs.
- On macroscopic examination, the brain shows *intense edema and vascular congestion.*
- On microscopic examination, there is *widespread neuronal degeneration* and an *inflammatory reaction* that is most severe in the *rhombencephalon* (midbrain, and floor of the fourth ventricle, particularly in the medulla).
- The basal ganglia, spinal cord, and dorsal root ganglia may also be involved. Negri bodies, the *pathognomonic microscopic finding*, are cytoplasmic, round to oval, eosinophilic inclusions that can be found in pyramidal neurons of the hippocampus and Purkinje cells of the cerebellum, sites usually devoid of inflammation.

◈ *Harrison 19th/1301*

- Pathologic studies show *mild inflammatory changes* in the CNS in rabies, with *mononuclear inflammatory infiltration* in the leptomeninges, perivascular regions, and parenchyma, including *microglial nodules called Babes nodules.*
- *Degenerative neuronal changes* usually are not prominent, and there is little evidence of neuronal death; *neuronophagia is observed occasionally.* The pathologic changes are surprisingly mild in light of the clinical severity and fatal outcome of the disease.
- *The most characteristic pathologic finding in rabies is the Negri body*
- The lack of prominent degenerative neuronal changes has led to the concept that *neuronal dysfunction*—rather than neuronal death—is responsible for clinical disease in rabies.

Microglia

Microglia are mesoderm-derived cells whose primary function is to serve as a fixed macrophage system in the CNS. They express many surface markers in common with peripheral monocytes/macrophages (such as CR3 and CD68). They respond to injury by (1) proliferation; (2) developing elongated nuclei (*rod cells*), as in neurosyphilis; (3) forming aggregates about small foci of tissue necrosis *(microglial nodules)*; or (4) congregating around cell bodies of dying neurons *(neuronophagia)*.

50. Ans. c. Vessel thrombosis

[Ref: Robbins 9th/231-34; Harshmohan 7th/50]

Hyperacute Rejection

◈ *Harshmohan 7th/50*

- Appears within minutes to hours of placing the transplant
- It is mediated by preformed humoral antibody
- There are numerous neutrophils around dilated & obstructed capillaries which are blocked by fibrin & platelet thrombi

"In acute rejection there is *infiltration of T & B cell*" *(Harshmohan 7th/50)*

◈ *Robbins 9th/233*

- This form of rejection occurs *within minutes or hours* after transplantation and can sometimes be recognized by the surgeon just after the graft vasculature is anastomosed to the recipient's.
- In contrast to the nonrejecting kidney graft, which rapidly regains a normal pink coloration and normal tissue turgor and promptly excretes urine, a hyperacutely rejecting kidney rapidly becomes *cyanotic, mottled, and flaccid and may excrete a mere few drops of bloody urine.*

- Immunoglobulin and complement are deposited in the vessel wall, and electron microscopy discloses early endothelial injury together with *fibrin-platelet thrombi.*
- There is also a rapid accumulation of neutrophils within arterioles, glomeruli, and peritubular capillaries. These early lesions point to an antigen-antibody reaction at the level of vascular endothelium.
- Subsequently, these changes become diffuse and intense, the *glomeruli undergo thrombotic occlusion* of the capillaries, and fibrinoid necrosis occurs in arterial walls.

Acute Rejection

◈ *Robbins 9th/233*

- This may *occur within days* of transplantation in the untreated recipient or may appear suddenly months or even years later, after immunosuppression has been employed and terminated. As suggested earlier, acute graft rejection is a combined process in which both cellular and humoral tissue injuries contribute. In any one patient, one or the other mechanism may predominate.
- Histologically, humoral rejection is associated with vasculitis, whereas cellular rejection is marked by an interstitial mononuclear cell infiltrate.

Mechanisms of Recognition and Rejection of Allografts

◈ *Robbins 9th/231-32*

- Rejection is a process in which T lymphocytes and antibodies produced against graft antigens react against and destroy tissue grafts
- *Recognition of Graft Alloantigens by T and B Lymphocytes:* The major antigenic differences between a donor and recipient that result in rejection of transplants are differences in HLA alleles.

T Cell–Mediated Reactions

◈ *Robbins 9th/233*

- Acute cellular rejection, also called *acute T cell–mediated rejection*, is most commonly seen within the initial months after transplantation and is heralded by clinical and biochemical signs of organ failure.
- T cells also contribute to chronic rejection.

Antibody-Mediated Reactions

◈ *Robbins 9th/233*

- Although T cells are pivotal in the rejection of organ transplants, antibodies produced against alloantigens in the graft are also important mediators of rejection. Antibody mediated reactions can take three forms.
- Hyperacute rejection occurs when preformed antidonor antibodies are present in the circulation of the recipient. Such antibodies may be present in a recipient who has previously rejected a transplant.
- Acute antibody-mediated rejection is caused by antidonor antibodies produced after transplantation.
- Chronic antibody-mediated rejection usually develops insidiously, without preceding acute rejection, and primarily affects vascular components.

51. Ans. a. Diet should.... & c. Anti IgA....

[Ref: Robbins 9th/782-83; Harrison 19th/1940-42]

"*The presence of Antiendomysial antibody is 90-95% sensitive & 90-95% specific*" *(Harrison 19th/1941)*

Celiac Disease: Diagnosis

- Small intestinal biopsy (duodenal/jejunal)[Q] (*Characteristic but not diagnostic*)
  - Absence or reduced height of villi (*Flat appearence*)[Q]
  - *Crypt hyperplasia*[Q], *villous atrophy*[Q] (But *not mucosal atrophy-Overall mucosal thickness remains the same*)
  - Cuboidal appearance of epithelial cells & *increased intraepithelial lymphocytes*[Q]
  - Increased lymphocytes & plasma cells in lamina propria
- Antiendomysial antibodies
  - Antiendomysial antibody has *90-95% sensitivity & 90-95% specificity.*
  - Prompt clinical & histopathological response, together with disappearance of Ig antiendomysial antibodies following institution of a *gluten free diet is diagnostic*[Q].

Associated disease	Complication
Dermatitis Herpeteformis[Q], Diabetes mellitus type I, IgA deficiency[Q]	Increased incidence of both gastrointestinal & non -gastrointestinal neoplasm as well as intestinal lymphoma

Table: Etiology

Environmental factors	Immunogenic factors	Genetic factors
Intolerance to gliadin[Q] a component of gluten, present in ***wheat, barley, rye & oats***[Q]	IgA antibodies are present. IgA antiendomysial, IgA antitissue tranglutaminase Antiendomysial antibody has 90-95% sensitivity & 90-95% specificity	95% express ***HLA-DQ$_2$ allele***[Q]

"Celiac disease: An *immunologic* component to etiology is suspected. Serum antibodies—*IgA antigliadin, IgA antiendomysial, and IgA anti-tTG antibodies*—are present, but it is not known whether such antibodies are primary or secondary to the tissue damage. The *antiendomysial antibody has 90–95% sensitivity and 90–95% specificity*; the antigen recognized by the antiendomysial antibody is tTG. Antibody studies are frequently used to identify patients with celiac sprue; patients with these antibodies should undergo duodenal biopsy. This autoantibody has not been linked to a pathogenetic mechanism (or mechanisms) responsible for celiac sprue" *(Harrison 19th/1940-41)*

Gluten Containing Grain	Gluten Free Grains
Wheat	**Rice**
Oat	**Corn**
Barley	*Millet*
Rye	*Topioca*
Spelt	

PHARMACOLOGY

52. Ans. a. Enhan... & e. Inhibi....

[Ref: K. D. T 7th/419-21; Katzung 12th/413; Harrison 19th/2548, 2551-56]

Gabapentin *(K. D. T 7th/419-21, Katzung 12th/413)*

- *This lipophilic GABA derivative crosses to the brain & enhances GABA release, but does not act as agonist at GABAA receptor*
- *Recently it has been found to modulate a subset of neuronal voltage sensitive Ca^{2+} channels which contain α2δ-1 subunits. It is postulated that decreased entry of Ca2+ into the presy naptic neuron through these channels could reduce glutamate release, lowering neuronal excitability.*
- *However, whether α2δ-1 Ca^{2+} channel modulation or the GABA enhancing action is responsible for the anticonvulsant/ analgesic effect of gabapentin, is not known*
- In spite of their close structural resemblance to GABA, gabapentin *does not act directly on GABA receptors.* They may, however, *modify the synaptic or nonsynaptic release of GABA*. An increase in brain GABA concentration is observed in patients receiving gabapentin.
- Gabapentin is transported into the brain by the L-amino acid transporter. Gabapentin binds avidly to the α2δ subunit of voltage-gated Ca^{2+} channels. Gabapentin also act presynaptically to decrease the release of glutamate; this effect is probably dependent on reduced presynaptic entry of Ca^{2+} via voltage-activated channels.

Mechanisms of Action of Antiepileptic Drugs

Harrison 19th/2548

- Antiepileptic drugs appear to act primarily by blocking the initiation or spread of seizures. This occurs through a variety of mechanisms that modify the activity of ion channels or neurotransmitters, and in most cases, the drugs have pleiotropic effects.
- The mechanisms include inhibition of Na+-dependent action potentials in a frequency-dependent manner (*e.g.*, phenytoin, carbamazepine, lamotrigine, topiramate, zonisamide, lacosamide, rufinamide), inhibition of voltage-gated Ca2+ channels (phenytoin *gabapentin* pregabalin), facilitating the opening of potassium channels (ezogabine), attenuation of glutamate activity (lamotrigine, topiramate, felbamate), potentiation of GABA receptor function (benzodiazepines and barbiturates), increase in the availability of GABA (valproic acid, *gabapentin,* tiagabine), and modulation of release of synaptic vesicles (levetiracetam). The two most effective drugs for absence seizures, ethosuximide and valproic acid, probably act by inhibiting T-type Ca^{2+} channels in thalamic neurons.

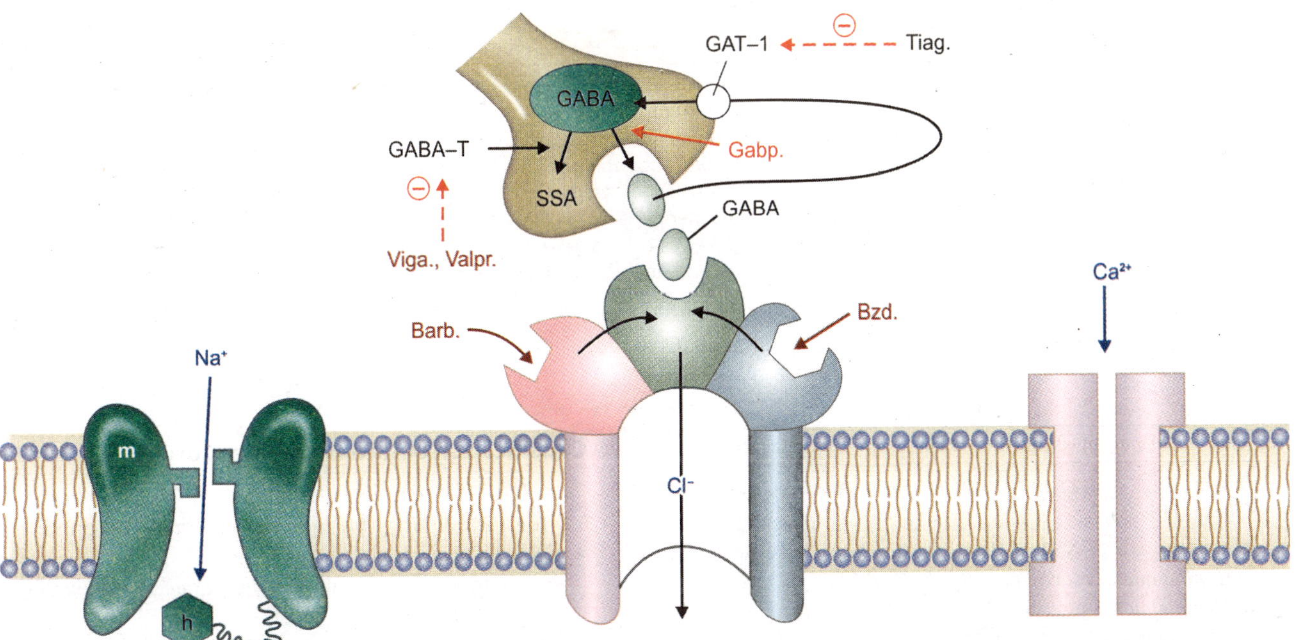

Fig: Major mechanism of anticonvulsant action

Prolongation of Na^+ Channel Inactivation	Facilitation of GABA Mediated Cl^- Channel Opening	Inhibition of 'T' Type Ca^{2+} Current
Phenytoin	Barbiturate (Barb)	Ethosuximide
Carbamazepine	Benzodiazepine (Bzd.)	Zonisamide
Valproate	Vigabatrin (Viga.)	Valporate
Lamotrigine	Valporate (Valpr.)	
Topiramate	Gabapentin (Gabp.)	
Zonisamide; Lacosamide	Tiagabine (Tiag.)	

53. Ans. d. Cardia… & e. ↓salivary

[Ref: KDT 7th/100-103, 117; Katzung 12th/97-102]

Cardiac muscarinic receptors are predominantly M 2 type & mediate vagal bradycardia *(KDT 7th/101)*

Dicyclomine

◈ *Katzung 12th/118, 126; KDT 7th/1117*

- *It is antagonist of M1 & M3 (smooth muscle)- Katzung*
- *Short t1/2 but action lasts upto 6 hr*
- *It has direct smooth muscle relaxant action in addition to weak anticholinergic*
- *Indication are- Morning sickness, motion sickness, dysmenorrhoea, irritable bowel syndrome*

Muscarinic Actions

◈ *KDT 7th/103*

Heart

"At the A-V node & His-purkinje fibres refractory period (RP) is increased & conduction is slowed; PR interval increases & partial to complete A-V block may be produced"

Eye

"Contraction of circular muscle of iris→miosis"
"Contraction of ciliary muscle →spasm of accommodation, increased outflow facility, reduction in intraocular tension (especially in glaucomatous patients)"

Smooth Muscle

"Peristalsis in ureter is increased. The detrusor muscle contracts while the bladder trigone & sphincter relaxes →voiding of bladder"

Glands

"Secretion from all parasympathetically innervated glands is increased via M3 & some M2 receptors: sweating, salivation, lacrimation, increased tracheobronchial & gastric secretion"

Table *(KDT 7th/101)*: **Characteristics of important subtypes of muscarinic receptor**

	M_1	M_2	M_3
Location & Function served	Autonomic ganglia: Depolarisation (late EPSP) Gastric glands: Histamine release, acid secretions CNS: Learning, memory, motor functions	SA node: Hyperpolarisation, ↓rate of impulse generations AV node: ↓velocity of conduction Atrium: Shortening of APD, ↓contractility Ventricle: ↓contractility Cholinergic nerve ending: Ach release CNS: Tremor, analgesia Visceral smooth muscle: contraction	Visceral smooth muscle: contraction Iris: Constriction of pupil Ciliary muscle: contraction **Exocrine glands**: ***secretion*** Vascular endothelium: release of NO → vasodilation
Agonists	Oxotremorine	Methacholine	Bethanechol
Antagonists	Pirenzepine, telenzepine	Tripitramine	Darifenacin

54. Ans. c. Abatacept, d. Monoclonal….& e. Methotrexate

[Ref: K. D. T 7th/211-12, 871-72; Katzung 12th/642; Goodman & Gilman's 11th/1942]

Nabumetone is a NSAID. It possess analgesic, anti-pyretic & anti-inflammatory activities. It is effective in the treatment of rheumatoid & osteoarthritis as well as in soft tissue injury (K. D. T 7th/203)

"Naproxen: It is a NSAID used for rheumatoid arthritis & ankylosing spondylitis (K. D. T 7th/201)

Classification of Anti-rheumatoid drugs

◈ *K. D. T 7th/211*

I. Disease modifying Anti-rheumatoid drugs (DMARDs):

- Nonbiological drugs
  - Immunosuppressants: *Methotrexate*[Q], *Azathioprine, Cyclosporine*[Q]
  - Sulfasalzine[Q]
  - Chloroquine or Hydroxychloroquine
  - Leflunomide[Q]

- Biological agents
    - *TNF-α inhibitors: Etanercept, Infliximab, Adalimumab*
    - IL-1 antagnoists: Anakinra

B. Adjuvant drugs: Corticosteroids (Prednisolone & others)

(Gold & penicillamine are obsolete DMARDs)

Methotrexate is now considered the ***DMARD of first choice to treat rheumatoid arthritis*** and is used in up to 60% of patients. It is active in this condition at much *lower doses* than those needed in cancer chemotherapy *(K. D. T 7th/211)*

Monoclonal Antibodies (e.g., Rituximab)

◈ *K. D. T 7th/871-72*

- It is a chimeric monoclonal antibody that bind to the CD20 B-cell antigen expressed on the surface of B-lymphocyte & B-cell lymphoma
- It has shown benefit in the treatment of *rheumatoid arthritis refractory to anti-TNF agents*. Rituximab has been approved for the treatment of active rheumatoid arthritis when combined with methotrexate *Katzung 12th/646*

DMARDS

◈ *Katzung 12th/643-49*

- The effects of disease-modifying therapies may take 6 weeks to 6 months to become evident; that is, they are slow-acting compared with NSAIDs.
- These therapies include methotrexate, azathioprine, penicillamine, hydroxychloroquine and chloroquine, organic gold compounds, sulfasalazine, several other immune-modulating agents, and immunoadsorption apheresis.
- Abatacept can be used as monotherapy or in combination with other DMARDs in patients with moderate to severe rheumatoid arthritis who have had an inadequate response to DMARDs or TNF antagonists. It reduces the clinical signs and symptoms of rheumatoid arthritis, including slowing of radiographic progression.
- Other drugs used in RA- TNF α blocker: certolizumab, etanercept, golimumab, infliximab, adalimumab
- **Tocilizumab:** It is a newer biological humanized antibody & bound to IL-6. Indicated for those who had an inadequate response to TNF antagonist

Disease Modifying Anti-rheumatoid Drugs (DMARDs)/ Slow Acting Anti-rheumatoid Drugs (SAARDs)

◈ *K. D. T 7th/211*

- Suppress the rheumatoid process, bring about a remission & retard disease progression
- Onset of benefit takes place a few months of regular treatment & relapses occur a few months after cessation of therapy

55. Ans. a. Juvenile..., c. Genera...., d. Com... & e. Act ....

[Ref: K. D. T 7th/420-21; Katzung 13th/407, 12th/414; Harrison 19th/2552, 18th/3262; CMDT 2015/960-61]

"Mechanism of action not known. However, it may modify synaptic release of glutamate/GABA by binding to a specific synaptic protein labeled SV2A" (K. D. T 7th/420; Katzung 13th/407)

Focal seizure without impairment of consciousness (previously described as simple partial) & focal seizure with impairment of consciousness (previously described as complex partial) (CMDT 2015/960-61)

Levetiracetam

◈ *CMDT 2015/960-61, Katzung 12th/414*

- *Approved as adjuvant therapy for focal onset seizure*
- *Approved as adjuvant therapy for primary generalized tonic-clonic*

Levetiracetam

- It is a piracetam analog that is ineffective against seizures induced by maximum electroshock or pentylenetetrazol but has prominent activity in the kindling model.
- The drug is marketed for the adjuvant treatment of *partial seizures* in adults & children for *primary generalized tonic-clonic seizures & for the myoclonic seizures of juvenile myoclonic epilepsy*

Levetiracetam

◈ *K. D. T 7th/420-21*

- *Because of good tolerability,* levetiracetam is being increasingly used in *complex partial seizure, generalized tonic-clonic seizure & myoclonic epilepsy*, mainly as add-on drug.

"*Treatment of* Generalized tonic-clonic seizure & simple partial seizure: Levetiracetam is another close contender"- *(K. D. T 7th/423)*

"*Treatment of* Complex partial seizure: Levetiracetam may be added in refractory cases" *(K. D. T 7th/423)*

"*Myoclonic & atonic seizures:* Levetiracetam is generally added in nonresponsive cases"*(K. D. T 7th/423)*

Table *(Harrison 19th/2552)*: **Selection of Antiepileptic Drug**

Primary Generalized Tonic-Clonic	Focal	Typical Absence	Atypical Absence, Myoclonic, Atonic
First-Line			
Lamotrigine Valproic acid	Lamotrigine Carbamazepine Oxcarbazepine Phenytoin Levetiracetam	Valproic acid Ethosuximide Lamotrigine	Valproic acid Lamotrigine Topiramate
Alternatives			
Zonisamide[a] Phenytoin Carbamazepine Oxcarbazepine Topiramate Phenobarbital Primidone Felbamate	Topiramate Zonisamide *Valproic acid*[Q] Tiagabine Gabapentin Lacosamide Exogabine Phenobarbital Primidone Felbamate	Lamotrigine Clonazepam	Clonazepam Felbamate Clobazam Rufinamide

56. Ans. a. Methicillin, b. Cloxacillin & d. Dicloxacillin

[Ref: K. D. T 7th/721]

Penicillinase- Resistant Penicillins

◈ *K. D. T 7th/721*

- *These congeners have side chains that protect the β-lactam ring from attack by staphylococcal penicillinase*
- *Their only indication is infections caused by penicillinase producing staphylococci, for which they are drug of choice, except in areas where methicillin resistant staph. aureus (MRSA) has become prevalent*

Classification of Penicillins

◈ *K. D. T 7th/721*

- Acid resistant alternative to penicillin G: Phenoxymethyl penicillin (Pn V)
- Penicillinase- resistant penicillins: *Methicillin, cloxacillin, Dicloxacillin*
- *Extended spectrum penicllins*
  - *Aminopenicillins: Ampicillin, bacampicillin, amoxicillin*
  - *Carboxypenicillins: Carbenicillin*
  - *Ureidopenicillins: Piperacillin, mezlocillin*

β- lactamase *inhibitors: clavulanic acid, sulbactam & tazobactam*

Methicillin-Resistance Staphylococcus Aureus (MRSA)

◈ *KDT 6th/700*

MRSA have acquired a PBP which has very low affinity for β lactams antibiotics. MRSA are *insensitive to all penicillinase-resistant penicillin and to other β lactams as well as to erythromycin, aminoglycosides, tetracyclines,* etc.

57. Ans. a. Occu...., c. Aggrevation.... & e. Most...

[Ref: K.D.T 7th/720; CMDT 2015/1460; Harrison 19th/1140; Neena Khanna 4th/206; G & G 11th/1181; Ananthanarayan 9th/377, 384]

Jarisch-Herxheimer Reaction

◈ *Harrison 19th/1140*

- A dramatic although usually mild reaction consisting of fever, chills, myalgias, headache, tachycardia, increased respiratory rate, increased circulating neutrophil count, and vasodilation with mild hypotension may follow the initiation of treatment for syphilis.
- This reaction is thought to be a response to lipoproteins released by dying *T. pallidum* organisms. The Jarisch-Herxheimer reaction occurs in *50% of patients with primary syphilis, 90% of those with secondary syphilis, and a lower proportion of persons with later stage disease.*
- Defervescence takes place within 12–24 h. In patients with secondary syphilis, erythema and edema of the mucocutaneous lesions may increase.

JARISCH-HERXHEIMER REACTION *reaction may occur after institution of chloramphenicol therapy for syphilis, brucellosis & typhoid fever" (G & G 11th/1181.)*

"Solely on the basis of experience with venereal syphilis, it is thought that *doxycycline or tetracycline* (at doses appropriate for syphilis) are alternatives for patients allergic to penicillin. A Jarisch-Herxheimer reaction may follow treatment of endemic treponematoses" *(Harrison 19th)*

"**Relapsing fever:** *Tetracycline or erythromycin;* antibiotic treatment may lead to Jarisch-Herxheimer reaction with fever, rigor, hypotension within 2 h of initiation"- *Harrison 19th/1147*

"**Whipples disease:** The occurrence of a Jarisch-Herxheimer *reaction within 24 h* of treatment initiation has been described, with rapid resolution. The addition of glucocorticoids may be beneficial in the management of clearly documented IRIS." *(Harrison 19th/1094)*

Leptospirosis: After Pn treatment, mild Jarisch-Herxheimer reaction may occur in some *(Anathanarayan 9th/384)*

Jarisch-Herxheimer Reaction

◈ *K. D. T 7th/720*

- Penicillin injected in a syphilitic patient (particularly secondary syphilis) may *produce shivering, fever, myalgia, exacerbation of lesions, even vascular collapse*
- This is due to sudden release of spirochetal lytic products & *lasts for 12-72 hours*
- It does not recur & does not need interruption of therapy
- Aspirin & sedation afford relief of symptoms

Managing Jarisch–Herxheimer Reaction

◈ *CMDT 2015/1460*

- The Jarisch–Herxheimer reaction, *manifested by fever and aggravation of the existing clinical picture* in *the hours following treatment,* is ascribed to the sudden massive destruction of spirochetes and is not an IgE-mediated allergic reaction. It is most common in *early syphilis, particularly secondary syphilis* where it can occur in 66% of cases.
- Patients should be reminded that the reaction does not signify an allergy to penicillin.

58. Ans. b. Amingl.... & e. Chlo....

[Ref: K. D. T 7th/692-93; Katzung 12th/792, 816]

Resistant Organism: Can Broadly Divided into 3 Types

◈ *K. D. T 7th/692-93*

- **Drug destroying:** The resistant microbe elaborate an enzyme which inactivates the the drug
  - β- lactamases are produced by staphylococci, hemophilus, gonococci etc which inactivate penicillin G
  - *Chloramphenicol* acetyl transferase is acquired by resistant E. coli, H. influenzae & S. typhi
  - Many of aminoglycosides-resistant coliforms have been found to produce enzymes which adenylate/acetylate/phosphorylate specific *aminoglycosides antibiotics*
- **Drug tolerant:** Loss of affinity of the target biomolecules of the microorganism for a particular AMA *e.g.* rifampicin, trimethoprim, fluoroquinolone
- **Drug imperable/drug efflux:** *e.g.,* some aminoglycosides, tetracyclins, chloroquine, erythromycin, fluoroquinolone etc.

"Enterococcal resistance to *vancomycin* is due to a plasmid mediated alteration of the dipeptide target site, reducing its affinity for vancomycin" *(K. D. T 7th/757)*

"*Fluoroquinolone*- mechanism of resistance: Resistance noted so far is due to chromosomal mutation producing a *DNA gyrase or topoisomerase IV* with reduced affinity for FQs, or due to reduced permeability/increased efflux of these drugs across bacterial membrane" *(K. D. T 7th/710)*

59. Ans. b. Increased. appetite & c. Hypersomnia.

[Ref: K. D. T 7th/406; Niraj Ahuja 7th/51]

Benzodiazepine Withdrawal

- *K. D. T 7th/406*
- Withdrawal symptom is generally mild; may be more intense in case of ultra rapid elimination drugs
- *Anxiety, insomnia, restlessness, malaise, loss of appetite, bad dreams* is all that occurs in most cases
- *Agitation, panic reaction, tremors & delirium* are occasional; convulsions are rare

- *Niraj Ahuja 7th/51*
- It is characterized by marked *anxiety, irritability, tremors, insomnia, vomiting, weakness, automatic hyperactivity with postural hypotension & seizures*
- Depression, transient psychotic episode, suicidal ideation, perceptual disturbances & rarely delirium have also been reported in withdrawal period

60. Ans. a. Tetra..., c. Ampic... & d. Acyc...

[Ref: K. D. T 7th/735, 721; Katzung 12th/794]

"*Ampicillin: It is partly excreted in bile & reabsorbed-enterohepatic circulation occurs. However, primary channel of excretion is kidney" (K. D. T 7th/722)*

"*Acyclovir: It is primarily excreted unchanged in urine, both by glomerular filtration & tubular secretion"- (K. D. T 7th/799)*

"*Most tetracyclines are primarily excreted in urine by glomerular filtration; dose has to be reduced in renal failure; doxycyline is an exception" (K. D. T 7th/735)*

"*Rifampicin: It is metabolized in liver to an active deacetylated metabolite which is excreted mainly in bile, some in urine. Urine & secretions may become orange-red" (KDT 7th/768)*

"Rifampin is well absorbed after oral administration and *excreted mainly through the liver into bile.* It then undergoes enterohepatic recirculation, with the bulk excreted as a deacylated metabolite in feces and a small amount in the urine. Dosage adjustment for renal or hepatic insufficiency is not necessary"- *(Katzung 12th/841)*

"Pyrazinamide is extensively metabolized in liver & excreted in urine" *(KDT 7th/769)*

"*Pyrazinamide metabolites are renally cleared" (Katzung 12th/843)*

"*Aminoglycosides (streptomycin & amikacin) are not metabolized in body & are excreted unchanged in urine" (KDT 7th/746)*

'Penicillin is rapidly excreted by the kidneys; small amounts are excreted by other routes. About 10% of renal excretion is by glomerular filtration and 90% by tubular secretion. *Nafcillin is primarily cleared by biliary excretion.* Oxacillin, dicloxacillin, and cloxacillin are eliminated by both the kidney and biliary excretion; no dosage adjustment is required for these drugs in renal failure" *(Katzung 12th/794)*

61. Ans. b. Inhibit viral DNA gyrase

[Ref: K. D. T 7th/799; Katzung 12th/862-64]

Acyclovir

- *K. D. T 7th/799*
- *This deoxiguanosine analogue antiviral drug requires a virus specific enzyme for conversion to the active metabolite that inhibit DNA synthesis & viral replication (inhibit viral DNA polymerase)*
- *It is active only against herpes group of viruses*
- *It primarily excreted unchanged in urine, both by glomerular filtration & tubular excretion*

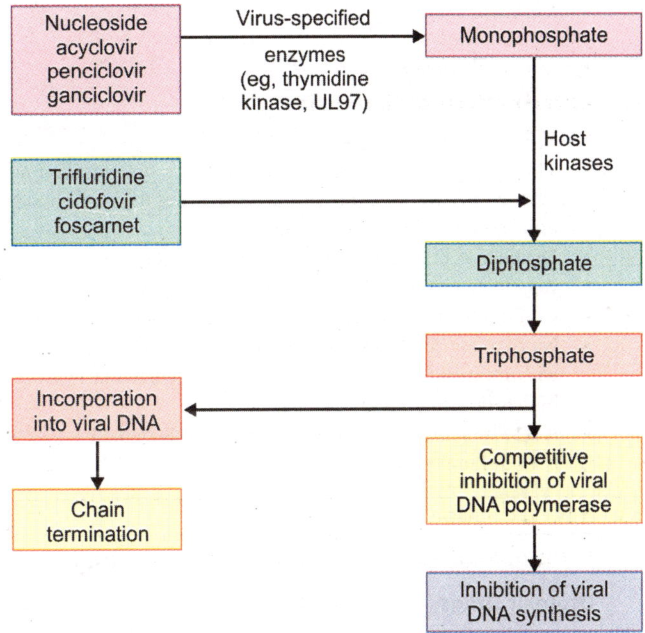

Fig: Mechanism of action of antiherpes agents

- *Katzung 12th/862-64*
- Acyclovir is an *acyclic guanosine derivative* with clinical activity against HSV-1, HSV-2, and VZV. In vitro activity against Epstein-Barr virus (EBV), cytomegalovirus (CMV), and human herpesvirus-6 (HHV-6) is present but comparatively weaker.
- Acyclovir *requires three phosphorylation steps for activation.* It is converted first to the monophosphate derivative by the virus-specified thymidine kinase and then to the di- and triphosphate compounds by host cell enzymes. Because it requires the viral kinase for initial phosphorylation, acyclovir is selectively activated, and the active metabolite accumulates, only in infected cells.

- Acyclovir triphosphate inhibits viral DNA synthesis by two mechanisms: competition with deoxy GTP for the *viral DNA polymerase*, resulting in binding to the DNA template as an irreversible complex; and chain *termination following incorporation into the viral DNA.*
- *Acyclovir is cleared primarily by glomerular filtration and tubular secretion.* The half-life is approximately 3 hours in patients with normal renal function and 20 hours in patients with anuria.

62. Ans. a. Ichthyosis, c. Skin pigmentation & d. Gastro-intestinal...

[Ref: K. D. T 7th/782; Katzung 12th/846; G & G 11th/1220; Neena Khanna 4th/268]

Side effects of Clofazimine

◈ *Neena Khanna 4th/268*

- *Ichthyosis*
- *Pigmentation*
- *Gastrointestinal side effects*

Adverse effects of Clofazimine

◈ *K. D. T 7th/782*

- The major disadvantage is *reddish-black discoloration of skin,* especially on exposed parts. Discoloration of hair & body secretions may also occur
- Dryness of skin & itching is often troublesome
- Acneform eruptions & phototoxicity have been noted
- Conjunctival pigmentation may create cosmetic problem
- Nausea, anorexia, abdominal pain, weight loss & enteritis with intermittent loose stools can occur, particularly when higher doses are used
- It is to be avoided during early pregnancy & in patients with liver or kidney damage

63. Ans. a. Cisplatin

[Ref: P. L. Dhingra 6th/33-34; K. D. T 7th/861; Katzung 12th/956]

Ototoxic Drugs

◈ *P. L. Dhingra 6th/33-34*

- Various drugs & chemical can damage the inner ear & cause sensorineural hearing loss, tinnitus & sometimes vertigo
- Cytotoxic drugs causing hearing loss are- nitrogen mustard (mechlorethamine), cisplatin & carboplatin

"***Cisplatin:*** Important toxicities are- renal impairment & emetogenic potential. Tinnitus, *deafness,* sensory neuropathy & hyperuricaemia are other problem" *(K. D. T 7th/861)*

"***Carboplatin:*** *Nephrotoxicity, ototoxicity & neurotoxicity are low as compared to cisplatin" (K. D. T 7th/861)*

Table *(Dhingra)*: **Ototoxic drugs**

A. Aminoglycoside antibiotics
Streptomycin
Dihydrostreptomycin
Gentamicin
Tobramycin
Neomycin
Kanamycin
Amikacin
Netilmycin
Sisomycin
B. Diuretics
Furosemide
Ethacrynic acid
Bumetanide
C. Antimalarials
Quinine
Chloroquine
Hydroxychloroquine
D. Cytotoxic drugs
Nitrogen mustard (Mechlorethamine)
Cisplatin
Carboplatin
E. Analgesics
Salicylates
Indomethacin
Phenylbutazone
Ibuprofen
F. Chemicals
Alcohol
Tobacco
Marijuana
Carbon monoxide
Poisoning
G. Miscellaneous
Erythromycin
Ampicillin
Propranolol
Propylthiouracil
Deferoxamine

64. Ans. a. Weight gain, b. Agranulocytosis & c. Sedation

[Ref: K. D. T 7th/441; Katzung 12th/509]

Haloperidol

◈ *K. D. T 7th/441*
- *It produces few autonomic effects, is less epileptogenic, does not cause weight gain, jaundice is rare*
- *Severe extrapyramidal syndrome- Katzung 12th/509*
- *It is preferred drug for acute schizophrenia*

Clozapine

◈ *K. D. T 7th/441*
- It *produces few or no extrapyramidal symptoms*; tardive dyskinesia is rare & prolactin level does not rise
- It is *quite sedative sedating*, moderately potent anticholinergic, but paradoxically induces hyperventilation
- Its major limitation is *higher incidence of agranulocytosis* (0. 8%) & other blood dyscrasias; weekly monitoring of leucocyte count is required
- Metabolic complication like weight gain, hyperlipidemia & precipitation of diabetes is *another major limitation*
- *High dose can induce seizures even in non-epileptics*
- Other side-effects are sedation, unstable B. P, tachycardia & urinary incontinence
- Few cases of myocarditis have been reported which start like flu but may progress to death

65. Ans. a. Old age

[Ref: Niraj Ahuja 7th/188; G & G 11th/784; Kaplan & Sadock's 11th/10120; Katzung 13th/524-26]

Note: *I could only get old age in spite of exhaustive searching (at least searching of 10 books). Please search for other options.*

"Cases of SSRI-associated hyponatremia *& the syndrome of inappropriate antidiuretic hormone have been seen in some patients, especially those who are older or treated with diuretics*"- *Kaplan & Sadock's 11th/10120*

Syndrome of Inappropriate Secretion of Antidiuretic Hormone (SIADH)

◈ *G & G 11Th/507*
- SIADH is a disease of impaired water excretion with accompanying hyponatremia and hypoosmolality caused by the inappropriate secretion of vasopressin. The clinical manifestations of plasma hypotonicity resulting from SIADH may include lethargy, anorexia, nausea and vomiting, muscle cramps, coma, convulsions, and death.
- A multitude of disorders can induce SIADH, including malignancies, pulmonary diseases, CNS injuries/diseases (*e.g.*, head trauma, infections, and tumors), and general surgery. The three drug classes most commonly implicated in drug induced SIADH include psychotropic medications *(e.g., fluoxetine, haloperidol, and tricyclic antidepressants)*, sulfonylureas (*e.g.*, chloropropamide), and vinca alkaloids *(e.g., vincristine and vinblastine)*.

Table *(Niraj Ahuja 7th/188)*: **Side effect of antidepressant drug**

S/E	Probable cause	Maximum with	Minimum with	Management
Hyponatremia	Probably SIADH	SSRIs; SNRIs	Not known, Probably MAOIs	***Risk higher in elderly***; avoid co-prescribing other drugs that cause hyponatremia (such as diuretics); monitor closely

66. Ans. a. Diabetes..., c. Haemophilia A & d. Von...

[Ref: K. D. T 7th/596-97, 616; Katzung 12th/616, 674, 677; G & G 11th/784-86]

Desmopressin

◈ *K. D. T 7th/596-97*
- This is selective V2 agonist
- Use- *diabetes insipidus, bedwetting in children & nocturia in adults, renal concentration test, Haemophilia & Von Willebrand disease*

"Bleeding esophageal varices: *drug used are vasopressin & terlipressin (both by its action through V1 receptor), octreotide*"- *(K. D. T 7th/597)*

◈ *G & G 11th/784-86*
- The V2-selective agonist, 1-deamino-8-D-arginine vasopressin, also called *desmopressin* (DDAVP), has ~3000 times greater antidiuretic - to - vasopressor ratio than vasopressin and is the preferred drug for the treatment of central diabetes insipidus.
- Central DI can be distinguished from nephrogenic DI by administration of desmopressin, which will increase urine osmolality in patients with central DI but have little or no effect in patients with nephrogenic DI.
- Antidiuretic peptides are the primary treatment for central DI, with *desmopressin being the preferred peptide.*
- V2 receptor agonists (*e.g.*, desmopressin) are *also used in bleeding disorders.*
- In most patients with type I von Willebrand's disease (vWD) and in some with type IIn vWD, desmopressin will elevate von Willebrand factor and shorten bleeding time.
- Desmopressin also increases factor VIII levels in patients with mild-to-moderate *hemophilia A.*
- Desmopressin is not indicated in *patients with severe hemophilia A, those with hemophilia B, or those with factor VIII antibodies.*
- Another V2 receptor-mediated application is the use of desmopressin fsor *primary nocturnal enuresis.*
- Desmopressin also relieves *post–lumbar puncture headache*, probably by causing water retention and thereby facilitating rapid fluid equilibration in the CNS.

Clinical application of Desmopressin

◈ *Katzung 12th/677*
- *Pituitary diabetes insipidus*
- *Peditric primary nocturnal enuresis*
- *Haemophilia A*
- *Von Willebrand disease*

67. Ans. b. Amino..., c. Carb..., d. Retinoic acid & e. Phenytoin

[Ref: K. D. T 7th/89, 831; Katzung 10th/975; Katzung 12th/1042-43; G & G 11th/; Drug in Pregnancy & Lactation by G. Briggs 6th/339]

"Quinine continues to be the drug of choice for severe falciparum during 1st trimester of pregnancy, because safety of artemisinins is not yet proven" (K. D. T 7th/831)

"Artesunate: Use is limited in second & third trimesters of pregnancy only when other drugs are found resistant" (Dutta Obs 8th/345; Katzung 13th/892 (Embryopathic effect proven only in animal studies, not in human)

"Avoid aminoglycosides during pregnancy: Risk of foetal ototoxicity" (K. D. T 7th/89)

"A recent report indicates 2. 7 fold higher malformation rate in fetuses exposed to ACE inhibitors in first trimester. ACE inhibitors must be stopped when women conceives"-(K. D. T 7th/89)

"Prophylactic folic acid administration is given during pregnancy to reduce the risk of neural tube defect" *(KDT 6th/592)*

Drugs	Congenital malformation
• *Penicillamine*[Q]	• *Cutis laxa*[Q]
• *Warfarin (Oral anticoagulants)*[Q]	• *Contradi syndrome*[Q] *(Chondrodysplasia punctata)*
• *Chlorambucil*	• *Genitourinary anomaly*[Q] *(Renal agenesis)*
• *Valproic acid*[Q]	• *Neural tube defect*[Q]
• *Carbamezapine*	• *Cleft lip and palate, Cardiac defect*[Q]
• *Corticosteroid*[Q]	• *Congenital heart disease, cleft lip and palate*[Q]
• *Barbiturates*	• *Respiratory depression*
• *Carbimazole*	• *Fetal Aplasia Cutis*[Q]
• *Lithium*[Q]	• *Ebstein anomaly, fetal goiter.*
• *DES*	• *Vaginal adenosis*[Q] *(Clear cell Ca)*
• *Thalidomide*[Q]	• *Phocomelia*[Q]
• *Chloramphenicol*	• *Grey baby syndrome*[Q]
• *Androgens*	• *Virilization; Limb, oesophagus and cardiac defects*
• *Isotretinoin*	• *Craniofacial defect, Heart anomaly, Abortion*
• *Indomethacin*	• *Premature closure of DA*
• *Tamoxifen*[Q]	• *Risk of Abortion and Fetal damage*
• *Cyclophosphamide*[Q]	• ***Multiple abnormalties***[Q] *(Drug in Pregnancy & Lactation by G. Briggs 6th/339)*

Table: Some drugs reported to have adverse effects on human fetal development

Agent	Effect (s)	Teratogenicity
Retinoids	Hydrocephalus etc.	K (known teratogen)

Table *(Katzung 12th/1042-43)*: **Drugs with significant adverse effects on the fetus (Partial list)**

Drug	Trimester	Effect
ACE inhibitors	All, especially second and third	Renal damage

Contd...

Drug	Trimester	Effect
Carbamazepine	First	Neural tube defects
Chlorpropamide	All	Prolonged symptomatic neonatal hypoglycemia
Cyclophosphamide	First	Various congenital malformations
Cytarabine	First, second	Various congenital malformations
Diazepam	All	Chronic use may lead to neonatal dependence
Isotretinoin	All	Extremely high risk of CNS, face, ear, and other malformations
Lithium	First	Ebstein's anomaly
Methotrexate	First	Multiple congenital malformations
Methylthiouracil	All	Hypothyroidism
Metronidazole	First	May be mutagenic (from animal studies; there is no evidence for mutagenic or teratogenic effects in humans)
Phenytoin	All	Fetal hydantoin syndrome
Propylthiouracil	All	Congenital goiter
Streptomycin	All	Eighth nerve toxicity
Tamoxifen	All	Increased risk of spontaneous abortion or fetal damage
Tetracycline	All	Discoloration and defects of teeth and altered bone growth
Thalidomide	First	Phocomelia (shortened or absent long bones of the limbs) and many internal malformations
Trimethadione	All	Multiple congenital anomalies
Valproic acid	All	Neural tube defects, cardiac and limb malformations
Warfarin	First	Hypoplastic nasal bridge, chondrodysplasia
	Second	CNS malformations
	Third	Risk of bleeding. Discontinue use 1 month before delivery.

68. **Ans. d. More potent & e. Gluco…**

[Ref: K. D. T 7th/289; Katzung 12th/700, 703, 712]

Triamcinolone

- *K. D. T 7th/289*
- *Slightly more potent than prednisolone but highly selective glucocorticoid; 4-32 mg/day oral; 5-40 mg i. m, intraarticular injection*
- *Also used topically*

Table *(K. D. T 7th/289)*: **Relative activities of systemic corticosteroids**

Compound	Glucocorticoid activity	Mineralocorticoid activity	Equivalent dose (anti-inflammatory)
Hydrocortisone	1	1	20 mg
Triamcinolone	5	0	4 mg

Table *(Katzung 12th/703)*: **Some commonly used natural and synthetic corticosteroids for general use**

Agent	Activity[1]			Equivalent Oral Dose (mg)	Forms available
	Anti-Inflammatory	Topical	Salt-retaining		
Short-to-medium acting glucocorticoids					
Hydrocotisone	1	1	1	20	Oral, injectable, topical
Cortisone	0. 8	0	0. 8	25	Oral
Prednisone	4	0	0.3	5	Oral
Prednisolone	5	4	0.3	5	Oral, injectable
Methylprednisolone	5	5	0	4	Oral, injectable
Meprednisone[2]	5		0	4	Oral, injectable
Intermediate-acting glucocorticoids					
Triamcinolone	5	5[3]	0	4	Oral, injectable, topical
Paramethasone[2]	10		0	2	Oral, injectable
Fluprednisolone[2]	15	7	0	1. 5	Oral
Long-acting glucocorticoids					
Betamethasone	25-40	10	0	0. 6	Oral, injectable, topical
Dexamethasone	30	10	0	0. 75	Oral, injectable, topical
Mineralocorticoids					
Fludrocortisone	10	0	250	2	Oral
Desoxycorticosterone acetate	0	0	20		Injectable, pellets

[1] Potency relative to hydrocortisone

MICROBIOLOGY

69. **Ans. a. Cystic fibrosis & c. Chron….**

[Ref: Ananthanarayan 9th/316; Medical microbiology by Greenwood 16th/286-88; Jawetz Microbiology 27th/248-49]

"Burkholderia cepacia is increasingly being recognized as an opportunist environmental pathogen, particularly in those with cystic fibrosis or chronic granulomatous disease, in whom it causes fatal necrotizing pneumonia" (Ananthanarayan 9th/316; Greenwood 16th/286-88)

"Myeloperoxidase deficiency: Patients are particularly liable to Candida albicans" (Ananthanarayan 9th/175)

Burkholderia Cepacia

- *Jawetz 27th/248-49*
- *Burkholderia cepacia* is an environmental organism that is able to grow in water, soil, plants, animals, and decaying vegetable materials.

- In hospitals, *B cepacia* has been isolated from a wide variety of water and environmental sources from which it can be transmitted to patients.
- *Patients with cystic fibrosis are vulnerable to B cepacia infection*. They may have asymptomatic carriage, progressive deterioration over a period of months, and rapidly progressive deterioration with necrotizing pneumonia and bacteremia. Although a relative small percentage of cystic fibrosis patients become infected, the association with progressive disease makes *B cepacia* a major concern for these patients.
- It is likely that *B cepacia* can be transmitted from one cystic fibrosis patient to another by close contact.
- *B cepacia* grows on most media used in culturing patients' specimens for gram-negative bacteria. Selective media containing colistin also can be used. *B cepacia* grows more slowly than enteric gram-negative rods, and it may take 3 days before colonies are visible.

70. Ans. b. 4...., c. Uter.... & e. Egg....

[Ref: Paniker's Parasitology 7th/121; Medical microbiology by Greenwood 16th/610-11]

Both T. saginata & T. solium contains 4 suckers in head (scolex) but it may be pigmented in former & not pigmented in later (Panikar 7th/120-21)

Table (*Panikar 7th/121*): **Difference between Taenia saginata and Taenia solium**

	Taenia saginata	Taenia solium
Length	5-10 m	2-3 m
Scolex	Large quadrate	Small and globular
	Rostellum and hooks are absent	Rostellum and hooks are present
	Suckers may be pigmented	Suckers not pigmented
Neck	Long	Short
Proglottids	1, 000-2, 000	Below 1, 000
Measurement (gravid segment)	20 mm × 5 mm	12 mm × 6 mm
Expulsion	Expelled singly	Expelled passively in chains of 5 or 6
Uterus	Lateral branches15-30 on each side; thin and dichotomous	Lateral branches 5-10 on each side; thick and dendritic
Vagina	Present	Absent
Accessary lobe of ovary	Absent	Present
Testes	300-400 follicles	150-200 follicles
Larva	Cysticercus bovis; present in cow not in man	Cysticercus cellulosae; present in pig and also in man
Egg	Not infective to man	Infective to man

71. Ans. a. α -toxin .... c. Low .... & d. Devitalized tissue...

[Ref: Ananthanarayan 9th/257-59; Harrison 19th/990-94; Greenwood 16th/231

Clostridium intestinale cause bacteremia (*http://www. ncbi. nlm. nih. gov/pmc/articles/PMC1081394/)*

Gas Gangrene

◈ *Greenwood 16th/232-33*

- The presence of devitalized or dead tissue, blood clot, extravasated fluid, foreign bodies & co-incident pyogenic infection are all that promote the occurrence of gas gangrene in a wound
- Predisposing host factors include debility, old age & diabetes
- When clostridial infection has been initiated in a focus of devitalized anaerobic tissue, the organism multiply rapidly & produce a range of toxins & aggression. These damage tissue by various necrotizing effects. They spread into adjacent viable tissue, particularly muscle, kill it & render it anaerobic & vulnerable to further colonization, with production of more toxins & aggressins
- *α -toxin is generally considered to be the main cause of the toxaemia associated with gas gangrene*

"α -toxin: *This is the most important toxin biologically & is responsible for profound toxaemia of gas gangrene"* (Ananthanarayan 9th/254)

◈ *Ananthanarayan 9th/257*

- Gas *gangrene results only if the condition favourable for clostridium multiplication exist in wound*
- *The most important of these is low oxygen tension*
- *The ionized calcium salts & silicic acid in soil cause necrosis*
- *Crushing tissue or tearing of arteries produce anoxia of muscle*
- *The Eh & pH of the damaged tissue fall & these change along with the chemical change that occur in damaged & anoxic muscle, provide ideal pabulum for the proliferation of anaerobes*
- *Clostridium multiply & elaborate toxins which cause further damage. These include- lecithinase, collagenase, α -toxin etc*

Gas Gangrene (Clostridial Myonecrosis)

- Gas gangrene is characterized by *rapid and extensive necrosis of muscle*[Q] accompanied by gas formation and systemic toxicity and occurs when bacteria invade healthy muscle from adjacent traumatized muscle or soft tissue
- The incubation period of gas gangrene is usually short: almost always <3 days [Q] and frequently <24 h. *Some 80% of cases are caused by C. perfringens, while C. novyi, C. septicum, and C. histolyticum cause most of the remaining cases*
- An essential factor in the genesis of gas gangrene appears to be *trauma*[Q], particularly involving deep muscle laceration. The entity of clostridial myonecrosis is relatively uncommon after simple, through-and-through bullet wounds without shattering of bone and is relatively common after shrapnel fragmentation wounds, particularly when deep muscle is involved
- Cl. Perferingens has *at least 17 possible virulence factors including 12 active tissue toxin and enterotoxin*[Q].

- The α-toxin is a phospholipase C (lecithinase) that splits lecithin into phosphorylcholine and diglyceride. It has been associated with *gas gangrene and is known to be hemolytic*[Q] to destroy platelets and polymorphonuclear leukocytes (PMNs), and to cause widespread capillary damage. When injected IV, it causes massive intravascular hemolysis and damages liver mitochondria.
- The α *toxin* may be important in the initiation of muscle infections that can progress to gas gangrene.

The Gas Gangrene

◈ *Ananthanarayan 8th/256*

- *Established pathogen: Cl. perfringens, Cl. septicum, Cl. novyi*
- *Less pathogenic: Cl. histolyticum, Cl. fallax*
- *Doubtful pathogen: Cl bifermentans, Cl sporogenes*

72. Ans. b. Interfe..., d. Inhibi.... & e. Acton...

[Ref: K. D. T 7th/99-100, 121; Ananthanarayan 9th/264]

Muscuranic receptors are also present in CNS (*K. D. T 7th/100*)

Botulinum Toxin

◈ *K. D. T 7th/99-100, 121*

- *"Two toxins interfere with cholinergic transmission* by affecting release: *botulinum toxin inhibit release, while black widow spider toxin induces massive release & depletion"- K. D. T 7th/99*
- *A localized injection can be used in treatment of a number of spastic & other neurological conditions due to overactivity of cholinergic nerves like blepharospasm, spastic cerebral palsy, strabismus, spasmodic torticollis, nystagmus, hemifacial spasm, poststroke spasticity, spasmodic dysphonia, axillary hyperhydrosis etc*
- However its incorrect injection or overdose can be dangerous

◈ *Ananthanarayan 9th/264*

- It acts by *blocking the production or release of acetylcholine* at the synapses & neuromuscular junctions
- Onset is marked by diplopia, dysphagia & dysarthria due to *cranial nerve involvement*
- A *symmetric descending paralysis* is the characteristic pattern, ending in death by respiratory paralysis

73. Ans. a. HIV-2...., d. More....... & e. Mode....

[Ref: Ananthanarayan 9th/573, 194-95; Harrison 19th/1216, 1222; Greenwood 16th/527]

HIV 2

◈ *Ananthanarayan 9th/573*

- HIV strains first isolated from *West Africa in 1986*, which react with HIV type 1 antiserum very weakly or not at all have been termed HIV type 2
- *HIV 2 has only 40% genetic identity with HIV 1.*
- *It is more closely related to simian immunodeficiency virus than to HIV 1*
- It is much *less virulent than HIV 1*
- It is largely confined to West Africa, through isolations have been reported from some other areas, including western & southern India
- *HIV-2 is transmitted by same routes as HIV-1- Greenwood 16th/535*
- Line immune assays (LIAs): These assays allow for application of antigens from more than one virus, thereby allowing them to act as combination assays & to differentiate infection by HIV 1 & HIV 2- *Ananthanarayan 9th/580*

The Blood Banks who intend to supply the blood units/components shall test the following mandatory tests before supplying to Blood Storage Centres. (http://cdsco. nic. in/html/guideline. html)

- Blood Grouping
- Anti Body Testing
- *Hemoglobin Content*
- *HIV I & II Antibodies*
- *Hepatitis B Surface antigen*
- *Hepatitis C Antibody*
- *Malarial Parasite*
- *Syphillis or VDRL*

◈ *Harrison 19th/1216, 1222*

- *HIV-2 was first identified in 1986 in West African patients and was originally confined to West Africa.*
- HIV-1 viruses likely came from chimpanzees and/or gorillas, and HIV-2 from sooty mangabeys.
- *The screening of blood donations for antibodies to HIV-1 and HIV-2* are done to reduce chance of infection.

74. Ans. b. Oral..., c. Candidiasis

[Ref: Park 23rd/349; Ananthanarayan 9th/575; Harrison 19th/1215-16, 1257]

Note: As Q do not specifically mentioned CDC or WHO criteria for staging, so we would decide answer on applying both criteria

Option	Stage 3 criteria	Why included/excluded from answer
A	>1 month duration (WHO)	As in option duration is not mentioned, so it is excluded from answer
B	Oral hairy leukoplakia (WHO)	So, Included in answer
C	Candidiasis (WHO & CDC)	So, Included in answer
D	Chronic diarrhea > 1 month (WHO)	As in option duration is – 20 days, so excluded from the answer
E	CD4 count <14% in adult (CDC)	So excluded from the answer

HIV Stages

◈ *Harrison 19th/1215-16*

- The current U. S. CDC classification system for HIV infection and AIDS categorizes people on the basis of clinical conditions associated with HIV infection and CD4+ T lymphocyte measurement.

- A confirmed HIV case can be *classified in one of five HIV infection stages (0, 1, 2, 3, or unknown).*
- If there was a negative HIV test within 6 months of the first HIV infection diagnosis, the stage is 0, and remains 0 until 6 months after diagnosis.
- *Advanced HIV disease (AIDS) is classified as stage 3* if one or more specific opportunistic illness has been diagnosed. Otherwise, the stage is determined by CD4 test results and immunologic criteria
- If none of these criteria apply (*e.g.,* because of missing information on CD4 test results), the stage is U (unknown).
- The definition and staging criteria of AIDS are complex and comprehensive and were *established for surveillance purposes* rather than for the practical care of patients. Thus, the clinician should not focus on whether the patient fulfills the strict definition of AIDS, but should view HIV disease as a spectrum ranging from primary infection, with or without the acute syndrome, to the asymptomatic stage, to advanced stages associated with opportunistic diseases.

Table *(Harrison 19th/1215)*: **CDC stage 3 (AIDS)- defining Opportunistic illness in HIV infection**

- Bacterial infections, multiple or recurrent[a]
- ***Candidiasis*** of bronchi, trachea, or lungs
- ***Candidiasis*** of esophagus
- Cervical cancer, invasive[b]
- Coccidioidomycosis, disseminated or extrapulmonary
- Cryptococcosis, extrapulmonary ***Cryptosporidiosis, chronic intestinal (>1 month's duration)***
- Cytomegalovirus disease (other than liver, spleen, or nodes), onset at age >1 month
- Cytomegalovirus retinitis (with loss of vision)
- Encephalopathy attributed to HIV
- **Herpes simplex:** chronic ulcers (>1 month's duration) or bronchitis, pneumonitis, or esophagitis (onset at age >1 month)
- Histoplasmosis, disseminated or extrapulmonary
- Isosporiasis, chronic intestinal ***(>1 month's duration)***
- Kaposi's sarcoma
- Lymphoma, Burkitt's (or equivalent term)
- Lymphoma, immunoblastic (or equivalent term)
- Lymphoma, primary, of brain
- *Mycobacterium avium* complex or *Mycobacterium kansasii*, disseminated or extrapulmonary
- *Mycobacterium tuberculosis* of any site, pulmonary, disseminated, or extrapulmonary
- Mycobacterium, other species or unidentified species, disseminated or extrapulmonary
- *Pneumocystis jirovecii* (previously known as *Pneumocystis carinii*) pneumonia
- Pneumonia, recurrent*b*
- Progressive multifocal leukoencephalopathy
- *Salmonella* septicemia, recurrent
- Toxoplasmosis of brain, onset at age >1 month
- Wasting syndrome attributed to HIV*a*
- Only among children age <6 years.
- Only among adults, adolescents, and children age ≥6 years.

"Fungal infections may also be a cause of *diarrhea* in patients with HIV infection. *Histoplasmosis, coccidioidomycosis, and penicilliosis* have all been identified as a cause of fever and diarrhea in patients with HIV infection. Cryptosporidia, microsporidia, and *Isospora belli* are the most common opportunistic protozoa that infect the GI tract and cause diarrhea in HIV-infected patients"- *Harrison 19th/1257*

WHO Clinical Staging system for HIV infection and HIV related disease

Park 23rd/349

- WHO has developed a clinical staging system based on clinical criteria
- Clinical condition or performance score, which is the higher, determines whether a patient is at clinical stage 1, 2, 3 or 4
- Clinical stage is important as a criteria for starting antiretroviral therapy (ART)

Table: *(Harrison 19th/1216): CDC HIV Infection Stages 1-3 bases on Age-Specific CD4+ T Lymphocyte count or CD4+ T Lymphocyte percentage of total lymphocytesa*

	Age on Date of CD4T+ Lymphocyte Test					
	<1 year		1-5 Years		6 Years Through Adult	
Stage[a]	Cells/µL	%	Cells/µL	%	Cells/µL	%
1	>1, 500	>34	>1, 000	>300	>500	>26
2	70-1, 499	26-33	500-999	22-29	200-499	14-25
3	<750	<26	<500	<22	<200	<14

[a]*The stage is bases primarily on the CD4+ T-Lymphocyte count; the CD4+ T-lymphocyte count takes precedence over the CD4 T-lymphocyte percentage, and the percentage is considered only if the count is missing.*

Table *(Park 23rd/349)*: **WHO Clinical staging of HIV disease**

Clinical stage 1
Asymptomatic
Persistent generalized lymphadenopathy
Clinical stage 2
Moderate unexplained weight loss (under 10% of presumed or measured body weight)
Recurrent respiratory tract infections (sinusitis, tonsillitis, otitis media, pharyngitis)
Herpes zoster
Angular cheilitis
Recurrent oral ulcerations
Papular pruritic eruptions
Seborrhoeic dermatitis
Fungal nail infections
Clinical stage 3
Unexplained severe weight loss (over 10% of presumed or measured body weight)
Unexplained chronic diarrhea for longer than 1 month
Unexplained persistent fever (intermittent or constant for longer than 1 month)
Persistent oral candidiasis
Oral hairy leukoplakia
Pulmonary tuberculosis
Severe bacterial infections (*e.g.*, pneumonia. Empyema, meningitis, pyomyositis, bone or joint infection bacteraemia, servere pelvic inflammatory disease)
Acute necrotizing ulcerative stomatitis, gingivitis or periodontitis
Unexplained anaemia (below 8 g/dl), neutropenia (below 0. 5 × 10^9/1) and/or chronic thrombocytopenia (below 50 × 10^9/1)
Clinical stage 4
HIV wasting syndrome
Pneumocystis jiroveci pneumonia
Recurrent severe bacterial pneumonia
Chronic herpes simplex infection (orolabial, genital or anorectal of more than 1 month's duration or visceral at any site)
Oesophageal candidiasis (or candidiasis of trachea, bronchi or lungs)
Extrapulmonary tuberculosis
Kaposi sarcoma
Cytomegalovirus disease (retinitis or infection of other organs, excluding liver, spleen and lymph nodes)
Central nervous system toxoplasmosis
HIV encephalopathy
Extrapulmonary cryptococcosis including meningitis
Disseminated non-tuberculous mycobacteria infection
Progressive multifocal leukoencephalopathy
Candida of the trachea, bronchi, or lungs
Chronic cryptosporidiosis (with diarrhea)
Chronic isosporiasis
Disseminated mycosis (*e.g.*, histoplasmosis, coccidioidomycosis, penicilliosis)
Recurrent nontyphoidal Salmonella bacteremia
Lymphoma (cerebral or B-cell non-Hodgkin)
Invasive cervical carcinoma
Reactivation of American trypanosomiasis (meningoencephalitis or myocarditis)

Contd...

75. Ans. a. Sulphu..., c. Petechi....& d. Cor....

[Ref: Ananthanarayan 9th/392; Harrison 19th/979; Greenwood 16th/189-90]

*"Isolation in culture: **Sulphur granules** or pus containing **actinomycetes** are washed & inoculated" (Ananthanarayan 9th/392)*

***"Petechial lesion: Meningococci** may sometimes be demonstrated in petechial lesions by microscopy & culture" (Ananthanarayan 9th/230)*

"Throat samples should be submitted to the laboratory for culture with the notation that diphtheria is being considered. This information should prompt cultivation on special selective medium and subsequent biochemical testing to differentiate C. diphtheriae from other nasopharyngeal commensal corynebacteria." *(Harrison 19th/979)*

*"The **diphtheria bacilli within the membrane** continue to produce toxin actively" (Park 23rd/161)*

*"**Rheumatic valvulitis** is manifestation of rheumatic heart disease. Rheumatic fever is an acute, **immunologically mediated, multisystem inflammatory disease** classically occurring a few week after an episode of group A streptococcal infection" (Robbins 9th/557-59)*

"Acute rheumatic fever: *This occur after 1-3 week after acute infection of S. pyogenes so that organism may not be detectable when sequelae set in. Essential lesion is characterized by Aschoff nodules" (Ananthanarayan 9th/214)*

76. Ans. d. Typically....

[Ref: Ananthanarayan 9th/331; Robbins 9th/370; Harrison 19th/1012-13; Greenwood 16th/309]

Haemophilus Ducreyi

◈ *Ananthanarayan 9th/331*

- *Chancroid or soft sore is characterized by tender non-indurated irregular ulcers on the genitalia*
- *The infection remains localized, spreading only to the regional lymph nodes which are enlarged & painful*
- *"**Haemophilus ducreyi:*** After an incubation period of 4-7 days, the initial lesion—a papule with surrounding erythema—appears. In 2 or 3 days, the papule evolves into a pustule, which spontaneously ruptures and forms a sharply circumscribed ulcer that is generally *not indurated.* The *ulcers are painful and bleed easily;* little or no inflammation of the surrounding skin is evident. Approximately half of patients develop enlarged, *tender inguinal lymph nodes,* which frequently become fluctuant and spontaneously rupture" *(Harrison 18th)*

Table *(Harrison19th/880)*: **Clinical Features of Genital Ulcers**

Feature	Syphillis	Herpes	Chancroid	Lymphogranuloma Venereum	Donovanosis
Incubation period	9–90 days	2–7 days	1– 14 days	3 days–6weeks	1–4 weeks (up to 6 months)
Early primary lesions	Papule	Vesicle	Pustule	Papule, pustule, or vesicle	Papule
No. of lesions	Usually one	Multiple	Usually multiple, may coalesce	Usually one; often not detected, despite lymphadenopathy	Variable
Diameter	5–15 mm	1–2 mm	Variable	2–10 mm	Variable
Edges	Sharply demarcated, elevated, round, or oval	Erythematous	Undermined, ragged, irregular	Elevated, round, or oval	Elevated, irregular
Depth	Superficial or deep	Superficial	Excavated	Superficial or deep	Elevated
Base	Smooth, nonpurulent, relatively nonvascular	Serous, erythematous, nonvascular	Purulent, bleeds easily	Variable, nonvascular	Red and velvety, bleeds readily
Induration	Firm	None	Soft	Occasionally firm	Firm
Pain	**Uncommon**	**Frequently tender**	**Usually very tender**	**Variable**	**Uncommon**
Lymphadenopathy	Firm, nontender, bilateral	Firm, tender, often bilateral with initial episode	Tender, may suppurate, loculated, usually unilateral	Tender, may suppurate, loculated, usually unilateral	None; pseudobuboes

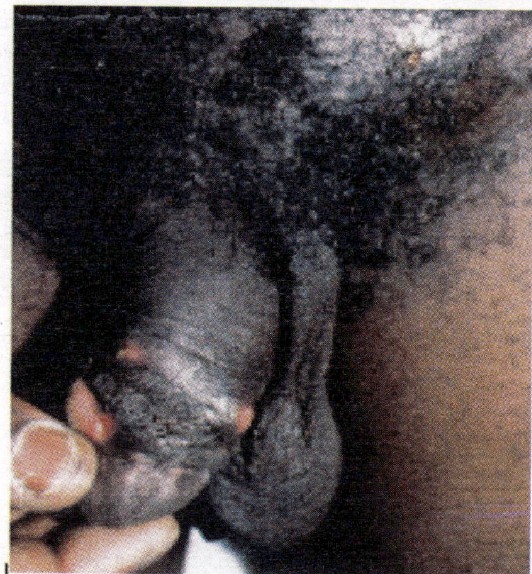

Fig: Chancroid with characteristic penile ulcers and associated left inguinal adenitis (bubo)

77. Ans. a. Seasonal spread., c. Tetracycline.......& e. All....

[Ref: Ananthanarayan 9th/321-24; Park 23rd/292-97; Harrison 19th/1070-75; Greenwood 16th/329-32]

Plague

- *Ananthanarayan 9th/321-24*
- *Epidemic generally occur in cool, humid seasons that favour the multiplication of fleas, leading to higher flea index*
- *Fleas do not thrive in hot, dry weather & the transmission of infection is interrupted*
- Two *types of vaccine* have been in use- *Killed vaccine (prepared at the Haffkine Institute, Mumbai) & live vaccine (it is no longer recommended)*
- *Streptomycin, doxycycline & chloramphenicol are effective*
- *Park 23rd/292-97)*
- Outbreaks of plague are *usually seasonal in nature.* In northern India, the plague season starts from September until may. The disease tends to die out with the onset of hot weather.
- On the contrary, in south India, there was no definite plague season
- Temperature & humidity: A mean temperature of 20 to 25 deg. C, & a relative humidity of 60% & above are considered favourable for spread of plague
- Agent: Y. pestis- *a gram negative, non-motile, cocco-bacillus* that exhibit bipolar staining with special stains (e. g Wayson'd stain)
- Source of infection: Infected rodents & fleas & case of pneumonic plague

- Age & sex: *All ages & both sexes are susceptible*
- Commonest & most efficient vector is- the rat flea, X. cheopis
- There are 3 main clinical forms: Bubonic, pneumonic & septicaemic plague
- Immunization is a valuable preventive measure
- **Chemoprophylaxis:** The drug of choice is tetracycline. A cheaper alternative is sulfonamide
- Treatment: The drug of choice is streptomycin. Tetracycline is an alternative drug. Other drugs used are- gentamycin, sulfonamide etc

78. Ans. a. Polio virus, b. Coxasa.... & c. Rhinovirus

[Ref: Ananthanarayan 9th/484-85, 440; Harrison 19th/1289-95; Jawetz 27th/514]

Rheovirus belongs to reoviridae family (*Ananthanarayan 9th/441*)

Corona virus *belongs to coronaviridae* (*Ananthanarayan 9th/441*)

"The family picornaviridae *contains 4 genera of medical importance- enterovirus (polio, coxsackie A & B, echovirus, entrovirus 68-71), rhinovirus, hepatovirus (Hepatitis A) & parechovirus"* (*Ananthanarayan 9th/484–851*)

"Enteroviruses, members of the family Picornaviridae, are so designated because of their ability to multiply in the gastrointestinal tract. Despite their name, these viruses are not a prominent cause of gastroenteritis. Enteroviruses encompass more than ***100 human serotypes****: 3 serotypes of poliovirus, 21 serotypes of coxsackievirus A, 6 serotypes of coxsackievirus B, 28 serotypes of echovirus, enteroviruses 68–71, and multiple new enteroviruses (beginning with enterovirus 73) that have been identified by molecular techniques. Human enteroviruses have been reclassified into four species designated A–D. Echoviruses 22 and 23 have been reclassified as parechoviruses 1 and 2 on the basis of low nucleotide homology and differences in viral proteins."* (*Harrison 19th/1289*)

"The Picornaviridae *family contains 12 genera, including Enterovirus (enteroviruses, rhinoviruses), Hepatovirus (hepatitis A virus), Kobuvirus (Aichi vius), Parechovirus (parechoviruses), Cardiovirus (cardioviruses) & Aphthovirus (foot-and-mouth disease viruses). The first five groups contain important human pathogens. Rhinoviruses historically were placed in separate genus but are now considered to be members of Enterovirus genus"* (*Jawetz 27th/514*)

79. Ans. c. Affected child can survives

[Ref: Ananthanarayan 9th/174-75; Robbins 9th/239-40]

Severe Combined Immunodeficiency

◈ *Ananthanarayan 9th/174-75*

- *Adenosine deaminase deficiency: This the first immunodeficiency disease associated with an enzyme deficiency*
- *Deficiency of both humoral & CMI response*

Table (*Ananthanarayan 9th/174; 8th/156*)**: Disorder of specific immunity**

Humoral immunodeficiency (B cell defect)	Cellular immunodeficiency (T cell defect)	Combined immunodeficiency (B & T cell defect)
• X-linked Agammaglobulinemia • Common variable Immunodeficiency • Selective Ig deficiency	• DiGeorge Syndrome • Chronic mucocutaneous candidiasis	• Nezelay of Syndrome • Ataxia Telangiectasia • Wiskott-Aldrich syndrome • Severe Combined Immunodeficiency (SCID)

Severe Combined Immunodeficiency

◈ *Robbins 9th/239-40*

- Persons with SCID are extremely susceptible to recurrent, severe infections by a wide range of pathogens, including *Candida albicans*, *Pneumocystis jiroveci*, *Pseudomonas*, cytomegalovirus, varicella, and a whole host of bacteria.
- Without HSC transplantation, *death occurs within the first year of life.*
- The most common form, accounting for 50% to 60% of cases, is X-linked, and hence SCID is more common in boys than in girls. The genetic defect in the X-linked form is a **mutation in the common γ-chain (γc) subunit of cytokine receptors**
- Autosomal recessive SCID: The remaining forms of SCID are autosomal recessive disorders. The most common cause of autosomal recessive SCID is a deficiency of the enzyme adenosine deaminase (ADA). Other is Mutations of an intracellular kinaseJak3 & Mutations in recombinase-activating genes (RAG)
- Although the mechanisms by which ADA deficiency causes SCID are not entirely clear, it has been proposed that deficiency of ADA leads to accumulation of deoxyadenosine and its derivatives (*e.g.,* deoxy-ATP), which are toxic to rapidly dividing immature lymphocytes, especially those of the T-cell lineage. Hence there may be a greater reduction in the number of T lymphocytes than of B lymphocytes.
- *Currently, HSC transplantation is the mainstay of treatment*, but X-linked SCID is the first human disease in which gene therapy has been successful.

Severe Combined Immunodeficiency

- The SCID syndrome is characterized by gross functional impairment of both *humoral and cell-mediated immunity* and by susceptibility to devastating fungal, bacterial, and viral infections.
- The syndrome is inherited either as an *X-linked or autosomal recessive defect*, and affected infants rarely survive beyond 1 year without treatment.
- The syndrome has been associated with mutations in one of several genes whose products are necessary for the normal differentiation of *T, B, and sometimes, NK cells.*

80. Ans. e. No role in cell mediated immunity

[Ref: Ananthanarayan 9th/137; Robbins 9th/192; Medical microbiology by Greenwood 16th/129; Harrison 19th/372e6-7]

NK Cell

◈ *Robbins 9th/192*

- The function of NK cells is to destroy irreversibly stressed and abnormal cells, such as virus-infected cells and tumor cells.
- NK cells make up approximately 5% to 10% of peripheral blood lymphocytes.
- NK cells are endowed with the ability to kill a variety of *virus-infected cells and tumor cells*, without prior exposure to or activation by these microbes or tumors. *This ability makes NK cells an early line of defense against viral infections and, perhaps, some tumors*

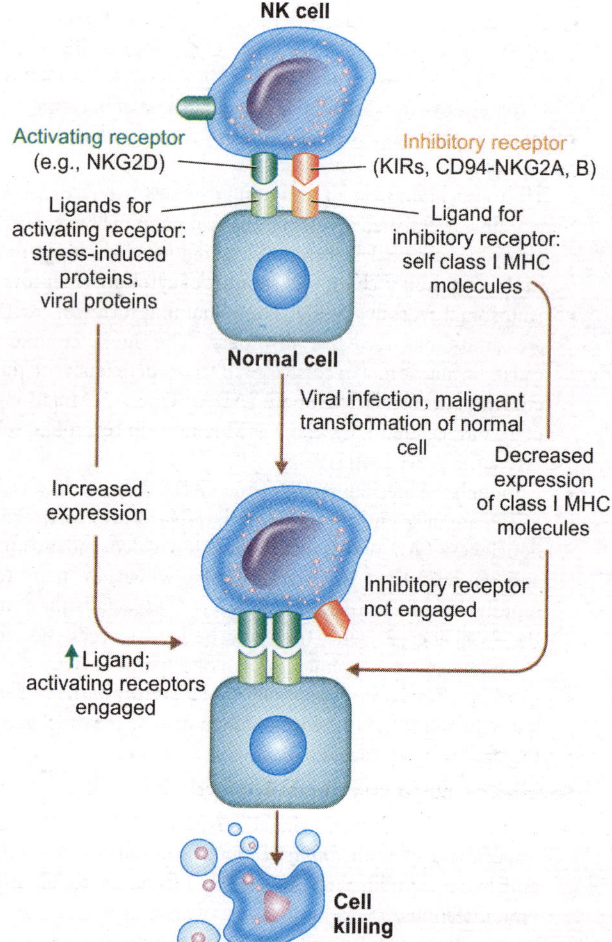

Fig: Schematic representation of NK-cell receptors and killing. NK cells express activating and inhibitory receptors; some examples of each are indicated. Normal cells are not killed because inhibitory signals from normal MHC class I molecules override activating signals. In tumor cells or virus-infected cells, there is increased expression of ligands for activating receptors, and reduced expression or alteration of MHC molecules, which interrupts the inhibitory signals, allowing activation of NK cells and lysis of target cells. KIR, killer cell Ig-like recepors.

"NK cell: They have CD 16 & CD 56[Q] *on their surface. They release several cytolytic factors; one of these, perforins, which resembles complement C9, cause transmembrane pores through which cytotoxic factor enter the cell. NK cell activity is augmented by interferon*[Q]*"* (Ananthanarayan 9th/137)

" N K cell: Form part of innate immunity as it does not require prior sensitisation by antigen. Their cytotoxicity is not antibody dependent or MHC restricted" (Ananthanarayan 9th/137)

Large Granular Lymphocytes/Natural Killer Cells

◈ *Harrison 19th/372e6-7*

- Large granular lymphocytes (LGLs) or NK cells account for~5–15%of peripheral blood lymphocytes. NKs cells are nonadherent, nonphagocytic cells with large azurophilic cytoplasmic granules.
- NKs cells express surface receptors for the Fc portion of IgG (*CD16*) and for NCAM-I (*CD56*)[Q], and many NK cells express some T lineage markers, particularly CD8, and proliferate in response to IL-2.
- NK cells arise in both bone marrow and thymic microenvironments.
- Functionally, NK cells share features with both monocytes-macrophages and neutrophils in that *they mediate both antibody-dependent cellular cytotoxicity (ADCC) and NK cell activity.*
- NK cell activity may play an *important role in immune surveillance and destruction of malignant and virally infected host cells*[Q]
- The ability of NK cells to kill target cells is *inversely related to target cell expression of MHC class I* molecules.
- *To eliminate malignant and virally infected cells,* NK cells also require activation through recognition of NK activation molecules on the surface of target cells.
- Recent evidence suggests that NK cells, though not possessing rearranging immune recognition genes, may be able to mediate recall responses for certain immune reactions such as *contact hypersensitivity.*
- Some NK cells express CD3 and are termed NK/T cells[Q].

81. Ans. b. Ostelma… & c. Zanam…

[Ref: Park 23rd/156-59; Ananthanarayan 9th/503]

Swine influenza

◈ *Ananthanarayan 9th/503*

- It emerged in march 2009 as new H1N1 virus disease
- Also called as *swine origin influenza*
- It spread from person to person & caused a pandemic

Pandemic influenza A (H1N1) 2009

◈ *Park 23rd/156-59*

- Currently susceptible to *oseltavir & zanamivir* but resistant to amantadine or rimantadine
- Treatment: oseltavir adult oral dose is 75 mg twice daily for 5 days. Zanamivir dose is two inhalation (2 × 5 mg) twice daily for 5 days
- **Chemoprophylaxis:** Oseltavir is drug of choice for chromoprophylaxis. It should be given till 10 days after last exposure

- Influenza vaccine only become *effective about 14 days after vaccination.* Those infected shortly before (1-3 days) or shortly after immunization can still get the disease.
- Vaccinated individuals can also get influenza caused by a *different strain of influenza virus*, for which the vaccine does not provide protection

82. Ans. a. HBsAg, c. Anti-HBe & d. Ant...

[Ref: Ananthanarayan 9th/546-48; Park 23rd/215; Harrison 19th/2016-18]

Table *(Harrison 19th/2017)*: **Commonly Encountered Serologic Patterns of Hepatitis B Infection**

HBsAg	Anti-HBs	Anti-HBc	HBeAg	Anti-HBe	Interpretation
+	–	IgM	+	–	Acute hepatitis B, high infectivity
+	–	IgG	+	–	Chronic hepatitis B, high infectivity
+	–	IgG	–	+	1. Late acute or chronic hepatitis B, low infectivity 2. HBeAg-negative ("precore- mutant") hepatitis B (chronic or, rarely, acute)
+	+	+	+/–	+/–	1. HBsAg of one subtype and heterotypic anti-HBs (common) 2. Process of seroconversion from HBsAg to anti-HBs (rare)
–	–	IgM	+/–	+/–	1. Acute hepatitis B 2. Anti-HBc "window"
–	–	IgG	–	+/–	1. Low-level hepatitis B carrier 2. Hepatitis B in remote past
–	+	IgG	–	+/–	Recovery from hepatitis B
–	+	–	–	–	1. Immunization with HBsAg (after vaccination) 2. Hepatitis B in the remote past (?) 3. False-positive

Hepatitis B: Serologic and Virologic Markers

Harrison 19th/2016-18

- The first[Q] virologic marker detectable in serum within 1-12 weeks[Q], usualy between 8-12 weeks, is *HBsAg.* [Q]
- In typical case, HBsAg becomes undetectable 1-2 months after the onset of jaundice and rarely persists beyond 6 months. After HBsAg disapperars, *antibody to HBsAg (anti-HBs)* detectable in serum and remains detectable indefinitely thereafter.
- Testing for IgM anti-HBc may be useful to distinguish between acute or recent infection (IgM anti-HBc-positive) and chronic HBV infection (IgM anti-HBc-negative, IgG anti-HBc-positive).
- Another serologic marker that may be of value in patients with hepatitis B is HBeAg. Its principal clinical usefulness is as an indicator of relative infectivity. Because *HBeAg is invariably present during early acute* hepatitis B, HBeAg testing is indicated primarily during follow-up of chronic infection
- Anti-HBs is rarely detectable in the presence of HBsAg in patients with *acute* hepatitis B, but 10–20% of persons with *chronic* HBV infection may harbor low-level anti-HBs
- Like HBeAg, serum HBV DNA is an indicator of HBV replication, but tests for HBV DNA are more sensitive and quantitative.

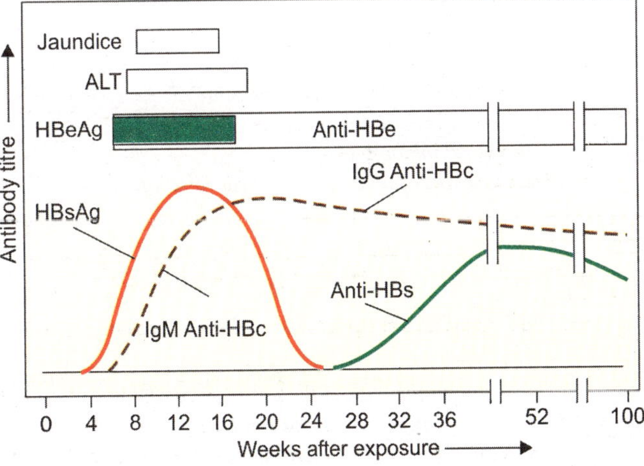

Fig: Scheme of typical clinical and laboratory features of acute hepatitis B

83. Ans. c. Vagal....

[Ref: Reddy 33rd/339; Parikh 6th/3.40]

Hanging: Causes of Death

◈ *Reddy 33rd/339*
- ***Asphyxia:*** *A tension of 15 kg on ligature blocks the trachea*
- ***Venous congestion:*** *The jugular veins are blocked by a tension in the rope of 2 kg*
- ***Combined asphyxia & venous congestion:*** *Commonest cause*
- ***Cerebral anaemia:*** *A tension 0f 4-5 kg on ligature blocks carotid arteries & the 20 kg, the vertebral arteries*
- ***Reflex vagal inhibition***
- Fracture of dislocation of the cervical vertebrae (injury to spinal cord)

Note: *"Contrary to popular belief, the more common cause of death by hanging in most instances is compression of neuro-vascular bundles in the neck & not asphyxia by airway obstruction" (Parikh 6th/3. 40)*

Delayed Death in Hanging: Death Delayed for Several Days is Rare. It Occurs Due to

◈ *Reddy 33rd/339*
- *Aspiration pneumonia*
- *Infections*
- *Oedema of lungs*
- *Oedema of larynx*
- *Hypoxic encephalopathy*
- *Infarction of brain*
- *Abscess of brain*
- *Cerebral softening*

Strangulation: Causes of death

◈ *Reddy 33rd/347*
- *Asphyxia*
- *Cerebral anaemia or Venous congestion*
- *Combined asphyxia & venous congestion*
- *Reflex vagal inhibition*
- *Fracture of dislocation of the cervical vertebrae (rare)*

84. Ans. d. Bulle...

[Ref: Reddy 33rd/224, 32nd/205, 235; Parikh 6th/4.43-44]

Smudge ring/Lead ring/Grease collar/Dirt collar

◈ *Parikh 6th/4.44*
- *This is due to the wipe of the soft metal of the bullet, or dirt present on it, or grease carried from the barrel & is deposited round the entrance wound internal to the abraded collar*
- *The smudge ring may therefore be absent when the jacketed bullet has passed through clothing*
- *The smudging in case of lead shot or unjacketed bullets can be detected microchemically on the target (skin/cloth)*
- *The forensic value of bullet wipe is to establish a hole as a bullet hole, to determine the entry site, & on occasion the sequence of shots or bullet's passage through multiple objects.*

Gutter fracture: *They are formed when part of the thickness of the bone is removed so as to form a gutter, e.g., in oblique bullet wound"- Reddy 33rd/247; 32nd/235*

"Abrasion collar (Marginal abrasion): *Abrasion collar surrounds the dirt collar. The abraded collar is reddish at first, but becomes reddish brown as it dries. Some contusion is present in abraded collar & as such, it is also called "contusion collar". These two features are proof of an entrance firearm wound" (Reddy 32nd/213)*

Firearm Wound

◈ *Reddy 32nd/205*
- They are recognized without difficulty
- Wounds produced by rifled weapon may simulate wounds inflicated by a red hot poker or a burning pointed stick
- Glancing wounds (striking someone or something at an angle rather than directly and with full force) ***may simulate incised or lacerated wounds.***
- A bullet that pass through glass or some other object & then strikes the body may produce a *wound resembling a laceration*
- Firearm wounds cause crushing of the tissues & produce an actual hole

Firearm injuries

◈ *Parikh 6th/4.39-40*
- Firearm injuries are wounds caused to the body tissue due to impact, entry & passage of a missile discharged from a firearm. They generally *simulate contused wounds*
- When a missile pass tangentially, the wound *may simulate an abrasion or a gutter*
- Slit like exit wounds are occasionally encountered. They are due to the bullet exiting on its board side or due to exit of a fragmented bone. Such injuries *may simulate incised wounds or stab wounds*

85. Ans. a. Pattern, b. Imprint, c. Graze & e. Scratch

[Ref: Reddy 33rd/181-82; Parikh 6th/4.2-4.3, 4. 10]

Abrasions or Gravel Rash

◈ *Reddy 33rd/181-82; Parikh 6th/4.2-4.3*

It is a destruction of the skin, which usually involves the superficial layers of the epidermis only. They are caused by friction against a rough surface or by compression. Some pressure & movement by agent on the surface of the skin is essential

Types: Abrasions are of four types

- Scratches (linear abrasions): *It is an abrasion with length but no significant width. Subtype-point scratch & fingernail abrasions*
- Grazes (sliding, scraping or grinding abrasion): *They are the most common type. They occur when there is movement b/w the skin & some rough surface in contact with it. Subtype-brush burn, friction burn etc.*
- Pressure abrasion (crushing or friction abrasions): *e.g., ligature mark in case of hanging & strangulation & the teethbite marks*
- Impact abrasion (contact or imprint abrasion): *caused by a rough object at or near right angle to the skin surface.*
- Pattern abrasion: *Impact abrasion & pressure abrasion*

ALSO KNOW

- *Lacerations types:* Split laceration (subtype-incised like wound), *stretch laceration,* avulsion, tears, cut lacerations etc *(Reddy 33rd/190-91; Parikh 6th/4. 10)*

86. Ans. e 325 I. P. C

[Ref: Reddy 33rd/294-95, 292; Parikh 6th/4. 59-4. 60]

I. P. C Related to injury

◈ *Reddy 33rd/294-95*

S.321, I. P. C: voluntarily causing hurt
S.322, I. P. C: voluntarily causing grievous hurt
S.323, I. P. C: Punishment for voluntarily causing hurt: imprisonment up to one year, or fine up to Rs 1000 or both
S.324, I. P. C: voluntarily causing hurt by dangerous weapons or means (3 year imprisonment)
S.325, I. P. C: *Punishment for voluntarily causing grievous hurt: Imprisonment for a term extending to seven years & also fine.*
S.326, I. P. C: Voluntarily causing grievous hurt by dangerous weapons or means. Imprisonment up to ten years & also fine

Grievous Injury[Q] (Sec 320 IPC[Q])

1. **Emasculation**[Q] (cutting off penis, castration, or causing loss of power of erection due to spinal injury)
2. Permanent privation of either eye[Q]
3. Permanent privation of either ear[Q]
4. **Privation of any member**[Q] (part, organ or limb) or joint
5. Permanent disfiguration of head or face[Q]
6. Fracture or dislocation of bone or a tooth[Q]
7. Destruction or permanent impairing of powers of any member or joint[Q]
8. **Any hurt which endangers life[Q], or which causes the sufferer to be, during the space of *20 days*[Q], *in severe body pain, or unable to follow his daily routine*[Q]**

87. Ans. c. Stry..., d. Sun... & e. Chol...

[Ref: Reddy 33rd/155; Parikh 6th/3. 8-3. 9]

Post- Mortem Caloricity

◈ *(Reddy 33rd/155, Parikh 6th/3. 8-3. 9, http://ourforensicmedicine.blogspot. in/2010/02/23-causes-of-post-mortem-caloricity. html)*

- In this condition, the temperature of the body remains raised for the first two hours or so after death
- This occur
  - *When the regulation of heat production has been severely disturbed before death, as in sunstroke & in some nervous disorder*
  - *When there has been a great increase in heat production in the muscle due to convulsions, as in tetanus & strychnine poisoning etc*
  - *When there has been excessive bacterial activity, as in septicaemic condition, cholera & other fevers*
- *Pontine haemorrhage & sunstroke*
- *Tetanus & strychnine poisoning*
- *Acute viral or viral infections such as lobar pneumonia, typhoid fever, encephalitis & encephalomyelitis*

"Factor affecting cooling of body (Algor mortis): Build of cadaver: Children & old people cool more rapidly than adult"-(Reddy 33rd/155)

- Post mortem Glycogenolysis
  - This is a normal phenomenon and the rise is 3. 6°F or 2°C
- Various causes of death such as
  - Septicaemia
    - Infectious diseases
    - Bacteremia
    - Tetanus, rabies, yellow fever
- Asphyxial conditions
- Severe convulsions
  - Tetanus
  - Strychnine
- Hyperpyrexia at death
  - Heat stroke (sun stroke)
  - Pontine Haemorrhage
- High atmospheric temperature
- Peritonitis, meningitis, nephritis
- Alcohol poisoning

88. Ans. a. Dry air & e. Warm air

[Ref: Reddy 33rd/172-73; Parikh 6th/3.31]

Factor Necessary for the Production of Mummification

◈ *Reddy 33rd/172*

- The absence of moisture in the air
- The *continuous action of dry or warmed air*

"Mummification: *Chronic arsenic or antimony poisoning is said to favour the process of mummification in dry & warm climate" (Parikh 6th/3.31)*

89. Ans. e. Ethanol

[Ref: Reddy 33rd/519, 515-17; Reddy 27th/456; Parikh 6th/8. 17; CMDT 2016/1560; Handbook of dialysis by Daugirdas 4th/302-315]

Note:
- *Theophylline, ethylene glycol & phenobarbitone (barbiturates) are cleared by both, activated charcoal & haemodialysis*
- *Benzodiazepines are cleared only by activated charcoal*
- *Ethanol is removed only by haemodialysis not by activated charcoal (so obviously the answer)*

Hemodialysis

◈ *Reddy 33rd/519*

- It is very useful for removing ethanol, methanol, ethylene glycol, chloral hydrate, lithium, trivalent arsenic, acetaminophen, bromide, Phenobarbital, salicylate, fluoride, sodium chlorate, digitalis, methaqualone, boric acid & thiocynate

"Haemodialysis has been employed for removing barbiturates[Q], boric acid, glutethimide, methyl alcohol[Q], salicylates[Q] and thiocyanates from the blood. Haemperfusion is superior to haemodialysis for removal of lipid soluble drugs. Exchange transfusion is only feasible with small children and has been applied to poisonings by salicylates, barbiturates, iron salts, carbon monoxide, etc. All toxic substances, including non-dialysable ones, are removed by this technique" *(Parikh 6th/8.17)*

"Ethylene glycol poisoning treatment: Activated charcoal, gastric lavage & haemodialysis" (Reddy 33rd/583)

Table *(CMDT 16/1560)*: **Recommended use of hemodialysis in poisoning**

Poison	Indications
Carbamazepine	Seizures, severe cardiotoxicity; serum level > 60 mg/L
Ethylene glycol	Acidosis, serum level > 50 mg/dL
Lithium[Q]	Severe symptoms; level > 4 mEq/L more than 12 hours after last dose
Methanol[Q]	Acidosis, serum level > 50 mg/dL
Phenobarbital	Intractable hypotension, acidosis despite maximal supportive care
Salicylate[Q]	Sever acidosis, CNS symptoms, level > 100 mg/dL (acute overdose) or > 60 mg/dL (chronic intoxication)
Theophylline[Q]	Serum level > 90-100 mg/L (acute) or seizures and serum level > 40> mg/L (chronic)
Valproic acid	Serum level > 900-1000 mg/L or deep coma, severe acidosis

"Activated charcoal as physical antidote: *Barbiturates, atropine, benzodiazepine, opiates, quinine, strychnine, phenothiazines, digitalis, amphetamines, antidepressant, antiepileptics, antihistamines, chloroquine, cimetidine, tetracyclines, theophyllines, pyrethrins, aluminium phosphide are well absorbed. Phenol, salicylates, kerosene, paracetamol are moderately absorbed. It is* not useful *in poisoning with corrosive, heavy metals, cyanides, hydrocarbons & alcohol" (Reddy 33th/517)*

"Charged (ionized) chemicals such as mineral acids, alkalis, and highly dissociated salts of cyanide, fluoride, iron, lithium, and other inorganic compounds are not well adsorbed by charcoal"

90. Ans. b. First…., c. Canni…., d. Cann….

[Ref: Reddy 33rd/68-71; Parikh 6th/2. 7]

Table *(Reddy 33rd/71; Parikh 6th/2.7)*: **Eruption of deciduous teeth**

Tooth	Eruption
Central incisor (lower)	6 to 8 months
Central incisor (upper)	7 to 9 months
Lateral incisor (upper)	7 to 9 months
Lateral incisor (lower)	10-12 months
First molar	12 to 14 months
Canine	17 to 18 months
Second molar	20 to 30 months

Table *(Reddy 33rd/71; Parikh 6th/2.7)*: **Eruption of permanent teeth**

Tooth	Eruption
First molar	6 to 7 years
Central incisor	6 to 8 years
Lateral incisor	7 to 9 years
First bicuspid	9 to 11 years
Second bicuspid	10 to 12 years
Canine	11 to 12 years
Second molar	12 to 14 years
Third molar	17 to 25 years (17-21 *in Parikh 6th/2. 7*)

PSM

91. Ans. a. BCG, b. Oral polio vaccine & c. Measles

[Ref: Park 23rd/103, 216; Ananthanarayan 9th/83; Park 19th/97-98, 162, 170, 179; Harrison 17th/779; Asma Rahim community medicine 1st/141]

C/I for Vaccines

- Live vaccines should not be administered to persons with immunodeficiency disease[Q] or to persons whose immune response may be suppressed because of leukemia, lymphoma or malignancy or because of therapy with cortiocosteriods, alkylating agents, antimetabolic agents or radiation
- Pregnancy[Q] is another C/I, for live vaccines unless the risk of infection exceeds the risk of harm to the foetus of some live vaccines
- The only absolute C/I for killed vaccine is severe local or general reaction to a previous dose.

BCG C/I

◈ *Park 23rd/197*

- Unless specifically indicated, BCG should not be given to patients suffering from generalized eczema[Q], infective dermatosis[Q], hypogammaglobulinaemia, to those with a history of deficient immunity[Q] (symptomatic HIV infection, known or suspected congenital immunodeficiency, leukemia, lymphoma or generalized malignant disease), patient under immunosuppressive treatment (corticosteriods, alkylating agents, antimetabolites, radiation) & pregnancy[Q]

DPT C/I

◈ H 19th/789, 17th/779

- Severe allergic reaction to a previous dose or a vaccine component
- Encephalopathy[Q] (*e.g.*, coma, decreased level of consciousness, prolonged seizures) within 7 days of a previous dose of DPT
- Progressive neurological disorder, including infantile spasm, uncontrolled epilepsy, progressive encephalopathy[Q]

Hepatitis B C/I

◈ *Park 23rd/216*

- Individuals with a history of allergic reactions to any of the vaccines components
- Neither pregnancy or lactation is a C/I for use of this vaccine.

OPV C/I

◈ *Park 19th/170, Asma Rahim community medicine 1st/141*

- Immunocompromised, immune deficiency[Q], HIV disease[Q] & active viral infection
- Acute infectious diseases, fever, diarrhoea & dysentery

Table *(Park 23rd/103)*: **Commonly used Immunizing agent**

Live attenuated vaccines	BCG; Typhoid oral	Bacterial
	Oral polio; Yellow fever; Measles Rubella; Mumps; Chicken pox; Influenza	Viral
	Epi. Typhus	Rickettsial
Inactivated or killed vaccines	Typhoid; Cholera; Pertussis; C. S. meningitis; Plague	Bacterial
	Rabies; Salk (polio); *Influenza;* **Hepatitis B**; Hepatitis A; Japanese encephalitis; KFD	Viral
Toxoids	Diphtheria; Tetanus	Bacterial

92. Ans. e Hepatitis B

[Ref: Above Q; Park 23rd/103, 197, 216; Ananthanarayan 9th/83]

Live Attenuated Vaccines[Q]

◈ *Park 23rd/103*

- Live vaccines (*e.g., BCG, measles, oral polio*) are prepared from live (generally attenuated) organisms.
- These organisms have been passed repeatedly in the laboratory in tissue culture or chick embryos and have lost their capacity to induce full-blown disease but retain their immunogenicity.
- In general, live vaccines are more potent immunizing agents than killed vaccines.
- Live vaccines should not be administered to persons with *immune deficiency disease* or to persons whose immune response may be suppressed because of therapy with *corticosteroids, alkylating agents, antimetabolic agents, or radiation*
- *Pregnancy is another contraindication* unless the risk of infection exceeds the risk of harm to the foetus of some live vaccines.

MMR C/I

◈ *H 17th/779*

- Known severe immunodeficiency[Q] (*e.g.*, hematological & solid tumours, congenital immunodeficiency, long term immunosuppressive therapy[Q], or severely symptomatic HIV infection)
- Severe allergic reaction to a previous dose or a vaccine component
- Pregnancy[Q]

93. Ans. b. Refere.... & d. Referen....

[Ref: Park 23rd/632]

Reference Indian Adult Man

◈ *Park 23rd/632*

- Reference man is *aged b/w 18-29 years & weighs 60kg with a height of 1. 73 meter & a BMI of 20.3*; is free from disease & physically fit for active work
- On each working day, he is *engaged in 8 hours of occupation which usually involves moderate activity;* while when not at work he spends 8 hours in bed, 4-6 hours in sitting & moving about, 2 hours in walking & in active recreation or household duties

Reference Indian Adult Woman

◈ *Park 23rd/632*

- Reference *woman is aged b/w 18-29 years, non-pregnant non-lactating (NPNL) & weighs 55 kg* with a *height of 1. 61 meter & a BMI of 21.2,* is free from disease & physically fit for active work.
- On each working day she is *engaged in 8 hour of occupation,* which usually involves moderate activity, while when not at work she spends 8 hours in bed, 4-6 hours in sitting & moving about, 2 hours in walking & in active recreation or household duties

94. Ans. c. In 8th 5 -yr...

[Ref: Park 23rd/706; National Health Programmes of India by Jugal Kishore 7th/457-63, http.//www. nih. ernet. in/rbis/india_information/ drinking. htm]

Note: *8th 5-year plan was implemented b/w 1992-1997*

Water Requirement

◈ *Park 23rd/706*

- The consumption of water depends upon climate conditions, standard of living & habits of people
- A daily supply of *150-200 liters per capita is considered as an adequate supply to meet the needs for all urban domestic purpose*
- In India *40 liters of water supply per capita per day was the set target to be achieved in rural areas*

Recommeded Norms for Water Supply

- *http://www. nih. ernet. in/rbis/india_information/drinking. html*

S. N.	Population	Recommended water supply norm (lpcd)
1	Less than 20, 000	
	a. Population served by stand posts	40
	b. Population provided with pipe connections	70
2	20, 000 to less than 100, 000	100
3	100, 000 to less than 1, 000, 000	100 (with no sewerage system)
		135 (with sewerage system)
4	1, 000, 000 and above	150
5	Rural and hills (per elevation difference of 100 m)	*40 or one hand-pump for 250 persons within a walking distance of 1. 6 km*
6	Rural – additional water for cattle in Desert Development Programme (DDP) areas.	30

Source: *(WG (1999) and Planning Commission (2006).*

New Initiative in 12th Five Year Plan (2012-2017)

- *Enhancement of service levels for rural water supply from the norms of 40 lpcd to 55 lpcd for designing of system*
- *Target being at least 50% of rural population in the country to have access to water within their household premises or within 100 meters radius, with at least 30% having individual household connection, as against 13% today*

National Rural Drinking Water Programme (NRDWP)

- *http://www. gktoday. in/national-rural-drinking-water-programme*

- NRDWP is a flagship programme of the Government and a component of the Bharat Nirman with the objective of ensuring provision of safe and adequate drinking water supply through handpumps, piped water supply etc. to all rural areas, households and persons.
- This programme was launched after merging the three erstwhile programmes on: Accelerated Rural Water Supply Programme- ARWSP, Swajaldhara & National Rural Water Quality Monitoring & Surveillance.
- Objectives/Norms for providing drinking water The Objectives of this programme is to provide: *40 liters per capita per day (lpcd) of safe drinking water for human beings.30 lpcd additional for cattle in the Desert Development Programme Areas. One hand-pump or stand post for every 250 persons. The water source should exist within the habitation/within 1. 6 km in the plains and within 100 mtrs. elevation in the hilly areas*

"The National Commission on Urbanization, Govt. of India, has suggested minimum norms for use of water. According to the commission, even in the worst drought conditions and even in the poorest colonies, at least 70 liters of water must be delivered per day to sustain the human life at a minimum standard of hygiene" Different organizations and individuals have given different norms for water supply in cities and rural areas. The figure adopted by the NCIWRD (1999) were 220 liter per capita per day (lpcd) for classes I cities. For the cities other than class I, the norms are 165 lpcd for year 2025 and 220 lpcd for the year 2050. For rural areas, 70 lpcd and 150 lpcd have been recommended for the year 2025 and 2050. Based on these norms and projection of population, it is estimated that by the year 2050, the water requirements per year for domestic use will be 90 km3 for low demand scenario and 111 km3 for high demand scenario. It is expected that surface and ground water sources will meet about 70% of urban water requirement and 30% of rural water requirement"

Water Supply for Residence

- *https://law. resource. org/pub/in/bis/S03/is. 1172. 1993. html*

- A minimum of 70 to 100 litres per head per day may be considered adequate for domestic needs of urban communities, apart from non domestic needs as flushing requirements. As

NOTE *The value of water supply given as 150–200 litres per head per day may be reduced to 135 litres per head per day for houses for Lower Income Groups (LIG) and Economically Weaker Section of Society (EWS), depending upon prevailing conditions.*

The rural water supply programme guidelines have been modified as the National Rural Drinking Water Programme, and made effective from 01. 04.2009, with an aim to address the concerns of the sector. The major changes in approach are as follows:

Goals – Strategic Plan (2011-2022) *(http://mdws. gov. in/sites/upload_files/ddws/files/pdf/NRDWP_ Guidelines_2013. pdf)*

- **The Goal of the Strategic Plan is:** *To ensure, that every rural person has enough safe water for drinking, cooking and other domestic needs as well as livestock throughout the year including during natural disasters and, by 2022, every rural person in the country will have access to 70 lpcd within their household premises or at a horizontal or vertical distance of not more than 50 meters from their household without barriers of social or financial discrimination. Individual States can adopt higher quantity norms, such as 100 lpcd*
- **Paradigm shift:** *In the Eleventh Five year Plan the basis of coverage under the rural water supply programme telescoped from habitations to households i.e. ensuring drinking water supply to all households in the community. Hitherto rural water supply was predominantly provided through hand pumps. In the Twelfth Five Year Plan, there will be a major shift of emphasis towards piped water supply with the goal of providing at least 50% of the rural population with at least 55 lpcd within the household premises or at a horizontal or vertical distance of not more than 100 metres from their household without barriers of social or financial discrimination.*
- **Enhancement of service levels** *for rural water supply from the norm of 40 lpcd to 55 lpcd for designing of systems The basic minimum service level of potable drinking water supply service in rural areas that was adhered to since the inception*

of ARWSP was 40 lpcd. The minimum level should be 55 lpcd in Twelfth Five Year Plan

- **Highest priority should be given to habitations** *with 0-15 lpcd, then to habitations with 15-30 lpcd, then 30-40 lpcd and finally to these with 40-55 lpcd.*

95. Ans. a. Education & b. Income & e. Physi....

[Ref: en. wikipedia. org/wiki/Multiple_deprivation_index; www. slideshare. net/garrysimmons/what-is-multiple-deprivation; www. prsindia. org/ billtrack/cover-note-on-higher-education-1360/]

"Address disparities of income, gender, region by creating deprivation index" *[http://www. prsindia. org/billtrack/cover-note-on-higher-education-1360/]*

Deprivation Index

◈ *http://archive. indianexpress. com/news/use-deprivation-index-to-help-more-sections-suggests-panel/20054/*

- The National Knowledge Commission (NKC) has proposed a Deprivation Index formula to assess the backwardness of students.
- The formula will be used to quantify deprivation of various kinds to introduce affirmative action and make higher education as "inclusive" as possible.
- This is apart from the existing reservation for SC/ST and Backward classes.
- The Deprivation Index proposes to look at *the "social background, caste, religion and gender, family education history, family income, type of school, place of residence (distinguishing between urban and rural areas, and accounting for regional deprivation) and physical disability."*

Indices of deprivation 2007 (ID 2007)-*en.wikipedia.org; www. graham-center.org*

- The **Indices of deprivation 2007 (ID 2007)** is a deprivation index at the small area level, created by the British Department for Communities and Local Government (DCLG) and released on 12 June 2007.
- It follows the Indices of deprivation 2004 (ID2004) and because much of the datasets are the same or similar between indices, it allows for a comparison of 'relative deprivation' of an area between the two indices
- The Index is made up of seven distinct dimensions of deprivation called Domain Indices.
  - **Income**
  - **Employment**
  - **Health and disability**
  - **Education, skills and training**
  - **Barriers to housing and services**
  - **Living environment**
  - **Crime**

96. Ans. c. Breast

[Ref: Park 23rd/382-84; Harshmohan 7th/198]

Note:
- *ICMR recent report is "3 year report (2009-11) of population based cancer registry" from 25 PBCR in India"-mhjfbmdgcfjbbpaeojofohoefgiehjai/index. html*
- *According to park (ICMR 2012 data) breast cancer is most common cancer in women in india*

Cancer

◈ *Park 23rd/382-84*

- *In India, the national cancer registry programme of the ICMR provides data on incidence, mortality & distribution of cancer from 25 population-based registries & 5 hospitals based registries*
- *The five most frequent cancers in men (2012) were cancer lung, lip & oral cavity, stomach, colorectum & other pharynx*
- *The five most frequent cancers in women (2012) were breast, cervix uteri, colorectum, ovary, lip & oral cavity*
- *"Breast cancer: It is the most common cancer both in developed & developing countries. It is estimated that during the year 2012, about 144937 new cases of breast cancer in women occurred, which accounts for 27% of malignant cases in women (an incidence of 25. 8 per lac)" (23rd/389)*
- *Cancer of cervix: In india, it is second most common killer cancer among women. It is estimated during 2012, 122644 new cases of cancer cervix occurred in the country (an incidence rate 22 per lac)" (23rd/388)*

Table *(Park 23rd/384)*: **Women—Estimated Incidence & Prevalence of cancer (Partial list) in India, 2012**

Cancer	Incidence (% of total)	Incidence (age standardized rate)	5 yr Prevalence (% of total)	5 yr Prevalence (Proportion per lac population)
Breast	27.0	25. 8	35.3	92. 6
Cervix uteri	22. 9	22. 0	27.4	72. 0

Table *(Park 23rd/384)* **Men—Estimated Incidence & Prevalence of cancer (Partial list) in India, 2012**

Cancer	Incidence (% of total)	Incidence (age standardized rate)	5 yr Prevalence (% of total)	5 yr Prevalence (Proportion per lac population)
Lung	11.3	11. 0	3. 7	5.4
Lip & oral cavity	11.3	10. 1	12. 6	18. 5

Table *(Park 23rd/384)*: **Both Sexes—Estimated Incidence & Prevalence of cancer (Partial list) in India, 2012**

Cancer	Incidence (% of total)	Incidence (age standardized rate)	5 yr Prevalence (% of total)	5 yr Prevalence (Proportion per lac population)
Breast	14.3	25. 8	22.2	92. 6
Cervix uteri	12. 1	22. 0	17.3	72. 0

97. Ans. a. Child. sex ratio..., d. CDR-... & e. 18 y...

[Ref: Park 23rd/490; Ananthanarayan 9th/; Indian Year Book 2015/9; Indian Economy by Ramesh Singh 6th/Census 2011; Reddy 27th/73; Parikh 6th/2. 13]

> *Note: Child sex ratio according to provisional data (914) & final revised data (919). So 914 given in option can be taken as correct*

***General fertility rate**- 80.3 (2012) (Park 23rd/490)*
***Total fertility rate**- 2.4 (2012) (Park 23rd/490)*
***General marital fertility rate**- 114. 9 (2012) (Park 23rd/490)*
***Total marital fertility rate**- 4.4 (2012) (Park 23rd/490)*
***Crude birth rate**-22. 1 per 1000 (2010); 21. 6 per 1000 (2012) (Park 23rd/490)*
***Crude death rate**- 7.2 per 1000 (2010); 7. 0 per 1000 (2012) (Park 23rd/490)*
***Gross reproductive rate**- 1. 1 (2012) (Park 23rd/490)*

"**The Crude Birth Rate (CBR)** at the national level during 2013 stands at 21.4, a decline of 0.2 points over 2012. The maximum CBR has been reported in Bihar (27.6) and the minimum in Kerala (14.7)," *(Sample Registration System (SRS) survey)*

Table *(http://www. censusindia. gov. in/vital_statistics/SRS_Reports_2013. html)* **Data from SRS, 2013**

CBR	21.4
CDR	7. 0
General fertility rate	78. 5
Total fertility rate	2.3
Infant mortality rate	40

Indian Majority Act (1875, Sec 3)

- "A person ***attains majority on the completion of 18 years***[Q], but when a person is under the **guardianship of court of Wards,** or is under a guardian appointed by the Courts, he attains majority on the ***completion of 21 years***[Q]" *(Reddy 27th/73)*
- Child Marriage Restrain Act, 1978: A female ***under 18 years and a male under 21 years***[Q], cannot contract marriage *(Reddy 27th/73)*

2011 Census

- *The provisional figures of census 2011 were released by the ministry of Home affairs on 31st march, 2011*
- *The final data were released in may 2013 (some modification of data)*
- *Child Sex ratio (2011)- 919 Indian Year Book 2015/9*

Provisional data from the census was released on 31 March 2011 *(and was updated on 20 May 2013).*

Population	Total	1, 210, 726, 932
	Males	623, 121, 843
	Females	587, 447, 730
Literacy	Total	74%
	Males	82. 10%
	Females	65. 50%
Density of population	per km2	382
Sex ratio	per 1000 males	940 females
Child sex ratio (0–6 age group)	per 1000 males	919 females

98. Ans. b. Denomi... & d. Numer....

[Ref: Park 23rd/139; Biostatistics by Rao 2nd/70-71, 418; https://onlinecourses. science. psu. edu/stat507/node/71; http://en. wikipedia. org/wiki/Positive_and_negative_predictive]

> *Note: In PPV, numerator contains only true positive (not all positive) & denominator contains all positive*

"The positive and negative predictive values (PPV and NPV respectively) are the proportions of positive and negative results in statistics and diagnostic tests that are true positive and true negative results. The PPV and NPV describe the performance of a diagnostic test or other statistical measure. A high result can be interpreted as indicating the accuracy of such a statistic. The PPV and NPV are not intrinsic to the test; they depend also on the prevalence. The PPV can be derived using Bayes' theorem." *(http://en. wikipedia. org/wiki/Positive _and_negative_predictive_values)*

Table *(Park 23rd/139)*: **Screening Test Result by diagnosis**

Screening Test Result	Diagnosis		Total
	Disease	Not disease	
Positive	A (true positive)	B (False positive)	A+B
Negative	C (False Negative)	D (True negative)	C+D
Total	A+C B+D		A+B+C+D

- *Sensitivity* $= A/(A + C) \times 100$
- *Specificity* $= D/(B + D) \times 100$
- *Predictive value of positive test* $= A/(A + B) \times 100$

A & E

- *Predictive value of negative test = D/(C+D) X 100*
- *Percentage of false negative = C/(A+C) X 100*
- *Percentage of false positive = B/(B+D) X 100*

$$\text{Positives predictive value} = \frac{\text{number of true positives}}{\text{number of true positives + number of false positives}}$$

PPV & NPP

◈ *https://onlinecourses. science. psu. edu/stat507/node/71*

- *Positive and negative predictive values are influenced by the prevalence* of disease in the population that is being tested. If we test in a high prevalence setting, it is more likely that persons who test positive truly have disease than if the test is performed in a population with low prevalence...
- Using the same test in a population with higher prevalence increases *positive predictive value. Conversely, increased prevalence results in decreased negative predictive value.*
- *When considering predictive values of diagnostic or screening tests, recognize the influence of the prevalence of disease.* The figure below depicts the relationship between disease prevalence and predictive value in a test with 95% sensitivity and 95% specificity:

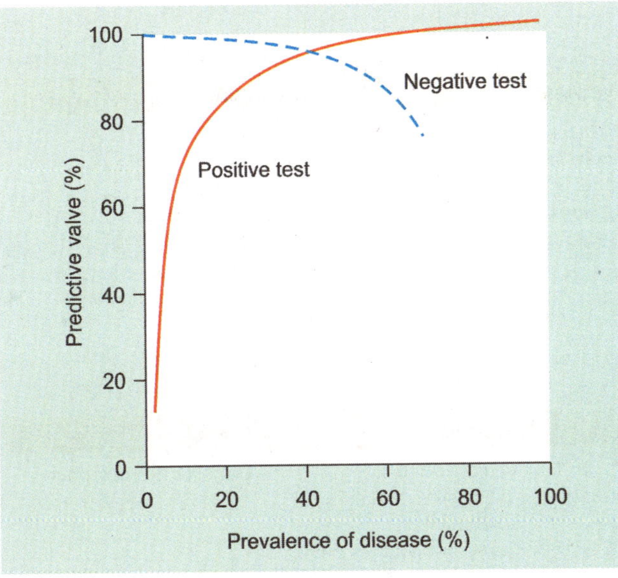

Fig: Relationship between disease prevalence and predictive value in a test with 95% sensitivity and 85% specificity.

99. Ans. a. Polio, b. Diphtheria., c. Anthrax & e. Hepatitis B

[Ref: Park 23rd/95-96; Ananthanarayan 9th/72]

◈ *(Park 23rd/96: Writes)*

- *Incubatory carriers*: Measles, mumps, polio, pertussis, influenza, diphtheria and hepatitis B
- *Convalescent carriers: Typhoid fever, dysentery (bacillary and amoebic), cholera,* diphtheria and whooping cough.
- *Healthy carriers: Poliomyelitis, cholera, meningococcal meningitis, salmonellosis, and diphtheria*
- Temporary carriers: May be included the incubatory, convalescent and healthy carries.
- Chronic carriers: Typhoid fever, hepatitis B, dysentery, cerebro-spinal meningitis, malaria & gonorrhoea

100. Ans. a. Stap...., c. Hepa...., d. Typhoid. & e. Hem....

[Ref: Park 23rd/95-96; Ananthanarayan 9th/72, 203-05, 330, 216, 296, 545]

[Refer Q 99 for explanation]

"*Staphylococcus carriage starts early in life*, colonization of umbilical stump being very common in babies born in hospitals. Some carriers, called 'shedders' disseminate very large number of cocci for prolonged periods" *(Ananthanarayan 9th/203-04)*

Hemophilus influenza: Carriage in upper respiratory tract is common, particularly in young children, but such strains are usually non-capsulated & not responsible for acute invasive infection. Rifampicin is given to eradicate the carrier state" (Ananthanarayan 9th/330)

101. Ans. a. Birefri...., b. Fib..., d. Impa... & e. Notif.....

[Ref: Park 23rd/806; Harrison 19th/1688]

Silicosis

◈ *Park 23rd/806*

- *The longer the duration of exposure, the greater the risk of developing silicosis*
- *It is found that the incubation period may vary from a few month up to 6 years of exposure, depending upon the above factors*
- *Pathologically, silicosis is characterized by a dense nodular fibrosis, the nodule ranging from 3 to 4 mm in diameter*
- *Some of the early manifestations are irritant cough, dyspnea on exertion & pain in chest*
- *With more advanced disease, impairment of total lung capacity (TLC) is commonly present*
- *A X-ray of chest shows "snow storm" appearance in the lung fields*
- *Silicosis is progressive & what is more important is that silicotics are prone to pulmonary tuberculosis, a conditional called "silico-tuberculosis"*
- *There is no effective treatment for silicosis. Fibrotic change that have already taken place cannot be reversed*
- *It was made notifiable disease under the Factories Act 1948 & Mines act 1952*

"Characteristic lung tissue pathology in nodular silicosis consists of fibrotic nodules with concentric "onion-skinned" arrangement of collagen fibers, central hyalinization, and a cellular peripheral zone, with ***lightly birefringent particles*** *seen under polarized light" (http://www. askdrwiki. com/mediawiki/index. php?title = Silicosis#Pathology)*

Table *(Harrison 19th/1688)*: **Categories of Occupational Exposure and Associated Respiratory Conditions**

Occupational Exposures	Nature of Respiratory Responses	Comment
Inorganic Dusts		
Asbestos: mining, processing, construction, ship repair	***Fibrosis (asbestosis), pleural disease, cancer, mesothelioma***[Q]	Virtually all new mining and construction with asbestos done in developing countries
Silica: mining, stone cutting, sandblasting, quarrying	Fibrosis (silicosis), PMF, cancer, silicotuberculosis[Q], COPD	Improved protection in United States, persistent risk in developing countries

102. Ans. a. Gonorrhoea & b. Pertussis

[Ref: Ananthanarayan 9th/684; Ananthanarayan 8th/381, 322; Medical Parasitology by Paniker 6th/214; Park 23th/93, 276, 788

"The term enteric fever includes typhoid fever caused by S. typhi & paratyphoid fever caused by S. paratyphi A, B & C. While Salmonella paratyphi A occur only in human beings, S. paratyphi B can infect animals such as dogs or cows, which may acts as source of human disease"- Ananthanarayan 9th/296

Zoonosis: (Infection of animals communicable to man)

*Zoonosis is defined as an infection or infectious disease that is transmissible under natural conditions from vertebrate animals to man Zoonotic disease may be due to infections with **viruses, bacteria, protozoa, helminths, fungi or arthropods.***

Zoonosis: 4 Categories

1. *Direct zoonosis*
2. *Cyclozoonosis*
3. *Metazoonosis e.g., arbovirus infection*
4. *Saprozoonosis*

Table: *(Park 23th/93)*: **Partial List of Zoonosis**

Bacterial	Viral	Protozoan	Helminthic
Anthrax *Brucellosis* *Q fever (Soft tick)* *Leptospirosis* *Tuberculosis* *Plague*[Q]	Cowpox Monkey pox Westernequine encephalitis Ross river fever Yellow fever (Mosquito) Japanense encephalitis[Q] Lassa fever Rabies	Leishmaniasis Toxoplasmosis Trypnosomiasis Babesiosis	Clonorchiasis Fasciopsis Echistosomiasis Taeniasis Trichinellosis

Table (Ananthanarayan 9th/684): Common Zoonotic disease

Bacterial	Rickettsia	Virus	Parasite	Fungus
Anthrax Brucellosis Leptospirosis Salmonellosis Plague[Q]	Scrub typhus Murine typhus Tick typhus Q fever	Yellow fever Japanense encephalitis KFD Chikungunya Rabies	Echinococcosis Taeniasis Leishmanisis Toxoplasmosis	Zoophilic dermatophytes

OPHTHALMOLOGY

103. Ans. e. Sutures lines

[Ref: Gray's 40th/656-58; ; Parson 22nd/483; Snell's 9th/554; https://en. wikipedia. org/wiki/Orbital_fascia; BDC 6th/Vol. III/205]

"**Periorbita:** It is the periosteal lining of orbital walls. The periorbita is attached to the ***suture lines, fissures and foramina of the orbit.*** Posteriorly the periorbita is continuous with the optic nerve sheath"*(http://www. drtbalu. co. in/orbit. html)*

Orbital Fascia

◈ *https://en. wikipedia. org/wiki/Orbital_fascia; BDC 6th/Vol. III/205*

- The Orbital Fascia forms the periosteum of the orbit. It is *loosely connected* to the bones and can be readily separated from them.
- Behind, it is united with the dura mater by processes which pass through the optic foramen and superior orbital fissure, and with the sheath of the optic nerve.
- In front, it is connected with the periosteum at the margin of the orbit, and sends off a process which assists in forming the orbital septum.

- From it two processes are given off; one to enclose the lacrimal gland, the other to hold the pulley of the Obliquus superior in position.

Periosteum

◈ *Gray's 40th/656-58*

- The periosteum of the orbit is only loosely attached to bone. Behind, it is united with the dura mater surrounding the optic nerve and in front it is continuous with the periosteum of the orbital margin, where it gives off a stratum which contributes to the *orbital septum*.
- It also attaches to the trochlea, and, as the lacrimal fascia, forms *the roof and lateral wall of the fossa* for the nasolacrimal sac.

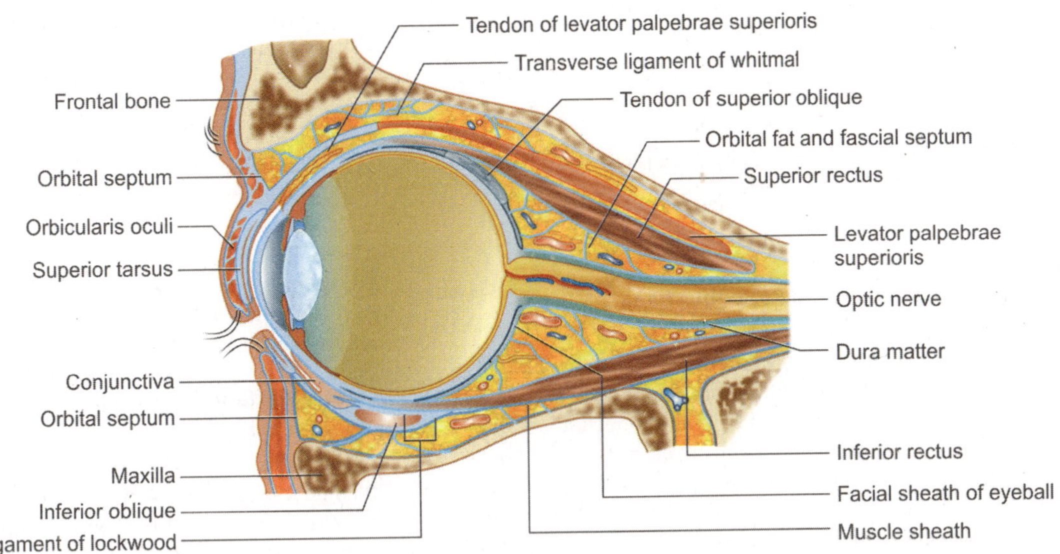

Fig: The contents of the orbit-sagittal section

104. Ans. a. >4…, c. Asso…, d. Undiff… & e. Scle…

[Ref: A. K. Khurana 6th/306-07; Parson 22nd/379-80; Robbins 9th/1339]

> *Note: Regarding option A : as 3mm size of tumor is deciding factor for small (<3mm, group A –best prognosis) & large (>3mm, group B, poorer prognosis) tumor. So option A (>4mm size of tumor) might have poor prognosis*

Earlier Reese & Ellsworth developed a classification of intraocular retinoblastoma, which was of prognostic significance for control of local disease. But it has become irrelevant with availability of newer chemotherapeutic agents & modes of therapy" *(A. K. Khurana 6th/306; Parson 22nd/378-79)*

Prognosis of Retinoblastoma

◈ *A. K. Khurana 6th/307*

- If untreated the prognosis is almost always bad and the patient invariably dies. Rarely *spontaneous regression* with resultant cure and shrinkage of the eyeball may occur due to necrosis followed by calcification; suggesting role of some *immunological phenomenon.*
- Prognosis is fair (survival rate 70-85%) if the eyeball is enucleated before the occurrence of extraocular extension.
- ***Poor prognostic factors are:*** *Optic nerve involvement, undifferentiated tumour cells and massive choroidal invasion*

"The prognosis of retinoblastoma, if untreated, is always bad & the patient invariably dies. Success with chemotherapy for retinoblastoma, defined as avoidance of external beam radiation & enucealtion, was 100% for group A, 93% for group B, 90% for group C & 47% for group D in the international classification - Parson 22nd/382

Table: International classification of Retinoblastoma

Group	Quick Reference	Specific Features
A	Small tumour	Rb < 3 mm
B	Larger tumour	Rb > 3 mm or
	Macula	Macula Rb location (< mm to foveola)
	Juxtapapillary	Juxtapapillary Rb location (< 1. 5 mm to disc)
	Subretinal fluid	Subretinal fluid < 3 mm from margin
C	Focal seeds	Rb with
		Subretinal seeds < 3mm from Rb
		Vitreous seeds < 3mm from Rb
		Both subretinal and vitreous seeds < 3mm from Rb
D	Diffuse seeds	Rb with
		Subretinal seeds > 3 mm from Rb
		Vitreous seeds > 3mm from Rb

Contd...

Group	Quick Reference	Specific Features
		Both subretinal and vitreous seeds > 3mm from Rb
E	Extensive Rb	Massive Rb with anatomic or functional destruction of the eye and/or Neovascular glaucoma
		Opaque media from haemorrhage in anterior chamber, vitreous or subretinal space
		Invasionof post-laminar optic nerve, choroid (>2 mm), sclera, orbit, anterior chamber
		Tumour touching lens
		Diffuse infiltrating tumour
		Phthisis or pre-phthisis

Prognosis and Survival for Retinoblastoma

◈ *https://www. cancer. ca/en/cancer-information/cancer*

- **Cancer spread:** Children with retinoblastoma that has not spread outside the eye (intraocular retinoblastoma) have a better prognosis than children with retinoblastoma that has spread outside the eye or to other parts of the body (extraocular retinoblastoma or metastatic retinoblastoma).
- The International Classification for Intraocular Retinoblastoma classifies each eye separately. *Children in group A have the most favourable prognosis and are most likely to be able to see after treatment.*
- In the Reese-Ellsworth staging system, children in *group I (very favourable stage) are most likely to be able to see after treatment.*
- In the TNM staging system, the lower the stage of retinoblastoma, the better the expected outcome.
- Children who have a lower grade of retinoblastoma or a well-differentiated tumour have a more favourable prognosis than children with a higher grade or *poorly differentiated tumour.*
- *Younger children* tend to have a *better prognosis* than older children. When retinoblastoma is caught at an earlier age, the chances of survival and saving the eye are better.
- ***Glaucoma*** is a condition that is characterized by increased pressure in the eye. Children with retinoblastoma who develop glaucoma tend to have a worse prognosis than children who don't develop glaucoma.

105. Ans. a. The terms 'A'... & d. Usually....& e. Obliqu....

[Ref: A. K. Khurana 6th/348, 357; Parson 22nd/427-29]

Squint or strabismus

◈ *A. K. Khurana 6th/344, 348, 353*

- Normally visual axis of the two eyes are parallel to each other in the 'primary position of gaze' and this alignment is maintained in all positions of gaze. A *misalignment of the visual axis of the two eyes is called squint or strabismus.*
- Classification of strabismus

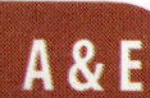

- Apparent squint or pseudostrabismus:
  - *Pseudoesotropia* or apparent convergent squint &
  - *Pseudoexotropia* or apparent divergent squint
- Latent squint (Heterophoria):
  - Esophoria.
  - Exophoria.
  - Hyperphoria.
  - Cyclophoria
- Manifest squint (Heterotropia)
  - Concomitant squint:
    - Convergent squint (esotropia)
    - Divergent squint (exotropia),
    - Vertical squint (hypertropia)
- Incomitant squint:
  - Paralytic,
  - A & V pattern heterotropias
  - Restrictive

"A-V patterns may be observed in horizontal strabismus. When A-V patterns are associated, the horizontal concomitant strabismus becomes vertically incomitant" (A. K. Khurana 6th/348)

'A' and 'V' Pattern Heterotropia

◈ *A. K. Khurana 6th/357*

- The terms 'A' or 'V' pattern squint are labelled when the amount of deviation in squinting eye varies by more than 10° and 15°, respectively, between upward and downward gaze.
- ***'A' and 'V' esotropia:*** In 'A' esotropia the amount of deviation increases in upward gaze and decreases in downward gaze. The reverse occurs in 'V' esotropia.
- ***'A' and 'V' exotropia:*** In 'A' exotropia the amount of deviation decreases in upward gaze and increases in downward gaze. The reverse occurs in 'V' exotropia.
- ***Etiology:*** Oblique muscle dysfunction is the commonest cause of AV pattern. Other causes include horizontal rectus muscle dysfunction, vertical muscle dysfunction & certain orbital factors
- ***Clinical presentations:*** A and V pattern heterophoria essentially refer to vertically incomitant horizontal strabismus. Thus, the horizontally comitant esotropias and exotropias may be associated with A or V patterns.

◈ *Parson 22nd/427-29*

- A tendency for eye to diverge on elevation is physiological. Any squint can show a variation in deviation in upward & downward gaze & depending on the nature of the squint, An A & V pattern can be recognised
- The A & V phenomenon should be assessed by the cover test in 25^0 upward & downward gaze. This test is carried out for near & distance fixation
- In general it is found that oblique muscle are more important in production of A & V phenomenon than the vertical recti.
- Usually, overaction of the inferior oblique or weakness of superior oblique leads to a V pattern & overaction of the superior oblique or weakness of inferior oblique to an A pattern

- If there is no definite overaction of the obliques, then the vertical recti are shifted

106. Ans. b. Amblyopi.... & c. Angl....

[Ref: A. K. Khurana 6th/348; Parson 22nd/428-29; Kanski 5th/543]

Infantile Esotropia (Previously Called Congenital Esotropia)

◈ *A. K. Khurana 6th/348*

- Age of onset, is usually 1-2 months of age, but occur any time in first 6 months of life.
- Angle of deviation is usually constant & fairly large (> 30o),
- **Fixation pattern:** Binocular vision does not develop & there is alternate fixation in primary gaze and crossed fixation in lateral gaze.
- ***Amblyopia*** develops in 25-40% of cases
- Associations include inferior oblique overaction (usually developing after 1 year of age), dissociated vertical deviation (DVD) in about 70-90% cases & latent horizontal nystagmus
- **Treatment:** Surgery is treatment of choice
  - Time of surgery: Surgery should be *done b/w 6 months to 2 years* (preferably before 1 yr of age)
  - Amblyopia treatment by patching the normal eye should always be done before performing the surgery
  - Recession of both medial recti is preferred over unilateral recess-resect procedure

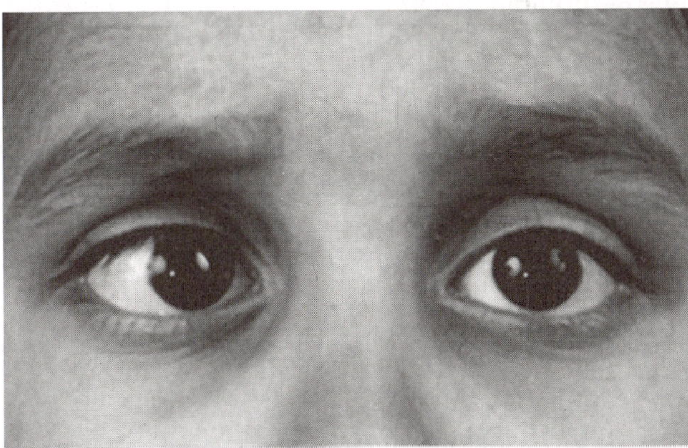

Fig: Right Esotropia

107. Ans. a. Avascular, b. Growt.... & d. Transparent & e. Ecto.....

[Ref: A. K. Khurana 6th/179-81; Parson 22nd/261-62; I. B. Singh Embryology 10th/356]

"The lens of the eye is developed from a thickened area of surface ectoderm, the lens placode" (I. B. Singh Embryology 10th/356)

"The lens grow in size continuously throughout life & in this respect it is unique among the organs of the body. At birth its weight is about 65 mg & by 80 years of age it has been found to weigh 258 mg" (Parson 22nd/261)

Lens

◈ *A. K. Khurana 6th/179-81*

- It is a *transparent,* biconvex, crystalline structure placed between iris and the vitreous in a saucer shaped depression the patellar fossa.
- Its diameter is 9-10 mm and thickness varies with age from 3. 5 mm (at birth) to 5 mm (at extreme of age).
- **It has got two surfaces:** The anterior surface is less convex (radius of curvature 10 mm) than the posterior (radius of curvature 6 mm).
- Its refractive index is 1.39 and total power is 15-16 D.

Structure of lens

- ***Lens capsule:*** It is a thin, *transparent,* hyaline membrane surrounding the lens which is thicker over the anterior than the posterior surface. The lens capsule is thickest at pre-equator regions (14 μ) and thinnest at the posterior pole (3 μ).
- ***Lens fibres:*** The epithelial cells elongate to form lens fibres which have a complicated structural form. Mature lens fibres are cells which have lost their nuclei. *As the lens fibres are formed throughout the life, these are arranged compactly as nucleus and cortex of the lens*
- ***Nucleus:*** It is the central part containing the oldest fibres.
- *"Lens requires a continuous supply of energy* (ATP) for active transport of ions and amino acids, maintenance of lens dehydration, and for a continuous protein and GSH synthesis"
- ***Source of nutrient supply:*** The crystalline lens, being an *avascular structure* is dependent for its *metabolism on chemical exchanges with the aqueous humour.*

108. Ans. c. More.... & d. Disc edema.

[Ref: A. K. Khurana 6th/286; Parson 22nd/517-18]

Ocular Ischaemic Syndrome

◈ *A. K. Khurana 6th/286*

- Ocular ischaemic syndrome refers to a rare condition resulting from chronic ocular hypoperfusion secondary to carotid artery stenosis (90% stenosis)
- *Risk factors* include male gender, old age (60-90 years), smoking, for carotid stances hypertension, diabetes mellitus and hyperlipidaemia.
- The *manifestations* of carotid occlusive disease include: ***Amaurosis fugax*** (transient retinal ischaemic attack), Retinal artery occlusion (due to embolus), Transient cerebral ischaemic attacks (TIA), Stroke, and Asymetrical diabetic retinopathy.
- Ocular ischaemic syndrome is usually unilateral (80%), affecting elderly males more commonly than females.
- ***Symptoms included:***
  - *Loss of vision,* which usually progresses gradually over several weeks or months.
  - *Transient black outs* (amaurosis fugax) may be noted by some patients.

- *Pain*-ocular or periorbital— may be complained by some patients.
- *Delayed dark adaptation* may be noted by a few patients.

- ***Signs include:***
  - *Cornea* may show oedema and striae.
  - *Anterior chamber* may reveal faint aqueous flare with few, if any, cell (ischaemic pseudoiritis).
  - *Pupil* may be mid dilated and poorly reacting.
  - *Iris* shows rubeosis iridis (in 66% cases) and atrophic patches.
  - *Cataract* may occur as a complication in advanced cases.
  - *Neovascular glaucoma* is a frequent sequelae to anterior segment neovascularization.
  - *Fundus examination* may reveal:
    - *Venous dilatation* with irregular caliber but no or only mild tortuosity.
    - *Retinal arterial* narrowing is present.
    - *Retina* show *midperipheral dot and blot haemorrhages, microaneurysms and cotton wool spots.*
    - *Retinal neovascularization* is noted in 37% cases, which may be in the form of NVD and occasionally NVE.
    - *Macular oedema* is a common complication.

"Ocular ischemic syndrome: *The fundoscopic findings may mimic other vascular retinal disorders and involutive changes seen in elderly population: constriction, straightening and narrowing of the arteries, dilated retinal veins, but without accentuated tortuosity commonly seen in vein occlusions. Venous beading may resemble features of proliferative diabetic retinopathy. In the majority of cases there are dot and blot retinal hemorrhages distributed diffusely around the periphery, but they can spread onto the posterior pole. The other features of retinal ischemia may also be present: cherry red spot appearance, cotton wool exudates, optic atrophy and edema"* (Advances in Opthalmology by S. Rumelt 2012/Retina)

109. Ans. d. CRVO

[Ref: A. K. Khurana 6th/437-38; Parson 22nd/399]

Central retinal vein occlusion **(CRVO):** *Observation & monitoring is all that is required in patients with mild to moderate visual loss, as the condition (especially non-ischemic CRVO), in more than 50% cases of CRVO resolves with almost normal vision"* (A. K. Khurana 6th 272)

"Sympathetic ophthalmitis: *Though rare, the disease is potentially sight threatening. Prompt recognition with early institution of steroid therapy helps to salvage vision"* (Parson 22nd/399)

"The eye being small & delicate structures, sometimes even apparently minor trauma can have devasting effects.

First aid at primary care level for chemical burns is important. The eye must be thoroughly irrigated with water or physiological solutions like saline or ringer lactate. In case of lacerating injuries, after giving primary aid, person should be urgently referred to nearest eye specialist" *(Parson 22nd/399)*

"Retinal artery occlusion (RAO) *represents an ophthalmologic emergency"* (Advances in Opthalmology by S. Rumelt 2012/Retina)

"Bacterial endophthalmitis: It is an emergency and should be managed energetically (A. K. Khurana 6th/214)

"Acute primary angle-closure glaucoma: An attack of acute primary angle closure glaucoma occurs due to a sudden total angle closure leading to severe rise in IOP. It usually does not terminate of its own and thus if not treated lasts for many days. This is sight threatening emergency" (A. K. Khurana 6th/244)

"An early diagnosis and vigorous therapy is the hallmark of the treatment of endophthalmitis. Following therapeutic regime is recommended for suspected bacterial endophthalmitis" (A. K. Khurana 6th/171)

"Treatment of central retinal artery occlusion is unsatisfactory, as retinal tissue cannot survive ischaemia for more than 90-100 minutes. The emergency treatment should include: Immediate lowering of intraocular pressure by intravenous mannitol & acetazolamide, paracentesis of anterior chamber and intermittent ocular massage; Vasodilators and inhalation of a mixture of 5% carbon dioxide and 95% oxygen; Intravenous steroids; fibrinolytic therapy; laser photodisruption of embolus" (A. K. Khurana 6th/270)

"Papilloedema: *It is a neurological emergency and requires immediate hospitalisation. As a rule unless the causative disease is treatable or cerebral decompression is done, the course of papilloedema is chronic and ultimate visual prognosis is bad"* (A. K. Khurana 6th/325)

110. Ans. d. Corn....& e. Rich....

[Ref: A. K. Khurana 6th/95-97; Parson 22nd/191-93; Cornea by Krachmer 2th/3, 729-31]

"Oxygen is derived directly from air through the tear film. This is an active process undertaken by the epithelium. Therefore, corneal hypoxia may occur with over wear of contact lesnses" *(A. K. Khurana 6th/97)*

"The endothelial cells contain 'active-pump' mechanism which keeps cornea dehydrated" *(A. K. Khurana 6th/96)*

Corneal Transparency:

The transparency is the result of: *(A. K. Khurana 6th/97)*

- Peculiar arrangement of corneal lamellae (lattice theory of Maurice),
- Peculiar refractive index of corneal lamellae (Goldmann & Benedek theory)
- Avascularity of cornea
- Relative state of dehydration (78% water content), which is maintained by barrier effects of epithelium and endothelium and the active Na+ K+ ATPase pump of the endothelium.
- Swelling pressure of stroma which counters the imbibitions effect of intraocular pressure

For these processes, cornea needs some energy.

Cornea

- *Parson 22nd/191-93*

- The normal healthy cornea is avascular & devoid of lymphatic channels

- Corneal cell derive nourishment by diffusion from the aqueous, the capillaries at the limbus & oxygen dissolved in the tear film
- Corneal thickness is more in periphery than at center
- Cornea is most important refractive surface of the eye

"Histologically, the cornea consists of 6 distinct layers. From anterior to posterior these are: epithelium, Bowman's membrane, substantia propria (corneal stroma), Pre-Descemet's membrane (Dua's layer), Descemet's membrane and endothelium"- *(A. K. Khurana 6th/95)*

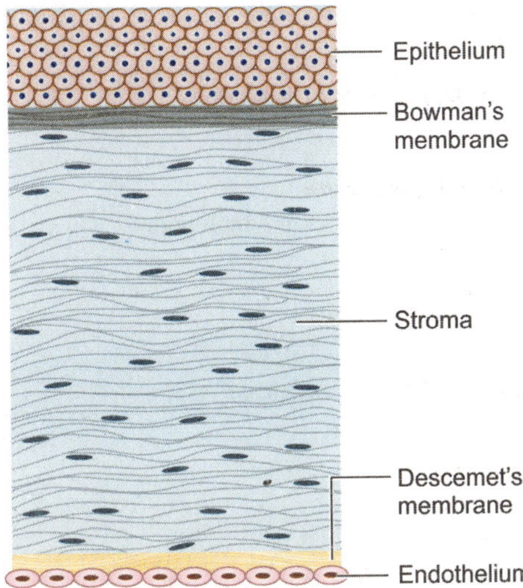

Fig: Layers of cornea

Different Layers of Cornea

- *Transparent*[Q], *avascular*[Q] & watch glass like structure
- Forms anterior 1/6th of the outer fibrous coat of the eyeball
- Thickness is more in the periphery than in the centre
- Oxygen is mostly derived directly from the air through *tear film* with a small contribution from the limbal capillaries
- Glucose supply for corneal metabolism is *mainly (90%) derived from the aqueous*[Q] & supplemented (10%) by the limbal capillaries.
- Refractive power of the cornea is about *45D*[Q] which is 3/4th of total refractive power of the eye (60D) [Q]
- "The transparency of the cornea is due to its *relatively dehydrated state*[Q], *absence of blood vessels*[Q] *& pigment, uniform refractive index of all the layers & uniform spacing of the collagen fibrils*[Q] *in the stroma" (Parson 20th/182)*
- The adult human cornea measures *11 to 12 mm horizontally*[Q] & *9 to 11 mm vertically*[Q]

ENT

111. Ans. a. Small..., c. Healin.... & d. It is ....

[Ref: P. L. Dhingra 6th/65; Logan Turner 10th/438-39]

Secretory Otitis Media

◈ *Logan Turner 10th/438-39*

- *The question of whether or not to insert a grommet tube to ventilate the middle-ear cavity after routine myringotomy & aspiration is debated in literature. Shah examined a series in whom a grommet had been inserted anteriorly in one year & he found in period b/w 6week & 6 months postoperatively that 80% of the ears with the grommet had normal hearing compared with 20% of cases with no grommet*
- *If a grommet is inserted it may be placed posteriorly or anteriorly depending upon the preference of the surgeon*
- *Those who place it anteriorly regard this as being more physiological because air normally enters the tympanum through an anterior orifice & it is in the anterior part of the tympanum that the secretory cells abound & have to be dried off*
- *While the tube remains in place (from 2month to 2 years & the period is longer with the anteriorly placed tube), care must be taken to avoid water entering the middle ear through the grommet*
- *The grommet is either rejected spontaneously or may be removed, preferably under an anaesthetic because this is momentarily painful. Healing occurs more quickly after extrusion than after removal*
- Thin scars on the tympanic is more frequent in the ears that had had grommets which suggests that grommets may inhibit healing
- *Recurrence (after initial myringotomy, aspiration & grommet insertion) are once again treated by myringotomy & at the second or certainly at the third myringotomy, most surgeon will insert a grommet. Maswon reports that 35% of cases require a second grommet & 11% need a third*
- ***Tympanoscelerosis*** *is seen much more frequently in children since secretory otitis media became prevalent & it appears to occur more often if grommets are inserted*

Grommet Insertion

◈ *P. L. Dhingra 6th/65*

- If myringotomy & aspiration combined with medical measures have not helped & fluid recurs, a grommet is inserted to provide continued aeration of middle air
- It is left in place for weeks or months or till it is spontaneously extruded

"Ventilating tubes can be placed within an atelectatic TM in an attempt to equalize the pressure and allow the TM to return to its normal anatomic position. Fifty percent of patients with pressure equalization tubes experience at least one episode of otorrhea, and 3% will have symptoms persisting beyond 6 weeks. After extrusion of the tube, the majority of iatrogenic TM perforations will heal. Residual perforation rates are 2 to 3% for button or grommet tubes but as high as 47% for T tubes" (Ballenger Head & Neck Surgery 16th/Chap 10)

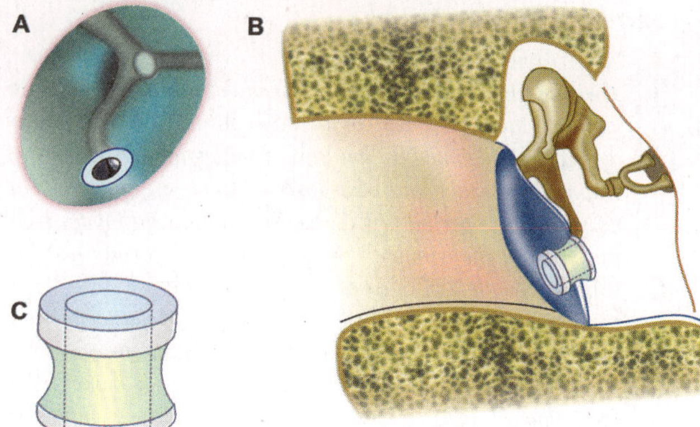

Fig: Grommet in tympanic membrane (A & B), the grommet (C)

112. Ans. b. Clinica…., c. Nasal…, d. Hyper…. & e. Anti-….

[Ref: P. L. Dhingra 6th/170; Logan Turner 10th/40, 373; Ballenger Head & Neck Surgery 16th/Chap 33]

Vasomotor Rhinitis (VMR)

◈ *P. L. Dhingra 6th/170*

- *It is nonallergic rhinitis but clinically simulating nasal allergy with symptom of nasal obstruction, rhinorrhoea & sneezing*
- Autonomic nervous system is unstable in case of VMR. Nasal mucosa is also hyper-reactive & responds to several non-specific stimuli e.g., change in temperature, humidity, blasts of air, small amount of dust or smoke
- *The condition usually persists throughout the year & all the tests of nasal allergy are negative*
- *"VMR: Swelling (or hypertrophy) of inferior turbinate is frequently seen & may appear as most obvious cause of obstruction"*
- ***Symptom:*** *Paroxysmal sneezing, excessive rhinorrhoea, nasal obstruction & postnasal drip*
- ***Sign:*** *Nasal mucosa over the turbinates is generally congested & hypertrophic. In some, it may be normal*
- ***Complication:*** *Long standing cases develop nasal polyp, hypertrophic rhinitis & sinusitis*
- ***Medical treatment:*** *Avoidance of physical factor which provoke symptoms; anti-histaminics & oral nasal decongestant; systemic steroid*
- ***Surgical treatment:*** *Relieving of nasal obstruction (reduce size of nasal turbinates, correction of deviated nasal septum & removal of nasal polyp) & vidian neurectomy*

Idiopathic (Vasomotor) Rhinitis

◈ *Ballenger Head & Neck Surgery 16th/Chap 33*

- The term "idiopathic rhinitis" relates to any inflammation of the nose the cause of which is unknown.
- It is the *diagnosis of exclusion* as underlying causative or contributory factors can often be found if carefully sought.
- *Therapy may encompass avoidance of obvious triggers*, but most patients require medication, the mainstays of which are topical *corticosteroids* that are safe for long-term use.
- Surgery has a limited role to play. Vidian neurectomy has had a vogue but has largely been abandoned as the effects are unpredictable and at best short-lived. *Correction of septal deformity and/or turbinate hypertrophy is occasionally indicated if medication fails.*

113. Ans. b. Carotid Artery & d. Brachial plexus

[Ref: P. L. Dhingra 6th/388-89; P. L. Dhigra 5th/396; CSDT11th/1301; L & B 26th/705, 25th/733]

Classical Radical Neck Dissection

◈ *L & B 26th/705, 25th/733*

Structures Removed are

- Cervical lymphatics and lymph node
- *Internal jugular vein*
- *Accessory nerve*[Q]
- *Submandibular gland*[Q]
- *Sternocleidomastiod muscle*
- *Tail of parotid* (*P. L. Dhigra 5th/396*)
- Omohypoid muscle

Structure Saved are

◈ *P. L. Dhigra 5th/396*

- Carotid artery
- Brachial plexus, phrenic nerve, *vagus nerve*, cervical sympathetic chain, marginal mandibular br. of facial, lingual & hypoglossal nerves

"RND does not removes nodes of postauricular, suboccipital, parotid (except those in tail), facial, retropharyngeal & pretracheal regions" (P. L. Dhigra 5th/396.)

Modified Radical Neck dissection

◈ *L & B 26th/705, 25th/733*

Structures preserved are one or more of the followings–

- Accessory nerve
- Sternocleidomastiod muscle
- Internal jugular vein

114. Ans. b. Perforat…, c. Persistant sinus & d. Crust….

[Ref: Harrison 19th/2182-84; P. L. Dhingra 6th/159-60; Logan Turner 10th/60; Ballenger Head & Neck Surgery 16th/Chap 33]

> *Note: Wegener's granulomatosis is not mentioned as aetiology of nasal polyp (P. L. Dhingra 6th/ 171)*

Granulomatosis with Polyangiitis (Wegener's)

◈ *P. L. Dhingra 6th/159-60*

- *Granulomatosis with polyangiitis (Wegener's)* is a distinct clinicopathologic entity characterized by granulomatous vasculitis of the *upper and lower respiratory tracts together with glomerulonephritis.*

- In addition, variable degrees of disseminated vasculitis involving both small arteries and veins may occur.
- Lung involvement typically appears as multiple, bilateral, nodular cavitary infiltrates, which on biopsy almost invariably reveal the typical necrotizing granulomatous vasculitis.

◈ *Harrison 19th/2182-84*

- *Early symptoms includes clear or blood-stained nasal discharge which later become purulent. The patient often complains of persistent cold or sinus*
- *Nasal findings include crusting, granulations, septal perforation & a saddle nose*
- *Destruction may also involve eye, orbit, palate, oral cavity, or oropharynx*
- "In the nose, the swollen, inflamed mucosa produces blockage and blood-stained crusting. There may be destruction of the septum with a *characteristic implosion of the nasal bridge*. The nasopharynx, ears, mouth, larynx, trachea, cranial nerves, and orbit may all be involved" *(Ballenger Head & Neck Surgery 16th/Chap 33)*

"The nose and paranasal sinuses are involved in over 90% of cases of Wegener granulomatosis. It is often not realized that involvement at these sites is more common than involvement of lungs or kidneys. Examination shows bloodstained crusts and friable mucosa" (CMDT 2015/222)

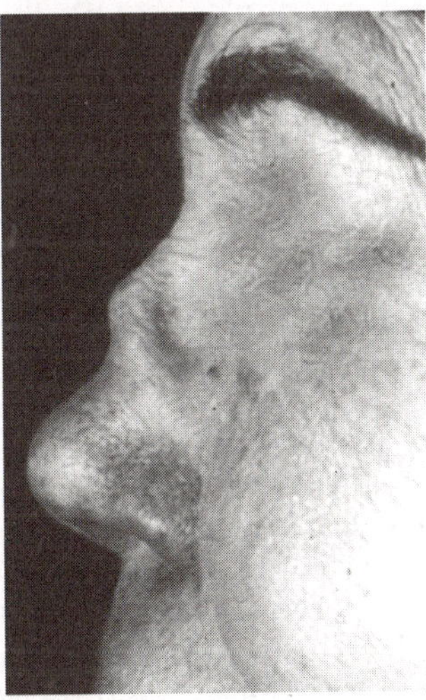

Fig: Photograph showing typical collapse of the nasal bridge in a patient with Wegener's granulomatosis

115. Ans. a. U/l hearing... c. Most..... & d. Sens.....

[Ref: P. L. Dhingra 6th/112-14; Logan Turner 10th/339-44]

Vestibular Schwannoma (Acoustic Neuroma)

◈ *P. L. Dhingra 6th/112-14*

- It accounts for 80% of all cerebellopontine angle tumours & 10% of all the brain tumours
- It is a benign, encapsulated, extremely slow-growing tumour of the VIIIth nerve. Bilateral tumours are seen in patients with neurofibromatosis
- This tumour always arise from the Schwann cells of the vestibular, but rarely from the cochlear division of VIIIth nerve within the internal auditory canal. As it expand, it causes widening & erosion of canal & then appears in the cerebellopontine angle. Here, it may grow anterosuperiorly to involve Vth nerve or inferiorly to involve IXth, Xth & XIth cranial nerves
- **Age & Sex:** It is mostly seen in age group of 40-60 years. Both sex are equally affected

◈ *Logan Turner 10th/339*

- 90% are unilateral
- Commonest presenting symptoms are *unilateral deafness or tinnitus* or a combination of both
- Commonest nerve of origin is the superior vestibular, followed by inferior vestibular & rarely the cochlear
- They are commoner in females than males in the ratio of 3: 2 (c. f Dhingra, equal incidence) & usually present in fourth decade or above

◈ *CMDT 2015/212-13*

- Eighth cranial nerve schwannomas are among the most common intracranial tumors. *Most are unilateral*, but about 5% are associated with the hereditary syndrome, neurofibromatosis type 2, in which bilateral eighth nerve tumors may be accompanied by meningiomas and other intracranial and spinal tumors.
- These benign lesions arise within the internal auditory canal and gradually grow to involve the *cerebellopontine angle*, eventually compressing the pons and resulting in hydrocephalus.
- Their typical auditory symptoms are *unilateral hearing loss* with a deterioration of speech discrimination exceeding that predicted by the degree of pure tone loss.
- Nonclassic presentations, such as sudden unilateral hearing loss, are fairly common. Any individual with a unilateral or asymmetric *sensorineural hearing loss* should be evaluated for an intracranial mass lesion. Vestibular dysfunction more often takes the form of continuous dysequilibrium than episodic vertigo.
- **Diagnosis** is made by enhanced MRI.
- **Treatment** consists of observation, microsurgical excision, or stereotactic radiotherapy, depending on such factors as patient age, underlying health, and size of the tumor at presentation.

116. Ans. b. Thyroarytenoid & e. Cricothyroid

[Ref: P. L. Dhingra 6th/283; Logan Turner 10th/146; BDC 4th/Vol. III 243]

Muscle of Larynx

- Abductor Posterior cricoarytenoid[Q]
- Adductor (3 muscle given in Dhingra): Lateral cricoarytenoid, Interarytenoid (Transverse arytenoids) & thyroarytenoid[Q]

Note: 4th muscle given in BDC not in Dhingra !!: Cricothyroid

- Tensor Cricothyroid & vocalis[Q] (internal part of thyroarytenoid)
  - *All muscle of larynx are supplied by Recurrent Laryngeal nerve*[Q] except the cricothyroid muscle. The latter receive its innervation from External Laryngeal nerve[Q] - a branch of superior Laryngeal nerve
- **Sensory**
  - Above vocal cords - Internal Laryngeal nerve a branch of *Superior Laryngeal nerve*[Q]
  - Below vocal cords - *Recurrent Laryngeal nerve*[Q]s

117. Ans. b. Commonly occur at Junction of middle & posterior 1/3

[Ref: P. L. Dhingra 6th/303-04; Logan Turner 10th/166-67; L & B 26th/695-96]

Vocal Nodules (Singer's or Screamer's Nodes)

◈ *P. L. Dhingra 6th/303-04*

- Their size varies from that of pin-head to half a pea
- They are the result of vocal trauma when person speaks in unnatural low tones for prolonged periods or at high intensities
- They mostly affect teachers, actors, vendors or pop singers. They are also seen in school going children who are too assertive & talkative
- Patients complains of hoarseness. Vocal fatigue & pain in the neck on prolonged phonation are other common symptoms
- Early cases of vocal nodules can be treated conservatively by educating the patient in proper use of voice. With this treatment, many nodules in children disappear completely
- Surgery is required for large nodules or nodules of long standing in adults. They are excised with precision under operating microscope either with cold instruments or laser avoiding any trauma to the underlying vocal ligament
- Speech therapy & re-education in voice production are essential to prevent their recurrence

Vocal nodules (Singer's or Screamer's nodes): They appear symmetrically on the free edge of vocal cord, at the junction of anterior one-third, with the posterior two-third, as this is the area of maximum vibration of cord & thus subject to maximum trauma" (P. L. Dhingra 6th/303)

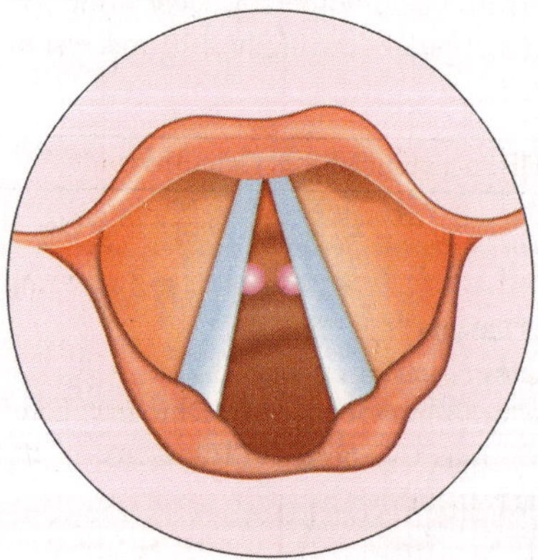

Fig: Vocal nodules. Typically, they form at the junction of anterior one-third with posterior two-thirds of vocal cords

118. Ans. a. Fun…, c. Aller…. & e. Surgi…

[Ref: P. L. Dhingra 6th/196; Logan Turner 10th/51-52; Ballenger's Otorhinolaryngology 16th/764, 770]

Allergic Fungal Sinusitis

◈ *P. L. Dhingra 6th/196*

- It is an *allergic reaction* to the causative fungus & presents with sinunasal polyposis & mucin. The latter contains eosinophils, Charcot-Leyden crystals & fungal hyphae
- There is *no invasion of the sinus mucosa with fungus*
- Usually more than one sinus are involved on one or both sides
- CT scan shows *mucosal thickening with hyperdense areas*
- There may be expansion of the sinus or bone erosion due to pressure, *but no fungal invasion*
- Treatment is endoscopic surgical clearance of the sinuses with provision of drainage & ventilation. This is combined with pre & postoperative systemic steroids

Four Different Varieties of Fungal Infection of Sinuses are Seen

◈ *P. L. Dhingra 6th/196*

- Fungal ball
- Allergic fungal sinusitis
- Chronic invasive sinusitis
- Fulminant fungal sinusitis

◈ *Ballenger's Otorhinolaryngology 16th/764, 770*

- Most patients with AFS are immunocompetent and present with features of refractory sinusitis and nasal polyposis. *Many also have a history of atopy or asthma.*
- The pathogenesis of AFS is incompletely understood, but evidence supports a Gell and Coombs *type I (IgE-mediated) immune response to fungal antigens. Type III and IV immune responses may also be involved.*
- The pathologic hallmark of AFS is "allergic mucin, " consisting of eosinophils, Charcot-Leyden crystals, and *scattered fungal hyphae.* Although AFS is not thought to be invasive, bony erosion is seen on computed tomographic (CT) scans in 20% of reported cases.
- Laboratory abnormalities include eosinophilia, elevated total serum IgE, and elevated IgE radioallergosorbent test (RAST) titers to specific fungi. The *diagnosis of AFS is confirmed by demonstration of allergic mucin and culture of the fungus.*
- It is treated by surgical débridement and aeration of the involved sinus followed by the *use of systemic and topical intranasal corticosteroids.*
- Recurrence is common and may be heralded by rising serum total IgE levels.
- Specific immunotherapy with multiple relevant fungal and nonfungal antigens has reduced the necessity for corticosteroid therapy, while preventing recurrence of the disease and the need for repeat surgery

119. Ans. b. Cholestetoma., d. Perfo…. & e. Sero….

[Ref: P. L. Dhingra 6th/29-34; Logan Turner 10th/323-25]

"Acoustic neuroma & presbycusis causes sensorineural HL" *(P. L. Dhingra 6th/32)*

Characteristic of Conductive HL

- Negative Rinne test i. e BC>AC
- Weber lateralized to poorer ear
- Normal absolute bone conduction
- Low frequencies affected more
- Loss is not more than 60 dB
- Speech discrimination is good
- Audiometry shows bone conduction better than air conduction with air-bone gap. Greater the air-bone gap, more is the conductive loss

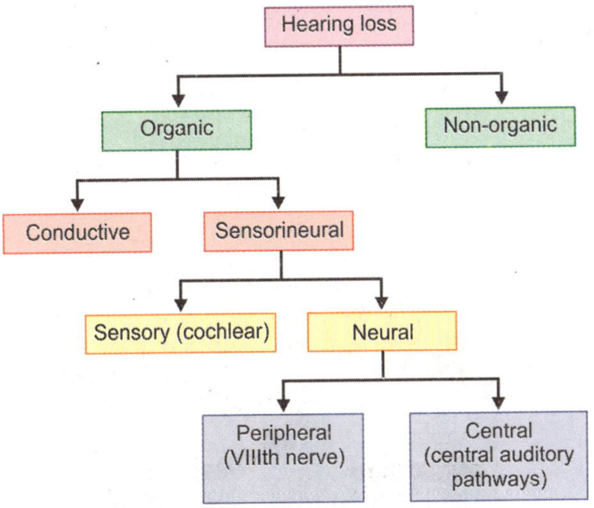

Fig: Classification of HL

Table: Congenital causes of conductive hearing loss

- Meatal atresia
- Fixation of stapes footplate
- Fixation of malleus head
- Ossicular discontinuity
- Congenital cholesteatoma

Table: Acquired causes of conductive hearing loss

External ear	Any obstruction in the ear canal, *e.g.,* wax, foreign body, furuncle, acute inflammatory swelling, benign or malignant tumour or atresia of canal.
Middle ear	• Perforation of tympanic membrane, traumatic or infective
	• Fluid in the middle ear, *e.g.,* acute otitis media, serous otitis media or haemotympanum
	• Mass in middle ear, *e.g.,* benign or malignant tumour
	• Disruption of ossicles, *e.g.,* trauma to ossicular chanin, chronic suppurative otitis media, cholesteatoma
	• Fixation of ossicles, *e.g.,* otosclerosis, tympanosclerosis, adhesive otitis media
	• Eustachian tube blockage, *e.g.,* retracted tympanic membrane, serous otitis media

120. Ans. a. Occur..., b. Hemi... & d. Tre....

[Ref; www. ncbi. nlm. nih. gov/pubmed/68222; Ballenger's Otorhinolaryngology 16th/962, 963f, 964]

Defects of the Anterior Mandibular Arch

◈ *Ballenger's 16th/962, 963f, 964*

- *Defects of the anterior mandibular arch* cause severe problems that cannot be reversed without formal reconstruction. These problems combine to produce the classic *"Andy Gump" deformity*, named after the 1917 comic strip character whose appearance suggests loss of the anterior mandibular arch.
- When the anterior mandibular arch is removed, there is usually an associated soft tissue deficit too large to close primarily. A *mandibular reconstruction plate* can be used to secure the remaining mandibular bodies and restore continuity to the arch.
- As the plate and screws used for reconstruction of the anterior mandibular arch are subject to multiplanar shear, torsion, bending, and loading, the high failure rate of plates not secured to a continuous bony arch is not surprising.
- Functionally, resection of the anterior arch of the mandible results in disabilities, including drooling and interference with eating, directly related to the amount of bone removed. Aesthetically, this "Andy Gump" deformity results in an inferior cosmetic appearance.
- For instance, *resection of the anterior mandibular arch produces the "Andy Gump" deformity*, which is a complete loss of anterior oromuscular support and oral competence. Because this is such a debilitating functional and esthetic problem, it is important to reconstruct this defect at the time of resection.

Andy Gump" deformity: *(From various internet sites http://www.headandneckcancerguide. org/glossary/andy-gump-deformity/)*

"Named after a character in an early 20th-century comic strip who had an altered facial profile ***due to a missing lower jawbone, or mandible****. The character was likely modeled after a patient who had undergone an early surgery for head and neck cancer that involved the removal of the lower jaw. Not only did patients have a different facial profile as the result of such a surgery, but they* ***also had problems with eating and drooling****" (http://www.headandneckcancerguide. org/glossary/andy-gump-deformity/)*

"Resecting the anterior arch of the mandible beyond the midline without reconstructing the bone with loss of the anterior attachments of the suprahyoid muscles (digastric, geniohyoid, mylohyoid, genioglossus) leads to an Andy Gump deformity with loss of oral competence, drooling, and a very poor cosmetic outcome. The mandible forms the peripheral border of the floor of mouth, and may be involved by floor of mouth tumours or may have to be divided (mandibulotomy) or resected (alveolectomy/marginal mandibulectomy/segmental mandibulectomy/hemimandibulectomy)" *(https://vula. uct. ac. za/access/content/group)*

Types of Mandibulectomy

◈ *https://books. google. co. in/books?id=sMJVzFZGFkcC&pg*

- Marginal mandibulectomy- where the alveolar part is removed, preserving lower border (so can prevent Andy Gump deformity)

- Segmental mandibulectomy
- Arch preserving mandibulectomy (Also can prevent Andy Gump deformity)
- Hemi mandibulectomy

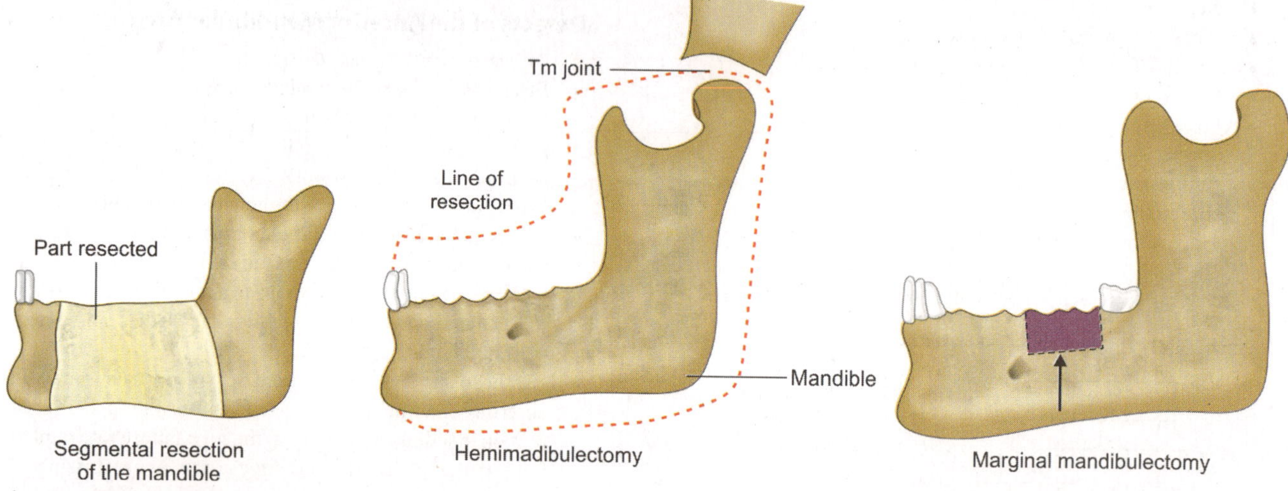

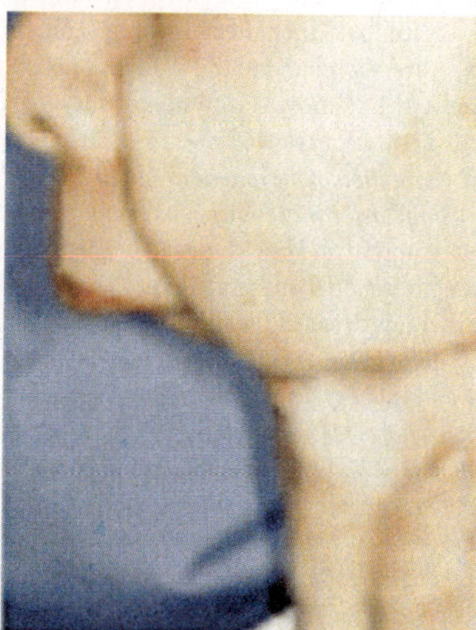

Fig: Unreconstructed mandibulectomy defect

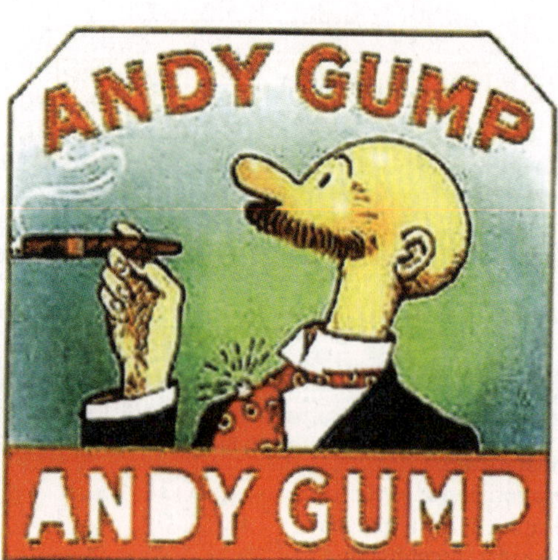

Fig: "Andy Gump" deformity

121. Ans. a. Bronchiectasis, b. Atelectasi, c. Subcutaneous...... & d. Pneumothorax

[Ref: P. L. Dhingra 6th/321-22, 440, P. J. Mehta 20th/143]

Collapse/Atelectasis of lung: *Caused by obstruction, compression or loss of surfactant" (P. J. Mehta 20th/143)*

"Emphysematous bullae may rupture causing spontaneous pneumothorax. A foreign body may shift from one side to other causing change in physical sign. A retained foreign body may later give rise to pneumonitis, bronchiectasis or lung abscess" (P. L. Dhingra 6th/321)

"Bronchiectasis is an abnormal & permanent dilation of one or more bronchi. It may be due to cystic fibrosis, infection etc" *(P. J. Mehta 20th/175)*

Table *(P. L. Dhingra 6th/321)*: **Symptoms & sign of foreign bodies at different level**

Site of foreign bodies	Symptoms & sign
Larynx	Complete obstruction leading to death Partial obstruction: stridor, hoarseness, cough, respiratory difficulty
Trachea	Choking, stridor, wheeze, cough, palpatory thud, audible slap
Bronchi	Cough, wheeze & diminished air entry to lung forms a triad Respiratory distress with swelling of foreign body ***Lung collapse, emphysema, pneumonitis, bronchiectasis or lung abscess*** are late feature

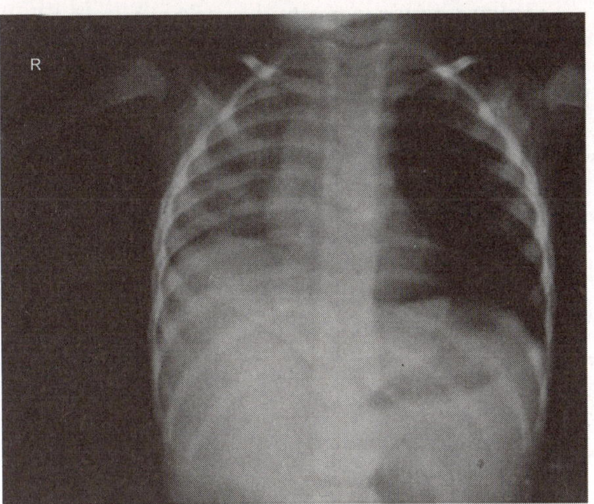

Fig: PA Chest in a child with a radiolucent foreign body (a peanut) in right bronchus. (i) collapse of right lung and shift of mediastinum to the same side. (ii) Raised dome of diaphragm on the right (iii) Emphysema left lung

MEDICINE

122. Ans. c. TOF

[Ref: Harrison 19th/1521-22, 1526; O. P. Ghai 8th/415; P. J. M 20th/437]

"**VSD:** Increased pulmonary arterial pressure *results from increased pulmonary blood flow and/or resistance, the latter usually the result of obstructive, obliterative structural changes within the pulmonary vascular bed" (Harrison 19th/1522)*

"**ASD:** *Examination usually reveals a prominent RV impulse and palpable pulmonary artery pulsation. The first heart sound is normal or split, with accentuation of the tricuspid valve closure sound. Increased flow across the pulmonic valve is responsible for a midsystolic pulmonary outflow murmur." (Harrison 19th/1521)*

"**TOF:** *When the RV outflow obstruction is severe, pulmonary blood flow is reduced markedly, and a large volume of desaturated systemic venous blood shunts right-to-left across the VSD. Severe cyanosis and erythrocytosis occur, and symptoms of systemic hypoxemia are prominent" (Harrison 19th/1526)*

VSD

◈ *O. P. Ghai 8th/415*

- There is increased flow of blood across pulmonary valve producing ejection systolic murmur at pulmonary valve.
- The large volume of blood passing through the lungs is recognized in the chest X-ray as pulmonary plethora

P. J. M 20th/437: Writes

Pulmonary oligmeia: Fallot's tetrad & triad, Truncus arteriosus, severe pulmonary stenosis

Pulmonary plethora: Left ventricular failure, valvular heart disease (MS, MR, AS, AR)

◈ *(https://quizlet. com/1255665/defects-with-increased- pulmonary-blood-flow-flash-cards/)*

- The common manifestations of defects with increased pulmonary blood flow: tachypnea, tachycardia, and CHF
- The three most common types of defects are: VSD, ASD, and PDA

"Congenital heart defects may cause cyanosis. Often, an obvious cardiac reason for cyanosis is decreased PBF; however, several congenital heart defects cause systemic cyanosis with increased PBF, such as TGA, truncus arteriosus, and TAPVR"

123. Ans. b. Knee jerk..., c. Motor... & e. Root...

[Ref: Harrison 19th/115, 1791, 2651; Robbins 9th/; P. J. M 20th/336; L & B 26th/; CMDT 2015/1670]

Note: Ankle jerk may lost in both

Cauda Equina Syndrome

◈ *CMDT 2015/1670*

- It often presents with bowel or bladder symptoms (or both) and is an emergency.
- It is suggested by *urinary retention or incontinence, saddle anesthesia, decreased anal sphincter tone or fecal incontinence, bilateral lower extremity weakness, and progressive neurologic deficits.*

Table *(P. J. M 20th/336)*: **Differences b/w Conus medullaris & Cauda equina**

Features	Conus medullaris	Cauda equine
1. Root pains	Absent	Present
2. Sensory change	Saddle shaped distribution with perianal anesthesia, Usually symmetrical	May invoke any part of the lower limbs asymmetrically
3. Motor changes	Absent	Marked motor changes with wasting-asymmetrical
4. Sphincters	Always involved (yearly)	May be involved (late)
5. Reflexes	Knee jerk normal; ankle jerk lost; plantar extensor	Knee & ankle jerks may be lost
6. Impotence	Frequent	Less frequent

"Cauda equina syndrome is characterized by low back pain; diminished sensation over the buttocks, posterior-superior thighs, and perineal area in a saddle distribution; *rectal and bladder dysfunction*; sexual impotence; *absent bulbocavernous, patellar, and Achilles'* reflexes; and variable amount of lower-extremity weakness. This reflects compression of nerve roots as they form the cauda equina after leaving the spinal cord. The majority of cauda equina tumors are primary tumors of glial or nerve sheath origin; metastases are very rare" *(Harrison 19th/1791)*

"The conus medullaris is the tapered caudal termination of the spinal cord, comprising the sacral and single coccygeal segments. The distinctive conus syndrome consists of bilateral saddle anesthesia (S3-S5), *prominent bladder and bowel dysfunction (urinary retention and incontinence with lax anal tone),* and impotence. The bulbocavernosus (S2-S4) and anal (S4-S5) reflexes are absent. Muscle strength is largely preserved. By contrast, lesions of the cauda equina, the nerve roots derived from the lower cord, are characterized by low back and radicular pain, asymmetric leg weakness and sensory loss, variable areflexia in the lower extremities, and *relative sparing of bowel and bladder function.* Mass lesions in the lower spinal canal often produce a mixed clinical picture with elements of both cauda equina and conus medullaris syndromes" *(Harrison 19th/2651)*

124. Ans. a. Increase... & e. Analgesics...

[Ref: Harrison 19th/110; Emergency Medicine by SN Chugh 4th/235-38; CMDT 2015/957; L & B 26th/605]

"Headache due to intracranial pathology or raised intracranial tension worsens during coughing, straining or adopting the head in low posture" (Emergency Medicine by SN Chugh 4th/237)

"Unilateral pulsating/throbbing headache are usually vascular such as migraine & cluster headaches" (Emergency Medicine by SN Chugh 4th/237)

"Acute severe headache commonly suggests subarachnoid haemorrhage & meningitis. Progressive worsening headache suggests raised ICP" (Emergency Medicine by SN Chugh 4th/235)

"Analgesics & simple analgesic combinations are more useful for mild to moderate headache such as migraine, tension-type or cluster headache. Corticosteroid are recommended in acute headache due to raised ICP" (Emergency Medicine by SN Chugh 4th/235-38)

Raised CSF Pressure Headache

Harrison 19th/110

- Raised CSF pressure is well recognized as a cause of headache. Brain imaging can often reveal the cause, such as a space-occupying lesion. NDPH due to raised CSF pressure can be the presenting symptom for patients with idiopathic intracranial hypertension (pseudotumor cerebri) without visual problems, particularly when the fundi are normal. Persistently raised intracranial pressure can trigger chronic migraine.
- These patients typically present with a history of *generalized headache that is present on waking and improves as the day goes on.* It is *generally worse with recumbency.*
- Visual obscurations are frequent.
- The diagnosis is relatively straightforward when papilledema is present, but the possibility must be considered even in patients without funduscopic changes. Formal visual field testing should be performed even in the absence of overt ophthalmic involvement.
- *Headache on rising in the morning or nocturnal headache is also characteristic of obstructive sleep apnea or poorly controlled hypertension.*
- *Management: Riased ICT needs diagnostic evaluation by CT scan or MRI. For control, I. V mannitol or steroids may be helpful- (Emergency Medicine by SN Chugh 4th/239)*

ALSO KNOW

Arterial Hypertension

Ballenger Head & Neck Surgery 16th/Chap 35

- *Arterial hypertension can be acute or chronic. Chronic hypertension is not typically associated with headache. On the other hand, acute hypertension certainly may cause cephalalgia.*
- *Typically, headache begins with diastolic pressures greater than 115 mm Hg. It is throbbing, associated with nausea, and does not respond to analgesics.*

125. Ans. d. AR & e. PR

[Ref: Harrison 19th/Chap 51e- 11536, 1550, 1449; P. J. M 20th/199-200]

"Early Diastolic Murmurs: Chronic AR results in a highpitched, blowing, decrescendo, early to mid-diastolic murmur that begins after the aortic component of S2 (A2) and is best heard at the second right interspace" (Harrison 19th/Chap 51e-1)

"Pulmonic regurgitation (PR) results in a decrescendo, early to middiastolic murmur (Graham Steell murmur) that begins after the pulmonic component of S2 (P2), is best heard at the 2nd left interspace, and radiates along the left sternal border" (Harrison 19th/Chap 51e-1)

Table: *(Harrison 19th/Chap 51e-1)*

Early Diastolic Murmurs

Aortic Regurgitation

- **Valvular:** Congenital (bicuspid valve), rheumatic deformity, endocarditis, prolapse, trauma, post-valvulotomy
- **Dilation of valve ring:** aorta dissection, annuloaortic ectasia, cystic medial degeneration, hypertension, ankylosing spondylitis
- **Widening of commissures:** syphilis

Pulmonic Regurgitation

- **Valvular:** Post-valvulotomy, endocarditis, rheumatic fever, carcinoid
- **Dilation of valve ring:** Pulmonary hypertension; Marfan syndrome
- **Congenital:** Isolated or associated with tetralogy of Fallot, VSD, pulmonic stenosis

Mid-Diastolic Murmurs

- Mitral: Mitral stenosis; Carey-Coombs murmur (mid-diastolic apical murmur in acute rheumatic fever); Increased flow across nonstenotic mitral valve (*e.g.,* MR, VSD, PDA, highoutput states, and complete heart block)
- Tricuspid: Tricuspid stenosis; Increased flow across nonstenotic tricuspid valve (*e.g.,* TR, ASD, and anomalous pulmonary venous return)
- Left and right atrial tumors (myxoma)
- Severe AR (Austin Flint murmur)

Diastolic murmur *(P. J. M 20th/199-200)*

- *These are the murmurs which occur b/w the second heart sound & the first heart sound, during any part of diastole*
- *Early diastolic murmur: AR, PR, Graham Steel's murmur (in PR due to pulmonary hypertension)*
- *Mid diastolic murmur: MS, TS, Carey Coombs murmur, Austin Flint murmur, Flow murmur (ASD, VSD, PDA, MR, TR)*
- Late diastolic or presystolic murmur: MS, TS, Left atrial myxoma, right atrial myxoma

Systolic Murmur *(P. J. M 20th/199)*

- TOF- Mid-systolic or ejection systolic

126. Ans. a. Used. in..., b. Efficacy... & c. Can...

[Ref: Harrison 19th/2590-93; Emergency Medicine by SN Chugh 4th/238-39; KDT 7th/177-79; CMDT 2015/954-56; Katzung 13th/283-85]

Drug Therapy of Migraine

◈ *KDT 7th/177-79*

- *"The use of triptans should be restricted to treatment of acute attacks of moderate to severe migraine not responding to analgesics or their combinations"- (KDT 7th/179)*
- *Ergotamine & sumatriptan should not be administered within 24 hours of each others"- (KDT 7th/179)*

Table *(KDT 7th/177)*: **Drug therapy of migraine**

Severity	Drug Therapy
Mild	Simple analgesics/NSAIDS or their combinations (±antiemetics)
Moderate	NSAIDS combinations/a triptans/ergot alkaloids (+ antiemetics)
Severe	a triptans/ergot alkaloids (+ antiemetics) + prophylaxis (propranolol/other β blockers; Amitriptyline/other tricyclic antidepressants; Flunarizine/other Ca^{2+} channel blockers; Valproate/topiramate

"Triptans are rapidly effective agent for *aborting attacks*. Triptans may cause nausea and vomiting. They should probably be avoided in women who are pregnant, in patients with hemiplegic or basilar migraine, and in patients with risk factors for stroke (such as hypertension, prior stroke or transient ischemic attack, diabetes mellitus, hypercholesterolemia, obesity). Triptans are contraindicated in patients with coronary or peripheral vascular disease. Patients often experience greater benefit when the *triptan is combined with naproxen (500 mg)" (CMDT 2015/955)*

5-HT1B/1D Receptor Agonists

◈ *Harrison 19th/2590-91*

- Oral Stimulation of 5-HT1B/1D receptors can stop ***an acute migraine*** *attack.*
- Ergotamine and dihydroergotamine are nonselective receptor agonists, whereas the triptans are selective 5-HT1B/1D receptor agonists.
- A variety of triptans, 5-HT1B/1D receptor agonists—sumatriptan, almotriptan, eletriptan, frovatriptan, naratriptan, rizatriptan, and zolmitriptan—are now available for the treatment of migraine.
- Unfortunately, ***monotherapy with a selective oral 5-HT-1B/1D receptor agonist does not result in rapid, consistent, and complete relief of migraine in all patients.***
- Because the clinical studies demonstrating the efficacy of ergotamine in migraine predated the clinical trial methodologies used with the triptans, it is difficult to assess the clinical efficacy of ergotamine versus the triptans. ***In general, ergotamine appears to have a much higher incidence of nausea*** *than triptans but less headache recurrence.*
- The drugs that have been approved by the FDA for the **prophylactic treatment** of migraine include ***propranolol, timolol, sodium valproate, topiramate, and methysergide*** (not available). In addition, a number of other drugs appear to display prophylactic efficacy. This group includes ***amitriptyline, nortriptyline, flunarizine, phenelzine, gabapentin, and cyproheptadine.***

127. Ans. a. ACE... & d. Excision...

[Ref: Harrison 19th/1628- 29, 1618; P. J. M 20th/52; CMDT 2015/908-09]

"ACE inhibitors *are useful in renovascular hypertension. They are C/I in bilateral renal artery stenosis. These drugs are useful in hypertensive diabetics because of neutral effect of carbohydrate metabolism. In addition they decreases microalbuminuria" (P. J. M 20th/52)*

Renal Aretry Stenosis: Treatment *(CMDT 2015/908-09, CMDT 2015/908-09, CMDT 2015/909, CMDT 2015/908)*

- While restoring renal blood flow and perfusion seems intuitively beneficial for high-grade occlusive lesions, revascularization procedures also pose hazards and expense.
- Patients with FMD are commonly younger females with otherwise normal vessels and a long life expectancy. These patients often respond well to *percutaneous renal artery angioplasty*. If BP can be controlled to goal levels and kidney function remains stable in patients with ARAS, it may be argued that medical therapy with follow-up for disease progression is equally effective.
- Medical therapy should include *blockade of the renin-angiotensin system, attainment of goal BPs, cessation of tobacco, statins, and aspirin.*
- *Renal revascularization is now often reserved for patients failing medical therapy or developing additional complications.*
- Although renal blood flow usually can be restored by endovascular stenting, recovery of renal function is limited to about 25% of cases, with no change in 50% and some deterioration evident in others.
- When hypertension is refractory to effective therapy, revascularization offers real benefits.

"ARF is precipitated by ACE inhibitors in patients with b/l renal stenosis due to dilation of efferent arterioles & fall in glomerular filtration pressure. ACE inhibitors are contraindicated" (KDT 7th/502)
"The ACE inhibitors are one of the first choice drugs in all grades of essential as well as renovascular hypertension (except those with b/l renal stenosis)" (KDT 7th/502)

- Treatment of atherosclerotic ischemic renal disease is controversial. Options include medical management, *angioplasty with or without stenting, and surgical bypass.* A 2009 study has shown that intervention is no better than optimal medical management in typical patients in whom renal artery stenosis was diagnosed via gold-standard mechanisms.
- Angioplasty might reduce the number of antihypertensive medications but does not significantly change the

progression of kidney dysfunction in comparison to patients medically managed. *Stenting produces significantly better angioplastic results.* However, blood pressure is equally improved, and serum creatinines are similar at 6 months of observation compared with both angioplasty and stents. Angioplasty is equally as effective as, and safer than, surgical revision.

- **Essentials of Diagnosis**
  - *Produced by atherosclerotic occlusive disease (80–90% of patients) or fibromuscular dysplasia (10–15%),*
  - *Hypertension &*
  - *Acute renal failure in patients starting therapy with an ACE inhibitor.*
- *Atherosclerotic is chemic renal disease accounts for nearly all cases of renal artery stenosis. Fibromuscular dysplasia can also cause renal artery stenosis.*
- Three prevailing methods used for screening are *Doppler ultrasonography, captopril renography, and magnetic resonance angiography (MRA).*
- Renal angiography is the gold standard for diagnosis.

128. Ans. a. DM… b. Amyloidosis… & d. ACE…

[Ref: Harrison 19th/293; KDT 7th/505; Robbins 9th/898, 262; O. P. Ghai 8th/473; CMDT 2015/890-91]

"Albuminuria remain stable in those treated with ACE inhibitors, but aggravates in untreated diabetics. ACE inhibitor reduce proteinuria in nondiabetic case also" (KDT 7th/505)

"Amyloidosis: Renal involvement gives rise to proteinuria that may be severe enough to cause the nephritic syndrome" (Robbins 9th/262)

"Systemic disease with glomerular involvement: amyloidosis, DM, SLE, Goodpasture syndrome" (Robbins 9th/900)

Proteinuria

◈ *CMDT 2015/890-91*

- Proteinuria is defined as excessive protein excretion in the urine, generally greater than 150–160 mg/24 h in adults. Significant proteinuria is a sign of an underlying renal abnormality, usually glomerular in origin when greater than 1 g/d. There are four primary reasons for development of proteinuria:
  - Functional proteinuria is a benign process stemming from stressors such as acute illness, exercise, and "orthostatic proteinuria."
  - Overload proteinuria can result from overproduction of circulating, filterable plasma proteins (monoclonal gammopathies), such as *Bence Jones proteins associated with multiple myeloma.* Urinary protein electrophoresis will exhibit a discrete protein peak. Other examples of overload proteinuria include *myoglobinuria in rhabdomyolysis and hemoglobinuria in hemolysis.*
  - Glomerular proteinuria results from *effacement of epithelial cell foot processes and altered glomerular permeability with an increased filtration fraction of normal plasma proteins.* Glomerular diseases exhibit some degree of proteinuria.
  - Tubular proteinuria occurs as a result of faulty reabsorption of normally filtered proteins in the proximal tubule, such as *β_2-microglobulin and immunoglobulin light chains.* Causes include *acute tubular necrosis, toxic injury (lead, aminoglycosides), drug-induced interstitial nephritis, and hereditary metabolic disorders (Wilson disease and Fanconi syndrome).*

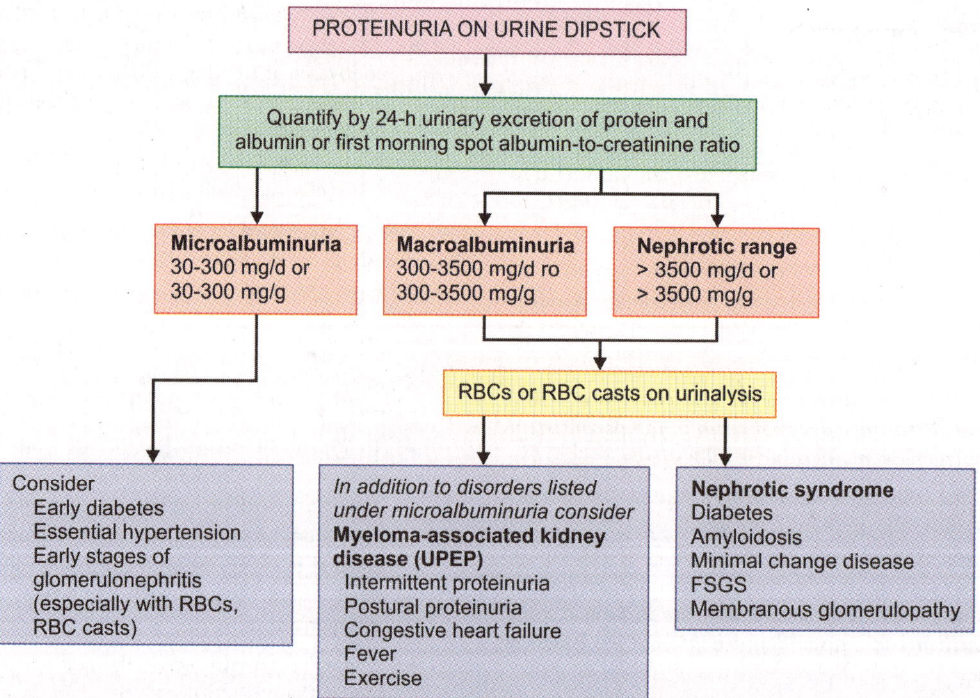

Fig: Approach to the patient with proteinuria

Table *(O. P. Ghai 8th/473)*: **Conditions presenting with proteinuria**

Glomerular proteinuria
Nephrotic syndrome (minimal change disease, focal segmental glomerulosclerosis, congenital nephritic syndrome)
Membranoproliferative glomerulonephritis, membranous nephropathy
Hepatitis B and C nephropathy, HIV nephropathy
Reflux nephropathy
Amyloidosis
Associated hematuria: Postinfectious glomerulonephritis, IgA, nephropathy, Henoch-Schonlein nephritis, lupus nephritis, Alport syndrome
Tubular Proteinuria
Drug induced nephropathy (analgesics)
Heavy metal nephropathy (*e.g.,* gold, lead, cadmium)
Renal tubular acidosis
Interstitial nephritis, pyelonephritis
Intermittent or transient proteinuria
Postural (orthostatic)
Fever
Exercise

129. Ans. b. Cutoff... & c. Cutoff...

[Ref: Harrison 19th/1718; P. J. M 20th/142-43; CMDT 2015/310, 1633; https://books. google. co. in/books?isbn=1493922238]

"**Chylothorax:** *Pleural fluid- milky white, triglyceride levels > 110 mg/dL" (P. J. M 20th/142-43)*
Chylothorax: *Pleural fluid triglyceride concentration can be less than 110 mg/dl in 15% of cases. A microscopic examination that shows chylomicrons is also diagnostic of a chylothorax & can be used as a confirmatory test if the triglyceride levels are equivocal. On microscopy, fat globule will clear with alkali or ether & will stain with Sudan III" (https://books. google. co. in/ books?isbn=1493922238)*
"Staining for fatty acids, triglycerides, lipoproteins, and other lipids is done through the use of lysochromes (fat-soluble dyes). These dyes can allow the qualification of a certain fat of interest by staining the material a specific color. Some examples: *Sudan IV, Oil Red O, and Sudan Black B" (http://en. wikipedia. org/wiki/ Triglyceride#Staining)*

Chylothorax

◈ *Harrison 19th/1718*

- A chylothorax occurs when the thoracic duct is disrupted and chyle accumulates in the pleural space. The most common *cause of chylothorax is trauma (most frequently thoracic surgery), but it also may result from tumors in the mediastinum.*
- Patients with chylothorax present with dyspnea, and a large pleural effusion is present on the chest radiograph. Thoracentesis reveals milky fluid, and biochemical analysis reveals a triglyceride level that exceeds 1.2 mmol/L *(110 mg/dL).*

130. Ans. a. TB, b. Malignancy & d. Thoracic...

[Ref: Kundu 4th/55; Harrison 19th/1718; P. J. M 20th/142; CMDT 2015/310, 1633]

Chylous (Milky) Effusion

◈ *Kundu 4th/55; P. J. M 20th/142*

- *T. B*
- *Malignancy*
- *Lymphoma*
- *Filariaisis*
- *Myxoedema*
- *Trauma*

Chylothorax

- *Chylothorax* is an accumulation of milky fluid, usually of lymphatic origin, in the pleural cavity. Chyle is milky white because it contains finely emulsified fats.
- *It may be bilateral but is more often confined to the left side.* The volume of fluid is variable but rarely assumes the massive proportions of hydrothorax.
- Chylothorax is most often caused by *thoracic duct trauma or obstruction* that secondarily causes rupture of major lymphatic ducts. This disorder is encountered in *malignant conditions* arising within the thoracic cavity that cause obstruction of the major lymphatic ducts. *More distant cancers may metastasize* via the lymphatics and grow within the right lymphatic or thoracic duct to produce obstruction.

Table: Pleural Space Fluid Accumulations

Condition	Type of Fluid	Common Associations
Inflammatory		
Serofibrinous pleuritis	Serofibrinous exudates	Inflammation in adjacent lung Collagen vascular disease
Suppurative pleuritis (empyema)	Pus	Suppurative infection in adjacent lung
Hemorrhagic pleuritis	Bloody exudates	Tumor
Noninflammatory		
Hydrothorax	Transudate	Congestive heart failure
Hemothorax	Blood	Ruptured aortic aneurysm, trauma
Chylothorax	***Chyle (lymph)***	***Tumor obstruction of normal lymphatics***

131. Ans. c. Intention...

[Ref: Harrison 19th/2609-11; CMDT 2015/988-91]

Note: *Intention tremor is seen in cerebellar lesion*

Parkinson's Disease (PD) and Related Disorders

◈ *Harrison 19th/2609*

- PD is the second commonest neurodegenerative disease, exceeded only by Alzheimer's disease (AD).

- PD affects men and women of all races, all occupations, and all countries.
- The *mean age of onset is about 60 years*, but cases can be seen in patients in their 20s, and even younger.
- Clinically, PD is characterized by *rest tremor, rigidity, bradykinesia, and gait impairment,* known as the "cardinal features" of the disease.
- Additional features can include *freezing of gait, postural instability, speech difficulty, autonomic disturbances, sensory alterations, mood disorders, sleep dysfunction, cognitive impairment, and dementia,* all known as nondopaminergic features because they do not fully respond to dopaminergic therapy.

Table *(Harrison 19th/2609)*: **Clinical Features of Parkinson's Disease**

Cardinal Features	Other Motor Features	Nonmotor Features
Bradykinesia Rest tremor Rigidity Gait disturbance/ postural instability	Micrographia ***Masked facies (hypomimia) equalize*** Reduced eye blink Soft voice (hypophonia) Dysphagia Freezing	Anosmia. Sensory disturbances (*e.g.,* pain) Mood disorders (*e.g.,* depression) Sleep disturbances Autonomic disturbances Orthostatic hypotension Gastrointestinal disturbances Genitourinal disturbances Sexual dysfunction Cognitive impairment/ Dementia

132. Ans. a. CLL d. Gaucher's...

[Ref: Harrison 19th/412, 18th/471; P. J. M 20th/68]

Table *(Harrison 19th/412; 18th/471)*: **Diseases Associated with Massive Spleenomegaly**

Chronic Myeloid Leukemia[Q]	Gaucher's disease[Q]
Lymphomas	Chronic lymphocytic leukemia[Q]
Hairy cell leukemia[Q]	Sarcoidosis[Q]
Myelofibrosis with myeloid metaplasia	Autoimmune hemolytic anemia
Polycythemia vera	Diffuse splenic hemangiomatosis

[a]*The spleen extends greater than 8 cm below left costal margin and/or weighs more than 1000 g.*

133. Ans. a. Pituitary... & d. Pheochromoc...

[Ref: Harrison 19th/2314; CMDT 2015/1147-51]

General Considerations

◈ *CMDT 2015/1147*

- The term Cushing "syndrome" refers to the manifestations of excessive corticosteroids, commonly due to supraphysiologic doses of corticosteroid drugs and rarely due to spontaneous production of excessive corticosteroids by the adrenal cortex.
- Overall, the medical use of glucocorticoids for immunosuppression, or for the treatment of inflammatory disorders, is the most common cause of Cushing's syndrome.
- About 40% of cases are due to Cushing "disease, " by which is meant the manifestations of hypercortisolism due to ***ACTH hypersecretion by the pituitary***. Cushing disease is caused by a benign pituitary adenoma that is typically very small (< 5 mm) and usually located in the anterior pituitary (98%) or in the posterior pituitary (2%).
- About ***10% of cases are due to nonpituitary ACTH secreting neoplasms*** (*e.g.,* small cell lung carcinoma), which produce excessive amounts of ectopic ACTH.
- About 15% of cases are due to ACTH from a source that cannot be initially located.
- About 30% of cases are due to excessive autonomous secretion of cortisol by the adrenals—independently of ACTH, serum levels of which are usually low. Most such cases are due to a ***unilateral adrenal tumor***.

Table *(Harrison 19th/2314)*: **Causes of Cushing's Syndrome**

Causes of Cushing's Syndrome	Female; Male Ratio	%
ACTH-Dependent Cushing's		90
Cushing's disease (= ACTH-producing pituitary adenoma)	4: 1	75
Ectopic ACTH syndrome (due to **ACTH secretion by bronchial or pancreatic carcinoid tumors, small cell lung** cancer, medullary thyroid carcinoma, pheochromocytoma and others)	1: 1	15
ACTH-Independent Cushing's	4: 1	10
Adrenocortical adenoma Adrenocortical carcinoma		5-10 1%
Rare causes: PPNAD, primary pigmented nodular adrenal disease; AIMAH, ACTH-independent massive adrenal hyperplasia; McCune-Albright syndrome		<1%

Abbreviations: AIMAH, ACTH-independent macronodular hyperplasia; PPNAD, primary pigmented nodular adrenal disease

134. Ans. a. Hyperglycemia., c. Dehydration & d. Coma.

[Ref: Harrison 19th/2417, 2420]

Hyperglycemic Hyperosmolar State (HHS)

◈ *Harrison 19th/2420*

- The prototypical patient with HHS is an elderly individual with type 2 DM, with a several-week history of polyuria, weight loss, and diminished oral intake that culminates in mental confusion, ***lethargy, or coma.***

A & E

- The physical examination reflects ***profound dehydration and hyperosmolality*** and reveals hypotension, tachycardia, and altered mental status.
- Notably **absent** are symptoms ***of nausea, vomiting, and abdominal pain and the Kussmaul respirations*** characteristic of DKA.
- HHS is often precipitated by a serious, concurrent illness such as myocardial infarction or stroke. Sepsis, pneumonia, and other serious infections are frequent precipitants and should be sought.
- ***Relative insulin deficiency and inadequate fluid intake are the underlying causes of HHS.*** Insulin deficiency increases hepatic glucose production (through glycogenolysis and gluconeogenesis) and impairs glucose utilization in skeletal muscle (see above discussion of DKA).
- Hyperglycemia induces an osmotic diuresis that leads to intravascular volume depletion, which is exacerbated by inadequate fluid replacement.
- The ***absence of ketosis in HHS is not understood.*** Presumably, the insulin deficiency is only relative and less severe than in DKA.

Table *(Harrison 19th/2417)*: **Laboratory Values in Diabetic Ketoacidosis (DKA) and Hyperglycemic Hyperosmolar State (HHS) (Representative Ranges at Presentation)**

	DKA	HHS
Glucose, mmol/L (mg/dL)	13. 9–33.3 (250–600)	33.3–66. 6 (600–1200)
Sodium, meq/L	125–135	135–145
Potassium	Normal to ↑	Normal
Magnesium	Normal	Normal
Chloride	Normal	Normal
Phosphate	Normal	Normal
Creatinine	Slightly ↑	Moderately ↑
Osmolality (mOsm/mL)	300–320	330–380
Plasma ketones	++++	+/–
Serum bicarbonate, meq/L	<15 meq/L	Normal to slightly ↓
Arterial pH	6. 8–7.3	>7.3
Arterial PCO_2, mmHg	20–30	Normal
Anion gapa[Na – (Cl + HCO3)]	↑	Normal to slightly ↑

135. Ans. c. Surgery..., d. Prior... & e. Prior...

[Ref: Harrison 19th/2329-31; Robbins 9th/1134-36]

"Sestambi scanning is the preferred way in which to localize diseased parathyroid glands prior to operation" (*http://www.endocrineweb. com/conditions/parathyroid/sestamibi-scanning)*

Treatment: Pheochromocytoma

◈ *Harrison 19th/2330-31*

- ***Complete tumor removal is the ultimate therapeutic goal,*** can be achieved by partial or total adrenalectomy
- Preoperative patient preparation is essential for safe surgery.
- ***α-Adrenergic blockers (phenoxybenzamine)*** should be initiated at relatively low doses (*e.g.,* 5–10 mg orally three times per day) and increased as tolerated every few days. Adequate alpha blockade generally requires 7 days, with a typical final dose of 20–30 mg phenoxybenzamine three times per day.
- Beta blockers (*e.g.,* 10 mg propranolol three to four times per day) can be ***added after starting alpha blockers*** and increased as needed if tachycardia persists.
- ***Nitroprusside infusion*** is useful for intraoperative hypertensive crises, and hypotension usually responds to volume infusion.
- Although laparotomy was the traditional surgical approach, ***endoscopic surgery,*** using either a transperitoneal or a retroperitoneal approach, is associated with fewer complications, a faster recovery, and optimal cosmetic results. Atraumatic endoscopic surgery has become the method of choice.

Pheochromocytoma

◈ *Review of facts*

- It is catecholamine[Q] producing tumour of sympathetic or Parasympathetic nervous system
- Pheochromocytomas usually subscribe to a convenient "**rule of 10**" (*Robbins, Harrison & CMDT*)
  - 10% are bilateral[Q]
  - 10% are malignant[Q]
  - **10% are extra adrenal**[Q]
  - 10% are associated with familial syndrome[Q]
  - 10% arise in childhood
  - Approximately 10% are in thorax
  - Most are < 10 cm in diameter
  - 10% not associated with Hypertension
  - About 10% tumour involves both adrenal gland
  - 10% extradrenal tumour are extra abdominal

Table *(Harrison)*: **Biochemical and Imaging Methods Used for Pheochromocytoma and Paraganglioma Diagnosis**

Diagnostic Method

24-h urinary tests

- Vanillylmandelic acid
- Catecholamines
- Fractionated metanephrines
- Total metanephrines

Plasma tests

- Catecholamines
- Free metanephrines
- CT
- MRI
- MIBG scintigraphy
- Somatostatin receptor scintigraphy
- Dopa (dopamine) PET

136. Ans. a. Sterioid, b. 5-Aminosal..., c. Azathioprine & e. Adalimumab.

[Ref: Harrison 19th/1959-64; CMDT 2015/640]

"Daclizumab is used to prevent renal & other transplant rejection reaction"-(KDT 7th/884)

Specific Drug Therapy: Crohn Disease

◈ *CMDT 2015/640*

- **5-aminosalicylic acid agents:** Mesalamine (Asacol 2.4–4.8 g/d orally; Pentasa 4 g/d orally) has long been used as initial therapy for the treatment of mild to moderately active colonic and ileocolonic Crohn disease.
- **Antibiotics**: Antibiotics also are widely used by clinicians for the treatment of active luminal Crohn disease
- **Corticosteroids:** Approximately one-half of patients with Crohn disease require corticosteroids at some time in their illness.
- **anti-TNF therapies**: ***Infliximab, adalimumab, and certolizumab*** are used for the treatment of patients with moderate to severe Crohn disease (including fistulizing disease) with an inadequate response to mesalamine, antibiotics, corticosteroids or immunomodulators.
- **Immunomodulating drugs**: ***azathioprine, mercaptopurine, or methotrexate***—Immunomodulating agents are used in patients with Crohn disease who have not responded to corticosteroids or who require repeated courses of long-term corticosteroids to control symptoms.

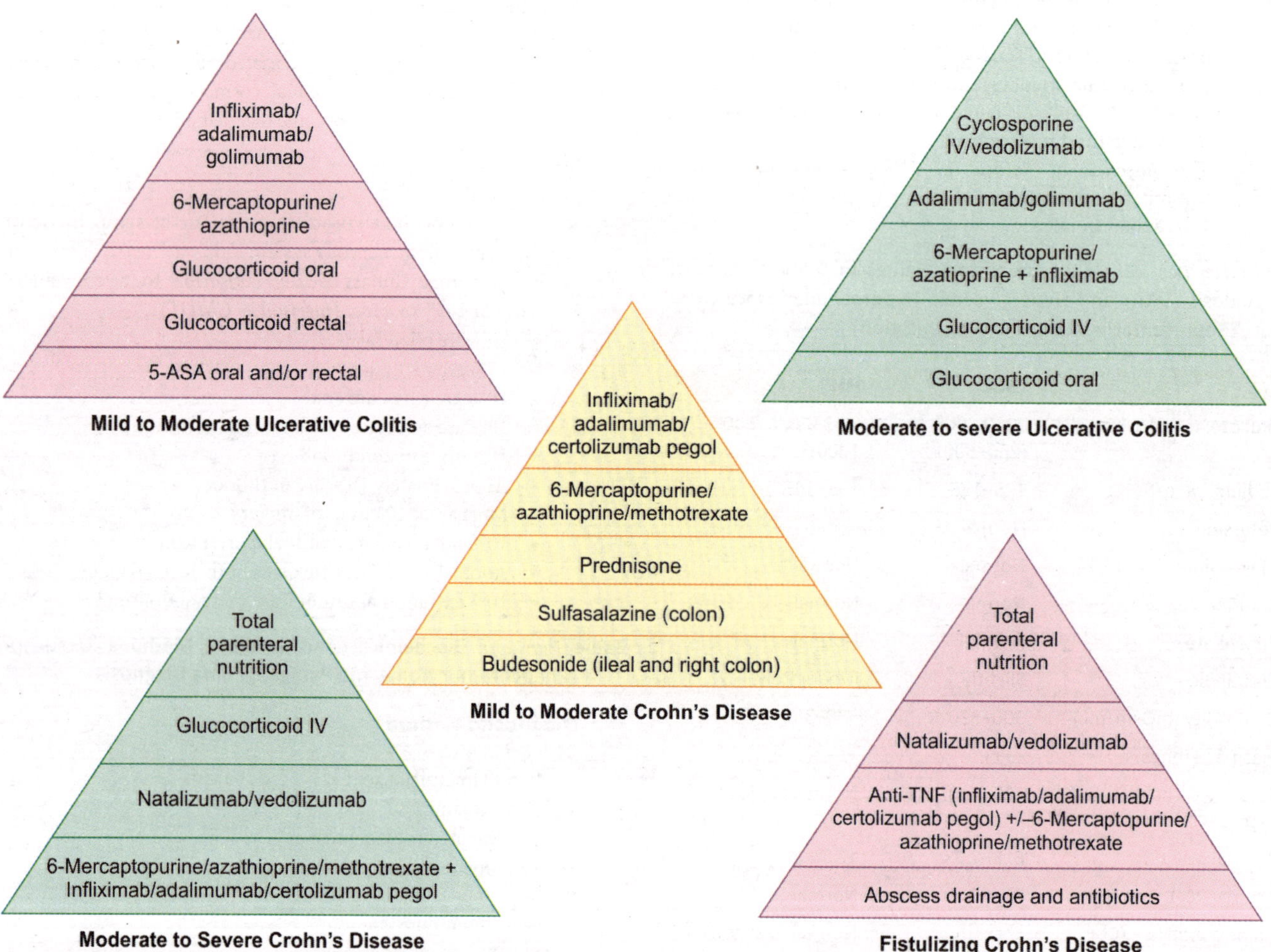

Fig: (Harrison): Medical management of inflammatory bowel disease. 5-ASA, 5-aminosalicylic acid; CD, Crohn's disease; UC, ulcerative colitis

137. Ans. d. Monophasic...

[Ref: Ajay Yadav 5th/259]

*"**2010 AHA guideline for CPR**: Contrary to previous recommendation of 3 successive shocks (200, 300, 360 J) nowadays **1st & all subsequent shocks are of 360 Joules with monophasic & 120-200 Joules with biphasic**" (Ajay Yadav 5th/259)*

138. Ans. d. Tabes... & e. Gumma...

[Ref: Harrison 19th/1134-38; Robbins 9th/379; CMDT 2015/1462-64, 654-55]

*"With secondary syphilis, **condylomata lata** (pale-brown, flat verrucous lesions) may be seen, with secretion of foul-smelling mucus. Condylomata acuminata (warts) are a significant cause*

of anorectal symptoms. Caused by the human papillomavirus (HPV), they may occur in the perianal area, the anal canal, or the genitals. (CMDT 2015/654-55)

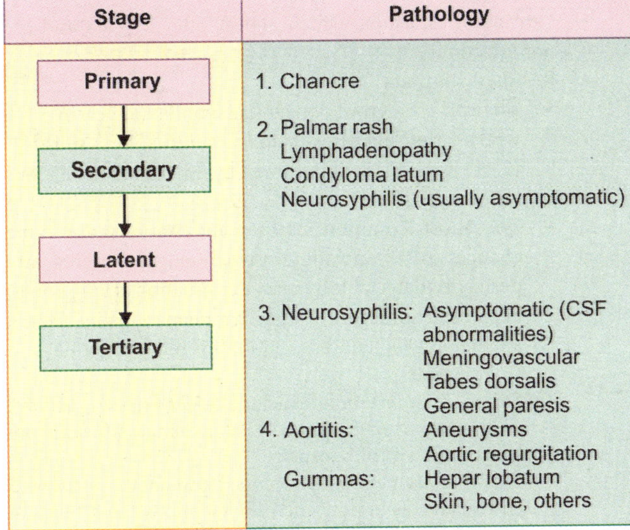

Late (Tertiary) Syphilis: Essentials Of Diagnosis (CMDT)

- Infiltrative tumors of skin, bones, liver (gummas).
- Aortitis, aneurysms, aortic regurgitation.
- Central nervous system disorders, including meningovascular and degenerative changes, paresthesias, shooting pains, abnormal reflexes, dementia, or psychosis.

Secondary Syphilis

◈ *Harrison 19th/1135*

- The protean manifestations of the secondary stage usually include localized or diffuse ***mucocutaneous lesions and generalized nontender lymphadenopathy***. The ***healing primary chancre is still present in 15% of cases***, and the stages may overlap more frequently in persons with concurrent HIV infection than in those without this co-infection.
- The skin rash consists of ***macular, papular, papulosquamous, and occasionally pustular syphilides***; often more than one form is present simultaneously. Rarely, severe necrotic lesions (*lues maligna*) may appear.
- In warm, moist, intertriginous areas (commonly the perianal region, vulva, and scrotum), papules can enlarge to produce broad, moist, pink or gray-white, highly infectious lesions ***(condylomata lata)*** in 10% of patients with secondary syphilis.

139. Ans. a. Foetus..., b. Syphilis..., d. If infant... & e. Foetus...

[Ref: Dutta's Obstetrics 8th/342-44; Harrison 19th/1136-37; Robbins 9th/379; CMDT 2015/1465-66]

"When the mother is suffering from from syphilis, infection of foetus does not occur before the 4th month; ***it is most likely to occur after 6th month*** *by which time the Langhan's cell layer has completely atrophied. Infection of foetus is* ***most likely to occur when the mother is suffering from primary or secondary stages of syphilis than late stage****" (Park 23rd/528)*

Syphilis

◈ *O. P. Ghai 8th/182)*

- *If the mother is diagnosed to have syphilis & she received adequate treatment at least one month before delivery, the infant does not require any treatment*
- *If the mother did not receive any treatment or inadequate treatment or her treatment status is not known & the* **neonate does not have any signs of congenital syphilis**, *the* ***infant should be treated with procaine or benzathine penicillin***. *Along with the baby, the mother & her partner should also be treated*
- *If the* **infant shows sign of congenital syphilis**, ***he/she should be treated with crystalline penicillin for the 10 days***

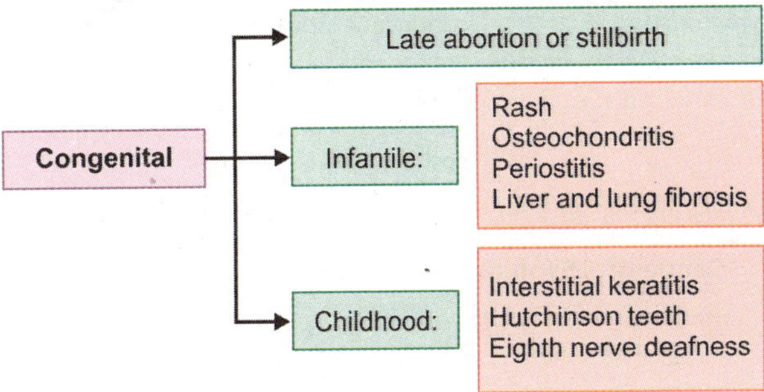

Syphilis in Pregnancy

◈ *CMDT 2015/1465; Harrison 19th/1136*

- All pregnant women should have a nontreponemal serologic test for syphilis at the time of the first prenatal visit. In women who may be at increased risk for syphilis or for populations in which there is a high prevalence of syphilis, ***additional nontreponemal tests should be performed during the third trimester at 28 weeks and again at delivery.***
- ***The only acceptable treatment for syphilis in pregnancy is penicillin in dosage schedules appropriate for the stage of disease***
- **Penicillin prevents congenital syphilis in 90% of cases, even when treatment is given late in pregnancy.** Tetracycline and doxycycline are contraindicated in pregnancy.
- Transmission of *T. pallidum* across the placenta from a ***syphilitic woman to her fetus may occur at any stage of pregnancy, but fetal damage generally does not occur until after the fourth month of gestation, when fetal*** immunologic competence begins to develop.
- The risk of fetal infection during untreated ***early maternal syphilis is ~75–95%, decreasing to ~35% for maternal syphilis of >2 years' duration. Adequate treatment of the woman before the 16th week of pregnancy should prevent fetal damage, and treatment before the third trimester should adequately treat the infected fetus.***
- Untreated maternal infection may result in *a rate of fetal loss of up to 40%* (with stillbirth more common than abortion because of the late onset of fetal pathology), prematurity, neonatal death, or nonfatal congenital syphilis.

Table *(Harrison 19th/1139)*: **Recommendations for the Treatment of Syphilisa**

Stage of Syphilis	Patients without Penicillin Allergy
Primary, secondary, or early latent	*CSF normal or not examined*: Penicillin G benzathine (single dose of 2.4 mU IM) *CSF abnormal:* Treat as neurosyphilis
Late latent (or latent of uncertain duration), cardiovascular, or benign tertiary	*CSF normal or not examined*: Penicillin G benzathine (2.4 mU IM weekly for 3 weeks) *CSF abnormal:* Treat as neurosyphilis
Neurosyphilis (asymptomatic or symptomatic)	Aqueous crystalline penicillin G (18–24 mU/d IV, given as 3–4 mU q4h or continuous infusion) for 10–14 days *or* Aqueous procaine penicillin G (2.4 mU/d IM) plus oral probenecid (500 mg qid), both for 10–14 days
Syphilis in pregnancy	According to stage

Congenital Syphilis

◈ *Harrison 19th/1136*

- Transmission of *T. pallidum* from a syphilitic woman to her fetus across the placenta may occur at any stage of pregnancy, but fetal damage generally ***does not occur until after the fourth month of gestation, when fetal immunologic competence begins to develop.***

Manifestations: Divided into three types according to their timing:

- **Early manifestations**, which appear within the first 2 years of life (often at 2–10 weeks of age), are infectious, and resemble the manifestations of severe secondary syphilis in the adult;
- **Late manifestations**, which appear after 2 years and are noninfectious;
- **Residual stigmata**
  - The earliest sign of congenital syphilis (appearing 2–6 weeks after birth) is ***usually rhinitis, or "snuffles"*** (23%), which is soon followed by other mucocutaneous lesions (35–41%).
  - The most common early manifestations are bone changes (61%), including osteochondritis, osteitis, and periostitis detectable by x-ray examination of long bones; hepatosplenomegaly (50%); lymphadenopathy (32%); anemia (34%); jaundice (30%); thrombocytopenia; and leukocytosis.
  - Other manifestations include *eighth-nerve deafness and recurrent arthropathy.* Bilateral knee effusions are known as **Clutton's joints.**
  - Gummatous periostitis occurs between the ages of 5 and 20 and, as in nonvenereal endemic syphilis, tends to cause ***destructive lesions of the palate and nasal septum.***
  - Classic stigmata include ***Hutchinson's teeth*** (centrally notched, widely spaced, peg-shaped upper central incisors), ***"mulberry" molars*** (sixth-year molars with multiple, poorly developed **cusps**), ***saddle nose, and saber shins.***

140. Ans. b. CHF

[Ref: Harrison 19th/287; P. J. M 20th/70; CMDT 2015/585-86]

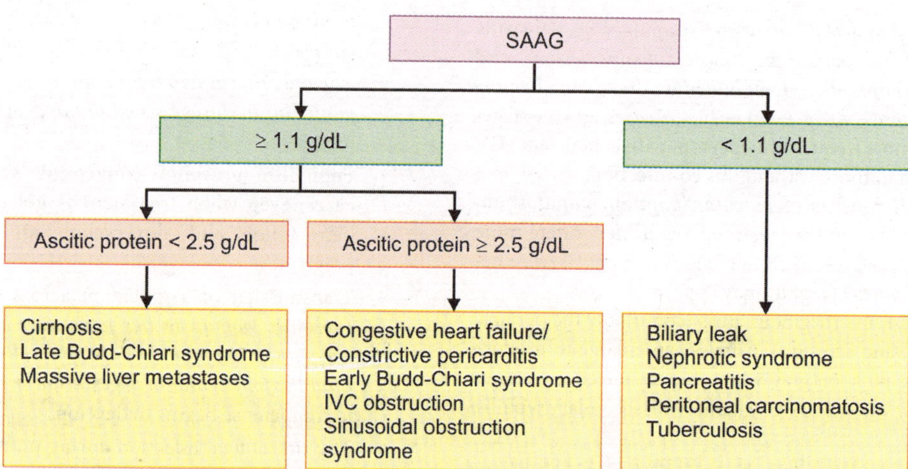

Fig: *(Harrison 19th/287)*: Algorithm for the diagnosis of ascites according to the serum-ascites albumin gradient (SAAG). IVC, inferior vena cava

Evaluation of Ascites

◈ *Harrison 19th/287*

- *Serum-ascites albumin gradient (SAAG)* is useful for distinguishing ascites caused by portal hypertension from nonportal hypertensive ascites The SAAG reflects the pressure within the hepatic sinusoids and correlates with the hepatic venous pressure gradient.
- The SAAG is calculated by subtracting the ascitic albumin from the serum albumin and does not change with diuresis.
- A **SAAG ≥1. 1 g/dL** reflects the presence of portal hypertension and indicates that the ascites is from an increased pressure in the hepatic sinusoids.
- A **SAAG <1. 1 g/dL** indicates that the ascites is not related to portal hypertension as in tuberculous peritonitis, peritoneal carcinomatosis, or pancreatic ascites.

- For high-SAAG (≥1.1) ascites, the **ascitic protein level** can provide further clues to the etiology. An ascitic **protein level of ≥2. 5 g/dL** indicates that the hepatic sinusoids are normal and allows passage of protein into the ascites, as occurs in cardiac ascites, sinusoidal obstruction syndrome, or early Budd-Chiari syndrome.
- An ascitic **protein level <2.5 g/dL** indicates that the hepatic sinusoids have been damaged and scarred and no longer allow passage of protein, as occurs with cirrhosis, late Budd-Chiari syndrome, or massive liver metastases.

141. Ans. c. Water..., d. Pulsus... & e. Collapsing...

[Ref: Harrison 19th/1445-46; Kundu 4th/295-97; P. J. M 20th/40-42]

Table *(P. J. M 20th/40-42; Kundu 4th/295-97)*: **Different types of pulse**

Pulse type	Condition
Anacrotic pulse	Aortic stenosis
Pulsus bisferiens	Idiopathic hypertrophic subaortic stenosis; Severe AR with mild AS
Dicrotic pulse	Fever like typhoid fever, congestive cardiac failure, cardiac temponade, following open heart surgery
Pulsus parvus Et Tardus	Severe AS
Pulsus alternans	LVF, Toxic myocarditis, Paroxymal tachycardias
Pulsus paradoxus	SVC obstruction; Lung conditions-asthma, emphysema, airway obstruction; Cardiac-pericardial effusion, constrictive pericarditis, severe CCF
Pulsus bigeminus	A. V block, sinoatrial block with ventricular escape
Thready pulse	Shock especially cardiogenic
Waterhammer pulse (High volume collapsing pulse)	High output states like anaemia, beri-beri, thyrotoxicosis; Cardiac lesions- AR, PDA, Rupture of sinus of valsalva into the heart chambers, aortopulmonary window

142. Ans. c. Codeine & e. Tramadol

[Ref: L & B 26th/245; http://www. paincommunitycentre. org/article/who-analgesic-ladder; http://www. who. int/cancer/palliative/painladder/en/]

Pain control in Malignant Disease

◈ *L & B 26th/245*

The World Health Organization's booklet advises use of a '**pain step ladder**':

- **First step: Simple analgesics**: aspirin, paracetamol, nonsteroidal anti-inflammatory agents, tricyclic drugs or anticonvulsant drugs.
- **Second step: Intermediate strength opioids**: codeine, tramadol or dextropropoxyphene.
- **Third step: Strong opioids**: morphine (pethidine has now been withdrawn).
- Oral opiate analgesia is necessary when the less powerful analgesic agents no longer control pain on movement, or enable the patient to sleep.
- **Oral morphine,** often used for chronic pain, can be prescribed in short-acting liquid or tablet form and should be administered regularly every 4 hours until an adequate dose of drug has been titrated to control the pain over 24 hours.
- Additional short-acting opioids (**morphine/fentanyl**) can then be used to cover episodes of breakthrough pain.

*"The analgesic ladder can be described as a **three-step approach** of sequential use of pharmacologic agents commensurate with the pain level as reported by the patient. Moving up from no treatment, the patient can be started on non- opioids (e.g., aspirin, paracetamol or non-steroidal anti-inflammatory drugs (NSAIDS)) for mild pain, then increasing to weak opioids like codeine and its derivatives for moderate pain and finally escalating to **strong opioids** like **morphine**, oxycodone, hydrocodone, methadone and **fentanyl** for the **highest level of pain (i. e step 3)**" (http://www. paincommunitycentre. org/article/who-analgesic-ladder)*

WHO's Cancer Pain Ladder for Adults;

◈ *(http://www. who. int/cancer/palliative/painladder/en/)*

- If pain occurs, there should be prompt oral administration of drugs in the following order: *nonopioids (aspirin and paracetamol); then, as necessary, **mild opioids (codeine)**; then **strong opioids such as morphine**,* until the patient is free of pain.
- To maintain freedom from pain, drugs should be given "by the clock", that is every 3-6 hours, rather than "on demand"
- This three-step approach of administering the right drug in the right dose at the right time is inexpensive and 80-90% effective.

WHO's Pain Relief Ladder

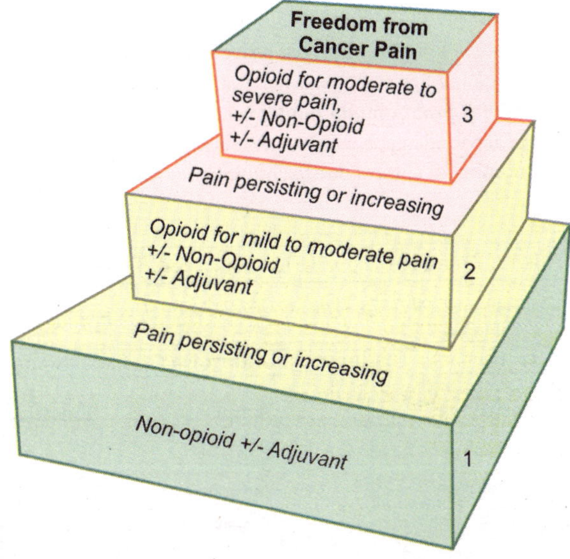

143. Ans. a. H. pylori..., b. Eradcation..., c. Eradication... & d. Duodenum...

[Ref: Harrison 19th/1911-21; CMDT 2015/607-12]

"Ulcer disease will develop in an estimated 10% of infected patients. The ***prevalence of H. pylori infection in duodenal ulcer patients is 75–90%. The association with gastric ulcers is lower,*** but H. pylori is found in most patients in whom NSAIDS cannot be implicated. Infection with cag-A positive strains of *H pylori* is associated with an ***18-fold and 2. 9-fold increased risk of duodenal and gastric ulcer, respectively***" (CMDT 2015/608)

Peptic Ulcer Disease

◈ *Harrison 19th/1911-21*

- Gastric infection with the bacterium *H. pylori* accounts for the majority of PUD
- *H. pylori* and NSAID-induced injury account for the majority of **DUs**
- As in DUs, the majority of GUs can be attributed to either *H. pylori* or NSAID-induced mucosal damage
- Although acid secretion is still important in the pathogenesis of PUD, ***eradication of H. pylori and therapy/prevention of NSAID-induced disease is the mainstay of treatment***
- The physician's goal in treating PUD is to provide relief of symptoms (pain or dyspepsia), promote ulcer healing, and ultimately prevent ulcer recurrence and complications. The greatest impact of understanding the role of *H. pylori* in peptic disease has been the ability to prevent recurrence.
- ***Documented eradication of H. pylori in patients with PUD is associated with a dramatic decrease in ulcer recurrence to <10–20% as compared to 59% in GU patients and 67% in DU patients when the organism is not eliminated.***
- Eradication of the organism may lead to diminished recurrent ulcer bleeding. The impact of its eradication on ulcer perforation is unclear.

H pylori Eradication Therapy

◈ *CMDT 2015/610*

- Eradication of *H pylori* has proved difficult.
- Combination regimens that use ***two or three antibiotics with a proton pump inhibitor*** or bismuth are required to achieve adequate rates of eradication and to reduce the number of failures due to antibiotic resistance.

Table *(Harrison 19th/1920)*: **Drugs Used in the Treatment of Peptic Ulcer Disease**

Drug Type/Mechanism	Examples
Acid-suppressing drugs	
Antacids	Mylanta, Maalox, Tums, Gaviscon
H_2 receptor antagonists	Cimetidine
Proton pump inhibitors	Omeprazole; Lansoprazole; Rabeprazole; Pantoprazole; Esomeprazole
Mucosal protective agents	
Sucralfate	Sucralfate
Prostaglandin analogue	Misoprostol
Bismuth-containing compounds	Bismuth subsalicylate (BSS)

Table *(Harrison 19th/1922)*: **Regimens Recommended for Eradication of H. Pylori Infection**

Drug	Dose
Triple Therapy	
1. Bismuth subsalicylate plus	2 tablets qid
Metronidazoleplus	250 mg qid
Tetracyclinea	500 mg qid
2. Ranitidine bismuth citrate plus	400 mg bid
Tetracyclineplus	500 mg bid
Clarithromycin or metronidazole	500 mg bid
3. Omeprazole (lansoprazole) plus	20 mg bid (30 mg bid)
Clarithromycinplus	250 or 500 mg bid
Metronidazoleb or	500 mg bid
Amoxicillinc	1 g bid
Quadruple Therapy	
Omeprazole (lansoprazole)	20 mg (30 mg) daily
Bismuth subsalicylate	2 tablets qid
Metronidazole	250 mg qid
Tetracycline	500 mg qid

144. Ans. a. Prominent..., b. Pericardial... & d. Thickened...

[Ref: Harrison 19th/1573, 17th/1497; CMDT 2015/415, 422]

Table *(Harrison 18th)*: **Features that Distinguish Cardiac Tamponade from Constrictive Pericarditis and Similar Clinical Disorders**

Characteristic	Tamponade	Constrictive Pericarditis	Restrictive Cardiomyopathy	RVMI
Clinical				
Pulsus paradoxus[Q]	Common[Q]	Usually absent[Q]	Rare	Rare
Jugular veins				
Prominent y descent [Q]	Absen[Q]	Usually present[Q]	Rare	Rare

Characteristic	Tamponade	Constrictive Pericarditis	Restrictive Cardiomyopathy	RVMI
Prominent x descent [Q]	Present[Q]	Usually present[Q]	Present	Rare
Kussmaul's sign[Q]	Absent	Present	Absent	Present
Third heart sound	Absent	Absent	Rare	May be present
Pericardial knock	Absent	Often present	Absent	Absent
Electrocardiogram				
Low ECG voltage[Q]	May be present	May be present	May be present	Absent
Electrical alternans[Q]	May be present	Absent	Absent	Absent
Echocardiography				
Thickened pericardium	Absent	Present	Absent	Absent
Pericardial calcification	Absent	Often present	Absent	Absent
Pericardial effusion	Present	Absent	Absent	Absent
RV size	Usually small	Usually normal	Usually normal	Enlarged
Myocardial thickness	Normal	Normal	Usually increased	Normal
Right atrial collapse and RVDC	Present	Absent	Absent	Absent
Increased early filling, mitral flow velocity	Absent	Present	Present	May be present
Exaggerated respiratory variation in flow velocity	Present	Present	Absent	Absent
CT/MRI				
Thickened/calcific pericardium	Absent	Present	Absent	Absent
Cardiac catheterization				
Equalization of diastolic pressures	Usually present	Usually present	Usually absent	Absent or present
Cardiac biopsy helpful?	No	No	Sometimes	No

Abbreviations: RV, right ventricle; RVMI, right ventricular myocardial infarction; RVDC, right ventricular diastolic collapse; ECG, electrocardiograph.

Table *(Harrison 19th/1573)*: **Features that Distinguish Cardiac Tamponade from Constrictive Pericarditis and Similar Clinical Disorders**

Characteristic	Tamponade	Constrictive Pericarditis	Restrictive Cardiomyopathy	RVMI	Effusive Constrictive Pericarditis
Clinical					
Pulsus paradoxus	+++	+	+	+	+++
Jugular veins					
Prominent y descent	–	++	+	+	–
Prominent x descent	+++	++	+++	+	+++
Kussmaul's sign	–	+++	+	+++	++
Third heart sound	–	–	+	+	+
Pericardial knock	–	++	–	–	–
Electrocardiogram					
Low ECG voltage	++	++	++	–	++
Electrical alternanas	++	–	–	–	+
Echocardiogram					
Thickened pericardium	–	+++	–	–	++
Pericardial calcification	–	++	–	–	
Pericardial effusion	+++	–	–	++	
RV size	Usually small	Usually normal	Usually normal	Enlarged	
RA and RV	+++	–	–	–	

A& E

Characteristic	Tamponade	Constrictive Pericarditis	Restrictive Cardiomyopathy	RVMI	Effusive Constrictive Pericarditis
Exaggerated respiratory	+++	+++	–	+++	
CT/MRI					
Thickened pericardium	–	+++	–	++	
Cardiac catheterization					
Equalization of diastolic	+++	+++	–	++	

145. Ans. a. Confusion, b. Uremia. & c. Resipratory...

[Ref: Harrison 19th/806-07; CMDT 2015/270]

Site of Care

◈ *Harrison 19th/806-07*

- There are **currently two sets of criteria**: The *Pneumonia Severity Index (PSI), a prognostic model used to identify patients at low risk of dying; and the CURB-65 criteria, a severity-of-illness score.*
- The **CURB-65 criteria** include five variables: confusion (C); ***urea >7 mmol/L*** (U); respiratory rate ≥30/min (R); ***blood pressure, systolic ≤90 mmHg*** or diastolic ≤60 mmHg (B); and ***age ≥65 years*** (65). Patients with a score of 0, among whom the 30-day mortality rate is 1. 5%, can be treated outside the hospital. ***With a score of 2, the 30-day mortality rate is 9.2%, and patients should be admitted to the hospital.*** Among patients with scores of ≥3, mortality rates are 22% overall; these patients may require admission to an ICU.

When to Admit

◈ *CMDT 2015/270*

There are two widely used clinical prediction rules available to guide admission and triage decisions, the ***Pneumonia Severity Index (PSI) and the CURB-65.***

- The CURB-65 assesses five simple, independent predictors of increased mortality (***confusion, uremia, respiratory rate, blood pressure, and age > 65***) to calculate a 30-day predicted mortality. Compared with the PSI, the simpler CURB-65 is less discriminating at low mortality but excellent at identifying patients with high mortality who may benefit from ICU level care.
- A modified version (CRB-65) dispenses with serum blood urea nitrogen and eliminates the need for laboratory testing.

146. Ans. b. ↓FEV1/FEV6, c. ↑RV, d. ↑TLC & e. ↓Peak...

[Ref: Harrison 19th/1662, Chap306e; Robbins 9th/674; CMDT 2015/257-58; http://www. ncbi. nlm. nih. gov/pubmed/19349398]

"The conventional FEV (1)/FVC test is the "gold standard" to quantitate airway obstruction, but elderly subjects or patients with severe respiratory diseases quite frequently cannot make such an effort. Many studies have investigated the usefulness of **FEV (1)/forced expired volume in 6 s (FEV (6))** measurements as an alternative for FEV (1)/FVC for ***diagnosis of airway obstruction.*** FEV (1)/FEV (6) is a ***sensitive and specific test*** for the diagnosis of airway obstruction. FEV (1)/FEV (6) can be used as a valid alternative for FEV (1)/FVC in the diagnosis of airway obstruction"- *http://www. ncbi. nlm. nih. gov/pubmed/19349398*

"The data from the current study indicate that FEV1/FEV6, 73% and FEV6, 82% predicted can be used as a valid alternative for the FEV1/FVC, 70% and FVC, 80% pred cut-off points for the detection of obstruction and restriction, respectively" (http://erj. ersjournals. com/content/27/2/378. full. pdf)

Table Difference b/w obstructive & Restrictive lung diseases

	Obstructive lung disease (e. g emphysema)	Restrictive lung disease
Residual volume	***Increase***[Q]	Decrease[Q]
FRC	Increase[Q]	Decrease[Q]
Total lung capacity	***Normal to increase***[Q]	Decrease
Diffusion capacity·	Normal[Q] (Except emphysema)	Decreased[Q]
Vital capacity	Decrease[Q]	Decrease
FEF 25-75%	Decrease	Normal
FEV_1/FVC	Decrease[Q]	Normal to increase[Q]

Table *(Harrison)*: **Common abnormalities of pulmonary function. Pulmonary function values are expressed as a percentage of normal predicted values**

	Restriction due to increased lung elastic recoil (pulmonary fibrosis)	Restriction due to chest wall abnormality (moderate obesity)	Restriction due to respiratory muscle weakness (myasthenia gravis)	Obstruction due to airway narrowing (acute asthma)	Obstruction due to decreased elastic recoil (severe emphysema)
TLC	60%	95%	75%	100%	130%
FRC	60%	65%	100%	104%	220%
RV	60%	100%	120%	120%	310%
FVC	60%	92%	60%	90%	60%

Contd...

	Restriction due to increased lung elastic recoil (pulmonary fibrosis)	Restriction due to chest wall abnormality (moderate obesity)	Restriction due to respiratory muscle weakness (myasthenia gravis)	Obstruction due to airway narrowing (acute asthma)	Obstruction due to decreased elastic recoil (severe emphysema)
FEV1	75%	92%	60%	35% pre-b. d. 75% post-b. d	35% pre-b. d. 38% post-b. d.
Raw	1. 0	1. 0	1. 0	2. 5	1. 5
DLCO	60%	95%	80%	120%	40%

147. Ans. All

[Ref: Harrison 19th/1268-70; Robbins 9th/253-54; CMDT 2015/145, 1309]

Kaposi Sarcoma

◈ *Robbins 9th/253-54*

- Kaposi sarcoma, a vascular tumor, is the ***most common neoplasm in patients with AIDS.***
- ***HHV-8 (KSHV) has been strongly implicated as a viral cofactor*** in the pathogenesis of KS.
- The lesions of KS are **characterized by** the proliferation of spindle-***shaped cells that express markers of both endothelial cells (vascular or lymphatic) and smooth muscle cells.*** There is also a profusion of slitlike vascular spaces, suggesting that the lesions ***may arise from primitive mesenchymal precursors of vascular channels.***

General Considerations

◈ *CMDT 2015/145, 1309*

- Kaposi sarcoma continues to occur largely in homosexual men with HIV infection as an AIDS-defining illness.
- ***Human herpes virus 8 (HHV-8), or Kaposi sarcoma-associated herpes virus (KSHV), is universally present in all forms of Kaposi sarcoma.***

Treatment

- For Kaposi sarcoma in the elderly, palliative local therapy with ***intralesional chemotherapy or radiation is usually all that is required.***
- In the setting of iatrogenic immunosuppression, the treatment of Kaposi sarcoma is primarily reduction of doses of immunosuppressive medications.
- ***In AIDS associated Kaposi sarcoma, the patient should first be given effective anti-HIV antiretrovirals*** because in most cases this treatment alone is associated with improvement.
- Other therapeutic options include ***cryotherapy or intralesional vinblastine*** (0. 1–0. 5 mg/mL) for cosmetically objectionable lesions; ***radiation therapy*** for accessible and space-occupying lesions; and ***laser surgery*** for certain intraoral and pharyngeal lesions.
- Systemic therapy is indicated in patients with rapidly progressive skin disease. It includes Liposomal doxorubicin, Alpha-interferon, Paclitaxel and other taxanes

148. Ans. c. Torsade..., d. Tetany & e. Calcium...

[Ref: Harrison 19th/2461-62, 463-e4; CMDT 2015/878-79]

"It is important to consider the need for calcium, potassium, and phosphate supplementation in patients with hypomagnesemia. In severely hypomagnesemic patients with concomitant hypocalcemia and hypophosphatemia, administration of IV magnesium alone may worsen hypophosphatemia, provoking neuromuscular symptoms or rhabdomyolysis, due to rapid stimulation of PTH secretion. This is avoided by ***administering both calcium and magnesium***" *(Harrison 19th/2462)*

*"The electrolyte disturbances that have been reported to precipitate **torsade** include hypokalemia and hypomagnesemia"- http://emedicine. medscape*

Hypomagnesemia: Clinical Findings

◈ *(CMDT 2015/878-79)*

- Common symptoms are those of hypokalemia and hypocalcemia, with weakness and muscle cramps. Marked neuromuscular and central nervous system hyperirritability may produce *tremors, athetoid movements, jerking, nystagmus, Babinski response, confusion, and disorientation.*
- Cardiovascular manifestations include ***hypertension, tachycardia,*** and ventricular arrhythmias.
- Hypomagnesemia may cause generalized alterations in neuromuscular function, including ***tetany,*** tremor, seizures, muscle weakness, ataxia, nystagmus, vertigo, apathy, depression, irritability, delirium, and psychosis.
- Cardiac arrhythmias may occur, including sinus tachycardia, other supraventricular tachycardias, and ventricular arrhythmias.
- **Electrocardiographic abnormalities** may include prolonged PR or QT intervals, T-wave flattening or inversion, and ST straightening.
- Other electrolyte abnormalities often seen with hypomagnesemia, including ***hypocalcemia*** (with hypocalciuria) and ***hypokalemia,*** may not be easily corrected unless magnesium is administered as well.

149. Ans. b. Transient..., c. Depression... & e. T wave...

[Ref: Harrison 19th/1593-98; CMDT 2015/361-63]

Unstable Angina (UA)

◈ *Harrison 19th/1593-98*

- In UA, ***ST-segment depression, transient ST-segment elevation, and/or T-wave inversion occur in 30 to 50% of patients.***
- In patients with the clinical features of UA, the presence of ***new ST-segment deviation,*** even of only 0. 05 mV, is an important predictor of adverse outcome. T-wave changes

are sensitive for ischemia but less specific, unless they are new, ***deep T-wave inversions*** (0.3 mV).

- **UA** is defined as angina pectoris or equivalent ischemic discomfort ***with at least one of three features: (1) it occurs at rest (or with minimal exertion), usually lasting >10 minutes; (2) it is severe and of new onset (i.e., within the prior 4–6 weeks); and/or (3) it occurs with a crescendo pattern (i.e., distinctly more severe, prolonged, or frequent than previously).***
- The diagnosis of **NSTEMI** is established if a patient with the clinical features of UA develops evidence of myocardial necrosis, as reflected in ***elevated cardiac biomarkers.***
- UA/NSTEMI is most commonly caused by a reduction in oxygen supply and/or by an increase in myocardial oxygen demand superimposed on a lesion that causes coronary arterial obstruction, usually an atherothrombotic coronary plaque.

Unstable angina & NSTMI: Treatment

◈ *Harrison 19th/1595-98*

- "In order to provide relief and prevention of recurrence of chest pain, initial treatment should include ***bed rest, nitrates, and beta blockers.***"
- **Nitrates** should first be given sublingually or by buccal spray (0.3–0. 6 mg) if the patient is experiencing ischemic pain. If pain persists after three doses given 5 min apart, intravenous nitroglycerin (5–10 µg/min using nonabsorbing tubing) is recommended

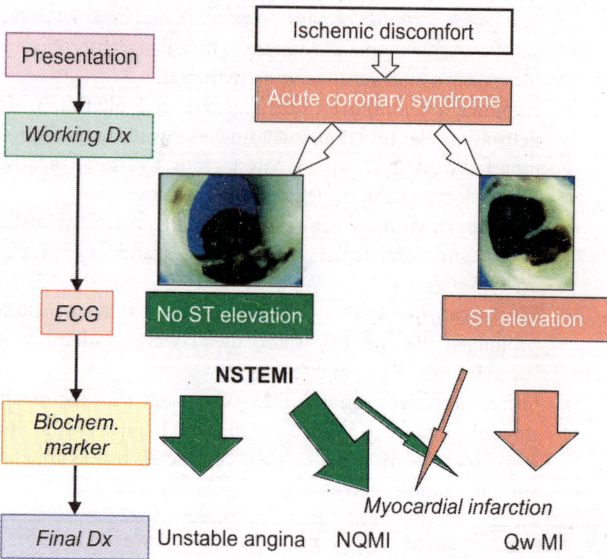

Fig: Acute coronary syndrome

150. Ans. a. Also found..., b. May... & c. It is...

[Ref: Harrison 19th/2143; CMDT 2015/816-20; Harshmohan 7th/66]

*"IgM, IgG, and IgA isotypes of RF occur in sera from patients with RA, although the **IgM isotype is the one most frequently measured** by commercial laboratories. **Serum IgM RF has been found in 75–80% of patients with RA**; therefore, a negative result does not exclude the presence of this disease. It is also found in other connective tissue diseases, such as primary **Sjögren's syndrome**, systemic lupus erythematosus, and type II mixed essential cryoglobulinemia, as well as chronic infections such as subacute bacterial endocarditis and hepatitis B and C. Serum **RF may also be detected in 1–5% of the healthy population**" (Harrison 19th/2143)*

*"Detection of serum RF and anti-CCP antibodies is important in differentiating RA from other polyarticular diseases, although. **RF lacks diagnostic specificity** and may be found in association with other chronic inflammatory diseases in which arthritis figures in the clinical manifestations" (Harrison 19th/2143)*

*"**Sjogren's syndrome**: Positive Rheumatoid factor in 25% of cases (Harshmohan 7th/66)*

"Rheumatoid factor and antibodies to cyclic citrullinated peptides (anti-CCP) are present in 70–80%" (CMDT 2015/817)

Rheumatoid Arthritis: Laboratory Findings

◈ *CMDT 2015/817-18*

- Anti-CCP antibodies and rheumatoid factor, an ***IgM antibody directed against the Fc fragment of IgG***, are present in 70–80% of patients with established rheumatoid arthritis.
- **Rheumatoid factor** has a ***sensitivity of only 50% in early disease. Anti-CCP antibodies are the most specific blood test for rheumatoid arthritis (specificity ~95%).***
- Rheumatoid factor can occur in ***other autoimmune disease and in chronic infections, including hepatitis C, syphilis, subacute bacterial endocarditis, and tuberculosis***. The prevalence of rheumatoid factor positivity also ***rises with age in healthy individuals.*** Approximately 20% of rheumatoid patients have antinuclear antibodies.
- The ESR and levels of C-reactive protein are typically elevated in proportion to disease activity. A moderate hypochromic normocytic anemia is common.
- The white cell count is normal or slightly elevated, but leukopenia may occur, often in the presence of splenomegaly (*e.g.*, Felty syndrome). The platelet count is often elevated, roughly in proportion to the severity of overall joint inflammation.

SURGERY

151. Ans. b. Discolouration... & C Boggy...

[Ref: Manipal Surgery 4th/1040; S. Das Textbook 6th/543]

Posterior Cranial Fossa Fracture

◈ *Manipal Surgery 4th/1040; S. Das Textbook 6th/543*

- *Extravasation of blood in the suboccipital region causing **boggy swelling in the nape of the neck***
- *9th, 10th & 11th cranial nerves may be involved*
- ***Battle sign: Discolouration of skin & collection of blood occur in the region of mastoid process***

Anterior Cranial Fossa Fracture

◈ *Manipal Surgery 4th/1040; S. Das Textbook 6th/543*

- In this fracture there will be haemorrhage from the nose (epistaxis) &/or escape of CSF (***CSF Rhinorrhoea***) & even brain matter through nose
- There may be subconjunctival haemorrhage
- Olfactory nerve is frequently torn. Optic nerve usually escapes injury.3rd, 4th & Ist division of 5th & 6th cranial nerve may be injured at sphenoidal fissure

Middle Cranial Fossa Fracture

◈ *Manipal Surgery 4th/1040; S. Das Textbook 6th/543*

- Haemorrhage & escape of cranial content (CSF & brain matter) may be ***expected from the ear (CSF otorrhoea)*** & the mouth
- Occasionally there may be epistaxis when the nasal sinuses are affected
- 7th, 8th & occasionally 6th cranial nerve may be injured

152. Ans. b. Nocturia. & e. Urgency

[Ref: L & B 26th/1315; Nelson 19th/1848-49; S. Das 6th/1251-52]

Overactive Bladder

◈ *https://en. wikipedia. org/wiki/Overactive_bladder*

- Overactive bladder is characterized by a group of four symptoms: ***urgency, urinary frequency, nocturia, and urge incontinence***. Urge incontinence is not present in the "dry" classification.
- **Urgency** is considered the hallmark symptom of overactive bladder
- **Urinary frequency** is considered abnormal if the person urinates more than eight times in a day.
- **Nocturia** is a symptom where the person complains of interrupted sleep because of an urge to void
- **Urge incontinence** is a form of urinary incontinence characterized by the involuntary loss of urine occurring for no apparent reason

The Overactive Bladder

◈ *L & B 26th/1315*

- Phasic increases in pressure give rise to ***urgency and urge incontinence*** (detrusor overactivity). This abnormality is found in patients with neurogenic bladder dysfunction, when it is known as detrusor hyperreflexia.
- About 50 per cent of men with bladder outflow obstruction have detrusor instability, and in about half of them the instability resolves after prostatectomy.

Urge Incontinence

◈ *Schwartz 8th/Chap 39*

- An **overactive bladder** is characterized by involuntary detrusor contractions. If these involuntary contractions generate sufficient pressure to overcome the urethral resistance, ***urinary incontinence*** results.
- Two terms distinguish the **etiology of overactive bladders. Involuntary bladder contractions** secondary to an upper tract neurologic insult, such as a stroke or spinal cord injury, is referred to as ***detrusor hyperreflexia***. Involuntary contractions resulting from irritation of the bladder itself is termed ***detrusor instability.***
- When possible, the underlying etiology for an ***overactive bladder*** should be addressed. For example, if stress incontinence is the primary problem, the urge incontinence will resolve in more than half of patients after surgical treatment for stress incontinence.
- The vast majority of patients with ***overactive bladders*** do not have a clearly identifiable cause and symptomatic treatment is employed.
- Anticholinergics are effective, particularly when combined with timed voiding. Various biofeedback programs are effective for motivated patients with milder symptoms. A permanent sacral nerve stimulator can be implanted to inhibit bladder contractions and help prevent urinary incontinence.

Overactive Bladder (OAB) Symptoms

◈ *http://www. medicinenet. com/overactive_bladder/article. htm*

Symptoms of overactive bladder (OAB) result from sudden and involuntary contractions of the bladder muscles, leading to a

- Sudden need to urinate (urinary urgency) and/or
- Urinary incontinence (leakage of urine)
- In addition to urinary urgency and incontinence, symptoms of overactive bladder can include- urinary frequency (having to urinate often) & nocturia (urinating frequently at night).

153. Ans. e Orchidectomy...

[Ref: L & B 26th/1377-79; 25th/1377-79; CSDT11th/1338-39]

Incompletely Descended Testis

◈ *L & B 26th/1377-79*

- About 4 per cent of boys are born with one or both testes incompletely descended. About two thirds of these reach the scrotum during the first three months of life, but full descent after that is uncommon. The ***incidence of testicular maldescent at the age of one year is around 1 per cent.***
- The condition is more common on the right and is bilateral in 20 per cent of cases.
- Microscopic changes are apparent from 1–2 years, including ***loss of Leydig cells, degeneration of Sertoli cells and decreased spermatogenesis***.
- The **cancer risk** for adults after cryptorchidism in childhood is ***5–10 times greater than normal.***
- **Orchidopexy** is usually performed before the boy reaches 12 months of age in an attempt to prevent the consequences The testis and ***spermatic cord are mobilized and the testis is repositioned in the scrotum***.
- Orchidectomy should be considered if the incompletely descended testis is atrophic, particularly in the post-pubertal boy if the other testis is normal

"About 4% of boys are born with one or both testes incompletely descended have increased liability to malignant disease; cancer is more common in an incompletely descended testes. ***Orchidopexy*** *may or may not diminish the risk but it does improve the prospect of early diagnosis.* ***Orchidopexy is usually performed after the***

age of 1 year to avoid the risks of operating on a tiny patient. ***Testes should be brought down into the scrotum before the boy starts school"*** *(L & B 26th/1377-79, 25th/1377-78)*

Undescended Testis (Cryptorchidism)

◈ *CSDT11th/1338-39*

- The incidence of ***undescended or partially descended testis is 1–2% in full-term*** infants and up to ***30% in premature babies.*** The right testis is affected in 45% of cases, the left testis in 30%, and both testes in 25%.
- ***Operation is indicated after 12–18 months*** since degenerative changes begin to take place in these testes that may impair spermatogenesis and lead to malignant transformation.
- ***Orchidopexy is the surgical method for mobilizing the testis***

154. Ans. a. Hip..., c. Presented..., d. T. B can... & e. Causes referred...

[Ref: L & B 26th/985; Sabiston 19th/1108-09; CSDT 11th/526; Manipal 4th/661]

"Psoas abscesses may be primary or secondary. ***Primary psoas abscesses, which occur without associated disease of other organs, are caused by hematogenous spread of Staphylococcus aureus*** from an occult source and are predominantly seen in children and young adults. Secondary psoas abscesses result from spread of infection from adjacent organs, principally from the intestine, and are therefore most often polymicrobial. The ***most common cause is Crohn's disease.*** The pyogenic bacteria (*E coli*, bacteroides, proteus, klebsiella) have replaced *Mycobacterium tuberculosis* as the major causative organism. A positive blood culture—especially with *Bacteroides*—is an ominous finding" *(CSDT 11th/526)*

Retroperitoneal (Psoas) Abscess

◈ *L & B 26th/985*

- The retroperitoneal space can also be a site for abscess formation which for practical purposes is ***almost synonymous with psoas abscess.***
- With the decline of *Mycobacterium tuberculosis* as a major pathogen in developed countries a psoas abscess was mostly found secondary to direct spread of infection from the inflamed ± perforated digestive or urinary tract.
- Clinical presentation is with **back pain, lassitude and fever.** A swelling may point to the groin as it tracks along ileopsoas.
- Pain may be elicited by ***passive extension of the hip or a fixed flexion of the hip*** evident on inspection.

Retroperitoneal Abscesses

◈ *Sabiston 19th/1108-09*

- The bacteriology of retroperitoneal abscesses is related to the etiology. Infections originating from the **kidney** are often monomicrobial, involving gram-negative rods such as ***Proteus mirabilis* and *E. coli*.** Abscesses associated with diseases of the **gastrointestinal tract** involve *E. coli, Enterobacter* **species, enterococci, and anaerobic species such as** *Bacteroides*.
- These infections are multimicrobial, involving species such as gram-negative bacilli, enterococci, and anaerobic species. ***Infections from hematogenous spread are usually monomicrobial and related to staphylococcal species.*** **Tuberculosis** of the spine is an important cause of retroperitoneal abscesses in immunocompromised individuals and those immigrating from underdeveloped countries.
- The **most common symptoms** of retroperitoneal abscesses include ***abdominal or flank pain (60%-75%), fever and chills (30%-90%), malaise (10%-22%), and weight loss (12%).*** Patients with psoas abscesses may have ***referred pain to the hip, groin, or knee.***

155. Ans. b. Commonly..., c. Pain... & d. Pain...

[Ref: L & B 26th/877-78, 25th/899; Sabiston 19th/1727-28; CSDT 11th/815-16; Textbook of Surgery by S. Das 5th/151]

Intermittent Claudication

◈ *L & B 26th/877-78*

- Intermittent claudication is a ***cramp-like pain*** felt in the muscles that is:
  - Brought on by walking;
  - Not present on taking the first step (unlike osteoarthritis);
  - Relieved by standing still (unlike nerve compression from a lumbar intervertebral disc prolapse or osteoarthritis of the spine or spinal stenosis).
- The ***pain of claudication is usually felt in the calf*** because the superficial femoral artery is the most commonly affected (70 per cent of cases). Aortoiliac disease (30 per cent of cases) may cause

◈ *CSDT 11th/815-16*

- It refers to pain or fatigue in muscles of the lower extremity ***caused by walking and relieved by rest.***
- Patients occasionally describe "cramping" or "tiredness" in the muscle. Typically, symptoms are completely relieved after 2–5 minutes of inactivity.
- Claudication is distinguished from other types of pain in the extremities in that some exertion is always required before it appears; it is reproducible; it does not occur at rest; and it is ***relieved by cessation of walking.***
- Relief of symptoms ***is not dependent upon sitting or other positional change.*** The distance a patient can walk varies with the rate of walking, the level of incline, and the degree of arterial obstruction.
- Regardless of which arterial segment is involved, ***claudication most commonly involves the calf muscles due to their high workload with normal walking.***
- The correct diagnosis should be easily established by determining the *location of pain (calf), the quality of the pain, the length of time required for relief of symptoms, the reproducibility of symptoms, the distance walked before symptoms begin* ***(initial claudication distance)****, and the type of rest or position required for symptom relief.*

156. Ans. c. Typical... & e. Treatment...

[Ref: L & B 26th/894- 99; Sabiston 19th/1697-99 Sabiston 18th/1906-20; CSDT 11th/829-35; Manipal 4th/1031-32; Harrison 19th/1639-40, 17th/1564-65; Robbins 9th/503, 7th/531-32]

"Most AAAs rupture into the retroperitoneal cavity, which results in the ***classical triad of pain, hypotension, and a pulsatile mass. However, this triad is seen in only 25–50% of patients***"- *http://www. ncbi. nlm. nih. gov/pubmed*

Abdominal Aortic Aneurysm (AAA)

◈ *Harrison 19th/1639-40; 17th/1564-65*

- The classic presentation of a ruptured AAA is the **triad** of ***sudden-onset midabdominal or flank pain, shock, and the presence of a pulsatile abdominal mass.*** However, ***only one third of patients with ruptured AAA present with this triad.***
- The pain may radiate into the groin or thigh and is usually severe, constant, and unaffected by position. It is more commonly located on the left side.

◈ *L & B 26th/894-99*

- Abdominal aortic aneurysm is by far the most common type of large vessel aneurysm and is found in 2 per cent of the population at autopsy; ***95 per cent have associated atheromatous degeneration and 95 per cent occur below the renal arteries.***
- An asymptomatic abdominal aortic aneurysm in an otherwise fit patient should be ***considered for repair if >55 mm in diameter*** (measured by ultrasonography).
- **Endovascular aneurysm repair** (EVAR) is now established in clinical practice and has been shown to have reduced mortality compared to ***open repair*** over the first six years. Currently, about 50 per cent of infrarenal aneurysms are suitable for EVAR which is dependent on the morphology of the aneurysm when assessed by CT scan.
- Less than 50 per cent of patients with rupture survive to reach hospital. Ruptured abdominal aortic aneurysm is a surgical emergency; it should be suspected in a patient with the ***triad of severe abdominal and/or back pain, hypotension and a pulsatile abdominal mass.***

◈ *Harrison 19th/1639-40; 17th/1564-65*

- Atleast 90% of abdominal aortic aneurysm (AAA) of ***size > 4cm***[Q] in diameter is due to atherosclerosis.
- ***Male*** are more frequently affected than female.
- The aneurysm **most commonly** arises *below the level of renal artery*[Q].
- Prognosis of abdominal aortic aneurysm is depends on size of the aneurysm and the severity of co-existing coronary artery and cerebrovascular disease. Most of the time they are asymptomatic

"**Operative repair**[Q] *of the aneurysm and insertion of a prosthetic graft are indicated for abdominal aortic aneurysms of any size that are expanding rapidly or are associated with symptoms. For asymptomatic aneurysms, operation is indicated if the diameter is >5. 5 cm.* ***Endovascular repair with stent placement is an emerging approach*** *but, at the current time, is associated with a mortality rate of approximately 40%."* (Harrison 19th/1640, 17th/1564)

"Obstruction of a vessel, particularly of the iliac, renal, mesenteric, or vertebral branches that supply the spinal cord leading to ischemic tissue injury. The ***treatment*** *of abdominal and thoracic arortic aneurysms is evolving toward* ***endoluminal approaches using stent grafts*** *(expandable wire frames covered by a cloth sleeve) rather than surgery for some patients"* (Robbins 9th/503, 7th/532)

"Approx.40-60% pt. have suitable anatomy & are candidate for endoluminal repair with stent placement" *(Fisher Mastery of Surgery 5th/2052)*

"Ninety percent of aneurysms *of the abdominal aorta involve the segment of the* ***aorta between the takeoff of the renal arteries and the aortic bifurcation****, but may include variable portions of the common iliac arteries"* (CSDT 11th/830)

*"****AAA:*** *95% have associated atheromatous degeneration &* ***95% occur below the renal arteries****"* (L&B 25th/918)

157. Ans. a. Incidence..., c. More..., d. Commonly... & e. May...

[Ref: L & B 26th/964-65; Sabiston 19th/1128-29; CSDT 11th/792-93; Manipal 4th/867]

Factor which Precipitate Incisional Hernia

◈ *Manipal 4th/867*

- ***Anatomical site:*** *The* ***midline is*** *especially weak in lower abdomen because of absence of posterior rectus sheath below the arcuate line of or semilunar line. That is the reason why many cases of incisional hernia after gynaecological operations*
- *Lumbar incision,* ***lower midline incision*** *& large transverse incisions often give rise to incisional hernias*

"Incisional hernias ***account for 15% to 20% of all abdominal wall hernias;*** *umbilical and epigastric hernias constitute 10% of hernias.* ***Incisional hernias are twice as common in women as in men.*** *"* (Sabiston 19th/1129)

Incisional Hernia

◈ *L & B 26th/964-65*

- These arise through a defect in the musculofascial layers of the abdominal wall in the region of a ***postoperative scar.*** Thus they may appear anywhere on the abdominal surface.
- Incisional hernias have been reported in ***10–50 per cent of laparotomy incisions*** and 1–5 per cent of laparoscopic port-site incisions.
- Factors predisposing to their development are patient factors (***Obesity***, general poor healing due to malnutrition, immunosuppression or steroid therapy, chronic cough, cancer), wound factors (poor quality tissues, wound infection) and surgical factors (inappropriate suture material, incorrect suture placement).

◈ *L & B 26th/964*

- Incidence ***10–50 per cent after surgery***
- Causation due to patient, wound and surgeon factors
- Wide variation in size
- Often multiple defects within the same scar
- Obstruction is common but strangulation is rare
- Open and laparoscopic repairs possible
- ***About 10% of abdominal operations result in incisional hernias.***
- *"**Incisional hernias** occur as a result of excessive tension and **inadequate healing of a previous incision**, which is often associated with surgical site infection. **Obesity**, advanced age, malnutrition, ascites, pregnancy, and conditions that increase intra-abdominal pressure are factors that predispose to the development of an incisional hernia. (Sabiston 18th/1173)*

Incisional Hernia (Ventral Hernia)

◈ *CSDT 11th/792-93*

Etiology

- Poor surgical technique. Inadequate fascial bites, tension on the fascial edges, or too tight a closure are most often responsible for incisional failure.
- Postoperative wound infection.
- Age. Wound healing is usually slower and less solid in older patients.
- **Obesity.** Fat patients frequently have increased intra-abdominal pressure. The presence of fat in the abdominal wound masks tissue layers and increases the incidence of seromas and hematomas in wounds

158. Ans. b. 5 Node..., c. T1N2M0... & e. Any tumour...

[Ref: L & B 26th/1048-49; Sabiston 19th/1207-08]

Staging of Gastric Carcinoma

◈ *L & B 26th/1048*

- In an attempt to reflect the current evidence base and to improve outcome prediction for individual patients ***all gastric tumours whose epicentre is within 5 cm of the gastrooesophageal junction and extend into the oesophagus are now classified according to the oesophageal system.***
- ***Tumours whose epicentre is within 5 cm of the gastro-oesophageal junction but do not extend into the oesophagus, and all other gastric cancers are staged using the revised gastric staging system.***
- In addition, any tumour that perforates the serosa is now classified as T4 disease.

Direct spread: *The tumour penetrates the muscularis, serosa and ultimately adjacent organs such as the pancreas, colon and liver. (L & B 26th/1048)*

Table *(L & B 26th/1048)*: **International Union Against Cancer (UICC) staging of gastric cancer.**

T1	*Tumour involves lamina propria, submucosa*
	T1a lamina propria
	T1b submucosa
T2	*Tumour invades muscularis propria*
T3	*Tumour involves subserosa*
T4a	*Tumour perforates serosa*
T4b	*Tumour invades adjacent organs*
N0	*No lymph nodes*
N1	*Metastasis in 1–2 regional nodes*
N2	*Metastasis in 3–6 regional nodes*
N3a	*Metastasis in 7–15 regional nodes*
N3b	*Metastasis in more than 15 regional nodes*
M0	*No distant metastasis*
M1	*Distant metastasis (this includes peritoneum and distant lymph nodes)*

Table *(Harrison 19th/535)*: **Staging System for Gastric Carcinoma**

Stage	TNM	Features
0	T_{is}N0M0	Node negative; limited to mucosa
IA	T1N0M0	Node negative; invasion of lamina propria or submucosa
IB	T2N0M0 T1N1M0	Node negative; invasion of muscularis propria
II	T1N2M0 T2N1M0	Node positive; invasion beyond mucosa but within wall
	T3N0M0	Node negative; extension through wall
IIIA	T2N2M0 T3N1-2M0	Node positive; invasion of muscularis propria or through wall
IIIB	T4N0-1M0	Node negative; adherence to surrounding tissue
IIIC	T4N2-3M0 T3N3M0	>3 nodes positive; invasion of serosa or adjacent structures 7 or more positive nodes; penetrates wall without invading serosa or adjacent structures
IV	T4N2M0	Node positive; adherence to surrounding tissue
	T1-4N0-2 M1	Distant metastases

159. Ans. **b. PPI is...**

[Ref: L & B 26th/1039-40; Sabiston 19th/1203]

Early and Late Dumping

◈ *L & B 26th/1039-40*

Although considered together because the symptoms are similar, early and late dumping have different aetiologies. ***A common feature, however, is early rapid gastric emptying.*** Many patients have both early and late dumping.

Early Dumping

◈ *L & B 26th/1039*

- It consists of abdominal and vasomotor symptoms that are found in about 10 per cent of patients following gastrectomy or vagotomy and drainage.
- The small bowel is filled with foodstuffs from the stomach, which have a high osmotic load, and this leads to the sequestration of fluid from the circulation into the gastrointestinal tract. This can be observed by the rise in the packed cell volume while the symptoms are present.
- The principal treatment is dietary manipulation. ***Small, dry meals are best***, and ***avoiding fluids with a high carbohydrate content also helps***.
- Fortunately, following operation, the syndrome tends to improve with time. For some reason, however, there is a group of patients who suffer intractable dumping regardless of any of these measures.
- The ***somatostatin analogue octreotide*** given before meals has been shown to be useful in some individuals and the long-acting preparation may also be useful.
- Revisional surgery may be occasionally required.

Late Dumping

◈ *L & B 26th/1039*

- This is reactive hypoglycaemia. The carbohydrate load in the small bowel causes a rise in the plasma glucose, which, in turn, causes insulin levels to rise, causing a secondary hypoglycaemia.
- This can be easily demonstrated by serial measurements of blood glucose in a patient following a test meal.
- The *treatment is essentially the same as for early dumping*. Octreotide is very effective in dealing with this problem.

Table *(L & B 26th/1039)*: **Features of early and late dumping**

	Early	Late
Incidence	5-10%	5%
Relation to meals	Almost immediate	Second hour after meal
Durations of attack Relief	30-40 minutes lying down	Food
Aggravated by	More food	Exercise
Precipitating factor	Food, especially carbohydrate-rich and wet	As early dumping
Major symptoms	Epigastric fullness, sweating light headedness, tachyoardia, colic sometimes diarrhea	Tremor, faintness prostration

Early form of Dumping Syndrome

◈ *Sabiston 19th/1203*

- The early form of dumping syndrome usually occurs within ***20 to 30 minutes after ingestion of a meal and is accompanied by both GI and cardiovascular symptoms.***
- The symptoms characteristically occur while the ***patient is seated at the table eating or shortly after eating.***
- Although the exact sequence of events responsible for this syndrome remains to be fully defined, it is generally agreed that it ***occurs because of the rapid passage of food of high osmolarity from the stomach into the small intestine.***
- Most patients subjected to gastric surgery complain of some dumping-like symptoms after surgery. Most, ***however, experience spontaneous relief and require no specific therapy.***
- In those situations in which symptoms are prolonged, ***dietary measures are usually sufficient.*** These **dietary measures include** ***avoiding foods containing large amounts of sugar, frequent feeding of small meals rich in protein and fat, and separating liquids from solids during a meal.***

Late Dumping

◈ *Sabiston 19th/1203*

- The syndrome of late dumping appears ***2 to 3 hours after a meal*** and is far less common than early dumping. The ***basic defect in this order is also rapid gastric emptying***; however, ***it is related specifically to carbohydrates being delivered rapidly into the proximal intestine.***
- These patients should be ***advised to ingest frequent small meals and to reduce their carbohydrate intake.*** Some patients have found benefit with pectin either alone or in combination with acarbose, an α-glucoside hydrolase inhibitor that delays carbohydrate absorption through impairment of intraluminal starch and sucrose digestion.

160. Ans. **All**

[Ref: L & B 26th/992-93; Sabiston 19th/1043- 46, 18th/1082-85; Harrison 19th/98, 1910, 17th/1854]

"Gastrointestinal disorders are the most common cause of nontraumatic chest discomfort and often produce symptoms that are difficult to discern from more serious causes of chest pain, ***including myocardial ischemia.*** Esophageal disorders, in particular, may simulate angina in the character and location of the pain. Chest pain can result from injury to the esophagus, such as a Mallory-Weiss tear or ***even an esophageal rupture (Boerhaave syndrome) caused by severe vomiting***" *(Harrison 19th/98)*

Boerhaave's Syndrome

◈ *Sabiston 19th/1043-46*

- It has since been elucidated that recurrent emesis disrupts the normal vomiting reflex that enables sphincter relaxation, ***resulting in an increase in intrathoracic esophageal pressure and perforation.***
- Postemetic rupture of the esophagus, now known as *Boerhaave's syndrome,* is only one of many causes of esophageal rupture

- Signs of perforation change as time progresses. Early on, a patient may present with tachypnea, tachycardia, and a low-grade fever but have no other overt signs of perforation. With increased mediastinal and pleural contamination, patients progress toward hemodynamic instability and shock.
- Diagnosis of an esophageal perforation may be made radiographically. A chest roentgenogram may ***demonstrate a hydropneumothorax***.
- ***Most perforations are found above the GEJ on the left lateral wall of the esophagus,*** which results in a 10% false-negative rate in the contrast esophagram if the patient is not placed in the lateral decubitus position.
- Chest CT shows ***mediastinal air and fluid*** at the site of perforation
- Esophageal barotrauma or Boerhaave syndrome or spontaneous perforation of the esophagus is usually due to severe barotrouma when a person vomits against a closed glottis. The pressure in the esophagus rapidly increases & it ***bursts at its weakest point in the lower third***[Q]. The second MC site of perforation is at the ***midthoracic esophagus on the right side at the level of the azygos vien.***
- **C/F:** - The most serious type of perforation, because of the *volume of infected material that is released under pressure.*
    - Presented with ***severe pain in the chest or upper abdomen***[Q] following a meal or a bout of drinking.
    - Vomiting, hematemesis, or dysphagia also may accompany them.
    - Many cases may be ***misdiagnosed as myocardial infarction or as perforated peptic ulcer or pancreatitis***[Q].
    - There may be surprising amount of rigidity on examination of the upper abdomen.

> ***Pneumomediastinum (Oesophageal perforation)***: *The physical examination usually reveals subcutaneous emphysema in the suprasternal notch and* ***Hamman's sign***[Q]*, which is a* ***crunching or clicking noise synchronous with the heartbeat***[Q] *and best heard in the left lateral decubitus position (Harrison 19th/1910, 17th/1661)*

161. Ans. a. Presents…, c. Associated… & d. Fibrosis…

[Ref: L & B 26th/771; Robbins 9th/231; Sabiston 19th/896; Harshmohan 7th/796; Harrison 19th/2299, 291e-1t]

"Despite extensive fibrosis, ***thyroid dysfunction is uncommon.*** *There is association b/w Reidel's thyroiditis & IgG4 –related systemic diseases causing idiopathic fibrosis at other sites (retroperitoneum, mediastinum, biliary tree, lung & orbit" (Harrison 19th/2299)*

Riedel's thyroiditis or Invasive Fibrous Thyroiditis or Riedel's Struma

L & B 26th/771; Harshmohan 7th/796

- It is a rare disorder that typically occurs in middle-aged women. It presents with an insidious ***painless goiter*** with local symptoms due to compression of the esophagus, trachea, neck veins, or recurrent laryngeal nerves.
- ***Dense fibrosis*** disrupts normal gland architecture and can extend outside the thyroid capsule. Despite these extensive histologic changes, ***thyroid dysfunction is uncommon.***
- Diagnosis requires open biopsy as FNA biopsy is usually inadequate.
- Treatment is directed to surgical relief of ***compressive symptoms***. Tamoxifen may also be beneficial. There is an association between Riedel's thyroiditis and idiopathic fibrosis at other sites (retroperitoneum, mediastinum, biliary tree, lung, and orbit).

Riedel's Struma

Sabiston 19th/896

- Riedel's thyroiditis (struma) is a rare entity characterized by a firm thyroid secondary to a chronic inflammatory process involving the entire gland.
- Surgical pathology reveals ***dense fibrous tissue*** and nearly total obliteration of normal follicular architecture.

IgG4-Related Disease

Robbins 9th/231

- IgG4-related disease (IgG4-RD) is a newly recognized constellation of disorders characterized by tissue infiltrates dominated by IgG4 antibody-producing plasma cells and lymphocytes, particularly T cells, storiform fibrosis, obliterative phlebitis, and ***usually increased serum IgG4.***
- Although recognized only recently, IgG4-related disease has now been described in virtually every organ system: the biliary tree, salivary glands, periorbital tissues, kidneys, lungs, lymph nodes, meninges, aorta, breast, prostate, thyroid, pericardium, and skin. Many medical conditions long viewed as confined to single organs are part of the IgG4-RD spectrum.
- These include Mikulicz syndrome (enlargement and fibrosis of salivary and lacrimal glands), ***Riedel thyroiditis***, idiopathic retroperitoneal fibrosis, autoimmune pancreatitis, and inflammatory pseudotumors of the orbit, lungs, and kidneys, to name a few.

162. Ans. a. Normal…, b. T4 to… & e. Increased…

[Ref: CMDT 2015/1096; Harrison 19th/2299-2300]

Sick Euthyroid Syndrome

Harrison 19th/2299-2300

- Any acute, severe illness can cause abnormalities of circulating TSH or thyroid hormone levels in the absence of underlying thyroid disease, making these measurements potentially misleading. The major cause of these hormonal changes is the release of cytokines such as IL-6. Unless a thyroid disorder is strongly suspected, the routine testing of thyroid function should be avoided in acutely ill patients.
- The most common hormone pattern in sick euthyroid syndrome (SES) is a ***decrease in total and unbound T_3 levels (low T_3 syndrome) with normal levels of T4 and TSH.***
- The magnitude of the fall in T_3 correlates with the severity of the illness. ***T_4 conversion to T_3 via peripheral deiodination is impaired, leading to increased reverse T_3 (rT_3).***

- Despite this effect, decreased clearance rather than increased production is the major basis for increased T_3. Also, T_4 is alternately metabolized to the hormonally inactive T_3 sulfate.
- It is generally assumed that this low T_3 state is adaptive, because it can be induced in normal individuals by fasting. Teleologically, the fall in T_3 may limit catabolism in starved or ill patients.

163. Ans. d. Parotid. tumours...

[Ref: L & B 26th/722, 728, 732-33; Sabiston 19th/811-13; Textbook of Surgery by S. Das 5th/607-60]

"**Tumours of minor salivary glands** *are histologically similar to those of major glands; however, up to* ***90 per cent of minor salivary gland tumours are malignant***" *(L & B 26th/722)*

"**Warthin tumour** *(papillary cystadenoma Lymphomatosum):* ***It arise almost always***[Q] ***in the parotid gland*** *(the only tumour virtually restricted to the parotid & occur more commonly in male*[Q] *than in female (other tumour more common in female). Oncocytes*[Q] *that are epithelial cell stuffed with mitochondria are found in warthin tumour. (Robbins 9th/745, 7th/792-93)*

"*The* ***parotid gland*** *is the* ***most common site for salivary tumours****. Most tumours arise in the superficial lobe and present as slow growing, painless swellings below the ear, in front of the ear or in the upper aspect of the neck" (L & B 26th/732)*

"*Tumours involving the* ***sublingual gland*** *are extremely rare and are usually (85 per cent) malignant. Treatment requires wide excision involving the overlying mucosa and simultaneous neck dissection" (L & B 26th/725)*

"*Tumours of the* ***submandibular gland*** *are uncommon and usually present as a slow-growing, painless swelling within the submandibular triangle. Only 50 per cent of submandibular gland tumours are benign, in contrast to 80–90 per cent of parotid gland tumours" (L & B 26th/728)*

Table *(L & B 26th/728)*: **Salivary gland tumours – frequency and distribution.**

Type	Location	Frequency	Malignant (%)
Major	Parotid	Common	10-20
	Submandibular	Uncommon	50
	Sublingual	Very rate	85
Minor	Upper aerodigestive tract	Rare	90

Pleomorphic Adenoma (Mixed Tumour)

- This is the commonest tumour[Q] of the major salivary glands
- This tumour most *commonly*[Q] *occur in the parotid & about 90% is seen in this gland*; 7% is seen in submandibular gland. In the parotid the commonest location is the tail of parotid[Q].
- **Age**: It is more frequent around 40 years of age, but it is also seen in children
- **Sex**: Slightly higher incidence in *woman*[Q] has been noticed
- **Symptom**: The patients complains of a painless swelling of the side of the face which has been present for months or years. It is a slow growing tumour[Q] & gradually increases in size.
- This tumour is *radioresistant*[Q], so excision is the treatment of choice.
- *Superficial parotidectomy*[Q] *is the treatment of choice*[Q]. This operation is also known as **patey's operation** *(S. Das 5th/609)*
- In case of submandibular gland neoplasms, the whole gland is excised with particular care to preserve the lingual & hypoglossal nerve[Q].

164. Ans. a. Prevention..., b. Main indication... & c. Reduce...

[Ref: Sabiston 19th/1435-38, 18th/1535-40; Harrison 19th/1890-91, 2063-64, 18th/2599; L & B 26th/1075- 76, 25th/1090; CMDT 2016/604-07; CSDT11th/585-87; Manipal Surgery 3rd/461-62]

Surgical Shunts for Variceal Haemorrhage

◈ *L & B 26th/1076*

- The increasing availability of liver transplantation and TIPSS has greatly reduced the indications for surgical shunts. It is rarely considered for the acute management of variceal haemorrhage, as the morbidity and mortality in these circumstances are high.
- The **main current indication for a surgical shunt** is a patient with ***Child's grade A cirrhosis, in whom the initial bleed has been controlled by sclerotherapy.*** Long-term β-blocker therapy and chronic sclerotherapy or banding are the main alternatives.
- ***Surgical shunts are an effective method of preventing rebleeding from oesophageal or gastric varices, as they reduce the pressure in the portal circulation by diverting the blood into the low-pressure systemic circulation.***
- Shunts may be divided into ***selective (e.g., splenorenal) and non-selective*** *(e.g.,* ***portocaval****)*, the former attempting to ***preserve blood flow to the liver*** while decompressing the left side of the portal circulation responsible for giving rise to the oesophageal and gastric varices.
- Selective shunts may be associated with a lower incidence of portal systemic encephalopathy (PSE)

"**Portosystemic surgical shunts are:** ***End to side portocaval shunt, Side to side portocaval shunt, mesentericocaval shunt, proximal splenorenal & distal splenorenal shunt***" *(Manipal Surgery 3rd/461-62)*

Variceal Hemorrhage

◈ *Harrison 19th/2063-64*

- Treatment for variceal hemorrhage as a complication of portal hypertension is divided into two main categories: (1) primary prophylaxis and (2) prevention of re-bleeding once there has been an initial variceal hemorrhage primary prophylaxis can be achieved either through nonselective beta blockade or by variceal band ligation
- Once patients have had an acute bleed and have been managed successfully, attention should be paid to preventing recurrent bleeding. ***This usually requires repeated variceal band ligation until varices are obliterated***. Beta blockade may be of adjunctive benefit in patients who are having recurrent variceal band ligation; however, once varices have been obliterated, the need for beta blockade is lessened.
- ***Portosystemic shunt surgery is less commonly performed with the advent of TIPS***

Esophageal Varices

◈ *Harrison 19th/2063-64*

- Two complementary strategies guide therapy of bleeding varices: ***local treatment of the bleeding varices and treatment of the underlying portal hypertension.***
- Local therapies, including ***endoscopic variceal band ligation, endoscopic variceal sclerotherapy***, and balloon tamponade with a Sengstaken-Blakemore tube, effectively control acute hemorrhage in most patients
- **Endoscopic variceal ligation (EVL)** is indicated for the prevention of a ***first bleed (primary prophylaxis)*** from large esophageal varices, particularly in patients in whom beta blockers are contraindicated or not tolerated. EVL is also the preferred endoscopic therapy for control of active esophageal variceal bleeding and for subsequent eradication of esophageal varices ***(secondary prophylaxis).***
- **EVS** also controls acute hemorrhage in most patients, but it is generally ***used as salvage therapy when band ligation fails because of its higher complication rate compared to EVL.*** These techniques are used when varices are actively bleeding during endoscopy or (more commonly) when varices are the only identifiable cause of acute hemorrhage

Portosystemic Shunts

◈ *Sabiston 19th/1435-38; 18th/1535-40*

- Portosystemic shunts are ***clearly the most effective means of preventing recurrent hemorrhage*** in patients with portal hypertension. These procedures are effective because they all, to some degree, decompress the portal venous system by ***shunting portal flow into the low-pressure systemic venous system.***
- Depending on whether they completely decompress, compartmentalize, or partially decompress the portal venous circulation, portosystemic shunts can be **classified as *nonselective, selective, or partial.***
- In addition to variceal decompression, the goal of selective and partial portosystemic shunts is preservation of ***hepatic portal perfusion,*** thereby preventing or minimizing the adverse consequences of these procedures.

165. Ans. d. Unilateral cases...

[Ref: L & B 26th/634-38; Manipal 4th/297; L & B 25th/658-668; CSDT 11th/1257-58; Sabiston 18th/2138]

Cleft lip & Palate

◈ *L & B 26th/638, 25th/657*

- "**Cleft lip** repair is commonly performed ***between three and six months of age,*** whereas cleft palate repair is frequently performed between six and 18 months" *(L & B 26th/638)*
- The typical distribution of cleft types is:
  - ***Cleft lip alone: 15 per cent;***
  - ***Cleft lip and palate: 45 per cent;***
  - ***Isolated cleft palate: 40 per cent.***

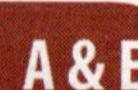

- Cleft lip/palate predominates in males, whereas cleft palate alone appears to be more common in females. ***In unilateral cleft lip, the deformity affects the left side in 60 per cent of cases***

◈ *Manipal 4th/297*

- C. lip results from abnormal development of the median nasal & maxillary process
- Cleft palate results from a failure of fusion of the two palatine process
- In 80% of the cases, cleft lip is unilateral & in about 60% of the cases it is associated with cleft palate

Table *(L & B 26th/638, 25th/657)*: **Timing of primary cleft lip and palate procedures (after Delaire)**

Cleft lip alone	
Unilateral (one side) One operation at 5–6 months	
Bilateral (both sides) One operation at 4–5 months	
Cleft palate alone	
Soft palate only:	One operation at 6 months
Soft and hard palate:	Two operations Soft palate at 6 months Hard palate at 15–18 months
Cleft lip and palate	
Unilateral: Two operations—	Cleft lip and soft palate at 5–6 months Hard palate and gum pad with or without lip revision at
Bilateral: Two operations—	Cleft lip and soft palate at 4–5 months Hard palate and gum pad with or without lip revision at 15–18 months

"The timing of cleft repair is important, and a general recommendation is ***lip repair at 3 months, palate repair by 12 months, and alveolar bone grafting at about 9 years*** which coincides with partial eruption of the canine teeth" *(Sabiston 18th/2138)*

166. Ans. b. First..., d. CVP...

[Ref: L & B 26th/303-06; CSDT 11th/238; Manipal 4th/173; Oxford surgery 5th/367-73]

Trauma Care

◈ *Oxford surgery 5th/367-73*

- Hypovolemic shock is the most common type of shock seen in trauma patient & occurs secondary to acute blood loss
- Therapy is restoration of intravascular volume. Thus, the patient should have two large-bore intravenous lines placed (14 or 16 gauges). The antecubital veins are preferred sites. If there is peripheral venous collapsed, then cannula is inserted into femoral vein.
- The ***subclavian & internal jugular vein*** should be reserved for those patients in whom major venous intra-abdominal injuries or pelvic fractures prevent effective use of femoral approach
- A blood specimen should be simultaneously obtained for cross matching
- Resuscitation consists of an initial bolus of 2 L of crystalloid solution
- If time has not allowed proper cross-matching, ***type O blood should be used***

- If a patient is fairly stable & access to CT is readily available, head & abdomen/pelvis CT scans can be obtained

Vascular Access

◈ *CSDT 11th/238*

- All patients with significant trauma should have large-caliber peripheral intravenous catheters inserted immediately for administration of crystalloid fluids as needed. If any degree of shock is present, at least two 14–16 gauge percutaneous intravenous lines should be established, usually in the antecubital fossa.
- If severe shock, hypovolemic cardiac arrest, or major vascular lesions are present, three intravenous lines are necessary, and one of the venous lines should be placed so that ***central venous pressure can be monitored as fluids are administered.***
- ***A blood sample for type and crossmatch*** should be sent from the venous line, if not already drawn.
- As soon as the first intravenous line is inserted, rapid crystalloid infusion should begin. Adult patients should be given 2 L of Ringer's lactate or normal saline. An additional 2 L of crystalloid may be administered if there is no improvement in blood pressure or only a transient response.
- ***Beyond this amount, packed red blood cells must also be given in combination with crystalloid solutions to avoid excessive hemodilution.***
- ***Group O, Rh-negative packed red blood cells*** should be immediately available for any patient with impending cardiac arrest or massive hemorrhage. Type-specific blood should be available within 15 minutes of patient arrival to the hospital.

ABCDE of Trauma Care

◈ *L & B 26th/303*

- Airway with cervical spine protection
- Breathing and ventilation
- Circulation with haemorrhage control
- Disability: Neurological status
- Exposure: Completely undress the patient and assess for other injuries

167. Ans. d. Ultrasound. is...

[Ref: L & B 26th/1200-08; Manipal 4th/828; L & B 25th/1205-12; Harrison 19th/1985-88, 18th/2516-18; CSDT11th/669]

Investigation

◈ *L & B 26th/1206*

- The diagnosis of acute appendicitis is essentially clinical
- The premise that it is better to remove a normal appendix than to delay diagnosis does not stand up to close scrutiny, particularly in the elderly. A number of clinical and laboratory-based scoring systems have been devised to assist diagnosis. The most widely used is the Alvarado score. A score of 7 or more is strongly predictive of acute appendicitis.
- In patients with an equivocal score (5–6), ***abdominal ultrasound*** or ***contrast-enhanced CT examination*** further reduces the rate of negative appendicectomy. Abdominal ultrasound examination is more useful in children and thin adults, particularly if gynaecological pathology is suspected, with a diagnostic accuracy in excess of 90 per cent
- ***Contrast-enhanced CT scan is most useful in patients in whom there is diagnostic uncertainty,*** particularly older patients, in whom acute diverticulitis, intestinal obstruction and neoplasm are likely differential diagnoses. Selective use of CT scanning may be cost-effective by reducing both the negative appendicectomy rate and the length of hospital stay

Imaging

◈ *Harrison 19th/1987-88*

- The effectiveness of **ultrasonography** as a tool to diagnosis appendicitis is highly operator dependent. Even in very skilled hands, the appendix may not be visualized. Its overall sensitivity is 0. 86, with a specificity of 0. 81.
- Ultrasonography, especially intravaginal techniques, appears to be most useful for identifying pelvic pathology in women. Ultrasonographic findings suggesting the presence of appendicitis include wall thickening, an increased appendiceal diameter, and the presence of free fluid.
- The sensitivity and specificity of **computed tomography (CT)** are 0. 94 and 0. 95, respectively. ***Thus, CT imaging, given its high negative predictive value, may be helpful if the diagnosis is in doubt,*** although studies performed early in the course of disease may not have any typical radiographic findings.

*"Pain is initially felt in umbilical region. **After a few hours, the pain localizes to the right iliac fossa.** This is called shifting pain of acute appendicitis" (Manipal 4th/828)*

*"**Lymphoid hyperplasia** narrows the lumen of the appendix, leading to luminal obstruction & later culminates to **acute appendicitis**" (L & B 26th/1202)*

Symptoms of Appendicitis

◈ *L & B 26th/1203*

- Periumbilical colic
- Pain shifting to the right iliac fossa
- Anorexia
- Nausea

Children

◈ *L & B 26th/1203*

- The diseases most commonly mistaken for acute appendicitis are acute gastroenteritis and mesenteric lymphadenitis. In mesenteric lymphadenitis, the pain is colicky in nature and cervical lymph nodes may be enlarged.
- ***It may be impossible to clinically distinguish*** Meckel's diverticulitis from acute appendicitis. The pain is similar; however, signs may be central or left sided. Occasionally, there is a history of antecedent abdominal pain or intermittent lower gastrointestinal bleeding.

*"**The sequence of abdominal discomfort and anorexia associated with acute appendicitis is pathognomonic**. The pain is described as being located in the periumbilical region initially and then migrating to the right lower quadrant. This classic sequence of symptoms occurs in only 66% of patients" (Harrison 18th/2516)*

*"The classical features of acute appendicitis begin with **poorly localised colicky abdominal pain**. This is due to mid-gut visceral discomfort in response to appendiceal inflammation and obstruction. **The pain is frequently first noticed in the periumbilical region** and is similar to, but less intense than, the colic of small bowel obstruction. " (L & B 25th/1208-09)*

Table *(L & B 26th)*: **The Alvarado (MANTRELS) score**

		Score
Symptoms	Migratory RIF pain	1
	Anorexia	1
	Nausea and vomiting	1
Signs	Tenderness (RIF)	2
	Rebound tenderness	1
	Elevated temperature	1
	Leukocytosis	2
	Shift to left	1
Total		10

168. Ans. a. Obesity..., c. ↑Incide... & e. Chronic...

[Ref: L & B 26th/1004-07; Robbins 9th/758-59, 7th/807; Harrison 19th/532-33, 18th/764]

*"**Adenocarcinoma of esophagus** most commonly produce mucin & form glands, often with **intestinal-type** morphology. In contrast to adenocarcinoma, half of squamous cell carcinoma occur in middle third of the esophagus. **Squamous cell carcinoma** begins as an in situ lesion termed **squamous dysplasia**" (Robbins 9th/758-59)*

Esophageal Adenocarcinoma

◈ *Robbins 9th/758, 8th/772*

- Adenocarcinoma now represents more than half of all esophageal cancers reported in the United States
- ***The majority of cases arise from the Barrett mucosa***. In rare instances, adenocarcinoma originates from heterotopic gastric mucosa or submucosal glands.
- The lifetime risk for cancer development from Barrett esophagus is approximately 10%.
- ***Tobacco use, radiation exposure and obesity are risk factors***, but there is no close association between alcohol ingestion and the development of adenocarcinoma of the esophagus. *Helicobacter pylori* infection may be a contributing factor, but there is no general agreement about this issue.
- **Adenocarcinomas arising** in the setting of Barrett esophagus are usually located in the ***distal third of esophagus and may invade the adjacent gastric cardia.***
- ***Adenocarcinomas arising in Barrett esophagus*** chiefly occur in patients over age 40, with a median age in the sixth decade. Similar to Barrett esophagus, adenocarcinoma is ***more common in men than in women***, and whites are affected more frequently than blacks, in contrast to squamous cell carcinomas.

Esophageal Cancer

◈ *Harrison 19th/532-33*

- Worldwide, squamous cell carcinoma is the more common cell type, having an incidence that rises strikingly in association with geographic location
- Whereas squamous cell cancers comprised the vast majority of esophageal cancers in the United States as recently as 40–50 years ago, ***more than 75% of esophageal tumors are now adenocarcinomas***, with the incidence of this histologic subtype continuing to increase rapidly.
- ***About 5% of esophageal cancers occur in the upper third of the esophagus (cervical esophagus), 20% in the middle third, and 75% in the lower third***

Table *(Harrison 19th/533)*

Some etiologic factors associated with adenocarcinoma of esophagus
Chronic gastroesophageal reflux
Obesity
Barrett's esophagus
Male sex
Cigarette smoking

169. Ans. a. May be..., c. Neostigmine...

[Ref: L & B 26th/1197; Harrison 19th/1982]

Pseudo-Obstruction

◈ *L & B 26th/1197*

- This condition describes an obstruction, usually of the colon, that occurs in the absence of a mechanical cause or acute intra abdominal disease. It is associated with a variety of syndromes in which there is an underlying neuropathy and/or myopathy and a range of other factors

Small Intestinal Pseudo-Obstruction

- This condition may be primary (i.e. idiopathic or associated with familial visceral myopathy) or secondary.
- The clinical picture consists of recurrent subacute obstruction. The diagnosis is made by the exclusion of a mechanical cause.
- Treatment consists of initial correction of any underlying disorder. ***Metoclopramide and erythromycin may be of use.***

Colonic Pseudo-Obstruction

- This may occur in an acute or a chronic form. The former, also known as Ogilvie's syndrome, presents as acute large bowel obstruction.
- ***The absence of a mechanical cause requires urgent confirmation by colonoscopy*** or a single-contrast water-soluble barium enema or CT. Once confirmed, pseudo-obstruction requires treatment of any identifiable cause.

- If this is ineffective, ***intravenous neostigmine*** should be given (1 mg intravenously), with a further 1 mg given intravenously within a few minutes if the first dose is ineffective.
- During this procedure, it is best to sit the patient on a commode. ECG monitoring is required and atropine should be available.
- If neostigmine is not effective, ***colonoscopic decompression should be performed***.

Trychobezoars and Phytobezoars

- These are firm masses of undigested hair ball and fruit/vegetable fibre, respectively. These causes bolus obstruction of intestine (not pseudo-obstruction) *(L & B 26th/1183)*

Table *(L & B 26th/1197)*: **Factors associated with pseudo-obstruction**

Metabolic
▪ Diabetes
▪ Hypokalaemia
▪ Uraemia
▪ Myxodoema
Severe trauma (especially to the lumbar spine and pelvis)
Shock
▪ Burns
▪ Myocardial infarction
▪ Stroke
▪ Idiopathic
▪ Septicaemia
▪ Postoperative (for example, fractured neck of femur)
Retroperitoneal irritation
▪ Blood
▪ Urine
▪ Enzymes (pancreatitis)
▪ Tumour
Drugs
▪ Tricyclic antidepressants
▪ Phenothiazines
▪ Laxatives
Secondary gastrointestinal involvement
▪ Scleroderma
▪ Chagas' disease

Table *(Harrison 19th/1982)*: **Most common causes of ileus (functional or pseudo-obstruction of the intestine**

- Intra abdominal procedures, lumbar spinal injuries, or surgical procedures on the lumbar spine and pelvis
- Metabolic or electrolyte abnormalities, especially hypokalemia and hypomagnesemia, but also hyponatremia, uremia, and severe hyperglycemia
- Drugs such as opiates, antihistamines, and some psychotropic (*e.g.*, haloperidol, tricyclic antidepressants) and anticholinergic agents
- Intestinal ischemia
- Intraabdominal or retroperitoneal inflammation or hemorrhage
- Lower lobe pneumonias
- Intraoperative radiation (likely due to muscle damage)
- Systemic sepsis
- Hyperparathyroidism
- Pseudo-obstruction (Ogilvie's syndrome)
- Ileus secondary to hereditary or acquired visceral myopathies and neuropathies that disrupt myocellular neural coordination
- Some collagen vascular diseases such as lupus erythematosus or scleroderma

170. Ans. a. Most..., c. Treatment... & d. Most...

[Ref: L & B 26th/1184-85, 1188; 25th/1194-95; Sabiston 19th/1314-16; 18th/1369-71]

"The increased incidence of volvulus in volvulus belt (an area extending along south America, Africa, Middle East, India & Russia) has been attributed to a ***diet high in fiber*** and vegetables" *(Sabiston 19th/1314)*

Volvulus

◈ *L & B 26th/1185*

- May involve the small intestine, caecum or sigmoid colon; neonatal midgut volvulus secondary to midgut malrotation is life-threatening
- The ***most common spontaneous type in adults is sigmoid***
- Sigmoid volvulus can be relieved by decompression per anum
- Surgery is required to prevent or relieve ischaemia

Sigmoid Volvulus

◈ *L & B 26th/1188*

- The symptoms are of large bowel obstruction. Presentation varies in severity and acuteness, with younger patients appearing to develop the more acute form.
- Abdominal distension is an early and progressive sign, which may be associated with hiccough and retching. Constipation is absolute. In the elderly, a more chronic form may be seen. In some patients, the ***grossly distended torted left colon*** is visible through the abdominal wall.

Colonic Volvulus

◈ *Sabiston 19th/1314-16; 18th/1369-71*

- The condition most commonly affects the colon & ***most common site is sigmoid colon, with less frequent occurrences involving the right colon and terminal ileum***
- ***Sigmoid volvulus accounts for two thirds to three fourths of all cases of colonic volvulus.***
- Predisposing factors include ***chronic constipation and aging, with the average age of presentation being in the seventh to eighth decade of life.***
- Sigmoid volvulus may present as ***acute or subacute intestinal obstruction*** with signs and symptoms indistinguishable from those caused by cancer of the distal colon...
- CT reveals a characteristic mesenteric whorl.
- A contrast enema typically demonstrates the point of obstruction with the pathognomonic "***bird's beak***" deformity revealing the twist that obstructs the sigmoid lumen
- **Treatment of the sigmoid volvulus** begins with appropriate resuscitation and in most cases involves nonoperative decompression. Decompression relieves the acute problem and allows resection as an elective procedure, which can be accomplished with reduced morbidity and mortality.
- Patients with signs of colonic necrosis are not eligible for nonoperative decompression.
- Even if detorsion of the sigmoid is successful, ***elective sigmoid resection*** is indicated in most cases because of the extremely high recurrence rate (approaching 70%).

171. Ans. b. Sign &... c. Profuse..., & d. Sigmoid...

[Ref: L & B 26th/1170-71; Sabiston 19th/1309]

Diverticular Disease of the Large Intestine

◈ *Sabiston 19th/1309-14*

- ***Diverticula most commonly affect the sigmoid colon*** & are confined to the sigmoid colon in approx. 50% of patients with diverticulosis. The next most common area involved is the descending colon (approax. 40% of affected individuals) & the entire colon has diverticula in 5% to 10% of patients with diverticulosis

Diverticular disease of the Large Intestine

◈ *L & B 26th/1170-71*

- Diverticula are ***found in the left colon in around 75 per cent*** of over 70 year olds in the Western world. The condition is overwhelmingly found in the sigmoid, but diverticula are found in the caecum and can affect the whole colon (but not the rectum).
- Interestingly, in South-East Asia, right-sided diverticular disease is more common. Diverticula are most often ***asymptomatic (diverticulosis)*** and found incidentally, but can present ***clinically with sepsis or haemorrhage.***
- Epidemiology supports the widely held view that diverticular disease is a consequence of a ***refined Western diet deficient in dietary fibre.*** Diverticular disease is rare in Africa and Asia where the diet is high in natural fibre.

Complications of Diverticular Disease

◈ *L & B 26th/1170*

The majority of patients with diverticula are asymptomatic; historical studies suggest somewhere between 10 and 30 per cent will have symptomatic complications These complications are:

- **Pain and inflammation** (Diverticulitis).
- **Perforation**: Most often contained leading to pericolic abscess formation, but occasionally free leading to generalized peritonitis.
- **Intestinal obstruction**: Progressive fibrosis can cause stenosis of the sigmoid and large bowel obstruction or loops of small intestine can adhere to an inflamed sigmoid resulting in small bowel obstruction.
- **Haemorrhage:** Diverticulitis may present with profuse colonic haemorrhage.
- **Fistula formation:** (Colovesical, colovaginal, enterocolic, colocutaneous) occurs in 5 per cent of cases, colovesical.

Clinical Features

◈ *L & B 26th/1171*

- ***In mild cases, symptoms such as distension, flatulence and a sensation of heaviness in the lower abdomen may be indistinguishable from those of irritable bowel syndrome.*** These symptoms are thought to result from a combination of increased luminal pressure affecting wall tension and increased visceral hypersensitivity.
- The **difficulty in distinguishing** between otherwise uncomplicated diverticular disease and irritable bowel syndrome is such that surgical treatment is rarely, if ever, appropriate for diverticular disease in the absence of complications.
- Diverticulitis typically presents as persistent lower abdominal pain, usually in the left iliac fossa accompanied by loose stools or indeed constipation. Fever, malaise and leukocytosis can differentiate diverticulitis from painful diverticulosis.
- The lower abdomen is tender, especially on the left, but occasionally also in the right iliac fossa, if the sigmoid loop lies across the midline.
- ***Hemorrhage from colonic diverticula is typically painless & profuse***

172. Ans. a. May be..., b. Lymphoedema... & c. Condition...

[Ref: L & B 26th/926-29; Sabiston 19th/1821-23]

Primary Lymphoedema

◈ *L & B 26th/928-29*

- It has been proposed that all cases of primary lymphoedema are due to ***an inherited abnormality of the lymphatic system, sometimes termed 'congenital lymphatic dysplasia'.***
- However, it is possible that many sporadic cases of primary lymphoedema occur in the presence of a (near-)normal lymphatic system and are actually examples of secondary lymphoedema for which the triggering events have gone unrecognised.

- Primary lymphoedema is much ***more common in the legs than the arms.*** This may be because of gravity and a bipedal posture, the fact that the lymphatic system of the leg is less well developed, or the increased susceptibility of the leg to trauma and/or infection.
- Furthermore, loss of the venoarteriolar reflex (VAR), which protects lower limb capillaries from excessive hydrostatic forces in the erect posture, with age and disease (CVI, diabetes), may be important.
- Primary lymphoedema is usually classified on the basis of apparent genetic susceptibility, age of onset or lymphangiographic findings.
- **Lymphoedema congenita** (Onset at or within two years of birth) is more common in males and is more likely to be bilateral and involve the whole leg.
- Lymphoedema praecox (onset from 2 to 35 years) is three times more common in females, has a peak incidence shortly after menarche, is three times more likely to be unilateral than bilateral and usually only extends to the knee.
- Lymphoedema tarda develops, by definition, after the age of 35 years and is often associated with obesity, with lymph nodes being replaced with fibrofatty tissue. The cause is unknown. Lymphoedema developing for the first time after 50 years should prompt a thorough search for underlying (pelvic, genitalia) malignancy. It is worth noting that, in such patients, lymphoedema often commences proximally in the thigh rather than distally
- Physical therapy for lymphoedema comprising bed rest, elevation, bandaging, compression garments, ***massage and exercises***

Table *(L & B 26th/926)*: **Aetiological classification of lymphoedema**

Primary lymphoedema	Congenital (onset <2 years old): sporadic; familial (Nonne-Milroy's disease) Praecox (onset 2-35 years old); sporadic; familial (Latessier-Meige's disease) Tarda (onset after 35 years old)
Secondary lymphoedema	Parasitic infection (filariasis) Fungal infection (Tinea pedis) Exposure to foreign body material (silica particles) Primary lymphatic malignancy Metastatic spread to lymph nodes Radiotherapy to lymph nodes Surgical excision of lymph nodes Trauma (particularly 7 degloving injuries) Superficial thrombophlebitis Deep venous thrombosis

173. Ans. c. Symptomatic. cases...

[Ref: Harrison 19th/123e1-2; L & B 26th/868]

"Diagnosis & treatment are best achieved by complete thymectomy, which is usually performed as a median sternotomy" *(L & B 26th/868)*

Thymoma

◈ *Harrison 19th/123e1-2*

- Thymoma ***is the most common cause of an anterior mediastinal mass in adults, accounting for ~40% of all mediastinal masses.***
- Thymomas are most common in the fifth and sixth decades, are uncommon in children, and are distributed evenly between men and women.
- ***About 40–50% of patients are asymptomatic;*** masses are detected incidentally on routine chest radiographs.
- When symptomatic, patients may have ***cough, chest pain, dyspnea, fever, wheezing, fatigue, weight loss, night sweats, or anorexia.*** Occasionally, thymomas may obstruct the superior vena cava. Pericardial effusion may be present.
- About 40% of patients with thymoma have another systemic autoimmune illness related to the thymoma. ***About 30% of patients with thymoma have myasthenia gravis,*** 5–8% have pure red cell aplasia, and ~5% have hypogammaglobulinemia.
- Thymoma with hypogammaglobulinemia also is called Good's syndrome. Among patients with myasthenia gravis, ~10–15% have a thymoma.
- ***Thymoma more rarely may be associated with polymyositis, systemic lupus erythematosus, thyroiditis, Sjögren's syndrome, ulcerative colitis, pernicious anemia, Addison's disease, stiff person syndrome, scleroderma, and panhypopituitarism.***

174. Ans. a. Benign..., b. May be... & d. Malignant...

[Ref: Harrison 19th/123e1-2; L & B 26th/868; Robbins 9th/626-27; Sabiston 19th/1603]

Histologic Subtypes of Thymomas

◈ *Robbins 9th/627*

- Tumors that are cytologically benign and noninvasive
- Tumors that are cytologically ***benign but invasive or metastatic***
- Tumors that are cytologically ***malignant (thymic carcinoma)***

Invasive Thymoma

◈ *Robbins 9th/627*

- **Invasive thymoma** refers to a tumor that is ***cytologically benign but locally invasive.***
- These tumors are ***much more likely to metastasize.***
- The ***epithelial cells are most commonly of the cortical variety,*** with abundant cytoplasm and rounded vesicular nuclei, and are usually mixed with numerous thymocytes.
- These tumors account for about 20% to 25% of all thymomas.
- **By definition, invasive thymomas penetrate through the capsule into surrounding structures.** The extent of invasion has been subdivided into various stages.

Noninvasive Thymomas

◈ *Robbins 9th/627*

- **Noninvasive thymomas** are most often composed of ***medullary-type epithelial cells*** or a mixture of medullary and cortical type epithelial cells. The medullary type epithelial cells are elongated or spindle-shaped

- The medullary and mixed patterns together account for about 50% of all thymomas.

Thymic Carcinoma

◈ *Robbins 9th/627*

- It represents about 5% of thymomas. Macroscopically, they are usually fleshy, obviously invasive masses, sometimes accompanied by metastases to sites such as the lungs.
- Microscopically, most are **squamous cell carcinomas**. The next most common variant is **lymphoepithelioma like carcinoma**
- About 50% of lymphoepithelioma like carcinomas ***contain monoclonal EBV genomes, consistent with a role for EBV in their pathogenesis.***

Thymomas: Pathology and Etiology

◈ *Harrison 19th/123e1-2*

- Thymomas are epithelial tumors, and all of them have malignant potential. It is ***not worthwhile to try to divide them into benign and malignant forms***; the key prognostic feature is whether they are ***noninvasive or invasive.***
- **About 65% of thymomas are encapsulated and noninvasive,** and ***about 35% are invasive.*** They may have a variable percentage of lymphocytes within the tumor, but genetic studies suggest that the ***lymphocytes are benign polyclonal cells.***
- The **epithelial component of the tumor** may consist primarily of round or oval cells derived mainly from the cortex or spindle-shaped cells derived mainly from the medulla or combinations of the two types. Cytologic features are not reliable predictors of biologic behavior.
- ***Thymic carcinomas are invasive and have a poor prognosis.***
- ***Some data suggest that Epstein-Barr virus may be associated with thymom***
- Treatment is determined by the stage of disease.

Differentiation Between Benign and Malignant Disease

It is determined by the presence of gross invasion of adjacent structures, metastasis, or microscopic evidence of capsular invasion. 15–65% of thymomas are benign. The relative percentage is partially related to early surgical treatment of myasthenia gravis; when thymectomy is performed early in the course of myasthenia gravis, a greater percentage of thymomas are benign.

Table: Staging of thymoma

Stage I:	Tumor is well encapsulated without evidence of gross or microscopic capsular invasion.
Stage II:	Tumor exhibits pericapsular growth into adjacent fat or mediastinal pleura or microscopic invasion of the thymic capsule.
Stage III:	Tumor invades adjacent organs.
Stage IVa:	Intrathoracic metastatic spread occurs.
Stage IVb:	Extrathoracic metastatic spread occurs (uncommon).

175. Ans. b. Usually..., c. Rare..., d. Treatment...

[Ref: L & B 26th/807; Sabiston 19th/845; CSDT 11th/342; Schwartz 8th/ Chap 16; Manipal 4th/383]

"***Tumors rarely involve the nipple-areola complex*** or ulcerate to the skin" *(http://emedicine. medscape. com/article/188728)*

Phyllodes Tumour

◈ *L & B 26th/807; CSDT 11th/342*

- These benign tumours, previously sometimes known as serocystic disease of Brodie or cystosarcoma phyllodes, ***usually occur in women over the age of 40 years*** but can appear in younger women.
- They present as a large, sometimes massive, tumour with an unevenly bosselated surface. Occasionally, ulceration of overlying skin occurs because of pressure necrosis.
- Phyllodes tumor is a fibroadenoma-like tumor with cellular stroma that grows rapidly. It may reach a large size and if inadequately excised will recur locally. The ***lesion can be benign or malignant.***
- Despite their size they *remain mobile on the chest wall.*
- There is no nipple retraction (differentiated from breast carcinoma" *(Manipal 4th/383)*
- Histologically, there is a wide variation in their appearance, with ***some of low malignant potential*** resembling a fibroadenoma and ***others having a higher mitotic index, which are histologically worrying.*** The latter may recur locally but, despite the name of cystosarcoma phyllodes, they are rarely cystic and only very rarely develop features of a sarcomatous tumour. These may ***metastasise via the bloodstream.***
- Treatment for the **benign type** is enucleation in young women or ***wide local excision***. Massive tumours, recurrent tumours and those of the **malignant type** will ***require mastectomy***

Phyllodes Tumors

◈ *Sabiston 19th/845*

- First called *cystosarcoma phyllodes*, the name has been changed to *phyllodes tumor* in recognition of its usually benign course.
- However, with increasing cellularity, an invasive margin, and truly sarcomatous appearance, these tumors may be classified as ***malignant phyllodes tumors.***
- **Benign phyllodes** tumors are recognized as firm, lobulated masses between 2 and up to 40 cm in size, with an average size of about 5 cm (larger than average fibroadenomas).

Phyllodes Tumors

◈ *Schwartz 8th/Chap 16*

- These tumors are classified as benign, borderline, or malignant. Borderline tumors have a greater potential for local recurrence.
- Most malignant phyllodes tumors contain liposarcomatous or rhabdomyosarcomatous elements rather than fibrosarcomatous elements. Small phyllodes tumors are excised with a 1-cm margin of normal-appearing breast tissue.

- When the diagnosis of a phyllodes tumor with suspicious malignant elements is made, re-excision of the biopsy site to insure complete excision of the tumor with a 1-cm margin of normal-appearing breast tissue is indicated. ***Large phyllodes tumors may require mastectomy.*** Axillary dissection is not recommended as axillary lymph node metastases rarely occur.

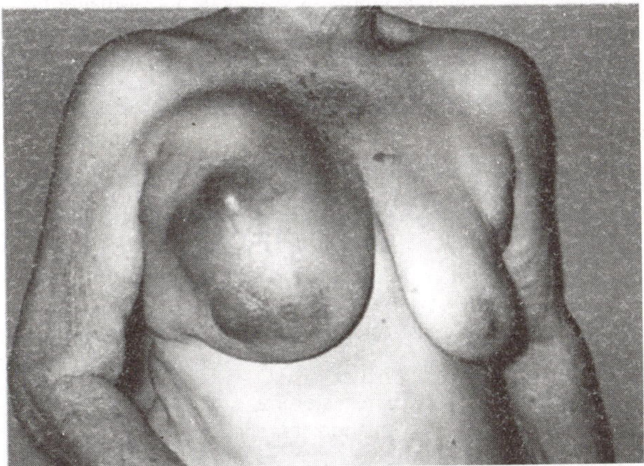

Fig: Malignant phyllodes tumor (cystosarcoma phyllodes)

176. Ans. c. Rupture..., d. Common... & e. Drainage...

[Ref: L & B 26th/1259-60; Sabiston 19th/1392-93; S. Das 5th/1073; Manipal 4th/798-99; Sabiston 18th/1445-47; CSDT 11th/771]

*"Anorectal abscess can rupture inside as well as outside resulting in a **fistula**" (Manipal 4th/799)*

ANORECTAL ABSCESSES

◈ *L & B 26th/1259-60*

"Classification of anorectal abscess: There are four types of abscess-perianal, ischiorectal, submucous & pelvirectal. Of these ***perianal (60%) & ischiorectal (30%) are common abscesses****" (S. Das 5th/1073)*

◈ *L & B 25th/1262*

- Usually produces a painful, throbbing swelling in the anal region. The patient often has swinging pyrexia
- Subdivided according to anatomical site into ***perianal, ischiorectal, submucous and pelvirectal***
- Underlying conditions include fistula-in-ano (most common), Crohn's disease, diabetes, immunosuppression
- **Treatment** is ***drainage of pus in first instance, together with appropriate antibiotics***
- Always look for a potential underlying problem

*"**Infection originates in the intersphincteric plane,** most likely in one of the anal glands. This may result in a simple intersphincteric abscess, or it may extend vertically either upward or downward, horizontally or circumferentially, resulting in a number of clinical presentations." (Sabiston 18th/1445)*

*"Anorectal abscesses should be **treated by drainage as soon as the diagnosis is established**. If the diagnosis is in question, an examination under anesthesia is often the most expeditious way both to confirm the diagnosis and to treat the problem. Delayed or inadequate treatment may occasionally cause extensive and life-threatening suppuration with massive tissue necrosis and septicemia. **Antibiotics are only indicated if there is extensive overlying cellulitis** or if the patient is immunocompromised, has diabetes mellitus, or has valvular heart disease. **Antibiotics alone are ineffective at treating perianal or perirectal infection**" (Sabiston 18th/1446)*

*"As an abscess enlarges, it spreads in one of several directions. A **perianal abscess is the most common manifestation** and appears as a painful swelling at the anal verge. Spread through the external sphincter below the level of the puborectalis produces an ischiorectal abscess. These abscesses may become extremely large and may not be visible in the perianal region. Digital rectal exam will reveal a painful swelling laterally in the ischiorectal fossa" (Sabiston 18th/1446)*

177. Ans. a. Albumin, b. Alanine..., c. Asparate... & d. Lactate...

[Ref: Textbook of Emergency Medicine by SN Chugh 4th/84; L & B 26th/1129; CMDT 2015/708-09; Schwartz 8th/1239]

Assessment of Severity

◈ *L & B 26th/1129*

- On account of the difference in outcome between patients with mild and severe disease, it is important to define that group of patients who will develop severe pancreatitis.
- Various scoring systems have been introduced, such as the Ranson and Glasgow scoring systems
- At 48 hours after the onset of symptoms, a Glasgow score of 3 or more, a C-reactive protein level greater than 150 mg/L and a worsening clinical state with sepsis or persisting organ failure indicate a severe attack.

Table *(L & B 26th/1129)*: **Scoring systems to predict the severity of acute pancreatitis: in both systems, disease is classified as severe when three or more factors are present**

Ranson score	Glasgow scale
On admission	**On admission**
Age > 55 years	Age > 55 years
White blood cell count > 16 × 10^9/L	White blood cell count > 15 × 10^9/L
Blood glucose > 10 mmol/L	Blood glucose > 10 mmol/L (no history of diabetes)
LDH > 700 units/L	Serum urea > 16 mmol/L (no response to intravenous fluid)
Within 48 hours	**Within 48 hours**
AST > 250 Sigma Frankel units per cent	Arterial oxygen saturation (PaO2) < 8 kPa[60 mmHg]
Within 48 hours	**Within 48 hours**
Blood urea nitrogen rise > 5 mg per cent	Serum calcium < 2. 0 mmol/L

Contd...

Arterial oxygen saturation (PaO2) < 8 kPa[60 mmHg]	Serum albumin < 32 g/L
Serum calcium < 2. 0 mmol/L	LDH > 600 units/L
Fluid sequestration > 6 litres	AST/ALT > 600 units/L

ALT, alanine aminotransferase; AST, aspirate aminotransferase; LDH, lactate dehydrogenase; PaO_2, arterial oxygen tension.

Table *(Schwartz)*: **Ranson's Prognostic Signs of Pancreatitis**

Criteria for acute pancreatitis not due to gallstones	
At admission	**During the initial 48 h**
Age >55 yrQ	Hematocrit fall >10 points
WBC >16, 000/mm³	BUN elevation >5 mg/dL
Blood glucose >200 mg/dL	Serum calcium <8 mg/dL
Serum LDH >350 IU/LQ	Arterial PO2 <60 mm Hg
`Serum AST >250 U/dL	Base deficit >4 mEq/L
	Estimated fluid sequestration >6 L
Criteria for acute gallstone pancreatitis	
At admission	**During the initial 48 h**
Age >70 y	Hematocrit fall >10 points
WBC >18, 000/mm³	BUN elevation >2 mg/dL
Blood glucose >220 mg/dL	Serum calcium <8 mg/dL
Serum LDH >400 IU/L	Base deficit >5 mEq/L
Serum AST >250 U/dL	Estimated fluid sequestration >4 L

Glasgow Criteria

◈ *Textbook of Emergency Medicine by SN Chugh 4th/84*

- P - PaO_2 <8kPa
- A - Age >55 year old
- WBC >15x10⁷/L
- C - Calcium <2 mmol/L
- R - Renal function, Urea >16 mmol/L
- E - Enzymes: LDH >600IU/L; AST >200IU/L
- A - Albumin <32g/L (serum)
- S - Sugar: blood glucose >10 mmol/L

OBSTETRICS & GYNAECOLOGY

178. Ans. **c. High..., e. E2...**

[Ref: Shaw's Gynaecology 16th/430-34; Dutta Gynaecology 5th/440, 450]

"PCOD: Infertility is due to anovulatory cycles"- Shaw's Gynaecology 16th/432

Stein-Leventhal Syndrome or PCOD or PCOS

◈ *Shaws Gynaecology 16th/430*

- PCOS includes chronic nonovulationQ, hyperandrogenismQ associated with normal or raised oestradiol level (E2), raised LHQ & low FSH/LH ratioQ.
- The patients are mostly 15-25 years of age. The disease has genetic & familial tendency & may be autosomal dominant inherited.

Table: Presentations of PCOD

Clinical Features	Hormonal	Sequelae
• Young womanQ	• E_2 levelQ	Diabetes (15%)Q
• Central obesity	• FSH normal; LH > 10 IU/ml	CVS disorder
• BMI > 30 kg/cm²	• FSH/LH ratio	Lipidaemia
• Waist line >88 cm (35")	• AndrogensQ	Hypertension
• Oligomenorrhoea, amenorrhoea	• ↑Testosterone, epiandrostenedione,	Endometrial cancer
• Infertility (20%)Q	• Dehydroepiandros-terone	Breast cancer
• HirsutismQ	• 17-alpha-hydroxy progesterone > 300 ng/dl	Premature ovarian failure following surgery
• Acanthosis nigraQ due to insulin resistance. Thick pigmented skin over the nape of neck, inner thigh and axilla. • Most androgen from ovary • Fasting insulin >10mIU/L	• Testosterone > 2 ng/ml • Most androgens from ovary • Prolactin • Sex hormone binding globulin (SHBG) ¯ • ↓ E_2/oestrone (E_1) ratio • F. blood glucose/fasting insulin ratio < 4. 5	

Diagnosis

Diagnosis is based upon the presence of any two of the following three criteria

- Oligomenorrhoea &/or anovulationQ
- HyperandrogenismQ (Clinical &/or biochemical)
- Polycystic ovariesQ (Ultrasound finding)

Possible Late Sequelae of PCOD are:

- Risk of developing diabetes mellitus (15%) due to insulin resistance
- Risk of developing endometrial carcinomaQ due to elevated level of oestrogen.
- Risk of hypertension & cardiovascular disease due to abnormal lipid profile (dyslipidaemia)
- Breast cancer

179. Ans. **d. Common in...**

[Ref: Shaws Gynaecology 16th/409-420; Dutta Gynaecology 6th/304-09]

***"Laproscopy is the gold standard in diagnosis of endometriosis.** It is both diagnostic & therapeutic" (Shaws Gynaecology 16th/415)*

***"Sampson gave implantation theory of endometriosis** in 1922"* (Shaws Gynaecology 16th/409)

"Endometriosis *possibly* ***interferes with tubal motility and function.*** *It may* ***inhibit ovulation*** *and because of dyspareunia there is reduced frequency of sexual intercourse. Other causes of infertility are* ***luteinized unruptured follicular (LUF) syndrome, increased prolactin and corpus luteal phase defect, non-ovulation and tubal blockage. Prostaglandin affects the tubal motility & causes corpus luteolysis too. The macrophages in the peritoneal fluid engulf the sperms or immobilize them"*** (Shaw 16th/414)

"Dysmenorrhoe is the most common symptom" (Shaw 16th/413)

Endometriosis

- Occurrence of functioning endometrial tissue (both glands + stroma)[Q] outside the cavity of uterus.
- ***Age group: 30 -40 years (Most common)***[Q] *(Jeffcoate 7th/368)*
- Seen in high socio-economic status because of late marriage[Q] & late child bearing[Q].
- Most common in nulliparous females[Q]. *(Jeffcoate 7th/369-370; Shaw 14th/420)*
- Familial predisposition (risk is seven times higher if a ***first degree relative has diseases***. Risk is further increased in homozygous twins).
- It is a hormone dependant condition (Estrogen dependant[Q].

Site: It can occur anywhere in the body. Most common site is ovary (30-40%, 2nd most common site is pouch of douglas[Q]

Pathology

Peritoneum: *Earliest lesion is red petechial, later becoming cystic, dark brown, blue black in appearance called as Powder burn appearance/Gun shot appearance.*

Ovary: *Characteristic* ***bilateral***[Q] ***cyst***[Q] ***or endometrioma (which is a true cyst***[Q] ***with columnar lining epithelium)***[Q]*. Beneath the epithelium are large cells with brown cytoplasm due to ingested pigments like hemosiderin called as Pseudoxanthoma cells. Cyst contains tarry brown fluid*[Q]*. Shaw 14/e, p 421*

Peritoneal cavity: *Contains yellow brownb fluid which has prostaglandin responsible for the pain of brown endometriosis.*

Symptoms: Patients Present with a Characteristic Triad of

- Infertility[Q]
- Progressively increasing dysmenorrhea[Q]
- Dyspareunia[Q]

Dyspareunia: *Occurs when POD and rectovaginal septum are involved.*

Menstrual irregularities: *Like menorrhagia, polymenorrhea are seen.*

Premenstrual spotting *may occur and is more likely to be associated with endometriosis than with luteal phase inadequacy*

Other symptom: *Chronic pelvic pain, pain during defecation. Intermittent pyrexia and urinary symptoms.*

180. Ans. a. A woman...

[Ref: Park 23rd/508-09; Shaws Gynaecology 16th/281-82; Dutta obstetrcis 8th/638, 633; Dutta Gynaecology 6th/494-600]

Female Sterilization

◈ *Shaws Gynaecology 16th/281-82*

- *Tubal ligation can be done at any convenient time to the patient.* **Postpartum ligation** *is done within the first week of delivery when the patient is already hospitalized.* ***Interval sterilization*** *is done when the woman is not pregnant or any time after 6 weeks of delivery. It can be combined with caesarean section*
- Indications
  - *Multiparity*
  - *Need of permanent method*
  - *Obstetrics- Three caesarean deliveries*
  - *Medical diseases at high risk of pregnancy*
  - *Pyschiatric problems*
  - *Breast cancer*
  - *Eugenic conditions: Repeat fetal malformations such as hemophilia, Rh incompatibility, Wilson's disease, Tay-Sachs disease & Marfan syndrome*
- Contraindication
  - ***Young women less than 25 years*** *(as dictated by GOI)*
  - ***Parity less than two children*** *(as per the government rule)*
  - ***Local infection***
  - *Prolapse- tubectomy can be done at the time of repair surgery*

Government Guidelines for Sterilization

◈ *Park 23rd/508-09*

- The **age of the husband** should ***not ordinarily be less than 25 years nor should it be over 50 years***
- The ***age of the wife should not be less than 20 years or more than 45 years***
- The motivated couple ***must have 2 living children at the time of operation***
- If the couple has 3 or more living children, the lower limit of age of the husband or wife may be relaxed at the discretion of the operating surgeon
- It is sufficient if the ***acceptor declares having obtained the consent of his/her spouse to undergo sterilization operation without outside pressure, inducement or coercion*** & that he/she knows that for all practical purposes, the operation is irreversible, & also that the spouse has not been sterilized earlier

181. Ans. c. Breast..., d. Ovarian..., e. Endo...

[Ref: Shaws Gynaecology 16th/458, 485, 522; Dutta Gynaecology 5th/325]

*"**Breast Cancer: Nulliparity,** late first pregnancy after 30 years of age & nonlactation are the high risk factors" (Shaws Gynaecology 16th/458)*

*"Risk factor for **ovarian cancer**: **Nulliparous or of low parity;** age b/w 45 & 60 years; late menopause" (Shaws Gynaecology 16th/522 (Table))*

*"**Cancer cervix**: High risk women are: Coitus before the age of 18; multiple sexual partner; delivery of first baby before the age of 20 years; multiparity with poor birth spacing b/w pregnancies" (Shaws Gynaecology 16th/485)*

"Risk factor for **endometrial cancer**: ***Nulliparity,*** *low parity, early menarche, late menopause" (Shaws Gynaecology 16th/509)*

*"***Vaginal cancer***: It occur in elderly women after over 70 year of age when sexual activity has generally ceased" (Shaws Gynaecology 16th/481)*

182. Ans. b. MSAFP..., d. Unconjugated... & e. β -hCG

[Ref: Dutta's Obstetrics 8th/128-29, 567-68; William's Obstetrics 23rd/292-93; Fernando Arias 3rd/44-45; Nelson 18th/508; O. P. Ghai 7th/614]

Screening Methods: First Trimester

Screening Parameters are

Biophysical: *(i) ultrasound measurement of nuchal transluceny (NT), (ii) nasal bone*

Biochemical: *(i) free β -hCG, (ii) PAPP-A (Pregnancy associated plasma protein-A)*

Time of Test: ***b/w 11 weeks & 14 weeks***

Values: *PAPP-A- reduced; β -hCG- increased; NT- measurement increased in trisomy 21*

> *Note:*
> - *NT is the fluid-filled space (detected by USG) b/w the fetal skin & the underlying soft tissue at the region of fetal neck. NT ≥ mm is abnormal. Combined tests can detect trisomy 21 in 92% cases with a false-positive rate of 5%*
> - *First trimester screening is either equal or even superior to second trimester screening*

Screening Methods: Second Trimester

- *It is done b/w 15 weeks & 22 weeks*
- *MSAFP: Low level are found in down syndrome*
- ***Triple test:*** *It is a combine test which includes MSAFP, hCG & uE3 (unconjugated estriol). It is used for detection of down syndrome. In an affected pregnancy, levels of MSAFP & uE3 tend to low while that of hCG is high*
- ***Quadruple (Quad) screening include four biochemical analytes:*** *MSAFP, hCG, uE3 & dimeric inhibin-A. It can detect trisomy 21 in 85% cases. Level of serum analytes in cases with trisomy 21: MSAFP-reduced, hCG-increased, uE3-reduced & dimeric inhibin-A- elevated*

> *Note: Best screening procedure is combined first & second trimester procedures*

*"All women should be offered screening for Down syndrome in their second trimester by means of 3 maternal serum tests (***free β-hCG, unconjugated estriol, and α-fetoprotein***). Even more efficient, with a detection rate of 95%, is a method of screening using maternal age and fetal nuchal* ***translucency (NT) thickness along with maternal serum β-hCG, PAPP-A (pregnancy-associated plasma protein-A), unconjugated estriol, and α-fetoprotein.*** *Increased levels of maternal serum α-fetoprotein (MSAFP) are also linked to other abnormal fetal conditions, including open neural tube defects and defects of the gastrointestinal system and genitourinary system." (Nelson 18th/508)*

"Patient who wish to get a prenatal diagnosis have a number of options. They can directly get a fetal karyotype by chorionic villus sampling or amniocentesis. Alternatively (if parents do not want invasive testing) an initial screening may be performed with maternal serum markers-PAAP-a & ***free β-hCG in first trimester & serum α-fetoprotein, human chorionic gonadotropin, unconjugated estriol & inhibin A in second trimester"*** *(O. P. Ghai 7th/614)*

Table *(William's Obstetrics 23rd/293)*: **Selected Down Syndrome Screening Strategies**

Strategy	Analytes	Detection Rate[a] (%)
First-trimester screen NT (First trimester)	NT, PAPP-A, hCG or free b-hCG NT	79-87 64-70
Triple test	MSAFP, hCG or free b-hCG, mE3	60-69
Quadruple (Quad) test	MSAFP, hCG or free b-hCG, mE3, inh	67-81
Integrated screen	First-trimester screen & Quad test-results withheld until Quad test completed	94-96
Stepwise sequential screen	First-trimester screen & Quad test	90-95
	1% offered diagnostic test after first trimester screen	
	99% proceed to Quad test, results withheld until, Quad test completed	
Contingent sequential screen	First-trimester screen & Quad test	88-94
	1% offered diagnostic test after first trimester screen	
	15% proceed to Quad test, results withheld until, Quad test completed	
	84% have no additional test after first-trimester screen	

183. Ans. a. > 50%...., c. ~ 0. 5 ng... & e. Daily...

[Ref: Shaws Gynaecology 16th/43-44; Dutta Gynaecology 6th/571]

Testosterone

- *Shaws Gynaecology 16th/43-44*
- ***50% testosterone comes from the ovaries% the rest from adrenal gland***
- *Ovarian stromal tissue secrete androgenic products, namely testosterone, dehydroepiandrosterone (DHEA) & androstenedione*
- *The normal increase in stromal tissue at ovulation causes a slight increase in the secretion of these hormones*
- *After the menopause, the increased ovarian stroma is responsible for the rise in these hormones & the development of hirsutism in some postmenopausal women*
- ***Total daily production of testosterone is 0.2-0.3% mg & the plasma level is 0.2-0. 8 ng/ml***
- 80-85% androgen are bound to SHBP & 10-15% to albumin
- 1-2% free testosterone remains biologically active & acts at the peripheral targets, i. e hair growth & acne by conversion to dihydrotestesterone by hydroxylase enzyme

A & E

- Clinically, administration of androgen causes follicular atresia & anovulation

184. Ans. c. Remain..., d. Spermicidal..., e. Causes...

[Ref: Shaws Gynaecology 16th/266; Novak's Gynaecology 14th/257; Park 23rd/495; Dutta Gynaecology 6th/476]

Nonoxynol-9

◈ *Shaws Gynaecology 16th/266*
- This ***spermicidal agent*** kills the sperm before the latter gain access to the cervical canal
- Used alone, ***failure rate is high***, approximately 30 per 100 women years
- This remain effective for 1-2 hr after the application
- By causing irritation & abrasion in chronic use, they can cause vaginal ulceration & perhaps increase the risk of HIV spread rather than prevent it. Therefore, spermicidal agents should not be recommended to HIV couples
- Concern have been raised about possible teratogenicity- *(Novak's Gynaecology 14th/257)*
- It is toxic to lactobacilli that normally colonize the vagina. Women who use spermicide regularly have increased vaginal colonization with the bacterium E. Coli & may be predisposed to E. Coli bacteriuria after intercourse *(Novak's Gynaecology 14th/257)*

185. Ans. a. Stead... & d. Intervals...

[Ref: Dutta's Obstetrics 8th/137; William's Obstetrics 23rd/390]

False Labor Pain

◈ *Dutta's Obstetrics 8th/137*
- *Dull in nature*
- *Confined to lower abdomen & groin*
- *Not associated with hardening of the uterus*
- *They have no other features of true labor pain*
- *Usually relieved by enema or sedative*

Characteristic of True & False Labor

◈ *William's Obstetrics 23rd/390*

True Labor
- Contractions occur at regular intervals.
- Intervals gradually shorten.
- Intensity gradually increases.
- Discomfort is in the back and abdomen.
- Cervix dilates.
- Discomfort is not stopped by sedation.

False Labor
- Contractions occur at irregular intervals.
- Intervals remain long.
- Intensity remains unchanged.
- Discomfort is chiefly in the lower abdomen.
- Cervix does not dilate.
- Discomfort usually is relieved by sedation.

TRUE LABOUR PAINS: *The features of true labour pains are: (Dutta's Obstetrics 8th/137)*
- Painful uterine contractions (labour pains) at regular intervals
- Contraction with increasing intensity and duration
- "Show"
- Progressive effacement and ***dilation of the cervix***
- Formation of the "bag of waters"
- ***Labour pains:*** *Throughout pregnancy, painless Braxton Hicks contractions with simultaneous hardening of the uterus occur. These contractions change their character, become more powerful, intermittent and are associated with pain. The pains are more often* ***felt in front of the abdomen or radiating towards the thighs.***
- ***Show:*** *With the onset of labour, there is profuse cervical secretion. Simultaneously, there is slight oozing of blood from rupture of capillary vessels of the cervix and from the raw decidual surface caused by separation of the membranes due to stretching of the lower uterine segment.* ***Expulsin of cervical mucus plug, mixed with blood is called "show".***
- ***Dilation of internal os:*** *With the onset of labour pain, the* ***cervical canal begins to dialte*** *more in the upper part than in the lower, the former being accompained by corresponding stretchng of the lower uterine segment.*

186. Ans. a. Karyotype..., c. βHCG... & e. Immunostaining...

[Ref: Shaws Gynaecology 16th/311-16; Dutta Gynaecology 5th/; Shaw's Gynaecology 15th/250-56, 14th/226-232; Dutta Obstetrics 8th/22-30; Williams obstetrics 23th/260]

Partial or Incomplete Mole

◈ *Dutta Obstetrics 8th/30*
- There is fetus or at least an amniotic sac
- The karyotype is triploid either 69XXY or 69XYY with one maternal but usually two paternal haploid chromosome
- Malignant potential is low

Table *(Dutta Obstetrics 8th/230)*: **Features of complete and partial mole**

Features	Complete mole	Partial mole
Embryo/Fetus[Q]	Absent[Q]	Present
Hydropic degeneration of villi	Pronounced & diffused	Variable & Focal
Trophoblactic hyperplasia	Diffuse	Focal
Uterine size	More than the date (30-60%)	Less than the date
Karyotype	46 XX (85%), paternal in origin	Triploid (90%), diploid (10%)
Thecan lutein cysts	Common (25-50%)	Uncommon
Classic clinical symptom	**Common**	**Rare**
Beta-hCG level[Q]	High (>50, 000)	Slight elevation (<50, 000)
Risk of persistent GTN	**20%**	**<5%**
Immunostaining ($p57^{KIP2}$)	**Negative**	**Positive**

***H. mole**: (Short Review)*

It is prevalent among teenaged & elderly patients with high parity

Symptoms

- Vaginal bleeding (Commonest, in 90%, "***white currant in red currant juice***")[Q]
- Varying degrees of lower abdominal pain
- Constitutional symptoms like excessive vomiting, breathlessness, thyrotoxicosis, features of tremors or tachycardia
- ***Expulsion of grape like vesicles per vaginum is diagnostic of vesicular mole***[Q]
- History of quickening is absent.

Signs

- Ill looking patient, prominent pallor
- ***Features of pre-eclampsia*** (hypertension, oedema & or proteinuria).
- ***The size of the uterus is more than that expected for the period of amenorrhorea***[Q]
- Doughy, firm elastic feel of the uterus
- ***Fetal parts are neither felt nor fetal movements***

Absence of Fetal Heart Sound

- ***High HCG in urine*** (positive pregnancy test) diluted upto 1: 200 to 1: 500 beyond 100 days of gestation is very much suggestive. Rapidly increasing value of serum HCG > 100, 000 mIU/ml, are usual with molar pregnancy. Normal pregnancy values are below 60, 0000 mIU/ml. *(there is no mention of doubling time)*

187. Ans. b. Selheim, c. Kronig

[Ref: Dutta Obstetrics 8th/672; William's Obstetrics 23rd/549; http://emedicine. medscape. com/article/263424-overview#a15]

Techniques of Cesarean Section

◈ *William's Obstetrics 23rd/549*

- **Abdominal incisions:** Usually midline vertical or a suprapubic transverse incision (*Pfannenstiel incision, Maylard incision,* Joel Cohen incision) is used. Only in special circumstances would a paramedian or midtransverse incision be employed
- Uterine Incisions
  - Most often the incision is made in the ***lower uterine segment transversely*** as described by **Kerr** in 1926.
- Occasionally, a ***low-segment vertical incision as described by Krönig in 1912*** may be used.
- The so-called *classical incision* is a vertical incision into the body of the uterus above the lower uterine segment and reaching the uterine fundus. This incision is seldom used today.
- For most cesarean deliveries, the transverse incision is the operation of choice. Its advantages are that it
  - Is easier to repair,
  - Is located at a site least likely to rupture during a subsequent pregnancy, and
  - Does not promote adherence of bowel or omentum to the incisional line. If the fetus is not presenting by the vertex, if there are multiple fetuses, or if the fetus is very immature and the woman has had no labor, a lower-segment vertical or even a classical incision may, at times, prove to be advantageous.

"In more than 90% of cesarean deliveries, ***a low transverse (Monroe-Kerr) incision*** *is made. The incision is made 1-2 cm above the original upper margin of the bladder with a scalpel. The initial incision is small and is continued into the uterine wall until either the fetal membranes are visualized or the cavity is entered (with care taken not to injure the underlying fetus, especially in well-labored patients with thinned out lower uterine segments)" (http://emedicine. medscape. com/article/263424-overview#a15)*

Uterine Incision

◈ *https://books. google. co. in/books?id=suuA*

- Classical: More likely to rupture in the next pregnancy
- **Low vertical (Kronig):** May tear through cervix
- Low transverse (Kerr) incision: Less blood loss, easiest to repair, located at site least likely to rupture in next pregnancy

The Lower Uterine Segment Incision:

(https://books. google. co. in/books?id = suuA_qR7CU0C&pg = PA131&lpg = PA131&dq = incision + %28Kronig/Sellheim)

- It is the most commonly performed. It has the advantage of:
  - Having less bleeding unless extended (as the lower segment is less vascular and away from implantation),
  - The scar is stronger and less incidence of subsequent rupture (0.2-0.4%).
  - Less ileus, stomach dilatation,
  - Infection and adhesions is anticipated with lower segment incisions compared to upper segment incisions.
- Low cervical incision may be a ***low cervical transverse (LCT) incision (Monroe/Kerr) or a low cervical vertical (LCV) incision (Kronig/Selheim).***
- In general, the LCV incision tends to have increased blood loss because it extends into the upper uterine segment and has been thought to have a greater incidence of rupture during subsequent pregnancies when compared with the LCT incision, although this has not been substantiated. Its main disadvantage is possible downward extension with bladder injury. On the other hand, the LCT uterine incision has a greater tendency to extend laterally into the uterine vessels at the time of operation

Transverse Incision (Kerr)

◈ *https://quizlet. com/32389595/maternity-final-quizlet-high-risk-flash*

"Lowest & narrowest part of abdomen just below pubic hair line, doesn't allow for any extension of this incision, can be done if time is not a factor"

Vertical Incision (Sellheim)

◈ *https://quizlet. com/32389595/maternity-final-quizlet-high-risk-flash-cards/*

"Between symphysis pubis and navel, quicker, used for emergencies or with fetal distress with rapid birth, with preterm or macrosomic infants or obese mothers"

188. Ans. a. Immediately..., b. 1 week..., c. Post... & e. Any time...

[Ref: Shaws Gynaecology 16th/270; Park 23rd/497-98; Dutta Gynaecology 6th/480-81]

Timing of Insertion of IUCD

◈ *Shaws Gynaecology 16th/270*

- It is advisable to insert IUCD ***during or soon after menstruation & after abortion or MTP***
- Lately, **immediate postpartum** insertion within 10 min of placental expulsion or within 24 hr of delivery is practiced & is found effective. This save the woman second visit to the clinic. There is no clinical evidence of increase in perforation, expulsion etc

◈ *Park 23rd/497-98*

- Although the IUCD can be inserted at almost any time during a women's reproductive years (except during pregnancy), the most propitious time for insertion is during menstruation or within 10 days of the beginning of a menstrual period (because diameter of cervical canal is greater)
- IUCD insertion can also be taken up during the first week after delivery before the women leaves the hospital (immediate postpartum insertion), but carries risk of perforation & high expulsion
- A convenient time for insertion is 6-8 weeks after delivery (post-puerperal insertion). It has several advantage
- IUCD insertion can also be taken up immediately after a legally induced first trimester abortion. But IUCD insertion immediately after a second trimester abortion is not recommended (high risk of infection)

◈ *Dutta Gynaecology 6th/480-81*

- ***Interval*** *(When the insertion is made in the interconceptional period beyond 6 week following childbirth or abortion)- It is preferable to insert 2-3 days after the period is over. During lactational amenorrhoea, it can be inserted at any time*
- ***Postabortal:*** *Immediately following termination of pregnancy*
- ***Postpartum:*** *Can be done before patients are discharged from the hospital. Because of high rate of expulsion, it is preferable to withhold insertion for 6 week when the uterus will be involuted to near normal size*
- ***Postplacental*** *delivery- Insertion immediately following delivery of the placenta could be done. But the expulsion rate is high*

189. Ans. a. Pelvi... & d. HIV...

[Ref: Shaws Gynaecology 16th/273-74; Dutta Gynaecology 6th/485-491; Dutta Obsterics 8th/622-27; Novak's Gynaecology 14th/274; Harrison 19th/2391]

*'The proportion of women becoming pregnant **within 2 months of discontinuing the pill** may be range from 15-35%" (Park 23rd/502)*

Combined Oral Contraceptive

◈ *Shaws Gynaecology 16th/273-74*

- In a non-lactating woman, COC can be started after 3 weeks of delivery, but can be given soon after an abortion, MTP or an ectopic pregnancy
- ***HIV antiviral reduce effectiveness of COC*** but when combined with condoms, COC are protective against pregnancy
- "99% of women will have normal menstrual cycles within 6 months of stopping COC but return of fertility may be slightly delayed due to delayed return of ovulation"
- "Ovulation return within 3 months of withdrawl of drug in 90% cases" *(Dutta Gynaecology 6th/490)*
- "**IUCD:** About 75% women conceive within 6 months of its removal & almost 90% conceive within a year" *(Shaws Gynaecology 16th/272)*
- 90% ovulate within 3 months of stopping the drug
- *"**Use of COC generally is not advised during lactation** because they reduce the amount & quality of breast milk. It can be used after 6 weeks, once milk production is established. Progestin-only pills, implants & injectable contraception do not affect milk quality or quantity" (Novak's 14th/254)*

Combined Oral Contraceptive

◈ *Dutta Gynaecology 6th/485-491*

- ***Selection of patient:*** *History & general examination should be thorough, taking special care to screen cases for contraindications (headach, migraine). Examination of breasts for any nodules, weight & blood pressure are to be noted. **Pelvic examination to exclude cervical pathology, is mandatory**. Cervical cytology to exclude abnormal cells, is to be done*
- ***Follow up:*** *The patient should be examined after 3 month, then after 6 months & then yearly. The patient above the age of 35 year should be checked more frequently. Examination of breasts, weight & blood pressure recording & **Pelvic examination including cervical pathology, to be done** & compared with the previous records*

*"**Combined oral pills** are highly effective, **protect against ovarian and endometrial cancer.** Although there remains controversy, most data suggest that **no link exists between COC use and breast cancer risk** yet **COC should not be given to female suffering from breast carcinoma**" (Novak's Gynaecology 14th/274)*

Table *(Harrison 19th/2391)*: **Oral Contraceptives Dis- ease Risk**

Cervical cancer—	*Relative risk 2–4 times[Q]*
Ovarian cancer—	*50% reduction in risk[Q]*
Endometrial cancer—	*40% reduction in risk[Q]*

190. Ans. c. Life span...

[Ref: Dutta Obstetrics 7th/550-51; Dutta Gynaecology 6th/628-29; Park 23rd/505]

Implanon

◈ *Dutta Obstetrics 7th/550-51*

- It is a progestin only delivery system containing ***etonorgestrel.***
- It is a long term (***upto 3 years***) reversible contraception
- It consists of single closed capsule & contain ***68 mg of etonorgestrel.***
- It releases the hormone about ***60 μg, gradually reduced to 30 μg per day over 3 years***
- It does not cause decrease in bone mineral density
- It inhibit ovulation in 90% of the cycles for the first year
- It has got supplementary effect on endometrium (atrophy) & cervical mucous (thick) as well

- Efficacy is extremely high with pearl index of 0. 01
- This safe & effective method is considered as reversible sterilization
- Advantage are same as DMPA
- **Drawback:** Frequent irregular menstrual bleeding, spotting & amenorrhoea are common
- Contraindication are similar to POP

◈ *Johns Hopkins Manual of Gynecology and Obstetrics 3rd/Chap 28*

- Progestin-only implants prevent pregnancy by suppressing ovulation, thickening cervical mucus, and altering the endometrium (atrophy).
- A single rod implant (Implanon was approved in the United States in July, 2006. This 4 cm Ã— 2 mm implant releases etonogestrel, the active metabolite of desogestrel, and is placed under the skin of the upper arm is effective for 3 years.
- Effectiveness. Fewer than 1 pregnancy per 100 women over 1 year.
- Advantages. Highly effective, long-acting.

*"Nexplanon/**Implanon** consists of **a single rod** made of ethylene vinylacetate copolymer that is 4cm long and 2mm in diameter. It is similar to a matchstick in size. The rod contains 68 mg of etonogestrel (sometimes called 3-keto-destrogestrel), a type of progestin. Serum levels maintain relatively stable through 36 months, which implies that the method may be effective for longer than 3 years" (http://en. wikipedia. org/wiki)*

191. Ans. a. Weight..., b. Cause..., c. It can...

[Ref: Shaws Gynaecology 16th/275-76; Dutta Gynaecology 6th/491; Jeffcoate's Priciples of Gynecology 7th/821, 822, Novak's Gynecology 14th/254]

Progestogen only Pill (POP)/Minipil

◈ *Shaws Gynaecology 16th/275-76*

- Minipill does not have some of the major side effects of the combined pills & it is well suited for lactating women; some progestogens, in fact, increases milk secretion
- ***Side-effect:*** *weight gain, irregular menstrual bleeding, depression, breast cancer, thromboembolism*
- ***Advantage:*** *They can be recommended to – lactating women, women over 35 years, those with focal migraine, those intolerant to estrogen or oestrogen contraindicated, diabetic, hypertensive & sickle cell anemia*
- *As regards to return of fertility, it is faster than in COC users because ovulation is not suppressed in all cases (suppressed in 40%)*
- ***Contraindication:*** *C/I to POP are previous are previous ectopic pregnancy, ovarian cyst, breast & genital cancer,* abnormal *vaginal bleeding, active liver & arterial disease, porphyria, liver tumor*
- *Because of osteopenia, it is contraindicated in adolescents & young women*

***"Progestin-only pill is started 21 day postpartum[Q] & soon after abortion. The tablet is taken daily without a break"**- (Shaw's Gynecology 14th/210)*

***"Progestin-only pill can be started 2 to 3 days postpartum[Q]**, whereas depot medroxyprogesterone acetate (Depo provera) injections or implants can begin at 6 weeks" (Novak's Gynecology 14th/254)*

192. Ans. d. Unilateral..., e. Constitute...

[Ref: Shaws Gynaecology 16th/441-42; Dutta Gynaecology 6th/381-82; Shaw's Gynaecology 14th/338]

***"It may co-exist with pregnancy (20-30%)"** (Dutta Gynaecology 5th/367)*

*"**Germ cell tumour** accounts for 15-20% of all ovarian tumor. The majority of tumours (about 95%) are benign cystic teratoma, also called dermoids. Below the age of 20 years, 60% of tumour are of germ cell origin & in girls under the age of 10 years, almost 85% belong to this group & are invariably malignant. Dysgerminoma accounts for 3-5% of all ovarian tumour" (Shaws Gynaecology 16th/439)*

***"Dysgerminoma[Q] is b/l in only 10% cases[Q] (Shaws, 10-15%-Novak's) In fact, dysgerminoma is the only germ cell malignancy that has significant rate of bilaterality, other germ cell tumors are rarely bilateral"** (Shaws Gynaecology 16th/441& Novak's 14th/1508)*

***"Dysgerminoma is the commonest (30-40%) malignant germ cell tumour"** (Dutta Gynaecology 6th/381)*

*"**Treatment:** Majority (75%) of tumor is confined to one ovary & are stage I at time of diagnosis. In young patient where preservation of fertility is desired, laparotomy for surgical staging & **unilateral salpingo-oophorectomy** is done. If there is any suspicion of involvement to the other ovary, bisection of contralateral ovary & excisional biopsy should be done. Tumor is sensitive to both chemotherapy & radiotherapy"- (Dutta Gynaecology 6th/381-82)*

***"It usually arises in young women[Q] or in children, with an average incidence at the age of 20"** (Shaws.16th/441)*

Dysgerminoma

- "Dysgerminoma is the *most common*[Q] *malignant germ cell tumor*, accounting for about 30-40% of all ovarian cancers of germ cell origin.
- They accounts for only 1-3% of all ovarian cancers (Novak's, 3-5% - Shaw's), but they represent as many as 5-10% of ovarian cancer in patients younger than 20 years" – *(Novak's 14th/1506)*
- They are ***very sensitive to radiation therapy***[Q]. Loss of fertility is a problem with radiation therapy
- "There have been numerous reports of successful control of metastatic dysgerminoma with systemic chemotherapy & this technique should now be regarded as the treatment of choice. The obvious advantage is the preservation of fertility" *(Novak's 14th/1509)*
- It corresponds to the *seminoma of the testis*[Q]
- It usually arise in young woman with an average incidence at age of 20yr. 75% of dysgerminoma occur b/w the ages of 10 & 30 years[Q].
- The tumor is ***neutral*** & does not secrete either male or female sex hormones but *secrete placental alkaline phosphatase, lactate dehydrogenase & β-HCG.*

- The treatment of patient with early dysgerminoma is *primarily surgical.* Chemotherapy or radiation is administered to patients with metastatic disease

193. Ans. a. Pre-eclampsia..., b. Common... & d. Premature...

[Ref: Dutta's Obstetrics 8th/294, 7th/252-258; William's Obstetrics 23rd/761-75]

*"**Prior abruption: Risk of recurrence** for a woman with previous abruption varies between **5 to 17 percent**" (Dutta's Obstetrics 7th/253)*

*"Character of blood in abruption placentae- **dark coloured** (c. f bright red in placenta praevia)" (Dutta's Obstetrics 7th/246)*

*"Prevalence of **Abruptio placentae is more with high birth order (pregnancies with gravida 5 or more)"** (Dutta's Obstetrics 7th/252)*

*"**Hypertension in pregnancy** is the most important predisposing factor. **Pre-eclampsia**, gestational hypertension & essential hypertension, all are associated with placental abruption" (Dutta's Obstetrics 7th/252)*

Recurrent Abruption

◈ *William's Obstetrics 23rd/764-65*

- Pritchard and co-workers (1970) identified a ***recurrence rate of severe abruption in 1 in 8 pregnancies.***
- Furuhashi and colleagues (2002) analyzed subsequent pregnancy outcomes from 27 women who had a prior placental abruption. Of the six (***22%***) recurrences, four were at a gestational age 1 to 3 weeks earlier than the first abruption.

Abruptio Placentae (AP)

◈ *Johns Hopkins Manual of Gynecology and Obstetrics, 3rd*

- ***Abruptio placentae (AP) is the premature separation of the normally implanted placent*** a from the uterine wall due to uterine vessel hemorrhage into the decidua basalis.
- Placental abruption accounts for one-third of all antepartum bleeding.
- AP has a recurrence rate of ***5% to 17%*** after an episode in one previous pregnancy and ***25%*** after an episode in two previous pregnancies.
- When the abruption results in a stillbirth, there is a 7% incidence of a stillbirth in future pregnancies
- Although many cases continue to be idiopathic, AP is associated with maternal hypertension, ***advanced maternal age, multiparity***, cocaine use, tobacco use, chorioamnionitis, and trauma.
- Patients with chronic hypertension, superimposed ***pre-eclampsia, or severe pre-eclampsia*** have a fivefold increased risk of severe abruption compared to normotensive counterparts.

Table *(William Obs.)*: **Risk Factors for Placental Abruption**

Risk Factor	Relative Risk
Increased age and parity	1.3–1. 5
Preeclampsia	2. 1–4. 0
Chronic hypertension	1. 8–3. 0
Preterm ruptured membranes	2.4–4. 9
Multifetal gestation	2. 1
Hydramnios	2. 0
Cigarette smoking	1.4–1. 9
Thrombophilias	3–7
Cocaine use	NA
Prior abruption	10–25
Uterine leiomyoma	NA

194. Ans. b. Fractional..., c. Aspiration... & d. Hyster...

[Ref: Shaw's Gyanecology 16th/510, 14th/60-62; Novak's Gynaecology14th/490-93; Dutta's Gynaecology 6th/356-57]

*"**Colposcopy is used for cervical cancer:** Aim- To study cervix when pap smear detects abnormal cells, to locate abnormal areas & take a biopsy, to study the extent of abnormal lesions, conservative surgery under colposcopic guidance & follow-up of conservative therapy cases" (Shaw's Gyanecology 16th/490)*

*"**Endometrial carcinoma:** Pap smear is only 50% sensitive & not reliable" (Shaw's Gyanecology 16th/510)*

*"**Endometrial carcinoma:** PET-CT reveals metabolic activity in the tissue & **is a gold standard for staging**" (Shaw's Gyanecology 16th/510)*

Investigation for Endometrial carcinoma

◈ *Summarised from the text Shaw's 16th/510*

- ***Pap smear (only 50% sensitive & not reliable)***
- Aspiration cytology from uterine cavity (6 monthly screening)
- Fractional curettage (Histological study & extent of lesion)
- Hysteroscopic inspection & selective biopsy (biopsy from suspicious area)
- USG
- Doppler USG
- CT, PET-CT & MRI
- Cystoscopy & Proctoscopy
- X-ray lung, bone & liver
- CA-125
- Sonosalpingography (useful in detecting endometrial polyp which could be malignant)

Diagnosis of Endometrial carcinoma

◈ *Dutta's Gynaecology 6th/356-57*

- Papanicolaou smear is not a reliable diagnostic test for endometrial carcinoma (positive only in 30% cases)
- **Endometrial biopsy:** Using curette or cannula has been done with reliability (90%). Histology is the definitive diagnosis
- USG & color Doppler
- Hysteroscopy
- **Fractional curettage:** It is not only the definite method of diagnosis but can detect the extent of growth
- **CT scan of pelvis & abdomen:** To detect L. N metastases
- **MRI:** Can detect myometrial invasion
- PET scan

195. Ans. a. Leg are... & c. Gynaecomastia.

[Ref: Robbins 9th/165; Shaws Gynaecology 16th/147; Dutta Gynaecology 5th/424; Harrison 19th/2350; Shaw's 14th/183-85]

"Sole to pubic length is more than normal" *- (Shaws Gynaecology 16th/147)*

Klinefelter Syndrome (47XXY)

Pathophysiology

- The classic form of KS (47, XXY) occurs following meiotic nondisjunction of the sex chromosomes during gametogenesis (40% during spermatogenesis, 60% during oogenesis)

Clinical Features

- KS is characterized by *small testes, infertility, **gynecomastia,** eunuchoid proportions, and poor virilization in phenotypic males.*
- It has an incidence of at least 1 in 1000 men, but many are not diagnosed. In severe cases, individuals present prepubertally with small testes, or with impaired androgenization and gynecomastia at the time of puberty. Developmental delay and learning disabilities may be a feature. Later in life, eunuchoid features or infertility lead to the diagnosis.
- Testes are small and firm[median length 2. 5 cm (4 mL volume); almost always <3. 5 cm (12 mL)], and typically seem inappropriately small for the degree of androgenization.
- ***Plasma concentrations of FSH and luteinizing hormone (LH) are increased in most patients with 47, XXY*** (90 and 80%, respectively) and plasma testosterone is decreased (50–75%), reflecting primary gonadal failure. Estradiol is often increased because of chronic Leydig cell stimulation by LH

Treatment

- Gynecomastia should be treated by surgical reduction if it causes concern
- Androgen supplementation improves virilization, libido, energy, hypofibrinolysis, and bone mineralization in underandrogenized men but may occasionally worsen gynecomastia
- Fertility has been achieved ***using in vitro fertilization in men with oligospermia or with intracytoplasmic sperm injection (ICSI)*** following retrieval of spermatozoa by testicular sperm extraction techniques. In specialized centers, successful spermatozoa retrieval using this technique is possible in >50% of men with non-mosaic KS.
- Following **ICSI and embryo transfer,** successful pregnancies can be achieved in ~50% of these cases. The risk of transmission of this chromosomal abnormality needs to be considered, and preimplantation screening may be desired.

PAEDIATRICS

196. Ans. b. β-Thalassemia., d. G6PD... & e. Rh...

[Ref: O. P. Ghai 8th/173, 312; Nelson 19th/1376-77]

"Sickle cell anaemia: HbF inhibits the polymerization of HbS even more than HbA; hence, infants do not become symptomatic until they reach 5 or 6 months of age, when the level of HbF normally falls" (Robbins 9th/635

"Sepsis causes unconjugated hyperbiliruninemia & neonatal cholestasis" (Nelson 19th/1376-77)

Important causes of Jaundice in neonate

◈ *O. P. Ghai 8th/173*

- **Hemolytic:** ***Rh incompatibility,*** ABO incompatibility, ***G6PD deficiency, thalassemias,*** hereditary spherocytosis
- **Non-hemolytic:** Prematurity, extravasated blood, inadequate feeding, polycythemia, idiopathic, breast milk jaundice

Neonatal Cholestasis

◈ *Nelson 18th/1668-72*

- It is defined as prolonged elevation of serum levels of conjugated bilirubin beyond the 1st 14 days of life. Jaundice that appears after 2 wk of age, progresses after this time, or does not resolve at this time should be evaluated and a conjugated bilirubin level determined.
- Cholestasis in a newborn can be due to infectious, genetic, metabolic, or undefined abnormalities giving rise to *mechanical* obstruction of bile flow or to *functional* impairment of hepatic excretory function and bile secretion
- Functional impairment of bile secretion can result from congenital defects or damage to liver cells or to the biliary secretory apparatus. Neonatal cholestasis can be divided into extrahepatic and intrahepatic disease
- **Aagenaes syndrome** is a form of idiopathic familial intrahepatic cholestasis associated with lymphedema of the lower extremities.
- **Alagille syndrome** (arteriohepatic dysplasia) is the most common syndrome with intrahepatic bile duct paucity.

197. Ans. b. Swap..., c. Can... & d. Can...

[Ref: O. P. Ghai 8th/50; Nelson 19th/27-31]

"Child can transfer objects from one hand to other by 6-7 month" *(O. P. Ghai 8th/49)*

*"**At 3 month:** Prone-Lifts head and chest with arms extended; head above plane of body on ventral suspension"- (Nelson 19th/28)*

*"**Prone**: At 6 month, he can lift his head & the greater part of chest while supporting weight on the extended arm" (Ghai 8th/46*

"Pincer grasp approach to small object (index finger & thumb)" (O. P. Ghai 8th/50)

By about nine months, your baby should be able to point at things with his index fingers and begin trying to pick up Cheerios using only his thumb and index finger. *(http://www. early intervention support. com/fine-motor-skills-development-babies-7-12-months/)*

"Between 6 & 7 months, the infant can hold a bottle securely & willingly drop any grasped object" (https://books. google. co. in/ books?id)

Table *(O. P. Ghai 8th/50)*: **Key fine motor developmental milestone**

Age	Milestone
4 month	Bidextrous reach (reaching out for objects with both hands)
6 month	Unidextrous reach (reaching out for objects with one hands); transfers object
9 month	Immature pincer grasp; probes with forefinger
12 month	Pincer grasp mature

Table *(Nelson)*: **Developmental Milestones in the First 2 Yr of Life**

Milestone	Average Age of Attainment (Month)
GROSS MOTOR	
Holds head steady while sitting[Q]	2
Pulls to sit, with no head lag	3
Brings hands together in midline	3
Asymmetric tonic neck reflex gone[Q]	4
Sits without support[Q]	6
Rolls back to stomach	6. 5
Walks alone[Q]	12
Runs[Q]	16
FINE MOTOR	
Grasps rattle[Q]	3. 5
Reaches for objects	4
Palmar grasp gone	4
Transfers object hand to hand	5. 5
Thumb-finger grasp	8
Turns pages of book	12
Scribbles	13
Builds tower of 2 cubes[Q]	15
Builds tower of 6 cubes	22
Communication and Language	
Smiles in response to face, voice	1. 5
Monosyllabic babble[Q]	6
Inhibits to "no"	7
Follows one-step command with gesture	7
Follows one-step command without at gesture	10
Says "mama" or "dada"	10
Points to objects	12
Speaks first real word[Q]	15
Speaks 4-6 words	18
Speaks 10-15 words	19
Speaks 2 word sentences[Q] (*e.g.*, "Mommy shoe")	
Cognitive	
Stares momentarily at spot where object disappeared	2
Stares at own hand	4
Bangs 2 cubes	8
Uncovers toy (after seeing it hidden)	8
*Egocentric symbolic play (**e.g.,** pretends to drink from cup)*	12
Uses stick to reach toy	17
Pretend play with doll (*e.g.*, gives doll bottle)	17

AT 3 MO	
Prone:	Lifts head and chest with arms extended; ***head above plane of body on ventral suspension***[Q]
Supine:	Tonic neck posture predominates; reaches toward and misses objects; waves at toy
Sitting:	Head lag partially compensated when pulled to sitting position; early head control with bobbing motion[Q]; back rounded
Reflex:	Typical Moro response has not persisted; makes defensive movements or selective withdrawal reactions
Social:	Sustained social contact; listens to music; says" aah, ngah"

◈ *O. P. Ghai: Milestone*

Age	Milestone
5-7 months	Transfers objects from one hand to other[Q]
7 months	Palmar grasp[Q]
9 months	Pincer grasp[Q]

198. Ans. a. It is..., b. More... & c. May be...

[Ref: Harison 19th/1520-21; O. P. Ghai 8th/413; Nelson 19th/1554; Robbins 9th/534]

Atrial Septal Defect

◈ *Robbins 9th/534*

- *Secundum ASD (90% of all ASD)*
- *Primum anomalies (5% of all ASD) occur adjacent to the AV valve & are often associated with AV valve abnormalities &/ or a VSD*

◈ *Harison 19th/1520-21*

- Atrial septal defect (ASD) is a common cardiac anomaly that may be first encountered in the adult and occurs more frequently in females.
- **Sinus venosus ASD** occurs high in the atrial septum near the entry of the superior vena cava into the right atrium and is associated frequently with anomalous pulmonary venous connection from the right lung to the superior vena cava or right atrium
- **Ostium primum ASDs** lie adjacent to the atrioventricular valves, either of which may be deformed and regurgitant.
- ***Ostium primum ASDs are common in Down's syndrome***, often as part of complex atrioventricular septal defects with a common atrioventricular valve and a posterior defect of the basal portion of the interventricular septum.
- The **most common ostium secundum ASD** involves the ***fossa ovalis*** and is midseptal in location; this should not be confused with a patent foramen ovale.
- The left-to-right shunt causes *diastolic overloading of the RV* and increased pulmonary blood flow. Patients with ASD are usually asymptomatic in early life, although there may be some physical underdevelopment and an increased tendency for respiratory infections; cardiorespiratory symptoms occur in many older patients.

199. Ans. a. Peak incidence..., d. Selective...

[Ref: Robbins 9th/917-18; O. P. Ghai 8th/477-78]

Minimal Change Disease

◈ *O. P. Ghai 8th/477-78*

- ***Age at onset: 2-6 yr***
- ***Response to steroid: Remission in >95%***
- ***Selectivity of proteinuria: High***
- ***Prognosis: Good, relapse stop by second decade.***
- *In contrast,* **steroid resistant form of nephritic syndrome** *(usually associated with significant glomerular lesions) has less satisfactory course & a* ***significant proportion progress to chronic renal failure***

◈ *Robbins 9th/917-18*

- This relatively benign disorder is the ***most frequent cause of nephrotic syndrome in children,*** but it is less common in adults. *It is characterized by diffuse effacement of foot processes of epithelial cells in glomeruli that appear virtually normal by light microscopy.*
- The ***peak incidence is between 2 and 6 years of age.*** The disease sometimes follows a respiratory infection or routine prophylactic immunization. *Its most characteristic feature is its usually dramatic response to corticosteroid therapy.*
- The glomeruli are normal by light microscopy. By electron microscopy, the basement membrane appears normal, and no electron-dense material is deposited. **The principal lesion is in the visceral epithelial cells, which show a uniform and diffuse effacement of foot processes,** these being replaced by a rim of cytoplasm often showing vacuolization, swelling, and hyperplasia of villi.
- Despite massive proteinuria, renal function remains good, and there is commonly no hypertension or hematuria. The proteinuria usually is highly selective, most of the protein consisting of albumin.
- ***Most children (more than 90%) with minimal change disease respond rapidly to corticosteroid therapy.*** However, the nephrotic phase may recur, and some patients may become steroid dependent or resistant. Nevertheless, the ***long-term prognosis for patients is excellent, and even steroid-dependent disease resolves when children reach puberty. Although adults are slower to respond, the long-term prognosis is also excellent.***

200. Ans. a. Micturating... & b. Radioisotope...

[Ref: Nelson 19th/1836; L & B 26th/1273-75; O. P. Ghai 8th/485; S. Das 6th/1161]

"***Micturating cystography and radioisotope renography*** are helpful in excluding vesicoureteric reflux and renal scarring. Treatment aims to relieve symptoms, correct causes and prevent renal scarring. Vesicoureteric reflux may resolve spontaneously, some may need antibiotic prophylaxis or, in a very small number of cases, an endoscopic treatment or a reimplantation of the ureter"- *(L & B)*

Vesicoureteric Reflex

◈ *O. P. Ghai 8th/485*

- *Two techniques are commonly used to detect VUR. The* ***radiocontrast MCU*** *is commonly used since in additional to showing VUR it provide excellent anatomical detail*
- ***Isotope radionuclide cystography*** *is more sensitive for detecting VUR & causes less radiation exposure but provides less anatomical detail*

◈ *Nelson 19th/1836*

- Retrograde flow of urine from the bladder to the ureter and renal pelvis is referred to as **vesicoureteral reflux.**
- **Diagnosis of reflux** usually requires catheterization of the bladder, instillation of a solution containing iodinated contrast or a radiopharmaceutical, and radiologic imaging of the lower and upper urinary tract—a ***contrast VCUG or radionuclide VCUG, respectively.***
- Radiation exposure during radionuclide VCUG is significantly less than that from a contrast VCUG. However, the contrast study provides more anatomic information, such as demonstration of a duplex collecting system, ectopic ureter, paraureteral (bladder) diverticulum, bladder outlet obstruction in boys, upper urinary tract stasis, and signs of voiding dysfunction, such as a "spinning top" urethra in girls.
- The reflux grading system is based on the appearance on VCUG. ***Consequently, the VCUG is used as the initial study in most centers.*** For follow-up evaluation, the radionuclide cystogram often is preferred because of the lower radiation exposure
- **Indirect cystography** is a technique of detecting reflux without catheterization that involves injecting an intravenous radiopharmaceutical that is excreted by the kidneys, waiting for it to be excreted into the bladder, and imaging the lower urinary tract while the patient voids. This technique detects only 75% of reflux cases, however.
- Another technique, which avoids radiation exposure, involves the instillation of sonographic contrast medium through a urethral catheter. The ***kidneys are imaged sonographically.*** The advantage of this technique is the absence of radiation, but it is less accurate than contrast VCUG and reflux cannot be graded.

201. Ans. a. Penis... & c. Scanty hair...

[Ref: O. P. Ghai 8th/63-64; Shaws Gynaecology 16th/55-58; Dutta Gynaecology 6th/50]

"Peak growth velocity in girls occur before attainment of menarche (stage 3) in girls whereas boys have their peak growth velocity during later stages of puberty (stages 4-5)"(O. P. Ghai 8th/64)

Table: Tanner Classification of Female Adolescent Development

Stage	Breast Development	Pubic Hair Development
I	Papillae elevated (preadolescent), no breast buds	None
II	Breast buds and papillae slightly elevated	Sparse, long, slightly pigmented
III	Breasts and areolae confluent, elevated	Darker, coarser, curly
IV	Areolae and papillae project above breast	Adult–type pubis only
V	Papillae projected, mature	Lateral distribution

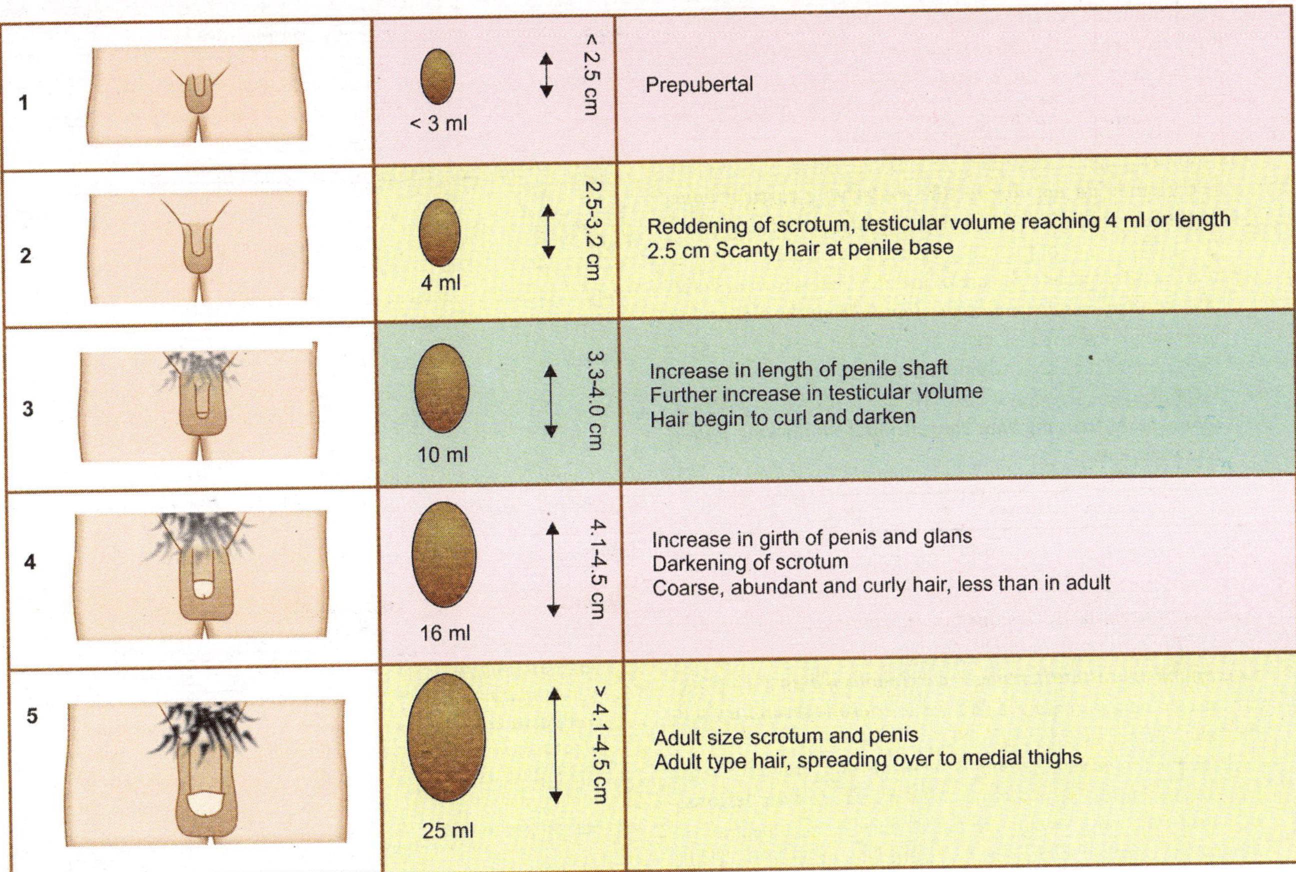

Fig: Sexual maturity rating

ORTHOPAEDICS

202. Ans. b. Can be... & d. Mechanically...

[Ref: Maheswari 5th/32-33; Apley 9th/701-03315-16]

Locking Compression Plate

◈ *Maheswari 5th/32-33*

- *The latest development in plating technique is locking compression plate (LCP)*
- *It has rigid plate: Screw construct,* ***which has been found to be mechanically superior to a conventional plate***
- ***LCP can be used as compression plate****, as neutralization plate,* ***as a buttress plate****, as a bridging plate & as a locked plate*
- ***It is particularly suitable for periarticular fractures & fractures in osteoporotic bones***

Types of Plate

◈ *Maheswari 5th/32-33*

- Conventional plate
- **Bridging plate:** The fracture is stabilized without touching the small communicated pieces of bone
- Low contact dynamic compression plate (modification of conventional plate)
- Locking compression plate
- Carbon plates (not widely accepted)

When do Locking Plates Work Best?

◈ *tchealth. org/.../Locking%20 Plates%20-%20Advantages%20&%20 Indicat.*

- *Osteopenic bone*
- *Metaphyseal areas*
- *Periprosthetic fractures*
- *Failed fixation (nonunion)*
- *Screw strippage*

Locking Plates & Screws

◈ *tchealth. org/.../Locking%20Plates%20-%20 Advantage*

- **Anatomic Reduction:** Locked plate design allows lag screw and compression plating techniques
- **Stable Internal Fixation:** Locking screws increase stability in osteoporotic and metaphyseal bone
- **Preservation of Blood Supply:** Limited bony contact stabilizes fracture without plate-to-bone compression
- ***Tapered tip allows submuscular plate insertion, decreasing tissue destruction***
- ***Early Active Pain Free Mobilization***

Locking versus nonlocking plates

◈ *www2. aofoundation. org*

There are several advantages to a locking plate/screw system:

- Conventional plate/screw systems require precise adaptation of the plate to the underlying bone. Without this intimate contact, tightening of the screws will draw the bone segments toward the plate, resulting in alterations in the position of the osseous segments and the occlusal relationship. Locking plate/screw systems offer certain advantages over other plates in this regard.

- Another potential advantage in locking plate/screw systems is that they ***do not disrupt the underlying cortical bone perfusion as much as conventional plates***, which compress the undersurface of the plate to the cortical bone.
- A third advantage to the use of locking plate/screw systems is that the ***screws are unlikely to loosen from the plate***. This means that even if a screw is inserted into a fracture gap, loosening of the screw will not occur.
- Locking plate/screw systems have been shown to ***provide more stable fixation than conventional nonlocking plate/screw systems.***

203. Ans. a. Prostate & b. Breast

[Ref: Robbins 9th/1207; Maheswari 5th/247; Apley 9th/216]

"Metastases are usually osteolytic & pathological fractures are common. **Osteoblastic lesions** *are uncommon, they usually occur in* ***prostatic carcinoma****" (Apley 9th/216)*

Carcinoma of prostate in males & carcinoma of breast *in female are the commonest tumous to give rise to* ***sclerotic secondary's*** *in the bone" (Maheswari 5th/247)*

"The radiographic manifestations of metastases may be purely lytic, purely blastic, or mixed lytic and blastic. In **lytic lesions**, *the metastatic cells secrete substances such as prostaglandins, interleukins, and PTHRP, which stimulate osteoclastic bone resorption; the tumor cells themselves do not directly resorb bone.* ***Carcinomas of the kidney, lung, and gastrointestinal tract and malignant melanoma produce this type of bone destruction.*** *Similarly, metastases that elicit a* **sclerotic response**, *particularly* ***prostate adenocarcinoma***, *do so by stimulating osteoblastic bone formation. Most metastases induce a mixed lytic and blastic reaction" (Robbins 9th/1207)*

204. Ans. a. Vascular... & b. Neuro...

[Ref: Maheswari 5th/42-43; Apley 9th/711-12]

Complications of Fractures

◈ *Maheswari 5th/42-43*

- ***Immediate complications: Occurring at the time of the fracture***
- Early complications: Occurring in the initial few days after the fracture
- Late complications: Occurring a long time after the fracture

"Fracture & dislocation are the commonest cause of peripheral nerve injuries" *(Maheswari 5th/62)*

Table *(Maheswari 5th/42-43)*: **Immediate complications**

Systemic	Hypovolaemic shock
Local	*Injury to major vessels* *Injury to muscles & tendon* *Injury to joints* *Injury to viscera*

Table *(Maheswari 5th/42-43)*: **Early complications**

Systemic	*Hypovolaemic shock; ARDS; Fat embolism syndrome; DVT & Pulmonary embolism; Aseptic traumatic fever; Septicemia; Crush syndrome*
Local	*Infection;* ***Compartment syndrome***

Table *(Maheswari 5th/42-43)*: **Late complications**

Imperfect union of the fracture	Delayed union; Non-union; Malunion; Cross union
Others	Avascular necrosis; Shortening; Joint stiffness; Sudeck's dystrophy; Osteomyelitis; Ischaemic contracture; Myositis ossificans; Osteoarthritis

Local complications can be divided into early (those that arise during the first few weeks following injury) & late (Apley 9th/711)

Table *(Apley 9th/712)*: **Local complications of fracture**

Urgent	Less urgent	Late
1. Local visceral injury 2. ***Vascular injury*** 3. ***Nerve injury*** 4. ***Compartment syndrome*** 5. Haemathrosis 6. Infection 7. Gas gangrene	1. Fracture blister 2. Plaster sore 3. Pressure sore 4. Nerve entrapment 5. Myositis ossificans 6. Ligament injury 7. Tendon lesions 8. Joint stiffness 9. Algodystrophy	1. Delayed union 2. Malunion 3. Non-union 4. Avascular necrosis 5. Muscle contracture 6. Joint instability 7. Osteoarthritis

205. Ans. c. Bone... & e. Proper...

[Ref: Maheswari 5th/11-12; Apley 9th/689-9, 716-70]

Infection: Both biology & stability are hampered by active infection*; not only is there bone lysis, necrosis & pus formation, but implants which are used to hold the fracture tend to loosen" (Apley 9th/716)*

Bone grafting is used in treatment of malunion (Maheswari 5th/50)

Factors Affecting Fracture Healing

◈ *Maheswari 5th/11-12*

- **Age of the patient:** Fractures unite faster in children. On an average, bones in children unite in half the time compared to that in adult
- **Type of bone:** Flat & cancellous bones unite faster than tubular & cortical bones
- **Pattern of fracture:** Spiral fracture unite faster, which in turn unite faster than transverse fracture. Comminuted fractures heal slower
- **Disturbed pathoanatomy:** ***Soft tissue interposition*** & ischemic fracture ends hinder healing
- **Type of reduction:** *Good apposition of fracture results in faster union*
- **Immobilisation:** It is not necessary to immobilize all fractures (*e. g.*, fracture ribs, scapula etc). They heal anyway.

Some fracture need strict immobilization (*e.g.*, fracture of the neck of the femur) & may still not heal

- ***Open fracture:*** *Often go into delayed union & non-union*
- **Compression at fracture site:** Compression enhances the rate of union in cancellous bone

In cortical bones, compression at the fracture site enhances rigidity of fixation & possibly results in primary bone healing

206. Ans. a. Foot..., c. Difficult..., d. May... & e. May...

[Ref: Maheswari 5th/210-18; Apley 9th/591-95; http://link. springer. com/ chapter/10. 1007/978-1-4613-9269-9_13; CSDT 11th/1195-96; Apley 8th/488; Nelson 19th/2336, 18th/2777-78]

Atypical Idiopathic Clubfoot

◈ *http://link. springer. com/chapter/10. 1007/978-1-4613-9269-9_13*

- It occurs in a very small percentage of congenital clubfeet.
- At birth, it appears to be a typical clubfoot with no associated abnormalities and without any stigmata of neurological or genetic syndromes. The main difference is that it ***responds altogether differently to both operative and nonoperative treatment.***
- Results with early soft tissue surgery are unpredictable and, unlike the more common typical idiopathic clubfoot, early surgery usually ***results in a grotesque, overcorrected severe flatfoot.***

Features of Atypical/Complex Clubfoot

◈ *http://www. kaahe. org/health/en*

- A short and fat or swollen foot.
- The big toe is short and points upward
- A *crease runs across the bottom (sole) of the foot from side to side.*
- There is a *deep crease in the skin above the heel.*
- The heel area is rigidly tilted inward.
- The *foot is rigidly flexed downward* and the heel cord is very tight, wide, and long.
- The calf muscle is very small and bunched up under the back of the knee.

"**Atypical clubfoot**: *Some clubfoot are more difficult to correct. These resistant clubfeet may be a variant that is unusually stiff. In others, the clubfoot are complex because they were treated by non-Ponseti methods. Such treatment often creates additional deformity that makes management more difficult. Evaluation Examination often demonstrates* ***severe plantar flexion of all metatarsals, a deep crease just above the heel and across the sole of the midfoot****, and a* ***short hyperextended big toe****" (http:// www. global-help. org/publications/books/help_cfponseti. pdf)*

"Clubfoot are associated with arthrogryposis multiplex congenital, ***spina bifida****, myelomeningocele, neurofibromatosis & chondrodysplasia punctata" (Danhert Radiology 5th/25)*

"CTEV: Cause could be a genetic defect, or a form of arrested development. Its occurrence in ***neurological disorders & neural tube defects (myelomeningocele & spinal bifida)***[Q] *points to a neuromuscular disorder" (Apley 8th/488)*

Clubfoot or Talpes Equinovarus

- It is **most commonly** an ***idiopathic congenital condition***[Q]
- It occurs twice as often in boys and is bilateral half the time. There is a familial tendency, with a 5% chance that a sibling will also be affected.
- In congenital clubfoot, there is more or less rigid ***inversion of the hindfoot, adduction of the forefoot, and limited dorsiflexion***—an equinovarus deformity.

207. Ans. b. Osteosarcoma.

[Ref: Maheswari 5th/239; Apley 9th/207; Harrison 19th/712]

Osteosarcoma *is the second most common tumour. These tumours occur b/w the ages of 15-25 years, constituting the commonest musculo-skeletal tumour at that age (Maheswari 5th/239)*

"**Osteoid osteoma**: *It is the commonest true benign tumour of the bone" (Maheswari 5th/235)*

"Of the primary bone malignancies, multiple myeloma is the commonest. ***Osteochondroma*** *is the commonest benign tumour of the bone. Most primary malignant bone tumours occur in children & young adult" (Maheswari 5th/235)*

"**Ewing sarcoma**: *This is highly malignant tumour occurring b/w the age of 10-20 years, sometimes up to 30 years" (Maheswari 5th/239)*

Giant cell tumour: *The tumour is seen commonly in the age group of 20-40 years" (Maheswari 5th/237)*

Chondrosarcoma: *It occurs commonly in adults b/w 30-60 years of age & is rare in children (Maheswari 5th/246)*

"The peak incidence of ***osteogenic sarcoma*** *is during* ***adolescence****, correlating with the rapid bone growth; it is* ***rare below the age of 5-year****" (O. P. Ghai 7th/593)*

"**Primary osteosarcoma** *occur in age group of* ***15-25 years****. The* ***secondary osteosarcoma*** *occur in older age (****45 yr*** *onward)" (Maheswari 4th/218)*

"**Multiple Myeloma** *increases in incidence with age. The* ***median age at diagnosis is 70 years****; it is uncommon under age 40. Males are more commonly affected than females" (Harrison 19th/712)*

208. Ans. d. E coli is...

[Ref: Maheswari 5th/175-78; Apley 9th/43-45; Nelson 18th/2846; Maheswari 3rd/163]

Complication: Damage to the cartilaginous physis or the epiphysis in the growing child is the most serious complication. Sequelae include retarded growth, partial or complete destruction of epiphysis, deformity of the joint, epiphyseal osteonecrosis, acetabular dysplasia & psuedoarthrosis of the hip"*(Apley 9th/45)*

"***Aspirate the joint*** *& examine the fluid. A WBC & gram stain should be carried out immediately. Sample of fluid are also sent for full microbiological examination & tests for antibiotic sensitivity" (Apley 9th/44)*

Septic Arthritis

◈ *Maheswari 5th/175-78; 3rd/163*

- ***It is more common in children & males are more susceptible. Staphylocoocus aureus is the commonest causative organism, other organisms are strepto-pneumo & Gonococcus.***
- **The organism reach the joint by one of the following routes:**
    - **Haematogenous:** This is the commonest route
    - Secondary to nearby osteomyelitis: This is a particularly common route in joints with intra-articular metaphysic
    - Penetrating wounds
    - Iatrogenic
    - Umbilical cord sepsis

Pathogenesis

◈ *Nelson 18th/2846*

- Suppurative arthritis ***primarily occurs as a result of hematogenous seeding of the synovial space***. Less often, organisms enter the joint space by direct inoculation or extension from a contiguous focus.
- The synovial membrane has a rich vascular supply and lacks a basement membrane, providing an ideal environment for hematogenous seeding.

Table *(Maheswari 5th/177)*: **Synovial joint examination**

Points	Normal	Non-inflammatory	Inflammatory	Septic
Gross examination Volume (ml)	Often < 3. 5 ml	Often > 3. 5 ml	Often > 3. 5 ml	> 3. 5 ml
• Viscosity	High	High	Low	Variable
• Colour	Colourless	Straw yellow	Yellow	Variable
• Clarity	Transparent	Transparent	Translucent	Opaque
Examination in lab.				
• WBC count	< 200	200-2000	2000-7500	> 10000
• PMN leucocytes	< 25%	< 25%	> 50%	>75%
• Culture	–	–	–	+
• Mucin clot	Firm	Firm	Friable	Friable
• Glucose level	Equal to blood glucose	Nearly equal to blood glucose	< 25 mg% of blood glucose	> 25 mg% of blood glucose
• Crystal examination: Positive in Gout–Sodium biurate,			Positive in Pseudogout-Ca pyrophosphate	

209. Ans. b. Hypoxia., d. Tachypnoea. & e. Petechial...

[Ref: Maheshwari 5th/43-44; Apley 9th/681]

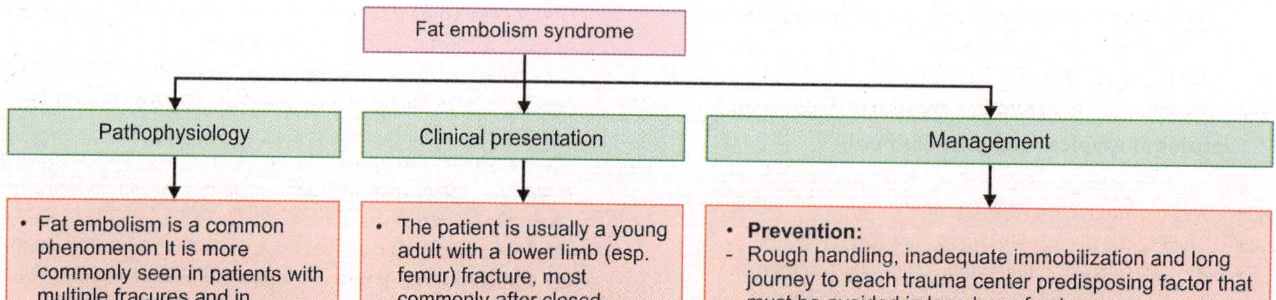

Pathophysiology

- Fat embolism is a common phenomenon It is more commonly seen in patients with multiple fracures and in fractures (involving **lower limb** especially **femur**[Q]
- Fat originates from the site of trauma, particularly from the injured marrow of the fractured bones and the suggestion that the fat arises from the the plasma as a result of agglutination of chylomicrons is not supported by th vivo experiments.
- Circulating **fat globules >** *10mm in diameter* occur in most adults after close fracture of *long bones*[Q] and histological traces of fat can be found in the lungs and other internal organs.
- Few of these patients develop clinical features similar to ARDS and are k/a **fat embolism syndrome**

Clinical presentation

- The patient is usually a young adult with a lower limb (esp. femur) fracture, most commonly after closed fractures of **long bone** (esp *shaft femur)* and more so when fractures are *multiple*[Q].
- It usually manifests itself within **24-48 hours**[Q], but occasionally the onset may be delayed for several days.
- Early warning signs (within 72 hours of injury) are a slight rise in temperature ***(pyrexia)*** *and pulse rate* **(tachycardia)**[Q]
- In more pronounced cases there is breathlessness, mild mental confusion or ***restlessness***[Q], ***pectechiac***[Q] on chest, axillae, retina & conjuctival folds; progressing to marked ***respiratory distress*** & coma in severe cases.

Management

- **Prevention:**
- Rough handling, inadequate immobilization and long journey to reach trauma center predisposing factor that must be avoided in long bone fractures
- Fracture statbilization by IM nail
- Stopping the emboli from reaching main circulation by tieing profunda vein (? of doubtful value)
- Removing fat emboli from circulation by
- Lipolytic agents as heparin[Q] (serum lipase activity)
- Hypertonic glucose (decrease FFA production)
- **Offset its effect by**
- Vasodilation e.g. phenxybenzamine
- Prompt correction of hypovlemia
- Prophylactic use of O_2
- *Dextran*[Q] (expand plasma volume, reduce RBC aggregation and platelet adherence)
- Aprotinin (this protease inhibitor) decrease platelet aggregation and serotonin release)
- Alcohol has vasodilator & lipolytic effect.
- **Treatment of established Case**
- The aim of treatment is maintaining adequate oxygen level in the ventilation.
- **Oxygen** is the only therapeutic tool of proven use[Q]. It should be administered in sufficient amount to maintain arterial PO_2 > 80mm Hg
- O_2 toxicity (pneumonitis) is avoided by using O_2 conc. below 40%.
- **Steroids** are given to avoid chemical pneumonitis resulting from break down of pulmonary fat emboli into FFA.
- Surface cooling will diminish O_2 demand.

Fig: Fat emabolism syndrome

Fat Embolism Syndrome

◈ *Maheshwari 5th/43-44*

- Tachycardia
- Slight rise of temperature
- Breathlessness
- Hypoxia from involvement of lung
- Tachypnoea
- Petechial rash
- Respiratory failure
- Drowsy
- Restless
- Coma

210. Ans. d. Prolapsed... & e. Sciatica.

[Ref: Maheshwari 5th/260, 221; Apley 9th/255-56; S. Das Textbook 6th/514-15; Hutchison's Clinical method 21st/205; L & B 26th/443, 472]

"Pain & limitation of Straight leg raising (SLR) is a feature of prolapsed intervertebral disc when there is irritation or compression of one of the roots of the sciatic nerve" *(Hutchison's Clinical method 21st/205)*

Straight leg raising: This test is useful in patients with sciatica" *(Hutchison's Clinical method 21st/280)*

Straight leg raising test: *This is a test to detect nerve root compression" (Maheshwari 5th/260)*

"**Trendelenburg's test**: *This is a test to establish the stability of the hip. Positive test occur in* **CDH**. *This test is performed in an older child. The child asked to stand on the affected side. The opposite anterior superior iliac spine (that of the normal side) dips down" (Maheshwari 5th/221)*

Straight Leg Raising Test

◈ *S. Das Textbook 6th/514-15*

- *If the pain is evoked under 40° it suggests impingement of the* ***protruding intervertebral disc*** *on a nerve root. If the pain evoked at an angle above 40° it indicates tension on nerve root that is abnormally sensitive from a cause not necessarily an intervertebral disc protrusion*
- *At the angle when the patient experiences first twinge of pain, the ankle is passively dorsiflexed. This cause aggravation of the pain due to* ***additional traction to the sciatic nerve (Bragard's sign)****. It suggests irritation of one or more nerve roots either by disc protrusion or from some other space occupying lesions. The second part of the test is important to differentiate sciatica from the diseases of the sacroiliac joint. In the latter condition SLRT will be positive but there will be no aggravation of pain during passive dorsiflexion of the ankle*

Special Tests

◈ *L& B 26th/443*

- Lasègue's straight leg raise test. This test increases tension along the sciatic nerve (L5 and S1 nerve roots). With the patient supine, elevate the leg with the knee bent to check pain-free movement of the hip. Then, straighten the knee and note the angle which the hamstrings allow the hip to flex. Finally, allow the hip to extend until tension is removed from the hamstring muscles and then the ankle is dorsiflexed firmly, tugging on the sciatic nerve. If the patient experiences pain running down the leg, then the test is positive.
- Contralateral stretch test. Elevate the asymptomatic leg; if pain is reproduced in the other leg the test is considered positive

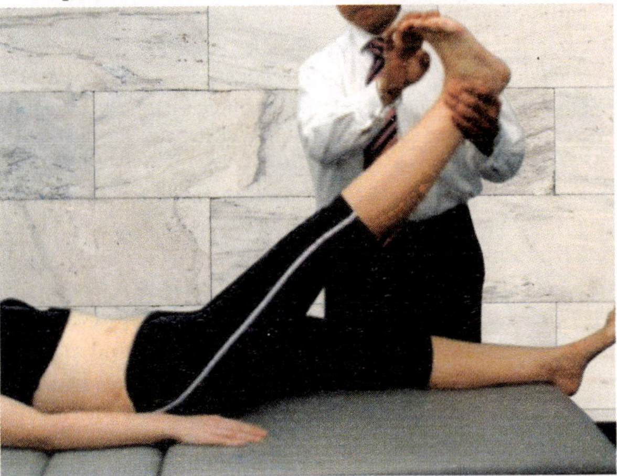

Fig: Lasègue's straight leg test

211. Ans. d. Positive Romberg...

[Ref: Maheshwari 5th/260, 348; Harrison 19th/162-64; P. J. M 20th/281]

"In sensory ataxia the patient is able to maintain the upright position while the eyes are open, but when the eyes are closed he sways. This is a ***positive Romberg sign***' *(P. J. M 20th/281)*

Abnormal Gaits

◈ *http://en. wikipedia. org/wiki/Gait Maheshwari 5th/260, 348*

- **Antalgic gait**: ***occurs in painful conditions of the lower limb***
- **Charlie-Chaplin gait:** Occurs in tibial torsion.
- **Circumduction gait:** Occurs in hemiplegia
- **Waddling gait:** Occurs in bilateral congenital hip dislocation
- **High stepping gait:** Occurs in foot drop
- **Scissoring gait:** Occurs in cerebral palsy
- **Stiff hip gait:** Occurs in ankylosis of the hip
- **Trendelenburg gait:** Occurs in unstable hip due to ***congenital dislocation of hip***, gluteus medius muscle weakness

Sensory Ataxia

◈ *Harrison 19th/163*

- As reviewed earlier in this chapter, balance depends on high-quality afferent information from the visual and the vestibular systems and proprioception. When this information is lost or degraded, balance during locomotion is impaired and instability results.
- The ***sensory ataxia*** of tabetic neurosyphilis is a classic example. The contemporary equivalent is the patient with neuropathy affecting large fibers. Vitamin B 12 deficiency is a treatable cause of large-fiber sensory loss in the spinal cord and peripheral nervous system. Joint position and vibration sense are diminished in the lower limbs. The stance in such

patients is destabilized by eye closure; they often look down at their feet when walking and do poorly in the dark.

"Observation of gait is an important aspect of diagnosis that may provide information about several musculoskeletal and neurological conditions. In particular, there are **eight basic pathological gaits** that can be attributed to neurological conditions: ***hemiplegic, spastic diplegic, neuropathic, myopathic, Parkinsonian, choreiform, ataxic (cerebellar) and sensory***. http://stanfordmedicine25. stanford. edu/the25/gait. html

Sensory Gait

◈ *http://stanfordmedicine25. stanford. edu/the25/gait. html*

- As our feet touch the ground, we receive propioreceptive information to tell us their location. The sensory ataxic gait occurs when there is loss of this propioreceptive input. In an effort to know when the feet land and their location, the patient will slam the foot hard onto the ground in order to sense it.
- A key to this gait involves its exacerbation when patients cannot see their feet (i.e. in the dark). This gait is also sometimes referred to as a stomping gait since patients may lift their legs very high to hit the ground hard.
- This gait can be seen in disorders of the *dorsal columns (B12 deficiency or tabes dorsalis) or in diseases affecting the peripheral nerves (uncontrolled diabetes)*. In its severe form, this gait can cause an ataxia that resembles the cerebellar ataxic gait.

Table *(Harrison 19th/164)*: **Features of Cerebellar Ataxia, Sensory Ataxia, and Frontal Gait Disorders**

	Cerebellar Ataxia	Sensory Ataxia	Frontal Gait
Base of support	Wide-based	Narrow base, looks down	Wide-based
Velocity	Variable	Slow	Very slow
Stride	Irregular, lurching	Regular with path deviation	Short, shuffling
Romberg	+/–	Unsteady, falls	+/–
Heel shin	Abnormal	+/–	Normal
Initiation	Normal	Normal	Hesitant
Turns	Unsteady	+/–	Hesitant, multistep
Postural instability	+	+++	++++; Poor postural synergies getting up from a chair
Falls	Late event	Frequent	Frequent

Frontal Gait Disorder

◈ *Harrison 19th/163*

- Frontal gait disorder, sometimes known as *gait apraxia*, is common in the elderly and has a variety of causes.
- The term is used to describe a shuffling, freezing gait with imbalance and other signs of higher cerebral dysfunction. Typical features include a wide base of support, a short stride, shuffling along the floor, and difficulty with starts and turns.

ANESTHESIA

212. Ans. a. N2O… & c. Sevoflurane…

[Ref: Ajay Yadav 5th/70-87; Morgan's clinical aneasthesia 5th/163-70]

Nitrous Oxide

◈ *Ajay Yadav 5th/76-78*

- Nitrous oxide is good analgesia
- It is not complete anaesthesia (used as a ***supplement to anesthesia***)
- When given along with other inhalational agent it increases the alveolar concentration of that agent (second gas effect)
- Not a muscle relaxant
- C/I in pneumothorax, pneumoperitoneum, middle ear surgery, tympanoplasty

Halothane

◈ *Ajay Yadav 5th/79-81*

- Widely used inhalational agent
- Stored in amber coloured bottle & contains thymol 0. 01% as preservative (To prevent decomposition by light)
- Not a good analgesic
- It is a potent bronchodilator
- It cause hepatitis. Risk factor includes- multiple exposure, hypoxia, middle age, obesity, female & patient with other autoimmune disease

Sevoflurane

◈ *Ajay Yadav 5th/82-83*

- *Odour is sweet so induction is smooth*
- *Faster, pleasant & smooth induction with no significant systemic toxicity* ***makes sevoflurane as the agent of choice for induction in children***
- *Because of bronchodilation it is the inhalational agent of choice for asthmatics in present day practice*

Isoflurane

◈ *Ajay Yadav 5th/81-82*

- Pungent ethereal odor so induction is not smooth
- Not a good analgesic
- Hypotension is maximum (It is the inhalational agent of choice for controlled hypotension)
- It can cause coronary steal phenomenon (but concern is only theoretical)
- Isoflurane's cardiac stability makes it the agent of choice for cardiac patients (except myocardial ischemia)
- It is also agent of choice for neurological procedure

213. Ans. d. Thiopentone…

[Ref: Ajay Yadav 5th/133-35; Miller 7th/1187-89; Lee 13th/353; Morgan's clinical aneasthesia 4th/945-950; Wylie's Anaesthesia 7th/365, 367]

Malignant Hyperthermia

◈ *Ajay Yadav 5th/133-35*

- It is due to abnormality of ***type I Ryanodine receptor*** which is calcium releasing channel of sarcoplasmic reticulum
- The abnormality leads to excessive accumulation of calcium in sarcoplasmic reticulum which causes sustained contraction of muscle
- It is a genetic disease ***usually autosomal dominant*** but can be recessive also
- **Screening/evaluation of suspected individual:** All high risk patient must undergo blood creatinine kinase level. Patients with elevated CK levels in normal resting conditions should be managed as susceptible & does not require further testing.
- Patient with normal CK levels should undergo muscle biopsy studies (where muscle is subjected to triggering factors like halothane & suxamethonium).
- If the biopsy studies are negative then only the patient can be considered non susceptible

◈ *Barash Clinical Anesthesia 6th/Chapter 24*

- The ***gold standard test for diagnosis of MH susceptibility is the caffeine-halothane contracture test*** (of freshly biopsied muscle) wherein muscle is exposed to incremental doses of caffeine or to halothane.
- MH susceptibility is inherited in an ***autosomal dominant pattern in humans.***
- MH has been associated with mutations in three genes, most frequently the ***ryanodine receptor gene (RYR1)***, rarely the dihydropyridine receptor gene, and the gene that elaborates the sodium channel of muscle.

"**Increased ETCO$_2$** (may rise to >100 mmHg) is most sensitive early sign of ***malignant hyperthermia***" *(Ajay Yadav 1st/102)*

"***Clinical feature:*** *Hypoxia, cyanosis,* ***tachycardia, hypertension & cardiac arrhythmia***" *(Ajay Yadav 2nd/102)*

Drug known to trigger MH:

- Ether
- Cyclopropane
- *Halothane*[Q]
- Methoxyflurane
- Enflurane
- Isoflurane
- Desflurane
- Sevoflurane
- *Succinyl choline*[Q]

Safe Anaesthetic drug in patient who are susceptible to MH

- **Thiopentone sodium**[Q]
- Pancuronium
- *Nitrons oxide*
- Propofol[Q]
- Etomidate
- *Benzodiazepines*
- *Ketamine*
- Opiates
- Droperidol

---

214. Ans. **a. Most..., b. Most... & d. In Children...**

[Ref: Ajay Yadav 5th/43-46; Lee 13th/209; Miller 7th/Chap50; Morgan's clinical aneasthesia 5th/321]

"The size of the tracheal tube is normally described as the internal diameter (ID) in millimeters. ***Tracheal tube sizes of 8 mm (ID) for males and 7.5 mm (ID) for females are often used.*** Tracheal tubes used in adult patients have a cuff near the distal end that is inflated to provide a seal against the tracheal wall to protect the lungs from pulmonary aspiration and to ensure that the tidal volume delivered ventilates the lungs rather than escapes into the upper airway. Cuffs are normally inflated with air and have an inflation tube with a pilot balloon that indicates cuff inflation"- *Miller 7th/Chap50*

Endotracheal Tube

◈ *Ajay Yadav 5th/43-46*

- Two types- red rubber (reusable, costlier, non-transparent) & ***PVC (disposable,*** cheap, transparent)
- May be cuffed or uncuffed
- Cuff pressure should be less than 30 cm of H_2O to prevent tracheal ischemia
- In a normal healthy male usually 9 number tube is used & for normal healthy female usually 8 number tube is used
- In children less than 10 years of age uncuffed tube should be used & there should be slight leak to avoid barotraumas if inspiratory pressure exceeds above 30 cm H_2O

◈ *Lee 13th/209*

- ***Cuffs prevent leakage b/w the ETT & the trachea***- both leakage of gas outwards during IPPV & of gastric contents, blood & mucus into the lungs
- Overinflation may cause sore throat or at worst, necrosis of the tracheal mucosa

---

215. Ans. **d. Hypotension...**

[Ref: Ajay Yadav 5th/155-61; Lee 13th/479; Oxford Handbook of Anesthesia 3rd/832]

> ***Note:*** *Due to associated serious complications (many are life threatening), it must not be given by unskilled doctors*

Preparation for Subarachnoid Block (Spinal Anesthesia)

◈ *Lee 13th/479*

- ***Obtaining venous access***
- *Commencing intravenous infusion (to minimize post spinal hypotension)*

Subarachnoid Block (Spinal Anesthesia)

◈ *Ajay Yadav 5th/155-61*

- *It is most commonly used anaesthetic technique*
- *In adult level is usually L3-4*
- **Indications:** Orthopaedics surgery, general surgery (pelvic & perineal), gynecological & obstetrical surgery, urological surgeries etc
- Most commonly drugs used in India are- xylocaine (lignocaine) & Sensoricaine (bupivacine)

- ***Hypotension is most common side-effect:*** It is managed by preloading & intraoperative fluids & vasopressors. ***For this good i. v acess is very important***
- Other side-effects & complications are- bradycardia, apnoea, nausea & vomiting, cardiac arrest, high spinal, post spinal headache, meningitis, spinal cord ischemia etc

Subarachnoid Block (Spinal Anesthesia) in Children

◈ *Ajay Yadav 5th/161*

- In ***children it should be given in lower space (L4-5)***
- As children are usually free of haemodynamic side effects therefore preloading is not required till the age of 8 years
- Due to more CSF volume, dose of local anaesthetics required is more & duration of block is less

216. Ans. a. CVP…, b. Prior…, c. For… & e. For giving…

[Ref: Ajay Yadav 5th/59; Morgan's clinical aneasthesia 5th/100]

Indication of CVP

◈ *Ajay Yadav 5th/59; Morgan's clinical aneasthesia 5th/100*

- ***Major surgeries*** where large fluctuations in haemodynamics are expected
- Open heart surgeries
- ***Fluid management in shock***
- As a venous access in patient with poor peripheral veins
- Parenteral nutrition
- Aspiration of air embolism
- Cardiac pacing

Central Venous Catheters

- The term *central venous catheter* refers to a catheter that is designed for cannulation of the subclavian vein, the internal jugular vein, or the femoral vein.
- As indicated in Table 6.2, these catheters are much longer than the catheters used to cannulate peripheral veins and are typically 15 to 25 cm (6 to 10 inches) in length. They also are available with two or three separa

SKIN

217. Ans. c. Bacterial infection e. Usually…

[Ref: Neena Khanna 4th/141-42]

Acute Paronychia

◈ *Neena Khanna 4th/141-42*

- Paronychia is inflammation of ***nail folds*** & could be acute or chronic
- Etiology: ***Staphylococcus*** enter the nail fold (through breaks in the skin of nail fold or cuticle)
- Predisposing factors: including chronic paronychia, nail biting & hang nails
- Clinical feature: Nail fold is swollen, red & tender. Pus may be visible under the nail fold or on the nail bed. May be associated with lymphadenopathy & constitutional symptoms
- Treatment: Systemic antistaphylococcal antibiotics (erythromycin & cloxacillin). If need be, surgical drainage

◈ *Neena Khanna 4th/142*

- *It is an inflammatory dermatosis of nail folds with secondary effects on the nail matrix & nail growth*
- ***Etiology:*** *Microbial colonization: the space b/w nail plate & proximal nail fold is colonized by* ***candida***, Staphylococcus & gram negative bacteria
- ***Predisposing factor:*** *wet work, finger sucking, DM, candidal vulvovaginitis*
- ***Clinical features:*** *Nail fold is swollen & rolled. Adjacent nail plate becomes riged & disclored. Sometime a bead of pus can be expressed from under the nail fold*
- ***Treatment:*** *Topical antibiotics (gentamycin, ciprofloxacin) & antifungal (clotrimazole); Systemic antibiotics (may help in more inflamed lesions) & weekly fluconazole (in recurrent disease)*

218. Ans. a. Benign, c. Proliferation… & e. Cherry…

[Ref: L & B 26th/599; http://www. dermishealth. com/campbell-de-morgan-spots. html; http://www. pcds. org. uk/clinical-guidance/cherry-angioma-syn. -campbell-de-morgan-spot]

Campbell De Morgan spots

◈ *L & B 26th/599*

"These are arteriovenous fistulae at the dermal capillary level that usually, although not exclusively, occur in skin on the trunk of older patients. Multiple lesions are associated with liver disease"

◈ *http://www. patient. co. uk/doctor/Campbell-de-Morgan-Spot. htm*

Aetiology

Their cause remains unknown:

- Chemical exposure (mustard gas, 2-butoxyethanol) causes multiple lesions to develop.
- ***Pregnancy and prolactinomas*** are associated with the development of lesions, implicating hormonal mediators.

Epidemiology

- These are the ***most common cutaneous vascular proliferation***. Few reports have been published recently but there is evidence showing 75% of those over 75 years old may have them
- They increase in frequency and size with age.
- The most common age of onset is in the third and fourth decades of life.
- They are seen across all races and sexes.

Visual Appearance

- 1-3 mm diameter macules which may become larger papules over time.
- ***Typical bright cherry red colour*** but can appear violaceous.
- They are non-blanching.

Campbell de Morgan Spots

◈ *http://www. dermishealth. com/campbell-de-morgan-spots. html http:// www. pcds. org. uk/clinical-guidance/cherry-angioma-syn. -campbell-de-morgan-spot*

- Campbell de Morgan spots, also known as campbell de morgan angiomas, cherry angiomas, cherry spots and senile angiomas, are ***benign (non-cancerous) skin growths made of blood vessels.***
- They get their name from the name of an English surgeon. The growths are bright red, often described as "***cherry-red***" (hence they are often referred to as cherry angiomas). They can appear anywhere on the body, but ***most often appear on the torso.***
- They range in size from the size of a pinhead to a quarter inch in diameter. They may be flat or dome-shaped, sticking out from the skin. They are ***usually painless. Often only one growth*** is seen but sometimes there are multiple growths.
- **What Causes Campbell de Morgan Spots?:** No one knows for sure, but they may be ***hereditary***. Some medical professionals think ***hormonal changes***, like those that occur ***during pregnancy***, can trigger the spots to appear. That's certainly not the only thing that causes them, though, since men can get them, too. They appear ***most commonly in adults over the age of 30*** but people of any age can get them.
- **How Are Campbell de Morgan Spots Diagnosed?:** A doctor can usually make the diagnosis just by looking at the spots. If there is a question about the diagnosis, a biopsy may be recommended. While cherry angiomas are ***non-cancerous***, it's important to make sure you're not dealing with something more serious or even cancerous.
- Treatment is not normally required
- Lesions that catch/bleed can be removed by curettage and sent for histology

219. Ans. a. Lichen planus, c. Sjo…

[Ref: Neena Khanna 4th/56; Harrison 19th/2041; Roxburg 16th/; Hepatology by Kuntz 2nd/443]

"Lichen planus: Hepatitis C infection" *(Neena Khanna 4th/56)*

Hepatitis C Associated Disease

◈ *Harrison 19th/2041)*

- Attention has been drawn as well to associations between hepatitis C and such cutaneous disorders as ***porphyria cutanea tarda and lichen planus.***
- **Immune complex:** Mediated extrahepatic complications of chronic hepatitis C are less common than in chronic hepatitis B (despite the fact that assays for immune complexes are often positive in patients with chronic hepatitis C), with the exception of ***essential mixed cryoglobulinemia***, which is linked to cutaneous vasculitis and membranoproliferative glomerulonephritis as well as lymphoproliferative disorders such as B-cell lymphoma and unexplained monoclonal gammopathy.
- In addition, chronic hepatitis C has been associated with extrahepatic complications unrelated to immune-complex injury. These include ***Sjögren's syndrome, lichen planus, porphyria cutanea tarda, type 2 diabetes mellitus, and the metabolic syndrome (including insulin resistance and steatohepatitis)***

Extrahepatic Manifestations in Viral Hepatitis C:

◈ *Hepatology by Kuntz 2nd/443*

- *Agranulocytosis*[Q]
- *Aplastic anaemia*
- *Corneal ulceration*
- *Cryoglobulinaemia*[Q]
- *Diabetes mellitus (type I)*
- Erythema exsudativum multiforme
- *Glomerulonephritis*[Q]
- *Guillain-Barre syndrome*
- *Hyperlipasaemia*
- *Lichen planus*[Q]
- *Non-Hodgkin lymphoma*
- *Polyarteristis nodosa*[Q]
- *Polyarthritis*[Q]
- *Polyneuritis*
- *Porhyria cutanea tarda*[Q]
- *Sialadenitis*
- *Sjogren's syndrome/Sicca syndrome*
- *Thrombocytopenia*
- *Thyroditis*

220. Ans. c. Itching…

[Ref: Neena Khanna 4th/341-44, 3rd/297; Harrison 19th/2744-45; KDT 6th/863-64]

*"The **number of mites** normally present in an individual patient varies, being **less than 7-8 in an adult**. Most lesions in scabies are due to hypersensitivity" (Neena Khanna 4th/341)*

"Scabicides used are: Permethrin cream[Q] ***(5%), Gamma benzene hexachloride (G-BHC1%), Crotamiton (10%),*** *Benzyl benzoate (25%) & Ivermectin (single oral dose 200 μg/kg)" (Neena Khanna 3rd/297)*

Scabies (Sarcoptes scabiei var. hominis)

- **Morphology:** ***Pruritic***[Q]***, erythematous papules, burrows, and vesicles in web spaces, volar wrists, waist, genitals and axillae***
- ***Scalp, face, palm & soles are characteristically involved in infants/children***
- The itching and rash associated with scabies derive from a sensitization reaction directed against the excreta that the mite deposits in its burrow. Burrows become surrounded by infiltrates of eosinophils, lymphocytes, and histiocytes, and a generalized hypersensitivity rash later develops in remote sites
- Hyperinfestation with thousands of mites, a condition known as ***crusted scabies or Norwegian scabies***, may result from glucocorticoid use, immunodeficiency, and neurologic and psychiatric illnesses that limit itching and scratching.
- Intense itching worsens at ***night and after a hot shower***[Q]

Scabies: Treatment

◈ *Harrison 19th/2744-45*

- **Permethrin cream** (5%) is less toxic than ***1% lindane (G-BHC)*** preparations and is effective against lindane-tolerant infestations.

- Successful treatment of crusted scabies requires pre-application of a ***keratolytic agent such as 6% salicylic acid*** and then of scabicides to the scalp, face, and ears.
- Although ivermectin, a single oral dose (200 μg/kg) effectively treats scabies in otherwise-healthy persons; patients with crusted scabies may require two doses separated by an interval of 1–2 weeks.
- Antihistamines, salicylates, and calamine lotion relieve itching during treatment, and topical glucocorticoids are useful for pruritus.
- To prevent reinfestations, bedding and ***clothing should be washed and/or dried on high heat or heat-pressed,*** and close contacts, even if asymptomatic, should be treated simultaneously.

221. Ans. b. Drug..... & d. caused. by....

[Ref: Neena Khanna 4th/53; Harrison 19th/347-49; CMDT 2015/107-08]

Pityriasis Rosea

◈ *Neena Khanna 4th/53*

Etiology

Unknown. A virus (HHV-7 more frequently, HHV-6 less frequently) has often been incriminated, but Pitryiasis rosea is not contagious

Epidemiology

Age: Usually b/w ages of 10-35 years
Sex: No gender predilection
Season: Incidence lowest in summer

Morphology

Herald patch, Fir tree or Christmas tree appearance

Site

Trunk along line of cleavage; sometimes (20%) lesions occur predominantly on extremities & neck (inverse pattern)

◈ *CMDT 2015/107-08*

Essentials of Diagnosis

- Oval, fawn-colored, scaly eruption following cleavage lines of trunk.
- ***Herald patch precedes eruption by 1–2 weeks.***
- Occasional pruritus.

General Considerations

- This is a common mild, acute inflammatory disease that is 50% more common in females. Young adults are principally affected, mostly in the spring or fall. Concurrent household cases have been reported.
- ***Itching is common*** but is usually mild.
- The diagnosis is made by finding one or more classic lesions. The lesions consist of oval, fawn-colored plaques up to 2 cm in diameter. The centers of the lesions have a crinkled or ***"cigarette paper" appearance*** and a collarette scale, ie, a thin bit of scale that is bound at the periphery and free in the center.
- Only a few lesions in the eruption may have this characteristic appearance, however. Lesions follow cleavage lines on the trunk (so-called ***Christmas tree pattern***), and the proximal portions of the extremities are often involved. A variant that affects the flexures (axillae and groin), so-called inverse pityriasis rosea, and a papular variant, especially in black patients, also occur.
- An initial lesion ("***herald patch***") that is often larger than the later lesions often precedes the general eruption by 1–2 weeks. The eruption usually lasts 6–8 weeks and heals without scarring
- Pityriasis rosea often requires no treatment.
- Pityriasis rosea is usually ***an acute self-limiting illness that disappears in about 6 weeks.***

PSYCHIATRY

222. Ans. b. OCD & c. Phobia.

[Ref: Ahuja 7th/94, 214-15, 80; Kaplan & Sadock 11th/425, 1266-67]

"The principal behavioral **approaches in OCD** are ***exposure and response prevention.*** Desensitization, thought stopping, flooding, implosion therapy, and aversive conditioning have also been used in patients with OCD. In behavior therapy, patients must be truly committed to improvement" *(Kaplan & Sadock 11th/425)*

"**Phobia**: *If properly planned, behavior therapy (flooding; systemic desensitization;* ***exposure & response prevention*** *& relaxtion technique) is usually successful" (Ahuja 7th/94)*

223. Ans. d. PTSD & e. Acute...

[Ref: Ahuja 7th/111-12; Kaplan & Sadock 11th/437-40, 449]

Acute stress reaction: *In this disorder there is an immediate & clear temporal relationship b/w an exceptional stressor (such as death of a loved one,* ***natural catastrophe, accident****, rape) & the onset of symptoms. The symptoms range from a dazed condition, anxiety, depression, anger, despair, overactivity or withdrawl & constriction of field of consciousness. The symptoms* ***resolve rapidly (within few hours usually),*** *if removal from the stressful environment is possible. If stress continues or cannot be reversed, the* **resolution of symptoms begin after 1-2 days & is usually minimal after about 3 days"** *(Ahuja 7th/111-12)*

Posttraumatic stress disorder (PTSD)*: This disorder arises as a delayed &/protracted response to an exceptionally stressful or catastrophic life event or situation, which is likely to cause pervasive distress in almost any person (e. g disasters, war, rape or torture, serious accident. The symptoms of PTSD may develop, after a period of latency, within six months after the stress or may be delayed beyond this period"- Ahuja 7th/112*

Trauma & Stress Related Disorders

◈ *Kaplan & Sadock 11th/437-38, 449*

- ***Posttraumatic stress disorder (PTSD)*** & ***acute stress disorder*** are marked by increased stress & anxiety following exposure to a traumatic or stressful events
- The stressors causing both acute stress disorder and PTSD are sufficiently overwhelming to affect almost anyone.

They can arise from experiences in war, torture, natural catastrophes, assault, rape, and serious accidents, for example, in cars and in burning buildings.

- Persons re-experience the traumatic event in their dreams and their daily thoughts; they are determined to evade anything that would bring the event to mind and they undergo a numbing of responsiveness along with a state of hyperarousal. Other symptoms are depression, anxiety, and cognitive difficulties, such as poor concentration.
- The lifetime incidence of PTSD is estimated to be 9 to 15% and the lifetime prevalence of PTSD is estimated to be about 8% of the general population
- The presence of a stressor is a requirement in the diagnosis of adjustment disorder, PTSD, and acute stress disorder. PTSD and acute stress disorder have the nature of the stressor better characterized and are accompanied by a defined constellation of affective and autonomic symptoms.
- In contrast, the stressor in adjustment disorder can be of any severity, with a wide range of possible symptoms. When the response to an extreme stressor does not meet the acute stress or posttraumatic disorder threshold, the adjustment disorder diagnosis would be appropriate.

224. Ans. a. Post-partum...

[Ref: Dutta Obstetrics 8th/512; Ahuja 7th/145-46; William's Obstetrics 23rd/655-56]

"It is no surprise that 25-50% of all women can develop psychological symptoms in the puerperal period. The commonest type of presentation is mild depression & irritability, often known as **post-natal blues**. These blues pass off ***within a few days***. Severe psychiatric symptoms include-depressive episode with psychotic symptoms (most common), schizophrenia like symptoms, manic episode & delirium (least common)" *(Ahuja 7th/145)*

Psychiatric Disorders During Puerperium

◈ *Dutta Obstetrics 8th/512*

In the first 3 month after delivery, the incidence of mental illness is high. Overall incidence is about 15-20%

Puerperal Blues

- It is a transient state of mental illness observed 4-5 days after delivery & it last for a few days
- Nearly 50% of the postpartum women suffer from the problem
- **Manifestation:** Depression, anxiety, tearfulness, insomnia, helplessness & negative feeling toward the infant
- Treatment is reassurance & psychological support by the family members

Postpartum Depression

- *It is observed in 10-20% of mothers*
- *It is more gradual in onset over the first 4-6 months following delivery or abortion*
- *Manifested by loss of energy & appetite, insomnia, social withdrawl, irritability & even suicide attitude*
- ***Treatment:*** *Fluoxetine & other SSRI; estrogen patch & psychiatric consulation*

Postpartum Psychosis (Schizophrenia)

- Observed in about 0. 14-0.26% of mothers
- Manifested by fear, restlessness, confusion followed by hallucinations, delusions & disorientation. Suicidal & infanticidal impulse may be present
- ***Treatment:*** *A psychiatrist must be consulted urgently. Chlorpromazine, estradiol, Lithium & ECT may be used*

Depression

◈ *William's Obstetrics 23rd/655-56*

- It is fairly common for a mother to exhibit some degree of depressed mood a few days after delivery. This situation is termed *postpartum blues,* and it likely is the consequence of a number of factors
- In the great majority of cases, effective treatment need be nothing more than anticipation, recognition, and reassurance. ***This mild disorder is self-limited and usually remits after 2 to 3 days***, although it sometimes persists for up to 10 days. Should postpartum blues persist or worsen, a careful search should begin for symptoms of major depression, which can occur in almost 20% of puerperal women. If severe, prompt consultation is carried out
- Similarly, suicidal or infanticidal ideation is dealt with emergently.

Emotional Reactions

◈ *COGDT 10th/Chap12*

- These reactions range from the common, physiologic, relatively mild and transient "***maternity blues***," ***which affect some 50–70% of postpartum women, to more severe reactions including depression and rare puerperal psychosis.***
- Postpartum blues or maternity blues occurs in ***up to 70% of postpartum women and appear to be a normal psychological adjustment or response***. It is generally characterized by tearfulness, anxiety, irritation, and restlessness.
- This symptomatology can be quite diverse and may include *depression, feelings of inadequacy, elation, mood swings, confusion, difficulty concentrating, headache, forgetfulness, insomnia, depersonalization, and negative feelings toward the baby.*
- These ***transient symptoms usually occur within the first few days after delivery and cease by postpartum day 10***, although bouts of weeping may occur for weeks after delivery. The blues are self-limiting, but the distress can be diminished by physical comfort and reassurance.

RADIOLOGY

225. Ans. a. Hydatid...

[Ref: Review of Radiology by Sumer Sethi 6th/59; Danhert Radiology manual 5th/493]

Hydatid Lung

◈ *Review of Radiology by Sumer Sethi 6th/59*

- No or rare calcification in lung
- ***Water lily sign*** or Camalote sign (in chest X-ray)

Lung Echinococcosis

◈ *Danhert Radiology manual 5th/493*

- ***Water lily sign***: Completely collapsed crumpled cyst membrane floating on the cyst fluid
- Sign of Camalotte
- Serpent sign
- Cumbo sign
- Meniscus sign
- Crescent sign

Hemartoma lung: *Carney's triad & calcification (Danhert Radiology manual 5th/489)*

Silicosis: eggshell calcification: *WHO Manual of Radiological (Interpretation 1st/75)*

226. Ans. a. MRI & c. USG

[Ref: L & B 26th/174; Review of Radiology by Sumer Sethi 6th/5, 9; Danhert Radiology manual 5th/1070-71]

Ultrasound

◈ *L & B 26th/174-75*

- Ultrasound is the second commonest method of imaging. It relies on high-frequency sound waves generated by a transducer containing piezoelectric material.
- The generated sound waves are reflected by tissue interfaces and, by ascertaining the time taken for a pulse to return and the direction of a pulse, it is possible to form an image.
- Medical ultrasound uses frequencies in the range 3–20 MHz.

Magnetic Resonance Imaging

◈ *L & B 26th/177-78*

- Over the last 20 years, MRI has become an integral part of the imaging arsenal with ever-expanding indications.
- MRI relies on the fact that nuclei containing an odd number of protons or electrons have a characteristic motion in a magnetic field (precession) and produce a magnetic moment as a result of this motion.
- In a strong uniform magnetic field such as a MRI scanner, these nuclei align themselves with the main magnetic field and result in a net magnetic moment. A brief radiofrequency pulse is then applied to alter the motion of the nuclei.

Table *(L & B 26th/174)*: **Typical effective doses from diagnostic medical exposures**

Diagnostic procedure	Typical effective dose (mSv)	Equivalent no. of chest radio-graphs	Approximately equivalent period of natural background radiation
Radiographic examinations			
Limbs and joints (except hip)	< 0. 01	< 0. 5	< 1. 5 days
Chest (single posteroanterior film)	0. 02	1	3 days
Skull	0. 07	3. 5	11 days
Thoracic spine	0. 7	35	4 months
Lumbar spine	1.3	65	7 months
Hip	0.3	15	7 weeks
Pelvis	0. 7	35	4 months
Abdomen	1. 0	50	6 months
Intravenous urography (IVU)	2. 5	125	14 months
Barium swallow	1. 5	75	8 months
Barium meal	3	150	16 months
Barium follow-through	3	150	16 months
Barium enema	7	350	3.2 months
CT head	2.3	115	1 year
CT chest	8	400	3. 6 year
CT abdomen of pelvis	10	500	4. 5 year
Radionuclide studies			
Lung ventilation (^{133}Xe)	0.3	15	7 weeks
Lung perfusion (^{99m}TC)	1	50	6 months
Kidney (^{99m}TC)	1	50	6 months
Thyroid (^{99m}TC)	1	50	6 months
Bone (^{99m}TC)	4	200	1. 8 years
Dynamic cardiac (^{99m}TC)	6	300	2. 7 years
PET head (18F-FDG)	5	250	2.3 years

Contd...

227. Ans. d. Microwave

Ref: Robbins 9th/428; Review of Radiology by Sumer Sethi 6th/166; L & B 26th/172]

Injury Produced by Ionizing Radiation

◈ *Robbins 9th/428*

- *Radiation* is energy that travels in the form of waves or high-speed particles. Radiation has a wide range of energies that span the electromagnetic spectrum; it can be divided into nonionizing and ionizing radiation. The energy of **nonionizing radiation** such as ***UV and infrared light, microwave, and sound waves***, can move atoms in a molecule or cause them to vibrate, but is not sufficient to displace bound electrons from atoms.

- By contrast, *ionizing radiation* has sufficient energy to remove tightly bound electrons. Collision of electrons with other molecules releases electrons in a reaction cascade, referred to as ionization. The main sources of ionizing radiation are **x-rays *and* gamma rays** (electromagnetic waves of very high frequencies), ***high-energy neutrons, alpha particles*** (composed of two protons and two neutrons), and *beta particles*, which are essentially electrons.
- At equivalent amounts of energy, alpha particles induce heavy damage in a restricted area, whereas x-rays and gamma rays dissipate energy over a longer, deeper course, and produce considerably less damage per unit of tissue. About 50% of the total dose of ionizing radiation received by the U. S. population is human-made, mostly originating from medical devices and radioisotopes. In fact, the exposure of patients to ionizing radiation during radiologic imaging tests roughly doubled between the early 1980s and 2006, mainly because of much more widespread use of CT scans.
- Ionizing radiation is a double-edged sword. It is indispensable in medical practice, being used in the treatment of cancer, in diagnostic imaging, and in therapeutic or diagnostic radioisotopes, but it also produces adverse short- and long-term effects such as *fibrosis, mutagenesis, carcinogenesis*, and *teratogenesis*.

228. Ans. a. String..., d. Air... & e. Valvulae...

[Ref: BDC 6th/Vol. II 438; Review of Radiology by Sumer Sethi 6th/123; Grainger & Allison's Diagnostic Radiology 6th/598, 602; Danhert Radiology manual 5th/767; L & B 26th/1143-44]

"Dilated loop of small intestine are readily identified if they are gas filled on supine radiograph. The ***strings of beads sign, caused by a line of gas bubbles trapped b/w the valvulae conniventes,*** *is seen only when very dilated small bowel is almost completely filled with fluid & is virtually diagnostic of small bowel obstruction"- Allison's Diagnostic Radiology 6th/598*

Jejunal & ileal obstruction

◈ *Danhert Radiology manual 5th/751*

- Candy crane sign appearance in erect position= > 3 distended small bowel loops > 3 cm with gas–fluid level (>3-5 hr after onset of obstruction
- Stretch sign= ***erectile valvulae conniventes*** completely encircle bowel lumen
- Stepladder appearance in low obstruction (the greater the number of dilated bowel loops, the more distal the site of obstruction)
- String of beads

Duodenal Obstruction

◈ *Danhert Radiology manual 5th/751*

- **Double-bubble sign:** Air fluid level in stomach + duodenum

Small bowel obstruction

◈ *Review of Radiology by Sumer Sethi 6th/123*

- ***Multiple centrally placed*** loops with valvulae connvinates in jejunum & diameter 3-5 cm
- May show strings of beads appearance due to air trapped within valvulae & rest of loop being fluid filled

Large bowel Obstruction

◈ *Review of Radiology by Sumer Sethi 6th/123*

- ***Few peripherally placed loops with haustra*** & diameter 5 cm+ & showing fecal matter within dilated loop
- A caecal diameter of > 9cm implies impending perforation
- Demonstration of the air in rectum implies a paralytic ileus rather than mechanical obstruction

Summary Box: Anatomy of the small and Large Intestine

◈ *L & B 26th/1143*

- **Small intestine:** Comprises jejunum and ileum & has valvulae conniventes
- **Large intestine:** Comprises caecum, ascending, transverse, descending and sigmoid colon has appendices epiploicae and taenia coli

"Distended small and large intestine can be distinguished on an abdominal radiograph as the small bowel has complete transverse markings caused by the valvulae conniventes, while the colon has incomplete lines from the sacculation caused by the taeniae" (L & B 26th/1144)

"The jejunum tends to have a wider diameter and a thicker wall, with more prominent mucosal folds (**valvulae conniventes**), while the ileum has a thicker, more fatty mesentery with more complex arterial arcades" *(L & B 26th/1143)*

Imaging

◈ *L & B 26th/1189-90*

- **In intestinal obstruction**, fluid levels appear later than gas shadows as it takes time for gas and fluid to separate. These are most prominent on an erect film. In adults, two inconstant fluid levels – one at the duodenal cap and the other in the terminal ileum – may be regarded as normal.
- When fluid levels are pronounced, the obstruction is advanced. In the small bowel, the ***number of fluid levels is directly proportional to the degree of obstruction and to its site, the number increasing the more distal the lesion.***
- In contrast, **low colonic obstruction** does not commonly give rise to small bowel fluid levels unless advanced, whereas high colonic obstruction may do so in the presence of an incompetent ileocaecal valve. Colonic obstruction is usually associated with a large amount of gas in the caecum. A limited water-soluble enema should be undertaken to differentiate large bowel obstruction from pseudo-obstruction.

Radiological Features of Obstruction

◈ *L & B 26th/1189*

- The obstructed small bowel is characterised by straight segments that are ***generally central and lie transversely***. No gas is seen in the colon
- The jejunum is characterised by its ***valvulae conniventes***, which completely pass across the width of the bowel and are regularly spaced, giving a 'concertina' or ladder effect
- **Ileum:** The distal ileum has been piquantly described by Wangensteen as featureless

- **Caecum:** A distended caecum is shown by a rounded gas shadow in the right iliac fossa
- Large bowel, except for the caecum, shows haustral folds, which, unlike valvulae conniventes, are spaced irregularly, do not cross the whole diameter of the bowel and do not have indentations placed opposite one another

229. Ans. a. Brachytherapy

[Ref: Radiology by Sumer Sethi 6th/176; Grainger & Allison's Diagnostic Radiology 6th/1737- 44; Brachytherapy Applications & Technique 2007 by M. Devlin; Perez & Brady's Radiation Oncology 5th/54; Harrison 19th/103e4-5]

Types of Radiotherapy

◈ *Grainger & Allison's Diagnostic Radiology 6th/1737-44*
- **External beam radiotherapy:** *It refer to any situation where the source of the radiation is located at a distance from the patient & the beam of radiation is then directed towards a defined treatment area. Approximately 85% of all therapeutic radiation exposures are delivered using external beam techniques.*
- *Conventional external beam radiotherapy*
- *Three dimensional conformal radiotherapy*
- **Intensity-modulated radiotherapy:** *In this the intensity of radiation beam is modulated across each treatment beam*
- ***Stereotactic body radiotherapy:*** *The distribution of radiation beam is in 3-dimensions & not in two as in traditional radiotherapy*
- **Brachytherapy:** *It refers to situation in which a radioisotope is placed onto or inside the patient. The source can be placed into the target tissues or tumour itself such as prostate or breast (interstitial brachytherapy, into a body cavity such as the uterine cavity, oesophagus or bronchus (intracavity/intraluminal brachytherapy) or onto the skin surface to treat a cutaneous malignancy*
- **Particle therapy:** Also known as Hadron therapy. It is an external beam radiation technique in which highly energetic particle such as protons, neutrons or positive ions are directed at the tumor

Teletherapy: Treatment in which the radiation source is at a distance from the body. Linear accelerators & cobalt machines are used in teletherapy. Also called external beam therapy"-

"**Brachytherapy:** A type of radiation therapy is which radioactive materials are placed in direct contact with the tissue being treated. Broadly it is of two types- interstitial or intracavity" *(Review of Radiology by Sumer Sethi 6th/176)*

Types of Brachytherapy

- **Mold brachytherapy**[Q] : Superficial tumours can be treated using sealed sources placed close to the skin
- **Interstitial brachytherapy**[Q] : Here the sources are inserted into tissue
- **Intracavitary brachytherapy**[Q]: Places the sources inside a pre-existing body cavity
- **Intravascular brachytherapy:** Places a catheter inside the vasculature through which sources are sent and returned
- **Electronic brachytherapy:** Places a miniature low energy (< 50kVp) X-ray tube source into a pre-positioned applicator within body/tumor cavities to rapidly deliver high doses to target tissues while maintaining low doses to distant non-target tissues

Therapeutic Radiation

◈ *Harrison 19th/103e4-5*
- ***Therapeutic radiation is delivered in three ways:***
  - *Teletherapy*, with focused beams of radiation generated at a distance and aimed at the tumor within the patient;
  - *Brachytherapy*, with encapsulated sources of radiation implanted directly into or adjacent to tumor tissues; and
  - *Systemic therapy*, with radionuclides administered, for example, intravenously but targeted by some means to a tumor site.
- **Teletherapy** with X-ray or gamma-ray photons is the most commonly used form of radiation therapy.

230. Ans. a. Pineal..., b. Choroids... & d. Duramater...

[Ref: Review of Radiology by Sumer Sethi 6th/137; Danhert Radiology manual 5th/230]

Normal Intracranial Calcification

◈ *Review of Radiology by Sumer Sethi 6th/137*
- ***Pineal, habenulae***
- ***Choroids plexus***
- ***Dura (falx, tentorium, over vault)***
- ***Ligamnets (petroclinoid & interclinoid)***
- ***Pacchionian bodies***
- ***Basal*** ganglia & dentate nucleus
- ***Pituitary***
- ***Lens***

Physiological Intracranial Calcification

◈ *Danhert Radiology manual 5th/230*
- *Pineal calcification: Present 2/3 of adult population*
- *Habenula: Approximately 1/3 population*
- *Choroid plexus*
- *Dura, falx cerebri, falx cerebella, tentorium- 10% population*
- *Petroclinoid ligament*
- *Interclinoid ligament*
- *Arteriosclerosis*
- ***Basal ganglia***

Basal Ganglia Calcification

◈ *Review of Radiology by Sumer Sethi 6th/137*
- *Idiopathic*
- *Pseudohypoparathyroidism*
- *Familial*
- *Hypoparathyroidism*
- *Fahr's syndrome*
- *Cockaynes syndrome*
- *CO, Pb poisoning*
- *Toxoplasmosis*

Note: *Calcification is periventricular in congenital CMV infection while it is scattered in toxoplasmosis*

ANSWER SHEET

1 – 50		51 – 100		101 – 150		151 – 200		201 – 250	
1	A B C D E	51	A B C D E	101	A B C D E	151	A B C D E	201	A B C D E
2	A B C D E	52	A B C D E	102	A B C D E	152	A B C D E	202	A B C D E
3	A B C D E	53	A B C D E	103	A B C D E	153	A B C D E	203	A B C D E
4	A B C D E	54	A B C D E	104	A B C D E	154	A B C D E	204	A B C D E
5	A B C D E	55	A B C D E	105	A B C D E	155	A B C D E	205	A B C D E
6	A B C D E	56	A B C D E	106	A B C D E	156	A B C D E	206	A B C D E
7	A B C D E	57	A B C D E	107	A B C D E	157	A B C D E	207	A B C D E
8	A B C D E	58	A B C D E	108	A B C D E	158	A B C D E	208	A B C D E
9	A B C D E	59	A B C D E	109	A B C D E	159	A B C D E	209	A B C D E
10	A B C D E	60	A B C D E	110	A B C D E	160	A B C D E	210	A B C D E
11	A B C D E	61	A B C D E	111	A B C D E	161	A B C D E	211	A B C D E
12	A B C D E	62	A B C D E	112	A B C D E	162	A B C D E	212	A B C D E
13	A B C D E	63	A B C D E	113	A B C D E	163	A B C D E	213	A B C D E
14	A B C D E	64	A B C D E	114	A B C D E	164	A B C D E	214	A B C D E
15	A B C D E	65	A B C D E	115	A B C D E	165	A B C D E	215	A B C D E
16	A B C D E	66	A B C D E	116	A B C D E	166	A B C D E	216	A B C D E
17	A B C D E	67	A B C D E	117	A B C D E	167	A B C D E	217	A B C D E
18	A B C D E	68	A B C D E	118	A B C D E	168	A B C D E	218	A B C D E
19	A B C D E	69	A B C D E	119	A B C D E	169	A B C D E	219	A B C D E
20	A B C D E	70	A B C D E	120	A B C D E	170	A B C D E	220	A B C D E
21	A B C D E	71	A B C D E	121	A B C D E	171	A B C D E	221	A B C D E
22	A B C D E	72	A B C D E	122	A B C D E	172	A B C D E	222	A B C D E
23	A B C D E	73	A B C D E	123	A B C D E	173	A B C D E	223	A B C D E
24	A B C D E	74	A B C D E	124	A B C D E	174	A B C D E	224	A B C D E
25	A B C D E	75	A B C D E	125	A B C D E	175	A B C D E	225	A B C D E
26	A B C D E	76	A B C D E	126	A B C D E	176	A B C D E	226	A B C D E
27	A B C D E	77	A B C D E	127	A B C D E	177	A B C D E	227	A B C D E
28	A B C D E	78	A B C D E	128	A B C D E	178	A B C D E	228	A B C D E
29	A B C D E	79	A B C D E	129	A B C D E	179	A B C D E	229	A B C D E
30	A B C D E	80	A B C D E	130	A B C D E	180	A B C D E	230	A B C D E
31	A B C D E	81	A B C D E	131	A B C D E	181	A B C D E	231	A B C D E
32	A B C D E	82	A B C D E	132	A B C D E	182	A B C D E	232	A B C D E
33	A B C D E	83	A B C D E	133	A B C D E	183	A B C D E	233	A B C D E
34	A B C D E	84	A B C D E	134	A B C D E	184	A B C D E	234	A B C D E
35	A B C D E	85	A B C D E	135	A B C D E	185	A B C D E	235	A B C D E
36	A B C D E	86	A B C D E	136	A B C D E	186	A B C D E	236	A B C D E
37	A B C D E	87	A B C D E	137	A B C D E	187	A B C D E	237	A B C D E
38	A B C D E	88	A B C D E	138	A B C D E	188	A B C D E	238	A B C D E
39	A B C D E	89	A B C D E	139	A B C D E	189	A B C D E	239	A B C D E
40	A B C D E	90	A B C D E	140	A B C D E	190	A B C D E	240	A B C D E
41	A B C D E	91	A B C D E	141	A B C D E	191	A B C D E	241	A B C D E
42	A B C D E	92	A B C D E	142	A B C D E	192	A B C D E	242	A B C D E
43	A B C D E	93	A B C D E	143	A B C D E	193	A B C D E	243	A B C D E
44	A B C D E	94	A B C D E	144	A B C D E	194	A B C D E	244	A B C D E
45	A B C D E	95	A B C D E	145	A B C D E	195	A B C D E	245	A B C D E
46	A B C D E	96	A B C D E	146	A B C D E	196	A B C D E	246	A B C D E
47	A B C D E	97	A B C D E	147	A B C D E	197	A B C D E	247	A B C D E
48	A B C D E	98	A B C D E	148	A B C D E	198	A B C D E	248	A B C D E
49	A B C D E	99	A B C D E	149	A B C D E	199	A B C D E	249	A B C D E
50	A B C D E	100	A B C D E	150	A B C D E	200	A B C D E	250	A B C D E

NAME OF THE CANDIDATE	ROLL NO.	CENTRE NO.	QUESTION BOOKLET NO.	BOOKLET CODE
CATEGORY SC ○ ST ○ OBC ○ GEN ○ CW ○ PH ○	0 0 0 0 0 1 1 1 1 1 2 2 2 2 2 3 3 3 3 3 4 4 4 4 4 5 5 5 5 5 6 6 6 6 6 7 7 7 7 7 8 8 8 8 8 9 9 9 9 9	0 0 1 1 2 2 3 3 4 4 5 5 6 6 7 7 8 8 9 9	0 0 0 0 0 1 1 1 1 1 2 2 2 2 2 3 3 3 3 3 4 4 4 4 4 5 5 5 5 5 6 6 6 6 6 7 7 7 7 7 8 8 8 8 8 9 9 9 9 9	A B C D

INSTRUCTIONS FOR FILLING THE SHEET

1. This sheet should not be folded or crushed.
2. Use only blue/black ball pen to fill the circles.
3. Use of pencil is strictly prohibited.
4. Circles should be darkened properly and completely.
5. Cutting & erasing on this sheet is not allowed.
6. Do not use any stray marks on the sheet.
7. Do not use marker, white fluid or any other device to hide the shading already done.

WRONG METHOD ⊗ ● ✓ ○ ○

CORRECT METHOD ○ ○ ○ ● ○

CANDIDATE'S SIGNATURE
(in ball - point pen)

INVIGILATOR'S SIGNATURE
(in ball - point pen)

NOVEMBER

2014

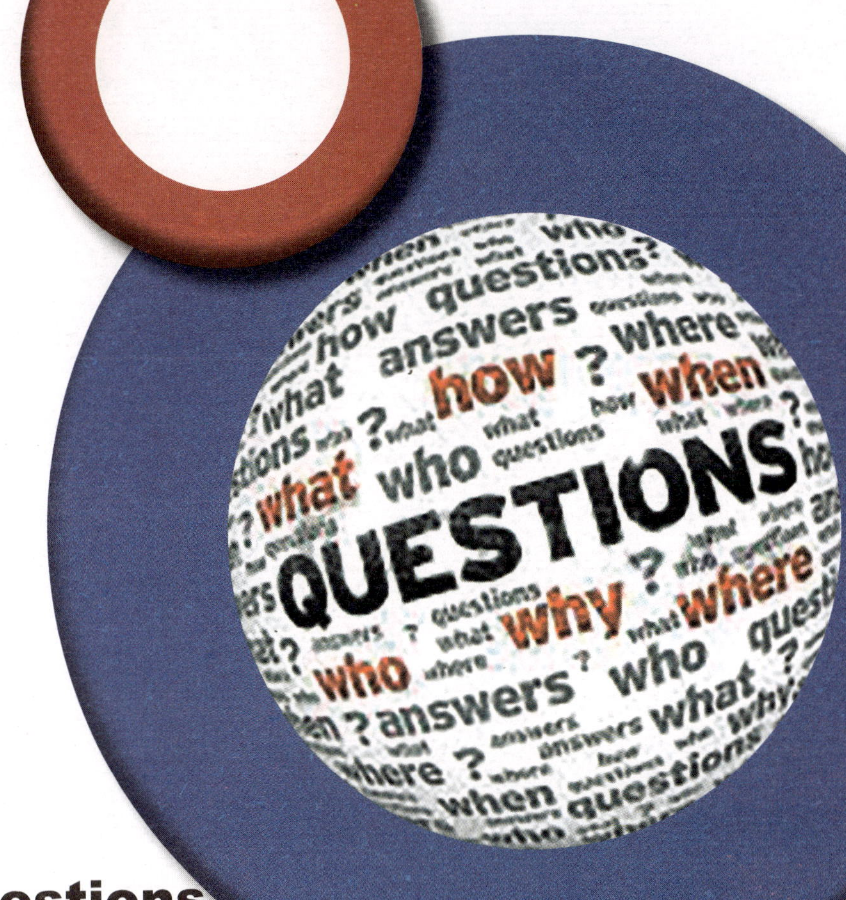

Multiple Choice Questions

Answers & Explanations

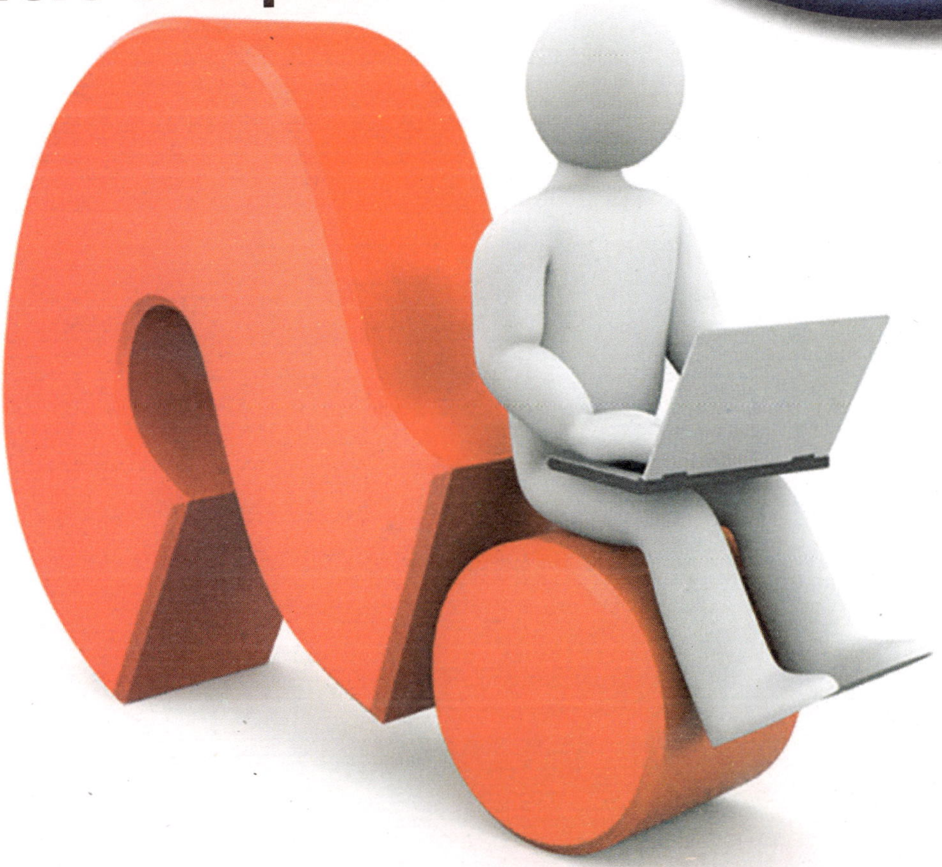

NOVEMBER 2014 MULTIPLE CHOICE QUESTIONS

ANATOMY

1. **Which of the following statement is true about pinna except:**
   a. In Treacher-Collins syndrome malformed pinna may be present
   b. Made up of elastic cartilage
   c. Develop from 1st pharyngeal cleft only
   d. Help in localization of sound
   e. May involves in relapsing perichondritis
2. **Paired laryngeal cartilage (s) is/are:**
   a. Thyroid
   b. Arytenoid
   c. Corniculate
   d. Cricoid
   e. Cuneiform
3. **All are true about mediastinum except:**
   a. Heart passes through superior mediastinum
   b. Heart passes through middle mediastinum
   c. Thymus remnant may present in middle mediastinum
   d. Posterior boundary of posterior mediastinum corresponds to T1-T4 vertebrae
   e. Lower border of anterior mediastinum is extended more than posterior mediastinum
4. **True about medial meniscus:**
   a. Made up of hyaline cartilage
   b. Injury of lateral meniscus is more frequent than medial meniscus
   c. C shaped
   d. Fixed to medial collateral ligament
   e. Inner part is more avsacular
5. **Which of the following statement is/are true about oculomotor nerve:**
   a. Arise from pons
   b. Edinger-Westphal nucleus gives rise to parasympathetic supply of oculomotor nerve
   c. Arise from medulla
   d. Passes through interpeduncular fossa
   e. Related to medial wall of cavernous sinus
6. **Derivative (s) of mesonephric duct includes:**
   a. Some part of prostatic Urethra
   b. Seminal vesicle
   c. Round ligament of uterus
   d. Vas deferens
   e. Ductus deferens
7. **All are true regarding Uterus except:**
   a. Lymph vessels from fundus drain to para-aortic lymph nodes
   b. Broad ligament provides primary support to uterus
   c. Mainly supplied by uterine arteries
   d. Posterior surface is related to intestine

PHYSIOLOGY

8. **Which of the following statement is/are true regarding Fick principle of measurement of cardiac output:**
   a. Cardiac output is calculated by amount of oxygen consumed by whole body per unit mass divided by A-V Oxygen difference across the lung
   b. Oxygen concentration in artery is measured by passing catheter to Pulmonary artery
   c. Mixed venous blood is measured by inserting catheter into pulmonary artery
   d. Rate of oxygen absorption by the lungs is measured by spirometry
   e. For oxygen content of artery, any artery of body can be chosen
9. **Feature (s) of hyperprolactinemia is/are all except:**
   a. Amenorrhoea
   b. Decrease milk production
   c. Galactorrhoea
   d. Hypogonadotropic hypogonadism
   e. Hypothyroidism may cause hyperprolactinemia
10. **True about Oxytocin:**
    a. Secreted from anterior pituitary
    b. Secreted by posterior pituitary
    c. Decapeptide
    d. Gonadotropin releasing hormone (GnRH) stimulate its secretion
    e. Cause milk ejection by contraction of myoepithelium of breast
11. **True statement relating to compliance of lung:**
    a. Increased by surfactant
    b. Decreased in emphysema
    c. At height of inspiration compliance is less
    d. It can be measured by measuring intrapleural pressure at different lung volume
12. **Which of the following is true regarding GLUT-5:**
    a. Present in brain
    b. Present in Adipose tissue, skeletal muscle & skin
    c. Insulin mediated transporter
    d. Sodium independent transport
    e. Present in RBC
13. **True about hormone sensitive lipase:**
    a. Activity is increased by insulin
    b. Found intracellular
    c. Activated by Epinephrine
    d. Located in wall blood capillaries

Answer

1. c. 2. b, c, e. 3. a, c, d, e. 4. c, d, e. 5. b, d. 6. a, b, d, e. 7. b.
8. a, c, d, e. 9. b. 10. b, e. 11. a, c, d. 12. d. 13. b, c.

14. Which of the following is/are Pain scale:
a. McGill Pain Questionnaire
b. Visual analogue scale
c. Coloured Analogue Scale

BIOCHEMISTRY

15. True statement regarding Lactate dehydrogenase deficiency:
a. Fumarate level increases
b. Exercise intolerance
c. Muscle cramps may occur
d. It operate in anaerobic condition
e. It is key enzyme of Kreb cycle

16. Hyaluronic acid is composed of:
a. N-acetyl glucosamine
b. N-acetyl galactosamine
c. Glucuronic acid
d. N-acetylneuramic acid
e. Iduronic acid

17. All are feature of Refsum disease except:
a. Deficiency of α-hydroxylase
b. Defect in β oxidation
c. Accumulation of phytanic acid
d. Peripheral neuropathy
e. Treated by removing phytanic acid precursors from diet

18. Which of the following enzyme (s) participate in protein synthesis:
a. DNA ligase
b. DNA Helicase
c. Peptidase
d. Peptidyl transferase
e. DNA polymerase

19. True about peptide bond formation:
a. The NH2 group of new aminoacyl t -RNA at 'A' site combine with the – COOH group of Met-t -RNA occupying the 'P' site
b. The NH2 group of new aminoacyl t – RNA at 'P' site combine with the – COOH group of Met-t-RNA occupying the 'A' site
c. Reaction is catalyzed by peptidyl transferase
d. Peptide bond formation require energy

20. All are true regarding Urea cycle except:
a. Urea formed from ammonia
b. Rate limiting enzyme is ornithine transcarbamoylase
c. Require Energy expenditure
d. Malate is byproduct of urea cycle
e. One nitrogen of urea comes from for aspartate

21. Which of the following is true regarding phenylketonuria:
a. Dietary phenylalanine restriction is used in treatment
b. Occur due to deficiency of Phenylalanine hydroxylase enzyme
c. Occur due to increase activity of phenylalanine hydroxylase enzyme
d. Tyrosine must be supplied in diet
e. Diet should contain high phenylalanine containing food items

22. In Benedict test, red colour is/are produced by:
a. Sucrose
b. Inositol
c. Fructose
d. Lactose
e. Maltose

23. True statements are:
a. Vitamin A in dose 20, 000 unit may be used during lactation to prevent Vit A deficiency to infants
b. High dose of Vitamin C may cause renal stone
c. Vitamin E reduces risk of atherosclerosis
d. Folic acid deficiency cause microcytic anaemia
e. Banana is a rich source of Vit. B6

24. Thiamine act as co-enzyme for:
a. Transketolase
b. Pyruvate dehydrogenase
c. Alcohol dehydrogenase
d. Transaminase

25. Thiamine deficiency cause (s):
a. Glossitis
b. Polyneuropathy
c. Pellagra
d. Angular stomatitis
e. Cardiomegaly

26. Feature (s) of Korsakoff psychosis:
a. Confabulation
b. Retrograde amnesia
c. Ophthalmoplegia
d. Delirium

27. Glycogen storage disorder (s) is/are:
a. Niemann-Pick disease
b. Gaucher disease
c. Tay-Sachs Disease
d. Pompe's disease
e. McArdles disease

IMMUNOGENETICS & MOLECULAR BIOLOGY

28. True about DNA hyperchromatism:
a. It is increase of absorbance
b. Measured by absorbance at 260 nm (in a spectrophotometer)
c. It occurs when the DNA duplex is denatured
d. Double stranded DNA is more hyperchromic than ssDNA

29. All are true about DNA methylation except:
a. It usually occurs in the cytosine
b. Can alters the gene expression pattern in cells
c. Role in genomic imprinting
d. No role in carcinogenesis
e. Essential for normal development

30. All are true regarding epigenetics mechanism except:
a. Non-heritable
b. Acetylation of Histone
c. Hereditary
d. Methylation of DNA
e. X chromosome inactivation

Answer

14. All	15. b, c, d.	16. a, c.	17. b.	18. d.	19. a, c.	20. b, d.
21. a, b, d.	22. c, d, e.	23. a, b, c, e.	24. a, b.	25. b, e.	26. a, b, c.	27. d, e.
28. a, b, c.	29. d.	30. a.				

31. **Which of the following is true regarding DNA double-strand breaks repair pathway:**
    a. Homologous recombination require a long homologous sequence to guide repair
    b. Non-homologous end-joining does not require a long homologous sequence to guide repair
    c. Homologous recombination repairs DNA before the cell enters mitosis
    d. Non-homologous end-joining repairs DNA before the cell enters mitosis
    e. Non-homologous end joining is prominent DSB repair mechanism in mammals
32. **Group of alleles that are closely linked together at a genomic locus & inherited together as a cluster is/are:**
    a. Idiotype
    b. Haplotype
    c. Genotype
    d. Phenotype
33. **The size of Microsatellite repeat sequence is:**
    a. <1 kb
    b. 2-6 bp
    c. 1-3 kb
    d. >3 kb
    e. 5-20 bp

PATHOLOGY

34. **Feature of Von Hippel Lindau syndrome:**
    a. Mutation in chromosome 13
    b. Mutation in chromosome 3
    c. Pancreatic cyst
    d. Cerebellar hemangioblastoma
35. **All are the feature (s) of Hermansky-pudlak syndrome except:**
    a. Autosomal dominant inheritance
    b. Oculocutaneous albinism
    c. Bleeding disorder
    d. Pulmonary fibrosis
36. **Difference between active & resting cell depend on which phase of cell cycle:**
    a. G0
    b. G1
    c. G2
    d. M
    e. S
37. **Not feature (s) of apoptosis:**
    a. Mediated by Caspases
    b. Inhibition of Endonuclease activity
    c. Membrane bleb are seen
    d. Chromatin condensation
    e. Association with inflammation
38. **All are true about Mitochondrial DNA except:**
    a. Contains 37 gene
    b. Transmit from mother to offsprings
    c. Transmit in classical mendelian fashion
    d. Cause Leber hereditary optic neuropathy
39. **True about Intravascular hemolysis:**
    a. Increased serum haptoglobin
    b. Increase Stercobilin in urine
    c. Increase plasma myoglobin
    d. Increased fecal excretion of urobilin
    e. Hemosiderinuria
40. **Cause (s) of conjugated hyperbilirubinemia:**
    a. Crigler–Najjar syndrome
    b. Hemochromatosis
    c. Large hematoma
    d. Gilbert syndrome
    e. Rotor's syndrome
41. **Feature (s) of Rheumatic heart disease is/are:**
    a. Endocarditis
    b. Constructive pericarditis
    c. Most commonly involve tricuspid valve
    d. Bread butter pericarditis
    e. Pancarditis
42. **Cystic fibrosis is/are associated with:**
    a. Pectus excavatum
    b. Aniridia
    c. Mucous plug syndrome
    d. Decrease sodium content in sweet
    e. Steatorrhoea
43. **Percutaneous liver biopsy is/are contraindicated in:**
    a. Ascites
    b. Hemangioma of liver
    c. Platelet count <60000/μl
    d. Hepatic metastasis
    e. Echinococcus cyst in liver
44. **True about Alcoholic cirrhosis:**
    a. Predominantly macronodular pattern
    b. Bile duct proliferation
    c. Mallory body hardly seen
    d. Disturbed normal architecture
45. **All are true about Lesch-Nyhan syndrome except:**
    a. Hyperuricemia
    b. Mental retardation
    c. Stone production
    d. Occur equally in both sexes
    e. X-linked
46. **Marker (s) of Langerhans cell histiocytosis:**
    a. CD1a
    b. S 100
    c. CD 3
    d. CD 5
    e. CD 30
47. **Breast cancer is/are associated with:**
    a. Familial adenomatous polyposis
    b. Ataxia-telangiectasia
    c. Peutz-Jeghers syndrome
    d. Cowden disease
    e. Von Hippel Lindau syndrome

Answer

31. a, b, c, e.	32. b.	33. b.	34. b, c, d.	35. a.	36. a.	37. b, e.
38. c.	39. d, e.	40. e.	41. a, d, e.	42. c, e.	43. a, b, c, e.	44. b, c, d.
45. d.	46. a, b.	47. b, c, d.				

48. Hyperglycemia is/are associated with:
a. Cushing disease
b. Addison disease
c. Pheochromocytoma
d. Hyperthyroidism
e. Acromegaly

49. Hypercalcemia in malignancy is/are caused by:
a. Small cell carcinoma of lung
b. Ovarian carcinoma
c. Breast carcinoma
d. Renal carcinoma
e. Osteosarcoma

50. Calcium level is increased in:
a. Parathyroid adenoma
b. Thiazide diuretics
c. Chronic renal failure
d. Hypervitaminosis D

51. Cause (s) of megaloblastic anaemia include:
a. Anticonvulsant drugs
b. Pregnancy
c. Resection of ileum
d. Gastrectomy
e. Crohn's disease

52. Feature (s) of fibroadenoma of breast include:
a. Clearly defined edge on palpation
b. Hormone responsive tumor
c. Contain both epithelial & stromal elements
d. Well-encapsulated
e. Common after menopause

53. True about Neutrophil:
a. Engulf bacteria
b. Multilobed
c. Neutrophil granules are slightly basic and stain weakly with the azurophilic component of Romanowsky stains
d. Neutrophilia occur in acute bacterial infection
e. Primary granules is also called specific granules

54. All are true about Histamine except:
a. Secreted by macrophage
b. Vasoconstriction of arterioles
c. Smooth muscle contraction
d. Mediate inflammation

55. Which of the following statement (s) is/are true:
a. In Robertsonian translocation the breaks occur close to the centromeres of each chromosome
b. Aneuploidy is abnormal chromosome number caused by either gain or loss of chromosome
c. Comparative genomic hybridisation (CGH) is a technique that permits the detection of chromosomal copy number
d. Haploid is normal number & composition of chromosome

56. All of the the following statement (s) is/are true except:
a. Denver group F-contain X chromosome
b. Denver group C-contain X chromosome
c. Denver group G-contain acrocentric chromosome
d. Bar body is inactive X chromosome
e. In normal females generally one of the chromosomes undergoes X inactivation in somatic cells

PHARMACOLOGY

57. Fomepizole can be used in:
a. Methanol poisoning
b. Organophosphorus poisoning
c. Ethylene glycol poisoning
d. Barbiturate poisoning

58. Which of the following drug interact with Warfarin:
a. ACE inhibitor
b. Azithromycin
c. Fluconazole
d. Aspirin
e. Benzodiazepine

59. All of the following is true about hydroxyurea except:
a. Cause myelosuppression
b. Oral bioavailability is very less
c. Used in CML
d. Act as radiosensitizer
e. Used in sickle cell anaemia

60. All are true about hydrochlorothiazide except:
a. Cause hyperglycemia
b. Inhibit Na-Cl symport
c. Increases calcium excretion in urine
d. Cause hyperuricaemia
e. Used in treatment of renal stone

61. ATT drug with significant renal excretion is/are:
a. INH
b. Rifampicin
c. Pyrazinamide
d. Amikacin
e. Streptomycin

62. Which of the following statement about proton pump inhibitors is/are true except:
a. Hit & run drug
b. Acidic medium is essential for activity
c. Act on H+/K+ ATPase
d. Forms an integral component of anti-H.pylori regimens
e. Act best in alkaline medium

63. True about amphotericin B:
a. Liposomal preparation is available
b. Orally absorbed
c. Used only in intravenous form
d. Protein synthesis inhibitor

64. Antibiotic which acts through cell wall inhibition:
a. Penicillin
b. Daptomycin
c. Aminoglycoside
d. Cephalosporin
e. Imipenam

65. Which of following statement is true about canagliflozin:
a. SGLT-2 inhibitor
b. Blocks Na/glucose symport..
c. Causes glycosuria & polyuria
d. Increases chance of vaginal infections

Answer

48. a, b, c, d, e.	49. b, c, d.	50. All	51. All	52. a, b, c, d.	53. a, b, c, d.	54. a, b.
55. a, b, c.	56. a.	57. a, c.	58. c, d.	59. b.	60. c.	61. a, c, d, e.
62. e.	63. a.	64. a, d.	65. a, c, d.			

66. Which of following is/are true about metformin:
a. Cause lactic acid
b. PPAR γ agonist
c. Contraindicated in Renal failure
d. Cause hypoglycemia
e. GI disturbances are common side effect

67. Peripheral neuropathy is/are caused by:
a. Vincristine
b. Sulfonamide
c. Amiodarone
d. Paclitaxel

68. Common action (s) of epinephrine & norepinephrine includes:
a. Skin vasodilation
b. Bronchial muscle contraction
c. Increase systolic BP
d. Increase HR
e. Renal vasoconstriction

69. Valid drug combinations are:
a. Sulfamethoxazole +trimethoprim
b. Penicillin + Tetracycline/chloramphenicol: Pneumococci
c. Piperacillin-Tazobactam
d. Enalapril-Hydrochlorothiazide
e. Ibuprofen & serratiopeptidase

70. A Patient presented in emergency room with severe malaria. He was given artusunate at 0 hr, 12 hr, 24 hr & then once a day till 3 day. Which of the following statement (s) is/are correct regarding further management of the patient:
a. Patient may later switched to oral drug if patient able to tolerate
b. Dextrose drip should be started
c. Artesunate should never be given singly
d. Steroid is beneficial

71. Which of the following is/are true regarding plasma concentration time curve of a drug:
a. Peak concentration determine bioavailability
b. Intramuscular administration have curve different from oral administration
c. Area under curve determine therapeutic response
d. Bioavailability of an orally administered drug can be calculated by comparing the area under curve after oral & after I.V. administration
e. Changes in the rate of absorption and extent of bioavailability can influence both the duration of action and the effectiveness of the same total dose of a drug administered in different formulations

72. Not indicated for anaerobic colitis treatment:
a. Metronidazole
b. Aminoglycoside
c. Amikacin
d. Piperacillin-tazobactam
e. Imipenem

MICROBIOLOGY

73. True about Ebola virus:
a. Belongs to family filoviridae
b. Transmission may occur from dead bodies
c. Transmitted by sexual contact
d. Incubation period is less than 48 hr
e. Contains single-stranded RNA

74. All are true about Toxoplasma infection except:
a. May occur due to ingestion of oocyst from cat's faeces
b. May spread by organ transplantation
c. Toxoplasmosis is usually symptomatic in immunocompetent person
d. Infection is severe & progressive in immunocompromised host
e. Human infection is dead end for parasite

75. Which of the following disease (s) is/are not toxin mediated:
a. Diphtheria
b. Tetanus
c. Pertussis
d. Anthrax
e. Syphilis

76. Commonly used stain (s) for identifying fungus include (s):
a. Periodic acid-Schiff (PAS) stain
b. Von Kossa stain
c. Muramine silver stain
d. Gomori's methenamine silver
e. Giemsa stain

77. Non-treponemal test includes:
a. RPR
b. VDRL
c. FTA-ABS
d. TPHA
e. TPI

78. Which of following Culture media combination is/are true except:
a. Thayer-Martin media: Gonorrhoea
b. Chocolate agar-: enriched media
c. Lowenstein-Jensen Medium: Mycobacterium tuberculosis
d. Muller-Hinton agar: Corynebacterium diphtheriae
e. Mac Conkey's agar: Non lactose fermenters form colourless colonies

79. All of the following are true regarding legionella except:
a. Cause Pontiac fever
b. Aerobic gram negative bacilli
c. Can grow on simple medium
d. Grow on BCYE agar
e. Communicable from infected patients to others

80. All are true about gonorrhea except:
a. Gonorrhoea means flow of seed
b. Discharge may contain neutrophil
c. Initially discharge is scanty & mucoid in urethritis
d. Caused by gram positive cocci
e. Symptom is more severe in female than males

Answer

66. a, c, e. 67. a, c, d. 68. c, e. 69. a, c, d, e. 70. a, b, c. 71. b, d, e. 72. b.
73. a, b, c, e. 74. c. 75. e. 76. a, d. 77. a, b. 78. d. 79. c, e.
80. d, e.

81. All are true about H.pylori except:
a. Spiral rod in shape & flagellated
b. Gram –ve bacillus
c. Urease activity is essential for colonization in gastric mucosa
d. Grow under microaerophilic conditions
e. Culture of endoscopic biopsy material is gold standard

82. All statements are true about mycetoma except:
a. Eumycetoma is caused by bacteria
b. Surgery is important component of treatment
c. Usually painless
d. Diagnosis can be made by examination of lesion
e. Can affect lower & upper extremities

83. Stain used for mycobacterium:
a. Ziehl-Neelsen stain
b. Kinyoun stain
c. Auramine -rhodamine
d. Gomori methenamine silver stain

84. True about non-industrial anthrax:
a. May occur in butcher
b. Animal hair is a source of infection
c. Commonly occurs in factory worker
d. Stomoxys calcitrans insect may transmit the infection
e. It is a zoonosis

85. Zoonotic diseases are all except:
a. Leptospirosis
b. Guinea worm
c. Rabies
d. Plague
e. Japanense encephalitis

86. All of the following is/are true regarding candidiasis:
a. Commonly involve mucosa & skin
b. Not involve nails
c. Caused by yeast like fungus
d. Diabetes is most important risk factor
e. Causes meningitis in immunocompromised persons

87. Feature (s) of Taenia capitis is/are all except:
a. May presents as a boggy swelling
b. Most commonly occurs in elderly
c. May present as black dot
d. Caused by trichophyton & microsporum but not by epidermophyton
e. Scutulum formation

88. Which of the following is/are true about pasteurerlla multiocuda:
a. May cause meningitis
b. Transmitted by unpasteurized milk
c. Cause disease exclusively in human
d. Gram-negative coccobacillus

89. Which of the following has incubation period of < 5 day:
a. Salmonella typhi
b. Vibrio parahaemolyticus
c. Campylobacter jejuni
d. Shigella dyseneteriae
e. Yersinia pestis

90. Verruga peruana is caused by:
a. B. Bacilliformis
b. B.Henselae
c. B.Quintana
d. B.Elizabethae
e. B. Grahamil

91. Which of the following statement is/are true about Staphylococcus aureus:
a. Contains nuc gene
b. Causes community acquired pneumonia
c. Expression of methicillin resistance increases when it is incubated at 37°C on blood agar
d. Coagulase enzyme is a virulence factor
e. Causes food poisoning

FORENSIC MEDICINE

92. Gun shot injury may cause (s):
a. Abrasion collar
b. Gutter fracture
c. Rail track injury
d. Incised like injury
e. Lacerated like injury

93. Not characteristics of poisonous snake:
a. Small scales on head
b. Large scales on belly & cover entire breadth
c. Short & solid fangs
d. Compressed tail
e. Usually nocturnal in habit

94. Which of the following is not component of typical embalaming agent:
a. Na citrate
b. Na borate
c. Formaldehyde
d. Glycerine

95. True about Pugilistic attitude:
a. Flexion of hip & knee
b. Occur due to coagulation of protein by burning
c. Extension of elbow
d. Flexion of fingers

96. Which of the following can be ground for divorce:
a. Sterile female
b. Impotent man
c. Diabetes
d. Premature ejaculation
e. Pre-existing incurable mental disorder

97. Not true regarding Voyeurism:
a. S. 354C, IPC define punishment
b. For first offence imprisonment of 1-3 year with fine
c. For repeat offence imprisonment may extend to 5-10 year
d. Cognizable offence
e. Repeat offence is considered as non-bailable offence

Answer

81. e.	82. a.	83. a, b, c.	84. a, b, d, e.	85. b.	86. b.	87. b.
88. a, d.	89. b, c, d.e.	90. a.	91. a, b, d, e.	92. a, b, d, e.	93. c.	94. None
95. a, b, d.	96. b, e.	97. c.				

PSM

98. Which of the following viral exanthema combination is/are correct except:
- a. Varicella-no relation of rash with fever
- b. Rubella-palatal petechiae may occur
- c. Roseola -rash appear after fever subsides
- d. Measles-rash occurs behind the ears along hair line
- e. Chickenpox-pleomorphic rashes occur

99. Which of the following act is/are passed after independence:
- a. ESI act
- b. Factory act
- c. MTP act
- d. Epidemic disease act
- e. SARDA act

100. Which of the following is/are true about leprosy:
- a. Positive skin smear at any site is considered multibacillary leprosy
- b. Grenz zone is seen in lepromatous spectrum
- c. It is eradicated from India in 2000
- d. 12 month of MDT is recommended for multibacillary leprosy
- e. Multidrug therapy is given

101. Which of the following is/are features of septic tank:
- a. Minimum capacity should be 500 gallons
- b. Water tight seal
- c. Recommended for large communities
- d. Seeded with ripe sludge drawn from another septic tank
- e. Anaerobic process takes place

102. True about Standard deviation:
- a. 1 SD covers 95% population
- b. Normal standard deviate deviation from the mean in a normal distribution
- c. Represent measurement of dispersions
- d. It is better indicator of variability than range

103. Wild polio is still endemic in:
- a. India
- b. Pakistan
- c. Afghanistan
- d. Bangladesh
- e. Nigeria

104. True about census in India:
- a. First census conducted in 1851
- b. Director General of Health Services of India (DGHS) is supreme officer for conducting census
- c. Literacy rate is also included in census
- d. Conducted in accordance to Census act, 1948
- e. Conducted in Mid year

105. Which of the following carcinoma is caused by asbestos:
- a. Mesothelioma
- b. Bronchial carcinoma
- c. Laryngeal carcinoma
- d. Breast cancer

OPHTHALMOLOGY

106. Lateral wall of orbit is/are formed by:
- a. Lesser wing of sphenoid
- b. Frontal process of zygomatic bone
- c. Greater wing of sphenoid
- d. Lacrimal bone
- e. Maxilla

107. True about Leber optic neuropathy:
- a. X-linked disease
- b. Primarily affects male
- c. Disc become pale & atrophic
- d. Transmitted from mother to child
- e. Mitochondrial inheritance

108. Risk factor for cystoid macular edema include (s) all except:
- a. Hypertensive retinopathy
- b. Vitreous loss
- c. Diabetes mellitus
- d. Cataract surgery is an important cause
- e. Lower incidence with intracapsular cataract extraction than extracapsular cataract extraction

109. All are true regarding congenital ptosis except:
- a. Levator palpebrae superioris dystrophy may present
- b. Associated with diplopia
- c. Lid crease is decreased
- d. Amblyopia can occur

110. Feature (s) of Infantile glaucoma is/are except:
- a. Aniridia may be associated
- b. Treatment includes trabeculotomy
- c. Buphthalmos can occur
- d. Cornea is thin & clear
- e. May be associated with Sturge-weber syndrome

111. True about Arcus senilis:
- a. Fatty infiltration
- b. Axial corneal degeneration
- c. Deposition occur in stroma of peripheral cornea
- d. Amyloid deposit
- e. Involve limbus

112. True about moderate flare uveitis:
- a. Categorised as grade 1+
- b. Categorised as grade 2+
- c. Categorised as grade 3+
- d. Hazy cornea
- e. Clear iris detail

113. Not true about Ectopia lentis in marfan syndrome:
- a. Inferior nasal displacement of lens
- b. Lens is displaced down and outward
- c. Lens displaced upwards and temporally
- d. Anterior dislocation of the lens into the pupil or anterior chamber may cause pupillary block with acute glaucoma
- e. Posterior dislocation can cause harmful vitreous traction on the retina

Answer

98. a. | 99. a, b, c. | 100. a, b, d, e. | 101. a, b, d, e. | 102. b, c, d. | 103. b, c, e. | 104. c, d.
105. a, b, c. | 106. b, c. | 107. b, c, d, e. | 108. e. | 109. b. | 110. d. | 111. a, c.
112. b, e. | 113. a, b.

ENT

114. True about croup:
a. Caused by H.influenzae
b. X-ray PA view shows steeple sign of subglottic narrowing
c. Stridor is present
d. Supraglottic edema is present
e. Commonly present in 6 month-3 year age group

115. True about Mobius syndrome:
a. 10th CN involvement
b. 7th CN involvement
c. Abduction defect
d. Esotropia
e. 6th CN involvement

116. All are true about nasopharyngeal fibroma except:
a. Most common age of presentation is 20-50 yr
b. Radioresistant tumour
c. Highly vascular
d. Benign in nature
e. Surgery is treatment of choice

117. Which of the following feature (s) of rhinoscleroma is/are true except:
a. Atrophy of nasal mucosa
b. Caused by fungus
c. Treatment by antifungal drug
d. Caused by bacteria
e. Causative organism may be cultured from biopsy material

118. True about choanal atresia:
a. Unilateral atresia should be operated within 6 month of age
b. Occur d/t persistence of bucconasal membrane
c. B/l atresia usually presents with respiratory difficulties
d. Bilateral atresia may cause cyanosis
e. Diagnosed by failure to pass a catheter from nose to pharynx

119. Which of the following is true regarding mandibular fracture:
a. Inferior alveolar nerve damage may occur
b. Panorex radiograph is very helpful in management
c. Ramus is the most common site of fracture
d. Condylar fracture heals spontaneously & require no active intervention
e. Condylar fracture is most common site

120. Complication of modified radical mastoidectomy include (s):
a. Conductive hearing loss
b. Facial nerve injury
c. Change in taste sensation
d. Sensory hearing loss

121. True about Ethmoidal sinus:
a. Fully developed by 25 yr
b. Consists of 3-18 sinus on each side
c. Absent at birth
d. Lamina papyracea separate from orbit
e. Anterior ethmoidal group cells-open into superior meatus

122. Which of the following statement (s) is/are true about labyrinthitis:
a. Initially quick component of nystagmus occur toward diseased ear but in later stage shift toward healthy ear
b. May occur as a complication of chronic suppurative otitis media
c. Resolve spontaneously in 1-6 wk
d. Medical treatment alone is sufficient
e. Vertigo may be present

123. Which of the following is not self retaining retractor:
a. Mollison's mastoid retractor
b. Jansen's mastoid retractor
c. Lempert's endaural retractor
d. Davis Retractor

MEDICINE

124. Feature (s) of ↑ICT include:
a. Constricted pupil
b. Tachycardia
c. Bradycardia
d. Hypertension
e. Respiratory depression

125. Which of the following is/are true regarding Asthma & COPD:
a. COPD shows less reversibility to bronchodilators while asthma shows significant improvement
b. Asthma has a gradual progression of dyspnea on exertion, punctuated by acute exacerbations of shortness of breath. while most COPD patients have normal breathing the majority of the time
c. COPD patients may have acute exacerbations while asthmatic patients have recurrent episode
d. Steroid therapy is more beneficial to asthma patients than COPD patients
e. Neutrophils have primary a role in pathogenesis of asthma & eosinophils have primary role in COPD

126. Which of the following is/are true about Subarachnoid Hemorrhage (SAH):
a. Saccular aneurysm is most common cause of SAH after head trauma
b. Severe headache may present
c. CT angiography help in localizing aneurysm
d. CT scan is investigation of choice for acute SAH
e. Digital subtraction angiography is better than CT angiography for SAH

127. All are true about Granulomatosis with Polyangitis except:
a. Kidney involvement
b. Lung involvement
c. Mainly involve small & medium sized vessel
d. Good prognosis
e. More common in female

Answer

114. a, b, c, e.	115. b, c, d, e.	116. a, b.	117. b, c.	118. b, c, d, e.	119. a, b, e.	120. All
121. b, d.	122. a, b, e.	123. d.	124. c, d, e.	125. a, c, d.	126. a, b, c, d.	127. c, d, e.

128. All are true regarding renal artery stenosis except:
- a. Most common cause is atherosclerosis
- b. Arterioles in the involved kidney shows more significant arteriolosclerosis than uninvolved kidney
- c. Fibromuscular dysplasia is common in young women
- d. Involved kidney may become contracted
- e. Show elevated plasma rennin level

129. ECG change (s) in pulmonary embolism may includes:
- a. ST elevation in V1 & aVR
- b. T wave inversion in V1 to V4
- c. S1Q3T3 pattern
- d. Left axis deviation
- e. Right bundle branch block

130. A patient has short h/o increased jugular venous pressure, weak peripheral pulse & low B.P. Likely condition (s) may be:
- a. Tension pneumothorax
- b. Venous gas embolism
- c. Pulmonary embolism
- d. Cardiac temponade
- e. Septic shock

131. All are true about insulinoma except:
- a. Symptomatic hypoglycemia may be present
- b. Most common endocrine tumor of pancreas
- c. Associated with MEN 2
- d. Benign lesion with no malignant potential
- e. More common in head of pancreas

132. Which of the following is true regarding pseudobulbar palsy:
- a. Dysphagia
- b. Jaw jerk brisk
- c. Absent gag reflex
- d. Tongue fasciculation present
- e. Plantar reflex is extensor

133. A patient presented with high pH, low arterial CO2 & low plasma HCO3-level. Which of the following statement is true regarding the presentation & various causes:
- a. Compensated respiratory alkalosis
- b. Chronic renal failure
- c. Persistent vomiting
- d. Cerebro-vascular accident
- e. Hepatic failure

134. Which of the following is true about treatment of asthma:
- a. Long acting β2 agonist for acute attack
- b. Long acting β2 agonist for long term treatment
- c. Short acting β2 agonist for acute attack
- d. I.V Steroid for severe asthma exacerbation
- e. Inhaled steroid for persistent asthma

135. Side-effect (s) of inhalational steroid is/are all except:
- a. Adrenal suppression
- b. Cataract
- c. Osteoporosis
- d. Hypoglycemia
- e. Skin thinning

136. All are true about true about syncope except:
- a. Consciousness is lost
- b. More common in standing than lying postion
- c. Vasovagal type is common
- d. Return of consciousness is slow & take hours
- e. Short duration

137. Feature (s) of factor VIII deficiency:
- a. X linked recessive inheritance
- b. ↑Clotting time
- c. ↑Bleeding time
- d. Intrinsic pathway affected
- e. ↑aPTT

138. Unequal pulse in upper & lower extremities (i.e., radio-femoral delay) is/are seen in:
- a. Aortic dissection
- b. Post-ductal coarctation of aorta
- c. Supra-valvular Aortic stenosis
- d. Sub-valvular Aortic stenosis
- e. Takayasu's syndrome

139. Drug (s) given in thyroid crisis:
- a. Esmolol
- b. Iodine
- c. Hydrocortisone
- d. Aspirin
- e. Propylthiouracil

140. Which of the following dyads of disease-neurotransmitter is correct:
- a. Myasthenia gravis-Acetylcholine receptor
- b. Spasticity-GABA
- c. Lambert-Eaton myasthenic syndrome –Acetylcholine
- d. Stiff-person syndrome-Glycine
- e. Parkinson's disease –Dopamine

141. All are true about Menetrier's disease except:
- a. Increased gastric acid secretion
- b. Protein-losing gastropathy
- c. Mainly affects body & fundus
- d. No malignant potential
- e. Transforming growth factor-α is overexpressed

142. According to Surviving Sepsis Guidelines 2013, which of the following is/are correct regarding sepsis & septic shock treatment guideline:
- a. Urine output should be > 2ml/kg
- b. Mean arterial pressure goal should be ≥ 65 mm Hg
- c. Dopamine as the first choice vasopressor
- d. Colloid is initial fluid of choice in the resuscitation
- e. Administration of effective intravenous antimicrobials within the first hour of recognition

143. Brain death can be assessed by:
- a. Apnoea test
- b. CT scan
- c. MRI scan
- d. Cerebral angiography
- e. Transcranial Doppler

Answer

128. b.	129. a, b, c, e.	130. a, b, c, d.	131. c, d, e.	132. a, b, e.	133. a, d, e.	134. b, c, d, e.
135. d.	136. d.	137 a, b, d, e.	138. b.	139. a, b, c, e.	140. a, c, e.	141. d.
142. b, e.	143. a, d, e.					

144. Presentation (s) of Bechet syndrome may include:
- a. Erosive arthritis
- b. Recurrent aphthous ulcers of the mouth
- c. Uveitis
- d. Genital ulcer
- e. Pathergy test

145. All are true about pheochromocytoma except:
- a. 90% malignant
- b. Surgery is definitive treatment
- c. Highly vascular
- d. Needle biopsy should be avoided
- e. Increased urinary excretion of metanephrines

146. MIBG (metaiodobenzyl guanithidine) is analogue to:
- a. Epinephrine
- b. Adenine
- c. Norepinephrine
- d. Guanine
- e. Phenylephrine

147. Which of the following is true regarding adrenocortical carcinomas:
- a. Increased urinary excretion of VMA
- b. Does not cause metastasis
- c. Surgery is mainstay treatment
- d. Associated with Li-Fraumeni syndrome

148. A 40 year old lady from Himachal Pradesh has fever & eschar on body. Blood investigation revealed: Hb=12 gm%, TLC=9800/μl, Platelet 80000. Which of the following drug (s) may be used in her treatment:
- a. Oral Doxycycline
- b. Meropenem
- c. Azithromycin
- d. Tetracycline
- e. Chloramphenicol

149. All are true about "a" wave except:
- a. It is often the largest positive wave visible
- b. Giant wave in atrial fibrillation
- c. Tricuspid stenosis produces gaint wave
- d. Heart block diminish magnitude of a wave
- e. Produced by right atrial contraction

150. Which of the condition cause pericarditis due to hypersensitivity:
- a. SLE
- b. Rheumatic fever
- c. Dressler syndrome
- d. Uraemia
- e. Myxedema

151. All are true about acute radiation pneumonitis except:
- a. Fever not present
- b. Steroid is beneficial
- c. X-ray chest finding correlates poorly with symptom
- d. Develop immediately after radiotherapy

152. True about Kallman syndrome:
- a. Amenorrhoea
- b. Hypergonadotrophic state
- c. Anosmia
- d. Failure of secondary sexual development

SURGERY

153. Glasgow coma scale E3M4V5 represents:
- a. Spontaneous eye opening
- b. Eye opening with pain stimulus
- c. Incomprehensible sound
- d. Oriented conversation
- e. Decorticate posturing

154. Complication (s) of Salivary gland operation:
- a. Subcutaneous fistula
- b. Opposite gland compensatory hypertrophy
- c. Gustatory sweating
- d. Facial Nerve damage

155. Punched out ulcer is/are seen in:
- a. Arterial ulcer
- b. Venous ulcer
- c. Tubercular ulcer
- d. Basal cell carcinoma
- e. Gummatous ulcer

156. Which of the following is/are true regarding renal transplanatation except:
- a. Curvilinear incision is made in lower quadrant
- b. Transplanted kidney is placed in retroperitoneal position
- c. Recipients kidney is first removed from renal fossa to make space for donor kidney
- d. Anastomosis of external iliac artery with renal artery
- e. Donor renal vein is anastomosed with external iliac vein

157. Which of the following plan of management is/are correct with regard to Cleft lip & cleft palate in children:
- a. Unilateral lip only-1 year of age
- b. Bilateral lip-1 year of age
- c. Bilateral lip should be repaired at 5 month
- d. Both soft & hard palate at 1 year in one setting
- e. Cleft lip and soft palate at 5–6 months & hard palate at 15-18 months of age

158. Suture number 2-0 corresponds to diameter of:
- a. 0.21 mm
- b. 0.24 mm
- c. 0.27mm
- d. 0.30 mm
- e. 0.33 mm

159. Which of the following is/are correct regarding eczema of breast & Paget's disease of nipple:
- a. Generally eczema is unilateral whereas paget's disease is bilateral
- b. Eczema may be associated with lactation
- c. Nipple may be destroyed in Paget's disease while it normally intact in eczema
- d. Inversion of nipple may occur in Paget's disease
- e. Associated with breast lump in eczema

Answer

144. b, c, d, e	145. a.	146. c.	147. c, d.	148. a, c, d, e.	149. b, d.	150. a, b, c.
151. a, d.	152. a, c, d.	153. d.	154. a, c, d.	155. a, e.	156. c.	157. c, e.
158. d.	159. b, c, d.					

160. Correct combination (s) of Hernia with their content:

a. Littre hernia: Meckle's diverticulum
b. Richter's hernial-small intestine
c. Pantaloon-hernial sac on either side of inferior gastric artery
d. Hernia-en-glissade-urinary bladder
e. Maydl's hernia-intestine

161. Which of the following is true about esophagus except:

a. Serosa not present
b. Middle & lower third made up of striated muscle
c. Lower oesophageal sphincter is a zone of relatively high pressure
d. In achalasia cardia LOS tone is increased so that food can not pass below
e. It has side to side & anteroposterior curvatures

162. Which of the following is true about rectal prolapse:

a. Submucous type is more common in adult
b. Submucous type is more common in children
c. Prolapse is often full thickness in adult
d. Operation is generally required in complete prolapse

163. True about Hypospadias:

a. Glandular & coronal variety is most common
b. Circumcision should be avoided
c. In distal type chordee frequently occurs
d. Curvature of penis is normal in all types
e. More proximal hypospadias is corrected for mainly cosmetic reasons

164. All are true about BPH except:

a. Submucosal gland hyperplasia in transition zone
b. Penile uretha elongation
c. Prostatic urethra may be compressed
d. Less than 20ml/second peak flow rate is strong indication for TURP
e. BPH occur due to growth in peripheral zone of prostate

165. True statement (s) about laproscopic cholecystectomy:

a. Cosmetically better
b. Bleeding is more common in open cholecystectomy than laproscopic cholecystectomy
c. Veress needle is used in closed technique
d. Laparoscope with attached video camera is inserted through umbilical port
e. Previous abdominal surgery is absolute contraindication

166. Which of the following is true about digital rectal examination:

a. Index finger is used
b. In BPH rectal mucosa is free whereas in in prostate cancer mucosa of rectum is adhered
c. Puborectalis is felt anteriorly
d. Anal sphincter length can not be assessed

167. Which of the following increases risk of urinary stones:

a. Increased urinary citrate
b. ↑ Calcium level in blood
c. Hypervitaminosis A
d. Hypoparathyroidism
e. Decrease in urinary colloid

168. True about duodenal diverticula:

a. Most common of the GIT diverticula
b. Commonly occur on medial border
c. Often present in periampullary region
d. It should be treated aggressively due to high malignant potential
e. It can cause pancreatitis by producing obstruction at the opening of the duct

169. Psammoma bodies is/are seen in:

a. Medullary carcinoma of thyroid
b. Ependymoma
c. Papillary carcinoma thyroid
d. Follicular carcinoma of thyroid
e. Meningioma

170. Which of the following is/are true about primary hyperparathyroidism:

a. Associated with MEN I & II
b. Increase risk of renal stone
c. About 50 gram of gland tissue can be left during surgery to prevent hypocalcemia
d. Cause benign hypertension
e. Mc sporadic cause is hyperplasia

171. Which of the following is/are features of Testicular torsion which is not present in epididymo-orchitis:

a. Redness of skin
b. Elevation of testis worsen pain
c. Doppler ultrasound scan show absence of the blood supply to the affected testis
d. Fever
e. Dysuria

172. True about Typhoid ulcer:

a. Perforation is common in 2nd & 3rd week after onset of typhoid fever
b. Perforation may present at multiple site
c. Commonly involve jejunum
d. Commonly involve ileum
e. Peritoneal lavage is contraindicated for perforated ulcer

173. Feature of third degree burn:

a. Pain present
b. Transudation of fluid present
c. Whole dermis destroyed
d. Erythematous in appearance
e. Blister formed

Answer

160. All	161. b.	162. b, c, d.	163. a, b.	164. b, d, e.	165. a, c, d.	166. a, b.
167. b, c, e.	168. b, c, e.	169. c, e.	170. a, b, c.	171. b, c.	172. a, b, d.	173. c.

174. A patient has h/o hypertension & diabetes. The mechanism of higher chance of ulcer in this patient is due to:
a. Hyperglycemia suppress immunity
b. Vascular insufficiency
c. Atherosclerotic changes
d. Venous stasis
e. Trophic skin changes

OBSTETRICS & GYNAECOLOGY

175. Cause (s) of still birth:
a. Prematurity
b. Syphilis
c. Abruptio placentae
d. Diabetes

176. Which of the following is true about endometrial carcinoma:
a. Less aggressive in post menopausal women
b. More common in diabetes
c. Common after 40 yr of age
d. Associated with PCOD
e. Associated with hereditary nonpolyposis colorectal cancer syndrome (HNPCC)

177. High level of hCG found in:
a. Twin
b. Down syndrome
c. Choriocarcinoma
d. Colon carcinoma
e. Ectopic pregnancy

178. All of the following is true about Abruptio placentae except:
a. Premature separation of normal attached placentae
b. Bright red blood
c. Risk of recurrence is about 15% with previous abruption
d. More common in multigravida
e. Pre-eclampsia is a risk factor

179. True about Trichomonas vaginitis:
a. Important cause of recurrent abortion
b. T.vaginalis is a flagellated protozoa
c. Metronidazole is used for treatment
d. Strawberry cervix
e. Curdy discharge

180. True about Mirena:
a. Effective life is 2yr
b. LNG containing IUD
c. Cause endometrial hyperplasia
d. Suppression of endometrium
e. No significant effect on ovaries

181. All are true about LNG except:
a. Cause Endometrial suppression
b. Can be used in emergency contraception
c. Can not be given to lactating women
d. Devoid of estrogenic side-effects

182. True about amniotic fluid:
a. Same concentration of plasma throughout pregnancy
b. Forms from transudation of plasma through fetus skin before 20 wk of gestation
c. Fetus swallows amniotic fluid
d. Protects fetus from injury
e. Main channel for gaseous exchange

183. True about obstetrical outlet:
a. Posterior wall is deficient
b. Bounded above by the plane of least pelvic dimensions
c. Anterior wall is formed by ischial bones
d. Minimum obstetric diameter
e. Its plane is plane of least pelvic dimensions

184. Which of the following is/are criteria for the expectant management in pre-eclampsia except:
a. Platelet count <100000/micro litre
b. B.P > 140/90 mm Hg
c. Urine output < 400ml/day
d. Persistent headache
e. Visual disturbances

185. IUCD is absolutely contraindicated in:
a. HIV positive women
b. Previous ectopic tubal pregnancy
c. Mild anaemia
d. Undiagnosed vaginal bleeding

186. True statement regarding use of ACE inhibitors in pregnancy:
a. Cause polyhydramnios
b. Cause renal agenesis
c. Cause pulmonary hypoplasia
d. Use during first 3 month is safe
e. Safe in last trimester

187. True about ovulation & menstruation:
a. Temperature decrease at time of ovulation
b. Estrogen have a role in proliferative phase
c. LH surge occurs before ovulation
d. 100 ml blood loss is normal

PAEDIATRICS

188. Preterm babies have increased chance of:
a. Heart disease
b. Respiratory distress syndrome
c. Necrotising colitis
d. Meconium aspiration syndrome

189. Which of the following can presents with cyanosis at birth:
a. Tetralogy of Fallot
b. TGA
c. PDA
d. VSD
e. Atrial septal defect (ASD)

Answer

174. a, b, c, e.	175. All	176. b, c, d, e.	177. a, b, c.	178. b.	179. b, c, d.	180. b, d, e.
181. c.	182. b, c, d.	183. b, e.	184. b.	185. b, d.	186. b, c.	187. b, c, d.
188. a, b, c.	189. a, b.					

190. Which of the following is/are true regarding development of child during 6 to 12 yr of age:
a. Weight increases by 1-2 kg/yr
b. Head grow at the rate of 2-3 cm/yr
c. Growth occur continuously
d. Growth occur in spurts
e. Height increases at rate of 6-7 cm/yr

191. True about Asperger syndrome:
a. More common in girl
b. Repetitive activity pattern
c. Subnormal intelligence is consistent feature
d. Severe language impairments is characteristic

192. True bout Autistic disorder:
a. Quality decrease in social interaction
b. All affected children have subnormal intelligence
c. Treatment should targeted toward Speech development
d. Seen only after 3 yr of age
e. Stereotyped patterns of behavior

193. True about HIV infection in infants:
a. Mainly occur through horizontal transmission
b. HIV DNA PCR positive at 3 month confirms diagnosis
c. Positive antibody test for IgG antibody at 3 month confirm infected infant
d. Passive transfer of maternal body generally persists for 12 month

194. Common feature of marfan syndrome & Homocystinuria:
a. Arm span > Height
b. Ectopia lentis
c. Hypermobility of joint
d. Mental retardation
e. Arachnodactyly

ORTHOPAEDICS

195. Distal interphalangeal joint involvement occur in:
a. Boutonniere deformity
b. Swan neck deformity
c. Mallet finger
d. Trigger finger
e. Dupuytren's contracture

196. All are true about Slipped capital femoral epiphysis except:
a. Avascular necrosis may occur
b. Usually occur after 10 year of age
c. Obesity is a risk factor
d. Frog-leg lateral view is helpful
e. More common in girls

197. Pathological fracture not found in:
a. Bone cyst
b. Osteoporosis
c. Chronic osteomyelitis
d. Osteochondroma
e. Osteogenesis imperfecta

198. Commonest cause of acute osteomyelitis:
a. Trauma
b. Surgery
c. Fungal infection
d. Hematogenous route
e. Tubercular infection

199. True about Osteosarcoma:
a. Primary osteosarcoma is most commonly occur in age group of less than 20 yr
b. Periosteal reaction is present
c. Present as elevated soft tissue mass
d. Commonly associated with osteiod osteoma
e. Formation of bone by the tumor cells is characteristic

200. True about Clubfoot:
a. Abduction of forefoot
b. Associated with breech presentation
c. Dennis-Brown splint used
d. Adduction of forefoot
e. Associated with spina bifida

201. All are true about Pott's spine except:
a. Thoracic vertebrae T6-T8 is most commonly affected site
b. Paradiscal is commonest variety
c. Muscular rigidity & stiffness is common
d. Posterior part of vertebrae is more affected than anterior part
e. Back pain is the commonest presenting symptom

ANAESTHESIA

202. A Patient has hypersensitivity to neostigmine. He has to undergo upper abdominal surgery. Muscle relaxant of choice is:
a. Pancuronium
b. Rapacuronium
c. Vecuronium
d. Atracurium
e. Piperacurium

203. Which of the following condition (s) can cause exaggerated hyperkalemia in patients with use of succinylcholine:
a. Burn
b. Spinal cord injury
c. Muscular dystrophy
d. Tetanus
e. Abdominal organ injury

204. Which of the following does not increase intracranial pressure:
a. Sodium thiopentone
b. Desflurane
c. Mannitol
d. Sevoflurane
e. Propofol

205. Mechanism of action of general anesthesia is/are:
a. GABA-A receptor
b. GABA-B receptor
c. NMDA receptor
d. Na+ channel blockage

Answer

190. d, e.	191. b.	192. a, c, e.	193. b, d.	194. b, e.	195. a, b, c.	196. e.
197. None	198. d.	199. a, b, c, e.	200. c, d, e.	201. a, d.	202. d.	203. a, b, c, d.
204. a, c, e.	205. a, c.					

206. Which of the following statement is correct regarding mechanism of action of local anaesthesia:
a. Blockage of resting sodium channel is more than activated sodium channel
b. Faster conducting fibers blocked easily
c. Block Na-K ATPase channel
d. Fine touch goes before pain
e. In regional block I.V injection is used

SKIN

207. Feature (s) of Hailey Hailey disease is/are:
a. A bullous disorder
b. Crusted erosion
c. Most commonly present in infant
d. Also called as familial benign pemphigus
e. Intraepidermal bullous disorder

208. Skin lesion of chronic liver disease:
a. Terry nail
b. Palmar erythema
c. Purpura
d. Spider naevi

209. Nail changes of lichen planus includes:
a. Pterygium
b. Salmon patch
c. Subungual hyperkeratosis
d. Splinter haemorrhage
e. Thinning of nail plate

PSYCHIATRY

210. Feature (s) of Schizophrenia is/are:
a. 1st rank symptom is helpful in making diagnosis
b. Depression may be present
c. Brain ventricle enlargement may be present
d. Onset occur only after age of 40 yr
e. Usually onset occur later in women as compared to men

211. Which of following is perception disorder:
a. Delusion
b. Hallucination
c. Obsession
d. Depersonalization
e. Illusion

212. Which of the following modality is/are not included in behaviour therapy:
a. Role playing
b. Scheduling activities
c. Graded task assignment
d. Identifying maladaptive assumptions

213. Diazepam can be used for:
a. Agitation in emergency room
b. Long term treatment of epilepsy
c. Status epilepticus
d. Convulsion in tetanus

214. Benzodiazepines used in seizure treatment:
a. Lorazepam
b. Temazepam
c. Alprazolam
d. Clobazam
e. Midazolam

RADIOLOGY

215. True statement regarding Iodine-131:
a. It is the only isotope of iodine used for thyroid
b. Contraindicated in pregnancy
c. Emits α rays
d. Emits β rays
e. Emits γ rays

216. Side-effects (s) of Pituitary irradiation:
a. Hypopituitarism
b. Decrease risk of secondary tumor
c. Optic nerve damage
d. Increased risk of cerebrovascular accident

217. False increase in size of heart on chest x-ray PA view is/are seen in:
a. Rotation of patient
b. Supine view
c. Film taken in expiration
d. Pneumonia

218. Radiographic feature (s) of left atrial enlargement:
a. Carinal angle splaying
b. Straight left border
c. Double atrial shadow
d. Boot shaped
e. Apex shifted outward

219. All are true regarding PET scan except:
a. Help in assessment of both anatomical & functional status of tissue
b. Do not pose any radiation exposure to patient
c. Superior to CT for anatomical detail
d. FDG is used

220. Which of the following is true regarding MRI:
a. MRI is better than CT scan for bony lesion
b. Grey matter is grey on T1WI
c. Uses dye gadolinium
d. Gadolinium is safer than iodine based contrast agent
e. Can be used in multiple plain

221. Radioactivity is/are measures by:
a. Sievert
b. Curie
c. Gray
d. Rad
e. Bequeral

MCQs

Answer

206. e. 207. a, b, d, e. 208. a, b, d. 209. a, e. 210. a, b, c, e. 211. b, e. 212. d.
213. a, c, d. 214. a, d. 215. b, d, e. 216. a, c, d. 217. a, b. 218. a, b, c. 219. b, c.
220. b, c, d, e. 221. b, e.

ANATOMY

1. **Ans. c. Develop...**

[Ref: B. D. C. 6th/Vol. III 272; Gray's 40th/618, 650, 653; L & T 10th/409, 412]

Note: *Pinna develop from both 1st & 2nd pharyngeal cleft (so option C is incorrect)*

"Treacher–Collins syndrome: The pinnas lies lower than usual & may be normal or underdeveloped, while the external meatus may be normal or stenosed" *(L & T 10th/412)*

"**Treacher–Collins syndrome (mandibulofacial dysostosis):** malformed pinna & meatal atresia" *(P. L. Dhingra 5th/129)*

"Pinna helps to collect sound waves & to localize the source of the sound" *(A. K. Jain 5th/1105)*

"The greater part of **pinna/auricle** is made up of a single crumpled plate of ***elastic cartilage***" *(B. D. C. 6th/Vol. III 272)*

"The auricle is **formed from** about six mesodermal thickenings (called tubercles or hillocks)that appear on the mandibular & hyoid arches, around the opening of the dorsal part of the ***first ectodermal cleft*** (*i.e.,* around the opening of the external acoustic meatus" *(I. B. Singh Embryology 8th/317)*

"Pinna **develop from** 6 auricle hillocks. A hillock from the ***1st arch forms tragus***, while remainder part of pinna develops by fusion of other tubercles from the both the ***1st & 2nd arches***" *(L & T 10th/409)*

"The 6 hillocks is formed around the margins of the dorsal portion of the ***1st pharyngeal cleft*** of the six, three on the caudal edge of the 1st pharyngeal (mandibular)arch & three on cranial edge of the ***2nd pharyngeal*** (hyoid) arch" *(Gray's 40th/653)*

"**Relapsing perichondritis:** It is a rare autoimmune disorder involving ***cartilage of pinna.*** Other cartilages, septal. Laryngeal, tracheal, costal may also be involved" *(P. L. Dhingra 5th/56)*

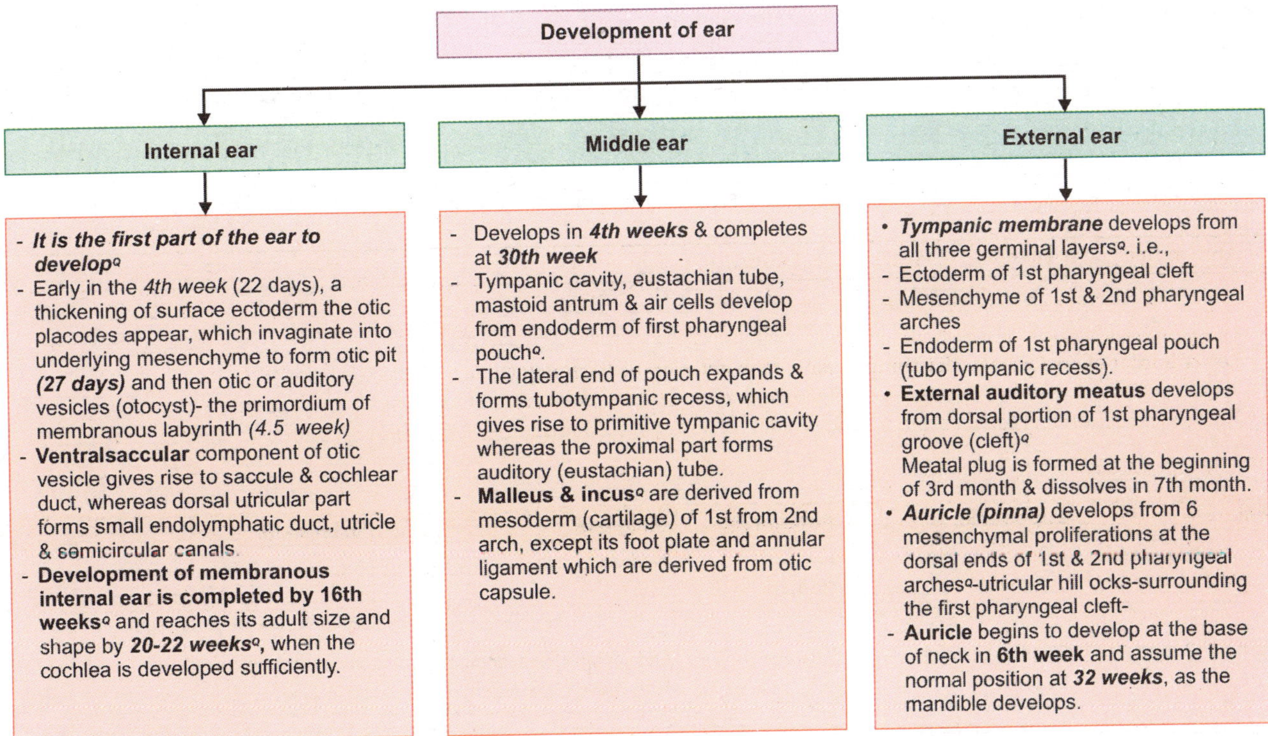

2. Ans. b. Arytenoid... c. Corniculate e. Cuneiform

[Ref: BDC 6th/Vol. III 253; Snell's Clinical Anatomy 8th/802-03; Gray's Anatomy 39th/633-646; Moore Clinical oriented Anatomy5th/1089-99; Snell's Clinical Anatomy 8th/35-36]

Table: Laryngeal Cartilage

Unpaired	Paired
Thyroid[Q]	Arytenoid[Q]
Cricoid	Corniculate[Q]
Epiglottis[Q]	Cuneiform[Q]

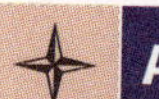

ALSO KNOW

- *Cricoid cartilage is the only cartilage that forms complete ring*[Q]
- *Thyroid cartilage (Adams apple) is the largest cartilage of the larynx*

Hyaline Cartilage	Elastic Cartilage
Thyroid [Q]	Epiglottis[Q]
Cricoid	Corniculate
Basal part of arytenoid cartilage	Cuneiform
Trachea[Q]	Process of arytenoids

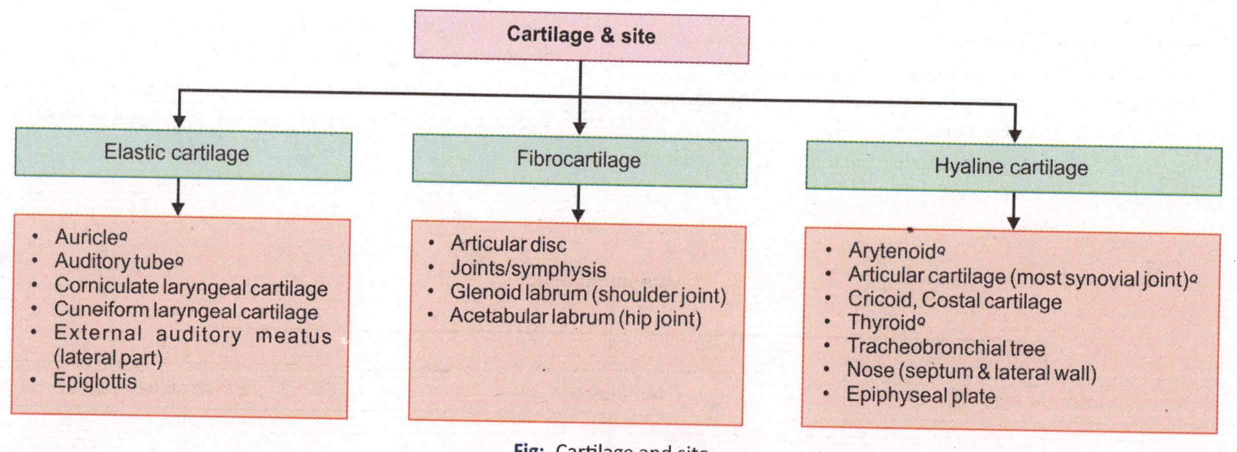

Fig: Cartilage and site

3. Ans. a. Heart..., c. Thymus... d. Posterior... e. Lower...

[Ref: B. D. C. 6th/Vol. I 245-47; Snell's Anatomy 8th/79-80]

Lower border of posterior mediastinum is ***more than anterior mediastinum*** (shown in diagram below)
"**Heart** enclosed in pericardium passes through *middle part of the inferior mediastinum or middle mediastinum*" *(B. D. C. 6th/Vol. I 245)*
"Inferior mediastinum is divided into-anterior, middle & posterior mediastinum" *(B. D. C. 6th/Vol. I 246)*

Feature	Superior M.	Anterior M.	Middle M.	Posterior M.
Anterior Boundary	Manubrium sterni	Body of sternum	Posterior surface of sternum	Pericardium, bifurcation of trachea, pulmonary vessel, Posterior part of the upper surface of diaphragm
Posterior Boundary	Upper 4 vertebrae (T1-T4)	Pericardium	Oesophagus, descending thoracic aorta & azygos	Lower 8 thoracic vertebrae
Important contents	Trachea, Oesophagus, arch of aorta, ***Thymus,*** thoracic aorta	Lowest part of thymus	Heart enclosed in pericardium, Ascending aorta, Pulmonary trunk, Two pulmonary arteries, bifurcation of trachea, Left & right bronchi	Oesophagus, descending thoracic aorta, Azygos & hemiazygos vein

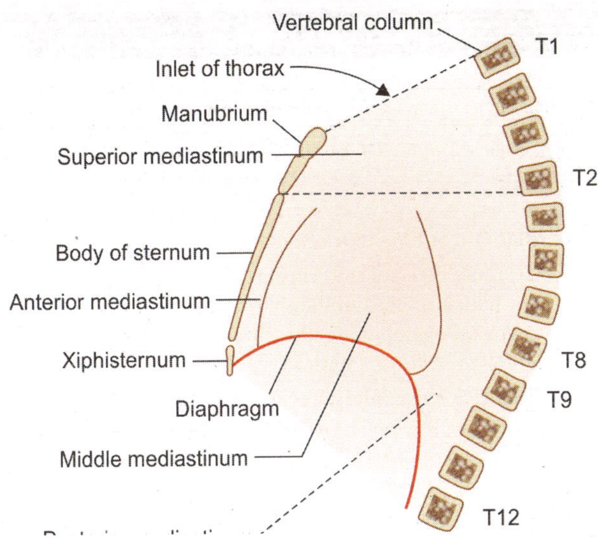

Fig: Subdivisions of the mediastinum

4. Ans. c. C shaped..., d. Fixed..., e. Inner...,

[Ref: BDC 6th/Vol. II 143, 4th/Vol. II 145-46; Gray's 40th/1397-98; Snell's 8th/629]

"The menisci are C-shaped sheets of fibrocartilage" (Snell's 8th/629)
"The **medial meniscus** is ***torn more frequently*** because it is ***less mobile*** (being ***fixed to the medial collateral ligament)***" *(Maheshwari 3rd/129)*

Menisci (Semilunar Cartilages)

◈ *B. D. C. 6th/Vol. II 143, 4th/Vol. II 145-46*

- "The menisci (semilunar cartilages) have crescentic shape, intracapsular & fibrocartilaginous in nature"
- "Their **peripheral** attached borders are thick & convex; their free, **inner borders** are thin & concave. Their peripheries are vascularized by capillary loops from the fibrous capsule & synovial membrane, while their inner regions are avascular"
- **"Tears of menisci are common**. Most occur in avascular inner zone & seldom heal spontaneously. Peripheral zone (vascularized zone) have the potential to heal spontaneously"
- "The **medial meniscus** is more vulnerable than lateral because of its fixity to the tibial collateral ligament & because of greater excursion during rotatory movement. Lateral meniscus is protected by popliteus"*(B. D. C. 6th/Vol. II 147)*
- *"**Medial meniscus**: Its peripheral border is attached to the fibrous capsule & the deep surface of the **medial collateral ligament**. The tibial attachment of the meniscus is known as the coronary ligament" (Gray's 40th/1398)*

5. Ans. b. Edinger-Westphal... & d. Passes...

[Ref.: BDC 6th/Vol. III 360-62; Snells' Anatomy 8th/757; Gray's 40th/666]

Cranial Nerves Origins from the Brainstem

◈ *http: //www.usmle-forums.com/*

- III and IV from the midbrain
- V, VI, VII & VIII from the pons
- IX, X, XI & XII from the medulla

Oculomotor Nerve

"The nerve passes b/w the superior cerebral & posterior cerebral arteries & runs forward in the ***interpeduncular cistern***, on the lateral side of the posterior communicating artery to reach cavernous sinus" *(B. D. C. 6th/Vol. III 361)*
"The nerve enter the **cavernous sinus** by piercing the posterior part of its roof on the lateral side of the posterior clinoid process. It descends to the ***lateral wall of the sinus*** where it lies above the trochlear nerve"*(B. D. C. 6th/Vol. III 362)*
"The nerve continues into middle cranial fossa in the ***lateral wall of the cavernous sinus.*** Intrinsic muscle of the eye is supplied by parasympathetic component of oculomotor nerve" *(Snells' Anatomy 8th/757)*
"The fibres for the constrictor papillae & for the ciliaris (*i.e.*, general visceral efferent or **parasympathetic branch**) arise from the ***Edinger Westphal nucleus*** which forms part of the oculomotor nuclear complex" *(B. D. C. 6th/Vol. III 360)*
"The ***nerve emerges at the midbrain,*** on the medial side of the crus of the cerebral peduncle & passes along the ***lateral dural wall of the cavernous sinus***, dividing into superior & inferior divisions which run beneath the trochlear & ophthalmic nerves" *(Gray's 40th/666)*

6. Ans. a. Some..., b. Seminal..., d. Vas..., e. Ductus...

[Ref: Embryology by I. B. Singh 8th/265, 237-45; Snells' Anatomy 8th/357]

*"The part of gubernaculum b/w uterus & the labius majus becomes the **round ligament of the uterus**" (Embryology by I. B. Singh 8th/264)*
"The **mesenchymal cells** occupying the core of the inguinal fold condense as another cord, the ***gubernaculums"*** *(Gray's 40th/1320)*

Mesonephric (or Wolffian) Duct

◈ *Snells' Anatomy 8th/357*

- *"In both sexes, the mesonephric (or Wolffian) duct gives origin on each side to the ureteric bud, which forms the **ureter, the pelvis of the ureter, the major & minor calyces & the collecting tubules of the kidney.** Its inferior end is absorbed into the developing bladder & forms the **trigone & part of the urethra"***
- In the male, its upper or cranial end is joined to the developing testis by the efferent ductules of the testis & so it becomes the **duct of the epididymis, the vas deferens & the ejaculatory duct**. From the latter, a small diverticulum arises that forms the seminal vesicle
- In the female, the mesonephric duct largely disappears. Only small remnants persists-as the duct of the epoophoron & the duct of the paroophoron. The caudal end may persists & extend from the epoophoron to the hymen as Gartner's duct

Fate of Mesonephric Duct

◈ *I. B. Singh 8th/264*

- Ureteric buds from which ureters, pelvis, calyces & collecting tubules of the kidneys are derived
- Trigone of the bladder
- Posterior wall of the part of the prostatic urethra, cranial to the opening of the ejaculatory ducts
- Epididymis
- *Ductus deferens*
- *Seminal vesicles*
- *Ejaculatory ducts*
- *Mesodermal part of prostate*
- *Appendix of epididymis*

Table *(I. B. Singh 8th/265)*

Structure	Male derivative	Female derivative
Mesonephric duct	***Appendix of epididymis, Epididymis, Ductus deferens, Ejaculatory duct, Seminal vesicles***	***Appendix of ovary Gartner's duct***
Paramesonephric duct	Appendix of testis, Utricle of prostate	Uterine tube, Uterus, Upper vagina
Mesonephric tubules	Vasa efferentia, Paradidymis	Epoophoron, Paroophoron

7. Ans. b. Broad..

[Ref: BDC 6th/Vol. II 387-92; Snells' Anatomy 8th/366]

Uterus

◈ *B. D. C. 6th/Vol. II 387-92*

- **Arterial supply:** Chiefly by the ***two uterine arteries*** which are markedly enlarged during pregnancy. Partly by the ovarian arteries
- **Lymphatic drainage are by:** Mainly *Aortic nodes & partly by superficial inguinal nodes (fundus & upper part of body), External iliac node (lower part of body) & external iliac, internal iliac, sacral nodes (cervix)*
- "Lymph vessel from the fundus drains into ***para-aortic nodes***" *(Snells' Anatomy 8th/366)*
- **"Posterior surface or intestinal surface:** *It is convex & is related to coils of the terminal ileum & to the sigmoid colon. It is covered with peritoneum & forms the anterior wall of the rectouterine pouch"*
- *"Anterior or vesical surface: It is flat & related to the urinary bladder"*
- Secondary supports: These are of ***doubtful value*** & are formed by peritoneal ligaments. These are provided by ***broad ligaments,*** uterovesical fold of peritoneum & rectovaginal fold of peritoneum"

PHYSIOLOGY

8. Ans. a. Cardiac..., c. Mixed..., d. Rate..., e. For...

[Ref: Ganong 25th/543-44, 24th/546-47; A.K. Jain 5th/356; Guyton 11th /244]

Cardiac Output Measurement

- Two methods of measuring output that are applicable to humans, in addition to Doppler combined with echocardiography, are the **direct Fick method** and the **indicator dilution method.**
- The **Fick principle** states that *the amount of a substance taken up by an organ (or by the whole body) per unit of time is equal to the arterial level of the substance minus the venous level **(A-V difference)** times the blood flow.*
- This principle can be applied, of course, only in situations in which the arterial blood is the sole source of the substance taken up. The principle can be used to determine **cardiac output** by measuring the ***amount of O_2 consumed by the body in a given period and dividing this value by the A-V difference across the lungs.***
- In applying this Fick procedure for measuring cardiac output in the human being, **mixed venous blood is usually obtained through a catheter inserted up the brachial vein of the forearm, through the subclavian vein, down to the right atrium and, finally, into the right ventricle or pulmonary artery.**
- And *systemic arterial blood* can then be obtained from any systemic artery in the body.
- The *rate of oxygen absorption* by the lungs is measured by the rate of disappearance of oxygen from the respired air, using any type of oxygen meter (e.g ***close circuit spirometry***)
- Because systemic arterial blood has the same O_2 content in all parts of the body, ***the arterial O_2 content can be measured in a sample obtained from any convenient artery.*** A sample of venous blood in the pulmonary artery is obtained by means of a cardiac catheter.
- An example of the calculation of cardiac output using a typical set of values is as follows:

Output of Left Ventricle

$$= \frac{O_2 \text{ consumption (mL/min)}}{[A_{O2}] - [V_{O2}]}$$

$$= \frac{250 \text{ mL/min}}{90 \text{ mL/L arterial blood - 140 mL venous blood in pulmonary artery}}$$

$$= \frac{250 \text{ mL/min}}{50 \text{ mL/L}}$$

$$= 5\text{L/min}$$

ALSO KNOW

- *"In the indicator dilution technique, a known amount of a substance such as a dye or, more commonly, a radioactive isotope is injected into an arm vein and the concentration of the indicator in serial samples of arterial blood is determined." -Guyton 11th /244*

9. Ans. b. Decreas..

[Ref: Ganong 25th/331-33, 24th/334-35; A.K. Jain 5th/695-96; Guyton 11th /907, 918-921, 1039-40;CMDT 2016/1096-97, 06/1113-14]

"**Hypothyroidism & cirrhosis** can ***cause hyperprolactinemia***" *(CMDT 2016/1096)*

"**Hyperprolactinemia** due to any cause may result in ***hypogonadotropic hypogonadism.*** Women may note ***oligomenorrhoea or amenorrhoea. Galactorrhoea, defined as lactation in absence of nursing, is common***" *(CMDT 2016/1097, 06/1114)*

"**Primary hypothyroidism** is associated with mild ***hyperprolactinemia,*** probably because of compensatory TRH secretion"

"**Prolactin deficiency** inhibits ***postpartum lactation***"

"**Hypogonadotropic hypogonadism** often develops in patients with ***hyperprolactinemia***; it may be reversed with treatment of the hyperprolactinemia"

Prolactin

◈ *Ganong 25th/331-33, 24th/334-35*

- Prolactin causes milk secretion from the breast after estrogen and progesterone priming. Its effect on the breast is increased production of casein and lactalbumin.
- Prolactin also inhibits the effects of gonadotropins, possibly by an action at the level of the ovary.
- The function of prolactin in normal males is unsettled, but excess prolactin secreted by tumors causes impotence.
- PRL is unique among the pituitary hormones in that the predominant central control mechanism is inhibitory, reflecting dopamine-mediated suppression of PRL release
- PRL acts to induce and maintain *lactation, decrease reproductive function and suppress sexual drive.* These functions are geared toward ensuring that maternal lactation is sustained and not interrupted by pregnancy.
- Thyrotropin-releasing hormone (TRH) (pyro Glu-His-Pro-NH_2) is a hypothalamic tripeptide that elicits prolactin release within 15–30 min after intravenous injection. The physiologic relevance of TRH for PRL regulation is unclear and it appears primarily to regulate TSH
- *Vasoactive intestinal peptide* (VIP) also induces PRL release, whereas glucocorticoids and thyroid hormone weakly suppress PRL secretion.
- ***The hyperprolactinemia may cause galactorrhea, but in many individuals there are no demonstrable endocrine abnormalities.***
- Prolactin may produce amenorrhea by blocking the action of gonadotropins on the ovaries.

10. Ans. b. Secreted..., e. Cause...

[Ref: Ganong 25th/311-13, 24th/311-13; Guyton 11th /918, 1040-41, 928]

Gonadotropin-releasing hormone (GnRH): It is secreted from hypothalamus & stimulates secretion of ***FSH & LH***" *-Guyton 11th /921*

"**Oxytocin** *stimulate* ***contraction of the smooth muscle cell (myoepithelium)*** *lining the duct of mammary glands; therefore, cause* ***milk ejection*** *from lactating breast" (A. K. Jain 5th/699)*

Oxytocin

◈ *Ganong 25th/311-13, 24th/311-13; Guyton 11th /918, 1040-41, 928It is secreted by posterior pituitary*

- Oxytocin stimulates postpartum milk letdown in response to suckling
- Oxytocin is also a ***nonapeptide (9 amino acids) a***nd it differs from AVP only at positions 3 and 8. However, it has relatively little antidiuretic effect and seems to act mainly on mammary ducts to facilitate milk letdown during nursing.
- It also may help initiate or facilitate labor by stimulating contraction of uterine smooth muscle, but it is not clear if this action is physiologic or necessary for normal delivery.

11. Ans. a. Increased..., c. At..., d. It can...

[Ref: Ganong 25th/629-32, 24th/629-33; Guyton 11th /473-75; A. K. Jain 5th/437]

"**Compliance of lung**: It can be measured by ***measuring intrapleural pressure at different lung volume.*** intrapleural pressure indicates distensibility of lungs" *(A. K. Jain 5th/437)*

Factor Affecting Lung Compliance

◈ *A. K. Jain 5th/437*

- "If surface tension is high as in deficiency of surfactant, more pressure is required to distend the lungs, therefore compliance is decreased" (*i.e.,* ***deficiency of surfactant-less compliance; more surfactant-more compliance***)
- "**Phase of respiratory cycle**: Compliance is slightly greater when measured during deflation than when measured during inflation. ***Compliance decreases with the inflation*** of the lungs as more pressure is required to distend the already distended lung"
- **Lung volume:** An individual with only one lung has approximately ½ the change in volume (Δ V) for a given change in pressure (ΔP)
- Effect of gravity: In the standing position compliance is less at the apices of the lung as there are more distended alveoli at the apex

Compliance of the Lungs

◈ *Guyton 11th /473-75*

- The change in lung volume per unit change in airway pressure ($\Delta V/\Delta P$) is the **stretchability (compliance)** of the lungs and chest wall. It is normally measured in the pressure range where the relaxation pressure curve is steepest and the normal value is approximately 0.2 L/cm H_2O. However, ***compliance depends on lung volume***; an individual with only one lung has approximately half the ΔV for a given ΔP.

- **Compliance** is also slightly greater when measured during deflation than when measured during inflation. Consequently, it is more informative to examine the whole pressure-volume curve.
- The curve is shifted downward and to the right (**compliance is decreased**) by ***pulmonary congestion and interstitial pulmonary fibrosis***; pulmonary fibrosis is a progressive disease of unknown cause in which there is stiffening and scarring of the lung.
- The curve is shifted upward and to the **left (compliance is increased)** in ***emphysema.***
- An important factor affecting the compliance of the lungs is the **surface tension** of the film of fluid that lines the alveoli.

12. Ans. d. Sodium...

[Ref: Ganong 25th/435, 24th/435; Harper 30th/191, 28th/171; Lippincott Biochemistry 4th/97]

*"**GLUT-5** is unusual in that it is the primary transporter for **fructose (instead of glucose)** in small intestine & the testes" (Lippincott Biochemistry 4th/97)*

*'**GLUT-5 is sodium independent facilitated diffusion mechanism**" (Lippincott Biochemistry 4th/97)*

Table *(Ganong 25th/433)*: **Glucose transporter in mammals**

	Function	Major Sites of Expression
Secondary active transport (Na-glucose cotransport)		
SGLT 1	Absorption of glucose	Small intestine, renal tubules
SGLT 2	Absorption of glucose	Renal tubules
Facilitated diffusion		
GLUT 1	Basal glucose uptake	Placenta, blood-brain barrier, brain, red cells, kidneys, colon, many other organs
GLUT 2	B-cell glucose sensor; transport out of intestinal and renal epithelial cells	B cells of islets, liver, epithelial cells of small intestine, kidneys
GLUT 3	Basal glucose uptake	Brain, placenta, kidneys, many other organs
GLUT 4	Insulin-stimulated glucose uptake	Skeletal and cardiac muscle, adipose tissue, other tissues
GLUT 5	Fructose transport	Jejunum, sperm
GLUT 6	None	Brain, Spleen & Leukocytes
GLUT 7	Glucose 6-phosphate transporter in endoplasmic reticulum	Liver,

Contd...

Table *(Harper 30th/191, 28th/171)*: **Major Glucose Transporters**

	Tissue Location	Function
Facilitative bidirectional transporters		
GLUT 1	Brain, kidney, colon, placenta, erythrocytes	Glucose uptake
GLUT 2	Liver, pancreatic β-cell, small intestine, kidney	Rapid uptake or release of glucose
GLUT 3	Brain, kidney, placenta	Glucose Uptake
GLUT 4	Heart and skeletal muscle, adipose tissue	Skeletal and cardiac muscle, adipose tissue, other tissues
GLUT 5	Small intestine	Absorption of glucose
Sodium-dependent unidirectional transporter		
SGLT-1	Small intestine and kidney	Active uptake of glucose against a concentration gradient

13. Ans. b. Found..., c. Activated...

[Ref: Ganong 23rd/27; Harper 28th/220, 215]

"Lipoprotein lipase is located on the walls of ***blood capillaries***, anchored to the endothelium by negatively charged proteoglycan chains of heparan sulfate. It has been found in heart, adipose tissue, spleen, lung, renal medulla, aorta, diaphragm and lactating mammary gland, although it is not active in adult liver"*(Harper 30th/257, 28th/215)*

Free Fatty Acid Metabolism

◈ *Ganong 25th/28, 23rd/27*

- The supply of FFA to the tissues is regulated by two lipases- Lipoprotein lipase & Hormone-sensitive lipase
- Lipoprotein lipase on the ***surface of the endothelium of the capillaries*** hydrolyzes the triglycerides in chylomicrons and VLDL, providing FFA and glycerol, which are reassembled into new triglycerides in the fat cells.
- The intracellular hormone-sensitive lipase of adipose tissue catalyzes the breakdown of stored triglycerides into glycerol and fatty acids, with the latter entering the circulation.
- The hormone-sensitive lipase is converted from an inactive to an active form by cAMP via protein kinase A. The adenylyl cyclase in adipose cells is in turn activated by glucagon. It is also activated by the catecholamines norepinephrine and epinephrine

- Growth hormone, glucocorticoids and thyroid hormones increase the activity of the hormone-sensitive lipase, but they do it by a slower process that requires synthesis of new protein..
- On the other hand, insulin and prostaglandin E decrease the activity of the hormone-sensitive lipase, possibly by inhibiting the formation of cAMP.
- Activity of the hormone-sensitive lipase is increased by fasting and stress and decreased by feeding and insulin. Conversely, feeding increases and fasting and stress decrease the activity of lipoprotein lipase.

Lipolysis Is Controlled by Hormone-Sensitive Lipase

◈ *Harper 30th/261-62, 28th/220*

- Triacylglycerol undergoes hydrolysis by a **hormone-sensitive lipase** to form free fatty acids and glycerol. This lipase is distinct from lipoprotein lipase, which catalyzes lipoprotein triacylglycerol hydrolysis before its uptake into extrahepatic tissues
- **Hormone-sensitive lipase is activated** by ***ACTH, TSH, glucagon, epinephrine, norepinephrine and vasopressin and inhibited by insulin, prostaglandin E_1 and nicotinic acid***

14. Ans. All (a b c)

[Ref: www.merckmanuals.com/professional/neurologic_disorders /pain/ evaluation_of_pain.html]

"A **pain scale** measures a patient's pain intensity or other features. Pain scales are based on self-report, observational (behavioral), or physiological data. Self-report is considered primary and should be obtained if possible. Pain scales are available for neonates, infants, children, adolescents, adults, seniors and persons whose communication is impaired. Pain assessments are often regarded as **"the 5th Vital Sign."**

Table Examples of pain scales

	Self-report	Observational	Physiological
Infant	—	Premature Infant Pain Profile; Neonatal/Infant Pain Scale	—
Child	Faces Pain Scale -Revised; Wong-Baker FACES Pain Rating Scale; *Coloured Analogue Scale*	FLACC (Face Legs Arms Cry Consolability Scale); CHEOPS (Children's Hospital of Eastern Ontario Pain Scale)	Comfort
Adult	***Visual Analog Scale*** **(VAS)**; Verbal Numerical Rating Scale (VNRS); Verbal Descriptor Scale (VDS); Brief Pain Inventory	—	

List of Pain Measurement Scales

- Alder Hey Triage Pain Score
- Behavioral Pain Scale (BPS)
- Brief Pain Inventory (BPI)
- A More Objective and Better Defined Pain Scale from Remote Medicine Ireland.
- Checklist of Nonverbal Pain Indicators (CNPI)
- Clinical Global Impression (CGI)
- Critical-Care Pain Observation Tool (CPOT)
- COMFORT scale
- Dallas Pain Questionnaire
- Descriptor differential scale (DDS)
- Dolorimeter Pain Index (DPI)
- Edmonton Symptom Assessment System
- Faces Pain Scale -Revised (FPS-R)
- Face Legs Activity Cry Consolability scale
- **Lequesne algofunctional index:** A composite measure of pain and disability, with separate self-report questionnaires for hip and knee OA (osteoarthritis):
- McGill Pain Questionnaire (MPQ)
- Neck Pain and Disability Scale –NPAD
- Numerical 11 point box (BS-11)
- Numeric Rating Scale (NRS-11)
- Oswestry Index
- Palliative Care Outcome Scale (PCOS)
- Roland-Morris Back Pain Questionnaire
- Support Team Assessment Schedule (STAS)
- Wong-Baker FACES Pain Rating Scale
- Visual analog scale (VAS)

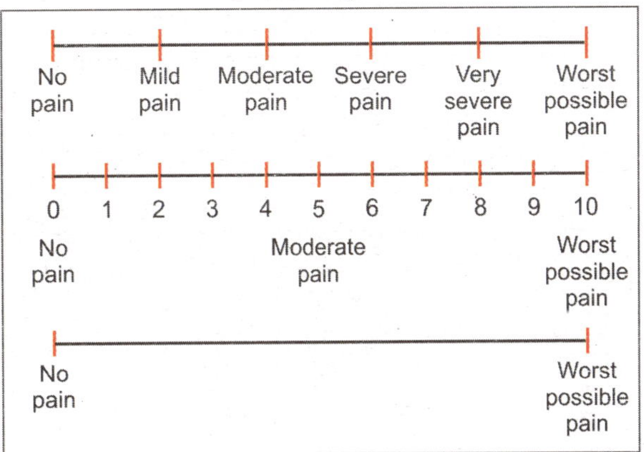

Fig: Visual analog scale

BIOCHEMISTRY

15. Ans. b. Exercise..., c. Muscle..., d. It operate...

[Ref: Harper 30th/171, 69, 28th/149-151; Harrison 19th/433e2; Lippincott 4th/103, 111; Chatterjea & Shinde 7th/313]

*"**Fumarate** is converted **to malate** by fumarase enzyme in **Kreb cycle (so fumarate level increases in defective enzyme functioning in Kreb's cycle, not in abnormality of glycolysis** i.e., **lactate dehydrogenase deficiency**" (Harper 28th/145)*

"**Lactate dehydrogenase** *catalyse conversion of* ***pyruvic acid to lactic acid*** *(Chatterjea & Shinde 7th/313)*

Glycolysis & Oxidation of Pyruvate

◈ *Harper 30th/171, 28th/149-150*

- The redox state of the tissue now determines which of two pathways (aerobic & anaerobic) are followed for metabolism of pyruvate
- Under **anaerobic conditions**, the NADH cannot be reoxidized through the respiratory chain to oxygen. Pyruvate is reduced by the NADH to lactate, catalyzed by **lactate dehydrogenase.** There are different tissue specific isoenzymes lactate dehydrogenase that have clinical significance.
- The reoxidation of NADH via lactate formation allows glycolysis to proceed in the absence of oxygen by regenerating sufficient NAD^+ for another cycle of the reaction catalyzed by *glyceraldehydes-3-phosphate dehydrogenase.*
- Under **aerobic conditions,** ***pyruvate is taken up into mitochondria*** and after oxidative decarboxylation to acetyl-CoA is oxidized to CO_2 by the citric acid cycle. The reducing equivalents from the NADH formed in glycolysis are taken up into mitochondria for oxidation via one of the two shuttles.

Tissues That Function under Hypoxic Conditions Produce

◈ *Lactate Harper 28th/150-51*

- This is true of skeletal muscle, particularly the white fibers, where the rate of work output and hence the need for ATP formation, may exceed the rate at which oxygen can be taken up and utilized. Glycolysis in erythrocytes always terminates in lactate, because the subsequent reactions of pyruvate oxidation are mitochondrial and erythrocytes lack mitochondria.
- Other tissues that normally derive much of their energy from glycolysis and produce lactate include brain, gastrointestinal tract, renal medulla, retina and skin. The liver, kidneys and heart usually take up lactate and oxidize it but will produce it under hypoxic conditions.

What is Lactate Dehydrogenase Deficiency?

◈ *http: //ghr.nlm.nih.gov/condition/lactate-dehydrogenase-deficiency*

- Lactate dehydrogenase deficiency is a condition that affects how the body breaks down sugar to use as energy in cells, primarily muscle cells.
- **There are two types of this condition:** lactate dehydrogenase-A deficiency (sometimes called glycogen storage disease XI) and lactate dehydrogenase-B deficiency.
- People with lactate dehydrogenase-A deficiency experience ***fatigue, muscle pain and cramps during exercise (exercise intolerance).***

Table *(Harrison 19th/433e2)*: **Features of Glycogen Storage Diseases and Galactose and Fructose Disorders**

Type/Common Name	Basic Defect	Clinical Features
Lactate dehydrogenase deficiency	Lactate dehydrogenase -M subunit	Exercise intolerance, muscle cramps, myoglobinuria on strenuous exercise, increased CK, erythematous skin eruption and uterine stiffness resulting in childbirth difficulty in female

16. Ans. a. N-acetyl..., c. Glucuronic...

[Ref: Harper 30th/156, 159, 637, 640, 28th/119, 534-39; Lippincott 4th/159, 163; Chatterjea & Shinde 7th/38]

"**Composition of Hyaluronic Acid**: It is composed of repeating units of ***N-acetyl glucosamine & D-Glucuronic acid***. On hydrolysis, it yields equimolecular quantities of D-Glucosamine, D-Glucuronic acid & acetic acid"- *(Chatterjea & Shinde 7th/38)*

Hyaluronic Acid

◈ *Harper 30th/637, 28th/535*

- Hyaluronic acid consists of an unbranched chain of repeating disaccharide units containing GlcUA and GlcNAc.
- Hyaluronic acid is present in bacteria and is widely distributed among various animals and tissues, including synovial fluid, the vitreous body of the eye, cartilage and loose connective tissues.
- **Hyaluronic acid** is especially high in concentration in embryonic tissues and is thought to play an important role in permitting **cell migration** during morphogenesis and wound repair. Its ability to attract water into the extracellular matrix and thereby "loosen it up" may be important in this regard. The high concentrations of hyaluronic acid and chondroitin sulfates present in **cartilage** contribute to its

17. Ans. b. β oxidation...

[Ref: Harper 30th/231, 614, 28th/191, 493; Lippincott 4th/195; Harrison 19th/2681, 18th/3456, 236]

"**Refsum disease** is a rare autosomal recessive disorder caused by a deficiency of α-hydroxylase" *(Lippincott 4th/195)*

"**Refsum's disease:** ***Alpha oxidation*** *does not occur. Alpha oxidation is mainly used for fatty acids that have a methyl group at beta-carbon, which* ***block beta-oxidation.*** *This process occur mainly in* ***endoplasmic reticulum*** *& some also in peroxisomes "* *(Vasudevan Biochemistry 5th/137)*

"**Refsum's disease** is a rare neurologic disorder due to a metabolic defect that results in the ***accumulation of phytanic acid***, which is found in dairy products and ruminant fat and meat. Phytanic acid is thought to have pathological effects on *membrane function, protein prenylation and gene expression" (Harper 30th/231, 28th/191)*

Refsum Disease

◈ *Harrison 19th/2681, 18th/3456*

- Refsum disease can manifest in infancy to early adulthood with the classic **tetrad** of *(1)* ***peripheral neuropathy****, (2) retinitis pigmentosa, (3) cerebellar ataxia and (4) elevated CSF protein concentration.*
- Most affected individuals develop progressive distal sensory loss and weakness in the legs leading to footdrop by their 20s.
- Subsequently, the proximal leg and arm muscles may become weak.
- Patients may also develop sensorineural hearing loss, cardiac conduction abnormalities, ichthyosis and anosmia.
- Serum phytanic acid levels are elevated.
- Nerve biopsy demonstrates a loss of myelinated nerve fibers, with remaining axons often thinly myelinated and associated with onion bulb formation.
- Refsum disease is genetically heterogeneous but autosomal recessive in nature. Classical Refsum disease with childhood or early adult onset is caused by mutations in the gene that encodes for ***phytanoyl-CoA α-hydroxylase*** *(PAHX)*.
- These mutations lead to the accumulation of phytanic acid in the central and peripheral nervous systems.
- Refsum disease is treated by **removing phytanic precursors** ***(phytols: fish oils, dairy products and ruminant fats)*** from the diet.

18. Ans. d. Peptidyl...

[Ref: Harper 30th/422-24, 28th/359-66, 323; Lippincott 4th/438-42; Chatterjea & Shinde 7th/248-50]

Enzyme Required for Translation

◈ *Chatterjea & Shinde 7th/248-50*

- **Amino-acyl-t-RNA synthetase:** Enzyme required for activation of amino acids
- Peptide synthetase (***peptidyl transferase***)

Peptide Bond Formation

" The ***NH_2 of new aminoacyl t - RNA (A_1) in 'A' site combine with the - COOH group of Met - t -RNA*** occupying the 'P' site. The reaction is catalyzed by peptidyl tranferase" *(Chatterjea & Shinde 7th/251)*

*"**Peptidases** degrades proteins to amino acids"-(Harper 30th/288, 28th/239)*

Table *(Harper 30th/382, 28th/323)*: **Classes of Proteins Involved in Replication**

Protein	Function
DNA polymerases	Deoxynucleotide polymerization
Helicases	Processive unwinding of DNA
Topoisomerases	Relieve torsional strain that results from helicase-induced unwinding
DNA primase	Initiates synthesis of RNA primers
Single-strand binding proteins	Prevent premature reannealing of dsDNA
DNA ligase	Seals the single strand nick between the nascent chain and Okazaki fragments on lagging strand

19. Ans. a. The NH2..., c. Reaction...

[Ref: Harper 30th/422-25, 28th/359-66; Lippincott 4th/438-42; Chatterjea & Shinde 7th/248-50]

"Peptidyl transferase ***catalyses peptide bond formation"****-* *Harper 30th/422, 28th/362*

Peptide Bond Formation

- The ***α-amino group of the new aminoacyl-tRNA in the A site*** carries out a nucleophilic attack on the esterified ***carboxyl group of the peptidyl-tRNA occupying the P site*** (peptidyl or polypeptide site). At initiation, this site is occupied by aminoacyl-tRNA met^{i}.
- This reaction is catalyzed by a **peptidyltransferase,** a component of the 28S RNA of the 60S ribosomal subunit. This is another example of ribozyme activity and indicates an important—and previously unsuspected—direct role for RNA in protein synthesis.
- Because the amino acid on the aminoacyl-tRNA is **already "activated,"** ***no further energy source is required for this reaction***. The reaction results in attachment of the growing peptide chain to the tRNA in the A site.

Materials Required for Protein Synthesis *(Shinde)*

- *Amino acias*[Q]
- *DNA & 3 RNAs (m-RNA, t-RNA, r-RNA)*
- *Polyribosomes (polysomes)*[Q]
- ***Enzymes****: Aminoacyl-t-RNA synthetase, peptidyl transferase*
- ***Factors***
    - ***Initiation facors****-IF1 to 3 (For prokaryotes)*
    - *10 eIF (eIF-1, eIF-2, eIF-3, eIF-4A, eIF-4B, eIF-4G, eIF-4E, elf-5*[Q]*,* ***for eukaryotes)***
    - ***Elongation factors****-EF1 & EF2*[Q]
    - ***Release factors*** *R1 & R2*
    - ***Coenzymes & cofactors;*** *FH4 Mg^{2+}*
- Energy
    - *ATP, GTP*[Q]

Steps of Translation (Protein synthesis)

- Activation of amino acids
- Initiation
- Elongation
- Termination
- Post-translational processing

20. Ans. b. Rate limiting..., d. Malate...

[Ref; Harrison 19th/434e3-5, 18th/3216, 3219;17th/2472-74; Harper 30th/290-96, 28th/243;Shinde 7th/450-51; Vasudevan 5th/180-81]

Urea Cycle: 5 Steps (Given in Fig.)

- Synthesis of carbamoyl-phosphate
- Synthesis of citrulline
- Synthesis of argininosuccinate
- Cleavage of argininosuccinate
- Cleavage of arginine to form ornithine & urea

"**Urea** *has two amino groups,* ***one derived from ammonia & other from aspartate****. Carbon atom is supplied from carbon dioxide" (Satyanarayan 3rd/337)*

Urea Cycle

$NH_3 + CO_2 +$ Aspartate → Urea + Fumarate

Fumarate *is converted into malate & then to oxaloacetate in* ***TCA cycle****- (Satyanarayan 3rd/339)*

"Rate-limiting enzyme (pacemaker enzyme) of Urea cycle: ***Carbamoyl phosphate synthetase I*** (CPS II is involved in pyrimidine synthesis)"*(Harper 28th/245)*

"**Significance of urea cycle:** ***detoxication of ammonia to urea*** & biosynthesis of arginine (arginine is used in protein synthesis)" *(Shinde 7th/450)*

Synthesis of **1 mol of urea**[Q] requires ***3 mol of ATP plus 1 mol each of ammonium ion & of the α-amino nitrogen of aspartate***[Q] *(Harper 30th/292, 28th/243)*

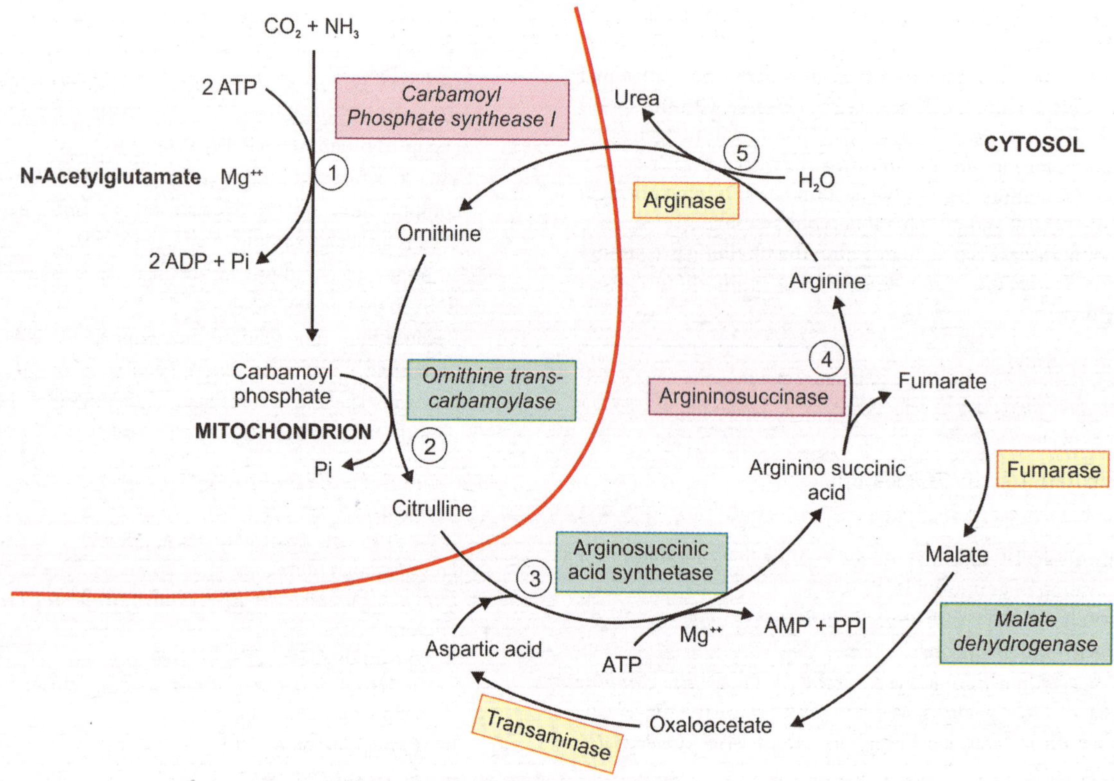

Fig: Biosynthesis of urea or Ornithine–Urea Cycle

Rate Limiting Enzymes for Various Pathways/Cycles

◈ *http: //quizlet.com/16921488/rate-limiting-enzymes-and-diagnoses-flash-cards/*

- **Rate-limiting enzyme of Glycolysis:** Phosphofructokinase-1 (PFK-1)
- **Rate-limiting enzyme of Gluconeogenesis:** Fructose-1, 6, biphosphatase
- **Rate-limiting enzyme of TCA cycle:** Isocitrate dehydrogenase
- **Rate-limiting enzyme of Glycogen Synthesis:** Glycogen synthase (not too hard there)
- **Rate-limiting enzyme of Glycogenolysis:** Glycogen phophorylase (phophorylase breaks phosphate bond, which means activated glycogen releases a lot of energy)
- **Rate-limiting enzyme of HMP Shunt:** Glucose-6-Phosphate dehydrogenase (bad to lose this in RBCs)
- **Rate-limiting enzyme of de novo pyrimidine synthesis:** Carbamoyl phosphate synthase II (CPS I is involved in urea cycle)

- **Rate-limiting enzyme of de novo purine synthesis:** Glutamine-PRPP amidotransferase
- **Rate-limiting enzyme of Urea cycle:** ***Carbamoyl phosphate synthetase I*** (CPS II is involved in pyrimidine synthesis) *(Harper 30th/294, 28th/245)*
- **Rate-limiting enzyme of fatty acid synthesis:** Acetyl-CoA carboxylase (ACC)
- **Rate-limiting enzyme of fatty acid oxidation:** Carnitine acyltransferase I
- **Rate-limiting enzyme of Ketogenesis:** HMG-CoA synthase
- **Rate-limiting enzyme of Cholesterol synthesis:** HMG-CoA reductase

21. Ans. a. Dietary..., b. Occur..., d. Tyrosine...

[Ref: Harrison 19th/434e1-3, 18th/3217-18; Harper 30h/304-306, 28th/254; Lippincott 4th/270-72]

"In patients with ***PKU, tyrosine cannot be synthesized from phenylalanine*** *& therefore, it* ***becomes an essential amino acid*** *that* ***must be supplied in the diet****"-Lippincott 4th/270-*

Treatment: Phenylketonuria

◈ *Harrison 19th/434e1, 18th/3217-18*

- To prevent mental retardation, diagnosis and initiation of dietary treatment of classic phenylketonuria must occur before the child is 3 weeks of age. Abnormal values are confirmed using quantitative analysis of plasma amino acids.
- ***Dietary phenylalanine restriction*** is usually instituted if blood phenylalanine levels are >300 μmol/L (5 mg/dL).
- Treatment consists of a ***special diet low in phenylalanine*** and ***supplemented with tyrosine***, since tyrosine becomes an essential amino acid in ***phenylalanine hydroxylase deficiency.***
- About one-third of all patients with phenylketonuria and the majority of those with milder forms (phenylalanine <1200 μmol/L at presentation) show increased tolerance to dietary proteins and improved metabolic control when treated with tetrahydrobiopterin (5–20 mg/kg per day), an essential cofactor of phenylalanine hydroxylase. This drug should be used in addition to dietary therapy.
- Pregnancy risks can be minimized by continuing lifelong phenylalanine-restricted diets and assuring *strict phenylalanine restriction 2 months prior to conception and throughout gestation.*

Table *(Harrison 19th/434e2-3, 17th/2471-72)*: **Inherited Disorders of Amino Acid Metabolism**

Amino acid	Condition	Enzyme Defect	Clinical Findings
Phenylalanine[Q]	Phenylketonuria type I	Phenylalanine hydroxylase[Q]	Mental retardation[Q], microcephaly[Q], hypopigmented skin and hairs, eczema, "mousy" odor
	Phenylketonuria type II	Dihydropteridine reductase[Q]	Mental retardation, hypotonia, spasticity, myoclonus
	Phenylketonuria type III	6-Pyruvoyl-tetrahydropterin synthase[Q]	Dystonia, neurologic deterioration, seizures, mental retardation

Contd...

22. Ans. c. Fructose, d. Lactose, e. Maltose

[Ref: Lippincott 4th/84-85; Chatterjea & Shinde 7th/31; Satyanarayan 3rd/16]

- **Benedict test** is positive for ***lactose and maltose*** (but not for sucrose as it is a non reducing sugar

"**Inositol** is also called as ***muscle sugar***. Chemically it is hexa hydroxyl cyclohexane" *(Chatterjea & Shinde 7th/190)*

'**Reducing sugars** *can react with chromogenic agents (for e.g,* ***Benedict's reagent*** *or Fehling's solution or Barfoed's test) causing the reagent to be reduced & coloured, with anomeric carbon of the sugar becoming oxidized" (Lippincott 4th/84; Satyanarayan 3rd/16)*

"In **Benedict's test,** reaction of reducing sugar with Benedict's reagent produce ***red colour of cuprous oxide****" (Chatterjea & Shinde 7th/31)*

Benedict's Test for Reducing Sugars

- **Benedict's reagent** is a chemical reagent named after an American chemist, Stanley Rossiter Benedict.
- Benedict's test commonly used for the presence of reducing sugar (s), however other reducing substances also give a positive reaction. This includes ***all monosaccharides and many disaccharides, including lactose and maltose.***
- Even more generally, Benedict's test will detect the presence of aldehydes and alpha-hydroxy-ketones, including those that occur in certain ketoses. Thus, although the ketose fructose is not strictly a reducing sugar, it is an alpha-hydroxy-ketone and gives a positive test because it is converted to the aldoses glucose and mannose by the base in the reagent

What Is a Reducing Sugar?

- Sugars are classified as **reducing** or **non-reducing** based on their ability to act as a reducing agent during the Benedict's Test. A reducing agent donates electrons during a redox reaction and is itself oxidized.
- The **aldehyde functional group** is the reducing agent in reducing sugars. Reducing sugars have either an aldehyde functional group or have a ketone group -in an open chain form -which can be converted into an aldehyde.
- Reducing sugars are **simple sugars** and include all monosaccharides and most disaccarides. Some examples of monosaccharides are glucose, fructose and galactose. Examples of reducing disaccharides are ***lactose and maltose.***

23. Ans. a. Vitamin a...., b. High..., c. Vitamin e..., e. Banana...

[Ref: Harrison 19th/96e1-7, 18th/599; Harper 30th/547-62, 28th/471-78; Lippincott 4th/374]

"**Vit. C toxicity: Oxalate kidney stones** are of theoretic concern because ascorbic acid is metabolized to oxalate, but stone formation has not been frequently reported"*(CMDT06/1275)*

"**Prophylaxis against xerophthalmia**: *Lactating mothers should be given 20, 000 IU orally once at delivery or during the next 2 months. This will raise the concentration of vitamin A in the breast milk & therefore, help **to protect the breastfed infant**" (Khurana 5th/466)*

"Folic acid deficiency cause *megaloblastic anaemia (macrocytic)*"*(Lippincott 4th/374)*

"Vit. E *reduces the risk of atherosclerosis*" *(Vasudevan 5th/291)*

"Banana: It is a very good source of **vitamin-B6** (pyridoxine), provides about 28% of daily-recommended allowance"-*http: // www. nutrition-and-you.com/banana-fruit.html*

Table *(http: //www.whfoods.com/)*: **Banana, fresh1.00 medium, 118.00 grams, Calories: 105**

Nutrient	Amount	DRI/DV (%)	World's Healthiest Foods Rating
Vitamin B6	0.43 mg	25	Very good
Manganese	0.32 mg	16	Good
Vitamin C	10.27 mg	14	Good
Fiber	3.07 g	12	Good
Potassium	422.44 mg	12	Good
Biotin	3.07 mcg	10	Good
Copper	0.09 mg	10	Good

Toxicity of Vitamin C

◈ *Harrison 19th/96e5, 18th/599*

- Since vitamin C may be metabolized to oxalate, it is feared that chronic high-dose Vitamin C supplementation could result in an increased prevalence of ***kidney stones.***
- However, this has not been borne out in several trials, except in patients with preexisting renal disease. Thus, *it is reasonable to advise patients with a past history of kidney stones not to take large doses of vitamin C.*

24. Ans. a. Transketolase, b. Pyruvate...

[Ref: Harper 30th/555, 28th/52; Chatterjea & Shinde 7th/166-67]

"NAD+ (by vitamin B 3) acts as coenzyme for alcohol dehydrogenase"*(Chatterjea & Shinde 7th/171)*

"Pyridoxal phosphate (by vitamin pyridoxine, B6) acts as coenzyme for transaminases like aminotransferase" *(Chatterjea & Shinde 7th/173)*

Thiamine (Vitamin B_1)

- Biologically active form is thiamine pyrophosphate (TPP)
- TPP acts as coenzyme in: Pyruvate dehydrogenase (oxidative decarboxylation), α-oxoglutarate dehydrogenase complex (oxidative decarboxylation), ***transketolase (transketolation reaction), tryptophan pyrrolase, pyruvate carboxylase*** (non-oxidative decarboxylation) *(Chatterjea & Shinde 7th/166-67)*

25. Ans. b. Polyneuropathy, e. Cardiomegaly

[Ref: Harrison 19th/96e-3, 18th/594-96; Harper 30th/555-56, 28th/468]

Thiamine Deficiency

◈ *Harrison 19th/96e-3, 18th/595-96*

- Thiamine deficiency in its early stage induces anorexia and nonspecific symptoms (*e.g.*, irritability, decrease in short-term memory). Prolonged thiamine deficiency causes beriberi, which is classically categorized as wet or dry, although there is considerable overlap. In either form of beriberi, patients may complain of pain and paresthesia.
- *Wet beriberi* presents primarily with cardiovascular symptoms, due to impaired myocardial energy metabolism and dysautonomia and can occur after 3 months of a thiamine-deficient diet. Patients present with an ***enlarged heart, tachycardia, high-output congestive heart failure, peripheral edema and peripheral neuritis.***
- Patients with *dry beriberi* present with a ***symmetric peripheral neuropathy of the motor and sensory systems with diminished reflexes***. The neuropathy affects the legs most markedly and these patients have difficulty rising from a squatting position.
- Alcoholic patients with chronic thiamine deficiency also may have central nervous system (CNS) manifestations known as *Wernicke's encephalopathy*, ***consisting of horizontal nystagmus, ophthalmoplegia (due to weakness of one or more extraocular muscles), cerebellar ataxia and mental impairment***. When there is an additional loss of memory and a confabulatory psychosis, the syndrome is known as ***Wernicke-Korsakoff syndrome***. Despite the typical clinical picture and history, Wernicke-Korsakoff syndrome is underdiagnosed.

Table *(Harrison 19th/96e-1)*: **Principal Clinical Findings of Vitamin Malnutrition**

Nutrient	Clinical Finding	Contributing Factors to Deficiency
Thiamine	**Beriberi:** Neuropathy, muscle weakness and wasting, cardiomegaly, edema, ophthalmoplegia, confabulation	Alcoholism, chronic diuretic use, hyperemesis
Riboflavin (B_2)	Magenta tongue (***Painful glossitis***[Q], the tongue assuming a red purple colour-Chatterjea & Shinde 7th/169), angular stomatitis, seborrhea, cheilosis	—

Contd...

Nutrient	Clinical Finding	Contributing Factors to Deficiency
Niacin	**Pellagra:** Pigmented rash of sun-exposed areas, bright red tongue, diarrhea, apathy, memory loss, disorientation	Alcoholism, vitamin B_6 deficiency, riboflavin deficiency, tryptophan deficiency
Vitamin B6	Seborrhea, glossitis convulsions, neuropathy, depression, confusion, microcytic anemia	Alcoholism, isoniazid
Folate	Megaloblastic anemia, atrophic glossitis, depression, ↑homocysteine	Alcoholism, sulfasalazine, pyrimethamine, triamterene
Vitamin B12	Megaloblastic anemia, loss of vibratory and position sense, abnormal gait, dementia, impotence, loss of bladder and bowel control, ↑homocysteine, ↑methylmalonic acid	Gastric atrophy (pernicious anemia), terminal ileal disease, strict vegetarianism, acid reducing drugs (*e.g.,* H2 blockers)
Vitamin C	**Scurvy:** Petechiae, ecchymosis, coiled hairs, inflamed and bleeding gums, joint effusion, poor wound healing, fatigue	Smoking, alcoholism
Vitamin A	Xerophthalmia, nightblindness, Bitot's spots, follicular hyperkeratosis, impaired embryonic development, immune dysfunction	Fat malabsorption, infection, measles, alcoholism, protein-energy malnutrition
Vitamin D	**Rickets:** Skeletal deformation, rachitic rosary, bowed legs; osteomalacia	Aging, lack of sunlight exposure, fat malabsorption, deeply pigmented skin
Vitamin E	Peripheral neuropathy, spinocerebellar ataxia, skeletal muscle atrophy, retinopathy	Occurs only with fat malabsorption, or genetic abnormalities of vitamin E metabolism/transport
Vitamin K	Elevated prothrombin time, bleeding	Fat malabsorption, liver disease, antibiotic use

26. Ans. a. Confabulation, b. Retrograde, c. Optha...

[Ref: Harrison 19th/96e-3, 18th/597, 2260;Harper 30th/556, 28th/473; Lippincott 4th/129-34; Kaplan & Saddock's Synopsis of Psychiatry 10th/345-50; Ahuja 6th/41-42]

Note: As Q is specially asking about korsakoff psychosis (not Wernicke-Korsakoff syndrome), so answer should not include ophthalmoplegia

Korsakoff 's Syndrome

"Because the ***chronic memory loss*** of **Korsakoff syndrome** often follows an episode of Wernicke encephalopathy, the chronic disorder is sometimes known as Wernicke-Korsakoff syndrome. ***But Korsakoff syndrome can also develop in individuals who have not had a prior episode of Wernicke encephalopathy***. http: //www.alz.org/dementia.

There are Six Major Symptoms of Korsakoff's Syndrome

◈ *http: //en. wikipedia.org /wiki*

- ***Anterograde amnesia:*** *Inability to form new memories*
- ***Retrograde amnesia:*** *Severe loss of memories formed before the onset of the condition*
- ***Confabulation:*** *That is, invented memories which are then taken as true due to gaps in memory sometimes associated with blackouts*
- *Minimal content in conversation*
- *Lack of insight*
- ***Apathy:*** *The patients lose interest in things quickly and generally appear indifferent to change.*

"Alcoholic patients with chronic thiamine deficiency also may have central nervous system (CNS) manifestations known as *Wernicke's encephalopathy*, consisting of horizontal nystagmus, ophthalmoplegia (due to weakness of one or more extraocular muscles), cerebellar ataxia and mental impairment. ***When there is an additional loss of memory and a confabulatory psychosis***, the syndrome is known as ***Wernicke-Korsakoff syndrome***. Despite the typical clinical picture and history, Wernicke-Korsakoff syndrome is underdiagnosed" *(Harrison 19th/96e-3, 18th/597)*

Wernicke's Encephalopathy

◈ *Robbins 9th/1304, 8th/1328*

- *Thiamine (vitamin B_1) deficiency* causes Wernicke's encephalopathy
- With time, there is infiltration of macrophages and development of a cystic space with hemosiderin-laden macrophages as a permanent sign of the process. These chronic hemosiderin-laden lesions predominate in patients with ***Korsakoff syndrome.***
- Lesions in the medial dorsal nucleus of the ***thalamus*** appear to be the best correlate of the memory disturbance and confabulation.
- **Ocular motor abnormalities** include horizontal nystagmus on lateral gaze, lateral rectus palsy (usually bilateral), conjugate gaze palsies and rarely ptosis.
- **Gait ataxia** probably results from a combination of polyneuropathy, cerebellar involvement and vestibular paresis. The pupils are usually spared, but they may become miotic with advanced disease.
- As these symptoms recede, an amnestic state with impairment in recent memory and learning may become more apparent (*Korsakoff's psychosis*). ***Korsakoff's psychosis is frequently persistent; the residual mental state is characterized by gaps in memory, confabulation and disordered temporal sequencing.***
- Without treatment patient may develop korsakoff psychosis

Note: Wernicke's Disease[Q]: The characteristic clinical triad is that of ophthalmoplegia, ataxia and global confusion

27. **Ans.** **d. Pompe's..., e. McArdles...**

[Ref: Harper 30th/179, 28th/160; Lippincott 4th/129-34]

"Niemann-Pick disease, Tay-sachs disease & Gaucher's disease are lysosomal storage diseases"

Table *(Harper 30th/179, 28th/160)*: **Glycogen Storage Diseases.**

Type	Name	Enzyme Deficiency	Clinical Features
0	–	Glycogen synthase	Hypoglycemia; hyperketonemia; early death
I	Von Gierke disease	Glucose 6-phosphatase	Glycogen accumulation in liver and renal tubule cells; hypoglycemia; lactic acidemia; ketosis; hyperlipemia
II	Pompe disease	Lysosomal α1→4 and α1→6 glucosidase (acid maltase)	**Accumulation of glycogen in lysosomes:** Juvenile onset variant, muscle hypotonia, death from heart failure by age 2; adult onset variant, muscle dystrophy
III	Limit dextrinosis, Forbe's or Cori's disease	Debranching enzyme	Fasting hypoglycemia; hepatomegaly in infancy; accumulation of characteristic branched polysaccharide
IV	Amylopectinosis andersen's disease	Branching enzyme	Hepatosplenomegaly; accumulation of polysaccharide with few branch points; death from heart or liver failure in first year of life
V	Myophosphorylase deficiency, McArdle's syndrome	Muscle phosphorylase	Poor exercise tolerance; muscle glycogen abnormally high (2.5–4%); blood lactate very low after exercise
VI	Hers' disease	Liver phosphorylase	Hepatomegaly; accumulation of glycogen in liver; mild hypoglycemia; generally good prognosis
VII	Tarui's disease	Muscle and erythrocyte phosphofructokinase 1	Poor exercise tolerance; muscle glycogen abnormally high (2.5–4%); blood lactate very low after exercise; also hemolytic anemia
VIII	–	Liver phosphorylase kinase	Hepatomegaly; accumulation of glycogen in liver; mild hypoglycemia; generally good prognosis
IX	–	Liver and muscle phosphorylase kinase	Hepatomegaly; accumulation of glycogen in liver and muscle; mild hypoglycemia; generally good prognosis
X	–	cAMP-dependent protein kinase A	Hepatomegaly; accumulation of glycogen in liver

Table *(Harrison 19th/432e 2-3-Partial list)*: **Selected Lysosomal Storage Diseases**

Clinical Features										
Disorder[a]	Enzyme Deficiency (Specific Therapy)	Stored Material	Clinical Types (Onset)	Inheritance	Neurologic	Liver Spleen Enlargement	Skeletal Dysplasia	Ophthalmologic	Hematologic	Unique Features
Tay-Sachs disease	β Hexo-saminidase A	GM_2 gangliosides	Infantile Juvenile	AR	Mental retardation, seizures, later juvenile form	None	None	Cherry red spot in infantile form	None	Macrocephaly, hyperacusis in infantile form
Gaucher disease	Acid β-glucosidase (ET, SRT)	Gluco-sylcer-amide	Type 1 Type 2 Type 3	AR	None ++++ ++	++++ +++ ++++	++++ + ++++	None Eye,movements Eye movements	Gaucher cells in bone marrow, cytopenias	Adult form highly variable
Pompe disease	Acid α-glucosidase (ET)	Glycogen	Infantile late onset	AR	Neuro-muscular	±	None	None	None	Myocardiopathy

A & E

IMMUNOGENETICS & MOLECULAR BIOLOGY

28. Ans. a. It is..., b. Measured..., c. It occurs...

[Ref: Harper 30th/361, 28th/303; Satyanarayan 3rd/78; Lippincott 4th/397-98]

Hyperchromicity

◈ *Satyanarayan 3rd/78*

- It is the increase of absorbance (*optical density*) of a material. The most famous example is the hyperchromicity of DNA that occurs when the ***DNA duplex is denatured.***
- *"At a* **wavelength of 260 nm,** ***ssDNA has a higher relative absorbance than does double stranded DNA"*** *(Lippincott 4th/397-98)*
- The UV absorption is increased when the two single DNA strands are being separated, either by heat or by addition of denaturant or by increasing the pH level.
- The phosphodiester bonds are not broken by denaturation
- Loss of helical structure can be measured by increase in absorbance at 260 nm (in a spectrophotometer)
- The opposite, a decrease of absorbance is called **hypochromicity**
- Melting temperature (Tm) is defined as temperature at which half of the helical structure of DNA is lost
- **Renaturation (reannealing) is the process in which the separated complementary DNA strands can form a double helix**

The Denaturation (Melting) of DNA Is Used to Analyze Its Structure

◈ *Harper 30th/361, 28th/303*

- The double-stranded structure of DNA can be separated into two component strands (melted) in solution by increasing the temperature or decreasing the salt concentration. Not only do the two stacks of bases pull apart but the bases themselves unstack while still connected in the polymer by the phosphodiester backbone.
- Concomitant with this **denaturation of the DNA molecule** is an increase in the optical absorbance of the purine and pyrimidine bases—a phenomenon referred to as **hyperchromicity** of denaturation.

29. Ans. d. No role... ...

[Ref: Harper 30th/438; Harrison 19th/101e-4, 18th/668, 679; Robbins 9th/319-20, 893, 8th /306; Satyanarayan 3rd/359, 572; Lippincott 4th/460-62; Chatterjea & Shinde 7th/346, 426;en. wikipedia. org/wiki/ DNA_methylation]

"**Cytosine** in the sequence CG of DNA gets ***methylated to form 5'-methylcytosine.*** A major portion of CG (about 20%) in human DNA exists in methylated form. In general, methylation leads to loss of transcriptional activity & thus inactivation of genes" *(Satyanarayan 3rd/572)*

Genes & Epigenetic Changes: *Writes: Harrison 19th/101e-4, 18th/667-68*

- Gene silencing, an epigenetic change that leads to the loss of gene expression and occurs in conjunction with hypermethylation of the promoter and histone deacetylation, is another mechanism of tumor-suppressor gene inactivation.
- The preferential expression of a particular gene exclusively from the allele contributed by one parent is called parental imprinting and is thought to be regulated by covalent modifications of chromatin protein and DNA (often methylation) of the silenced allele.
- The role of epigenetic control mechanisms in the development of human cancer is unclear. However, a general decrease in the level of DNA methylation has been noted as a common change in cancer. In addition, numerous genes, including some tumor-suppressor genes, appear to become hypermethylated and silenced during tumorigenesis.
- Efforts are also under way to reverse the hypermethylation of CpG islands that characterizes many solid tumors.
- Drugs that induce DNA demethylation, such as 5-aza-2'-deoxycytidine, can lead to reexpression of silenced genes in cancer cells with restoration of function. However, 5-aza-2'-deoxycytidine has limited aqueous solubility and is myelosuppressive. Other inhibitors of DNA methyltransferases are in development. In ongoing clinical trials, inhibitors of DNA methylation are being combined with HDAC inhibitors. The hope is that by reversing coexisting epigenetic changes, the deregulated patterns of gene transcription in cancer cells will be at least partially reversed.

DNA Methylation Mechanism

◈ *en.wikipedia.org/wiki/DNA_methylation*

- After every cycle of DNA replication, several modifications occur in the DNA. *DNA methylation is one such post-synthesis modification.* DNA methylation has been proven by research to be manifested in a number of biological processes such as regulation of ***imprinted genes, X chromosome inactivation and tumor suppressor gene silencing in cancerous cells.***
- It also acts as a protection mechanism adopted by the pathogen DNA (mainly bacterial against the endonuclease activity that destroys any foreign DNA.)
- In ***DNA, methylation usually occurs in the CpG islands,*** a CG rich region, upstream of the promoter region. In humans, DNA methylation is carried out by a group of enzymes called ***DNA methyltransferases.***
- DNA methylation stably ***alters the gene expression pattern in cells*** such that cells can "remember where they have been" or decrease gene expression
- DNA methylation is ***essential for normal development*** and is associated with a number of key processes including genomic imprinting, X-chromosome inactivation, suppression of repetitive elements and carcinogenesis.

- Research has suggested that long-term memory storage in humans may be regulated by DNA methylation
- **Adenine *or* cytosine *methylation is part of the* restriction modification system *of many* bacteria,** in which specific DNA sequences are methylated periodically throughout the genome. Foreign DNAs (which are not methylated in this manner) that are introduced into the cell are degraded by sequence-specific restriction enzymes and cleaved.
- Within the bacterium, ***methylation protects the host DNA from cleavage by its own restriction enzyme. Unmethylated foreign DNA is not protected from cleavage.***

30. Ans. a. None..

[Ref: Harper 30th/438-39, 735, 28th/623, 344; Harrison 19th/101e-4, 18th /667-68; Robbins 9th/319-20, 8th /180-81, 307-08]

Epigenetic

"**Epigenetics** *is defined as the study of* **heritable** *chemical modification of DNA or chromatin that does not alter the DNA sequence itself. Example of such modification include the methylation of DNA & the methylation & acetylation of histones. Epigenetic modification is critical for normal development including-regulation of tissue specific gene expression,* ***X-chromosome inactivation*** *& genomic imprinting"* (Robbins 9th/319, 8th /180)

"An *epigenetic modification* refers to a change in the genome, ***heritable by cell progeny***, that does not involve a change in the DNA sequence. The ***inactivation of the second X chromosome*** in female cells is an example of an epigenetic silencing that prevents gene expression from the inactivated chromosome" *(Harrison 19th/101e-4, 18th /667-68)*

"There is also evidence that epigenetic mechanism (e.g, ***methylation/demethylation of cytosine in specific genes & acetylation of histones H3 & H4 affecting gene transcription)*** *may play a role in carcinogenesis. One area of interest regarding such changes are that they are potentially reversible"* (Harper 30th/735, 28th/623)

Epigenetic Influences on Cancer Gene Transcription

◈ *Harrison19th/102e-7, 18th/679*

- *Epigenetics* is defined as changes that alter the pattern of gene expression that *persist across at least one cell division but are not caused by changes in the DNA code.*
- Epigenetic changes **include** alterations of chromatin structure mediated by methylation of cytosine residues in CpG dinucleotides, modification of histones by acetylation or methylation, or changes in higher-order chromosome structure
- The transcriptional regulatory regions of active genes often contain a high frequency of CpG dinucleotides (referred to as *CpG islands*), which are normally unmethylated. Expression of these genes is controlled by transient association with repressor or activator proteins that regulate transcriptional activation.
- However, hypermethylation of promoter regions is a common mechanism by which ***tumor-suppressor loci are epigenetically silenced in cancer cells.***

31. Ans. a. Homologus..., b. Non-homologous..., c. Homologous..., e. Non-homologous...

[Ref: Harper 30th/389-91, Satyanarayan3rd/532; Robbins 9th/430-31, 8th /302; http: www.ncbi.nlm. nih.gov/pubmed/20192759]

"*Non-homologous end joining* (NHEJ) is the predominant type of DSB repair in mammalian cells, as opposed to lower eukaryotes"-*http: //www.nature.com/onc/journal*

DNA Double-strand Breaks Repair

◈ *Satyanarayan3rd/538*

- DSB in DNA are dangerous
- *They result in genetic recombination which may lead to chromosomal translocation, broken chromosome & finally cell death*
- *DSBs can be repaired by homologous recombination or non-homologous end joining*
- ***Homologous recombination occurs in yeasts while in mammals, non-homologous end joining dominates***

Double-Strand Breaks Repair Mechanism

◈ *http: //www.nature.com/onc/journal; http: //www.ncbi.nlm.nih.gov/pubmed/20192759*

- Double-strand breaks can be repaired through ***homologous recombination or through non-homologous end joining (NHEJ).***
- NHEJ is a DNA repair mechanism which, unlike homologous recombination, ***does not require a long homologous sequence to guide repair.***
- Whether homologous recombination or NHEJ is used to repair double-strand breaks is largely determined by the phase of cell cycle. ***Homologous recombination repairs DNA before the cell enters mitosis (M phase).***
- **DNA double-strand breaks** (DSB) are presumed to be the most deleterious DNA lesions as they disrupt both DNA strands.
- ***Homologous recombination (HR), single-strand annealing and non-homologous end-joining are considered to be the pathways for repairing DSB.***

32. Ans. b. Haplotype

[Ref: Harrison 19th/435, 18th /497, 505; Robbins 9th/195, 8th/177]

"The entire human genome now can be divided into blocks known as **haplotypes**, *which contain varying numbers of contiguous single nucleotide polymorphisms on the same chromosome that are in* ***linkage disequilibrium & hence inherited together as a cluster****"*-(Robbins 8th /177)

Haplotype

◈ *Harrison 19th/435, 18th /497*

- A *haplotype* refers to a ***group of alleles that are closely linked together at a genomic locus.***
- Haplotypes are useful for tracking the transmission of genomic segments within families and for detecting evidence of genetic recombination, if the crossover event occurs between the alleles.

- The presence or absence of certain haplotypes may also become relevant for the customized choice of medical therapies (pharmacogenomics) or for preventive strategies.

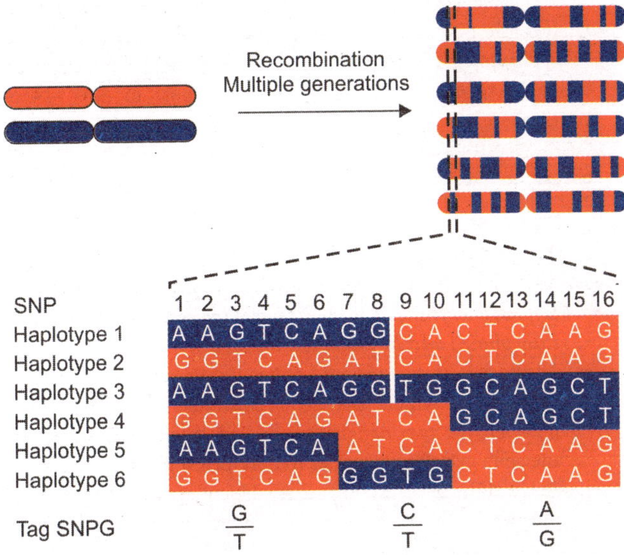

Fig: The origin of haplotypes is due to repeated recombination events occurring in multiple generations. Over time, this leads to distinct haplotypes. These haplotype blocks can often be characterized by genotyping selected Tag single-nucleotide polymorphisms, an approach that now facilitates performing genome-wide association studies (GWAS).

Genotypes and Phenotypes

◈ *Harrison 19th/435, 18th /497*

- An observed trait is referred to as a *phenotype*; the genetic information defining the phenotype is called the *genotype*.
- Alternative forms of a gene or a genetic marker are referred to as *alleles*.
- The normal or common allele is usually referred to as *wild type*.
- Genotypes describe the specific alleles at a particular locus.

"In immunology, an **idiotype** is a shared characteristic between a group of immunoglobulin or T cell receptor (TCR) molecules based upon the antigen binding specificity and therefore structure of their variable region. Idiotype describes the distinctive sequence and region that makes any immunoglobulin/TCR unique from others of the same type which is its variable region"-*wikipedia*

33. Ans. b. 2-6 bp...

[Ref: Harper 30th/377-78, 28th/319, 404]

"Microsatellite repeat sequences: Dispersed or group repeat sequences of 2–5 bp repeated up to 50 times. May occur at 50000–100000 locations in the genome"-*Harper 30th/377-78, 28th/404*

Microsatellite DNA Polymorphisms

◈ *Harper 30th/463, 28th/319*

- Short (*2–6 bp*), inherited, tandem repeat units of DNA occur about 50, 000–100, 000 times in the human genome.
- Because they occur more frequently—and in view of the routine application of sensitive PCR methods—they are replacing RFLPs as the marker loci for various genome searches.

PATHOLOGY

34. Ans. b. Mutation..., c. Pancr... d. Cerebellar...

[Ref: Robbins 9th/1317, 8th/1343; Harrison 18th/3384, 2051, 3078]

Von Hippel-Lindau Disease

◈ *Robbins 9th/1317, 8th/1343*

- This is an autosomal-dominant disease in which affected individuals develop tumors (capillary hemangioblastomas) within the ***cerebellar hemispheres, the retina and, less commonly, the brainstem and spinal cord***.
- Patients may also have **cysts** involving the ***pancreas, liver and kidneys and have a propensity to develop renal cell carcinoma of the kidney***
- The gene for von Hippel-Lindau disease, a tumor-suppressor gene, is located on **chromosome 3p25-26** and encodes a protein (pVHL) that appears to play a role in regulating several aspects of cellular function. The protein can serve as a component of a complex that functions in the ubiquitination pathway, contributing to protein degradation.
- The ***cerebellar capillary hemangioblastoma,*** the principal neurologic manifestation of the disease, is a highly vascular neoplasm that occurs as a mural nodule associated with a large fluid-filled cyst.
- Therapy is directed at the symptomatic neoplasms, including resection of the cerebellar hemangioblastomas and laser therapy for retinal hemangioblastomas. Partial nephrectomy is performed for renal carcinomas when these malignant neoplasms are bilateral.

Table *(Harrison 19th/599, 18th/3384)*: **Genetic Syndromes Associated with Primary Brain Tumors**

Syndrome	Inheritance	Gene/ Protein	Associated Tumors
Von Hippel–Lindau (VHL)	AD	Mutations in VHL gene	Hemangioblastomas Retinal angiomas, renal cell carcinoma, pheochromocytoma, pancreatic tumors and cysts, endolymphatic sac tumors of the middle ear

35. Ans. a. Autosomal...

[Ref: Harrison 19th/375e-2, 18th/970, 2477-78, e 39-2; emedicine.medscape.com/article]

Hermansky–Pudlak syndrome (HPS)

◈ *emedicine.medscape.com/article*

- It is a rare **autosomal recessive** disorder which results in **oculocutaneous albinism** (decreased pigmentation), bleeding problems due to a **platelet *abnormality*** (platelet storage pool defect) and storage of an abnormal fat-protein compound (lysosomal accumulation of ceroid lipofuscin).
- There are ***eight classic forms of*** the disorder, based on the genetic mutation from which the disorder stems.[3] A ninth type has also been described. This last type is due to a mutation in the gene Pallidin (PLDN).
- The course of HPS has been mild in rare instances of the disorder, however, the general prognosis is still considered to be poor.
- The disease can cause dysfunctions of the lungs, intestine, kidneys or heart. The major complication of most forms of the disorder is ***pulmonary fibrosis***
- The diagnosis of HPS is established by clinical findings of hypopigmentation of the skin and hair, characteristic eye findings and demonstration of absent dense bodies on whole mount electron microscopy of platelets.

Primary Immunodeficiencies Affecting Regulatory Pathways

◈ *Harrison 19th/375e-2, 18th/e 39-2*

- Several inherited disorders that lead to hemophagocytic lymphohistiocytosis (HLH) also have features that are important in terms of both diagnosis and prognosis. Three of these disorders—Griscelli syndrome, Chédiak-Higashi syndrome and the **Hermansky-Pudlak type II syndrome**—are characterized by partial albinism and silvery hair appearance that can facilitate diagnosis.
- Hermansky-Pudlak type II also can be a ***bleeding disorder*** if platelet aggregation is defective.

Table *(Harrison 18th/2478)*: **Primary Genetic Disorders Associated with Inflammatory bowel disease- Partial list**

Name	Genetic Association	Phenotype
Hermansky-Pudlak	Autosomal recessive chromosome 10q23	Granulomatous colitis, oculocutaneous albinism, platelet dysfunction, pulmonary fibrosis

36. Ans. a. G0...

[Ref: Robbins 9th/25, 8th/86-87;KDT 7th/875;Abeloff's Clinical Oncology 4th/428; Harrison 19th/427, 18th/673, Harrison 17th/516]

"The cell cycle consists of G_1 (presynthetic), *S* (DNA synthesis), G_2 (premitotic) and *M* (mitotic) phases. ***Quiescent cells are in a physiologic state called G_0***. Tissues may be composed primarily of quiescent cells in G_0, but most mature tissues contain some combination of continuously dividing cells, terminally differentiated cells, stem cells and quiescent cells that occasionally enter into the cell cycle" *(Abeloff's Clinical Oncology 4th/428)*

Phases of Cell Cycle

- The cell cycle consists of **four distinct phases**: ***G_1 phase, S phase (synthesis***[Q]***), G_2 phase (collectively known as interphase) and M phase (mitosis)***[Q].
- **M phase** is itself composed of two tightly coupled processes: ***mitosis***, in which the cell's chromosomes are divided between the two daughter cells and ***cytokinesis***, in which the cell's cytoplasm divides in half forming distinct cells.
- Activation of each phase is dependent on the proper progression and completion of the previous one. **Cells that have temporarily or reversibly stopped dividing are said to have entered a state of *quiescence* called G_0 *phase***[Q].

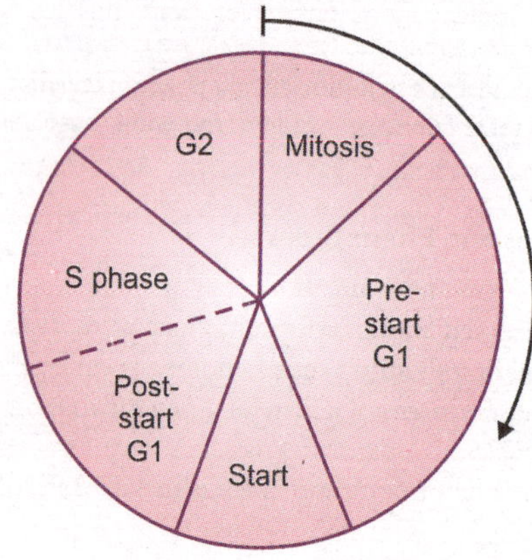

Fig: Sequence of events during the cell cycle

S Phase

- The ensuing ***S phase starts when DNA synthesis commences***[Q]; when it is complete, all of the chromosomes have been replicated, *i.e.*, each chromosome has two (sister) chromatids.
- During this phase, the amount of DNA in the cell has effectively doubled, though the ploidy of the cell remains the same.

State	Phase	Abbreviation	Description
Quiescent/ senescent	Gap 0	G0	A resting phase where the cell has left the cycle and has *stopped dividing*.
Interphase	Gap 1	G1	Cells increase in size in Gap 1. The G_1 *checkpoint* control mechanism ensures that everything is ready for DNA synthesis.

Contd...

State	Phase	Abbreviation	Description
	Synthesis	S	***DNA replication***[Q] occurs during this phase.
	Gap 2	G2	During the gap between DNA synthesis and mitosis, the cell will continue to grow. The G_2 checkpoint control mechanism ensures that everything is ready to enter the M (mitosis) phase and divide.
Cell division	Mitosis	M	Cell growth stops at this stage and cellular energy is focused on the orderly ***division into two daughter cells.*** A checkpoint in the middle of mitosis *(Metaphase Checkpoint)* ensures that the cell is ready to complete cell division.

37. Ans. b. Inhibition..., e. Association...

[Ref: Robbins 9th/40, 52-58, 8th/25-32, 13; Harrison 19th/85e-8, 18th/680, 2678-79]

Apoptosis	Intrinsic pathway/Phase (Mitochondrial pathway)	Cytochrome C, Apaf-1, AIF, Caspase9
	Extrinsic pathway/Phase (Death receptor initiated pathway)	TNF-Receptor-1, Fas (CD95), Caspase 8
	Execution phase	Caspases 3, 6, 7

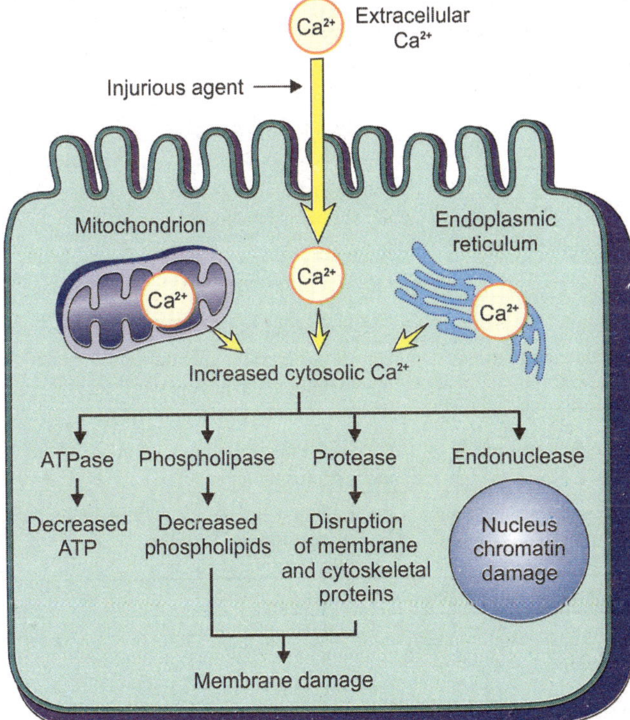

Fig: Sources and consequences of increased cytosolic calcium in cell injury

Apoptosis

- *"Condensation of chromatin, membrane bleb & cellular fragmentation takes place in apoptosis"-Robbins 9th/41, 8th/13*
- *"The **apoptotic cell** exhibit a characteristic breakdown of DNA into large 50-to 300-Kb pieces. Subsequently, there is **internucleosomal cleavage** of DNA into oligonucleosomes by Ca^{2+} & Mg^{2+} dependent **endonucleases**"-Robbins 7th/27*
- *"The **fundamental event in apoptosis** is the activation of enzymes called **Caspases** which are cysteine proteases involved in apoptosis by initiating apoptotic signals (via intrinsic or extrinsic pathway) & executing apoptotic program (via execution phase)"*
- The process of **apoptosis** is often accompanied by generation of reactive oxygen species, which bring about rapid ***oxidation of the fatty acids in phosphatidylserine*** before this lipid is externalized.
- Indeed, it is now apparent that only molecular species of ***phosphatidylserine*** with an oxidatively truncated *sn*-2 acyl group that incorporates terminal γ-hydroxy (or oxo)-α, β-unsaturated acyl moieties are recognized by scavenger receptors in macrophages as ***a prerequisite for engulfment of apoptotic cells.***

Table *(Robbins 9th/40, 8th/13)*: **Features of Necrosis and Apoptosis**

Feature	Necrosis	Apoptosis
Cell size	Enlarged (swelling)	Reduced (shrinkage)
Nucelus	Pyknosis → karyorrhexis → karyolysis	Fragmentation into nucleosome size fragments
Plasma membrane	Disrupted	Intact; altered structure, especially orientation of lipids
Cellular contents	Enzymatic digestion; may leak out of cell	Intact; may be released in apoptotic bodies
Adjacent inflammation	Frequent	No
Physiologic or pathologic role	Invariably pathologic (culmination of irreversible cell injury)	Often physiologic, means of eliminating unwanted cells; may be pathologic after some forms of cell injury, especially DNA damage

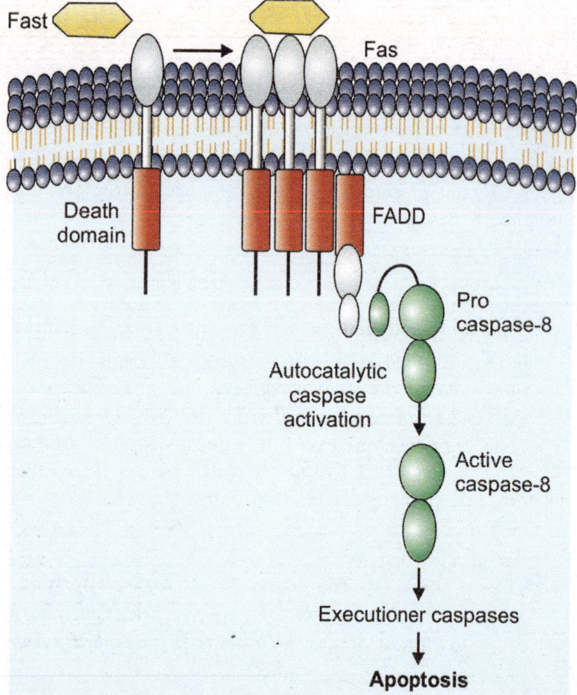

Fig: Extrinsic Pathway of Apoptosis

38. Ans. c. Transmit...

[Ref: Robbins 9t h/168, 171-72, 8th/171, 167;Harrison 19th/85e-6, 17th / Part 18 e-39; en.wikipedia. org/wiki]

Single-Gene Disorders with Nonclassic Inheritance

◈ *Robbins 9th/168, 8th/167*

It has become increasingly evident that transmission of certain single-gene disorders does not follow classic mendelian principles. This group of disorders can be classified into four categories:

- *Diseases caused by triplet-repeat mutations*
- ***Disorders caused by mutations in mitochondrial genes***
- *Disorders associated with genomic imprinting*
- *Disorders associated with gonadal mosaicism*

Mitochondria DNA

◈ *Harrison 17th /Part 18 e-39*

- The DNA sequence of mtDNA has been determined from a large number of organisms and individuals (including some organisms that are extinct) and the comparison of those DNA sequences represents a mainstay of phylogenetics, in that it allows biologists to elucidate the evolutionary relationships among species.
- ***Mothers transmit their mtDNA to both their sons and daughters,*** only the daughters are able to transmit the inherited mtDNA to future generations (***Maternal inheritance)***
- ***High somatic mtDNA mutation*** rate and the global effect on mitochondrial function counterbalance the reduced impact of the multiple copy number of each individual mtDNA mutation.
- This mtDNA sequence contains a total of ***37 genes, of which 13 encode mitochondrial protein components of the ETC. The remaining 22 tRNA-and 2 rRNA-encoding genes are dedicated to the process of translation of the 13 mtDNA-encoded proteins.***
- The accumulation of functional ***mtDNA deletions*** in a given tissue is expected to be associated with mitochondrial dysfunction, as reflected in an age-associated patchy and reduced cytochrome-c oxidase activity upon histochemical staining, especially in skeletal and cardiac muscle and brain.

Table *(Harrison 19th/85e-6, 17th /Part 18 e-39)*: **Mitochondrial Diseases Due to mtDNA Point Mutations and Large-Scale Rearrangements**

Disease	Phenotype
Leber hereditary optic neuropathy (LHON)	Loss of central vision leading to blindness in young adult life
NARP, Leigh's disease	Neuropathy, ataxia, retinitis pigmentosa, developmental delay, mental retardation, lactic acidemia
MELAS	Mitochondrial encephalomyopathy, lactic acidosis and stroke-like episodes; may manifest only as diabetes
MERRF	Myoclonic epilepsy, ragged red fibers in muscle, ataxia, increased CSF protein, sensorineural deafness, dementia
Deafness	Progressive sensorineural deafness, often induced by aminoglycoside antibiotics.
	Nonsyndromic sensorineural deafness
Chronic progressive external ophthalmoplegia (PEO)	Late-onset bilateral ptosis and ophthalmoplegia, proximal muscle weakness and exercise intolerance
Pearson syndrome	Pancreatic insufficiency, pancytopenia, lactic acidosis
Kearn-Sayre syndrome (KSS)	External ophthalmoplegia, heart-block, retinal pigmentation, ataxia

39. Ans. d. Increased..., e. Hemosiderinuria...

[Ref: Robbins 9th/631, 8th/641-42; Harrison 19th/649, 18th/881-83; CMDT06/490]

Intravascular Hemolysis

- Whatever the mechanism, intravascular hemolysis is manifested by (1) hemoglobinemia, (2) hemoglobinuria, (3) jaundice and (4) ***hemosiderinuria.***
- Free hemoglobin in plasma is promptly bound by an α_2-globulin (haptoglobin), producing a complex that is rapidly cleared by the mononuclear phagocyte system, thus preventing excretion into the urine. ***Decreased serum haptoglobin is characteristic of intravascular hemolysis.***
- When the liver is normal, jaundice is rarely severe. Excessive bilirubin excreted by the liver into the gastrointestinal tract leads to ***increased formation and fecal excretion of urobilin***

Hemolytic Anaemia

- The physiologic destruction of senescent red cells takes place within the mononuclear phagocytic cells of the spleen. In the great majority of hemolytic anemias, the premature destruction of red cells also occurs within the mononuclear phagocyte system (**extravascular hemolysis**), which undergoes a form of work-related hyperplasia marked by splenomegaly. Much less commonly, lysis of red cells within the vascular compartment (**intravascular hemolysis**) predominates.
- ***Intravascular hemolysis*** of red cells is caused by mechanical injury, complement fixation, infection by intracellular parasites such as falciparum malaria, or exogenous toxic factors.
- ***Extravascular hemolysis*** takes place whenever red cells are rendered "foreign" or become less deformable.

Table *(Harshmohan 6th/598)*: **Major differences b/w Unconjugated and Conjugated Bilirubin**

Feature	Unconjugated Bilirubin	Conjugated Bilirubin
Normal serum level	More	Less (less than 0.25 mg/dl)
Water solubility	Absent	Present
Affinity to lipids (alcohol solubility)	Present	Absent
Serum albumin binding	High	Low
Van den Bergh reaction	Indirect (Total minus direct)	Direct
Renal excretion	Absent	Present
Bilirubin albumin covalent complex formation	Absent	Present
Affinity to brain tissue	Present (Kernicterus)	Absent

Hemolytic Anemias Share the Following Features

- A shortened red cell life span (normal = 120 days); that is, premature destruction of red cells
- Elevated erythropoietin levels and increased erythropoiesis in the marrow and other sites, to compensate for the loss of red cells
- Accumulation of the products of hemoglobin catabolism, due to an increased rate of red cell destruction

Table *(Harrison 19th/649, 18th/873)*: **Some Common Features of Hemolytic Disorders**

Features	Findings
General examination	Jaundice, pallor
Other physical findings	Spleen may be enlarged; bossing of skull in severe congenital cases
Hemoglobin level	From normal to severely reduced
MCV, MCH	Usually increased
Reticulocytes	Increased
Bilirubin	Increased (mostly unconjugated)
LDH	Increased (up to 10x normal with intravascular hemolysis)
Haptoglobin	Reduced to absent (if hemolysis is part intravascular)

Table *(Harrison 19th/649, 18th/872)*: **Classification of Hemolytic Anemias**

	Intracorpuscular Defects	Extracorpuscular Factors
Hereditary	Hemoglobinopathies Enzymopathies Membrane- cytoskeletal defects	Familial (atypical) hemolytic uremic syndrome
Acquired	Paroxysmal nocturnal hemoglobinuria (PNH)	Mechanical destruction (microangiopathic) Toxic agents; Drugs; Infectious; Autoimmune

40. Ans. e. Rotor's...

[Ref: CMDT06/650; Robbins 9th/853, 8th/841; Harshmohan 6th/598; Harrison 19th/282, 18th/2532; O.P. Ghai 6th 170-171]

Table *(CMDT06/650)*: **Classification of jaundice**

Unconjugated hyperbilirubinemia (predominant indirect-reacting bilirubin)	Increased bilirubin production (*e.g.*, hemolytic anemias, hemolytic reactions, ***hematoma,*** pulmonary infarction) Impaired bilirubin uptake and storage (*e.g.*, posthepatitis hyperbilirubinemia, ***Gilbert syndrome, Crigler–Najjar syndrome,*** drug reactions)
Conjugated hyperbilirubinemia (predominant direct-reacting bilirubin)	• Hereditary cholestatic syndromes • Faulty excretion of bilirubin conjugates (*e.g.*, Dubin-Johnson syndrome, ***Rotor syndrome***) or mutation in genes coding for bile salt transport proteins (*e.g.*, progressive familial intrahepatic cholestasis syndromes, benign recurrent intrahepatic cholestasis and some cases of intrahepatic cholestasis of pregnancy)

Contd...

Conjugated hyperbilirubinemia (predominant direct-reacting bilirubin)	Hepatocellular Dysfunction
	Biliary epithelial damage (*e.g.,* hepatitis, hepatic cirrhosis)
	Intrahepatic cholestasis (*e.g.,* certain drugs, biliary cirrhosis, sepsis, postoperative jaundice)
	Hepatocellular damage or intrahepatic cholestasis resulting from miscellaneous causes (*e.g.,* spirochetal infections, infectious mononucleosis, cholangitis, sarcoidosis, lymphomas, industrial toxins)
	Biliary Obstruction
	Choledocholithiasis, biliary atresia, carcinoma of biliary duct, sclerosing cholangitis, choledochal cyst, external pressure on common duct, pancreatitis, pancreatic neoplasms

Table *(Robbins 9th/853, 8th/841)*: **Causes of jaundice**

Predominantly Unconjugated Hyperbilirubinemia

- Excess production of bilirubin[Q]
  - Hemolytic anemias
  - Resorption of blood from internal hemorrhage (*e.g.,* alimentary tract bleeding, hematomas).
  - Ineffective erythropoiesis syndromes (*e.g.,* pernicious anemia, thalassemia).
- Reduced hepatic uptake
  - Drug interference with membrane carrier systems
  - Some cases of Gilbert syndrome
- Impaired bilirubin conjugation[Q]
  - Physiologic jaundice of the newborn (decreased UGT 1A1 activity decreased excretion).
  - *Breast milk jaundice*[Q] *(β-glucuronidases in milk)*
  - Genetic deficiency of UGT 1A1 activity *(Crigler-Najjar's syndrome*[Q] types I and II).
  - *Gilberts' syndrome*[Q] (mixed etiologies)
  - Diffuse hepatocellular disease (*e.g.,* viral or drug-induced hepatitis, cirrhosis).

Predominantly Conjugated Hyperbilirubinemia

- Deficiency of canalicular membrane transporters
  - ***Dubin Johnson's syndrome***[Q]
  - ***Rotor's syndrome***[Q]
- Impaired bile flow

41. Ans. a. Endocarditis, d. Bread..., e. Pancarditis

[Ref: Robbins 9th/557-59, 8th/565-66; Harrison 19th/2149-54, 18th/2753]

Rheumatic Fever and Rheumatic Heart Disease

- Rheumatic fever (RF) is an acute, immunologically mediated, multisystem inflammatory disease that occurs a few weeks following an episode of group A streptococcal pharyngitis. ***Acute rheumatic carditis during the active phase of RF may progress to chronic rheumatic heart disease (RHD).***
- The ***most important consequence of RF*** are ***chronic valvular deformities,*** characterized principally by deforming fibrotic valvular disease (particularly **mitral stenosis**), which produces permanent dysfunction and severe, sometimes fatal, cardiac problems decades later.
- During acute RF, diffuse inflammation and Aschoff bodies may be found in any of the three layers of the heart—pericardium, myocardium, or endocardium—hence the lesion is called a **pancarditis**. In the pericardium, the inflammation is accompanied by a fibrinous or serofibrinous pericardial exudate, described as a **"bread-and-butter"** pericarditis, which generally resolves without sequelae.
- "If fibrinous pericarditis fails to resolve, it result in chronic adhesive pericarditis. Chronic adhesive pericarditis differ from chronic constrictive pericarditis in not embarrasing the function of heart" *(Harshmohan 7th/422, 438.)*
- The myocardial involvement-**myocarditis** takes the form of scattered Aschoff bodies within the interstitial connective tissue, often perivascular.
- Concomitant involvement of the **endocardium** and the left-sided valves by inflammatory foci typically results in fibrinoid necrosis within the cusps or along the tendinous cords on which sit small (1–2-mm) vegetations—verrucae—along the lines of closure. called **MacCallum plaques,** usually in the left atrium.
- **Chronic RHD** is characterized by organization of the acute inflammation and subsequent fibrosis. In particular, the valvular leaflets become thickened and retracted, causing permanent deformity. The cardinal anatomic changes of the mitral (or tricuspid) valve are **leaflet thickening, commissural fusion and shortening and thickening and fusion of the tendinous cords.**
- In chronic disease, the ***mitral valve is virtually always abnormal***, but involvement of another valve, such as the aortic, may be the most clinically important in some cases.
- ***RHD is overwhelmingly the most frequent cause of mitral stenosis (99% of cases).***
- In patients with RHD, the mitral valve alone is involved in 65%–70% of cases and mitral and aortic in about 25%; similar but generally less severe fibrous thickenings and stenoses can occur in the tricuspid valve and rarely in the pulmonic.
- Fibrous bridging across the valvular commissures and calcification create ***"fish mouth" or "buttonhole" stenoses.***
- RF is characterized by a constellation of findings that includes as major manifestations

- Migratory polyarthritis of the large joints,
- *Carditis,*
- *Subcutaneous nodules,*
- *Erythema marginatum of the skin and*
- *Sydenham chorea, a neurologic disorder with involuntary purposeless, rapid movements.*

42. Ans. c. Mucous..., e. Steatorrhoea

[Ref: Robbins 9th/466-71, 8th/465-71; Harrison 19th/1697-1700, 18th/2148-49; Nelson's 18th/1808; Robbins 7th/490-95]

Cystic Fibrosis (Mucoviscidosis)

- Autosomal recessive[Q] inheritance
- Appear at any point in life from before birth[Q] to much later in childhood or even in adolescence[Q]
- May leads to chronic lung disease[Q], pancreatic insufficiency[Q], ***steatorrhoea***[Q], malnutrition, hepatic cirrhosis, ***intestinal obstruction*** & male infertility[Q].
- "*In sweat glands duct, ENaC (Epithelial sodium channel) activity decreases as a result of CFTR mutation; therefore a hypertonic luminal fluid containing both high sweat chloride (the sine qua non of classic CF)& high sodium content is formed. This is the basis of the* ***salty sweat****; the mothers can often detect in their affected infant*"-(Robbins7th/490
- Biochemical studies indicate that the F_{508} *mutation*[Q] leads to improper processing and intracellular degradation of the CFTR protein.
- Diagnostic biophysical hallmark of CF is the raised transepithelial electric potential difference detected in airway epithelium

Table *(Robbins 9th/470, 8th/470)*: **Clinical Features of Cystic Fibrosis**

1. ***Chronic sinopulmonary disease*** manifested by
a. Persistent colonization/infection with typical cystic fibrosis *pathogens, including Staphylococcus aureus, nontypeable Hemophilus influenzae*, mucoid and nonmucoid *Pseudomonas aeruginosa, Burkholderia cepacia*
b. Chronic cough and sputum production
c. Persistent chest radiograph abnormalities (*e.g.,* bronchiectasis, atelectasis, infiltrates, hyperinflation)
d. Airway obstruction manifested by wheezing and air trapping
e. Nasal polyps; radiographic or computed tomographic abnormalities of paranasal sinuses
f. Digital clubbing
2. ***Gastrointestinal and nutritional abnormalities***, including
a. **Intestinal:** Meconium ileus, distal intestinal obstruction syndrome, rectal prolapsed
b. **Pancreatic:** Pancreatic insufficiency, recurrent pancreatitis
c. **Hepatic:** chronic hepatic disease manifested by clinical or histologic evidence of focal biliary cirrhosis, or multilobular cirrhosis
d. **Nutritional:** Failure to thrive (protein-calorie malnutrition), hypoproteinemia, edema, complications secondary to fat-soluble vitamin deficiency

Contd...

3. ***Salt-loss syndromes***: *Acute salt depletion, chronic metabolic acidosis*
4. ***Male urogenital abnormalities*** resulting in obstructive *azoospermia (congenital bilateral absence of vas deferens)*

"***Meconium plug syndrome*** *refers to a functional colonic obstruction in a newborn due to an obstructing meconium plug. It is usually transient and affects the left colon with meconium plugging the bowel distal to this segment.*
Associations: *May have a* higher prevalence with maternal diabetes; Hirschsprung's disease *in ~15% &* may be associated with cystic fibrosis" *(http: //radiopaedia. org/articles)*
"**Pectus excavatum** (a Latin term meaning *hollowed chest*) is the most common congenital deformity of the anterior wall of the chest, in which several ribs and the sternum grow abnormally. This produces a caved-in or sunken appearance of the chest. Pectus excavatum may occur in Marfan syndrome, Ehlers-Danlos Syndrome, spinal muscular atrophy & Celiac disease"
"**Aniridia** is the absence of the iris, usually involving both eyes. It can be congenital or caused by a penetrant injury. Aniridia in some individuals is associated with kidney nephroblastoma *(Wilms tumor), genitourinary anomalies, or intellectual disability and cerebellar ataxia (Gillespie syndrome), resulting in the* WAGR syndrome" *(en.wikipedia)*

43. Ans. a. Ascites, b. Hemangioma..., c. Platelet..., e. Echinococcus...

[Ref: http: //emedicine.medscape.com/; Harrison 19th/1998, 18th/2525-26, 2530-31; CMDT 2016/666, 688]

"***Hemangioma of liver****: Percutaneous biopsy of these lesions should be* ***avoided*** *as they are vascular lesions & may bleed profusely into the peritoneal cavity"-L & B 25th/1097*

Contraindications

◈ *http: //emedicine.medscape.com*

Contraindications to percutaneous liver biopsy are relatively few, but identifying contraindications is important to avoid the major complications associated with the procedure. Contraindications to liver biopsy include the following:

- Increased prothrombin time, international normalized ratio (INR) greater than 1.6
- ***Thrombocytopenia****, platelet count less than 60, 000*
- ***Ascites*** *(transjugular route preferred)*
- **Difficult body habitus** *(transjugular route preferred)*
- ***Suspected hemangioma***
- ***Suspected echinococcal infection***
- Uncooperative patient

Percutaneous Liver Biopsy

◈ *Harrison 19th/1998, 18th/2530-31*

- Liver biopsy is of proven value in the following situations: *(1) hepatocellular disease of uncertain cause, (2) prolonged hepatitis with the possibility of chronic active hepatitis, (3) unexplained hepatomegaly, (4) unexplained splenomegaly, (5) hepatic filling defects by radiologic imaging, (6) fever of unknown origin, (7) staging of malignant lymphoma.*

- **Contraindications** to performing a percutaneous liver biopsy include ***significant ascites and prolonged INR***. Under these circumstances, the biopsy can be performed via the transjugular approach.

44. Ans. b. Bile.., c. Mallory..., d. Distur...

[Ref: Robbins 9th /843-45, 827-28, 8th/857-60; Harrison 19th/2058-59, 18th/2592-93]

Microscopic Features of Alcoholic Cirrhosis

◈ *Harshmohan 6th/624*

- ***Nodular pattern:*** *Normal lobular architecture is effaced in which **central veins are hard to find** & is replaced with nodule formation*
- ***Fibrous septa:*** *Extend from central vein to portal region or portal tract to portal tract, or both*
- ***Hepatic parenchyma:*** *Form regenerative nodule*
- *"Necrosis, inflammation & bile duct proliferation: **The etiological clue to diagnosis in the form of Mallory bodies is hard to find in a fully-developed alcoholic cirrhosis**"*

Alcoholic Cirrhosis

◈ *Robbins 9th/827-28, 843, 8th/857-60*

- Regardless of the cause of cirrhosis, the pathologic features consist of the development of fibrosis to the point that there is ***architectural distortion*** with the formation of regenerative nodules.
- Chronic alcohol use can produce fibrosis in the absence of accompanying inflammation and/or necrosis. Fibrosis can be ***centrilobular, pericellular, or periportal.*** When fibrosis reaches a certain degree, there is ***disruption of the normal liver architecture*** and replacement of liver cells by regenerative nodules.
- In alcoholic cirrhosis, the nodules are usually <3 mm in diameter; this form of cirrhosis is referred to as ***micronodular.*** With cessation of alcohol use, larger nodules may form, resulting in a ***mixed micronodular and macronodular cirrhosis.***
- With time, the nodularity becomes more prominent; scattered larger nodules create a ***"hobnail" appearance*** on the surface of the liver. As fibrous septae dissect and surround nodules, the liver becomes more fibrotic, loses fat and shrinks progressively in size.
- Ischemic necrosis and fibrous obliteration of nodules eventually create broad expanses of tough, pale scar tissue ("***Laennec*** cirrhosis"). Bile stasis often develops.
- **Mallory bodies** are only rarely evident at this stage. Thus, **end-stage alcoholic cirrhosis comes to resemble, both macroscopically and microscopically, the cirrhosis developing from viral hepatitis and other causes.**

45. Ans. d. Occur...

[Ref: Robbins 9th/1215, 8th/144, 1243; Harrison 18th/491, 2386, 2383t; Danhert Radiology 5th/95; Nelson 18th/629-30]

Lesch-Nyhan Disease (LND)

◈ *Harrison 19th/431e-5, 18th/2386*

- This is a ***rare X-linked disorder*** of purine metabolism that results from HPRT deficiency. This enzyme is normally present in each cell in the body, but its highest concentration is in the brain, especially in the basal ganglia.
- **"Lesch –Nyhan syndrome can cause uric acid renal stone"** *(Harrison 18th/2386)*
- **Clinical manifestations** include hyperuricemia, intellectual disability, dystonic movement disorder that may be accompanied by choreoathetosis and spasticity, dysarthric speech and compulsive self-biting, usually beginning with the eruption of teeth
- The disorder appears in males; occurrence in females is extremely rare and ascribed to nonrandom inactivation of the normal X chromosome
- Those with classic LND rarely survive the 3rd decade because of renal or respiratory compromise
- ***"C/F of Lesch –Nyhan syndrome includes choreoathetosis, spasticity, mental retardation, self-mutilation of lips & fingertips"*** *(Danhert Radiology 5th/95)*
- "Most, but not all, persons with this deficiency have ***severe mental and physical problems throughout*** life"
- "A complete lack of HGPRT (hypoxanthine guanine phosphoribosyl transferase) occurs in the uncommon X-linked *Lesch-Nyhan syndrome,* **seen only in males** and characterized by ***hyperuricemia, severe neurologic deficits with mental retardation, self-mutilation and in some cases gouty arthritis***" *(Robbins 9th/1215, 8th/1243)*

Table *(Harrison 18th/2383t)*: **Major Causes of Renal Stones**

Stone Type and Causes	Ratio of M: F	Etiology	Diagnosis	Treatment
Lesch-Nyhan Syndrome	Males only	Hereditary	Reduced hypoxanthine-guanine phosphori-bosyltrans ferase level	Allopurinol

46. Ans. a. CD1a, b. S 100...

[Ref: Robbins 9th/621-22, 8th/631-32; Harrison 19th/135e-9, 18th/268, e 21-6; O.P. Ghai 7th/595]

Langerhans Cell Histiocytosis

- Langerhans cell histiocytosis is a disease of childhood that has been called ***histiocytosis X, Letterer-Siwe disease, Hand-Schuller-Christian disease and eosinophilic granuloma.*** Patients with Langerhans cell histiocytosis are at *increased risk of acute lymphoid leukemia or other lymphoid malignancy.*
- Three clinical syndromes are recognized. Solitary bone lesions, particularly those involving the skull, femur, pelvis, or ribs, are frequently called **eosinophilic granuloma.**

- The presence of multiple lesions affecting a single tissue, most often bone, is called **Hand-Schuller-Christian disease**. The presence of multiple lesions in multiple organs including bones, skin, liver, spleen and nodes is called **Letterer-Siwe disease.** The characteristic Birbeck granules are pathognomonic but only visible on electron microscopy.
- The clinical course tends to be inversely related to the number of lesions.
- Langerhans cells are bone marrow-derived and reside in the skin; their main function is to present antigen to T-cells. They are MHC class II, Fc receptor and ***S100 protein positive; they express CD4 and CD1a*** and they are not phagocytosing cells. They contain distinctive morphologic features such as ***Birbeck granules, rod or tennis racket-shaped structures*** of uncertain function.
- *"The **hallmark of LCH** is positivity for **S-100 protein & CD1a positivity**"(O.P.Ghai 7th/595)*

Table *(Robbins 7th /670)*: **Some Immune Cell Antigens Detected by Monoclonal Antibodies**

Antigen Designation	Normal Cellular Distribution
Primarily T-Cell Associated	
CD1	Cortical thymocytes and Langerhans histiocytes
CD3	Thymocytes, peripheral T cells
CD4	Helper subset of peripheral T cells, single positive medullary thymocytes and CD4/CD8 double positive thymocytes
CD5	T cells and a small subset of B cells
CD8	Cytotoxic subset of peripheral T cells, single positive medullary thymocytes, double positive cortical thymocytes and some NK cells
Primarily B-Cell Associated	
CD10	Marrow pre-B cells and germinal center B cells; also called CALLA
CD19	Marrow pre-B cells and mature B cells but not plasma cells
CD20	Marrow pre-B cells after CD19 and mature B cells but not plasma cells
CD21	EBV receptor; present on mature B cells and follicular dendritic cells
CD23	Activated mature B cells
CD79a	Marrow pre-B cells and mature B cells.
Primarily Monocyte or Macrophage Associated	
CD11c	Granulocytes, monocytes and macrophages; also expressed by hairy cell leukemias
CD13	Immature and mature monocytes and granulocytes
CD14	Monocytes
CD15	Granulocytes; also expressed by Reed-Sternberg cells and variants in classical Hodgkin lymphoma

Contd...

Antigen Designation	Normal Cellular Distribution
CD33	Myeloid progenitors and monocytes
CD64	Mature myeloid cells
Primarily NK-Cell Associated	
CD16	NK cells and granulocytes
CD56	NK cells and a subset of T cells
Primarily Stem Cell and Progenitor Cell Associated	
CD34	Pluripotent hematopoietic stem cells and progenitor cells of many lineages
Activation Markers	
CD30	Activated B cells, T cells and monocytes; also expressed by Reed-Sternberg cells and variants in classical Hodgkin lymphoma
Present on All Leukocytes	
CD45	All leukocytes; also known as leukocyte common antigen (LCA)
CD, cluster designation; NK, natural killer; CALLA, common acute lymphoblastic leukemia antigen; EBV, Epstein-Barr virus.	

47. Ans. b. Ataxia..., c. Peutz..., d. Cowden...

[Ref: Robbins 9th/1053-54, 8th/1077-78, 1343, 820-21; Harrison 18th/754; Schwartz 9th/436-40; Sabiston 18th/863; Harrison 17th/563-65]

Von Hippel Lindau syndrome is not associated with breast carcinoma *(Harrison 19th/2342, 18th/3384)*

"Familial adenomatous polyposis is associated with colorectal carcinoma & some other cancer but not breast cancer *(Robbins 8th/816)*

Table *(Schwartz)*: **Percent Incidence of Sporadic, Familial and Hereditary Breast Cancer**

Sporadic breast cancer	65–75%
Familial breast cancer	20–30%
Hereditary breast cancer	5–10%
BRCA-1	45%
BRCA-2	35%
p53 *(Li-Fraumeni syndrome)*	1%
STK11/LKB1 *(Peutz-Jeghers syndrome)*	<1%
PTEN *(Cowden disease)*	<1%
MSH2/MLH1 *(Muir-Torre syndrome)*	<1%
ATM *(Ataxia-telangiectasia)*	<1%
Unknown	20%

48. Ans. a. Cushing..., c. Phe.., d. Hyper.., e. Acrome..

[Ref; Harrison 19th/2399, 18th/2969]

Table *(Harrison 19th/2399, 18th/2969)*: **Etiologic Classification of Diabetes Mellitus-Partial list**

1. **Diseases of the exocrine pancreas**: Pancreatitis, pancreatectomy, neoplasia, cystic fibrosis, hemochromatosis, fibrocalculous pancreatopathy, mutations in carboxyl ester lipase
2. ***Endocrinopathies: Acromegaly, Cushing's syndrome, glucagonoma, pheochromocytoma***, hyperthyroidism, somatostatinoma, aldosteronoma
3. **Drug-or chemical-induced**: Glucocorticoids, vacor (a rodenticide), pentamidine, nicotinic acid, diazoxide, β-adrenergic agonists, thiazides, hydantoins, asparaginase, α-interferon, protease inhibitors, antipsychotics (atypicals and others), epinephrine
4. ***Infections***: Congenital rubella, cytomegalo virus, coxsackie virus
5. ***Uncommon forms of immune-mediated diabetes:*** "Stiff-person" syndrome, anti-insulin receptor antibodies
6. ***Other genetic syndromes*** sometimes associated with diabetes— Wolfram's syndrome, Down's syndrome, Klinefelter's syndrome, Turner's syndrome, Friedreich's ataxia, Huntington's chorea, Laurence-Moon-Biedl syndrome, myotonic dystrophy, porphyria, Prader-Willi syndrome

49. Ans. b. Ovarian..., c. Breast..., d. Renal...

[Ref: Robbins 9th/331, 8th/321, 1126-29; Harrison 19th/2476, 18th /3112, 3106; Williams Textbook of Endocrinology, 11th ed.]

Note: *Small cell carcinoma secretes calcitonin (cause hypocalcemia)*

Hypercalcemia

"Lung carcinoma, breast carcinoma and multiple myeloma account for more than 50% of all cases of malignancy-associated hypercalcemia. **Lung carcinomas** that produce hypercalcemia have ***squamous or large cell histology, whereas small cell carcinoma almost never causes hypercalcemia***. Among other solid tumors, the most common are *squamous* and *renal carcinomas. Gastrointestinal tumors and prostate carcinoma* are less common causes of hypercalcemia"-*Williams Textbook of Endocrinology, 11th ed*

Table *(Williams Textbook of Endocrinology11th ed.)*: **Malignancy-Associated Hypercalcemia**

Primary Site	No. (%) of Cases	Known Metastatic Disease (%)
Lung	111 (25.0)	62
Breast	87 (19.6)	92
Multiple myeloma	43 (9.7)	100
Head and neck	36 (8.1)	73
Renal and urinary tract	35 (7.9)	36
Esophagus	25 (5.6)	53
Female genitalia	24 (5.2)	81
Unknown primary	23 (5.2)	—
Lymphoma	14 (3.2)	91
Colon	8 (1.8)	—
Liver, biliary	7 (1.6)	—
Skin	6 (1.4)	—
Other	25 (5.6)	—
Total	444 (100)	

Table *(Robbins 9th/331, 8th/321)*: **Paraneoplastic Syndromes**

Clinical Syndromes	Major Forms of Underlying Cancer	Causal Mechanism
Hyper-calcemia	Squamous cell carcinoma of lung Breast carcinoma; Renal carcinoma Adult T-cell leukemia/ lymphoma Ovarian carcinoma	Parathyroid hormone-related protein (PTHRP), TGF-α, TNF, IL-1

Basic Pathophysiologic Mechanisms of Hypercalcemia

- ↑Ca^{2+} absorption form GIT e.g milk alkali syndrome, vit. intoxication.
- ↓ed renal excretion of Ca^{2+} *e.g.*, Renal failure
- ↑ed bone resorption *e.g.*, ↑ PTH, malignancy, hyperthyroidism etc.

Surgical causes **↑*Ca2+:***

- *Parathyroid adenomas*[Q]
- *MEN*[Q]
- *Pheochromocytoma*[Q]
- *Malignancies e.g., breast, Lung, kidney Ca,*

50. Ans. All (a b c d)

[Ref: Robbins 9th/1103, 8th/1126-29; Harrison 18th/3099]

Table *(Robbins 9th/1103, 8th/1129)*: **Causes of Hypercalcemia**

Raised PTH	Decreased PTH
Hyperparathyroidism	Hypercalcemia of malignancy
Primary (adenoma> hyperplasia)*	Osteolytic metastases (RANKL-mediated)
Secondary†	PTH-rP-mediated
Tertiary†	Vitamin D toxicity
Familial hypocalciuric hypercalcemia	Immobilization
	Thiazide diuretics
	Granulomatous disease (sarcoidosis)

Raised PTH	Decreased PTH
PTH-rP, Parathyroid hormone-related protein. RANKL, Receptor activator of nuclear factor κB ligand.	
* Primary hyperparathyroidism is the most common cause of hypercalcemia overall. Malignancy is the most common cause of symptomatic hypercalcemia. Primary hyperparathyroidism and malignancy account for nearly 90% of cases of hypercalcemia.	
† *Secondary and tertiary hyperparathyroidism are most commonly associated with progressive renal failure*	

Table *(H 19th/2470, 18th/3099)*: **Classification of Causes of Hypercalcemia**

I. Parathyroid-related
Primary hyperparathyroidism Adenoma (s) Multiple endocrine neoplasia Carcinoma
Lithium therapy
Familial hypocalciuric hypercalcemia
II. Malignancy-related
Solid tumor with metastases (breast)
Solid tumor with humoral mediation of hypercalcemia (lung, kidney)
Hematologic malignancies (multiple myeloma, lymphoma, leukemia)
III. Vitamin D—related
Vitamin D intoxication
↑1, 25 (OH)2D; sarcoidosis and other granulomatous diseases
Idiopathic hypercalcemia of infancy
IV. Associated with high bone turnover
Hyperthyroidism
Immobilization
Thiazides
Vitamin A intoxication
V. Associated with renal failure
Severe secondary hyperparathyroidism
Aluminum intoxication
Milk-alkali syndrome

51. Ans. All

[Ref: Robbins 9th/645-649, 8th/654-59; Harrison 19th/646, 18th/867]

"Crohn's disease cause cobalamine deficiency (megaloblastic anaemia)" *(Harrison 19th/646, 18th/867)*

Table *(Robbins 8th/655)*: **Causes of Megaloblastic Anemia**

Vitamin B_{12} Deficiency

Decreased Intake

- Inadequate diet, vegetarianism[Q]

Impaired absorption

- Intrinsic factor deficiency[Q]
  - Pernicious anemia, Gastrectomy
- Malabsorption states[Q]
  - Diffuse intestinal disease, *e.g.*, lymphoma, systemic sclerosis
  - Ileal resection[Q], ileitis
- Competitive parasitic uptake
  - Fish tapeworm infestation[Q]
- Bacterial overgrowth in blind loops[Q] and diverticula of bowel

Increased requirement

- Pregnancy, hyperthyroidism, disseminated cancer

Folic Acid Deficiency

Decreased Intake

- Inadequate diet–***alcoholism***[Q], infancy

Impaired absorption

- Malabsorption states; Intrinsic intestinal disease
- Anticonvulsants[Q], oral contraceptives[Q]

Increased loss

- Hemodialysis

Increased Requirement

- Pregnancy, infancy[Q], disseminated cancer, markedly increased
- Hematopoiesis

Impaired use

Folic acid antagonists[Q]

Unresponsive to Vitamin B_{12} or Folic Acid Therapy

Metabolic inhibitors of DNA synthesis and/or folate metabolism, e.g., methotrexate[Q]

52. Ans. a. Clear..., b. Hormone..., c. Contain..., d. Well...

[Ref: Robbins 9th/1069, 8th/1091-92; Sabiston 18th/866-67; L & B 25th/836, Danhert Radiology 5th/558; Harshmohan 6th/757-58]

Fibroadenoma

◈ *Harshmohan 6th/757-58*

- Unlike typical lumps from breast cancer, fibroadenomas are easy to move, with ***clearly defined edges***
- Fibroadenomas are sometimes called **breast mice or a breast mouse** owing to their high mobility in the breast

◈ *Robbins 9th/1069, 8th/1091-92*

- Most common benign breast tumor of female breast
- Most occur in women in their 20s & 30s and they are frequently multiple & bilateral
- Epithelium of fibroadenoma is hormonally responsive & increase during reproductive age (pregnancy & lactation). It regress after menopause
- It is an estrogen induced benign tumor-*Danhert Radiology 5th/558*

Fibroadenoma and Related Tumors

◈ *Sabiston 18th/866-67*

- Fibroadenomas are benign solid tumors composed of ***stromal and epithelial elements***. After carcinoma, fibroadenoma is the second most common tumor in the breast and is the ***most common tumor in women younger than 30 years.***

- In contrast to cysts, fibroadenomas appear in teenage girls and women during their early reproductive years; they are rarely seen as new masses in women after the age of 40 or 45.
- Clinically, they are firm tumors that may increase in size over a period of several months. They slip easily under the examining fingers and may be lobulated.
- On excision, fibroadenomas are ***well-encapsulated masses*** that may detach easily from surrounding breast tissue.
- ***Fibroadenomas do not have malignant potential***, although neoplasia may develop in the epithelial elements within them, just as in epithelium elsewhere in the breast.

53. Ans. a. Engulf..., b. Multilobed..., c. Neutrophil..., d. Neutrophilia...

[Ref: Robbins 9th/78, 82, 97, 8th/50-51, 53, 72, 184: Harrison 19th/415, 18th/472-76]

Routine Staining of Blood Smears

◈ *Wintrobe's Haematology 12th/Chap 1*

- Romanowsky stains have 2 component-methyl azure & eosin
- The Romanowsky stains differentially stain leukocyte granules, which aids in morphologic analysis of the cells. Thus, ***neutrophil granules are slightly basic and stain weakly with the azurophilic component***. The **eosinophils** contain a ***strongly basic spermine derivative and stain strongly with eosin***. In contrast, **basophil granules** contain predominately ***acidic proteins and stain a deep blue-violet***.

Neutrophil

◈ *Harrison 19th/413-15, 18th/472-76*

- 'Neutrophil contain ***primary or azurophil granules & secondary or specific granules***" *(Harrison 19th/415, 18th/472)*
- **"Neutrophilia** occur in ***acute bacterial infection***" *(Harrison 19th/418, 18th/477(Table))*
- The nucleus of neutrophils normally ***contains up to four segments***
- **Excessive segmentation** (more than five nuclear lobes) may be a manifestation of ***folate or vitamin B12 deficiency or the congenital neutropenia syndrome of warts, hypogammaglobulinemia, infections and myelokathexis (WHIM)***
- The neutrophil **granules** are of major importance for neutrophil function.
- On the basis of function and enzyme content, human neutrophil granules can be divided into three main types -***azurophil, specific and small storage granules.***
- Their function is not just to provide enzymes for hydrolytic substrate degradation -as in classical lysosomes --but also to kill ingested bacteria and, finally, to secrete their contents to regulate various physiological and pathological processes, including inflammation.
- Individual granule populations can be characterized morphologically (*e.g.*, ***azurophil granules*** are larger and contain more electron-dense material than *specific granules*), or biochemically using enzyme markers or other substances
- Neutrophil granules contain antimicrobial or cytotoxic substances, neutral proteinases, acid hydrolases and a pool of cytoplasmic membrane receptors.
- **Azurophil granules** function predominantly in the intracellular milieu (in the phagolysosomal vacuole), where they are involved in the killing and degradation of microorganisms. On the other hand, **neutrophil specific granules** are particularly susceptible to release their contents extracellularly and appear to have an important role in initiating inflammation.

Table: Neutrophil

	Surface marker	Characteristic
	Cd33, CD 13. ILCD 15, CD 14, CD 11b CD 10, CD 16	Condensed, multilobed nucleus

54. Ans. a. Release..., b. Vasoconstriction...

[Ref: Robbins 9th/83-84, 8th/57-58: Ananthanarayan 8th/165;Harrison 19th/2115, 18th/94]

- Histamine
- *"**Histamine** induces **smooth muscle contraction** in diverse tissues & organ, including vasculature, intestines, uterus & especially the bronchioles. It also stimulates secretions (secretagogue effect)" (Ananthanarayan 8th/165)*
- *Histamine* is widely distributed in tissues, the ***richest source being the mast cells*** that are normally present in the connective tissue adjacent to blood vessels. It is also found in blood basophils and platelets.
- Preformed histamine is present in mast cell granules and is released by mast cell degranulation in response to a variety of stimuli: (1) physical injury such as trauma, cold, or heat; (2) immune reactions involving binding of antibodies to mast cells; (3) fragments of complement called *anaphylatoxins* (C3a and C5a); (4) histamine-releasing proteins derived from leukocytes; (5) neuropeptides (*e.g.*, substance P); and (6) cytokines (IL-1, IL-8).
- In humans, histamine causes ***dilation of the arterioles and increases the permeability of venules*** (it, however, ***constricts large arteries***). It is considered to be the principal mediator of the immediate transient phase of increased vascular permeability, causing venular gaps, as we have seen.
- It acts on the microcirculation mainly via binding to H_1 receptors on endothelial cells

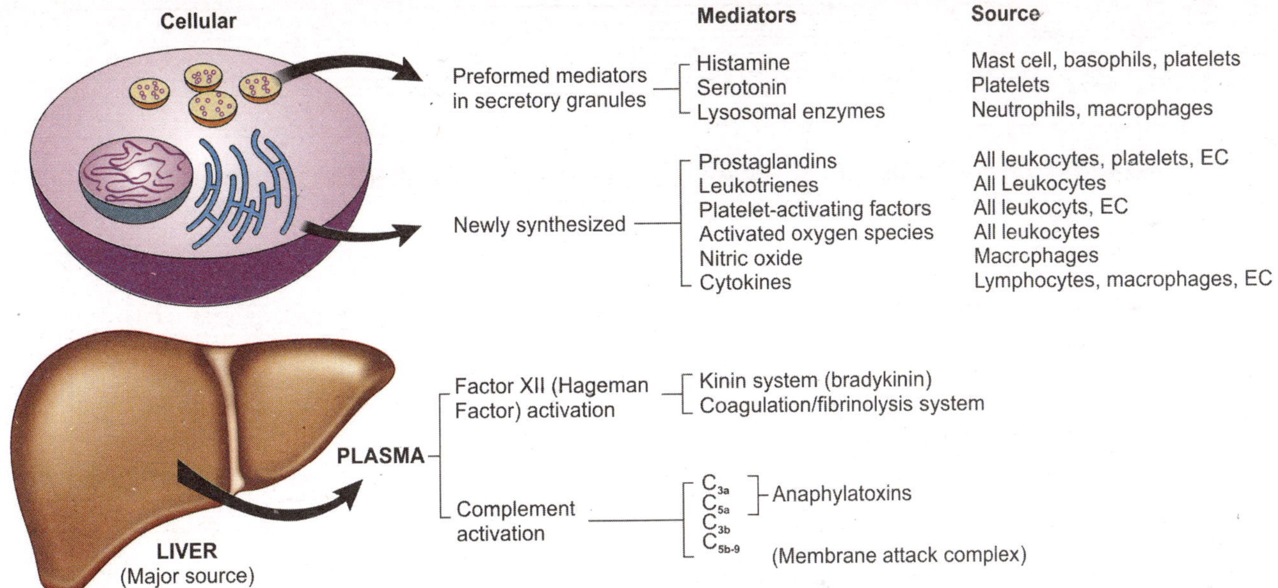

Fig: Chemical mediators of inflammation.

55. Ans. a. In Robertsonian..., b. Aneuploidy..., c. Comparative...

[Ref: Harrison 19th/83e 1-7, 18th /512-16, 517; Robbins 9th/160-61, 8th /159-62; Wintrobe's Clinical Hematology 12th /54]

Note: *Comparative genomic hybridisation (CGH) is a technique that permits the detection of chromosomal copy number changes without the need for cell culturing. It provides a global overview of chromosomal gains and losses throughout the whole genome of a tumour"-http: //www.ncbi.nlm.nih.gov/pmc*

Detects abnormalities in chromosomal Numbers *(Numerical Chr. Anomalies)*	Detects abnormalities in chromosomal Structure *(Structural Chr. Anomalies)*
Such as • *Aneuploidy* Q ▪ Trisomy, Tetrasomy • Polyploidy	Such as Translocations Q Deletions Inversions

Chromosomal Disorder

◈ *Robbins 9th/158-59, 8th/159*

- The normal chromosome complement is expressed as 46, XX for the female and 46, XY for the male. Any exact multiple of the haploid number is called ***euploid.*** If an error occurs in meiosis or mitosis, however and a cell acquires a chromosome complement that is not an exact multiple of 23, it is referred to as ***aneuploidy***.
- **Aneupoidy:** Chromosome which is not exact multiple of 23.
- "**Robertsonian translocation** (or centric fusion): It is a translocation between two acrocentric chromosomes. ***Typically the breaks occur close to the centromeres of each chromosome***. Transfer of the segments then leads to one very large chromosome and one extremely small one. Usually the small product is lost; however, because it carries only highly redundant genes (*e.g.*, ribosomal RNA genes), this loss is compatible with a normal phenotype"-*Robbins 9th/161, 8th/161*
- The usual causes for aneuploidy are *nondisjunction* and *anaphase lag*. The former occurs when a homologous pair of chromosomes fails to disjoin at the first meiotic division, or the two chromatids fail to separate either at the second meiotic division or in somatic cell divisions, resulting in two aneuploid cells. When nondisjunction occurs during gametogenesis, the gametes formed have either an extra chromosome (n+1) or one less chromosome (n-1). Fertilization of such gametes by normal gametes results in two types of zygotes—trisomic (2n+1) or monosomic (2n-1).
- **In anaphase lag,** one homologous chromosome in meiosis or one chromatid in mitosis lags behind and is left out of the cell nucleus. The result is one normal cell and one cell with monosomy. As seen subsequently, monosomy or trisomy involving the sex chromosomes, or even more bizarre aberrations, are compatible with life and are usually associated with variable degrees of phenotypic abnormalities.
- *Monosomy involving an autosome generally represents loss of too much genetic information to permit live birth or even embryogenesis, but a number of autosomal trisomies do permit survival.* With the exception of trisomy 21, all yield severely handicapped infants who almost invariably die at an early age.

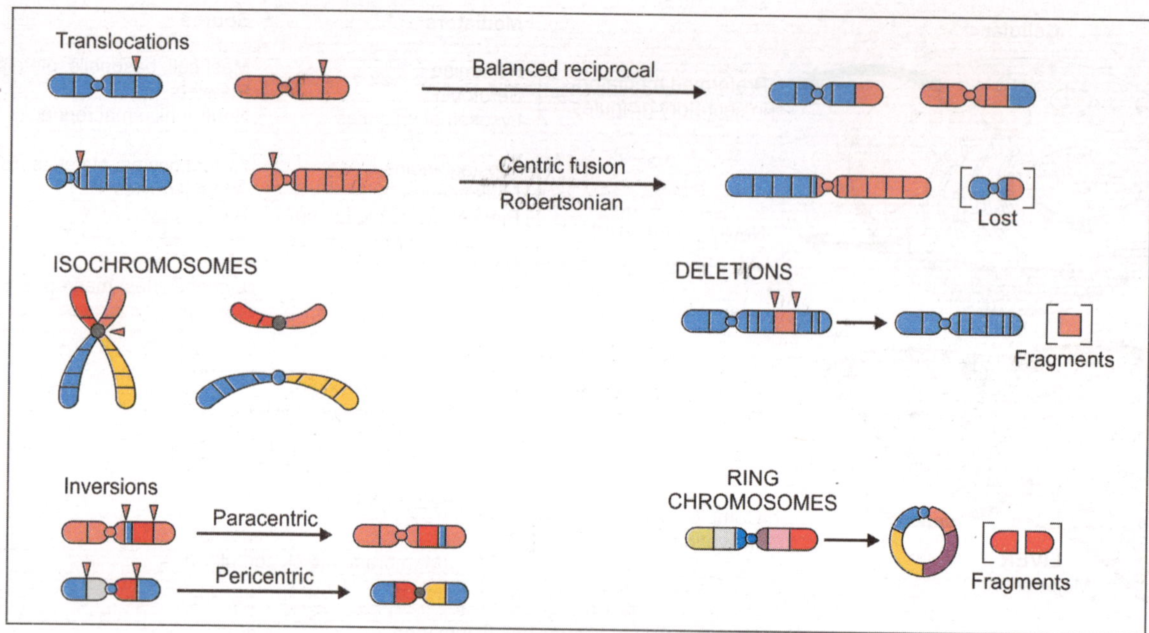

Fig: Chromosomal abnormalities

Table *(William's Haematology 7th)*: **Glossary of Cytogenetic Terminology**

Aneuploidy: An abnormal chromosome number caused by either gain or loss of chromosomes.

Centromere: The constriction along the length of the chromosome that is the site of the spindle fiber attachment. The position of the centromere determines whether chromosomes are metacentric (X-shaped, *e.g.*, chromosomes 1–3, 6–12, X, 16, 19, 20) or acrocentric (inverted V-shaped, *e.g.*, chromosomes 13–15, 21, 22, Y).

Diploid: Normal chromosome number and composition of chromosomes.

Haploid: Only one-half the normal complement, that is, 23 chromosomes.

Hyperdiploid: Additional chromosomes; therefore, the modal number is 47 or greater.

Hypodiploid: Loss of chromosomes with a modal number of 45 or less.

Inversion: Two breaks occur in the same chromosome with rotation of the intervening segment. If both breaks occur on the same side of the centromere, it is called a *paracentric inversion*. If they occur on opposite sides, it is called a *pericentric inversion*.

Isochromosome: A chromosome that consists of identical copies of one chromosome arm with loss of the other arm. Thus, an isochromosome for the long arm of chromosome 17 [i (17) (q10)] contains two copies of the long arm (separated by the centromere) with loss of the short arm of the chromosome.

Translocation: A break in at least two chromosomes with exchange of material. In a reciprocal translocation, there is no obvious loss of chromosomal material. Translocations are indicated by t; the chromosomes involved are noted in the first set of parentheses and the breakpoints in the second set of parentheses. For example, the Ph translocation is t (9; 22) (q34; q11.2).

56. Ans. a. Denver...

[Ref: Robbins 9th/159, 8th/159;Kumar and Clark 6th /172, 173; Harrison 19th/439, 18th/515;17th/411]

Denver Classification

The classification of human chromosomes on the basis of size and centromere position; the 23 pairs of chromosomes are classified in seven groups (A to G), in order of decreasing length. Used before it was possible to distinguish among the chromosomes of the groups

Chromosome Group (arranged in the following order in karyotype)	Chromosomes	Location Of Centromere
A	1-3	Metacentric
B	4-5	Submetacentric
D	13-15	Acrocentric
F	19-20	Metacentric
G	21-22, Y	Acrocentric
E	16-18	16 – Metacentric 17, 18 – Submetacentric
C	6-12, X	Submetacentric

Contd...

A & E

Metacentric	Group A, E (16), F
Submetacentric	Group B, C, E (17, 18)
Acrocentric	Group D, G

Metacentric Submetacentric Acrocentric Telocentric

Fig: Location of centromere

X-Inactivation

◈ *Harrison 19th/439, 18th/515;17th/411*

- In ***normal females***[Q], one of the chromosomes ***undergoes X inactivation***[Q] in somatic cells.
- The inactivation of the paternal or maternal X chromosome occurs randomly in each somatic cell and thereby serves as a mechanism of dosage compensation, ensuring that males and females have equal expression of most X-linked genes.
- Some genes on the X chromosome "escape" the inactivating mechanism and are expressed from both X chromosomes.
- In disorders such as Klinefelter syndrome, some genes may be expressed from both X chromosomes, resulting in its phenotypic features.
- "**Lyon hypothesis:** It states that (1) *only one of the X chromosomes is genetically active*, (2) ***the other X of either maternal or paternal origin undergoes heteropyknosis and is rendered inactive,*** (3) *inactivation of either the maternal or paternal X occurs at random among all the cells of the blastocyst on or about the 16th day of embryonic life* and (4) *inactivation of the same X chromosome persists in all the cells derived from each precursor cell.* Thus, the great preponderance of normal females are in reality mosaics and have two populations of cells, one with an inactivated maternal X and the other with an inactivated paternal X. Herein lies the explanation of why females have the same dosage of X-linked active genes as have males. The inactive X can be seen in the interphase nucleus as a darkly staining small mass in contact with the nuclear membrane known as the ***Barr body, or X chromatin***" *(Robbins 9th/164, 8th/164)*

PHARMACOLOGY

57. Ans. a. Metha.. & c. Ethyl..

[Ref: KDT 7th/395-96; Katzung 12th/398, 400, 1033]

Note: Fomepizole is drug of choice for methanol poisoning and ethylene glycerol poisoning.

Fomepizole

- It is a competitive inhibitor of the enzyme alcohol dehydrogenase, found in the liver. This enzyme plays a ***key role in the metabolism of ethylene glycol and methanol.***
- Fomepizole is most effective when given soon ***after ingestion of ethylene glycol or methanol***. Delaying the administration of fomepizole allows for the generation of harmful metabolites

Table *(Katzunng 12th/1033)*: **Examples of specific antidotes**

Antidote	Poison (s)
Acetylcysteine	Acetaminophen
Atropine	Anticholinesterases: Organophosphates, carbamates
Bicarbonate, sodium	Membrane-depressant cardiotoxic drugs (tricyclic antidepressants, quinidine, etc)
Deferoxamine	Iron salts
Esmolol	Theophylline, caffeine, metaproterenol
Ethanol	Methanol, ethylene glycol
Flumazenil	Benzodiazepines
Fomepizole	Methanol, ethylene glycol
Glucagon	β blockers
Naloxone	Narcotic drugs, other opioid derivatives
Physostigmine	Suggested for antimuscarinic anticholinergic agents; not for tricyclic antidepressants
Pralidoxime (2-PAM)	Organophosphate cholinesterase inhibitors

58. Ans. c. Fluconazole, d. Aspirin

[Ref: KDT 7th/623, 503; Katzung 12th/610]

"**Azithromycin:** *Interaction with theophylline, carbamazepine,* ***warfarin,*** *terfenadine & cisapride is* ***not likely****, but caution may be excercised" (KDT 7th/756)*

Drug Causing Enhanced Anticoagulant Action of Warfarin

◈ *KDT 7th/623*

- ***Aspirin:*** *Inhibit platelet aggregation & cause G.I bleeding*
- ***Newer cephalosporins (ceftriaxone, cefoperazone):*** *Cause hypoprothrombinemia*
- ***Broad spectrum antibiotics:*** *Inhibit gut flora & reduce vit. K production*

- ***Long acting sulfonamide, indomethacin, phenytoin & probenecid:*** *Displace warfarin from plasma protein binding*
- ***Chloramphenicol, erythromycin, celecoxib, cimetidine, allopurinol, amiodarone & metronidzole:*** *Inhibit warfarin metabolism*
- ***Tolbutamide & phenytoin:*** *Inhibit warfarin metabolism & vice versa*
- ***Liquid paraffin (habitual use):*** *Reduce vit. K absorption*

Drug Causing Reduced Anticoagulant Action of Warfarin

◈ *KDT 7th/623*

- **Barbiturates** (but not benzodiazepines), **carbamazepine, rifampin, & griseofulvin:** Induce the metabolism of oral anticoagulant
- **Oral contraceptive:** Increase blood levels of clotting factors

Drug Interactions

◈ *Katzung 12th/610*

- These interactions can be broadly divided into pharmacokinetic and pharmacodynamic effects
- Pharmacokinetic mechanisms for drug interaction with oral anticoagulants are mainly enzyme induction, enzyme inhibition and reduced plasma protein binding.
- Pharmacodynamic mechanisms for interactions with warfarin are synergism (impaired hemostasis, reduced clotting factor synthesis, as in hepatic disease), competitive antagonism (vitamin K) and an altered physiologic control loop for vitamin K (hereditary resistance to oral anticoagulants).
- The most serious interactions with warfarin are those that increase the anticoagulant effect and the risk of bleeding.
- The most dangerous of these interactions are the pharmacokinetic interactions with the pyrazolones phenylbutazone and sulfinpyrazone. These drugs not only augment the hypoprothrombinemia but also inhibit platelet function and may induce peptic ulcer disease
- Metronidazole, fluconazole and trimethoprim-sulfamethoxazole also stereoselectively inhibit the metabolic transformation of *S*-warfarin, whereas amiodarone, disulfiram and cimetidine inhibit metabolism of both enantiomorphs of warfarin.
- Aspirin, hepatic disease and hyperthyroidism augment warfarin effects-aspirin by its effect on platelet function and the latter two by increasing the turnover rate of clotting factors.
- The third-generation cephalosporins eliminate the bacteria in the intestinal tract that produce vitamin K and, like warfarin, also directly inhibit vitamin K epoxide reductase.
- Drugs with ***no*** significant effect on anticoagulant therapy include ethanol, phenothiazines, ***benzodiazepines***, acetaminophen, opioids, indomethacin and ***most antibiotics.***

Table *(Katzung 12th/610)*: **Pharmacokinetic and pharmacodynamic drug and body interactions with oral anticoagulants.**

Increased Prothrombin Time		Decreased Prothrombin Time	
Pharmacokinetic	Pharma-codynamic	Pharma-cokinetic	Pharma-codynamic
Amiodarone	Drugs	Barbiturates	Drugs
Cimetidine	Aspirin (high doses)	Cholestyramine	Diuretics
Disulfiram	Cephalosporins, third-generation	Rifampin	Vitamin K
Metronidazole	Heparin		Body factors
Fluconazole	Body factors		Hereditary resistance
Phenylbutazone	Hepatic disease		Hypothyroidism
Sulfinpyrazone	Hyper-thyroidism		
Trimethoprim-sulfamethoxazole			

59. Ans. b. Oral...

[Ref: KDT 7th/868; Katzung 12th/582]

Hydroxyurea

- Hydroxyurea is an analog of urea whose mechanism of action involves the inhibition of ***DNA synthesis*** by inhibiting the enzyme ribonucleotide reductase, resulting in depletion of deoxynucleoside triphosphate pools. This agent exerts its effects in the ***S phase of the cell cycle.***
- The drug is administered orally and has ***nearly 100% oral bioavailability.***
- It is mainly used in ***chronic myelogenous leukemia, blast crisis of acute myeloid leukemia,*** psoriasis & sickle cell anaemia
- However, it is also effective as an adjunct with radiation therapy (as ***radiosensitizer***) for head and neck cancer and in treating essential thrombocytosis and polycythemia vera.
- ***Myelosuppression is the dose-limiting toxicity,*** but nausea and vomiting, mucositis and diarrhea, headache and increased lethargy and a maculopapular skin rash with pruritus are also observed.

60. Ans. c. Increases...

[Ref: KDT 7th/584-86; Katzung 12th/260-61, 270]

Hydrochlorothiazide

- It ***inhibit Na^+-Cl^- symport*** predominantly in the DCT.
- In contrast to loop diuretics, which inhibit Ca^{2+} reabsorption, thiazides actually enhance Ca^{2+} reabsorption & ***decrease urine calcium excretion*** (causes ***hypercalcemia***).Thiazides are useful in the treatment of kidney stones caused by hypercalciuria.
- The major indications for thiazide diuretics are:
  - Hypertension
  - Heart failure
  - Nephrolithiasis due to idiopathic hypercalciuria and
  - Nephrogenic diabetes insipidus.

- "Thiazide cause carbohydrate intolerance & ***cause precipitation of diabetes***" *(KDT 7th/560)*

Toxicity

- **Hypokalemic metabolic alkalosis and hyperuricemia**
- **Impaired Carbohydrate Tolerance**
  Hyperglycemia may occur in patients who are overtly diabetic or who have even mildly abnormal glucose tolerance tests.
- **Hyperlipidemia** Thiazides cause a 5-15% increase in total serum cholesterol and low-density lipoproteins (LDL).
- Hyponatremia
  Hyponatremia is an important adverse effect of thiazide diuretics. It is due to a combination of hypovolemia-induced elevation of ADH, reduction in the diluting capacity of the kidney and increased thirst. It can be prevented by reducing the dose of the drug or limiting water intake.
- **Other Toxicities**
  Weakness, fatigability and paresthesias similar to those of carbonic anhydrase inhibitors may occur. Impotence has been reported but is probably related to volume depletion.
- **Contraindications**
  Excessive use of any diuretic is dangerous in hepatic cirrhosis, borderline renal failure, or heart failure

61. Ans. a. INH, c. Pyrazinamide, d. Amikacin, e. Streptomycin.

[Ref: KDT 7th/767; Katzung 12th/841]

*"**INH:** It is extensively metabolized in liver; most important pathway being N-acetylation by NAT2. The acetylated **metabolite is excreted in urine**" (KDT 7th/767)*

"Isoniazid metabolites and a small amount of unchanged drug are excreted mainly in the urine. The dose need not be adjusted in renal failure" *(Katzung 12th/841)*

*"**Rifampin:** It is metabolized in liver to an active deacetylated metabolite which is **excreted mainly in bile, some in urine.** Urine & secretions may become orange-red" (KDT 7th/768)*

"Rifampin is well absorbed after oral administration and ***excreted mainly through the liver into bile.*** It then undergoes enterohepatic recirculation, with the bulk excreted as a deacylated metabolite in feces and a small amount in the urine. Dosage adjustment for renal or hepatic insufficiency is not necessary" *(Katzung 12th/841)*

"Pyrazinamide is extensively metabolized in liver & excreted in urine" *(KDT 7th/769)*

"Pyrazinamide metabolites are renally cleared" *(Katzung 12th/843)*

*"**Aminoglycosides** (streptomycin & amikacin) are not metabolized*

62. Ans. e. (Act...)

[Ref: KDT 7th/34, 651-52; Katzung 12th/1085-89]

*"**Hit & run drugs** (whose effects last much longer than the drug itself), e.g., reserpine, guanethidine, MAO inhibitors, **omeprazole**" (KDT 7th/34)*

*"One of the PPIs is an integral component of all **anti-H.pylori regimens** along with 2 (triple drug) or 3 (quadruple drug) antimicrobial" (KDT 7th/657)*

"Since an acidic pH in the parietal cell acid canaliculi is required for drug activation & since food stimulates acid production, these drugs ideally should be given about 30 minutes before meal" (Goodmann & Gillmann 11th/969)

Proton Pump Inhibitors (PPI)

- ***PPI is inactive at neutral pH***, but at *pH<5 it rearranges to two charged cationic forms (a sulfenic acid & a sulphenamide configurations) that react covalently with -SH group of the H^+/K^+ ATPase enzyme & inactivate irreversibly*
- Proton pump inhibitors are administered as ***inactive prodrugs.*** To protect the acid-labile prodrug from rapid destruction within the gastric lumen, oral products are formulated for delayed release as acid-resistant, enteric-coated capsule or tablet formulations.
- After passing through the stomach into the alkaline intestinal lumen, the enteric coatings dissolve and the prodrug is absorbed.
- Bioavailability of all PPI is reduced by food
- At least 18 hours are required for synthesis of new ***H^+/K^+ ATPase*** pump molecules.
- Proton pump inhibitors undergo rapid first-pass and systemic hepatic metabolism and have negligible renal clearance.

63. Ans. a. Liposomal...

[Ref: KDT 7th/787-89; Katzung 12th/934, 849-52, 1066]

*"**AMB** is not absorbed orally, it can be given orally for intestinal candidiasis without systemic toxicity. **Administered I.V.** as suspension made from deoxycholate (DOC), it gets widely distributed in the body. It can be also **administered topically** for vaginitis, otomycosis etc." (KDT 7th/788)*

"**Liposomal AMB**: It has been produced to improve tolerability of I.V. infusion, reduce its toxicity & achieve targeted delivery. It delivers AMB particularly to reticuloendothelial cells in liver & spleen-especially valuable for kala azar & in immunocompromised" *(KDT 7th/788)*

Mechanism of Action

- **Amphotericin B** is selective in its fungicidal effect because it exploits the difference in lipid composition of fungal and mammalian cell membranes.
- **Ergosterol**, a cell membrane sterol, is found in the cell membrane of fungi, whereas the predominant sterol of bacteria and human cells is **cholesterol**.
- ***Amphotericin B binds to ergosterol and alters the permeability of the cell by forming amphotericin B-associated pores in the cell membrane.***
- Owing to its ***broad spectrum of activity*** and fungicidal action, amphotericin B remains a useful agent for nearly all life-threatening mycotic infections, although newer less toxic agents have begun to replace amphotericin B for many conditions.

- For treatment of systemic fungal disease, ***amphotericin B is given by slow intravenous infusion*** at a dosage of 0.5-1 mg/kg/d. It is usually continued to a defined total dose (*e.g.,* 1-2 g), rather than a defined time span, as used with other antimicrobial drugs.
- **Intrathecal therapy** for fungal meningitis is poorly tolerated and fraught with difficulties related to maintaining cerebrospinal fluid access.
- ***Local administration of amphotericin B*** has been used with success. Mycotic corneal ulcers and keratitis can be cured with topical drops as well as by direct subconjunctival injection. Fungal arthritis has been treated with adjunctive local injection directly into the joint.
- Candiduria responds to bladder irrigation with amphotericin B and this route has been shown to produce no significant systemic toxicity.

64. Ans. a. Penicillin, d. Cepha..

[Ref: KDT 7th/689-90; Katzung 12th/803]

Mechanism of Action of Drugs

- **Inhibit cell wall synthesis:** Penicillins, Cephalosporins, Cycloserine, Vancomycin, Bacitracin.
- **Cause leakage from cell membranes:** Polypeptides-Polymyxins, Colistin, Bacitracin. Polyenes-Amphotericin B, Nystatin, Hamycin.
- **Inhibit protein synthesis:** Tetracyclines, Chloramphenicol, Erythromycin, Clindamycin, Linezolid.
- **Cause misreading of m-RNA code and affect permeability: Aminoglycosides**-Streptomycin, Gentamicin, etc.
- **Inhibit DNA gyrase:** Fluoroquinolones -Ciprofloxacin and others.
- **Interfere with DNA function:** Rifampin.
- **Interfere with DNA synthesis:** Acyclovir, Zidovudine.
- **Interfere with intermediary metabolism:** Sulfonamides, Sulfones, PAS, Trimethoprim, Pyrimethamine, Metronidazole.

"**Daptomycin**: Its spectrum of activity is similar to that of vancomycin except that it is more rapidly bactericidal in vitro and it is active against vancomycin-resistant strains of enterococci and vancomycin-intermediate and -resistant strains of *S aureus*. The precise mechanism of action is not known, but it appears to ***bind to and depolarize the cell membrane, causing potassium efflux and rapid cell death***"*-Katzung 12th/803*

65. Ans. a. SGLT-2..., c. Causes..., d. Increases...

[Ref: KDT 7th/270; http: //www.diabetesincontrol.com]

Canagliflozin

- Canagliflozin is an antidiabetic drug used to improve glycemic control in patients with type 2 diabetes.
- It is a SGLT-2 inhibitor. Sodium-glucose co-transporter-2 (SGLT2) inhibitors are a new group of oral medications used for treating type 2 diabetes. The drugs work by helping the kidneys to lower blood glucose levels.
- Drugs in the SGLT2 inhibitors class include empagliflozin, canagliflozin, dapagliflozin, ipragliflozin (which has not yet been approved for use in the U.S.). At this time canagliflozin is the only drug in this class approved by the FDA for the treatment of type 2 diabetes.
- Canagliflozin produces beneficial effects on HDL cholesterol andsystolic blood pressure, but these effects are offset by ***increased LDL cholesterol***

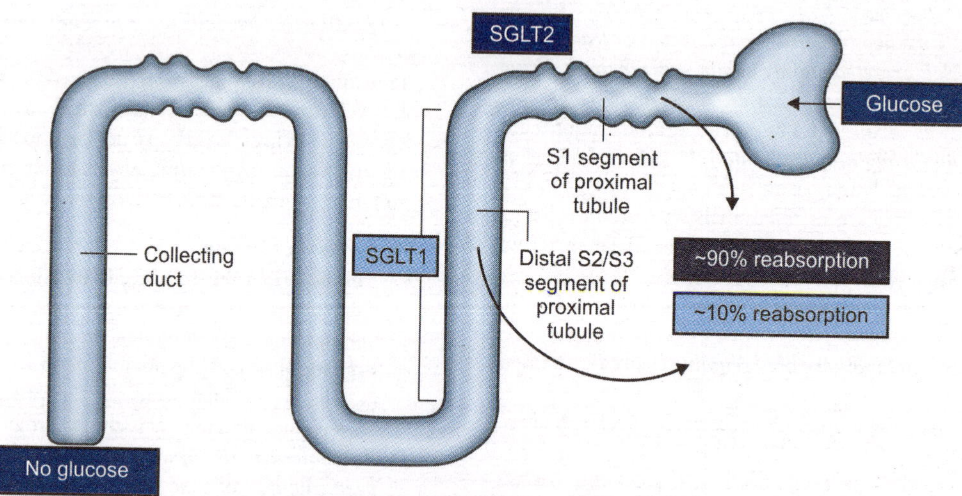

Fig: SGLT2 is a protein in humans that facilitates glucose reabsorption in the kidney. SGLT2 inhibitors block the reabsorption of glucose in the kidney, increase glucose excretion and lower blood glucose levels

- SGLT2 inhibitors have been approved for use as a treatment for diabetes since 2013. They are taken once a day with or without food.
- ***Vaginal yeast infections and urinary tract infections are the most common side effects*** associated with canagliflozin with the greatest risk being in female patients and those men who are uncircumcised.
- There is also an increased desire to urinate and the medication is not indicated in patients with type 1 diabetes, or patients with frequent ketones in their blood or urine, severe renal impairment, end stage renal disease or patients receiving dialysis. Patients should be advised to expect glucose to be in the urine and if they are using urine glucose strips that they will have a positive reading most of the time.
- ***Canagliflozin is less effective in patients with moderate renal failure and probably ineffective in severe renal failure and type 1 diabetes***

66. Ans. a. Cause..., c. Contraindicated..., e. GI...

[Ref: KDT 7th/275-76; Katzung 12th/757]

"**Thiazolidinedione (pioglitazone)** ***is PPAR γ agonist (peroxisome proliferator-activated receptor γ)***" *(KDT 7th/276)*

"**Biguanides (including metformin)** differ markedly from sulfonylureas: ***cause little or no hypoglycemia***[Q] in nondiabetics subject & even in diabetics episodes of hypoglycemia d/t metformin are rare" *(KDT 7th/275)*

*"**Metformin** is reported to **improve lipid profile as well in type II DM** (i.e ↓**LDL**)[Q]" (KDT 6th/275)*

Metformin (Biguanides)

◈ *Katzung 12th/757*

Mechanisms of Action

- These agents are more appropriately termed "euglycemic" agents.
- Currently proposed mechanisms of action includes
  - Reduced hepatic and renal gluconeogenesis
  - Slowing of glucose absorption from the gastrointestinal tract, with increased glucose to lactate conversion by enterocytes;
  - Direct stimulation of glycolysis in tissues, with increased glucose removal from blood; and
  - Reduction of plasma glucagon levels.

Toxicities

- The most common toxic effects of metformin are gastrointestinal (anorexia, nausea, vomiting, abdominal discomfort, diarrhea) and occur in up to 20% of patients.
- *Absorption of vitamin B_{12} appears to be reduced*[Q] during long-term metformin therapy and annual screening of serum vitamin B_{12} levels and red blood cell parameters has been encouraged by the manufacturer to determine the need for vitamin B_{12} injections.
- In the absence of hypoxia or renal or hepatic insufficiency, *lactic acidosis* is less common with metformin therapy than with phenformin therapy.
- Biguanides are ***contraindicated in patients with renal disease,*** alcoholism, hepatic disease, or conditions predisposing to tissue anoxia (*e.g.,* chronic cardiopulmonary dysfunction), because of an *increased risk of lactic acidosis*[Q] induced by biguanide drugs in the presence of these diseases.

Partial Table: Harrison 19th/2414, 17th/2299

Drug	Mechanism of Action	Examples	A1C Reduction (%)a	Agent-Specific Advantages	Agent-Specific Disadvantages	Contraindications/Relative Contraindications
Biguanides	↓Hepatic glucose production, weight loss, glucose, utilization, insulin resistance	Metformin	1–2	Weight loss	Lactic acidosis, diarrhea, nausea	Serum creatinine >1.5 mg/dL (men) >1.4 mg/dL (women), CHF, radiographic contrast studies, seriously ill patients, acidosis

"**Metformin** treats the root cause of ***PCOS,*** [Q] **rectifies endocrine & metabolic functions & improves fertility"** *(Shaw's Gynaecology 14th/332)*

"The insulin-sensitising drug **metformin** is useful in a variety of insulin-resistant and prediabetic conditions, including ***impaired glucose tolerance, obesity, polycystic ovary syndrome and metabolic abnormalities associated with HIV disease***" *(www.docguide.com/news)*

67. Ans. a. Vincristine, c. Amiodarone, d. Palitaxel

[Ref: Harrison 19th/2686-88, 18th/3463-66; KDT 7th/706]

Note: Sulfonamide not mentioned in list of drugs causing neuropathies (in Harrison)

Table: *(Harrison 19th/2686-88, 17th/2658)*: **Toxic Neuropathies**

	Circumstances of Toxicity	**Neuropathy**
Pharmaceutical agents		
Chloramphenicol	Mean cumulative dose 255 g, duration	S > M
Colchicine	Chronic dosing at 1.2 mg/d especially in the presence of renal dysfunction	Distal paresthesias and proximal weakness
Dapsone	200–400 mg/d over many months	Pure motor, especially upper limbs
Disulfiram	250–500 mg/d after several months used for alcoholism	SM
Ethambutol	>20 mg/kg per day over many months	Sensory neuropathy
Ethionamide	>15 mg/kg	Sensory neuropathy
Gold	Controversial, as rheumatoid arthritis can cause neuropathy Not dose dependent	S > M with myokymia
Isoniazid	>5 mg/kg over weeks or about 6 months, depending on acetylator status	Dose-dependent SM neuropathy
Metronidazole	Cumulative dose > 30 g	Sensory (small and large fiber)
Misonidazole	Cumulative dose > 18 g/m2	Sensory axonopathy
Nitrofurantoin	Standard dose of 200 mg/day over a few weeks	Mild SM neuropathy
Nitrous oxide	Dental surgery, anesthesia, substance abuse	S >> M
Nucleoside analogues (ddC, ddI, 4dT)	>12.5 mg/kg per day for ddI, 0.02 mg/kg per day for ddC and 0.5 mg/kg per day for 4dT	Painful sensory neuropathy
Pyridoxine	>200 mg a day over several months	Length-dependent axonopathy
Suramin[Q]	Peak serum concentration of 350 μg/mL	S > M; may be demyelinating
Taxol	Cumulative dose of >1500 mg/m2	S > M
Thalidomide	100 mg/d for 6 months.	S > M
Vincristine and other vinca alkaloids	Almost all patients	S > M but autonomic fibers also affected
Amiodarone	400 mg/day for 6–36 months, serum concentration of 2.4 mg/L	SM; dose-dependent
Perhexiline	Not dose-related	S (large fiber) and M, facial, autonomic
Polychlorinated biphenyls	Plasticizers, electrical insulators	SM
Suramin	Not dose-related	Demyelinating like subacute GBS
Trichloroethylene	Dry-cleaning, rubber, degreasing agent	Mainly cranial nerves: trigeminal, facial, oculomotor, optic
Platinum compounds, *e.g., cisplatin*	Cumulative dose more than 900 mg/m2	Large-fiber sensory
High-dose pyridoxine[Q]	Massive parenteral doses in grams over days	Sensory neuronopathy; gait ataxia, pseudoathetosis
Taxol	Single dose of ≥250 mg/m2	Sensory ataxia

Note: *S, sensory; M, motor; SM, sensorimotor; NCS, nerve conduction studies*

68. Ans. c. Increase..., e. Renal...

A & E

[Ref: KDT 7th/124-133; Goodman & Gillman 11th/244-248; Ganong 25th/353-56]

*"**Epinephrine cause bronchial muscle relaxation** (through β_2 receptor) whereas **norepinephrine has no action** (no action on β_2)"*

*"**Both epinephrine & norepinephrine increases renal vascular resistance & thus reduce renal blood flow**" (Goodman & Gillman 11th/244)*

Table *(KDT 7th/131)*: **Comparative effects of I.V. infusion of adrenaline, noradrenaline & isoprenaline**

Action	Adrenaline (Epinephrine)	Noradrenaline (Norepinephrine)	Isoprenaline
Heart rate	↑	↓	↑↑
Cardiac output	↑↑	–	↑↑
Blood pressure			
Systolic	↑↑	↑↑	↑
Diastolic	↓↑	↑↑	↓↓
Mean	↑	↑↑	↓
Blood flow			
Skin & mucus	↓	↓	-
mem.	↑↑	–, ↓	↑
Skeletal muscle	↓	↓	–
Kidney	↑↑	-	↑
Liver	↑	↑	↑
Coronary			
Bronchial muscle	↓↓	-	↓↓
Intestinal muscle	↓↓	↓	↓
Blood sugar	↑↑	–, ↑	↑

Table: *(KDT 7th/130)*

Adrenaline (Epinephrine)	$\alpha_1 + \alpha_2 + \beta_1 + \beta_2$ & weak β_3 action
Noradrenaline (Norepinephrine)	$\alpha_1 + \alpha_2 + \beta_1 + \beta3$ but no β_2 action
Isoprenaline	$\beta_1 + \beta_2 + \beta_3$ but no α action

69. Ans. a. Sulfa..., c. Pipera..., d. Enalapri..., e. Ibuprofe..

[Ref: KDT 7th/698-99, 725, 61-62; Katzung 12th/801]

Drugs & their Action

"***Tazobactam pharmacokinetics matches with piperacillin*** with which it has been combined for use in severe infections like peritonitis, pelvic/urinary/respiratory infections caused by β–lactamase producing bacilli" *(KDT 7th/725)*

"***ACE inhibitors/ARBs** are particularly synergistic with **diuretics**; this combination is very good for patients with associated CHF or LVH" (KDT 7th/571, 559)*

Serratiopeptidase is a proteolytic enzyme (protease) produced by enterobacterium *Serratia* sp.Brand name ***Nildol-SP (400+15)*** is combination of Serratiopeptidase & Ibuprofen (Royal Sapphire Remedies Tablet) *(http: //www.medindia.net/drug-price/serratiopeptidase)*

Example of Synergistic Action

◈ *(KDT & Katzung)*

- *Gentamycin or streptomycin + penicillins: Viridans streptococcal endocarditis* [Q], *enterococcal endocarditis*[Q]
- Ampicillin or amoxicillin + β–lactamase inhibitor clavulanic acid or sulbactam[Q]: β-lactamase producing *H.influenzae*, N. gonorrhoeae & other organism
- *Carbenicillin/ticarcillin+ gentamicin: Pseudomonas infection*[Q]*, especially in neutropenic patients*
- *Trimethoprim + sulfamethoxazole combination*[Q]*: Bacterial infections & Pneumocystis jiroveci pneumonia*
- *Rifampin + Isoniazid*[Q]*: Tuberculosis*[Q]
- *Ceftazidime + Ciprofloxacin: Pseudomonas* [Q]
- *Penicillin + Sulfonamide: Actinomycosis*[Q]
- *Streptomycin+ Tetracycline: Brucellosis*
- *Streptomycin + Chloramphenicol: K. pneumonia*
- *Rifampin + Dapsone: Leprosy*[Q]
- *Amphotericin B + Flucytosine: Cryptococcal meningitis*[Q]

Example of Antagonistic Action[Q]

- ***Penicillin + Tetracycline/chloramphenicol: Pneumococci***
- ***Penicillin + Erythromycin: Gr. A Streptococci***
- Nalidixic acid + Nitrofurantoin: E. coli

Combined use of Antimicrobials

◈ *KDT 7th/698-99*

- Penicillin/Ampicillin + Streptomycin/Gentamycin (Aminoglycosides): Additive/Synergistic
- ***Penicillin+Tetracycline/Chloramphenicol/Erythromycin: Antagonism***
- **Amphotericin B + Flucytosine: Synergistic**
- For empirical therapy of bacterial meningitis, vancomycin is usually combined with ceftriaxone/cefotaxime *-KDT 7th/757*
- *To overcome resistance, ceftriaxone has been combined with sulbactam or tazobactam (KDT 7th/728)*

70. Ans. a. Patient..., b. Dextrose..., c. Artesunate...

[Ref: KDT 7th/819-21; Park 23rd/262-67; Harrison 19th/1379-81, 18th/1698-1705]

> **Note:** "***Artemisin in derivatives never be given as monotherapy** for uncomplicated malaria. These rapidly acting drugs, if used alone, can lead to development of parasite resistance (Park 23rd/262, 21st/239)*

Severe Malaria Treatment: ACT

- ACT consists of artemisinin derivative combined with a long acting antimalarial drug (amodiaquine, lumefantrine, mefloquine or sulfadoxine-pyrimethamine)
- ***Artesunate:*** 2.4 mg/kg I.V. or I.M. given on admission (time=0), then at 12 hours & 24 hours, then once a day (dilute artesunate powder in 5% sodium bicarbonate provided in the pack)
- Once the patient can take oral therapy, patient ***should get full course of oral ACT***

Severe Malaria

◈ *Harrison 19th/1379-81, 18th/1701*

- Severe falciparum malaria constitutes a medical emergency requiring intensive nursing care and careful management. Ancillary drugs such as **high-dose glucocorticoids**, urea, heparin, dextran, desferrioxamine, antibody to tumor necrosis factor α and high-dose phenobarbital (20 mg/kg) have ***proved either ineffective or harmful in clinical trials and should not be used.***
- In acute renal failure or severe metabolic acidosis, hemofiltration or hemodialysis should be started as early as possible

- When the patient is unconscious, the **blood glucose level** should be measured every 4–6 h. ***All patients should receive a continuous infusion of dextrose and blood concentrations ideally should be maintained above 4 mmol/L.*** Hypoglycemia (<2.2 mmol/L or 40 mg/dL) should be treated immediately with bolus glucose.
- The parasite count and hematocrit level should be measured every 6–12 h. Anemia develops rapidly; if the hematocrit falls to <20%, then whole blood (preferably fresh) or packed cells should be transfused slowly, with careful attention to circulatory status. Renal function should be checked daily.
- Children presenting with severe anemia and acidotic breathing are often hypovolemic; in this situation, resuscitation with crystalloids or blood is indicated. Accurate assessment is vital

Table *(Harrison 19th/1378, 1380, 18th/1699)*: **Regimens for the Treatment of severe Falciparum Malaria**

Artesunatec (2.4 mg/kg stat IV followed by 2.4 mg/kg at 12 and 24 h and then daily if necessary)[g] *or, if unavailable, one of the following:* **Artemether**[c] (3.2 mg/kg stat IM followed by 1.6 mg/kg qd) or Quinine dihydrochloride (20 mg of salt/kg[h] infused over 4 h, followed by 10 mg of salt/kg infused over 2–8 h q8h[i]) or **Quinidine** (10 mg of base/kg[h] infused over 1–2 h, followed by 1.2 mg of base/kg per hour[i] with electrocardiographic monitoring)

Artemisinin and derivatives (artemether, artesunate)	Good oral absorption, slow and variable absorption of IM artemether; artesunate and artemether biotransformed to active metabolite dihydroartemisinin; all drugs eliminated very rapidly; t1/2: <1 h	Broader stage specificity and more rapid than other drugs; no action on liver stages; kills all but fully mature gametocytes of *P. falciparum*	Reduction in reticulocyte count (but not anemia); neutropenia at high doses	Anaphylaxis, urticaria, fever

71. Ans. b. Intramuscular..., d. Bioavailab..., e. Changes...

[Ref: KDT 7th/16-17; Katzung 12th/43-44]

Note: *Peak concentrations tells about therapeutic response & area under curve gives idea about bioavailability (explained through diagram)*

Blood Concentration-time Curve (AUC)

◈ *Goodman & Gilmann 11th/19*

- The **area under the blood concentration-time curve** (area under the curve, or AUC) can be used to calculate the ***clearance for first-order elimination.***
- *"Area under curve (blood concentration-time curve) can be used to calculate clearance. The AUC is also used as a **measure of bioavailability**"-Goodman & Gilmann 11th/19*
- The ***AUC is also used as a measure of bioavailability*** (defined as 100% for an intravenously administered drug).

Bioavailability will be <100% for orally administered drugs, mainly to incomplete absorption and first-pass metabolism and elimination. Thus, the therapeutic goal is to maintain steady-state drug levels within the therapeutic window. The application of pharmacokinetic monitoring to drug treatment in cases where the therapeutic index of a drug is narrow is beneficial since successful therapy is associated with a target blood level at steady-state.

Bioavailability

- Bioavailability is defined as the *fraction of unchanged drug reaching the systemic circulation following administration by any route.*
- The **area under the blood concentration-time curve (AUC)** is a common measure of the ***extent of bioavailability*** for a drug given by a particular route
- Incomplete bioavailability after s.c. or i.m. injection is less common, but may occur due to local binding of the drug
- For an intravenous dose of the drug, bioavailability is assumed to be equal to unity. For a drug administered orally, ***bioavailability may be less than 100%*** for two main reasons–***incomplete extent of absorption and first-pass elimination.***
- ***Bioavailability variation assumes practical significance for drugs with low safety margin (digoxin) or where dosage needs precise control (oral hypoglycaemics, oral hypocoagulants).***

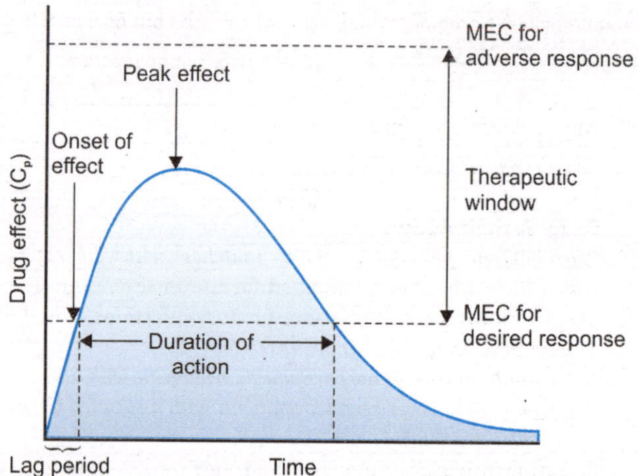

Fig: Temporal characteristics of drug effect and relationship to the therapeutic window (e.g., single dose, oral administration)

Table *(Katzung 12th/43)*: **Routes of administration, bioavailability and general characteristics**

Route	Bioavailability (%)	Characteristics
Intravenous (IV)	100 (by definition)	Most rapid onset
Intramuscular (IM)	75 to <100	Large volumes often feasible; may be painful

Contd...

Route	Bioavailability (%)	Characteristics
Subcutaneous (SC)	75 to <100	Smaller volumes than IM; may be painful
Oral (PO)	5 to <100	Most convenient; first-pass effect may be significant
Rectal (PR)	30 to <100	Less first-pass effect than oral
Inhalation	5 to <100	Often very rapid onset
Transdermal	80 to <100	Usually very slow absorption; used for lack of first-pass effect; prolonged duration of action

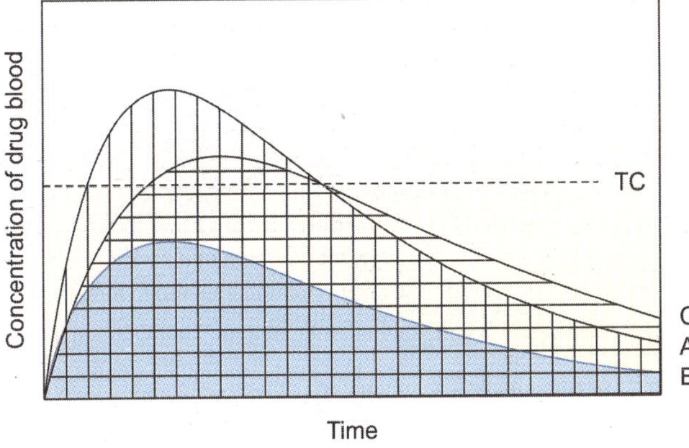

Fig: Blood concentration-time curves, illustrating how changes in the rate of absorption and extent of bioavailability can influence both the duration of action and the effectiveness of the same total dose of a drug administered in three different formulations. The dashed line indicates the target concentration (TC) of the drug in the blood

72. Ans. b. Aminoglycoside

[Ref: KDT 7th/838; Harrison 19th/1101, 18th/1338-39;Katzung 12th/904-05]

- "**Imipenem**: *Range of activity includes gram positive cocci, enterobacteriaceae, Ps aeruginosa, Listeria as well as* ***anaerobes like Bac. fragilis & Cl. difficile***" *(KDT 7th/731)*
- "**Anaerobic bacterial infection**: *They occur mostly after colorectal or pelvic surgery, appendectomy etc. Brain abscess & endocarditis may be caused by anaerobic organisms.* **Metronidazole** *is an effective drug for these. Other drug effective in anaerobic infection are* **clindamycin & chloramphenicol**" *(KDT 7th/838)*

Table *(Harrison 19th/1101)*: **Antimicrobial Therapy for Infections Involving Commonly Encountered Anaerobic Gram-Negative Rods**

Category 1 (<2% Resistance)	Category 2 (<15% Resistance)	Category 3 (Variable Resistance)	Category 4 (Resistance)
Carbapenems (imipenem, meropenem, doripenem) Metronidazole β-Lactam/β-lactamase inhibitor combination (ampicillin/sulbactam, ticarcillin/clavulanic acid, piperacillin/tazobactam) Chloramphenicol[b]	Tigecycline High-dose anti-pseudomonal penicillins	Cephamycins Clindamycin Penicillin Cephalosporins Tetracycline Vancomycin Erythromycin Moxifloxacin	Aminoglycosides Monobactams Trimethoprim-sulfamethoxazole

Note: [b]Chloramphenicol is probably not as effective as other category 1 antimicrobial agents in treating anaerobic infections.

Table *(Katzung 12th/904-05)*: **Empiric antimicrobial therapy based on microbiologic etiology.**

Suspected or Proved Disease or Pathogen	Drugs of First Choice	Alternative Drugs
Anaerobic bacteria		
Gram-positive (clostridia, Peptococcus, Actinomyces, Peptostreptococcus)	Penicillin, clindamycin	Vancomycin, carbapenems, chloramphenicol
Clostridium difficile	Metronidazole	Vancomycin, bacitracin
Bacteroides fragilis	Metronidazole	***Chloramphenicol, carbapenems, beta-lactam-beta-lactamase-inhibitor combinations,*** *clindamycin*
Fusobacterium, Prevotella, Porphyromonas	Metronidazole, clindamycin, penicillin	As for B fragilis

Anaerobic Infections

- *CMDT*
- Anaerobic bacteria comprise the majority of normal human flora. Normal microbial flora of the mouth (anaerobic spirochetes, prevotella, fusobacteria), the skin (anaerobic diphtheroids), the ***large bowel (bacteroides, anaerobic streptococci, clostridia)*** and the female genitourinary tract

(bacteroides, anaerobic streptococci, fusobacteria) produce disease when displaced from their normal sites into tissues or closed body spaces.

- In the **colon** there are upto 10^{11} anaerobes per gram of content—predominantly ***B fragilis, clostridia and peptostreptococci***. These organisms play a central role in most intra-abdominal abscesses following trauma to the colon, diverticulitis, appendicitis, or perirectal abscess and may also participate in hepatic abscess and cholecystitis, often in association with aerobic coliform bacteria.
- Agents that are active against ***B fragilis*** include ***metronidazole, chloramphenicol, moxifloxacin, tigecycline, ertapenem, imipenem, doripenem, ampicillin-sulbactam, ticarcillin-clavulanic acid and piperacillin-tazobactam***. Resistance to cefoxitin, cefotetan and clindamycin is increasingly encountered. Most third-generation cephalosporins have poor efficacy. Non-fragilis species of bacteroides may be less susceptible to the cephalosporins.

Table *(CMDT)*: **Treatment of anaerobic intra-abdominal infections.**

Oral therapy
• Moxifloxacin 400 mg every 24 hours
Intravenous therapy
• Moderate to moderately severe infections:
▪ Ertapenem 1 g every 24 hours or
▪ Ceftriaxone 1 g every 24 hours (or ciprofloxacin 400 mg every 12 hours, if penicillin allergic) plus metronidazole 500 mg every 8 hours or
▪ Tigecycline 100 mg once followed by 50 mg every 12 hours or
▪ Moxifloxacin 400 mg every 24 hours
• Severe infections:
▪ ***Imipenem***, 0.5 g every 6–8 hours; meropenem 1 g every 8 hours; doripenem 0.5 g every 8 hours; ***piperacillin/tazobactam*** 4.5 g every 8 hours

MICROBIOLOGY

73. Ans. a. Belongs..., b. Transm..., c. Tran..., e. Cont...

[Ref: Harrison 19th/1323-28, 18th/1633-36]

Ebola Virus

◈ *Harrison 19th/1323-28, 18th/1633-36*

- The family Filoviridae comprises two antigenically and genetically distinct genera: *Marburg virus* and *Ebola virus*.
- Typical filovirus particles contain a ***single linear, negative-sense, single-stranded RNA*** arranged in a helical nucleocapsid.
- After an **incubation period** of ***~7–10 days*** (range, ***3–16 days***), the patient abruptly develops fever, severe headache, malaise, myalgia, nausea and vomiting. Continued fever is joined by diarrhea (often severe), chest pain (accompanied by cough), prostration and depressed mentation. In light-skinned patients (and less often in dark-skinned individuals), a maculopapular rash appears around day 5–7 and is followed by desquamation.
- Bleeding may begin about this time and is apparent from any mucosal site and into the skin.
- Additional findings include edema of the face, neck and/or scrotum; hepatomegaly; flushing; conjunctival injection; and pharyngitis.

Characteristics of Ebola Virus

◈ *www.cdc.gov/vhf/ebola/about.htm*

- The length of time between exposure to the virus and the development of symptoms (incubation period) is between 2–21 days. Most often this is between 4–10 days..
- Between people, Ebola disease spreads only by ***direct contact with the blood or body fluids*** of a person who has developed symptoms of the disease. Body fluids that may contain ebola viruses include saliva, mucus, vomit, feces, sweat, tears, breast milk, úrine and semen.
- The WHO states that only people who are very sick are able to spread Ebola disease in saliva and whole virus has not been reported to be transmitted through sweat. Most people spread the virus through ***blood, feces and vomit.***
- Entry points for the virus include the nose, mouth, eyes, open wounds, cuts and abrasions.
- The Ebola virus may be able to persist for up to 8 ***weeks in the semen*** of survivors after they recovered, which could lead to ***infections via sexual intercourse.***
- Dead bodies remain infectious; thus, *people handling human remains in practices such as traditional burial rituals or more modern processes such as embalming are at risk.*
- The **natural reservoir** for Ebola has yet to be confirmed; however, **bats** are considered to be the most likely candidate species.
- The disease has a high risk of death, killing between 25% and 90% of those infected with the virus, averaging out at 50%. This is often due to low blood pressure from fluid loss and typically follows 6–16 days after symptoms appear.

74. Ans. c. Toxoplasmosis...

[Ref: Paniker Parasitology 6th/100: Harrison 19th/1398-1405, 18th/1722-26]

Toxoplasmosis

◈ *Harrison 19th/1398-1405*

- **Infective stage for man**: *Oocyst with sporozoites & tissue cyst with bradyzoites*
- Freshly passed oocyst is not infective (*needs development in the soil*)
- Human infection is ***dead end for the parasite***
- The principal source of human *Toxoplasma* infection remains uncertain.
- *Transmission usually takes place by the oral route* and can be attributable to ingestion of either sporulated oocysts from *contaminated soil or bradyzoites from undercooked meat*

- In addition to oral transmission, direct transmission of the parasite by blood or organ products ***during transplantation*** *takes place at a low rate*
- In persons whose immune systems are intact, acute toxoplasmosis is *usually asymptomatic and self-limited.* This condition can go unrecognized in 80–90% of adults and children with acquired infection
- In the **immunocompromised** or fetal host, the immune factors necessary to control the spread of tachyzoite infection are lacking. This altered immune state allows the persistence of tachyzoites and gives rise to progressive focal destruction that results in organ failure (*i.e.*, necrotizing encephalitis, pneumonia and myocarditis).
- ***Serologic testing has become the routine method of diagnosis.***
- Diagnosis of acute infection with *T. gondii* can be established by detection of the simultaneous presence of IgG and IgM antibodies to *Toxoplasma* in serum. The presence of circulating IgA favors the diagnosis of an acute infection.

Human infection is a dead end for the parasite. Human infection is obtained in the following ways

◈ *Paniker Parasitology 6th/100*

- Eating uncooked or undercooked infected meat containing tissue cysts.
- Ingestion of mature oocysts through food, water or fingers contaminated with cat feces directly or indirectly.
- Intrauterine infection from infected mother to babies.
- *Rarely by blood transfusion* or ***transplantation from infected donors.***

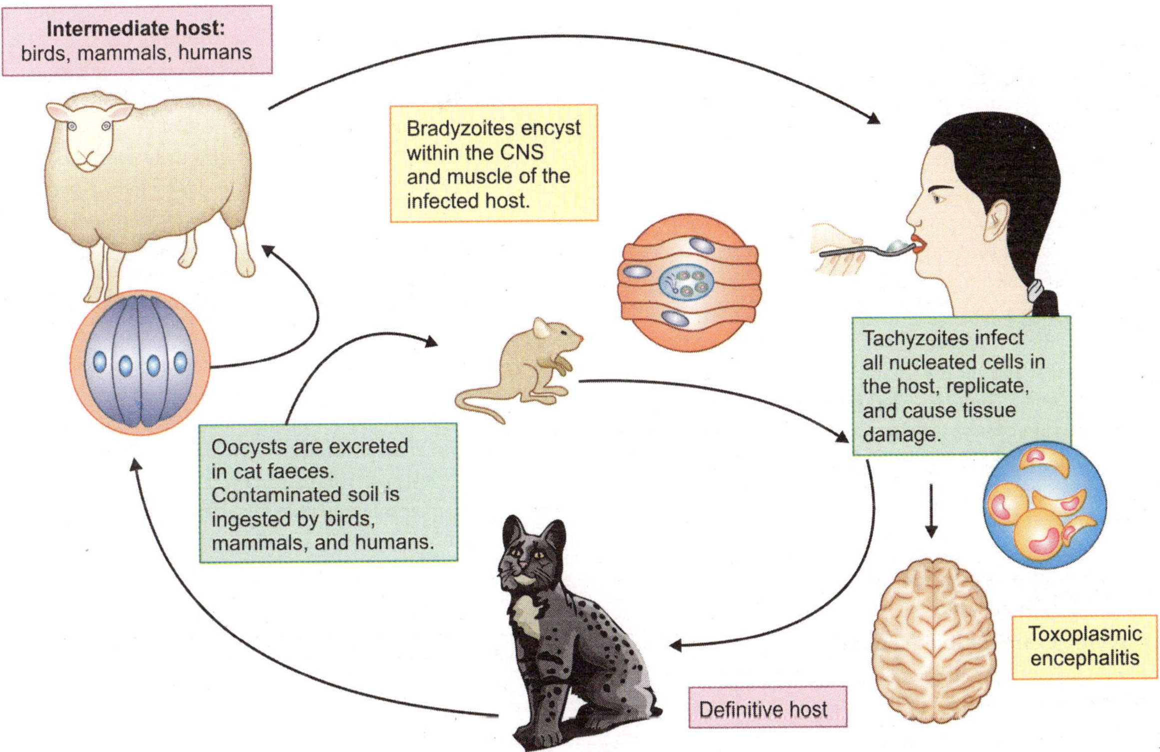

Fig: Life cycle of Toxoplasma gondii: The cat is the definitive host in which the sexual phase of the cycle is completed. Oocysts shed in cat feces can infect a wide range of animals, including birds, rodents, grazing domestic animals and humans. The bradyzoites found in the muscle of food animals may infect humans who eat insufficiently cooked meat products, particularly lamb and pork. Although human disease can take many forms, congenital infection and encephalitis from reactivation of latent infection in the brains of immunosuppressed persons are the most important manifestations

75. Ans. e. Syphilis...

[Ref: Ananthanarayan 8th/233, 317; Greenwood Microbiology 16th/91]

Virulent Strains

"Syphilis is caused by *Treponema pallidum*"-*Ananthanarayan 8th/372*

"Virulent strains of ***diphtheria*** *bacilli produce a very powerful* ***exotoxin.*** *The* ***pathogenic effects of the bacillus are due to toxin.*** *Almost all strains of gravis & intermedius (95-99%) are toxigenic, while only about 80-85% of mitis strains are so" (Ananthanarayan 8th/233)*

"Pertussis toxin (PT): *This is present only in* ***Bordetella pertussis.*** *It play an important role in the pathogenesis of*

***whooping cough**. PT toxoid is the major component of acellular pertussis vaccines" (Ananthanarayan 8th/336)*

*"The **anthrax toxin** is a complex of three fractions: the edema factor (OF or Factor I), the protective antigen factor (PA or Factor II) & the lethal factor (LF or Factor III)" (Ananthanarayan 8th/244 G)*

Note: • *Toxins inhibiting protein synthesis*
- *— Shigella dysenteriae I (Shiga toxin)*
- *— Diphtheria*
- *— Pseudomonas*
- *— Verotoxin I=Shiga like toxin of E.coli)*

76. Ans. a. Periodic..., d. Gomori's...

[Ref: Ananthanarayan 8th/601: Harrison 19th/1330, 18th/1637]

Stains & their Uses

"The ***PAS & methenamine silver*** stains are valuable methods for the demonstration of ***fungal elements*** in tissue section. The commonest culture media used in mycology are Sabouraud's glucose agar, Czapek-Dox medium & Corn meal agar" *(Ananthanarayan 8th/601)*

"The **von Kossa** stain is used to quantify mineralization in cell culture and tissue section" *(en.wikipedia.org/wiki)*

"The **auramine-rhodamine stain (AR)**, also known as the *Truant auramine-rhodamine stain*, is a histological technique used to visualize acid-***fast bacilli using*** fluorescence microscopy, notably species in the Mycobacterium genus"

"Giemsa stain is used in cytogenetics and for the histopathological diagnosis of malaria and other parasites"-*en.wikipedia.org/wiki*

"The stains most commonly used to identify fungi are ***periodic acid–Schiff and Gomori methenamine silver***. Candida, unlike other fungi, is visible on ***gram-stained tissue smears***. *Hematoxylin and eosin stain is not* sufficient to identify Candida in tissue specimens. When positive, an ***India ink preparation*** of cerebrospinal fluid (CSF) is diagnostic for cryptococcosis. Most laboratories now use calcofluor white staining coupled with fluorescent microscopy to identify fungi in fluid specimens" *(Harrison 19th/1330, 18th/1637)*

Microscopic Examination of Fungus

"Although specimens can be examined directly with KOH or ***calcofluor white stain***, the yeasts are rarely found. Even though they are sparse in tissue, the sensitivity of histopathologic sections is enhanced with routine fungal cell wall stains, such as ***Gomori's methenamine silver***, which stains the cell walls black, or the ***periodic acid-Schiff stain***, which imparts a red color to the cell walls"

77. Ans. a. RPR, b. VDRL

[Ref: Ananthanarayan 8th/375-76: Harrison 19th/1137-38, 18th/1384; CMDT 2016/1464; Greenwood Microbiology 16th/347]

Serologic Tests for Syphilis

◈ *CMDT 2016/1464*

There are two general categories of serologic tests for syphilis: (1) **Nontreponemal tests** detect antibodies to lipoidal antigens present in the host after modification by *T pallidum*. (2) **Treponemal tests** use live or killed *T pallidum* as antigen to detect antibodies specific for pathogenic treponemes.

Serologic Tests for Syphilis

◈ *Harrison 19th/1137-38, 18th/1384-85*

- There are two types of serologic test for syphilis: nontreponemal and treponemal. Both are reactive in persons with any treponemal infection, including yaws, pinta and endemic syphilis.
- The most widely used **nontreponemal antibody tests** for syphilis are the ***rapid plasma reagin (RPR) and Venereal Disease Research Laboratory (VDRL) tests***, which measure IgG and IgM directed against a cardiolipin-lecithin-cholesterol antigen complex.
- The **RPR test** is easier to perform and uses unheated serum; it is the test of choice for rapid serologic diagnosis in a clinical setting and can be automated. ***The VDRL test remains the standard for examining CSF.***
- The RPR and VDRL tests are recommended for screening or for quantitation of serum antibody. The titer reflects disease activity, rising during the evolution of early syphilis and often exceeding 1: 32 in secondary syphilis. *After therapy for early syphilis, a persistent fall by fourfold or more (e.g., a decline from 1: 32 to 1: 8) is considered an adequate response.*
- **Treponemal tests** measure antibodies to native or recombinant *T. pallidum* antigens and include the ***fluorescent treponemal antibody-absorbed (FTA-ABS) test and the T. pallidum particle agglutination (TPPA) test***, both of which are more sensitive for primary syphilis than the previously used hemagglutination tests.
- *When used to confirm positive nontreponemal test results, treponemal tests have a very high positive predictive value* for diagnosis of syphilis. In a screening setting, however, these tests give false-positive results at rates as high as 1–2%.
- Treponemal tests are likely to remain reactive even after adequate treatment and cannot differentiate past from current *T. pallidum* infection.

78. Ans. d. Muller-Hinton...

[Ref: Ananthanarayan 8th/39-43, 229]

Culture Media

*"**Thayer-Martin** is a useful **selective media for Neisseria gonorrhoeae**"-Ananthanarayan 8th/229*

"**Mueller-Hinton** *is **enriched media for Neisseria***"

"*C diphtheriae* and other corynebacteria grow aerobically on most ordinary laboratory media. On Loeffler's serum medium, corynebacteria grow much more readily than other respiratory organisms and the morphology of organisms is typical in smears"

"Lowenstein-Jensen Medium. It is used to ***culture tubercle bacilli***. It contains egg, malachite green and glycerol.

- Egg is an enrichment material which stimulates the growth of Tubercle bacilli,
- Malachite green inhibits growth of organisms other than mycobacteria

- Glycerol promotes the growth of *Mycobacterium tuberculosis* but not *Mycobacterium bovis*"

"**Chocolate Agar or Heated Blood agar:** Prepared by heating blood agar. It is used for culture of pneumococcus, gonococcus, meningococcus and Haemophilus. Heating the blood inactivates inhibitor of growths"

MacConkey Agar

- Most commonly used for enterobacteriaceae. It contains agar, peptone, sodium chloride, bile salt, lactose and neutral red. It is a selective and indicator medium.
- **Selective** as bile salt does not inhibit the growth of enterobactericeae but inhibits growth of many other bacteria.
- **Indicator** medium as the colonies of bacteria that ferment lactose take a pink colour due to production of acid. Acid turns the indicator neutral red to pink. These bacteria are called 'lactose fermenter', *e.g.*, Escherichia coli. Colourless colony indicates that lactose is not fermented, *i.e.*, the bacterium is non-lactose fermenter, *e.g.*, Salmonella. Shigella, Vibrio.

Laboratory Media

These are classified into **six types**: *(1) Basal media, (2) Enriched media, (3) Selective media, (4) Indicator media, (5) Transport media and (6) Storage media.*

- **Basal Media:** Basal media are those that may be used for growth (culture) of bacteria that do not need enrichment of the media. Examples: Nutrient broth, nutrient agar and peptone water. *Staphylococcus and Enterobacteriaceae* grow in these media.
- **Enriched Media:** The media are enriched usually by adding blood, serum or egg. Examples: Enriched media are *blood agar, chocolate agar and* ***Lowenstein-Jensen media.*** *Streptococci* grow in blood agar media.
- **Selective Media:** These media favour the growth of a particular bacterium by inhibiting the growth of undesired bacteria and allowing growth of desirable bacteria. Examples: ***MacConkey agar, Lowenstein-Jensen media,*** tellurite media
- **Indicator (Differential) Media:** An indicator is included in the medium. A particular organism causes change in the indicator, *e.g.*, blood, neutral red, tellurite. Examples: Blood agar and ***MacConkey agar*** are indicator media.
- **Transport Media:** These media are used when specimen cannot be cultured soon after collection. Examples: Cary-Blair medium, Amies medium, Stuart medium.
- **Storage Media:** Media used for storing the bacteria for a long period of time. Examples: Egg saline medium, chalk cooked meat broth.

79. Ans. c. Can..., e. Communicable...

[Ref: Ananthanarayan 8th/400-401: Harrison 19th/1014-17, 18th/1236-39; Greenwood 16th/320-21; CMDT 09/1278]

"Members of the Legionellaceae are aerobic gram-negative bacilli that do not grow on routine microbiologic media. ***Buffered charcoal yeast extract (BCYE) agar*** is the medium used to grow *Legionella*"-*Harrison 19th/1014, 18th/1236*

Pontiac fever[Q], ***caused by Legionella Pneumophila, is a milder, nonfatal influenza-like illness with fever, chills, myalgia & headache***- *(Ananthanarayan 8th/400)*

Important Features of Legionella

- Aerobic, Gram negative motile, non encapsulated bacilli[Q]
- Natural habitat are aquatic bodies such as stagnant water, mud, hot springs.
- Out breaks are associated with contaminated water source such as ***air conditioning cooling.***
- Multiple modes of transmission -***Aspiration (MC),*** Aerosolization, direct instillation etc.
- No man to man transmission[Q]
- No animal reservoir.

Table: Manifestations of Legionella Pneumophila

Pneumonia (Legionnaires' disease) [Q]	Pontiac fever[Q]
Atypical pneumonia Presents with high fever, diarrhoea, pneumonia	Acute febrile self limiting illness
Risk factors for Legionnaires disease: Cigarette smoking and other condition that impair mucociliary clearance Chronic lung disease; Advance age; Immunosuppression Surgery is predisposing factor in nosocomial infection with transplant recipient at highest risk.	

80. Ans. d. Caused..., e. Symptom...

[Ref: Harrison 19th/1005, 18th/1220-25; Ananthanarayan 8th/227-30, 7th/227-229; Greenwood Microbiology 16th/247-248; CMDT 09/1287]

"**Urethritis in male:** The discharge ***initially is scant and mucoid*** but becomes profuse and purulent within a day or two. Gram's stain of the urethral discharge may reveal PMNs and ***gram-negative intracellular monococci and diplococcic***"-*(Harrison 19th/1005, 18th/1222)*

"Clinical disease, ***as a rule, is less severe in women,*** *many of women may carry gonococci in the cervix without any symptoms.* ***Asymptomatic carriage of gonococci is rare in men****" (Ananthanarayan 8th/228)*

"The name ***gonorrhea*** *derives from the Greek words* ***gonos (seed) & rhoia (flow)*** *& described a condition in which semen flowed from the male organ without erection" (Greenwood Microbiology 16th/247)*

"The name gonorrhea ***(meaning flow of seed)*** *was first employed by Galen in 130 AD" (Ananthanarayan 8th/227)*

"Greek gonorrhoia ***flow of seed*** *(from the mistaken belief that the discharge contained semen)" (http: //www.thefreedictionary.com/)*

Gonococcal Infections

Male

- ***Acute urethritis***[Q] is the most common clinical manifestation of gonorrhoea in males & although some men remain asymptomatic.
- Urethral discharge & dysuria, usually without urinary frequency or urgency, are the major symptoms.

- **Other features:** Seminal vesiculitis[Q], inflammation or abscess of cowper's gland, urethral stricture & periurethral abscess or fistula (Watercan perineum[Q]), edema of penis & balanitis, prostatitis[Q] (rarely)
- Epididymitis[Q] (uncommon)

Female

- Initial infection involves urethra & cervix uteri
- ***Cervicitis** is MC*[Q] manifestation
- Vaginal mucosa is resistant[Q] due to stratified squamous epithelium but can involve ***(Vulvovaginitis)*** in anestrogenic women (prepubertal, postmenopausal)
- Infection spreads to endometrium, fallopian tube ***(salpingitis)***, bartholin gland, peritoneum with perihepatic inflammation ***(Fitz-Hugh-curtis syndrome)***[Q]

81. Ans. e. Culture...

[Ref: Ananthanarayan 8th/399: Harrison 19th/1040, 18th/1261-1264;Greenwood 16th/264]

Note: Culture is most specific but not gold standard

***"H. pylori** is a **gram negative spiral rod**[Q] **& grow under microaerophilic**[Q] **conditions with 5-20% CO_2**"-(Ananthanarayan 8th/399)*

Diagnosis of H.Pylori

Harrison 19th/1040, 18th/1261

- If endoscopy is performed, the most convenient biopsy-based test is the **biopsy urease test**. The presence of *H. pylori* urease leads to a pH alteration and therefore to a color change, which often occurs within minutes but can require up to 24 h.
- **Histologic examination** of biopsy specimens for *H. pylori* also is accurate, provided that a special stain (*e.g.*, a modified Giemsa or silver stain) permitting optimal visualization of the organism is used.
- **Microbiologic culture** is ***most specific but may be insensitive*** because of difficulty with *H. pylori* isolation.

H. pylori

Ananthanarayan 8th/399

- ***Gram –ve spiral rod***
- *H. pylori* is global, with a prevalence of ***30-60%, more in the developing*** than in the developed countries
- *H. pylori* cells normally possess a ***unipolar bundle of two to six sheathed flagella***
- **Urease** is central to *H. pylori* ***metabolism and virulence***, is ***necessary for its colonization of the gastric mucosa and is a potent immunogen that elicits a vigorous immune response.***

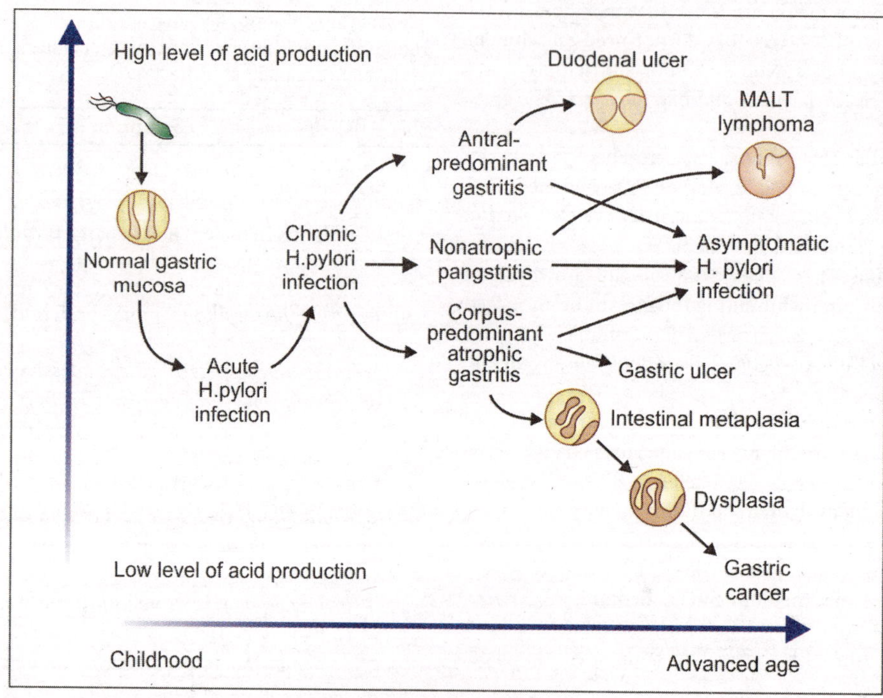

Fig: H. pylori infection

Table *(Harrison 19th/1040)*: **Tests Commonly Used to Detect Helicobacter pylori**

Test	Advantages	Disadvantages
Invasive (Based on Endoscopic Biopsy)		
Biopsy urease test[Q]	Quick, simple	Some commercial tests not fully sensitive before 24 h

Contd...

Test	Advantages	Disadvantages
Histology	May give additional histologic information	Sensitivity dependent on experience and use of special stains
Culture	Permits determination of antibiotic susceptibility	Sensitivity dependent on experience
Mycetoma or Madura Mycosis or Madura Foot		
Serology	Inexpensive and convenient	***Cannot be used for early follow-up***[Q]; some commercial kits inaccurate
13C or 14 C urea breath test	Inexpensive and simpler than endoscopy; ***useful for follow-up after treatment***[Q]	Low-dose irradiation in 14C test (although 14C is rarely used)
Stool antigen test	Inexpensive and convenient; useful for follow-up after treatment; may be useful in children	New test; role not fully established; appears less accurate than urea breath test, particularly when used to assess treatment success

82. Ans. a. Eumycetoma...

[Ref: Ananthanarayan 8th/393, 608: Harrison 19th/1355, 18th/258, 1667, 1329, e34-16f; Neena Khanna 1st/228; Greenwood 16th/223-224, 578]

Treatment of Lesion

"**Treatment of eumycetoma** involves both ***surgical extirpation of the lesion and use of antifungal agents***. Surgical removal of the lesions of eumycetoma is most effective if performed before extensive spread has occurred *(Harrison 19th/1355, 18th/1667)*

"Actinomycotic lesions may respond to sulphonamides & antibiotics but mycotic lesions are resistant & may ***require amputation***" *(Ananthanarayan 8th/608)*

"Mycetoma initially presents as a slowly progressive and ***painless subcutaneous swelling***, which is usually firm and rounded but it can also be soft and lobular. The ***lesions are painless except in the end stage where bone invasion may cause pain***"*-www.expertconsultbook.com*

Mycetoma or Madura Mycosis or Madura Foot

- Mycetomas are chronic, *slowly progressive* infections of the subcutaneous tissue, ***usually of the foot***[Q] & rarely of the other parts of the body like *hands*[Q], *gluteal region & thigh.*

Table: Etiological organisms of mycetoma

Actinomycetoma	Eumycetoma
• *Nocardia brasiliensis*[Q]	• *Madurella mycetomatis*[Q]
• *Streptomyces somaliensis*	• *Madurella grisea*
• *Actinomadura Madura*	• *Petriellidium boydii*

- Involvement of deeper tissue (bone of feet & hands) may cause deformities in long-standing cases *(Neena Khanna 1st/228)*
- The infection spreads throughout the foot, *invades bone* & is very destructive & disabling *(Roxburg/17th/43)*
- **Treatment**
  - *Actinomycetoma:* Respond to a 6-9 months course of combination of chemotherapeutic agents like Streptomycin + dapsone or co-trimoxazole etc
  - *Eumycetoma*: Ketoconazole, Itraconazole, Amphotericin B[Q]

- Most cases are reported from dry tropics & subtropics because of habit of walking barefoot

Mycetoma (Maduromycosis & Actinomycetoma)

◈ *CMDT*

- Mycetoma is a chronic local, slowly progressive destructive infection, usually involving the foot, that begins in subcutaneous tissues, frequently after localized trauma and then spreads to contiguous structures.
- ***Maduromycosis (also known as eumycetoma)*** is the term used to describe mycetoma caused by the true fungi and by phylogenetically diverse organisms.
- **Actinomycotic mycetoma** is caused by *Nocardia* and *Actinomadura* species.
- Tissue Gram stain reveals fine branching hyphae with actinomycotic mycetoma: Larger hyphae are seen with fungal mycetoma; the causative species can often be identified by the color of the characteristic grains within the infected tissues.
- *The prognosis is good for patients with actinomycetoma*, since they usually respond well to sulfonamides and sulfones, especially if treated early.
- The prognosis for maduromycosis is poor, though ***surgical debridement*** along with prolonged terbinafine or itraconazole therapy may result in a response rate of 70%. Amputation is necessary in far advanced cases.

83. Ans. a. Ziehl..., b. Kinyoun..., c. Auramine...

[Ref: Ananthanarayan 8th/348: Harrison 19th/1113-14, 18th/1350; Text Book of Diagnostic microbiology by Connie R. Mohan 3rd/691;Greenwood 16th/15]

"Ziehl-Neelsen method & phenol-auramine procedures are methods of great practical importance in diagnosis of mycobacterial diseases" *(Greenwood 16th/15)*

"The **Kinyoun method**, or **Kinyoun stain**, is an acid-fast procedure used to stain any species of the genus *Mycobacterium and Nocardia* species. It involves the application of a primary stain (carbol fuchsin), a decolorizer (acid-alcohol) and a counterstain (methylene blue)" *(http: //en.wikipedia.org/wiki/Kinyoun_stain)*

"**AFB Kinyoun Kit (Cold Method):** Method of staining acid-fast microorganisms, specifically mycobacterium. Procedure is similar to Ziehl-Neelsen stain, but does not involve heating the slides" *(http: //www.polysciences.com/Catalog)*

"In pathology, the **Grocott-Gomori's (or Gömöri) methenamine silver stain,** abbreviated **GMS**, is a popular staining method in histology. It is used widely as a screen for fungal organisms. Particularly useful in staining carbohydrates. It can be used to identify the yeast-like fungus *Pneumocystis jiroveci*[1] which causes a form of pneumonia called Pneumocystis Pneumonia (PCP) or Pneumocystosis." *(http: //en.wikipedia.org/ wiki/Grocott%27s _methenamine_silver_stain)*

"**T.B:** A presumptive diagnosis is commonly based on the finding of AFB on microscopic examination of a diagnostic specimen, such as a smear of expectorated sputum or of tissue (*e.g.*, a lymph node biopsy). Although inexpensive, AFB microscopy has relatively low sensitivity (40–60%) in culture-confirmed cases of pulmonary TB. The traditional method—light microscopy of specimens ***stained with Ziehl-Neelsen basic fuchsin dyes***—is nevertheless satisfactory, although time-consuming. Most modern laboratories processing large numbers of diagnostic specimens use ***auramine-rhodamine staining*** and fluorescence microscopy" *(Harrison 19th/1113, 18th/1350)*

Acid Fast Staining Techniques

- ***Ziehl–Neelsen stain*** (Classic and modified bleach types)
- ***Kinyoun stain***
- ***Fite stain:*** Fite-Faraco Staining & Wade Fite staining
- ***Ellis and Zabrowarny stain*** (no Phenol/carbolic acid)
- ***Auramine-rhodamine stain***
- ***Auramine phenol stain***

Acid Fast Organisms are

- ***All mycobacteria*** Q
  - *M.tuberculosis* Q; *M. Lepare* Q; ***Atypical mycobacteria***
- ***Nocordia*** Q
- **Spermatic head** Q
- ***Cryptosporidium parvum*** Q
- ***Isospora*** Q
- ***Cyclospora cyst*** Q
- ***Legionella micoadie*** Q
- ***Rhodococcus*** Q
- ***Bacterial spores*** Q

84. Ans. a. Can..., b. Animal..., d. Stomoxys..., e. It is...

[Ref: Ananthanarayan 8th/245: Greenwood Microbiology 16th/225-29; Harrison 19th/261e1-3, 18th/1768-70]

Anthrax

- It is zoonosis
- In humans, approximately 95% of cases are cutaneous anthrax and 5% are inhalation. Gastrointestinal anthrax is very rare.
- **Cutaneous anthrax** generally occurs on exposed surfaces of the arms or hands, followed in frequency by the face and neck. A pruritic papule develops 1–7 days after entry of the organisms or spores through a scratch.
- The papule rapidly changes into a vesicle or small ring of vesicles that coalesce and a necrotic ulcer develops. The lesions typically are 1–3 cm in diameter and have a characteristic central black eschar.
- Marked edema occurs. Lymphangitis and lymphadenopathy and systemic signs and symptoms of fever, malaise and headache may occur.
- After 7–10 days the eschar is fully developed. Eventually it dries, loosens and separates; healing is by granulation and leaves a scar. It may take many weeks for the lesion to heal and the edema to subside.
- In as many as 20% of patients, cutaneous anthrax can lead to sepsis, the consequences of systemic infection—including meningitis—and death.

Human Anthrax

◈ *Ananthanarayan 8th/245*

- *Human anthrax may be* **industrial** *or non-industrial (agriculture). The former is found in workers in industries such as* ***meat packing or wool factories***
- **Non-industrial** *is often an occupational disease in those who associate frequently with animals, such as* ***veterinarians, butchers & farmers****. It may also found in the* ***general population***
- Human anthrax may be in 3 forms-Cutaneous (Hide porter's disease), pulmonary (wool sorter's disease) & intestinal anthrax
- ***Cutaneous anthrax*** *used to be caused by shaving brushes made with* ***animal hair***
- **Stomoxys calcitrans** *& other bitings insects may* ***occasionally transmit infection*** *mechanically*

85. Ans. b. Guinea...

[Ref: Ananthanarayan 8th/381, 322; Medical Parasitology by Paniker 6th/214; Park 23rd/93, 276, 788 20th/238, 692, 262, 672]

Dracunculiasis

Dracunculiasis, also called guinea worm disease (GWD): Humans are definitive host. There is no animal reservoir" *(Medical Parasitology by Paniker 6th/214)*

(GWD), is an infection by the guinea worm. A person becomes infected when they drink water that contains water fleas infected with guinea worm larvae

Zoonosis: (Infection of Animals Communicable to Man)

Zoonosis is defined as an infection or infectious disease that is transmissable under natural conditions from vertebrate animals to man. Zoonotic disease may be due to infections with ***viruses, bacteria protozoa, helminths, fungi or arthropods.***

Zoonosis: 4 Categories

- Direct zoonosis
- Cyclozoonosis
- Metazoonosis e.g., arbovirus infection
- Saprozoonosis

Table (Park 23rd/788): **Important Zoonosis**

Bacterial	Viral	Protozoan	Helminthic
Anthrax Brucellosis[Q] fever (Soft tick) Leptospirosis Tuberculosis Plague[Q]	*Cowpox* *Monkey pox* *Western equine encephalitis* *Ross river fever* *Yellow fever (Mosquito)* *Japanense encephalitis*[Q] *Lassa fever* *Rabies*	Leishmanisis Toxoplasmosis Trypnosomiasis Babesiosis	Clonorchiasis Fasciopsis Echisto-somiasis Taeniasis Trichinellosis

86. Ans. b. Not...

[Ref: Ananthanarayan 8th/607-08: Harrison 19th/1342-44, 18th/1651-53]

Candidiasis (Candidosis, Moniliasis)

- Most common systemic mycosis
- It is an infection of ***skin, mucosa*** & rarely of internal organs
- It is caused by ***yeast like fungus, Candida albicans*** & occasionally by other candida species
- Ubiquitous in nature, these organisms are found on inanimate objects, in foods and on animals and are normal commensals of humans. They inhabit the gastrointestinal tract (including the mouth and oropharynx), the female genital tract and the skin.
- ***It is an opportunistic endogenous infection, the commonest predisposing factor being diabetes***
- Common mucosal lesions are- *Vaginitis & oral thrush*
- **Thrush** is characterized by white, adherent, painless, discrete or confluent patches in the mouth, tongue, or esophagus, occasionally with fissuring at the corners of the mouth
- **Vulvovaginal candidiasis** is accompanied by pruritus, pain and vaginal discharge that is usually thin but may contain whitish "curds" in severe cases.
- **Paronychia & onychia** are seen in occupations that lead to frequent immersion of hand in water
- *Septicemia, **endocrditis** & **meningitis*** may occur in person with ***prolonged immunosuppression***
- Other *Candida* skin infections include ***paronychia,*** a painful swelling at the nail-skin interface & ***onychomycosis,*** a fungal nail infection rarely caused by this genus.
- ***Generalized disseminated cutaneous candidiasis,*** another form of infection that occurs primarily in infants, is characterized by widespread eruptions over the trunk, thorax and extremities.
- Deeply invasive *Candida* infections may or may not be due to hematogenous seeding.

87. Ans. b. Most...

[Ref: Neena khanna 3rd/244; Ananthanarayan 8th/604-06: Greenwood 16th/574]

"**Scutulum:** The characteristic lesion of favus, appearing as a yellow saucershaped crust made up of hyphae and spores."-*dictionary.thefreedictionary.com*

Tinea Capitis and Tinea Barbae

◈ *Neena khanna 3rd/244*

- **T.capitis:** Caused by ***microsporum any species & Trichophyton most species****-Ananthanarayan 8th/606*
- Tinea capitis is dermatophytosis or ringworm of the scalp and hair.
- ***Age: Invariably a child***
- 3 Pattern are recognized:
  - Non-inflammatory (broken hair present as ***gray/black dot)***
  - Inflammatory (***kerion-present as a boggy swelling*** with multiple discharging sinus)
  - ***Favus*** (cause cicatrical alopecia)
- As the hair grows out of the follicle, the hyphae of **microsporum species** produce a chain of spores that form a sheath around the hair shaft (**ectothrix**). These spores impart a greenish to silvery fluorescence when the hairs are examined under Wood's light (365 nm).
- In contrast, ***T tonsurans,*** the chief cause of ***"black dot" Tinea capitis***, produces spores within the hair shaft **(endothrix).** These hairs do not fluoresce; they are weakened and typically break easily at the follicular opening. In prepubescent children, epidemic tinea capitis is usually self-limiting.
- Zoophilic species may induce a severe combined inflammatory and hypersensitivity reaction called a **kerion.**
- Another manifestation of *Tinea capitis* is **favus,** an acute inflammatory infection of the hair follicle caused by *T schoenleinii*, which leads to the ***formation of scutula (crusts) around the follicle***. In favic hairs, the hyphae do not form spores but can be found within the hair shaft.

Table: **Some Clinical Features of Dermatophyte Infection**

Skin Disease	Location of Lesions	Clinical Features	Fungi Most Frequently Responsible
Tinea corporis (ringworm)	Nonhairy, smooth skin.	Circular patches with advancing red, vesiculated border and central scaling. Pruritic.	T. rubrum, E. floccosum
Tinea pedis (athlete's foot)	Interdigital spaces on feet of persons wearing shoes.	Acute: itching, red vesicular. Chronic: itching, scaling, fissures.	T. rubrum, T. mentagrophytes, E. floccosum
Tinea cruris (jock itch)	Groin	Erythematous scaling lesion in intertriginous area Pruritic.	T. rubrum, T. mentagrophytes, E. floccosum

Contd...

Skin Disease	Location of Lesions	Clinical Features	Fungi Most Frequently Responsible
Tinea capitis	Scalp hair Endothrix: Fungus inside hair shaft. Ectothrix: Fungus on surface of hair	Circular bald patches with short hair stubs or broken hair within hair follicles. Kerion rare. Microsporum-infected hairs fluoresce.	T. mentagrophytes, M. canis
Tinea barbae	Beard hair	Edematous, erythematous lesion.	T. mentagrophytes
Tinea unguium (onycho-mycosis)	Nail	Nails thickened or crumbling distally; discolored; lusterless. Usually associated with *tinea pedis.*	T. rubrum, T. mentagrophytes, E. floccosum
Dermatophytid (ID reac-tion)	Usually sides and flexor aspects of fingers, palm, any site on body.	Pruritic vesicular to bullous lesions. Most commonly associated with tinea pedis.	No fungi present in lesion. May become secondarily infected with bacteria.

88. Ans. a. May..., d. Gram-negative...

[Ref: Ananthanarayan 8th/326: Greenwood Microbiology 16th/334-35;Park 23rd/655;Harrison 19th/183e-3, 18th/1235]

"Pasteurella multocida is not mentioned as milkborne infection" *(Park 23rd/655)*

Pasteurella Multocida

◈ *Harrison 19th/183e-3, 18th/1235*

- *P. multocida* is a bipolar-staining, ***gram-negative coccobacillus*** that colonizes the respiratory and gastrointestinal tracts of ***domestic animals;*** oropharyngeal colonization rates are 70–90% in cats and 50–65% in dogs.
- *P. multocida* can be transmitted to humans through bites or scratches, via the respiratory tract from contact with contaminated dust or infectious droplets, or via deposition of the organism on injured skin or mucosal surfaces during licking.
- Patients at the ***extremes of age*** or with serious underlying disorders (*e.g.*, cirrhosis, diabetes) are at increased risk for systemic manifestations, including ***meningitis***, peritonitis, osteomyelitis and septic arthritis, endocarditis and septic shock, but cases have also occurred in healthy individuals.
- If inhaled, *P. multocida* can cause acute respiratory tract infection, particularly in patients with underlying sinus and pulmonary disease.

Pasteurella Multocida (Formerly P. septica)

◈ *Ananthanarayan 8th/326; Greenwood Microbiology 16th/334-35*

- ***Pasteurella multocida*** is a Gram-negative, nonmotile, penicillin-sensitive coccobacillus belonging the Pasteurellaceae family.
- *P. multocida* is the cause of a ***range of diseases in mammals and birds***, including fowl cholera in poultry, atrophic rhinitis in pigs and bovine hemorrhagic septicemia in cattle and buffalo.
- It can also cause azoonotic infection in humans, which typically is a result of bites or scratches from domestic pets. Many mammals (including domestic cats and dogs) and birds harbor it as part of their normal respiratory microbiota.
- The bacteria may also cross the blood–brain barrier and cause ***meningitis***

89. Ans. b. Vibrio..., c. Campylobacter..., d. Shigella..., e. Yersinia...

[Ref: Ananthanarayan 8th/293, 299, 506, 312; Harrison 18th/1294; Greenwood 16th/300;]

"Vibrio parahaemolyticus: After an ***incubation period of 4 hr to 4 days,*** *symptoms develop & persists for a median period of 3 days" (Harrison 18th/1294)*

"Shigellae *cause bacillary dysentery. It has a short incubation period (1-7 days,* ***usually 48 hours)'*** *(Ananthanarayan 8th/285)*

"Campylobacter jejuni*: The incubation period is 1-7 days"- Ananthanarayan 8th/398*

"Enteric fever (Salmonella typhi): *The incubation period is usually* ***7-14 days*** *but may range 3-56 days" (Ananthanarayan 8th/293)*

"Salmonella gastroenteritis (caused by any salmonella other than s.typhi): Clinically the disease develops after short incubation period of ***24 hours or less,*** *with diarrhea, vomiting, abdominal pain & fever" (Ananthanarayan 8th/299)*

Plague (Yersinia Pestis)-incubation Period

◈ *Park 23rd/295*

- Bubonic: 2-7 days[Q]
- Septicemic: 2-7 days[Q]
- Pneumonic: 1-3 days

90. Ans. a. B. bacilliformis...

[Ref: Ananthanarayan 8th/411-12: Harrison 19th/1083, 1079, 18th/1319]

"Bartonellosis, or Carrión's disease, is caused by ***B. bacilliformis.*** The disease is characterized by two distinct phases: (1) an acute febrile hematic phase, known as Oroya fever; and (2) an eruptive phase manifested by cutaneous lesions, known as ***verruga peruana*** " *(Harrison 19th/1083, 18th/1319)*

"Verruga Peruana or Peruvian Wart: It is characterized by an eruptive phase, in which the patients develop a cutaneous rash produced by a proliferation of endothelial cells and is known as ***"Peruvian warts" or "verruga peruana"***. Depending of the size and characteristics of the lesions, there are three types: **miliary** (1–4 mm), **nodular** or **subdermic** and **mular** (>5mm). Miliary lesions are the most common. The most common findings are bleeding of verrugas, fever, malaise, arthralgias, anorexia, myalgias, pallor, lymphadeopathy and hepato-splenomegaly"

Table *(Harrison 17th/988)*: **Major Diseases Caused by Bartonella Species**

Disease	Organism	Risk Factor
Cat-scratch disease[Q]	*B. henselae* [Q]	Cat scratch or bite[Q]
Bacillary angiomatosis	B. quintana, B. henselae	Cat scratch or bite
Bacillary peliosis	B. henselae	Cat scratch or bite
Trench fever [Q]	*B. quintana* [Q]	Homelessness, body louse infestation, alcoholism
Endocarditis	B. quintana, B. henselae, B. elizabethae	As for cat-scratch disease and trench fever
Bartonellosis [Q]	B. bacilliformis	Sandfly bite [Q]

Table: Bartonella Pathophysiology in humans

Species	Human reservoir or incidental host	Animal reservoir	Pathophysiology	Distribution
B. bacilliformis	Reservoir		Causes Carrion's disease (Oroya fever, *Verruga peruana*)	Peru, Ecuador and Colombia
B. quintana	Reservoir		Causes trench fever, bacillary angiomatosis and endocarditis	Worldwide
B. clarridgeiae	Incidental	Domestic cat	Cat scratch disease	
B. elizabethae	Incidental	Rat	Endocarditis	
B. grahamii	Incidental	Mouse	Endocarditis and neuroretinitis	
B. henselae	Incidental	Domestic cat	Cat scratch disease, bacillary angiomatosis, peliosis hepatis, endocarditis, bacteremia with fever and neuroretinitis	Worldwide
B. koehlerae	Incidental	Domestic cat		
B. vinsonii	Incidental	Mouse, dog, domestic cat		
B. washoensis	Incidental	Squirrel	Myocarditis	
B. rochalimae	Incidental	Unknown	Carrion's disease-like symptoms	

91. Ans. a. Conta.., b. Cause.., d. Coagu..., e. Causes...

[Ref: Ananthanarayan 8th/195-202: Harrison 19th/805, 809, 18th/1160-70; Greenwood 16th/171]

Expression of methicillin resistance increases when it is incubated at 30°C *(Ananthanarayan 8th/197)*

Staphylococcus aureus causes ***both community acquired pneumonia & ventilator-associated pneumonia*** *(Harrison 19th/805, 809, 18th/2132, 2137)*

Staphylococcus Aureus

- *Staphylococcus aureus* is **coagulase-positive,** which differentiates it from the other species. *S aureus* is a major pathogen for humans.
- "A multiplex real-time polymerase chain reaction (RT-PCR) targeting the ***mecA and nuc genes*** was developed for the detection of methicillin resistance and identification of *Staphylococcus aureus*. Novel mecA and nuc primers and fluorescence resonance energy transfer hybridization probes specific for the mecA and nuc genes were evaluated". *(http: //jcm.asm.org/content/43/3/1361.full)*
- Staphylococci produce ***catalase***, which converts hydrogen peroxide into water and oxygen. The catalase test differentiates the staphylococci, which are positive, from the streptococci, which are negative
- **Food poisoning** due to staphylococcal enterotoxin is characterized by a ***short incubation period (1–8 hours);*** violent nausea, vomiting and diarrhea; and rapid convalescence. There is no fever.
- **Toxic shock syndrome** is manifested by an abrupt onset of high fever, vomiting, diarrhea, myalgias, a scarlatiniform rash and hypotension with cardiac and renal failure in the most severe cases.

92. Ans. a. Abrasion..., b. Gutt..., d. Incis..., e. Lace...,

[Ref: Reddy 32nd/205, 235; Parikh 6th/4.43-44]

- **Gutter fracture:** *They are formed when part of the thickness of the bone is removed so as to form a gutter, e.g., in oblique bullet wound"* (Reddy 32nd/235)
- **Abrasion collar (Marginal abrasion):** Abrasion collar surrounds the dirt collar. The abraded collar is reddish at first, but becomes reddish brown as it dries. Some contusion is present in abraded collar & as such, it is also called "contusion collar". These two features are proof of an ***entrance firearm wound"*** (Reddy 32nd/213)

Firearm Wound

◈ *Reddy 32nd/205*
- They are recognized without difficulty
- Wounds produced by rifled weapon may simulate wounds inflicated by a red hot poker or a burning pointed stick
- **Glancing wounds** (striking someone or something at an angle rather than directly and with full force) ***may simulate incised or lacerated wounds.***
- A bullet that pass through glass or some other object & then strikes the body may produce a ***wound resembling a laceration***
- Firearm wounds cause crushing of the tissues & produce an actual hole

Firearm Injuries

◈ *Parikh 6th/4.39-40*
- Firearm injuries are wounds caused to the body tissue due to impact, entry & passage of a missile discharged from a firearm. They generally ***simulate contused wounds***
- When a missile pass tangentially, the wound ***may simulate an abrasion or a gutter***
- Slit like exit wounds are occasionally encountered. They are due to the bullet exiting on its board side or due to exit of a fragmented bone. Such injuries ***may simulate incised wounds or stab wounds***

93. Ans. c. Short...

[Ref: Reddy 32nd/528; Parikh 6th/9.40-9.41]

Table *(Reddy 32nd/528)*: **Difference b/w Poisonous snake & Non-poisonous snake**

Trait	Poisonous snake	Non-poisonous snake
1. Head scales	*A- **small** (vipers)* *B- large &* *(a) |if there is an opening or pit b/w the eye & nostril (pit viper)* *(b) third labial touches the eye & nasal shields (cobra or coral snake)* *(c) No pits & third labial does not touch the nose & eye & central row of scales on back enlarged; undersurface of the mouth has only four infralabials, the fourth being the largest (kraits)*	***Large** with the exceptions as mentioned, under the poisonous snakes*
2. Belly scales	Large & cover entire breadth	Small like these on the back or moderately large, but do not cover the entire breadth
3. Fangs	Hollow like hypodermic needles	Short & solid
4. Teeth	Two long fangs	Several small teeth
5. Tail	Compressed	Not much compressed
6. Habits	Usually nocturnal	Not so

94. Ans. None

[Ref: Reddy 32nd/166; Parikh 6th/8.23]

Table *(Reddy 32nd/166)*: **A typical embalming fluid**

Ingredient	Proportion
Sodium borate (Buffer)	600 g
Sodium citrate (Anticoagulent)	900 g
Glycerine (Wetting agent)	600 ml
Sodium chloride (Control pH)	800 g
Eosin (Cosmetic)	30 mL
Soluble wintergreen (Perfume)	90 mL
Water (Vehicle)	Upto 10 litres
Formalin (Preservative)	1.5 litres

Contd...

Note: Formalin is aqueous solution of formaldehyde

A & E

95. Ans. a. Flexion..., b. Occur..., d. Flex...

[Ref: Reddy 32nd/307; 27th/286; Parikh 6th/4.156-4.157]

Pugilistic Attitude (Boxing, Fencing or Defence Attitute)

◈ *Reddy 27th/286; Reddy 32nd/307*

- It is the posture of a body which has been ***exposed to great heat***
- The ***legs are flexed at the hips and knees, the arms are flexed at elbows and wrists*** and held out in front of the body, head slightly extended, ***all fingers are hooked like claws.***
- **"Pugilistic attitude** *is present* ***whether a living or dead body*** *is burnt & has therefore no medico-legal significance" (Parikh 6th/4.156)*
- Contraction of paraspinal muscles often causes a marked opisthotonus, in an attitude commonly adopted by boxers.
- This stiffening is due to the ***coagulation of proteins of the muscles*** and dehydration which cause contraction. The flexor muscles being bulkier than extensors contract more due to which joints of all limbs are flexed
- ***It occurs whether the person was alive or dead at time of burning.***

96. Ans. b. Impo.., e. Pre-existing...

[Ref: http: //www.indidivorce.com/grounds-for-divorce-in-india.html; Reddy 32nd/; Parikh 6th/5.1, 5.24; Mr Himanshu Panshari, LLB, LLM (NALSA, Hyderabad)]

Note: • *Sterile female is not a ground for divorce*
• *Premature ejaculation, if leads to impotency then ground for divorce, otherwise not ground for divorce*

Impotent Man: A ground for divorce

◈ *http: //indiankanoon.org/docfragment /1317023/?formInput=impotence*

- "Impotency is a ground for annulling marriage. In *Parmaswami pillai v. Sornathammal AIR1969* it was held that the marriage of a woman with an impotent man is voidable"

"*Sirajmohmedkhan Janmohamadkhan v. Hafizunnisa Yasinkhan & Anr on 14 Sept 1981* HELD: Proved **impotence** of the husband and his inability to discharge his marital obligations amount to both legal and mental cruelty make it a just ground for the wife to refuse to live with the husband......... **impotence** under the civil law is a good ground for granting divorce or for refusing restitution of conjugal rights"

Premature Ejaculation: May be/may not be ground

◈ *http: //indiankanoon.org /doc/91736356/*

May be Ground for Divorce if it Leads to Impotency

"*In Ravi Luthravs Rekha on 7 May, 2013.* High Court of Delhi upheld the judgment of ADJ court. In the case it was alleged that husband was able to produce only a very feeble erection and some little ejaculation without penetration and then it would be followed by complete collapse leaving behind a trial of agony and frustration for the respondent/wife. The learned Additional District Judge has held that marriage between the parties was not consummated owing to **impotency** of the appellant/husband and the marriage between the parties has been annulled by a decree of nullity on the ground of **impotency** of the appellant/husband."

May not be Ground for Divorce

"It would not called impotency, as it is stress related disorder, which as per study majority of male has been suffering from"

Divorce

◈ *Parikh 6th/5.1, 5.24*

- *This means dissolution of a previously valid marriage. If the intrauterine age of the child is proved to be greater than the period of access b/w the parents, the dissolution of marriage is allowed by the court on* ***ground of adultery.***
- *The other grounds for divorce includes-(a) desertion (b) cruelty (c) criminal sex practices (e.g, rape, sodomy, or bestiality) & (d)* ***incurable insanity,*** *HIV infection, leprosy or venereal disease in a communicable form*

Following are the Grounds for Divorce in India Mentioned under the Hindu Marriage Act, 1955

◈ *http: //www.indidivorce.com/grounds-for-divorce-in-india.html*

- Adultery
- **Cruelty**
- **Desertion**
- **Conversion:** Incase either of the two converts himself/herself into another religion
- **Mental Disorder:** Mental disorder can become a ground for filing a divorce if the spouse of the petitioner suffers from ***incurable mental disorder and insanity*** and therefore cannot be expected from the couple to stay together.
- **Leprosy:** In case of a 'virulent and incurable' form of leprosy, a petition can be filed by the other spouse based on this ground
- **Venereal Disease:** If one of the spouses is suffering from a serious disease that is easily communicable, a divorce can be filed by the other spouse. The sexually transmitted diseases like AIDS are accounted to be **venereal Disease**
- **Renunciation**
- **Not Heard Alive**
- **No Resumption of Co-habitation**

The following are the grounds for divorce in India on which a petition can be filed only by the wife.

- If the husband has indulged in ***rape, bestiality and sodomy.***
- If the marriage is solemnized before the Hindu Marriage Act and the husband has again married another woman in spite of the first wife being alive, the first wife can seek for a divorce.
- A girl is entitled to file for a divorce if she was married before the age of fifteen and renounces the marriage before she attains eighteen years of age.
- If there is no cohabitation for one year and the husband neglects the judgment of maintenance awarded to the wife by the court, the wife can contest for a divorce.

97. Ans. c. For repeat...

[Ref: Reddy 32nd/394, 413; Parikh 6th/5.55; Reddy 27th/367; Criminal Amendment Bill, 2013]

Cognisable Offences (S.2 (c) Cr.P.C)

◈ *Reddy 32nd/6-7*

- *It is an offence in which a police officer can arrest a person without warrant from magistrate e.g., **rape, dowry death, ragging, death due to rape or negligent act**, etc.*
- *In such offences, the individual is sent by the police to the doctor for medical examination*

"Offence means any act or omission made punishable by any law (S.2 (n) Cr.P.C & S. 40, I.P.C). Offence are classified as **(1) Bailable & (2) Non-bailable.** *In bailable offences, the court cannot refuse bail & the police cannot keep the person in custody"-Reddy 32nd/6*

S.354C, I.P.C: *Voyeurism-Imprisonment of **not less than one year, may extend to 3 years & fine; for second & subsequent offences imprisonment of 3 to 7 years**"-Reddy 32nd/394*

Voyeurism or Scoptophilia

◈ *Reddy 32nd/413*

- *It is defined as one who, experiences recurrent, intense, sexually arousing fantasies, sexual urges or behaviours involving the act of observing an unsuspecting person who is naked, in the process of disrobing or engaged in sexual activity*
- Voyeurism or Scotophilia is defined as the desire to watch sexual intercourse or to observe genitals of others. Q
- *Most often the victim is stranger*
- *Masturbation at the scene or later to memories of watching the unsuspecting stranger is normally the source of sexual pleasure*
- *It is rare in female*

Table: Criminal Amendment Bill, 2013

354B	Assault or use of criminal force to woman with intent to disrobe.	Imprisonment of not less than 3 years but which may extend to 7 years and with fine.	Cognizable	Non-bailable	Any Magistrate
354C	Voyeurism	Imprisonment of *not less than 1 year but which ay extend to 3 years and with fine for* first conviction	Cognizable	Bailable	Any Magistrate
		Imprisonment of not less than 3 years but which may extend to 7 years and with fine for second or subsequent conviction	Cognizable	Non-bailable	Any Magistrate
354D	Stalking	Imprisonment up to 3 years and with fine for first conviction	Cognizable	Bailable	Any Magistrate
		Imprisonment up to 5 years and with fine for second or subsequent conviction	Cognizable	Non-bailable	Any magistrate

PSM

98. Ans. a. Varicella...

[Ref: Park 23rd/144-145, 148: O. P. Ghai 7th/185; Harrison 19th/1194, 18th/149, 153]

"An **exanthema** is a widespread erythematous rash that is accompanied by systemic symptoms such as fever, headache and malaise"

"Rubeola (measles): Eruptive phase is characterized by a typical, dusky-red, macular or macula-papular rash which begins ***behind the ears*** & spreads rapidly in a few hours over the face & neck"*(Park 23rd/148, 21st/138)*

"Rash usually appears as faint reddish *macules behind the ears, along the hairline & on the posterior aspects of cheeks" (Park 23rd/148)*

"Varicella (Chickenpox): A characteristic feature of rash is its ***pleomorphism*** i.e, all stage of rash (papules, vesicles & crusts) may be seen simultaneously at one time, in the same area. *Temperature rise with each fresh crop of rash" (Park 23rd/144-45)*

"Exanthem subitum (roseola) is caused by human herpes virus 6 and is most common among children <3 years of age. As in erythema infectiosum, the *rash usually appears after fever has subsided*. It consists of 2-to 3-mm rose-pink macules and papules that rarely coalesce, which occur initially on the trunk and sometimes on the extremities (sparing the face) and fade within 2 days" *(Harrison 19th/1194, 18th/148)*

"Rubella* (German measles)** also spreads from the hairline downward; unlike that of measles, however, the rash of rubella tends to clear from originally affected areas as it migrates and it may be pruritic. Forchheimer spots ***(palatal petechiae) may develop but are nonspecific because they also develop in mononucleosis and scarlet fever" *(Harrison 18th/148)*

Name	Number	Virus
Rubeola (Measles)	"First disease"	Measles virus
Rubella, (German Measles)	"Third disease"	Rubella virus
Erythema infectiosum	"Fifth disease"	Parvovirus B19
Roseola infantum	"Sixth disease"	HHV-6 and HHV-7

Table *(Harrison 19th/128, 18th/149)*: **Diseases Associated with Fever and Rash**

Disease	Description	Clinical Syndrome
Rubeola (measles, first disease)	Discrete lesions that become confluent as rash spreads from hairline downward, sparing palms and soles; lasts ≥3 days; Koplik's spots	Cough, conjunctivitis, coryza, severe prostration
Rubella (German measles, third disease)	Spreads from hairline downward, clearing as it spreads; Forchheimer spots	Adenopathy, arthritis
Exanthem subitum (roseola, sixth disease)	Diffuse maculopapular eruption over trunk and neck; resolves within 2 days	Rash following resolution of fever; similar to Boston exanthem (echovirus 16); febrile seizures may occur
Varicella (chicken-pox)	Macules (2–3 mm) evolving into papules, then vesicles (sometimes umbilicated), on an erythematous base ("dewdrops on a rose petal"); pustules then forming and crusting; lesions appearing in crops; may involve scalp, mouth; intensely pruritic	Malaise; generally mild disease in healthy children; more severe disease with complications in adults and immunocompromised children

99. Ans. a. ESI..., b. Factory..., c. MTP...

[Ref: Park 23rd/702, 21st/755, 647, 542]

Acts Passed

"Epidemic disease act *passed in* **1897"**-*Park 21st/647*

"As early as 1929, the **SARDA act** *was enacted forbidding the practice of child marriage"-Park 23rd/589*

"Child Marriage Restraint Act 1929 popularly known as the **Sarda Act** after its sponsor Rai Sahib Harbilas Sarda to the British India Legislature in India was passed on 28 September 1929, fixed the age of marriage for girls at 14 years and boys at 18 years. It came into effect six months later on April 1, 1930 and it applies to all of British India, not just to Hindus. It was a result of social reform movement in India. The legislation was passed by the British Indian Government."-*Internet*

"The ***prohibition of child marriage act,*** *2006 (PCMA) was enacted* ***repealing the child marriage restraint act of 1929*** *in order to prohibit child marriage rather than only restraining them" (Park 23rd/589, 21st/542)*

"ESI act passed in 1948 *(amended 1975, 1984 & 1989" (Park 23rd/815, 21st/756)*

"Indian factories act passed in 1948" *(Park 23rd/815, 21st/542)*

"Medical termination of pregnancy act was passed in 1971" *(Park 23rd/506, 21st/468)*

Note: *"The Vaccination Act, 1880: An Act to give power to prohibit inoculation and to make the vaccination of children compulsory in certain Municipalities and Cantonments"-http: //indiankanoon.org/doc/318197/*

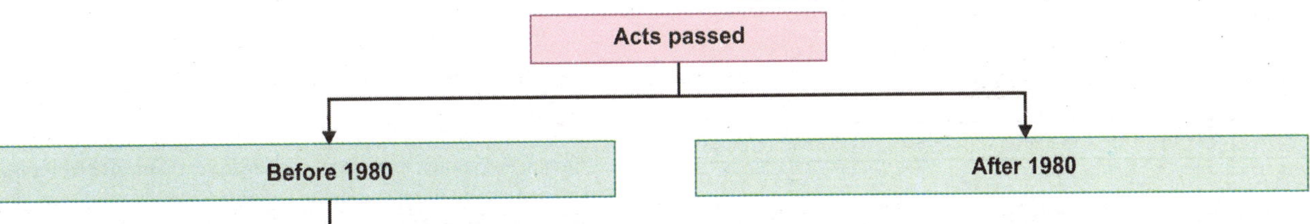

Before 1980

- **The Employees State Insurance Act (ESI), 1948[Q]** (Park 20th/720)
  The ESI Act passed in 1948 (amended in 1975, 1984 and 1989. It provides for certain cash and medical benefits to industrial employment injury.
- **The Factories Act. 1948** *(Park 20th/719)*
  The first indian factories Act dates as far back as 1881. The Act was revised and amended several times, the latest being the Factories (Amendment) Act, 1987.
- **The Prevention of Food Adulteration Act. 1954.** *(Park 20th/610)*
- **The Medical Termination of Pregnancy Act 1971[Q].** *(Park20th/610)*
- **The Employee's State Insurance Act, 1948** *(Park 20th/610)*
- **The Central maternity Benefit Act, 1969[Q].** *(Park 20th/610)*
- **The Children Act, 1960.** (Park 20th/610)
- **The Central Birth and Death Registration Act. 1969[Q].** *(Park 20th/610)*
- **Workmen's Compensation Act 1923** (Park20th/722)
- **Maternity benefit Act 1961** *(Park 20th/722)*

After 1980

- **Consumer Protection Act 1986** *(Park 20th/606)*
- **"The Air (Prevention and Control of Pollution) Act" 1981[Q]** *(Park 20th/645)*
- **The epidermic disease Act, 1897.** *(Park 20th/610)*
- **Juvenile justice Act 1986.** *(Park 20th/610)*
- **PNDT Act 1994[Q]**: An Act to provide for the regulation of the use of pre-natal diagnostic techniques for the purpose of etecting genetic or metabolic disorders or chromosomal abnormalities or certain congenital malformations or sex linked disorders and for the prevention of the misuse of such techniques of the purpose of *pre-natal* sex determination leading to female foeticide; and for matters connected there with or incidental there to (Internet)

Fig: Chart depicting acts passed before & after 1980

100. Ans. a. Positive..., b. Grenz..., d. 12 month..., e. Multidrug...

[Ref: Park 23rd/314-329. 21st/292-299; Harrison 19th/1122-27, 18th/1365-66, 17th/1022; Ananthanarayan 8th/364-69]

"Grenz zone occur in lepromatous leprosy" *(Neena Khanna 3rd/227)*

*"**Multibacillary leprosy:** with ≥ 6 skin lesions, as well as **all smear positive cases**" (KDT 7th/783)*

*"There is **no place for monotherapy** in treatment of leprosy"-(Neena Khanna 3rd/229)*

*"Slit skin smear: All patients who are AFB positive should be given **multibacillary treatment,** irrespective of the clinical presentation" (Neena Khanna 3rd/227)*

*33 state/UT we have achieved **elimination level** (prevalence rate <1 per 10, 000 population). Only 3 states/UT viz. Bihar, Chattisgarh & D & N Haveli has PR of 2-4 per 10, 000 population" (Park 23rd/316)*

"Paucibacillary leprosy: *A person having 1-5 skin lesions &/or only one nerve involvement*" *(Park 21st/292)*

"Multibacillary leprosy: *A person having 6 or more skin lesions &/or more than one nerve involvement*" *(Park 23rd/322)*

"Multibacillary leprosy: *MB blisterpacks for 12 months, within 18 month" (Park 23rd/324)*

Table *(KDT 7th/784)*: **National Leprosy Eradication Programme (2009) Classification of leprosy**

Paucibacillary (PB)	Multibacillary (MB)
• 1-5 skin lesions • No nerve/only one nerve involvement ± 1-5 skin lesions • Skin smear negative at all sites	• ***6 or more skin lesions*** • ***> 1 nerve involved irrespective of number of skin lesions*** • ***Skin smear positive at any one site***

101. Ans. a. Minimum..., b. Wate..., d. Seede.., e. Anae...

[Ref: Park 23rd/760, 21st/701]

Septic Tank

◈ *Park 23rd/760, 21st/701*

- The septic tank is ***water-tight masonry tank*** into which household sewage is admitted for treatment.
- It is a satisfactory means of disposing excreta & liquid wastes from individual dwellings, small groups of houses & institutions which have adequate water supplies but do not have access to a public sewerage system
- **Capacity:** The capacity of a septic tank will depend upon the number of users. ***A capacity of 20-30 gallons or 2.5 -5 c.ft. per person is recommended for household septic tanks. The minimum capacity of a septic tank should be at least 500 gallons***
- Septic tanks are ***not recommended for large communities***
- **Air space:** There should be a minimum air space of 30 cm b/w the level of liquid in the tank & the undersurface of the cover
- **Retention period:** Septic tanks are designed in this country to allow a *retention period of 24 hours*
- **Two stages** are involved in the purification of sewage. The **first stage, *anaerobic digestion*** take places in the septic tank proper & the **second stage,** aerobic ***oxidation takes*** place outside the septic tank, in sub-soil. Together, these two stages complete purification of sewage
- Newly built septic tanks are first filled with water up to the outlet level & then ***seeded with ripe sludge drawn from another septic tank,*** to provide the right type of bacteria to carry out the decomposition process

102. Ans. b. Normal..., c. Rep.., d. It is...

[Ref: Park 23rd/847-49, 21st/786;Biostatistics by BK Rao 2nd/54; Methods in Biostatistics by BK Mahajan 7th/57, 60-68; Basic & clinical Biostatistics 4th/30]

*"**Deviation from the mean in a normal distribution or curve is called relative or standard normal deviate or variate** & is given the symbol Z. It is measured in term of SDs & indicates how much an observation is bigger or smaller than mean in unit of SD. So Z will be a ratio"-BK Mahajan 7th/75*

Uses of SD

◈ *BK Mahajan 7th/57, 60*

- It summarises the deviations of a large distribution from mean in one figure used as a unit of variation
- Indicates whether the variation of difference of an individual from the mean is by chance, *i.e.,* natural or real due to some special reasons
- Helps in finding the standard error which determines whether the difference between means of two similar samples is by chance or real
- It also helps in finding the suitable size of sample for valid conclusion

*"**Range:** It has serious drawback. The notoriety of the range being dependent only on the minimum & maximum & not on the all the values, is a great disadvantage. **Standaerd deviation is universally accepted as an adequate measure of variability"** (Biostatistics by BK Rao 2nd/54)*

Measures of Central tendency	**Measures of Dispersion/Variation/Scatter for individual data** *(Methods in Biostatistics by BK Mahajan 7th/57)*
Mean Median	• Range
Mode	• ***Standard deviation*** • ***The mean Deviation*** • Coefficient of variation • Interquartile range

Standard deviation
This is a measure of spread of data about the mean $SD = \sqrt{\frac{\Sigma(x-\pi)^2}{n-1}}$

Contd...

Coefficient of variation (CV)

This is defined as the standard deviation divided by mean times 100%

$$CV = \frac{SD}{X} \times 100\%$$

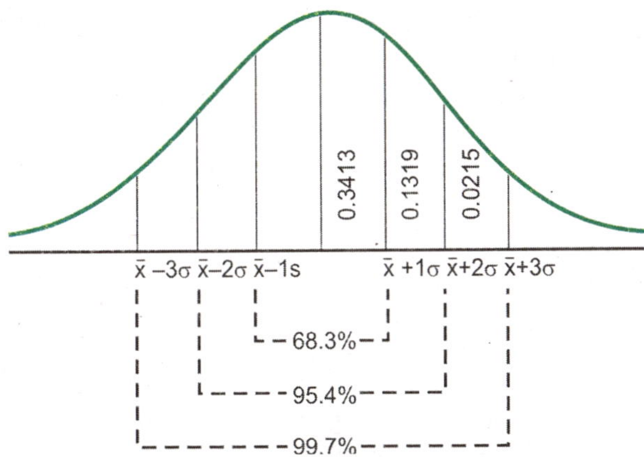

Although there is infinite no. of normal curves depending upon the mean & standard deviation, there is only one standardized normal curve.

The standard distribution curve (Normal distribution) is a perfectly ***symmetrical, bell shaped curve*** *such that the mean, median and mode, all have the same value and coincide at the centre*

Standard Distribution Curve (Normal)[Q]:

Mean = Median = Mode

Characteristic of Normal distribution Curve

- *Standard normal curve smooth*[Q]
- *Bell-Shaped*[Q]
- *Perfectly symmetrical*[Q]
- *Based on infinitely larger number of observation*
- *Total area of the curve is 1*[Q]
- *The mean is Zero*[Q]
- *Standard deviation is one*
- Mean, Median and mode all coincide
  - *Area in 1SD is 68.3%*
  - *Area in 2SD is 95.4%*[Q]
  - *Area in 3SD is 99.7%*

103. Ans. b.Pakistaan, c. Afganistan, e. Nigeria

[Ref: Park 23rd/203, 21st/182]

"**Till 2011,** polio was endemic in 4 countries-Pakistan, Afghanistan, **India** & Nigeria (Mnemonic-PAIN). But in ***2014, only 3 countries (Afghanistan, Nigeria and Pakistan;*** Mnemonic-PAN) ***remain polio-endemic, down from more than 125 countries in 1988***" *(http: //www.who.int/mediacentre/factsheets/fs114/en/)*

India Celebrates Victory Over Polio

◈ *http: //www.unicef. org/india/health*

"Completing three full years without reporting any case of polio, India celebrated a landmark achievement in public health on ***11 February 2014*** – the victory over polio. India has not reported any case of polio since a two-year old girl got polio paralysis on 13 January 2011 in Howrah district of West Bengal. India's victory over polio paves the way for polio-free certification of the South East Asia region of WHO in March end"

104. Ans. c. Literacy..., d. Conducted...

[Ref.: Park 23rd/840]

Census

◈ *Park 23rd/840*

- The first regular census in India was ***taken in 1881*** & conducted at regular interval of 10 year
- The census is usually ***conducted at the end of the first quarter of the first year in each decade,*** the reason being, most people are usually resident in their own homes during that period
- The legal basis of the census is provided by the ***census act of 1948***
- The supreme officer who directs, guides & operates the census is the ***Census Commissioner for India***
- Apart from demographic information, economic & social characteristic of population are also included in census (including ***literacy rate)***

105. Ans. a. Mesothelioma b. Bronchial..., c. Laryngeal

[Ref: Park 23rd/807, 21st/748; Robbins 9th/690-91; Harrison 19th/1688-89; Chapman 4th /536]

Carcinoma Associated with Asbestosis

◈ *Chapman 4th /536;Harrison 19th/1688-89*

- *"**Mesothelioma** have a strong association with crocidolite variety of **asbestos**"*
- ***Carcinoma bronchus** & Lung (squamous cell or adenocarcinoma)*[Q]
- *Pleural and peritoneal **mesotheliomas***[Q]
- *Gastrointestinal carcinoma (colon cancer)*
- ***Laryngeal carcinoma***[Q]
  - *Lung cancer*[Q] is the most frequent cancer associated with asbestos exposure.
  - The excess frequency of lung cancer (all histologic types) in asbestos workers is associated with a minimum latency of 15–19 years between first exposure and development of the disease.

Other Facts

- Benign pleural effusions may also occur. The fluid is typically a serous or bloody exudate.
- X-Ray shows "***ground glass" appearance***[Q]
- The sputum shows "***asbestos bodies"***[Q]

Table *(Harrison 19th/1688)*: **Categories of Occupational Exposure and Associated Respiratory Conditions**

Occupational Exposures	Nature of Respiratory Responses	Comment
Inorganic Dusts		
Asbestos: Mining, processing, construction, ship repair	Fibrosis (asbestosis), pleural disease, cancer, mesothelioma[Q]	Virtually all new mining and construction with asbestos done in developing countries
Silica: Mining, stone cutting, sandblasting, quarrying	Fibrosis (silicosis), PMF, cancer, ***silicotuberculosis***[Q], COPD	Improved protection in United States, persistent risk in developing countries
Coal dust: Mining	Fibrosis ***(coal workers' pneumoconiosis***[Q]***)***, PMF, COPD	Risk dropping in United States, increasing where new mines open
Beryllium: Processing alloys for high-tech industries	Acute pneumonitis, ***chronic granulomatous disease***[Q]***, lung cancer*** (highly suspect)	Risk in high-tech industries persists
Organic Dusts		
Cotton dust: Milling, processing	***Byssinosis***[Q] ***(an asthma-like syndrome***[Q]***)***, chronic bronchitis, COPD	Increasing risk in developing countries with drop in United States as jobs shift overseas
Grain dust: Elevator agents, dock workers, milling, bakers	Asthma, chronic bronchitis, COPD	Risk shifting more to migrant labor pool
Other agricultural dusts: Fungal spores, vegetable products, insect fragments, animal dander, bird and rodent feces, endotoxins, microorganisms, pollens.	Hypersensitivity pneumonitis ***(farmers' lung)***[Q], asthma, chronic bronchitis	Important in migrant labor pool but also resulting from in-home exposures

OPHTHALMOLOGY

106. Ans. b. Frontal..., c. Greater...

[Ref: BDC 4th/Vol. III 27; Khurana 6th/377; Khurana 5th/403; Gray's 40th /656]

*"Lateral wall of the orbit is formed by the orbital surface of the greater wing of the sphenoid posteriorly & the **frontal process of the zygomatic bone anteriorly**" (Gray's 40th /656)*

Bony Orbit

- *The bony orbits are quadrangular truncated pyramids situated between the anterior cranial fossa above and the maxillary sinuses below*
- *Each orbit is about 40 mm in height, width and depth and is formed by portions of* **seven bones:**
  - Frontal
  - Maxilla
  - Zygomatic
  - Sphenoid
  - Palatine,
  - Ethmoid and
  - Lacrimal. It has four walls (medial, lateral, superior and inferior), base and an apex.
- *The medial walls of two orbits are parallel to each other and, being thinnest, are frequently fractured during injuries as well as during orbitotomy operations and, it also accounts for ethmoiditis being the commonest cause of orbital cellulitis.*
- *The **orbital apex**: It is the posterior end of orbit. Here the four orbital walls converge. It has two orifices, the optic canal which transmits optic nerve and ophthalmic artery and the superior orbital fissure which transmits a number of nerves, arteries and veins*

***Orbital Wall**: Formed by*

- **Medial wall** of the orbit is formed by (from before backwards)
  - The frontal process of the maxilla[Q]
  - The lacrimal bone[Q]
  - Orbital plate of the ethmoid
  - Body of the sphenoid bone[Q]
- Lateral wall
  - Zygomatic (frontal process)
  - Greater wing of sphenoid
- Roof
  - Frontal[Q]
  - ***Lesser wing of sphenoid***
- Floor
  - Zygomatic
  - Palatine (orbital process)

107. Ans. b. Primar..., c. Disc..., d. Trans..., e. Mito...

[Ref: Khurana 5th/316; Parson 20th/319]

"Leber Congenital Amaurosis: *The **optic discs become pale,** the retinal vessel attenuated & macula affected"-Parson 20th/319*

Leber's disease or Leber's Hereditary Optic Neuropathy (LHON) or Leber optic atrophy

- It is a type of hereditary optic neuritis which ***primarily affects males around*** the age of 20 years.
- It is a ***mitochondrially inherited (transmitted from mother to offspring)*** degeneration of retinal ganglion cells (RGCs) and their axons that leads to an acute or subacute loss of central vision; this ***affects predominantly young adult males.***

- However, LHON is only transmitted through the mother as it is primarily due to mutations in the mitochondrial (not nuclear) genome and only the ovum contributes mitochondria to the embryo.
- It is transmitted by the ***female carriers.***
- The condition is characterised by progressive visual failure.
- The fundus is initially normal or in the acute stage disc may be mildly hyperaemic with telangiectatic microangiopathy. Eventually ***bilateral primary optic atrophy ensues.***
- **Leber hereditary optic neuropathy (LHON)** is an inherited form of vision loss. Although this condition usually begins in a person's teens or twenties, rare cases may appear in early childhood or later in adulthood. For unknown reasons, ***males are affected much more often than females.***
- Blurring and clouding of vision are usually the first symptoms of LHON.

108. Ans. e. Lower...

[Ref: Khurana 5th/212, 290; Parson 20th/268; CMDT06/1221, 164]

Risk Factors: Cystoid Macular Edema

◈ *http: //www.reviewofophthalmology.com/content/d/retinal_insider/c/46967/*

- The development of pseudophakic CME is influenced by pre-existing systemic and ocular conditions, as well as complications during surgery. It is important to identify risk factors for prophylaxis and treatment.
- ***Diabetes mellitus, even in the absence of diabetic retinopathy, has been shown to almost double pseudophakic CME incidence rates.*** The incidence of CME post-cataract surgery has also been reported higher in eyes with diabetic retinopathy. Optimally treating diabetic retinopathy and macular edema is advised prior to proceeding with cataract surgery.
- ***Uveitic eyes have a higher incidence of pseudophakic CME detected by OCT than non-uveitic eyes.*** Strict control of ocular inflammation for at least three months is recommended prior to cataract surgery. Other ocular conditions associated with a higher incidence of pseudophakic CME include epiretinal membrane, vitreomacular traction, retinal vein occlusion and topical prostaglandin use
- Before extracapsular cataract extraction technique, the rates of ***CME were higher with intracapsular cataract extraction.*** Despite advancements in phacoemulsification technique, surgical complications can still occur and increase the risk of CME. Retained lens fragments have a reported CME incidence up to 46%.
- ***Vitreous loss,*** vitreous to the wound, iris incarceration in the wound, posterior capsule rupture and YAG capsulotomy have all been reported to predispose to CME.
- Selection of the intraocular lens also plays a role in CME development. Iris-fixated IOLs have the highest reported rate of CME and anterior chamber intraocular lenses have a higher rate than posterior chamber intraocular lenses.

Cystoid Macular Edema (CME)

◈ *Khurana 5th/290*

It refers to collection of fluid in the outer plexiform (Henle's layer) and inner nuclear layer of the retina, centred around the foveola.

Etiology

- As postoperative complication following ***cataract extraction (Irvine-Gass syndrome)*** and penetrating keratoplasty.
- Retinal vascular disorders *e.g.,* ***diabetic retinopathy***, central retinal vein occlusion, branch retinal vein occlusion (BRVO), retinal telangiectasia (*e.g.,* Coat's disease), periphlebitis retinae (Eales disease) & ***hypertensive retinopathy***
- Intraocular inflammations *e.g.,* pars planitis, posterior uveitis, Behcet disease.
- As a side-effect of drugs *e.g.,* following use of adrenaline eyedrops, especially for aphakic glaucoma.
- Retinal dystrophies *e.g.,* retinitis pigmentosa.
- Vitreo macular traction
- **Miscellaneous causes:** Macular epiretinal membrane (ERM), intraocular tumors & collagen vascular disease

"**CME:** It most commonly occurs after ***cataract surgery.*** About 1-3% of those who have cataract extractions will experience decreased vision due to CME, usually within a few weeks after surgery. If the disorder appears in one eye, there is an increased risk (possibly as high as 50%) that it will also affect the second eye. Fortunately, however, most patients recover their vision with observation or treatment"-*http: //www.kellogg.umich.edu/*

◈ *Khurana 5th/212*

- Collection of fluid in the form of cystic loculi in the Henle's layer of macula is a frequent complication of cataract surgery. However, in most cases it is clinically insignificant, does not produce any visual problem and undergoes spontaneous regression. In few cases, clinically significant CME typically produces visual diminution 1–3 months after cataract extraction.
- In most cases it is associated with ***vitreous incarceration*** in the wound and mild iritis.

109. Ans. b. Associated...

[Ref: Khurana 5th/378; Parson 20th/435-38; Ptosis Surgery by Arnab Biswas 2010/77-80; Nelson 18th/2584-85]

Congenital Ptosis

◈ *Nelson 18th/2584-85*

- Congenital ptosis is usually a result of a ***localized dystrophy of the levator muscle*** in which the striated muscle fibers are replaced with fibrous tissue. The condition may be unilateral or bilateral and can be familial, transmitted as a dominant trait
- Parents often comment that the eye looks smaller because of the drooping eyelid. The ***lid crease is decreased or absent*** where the levator muscle would normally insert below the skin surface.

- If the ptosis is severe, affected children often attempt to raise the lid by lifting their brow or adapting a chin-up head posture to maintain binocular vision.
- **Marcus Gunn jaw-winking ptosis** accounts for 5% of ptosis in children. In this syndrome, an abnormal synkinesis exists between the 5th and 3rd cranial nerves; this causes the eyelid to elevate with movement of the jaw.
- **Amblyopia** may occur in children with ptosis. The amblyopia may be secondary to the lid's covering the visual axis (deprivation) or induced astigmatism (anisometropia). When amblyopia occurs, it should generally be treated before treating the ptosis.
- Ptosis can affect one eye or both eyes.
- Ptosis may be present at birth, or it may develop later in life. If a droopy eyelid is present at ***birth or within the first year of life, the condition is called congenital ptosis.***
- In most cases of congenital ptosis, the problem is isolated and does not affect the vision. Any ptosis that develops over a period of days or weeks can signal a serious medical problem and needs further neurologic and physical evaluation.
- It is associated with congenital w***eakness (maldevelopment) of the levator palpebrae superioris*** (LPS).
- **Complication:** ***Occlusion amblyopia,*** Astigmatism from the compression of the droopy eyelid & Ocular torticollis

It may occur in the following Forms

- ***Simple congenital ptosis*** *(not associated with any other anomaly)*
- ***Congenital ptosis with associated weakness of superior rectus muscle.***
- *As a part of* ***blepharophimosis syndrome***
- ***Congenital synkinetic ptosis*** *(Marcus Gunn jaw winking ptosis)*

110. Ans. d. Cornea...

[Ref: Khurana 5th/224-27; Parson 20th/284-85]

Primary Developmental/Congenital Glaucoma

◈ *Khurana 5th/224-27*
- True congenital glaucoma
- Infantile glaucoma
- Juvenile glaucoma

Clinical Feature

- ***Photophobia, blepharospasm, lacrimation and eye rubbing*** often occur together.
- ***Corneal signs:*** Corneal signs include its oedema, enlargement and Descemet's breaks.
    - *Corneal oedema:* It is frequently the first sign which arouses suspicion. At first it is epithelial, but later there is stromal involvement and ***permanent opacities*** may occur.
    - *Corneal enlargement:* It occurs along with enlargement of globe-***buphthalmos,*** especially when the onset is before the age of 3 years. Normal infant cornea measures 10.5 mm. A diameter of more than 13 mm confirms enlargement. Prognosis is usually poor in infants with corneal diameter of more than 16 mm.
    - *Tears and breaks in Descemet's membrane* (Haab's striae)
    - ***Sclera:*** becomes thin and appears blue due to underlying uveal tissue.
- ***Anterior chamber*** becomes deep.
- ***Iris*** may show iridodonesis and atrophic patches in late stage.
- ***Lens*** becomes flat due to stretching of zonules and may even subluxate.
- ***Optic disc*** may show variable cupping and atrophy especially after third year.
- ***IOP*** is raised which is neither marked nor acute.
- ***Axial myopia*** may occur

Surgical Procedures for Congenital Glaucoma

- ***Goniotomy***
- ***Trabeculotomy***
- ***Combined trabeculotomy and trabeculectomy: it*** is now-a-days the preferred surgery with better results.
- **Glaucoma drainage** device

Developmental Glaucomas with Associated Anomalies

- ***Glaucoma associated with iridocorneal dysgenesis:*** These include posterior embryotoxon characterised by a prominent Schwalbe's ring (Axenfeld anomaly), Rieger anomaly, Rieger syndrome, Peter's anomaly and combined Rieger syndrome and Peter's anomaly.
- *Glaucoma associated with* ***aniridia*** (50% cases).
- *Glaucoma associated with ectopia lentis syndromes,* which include Marfan's syndrome, Weil-Marchesani syndrome and homocystinuria.
- *Glaucoma associated with phakomatosis* is seen in ***Sturge-Weber syndrome*** (50% cases) and Von Recklinghausen's neurofibromatosis (25% cases).
- *Miscellaneous conditions.* Lowe's syndrome (oculo-cerebro-renal syndrome), Naevus of Ota, nanophthalmos, congenital ectropion uveae, congenital microcornea and rubella syndrome.

111. Ans. a. Fatty..., c. Deposition...

[Ref: Khurana 5th/117, 90; Parson 20th/201]

Arcus Senilis

- It refers to an annular ***lipid infiltration of corneal periphery.*** This is an age-related change occurring bilaterally in 60% of patients between 40 and 60 years of age and in nearly all patients over the age of 80.
- Sometimes, similar changes occur in young persons (arcus juvenilis) which may or may not be associated with hyperlipidemia.
- The arcus starts in the superior and inferior quadrants and then progresses circumferentially to form a ***ring*** which is about 1 mm wide.
- This ring of opacity is separated from the limbus by a clear zone (the lucid interval of Vogt). Sometimes there may be *double ring of arcus.*

◈ *http: //link.springer.com/article: Writes*

- Lipid accumulation is found in the peripheral corneal stroma, Bowman's membrane & Descemet's membrane as well as in perilimbal region of sclera
- The areas of the cornea & sclera near the limbus & perivascular areas of the sclera are never involved

Corneal Degenerations: Classification

[A] Depending upon Location

- Axial corneal degenerations
  - Fatty degeneration
  - Hyaline degeneration
  - Amyloidosis
  - Calcific degeneration (Band keratopathy)
  - Salzmann's nodular degeneration.
- Peripheral degenerations
  - Arcus senilis
  - Vogt's white limbal girdle
  - Hassal-Henle bodies
  - Terrien's marginal degeneration
  - Mooren's ulcer
  - Pellucid marginal degeneration
  - Furrow degeneration (senile marginal degeneration).

[B] Depending upon Etiology

- ***Age related degenerations:*** Arcus senilis, Vogt's white limbal girdle, Hassal-Henle bodies, Mosaic degeneration.
- ***Pathological degenerations:*** Fatty degeneration, amyloidosis, calcific degeneration, Salzmann's nodular degeneration, Furrow degeneration, spheroidal degeneration, Pellucid marginal degeneration, Terrien's marginal degeneration, Mooren's ulcer.

112. Ans. b. Categ..., e. Clear...

[Ref: Khurana 5th/151; Parson 20th/220]

Aqueous Flare

- It is due to leakage of protein particles into the aqueous humour from damaged blood vessels. It is demonstrated on the slit lamp examination by a point beam of light passed obliquely to the plane of iris
- In the beam of light, protein particles are seen as suspended and moving dust particles. This is based on the 'Brownian movements' or 'Tyndal phenomenon'. Aqueous flare is usually marked in nongranulomatous and minimal in granulomatous uveitis.
- ***The flare is graded from '0' to +4***
  - 0 = no aqueous flare,
  - +1 = just detectable;
  - ***+2 = moderate flare with clear iris details;***
  - +3 = marked flare (iris details not clear);
  - +4 = intense flare (fixed coagulated aqueous with considerable fibrin).

113. Ans. a. Infe... & b. Lens...

[Ref: Khurana 5th/214-16; Parson 20th/508, 215, 322; Nelson 18th/2890]

*"Marfan syndrome-**upward & outward lens dislocation (up & out)**" (http: //www.marfan.org/resource)*

Table *(Khurana 5th/214-16)*: **Dislocation of Lens**

Congenital lesion with Systemic anomalies	Spontaneous
• ***Marfan's syndrome (displaced upwards and temporarily)*** [Q] • ***Homocystinuria (subluxated downwards and nasally)*** [Q] • ***Weil-Marchesani syndrome (forward subluxation)*** [Q] • ***Ehler-Danlos syndrome (subluxation of lens and blue sclera)*** [Q] • ***Hyperlysinemia*** • ***Stickler syndrome*** • ***Sulphite oxidase deficiency***	• Hypermature cataract • Buphthalmos • High myopia • Staphyloma • Intra-ocular tumors • Uveitis

Ocular Features of Marfan Syndrome

◈ *http: //www.ima.org.il/FilesUpload/IMAJ/0/42/21399.pdf*

- Of the many ocular abnormalities seen in Marfan patients, so far the *most common is ectopia lentis*, occurring in 50–80% of affected individuals
- The most common cause of ectopia lentis is trauma, which accounts for nearly one half of all cases of lens dislocation.
- *Marfan syndrome is the most frequent cause of heritable ectopia lentis.* When associated with this syndrome, ectopia lentis is usually bilateral, symmetric and non-progressive
- The dislocation may be subtle and detectable only by observing phacodonesis or iridodonesis (tremulousness of the lens or iris, respectively) sometimes visible by gonioscopy. It may vary from an asymptomatic mild displacement seen only in *post-pupillary dilation*, to significant subluxation that places the equator of the lens in the pupillary axis and causes monocular diplopia (or quadropia if the condition is bilateral).
- A **forward dislocation of the lens into the pupil or anterior chamber** may cause pupillary block with acute glaucoma or chronic angle-closure glaucoma.
- **Posterior dislocation** can cause *harmful vitreous traction on the retina with leakage of lens proteins into the vitreous, which may cause chronic vitreitis and chorioretinal inflammation*

"Marfan syndrome: Upward displacement of the lens is common. It is usually not progressive but may contribute to the formation of cataracts. The ocular globe is frequently elongated and most patients are myopic but with adequate vision. Retinal detachment can occur" *(Harrison 19th/2513, 18th/3212)*

*"Marfan syndrome cause **sublaxation of lens, myopia & retinal detachment**"(Parson 20th/508)*

*"Marfan syndrome cause **vitreoretinal degeneration**" (Parson 20th/322)*

*"Marfan syndrome cause **blue sclera**" (Parson 20th/508)*

114. Ans. a. Caused..., b. X-ray..., c. Stridor..., e. Commonly...

[Ref: P.L. Dhingra 5th/307-09; Logan Turner 10th (1st Indian edition/390; Nelson 18th/1763]

Acute Laryngo-Tracheo-Bronchitis (or Croup or Acute Obstructive Subglottic Laryngitis)

◈ *P.L. Dhingra 5th/307-09; Logan Turner 10th/390*

- *Disease starts as upper respiratory infection with hoarseness & croupy cough*
- *Respiratory difficulty may gradually increase with signs of upper airway obstruction, i.e., suprasternal & intercostals recession*
- *This is a **disease of the subglottis***
- *Respirations are rapid & labored*
- *There is inspiratory stridor & expiratory wheeze*
- *The condition is diagnosed from acute epiglottitis by the **absence of supraglottic oedema**, the presence of sticky secretions & a normal lateral radiograph of the neck*
- ***X-ray PA view shows steeple sign of typical subglottic narrowing** (Nelson 18th/1763)*

Table: Differences between acute epiglottitis and acute laryngo-tracheo -bronchitis in children

	Acute epiglottitis	Acute laryngo-tracheo-bronchitis (or croup)
• Causative organism	Haemophilus influenzae type B[Q]	Parainfluenza virus type I and II[Q]
• Age	2-7 years[Q]	6 months – 3 years[Q]
• Pathology	Supraglottic larynx[Q]	Subglottic area
• Prodromal symptoms	Absent	Present
• Onset	Sudden	Slow
• Fever	High	Low grade or no fever
• Patient's look	Toxic	Non-toxic
• Cough	Usually absent[Q]	Present (Barking seal-like) [Q]
• Stridor	Present and may be marked[Q]	Present
• Odynophagia	Present with drooling of secretions	Usually absent
• Radiology	*Thumb sign on lateral view*[Q]	*Steeple sign on anteroposterior view of neck*[Q]
• Treatment	Humidified oxygen, third generation cephalosporin (ceftriaxone) or amoxicillin	Humidified O_2 tent, steroids

Diagnosis of Acute Epiglottitis

- Diagnosis is usually based **purely on history & clinical finding.** Lateral soft tissue radiograph may reveal the classic **'thumb sign.**[Q] of edematous epiglottis with a dilated hypopharynx. Transnasal fiberoptic laryngoscopy is most reliable & most commonly used technique to assess resolution of edema before extubation of tube in acute epiglotitis"-*Ballenger's otolaryngology*
- **Direct laryngoscopy** is the most important laryngeal investigation in general. It permits a close examination of laryngeal & pharyngeal structures" – *LT 10th/154*

115. Ans. b. 7th CN..., c. Abduction..., d. Esotro.. e. 6th CN...

[Ref: Nelson 18th/2450-51, 677, 2567, 2582; emedicine.medscape.com]

Mobius Syndrome

◈ *Nelson 18th/2450-51, 677, 2567, 2582*

- "It is characterized by ***bilateral facial weakness (i.e VII CN),*** which is often associated with ***abducens nerve paralysis (i.e. VI CN)"*** *(Nelson 18th/2450)*
- The facial palsy is commonly bilateral, frequently asymmetric and often incomplete, tending to spare the lower face and platysma.
- Ectropion, epiphora and exposure keratopathy may develop.
- The **abduction defect** may be unilateral or bilateral. ***Esotropia is common.***
- Whether the primary defect is maldevelopment of cranial nerve nuclei, hypoplasia of the muscles, or a combination of central and peripheral factors is unclear.
- ***Surgical correction of the esotropia*** is indicated and any attendant amblyopia should be treated.

Möbius Syndrome (also Spelled Moebius)

◈ *emedicine.medscape.com*

- It is an extremely rare congenital neurological disorder which is characterized by facial paralysis and the inability to move the eyes from side to side.
- Möbius syndrome results from the underdevelopment of the ***VI and VII cranial nerves.***
- The ***VI cranial nerve*** controls lateral eye movement and the ***VII cranial nerve*** controls facial expression. People with Möbius syndrome are born with facial paralysis and the inability to move their eyes laterally. Often, the upper lip is retracted due to muscle shrinkage.
- Occasionally, the cranial nerves V and VIII are affected. If cranial VIII is affected, the person experiences hearing loss.
- Children with Möbius syndrome may have delayed speech because of paralysis of muscles that move the lips, soft palate and tongue root.

"Moebius syndrome is a rare neurological disorder that is present at birth. It primarily affects the ***6th and 7th cranial nerves,*** leaving those with the condition unable to move their faces (they can't smile, frown, suck, grimace or blink their eyes) and ***unable to move their eyes laterally"*** *(http: //www. moebiussyndrome.com/)*

116. Ans. a. Most..., b. Radioresistant...

[Ref: P.L. Dhingra 5th/261-63; Logan Turner 10th (1st Indian edition/111-12]

Nasopharyngeal Fibroma (Juvenile Nasopharyngeal Angiofibroma)

- It is a rare tumour, though it is the ***commonest of all benign tumours of nasopharynx***
- It is locally invasive & destroys the adjoining structures
- Tumour is seen almost ***exclusively in males in age group of 10-20 years.*** Rarely, it may be seen in older people & females
- **Most common presentation:** ***Profuse & recurrent epistaxis***
- It is made up of ***vascular*** & ***fibrous tissue***. Mostly, the vessels are just endothelium-lined spaces with no muscle coat
- Surgical excision is now the treatment of choice
- **Radiotherapy** has been used as a ***primary mode of treatment***

117. Ans. b. Caused..., c. Treatment...

[Ref: P.L. Dhingra 5th/172-74; Logan Turner 10th (1st Indian edition)/61]

Rhinoscleroma

◈ *P.L. Dhingra 5th/172*

- It is a chronic granulomatous disease caused by **gram-negative bacillus** called *Klebsiella rhinoscleromatis or Frisch bacillus*
- Both sex of any age may be affected
- Disease runs with **3 stages**: ***Atrophic stage, granulomatous stage & cicatrical stage***
- Atrophic stage resemble atrophic rhinitis (*i.e.,* ***atrophy of nasal mucosa & turbinate bones)***
- The disease starts in the nose & extends to nasopharynx, oropharynx, larynx, trachea & bronchi
- **Biopsy:** Mikulicz cells & Russell bodies are diagnostic features of the disease
- Causative organisms can be ***cultured from the biopsy material***
- Both streptomycin & tetracycline are given together for a minimum period of 4-6 weeks & repeated, if necessary, after 1 month. Steroid can be combined to reduce fibrosis
- Surgical treatment may be required to establish the airway & correct nasal deformity

ALSO KNOW

Rhinosporidiosis

◈ *P.L. Dhingra 5th/174*

- *It is a fungal granuloma caused by Rhinosporidium seeberi*
- *The disease mostly affects nose & nasopharynx*
- *The disease is acquired through contaminated water of ponds, also frequently by animals*
- *Diagnosis is made on biopsy*
- *Treatment is complete excision of the mass with diathermy knife & cauterization of its base*
- *Not many drugs are effective against the disease. Dapsone has been tried with some success*

118. Ans. b. Occur..., c. B/l atresia..., d. Bilateral..., e. Diagnosed...

[Ref: P.L. Dhingra 5th/178, 458; O.P.Ghai 7th/336-37; Logan Turner 10th (1st Indian edition)/377-80; Nelson 18th/1743, 723]

Choanal Atresia

◈ *P.L. Dhingra 5th/178*

- *It is d/t **persistence of bucconasal membrane** & may be unilateral or bilateral, complete or incomplete, bony (90%) or membranous (10%)*
- *U/L atresia is more common & may remain undiagnosed until adult life.*
- ***B/L atresia*** *presents with* ***respiratory obstruction*** *as the newborn, being a natural nose-breather, does not breathe from mouth*
- *B/L atresia can present as a part of CHARGE association (coloboma, heart abnormalities, choanal atresia, retardation of growth & development, genitourinary defects & ear abnormalities)*
- *Diagnosis of choanal atresia can be made by (i) presence of mucoid discharge in the nose, (ii) absence of air bubbles in the nasal discharge, (iii)* ***failure to pass a catheter from nose to pharynx,*** *(iv) putting a few drops of a dye (methylene-blue) into the nose & seeing its passage into the pharynx, or (v) installing radio-opaque dye into the nose & taking a lateral film*
- *Emergency management may be required in bilateral choanal atresia to provide an airway*
- *A feeding nipple with a large hole provides a good oral airway* ***(McGovern's technique)*** *& obviates the need for tracheostomy.*
- *Definitive treatment consists of correction of atresia by transnasal or transpalatal approach. The latter is usually done at* ***one & a half years.***

◈ *Nelson 18th/1743, 723*

- When the obstruction is unilateral, the infant may be asymptomatic for a prolonged period, often until the 1st respiratory infection, when unilateral nasal discharge or persistent nasal obstruction may suggest the diagnosis.
- Infants with **bilateral choanal atresia** who have difficulty with mouth breathing make vigorous attempts to inspire, often suck in their lips and ***develop cyanosis.***
- Distressed children then cry (*which relieve the cyanosis*) and become calmer, with normal skin color, only to repeat the cycle after closing their mouths. Those who are able to breathe through their mouths at once experience difficulty when sucking and swallowing, becoming cyanotic when they attempt to feed.
- In **bilateral cases, *intubation or, less often, tracheotomy may be indicated.*** If the child is free of other serious medical problems, operative intervention is considered in the neonate; transnasal repair is the treatment of choice with the introduction of small magnifying endoscopes and smaller surgical instruments and drills. Stents are usually left in place for weeks after the repair to prevent closure or stenosis.

- **Operative correction of unilateral obstruction** may be ***deferred for several years***. In both unilateral and bilateral cases, restenosis necessitating dilation or reoperation, or both, is common.
- **Mitomycin C** has been used to help prevent the development of granulation tissue and stenosis.

119. Ans. a. Inferior..., b. Panor..., e. Condyl...

[Ref: P.L. Dhingra 5th/199-200; L & B 25th/331-32; CSDT 11th/1256; Washington Manual of Surgery 5th/481; Sabiston 18th/494-95, 2143]

"The **condylar neck** is the ***weakest part of the mandible*** and is the ***most frequent site of fracture***" *(L & B 25th/331)*

"Many patients with mandibular fractures experience trauma to the ***inferior alveolar nerve*** (a branch of the trigeminal nerve), which runs through a canal within the body of the mandible and terminates in the lower lip as the mental nerve. These patients may experience permanent numbness of the lower lip and teeth on the affected side. Fracture of the coronoid process of the mandible can result in ***trismus*** (inability to open the mouth) because the coronoid process normally passes beneath the zygomatic arch with mouth opening" *(Sabiston 18th/2143)*

Fracture of Mandible

- *P.L. Dhingra 5th/199-200*
- ***Condylar fractures are the most common.*** They are followed in frequency, by fracture of angle, body & symphysis (Mnemonics CABS). Fractures of the ramus, coronoid & alveolar processes are uncommon
- In fracture of condyle, if fragments are not displaced, pain & trismus are the main features & tenderness is elicited at the site of fracture. If fragments are displaced, there is in addition, malocclusion of teeth & deviation of jaw to the opposite side on opening the mouth
- X-rays useful in mandibular fractures are PA view of the skull (for condyle), right & left oblique view of mandible & ***panorex view***
- Both closed & open methods are used for reduction & fixation of the mandibular fractures

- *Washington Manual of Surgery 5th/481*
- ***Panorex radiographs*** are usually ***sufficient to diagnose mandible fracture*** & visualize postreduction
- Mandibualr fractures are not surgical emergencies & should be addressed after stabilization of patient. Fixation within 3 days has been shown to be result in more favourable outcome
- Complications includes *wound infection, maloculusion, non-union, tooth loss, temporomandibular joint ankylosis & paresthesis*

- *Sabiston 18th/494-95*
- Imaging techniques frequently used to identify and classify mandibular fractures include ***plain films, panoramic tomography (Panorex)*** and helical CT. A recent report has demonstrated the overall superiority of ***helical CT over Panorex*** in identifying and decreasing interpretation error in patients with mandibular fractures

- **Reduction and fixation of mandibular fractures** should be accomplished as precisely and expeditiously as possible because malocclusion is a major long-term complication.
- Condylar and subcondylar mandible fractures are most often treated by IMF alone. Surgical exposure of the temporomandibular joint places the facial nerve at risk and exposes the joint to possible injury and dysfunction.

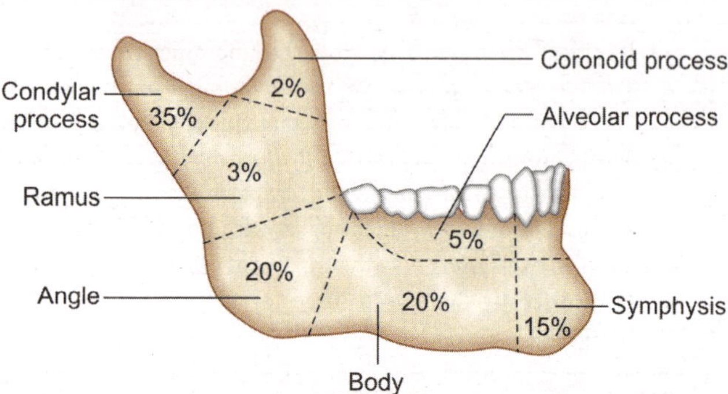

Fig: Fracture of mandible (Dingman's classification). Condylar fracture are the most common, followed by those of angle, body & symphysis of mandible

120. Ans. All (a, b, c, d)

[Ref: P.L. Dhingra 5th/414]

Complication of Radical Mastoidectomy/Modified Radical Mastoidectomy

- *P.L. Dhingra 5th/414*
- *Facial paralysis*
- *Perichondritis of pinna*
- *Injury to dura or sigmoid sinus*
- *Labyrinthitis, if stapes gets disclosed*
- ***Severe conductive deafness*** *of 50 dB or more. This is due to removal of all ossicles & tympanic membrane*
- ***Cavity problems:*** *25% of the cavities do not heal & continue to discharge, requiring regular after-care*

Complications of a Mastoidectomy Include

- *http: //www.healthline.com/)*
- ***Facial nerve paralysis or*** weakness (a rare complication caused by facial nerve injury)
- ***Sensorineural hearing loss*** (a type of inner ear hearing loss that may occur in up to 6% of patients)
- Vertigo (dizziness; it may persist for several days)
- ***Change in taste*** (food may taste metallic, sour, or otherwise "off"; this often resolves after a few months)
- Tinnitus (abnormal noises in the ear such as ringing, popping and hissing)

Complications do not Often Occur, but they may Include

- *www.surgery encyclopedia.com*
- Persistent ear discharge
- Infections, including meningitis or brain abscesses

- ***Hearing loss***
- ***Facial nerve injury*** (This is a rare complication.)
- Temporary dizziness
- ***Temporary loss of taste on the side of the tongue***

121. Ans. b. Consists..., d. Lamina...

[Ref: BDC 6th/Vol. III 245-46; P.L. Dhingra 5th/201-03; Logan Turner 10th (1st Indian edition)/9-10]

Ethmoidal Sinus

◈ *Dhingra 5th/201*

- Clinically, ethmoidal cells are divided into ***anterior ethmoidal group which opens into the middle meatus*** & posterior ethmoidal group, which opens into the superior meatus & sphenoethmoidal recess
- Their number varies from 3 to 18
- The thin paper like lamina of bone **(lamina papyracea)** ***separating air cells from the orbit*** can be easily destroyed leading to spread of ethmoidal infections into the orbit

Table *(P.L. Dhingra 5th/203)*: **Development and growth of paranasal sinuses**

	Status at birth	Growth	First radiologic evidence
Maxillary	Present at birth [Q]	Rapid growth from birth to 3 years and from 7-12 years. Adult size-15 years	4-5 months after birth
Ethmoid	Present at birth[Q] Anterior group: 5 × 2 × 2mm. Posterior group: 5 × 4 × 2mm.	Reach adult size by 12 years [Q]	1 year
Frontal	Not present	Invades frontal bone at the age of 4 years. Size increases until teens	6 years
Sphenoid	Not present	Reaches sella turcica by the age of 7 years, dorsum sellae by late teens and basisphenoid by adult age. Reaches full size between 15 years to adult age	4 years

Anatomy of PNS

◈ *P.L. Dhingra 5th/201*

Anterior group: This includes maxillary, frontal and anterior ethmoidal. They all open in the ***middle meatus***[Q] and their ostia lie anterior to basal lamella of middle turbinate.

Posterior groups: This includes posterior ethmoidal sinuses which open in the superior meatus and the ***sphenoid sinus which open in sphenoethmoidal recess***[Q].

122. Ans. a. Initially..., b. May..., e. Vertigo...

[Ref: P.L. Dhingra 5th/90-91; Logan Turner 10th (1st Indian edition/301-03]

Labyrinthitis

◈ *P.L. Dhingra 5th/90-91*

- This is a common complication of otitis media & if suspected, must be treated vigorously & promptly. Failure to do so may lead to total ***sensorineural deafness or meningitis***
- There are three types-
  - Circumscribed (fistula of labyrinth),
  - Diffuse serous &
  - Diffuse suppurative labyrinthitis
- ***Progression from circumscribed → diffuse serous → diffuse suppurative labyrinthitis***

Circumscribed

- **Circumscribed (paralabyrinthitis):** Most common type & least severe
- ***Chronic suppurative otitis media*** with cholesteatoma is the most common cause
- Patient complains of ***transient vertigo*** often induced by pressure on tragus, cleaning the ear or while performing valsalva manoeuvre
- **Treatment:** In chronic suppurative otitis media or cholesteatoma, ***mastoid exploration is often required to eliminate the cause***

Diffuse Serous

- Less common & more serious
- Most often it arise from pre-existing circumscribed labyrinthitis ***associated with chronic suppurative otitis media or cholesteatoma***
- Mild case complain of ***vertigo*** & nausea but in severe cases, vertigo is worse with marked nausea, vomiting & even spontaneous nystagmus
- ***Quick component of nystagmus is toward the affected ear***
- Cochlea is also affected with some degree of sensorineural hearing loss.
- If not checked, it may pass onto suppurative labyrinthitis with total loss of vestibular & cochlear function
- Antibacterial therapy is given in full dose to control infection
- **Surgical treatment includes:** Myringotomy (if labyrinthitis has followed acute otitis media & the drum is bulging), cortical mastoidectomy (in acute mastoiditis) & modified radical mastoidectomy (in chronic middle ear infection or cholesteatoma)

Diffuse Suppurative (Purulent)

- Least common & most dangerous variety which inevitably leads to a total & permanent loss of vestibular & auditory function
- Usually follow serous labyrinthitis
- There is severe vertigo with nausea & vomiting due to acute vestibular failure
- ***Spontaneous nystagmus will be observed with its quick component towards the healthy ear***
- There is total loss of hearing
- Treatment is same as for serous labyrinthitis

123. Ans. d. Davis...

[Ref: P.L. Dhingra 5th/463; http: //en.wikipedia.org/wiki/List_of_instruments_used_in_otorhinolaryngology]

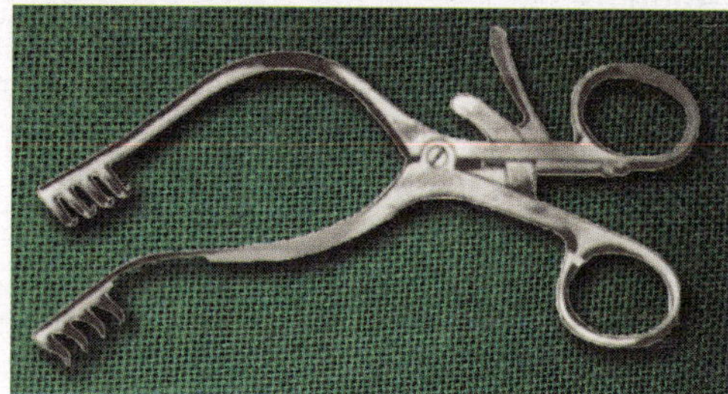

Fig: Mollison's mastoid retractor

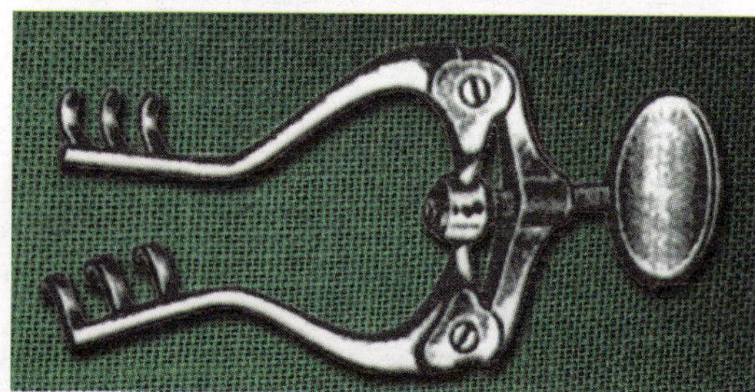

Fig: Jansen's self-retaining mastoid retractor

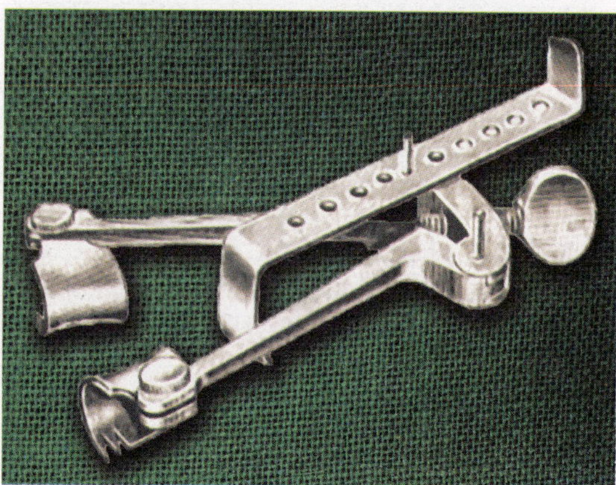

Fig: Lempert's endaural retractor

Surgical Retractors

◈ *http: //en.wikipedia.org/wiki/List_of_ instruments _used_in_ otorhinolaryngology,*

Mollison's mastoid retractor: *Used in mastoidectomy to retract soft tissue after incision & elevation of flaps. It is **self-retaining & haemostatic**"* (P.L. Dhingra 5th/463)

Jansen's self-retaining mastoid retractor: *used in mastoidectomy similar to Mollison's retractor"* (P.L. Dhingra 5th/463)

"Lempert's endaural mastoid retractor with third blade is a ***self-retaining retractor"*** *(books.google.co.in/books?id)*

Types of Retractors

There are 2 types of retractors on the basis of their functionality.

- Self retaining retractors
- Handheld retractors

Self Retaining Retractors

These retractors do not need an assistant to hold them in place. It hold tissue apart and lock it in place. Rib Spreaders come in this category. They hold the ribs apart during the abdominal surgery when the required organ is located inside the rib cage. Followings are the commonly used retractors:

Hand Held Retractors

These retractors require an assistant to hold them but the self retaining ones don't, once they are adjusted in position. The correct method of using a hand-held retractor is that it must be held by its handle properly so as to produce maximum exposure of the surgical area, maximum leverage and steady retraction.

◈ *http: //en.wikipedia.org/wiki*

- Hohmann retractor
- Lahey retractor
- Senn retractor
- Blair (Rollet) retractor
- Rigid rake
- Flexible rake
- Ragnell retractor
- Linde-ragnell retractor
- ***Davis retractor***
- Volkman retractor
- Kocher retractor
- Farabeuf retractor
- Mathieu retractor
- Jackson tracheal hook
- Crile retractor
- Meyerding finger retractor
- Little retractor
- Love nerve retractor
- Green retractor
- Goelet retractor
- Cushing vein retractor
- Langenbeck retractor
- Richardson retractor
- Richardson-eastmann retractor
- Kelly retractor
- Deaver retractor
- Doyen retractor
- Parker retractor
- Parker-mott retractor
- Roux retractor
- Mayo-collins retractor
- U.S. Army retractor
- Ribbon retractor
- Alm retractor
- Lone star retractor
- Gelpi retractor
- Gutow retractor
- Weitlaner retractor
- Beckman-weitlaner retractor
- Beckman-eaton retractor
- Beckman retractor
- Adson retractor
- Balfour retractor
- Finochietto retractor or rib spreader

MEDICINE

124. Ans. **c. Brady.. d. Hype..., e. Respir...**

[Ref: CSDT 11th/890;Harrison 19th/1778-80. 18th/1868, 2249, 2257, 232-33; Robbins 9th/1255, 8th/1383-84; CMDT 2016/993]

"**Blood pressure elevation** accompanied by ***bradycardia and respiratory slowing*** classically results from raised intracranial pressure. This "Cushing response, " however, usually appears only when intracranial hypertension is severe" *(CSDT 11th/890)*

"***Raised Intracranial Pressure and Herniation***: *Transtentorial (uncinate, mesial temporal) herniation* occurs when the medial aspect of the temporal lobe is compressed against the free margin of the **tentorium cerebelli**. With increasing displacement of the temporal lobe, the third cranial nerve is compromised, resulting in ***pupillary dilation and impairment of ocular movements on the side of the lesion***" *(Robbins 9th/1255, 8th/1383)*

Features of Increased ICT

- Loss of the normal autoregulation of blood pressure and pulse, called the ***Cushing's reflex, is a hallmark of severe brain injury or imminent crisis.*** This generally results in a *sudden rise in blood pressure and a slowing of the pulse.*
- Signs of increased ICP include decreasing level of consciousness, paralysis or weakness on one side of the body and ***a blown pupil, one that fails to constrict in response to light or is slow to do so.***
- **Cushing's triad, *a slow heart rate with high blood pressure and respiratory depression is a classic manifestation of significantly raised ICP.***
- **Anisocoria,** unequal pupil size, is another sign of serious traumatic brain injury
- ***Abnormal posturing, a characteristic positioning of the limbs caused by severe diffuse injury or high ICP, is an ominous***

125. Ans. **a. COPd..., c. COPD patients..., d. Steroid...**

[Ref: Harrison 19th/1661-62, 1676, 1702, 1707, 18th/2084-86, 2106, 2114; Robbins 9th/679, 8th/683; CMDT2016/262-63]

Comparison of COPD & Asthma

◈ *Harrison19th/1661-62, 18th/2084-86*

"Chronic obstructive pulmonary disease (COPD) is usually easy to differentiate from asthma as symptoms ***show less variability, never completely remit and show much less (or no) reversibility to bronchodilators***" *(Harrison 19th/1676, 18th/2109)*

"Patients with **COPD** has a gradual progression of dyspnea on exertion, punctuated by acute exacerbations of shortness of breath. In contrast, most **asthmatics** have normal breathing the majority of the time and have recurrent episodes of dyspnea usually associated with specific triggers, such as an upper respiratory tract infection or exposure to allergens"

"Of the obstructive lung diseases, asthma is most likely to have specific triggers related to sudden onset of dyspnea, although this can also be true of COPD"

"History as well as further testing can help distinguish among different obstructive diseases. ***COPD is almost exclusively seen in cigarette smokers. Asthmatics often show an acute response to inhaled bronchodilators*** *(e.g., albuterol)*"

"Apart from acute exacerbations, ***COPD is not generally responsive to oral corticosteroid therapy.*** Only 10–20% of stable outpatients with COPD given oral corticosteroids will have a greater than 20% increase in FEV_1 compared with patients receiving placebo" *(CMDT2016/262-63)*

"**Inhaled Corticosteroids** are by far the most effective controllers for asthma and their early use has revolutionized asthma therapy" *(Harrison 19th/1677, 18th/2111)*

"**COPD**: Available data suggest that inhaled glucocorticoids reduce exacerbation frequency by ~25%. The impact of inhaled corticosteroids on mortality rates in COPD is controversial. A meta-analysis and several retrospective studies suggest a mortality benefit, but in a recently published randomized trial, differences in mortality rate approached, but did not reach, conventional criteria for statistical significance. A trial of inhaled glucocorticoids should be considered in patients with frequent exacerbations, defined as two or more per year and in patients who demonstrate a significant amount of acute reversibility in response to inhaled bronchodilators." *(Harrison 19th/1705-06, 18th/2106)*

Inflammatory Cell in Asthma & COPD

"***Eosinophilic infiltration** is a **characteristic feature of asthmatic airways***"-*Harrison 19th/1693, 18th/2105*

"*In **COPD** there is macrophage activation & **neutrophil recruitment** in airway.* Concomitant cigarette smoke–induced loss of cilia in the airway epithelium and impaired macrophage phagocytosis predispose to bacterial infection with ***neutrophilia***" *(Harrison 19th/1701, 18th/2155)*

"**Asthma**: Many cells play a role in the inflammatory response, in particular eosinophils, mast cells, macrophages, T lymphocytes, neutrophils and epithelial cells" *(Robbins 9th/679, 8th/688)*

"**Asthma**: The clinical diagnosis is aided by the demonstration of an elevated eosinophil count in the peripheral blood and the finding of eosinophils in sputum" *(Robbins 9th/682, 8th/692)*

126. Ans. **a. Saccu..., b. Severe..., c. CT angi..., d. CT scan...**

[Ref: Harrison 19th/1784-87, 18th/2261-63; CMDT 2016/983;CSDT 11th/940; L & B 25th/303-06; emedicine.medscape. com/article/340527-overview Danhert Radiology Review Manual 5th/230;CSDT 11th/904;Chapman 4th/407; Brain's neurology 11th/834, 836]

"**Digital subtraction angiography;** It is useful in the diagnosis and treatment of arterial and venous occlusions, including carotid artery stenosis, pulmonary embolisms, acute limb ischaemia & Cerebral aneurysms and arterio-venous malformations (AVM). ***DSA is the gold standard investigation for renal artery stenosis. DSA*** is being used less and less routinely in imaging departments. ***It is being replaced by computed tomography angiography (CTA),*** which can produce 3D images through a test which is less invasive and stressful for the patient" *(emedicine.medscape.com/article)*

"**Dynamic contrast images** can be used to ***construct CT angiograms*** (CTAs) of vascular structures as well as physiologic maps of vascular perfusion. ***CTA has proved useful in assessment*** of the intracranial and extracranial carotid arteries, especially in acute stroke victims" *(Brain's neurology 11th /834)*

Subarachnoid Hemorrhage

◈ *Imaging CMDT 2016/983*

- A **CT scan** should be ***performed immediately*** to confirm that hemorrhage has occurred and to search for clues regarding its source. It is ***preferable to MRI*** because it is faster and more sensitive in detecting hemorrhage in the first 24 hours.
- **Cerebral arteriography** may be undertaken to determine the source of bleeding; it is not performed unless or until the patient's condition has stabilized and is good enough so that operative treatment is feasible.
- **MR angiography** may also permit these vascular anomalies to be visualized but is less sensitive than conventional arteriography.

Subarachnoid Hemorrhage

◈ *Harrison 19th/1784-86, 18th/2261-63*

- Excluding head trauma, the ***most common cause of SAH is rupture of a saccular aneurysm.***
- Sudden loss of consciousness may be preceded by a brief moment of ***excruciating headache,*** but most patients first complain of headache upon regaining consciousness.
- The patient often calls the **headache** "***the worst headache of my life***"
- The hallmark of aneurysmal rupture is blood in the CSF. ***More than 95% of cases have enough blood to be visualized on a high-quality noncontrast CT scan obtained within 72 h.***
- If the scan fails to establish the diagnosis of SAH and no mass lesion or obstructive hydrocephalus is found, a ***lumbar puncture should be performed*** to establish the presence of subarachnoid blood.
- Once the diagnosis of hemorrhage from a ruptured saccular aneurysm is suspected, ***four-vessel conventional x-ray angiography*** (both carotids and both vertebrals) is generally performed
- ***CT angiography is an alternative method for locating the aneurysm and may be sufficient to plan definitive therapy.***

Note: NCCT is indicated for head injury/stroke, acute haemorrhage & SAH-(Review of Radiology by Sumer Sethi 2nd/5)

Subarachnoid Hemorrhage

◈ *Review of Radiology by Sumer Sethi 2nd/6*
Acute SAH <48 hrs-CT investigation of choice
Chronic SAH >48 hrs-MRI investigation of choice

Table *(CMDT 2016/979)*: **Features of the SAH**

Clinical Features	Clinical Features
Present with sudden onset of worst headache of life, may lead rapidly to loss of consciousness; signs of meningeal irritation often present; etiology usually aneurysm or AVM, but 20% have no source identified.	CT to confirm diagnosis, but may be normal in rare instances; if CT negative and suspicion high, perform lumbar puncture to look for red blood cells or xanthochromia; angiography to determine source of bleed in candidates for treatment.

127. Ans. c. Mainly..., d. Good..., e. More...

[Ref: Harrison 19th/2182-85, 18th/2789 -92; Robbins 9th/511, 8th/516-17; CMDT 2016/843]

"**Wegener granulomatosis** (Granulomatosis with Polyangitis) is characterized in its full expression by ***vasculitis of small arteries, arterioles and capillaries,*** necrotizing granulomatous lesions of ***both upper and lower respiratory tract, glomerulonephritis*** and other organ manifestations. Without treatment, generalized disease is ***invariably fatal,*** with ***most patients surviving less than 1 year after diagnosis.*** It occurs most commonly in the fourth and fifth decades of life and ***affects men and women with equal frequency.***" *(CMDT 2016/843)*

Granulomatosis with Polyangitis (Wegener's)

◈ *Harrison 19th/2182-85, 18th/2789 -92*

- *Granulomatosis with polyangitis (Wegener's)* is a distinct clinicopathologic entity characterized by granulomatous vasculitis of the ***upper and lower respiratory tracts together with glomerulonephritis.*** In addition, variable degrees of disseminated vasculitis involving ***both small arteries and veins*** may occur.
- Granulomatosis with polyangitis (Wegener's) is an uncommon disease with an estimated prevalence of 3 per 100, 000. It is extremely rare in blacks compared with whites; the male-to-female ratio is 1: 1. The disease can be seen at any age.
- Lung involvement typically appears as multiple, bilateral, nodular cavitary infiltrates, which on biopsy almost invariably reveal the typical necrotizing granulomatous vasculitis.

Table *(Harrison 18th/2790)*

Granulomatosis with Polyangitis (Wegener's)
Kidney
Glomerulonephritis
Ear/nose/throat
Sinusitis; Nasal disease; Otitis media; Hearing loss
Subglottic stenosis; Ear pain; Oral lesions
Lung
Pulmonary infiltrates; Pulmonary nodules; Hemoptysis; Pleuritis
Eyes

128. Ans. b. Arterioles...

[Ref: Harrison 19th/1627-29, 18th/2375-76; Robbins 9th/940-41, 8th/951-52; CMDT 2016/916-17]

Renal Artery Stenosis

◈ *Robbins 9th/940-41, 8th/951-52*

- *"A large proportion of patients with renovascular hypertension have* ***elevated plasma or renal vein renin levels*** and almost all show a reduction of blood pressure when given competitive antagonists of angiotensin II"
- "The most common cause of renal artery stenosis (70% of cases) is occlusion by an atheromatous plaque at the origin of the renal artery. This lesion occurs more frequently in men and the incidence increases with advancing age and

A & E

diabetes mellitus. The plaque is usually concentrically placed and superimposed thrombosis often occurs"

- The second type of lesion leading to stenosis is so-called **fibromuscular dysplasia** of the renal artery. This is a heterogeneous group of lesions characterized by fibrous or fibromuscular thickening and may involve the intima, the media, or the adventitia of the artery. This is ***more common in women*** and tend to occur in younger age groups (*i.e.*, in the third and fourth decades).
- The ***ischemic kidney is usually reduced in size and shows signs of diffuse ischemic atrophy,*** with crowded glomeruli, atrophic tubules, interstitial fibrosis and focal inflammatory infiltrates.
- The ***arterioles in the ischemic kidney are usually protected from the effects of high pressure, thus showing only mild arteriolosclerosis. In contrast, the contralateral nonischemic kidney may exhibit more severe arteriolosclerosis,*** depending on the severity of the hypertension.

◈ *CMDT 2016/916*

Essentials of Diagnosis:

i. *Produced by **atherosclerotic occlusive disease** (80–90% of patients) or fibromuscular dysplasia (10–15%),*
ii. Hypertension &
iii. *Acute renal failure in patients starting therapy with an ACE inhibitor.*

- ***Atherosclerotic ischemic renal disease accounts for nearly all cases of renal artery stenosis. Fibromuscular dysplasia can also cause renal artery stenosis.***
- It occurs most commonly in those over 45 years of age with a history of atherosclerotic disease. Other risk factors include *renal insufficiency, diabetes mellitus, tobacco use and hypertension.*
- Fibromuscular ***dysplasia primarily affects young women.***
- Abdominal ultrasound discloses ***asymmetric kidney size*** when one renal artery is affected out of proportion to the other.
- Three prevailing methods used for screening are *Doppler ultrasonography, captopril renography and magnetic resonance angiography (MRA).*
- **Renal angiography** is the gold standard for diagnosis.

Macrovascular Disease of Kidney

◈ *Harrison 19th/1627-28, 18th/2375-76.*

- Because restoration of perfusion pressures can reverse these pathways, **renal artery stenosis** is considered a specifically treatable "secondary" cause of hypertension.
- **Fibromuscular dysplasia (FMD):** It may present clinically with ***hypertension in younger individuals*** (between age 15 and 50), ***most often women.***
- ***Atherosclerotic renal artery stenosis*** (ARAS) is ***common*** in the general population (6.8% of a community-based sample above age 65), a prevalence that increases with age

129. Ans. a. ST..., b. T wave..., c. Q1S3T3..., e. Right...

[Ref: The ECG Made Easy by Hampton 8th/148;Harrison 19th/1633, 18th/2172; CMDT 2016/294;CSDT 11th/880]

Possible ECG pattern in Pulmonary Embolism

◈ *The ECG Made Easy by Hampton 8th/148;*

- *Normal ECG with sinus tachycardia*
- *Peaked P wave*
- ***Right axis deviation***
- *Right bundle branch block*
- *Dominant R wave in lead V1 (i.e., R wave bigger than S wave)*
- ***Inverted T waves in lead V1-V3***
- *Deep S wave in lead V6*
- *Right axis deviation (S wave in lead I), plus Q waves & inverted T waves in lead III i.e., **S1Q3T3 sign***

Electrocardiogram in Pulmonary Embolism

◈ *Harrison 19th/1633, 18th/2172*

- The most frequently cited abnormality, in addition to sinus tachycardia, is the ***S1Q3T3 sign: an S wave in lead I, a Q wave in lead III and an inverted T wave in lead III.*** This finding is relatively specific but insensitive.
- Perhaps the most common abnormality is ***T-wave inversion in leads V_1 to V_4***

"**PE:** Electrocardiography may reveal *new-onset atrial fibrillation* or ischemic changes, but in most cases only ***acute sinus tachycardia and nonspecific ST and T wave changes*** are identified" *(CSDT 11th/880)*

"The **ECG** is abnormal in 70% of patients with PE. However, the most common abnormalities are sinus tachycardia and ***nonspecific ST and T wave changes,*** each seen in approximately 40% of patients. 5% or less of patients in the PIOPED I study had P pulmonale, right ventricular hypertrophy, right axis deviation and right bundle branch block" *(CMDT 2016/294)*

Electrocardiography

◈ *Hurst's The Heart, 12th Edition/Chapter 72*

- ECG findings in acute PE are generally nonspecific and include T-wave changes, ST-segment abnormalities, ***incomplete or complete right bundle-branch block,*** right axis deviation in the extremity leads and clockwise rotation of the QRS vector in the precordial leads.
- The **"classic" S_1 Q_3 T_3 pattern** is present in approximately 10% of PE cases.
- PE patients may present with finding of acute cor pulmonale, such as the ***S_1 Q_3 T_3 pattern, right bundle-branch block, a P-wave pulmonale, or right axis deviation.***
- It was recently suggested that a ***T-wave inversion in V_2 or V_3 is the most frequent ECG sign of massive PE.***

"The **$S_1Q_3T_3$ sign** (prominent S wave in lead I, Q wave and inverted T wave in lead III) is a sign of *acute cor pulmonale* (acute pressure and volume overload of the right ventricle because of pulmonary hypertension) and reflects right ventricular strain. Other ECG findings noted during the acute phase of a PE include ***new right bundle branch block*** (complete or incomplete), ***rightward shift of the QRS axis, ST-segment elevation in V_1 and aVR,*** generalized low amplitude QRS complexes, atrial premature contractions, sinus tachycardia, atrial fibrillation/flutter and ***T wave inversions in leads V_1-V_4.***"- *www.ncbi.nlm.nih.gov*

130. Ans. a. Tension..., b. Venous..., c. Pulm..., d. Cardi...

[Ref: Harrison 19th/1762, 18th/1972, 2171, 1976-77; Emergency Medicine by S.N.Chugh 8th/197]

"**Septic shock** *has* **low CVP** *(i.e., JVP)* **with high cardiac output**" *(Emergency Medicine by S.N.Chugh 8th/155)*

"**Compressive Cardiogenic Shock**: With extrinsic compression, the heart and surrounding structures are less compliant and therefore normal filling pressures generate inadequate diastolic filling and stroke volume. Blood or fluid within the poorly distensible pericardial sac may cause ***tamponade.*** Any cause of increased intrathoracic pressure such as ***tension pneumothorax,*** herniation of abdominal viscera through a diaphragmatic hernia, or excessive positive-pressure ventilation to support pulmonary function, can also cause compressive cardiogenic shock while simultaneously impeding venous return and preload" *(Harrison 18th/2221)*

"***Venous gas embolism****: It can cause acute cor pulmonale & cardiovascular collapse. Clinical sign includes hypotension, increased CVP, tachycardia etc."-Harrison 19th/1750, 18th/2221*

"***Tension pneumothorax:*** *There is decreased venous return to the heart & cardiac output falls leading to hypotension (cardiac temponade)" (Emergency Medicine by S.N.Chugh 8th/197)*

"***Cardiac temponade*** *(Pericardial effusion) should be considered in any patient with hypotension, low volume pulse & raised JVP" (Emergency Medicine by S.N.Chugh 8th/197)*

"***Large vessel pulmonary embolism*** *can cause hypotension/ shock & raised" (Emergency Medicine by S.N.Chugh 8th/27)*

"The three principal features of tamponade (*Beck's triad*) are ***hypotension, soft or absent heart sounds and jugular venous distention with a prominent x descent but an absent y descent. There a***re both limitation of ventricular filling and reduction of cardiac output. A high index of suspicion for cardiac tamponade is required since in many instances no obvious cause for pericardial disease is apparent and it should be considered in any patient with otherwise unexplained enlargement of the cardiac silhouette, hypotension and elevation of jugular venous pressure"*(Harrison 19th/1573, 18th/1972)*

Factors that Increase CVP Include

- *Hypervolemia*
- *Forced exhalation*
- *Tension pneumothorax*
- *Heart failure*
- *Pleural effusion*
- *Decreased cardiac output*
- *Cardiac tamponade*
- *Mechanical ventilation and the application of positive end-expiratory pressure (PEEP)*
- *Pulmonary Hypertension*
- *Pulmonary Embolism*

131. Ans. c. Associated..., d. Benign..., e. More...

[Ref: Harrison 19th/559, 569, 18th/3057, 3066-67; Robbins 9th/1121, 8th/1146-47; CMDT 2016/1232-35]

Insulinomas

◈ *Harrison 18th/3057, 3066-67*

- "**Insulinoma:** *About 90% are solitary & about 10% are multiple & are* ***always associated with MEN1. About 10% are malignant"*** *(L & B 25th/817)*
- *"****Majority of the insulinomas occur in the tail & body of pancreas*** *& majority of them are benign, one third are malignant & one-third are multiple" (Manipal manual of Surgery 3rd/501)*
- An insulinoma is an endocrine tumor of the pancreas that is thought to be derived from beta cells that ectopically secrete insulin, which results in ***hypoglycemia.***
- The average age of occurrence is 40–50 years old. The most common clinical symptoms are due to the effect of the ***hypoglycemia on the CNS (neuroglycemic symptoms)*** and include ***confusion, headache, disorientation, visual difficulties, irrational behavior and even coma.***
- Insulinomas are generally small (>90% <2 cm) and usually not multiple (90%); only ***5–15% are malignant*** and they almost invariably occur only in the pancreas, ***distributed equally in the pancreatic head, body and tail.***
- Insulinomas should be suspected in all patients with hypoglycemia, especially when there is a history suggesting that attacks are provoked by fasting, or with a family history of MEN1.
- The most reliable test to diagnose insulinoma is a fast up to 72 h with serum glucose, C-peptide, proinsulin and insulin measurements every 4–8 h.
- "**β-cell tumors (insulinomas)** are the ***most common of pancreatic endocrine neoplasms*** and may be responsible for the elaboration of sufficient insulin to induce clinically significant hypoglycemia. There is a characteristic clinical triad resulting from these pancreatic lesions:
  - Attacks of hypoglycemia occur with blood glucose levels below 50 mg/dL of serum;
  - The attacks consist principally of such ***central nervous system manifestations*** as confusion, stupor and loss of consciousness; and
  - The attacks are precipitated by fasting or exercise and are promptly relieved by feeding or parenteral administration of glucose" *(Robbins 9th/1121, 8th/1146)*

132. Ans. a. Dysphagia b. Jaw..., E Plantar...

[Ref: Harrison 19th/154, 18th/182; P.J.Mehta 15th/241; CMDT 2016/1016;Kundu 4th/275]

"Often the **gag reflex** *is preserved in* **pseudobulbar palsy**" *(Kundu 4th/276)*

"***Tongue*** *in pseudobulbar palsy: Spastic with pointed tip, there is* ***neither wasting nor any fasciculation seen*** *(Kundu 4th/275)*

"Plantar reflex is always extensor in pseudobulbar palsy& usually flexor in bulbar palsy" (Kundu 4th/275)

*"**Gag reflex:** The reflex is lost in lesions of 9th & 10th cranial nerve" (P.J.Mehta 15th/232)*

"With bilateral corticobulbar lesions, pseudobulbar palsy often develops: ***Dysarthria, dysphagia, dysphonia and emotional lability accompany bilateral facial weakness and a brisk jaw jerk.*** Spasticity accompanies upper motor neuron weakness but may not be present in the acute phase" *(Harrison 19th/154, 18th/182)*

Signs and Symptoms of Pseudobulbar Palsy Include

◈ *P.J.Mehta 15th/241; http: //en.wikipedia.org/wiki*

- Slow and indistinct speech
- Dysphagia (Difficulty in swallowing)
- Small, stiff and spastic tongue
- Brisk jaw jerk
- Dysarthria
- Labile affect
- Gag reflex may be normal, exaggerated or absent
- Examination may reveal upper motor neuron lesion of the limbs

Pseudobulbar Palsy

◈ *http: //www.patient.co.uk/*

Pseudobulbar palsy results from disease of the corticobulbar tracts. Bilateral tract damage must occur for clinically evident disease as the muscles are bilaterally innervated.

Presentation

- *Tongue -paralysed; no wasting initially and **no fasciculations;** 'Donald Duck' speech; unable to protrude.*
- *Palatal movements absent.*
- *Dribbling persistently.*
- *Facial muscles: May also be paralysed.*
- *Reflexes: exaggerated, eg jaw jerk.*
- *Nasal regurgitation may be present.*
- *Dysphonic*
- *Dysphagic*
- *Emotional lability may also be present.*

There may also be neurological deficits in the limbs, *e.g.,* increased tone, enhanced reflexes and weakness.

133. Ans. a. Compensated..., d. Cerebro..., e. Hepatic...

[Ref: CMDT 2016/895; Harrison 19th/315-24, 18th/365, 372]

*"**Chronic renal failure** causes **metabolic acidosis**" (Harrison 19th 1814, 18th/2312)*

*"**Vomiting causes metabolic alkalosis**" (CMDT06/891, Harrison 19th/321, 18th/369)*

Inferences from Data *given in*[Q]

High pH means-alkalosis

Decrease CO_2 means respiratory alkalosis

Low HCO_3^- level means metabolic acidosis

Here respiratory change is in accordance to pH, so it is primary part (& metabolic change-compensatory part)

Therefore it is a case of respiratory alkalosis with metabolic acidosis (Compensated respiratory alkalosis)

Normal Acid Base Homeostatsis

◈ *Harrison 19th/315-17, 18th/363*

- Systemic arterial pH is maintained between 7.35 and 7.45 by extracellular and intracellular chemical buffering together with respiratory and renal regulatory mechanisms. The control of arterial CO_2 tension ($PaCO_2$) by the central nervous system (CNS) and respiratory systems and the control of the plasma bicarbonate by the kidneys stabilize the arterial pH by excretion or retention of acid or alkali.
- Under most circumstances, CO_2 production and excretion are matched and the usual steady-state $PaCO_2$ is maintained at 40 mmHg.
- Underexcretion of CO_2 produces hypercapnia and overexcretion causes hypocapnia. Nevertheless, production and excretion are again matched at a new steady-state $PaCO_2$. Therefore, the Pa_{co2} is regulated primarily by neural respiratory factors and is not subject to regulation by the rate of CO_2 production. Hypercapnia is usually the result of hypoventilation rather than of increased CO_2 production. Increases or decreases in $PaCO_2$ represent derangements of neural respiratory control or are due to compensatory changes in response to a primary alteration in the plasma [HCO_3^-].

Respiratory Alkalosis

◈ *CMDT 2016/895*

"Respiratory alkalosis, or hypocapnia, occurs when hyperventilation reduces the PCO_2, which increases the pH. The most common cause of respiratory alkalosis is hyperventilation syndrome, but bacterial **septicemia** and **cirrhosis** are other common causes."

Table *(Harrison 19th/323, 18th/371)*

Respiratory Alkalosis

- **Central nervous system stimulation**
  - Pain
  - Anxiety, psychosis
  - Fever
  - Cerebrovascular accident
  - Meningitis, encephalitis
  - Tumor
  - Trauma
  - **Hypoxemia or tissue hypoxia**
  - High altitude
  - Pneumonia, pulmonary edema
  - Aspiration
  - Severe anemia
- **Drugs or hormones**
  - Pregnancy, progesterone
  - Salicylates
  - Cardiac failure
- **Stimulation of chest receptors**
  - Hemothorax
  - Flail chest
  - Cardiac failure
  - Pulmonary embolism
- **Miscellaneous**
  - Septicemia
  - Hepatic failure
  - Mechanical hyperventilation
  - Heat exposure
  - Recovery from metabolic acidosis

Table *(Harrison 19th/316, 18th/363)*: **Prediction of Compensatory Responses on Simple Acid-Base Disturbances and Pattern of Changes**

Disorder	Prediction of Compensation	pH	HCO_3^-	$PaCO_2$
Metabolic acidosis	$Paco_2 = (1.5X\ HCO_3^-) + 8 \pm 2$ or $Paco_2$ will ↓1.25 mmHg per mmol/L ↓in $[HCO_3^-]$ or $Paco_2 = [HCO_3^-] + 15$	Low	Low	Low
Metabolic alkalosis	$Paco_2$ will ↑0.75 mmHg per mmol/L ↑in $[HCO_3^-]$ or $Paco_2$ will ↑6 mmHg per 10 mmol/L ↑in $[HCO_3^-–]$ or $Paco_2 = [HCO_3^-] + 15$	High	High	High
Respiratory alkalosis	or	High	Low	Low
Acute	$[HCO_3^-]$ will ↓0.2 mmol/L per mmHg ↓in Pa_{co2}			
Chronic	$[HCO_3^-–]$ will ↓0.4 mmol/L per mmHg ↓in Pa_{co2}			
Respiratory acidosis		Low	High	High
Acute	$[HCO_3^-]$ will ↑0.1 mmol/L per mmHg ↑in Pa_{co2}			
Chronic	$[HCO_3^-]$ will ↑0.4 mmol/L per mmHg ↑in Pa_{co2}			

134. Ans. b. Long..., c. Short..., d. I.V..., e. Inhaled...

[Ref: Harrison 19th/1676-80, 18th/2109-2113; CMDT 2016/249-57]

"**Short-acting inhaled β_2-agonists,** including albuterol, levalbuterol, bitolterol, pirbuterol and terbutaline, are the most effective bronchodilators during ***exacerbations.*** All patients with acute symptoms should take one of these agents" *(CMDT 2016/254)*

"**Systemic corticosteroids** are effective primary treatment for patients with moderate to severe asthma exacerbations and for patients with exacerbations who do not respond promptly and completely to inhaled β_2-agonist therapy" *(CMDT 2016/254)*

"**Systemic corticosteroids** (oral or parenteral) are most effective in achieving prompt control of asthma ***during exacerbations*** or when initiating long-term asthma therapy in patients with severe symptoms"

"**Inhaled corticosteroids** are preferred, first-line agents for all patients with ***persistent asthma***"

Long-acting β2-agonists

◈ *CMDT 2016/249-50*

- It provide bronchodilation *for up to 12 hours after a single dose*
- They are **indicated** for *long-term prevention of asthma symptoms, nocturnal symptoms and for prevention of exercise-induced bronchospasm.*
- When added to standard doses of inhaled corticosteroids, long-acting β_2-agonists provide control equivalent to what is achieved by doubling the inhaled corticosteroid dose
- ***Should not be used for symptom relief or exacerbations. Use with inhaled corticosteroids.***

Short-acting β2-agonist

◈ *CMDT06/231*

"Mild asthma exacerbations: Many patients respond quickly and fully to an inhaled short-acting β_2-agonist alone"

Treatment of Asthma

◈ *Harrison 19th/1677, 18th/2111*

- ***"Inhaled Corticosteroids*** (ICSs) are by far the most effective controllers for asthma and their early use has revolutionized asthma therapy"-*Harrison 18th/2111*
- ***Corticosteroids are used intravenously*** *(hydrocortisone or methylprednisolone)* for the treatment of **acute severe asthma**

"**Systemic Corticosteroids**[Q]: Corticosteroids are used ***intravenously*** (hydrocortisone or methylprednisolone) for the treatment of acute severe asthma, although several studies now show that ***oral corticosteroids*** are as effective and easier to administer. A course of oral corticosteroids (usually prednisone or prednisolone 30–45 mg od for 5–10 days) is used to treat acute exacerbations of asthma; no tapering of the dose is needed. Approximately 1% of asthma patients may require maintenance treatment with oral corticosteroids; the lowest dose necessary to maintaining control needs to be determined" *(Harrison 19th/1677, 18th/2111)*

135. Ans. d. Hypoglycemia

[Ref: Harrison 19th/1677, 18th/2111;CMDT 2016/249;KDT 7th/230]

"**Systemic effects of long term inhaled glucocorticoids:** *Mood change, osteoporosis, growth retardation in children, bruising, petechiae, hyperglycemia & pituitary-adrenal suppression" (KDT 7th/230-31)*

Inhaled steroids are used in two form

◈ *KDT 6th/226*

- **Use drug in solution:** Metered dose inhaler, nebulizer[Q]
- **Use drug as dry powder:** Spinhaler, rotahaler

"The use of an inhalation chamber coupled with mouth washing after MDI use decreases local side effects (cough, dysphonia, oropharyngeal candidiasis) and systemic absorption. DPIs are not used with an inhalation chamber. Systemic effects (adrenal suppression, osteoporosis, skin thinning, easy bruising and cataracts) may occur with high-dose inhaled corticosteroid therapy" *(CMDT 2016/249)*

Side Effects of Inhaled Steroid

◈ *Harrison 19th/1677, 18th/2111*

- Local side effects include hoarseness (dysphonia) and oral candidiasis, which may be reduced with the use of a large-volume spacer device. There has been concern about systemic side effects from lung absorption
- At the highest recommended doses, there may be some suppression of plasma and urinary cortisol concentrations, but there is no convincing evidence that long-term treatment leads to impaired growth in children or to osteoporosis in adults.
- Indeed effective control of asthma with inhaled steroid reduces the number of courses of oral steroid that are needed and, thus, reduces systemic exposure to ICS.

136. Ans. d. Return...

[Ref: Harrison 19th/142-48, 18th/171-77; CMDT 2016/399; Emergency Medicine by S.N.Chugh 4th/242-43]

"A syncopal attack begins when the patient is usually in an upright position (sitting or standing).Period of unconsciousness is brief (seconds). Return of consciousness is prompt" *(Emergency Medicine by S.N.Chugh 4th/242-43)*

Vasomotor syncope: May be due to excessive vagal tone or impaired reflex control of the peripheral circulation. The most frequent type of vasodepressor syncope is vasovagal hypotension or the common faint, which is often initiated by a stressful, painful or claustrophic experience, especially in young women" *(CMDT 2016/399)*

Syncope

- Syncope is a transient, self-limited loss of consciousness due to acute global impairment of cerebral blood flow. The onset is rapid, duration brief and recovery spontaneous and complete.
- A syncopal prodrome (presyncope) is common, although loss of consciousness may occur without any warning symptoms. Typical presyncopal symptoms include dizziness, lightheadedness or faintness, weakness, fatigue and visual and auditory disturbances.
- The causes of syncope can be divided into three general categories:
  - Neurally mediated syncope (also called reflex syncope),
  - Orthostatic hypotension and
  - Cardiac syncope.
- Neurally mediated syncope comprises a heterogeneous group of functional disorders that are characterized by a transient change in the reflexes responsible for maintaining cardiovascular homeostasis. ***Episodic vasodilation and bradycardia occur in varying combinations, resulting in temporary failure of blood pressure control.***
- The ***upright posture imposes a unique physiologic stress upon humans; most, although not all, syncopal episodes occur from a standing position.*** Standing results in pooling of 500–1000 mL of blood in the lower extremities and splanchnic circulation. There is a decrease in venous return to the heart and reduced ventricular filling that result in diminished cardiac output and blood pressure.

137. Ans. a. X linked..., b. ↑Clotting..., d. Intrinsic...,e. ↑aPTT

[Ref: Harrison 19th/732-36, 18th/974-977; CMDT06/526;Robbins 9th/662-63, 8th/672; H17th/718-28]

Hemophilia

- Hemophilia is an **X-linked recessive hemorrhagic disease** due to mutations in the *F8* gene (hemophilia A or classic hemophilia) or *F9* gene (hemophilia B).
- ***Male subjects are clinically affected;*** women, who carry a single mutated gene, are generally asymptomatic. Clinically, hemophilia A and hemophilia B are indistinguishable.
- The disease phenotype correlates with the residual activity of FVIII or FIX and can be classified as severe (<1%), moderate (1–5%), or mild (6–30%).
- In the severe and moderate forms, the disease is characterized by bleeding into the joints (hemarthrosis), soft tissues and muscles after minor trauma or even spontaneously.
- Typically, the global tests of coagulation show only an isolated prolongation of the aPTT assay. Patients with hemophilia have normal bleeding times and platelet counts. The diagnosis is made after specific determination of FVIII or FIX clotting activity.

Table: Disease

Von-Willebrand Disease[Q]	↑ Bleeding time (Despite a normal platelet count)
	↑ PTT (Type 1 & 3)
Hemophilia A[Q]	Normal BT, platelet count & PT
	↑ PTT[Q]
Hemophilia B[Q]	Normal BT & PT[Q]
	↑ PTT
Henoch-schonlein purpura[Q]	Normal BT, PT, PTT & platelet count
Bernard –Sourlier syndrome[Q]	↑ BT

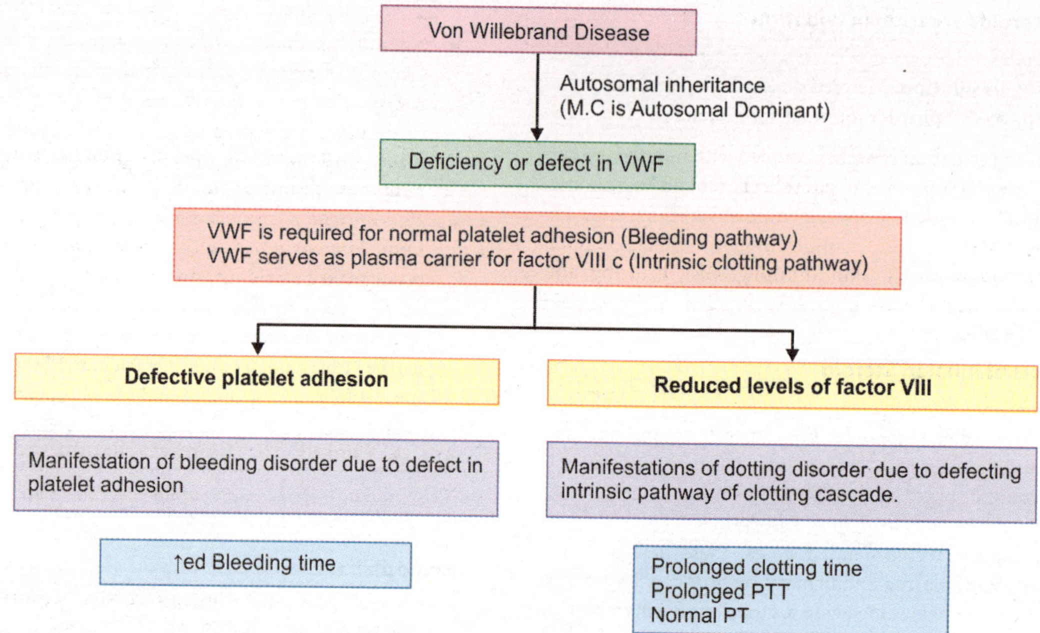

Fig: Chart depicting characteristics of Von Willebrand disease

Table: Characteristics of Haemophilia A & B

	Haemophilia A [Q] (Classical hemophilia)	Haemophilia B[Q] (Christmas disease)
Defect	Deficiency of coagulant subunit of factor *i.e.,* (VIII c) Factor VIII = VIIIc + VWF	Deficiency/absence of factor IX
Pathway of coagulation affected	Intrinsic Pathway[Q]	Intrinsic pathway[Q]
Whole blood clotting time	↑	↑
PTT[Q]	↑	↑
PT[Q]	N	N
BT[Q]	N	N
Platelet count[Q]	N	N
Tourniquet test[Q]	N	N

Table: Genetic and Laboratory Characteristics of Inherited Coagulation Disorders

Laboratory Abnormalitya					
Clotting Factor Deficiency	**Inheritance**	**aPTT**	**PT**	**TT**	**Treatment**
Factor VIII	**X-linked**	+	–	–	**FVIII concentrates**
Factor IX	X-linked	+	–	–	FIX concentrates

Prothrombin Time (PT)[Q]

◈ *Robbins 7th/649*

- This assay tests the extrinsic[Q] & common coagulation pathways [Q]
- A prolonged PT can results from deficiency or dysfunction of factor V, factor VII, factor X, prothrombin or fibrinogen

Partial Tromboplastin Time (PTT)[Q]

◈ *Robbins 7th/649*

- This assay tests intrinsic & common clotting pathways
- Prolongation of the PTT can be due to deficiency or dysfunction of factor V, VIII, IX, X, XI or XII, prothrombin or fibrinogen.

138. Ans. b. Post-ductal...

[Ref: Bedside Clinics in Medicine by Kundu 4th/294; P.J.Mehta 15th/41,182; Harrison 19th/1445, 18th/2064]

"Post-ductal coarctation of aorta causes *radio-femoral delay*" *(P.J.Mehta 15th/182)*

"Aortic dissection cause widening of pulse pressure" *(Harrison 19th/1641, 18th/2064)*

Causes of Radio-Femoral Delay

◈ *Kundu 4th/294*

- *Coarctation of aorta*
- Atherosclerosis of aorta
- Thrombosis or embolism of aorta
- Aortoarteritis

Inquality b/w Two Radial Pulse (Radio-Radial Delay)

◈ *Kundu 4th/294; P.J. Mehta 15th/41*

- Thoracic inlet syndrome (cervical rib, scalene syndrome)
- Aneurysm of aorta
- Takayasu's disease
- Pre-subclavian coarctation
- Supravalvular aortic stenosis
- Atherosclerosis of aorta

139. Ans. a. Esmolol b. Iodine c. Hydro.. e. Propy..

[Ref: Harrison 19th/2297, 18th/2927; Emergency Medicine by S.N.Chugh 4th/382; CMDT 2016/1113]

*"Blockade of peripheral effect of hormones: **Propranolol is drug of choice. Esmolol-an ultrashort acting betablocker is preferred in patients with CHF**" (Emergency Medicine by S.N.Chugh 4th/382(*

Thyroid Crisis or "Storm"

◈ *CMDT 2016/1113*

- This disorder, rarely seen today, is an extreme form of thyrotoxicosis that may occur with stressful illness, thyroid surgery, or RAI (Radioactive iodine) administration and is manifested by marked delirium, severe tachycardia, vomiting, diarrhea, dehydration and, in many cases, very high fever. The mortality rate is high.
- **A thiourea** drug is given (*e.g.*, **methimazole,** 15–25 mg orally every 6 hours or **propylthiouracil,** 150–250 mg orally every 6 hours).
- **Ipodate sodium** (500 mg/d orally) can be helpful if begun 1 hour after the first dose of thiourea. Iodide is given 1 hour later as Lugol solution (10 drops three times daily orally) or as sodium iodide (1 g intravenously slowly).
- **Propranolol** is given (cautiously in the presence of heart failure; see above) in a dosage of 0.5–2 mg intravenously every 4 hours or 20–120 mg orally every 6 hours.
- **Hydrocortisone** is usually given in doses of 50 mg orally every 6 hours, with rapid dosage reduction as the clinical situation improves.
- ***Aspirin is avoided*** since it displaces T4 from TBG, raising FT_4 serum levels. Definitive treatment with ^{131}I or surgery is delayed until the patient is euthyroid.

Thyrotoxic Crisis, or Thyroid Storm

◈ *Harrison 19th/2297, 18th/2927*

- *It* is rare and presents as a life-threatening exacerbation of hyperthyroidism, accompanied by fever, delirium, seizures, coma, vomiting, diarrhea and jaundice.
- The mortality rate due to cardiac failure, arrhythmia, or hyperthermia is as high as 30%, even with treatment.
- Large doses of **propylthiouracil** (600 mg loading dose and 200–300 mg every 6 h) should be given orally or by nasogastric tube or per rectum
- One hour after the first dose of propylthiouracil, stable **iodide** is given to block thyroid hormone synthesis via the Wolff-Chaikoff effect
- **Propranolol** should also be given to reduce tachycardia and other adrenergic manifestation. ***Although other β-adrenergic blockers can be used, high doses of propranolol decrease T_4 to T_3 conversion*** and the doses can be easily adjusted.
- Additional therapeutic measures include **glucocorticoids** (*e.g.*, dexamethasone, 2 mg every 6 h), **antibiotics** if infection is present, ***cooling, oxygen and intravenous fluids.***

140. Ans. a. Myasthenia..., c. Lambert e. Parkinson's..

[Ref: Harrison 19th/2701-03, 18th/3227, 3480, 3482, 2676, 3490]

"**Myasthenia gravis (MG)** is a neuromuscular disorder characterized by weakness and fatigability of skeletal muscles. The **underlying defect** is a decrease in the number of available ***acetylcholine receptors (AChRs)*** at neuromuscular junctions due to an *antibody-mediated autoimmune attack*" *(Harrison 19th/2701, 18th/3480)*

"**Lambert Eaton myasthenic syndrome** (LEMS) is caused by autoantibodies directed against ***P/Q-type calcium channels at the motor nerve terminals, which can be detected in ~85%*** of LEMS patients by radioimmunoassay. These autoantibodies result in ***impaired release of ACh from nerve terminals***"- *Harrison 19th/2703, 18th/3482*

"Pathologically, the hallmark features of **Parkinson's disease** are degeneration of ***dopaminergic neurons*** in the substantia nigra pars compacta (SNc), reduced striatal dopamine and intracytoplasmic proteinaceous inclusions known as Lewy bodies" *(Harrison 18th/3317)*

Table *(Harrison 19th/444e-3, 18th/3227)*: **Principal Classic Neurotransmitters**

Neurotransmitter	Clinical Aspects
Acetylcholine (ACh)	Acetylcholinesterases (nerve gases)
	Myasthenia gravis (antibodies to ACh receptor)
	Congenital myasthenic syndromes (mutations in ACh receptor subunits)
	Lambert-Eaton syndrome (antibodies to Ca channels impair ACh release)
	Botulism (toxin disrupts ACh release by exocytosis)
	Alzheimer's disease (selective cell death)
	Autosomal dominant frontal lobe epilepsy (mutations in CNS ACh receptor)
	Parkinson's disease (tremor)
Dopamine	Parkinson's disease (selective cell death)
	MPTP parkinsonism (toxin transported into neurons)
	Addiction, behavioral disorders
	Inhibits prolactin secretion
Norepinephrine (NE)	Mood disorders (MAOA inhibitors and tricyclics increase NE and improve depression)
	Anxiety
	Orthostatic tachycardia syndrome (mutations in NE transporter)
Serotonin	Mood disorders (SSRIs improve depression)
	Migraine pain pathway
	Pain pathway
γ-Aminobutyric acid (GABA)	***Stiff-person syndrome*** (antibodies to glutamic acid decarboxylase, the biosynthetic enzyme for GABA)
	Epilepsy (gabapentin and valproic acid increase GABA)
Glycine	***Spasticity***
	Hyperekplexia (myoclonic startle syndrome) due to mutations in glycine receptor
Glutamate	Seizures due to ingestion of domoic acid (a glutamate analogue)
Rasmussen's encephalitis (antibody against glutamate receptor 3)	
Excitotoxic cell death	

141. Ans. d. No malignant...

[Ref: Harrison 19th/1932, 18th/2459; Robbins 9th/768-69, 8th/782; CMDT 016/633]

"**Ménétrier's disease:** It is a rare isorder caused by excessive secretion of Transforming growth factor-α ***(TGF-α).*** The ***hypertrophic change*** may predominantly involve the ***body-fundus but antrum is generally spared.*** The gastric secretions contain excessive mucus and in many instances ***little to no hydrochloric acid*** due to glandular atrophy. In some patients, there may be sufficient ***protein loss in the gastric secretions*** to produce hypoalbuminemia and peripheral edema, thus constituting a form of *protein-losing gastroenteropathy*. Risk of ***gastric adenocarcinoma*** is increased in adults "*-Robbins 9th/768, 8th/782*

Ménétrier's Disease

◈ *Harrison 19th/1932, 18th/2459*

- The mucosal folds in Ménétrier's disease are often ***most prominent in the body and fundus.***
- The etiology of this unusual clinical picture is unknown. ***Overexpression of growth factors such as TGF-α may be involved in the process.***
- Epigastric pain, at times accompanied by nausea, vomiting, anorexia and weight loss, are signs and symptoms in patients with Ménétrier's disease. Occult GI bleeding may occur, but overt bleeding is unusual and, when present, is due to superficial mucosal erosions.
- 20–100% of patients (depending on time of presentation) develop a protein-losing gastropathy accompanied by ***hypoalbuminemia and edema. Gastric acid secretion is usually reduced or absent*** because of the replacement of parietal cells.
- Large gastric folds are readily detectable by either radiographic (barium meal) or endoscopic methods. Endoscopy with deep mucosal biopsy (and cytology) is required to establish the diagnosis and exclude other entities that may present similarly. A nondiagnostic biopsy may lead to a surgically obtained full-thickness biopsy to ***exclude malignancy.***
- Medical therapy with ***anticholinergic agents, prostaglandins, PPIs, prednisone and H_2 receptor antagonists*** yields varying results. Anticholinergics decrease protein loss. A high-protein diet should be recommended to replace protein loss in patients with hypoalbuminemia.

142. Ans. b. Mean..., e. Administration...

[Ref: http: //www.sccm.org/Documents/SSC-Guidelines.pdf; http: //www.survivingsepsis.org/; Harrison 19th/1756-58; Schwartz 8th]

"Crystalloids as the initial fluid of choice in the resuscitation of severe sepsis and septic shock"

*"**Norepinephrine as the first choice vasopressor** (grade 1B). Epinephrine (added to and potentially substituted for norepinephrine) when an additional agent is needed to maintain adequate **Dopamine as an alternative vasopressor agent to norepinephrine only in highly selected patients.**"*

Surviving Sepsis Guidelines 2013 Review & Update

◈ *http: //www.surviving sepsis.org/*

- The Surviving Sepsis Campaign launched in 2002 as a collaboration between the Society of Critical Care Medicine and the European Society of Intensive Care Medicine, with the shared goal of reducing deaths from sepsis and septic shock around the world.

- The Surviving Sepsis Campaign periodically publishes its Surviving Sepsis Guidelines, which many consider the standard of care for the treatment of severe sepsis and septic shock.
- The third edition of the Surviving Sepsis Guidelines were published in ***Critical Care Medicine*** in February 2013.

Early Goal-Directed Therapy for Severe Sepsis/Septic Shock

The goals during the **first 6 hours** of resuscitation should be **(Grade 1C):**

- ***Mean arterial pressure (MAP) ≥ 65 mm Hg;***
- ***Central venous pressure (CVP) 8-12 mm Hg*** *(12-15 mm Hg in patients receiving mechanical ventilation or with known preexisting decreased ventricular compliance);*
- ***Urine output ≥ 0.5 mL/kg/hr*** *(35 mL/hr for someone weighing 70 kg or 154 lbs);*
- ***Central venous oxygen saturation*** *(from the superior vena cava) ≥ 70%, or mixed venous oxygen saturation (from a pulmonary artery catheter) ≥ 65%.*

Regarding Fluid Management

- ***"Crystalloid is recommended for initial fluid resuscitation*** for severe sepsis and septic shock (Grade 1B).
- ***Hydroxyethyl starch*** (hetastarch) should not be used as therapy for sepsis, according to U.S. and European regulatory authorities (Grade 1B)"

Regarding use of Vasopressors

- Vasopressors should be begun within 6 hours for patients with hypotension despite aggressive initial fluid resuscitation (*i.e.*, septic shock), to maintain a mean arterial pressure ≥ 65 mm Hg **(Grade 1C).**
- ** **Hypoperfusion** is most often defined as hypotension after a challenge with IV fluid (2 liters crystalloid has been suggested for volume-replete patients) and/or blood lactate ≥ 4 mmol/L. Severe sepsis can also be defined by sepsis-induced organ dysfunction in the presence of a preserved blood pressure.*

Table *(http: //www.sccm.org/Documents/SSC-Guidelines.pdf):* **Antimicrobial therapy**

1. *Administration of effective **intravenous antimicrobials within the first hour of recognition of septic shock (grade 1B)** and severe sepsis without septic shock **(grade 1C)** as the goal of therapy.*
2. *Initial empiric anti-infective therapy of one or more drugs that have activity against all likely pathogens (bacterial and/or fungal or viral) and that penetrate in adequate concentrations into tissues presumed to be the source of sepsis **(grade 1B)**.*

Table *(http: //www.sccm.org/Documents/SSC-Guidelines.pdf)*: **Recommendations: Hemodynamic Support and Adjunctive Therapy**

Fluid Therapy of Severe Sepsis

1. ***Crystalloids*** *as the initial fluid of choice in the resuscitation of severe sepsis and septic shock* (grade 1B).

Contd...

2. ***Albumin*** *in the fluid resuscitation of severe sepsis and septic shock when **patients require substantial amounts of crystalloids*** (grade 2C).

Vasopressors

Vasopressor therapy initially to target a mean arterial pressure (MAP) of 65mm Hg (grade 1C).

Norepinephrine as the first choice vasopressor *(grade 1B).*

Epinephrine (added to and potentially substituted for norepinephrine) when an additional agent is needed to maintain adequate blood pressure (grade 2B).

Dopamine as an alternative vasopressor agent to norepinephrine only in highly selected patients *(e.g., patients with low risk of tachyarrhythmias and absolute or relative bradycardia) (grade 2C).*

143. Ans. a. Apnoea..., d. Cerebral..., e. Transcranial...

[Ref: Harrison 19th/1776, 18th/2252-53; Parikh 6th/3.1-3.10;Reddy Forensic 27th/119-20; Miller Anesthesiology 6th; CMDT 2016/1012]

Brain Death

◈ *Harrison 19th/1776, 18th/2252-53*

- Several sets of criteria have been advanced for the diagnosis of brain death
- Ideal criteria are simple, can be assessed at the bedside and allow no chance of diagnostic error. They contain three essential elements:
  - i. Widespread cortical destruction
  - ii. Global brainstem damage demonstrated by absent pupillary light reaction and by the loss of oculovestibular and corneal reflexes; and
  - iii. Destruction of the medulla, manifested by complete apnea.
- The heart rate is invariant and unresponsive to atropine. The pupils are usually midsized but may be enlarged; they should not, however, be small. Babinski signs are generally absent and the toe response is often flexor.
- Demonstration that **apnea** is due to irreversible medullary damage requires that the $PaCO_2$ be high enough to stimulate respiration during a test of spontaneous breathing. *Apnea testing* can be done safely by the use of diffusion oxygenation prior to removing the ventilator.
- "The **apnea test** (presence or absence of spontaneous respiratory activity at a $PaCO_2$ of at least 60 mm Hg) serves to determine whether the patient is capable of respiratory activity. Certain ancillary tests may assist the determination of brain death but are not essential. An ***isoelectric electroencephalogram,*** when the recording is made according to the recommendations of the American Electroencephalographic Society, may help in confirming the diagnosis. Alternatively, the demonstration of an absent cerebral circulation by ***intravenous radioisotope cerebral angiography or by four-vessel contrast cerebral angiography is confirmatory***"-CMDT 2016/1012
- Apnea is confirmed if no respiratory effort has been observed in the presence of a sufficiently elevated $PaCO_2$.
- An ***isoelectric EEG may be used as a confirmatory test for total cerebral damage. Radionuclide brain scanning, cerebral angiography, or transcranial Doppler***

measurements may also be included to demonstrate the absence of CBF but they have not been extensively correlated with pathologic changes.

"Brain death: Philadelphia Protocol: Lack of reflexus, pupil fixed & dilated, isoelectric EEG[Q] etc." *(Reddy Forensic 27th/119-20)*

Confirmatory Test but not Essential

- **An isoelectric ECG** done according to American noxious stimuli (unresponsive coma) [Q]
- Absence of cerebral circulation by ***IV radioisotope cerebral angiography or four vessel contrast cerebral angiography.***

Criteria for Brain Death

Harvard Criteria

- Unresponsively to intensely noxious stimuli (unresponsive)
- Total absence of spontaneous breathing.
- Absence of brainstem and spinal reflexes
- Absence of postural activity such as decerebration and
- A flat electroencephalogram (ECG)

Minnesota Criteria

The key element of the Minnesota criteria are:

- *Absence of spontaneous movement,*
- *Absence of spontaneous respirations over a four minute test period*
- *Absence of brain reflex as evidence by: fixed dilated pupils; absent gag, corneal and ciliospinal reflex; absent doll's eye movement; absent response to caloric stimulating and absent tonic neck reflex,*
- *Unchanged status for at least twelve hours and*
- *Responsible pathological process deemed irreparable.*

Other Criteria

President's Commission for the study Ethical problem in medicine and Behavioral Research, American Neurological Association etc.

Signs of Somatic or Clinical Death (Immediate Signs)

◈ *Parikh 6th/3.6*

These include:

- ***Insensibility and loss of EEG rhythm***[Q]
- ***Cessation of circulation, that is loss of ECG rhythm and***
- ***Cessation of respiration***[Q]**.**

144. Ans. b. Recurr..., c. Uveitis d. Genital..., e. Path..

[Ref: Harrison 19th/2194, 18th/2801-02; Neena Khanna 3rd/204-05; CMDT06/851]

Behçet Syndrome

◈ *Harrison 19th/2194, 18th/2801-02*

- Behçet's syndrome is a multisystem disorder presenting with recurrent oral and genital ulcerations as well as ocular involvement. The diagnosis is clinical and based on internationally agreed diagnostic criteria (given in table)
- ***"Non-deforming arthritis or arthralgias*** are seen in 50% of patients and affects the knees and ankles.
- Laboratory findings are mainly nonspecific indices of inflammation, such as leukocytosis and elevated erythrocyte sedimentation rate, as well as C-reactive protein levels."
- "Nonspecific skin inflammatory reactivity to any scratches or intradermal saline injection (pathergy test) is a common and specific manifestation."

Table *(Harrison 19th/2194, 18th/2801)*: **Diagnostic Criteria of Behçet's Disease**

Recurrent oral ulceration plus two of the following:
• Recurrent genital ulceration
• Eye lesions
• Skin lesions
• Pathergy test

Behçet Syndrome

◈ *CMDT06/851*

- **Essentials of Diagnosis:** Recurrent, painful aphthous ulcers of the mouth and genitals; additional cutaneous findings include *erythema nodosum*–like lesions, a follicular rash and the ***"pathergy" phenomenon*** (formation of a sterile pustule at the site of a needle stick).
- **Either anterior or posterior uveitis** posterior uveitis may be asymptomatic until significant damage to the retina has occurred & Variety of neurologic lesions that can mimic multiple sclerosis, particularly through involvement of the white matter of the brainstem.
- Essentially all of its protean manifestations, however, are believed to result from vasculitis that may involve all types of blood vessels: small, medium and large, on both the arterial and venous side of the circulation.
- The hallmark of Behçet disease is ***painful aphthous ulceration in the mouth.*** These lesions, which usually occur multiply, may be found on the tongue, gums and inner surfaces of the oral cavity
- Genital lesions, similar in appearance, are also common but do not occur in all patients.
- The **pathergy phenomenon** is frequently underappreciated (unless the patient is asked); in this phenomenon, sterile pustules develop at sites where needles have been inserted into the skin (*e.g.*, for phlebotomy) in some patients.

145. Ans. a. 90% malignant

[Ref: Harrison 19th/2329-32, 18th/2962-63; Robbins 9th/1134-36, 8th/1159-61; CMDT 2016/1159]

"Catastrophic hypertensive crisis and fatal cardiac arrhythmias can occur spontaneously or may be triggered by intravenous contrast dye or glucagon injection, ***needle biopsy of the mass***, anesthesia and surgical procedures" *(CMDT 2016/1159)*

Pheochromocytoma

- The mean age at diagnosis is about 40 years, although the tumors can occur from early childhood until late in life.
- The "rule of tens" for pheochromocytomas states that about ***10% are bilateral, 10% are extraadrenal and 10% are malignant***. However, these percentages are higher in the inherited syndromes.
- Pheochromocytomas and paragangliomas are ***well-vascularized tumors*** that arise from cells derived from the sympathetic (*e.g.*, adrenal medulla) or parasympathetic (*e.g.*, carotid body, glomus vagale) paraganglia

- Pheochromocytomas and paragangliomas synthesize and store catecholamines, which include ***norepinephrine (noradrenaline), epinephrine (adrenaline) and dopamine.*** Elevated plasma and urinary levels of catecholamines and the methylated metabolites, metanephrines, are the cornerstone for the diagnosis
- Immunoreactivity for *neuroendocrine markers* ***(chromogranin & synaptophysin)***[Q] is present in chief cells & while the peripheral sustentacular cells label with ***S-100***[Q]
- ***T_2 weighted MRI with gadolinium contrast is optimal for detecting pheochromocytoma*** & is somewhat better than CT for imaging extrarenal pheochromocytoma.
- Complete tumor removal is the ultimate therapeutic goal. Preoperative patient preparation is essential for safe surgery

Table *(Harrison 19th/2330)*: **Biochemical and Imaging Methods Used for Pheochromocytoma and Paraganglioma Diagnosis**

Diagnostic Method
24-h urinary tests
• Vanillylmandelic acid
• Catecholamines
• Fractionated metanephrines
• Total metanephrines
Plasma tests
• Catecholamines
• Free metanephrines
• CT
• MRI
• MIBG scintigraphy
• Somatostatin receptor scintigraphy
• Dopa (dopamine) PET

146. Ans. c. Norepinephrine

[Ref: http: //www.ncbi.nlm.nih. gov/; Robbins 9th/1134-35, 8th/1159-61; CMDT 2016/1161]

"***As an analogue of adrenergic neurotransmitter norepinephrine (NE),*** metaiodobenzylguanidine (MIBG) demonstrates high uptake both in normal sympathetically innervated tissues, such as the heart and salivary glands and in tumors that express the NE transporter (NET), specifically those of neural crest and neuroendocrine origin"-*http: //www.ncbi.nlm.nih.gov/*

"Pheochromocytoma can be localized using radioactive tracers including ***^{131}I-or ^{123}I-metaiodobenzylguanidine (MIBG),*** *^{111}In-somatostatin analogues, or ^{18}F-dopa (or dopamine)* ***Positron-emission tomography (PET).*** *Because these agents exhibit selective uptake in paragangliomas,* ***nuclear imaging is particularly useful in the hereditary syndromes"***

147. Ans. c. Surgery..., d. Associated...

[Ref: Harrison 19th/2321-23, 18th/2952-54; Robbins 9th/1132-33, 8th/1158; CMDT 2016/1155]

"Vanillylmandelic acid (VMA) is one of the metabolites of the catecholamines epinephrine (adrenaline) and norepinephrine. Increased VMA excretion into the urine can occur in ***Neuroblastomas, pheochromocytomas and other neuroendocrine tumors"*** *(Harrison 19th/2329-30, 18th/2963)*

Adrenocortical Carcinomas

◈ *Robbins 9th/1132-33, 8th/1158*

- These are rare neoplasms that can occur at any age, including childhood. They are more likely to be functional than adenomas are and carcinomas are therefore often associated with virilism or other clinical manifestations of hyperadrenalism.
- Two rare inherited causes of adrenal cortical carcinomas are ***Li-Fraumeni syndrome and Beckwith-Wiedemann syndrome***
- In most cases, adrenocortical carcinomas are large, invasive lesions, many exceeding 20 cm in diameter, that efface the native adrenal gland. The less common, smaller and better-circumscribed lesions may be difficult to distinguish from an adenoma.
- Microscopically, adrenocortical carcinomas may be composed of well-differentiated cells resembling those seen in cortical adenomas or bizarre, monstrous giant cells, which may be difficult to distinguish from those of an undifferentiated carcinoma metastatic to the adrenal.
- ***Metastases to regional and periaortic nodes are common,*** as is distant hematogenous spread to the lungs and other viscera. Bone metastases are unusual. The median patient survival is about 2 years

◈ *Harrison 19th/2321-23, 18th/2952-54*

- Adrenocortical carcinoma (ACC) is a rare malignancy
- ACC is generally considered a highly malignant tumor
- Germline *TP53* mutations are the cause of the ***Li-Fraumeni syndrome*** associated with multiple solid organ cancers including ACC and are found in 25% of pediatric ACC cases
- Although 60–70% of ACCs are biochemically found to overproduce hormones, this is not clinically apparent in many patients due to the relatively inefficient steroid production by the adrenocortical cancer cells.
- ***ACC carries a poor prognosis and cure can be achieved only by complete surgical removal.*** Capsule violation during primary surgery, ***metastasis at diagnosis*** and primary treatment in a nonspecialist center are major determinants of poor survival. If the primary tumor invades adjacent organs, en bloc removal of kidney and spleen should be considered to reduce the risk of recurrence.
- Surgery can also be considered in a patient with metastases if there is severe tumor-related hormone excess. This indication needs to be carefully weighed against surgical risk, including thromboembolic complications and the resulting delay in the introduction of other therapeutic options.

148. Ans. a. Oral..., c. Azithro... d. Tetra.. e. Chlo...

[Ref: Park 23rd/299-302, 21st/274-76; Harrison 19th/1154, 1159, 18th/1407, 1411-13; Ananthanarayan 8th/408-10; Medical microbiology by Greenwood 16th /372;Robbins 9th/384-85; CMDT 2016/1293, 06/1391-98]

Note: • *Most probably it is a rickettsial disease based on presentation of geographical region, fever, eschar, thrombocytopenia etc.*
• *Meropenem is not used in rickettsial disease (KDT 7th/731)*
• *"In Q fever there is no skin lesion" (Park 23rd/301)*

Rickettsial Diseases

◈ *Harrison 19th/1154, 18th/1407*

- The clinical manifestations of all the **acute presentations are similar during the first 5 days:** *fever, headache and myalgias with or without nausea, vomiting and cough.* As the course progresses, clinical manifestations—including occurrence of a macular, maculopapular, or vesicular rash; ***eschar;*** pneumonitis; and meningoencephalitis—vary from one disease to another
- Establishing the etiologic diagnosis of rickettsioses is very difficult during the acute stage of illness and definitive diagnosis usually requires the examination of paired serum samples after convalescence.
- Heightened clinical suspicion is based on epidemiologic data, history of exposure to vectors or reservoir animals, travel to endemic locations, clinical manifestations ***(sometimes including rash or eschar)*** and characteristic laboratory findings [including ***thrombocytopenia, normal or low white blood cell*** counts, elevated hepatic enzyme levels and hyponatremia].
- Such suspicion should be given prompt empirical treatment. ***Doxycycline is the drug of choice for most of these infections.***
- Clinical laboratory findings, such as ***thrombocytopenia*** (particularly in spotted fever and typhus rickettsioses, ehrlichioses, anaplasmosis and scrub typhus), normal or low WBC counts, mild to moderate serum elevations of hepatic aminotransferases and hyponatremia suggest some common pathophysiologic mechanisms.
- "**Murine typhus** (Endemic typhus): Successful isolation of causative agent was made from many part of India including ***shimla hills***"*(Park 21st/275)*
- ***"Tetracycline is drug of choice*** *for specific treatment of all rickettsial diseases. (Park 23rd/299)*
- ***Long acting (doxycycline, minocycline)*** now make single dose treatment possible"*(Park 23rd/299)*
- "Rickettsiae can be inhibited by ***tetracyclines or chloramphenicol.*** All early infections respond to treatment with these drugs" *(CMDT 2016/1293, 06/1391)*

Scrub Typhus (Chigger-Borne Typhus)

◈ *Harrison 19th/1159, 18th/1413*

- The classic case description includes an ***eschar where the chigger feeds (site of mite bite),*** regional lymphadenopathy and a maculopapular rash—signs that are seldom seen in indigenous patients. Fewer than 50% of Westerners develop an eschar and fewer than 40% develop a rash (on day 4–6 of illness).

Table *(Harrison 19th/1155)*: **Features of Selected Rickettsial Infections**

Disease	Organism	Rash%	Eschar%	L.N
Rocky Mountain spotted fever	Rickettsia rickettsii	90	<1	+
Mediterranean spotted fever	R. conorii	97	50	+
African tick-bite fever	R. africae	50	90	++++
Maculatum disease	R. parkeri	88	94	++
Rickettsialpox	R. akari	100	90	+++
Tick-borne lymphadenopathy	R. slovaca	5	100	++++
Flea-borne spotted fever	R. felis	80	15	—
Epidemic typhus	R. prowazekii	80	None	—
Murine typhus	R. typhi	80	None	—
Human monocytotropic ehrlichiosis	Ehrlichia chaffeensis	26	None	++
Ewingii ehrlichiosis	E. ewingii		None	
Human granulocytotropic anaplasmosis	Anaplasma phagocytophilum	Rare	None	—
Scrub typhus	Orientia tsutsugamushi	50	35	+++
Q fever	Coxiella burnetii	<1	None	—

149. Ans. b. Giant..., d. Heart...

[Ref: Harrison 19th/1443-44, 18th/1823; P.J.Mehta 15th/36-37; Hurst 12th/232]

JVP consists of 3 positive pulse waves (a, c & v) & two negative pulse waves (x & y)

A Wave

◈ *P.J.Mehta 15th/36-37*

- *It is produced by retrograde transmission of pressure pulse produced by right atrial contraction. In normal subjects the 'A' wave is* ***often the largest positive wave visible,*** *coinciding with the fourth heart sound*
- ***A wave is absent in atrial fibrillation***
- *A wave is diminished in: tachycardia & prolonged PR interval*
- **Large or giant wave: *tricuspid stenosis,*** *tricuspid atresia, pulmonary stenosis, right atrial myxoma, pulmonary hypertension*
- **Canon a wave:** ***Complete heart block,*** *ventricular tachycardia & ectopic beat*

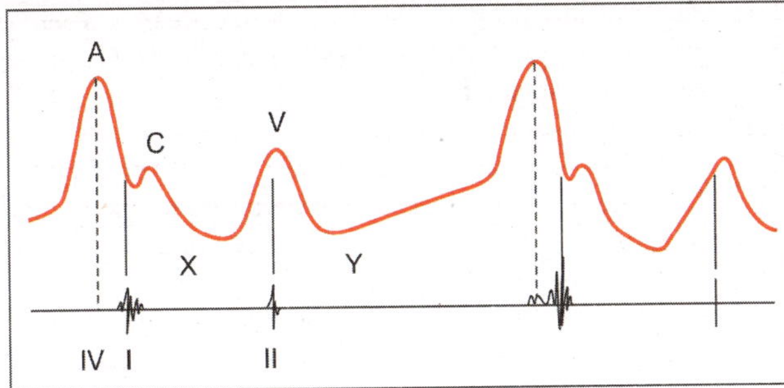

Fig: *(Harrison 19th/1444)* Jugular venous pulse

Table *(Harrison 18th/1823)*: **Jugular venous pulse**

A wave	A wave reflects ***right atrial presystolic contraction*** and occurs just after the electrocardiographic P wave, preceding the first heart sound (S_1). A **prominent *a* wave** is seen in patients with reduced right ventricular compliance; a cannon a wave occurs with atrioventricular (AV) dissociation and ***right atrial contraction against a closed tricuspid valve***. In a patient with a wide complex tachycardia, the appreciation of cannon a waves in the jugular venous waveform identifies the rhythm as ventricular in origin. The ***a wave is not present with atrial fibrillation.***
X wave	The X descent defines the fall in right atrial pressure after inscription of the a wave.
C wave	The C wave interrupts this x descent and is followed by a further descent.
V wave	The V wave represents atrial filling (atrial diastole) and occurs during ventricular systole. The height of the V wave is determined by right atrial compliance as well as the volume of blood returning to the right atrium either antegrade from the cavae or retrograde through an incompetent tricuspid valve In patients with TR, the V wave is accentuated and the subsequent fall in pressure (Y descent) is rapid. With progressive degrees of TR, the V wave merges with the c wave and the right atrial and jugular vein waveforms become "ventricularized."
Y wave	The Y descent, which follows the peak of the V wave, can become prolonged or blunted with obstruction to right ventricular inflow, as may occur with tricuspid stenosis (TS) or pericardial tamponade

150. Ans. a. SLE b. Rheumatic..., c. Dressler...

[Ref: Harrison 19th/1573, 18th/1972; Robbins 9th/574, 8th/581]

Table *(Harrison 19th/1571, 18th/1972)*: **III Pericarditis presumably related to hypersensitivity or autoimmunity**

A. Rheumatic fever

B. Collagen vascular disease (systemic lupus erythematosus, rheumatoid arthritis, ankylosing spondylitis, scleroderma, acute rheumatic fever, granulomatosis with polyangitis (Wegener's)

Contd...

C. Drug-induced (*e.g.,* procainamide, hydralazine, phenytoin, isoniazide, minoxidil, anticoagulants, methysergide)

D. Post-cardiac injury
1. Postmyocardial infarction (Dressler's syndrome)
2. Postpericardiotomy
3. Posttraumatic

Table *(Harrison 19th/1571, 18th/1972)*: **Etiologic Classification**

I. Infectious pericarditis

A. Viral (coxsackievirus A and B, echovirus, mumps, adenovirus, hepatitis, HIV)
B. Pyogenic (pneumococcus, streptococcus, staphylococcus, Neisseria, Legionella)
C. Tuberculous
D. Fungal (histoplasmosis, coccidioidomycosis, Candida, blastomycosis)
E. Other infections (syphilitic, protozoal, parasitic)

II. Noninfectious pericarditis

A. Acute myocardial infarction
B. Uremia
C. Neoplasia
1. Primary tumors (benign or malignant, mesothelioma)
2. Tumors metastatic to pericardium (lung and breast cancer, lymphoma, leukemia)

D. Myxedema
E. Cholesterol
F. Chylopericardium
G. Trauma
1. Penetrating chest wall
2. Nonpenetrating

H. Aortic dissection (with leakage into pericardial sac)
I. Postirradiation; J. Familial Mediterranean fever
K. Familial pericarditis; L. Whipple's disease M. Sarcoidosis

Table *(Robbins 9th/574, 8th/581)*

Presumably Immunologically Mediated
Rheumatic fever
Systemic lupus erythematosus
Scleroderma
Postcardiotomy
Postmyocardial infarction (Dressler) syndrome
Drug hypersensitivity reaction

151. Ans. a. Fever..., d. Develop...

[Ref: Harrison 19th/1797, 18th/2276; Robbins 9th/692-93, 8th/701; CMDT 2016/309, 06/298-99, 166]

Radiation Pneumonitis

- "Two phases of the pulmonary response to radiation are apparent: **an acute phase** (radiation pneumonitis) and a **chronic phase** (radiation fibrosis). ***Chest radiography, which correlates poorly with the presence of symptoms,*** usually demonstrates an alveolar or nodular infiltrate limited to the irradiated area. Air bronchograms are often observed.

Sharp borders of the infiltrate may help distinguish radiation pneumonitis from other conditions such as infectious pneumonia, lymphangitic spread of carcinoma and recurrent tumor" *(CMDT 2016/309, 06/298-99)*

◈ *Robbins 9th/692-93, 8th/701*

- It most often involves the lung within the radiation port but occasionally may extend to other areas of the same lung or even the contralateral lung.
- It occurs in acute and chronic forms. After clinical fractionated irradiation, *acute radiation pneumonitis* occurs in 10–20% of patients, 1 to 6 months after therapy, ***manifested by fever, dyspnea out of proportion to the volume of lung irradiated,*** pleural effusion and radiologic infiltrates that usually correspond to an area of previous radiation.
- ***With steroid therapy, these symptoms may resolve completely in some patients without long-term effects,*** while in others there is progression to *chronic radiation pneumonitis.*
- Morphologic changes are those of diffuse alveolar damage, including severe atypia of hyperplastic type II cells and fibroblasts. ***Epithelial cell atypia and foam cells within vessel walls are also characteristic of radiation damage***

◈ *Harrison 19th/1797, 18th/2276*

- Radiation pneumonitis usually develops from ***2–6 months after completion of radiotherapy.*** The clinical syndrome, which varies in severity, ***consists of dyspnea, cough with scanty sputum, low-grade fever and an initial hazy infiltrate on chest radiographs.***
- ***A lung biopsy*** may be necessary to make the diagnosis. Asymptomatic infiltrates found incidentally after radiation therapy need not be treated.
- However, ***prednisone*** should be administered to patients with fever or other symptoms. The dosage should be tapered slowly after the resolution of radiation pneumonitis, as abrupt withdrawal of glucocorticoids may cause an exacerbation of pneumonia.

152. Ans. a. Amen.. c. Anosmia d. Failure...

[Ref: Harrison 19th/2256, 18th/2878; CMDT 2016/1087, 06/1104, 1183]

Kallmann Syndrome

◈ *Harrison 19th/2256, 18th/2878*

- Kallmann syndrome results from defective hypothalamic ***gonadotropin-releasing hormone (GnRH)*** synthesis and is associated with ***anosmia or hyposmia*** due to olfactory bulb agenesis or hypoplasia.
- The syndrome also may be associated with ***color blindness, optic atrophy, nerve deafness, cleft palate, renal abnormalities, cryptorchidism and neurologic abnormalities such as mirror movements.***
- Genetic abnormalities, in addition to *KAL* mutations, also can cause isolated GnRH deficiency. GnRH deficiency prevents progression through puberty.
- Males present with delayed puberty and pronounced ***hypogonadal features,*** including micropenis, probably the result of low testosterone levels during infancy. ***Females present with primary amenorrhea and failure of secondary sexual development.***
- Kallmann syndrome and other causes of congenital GnRH deficiency are characterized by low LH and FSH levels and low concentrations of sex steroids (testosterone or estradiol). In sporadic cases of isolated gonadotropin deficiency, the diagnosis is often one of exclusion after other causes of hypothalamic-pituitary dysfunction have been eliminated. Repetitive GnRH administration restores normal pituitary gonadotropin responses, pointing to a hypothalamic defect.
- Long-term treatment of men with **human chorionic gonadotropin (hCG)** or testosterone restores pubertal development and secondary sex characteristics; women can be treated with cyclic estrogen and progestin.

SURGERY

153. Ans. d. Oriented...

[Ref: Harrison 19th/1730, 18th/3381-82; L & B 26th/312, 25th/301; Schwartz 8th/137; CSDT 11th/902]

Table: Glassgow Coma Scale

Feature	Score	Adults	Infants/Children
Eye opening[Q]	4	Spontaneous[Q]	Spontaneous
	3	To voice	To voice
	2	To pain	To pain
	1	None	None
Verbal Response	5	Oriented conversation	Alert, normal vocalization
	4	Confused	Cries, but consolable
	3	Inappropriate words	Persistently irritable
	2	Incomprehensible sounds	Restless, agitated, moaning
	1	None	None
Motor[Q] response	6	Obeys commands[Q]	Spontaneous purposeful
	5	Localizes pain	Localizes pain
	4	Withdraw[Q]	Withdraws
	3	Abnormal flexion (Decorticate posturing)	Abnormal flexion
	2	Abnormal extension *(Decerebrate posturing)*	Abnormal extension
	1	None	None

Maximum value of Glasgow Coma Scale is *15* and minimum is 3

- Scoring of *13-15* indicates ***mild head injury***[Q]
- Scoring of *9-12* indicates ***moderate head injury***[Q]
- Scoring of *less than 9* indicates ***severe head injury***[Q]

154. Ans. a. Subcuta..., c. Gustatory..., d. Facial...

[Ref: L & B 26th/734-735, 25th/763, 757; Schwartz 8th/; Sabiston 18th/834-36; S.Das 5th/615]

Note: *Opposite gland compensatory hypertrophy is not mentioned anywhere in above mentioned references*

Complications of Parotid Gland Surgery

◈ *L & B 25th/763*

Parotid gland surgery include following complications:

- Haematoma formation
- Infection
- Temporary facial nerve weakness
- Transection of the facial nerve and permanent facial weakness
- Sialocele
- Facial numbness
- Permanent numbness of the ear lobe associated with great auricular nerve transection
- Frey's syndrome (Gustatory sweating)

Complications of Submandibular Gland Excision

◈ *L & B 25th/757*

- Haematoma;
- Wound infection;
- Marginal mandibular nerve injury;
- Lingual nerve injury;
- Hypoglossal nerve injury;
- Transection of the nerve to the mylohyoid muscle producing submental skin anaesthesia.

Complications of parotidectomy

◈ *Manipal Manual of Surgery 3rd/271*

- Flap necrosis
- Facial nerve palsy
- Fluid collection
- Salivary fistula
- Frey's syndrome (Gustatory sweating)

"Parotid fistula: may occur as complication of superficial parotidectomy" *(S.Das 5th/615)*

***"Auriculotemporal syndrome (Frey's syndrome)** may occasionally follow superficial* parotidectomy" *(S.Das 5th/615)*

"Complications that may occur due to parotidectomy involve nerve dysfunction, ***Frey's syndrome*** (uncharacteristic sweating near glands), ***salivation from wound, numbness, facial asymmetry, necrosis (death of skin) near incision and tumor reappearance***" *(wiki)*

155. Ans. a. Arterial..., e. Gummatous...

[Ref: L & B 26th/917-18, 25th/933-35; Sabiston 18th/2148, 196; S.Das 5th/125-127]

***"Basal cell carcinoma** (Rodent ulcer) has **typical rolled edge**"* *(S.Das 5th/102)*

"Tubercular ulcer: Edge is undermined" *(S.Das 5th/129)*

"Puched out edge: *It is mostly seen in **gummatous ulcer or in a deep trophic ulcer.** The edge drop down at right angle to the skin surface as if it has been cut out with a punch" (Das 5th/125)*

"Arterial ulcer: *These ulcer tends to be **punched out"*** *(S.Das 5th/125)*

"Gummatous ulcers, *which occurs in tertiary syphilis, have **punched-out indolent edge"*** *(S.Das 5th/130)*

Arterial Ulceration

◈ *L & B 25th/935*

- ***It most commonly involves the toes. Any toe can be affected. Occasionally ulcers develop on the dorsum of the foot.***
- Ischemic ulcers are usually very ***painful*** and accompanied by rest pain in the foot. The margin of the ulcer is sharply ***demarcated or punched-out*** and the base is devoid of healthy granulation tissue. The surrounding skin is pale and mottled and signs of chronic ischemia are invariably present.

Venous Ulcer

◈ *L & B 26th/917-18, 25th/934-35*

- Venous disease is responsible for between 60% and 70% of all ulcers in the lower leg.
- ***"Almost all venous ulcers have surrounding lipodermatosclerosis.*** Another cause of ulceration should be considered if there is no evidence of lipodermatosclerosis or an ankle flare"
- ***"The venous ulcer of the leg characteristically develops in the skin of the gaiter region,*** the area between the muscles of the calf and the ankle.
- The majority of ulcers develop on the medial side of the calf but ulcers associated with lesser saphenous incompetence often develop on the lateral side of the leg."

156. Ans. c. Recipients...

[Ref: L & B 26th/1423-26, 25th/1422; Schwartz 8th; Sabiston 18th/692-707]

Renal Transplantation

◈ *Smith General Urology 17th/chap 36*

- While either iliac fossa is acceptable for the transplant, the ***right side*** is often preferred due to the longer and more horizontal segments of external iliac artery and vein compared to the left side.
- ***A lower quadrant curvilinear (Gibson) incision*** is made and the iliac vessels are exposed through a retroperitoneal approach.
- The renal-to-iliac-vein anastomosis is usually performed first, in an end-to-side fashion. The ***renal artery can be anastomosed end-to-end to the internal iliac.*** However, in older recipients and diabetics this vessel often has significant arterial plaque causing poor runoff.
- In addition, concern about compromising arterial flow to the penis via the pudendal artery with subsequent erectile

dysfunction limits this approach in older males. Because of these factors, an end-to-side anastomosis of the ***renal artery to the external iliac artery is*** more frequently done

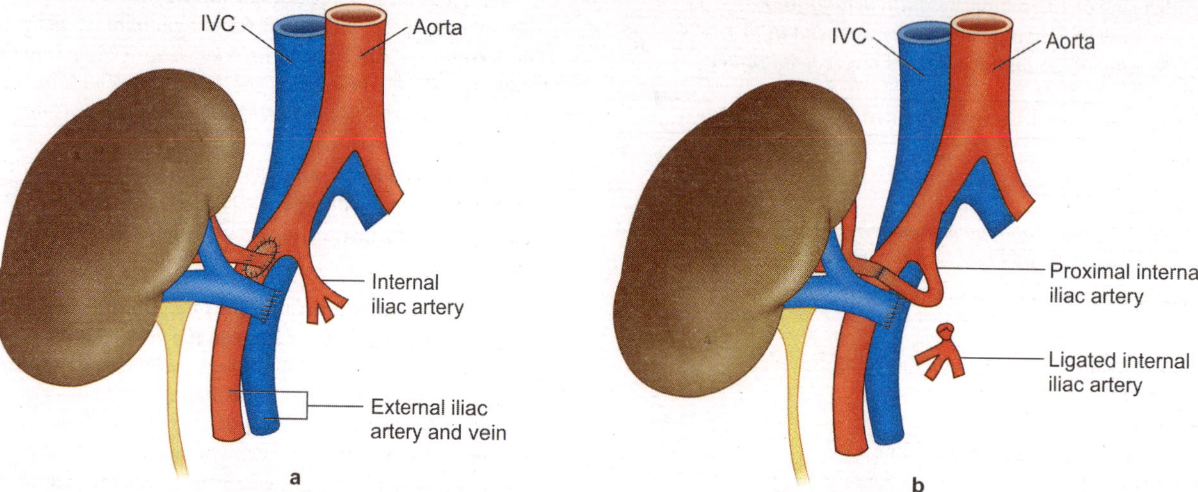

Fig: Implantation of a renal allograft. (a) The renal artery on a Carrel patch is anastomosed to the external iliac artery. (b) The renal artery is anastomosed end-to-end to the internal iliac artery.

Technique of Renal Transplantation

◈ *L & B 26th/424, 25th/1422*

- The transplant kidney is placed in the **iliac fossa in the retroperitoneal position** ***leaving the native kidneys in situ.***
- Using a retroperitoneal approach the donor ***renal vein is anastomosed end-to-side to the external iliac vein. The donor renal artery on a Carrel patch of donor aorta is anastomosed end-to-side to the external iliac artery***
- If the donor renal artery lacks an aortic patch, as in the case of a living donor transplant, it may be preferable to anastomose the ***donor artery end-to-end to the recipient internal iliac artery.***
- The **ureter,** which is kept reasonably short to avoid the risk of distal ischaemia, is then ***anastomosed to the bladder.***

Surgical Technique of Renal Transplantation

◈ *CSDT 11th/1378*

- The surgical technique of renal transplantation involves anastomoses of the renal artery and vein and ureter. The transplant kidney is ***placed in the iliac fossa through an oblique lower abdominal incision.*** The dissection is carried out by retracting the peritoneum medially so the kidney will lie in an extraperitoneal position. The iliac arteries and veins are mobilized as indicated for the proposed specific anastomoses.
- An **end-to-side anastomosis** is performed between ***renal vein and iliac vein; an end-to-side anastomosis is then performed between the renal artery and the iliac artery.***
- An alternative technique is to connect the ***renal artery end-to-end to the internal iliac artery,*** but this technique is more difficult in most patients. When multiple arteries are present there are several options.

Table *(L & B 25th/657)*: **Timing of primary cleft lip and palate procedures (after Delaire)**

Cleft lip alone	
Unilateral (one side): One operation at 5–6 months	
Bilateral (both sides): One operation at 4–5 months	
Cleft palate alone	
Soft palate only: One operation at 6 months	
Soft and hard palate:	Two operations Soft palate at 6 months Hard palate at 15–18 months
Cleft lip and palate	
Unilateral: Two operations	— Cleft lip and soft palate at 5–6 months hard palate and gum pad with or without lip revision at 15–18 months
Bilateral: Two operations	— Cleft lip and soft palate at 4–5 months Hard palate and gum pad with or without lip revision at 5–18 months

"The timing of cleft repair is important and a general recommendation is ***lip repair at 3 months, palate repair by 12 months and alveolar bone grafting at about 9 years*** which coincides with partial eruption of the canine teeth" *(Sabiston 18th/2138)*

The Typical Distribution of Cleft types is:

◈ *L & B 25th/657*

- **Cleft lip alone:** 15%
- **Cleft lip & palate:** 45%
- **Isolated cleft palate:** 40%

157. Ans. c. Bilateral..., e. Cleft...

[Ref: L & B 26th/637-38, 25th/658-668; CSDT 11th/1257-58; Sabiston 18th/2138]

158. Ans. d. (30 mm)

[Ref: L & B 26th/36, 25th/238-39; Sabiston 18th/271; CSDT11th/94-95]

The available sizes and Diameters of Suture are:

6-0 = 0.07 mm
5-0 = 0.10 mm
4-0 = 0.15 mm
3-0 = 0.20 mm
2-0 = 0.30 mm
0 = 0.35 mm
1 = 0.40 mm
2 = 0.5 mm

ALSO KNOW

Suture materials in common use in surgery: Absorbable (Suture--Tensile strength retention in vivo)

L & B 25th/238

- **Catgut (Plain):** *Lost within 7–10 days*
- **Catgut (Chromic):** *Lost within 21–28 days*
- ***Polyglactin: Approximately 60% remains at 2 weeks***
- ***Polyglyconate: Approximately 70% remains at 2 weeks***
- **Polyglycolic:** *Approximately 40% remains at 1 week 2 weeks*
- ***Polydioxanone: Approximately 70% remains at 2 weeks***
- **Polyglycaprone:** *21 days maximum*

Suture materials in common use in surgery: non-absorbable (Suture-Tensile strength)

L & B 25th/237

- **Nylon** ***(Polyamide polymer):*** *Loses 15–20% per year*
- **Polyester:** *Infinite (>1 year)*
- **Polybutester:** *Infinite (>1 year)*
- **Polypropylene:** *Infinite (>1 year)*

159. Ans. b. Eczem.., c. Nippl.., d. Inver..

[Ref: L & B 26th/810, 25th/838; S.Das 5th/716; http: //www.gponline.com/glance-pagets-disease-nipple-vs-eczema-Schwartz 8th; Sabiston 18th/858, 885]

Paget's Disease of the Nipple: Clinical Features

- Occurs almost exclusively in women.
- May occur at any age from 24 to 84, although it is most common around the menopause.
- Almost always associated with underlying carcinoma of the breast.
- ***Unilateral,*** persistent eczematous-type change of the nipple with erythema and scaling.
- Itching or burning sensation.
- Discharge and/or bleeding from the nipple.
- Ulceration.
- *Destruction of the nipple.*
- *Inversion of the nipple.*
- *Sometimes palpable breast lump*

"Paget's disease: Histologically, this disease is produced by ***intraductal carcinoma*** in the large sinuses just under the nipple. Clinically, this histologic variant produces a dermatitis that may appear eczematoid and moist or dry and psoriatic. ***It is usually confined to the nipple,*** although it can spread to the skin of the areola. Benign skin conditions such as eczema ***frequently begin on the areola*** whereas Paget's disease originates on the nipple and secondarily involves the areola"-*Sabiston 18th/885*

Eczema of Nipple: Clinical Features

- Often history of atopic eczema with personal or family history of hay fever or asthma.
- Allergic response to contact allergen.
- *May present during lactation.*
- *Bilateral.*
- Irritation.
- Acute inflammation, weeping vesicles or blisters.
- Chronic problems with dry, thickened areas.
- *Nipple preserved.*
- No breast lump.

Difference Between Paget's Disease and Eczema

Schwartz

- The biggest difference between Paget's disease and eczema is that ***Paget's disease always affects the nipple first whereas eczema usually first affects the area around the nipple which is known as the areola.***
- **Paget's disease of the nipple:** It frequently presents as a chronic, eczematous eruption of the nipple, which may be subtle, but may progress to an ulcerated, weeping lesion. *Paget's disease is usually associated with extensive DCIS and may be associated with an invasive cancer.*
- A palpable mass may or may not be present. Biopsy of the nipple will show a population of cells that are identical to the underlying DCIS cells (pagetoid features or pagetoid change).

160. Ans. All (a b c d e)

[Ref: L & B 26th.949-66, 25th/968-90; CSDT 11th/783-96; S.Das 5th/1122; radiopaedia.org/articles/pantaloon-hernia]

Hernia

"**Richter's hernia** is a hernia in which the sac contains only a portion of the ***circumference of the intestine*** (usually ***small intestine***). It usually complicates femoral and, rarely, obturator hernias"

Dual (Synonym: Saddle-bag, Pantaloon)

Hernia L & B 25th/975

This type of hernia consists of ***two sacs that straddle the inferior epigastric artery,*** one sac being medial and the other lateral to this vessel. The condition is not rare and is a cause of recurrence, one of the sacs having been overlooked at the time of operation.

Maydl's Hernia (Synonym: Hernia-in-W)

L & B 25th/976

Maydl's hernia is rare. The strangulated loop of the W lies within the abdomen, so local tenderness over the hernia is not marked. At operation, two comparatively ***normal-looking loops of intestine*** are present in the sac.

Sliding Hernia (Synonym: Hernia-en-glissade)

◈ *L & B 25th/977*

As a result of slipping of the posterior parietal peritoneum on the underlying retroperitoneal structures, the posterior wall of the sac is not formed of peritoneum alone, but by the ***sigmoid colon and its mesentery on the left, the caecum on the right and, sometimes, on either side by a portion of the bladder. It should*** be clearly understood that the caecum, appendix or a portion of the colon wholly within a hernial sac does not constitute a sliding hernia.

Table *(Schwartz)*: **Named Groin Hernia Syndromes**

Hernia	Definition
Cloquet	A femoral hernia perforating the aponeurosis of the pectineus and insinuating itself between this aponeurosis and the muscle, lying therefore behind the femoral vessels
Hesselbach's	Synonym for external femoral hernia
Laugier	Hernia passing through an opening in the lacunar ligament
Littré	A hernia containing a Meckel's diverticulum
Serafini's	The hernia sac passes behind the femoral vessels inside the sheath of the femoral vein

161. Ans. b. Middle...

[Ref: L & B 26th/987-88, 25th/1009-10; CSDT 11th/472-74; S.Das 5th/794-99]

Esophagus: Surgical Anatomy

*"In general the **oesophagus** is vertical, but shows slight curvature in following directions. There are **two side to side curvatures,** both towards the left. One is at the root of the neck & the other near the lower end. It also has **anteroposterior curvatures** that corresponds to the curvatures of the cervicothoracic spine"(BDC 6th/Vol. I 282)*

- The musculature of the upper oesophagus, including the upper sphincter, is striated. This is followed by a transitional zone of both striated and smooth muscle with the proportion of the latter progressively increasing so that, ***in the lower half of the oesophagus, there is only smooth muscle***
- The mucosal lining of the esophagus consists of stratified squamous epithelium that contains scattered mucous glands throughout. The esophagus has ***no serosal layer*** and, for this reason, does not heal as readily after injury or surgical anastomosis as other portions of the gastrointestinal tract.
- **The musculature of the esophagus** can be divided into an ***outer longitudinal and an inner circular layer.*** The ***upper 2 to 6 cm of the esophagus contain only striated muscle fibers.*** From there on, smooth muscle fibers gradually become more abundant. Most clinically significant esophageal motility disorders involve only the smooth muscle in the lower two thirds of the esophagus.
- When food passes through the UES, a contraction is initiated in the upper esophagus, which progresses distally toward the stomach. The wave initiated by swallowing is referred as **primary peristalsis.**
- Local stimulation by distention at any point in the body of the esophagus will elicit a peristaltic wave from the point of stimulus. This is called **secondary peristalsis** and aids esophageal emptying when the primary wave has failed to clear the lumen of ingested food or when the gastric contents reflux from the stomach.
- **Tertiary waves** are considered abnormal, but they are frequently seen in elderly subjects who have no symptoms of esophageal disease
- The ***LOS is a zone of relatively high pressure*** that prevents gastric contents from refluxing into the lower oesophagus
- ***Achalasia cardia:*** The physiological abnormalities are a non-relaxing LOS and absent peristalsis in the body of the oesophagus.

162. Ans. b. Submuc..., c. Prolapse..., d. Opera...

[Ref: L & B 26th/1219-21, 25th/1222; CSDT 11th/764-66]

Rectal Prolapse

◈ *L & B 26th/1220, 25th/1222*

- It may be mucosal or full thickness
- If full thickness, the whole wall of the rectum is included
- It commences as a rectal intussusception
- ***In children, the prolapse is usually mucosal and should be treated conservatively***
- ***In the adult, the prolapse is often full thickness and is frequently associated with incontinence***
- ***Surgery is necessary for full-thickness rectal prolapse***
- The operation is performed either via the perineum or via the abdomen

"In children: Mucosal prolapse often commences after an attack of diarrhoea, or from loss of weight and consequent loss of fat in the ischiorectal fossae. It may also be associated with fibrocystic disease, neurological causes and maldevelopment of the pelvis" *(L & B 25th/1222)*

"In adults: The condition in adults is often associated with third-degree haemorrhoids. In the female a torn perineum and in the male straining from urethral obstruction, predisposes to mucosal prolapse. In old age, both mucosal and full-thickness prolapse are associated with atony of the sphincter mechanism, but whether this is the cause of the problem or secondary to it is unknown" *(L & B 25th/1222)*

"The primary therapy for rectal prolapse is **surgery** and more than 100 different procedures have been described to treat this condition. Operations can be categorized as either *abdominal or perineal.* **Abdominal operations** have taken three major approaches:

- Reduction of the perineal hernia and closure of the cul-de-sac *(Moschowitz repair);*
- Fixation of the rectum, either with a prosthetic sling *(Ripsten and Wells rectopexy)* or by *suture rectopexy;* or
- Resection of redundant sigmoid colon. **Perineal approaches** have focused upon tightening the anus with a variety of prosthetic materials, reefing the rectal mucosa *(Delorme procedure),* or resecting the prolapsed bowel from the perineum *(perineal rectosigmoidectomy or Altemeier procedure)" (CSDT)*

A & E

163. Ans. a. Glan..., b. Circumcision...

[Ref: L & B 26th/1360, 25th/1362-63; CSDT 11th/1028; Textbook of Surgery by S.Das 5th/1322-23; Nelson 18th/2253-54]

"Circumcision should not be done in these patients, as the prepuce can be used later in surgical repair" *(CSDT 11th/1028)*

Hypospadias

- If the ***opening is glandular or coronal (85% of patients),*** the penis is usually functional both for micturition and procreation and repair is done ***primarily for cosmetic reasons***
- With more proximal displacement, chordee ***(ventral curvature of the penile shaft)*** frequently occurs and requires treatment or it will ***preclude straight erections and normal intercourse***
- Approximately 70% of hypospadias occur on the corona or distal shaft of the penis
- The goals of surgical treatment include correction of any penile curvature, moving the urethral opening to the tip of the glans and producing a cosmetically satisfactory result
- **Types:** Glandular, Coronal, Penile, Penoscrotal & Perineal
- The degree of hypospadias dictates the need for repair.
- Openings that are more proximal on the shaft require correction to allow voiding while standing, normal erection and proper sperm deposition during intercourse.
- Surgical plastic repair of hypospadias is currently accomplished by a variety of highly successful one-stage operations and is routinely performed *between 6 and 19 months of age.*
- ***"Denis-Browne's operation*** is still the *simple & most accepted operation"-Textbook of Surgery by S. Das 5th/1323*
- The most common complications of hypospadias surgery include meatal stenosis and fistula formation; however, improved techniques have decreased the incidence of these complications.

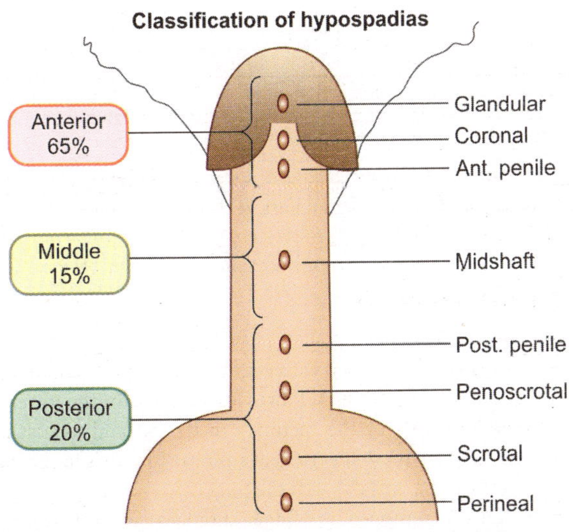

Fig: Classification of hypospadias and frequency by location of hypospadias

164. Ans. b. Penil.., d. Less.. & e. BPH..

[Ref: L & B 26th/1341-44, 25th/1344-46; CSDT 11th/1033-35; S.Das 5th/1259-70; Sabiston 18th/2271]

"BPH: The urethra become compressed laterally *so that it takes a shape of an anteroposterior slit due to enlargement of two lateral lobes of prostate " (S.Das 5th/1259)*

"Urinary flow rates *decrease* (for a voided volume > 200 ml, a peak flow ***rate of > 15 ml s–1 is normal,*** one of 10–15 ml s–1 is equivocal and one < 10 ml s–1 is low). A typical history and ***a flow rate < 10 ml s–1 will be sufficient for most urologists to recommend treatment"*** *(L & B 25th/1346, 1349)*

Benign Prostatic Hyperplasia (BPH)

"Transurethral resection of prostate (TURP) is a proven surgical technique that significantly improves lower urinary tract symptoms associated with BPH.This intervention is most commonly recommended in the patient with ***symptoms of bladder outlet obstruction and irritability that are moderate to severe, bothersome and interfere with the patient's quality of life.*** Although symptoms constitute the primary reason for recommending intervention, in patients with an obstructing prostate, there are some absolute indications. These are ***acute urinary retention, recurrent infection, recurrent hematuria and azotemia"*** *(Sabiston 18th/2271)*

"Prostate it is divided into the **peripheral zone (PZ),** which lies mainly posteriorly and from ***which most carcinomas arise*** and a central zone (CZ), which lies posterior to the urethral lumen and above the ejaculatory ducts as they pass through the prostate; the two zones are rather like an egg in an egg cup. There is also a ***periurethral transitional zone (TZ), from which most benign prostatic hyperplasia (BPH) arises"***

"BPH typically affects the submucous group of glands in the transitional zone, forming a nodular enlargement. Eventually, this overgrowth compresses the PZ glands into a false capsule and causes the appearance of the typical 'lateral' lobes"

"Urethra: The prostatic urethra is ***lengthened,*** sometimes to twice its normal length, but it is not narrowed anatomically. The normal posterior curve may be so exaggerated that it requires a curved catheter to negotiate it. When only one lateral lobe is enlarged, distortion of the prostatic urethra occurs"

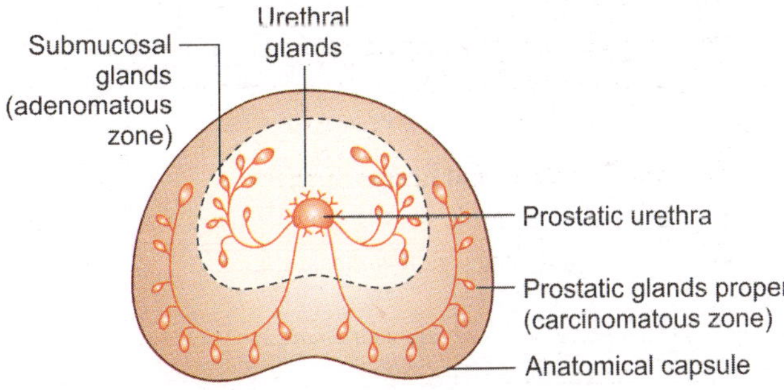

Fig: A transverse section of the prostate. The peripheral zone is the area from which most prostate cancers arise. The 'adenomatous' zone comprises the central and transitional zones

165. Ans. a. Cosm.., c. Veress.., d. Lapr...

[Ref: L & B 26th/1109-11, 98-100, 25th/247-55; Washington Manual of Surgery 5th/642-43; Maingot's Abdominal Operations; Mastery of Surgery 5th/1116; Manipal surgery 3rd/476]

Laparoscopic Cholecystectomy

- Initially, a ***small incision is made in the upper edge of the umbilicus.***
- With the **closed technique** a special hollow insufflation needle ***(Veress needle)*** that is spring-loaded with a retractable cutting outer sheath is inserted into the peritoneal cavity and used for insufflation. Once an adequate pneumoperitoneum is established, a 10-mm trocar is inserted through the supraumbilical incision.
- With the **open technique** the ***supraumbilical incision is carried through the fascia and into the peritoneal cavity.*** The open technique may initially appear time-consuming and even cumbersome; however, with practice, it is more efficient overall.
- A special blunt cannula **(Hasson cannula)** is inserted into the peritoneal cavity and anchored to the fascia. The laparoscope with the attached video camera is passed through the umbilical port and the abdomen inspected. Three additional ports are placed under direct vision
- Most of the dissection is carried out through the epigastric port using a dissector, hook, or scissors.
- ***Bleeding has been the most common cause for conversion to an open procedure.*** Bleeding plays a more important role in laparoscopic surgery because of factors inherent to the technique. These include a limited field that can easily be obscured by relatively small amounts of blood, magnification that makes small arterial bleeding appear to be a significant

Laparoscopic Cholecystectomy Procedure: *1 cm incision is made below the umbilicus, through which a pneumoperitoneum is maintained by CO_2 insufflation. Following this, a laparoscope in introduced & a camera is attached.* *Three small, 1 cm incision are made in epigastrium & in the right hypochondrium. These are used for suction, instrumentation, cauterization, dissection, retraction purpose-dissection port" (Manipal surgery 3rd/476)*

"Advantage: *Recovery is fast, pain is minimal &* ***acceptable & better cosmetic result"*** *(Manipal surgery 3rd/476)*

"Previous abdominal surgery is no longer a contraindication to laparoscopic surgery, *but preoperative evaluation is necessary to assess the type and location of surgical scars" (L B 25th/251)*

Limitations of Minimal Access Surgery

◈ *L& B*
- *Reliance on remote vision and operating*
- *Loss of tactile feedback*
- *Dependence on hand–eye coordination*
- *Difficulty with haemostasis*
- *Reliance on new techniques*
- *Extraction of large specimens*

"Laparoscopy surgery: *Massive abdominal distention* may result in an increased risk of iatrogenic bowel injury" *(Washington Manual of Surgery 5th/643)*

"C/I for **Laparoscopy are relative & includes uncorrectable coagulation defects, severe congestive heart failure, respiratory insufficiency, suspected acute & diffuse peritonitis & presence of distended bowel"** *(emedicine.medscape.com/article)*

"Absolute contraindications to Laparoscopy are few: Certainly, a patient who is unable to tolerate general anesthesia, a patient with gallbladder cancer (suspected or confirmed) and a patient with a frozen upper abdomen due to previous surgery or ***peritonitis*** are all individuals who should not undergo laparoscopy. In addition, **relative contraindications** include any ***previous right upper quadrant surgery,*** portal hypertension, coagulopathy, cholecystenteric fistula, advanced acute cholecystitis and ***pregnancy*** (during first and third trimesters)." *(Mastery of Surgery 5th/1116)*

Table: *(Maingot's):* **Contraindications to Laparoscopy**

Absolute
Unable to tolerate general anesthesia
Refractory coagulopathy
Suspicion of gallbladder carcinoma
Relative
Previous upper abdominal surgery
Cholangitis
Diffuse peritonitis
Cirrhosis and/or portal hypertension
Chronic obstructive pulmonary disease***/severe cardiopulmonary disease***
Cholecystoenteric fistula
Morbid obesity
Pregnancy

166. Ans. a. Index... & b. In BPH..

[Ref: L & B 26th/1345, 25th/1221, 1243; Manipal surgery 3rd/789]

"DRE in BPH: ***Enlarged lateral lobes can be easily felt. Rectal mucosa is free*** *(in an enlarged prostate gland, in case of carcinoma of prostate, the mucosa of rectum cannot be moved if it has infiltrated into the rectum" (Manipal surgery 3rd/789)*

Digital Examination

◈ *L & B 25th/1221*
- The index finger used with gentleness and precision remains a valuable test for rectal disease. Tumours in the lower and middle thirds of the rectum can be felt and assessed; by asking the patient to strain, even some tumours in the upper third can be 'tipped' with the finger.
- After it is removed, the finger should be examined for telltale traces of mucus, pus or blood. It is always useful to note the normal as well as the abnormal findings on digital examination, *e.g.*, the prostate in the male.

- Digital findings can be recorded as intraluminal (*e.g.*, blood, pus), intramural (*e.g.*, tumours, granular areas, strictures) or extramural (*e.g.*, enlarged prostate, uterine fibroids).

Digital Examination with the Index Finger

◈ *L & B 25th/1243*

- With an adequately lubricated index finger, the soft tissues around the anus are palpated for induration, tenderness and subcutaneous lesions. The index finger is then introduced gently into the anal canal along its ***posterior aspect.***
- At the apex of the canal, the ***sling of puborectalis is felt posteriorly;*** supralevator induration feels bony hard and is more easily appreciated if unilateral.
- The posterior surface of the prostate gland with its median sulcus can be palpated anteriorly in male patients; in female patients, the uterine cervix can be palpated. The presence of any distal intrarectal, intra-anal or extraluminal mass is recorded.
- ***Sphincter length, resting tone and voluntary squeeze are assessed.*** On withdrawal the examining finger is inspected for the presence of mucus, blood or pus and to identify stool colour.

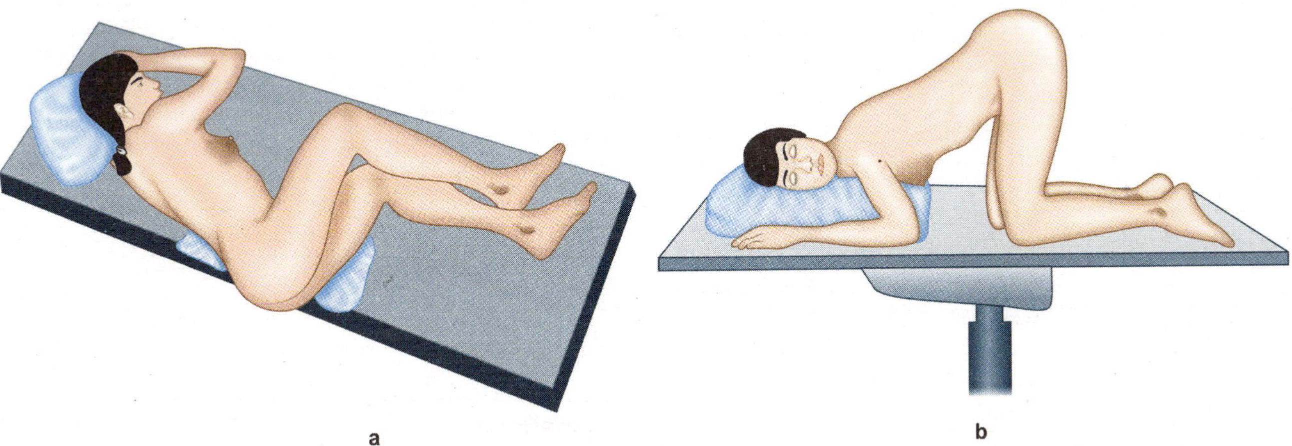

Fig: Positions for digital rectal examination. (a) Left lateral (Sims). (b) Knee–elbow

167. Ans. b. ↑ Calcium..., c. Hyperv..., e. Decrease...

[Ref: L & B 26th/1292, 25th/1295]

Aetiology of Renal Stone

◈ *L & B 25th/1295*

- ***Dietetic:*** Deficiency of vitamin A causes desquamation of epithelium. The cells form a nidus on which a stone is deposited.
- ***Altered urinary solutes and colloids:*** Dehydration increases the concentration of urinary solutes until they are liable to precipitate. Reduction of urinary colloids, which adsorb solutes, or mucoproteins, which chelate calcium, might also result in a tendency for crystal and stone formation.
- ***Decreased urinary citrate:*** The presence of citrate in urine, 300–900 mg 24 h–1 as citric acid, tends to keep otherwise relatively insoluble calcium phosphate and citrate in solution.
- ***Renal infection:*** Infection favours the formation of urinary calculi. Clinical and experimental stone formation are common when urine is infected with urea-splitting streptococci, staphylococci and especially *Proteus* spp.
- ***Inadequate urinary drainage and urinary stasis:*** Stones are liable to form when urine does not pass freely.
- ***Prolonged immobilization***
- ***Hyperparathyroidism:*** Hyperparathyroidism leading to hypercalcaemia and hypercalciuria is found in 5% or less of those who present with radiopaque calculi. In cases of recurrent or multiple stones, this cause should be eliminated by appropriate investigations

168. Ans. b. Common..., c. Often..., e. It can...

[Ref: L & B 25th/1158; CSDT 11th/622-23; Schawrtz]

Duodenal Diverticula

- Diverticula of the duodenum are relatively common, representing the ***second most common site for diverticulum formation after the colon.***
- Duodenal diverticula occur twice as often in women as in men and are rare in patients younger than age 40 years.
- They have been classified as congenital or acquired, true or false and intraluminal or extraluminal.
- ***Two thirds to three fourths of duodenal diverticula are found in the periampullary region (within a 2-cm radius of the ampulla) and project from the medial wall of the duodenum***
- The important thing to remember is that the majority of duodenal diverticula are asymptomatic
- Major complications of duodenal diverticula include ***obstruction of the biliary or pancreatic ducts*** that may contribute to cholangitis and ***pancreatitis,*** respectively; hemorrhage; perforation; and rarely, blind loop syndrome.
- ***Only those diverticula associated with the ampulla of Vater are significantly related to complications of cholangitis and pancreatitis.***

◈ *CSDT 11th/622-23*

"Duodenal diverticula usually arise on the ***medial aspect of the duodenum within 2 cm of the orifices of the bile duct*** and in some individuals the duct empties directly into a diverticulum"

◈ *CSDT 11th/562*

- Duodenal pulsion diverticula are acquired outpouchings of the mucosa and submucosa, ***90% of which are on the medial aspect of the duodenum.***
- They are rare before age 40. ***Most are solitary and within 2.5 cm of the ampulla of Vater.*** There is a high incidence of gallstone disease of the gallbladder in patients with juxtapapillary diverticula. Diverticula are not seen in the first portion of the duodenum, where diverticular configurations are due to scarring by peptic ulceration or cholecystitis.
- Serious complications are ***hemorrhage or perforation from inflammation, pancreatitis and biliary obstruction.***
- ***Surgical treatment is required for complications & rarely for persistent symptoms***

169. Ans. c. Papillary..., e. Meningioma

[Ref: Sabiston 18th/; Love & Bailey 26th/765, 25th/793-794, 24th/798-799; Harrison 19th/2305, 570,; Sabiston 18th/937-38; CSDT 11th/306; en.wikipedia. org/wiki/;www.ncbi.nlm.nih]

Psammoma Bodies Found in:

- P-papillary ca thyroid, paillary renal cell carcinoma, prolactinoma
- S-serous cyst adenoma of ovary
- A-appendiceal carcinoid (rare)
- M-meningioma

"Psammoma bodies are present in about 60% cases of papillary carcinoma of thyroid" *(CSDT 11th/306)*

Psammoma Bodies are Commonly seen in Certain Tumors such as:

◈ *en.wikipedia.org/wiki/*

- ***Papillary thyroid carcinoma***
- *Papillary renal cell carcinoma*
- *Micropapillary subtype of lung adenocarcinoma*
- *Ovarian papillary serous cystadenoma and cystadenocarcinoma*
- *Endometrial adenocarcinomas (Papillary serous carcinoma ~3%-4%)*
- ***Meningiomas,*** *in the central nervous system*
- *Peritoneal and Pleural Mesothelioma*
- *Somatostatinoma (pancreas)*
- Prolactinoma of the pituitary
- Mesothelioma, in membranes that line body cavities

170. Ans. a. Associated..., b. Incre..., c. About...

[Ref: L & B 26th/1771-74, 25th/800-805; CMDT 2016/1132-36; Sabiston 18th/960;CSDT 11th/308-09]

Primary Hyperparathyroidism

"**Primary hyperparathyroidism** is due to excess PTH secretion from a ***single parathyroid adenoma (83%),*** multiple adenomas (6%), hyperplasia (10%), or carcinoma (1%). Fewer abnormal parathyroid glands are identified at focal exploration"-*CSDT 11th/308*

"Although most cases of PHPT are sporadic, PHPT does occur within the spectrum of a number of inherited disorders such as ***MEN1, MEN2A, isolated familial HPT and familial HPT with jaw-tumor syndrome.*** All of these syndromes are inherited in an ***autosomal dominant*** fashion"

- Primary HPT is more commonly sporadic than familial
- Familial HPT occurs as part of the following genetically determined conditions: **MEN-1** (multiple endocrine neoplasia type 1; Werner's syndrome) & **MEN-2A** (Sipple's syndrome) and rarely **MEN-2B.**
- The majority (85%) of patients with sporadic primary HPT have a single adenoma, approximately 13% have hyperplasia affecting all four glands and about 1% will have more than one adenoma or a carcinoma. In familial disease, multiple gland enlargement is the norm.
- The **classic quartet** of '***stones, bones, abdominal groans and psychic moans***' is rarely observed in developed countries where the diagnosis is usually made on serum calcium estimation well before the full picture of severe bone disease (von Recklinghausen's disease), ***renal calculi and calcinosis,*** pancreatitis and psychiatric disorder develops.
- All abnormal glands are excised and, in the *event of sporadic four-gland disease, subtotal parathyroidectomy is carried out,* ***preserving approximately 50 mg of one gland.***

Table *(Schwartz)*: **Biochemical Features of Primary Hyperparathyroidism**

Serum Tests	Alternation
Calcium	***Increased,*** except in normocalcemic primary hyperparathyroidism
Intact PTH	Increased or inappropriately high
Chloride	Increased or high normal
Phosphate	Decreased or low normal
Chloride: Phosphate	Increased (usually >33)
Magnesium	Unchanged or decreased (in patients with osteitis fibrosa cystica)
Uric acid	Normal or increased
Alkaline phosphatase	Normal or increased (in the presence of bone disease)
Acid–base status	Mild hyperchloremic metabolic acidosis
Calcium: Creatinine clearance ratio	>0.02 (vs. <0.01 in BFHH)
1, 25-dihydroxy vitamin D	Normal or increased
Urine Tests	
24-Hour urinary calcium	Normal or increased

Table *(1990 NIH Consensus Conference Guidelines)*: **Indications for Parathyroidectomy in Patients with Asymptomatic Primary HPT**

At initial evaluation
• *Markedly increased serum calcium*
• *Episode of life-threatening hypercalcemic episode*
• *Reduced creatinine clearance*
• *Kidney stones on abdominal X-rays*
• *Markedly elevated 24-hour urinary calcium excretion*
• *Substantially decreased bone mass*
• *Age <50 years*

Contd...

Development of any of the following during follow-up

- *Typical skeletal, renal, or gastrointestinal symptoms*
- *Serum calcium >1–1.6 mg/dL above upper normal range*
- *A>30% decline in creatinine clearance*
- *Urinary calcium >400 mg/d*
- *Bone mass reduced to <2 SD below age-, gender- and race-matched controls*
- *Unwillingness or inability to undergo continued follow-up*

171. Ans. b. Elevation..., c. Doppler...

[Ref: L & B 26th/1379-80, 25th/1380; CSDT 11th/1040; S.Das 5th/1298]

Note: *Redness of scrotal skin & fever are found in both*

Acute Epididymo-orchitis

S.Das 5th/1304

- The initial symptom is pain & swelling of epididymis along with fever, malaise & chills
- Scrotal wall becomes red, oedematous & glossy

Testicular Torsion

S.Das 5th/1298

- ***The scrotum is swollen & tender. The scrotum may also be normal or red & oedematous. Sometimes it is difficult to differentiate it from acute epididymo-orchitis***
- ***Gradually within a few hours after onset the patient becomes pyrexic with slight leucocytosis***

Clinical Features of Testicular Torsion

L & B 25th/1380

- Testicular torsion is most common between 10 and 25 years of age although a few cases occur in infancy. Symptoms vary with the degree of torsion. Most commonly there is sudden agonising pain in the groin and the lower abdomen. The patient feels nauseated and may vomit.
- Torsion of a fully descended testis is usually easily recognised. The testis seems high and the tender twisted cord can be palpated above it. In mumps orchitis the cord is not particularly thickened.
- The ***onset of redness of the skin and a mild pyrexia*** may result in the condition being confused with epididymo-orchitis in the older patient; however, ***in epididymo-orchitis there will usually be dysuria associated with the accompanying urinary infection.***
- ***Elevation of the testis reduces the pain in epididymo-orchitis and makes it worse in torsion.*** Very occasionally, torsion can be convincingly mimicked by a small tense strangulated inguinal hernia compressing the cord and causing compression of the pampiniform plexus.
- **Doppler ultrasound scan** will confirm the absence of the blood supply to the affected testis, but performing this test may squander vital minutes.
- If there is any doubt about the diagnosis, the scrotum should be explored without delay. An empty oedematous hemiscrotum suggests that a tender lump at the external inguinal ring is a torted testis rather than a strangulated hernia.

172. Ans. a. Perforati..., b. Perforat..., d. Common...

[Ref: L & B 26th/1158, 25th/68-70;Harrison 19th/1051; CSDT 11th/695]

Note: *"Salmonella typhi may cause ulcers in the distal ileum or caecum" (CSDT 11th/695)*

Pathology of Typhoid Ulcer

L & B 25th/68-69

- Following ingestion of contaminated food or water, the organism colonises the Peyer's patches in the ***terminal ileum*** causing hyperplasia of the lymphoid follicles followed by necrosis and ulceration.
- The microscopic picture shows erythrophagocytosis with histiocytic proliferation. If the patient is left untreated or inadequately treated, the ***ulcers may lead to perforation and bleeding. The bowel may perforate at several sites including the large bowel.***
- **In the second or third week of the illness,** if there is severe generalised abdominal pain, this ***heralds a perforated typhoid ulcer.***
- The patient, who is already very ill, ***deteriorates further with classical features of peritonitis.***
- ***Laparotomy is then carried out.*** Thorough ***peritoneal lavage is essential.***

Treatment of Bowel Perforation from Typhoid

L & B 25th/70

- Manage in intensive care
- Resuscitate and give intravenous antibiotics
- Laparotomy– Choice of various procedures
- Commonest site of perforation is the terminal ileum
- Having found a perforation, always look for others
- In the very ill patient, consider some form of exteriorisation
- Close the peritoneum & leave the wound open for secondary closure

173. Ans. c. Whole...

[Ref: L & B 26th/389-90, 25th/381-83; Reddy 32th/305-06; CSDT 11th/267-72]

Full-thickness Burns (3° Burn)

L & B 25th/381

- The ***whole of the dermis is destroyed in these burns.***
- Clinically, they ***have a hard, leathery feel.*** The appearance can vary from that similar to the patient's normal skin to charred black, depending upon the intensity of the heat.
- There is *no capillary return.* Often, thrombosed vessels can be seen under the skin.
- These burns are ***completely anaesthetised:*** a needle can be stuck deep into the dermis without any pain or bleeding.

Burn

CSDT 11th/267-72

- Traditionally, burns have been classified as ***first-, second- and third-degree,*** but the current emphasis on burn healing has led to classification as ***partial-thickness burns, which can heal spontaneously and full-thickness burns,*** which require skin grafting, although deep partial-thickness burns are usually excised and grafted as well.

- A **first-degree burn** involves only the epidermis and is characterized by erythema and minor microscopic changes; tissue damage is minimal, protective functions of the skin are intact, skin edema is minimal and systemic effects are rare. Pain, the chief symptom, usually resolves in 48–72 hours and healing takes place uneventfully.
- **Second-degree or partial-thickness burns** are deeper, involving all of the epidermis and some of the corium or dermis. The systemic severity of the burn and the quality of subsequent healing are directly related to the amount of undamaged dermis. Superficial burns are often characterized by ***blister formation,*** while deeper partial-thickness burns have a ***reddish appearance*** or a layer of whitish nonviable dermis firmly adherent to the remaining viable tissue. Blisters, when present, continue to increase in size in the postburn period as the *osmotically active particles in the blister fluid attract water.*
- **Deep dermal burns** heal over a period of 25–35 days with a fragile epithelial covering that arises from the residual uninjured epithelium of the deep dermal sweat glands and hair follicles. Severe hypertrophic scarring occurs when such an injury heals; the resulting epithelial covering is prone to ***blistering and breakdown. Evaporative losses*** after healing remain high compared with losses in normal skin.
- **Full-thickness (third-degree) burns** have a characteristic white, waxy appearance and may appear to the untrained eye as unburned skin. Burns caused by prolonged exposure, with involvement of fat and underlying tissue, may be brown, dark red, or black. The diagnostic findings of full-thickness burns are ***lack of sensation in the burned skin, lack of capillary refill and a leathery texture*** that is unlike normal skin. All epithelial elements are destroyed, ***leaving no potential for reepithelialization.***

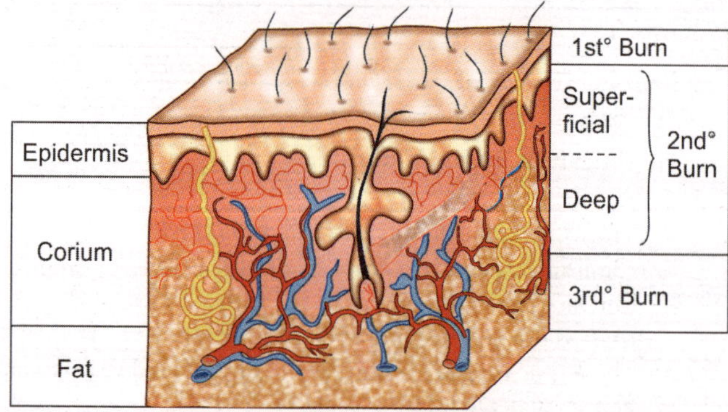

Fig: Layers of the skin showing depth of first-degree, second-degree and third-degree burns.

A & E

174. Ans. a. Hyperg..., b. Vasc..., c. Athero..., e. Trophic...

[Ref: Harrison 19th/2428, 18th/2987; L & B 26th/887, 25 /913, 537; CMDT 2016/1222]

Note: *"Hypertension can accelerates other complications of DM, particularly* ***cardiovascular disease & nephropathy.*** *Diabetic ulcer commonly result from decreased protective sensation. Diabetic ulcers are usually found on the plantar surface of foot over the metatarsal heads or heel" (Sabiston 18th/2148)*

Diabetic Gangrene

◈ *L & B 25th/913,*

- Diabetic gangrene is related to three factors: ***Trophic changes from peripheral neuropathy, ischaemia as a result of atheroma and low resistance to infection because of excess sugar in the Tissues.***
- The **neuropathy** impairs sensation and thus favours the neglect of minor injuries and infections.

Lower Extremity Complications

◈ *Harrison 19th/2428, 18th/2987*

- The reasons for the increased incidence of these disorders in DM involve the interaction of several pathogenic factors: ***neuropathy, abnormal foot biomechanics, peripheral arterial disease (PAD) and poor wound healing.***
- The **peripheral sensory neuropathy** interferes with normal ***protective mechanisms*** and allows the patient to sustain major or repeated minor trauma to the foot, often without knowledge of the injury. Disordered proprioception causes abnormal weight bearing while walking and ***subsequent formation of callus or ulceration.***
- ***Autonomic neuropathy*** results in anhidrosis and altered superficial blood flow in the foot, which promote ***drying of the skin and fissure formation. PAD and poor wound healing impede resolution*** of minor breaks in the skin, allowing them to enlarge and to become infected.
- Approximately 15% of individuals with type 2 DM develop a **foot ulcer** (great toe or MTP areas are most common) and a significant subset will ultimately undergo amputation (14–24% risk with that ulcer or subsequent ulceration).
- ***Risk factors for foot ulcers or amputation include: Male sex, diabetes >10 years' duration, peripheral neuropathy, abnormal structure of foot (bony abnormalities, callus, thickened nails), peripheral arterial disease, smoking, history of previous ulcer or amputation and poor glycemic control.*** Large calluses are often precursors to or overlie ulcerations.

Gangrene of Feet in DM

◈ *CMDT 2016/1222*

- The incidence of **gangrene of the feet** in diabetics is 30 times that in age-matched controls.
- The factors responsible for its development, in addition to ***peripheral vascular disease, are small vessel disease, peripheral neuropathy with loss of both pain sensation and neurogenic inflammatory responses and secondary infection.*** In two-thirds of patients with ischemic gangrene, pedal pulses are not palpable.
- Agents that reduce peripheral blood flow such as tobacco and propranolol should be avoided. ***Control of other risk factors such as hypertension is essential.***

- Cholesterol-lowering agents are useful as adjunctive therapy
- Improvement in peripheral blood flow with endarterectomy and bypass operations is possible in certain patients.

OBSTETRICS & GYNAECOLOGY

175. Ans. All (a, b, c, d)

[Ref: Dutta's Obstetrics 7th/607-08; William's Obstetrics 23rd/630-32, 3, 1211; Park 23rd/562-63]

"**Prematurity** *is a common cause of* ***still birth***" *(Reddy 32nd/417)*
"A stillbirth is the birth of newborn after ***28th completed*** *weeks (weighing 1000g or more when the baby does not breathe or show any sign of life after delivery" (Dutta's Obstetrics 7th/607)*
"In high prevalence areas, ***syphilis & malaria*** *in non-immune women are also* ***major causes of stillbirths****" (William's Obstetrics 23rd/1211)*

Table *(Dutta's Obstetrics 7th/608)*: **Important causes of stillbirths & main interventions**

Causes	Percent
Birth Asphyxia & trauma	30
*Pregnancy complications (**Placental abruption**, pre-eclampsia, **diabetes mellitus**)*	30
Fetal congenital malformations & chromosomal anomalies	15
Infection	5
Unknown cause	20

176. Ans. b. More..., c. Common..., d. Assoc..., e. Asso..

[Ref: Shaws 15th/416-20; Dutta Gynae 5th/341-47: Shaw's 14th/374: Novak's Gynaecology 14th/1344-45: Jeffcoates Gynaecology 7th/503]

"Women with **hereditary nonpolyposis colorectal cancer syndrome (HNPCC)** have a 40-60% lifetime risk for ***endometrial as well as colon cancer***" *(Novak's Gynaecology 14th/1345)*
"**Endometrial carcinoma:** Peak incidence is ***55-70 years***, 20-25% occur in ***perimenopausal women*** & only 5% develops in women below the age of 45 years" *(Shaws 15th/416)*
"Prognostic factor in endometrial carcinoma-Age at diagnosis ***(older the patient poorer the prognosis)****" (Dutta Gynae 5th/347, Novak's Gynaecology 14th/1362)*
"Endometrial cancer is a disease that occur ***primarily in postmenopausal women & increasingly virulent with advancing age****" (Novak's Gynaecology 14th/1344)*

Endometrial Ca-Risk Factors

- Unopposed & unsupervised administration of hormone replacement therapy (HRT) ***(Estrogen therapy)***[Q]
- Combined oral hormonal pills have a protective effect[Q]
- *Obesity*[Q], *Hypertension*[Q] & ***Diabetes***[Q]
- Chronic non-ovulatory cycles as seen in dysfunctional uterine bleeding
- Tamoxifen given to woman with breast Ca -Ca 2-3 times
- ***Nulliparous*** women have 2–3 times more risk than parous women
- Infertile women & women with ***polycystic ovarian disease***[Q] (on account of non-ovulation have high estrogen)
- In some families, a strong familial predisposition is noticed (Lynch II syndrome[Q])
- "Natural ***menopause***[Q] occuring after age of 52 years increases the risk for endometrial cancer 2.4 times compared with women who experienced menopause before 49 years of age, probably as a result of prolonged exposure of the uterus to progesterone deficient menstrual cycles" *(Novak's 14th/1344)*
- "More common in Jewesses than in women of other races" – *Jeffcoate's Gynaecology 7th/503*
- "Hypothyroidism have been associated with endometrial Ca, but a causal relationship has not been confirmed" *(Novak's 14th/1345)*

177. Ans. a. Twin, b. Down..., c. Choriocarcinoma

[Ref: Dutta's Obstetrics 7th/58-59; Shaw's 15th/42; William's Obstetrics 22nd/70; Nelson 18th/215 &, 2155; Harrison 19th/594, 609, 597]

HCG

*"High level of hCG could be detected in-****multiple pregnancy****, hydatidiform mole or* ***choriocarcinoma*** *& relatively high in pregnancy with a trisomy fetus* ***(Down syndrome). Plasma lower levels are found in ectopic pregnancies & in spontaneous abortion****" (Dutta's Obstetrics 7th/59)*
"hCG is produced by the syncytiotrophoblast[Q] of the placenta. Its value reach maximum levels ranging 100 IU & 200 IU/ml b/w 60-70 days of pregnancy[Q]. It can be detected in the maternal serum or urine as early as 8-9 days[Q] following ovulation. The rescue & maintenance of corpus luteum till 6 wk of pregnancy is the major biological function of hCG" *(Dutta obstetrics 6th/58)*

Table: Tumor Markers

Tumor Markers	Cancer	Non-Neoplastic Conditions
Hormones		
Human chorionic gonadotropin	Gestational trophoblastic disease, gonadal germ cell tumor	Pregnancy
Oncofetal Antigens		
Alphafetoprotein	Hepatocellular carcinoma, gonadal germ cell tumor	Cirrhosis, hepatitis[Q]
Carcinoembryonic antigen	Adenocarcinomas of the colon, pancreas, lung, breast, ovary	Pancreatitis, hepatitis, inflammatory bowel disease, smoking

hCG: Review of facts

- It is a glycoprotein[Q] consisting of a *hormone non-specific*[Q]*& a hormone specific β subunit*[Q].

- hCG is chemically & functionally similar to pituitary luteinising hormone[Q]. The α subunit is biochemically similar to LH, FSH & TSH where as the *β subunit is relatively unique*[Q] *to hCG.*
- It is produced by the *syncytiotrophoblast*[Q] of the placenta and secreted into the blood of both mother & fetus
- Half life of hCG is about 24 hours
- By radioimmunoassay it can be detected in the maternal serum or urine as early as 8-9 days[Q] following ovulation. In early pregnancy, the doubling time of hCG concentrations is plasma is 1.4-2 days[Q]. The blood & urine values reach maximum levels ranging 100 IU & 200 IU/ml b/w 60–70 days of pregnancy[Q]
- It is commercially obtained from the urine of pregnant women *(Shaws Gynaecology 14th/137)*
- The rescue & maintenance of corpus luteum till 6–7 weeks[Q] of pregnancy is the major biological function of hCG.

178. Ans. b. Bright

[Ref: Dutta's Obstetrics 7th/252-258; William's Obstetrics 23rd/761-75]

Abruption

***"Prior abruption: Risk of recurrence** for a woman with previous abruption varies between **5–17%**" (Dutta's Obstetrics 7th/253)*

*"Character of blood in abruption placentae- **Dark coloured** (c.f bright red in placenta praevia)" (Dutta's Obstetrics 7th/246)*

*"Prevalence of **Abruptio placentae is more with high birth order (pregnancies with gravida 5 or more)**" (Dutta's Obstetrics 7th/252)*

"Hypertension in pregnancy is the most important predisposing factor. ***Pre-eclampsia***, gestational hypertension & essential hypertension, all are associated with placental abruption" *(Dutta's Obstetrics 7th/252)*

Recurrent Abruption

◈ *William's Obstetrics 23rd/764-65*

- **Pritchard and co-workers (1970)** identified a ***recurrence rate of severe abruption in 1 in 8 pregnancies.***
- **Furuhashi and colleagues (2002)** analyzed subsequent pregnancy outcomes from 27 women who had a prior placental abruption. Of the six ***(22%)*** recurrences, four were at a gestational age 1–3 weeks earlier than the first abruption.

Abruptio Placentae (AP)

◈ *Johns Hopkins Manual of Gynecology and Obstetrics, 3rd*

- ***Abruptio placentae (AP) is the premature separation of the normally implanted placenta*** from the uterine wall due to uterine vessel hemorrhage into the decidua basalis.
- Placental abruption accounts for one-third of all antepartum bleeding.
- AP has a recurrence rate of ***5–17%*** after an episode in one previous pregnancy and ***25%*** after an episode in two previous pregnancies.
- When the abruption results in a stillbirth, there is a 7% incidence of a stillbirth in future pregnancies
- Although many cases continue to be idiopathic, AP is associated with maternal hypertension, ***advanced maternal age, multiparity,*** cocaine use, tobacco use, chorioamnionitis and trauma.
- Patients with chronic hypertension, superimposed ***pre-eclampsia, or severe pre-eclampsia*** have a fivefold increased risk of severe abruption compared to normotensive counterparts.

Table *(William Obs.)*: **Risk Factors for Placental Abruption**

Risk Factor	Relative Risk
Increased age and parity	1.3–1.5
Preeclampsia	2.1–4.0
Chronic hypertension	1.8–3.0
Preterm ruptured membranes	2.4–4.9
Multifetal gestation	2.1
Hydramnios	2.0
Cigarette smoking	1.4–1.9
Thrombophilias	3–7
Cocaine use	NA
Prior abruption	10–25
Uterine leiomyoma	NA

179. Ans. b. T.vaginali..., c. Metroni..., d. Strab...

[Ref: Shaws 15th/121; Dutta Gynaecology 5th/148; Novak's Gynaecology 14th/542-44; Harrison 17th/826; Shaw's Textbook of Gynaecology 14th /117-18130-33; William Obstetrics 23rd/226]

***"Candida vaginitis:** The discharge is thick & curdy white" (Dutta Gynaecology 5th/161)*

***"Trichomonas vaginitis:** It is caused by trichomonas vaginalis, a pear-shaped unicellular **flagellate protozoa**" (Dutta Gynaecology 5th/159)*

***"Trichomonas vaginitis:** On speculum examination, mucosa of the portio vaginalis part of cervix appear like **strawberry**" (Dutta Gynaecology 5th/160)*

***"Infection in genital tract** may be responsible for sporadic spontaneous abortion but its relation to recurrent abortion is inconclusive" (Dutta Obs. 7th/167)*

Table *(Harrison 19th/873)*: **Diagnostic Features and Management of Vaginal Infection**

Feature	Normal Vaginal Examination	Vulvovaginal Candidiasis	Trichomonal Vaginitis
Etiology	Uninfected; lactobacilli predominant	Candida albicans[Q]	Trichomonas vaginalis[Q]
Typical symptoms	None	Vulvar itching and/or irritation	Profuse purulent discharge; **vulvar itching**
Discharge			
Amount	Variable; usually scant	Scant	Often profuse
Color	Clear or slightly white	Curdy White	White or yellow
Consistency	Nonhomogeneous, floccular	Clumped; adherent plaques	Homogeneous
Inflammation of vulvar or vaginal epithelium	None	Erythema of vaginal epithelium, introitus; vulvar dermatitis, fissures common	***Erythema*** of vaginal and vulvar epithelium; colpitis macularis
pH of vaginal fluid	Usually ≤4.5	Usually ≤4.5	Usually ≥5.0
Amine ("fishy") odor with 10% KOH	None	None	May be present
Microscopy	Normal epithelial cells; lactobacilli predominant	Leukocytes, epithelial cells; mycelia or pseudomycelia in up to 80% of C. albicans culture-positive persons with typical symptoms	Leukocytes; motile trichomonads seen in 80–90% of symptomatic patients, less often in the absence of symptoms
Usual treatment	None	Azole cream, tablet, or suppository—*e.g.*, miconazole 100-mg vaginal suppository or clotrimazole 100-mg vaginal tablet, once daily for 7 days Fluconazole, 150 mg orally (single dose)	Metronidazole or tinidazole, 2 g orally (single dose) Metronidazole, 500 mg PO bid for 7 days

180. Ans. b. LNG..., d. Suppress..., e. No...

[Ref: Shaws 15th/121; Dutta Gynaecology 5th/148; Novak's Gynaecology 14th/542-44;Harrison 19th/873; Shaw's Textbook of Gynaecology 14th /117-18130-33;William Obstetrics 23rd/226]

Mirena

◈ *Shaws 15th/304-05*

- *It induces strong & uniform **suppression of endometrium.** Cervical mucous become very scanty" (Dutta Gynaecology 5th/459)*
- Total amount of LNG is 52 mg & it is released at the rate of 20 μg/day
- The LNG IUD can be used for at ***least 7 years*** & probably 10 years *(Park 21st/460)*
- *"LNG IUD device is to be **replaced every 5yr**" (Dutta obs 7th/538)*
- Mirena IUCD is employed to control menorrhagia
- It ***directly suppresses endometrium*** with minimal side effects
- ***It has no action on ovaries*** therefore, estrogen & progesterone level remain normal *(Shaws 15th/304)*
- Mirena IUS thickens the cervical mucus, thins the endometrial lining and may also alter tubal transport. The Mirena IUS is approved for 5 years of use and can also be used to treat menorrhagia and other menstrual disorders.
- **Advantages:** Highly effective at preventing pregnancy, immediately effective after insertion with prompt return of fertility after removal, offers long-term protection.
- Mirena IUS may also reduce menstrual blood loss and may decrease risk for endometrial cancer.
- **Disadvantage:** Slightly difficult to insert, take 3 months before it become effective, ***amenorrhoea occur*** in 20-25% which is not desirable in younger women etc.

181. Ans. c. Can...

[Ref: Shaws 15th/237; Dutta obstetrics 7th/549; Dutta Gynaecology 5th/459, 461]

Levonorgestrel (LNG) as Postcoital Contraceptive

- *"**LNG as Postcoital contraception:** One tablet (0.75 mg LNG) should be taken within 72 hours of unprotected intercourse & another within 12 hours later. Alternately two tablets can be taken as single dose"-Shaws 15th/237*

◈ *Shaws 15th/237*

- *LNG prevent ovulation & cause desynchronization of endometrium*
- *It can be offered to a lactating women*
- *It has no oestrogen & so no estrogen associated side effects*
- *It can be offered to hypertensive, cardiac & diabetic woman*

182. Ans. b. Forms..., c. Fetus..., d. Protects...

[Ref: Embryology by I. B. Singh 8th/75; Dutta Obstetrics 7th/39; Gray's 40th/181; William's Obstetrics 23rd/88-89; Langman's Embryology]

*"In **first half of pregnancy**, the composition of the fluid is **almost identical to a transudate of plasma.** But in **late pregnancy**, the composition is **very much altered mainly due to contamination of fetal urinary metabolites**" (Dutta Obstetrics 7th/39)*

"The **respiratory function of the placenta** makes the ***fetal oxygen supply and fetal carbon dioxide removal possible***"- *(Langman's Embryology)*

Amniotic Fluid

Embryology by I. B. Singh 8th/75

- *There is constant exchange of water b/w the amniotic fluid & maternal blood, the water being completely replaced every three hours.*
- *Sometime in fifth month the **fetus begins to swallow amniotic fluid***
- This fluid is absorbed (through the gut) into fetal blood & is transferred through the placenta to maternal blood
- When the fetal kidney start working the fetus passes urine into the amniotic fluid. This does not cause harm because fetal urine is made up mostly of water (metabolic wastes being removed from blood by the placenta & not through the kidneys)

Table: *(Dutta Obstetrics 7th/37)*

Production	Removal
• Transudation of maternal serum across the placental membranes • Transudation from fetal circulation across the umbilical cord or placental membranes • Secretion from amniotic epithelium • ***Transudation of fetal plasma through the highly permeable fetal skin before it is keratinized at 20th week*** • Fetal urine-daily output at term is about 400-1200 ml • ***Fetal lung fluid that enters the amniotic cavity to add to its volume***	• *Fetus swallows about 400-700 ml of liquor every day* • Intramembranous absorption of water & solutes (200-500 ml/day) from the amniotic compartment to fetal circulation through the fetal surface of the placenta

Langman's Embryology

- The amniotic cavity is filled with a clear, watery fluid that is produced in part by amniotic cells but is derived primarily from maternal blood.
- During the early months of pregnancy, the embryo is suspended by its umbilical cord in this fluid, which serves as a protective cushion. ***The fluid (a) Absorbs jolts, (b) Prevents adherence of the embryo to the amnion and (c) Allows for fetal movements.***
- The volume of amniotic fluid is replaced every 3 hours.

Amniotic Fluid: Composition

Dutta Obstetrics 7th/39

- **The composition includes: *Water (98-99%) & solid (1-2%)***
- **Solid**
  - Organic
    - Protein-0.3mg%
    - NPN-30mg%
    - Total lipids-50mg%
    - ***Glucose-20mg%***
    - Uric acid-4mg%
    - Hormones (prolactin, insulin & rennin)
    - Urea-30mg%
    - Creatinine-2mg%
  - **Inorganic:** Initially concentration of Na, Cl & K is almost the same as found in maternal blood. As pregnancy advances, there may slight fall in Na & K concentration, whereas the K concentration remains unaltered
  - Suspended particle
- It ***cushions the fetus against severe injury***; provides a medium in which the fetus can move easily; may be a source of fetal nutrients; and, in early pregnancy, is *essential for fetal lung development.*
- During late pregnancy, the amniotic fluid contains increasing quantities of particulate *material, including desquamated cells of fetal origin; lanugo and scalp hair; vernix caseosa; a few leukocytes; and small quantities of albumin, urates and other organic and inorganic salts.* The calcium content of amniotic fluid is low (5.5 mg/dL), but the electrolyte concentration is otherwise equivalent to that of maternal plasma.

183. Ans. b. Boun..., e. Its...

[Ref: Dutta's Obstetrics 7th/90-91; William's Obstetrics 23rd/32]

Obstetrical Outlet

Dutta's Obstetrics 7th/90-91

- *It is the segment of the pelvis **bounded above by the plane of least pelvic dimensions & below by the anatomical outlet***
- *Its **anterior wall is deficient** at the pubic arch; its **lateral walls** are formed by ischial bones & the **posterior wall** includes whole of the coccyx*
- ***Shape: It is antero-posteriorly oval***
- **Plane:** *The plane is otherwise known as **plane of least pelvic dimensions or narrow pelvic plane.** The plane extends from the lower border of the pubis symphysis to the tip of ischial spines & posteriorly to meet the tip of the 5th sacral vertebrae. It is narrowest plane in pelvis & roughly corresponds to the origin of levator ani muscle*
- **Diameters:** *Transverse (Syn-Bispinous 10.5 cm), Antero-posterior (11cm) & Posterior sagittal (5 cm)*

- **Axis:** *It is represented by a line joining the centre of the plane with the sacral promontory. Its direction is almost vertical*

184. Ans. **b. BP...**

[Ref: Dutta's Obstetrics 7th/220-228; William's Obstetrics 23rd/734, 708; CDTOG 10th/ch-19]

Note: B.P ≥ 160/110 is indication for active management

*"**Termination of pregnancy** is the only cure for preeclampsia. **Headache, visual disturbances or epigastric pain** is indicative that convulsion may be imminent & **oliguria** is another ominous sign. Severe preeclampsia demands anticonvulsant & usually antihypertensive therapy followed by delivery" (William's Obstetrics 23rd/729)*

Management of Preeclampsia Johns Hopkins

◈ *Manual of Gynecology and Obstetrics, The, 3rd Edition*

- In the management of preeclampsia, with few exceptions, maternal interests are best served by immediate delivery. However, this approach may not be in the best interest of the fetus. In the case of extreme prematurity, for example, the ***fetus may benefit from a period of expectant management*** during which corticosteroids are administered to accelerate fetal maturation.
- ***The decision to proceed with immediate delivery versus expectant management is based upon several factors, including disease severity, fetal maturity, maternal and fetal condition and cervical status.***
- For the purposes of management, preeclampsia may be classified as mild or severe
- Severe preeclampsia mandates hospitalization. Delivery is indicated if the gestational age is 34 weeks or greater, fetal pulmonary is confirmed, or evidence of deteriorating maternal or fetal status is seen. ***The goal of antihypertensive therapy is to achieve a systolic blood pressure < 160 mm Hg and a diastolic blood pressure < 105 mm Hg.***
- **Expectant management** is ***contraindicated in the presence of fetal compromise, uncontrollable hypertension, eclampsia, DIC, HELLP syndrome, cerebral edema, pulmonary edema, or evidence of cerebral or hepatic hemorrhage.***

"Criteria for Severe Pre-eclampsia

- A persistent SBP of ≥ 160 mm Hg systolic or DBP of ≥110 mm Hg
- Persistent severe epigastric pain
- Cerebral or visual disturbances
- ***Oliguria (<400ml/24hr***
- ***Protein excretion of > 5gm/day***
- Platelet count <100, 000/mm^3
- HELLP syndrome
- Retinal haemorrhage, exudates or papilledema
- ***Intrauterine growth restriction of the foetus***
- ***Pulmonary oedema"*** *(Dutta's Obstetrics 6th/226)*

Indications for Delivery with Early Onset Severe Preeclampsia

◈ *William's Obstetrics 23rd/729*

- Persistent severe headache or visual changes
- Eclampsia
- Shortness of breath
- Chest tightness with rales &/or SaO_2<94% breathing room air
- Pulmonary edema
- Uncontrolled severe hypertension despite treatment
- Oliguria <500 ml/24 hr or serum creatinine ≥ 1.5 mg/dl
- Persistent platelet counts <1, 00000/μ
- Suspected abruption, progressive labour &/or ruptured membrane

Table *(CDTOG)*: **Classification of Preeclampsia**

Mild Preeclampsia	Severe Preeclampsia
Blood pressure ≥140/90 mm Hg but < 160/110 mm Hg	Blood pressure ≥ 160 mm Hg systolic or ≥110 mm Hg diastolic on two occasions at least 6 hours apart while the patient is on bed rest
Proteinuria ≥300 mg/24 h but < 5 g/24 h	*Proteinuria* of 5 g or higher in 24-hour urine specimen or 3+ or greater on two random urine samples collected at least 4 hours apart
Asymptomatic	*Oliguria* < 500 mL in 24 hours
	Cerebral or visual disturbances
	Pulmonary edema or cyanosis
	Epigastric or right upper quadrant pain
	Impaired liver function; *Thrombocytopenia*
	Fetal growth restriction

Table *(William's Obstetrics 23rd/708)*: **Indications of Severity of Hypertensive Disorders during Pregnancy**

Abnormality	Mild	Severe
Diastolic blood pressure	< 100 mm Hg	110 mm Hg or higher
Proteinuria	Trace to 1+	Persistent 2+ or more
Headache	Absent	Present
Visual disturbances	Absent	Present
Upper abdominal pain	Absent	Present
Oliguria	Absent	Present
Convulsion (eclampsia)	Absent	Present
Serum creatinine	Normal	Elevated

Contd...

Abnormality	Mild	Severe
Thrombocytopenia	Absent	Present
Liver enzyme elevation	Minimal	Marked
Fetal growth restriction	Absent	Obvious
Pulmonary edema	Absent	Present

185. Ans. b. Previous..., d. Undiagnosed...

[Ref: Dutta Gyanaecology 5th/459; Park 20th/427, 19th/395; Dutta Obstetrics 6th/537; Shaw's Gynaecology 15th/228-29, 14th/205]

"IUCD can be inserted in HIV-positive woman on medication"- *(Shaw's Gynaecology 15th/229)*

Contraindications of IUCD

- *(Park)*

I- ABSOLUTE[Q]

- Suspected pregnancy
- *Pelvic Inflammatory disease (PID)*[Q]
- *Vaginal bleeding of undiagnosed aetiology*[Q]
- Cancer of the cervix, uterus or adnexal & other pelvic tumours
- *Previous ectopic pregnancy*[Q]

II- RELATIVE

- Anaemia
- Menorrhagia
- History of PID since last pregnancy
- Purulent cervical discharge
- Distortions of the uterine cavity due to congenital malformations, fibroids
- Unmotivated person

Other Contraindication

- *Dutta obstetrics 6th/537; Shaw's Gynaecology 14th/205*

- Nullipara[Q]
- *HIV (STD) positive women*[Q]
- Severe dysmenorrhoea
- Prolapse uterus because of chance of ascending infection
- Within 6 wks following caesarean section
- Dysfunctional uterine bleeding
- *Heart disease*: risk of infection
- Diabetic women who are not well controlled
- Levonorgestrel IUCD in breast cancer

The Ideal IUCD Candidate

- *Who has borne at least one child*[Q]
- *Has no history of pelvic disease*[Q]
- *Has normal menstrual periods*[Q]
- *Is willing to check the IUCD tail*

186. Ans. b. Cause r..., c. Cause pul..

[Ref: Dutta obstetrics 7th/507; Katzung 12th/185, 1042; William's Obstetrics 23rd/989, 313, 319; Nelson 18th/693]

"Fetal side effects of ACE inhibitors-*Oligohydramnios, IUGR, fetal renal tubular dysgenesis, neonatal renal failure & pulmonary hypoplasia*" *(Dutta obstetrics 7th/507)*

"The use of **ACE inhibitors** is ***contraindicated during the second and third trimesters of pregnancy because of the risk of fetal hypotension, anuria and renal failure, sometimes associated with fetal malformations or death.*** Recent evidence also implicates **first trimester** exposure to ACE inhibitors in increased teratogenic risk" *(Katzung 12th/185)*

Table *(Katzung 12th/1042)*: **Drugs with significant adverse effects on the fetus**

Drug	Trimester	Effect
ACE inhibitors	All, especially second and third	Renal damage

Angiotensin-Converting Enzyme Inhibitors

- *William's Obstetrics 23rd/319*

- These drugs disrupt the renin-angiotensin system, which has been shown to be ***essential for normal renal development.*** Interruption of angiotensin II type-1 receptor–mediated effects during embryogenesis in experimental animals results ***in renal papillary and tubular atrophy and a significant impairment in urinary concentrating ability***
- ACE inhibitors appear to have similar effects on human fetuses. In addition, they may provoke prolonged ***fetal hypotension and hypoperfusion,*** thus initiating a sequence of events leading to renal ischemia, renal tubular dysgenesis and then anuria.
- The resulting oligohydramnios prevents normal lung development and causes limb contractures. Reduced perfusion also causes growth restriction, relative limb shortening and maldevelopment of the calvarium.
- Because these changes occur during the fetal period, they are termed *ACE inhibitor fetopathy* (exposure must occur during a critical developmental period).

Exposure Must Occur During a Critical Developmental Period

Gestation is divided into three periods and syndromes resulting from teratogen exposure are named accordingly. Exposures within the first 8 weeks result in an *embryopathy* and after 8 weeks, a *fetopathy.*

- The *preimplantation period* is the 2 weeks from fertilization to implantation and has traditionally been called the "all or none" period.
- The *embryonic period,* from the second through the eighth week following conception, encompasses organogenesis and is thus the most crucial with regard to structural malformations.
- Maturation and functional development continue after 9 weeks and during this *fetal period,* certain organs remain vulnerable.

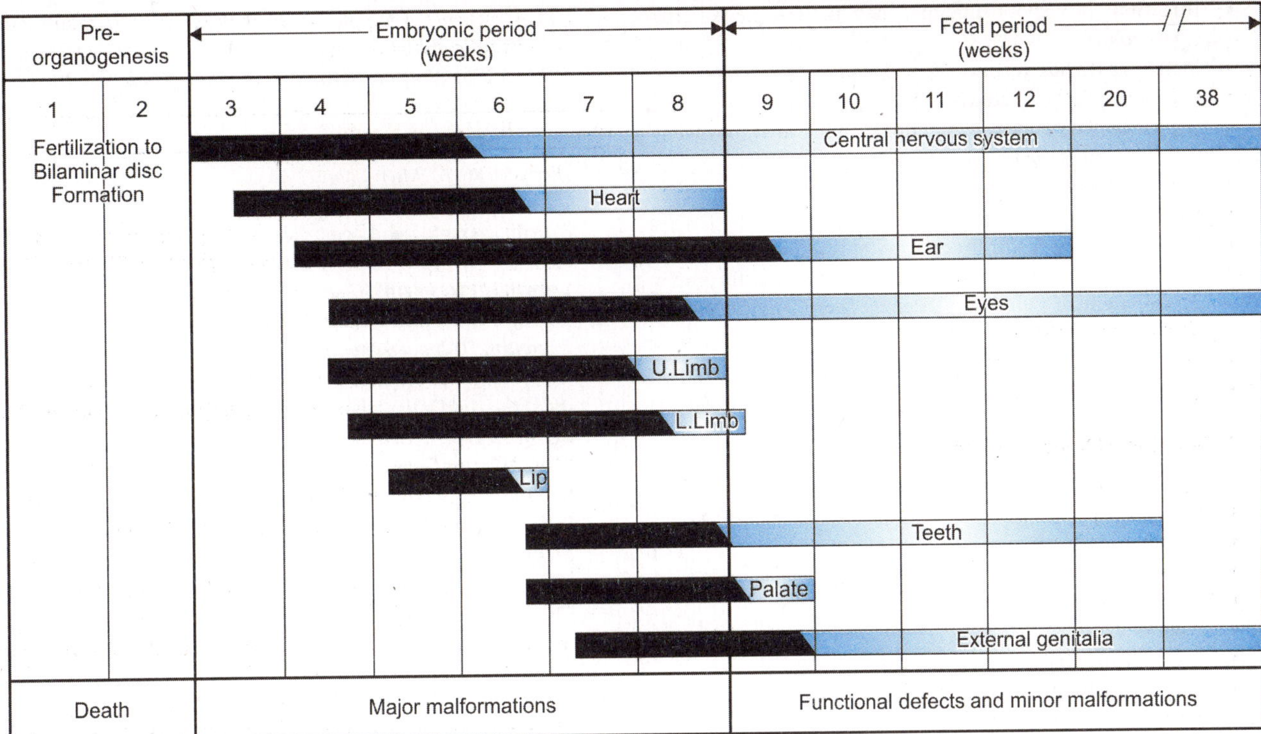

Fig: Development of fetus

187. Ans. b. Estrogen..., c. LH..., d. 100 ml...

[Ref: Ganong 25th/402Shaw 15th /30-32, 215-16, 222, 46-48; Dutta's Textbook of Gyanecology 5th/83; Johns Hopkins Manual of Gynecology and Obstetrics, The, 3rd Edition]

*"The **duration of bleeding** is about **3-5 days & estimated blood loss is between 50-200 ml**" (Shaw 15th /46)*

*"The phase of the **menstrual cycle** which starts when regeneration of menstruating endometrium is complete & lasts until the 14th day of cycle is referred to as the **proliferative phase or oestrogenic phase**" (Shaw 15th /32*

"The maximum peak of estrogen secretion is seen about 48 hours before ovulation, whereas the LH peak occurs about 24-36 hours before ovulation" *(Shaw 15th /46)*

*"A surge in LH secretion triggers ovulation, & **ovulation normally occurs about 9 hr after peak of LH surge** at midcycle" (Ganong 25th/402)*

"Ovulation normally occurs about 9 hours after the peak of the LH surge at midcycle. The ovum lives approximately 72 hours after it is extruded from the follicle but probably is fertilizable for less than half this time" *(Johns Hopkins Manual of Gynecology and Obstetrics, The, 3rd Edition*

Indicators of Ovulation

- *Johns Hopkins Manual*

- Knowing when during the menstrual cycle ovulation occurs is important in increasing fertility or, conversely, in contraception.
- A convenient but retrospective indicator of the ***time of ovulation is a rise in the basal body temperature.*** The cause of the temperature change at the time of ovulation is unknown but probably is due to the ***increase in progesterone secretion,*** as progesterone is thermogenic.
- A rise in urinary LH occurs during the rise in circulating LH that causes ovulation and this increase can be measured as another indicator of ovulation.

PAEDIATRICS

188. Ans. a. Hear.., b. Respi..., c. Necroti...

[Ref: Dutta's Obstetrics 7th/457-58; O.P.Ghai 7th/129; Nelson 18th/701-710]

*"**Necrotizing enterocolitis** occurs among **premature infants** under stress in the first week of life" (O.P.Ghai 7th/138)*

"Respiratory distress syndrome or hyaline membrane disease is common in preterm babies less than 34 weeks of gestation" *(O.P.Ghai 7th/143)*

"**Meconium aspiration syndrome** usually occurs in ***term or post term babies***" *(O.P.Ghai 7th/145)*

Preterm Neonate

- *Complication Dutta's Obstetrics 7th/457-58; O.P.Ghai 7th/129*

- **Respiratory syndrome:** Pulmonry oedema, Intra-alveolar haemorrhage, Idiopathic ***respiratory distress syndrome*** & Bronchopulmonary dysplasia

- **Infection:** Bronchopneumonia, meningitis & necrotizing enterocolitis
- Metabolic (hypoglycemia, hypocalcemia)
- Retinopathy of prematurity
- **Asphyxia:** Anatomical & functional immaturity, intraventricular haemorrhage
- Cerebral haemorrhage
- Hypothermia
- Fetal shock
- **Heart failure:** Precipitated by asphyxia with rapid development of pulmonary edema. There may be ***patent Ductus arteriosus***
- Jaundice
- Anaemia

IUGR Babies: Major Problems

◈ *O.P. Ghai 7th/129*

- Perinatal asphyxia
- Meconium aspiration
- Hypothermia
- Hypoglycemia
- Feed intolerance
- Polycythemia
- Growth retardation

Table *(Nelson 18th/705)*: **Neonatal Problems Associated with Premature Infants**

Respiratory

- **Respiratory distress syndrome** (hyaline membrane disease); Bronchopulmonary dysplasia; Pneumothorax, pneumomediastinum; interstitial emphysema Congenital pneumonia; Pulmonary hypoplasia; Pulmonary hemorrhage; Apnea

Cardiovascular

- Patent ductus arteriosus; Hypotension; Hypertension
- Bradycardia (with apnea); Congenital malformations

Hematologic

- Anemia (early or late onset)
- Subcutaneous, organ (liver, cranial, adrenal) hemorrhage[*]
- Hydrops—Immune or nonimmune

Gastrointestinal

- Poor gastrointestinal function—poor motility[*]
- Necrotizing enterocolitis
- Hyperbilirubinemia—direct and indirect[*]
- Congenital anomalies producing polyhydramnios
- Spontaneous gastrointestinal isolated perforation

Metabolic-Endocrine

- Hypocalcemia; Hypoglycemia; Hyperglycemia; Hypothermia

Central Nervous System

- Intraventricular hemorrhage; Periventricular leukomalacia; Hypoxic-ischemic encephalopathy; Retinopathy of prematurity; Hypotonia
- Congenital malformations; Kernicterus (bilirubin encephalopathy)

189. Ans. a. Tetralogy..., b. TGA

[Ref: Ghai 7th/401, 409, 413]

*"**TOF: Cyanosis may be present from birth** or make its appearance some years after birth" (Ghai 7th/409)*

*"**TGA:** Patients of complete TGA with intact ventricular septum are **cyanotic at birth**" (Ghai 7th/413)*

PDA, ASD & VSD are acyanotic condition (Ghai 7th/401)

190. Ans. d. Gro..., e. Height...

[Ref: Ghai 7th/6; Nelson 18th/57]

"On an average, a child gains about ***2 kg every year between the ages of 3 & 7 years & 3 kg per year after that till the pubertal growth spurts begin***" *(Ghai 7th/6)*

"**Length or height:** *The infant measures 50 cm at birth, 60 cm at 3 months, 70 cm at 9 months, 75 cm at 1 year & 90 cm at 2 years. A normal Indian child is 100 cm tall at age of 4 & ½ years. There after, the child gains **about 6 cm in height every year until the age of 12 years**" (Ghai 7th/6)*

"**Head circumference:** Head growth is rapid especially in the first half of infancy. The head growth slows considerably thereafter. Beginning at 33-35 cm at birth the head circumference gains 2 cm per month for first 3 month, 1 cm per month b/w 3-6 month & half cm per month for the rest of the first year of life. The mean head circumference is 40 cm at 3 month, 43 cm at 6 month, 46-47 cm at 1 year, 48 cm at 2 years. By ***12 years it is 52 cm***" *(Ghai 7th/6)*

Physical Development During Middle Childhood (6–11 yr of Age)

◈ *Nelson 18th/57*

- Growth during the period ***averages 3–3.5 kg (7 lb) and 6–7 cm (2.5 in) per year.***
- Growth occurs **discontinuously,** in 3–6 irregularly timed spurts each year, with each growth spurt lasting, on average, 8 wk.
- The ***head grows only 2–3 cm in circumference throughout the entire period,*** reflecting a slowing of brain growth. Myelinization is complete by 7 yr of age.

191. Ans. b. Repetitive...

[Ref: Nelson 18th/134, 136, 156; Kaplon Psychiatry 10th/1201-04]

Asperger Disorder

- "**Asperger syndrome:** It is ***four times more likely to occur in males than in females*** and usually is first diagnosed in children between the ages of 2 and 6" *(http: //www.webmd.com/brain/autism/mental-health-aspergers-syndrome)*
- The common characteristics include ***average or above-average intelligence***" *(http: //www.betterhealth.vic.gov.au/)*
- There is ***no clinically significant general delay in spoken or receptive language or cognitive development.*** Self-help skills, adaptive behavior and curiosity about the environment during the first 3 years should be at a level consistent with ***normal intellectual development***" *(Kaplon Psychiatry 10th/1204)*

◈ *Nelson 18th/136*

- Children with Asperger disorder have a qualitative impairment in the development of reciprocal social interaction, *often showing repetitive behaviors* and restricted, obsessional, idiosyncratic interests. They have deficits in nonverbal and pragmatic aspects of communication (facial expressions, gestures).

- They do not have the severe language impairments that characterize autism. They are awkward and clumsy and have unusual postures and gait.
- To meet the **diagnostic criteria** for Asperger syndrome, a child must manifest impairments in social interactions and show restrictive, ***repetitive patterns of behavior, interests,*** or achievements with other people; these disturbances must cause significant impairments in social or occupational functioning.
- **Unlike children with autism**, those diagnosed with Asperger syndrome have a history of ***normal language milestones,*** with single words used by age 2 yr and communicative phrases used by age 3 yr. There are often similar traits in family members.
- This disorder may represent a ***form of high-functioning autism*** (children with autism who do not have cognitive impairment), although this distinction remains controversial.

Table *(Nelson 18th/134)*: **Pervasive Developmental Disorders/ Autism Spectrum Disorders**

Autism	Asperger Syndrome	Rett Syndrome
Delayed and disordered communication	Similar to autism except language skills relatively intact	Almost always affects girls
Atypical social interaction	Usually not congnitively delayed	Regression in skills between 6 and 18 mo of age
Restricted range of interests		Repetitive hand movements
Onset before 3 yr of age		

192. Ans. a. Quality..., c. Treatment..., e. Stereotyped...

[Ref: Nelson 18th/133-36, 146; Ghai 7th/40-41; CPDT 18th/186, 187; Kaplan Synopsis of Psychiatry 10th/294, 1194]

Autistic Disorder

"Autistic disorder is characterized by symptoms from each of the following three categories: ***qualitative impairment in social interaction, impairment in communication and restricted repetitive and stereotyped patterns of behavior or interests"*** *(Kaplan Synopsis of Psychiatry 10th/1191)*

- ***"Autism i.e, marked impairment in reciprocal, social & interpersonal interaction"*** *(Ahuja 6th/177)*
- ***"Early measurable diagnostic symptoms and signs of*** autism ***include poor eye contact***[Q]***, little symbolic play***[Q]***, limited joint attention or orienting to one's name***[Q] ***and reliance on nonverbal communication with delay in use of words. Stereotypical body movements, a marked need for sameness*** *and a very narrow range of interests, are also common. The autistic child is often withdrawn and* ***spends hours in solitary play***[Q]***. Ritualistic behavior prevails,*** *reflecting the child's need to maintain a consistent, predictable environment" (Nelson 18th/133)*

"**Treatment of Autism**: There is compelling evidence that intensive behavioral therapy, beginning before 3 yr of age and ***targeted toward speech and language development,*** is successful in improving both language capacity and later social functioning" *(Nelson 18th/136)*

Typical Features of Autism: *Short Review*

- *Autism develops before 36 month*[Q] *of age and is typically diagnosable at 18 month of age*
- *Abnormal language and speech development (Abnormal communication)*
  - *Inability to develop normal* ***social skill***[Q] *(lack of eye contact gestures and facial expression)*
  - *Understand little or no language (therefore* ***fail to acquire speech***[Q]*)*
  - *Deficient comprehension and communicative use of* ***speech and gesture.***
- *Behavioural peculiarities such as ritualized repetitive or stereotyped behaviour and rigidity*
- ***Difficulty in concentration***[Q]
- *Severe deficit in social responsiveness and interpersonal skills*
  - *Intrusive sterotypes (repetitive behaviour) together with inability to concentrate may prevent children from engaging in meaningful activity or social interaction (difficulty in making friends)*[Q]
  - *Do not engage in pretended play (which starts before age of 2 in normal children)*
- *Mental retardation (about 75% of children with autism are mentally retarded)*[Q]
- *Epilepsy*[Q] *develops in one fifth to one third of autistic individuals*
- *EEG abnormalities*[Q] *are noted in half of the patients.*
- ***Treatment*** *is most successful when geared toward the individual's particular behavior patterns and language function. Parent education, training and support are always indicated and pharmacotherapy for certain target symptoms may be helpful.*

193. Ans. b. HIV..., d. Passive...

[Ref: Nelson 18th/1427-36; Dutta Obstetrics 7th/301]

Diagnosis of HIV Infection in Infants

◈ *Nelson 18th/1435-36*

- All infants born to HIV-infected mothers ***test antibody-positive at birth*** because of passive transfer of maternal HIV antibody across the placenta during gestation. Most uninfected infants ***lose maternal antibody between 6 and 12 month of age*** and are known as **seroreverters.**
- Because a small proportion of uninfected infants continues to test HIV ***antibody positive for up to 18 mo of age,*** positive IgG antibody tests, including the rapid tests, **cannot be used to make a definitive diagnosis of HIV infection**

in infants v The presence of IgA or IgM anti-HIV in the infant's circulation can indicate HIV infection, because these immunoglobulin classes ***do not cross the placenta;*** however, IgA and IgM anti-HIV assays have been both insensitive and nonspecific and therefore are not valuable for clinical use.

- In any child >18 months of age, demonstration of ***IgG antibody to HIV*** by a repeatedly reactive enzyme immunoassay (EIA) and confirmatory test ***(immunoblot or immunofluorescence assay)*** establishes the diagnosis of HIV infection.
- Viral diagnostic assays, such as ***HIV DNA or RNA PCR, HIV culture, or HIV p24 antigen immune-dissociated p24 (ICD-p24),*** are considerably more useful in young infants, allowing a definitive diagnosis in most infected infants by **1–6 months of age.**
- By **4–6 months of age,** the ***HIV culture and/or PCR identify all infected infants.*** *HIV DNA PCR is the preferred virologic assay in developed countries.* Almost 40% of infected newborns have ***positive test results in the 1st 2 days of life, with >90% testing positive by 2 wk of age.***
- **Plasma HIV RNA assays,** which detect viral replication, may be *more sensitive than DNA PCR* for early diagnosis, but data are limited.

Table *(Nelson 18th/1435)*: **Laboratory Diagnosis of HIV Infection**

Test	Comment
HIV DNA PCR	***Preferred test to diagnose HIV-1 subtype B infection in infants and children younger than 18 months of age;*** highly sensitive and specific by 2 wk of age and available; performed on peripheral blood mononuclear cells. False negatives can occur in non-B subtype HIV-1 infections
HIV p24 Ag	Less sensitive, false-positive results during 1 month of life, variable results; **not recommended**
ICD p24 Ag	Negative test result does not rule out infection; **not recommended**
HIV culture	Expensive, not easily available, requires up to 4 week to do test; **not recommended**
HIV RNA PCR	Not recommended for routine testing of infants and children younger than 18 months of age, because a negative result cannot be used to exclude HIV infection definitively. Preferred test to identify non-B subtype HIV-1 infections.

Transmission of HIV

◈ *Nelson 18th/1429*

- Transmission of HIV-1 occurs via sexual contact, parenteral exposure to blood, or ***vertical transmission from mother to child. The primary route of infection in the pediatric population is vertical transmission, accounting for almost all new cases.***
- **Vertical transmission** of HIV can occur before **(intra-uterine),** during **(intrapartum),** or after delivery (through **breast-feeding**).

194. Ans. b. Ectopia..., e. Arachnodactyly

[Ref: Khurana 5th/214-16; Parson 20th/507, 260; Harrison 19th/434e-2, 2512, 18th/1822, 3212, 3216; Nelson 18th/2890, 536-539, 2304]

"**Arachnodactyly:** This feature can occur on its own, with no underlying health problems. However, it can also be associated with certain medical conditions. Examples include: *Marfan syndrome, Ehlers-Danlos syndrome, Loeys–Dietz syndrome and homocystinuria. (wiki)*

"**Marfan syndrome:** Examination of the musculoskeletal system discloses dolichostenomelia (long, thin limbs) and the ***arm span substantially exceeds the height*** (>1.05 times height). The lower segment (distance from pubis to heel) is increased in comparison to the upper segment (height minus lower segment) and contributes to a diminished upper segment: lower segment ratio (U_s/L_s). Hand findings are nonspecific and include long, thin fingers ***(arachnodactyly)*** that are hyperextensible" *(Nelson 18th/2890)*

"**Marfan syndrome:** Tall stature with an abnormally low U_s/L_s ratio or an ***increased span-to-height ratio (i.e., >1.05)*** is the most consistent presenting feature" *(Nelson 18th/2890*

"Affected individuals with homocystinuria manifest *skeletal abnormalities* resembling those of Marfan syndrome; they are usually tall and thin, with elongated limbs and ***arachnodactyly***. Scoliosis, pectus excavatum or carinum, genu valgum, pes cavus, high arched palate and crowding of the teeth are commonly seen. These children usually have fair complexions, blue eyes and a peculiar malar flush. Generalized osteoporosis, especially of the spine, is the main roentgenographic finding" *(Nelson 18th/536)*

"***Arachnodactyly:*** It is elongated & slender tubular bones of the hands & feet. It is found in ***Marfan' syndrome & homocystinuria*** " *(Chapman Radiology 4th/57)*

"Patients with Marfan syndrome may have arachnodactyly and a positive "wrist" *(Harrison 19th/2512, 18th/1822)*

Marfan's Syndrome

◈ *Khurana 5th/214*

- It is an autosomal dominant mesodermal dysplasia. In this condition ***lens is displaced upwards and temporally (bilaterally symmetrical).***
- Systemic anomalies include arachnodactyly (spider fingers), long extremities, hyperextensibility of joints, high arched palate and dissecting aortic aneurysm.

Homocystinuria

◈ *Khurana 5th/214-15*

- It is an autosomal recessive, inborn error of metabolism. In it the lens is usually ***subluxated downwards and nasally (Inferotemporal displacement)*** *(Parson 20th/260)*
- Systemic features are fair complexion, malar flush, mental retardation, fits and poor motor control.
- Diagnosis is established by detecting homocystine in urine by sodium nitro-prusside test.

Table (Harrison 19th/434e-2, 18th/3216): **Inherited Disorders of Amino Acid Metabolism**

Amino acid (s)	Condition	Enzyme Defect	Clinical Findings
Homocystine	Homocystinuria	Cystathionine β-synthase	Lens dislocation, thrombotic vascular disease, mental retardation, osteoporosis

Comparison b/w Marfan & Homocystinuira

- *Inheritance*
    - **Marfan's:** Autosomal dominant
    - **Homocystinuria:** Autosomal recessive
- ***Aortic incompetence:***
    - **Marfan's:** Aortic incompetence may occur
    - **Homocystinuria:** Heart rarely affected
- ***Intellectual development:***
    - **Marfan's:** Normal
    - **Homocystinuria:** Mental retardation
- ***Other principle features:***
    - ***Marfan's:*** flat feet, herniae, scoliosis; there is a 50% reduction in life expectancy
    - ***Homocystinuria:*** osteoporosis, recurrent thromboembolism; characteristic laboratory features -plasma methionine and homocystine levels are elevated, homocystine is excreted in the urine, plasma cystine levels are reduced, positive urine cyanide-nitroprusside test; response to treatment with pyridoxine

ORTHOPAEDICS

195. Ans. a. Boutonniere..., b. Swan..., c. Mallet...

[Ref: www.jointpain.expert.net; Apley 8th/51-58; Maheswari 5th/288, 3rd/245-246, 257-58; Harrison 19th/2220, 17th/2086-87;Apley 8th/339]

"**Dupuytren's contracture:** ***Flexion of MP & PIP (DIP is not involved)"*** *(Maheswari 3rd/257)*

"**Mallet finger:** *The patient is unable to extend the terminal phalanx although the* ***distal interphalangeal joint can be extended passively"*** *(Guyton 40th/878)*

"**Mallet finger (baseball finger)** is an injury of the extensor digitorum tendon of the fingers at the ***distal interphalangeal joint (DIP).*** It results from hyperflexion of the extensor digitorum tendon and usually occurs when a ball (such as a softball, basketball, or volleyball), while being caught, hits an outstretched finger and jams it -creating a ruptured or stretched extensor digitorum tendon" *(orthoinfo.aaos.org/topic.cfm)*

Trigger Finger

"A disparity in size between the flexor tendon and the surrounding retinacular pulley system, most commonly at the level of the first annular (A1) pulley, results in ***difficulty flexing or extending the finger*** and the "triggering" phenomenon. The label of trigger finger is used because when the finger unlocks, it pops back suddenly, as if releasing a trigger on a gun"

"While difficulty extending the **proximal interphalangeal joint** may persist for months, it benefits from exercises to stretch the finger straighter" *(http: //en. wikipedia.org/wiki)*

"The initial complaint associated with **trigger finger** may be of a painless clicking with digital manipulation. Further development of the condition can cause the catching or popping to become painful with both flexion and extension and be related as occurring at ***either the metacarpophalangeal (MCP) or PIP joints"*** *(http: //www.ncbi.nlm.nih.gov/pmc/article)*

"**Boutonniere deformity**[Q] – *Flexion contracture of the PIP joints*[Q] *&* ***extension of the DIP joints"*** *(Guyton 40th/878; Maheswari 3rd/245-246)*

Swan Neck Deformity[q]

- It is a deformed position of the finger, in which the joint closest to the fingertip is permanently bent toward the palm while the nearest joint to the palm is bent away from it (***DIP hyperflexion with PIP hyperextension).***
- It is commonly caused by injury or inflammatory conditions like rheumatoid arthritis or sometimes familial (congenital, like ***Ehlers-Danlos syndrome)***

196. Ans. e. More...

[Ref: Nelson 18th/2808-10; Maheshwari 5th/323-324, 3rd/47; Apley 8th/426-30, 422, 427; http: //www1bpt.bridgeport.edu/~gwl/salter-harris classification. htm]

"**Slipped capital femoral epiphysis:** *It is virtually confined to children going through the pubertal growth spurt. Boys* ***(usually b/w 14 & 16 years)*** *are affected more than girls (who are, on average 2-3 year younger)" (Apley 8th/426)*

"**SCFE** is a hip disorder that affects adolescents, most often between ***12 and 15 yr of age*** and involves the displacement of the CFE from the metaphysis through the zone of hypertrophy layer of the physeal plate" *(Nelson 18th/2808)*

"Obesity is the most closely associated factor in the development of SCFE; about 65% of the patients are above the 90th percentile in weight-for-age profiles. There is a definite predilection for ***males to be affected more often than females*** and for the left hip to be affected more often than the right. Bilaterality has been reported in as many as 60% of cases, nearly half of which may be present at the time of initial presentation" *(Nelson 18th/2808)*

"Osteonecrosis and chondrolysis are the two most serious complications of SCFE. ***Osteonecrosis, or avascular necrosis,*** usually occurs as a result of injury to the retinacular vessels" *(Nelson 18th/2810)*

"**SCFE:** *Complication includes chondrolysis (7-10%) &* ***avascular necrosis of femoral head*** *(10-15%)" (ncbl.nlm.nib.gov)*

"**SCFE: Age:** ***Overweight 8-17 years old (mean age for boys 13, for girls 11 years); M: F 3: 1"*** *(Danhert Radilogy Manual 5th/72)*

Slipped Capital Femoral Epiphysis Radiopaedia.org

- The clinical symptoms and radiographic signs of SCFE vary according to the type of slip, but usually include pain in the groin, medial thigh, or knee and limitation of hip motion, especially internal rotation. Often when the hip is flexed the leg externally rotates in a *frog-leg position.*

- SCFE should be suspected in ***patients age 10–16*** who complain of vague knee pain, which may be referred pain from the hip.
- The diagnosis of SCFE usually is apparent from anteroposterior radiographs, but special views may be helpful.
- A cross-table, or true, lateral view can help determine the extent of posterior displacement of the epiphysis and a ***"frog-leg" lateral view*** best shows subtle slipping.

197. Ans. None

[Ref: Maheshwari 3rd/3-4; Apley's 8th/575-77]

Pathological Fractures

- *Maheshwari 3rd/3*
- A fractures is termed pathological when it occurs in a bone made weak by some disease
- Often, the bone breaks as a result of a trivial trauma or even spontaneously
- Osteoporosis is the commonest cause of pathological fracture; the bones most often affected are the vertebral bodies (thoracic & lumbar)

Table *(Maheshwari 3rd/3)*: **Causes of pathological fractures (Partial list)**

Localised Disease	Generalised Diseases
Inflammatory: *Pyogenic osteomyelitis, Tubercular osteomyelitis* **Neoplastic:** Giant cell tumour, osteosarcoma, Ewing's tumor **Miscellaneous:** Simple bone cyst, Aneurysmal bone cyst, Eosinophilic granuloma	**Hereditary:** *Osteogenesis imperfect,* **osteopetrosis** Acquired: ***Osteoporosis,*** Osteomalacia, rickets, scurvy, multiple myeloma, paget's disease, histiocytosis X, Gaucher's disease

"Osteochondromas are a relatively common imaging finding, accounting for 10-15% of all bone tumours and 20-50% of all benign bone tumours. Symptomatic presentation is either due to mechanical effects of the lesion, ***pathological fracture***, or malignant transformation" *(http: //radiopa edia.org/articles/osteo-chondroma; http: //www.patient.co.uk/doctor/bone-tumours; Danhert Radiology 5th/131)*

198. Ans. d. Hematogenous

[Ref: Maheshwari 5th/168, 3rd/157-162; Robbins 9th/1195, 8th/1221-23; Apley's 8th/28, 32]

"Acute osteomyelitis: This can be ***primary (haematogenous)*** *or secondary (following an open fracture or bone operation).* ***Haematogenous osteomyelitis is the commonest*** *& is often seen in children. Staphylococcus aureus is the commonest causative organism, others are streptococcus & pneumococcus" (Maheshwari 3rd/157)*

Acute Osteomyelitis

- Acute osteomyelitis is almost invariably a disease of children. The causal organism is usually **Staphylococcus aureus**[Q], less often one of the other gram-positive cocci, such as Streptococcus pyogenes or *S. pneumonia.*
- Patients with **sickle-cell disease** are prone to ***infection by salmonella***[Q]
- On X-ray, the earliest sign to appear is a periosteal new bone deposition **(Periosteal reaction)** at the **metaphysis.** It takes about 7-10 days to appear. Plain X-ray is unable to detect sequestra or sclerotic new bone for many weeks.
- *Bone scan with TC^{99} is earliest positive within 24 hours of onset of symptoms.*
- In acute osteomyelitis, metaphyseal infection is usual, the growth disc acts as a barrier to spread.

"All types of organisms, including viruses, parasites, fungi and bacteria, can produce osteomyelitis, but infections caused by ***certain pyogenic bacteria and mycobacteria are the most common"*** *(Robbins 8th/1221-23)*

"Pyogenic osteomyelitis is almost always caused by bacteria. Organisms may reach the bone by

- ***Hematogenous spread,***
- ***Extension from a contiguous site and***
- ***Direct implantation. Most cases of osteomyelitis are hematogenous in origin and develop in the long bones or vertebral bodies*** in otherwise healthy individuals. *Staphylococcus aureus* is responsible for 80% to 90% of the cases of pyogenic osteomyelitis in which an organism is recovered." *(Robbins 9th/1195, 8th/1221-23)*

199. Ans. a. Primary..., b. Periost..., c. Present..., e. Form...

[Ref: Maheshwari 5th/239-240, 3rd/218;Robbins 9th/1198-99, 8th/1225-27; Apley 8th/185-87]

Osteosarcoma

- *Maheshwari 3rd/218*
- On basis of clinical setting, this tumor is divided into 2 types-***Primary (age group 15-25 year) & Secondary (45 year onwards)***
- On basis of dominant histomorphology, this tumor is divided into-*osteoblastic, chondroid, fibroblastic & osteolytic/ telangiectatic*
- **Common sites of origin** (in decreasing order of frequency)- lower end of femur, upper end of the tibia & upper end of the humerus
- **X-ray:**
  - New bone formation in the matrix of the tumour,
  - ***Periosteal reaction,***
  - ***Cortex overlying the lesion is eroded,***
  - Codman's triangle,
  - Sun-ray appearance
- Sun-ray appearance

Osteosarcoma

- *Robbins 9th/1198-99, 8th/1221-23*
- Although the lesion can be either predominantly blastic or predominantly lytic, more commonly ***areas of bone***

production and bone destruction are present. If the tumor has broken through the cortex, a soft-tissue mass may be present at the time of diagnosis.

- Periosteal reaction may take the form of **"Codman's triangle, "** or it may have a "sunburst" or "hair on end" appearance.
- **Secondary osteosarcomas** occur at the site of another disease process. They rarely occur in young patients, but constitute almost half of the osteosarcomas in patients older than age 50 years. The most common factors associated with secondary osteosarcomas include ***Paget disease and previous radiation treatment.***
- Other **conditions** that have been reported to be associated with secondary osteosarcomas include ***fibrous dysplasia, bone infarcts, osteochondromas, chronic osteomyelitis, dedifferentiated chondrosarcomas, melorheostosis and osteogenesis imperfecta.***
- ***Cancerous cells produce bone matrix.***
- ***Osteosarcoma occurs in all age groups but has a bimodal age distribution; 75% occur in patients younger than age 20.*** The smaller second peak occurs in the elderly, who frequently suffer from conditions known to be associated with the development of osteosarcoma—Paget disease, bone infarcts and prior irradiation. Overall, men are more commonly affected than women (1.6: 1).
- The tumors frequently destroy the surrounding cortices and ***produce soft tissue masses.***
- **The formation of bone by the tumor cells is characteristic of osteosarcoma.**
- Osteosarcomas typically present as ***painful and progressively enlarging masses.*** Sometimes a sudden fracture of the bone is the first symptom.
- Radiographs of the primary tumor usually show a ***large, destructive, mixed lytic and blastic mass*** that has permeative margins.
- The tumor frequently ***breaks through the cortex and lifts the periosteum, resulting in reactive periosteal bone formation.***
- The triangular shadow between the cortex and raised ends of periosteum is known radiographically as *Codman triangle* and is characteristic but not diagnostic of this tumor.

200. Ans. c. Denni.., d. Addu..., e. Associ..

[Ref: Maheshwari 5th/216,; CSDT 11th/1195-96; Apley 8th/488; Nelson 18th/2777-78]

"Method of maintenance of the **clubfoot correction***: CTEV splints,* ***Denis-Brown splint*** *& CTEV shoes" (Maheshwari 3rd/198)*

"Clubfoot are associated with arthrogroposis multiplex congenital, ***spina bifida***, myelomeningocele, neurofibromatosis & chondrodysplasia punctata" *(Danhert Radiology 5th/25)*

"CTEV: Cause could be a genetic defect, or a form of arrested development. Its occurrence in ***neurological disorders & neural tube defects (myelomeningocele & spinal bifida)*** [Q] *points to a neuromuscular disorder" (Apley 8th/488)*

Clubfoot or Talipes Equinovarus

- It is **most commonly** an ***idiopathic congenital condition*** [Q]
- It occurs twice as often in boys and is bilateral half the time. There is a familial tendency, with a 5% chance that a sibling will also be affected.
- In congenital clubfoot, there is more or less rigid ***inversion of the hindfoot, adduction of the forefoot and limited dorsiflexion***—an equinovarus deformity.

Talipes Equinovarus (Clubfoot)

◈ *Nelson 18th/2777-78*

- Clubfoot is the term used to describe a deformity involving malalignment of the calcaneotalar-navicular complex. Components of this deformity may be best understood using the mnemonic CAVE (**cavus**, ***adductus***, **varus, equinus**).
- Although this is predominantly a hindfoot deformity, there are plantar flexion (cavus) of the 1st ray and adduction of the forefoot/midfoot on the hindfoot. The hindfoot is in varus and equinus.

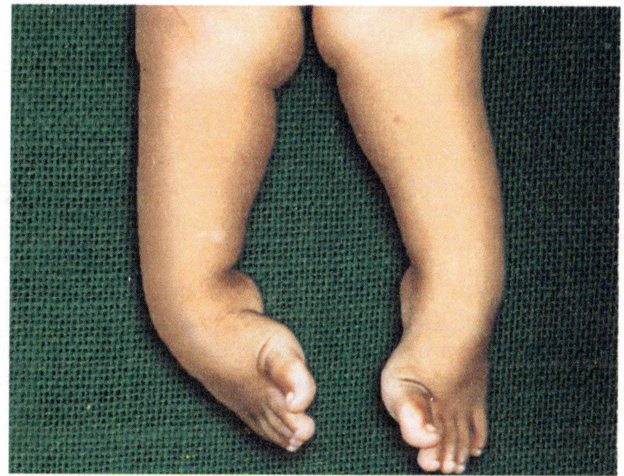

Fig: Clinical picture demonstrating clubfoot deformity.

201. Ans. a. Thoracic..., d. Poste...

[Ref: Maheswari 5th/186-187, 3rd/169-180; Apley 8th/44, 387-89; Children Orthopaedics & Fracture by Michael 2nd/159]

*"****Paradiscal is the commonest type.*** *In this, the contiguous areas of two adjacent vertebrae along with the intervening disc are affected" (Maheswari 3rd/172)*

"**Site affected in Pott's spine:** *Vertebral body (82%) with predilection for anterior part adjacent to superior/inferior endplate>> posterior elements" (Danhert Radiology 5th/170)*

"**Location of Pott's spine:** ***Upper lumbar+lower thoracic spine (L1 most common),*** *typically more than one vertebrae affected" (Danhert Radiology 5th/170)*

T.B Spine

◈ *Harrison 19th/1110-11, 18th/1347-48*

- While the ***upper thoracic spine is the most common site of spinal TB in children,*** the **lower thoracic and upper lumbar *vertebrae*** are usually affected in adults.

- From the ***anterior superior or inferior angle of the vertebral body, the lesion slowly reaches the adjacent body, later affecting the intervertebral disk.***
- With advanced disease, collapse of vertebral bodies results in kyphosis (*gibbus*). A paravertebral "cold" abscess may also form.

T.B. of the Spine & Pott's Paraplegia

◈ *Review of Important facts*

- The *spine is the commonest site*[Q] of bone & joint T.B.; the *dorso-lumbar*[Q] region being the one affected most frequently
- *Paradiscal type is commonest type*[Q] of vertebral T.B.
- *Back pain is the commonest presenting symptom*[Q] in pott's spine
- *Stiffness is a very early symptom* [Q] in T.B. of the spine & *reduction of disc space is the earliest sign*[Q] in the commoner paradiscal type.
- Pott's paraplegia occurs most commonly in T.B. of the *dorsal spine*[Q] because the spinal canal is narrowest in this part
- *Clonus (ankle or patellar) is most prominent early sign*[Q] in pott's paraplegia
- *Antero-lateral decompression (ALD) is most commonly*[Q] performed operation
- Usually, active spinal lesions involve a particular segment: Two vertebral bodies and the corresponding disc. Some authors have speculated that these areas are affected most often because of the generous arterial and venous supply and the high oxygen pressure requirement of the tuberculosis bacilli.
- A peridiscal presentation occurs in approximately 80% of patients, with the ***anterior vertebral body affected and contiguous progression through subligamentous burrowing (anterior longitudinal ligament) and eventual extension to the adjacent vertebrae.*** Less frequently, lesions occur centrally in the vertebral body.
- ***The posterior elements of the spine are rarely the only sites affected.***

ANAESTHESIA

202. Ans. d. Atracurium

[Ref: Ajay Yadav 5th/116-17; Lee 13th/189-95]

"Atracurium *undergo spontaneous degradation in plasma called as Hoffman degradation.* ***Atracurium is relaxant of choice if reversal agent is contraindicated"*** *(Ajay Yadav 5th/116-17)*

Other muscle relaxant: (mentioned in[Q]) require reversal with neostigmine (but ***we can not use neostigmine due to hypersensitivity***), so can not use in this patient

203. Ans. a. Burn b. Spinal..., c. Muscular..., d. Tetanus

[Ref: Ajay Yadav 5th/112-13; Lee 13th/190; KDT 7th/355; Barash Clinical Anesthesia 6th/MR]

"The **serum potassium** *may rise transiently by upto 0.5 mmol/L with suxamethonium, even in normal patient. This is exaggerated after* ***burns, tetanus & spinal cord injuries & also in patients with many other neurological & muscular disorders, such as stroke, cerebral palsy & muscular dystrophy.*** *This is due to the proliferation of extrajunctional receptors, which cause a massive outpouring of potassium when stimulated by suxamethonium" (Lee 13th/190)*

"Succinylcholine: Dangerous hyperkalemia can occur in patients with extensive burn & soft tissue injuries" *(KDT 7th/355)*

"Severe hyperkalemia, occasionally leading to cardiac arrest, has been described in patients *after major denervation injuries, spinal cord transection, peripheral denervation, stroke, trauma, extensive burns and prolonged immobility with disease* **a**nd may be related to potassium loss via a proliferation of extrajunctional receptors. Hyperkalemia has been reported with myotonia and muscle dystrophies and cardiac arrests have been reported in children before the diagnosis of the disease was made. Severe hyperkalemia after succinylcholine resulting in cardiac arrest has also been observed in acidotic hypovolemic patients" *(Barash Clinical Anesthesia 6th/MR)*

204. Ans. a. Sodium..., c. Mannitol e. Propofol

[Ref: Ajay Yadav 5th/86, 109; Lee 13th/643-45]

"Mannitol *is used in* **treatment** *of increased intracranial tension" (KDT 7th/591)*

Table *(Partial list)*: **Ajay Yadav 5th/86**

Agent	Effect on ICT
Sevoflurane	↑↑
Halothane	↑↑↑
Isoflurne	↑
Xenon	0
Nitrous oxide	↑
Enflurane	↑↑
Desflurane	↑↑

Table *(Partial list)*: **Ajay Yadav 5th/109**

Agent	Effect on ICT
Thiopentone	↓↓↓
Ketamine	↑↑↑
Propofol	↓↓↓
Diazepam	↓
Morphine	Variable (↓)

205. Ans. a. GABA-A..., c. NMDa...

[Ref: KDT 7th/372-73; Ajay Yadav 5th/71; Lee 13th/149; Miller 6th/721-22]

Mechanism of General Anaesthesia

◈ *KDT 7th/372-73*

- *Recent findings show that* ***ligand gated ion channel*** *(but not voltage sensitive ion channel) are the major targets of anaesthetic action*
- *The* ***$GABA_A$ receptor gated Cl-channel*** *is the most important of these: Many inhalational agents, barbiturates, benzodiazepines & propofol*
- *Action of* ***glycine*** *in the spinal cord & medulla is augmented by barbiturates, propofol & many inhalational anaesthetics*
- *Inhibition of excitatory type of* ***NMDA type of glutamate receptor:*** *Ketamine & N_2O*

Intravenous Anaestheisa

◈ *Lee 13th/149*

Those with actions at **γ-aminobutyric acid ($GABA_A$) receptor:** *Barbiturate, benzodiazepines, etomidate & propofol*

Which acts at the **N-methyl-D-aspartate (NMDA) receptor:** *Ketamine*

"Unlike the other IV anesthetics, ***ketamine does not interact with GABA receptors; however, it binds to non-NMDA glutamate receptors***[Q] and nicotinic, muscarinic, monoaminergic and opioid receptors. In addition, it also inhibits neuronal sodium channels (producing a modest local anesthetic action) and calcium channels (causing cerebral vasodilatation)" *(Miller 6th/744)*

"**Propofol:** Its mechanism of action is thought to be potentiation of ***γ-aminobutyric acid (GABA)***-induced chloride currents" *(Miller 6th/721-22)*

206. Ans. e. In regional...

[Ref: Ajay Yadav 5th/138-140, 149; Lee 13th/369-374]

Sequence of blockade of fibre C *(conduction velocity 0.5-2.3 m/s) >***B** *(conduction velocity 3-15m/s) >***A** *(conduction velocity 12-120 m/s) (Ganong 25th/94)* ***(It shows that slow conducting fibers blocks easily)***

"**Local anesthetic** *reversibily inhibit peripheral nerve conduction by blocking* ***voltage gated sodium & potassium channel.*** *The affinity of the sodium receptor is higher in* ***open or inactivated states*** *than in the resting state.* ***Blockade sequence*** *is-sympathetic> temperature (cold)> pain (prick) >proprioception (light touch with cotton)" (Lee 13th/374)*

Local Anesthesia

◈ *Ajay Yadav 5th/138-140, 149*

- Local anesthetics provide anesthesia and analgesia by blocking the transmission of pain sensation along nerve fibers
- The key target of local anesthetics is the ***voltage-gated sodium channel.*** The binding is intracellular and is mediated by hydrophobic interactions.
- Local anesthetics block voltage-gated sodium channels and thereby interrupt *initiation and propagation of impulses in axons*
- Among sensory fibers sequence of blockade is ***temperature (cold before hot) → pain→ touch → deep pressure → proprioception***
- Although LA can block sodium channel in any state but ***activated & inactivated channels (the channel with positive resting membrane potential but below threshold) are blocked more readily as compared to resting state channel*** (the channel with negative resting membrane potential)
- **Intravenous regional block** (Beir's Block)-After applying tourniquet 30 to 40 ml of 0.5% xylocaine, ***prilocaine is injected into a distal vein.*** Adequate tourniquet functioning is most vital in Bier's block

SKIN

207. Ans. a. A bullo..., b. Crust..., d. Also..., e. Intra...

[Ref: Neena Khanna 3rd/67; Roxburg 17th/255]

Hailey Hailey Disease (Familial Benign Pemphigus)

◈ *Neena Khanna 3rd/67*

- Pemphigus type of ***bullous disorder*** (***Intraepidermal lesion***)
- Autosomal dominant inheritance
- ***Presents in 3rd-4th decade***
- Presents as flaccid vesicles, ***crusted erosions*** & circinate plaques on erythematous base. May become hypertrophic & malodorous
- Major flexures (groins, perineum, axillae & side of neck)
- **Treatment includes:** Reduction of friction; keeping area dry. Combination of potent steroids with antibiotics (mainstay of treatment)

208. Ans. a. Tarry..., b. Palmar..., d. Spider...

[Ref: Neena Khanna 3rd/330, 148; Roxburg 17th/292-93]

Skin in Liver Disease

◈ *Neena Khanna 3rd/330*

Hepatic disease, especially when the patient has hepatic failure, is associated with:

- ***Pruritus:*** *Due to accumulation of bile salts, when there is* obstructive jaundice
- ***Yellowish pigmentation:*** *Due to accumulation of bile pigments*
- ***Spider nevi & palmar erythema:*** *Due to accumulation of estrogen & progesterone*
- ***White nails:*** *Due to hypoproteinemia*

"**Chronic Liver disease:** Other frequent findings include scleral icterus, *palmar erythema, spider angiomas,* parotid gland enlargement, digital clubbing, muscle wasting, or the development of edema and ascites. Men may have decreased body hair and gynecomastia as well as testicular atrophy, which may be a consequence of hormonal abnormalities or a direct toxic effect of alcohol on the testes"

White Nails (Terry's nails)

◈ *http://www.nhs.uk/conditions/nail-abnormalities/Pages/Introduction.aspx*

Terry's nails are typically white with reddened or dark tips and can be a sign of a wide range of medical conditions, including the following:

- ***Liver cirrhosis*** (about 80% of people with cirrhosis have Terry's nails)
- *Liver, kidney or heart failure*
- *Diabetes*
- *Iron-deficiency anaemia, which is a reduced number of red blood cells due to a lack of iron in the body*
- *Chemotherapy*
- Malnutrition

209. Ans. a. Pterygium e. Thinning...

[Ref: Neena Khanna 3rd/52-55; Harrison 19th/349, 17th/316]

"**Salmon patch:** *Commonest vascular malformation present at birth. Unlike other vascular malformation which persists, salmon patch involutes by the age of 1 year" (Neena Khanna 3rd/318)*

Nail Changes in Lichen Planus

◈ *Neena Khanna 3rd/54*

- *Seen in 15% of patients (less frequently in children)*
- *Thinning & distal splitting of nail plates*
- *Longitudinal grooves*
- *Tenting of nail plate*
- ***Pterygium formation*** *(which is diagnostic): The proximal nail fold is prolonged on to the nail bed, splitting & destroying the nail plate*

Nail Changes in Psoriasis

◈ *Neena Khanna 3rd/43*

- *10-50% of the patients with psoriasis have nail involvement*
- *Pitting*
- *Nail plate thickening*
- *Subungual hyperkeratosis*
- *Onycholysis*
- *Discolouration of nail plate*
- *Oil spots*

"**Splinter hemorrhages (or haemorrhages)** are tiny blood clots that tend to run vertically under the nails. Splinter hemorrhages are not specific to any particular condition and can be associated with *subacute infective endocarditis, scleroderma, trichinosis, systemic lupus erythematosus (SLE), rheumatoid arthritis, psoriatic nails, antiphospholipid syndrome, haematological malignancy and trauma" (wikipedia)*

Lichen Planus

◈ *Harrison 19th/349, 17th/316*

- The typical rash of lichen planus is well-described by the **"5 Ps"**: Well-defined ***pruritic, planar, purple, polygonal papules***[Q]. The commonly affected sites are near the wrist and the ankle.
- LP is a papulosquamous disorder that may affect the skin, scalp, nails and mucous membranes.
- Close examination of the surface of these papules often reveals a network of gray lines ***(Wickham's striae).***
- The skin lesions may occur anywhere but have a predilection for the wrists, shins, lower back and genitalia
- Involvement of the scalp, lichen planopilaris, may lead to scarring alopecia and nail involvement may lead to permanent deformity or loss of fingernails and toenails.
- ***LP commonly involves mucous membranes,*** particularly the buccal mucosa
- Additionally, LP may be associated with ***hepatitis C infection***[Q].

"**Nails pitting** may occur as a result of *imperfect nail plate formation in the matrix area.* It may be associated with ***psoriasis, lichen planus, alopecia areata, eczema or may occur even without diseases of the nails"*** *(www.skinatlas.com/pitting1.htm)*

Nail finding	Associated systemic conditions
Shape or growth change	
Clubbing	IBD, Ca lung, asbestosis, cirrhosis, congenital cyanotic heart disease, endocartitis, lung abscess
Koilonychia	Iron deficiency anemia
Onycholysis	Psoriasis, infection, hyperthyroidism, sacroidosis, trauma, amyloidosis, connective tissue disorders
Pitting	Psoriasis, alopecia areata, Lichen planus, Eczema.
Beau's lines	Any severe systemic illness that disrupts nail growth, Raynaud's disease, pemphigus trauma
Yellow nail	Lymphedema, bronchiectasis
Color change	
Terry's (white) nails	Hepatic failure, cirrhosis, diabetes mellitus, CHF, hyperthyroidis, malnutrition.
Azure lunula	Wilson's disease, silver poisoning, quinacrine therapy
Half-and-half nails	Specific for hypoalbuminemia
Muehrcke's lines	Arsenic poisoning
Mees' lines	Melanoma, benign nevus, chemical staining, normal variant in darkly pigmented people
Dark longitudinal streaks	Alopecia areata, vitiligo, atopic dermatitis, psoriasis
Longitudinal striations	Sub acute bacterial endocarditis, SLE, rheumatoid arthritis, Antiphospholipid syndrome, malignancies, trauma
Telangiectasia	Rheumatoid arthritis, SLE, dermatomyositis, scleroderma

PSYCHIATRY

210. Ans. a. 1st rank..., b. Dep.. c. Brain... e. Usua..

[Ref: Niraj Ahuja 6th/58-73; Kaplan & Saddok's Synopsis of Psychiatry 10th/467-75]

Note: *"Depression is a mood disorder that frequently co-exists with schizophrenia and which also needs treatment" (http://schizophrenia. com/deprssn.html)*

Schizophrenia

"Two common affective symptoms in **schizophrenia** are reduced emotional responsiveness, sometimes severe enough to warrant the label of anhedonia and overly active and inappropriate emotions such as extremes of rage, happiness and anxiety. Other feeling tones include perplexity, a sense of isolation, overwhelming ambivalence and ***depression***" *(Kaplan & Saddok's Synopsis of Psychiatry 10th/482)*

*"The **onset of schizophrenia** occurs **usually later in women & often runs a more benign course,** as compared to men" (Niraj Ahuja 6th/58)*

"Schneider's first rank symptoms of schizophrenia *though not specific but of **great help in making diagnosis & have significantly influenced the diagnostic criteria & classification** of schizophrenia. Second rank symptom of schizophrenia are considered less important for diagnosis of schizophrenia" (Niraj Ahuja 6th/58)*

*"Cranial CT scan, MRI scan & post-mortem studies show **enlarged ventricles** (not mounting to hydrocephalous) & mild cortical atrophy (with an overall reduction in brain volume & cortical grey matter by 5-10%) in some patients of schizophrenia" (Niraj Ahuja 6th/68)*

"Schneider's **First-rank symptoms are not specific for** schizophrenia & may be seen in other psychiatric disorders like ***mood disorders & organic psychiatric disorders"*** *(Niraj Ahuja 6th/58)*

Gender and Age

- *Kaplan & Saddok's Synopsis of Psychiatry 10th/468*

- Schizophrenia is equally prevalent in men and women: The two genders *differ, however, in the onset and course of illness.*
- ***Onset is earlier in men than in women:*** More than half of all male schizophrenia patients, but only one-third of all female schizophrenia patients, are first admitted to a psychiatric hospital before age 25.
- ***The peak ages of onset are 10–25 years for men and 25–35 years for women:*** Onset of schizophrenia before age 10 or after age 60 is extremely rare.

Cerebral Ventricles

- *Kaplan & Saddok's Synopsis of Psychiatry 10th/471*

"Computed tomography (CT) scans of patients with schizophrenia have consistently shown ***lateral and third ventricular enlargement*** and some reduction in cortical volume."

Table *(Kaplan 10th/467-68)*: **Kurt Schneider Criteria for Schizophrenia**

First-rank symptoms

- Audible thoughts
- Voices arguing or discussing or both
- Voices commenting
- Somatic passivity experiences
- Thought withdrawal and other experiences of influenced thought
- Thought broadcasting

- Delusional perceptions
- All other experiences involving volition made affects and made impulses

Second-rank symptoms

- Other disorders of perception
- Sudden delusional ideas
- Perplexity
- ***Depressive and euphoric mood changes***
- Feelings of emotional impoverishment

211. Ans. b. Hallu..., e. Illu...

[Ref: Niraj Ahuja 6th/14, 17; Kaplan & Sadock 10th/233, 281]

"Delusion *(false, unshakeable beliefs) are* ***content of thought disorder"*** *(Niraj Ahuja 6th/14)*

"Obsession is disorder of ***content of thought"*** *(Niraj Ahuja 6th/14)*

"Obsession *is an idea, impulse or image which intrudes into the conscious awareness repeatedly & patient tries to resist against it but is unable to " (Niraj Ahuja 6th/101)*

Perception

- *It is the process of being aware of a sensory experience & being able to recognize it by comparing it with previous experiences*
- *Perception disorders are-**hallucination, illusions & misinterpretations; depersonalization/derealization; somatic passivity phenomenon; autoscopy; abnormal vestibular sensations etc.***

212. Ans. d. Identifying...

[Ref: Niraj Ahuja 6th/85, 228-30; Kaplan & Saddok's Synopsis of Psychiatry 10th/953-959]

Note: Identifying maladaptive assumptions is a cognitive technique

Cognitive Techniques

- *Kaplan & Saddok's Synopsis of Psychiatry 10th/959*

"The therapy's cognitive approach includes **four processes:** *eliciting automatic thoughts, testing automatic thoughts,* ***identifying maladaptive underlying assumptions*** *and testing the validity of maladaptive assumptions"*

"Cognitive techniques: Recognizing & correcting negative automatic thoughts, teaching redistribution techniques, increasing objectivity in perspectives, ***identifying & testing maladaptive assumptions & decentering***" *(Niraj Ahuja 6th/230)*

Behavioral Techniques

◈ *Kaplan & Saddok's Synopsis of Psychiatry 10th/959*

- ***"Behaviour therapy for mood disorder:*** *This includes the various short-term modalities like social skills training; problem solving techniques, assertiveness training, self-control therapy,* ***activity scheduling*** *& decision-making techniques" (Niraj Ahuja 6th/85)*
- Behavioral and cognitive techniques go hand in hand; behavioral techniques test and change maladaptive and in- accurate cognitions. The overall purposes of such techniques are to help patients understand the inaccuracy of their cognitive assumptions and learn new strategies and ways of dealing with issues.
- Among the **behavioral techniques** in cognitive therapy are ***scheduling activities, mastery and pleasure, graded task assignments, cognitive rehearsal, self-reliance training, role-playing and diversion techniques.***
- One of the first things done in therapy is **scheduling activities** on an *hourly basis.* Patients keep records of the activities and review them with the therapist.

Behavior Therapy

◈ *Kaplan & Saddok's Synopsis of Psychiatry 10th/953-57*

- Behavior therapy involves changing the behavior of patients to reduce dysfunction and to improve quality of life.
- **Systematic desensitization** consists of three steps: relaxation training, hierarchy construction and desensitization of the stimulus.
- Therapeutic-graded exposure
- Flooding
- Participant modeling
- Assertiveness
- Aversion Therapy
- Eye Movement Desensitization and Reprocessing
- Positive Reinforcement

Table *(Kaplan 10th/957)*: **Some Common Clinical Applications of Behavior Therapy**

Disorder	Comments
Agoraphobia	Graded exposure and flooding
Alcohol dependence	Aversion therapy
Anorexia nervosa	Observe eating behavior; contingency management; record weight
Bulimia nervosa	Record bulimic episodes; log moods
Hyperventilation	Hyperventilation test; controlled breathing; direct observation
Other phobias	Systematic desensitization
Paraphilias	Electric shocks or other noxious stimuli

Contd...

Disorder	Comments
Schizophrenia	The token economy procedure & Social skills training methods.
Sexual dysfunctions	Sex therapy: It uses relaxation, desensitization and graded exposure as the primary techniques.
Shy bladder	Inability to void in a public bathroom; relaxation exercises
Type A behavior	Physiological assessment, muscle relaxation, biofeedback (on electromyogram [EMG]

Table *(Kaplan & Saddok's10th/959)*: **Cognitive Psychotherapy**

Goal	Identify and alter cognitive distortions that maintain symptoms
Selection criteria	Primarily used in dysthymic disorder
	Nonendogenous depressive disorders
	Symptoms not sustained by pathological family
Duration	Time-limited, usually 15–25 weeks, once-weekly meetings
Techniques	Collaborative empiricism
	Structured and directive
	Assigned readings
	Homework and behavioral techniques
	Identification of irrational beliefs and automatic thoughts
	Identification of attitudes and assumptions underlying negatively biased thoughts

213. Ans. a. Agitation..., c. Status..., d. Convulsion...

[Ref: KDT 7th/404-05; Niraj Ahuja 6th/209; Kaplan & Saddok's Synopsis of Psychiatry 10th/1018-20]

"Diazepam: *It has anticonvulsant activity in a variety of models but it is* ***not used for long term therapy of epilepsy*** *because of prominent sedative action & rapid development of tolerance to the anti-epileptic effect" (KDT 7th/418)*

"Diazepam use: To ***manage agitation in emergency room"*** *(Kaplan & Saddok's Synopsis of Psychiatry 10th/1020)*

Uses of Diazepam

◈ *KDT 7th/404-05, 418-19*

- It is oldest & all purpose BZD, used as anxiolytic, hypnotic, muscle relaxant, premedicant, anaesthetic & for emergency contol of seizure due to its broad spectrum activities *(KDT 7th/404-05)*
- It is a first line drug for ***emergency control of convulsions e.g., status epilepticus, tetanus,*** eclampsia, convulsant drug poisoning *(KDT 7th/418-19)*
- Rectal instillation OFdiazepam is now the preferred therapy for febrile convulsion in children *(KDT 7th/418-19)*

- ***Other use of BZD:*** *Before ECT, electrical cardioversion, endoscopies, in obstetrics & many minor procedures-diazepam i.v. has gained popularity because of its calming-amnesis-analgesic & muscle relaxant properties & relative safety*

Uses of Diazepam

- *Niraj Ahuja 6th/209*
- *Narco analysis or abreation*
- *Antipsychotic induced akathisia*
- *Treatment of alcohol withdrawl & other drug withdrawl syndromes*
- *Nightmares (diazepam also reduces the REM sleep duration)*
- *Insomnia*
- *Stage 4 NREM sleep disorders like enuresis, somnambulism (diazepam reduce duration of stage 4 NREM sleep)*
- *Agitated depression*

214. Ans. a. Lorazepam d. Clobazam

[Ref: KDT 7th/398, 412, 418-19; Niraj Ahuja 6th/207; Kaplan & Saddok's Synopsis of Psychiatry 10th/1018; Harrison 19th/2551-55, 18th/3262; O.P.Ghai 7th/528]

"Antiepileptic Benzodiazepines: *Clonazepam, diazepam, Lorazepam & clobazam" (KDT 7th/412)*

Table *(KDT 7th/398)*: **Benzodiazepines**

Hypnotic	Antianxiety	Anticonvulsant
Diazepam Flurazepam Nitrazepam Alprazolam Temazepam Triazolam	Diazepam Chlordiazepoxide Oxazepam Lorazepam Alprazolam	Clonazepam Diazepam Lorazepam clobazam

Febrile seizure: *Oral diazepam, midazolam* **&** ***clobazam*** **are effective prophylactics (Intermittent)"** *(O.P.Ghai 7th/528)*

RADIOLOGY

215. Ans. b. Contr..., d. Emits β..., e. Emits γ...

[Ref: Danhert Radiology manual 5th/1087-88; Review of Radiology by Sumer Sethi 2nd/101; Harrison 19th/263e-3, 18th/2937, 1790, 17th/1360;Dutta Gynaecology 5th/484, 4th /465; Merdith Radiation Physics & Nuclear Medicine/28]

"I-131 emits β & γ rays" *(Harrison 19th/263e-3, 18th/1790)*

"I-131 *is* ***contraindicated during pregnancy. Foetal thyroid will be destroyed*** *resulting in cretinism, other abnormalities if given during first trimester" (K.D.T 7th/256)*

"I-127 is stable isotope of iodine. Its radioactive isotope of medical importance is I-131 (role in hyperthyroidism due to Garve's disease & multinodular goiter; & in metastatic carcinoma of thyroid especially papillary or those cases of follicular carcinoma which concentrate iodine" *(K.D.T 7th/256)*

"I-123: ***It is agent of choice for thyroid imaging"*** *(Danhert Radiology manual 5th/1087)*

"For **radioactive iodine scanning I-131 & I-123** are used. ***For treatment of hyperthyroidism & thyroid cancer I-131 is used"*** *(CMDT06/1127)*

Table: Review of Radiology by Sumer Sethi 2nd/101

Radionuclide	Form in which used	Half-life	Radiation emitted	Method of administration
Iodine-131	Sodium iodide solution	8 days	Beta rays, Gamma rays	Oral

Table *(Dutta gynaecology 5th/484)*: **Radioisotopes commonly used in gynaecological malignancies brachytherapy are:**

Isotope	Energy (MeV)	Half life
Cesium 137 (Cs137)	0.662	30 years
Radium 226 (Ra226)	0.8	1620 years
Cobalt 60 (Co60)	1.173	5.3 years
Iridium 192 (Ir 192)[Q]	0.47[Q]	74 days
Gold 198 (Au 198)	0.411	2.96 days
Iodine 125 (I125)	0.027	60 days
Phosphorus 32 (P32)	0.698	14.3 days

Table: Merdith Radiation physics & nuclear medicine/28

Rays	Radioactive elements		t½
β	P-32 Sr-90 Y-90	Phosphorous Strontium Yttrium	14.3 days 28 years 2.54 days
β, γ	Ra-226 Au-198 *I – 131*[Q]	Radium Gold *Iodine (mainly b)*	1622 years[Q] 2.7 days 8 days
γ	Ir-192 Co-60[Q] Cs-137[Q] Xe-133 I-123 I-132 Tc-99 Ga-70 Tl-201 Rn-222 Cr-51 K-81 Se	Iridium Cobalt Cesium Xenon Iodine Iodine Technitium Gallium citrate Thallous chloride Radon Chromium Krypton Selenium	74.5 days 5.2 years 30 years 5.2 days 13 hours 2.3 hours 6 hours 3.2 days 3.1 days 3-6 days
N, γ	Cf – 252 Ta-182	Californium Tantulum	2.6 years 4 months

216. Ans. a. Hypo.. c. Optic..., d. Increased...

[Ref: Harrison 19th/2263-64, 18th/2886, 2879;CMDT 2016/1087, 06/1115; Devita 7th/1844; Leibel Philip 2nd/489]

S/E of Pituitary irradiation: ***Hypopituitarism,*** *some degree of memory impairment, increased long term risk of second tumor & small vessel ischemic episode" (CMDT 2016/1087, 06/1115)*

Radiation Therapy

◈ *Harrison 19th/2263, 18th/2886*

- Radiation is used either as a ***primary therapy*** for pituitary or parasellar masses or, more commonly, as an ***adjunct to surgery or medical therapy.***
- Because of its relatively slow onset of action, radiation therapy is usually reserved for ***postsurgical management.*** As an adjuvant to surgery, radiation is used to treat residual tumor and in an attempt to prevent regrowth.

Side Effects

◈ *Harrison 19th/2263-64, 18th/2886*

- In the short term, radiation may cause ***transient nausea and weakness. Alopecia and loss of taste and smell may be more long-lasting. Failure of pituitary hormone synthesis*** is common in patients who have undergone head and neck or pituitary-directed irradiation. More than 50% of patients develop loss of GH, ACTH, TSH and/or gonadotropin secretion within 10 years, usually due to hypothalamic damage. Lifelong follow-up with testing of anterior pituitary hormone reserve is therefore required after radiation treatment.
- ***Optic nerve damage*** with impaired vision due to optic neuritis is reported in about 2% of patients who undergo pituitary irradiation. **Cranial nerve damage is uncommon** now that radiation doses are <2 Gy (200 rad) at any one treatment session and the maximum dose is <50 Gy (5000 rad). The use of stereotactic radiotherapy may reduce damage to adjacent structures. Radiotherapy for pituitary tumors has been associated with adverse mortality rates, mainly from ***cerebrovascular disease.*** The cumulative risk of ***developing a secondary tumor*** after conventional radiation is 1.3% after 10 years and 1.9% after 20 years.

Cranial Irradiation

◈ *Harrison 19th/2256, 18th/2879*

"Cranial irradiation may result in long-term ***hypothalamic and pituitary dysfunction,*** especially in children and adolescents, as they are more susceptible to damage after whole-brain or head and neck therapeutic irradiation"

Types of Radiation Therapy for Pituitary Tumors

◈ *Devita 7th/1844*

Two types of radiation therapy are used to treat pituitary tumors:

- External beam radiation therapy
- Stereotactic radiosurgery

This therapy can be very effective, but it also has some drawbacks:

- It works slowly, so it can take months or years before the tumor growth and/or excess hormone production is fully controlled.
- It can damage the remaining normal pituitary. In most cases, normal pituitary function will be lost over time, requiring treatment with hormones.
- It may damage some normal brain tissue, particularly near the pituitary gland, which could affect mental function years later.
- The *optic nerves may be damaged, resulting in impaired vision.*
- The radiation may increase the *risk of developing a brain tumor later in life, although this risk is still likely to be low.*

217. Ans. a. Rotation..., b. Supine...

[Ref: WHO Radiographic Manual 2002/32-33; Basic Radiology (Lange) 2004/Heart imaging]

"Supine chest view: The ***heart appears enlarged*** & mediastinum may appear wide perhaps 10 cm" *(WHO Radiographic Manual 2002/32)*

"Chest X-ray should be taken in *full inspiration & correctly centered*: A film taken ***in expiration can cause confusion.*** It may simulate diseases *e.g.*, pulmonary congestion, ***cardiomegaly*** or a wide mediastinum" *(WHO Radiographic Manual 2002/32)*

Basic Radiology (Lange)

◈ *2004/Heart imaging: writes*

- With the patient in the **supine position**, there is normally a redistribution of blood flow to the upper lobe pulmonary veins (cephalization) and the ***heart may appear enlarged relative to its appearance on the upright PA radiograph,*** because of magnification
- If the patient has pulmonary disease such as ***emphysema, the heart may be enlarged,*** but because of the overinflation of the lungs, the cardiothoracic ratio may still be normal.

Thoracic Cage

◈ *http: //www.ncbi.nlm.nih.gov/books/NBK355/*

- ***Scoliosis and pectus excavatum*** can give a false impression of ***cardiomegaly*** due to a normal but displaced heart.
- Other causes of a false impression of cardiomegaly are the ***greater magnification of the heart on an AP film***

Mediastinal Widening

◈ *http: //radiologymasterclass.co.uk/tutorials/chest/chest_ pathology/ chest_ pathology _page9.html*

- Widening of the mediastinum is most often due to technical factors such as patient positioning or the projection used. ***Rotation, incomplete inspiration, or an AP view, may all exaggerate the width of the mediastinum, as well as heart size.***
- In the setting of trauma, patients are positioned **supine** while a chest X-ray is acquired, very often causing the ***mediastinum to appear wide spuriously.***

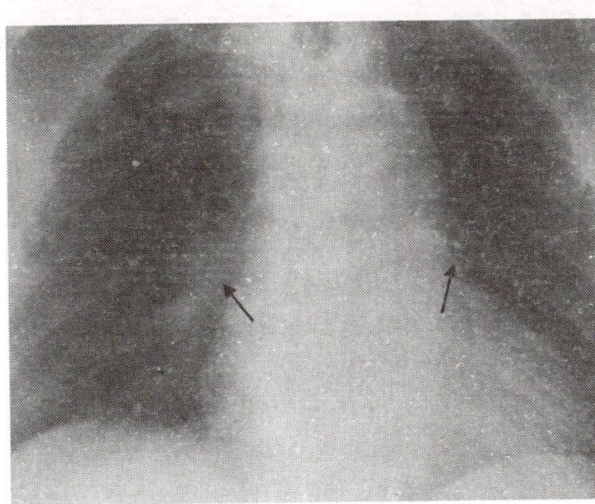

Fig: Supine AP chest radiograph showing apparent increase in heart size and prominent bronchovascular markings (arrows).

Braunwald's Heart Disease

- The standard chest radiograph is obtained with ***deep inspiration and the patient facing the film***. If patients are unable to stand, chest radiographs are generally obtained with their chest toward the tube and their back toward the film (*i.e.*, in the anteroposterior [AP] position). With the standard PA (posteroanterior) view, the heart appears smaller and its size and contour are more accurately depicted than on an AP view.
- Portable chest radiographs are obtained with patients positioned **supine or semisupine.** The degree of inspiration is therefore likely to be substantially less than with an erect film, making the ***heart appear relatively larger*** and providing less optimal visualization of the lungs, because they are not optimally expanded.
- As noted, the ***heart appears larger*** because of decreasing lung compliance with ***pectus excavatum*** have a narrowed AP diameter of the chest, increasing the transverse diameter.
- **Marked kyphosis or scoliosis** can also cause the heart or mediastinum to look abnormal. It is thus important to evaluate the spine and other bone structures systematically when looking at a chest radiograph.

218. Ans. a. Carinal..., b. Straight..., c. Double...

[Ref: Dahnert Radiology Review Manual 5th/575, 636-637; Harrison 17th/1467; P.J. Mehta 15th/160-61]

***"Boot shaped heart** is found in tetralogy of Fallot-Sumer Sethi 2nd/36; Radiology by Samarjit Bhadury 2nd/38)*

"Downward & outward extension of the apex is seen in left ventricle enlargement" *(Radiology by Samarjit Bhadury 2nd/38)*

Left Atrial Enlargement

◈ *Dahnert Radiology Review Manual 5th/575*

PA View Chest X-ray

- *Right retrocardiac double density*
- *>750 splaying of carina* with horizontal orientation of distal left mainstream bronchus
- Enlargement of left atrial appendages

Lateral View

- Increased convexity of postero-superior cardiac margin
- Posterior displacement of left upper lobe bronchus

Left Heart Enlargement

◈ *P.J. Mehta 15th/160*

- Double density seen through right upper border (AP view) (*i.e., **double atrial shadow**[Q])*
- Esophagus curving around the dilated left atrium
- ***Straightened left border***[Q]
- ***Splaying of mainstem bronchi***[Q] (*i.e.,* ↑ed carinal angle)
- Small aorta (due to decrease of forward cardiac output)
- Normal/Undersized LV

219. Ans. b. Do..., c. Superior...

[Ref: L & B 25th/136-37; Danhert Radiology manual 5th/1085; L &B 25th/136, Basic Radiology by Lange 2004; radiographics.rsna.org / content/23/2/315.full]

Table (*L & B 25th/130*): **Typical effective doses from diagnostic medical exposure in the 2000s**

Diagnostic procedure	Typical effective dose (mSv)	Equivalent no. of chest radiographs	Approximately equivalent period of natural background radiation$_a$
PET head (18F-FDG)	5	250	2.3 years

Positron Emission Tomography (PET)

◈ *L &B 25th/136 -37*

- PET is an extension of nuclear medicine, in which a positron-emitting substance such as ***18F is tagged*** and used to assess tissue metabolic characteristics.
- Nuclear medicine also differs from other means of imaging, ***which are largely anatomically based, as it also provides functional information.***
- The most commonly used radiolabelled tracer is ***18F-2-fluoro-2-deoxy-D-glucose (FDG),*** although other tracers can also be used in order to assess ***metabolic functions such as oxygen and glucose consumption and blood flow***.
- The **drawbacks** have been high cost, very limited availability and relatively low ***spatial resolution.*** The last of these has been addressed by PET/CT systems combining simultaneous PET imaging and CT, allowing the two sets of images to be registered so that the anatomical location of the abnormality can be localised more precisely.

Radionuclide Imaging

◈ *L &B 25th/137*

Strengths

- Allows ***functional imaging***
- Allows imaging of the ***whole body***
- Bone scan has a high sensitivity for metastatic bone disease, fractures and infection

- PET scanning is valuable in the detection of metastatic cancer

Weaknesses

- Specific agents are required for specific indications
- Often non-specific and an abnormal result may require further imaging
- Generally poor spatial resolution

Positron Emission Tomography

◈ *Basic Radiology by Lange 2004*

- At first glance, PET scans resemble CT scans. Images can be viewed on a TV monitor or on x-ray film. ***Areas of high metabolic activity (i.e., cerebral cortex, deep gray nuclei) demonstrate greater radiopharmaceutical uptake than do areas of low metabolic activity, such as white matter or cerebrospinal fluid. The bones of the skull and scalp soft tissues are, for the most part, invisible.***
- ***Anatomic resolution, although not as good as with CT or MR imaging,*** is better than with SPECT imaging. The major advantage of PET imaging is that it is extremely versatile, providing in vivo information about brain perfusion, glucose metabolism, receptor density and, ultimately, brain function.
- PET provides useful information in the setting of *stroke, epilepsy, dementia and tumors. At present, the two main indications are in the workup of patients with complex partial seizures and in identifying tumor recurrence in patients who have undergone surgery, radiation therapy, or both, for brain tumors.*
- *PET is an advanced imaging tool for diagnosis, staging and restaging of cancer. The method is based on identifying the increased glycolytic activity in malignant cells*
- It is possible to image the entire body in a single session, increasing the opportunity for finding unsuspected disease sites.
- *There are several sites of normal physiologic accumulation of FDG, hence FDG distribution is not limited to neoplastic tissues. The brain uses glucose as its primary substrate; consequently, accumulation is physiologically high in the cortex, basal ganglia, thalamus and cerebellum*

220. Ans. b. Grey..., c. Uses..., d. Gadolinium..., e. Can...

[Ref: Sumer Sethi 2nd/9-10; mriscans.cliniccompare.co.uk/mri-scan-with-contrast-dye; Danhert Radiology Review Manual 5th/1079; Bhadury 2nd/177; blog.radiology.ucsf.edu; www.diffen.com/difference / CT_ Scan_vs_ MRI]

"Grey matter is grey & white matter is white on T1WI & relationship is reversed on T2WI" *(Sumer Sethi 2nd/9)*

"The contrast dye used in these MRI Scans is generally ***gadolinium as complications are rarer in comparison to the Iodine origin dye*** used for X-rays and CT scans" *(mriscans.cliniccompare.co.uk/mri-scan-with-contrast-dye)*

*"At present, it could be argued that **all cranial cross-sectional studies,** except those for acute trauma or where there are known MRI contraindication, should be performed by MRI. **In spine, MRI is also the preferred option. A similar picure is emerging for musculoskeletal problems, for which MRI is nearly always the technique of choice"** (Grainger 2nd/97)*

*"**Within the chest, CT is still generally preferred.** For **abdominal & pelvic lesions** the choice b/w CT & MRI is not clear cut. Where clinical question concern just one anatomical region, a strong case for MRI can be made. Where a general survey of whole abdomen is needed, however, CT is still much to be preferred" (Grainger 2nd/97)*

- MR imaging has traditionally been used for ***neurologic indications, including brain tumors, acute ischemia, infection and congenital abnormalities.***
- More recently, MR imaging has been used for a number of non-neurologic indications, namely, ***spine, musculoskeletal, cardiac, hepatic, biliary, pancreatic, adrenal, renal, breast and female pelvis applications.***

"A **CT Scan** (or **CAT Scan**) and an MRI operate differently and are better suited for different types of diagnoses. ***An MRI suited for examining soft tissue, (e.g., ligament and tendon injury, spinal cord injury, brain tumors etc.)*** while a ***CT scan is better suited for bone injuries, lung and chest imaging and detecting cancers.*** CT scans are widely used in emergency rooms because the procedure takes less than 5 minutes. An MRI, on the other hand, can take up to 30 minutes.

An MRI typically costs more than a CT scan. One advantage of an ***MRI is that it does not use radiation while CT scans do.*** This radiation is harmful if there is repeated exposure"

Table: CT & MRI

	CT	MRI
Scope of application:	CT can outline bone inside the body very accurately.	MRI is more versatile than the X-Ray and is used to examine a large variety of medical conditions.
Application:	Suited for bone injuries, Lung and Chest imaging, cancer detection. Widely used in Emergency Room patient.	Suited for Soft tissue evaluation, *e.g.,* ligament and tendon injury, spinal cord injury, brain tumors etc.
Details of bony structures:	Provides good details about bony structures	Less detailed compared to X-ray
Details of soft tissues:	A major advantage of CT is that it is able to image bone, soft tissue and blood vessels all at the same time.	Much higher soft tissue detail as compare to CT scan.

Use & Advantage of MRI

- It is a non-invasive technique[Q]
- It is safe[Q] as it does not involve the use of ionising radiation
- Images can be readily produced in *any plane*[Q] *(multi planner capabilities) e.g.,* axial, sagittal or coronal without changing position of the patient
- It give high intrinsic contrast
- Lack of artefact from adjacent bones[Q]: This make MRI the modality of choice in areas such as the posterior fossa & pituitary fossa where the quality of CT image is degraded by artefact.

- MRI is imaging modality of *choice for most brain & spine disorders*[Q]

Limitations & Disadvantage of MRI

- Very high cost of imaging
- Inability to image bone & calcium[Q]
- It is unsuitable for patients with cardiac pacemakers[Q]& other ferromagnetic implants
- Imaging time is long, hence movement or motion artefacts are quite likely
- Highly operator dependent[Q], hence require technical expertise

221. Ans. b. Curie, e. Bequeral

[Ref: Sumer Sethi 2nd/18; Radiology by S. Bhadury 2nd/197; Harrison 19th/363e-1, 18th/1788; http: //www.nrc.gov/reading-rm/doc-collections/cfr]

Unit of Radioactivity Radiology

◈ *S. Bhadury 2nd/197: Writes*
- *It is measured by* ***Becquerel & Curie***
- *1Bq = 1 disintegration/second*[Q]
- *1 Curie (Ci) = 3.7 x 10^{10} disintegration/second*
- *1 Ci is equal to 37 gigabecquerel*

Unit of Biological Effectiveness or Equivalent Dose

◈ *Sumer Sethi 2nd/18*
- Rem
- SI unit = Sievert
- 1 Sievert = 100 Rem

Unit of Absorbed Radiation

◈ *Sumer Sethi 2nd/18*
- Rad
- SI unit = Gray
- 1 gray (Gy) = 100 rads

Unit of Radiation Exposure

◈ *Sumer Sethi 2nd/18*
- Roentgen
- SI unit= coloumb/kg

ANSWER SHEET

1 – 50	51 – 100	101 – 150	151 – 200	201 – 250
1 A B C D E	51 A B C D E	101 A B C D E	151 A B C D E	201 A B C D E
2 A B C D E	52 A B C D E	102 A B C D E	152 A B C D E	202 A B C D E
3 A B C D E	53 A B C D E	103 A B C D E	153 A B C D E	203 A B C D E
4 A B C D E	54 A B C D E	104 A B C D E	154 A B C D E	204 A B C D E
5 A B C D E	55 A B C D E	105 A B C D E	155 A B C D E	205 A B C D E
6 A B C D E	56 A B C D E	106 A B C D E	156 A B C D E	206 A B C D E
7 A B C D E	57 A B C D E	107 A B C D E	157 A B C D E	207 A B C D E
8 A B C D E	58 A B C D E	108 A B C D E	158 A B C D E	208 A B C D E
9 A B C D E	59 A B C D E	109 A B C D E	159 A B C D E	209 A B C D E
10 A B C D E	60 A B C D E	110 A B C D E	160 A B C D E	210 A B C D E
11 A B C D E	61 A B C D E	111 A B C D E	161 A B C D E	211 A B C D E
12 A B C D E	62 A B C D E	112 A B C D E	162 A B C D E	212 A B C D E
13 A B C D E	63 A B C D E	113 A B C D E	163 A B C D E	213 A B C D E
14 A B C D E	64 A B C D E	114 A B C D E	164 A B C D E	214 A B C D E
15 A B C D E	65 A B C D E	115 A B C D E	165 A B C D E	215 A B C D E
16 A B C D E	66 A B C D E	116 A B C D E	166 A B C D E	216 A B C D E
17 A B C D E	67 A B C D E	117 A B C D E	167 A B C D E	217 A B C D E
18 A B C D E	68 A B C D E	118 A B C D E	168 A B C D E	218 A B C D E
19 A B C D E	69 A B C D E	119 A B C D E	169 A B C D E	219 A B C D E
20 A B C D E	70 A B C D E	120 A B C D E	170 A B C D E	220 A B C D E
21 A B C D E	71 A B C D E	121 A B C D E	171 A B C D E	221 A B C D E
22 A B C D E	72 A B C D E	122 A B C D E	172 A B C D E	222 A B C D E
23 A B C D E	73 A B C D E	123 A B C D E	173 A B C D E	223 A B C D E
24 A B C D E	74 A B C D E	124 A B C D E	174 A B C D E	224 A B C D E
25 A B C D E	75 A B C D E	125 A B C D E	175 A B C D E	225 A B C D E
26 A B C D E	76 A B C D E	126 A B C D E	176 A B C D E	226 A B C D E
27 A B C D E	77 A B C D E	127 A B C D E	177 A B C D E	227 A B C D E
28 A B C D E	78 A B C D E	128 A B C D E	178 A B C D E	228 A B C D E
29 A B C D E	79 A B C D E	129 A B C D E	179 A B C D E	229 A B C D E
30 A B C D E	80 A B C D E	130 A B C D E	180 A B C D E	230 A B C D E
31 A B C D E	81 A B C D E	131 A B C D E	181 A B C D E	231 A B C D E
32 A B C D E	82 A B C D E	132 A B C D E	182 A B C D E	232 A B C D E
33 A B C D E	83 A B C D E	133 A B C D E	183 A B C D E	233 A B C D E
34 A B C D E	84 A B C D E	134 A B C D E	184 A B C D E	234 A B C D E
35 A B C D E	85 A B C D E	135 A B C D E	185 A B C D E	235 A B C D E
36 A B C D E	86 A B C D E	136 A B C D E	186 A B C D E	236 A B C D E
37 A B C D E	87 A B C D E	137 A B C D E	187 A B C D E	237 A B C D E
38 A B C D E	88 A B C D E	138 A B C D E	188 A B C D E	238 A B C D E
39 A B C D E	89 A B C D E	139 A B C D E	189 A B C D E	239 A B C D E
40 A B C D E	90 A B C D E	140 A B C D E	190 A B C D E	240 A B C D E
41 A B C D E	91 A B C D E	141 A B C D E	191 A B C D E	241 A B C D E
42 A B C D E	92 A B C D E	142 A B C D E	192 A B C D E	242 A B C D E
43 A B C D E	93 A B C D E	143 A B C D E	193 A B C D E	243 A B C D E
44 A B C D E	94 A B C D E	144 A B C D E	194 A B C D E	244 A B C D E
45 A B C D E	95 A B C D E	145 A B C D E	195 A B C D E	245 A B C D E
46 A B C D E	96 A B C D E	146 A B C D E	196 A B C D E	246 A B C D E
47 A B C D E	97 A B C D E	147 A B C D E	197 A B C D E	247 A B C D E
48 A B C D E	98 A B C D E	148 A B C D E	198 A B C D E	248 A B C D E
49 A B C D E	99 A B C D E	149 A B C D E	199 A B C D E	249 A B C D E
50 A B C D E	100 A B C D E	150 A B C D E	200 A B C D E	250 A B C D E

NAME OF THE CANDIDATE	ROLL NO.	CENTRE NO.	QUESTION BOOKLET NO.	BOOKLET CODE
CATEGORY	0 0 0 0 0	0 0	0 0 0 0 0	A
	1 1 1 1 1	1 1	1 1 1 1 1	B
SC ○	2 2 2 2 2	2 2	2 2 2 2 2	C
ST ○	3 3 3 3 3	3 3	3 3 3 3 3	D
OBC ○	4 4 4 4 4	4 4	4 4 4 4 4	
GEN ○	5 5 5 5 5	5 5	5 5 5 5 5	
CW ○	6 6 6 6 6	6 6	6 6 6 6 6	
PH ○	7 7 7 7 7	7 7	7 7 7 7 7	
	8 8 8 8 8	8 8	8 8 8 8 8	
	9 9 9 9 9	9 9	9 9 9 9 9	

INSTRUCTIONS FOR FILLING THE SHEET

1. This sheet should not be folded or crushed.
2. Use only blue/black ball pen to fill the circles.
3. Use of pencil is strictly prohibited.
4. Circles should be darkened properly and completely.
5. Cutting & erasing on this sheet is not allowed.
6. Do not use any stray marks on the sheet.
7. Do not use marker, white fluid or any other device to hide the shading already done.

WRONG METHOD

    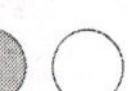

CORRECT METHOD

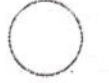 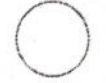 

CANDIDATE'S SIGNATURE
(in ball - point pen)

INVIGILATOR'S SIGNATURE
(in ball - point pen)

Vast and concise coverage of all important topics for proff exams as well a pg entrance exams. Presentation of topics are so arranged that are easy to remember via help of flowcharts and colourful diagrams. Detailed description of difficult questions helps to understand the concept. Topic wise practice questions helps to establish grip over the chapter topic by topic. IBQs are like cherry over the cake because IBQs are increasing in recent exam trends
Ankit Tiwari
Bundelkhand Medical College, Sagar

Question bank available for practice is good n enough comparing other books. Crisp concepts and brief explanations are given for quick revision to topics while solving questions. The volume of the book is tried to be kept as its minimum without compromising the quality. Language is student friendly even for hindi medium students and proper use of highlighting fonts n colours.
Naman Tiwari, GMC, Kota

SURGERY SIXER very nice book for PG preparation it contains all important points in all standard books like Sabiston ,Bailey ,Schwartz etc. Surgery Sixer book is very easy to prepare during last preparation & during last time revision best book is surgery sixer ,high yield one liners in all chapters was very nice clear image in all chapters with brief explanations ,this book is apt for all exam preparations ,image based questions was nice
Karthick Raja, GMC, Vilupuram

Excellent book written by one of the top faculty of Medicine. Fully – colored layouts and it is reader – friendly. Synopsis is given in the form of bullet points which help in easy revision. MCQs are explained in a way to eliminate the options and opt for the best choice.
Liyakat Ahmed
Navodaya Medical College, Raichur

WOW factor for me is Dr Deepak Marwah Sir. A must have book for every medical student due to its excellent content which is covered in a beautiful layout and presentation of colourful pages (best quality), soothing to eyes and conceptual boxes. Excellent presentation of theory part, way too many MCQs with logical references, not too much length to make it difficult to revise
Syed Aijaz Ahmad, GMC, Srinagar

Wow factors are point wise description of content, uses of tables and diagrams, all updates included, conceptual diagnostic algorithm.
Rashi Jain
JLN Medical College, Ajmer

Tables, Harrison updates and practice questions are the best part of the book. The number of practice questions are plenty for better preparation
P Harish
Kamineni Inst. Of Medical Sciences, Hyderabad

2019 Edition (May End)

Surgery Sixer book's One line creation is awesome to revise easily in last time. Recent advances, Bailey's update is correctly mentioned in this book... Image based questions with explanations are excellent. Surgery Sixer book is simplified book of Bailey & Love... The synopsis of this book are easily understood than any other book... It's easy to prepare
Theeran R, GMC, Villupuram

CBS Exam Books WOW! FACTORS of Previous Editions

Wow is its concise appearance, colorful, high quality smooth colour papers, Reading monotonous papers are really tiring. Nice layout and presentation. Two column concept is excellent. Concise content. IBQs are given sufficiently. Clear Radiology images. Above All, CRYSTAL CLEAR CONCEPTS.
Prithvi Raj, GMC, Thiruvarur

Surgery Sixer for NBE by R Rajamahendran is the most reffered MCQ book for surgery and so I got a copy of it. The book gives us a 15 day plan to complete it plus 5 days for revision just before the exam. The PGI section is sorted separately towards the end and the students not aspiring for that can skip that part. It also has MCQs on Instruments and image based questions which is the recent pattern in the entrance exams. Quick tables for last minute revision are also there making revision even more easy!!
Shivani Desai
(Feedback on CBS Exam Books FB Page)

MRP ₹1395/-

MRP ₹395/-

I should say whole book itself is a wow factor. The book is one of its kind so well explained, this is concise and adequate for undergraduates to prepare for entrance as well as for practical knowledge. I liked every bit of it the X Ray, CT Scan, USG all are so well explained in starting and here by disease wise. I think this is the best book for Radiology I have ever seen.
Shubhda Singh, Malda Medical College, Malda

Absolutely Stunning Book ..!! Surgery Presented in Easiest Way Possible. Colorful Presentations High Quality Paper, Seperate Boxes for Controversies, Bailey 27e Updates ..! Everything is Top Notch . No Second Thoughts . Go For it !!
Prithivi Raj
(Feedback on CBS Exam Books FB Page)

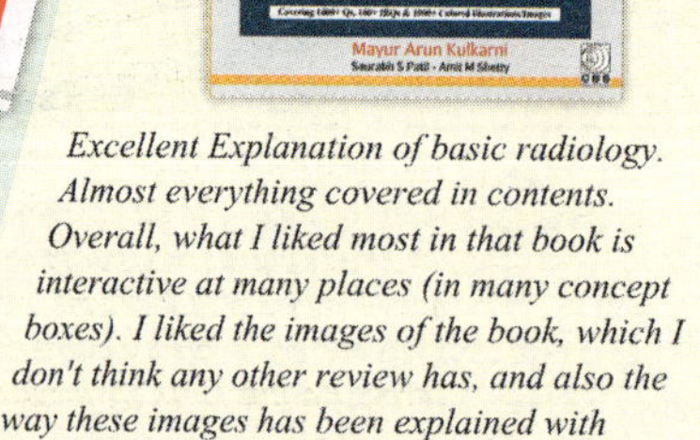

The book by Dr MAK is the best book in the subject for PG Aspirants. It covers many radiological images which have made understanding easy not only radiology but also related subjects. Extensive content and topic wise distribution of chapters have given the book an extra edge with such a great presentation. Radiology learning will be fun and interesting in SIR's way. The text in each chapter is very helpful to know the subject and then solving the practice questions is very helpful.
Mainak Mandal
KIMS, Bhubaneshwar

Concise matter that plays a vital role during revision. Centre of attraction in this book is separate column of bailley updates. Controversy desk as a column is a nice concept. I like it diagrammatic representation is best part of this book, practice questions by author are best selected questions from surgery. Helps in proff exams too. Hence, Undoubtedly best book for surgery in market. separate theory part is better for learning in comparison to other available surgery books in market.GIT in this book is so well presented that it made me fall for it. Correlated images favours it as best book of surgery. Instrument images and controversy desk leaves no stone unturned.
Shubham Jain, NSCB, Jabalpur

Excellent Explanation of basic radiology. Almost everything covered in contents. Overall, what I liked most in that book is interactive at many places (in many concept boxes). I liked the images of the book, which I don't think any other review has, and also the way these images has been explained with arrows, that makes concept more clear.
Ishtiyaq Ahmad Ganaie, ACOMS Jammu

The wow factor of the book is the content and the detailed explanation of the physics involved in each including the explanation of electromagnetic spectrum. Image based MCQs are amazing. All that is required for PG NEET is present in the book. Students need not refer to any additional source. The layout is presented well.
Apeksha, ESI Medical College, Bangaluru

Scan the QR Code to View Sample Pages of the Books